Pathophysiology
Adaptations and Alterations in Function

Pathophysiology
Adaptations and Alterations in Function
Fourth Edition

Barbara L. Bullock R.N., M.S.N., C.C.R.N.

Assistant Professor of Nursing
Houston Baptist University
Houston, Texas

with 9 contributors

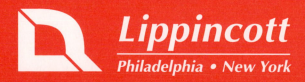

Lippincott
Philadelphia • New York

Acquisitions Editor: Lisa Stead
Editorial Assistant: Brian MacDonald
Project Editor: Amy P. Jirsa
Production Manager: Helen Ewan
Production Coordinator: Kathryn Rule
Senior Design Coordinator: Kathy Kelley-Luedtke
Interior Design: Arlene Putterman
Cover Design: Larry Didona
Indexer: Katherine Pitcoff

4th Edition

Library of Congress Cataloging in Publications Data

Bullock, Barbara L.
    Pathophysiology: adaptations and alterations in function /
Barbara L. Bullock; with 9 contributors. — 4th ed.
        p.   cm.
    Includes bibliographical references and index.
    ISBN 0-397-55164-9 (hardcover)
    1. Physiology. Pathological. I. Title.
    [DNLM: 1. Pathology. 2. Physiology.   QZ 4 B938p 1996]
RB113.B85 1996
616.07—dc20
DNLM/DLC
for Library of Congress   95-32143
                                                              CIP

Table 15-3: By permission of Mosby-Yearbook, Inc.

Flowcharts 25-1 and 25-3: By permission of Hutter AM Jr: Congestive
heart failure. Scientific American Medicine, Dale DC, Federman DD, Eds.
Section 1, Subsection II. © 1995 Scientific American, Inc. All rights
reserved.

Figure 25-10: By permission of DeSanctis RW, Dec GW:
Cardiomyopathies. Scientific American Medicine, Dale DC, Federman
DD, Eds. Section 1, Subsection XIV. © 1995 Scientific American, Inc. All
rights reserved.

Figures 32-11 and 40-16: From *Principles of Anatomy and Physiology*, 7th
Edition by Gerald J. Tortora and Sandra Reynolds Grabowski. Copyright ©
1993 by Biological Sciences Textbooks, Inc., A&P Textbooks, Inc., and
Sandra Reynolds Grabowski. Reprinted by permission of HarperCollins
Publishers, Inc.

*To my husband, Pete,
and children, Sheila, Brian, and Doug,
with my love and appreciation.*

Contributors

Roberta H. Anding, MS, RD/LD, CDE
Assistant Professor, School of Nursing
University of Texas Health Sciences Center
 at Houston
Houston, Texas

Barbara L. Bullock, RN, MSN, CCRN
Assistant Professor of Nursing
Houston Baptist University
Houston, Texas

Miguel F. da Cunha, PhD
Professor, School of Nursing
University of Texas Health Sciences Center
 at Houston
Houston, Texas

Darlene Hastie Green, RN, DSN
Clinical Researcher, Office of Clinical Practice
 Evaluation
University of Alabama Hospital
Birmingham, Alabama

Doris J. Heaman, DSN, RN
Assistant Professor, School of Nursing
The University of Alabama in Huntsville
Huntsville, Alabama

Reet Henze, DSN, RN
Associate Professor, School of Nursing
The University of Alabama in Huntsville
Huntsville, Alabama

Gretchen Schaefer McDaniel, RN, DSN
Health Care Education and Research
Hoover, Alabama

Sharron Patton Schlosser, DSN, RN
Professor of Nursing, Ida V. Moffett School of Nursing
Samford University
Birmingham, Alabama

Camille P. Stern, PhD, RN
Associate Professor
Armstrong State College, Department of Nursing
Savannah, Georgia

Joy H. Whatley, RN, DSN
Associate Professor, Ida V. Moffett School of Nursing
Samford University
Birmingham, Alabama

Reviewers

Sharon Ennis Axton, *RN, MS, PNP-CS*
Assistant Professor of Nursing
Houston Baptist University
Houston, Texas

Debra Berry, *RN, MS, FNP*
Assistant Professor of Nursing
Houston Baptist University
Houston, Texas

Miguel F. da Cunha, *PhD*
Professor, School of Nursing
University of Texas Health Sciences Center
   at Houston
Houston, Texas

Patricia Brown Dominguez, *RN, MSN*
Assistant Professor of Nursing
Houston Baptist University
Houston, Texas

Jack Keyes, *BA, PhD*
Professor of Biology
Linfield College, Portland Campus
Portland, Oregon

Bobbie Jean Low, *RN, MSN*
Assistant Professor of Nursing
Houston Baptist University
Houston, Texas

Peggy McCall, *RN, MSN, LNHA*
Assistant Professor of Nursing
Houston Baptist University
Houston, Texas
Owner/Director, Com for Care, Inc.
Houston, Texas

Kelly McKnight, *RN, BN, MSc*
Coordinator—Support for Nurses Program
Registered Nurses Association of Nova Scotia/Canada
Dartmouth, Nova Scotia, Canada

Kristen Oelman Miles, *RN, MS*
Instructor of Nursing
Houston Baptist University
Houston, Texas

Ainslie T. Nibert, *RN, MSN, CCRN*
Assistant Professor of Nursing
   and Department Chair, B.S.N. Division
Houston Baptist University
Houston, Texas

Annalee R. Oakes, *EdD, FAAN, CCRN*
Professor and Dean
Seattle Pacific University
Seattle, Washington

Dorothy Obester, *PhD, MSN, BSME, RN*
Professor of Nursing
Saint Francis College
Loretta, Pennsylvania

Olive Santavenere, *PhD, RN*
Associate Professor, Department of Nursing
Southern Connecticut State University
New Haven, Connecticut

Betty Souther, *RNC, PhD*
Associate Professor of Nursing,
   and Director, Center for Health Studies
Houston Baptist University
Houston, Texas

Nancy Yuill, *RN, PhD*
Dean, College of Nursing
Houston Baptist University
Houston, Texas

Pathophysiology is the study of the physiologic and biologic manifestations of disease and the adaptations that the body makes to the changes produced by the disease process. The fourth edition of *Pathophysiology: Adaptations and Alterations in Function* provides a basis for this study by expanding the student's knowledge in the sciences and exploring how alterations in structure (anatomy) and function (physiology) disrupt the human body as a whole. The concept of the body as a unit is central to the discussions in this book, because pathologic processes and responses are not isolated to one system, but rather affect the entire body as a whole.

Written for undergraduate and graduate students in nursing and other health-oriented disciplines, this text blends the conceptual and systems approaches. The overall mechanisms of disease are described first to set the stage for coverage of specific disease processes within each system.

Integral to the study of pathophysiology is an understanding of how the human body adapts to the stresses of life and to disease-causing stimuli. *Pathophysiology* begins its discussion of this adaptation at the cellular level. Because alterations cause a disruption in normal cellular processes, ultimately leading to tissue or organ alterations, the body's adaptive and compensatory mechanisms also occur at the cellular level. For this reason, cellular processes and alterations in these processes are discussed throughout the text. The concept of feedback and information sharing within the body is also explored in depth. In health the body functions in a negative feedback pattern that allows return to homeostasis. Some pathologic processes, however, establish a positive feedback pattern that, if unchecked, will result in death.

The understanding of disease processes is continually being updated and clarified by research. Continual advances in the study of disease and the human body's response provide a constant flow of new information to the field of Pathophysiology. In this edition of *Pathophysiology*, every attempt has been made to provide the most current information available. New concepts have been added and all of those retained from previous editions have been thoroughly edited and revised. All chap-

ters have been completely rewritten or updated to reflect current concepts. The contributors have taken great care to provide currency, detail, and concept synthesis for every topic in the book.

▼ ORGANIZATION

This edition retains many features of the first three editions, including the basic organization and presentation of topics. The organization of the text is intended to enhance the student's understanding of the effects of adaptation on the body as a whole. Both conceptual and systems approaches have been used. Physical and laboratory findings are emphasized in appropriate sections, but treatment regimens are included only to illustrate or clarify a process. Students are referred to the many current nursing and medical texts for information about treatment and nursing management.

Unit I provides a basis for understanding cellular dynamics and adaptation at the cellular level. Normal cellular structure, function, and organization is followed by alterations in cellular processes. Neoplasia has been added to this unit since it is basically a cellular alteration. Genetic principles and disorders complete this unit.

Unit 2 focuses on development through the life cycle. Chapters on development in reproduction, children, adults, and older adults provide a basis for understanding physiologic changes across the lifespan. A separate chapter on the effects of stress and sleep alterations throughout life has been added to this unit.

Unit 3 presents topics related to fluid, electrolytic, acid-base, and nutritional balance. Normal and altered balances are included in each chapter discussion. Shock is included in this unit because it affects the hemodynamic balances.

Unit 4 presents infectious diseases and the processes of inflammation and repair. The resolution of inflammation through the process of healing is included as well.

Unit 5 provides students with a basic understanding of immunity. Normal immunologic response, immune deficiency, and hypersensitivity responses are detailed in this unit.

Units 6 though 15 examine the physiology and pathophysiology of the major body systems. Systems presented include circulation, respiration, urinary excretion, endocrine regulation, digestion, musculoskeletal function, skin, neural control, and reproduction. For each system both normal and altered function are presented. The relationship between alterations in one system and the effect on other systems is consistently described.

Appendices are included to provide related useful information such as nutrition tables, dysrhythmias, and growth and development.

▼ *NEW TO THIS EDITION*

As with previous editions, all text and illustrations have been thoroughly reviewed, revised, and updated to reflect the most current information available.

New Chapters. Neoplasia has been moved from a unit to a chapter in the cellular dynamics unit. Coronary artery disease has been designated as a separate chapter. Concepts of stress and sleep have been recognized as a separate chapter to emphasize the importance of these topics.

Case Studies. Case studies have been added throughout the text to promote critical thinking and to help students apply the information presented in the text to actual clinical situations. Each case study is followed by analysis questions, with answers and further explanation provided in Appendix G.

Art Program. All of the illustrations and tables have been extensively reviewed and revised in order to provide clarity of textual material and to reflect the most recent accurate information. Over 100 new illustrations have been created especially for this edition.

Flowcharts. To clearly illustrate the physiology and pathophysiology of many processes, flowcharts have been added and revised from previous figures. These are included throughout the text.

Chapter Summaries. Brief chapter summaries are included at the end of each chapter. These learning devices are intended to emphasize key points of each chapter. Use of the chapter outlines and learning objectives also help students organize and structure study patterns.

References and Bibliography. Each chapter contains current references and each unit provides a thorough bibliography to allow the reader to pursue topics in greater depth.

▼ *INSTRUCTOR'S MANUAL, TEXT BANK, AND TRANSPARENCY MASTERS*

Pathophysiology: Adaptations and Alteration in Function, 4th edition, is accompanied by an Instructor's Manual designed to serve as a complement to the book for both students and instructors. The Instructor's Manual has been completely revised and updated. It contains lecture outlines, key terms and concepts, teaching strategies, and a bank of test questions. Transparency masters of select illustrations from the text can be used to enhance classroom presentation of material.

This text is intended to provide the reader with a comprehensive understanding of alterations and responses of the body when it is confronted with a variety of stimuli. The interrelationships among the various systems is emphasized. Attempts have been made to visualize the individual affected by thoses alterations so that a clinical focus can be made. This approach is used to provide the background necessary for health care providers.

Barbara L. Bullock, R.N., M.S.N.

Acknowledgments

Putting together a book of this magnitude requires contributions by many people. I gratefully acknowledge the contributors to previous editions. Their contributions provided the basis for the entire project. Contributors to previous editions are acknowledged below. The contributors to the fourth edition added new content and refined, updated, and expanded the third edition. Their diligence and attention to detail is greatly appreciated. With each successive edition, I am confronted with the vastness of the topics that are presented in this book. Concepts change as understanding and research progress. The struggle between keeping the text of a reasonable size and trying to cover the material adequately was the basis for some of the decisions regarding content retained and content deleted.

I also acknowledge the support and guidance provided by many talented persons at J.B. Lippincott Company, specifically, Lisa Stead, Associate Nursing Editor; Brian MacDonald, Nursing Editorial Assistant; and Amy Jirsa, Associate Managing Editor. Marcia Williams, Medical Illustrator, has handled all of the major art revisions, making many suggestions for wonderful changes. The results are truly outstanding.

Contributing authors to previous editions were Gaylene Altman, Gloria Anderson, Roberta H. Anding, Joseph L. Andrews, Jr., Pamela Appleton, Sue H. Baldwin, Anne Roome Bavier, Cheryl Bean, Carol Tull Bowdoin, Joan P. Bufalino, Martha Butterfield, Concepcion Y. Castro, Angela Smith Collins, Jules Constant, Miguel F. da Cunha, Virginia Earles, Ann Estes Edgil, Thomas Mark Fender, Shirley Freeburn, Dorothy Gauthier, Janet L. Gelein, Cherry Anderson Guinn, Doris J. Heaman, Reet Henze, Marcia Hill, Pamela Holder, Joan T. Hurlock, Karen E. Jones, Bonnie M. Juneau, June H. Larrabee, Carla A. Bouska Lee, Marianne T. Marcus, John A. R. Marino, Gretchen Schaefer McDaniel, M. S. Megahed, Frances Donovan Monahan, Jennie L. Moore, Emilie Musci, Betty Norris, Barbara R. Norwood, Leah F. Oakley, Donna Rogers Packa, Marilyn Nelsen Pase, Richard Pflanzer, Helen F. Ptak, Cammie M. Quinn, Darlene H. Renfroe, Pearl Philbrook Rosendahl, Sharron Patton Schlosser, Therese B. Shipps, Eileen Ledden Sjoberg, Carol A. Stephenson, Camille P. Stern, Metta Fay Street, Gloria Grissett Stuart, Margaret L. Trimpey, Joan M. Vitello, Joy H. Whatley, Linda Hudson Williams, and Joan W. Williamson.

My thanks also go to the expert reviewers for their helpful comments and suggestions. I imposed on the expert faculty to review major sections, and they took time from their busy schedules to help me.

I could not have completed this project without the continuing support of my husband, Pete. He xeroxed and mailed thousands of pages. He also provided encouragement and humor when it was sorely needed.

Contents

Unit 3 ▼ Fluid, Electrolyte, Acid–Base, Nutritional Balance, and Shock

SECTION TWO
Bodily Defense Mechanisms

Unit 4 ▼ Inflammation and Repair

SECTION 3
Organ and System Mechanisms: Adaptations and Alterations

Unit 8 ▼ Respiration

Unit 9 ▼ Urinary Excretion

Unit 12 ▼ Musculoskeletal Function

Unit 13 ▼ Protective Coverings of the Body

Unit 14 ▼ Neural Control

Unit 15 ▼ *Reproduction*

▼ Appendices

Pathophysiology

**Adaptations and Alterations
in Function**

Section One

Introduction to Pathophysiology: Adaptations and Alterations in Cellular Function

Cellular Dynamics

BECAUSE THE cell is the basis of life, it is appropriate to begin the study of pathophysiology with a review of normal cellular processes. An understanding of these processes is necessary for the understanding of concepts in every other unit of the text. The material can be found in many anatomy and physiology textbooks but is presented here as a convenient, accessible reference. After the presentation of normal cellular function are chapters relating to altered cellular function and the role of genetics in cellular activities.

Chapter 1 describes normal cellular function, with special emphasis on the cellular organelles, on movement of materials across the cell membrane, and on electrical properties of cells. Chapter 2 details the alterations in cells when they are exposed to a changing, hostile environment. Cellular adaptation, injury, and death are explored in terms of their effects on body function. Mechanisms

by which living balance can be maintained, even at the expense of altered intracellular metabolism, are explored. Altered cellular function ending in lethal change is described. Chapter 3 describes cell membrane changes and alterations in cellular function as a result of neoplasia. Discussions of carcinogenesis and the process of malignant growth and spread are included. Chapter 4 explains the principles of inheritance and relates them to the more common genetic disorders.

The reader is encouraged to use the learning objectives at the beginning of each chapter as a study guide outline for essential concepts. Chapter references are included to verify the research related to the specific topics. The bibliography at the end of the unit provides general and specific resources for further study.

Cells: Structure, Function, Organization

Barbara L. Bullock

▼ CHAPTER OUTLINE

Cellular Organelles
The Plasma Membrane
Mitochondria
   Formation of ATP
Endoplasmic Reticulum
Free Ribosomes
Golgi Complex
Lysosomes
Peroxisomes
The Cytoskeleton
Cilia and Flagella
Centrosomes and Centrioles
Nucleus
   Genes
   Protein Synthesis

Reproductive Ability of Cells
Regeneration of Cells
Reproduction of Cells
   Replication
   Mitosis
   Meiosis
Cellular Exchange
Passive Movement Across the Cell Membrane
   Diffusion
   Osmosis
   Filtration
   Facilitated Diffusion

Active Movement Across the Cell Membrane
   Active Transport
   Carrier-Mediated Transport Systems
   Endocytosis and Exocytosis
Electrical Properties of Cells
Cellular Movement
Ameboid Locomotion
Muscular Contraction
Cellular Organization
Epithelial Tissue
Muscular Tissue
Nervous Tissue
Connective Tissue
Chapter Summary

▼ LEARNING OBJECTIVES

1. Differentiate between intracellular and extracellular electrolyte composition.
2. Describe in detail the structure and function of the following organelles: cell membrane, mitochondria, ribosomes, endoplasmic reticulum, Golgi apparatus, lysosomes, microtubules, centrioles, nucleus, and nucleolus.
3. Explain the major ways by which adenosine triphosphate is formed.
4. Describe the process of protein synthesis, from DNA-RNA transcription to assembly of protein.
5. Compare the function of the smooth endoplasmic reticulum with that of the rough endoplasmic reticulum.
6. Explain briefly the negative feedback pattern seen with the reproduction of cells of the body.
7. Classify cells by their ability to regenerate.
8. Compare the processes of mitosis and meiosis.
9. Explain the mechanisms of transport across the cell membrane.
10. Identify carrier-mediated transport, according to its mechanism.
11. Explain the purpose of the sodium-potassium pump.
12. Compare receptor-mediated endocytosis, pinocytosis, and phagocytosis.
13. Describe the purpose of exocytosis.
14. Explain briefly the electrical properties of cells, including depolarization and repolarization.
15. Draw a cell exhibiting ameboid motion.
16. Describe the process of muscle contraction.
17. Compare smooth, cardiac, and skeletal muscle contraction.
18. Describe the differences in structure among four major types of cells in the human body.
19. Define the purposes of the three types of epithelial cells.
20. Differentiate among skeletal, cardiac, and smooth muscle on the basis of histologic appearance.
21. Describe briefly the components of the neuron.
22. Identify the structure and function of each type of connective tissue.

Barbara L. Bullock: PATHOPHYSIOLOGY: ADAPTATIONS AND ALTERATIONS IN FUNCTION, 4th ed.

4 © 1996 Lippincott-Raven Publishers

The cell is the structural and functional unit of the body that provides the basis for life. Understanding the biology of the human cell is essential to the study of pathophysiology. All pathophysiologic processes reflect changes in normal cellular function.

Cells make up the units of tissues, organs, and systems of the human body (Flowchart 1-1). The human body contains more than 75 trillion cells, each of which performs specific functions. These functions are determined by genetic differentiation and are controlled by a highly specific information system that directs the activity of cellular organelles.

Cells that have the major function of carrying out the activities of the organ are called *parenchymal cells*. This means that the parenchyma of an organ actually does its function. Some examples of parenchymal cells are hepatocytes, neurons, gastric parietal cells, osteocytes, and myocardial cells. Other cells, often called *stromal cells*, make it possible for the parenchymal cells to perform their functions by providing the supporting structure or architectural framework to hold the organ in place. Examples include neuroglia, gastric capillary endothelial cells, and cardiac connective tissue cells.

Although cells have different functions, they are alike in many ways. The similarities include how nutrients are used, what type of nutrients are needed, how oxygen is used, the disposition of excretory products, and the internal organization.

▼ Cellular Organelles

The cell is composed of many different structures that carry out its complex functions (Fig. 1-1). Within the cell are highly organized physical structures called *organelles*, which are suspended in the fluid medium called *cytoplasm*. This fluid surrounds the organelles and is external to the nucleus of a cell. The nucleus is essentially a storage area for nucleic acids, especially deoxyribonucleic acid (DNA), which codes for specific cellular proteins.

Cytoplasm is composed mostly of water with specific amounts of electrolytes, proteins, lipids, and carbohydrates. The intracellular electrolyte balance is closely regulated and differs from that of extracellular fluid (Table 1-1). Proteins function to maintain structural strength and form, provide for contractility of muscle tissue, and transport vital substances. Proteins also form the enzymes and many of the hormones necessary for regulation of intracellular reactions. Lipids make up a very small portion of the general cell and mainly join with proteins to keep the cell membranes insoluble in water. Carbohydrates constitute a very small amount of the cytoplasm and are used mainly in the formation of adenosine triphosphate (ATP) for energy.

THE PLASMA MEMBRANE

All cells are surrounded by a thin barrier, called the plasma membrane, that separates intracellular from extracellular fluids. Within the cell, some of the other organelles are bounded by a membrane that is similar in structure to the plasma membrane but named after the organelle (eg, mitochondrial membrane, lysosomal membrane).

The plasma membrane consists of a double layer of lipid molecules (the lipid bilayer) with proteins bound to the surface of each layer and also within the layers (Fig. 1-2). Lipids account for about half of the mass of the plasma membrane and consist of phospholipids, glycolipids, and others such as cholesterol. About 75% of the lipids are phospholipid molecules, which have a polar end and a nonpolar end. Phospholipids in the bilayer are arranged so their polar regions point toward the interior or exterior of the cell and their nonpolar regions are buried in the interior of the membrane. The polar region is *hydrophilic* and mixes with water, but the nonpolar region is *hydrophobic* and repels water. This arrangement allows the membrane to act as a barrier, restricting the loss of intracellular material and governing material entry. The lipid bilayer gives the membrane the ability to conform to the changing shape of the cell and to fill in the gaps between the proteins in the membrane.[3]

Proteins are anchored in or on the lipid bilayer. Those

Flowchart 1-1   The Human Body

The human body is composed of a complex interaction of subunits that join together to make a functioning whole.

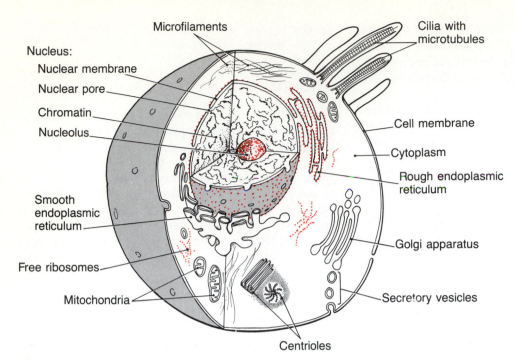

FIGURE 1-1 The general structure of the cell with its organelles.

bound to the inner or outer membrane surface are called *peripheral proteins*. Those partially or completely embedded in the lipid bilayer are called *integral or structural proteins*. Membrane proteins may have other types of molecules attached to them. Proteins on the outer membrane surface, for example, may have carbohydrates attached. These are called *glycoproteins*. Carbohydrates may also be attached to the polar regions of the phospholipid molecules, forming *glycolipids*. Membrane proteins not only form part of the molecular structure of the plasma membrane but have many functional roles, such as transportation and exchange of materials between the cell and its environment. Other proteins are enzymes that speed up or act as catalysts in chemical reactions.

The plasma membrane exists in a fluid state at body temperature, and the protein and lipid components move; that is, the structure of the plasma membrane is dynamic, not static. Both proteins and lipids can move from one area of the membrane to another. Because the membrane is fluid and resembles a patchwork or mosaic of proteins and lipids, this concept is often called the *fluid mosaic model* of membrane structure.

MITOCHONDRIA

Mitochondria (singular, mitochondrion) are membranous, rod-shaped organelles that synthesize ATP, a high-energy phosphate compound required by cells when they perform cellular work (eg, contraction, secretion, conduction, transport). In a sense, mitochondria

TABLE 1-1 *Composition of Extracellular (ECF) and Intracellular (ICF) Fluids*

Cellular Constituent	ECF	ICF
Sodium (Na$^+$)	140 ± 5 mEq/L	10 mEq/L
Potassium (K$^+$)	4 ± 0.5 mEq/L	140 mEq/L
Calcium (Ca^{++})	10 ± 1.0 mg/dL	<1 mg/dL
Magnesium (Mg^{++})	3 mEq/L	58 mEq/L
Chloride (Cl$^-$)	100 ± 10 mEq/L	4 mEq/L
Bicarbonate (HCO$_3^-$)	28 ± 3 mEq/L	10 mEq/L
Phosphates	4 ± 1 mEq/L	75 mEq/L
Glucose	90 ± 10 mg/dL	0–20 mg/dL
Amino Acids	30 mg/dL	200 mg/dL
pH	7.4 ± 0.5	7.0
Proteins	2 g/dL	16 g/dL

*Values are approximate and are meant to show the difference between ECF and ICF.

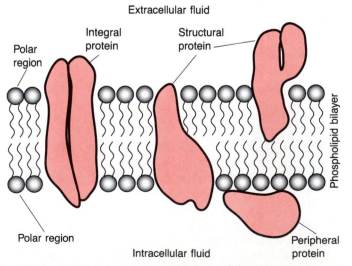

FIGURE 1-2 The structure and components of the lipid bilayer.

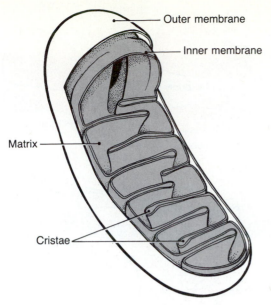

FIGURE 1-3 *Appearance and structure of a mitochondrion.*

are like batteries in a cell, providing energy in a form that allows the cell to function normally.

Mitochondria are bounded by a double membrane, the inner one of which is convoluted into a series of shelflike folds called *cristae* that project into the interior of

the organelle (Fig. 1-3). The folded inner membrane presents a large internal surface area on which enzymatic reactions that generate ATP take place. Cells that are very active and have a high energy requirement, such as skeletal muscle cells, have many mitochondria, whereas less active cells, such as bone or cartilage cells, have fewer mitochondria. Usually, within a given cell, mitochondria tend to be most numerous in areas that are highly energy dependent, such as around the contractile elements of the muscle cell or at the terminus of a nerve cell where transmission occurs.

Mitochondria are able to regenerate (replicate) themselves under conditions of increased energy need. They contain a type of DNA that is part of the mitochondrial structure. The replication process usually occurs at the time of cell division or when there is increased cellular need.

Formation of ATP

The process used by mitochondria to form ATP is called *oxidative phosphorylation*. It requires simple forms of carbohydrates, proteins, and fats. These substances enter the mitochondria and, with the help of oxidative enzymes, form ATP through the citric acid or Krebs' cycle (Fig. 1-4). High-energy phosphate radicals are formed

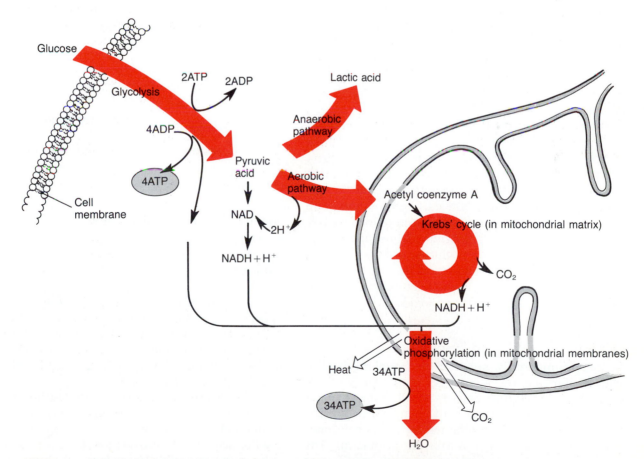

FIGURE 1-4 *Mechanism for the formation of adenosine triphosphate (ATP). ADP, adenosine diphosphate; NAD, nicotinamide-dinucleotide; NADH, reduced NAD.*

that later release their energy when ATP is catabolized or reduced to adenosine diphosphate (ADP). By reentering the mitochondria, and through an enzymatic reaction, ADP can receive another phosphate radical and form ATP anew. The process of catabolizing ATP to ADP results in energy release. The subsequent addition of the phosphate radical to the ADP is called *rephosphorylation.* The common intermediary in carbohydrate, protein, and fat metabolism is *acetyl coenzyme A* (acetyl CoA); its major source is glucose, but fats and proteins can also be metabolized to intermediates that can be fed into the Krebs' cycle.

Approximately 95% of ATP is formed in the mitochondria through a sequence of chemical reactions that require oxidative enzymes. The process involves glycolysis and then oxidation of the end product to form ATP. Important in the process is a coenzyme called *nicotinamide-adenine dinucleotide* (NAD), which functions to accept hydrogen ions. Normally, NAD picks up hydrogen and passes it to another acceptor to pick up more hydrogen. In the oxidative cycle, this acceptor is oxygen and the result is the formation of water.

A small amount of ATP can also be formed by glycolysis in the absence of oxygen, or anaerobic glycolysis. Figure 1-4 shows that glycolysis, itself, is an anaerobic process. Glycolysis proceeds to produce pyruvic acid (pyruvate). Without available oxygen, pyruvate is reduced to lactic acid. The system is inefficient, but it can keep certain cells viable for short periods of time. In the normal, unstressed cell, anaerobic metabolism provides less than 5% of the ATP requirements of the cell; the lactic acid that is formed diffuses out of the cell into the tissues and plasma. The glycolytic process occurs during periods of intense muscular exertion in which oxygen consumption exceeds oxygen supply. Cellular respiration does not produce enough ATP, and the resulting accumulation of lactic acid in the muscle causes pain. The process produces an *oxygen debt* of the muscle that requires deep breathing after exercise to restore the balance of ATP. The recovery time may be very short or up to several hours. This process has been termed *recovery oxygen consumption.* The lactic acid remaining in the muscle cell can be reconverted to glucose or pyruvic acid in the presence of oxygen. Lactic acid that leaves the cell during exercise is carried to the liver, where it is converted to glycogen and carbon dioxide.

ENDOPLASMIC RETICULUM

In some human cells, much of the cytoplasm is filled with an intricate, yet ordered, set of tubular or saclike channels called *cisternae* (Fig. 1-5). All of the channels are interconnected, giving rise to a netlike structure, the appearance of which is reflected by its name: endoplasmic reticulum (a net within the cytoplasm). The membranes of the endoplasmic reticulum (ER) are

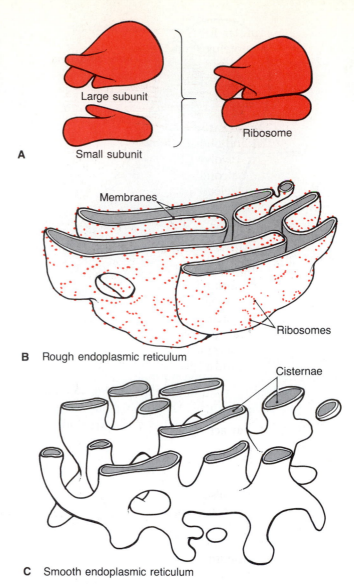

FIGURE 1-5 *Appearance of ribosomes and endoplasmic reticulum.* **A.** *Free ribosomes.* **B.** *Rough or granular endoplasmic reticulum.* **C.** *Smooth or agranular endoplasmic reticulum.*

continuous with the outer membrane of the nuclear envelope.

Much of the surface of the ER is covered with small particles or granules made up of ribonucleic acid (RNA) which synthesize protein. The particles, called *ribosomes,* give the outer membrane of the ER a rough or granular appearance; therefore, such endoplasmic reticulum is called *granular* or *rough ER.* Other surfaces of the endoplasmic reticulum are free of ribosomes and appear relatively smooth. This type of endoplasmic reticulum is called *agranular* or *smooth ER.*

The ER provides a large surface within the cell on which sequences of chemical reactions can occur. Enzymes and other substances are arranged in an assembly-line sequence to provide for efficient production of substances responsible for the metabolic functions of the cell.[2] The granular ER is involved primarily with the production of proteins. Proteins, such as hormones, that are destined to be secreted are put together on the ribosomes of the ER. Also, some of the proteins that form structural parts of the cell are produced here. The smooth ER is the site of formation of nonprotein substances, such as the fat-soluble triglycerides, fatty acids, steroids, and phospholipids. Enzymes within the smooth ER are involved in biotransformation of substances such as alcohol, pesticides, and carcinogens.[5] Calcium ions are released from sarcoplasmic reticulum, which is smooth ER in muscle cells (see pp. 835–836).

FREE RIBOSOMES

Some of the ribosomes within the cell are not bound to the ER. Instead, a number of ribosomes involved with the production of a specific protein molecule may be linked together, much like pearls on a string, forming a chain structure called a polyribosome (see Figure 1-1). Polyribosomes of several different lengths may be found in the cytoplasm, and all are involved with the formation or synthesis of protein molecules. Most of the proteins made on the polyribosomes are for the cell's own use in building cellular components (structural proteins) or in regulating cellular activities (enzymes).

GOLGI COMPLEX

The Golgi complex, also called the Golgi apparatus or the Golgi body, is a series of concentric, flattened saccules with membranes resembling those of the smooth ER (Fig. 1-6). In some cells, the Golgi membranes appear to be connected to the smooth ER and may be a specialized part of it. Membrane-bound vesicles are frequently observed near the Golgi membranes and represent either packaged chemicals arriving at the Golgi complex for further processing or packaged substances leaving the Golgi complex destined for secretion by way of exocytosis (see pp. 20–21).

The Golgi complex is predominant in various types of secretory cells, such as the pancreatic acinar cell, and plays several important roles in the process of secretion. Substances destined for secretion (eg, protein hormones) may be produced on the granular ER and then transported through the cisternae of the ER to the Golgi apparatus. The Golgi apparatus prepares the hormone for release by packaging it within a membranous vacuole, which then moves toward the plasma membrane, where the hormone is released to the exterior of the cell by exocytosis.

Other functions of the Golgi apparatus include production of some substances such as polysaccharides, chemical modification of molecules produced by the ER (eg, activation of enzymes), storage of synthesized molecules, and production of organelles called lysosomes.

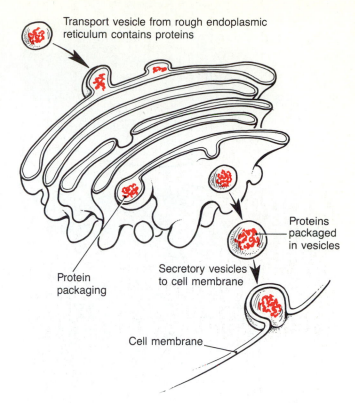

FIGURE 1-6 *Appearance and function of the Golgi apparatus.*

LYSOSOMES

Lysosomes are membrane-bound organelles that are spherical and contain digestive enzymes. They originate from the Golgi complex and ER and participate in intracellular digestive processes. Lysosomes contain a variety of hydrolytic enzymes that break down protein, nucleic acids, carbohydrates, and lipids. When a cell ingests material by endocytosis, lysosomes fuse their membranes with those of the endocytotic vesicle, forming a common membrane-bound vesicle in which digestion can occur (Fig. 1-7). The lysosomal membrane protects the other cellular organelles from the hydrolytic enzymes within the lysosome.

Lysosomes also digest "worn out" or damaged parts of the cell, thereby participating in the recycling of cellular constituents, a process called *autophagy*. However, when a cell dies, the lysosomes it contains rupture, releasing enzymes that cause the cell to self-destruct (*autolysis*). Normally, the lysosomal enzymes cannot break down the lysosomal membrane.

Numerous lysosomes are present in cells that are very active in ingesting matter by phagocytosis. In some of the leukocytes, for example, lysosomes are so numerous they give the cytoplasm a granular appearance. Lysosomes are a critical part of the body's defensive phagocytic cells that are responsible for destroying foreign proteins (see pp. 393–396). Lysosomal enzymes

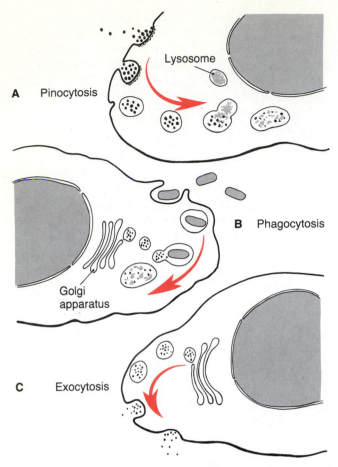

FIGURE 1-7 *A and B Endocytosis. Pinocytosis (A) allows for intake of certain substances through specific receptors on the cell surface. Phagocytosis (B) allows for intake and destruction of bacteria. **C.** Exocytosis is the process by which formed cellular elements are delivered to other areas of the body.*

in injured or dead tissue help prepare the affected area for repair.

PEROXISOMES

These intracellular organelles are smaller than lysosomes and contain oxidative enzymes that form hydrogen peroxide (H_2O_2). The H_2O_2 is involved with detoxification of potentially harmful substances, especially within the liver and kidney.[5]

THE CYTOSKELETON

The complex network of proteins that provide for cellular shape and, in some cases, the ability to carry out coordinated movement is called the cytoskeleton. It is composed of microfilaments, microtubules, and intermediate filaments. Microfilaments are different lengths of rodlike structures composed of actin, the thin filament of muscle tissue. Microfilaments are found both in muscle and in nonmuscular tissue.

Microtubules are nonmembranous, cylindrical organelles, the walls of which are composed of filaments of globular proteins called *tubulin* (Fig. 1-8). Microtubules, along with microfilaments, function to maintain the shape of a cell by providing structural support, to act as an internal conduit for the movement of materials from one part of the cell to another, and to provide for certain forms of cellular movement, such as ciliary motion.

Intermediate filaments are strong, tough proteins that provide structural reinforcement within cells. They also hold organelles in place and assist the microtubules in giving shape to the cell.[5]

CILIA AND FLAGELLA

Cilia are short protoplasmic extensions on the free surfaces of some cells that line body cavities or hollow viscera. The lining of the respiratory tract, for example, contains ciliated cells whose cilia move together to propel the mucus layer forward (see pp. 554–556). Cilia (singular, cilium) are microtubule-containing cylinders enclosed by an extension of the plasma membrane (Fig. 1-9). Usually, a single ciliated cell projects numerous cilia on its free surface, giving that portion of the cell surface a matlike appearance. One human cell type, the spermatozoon (sperm) or male reproductive cell, has a single, elongated cilium-like extension called a flagellum (plural, flagella). In cross section, a cilium or flagellum is bounded by a sheath that encloses an array of nine double microtubules arranged in a radial fashion, with two additional microtubules in the center. The compound tubular structure that is formed is called an *axoneme.*

Ciliary motion occurs when the microtubules, pow-

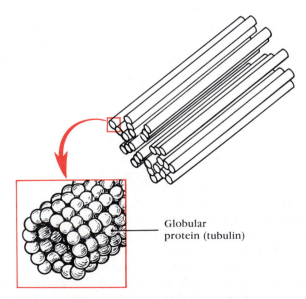

Globular protein (tubulin)

FIGURE 1-8 *Microtubules with filaments of globular proteins called tubulin. (Adapted from Snell, R.S. Clinical Histology for Medical Students. Boston: Little, Brown, 1984.)*

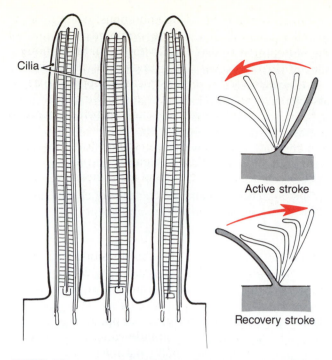

FIGURE 1-9 *Appearance of cilia on the surface of specific cells.*

ered by ATP, slide past one another. Cilia move with a swift forward movement and a slow backward stroke (like a whip). Their movement is coordinated so that stimulation is passed from one cilium to the next. On a sheet of ciliated cells, coordinated ciliary movement resembles the effect seen when wind ripples across a field of wheat. Ciliary movement in the upper respiratory tract is an important part of the body's defenses, helping to move inhaled particulate matter trapped in mucus toward the nasal and oral cavities, where it may be discharged or swallowed. Flagellar movement is undulating (wavelike), rather than whiplike. It is responsible for propelling sperm through body fluids at a rate of 1 to 4 mm per minute in a relatively straight line.

Microtubules, cilia, and flagella are nonmembranous organelles that are structurally related to the centriole. The centriole may be the source of microtubules, cilia, and flagella.

CENTROSOMES AND CENTRIOLES

Near the nucleus of many cells is a dense area of cytoplasm called the centrosome. It contains two hollow, cylindrical structures called centrioles which, like cilia, are composed of nine sets of microtubules arranged in a radial fashion, but without the central pair of tubules (9 + 0 pattern). Centrioles are often found near the nuclear envelope, with the long axis of one lying at right angles to the other (Fig. 1-10). The function of the centrioles is to form and organize a complex array of microtubules in nondividing cells. In dividing cells, it

forms the spindle apparatus, a structure needed to separate a single cell into two daughter cells when the cell divides (see p. 15). The microtubules that make up the wall of the centriole are arranged in sets of three, each set lying in the same plane and embedded in a dense granular substance.

NUCLEUS

The nucleus is a large, membranous organelle that is frequently located near the center of a cell. It contains large quantities of DNA, which form the *genes*. Cellular activities and structure are controlled through the genes. The nucleus is separated from the cytoplasm by a membranous structure called the *nuclear envelope* (Fig. 1-11). In contrast to the plasma membrane, it consists of two distinct membranes. The membranes are fused together periodically to form circular pores, through which material can pass in and out of the nucleus. The pores are about 10 times larger than those of the plasma membrane, allowing many protein molecules to pass through with relative ease. Most ions and water-soluble molecules also move easily between the nucleus and cytoplasm. The inner membrane of the nuclear envelope represents the actual nuclear membrane, and the outer

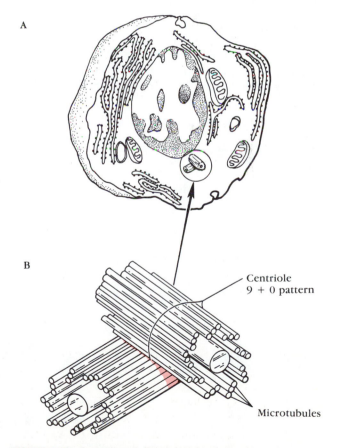

FIGURE 1-10 *Centrioles.* **A.** *Placement in relationship to the nucleus.* **B.** *Appearance and composition of the centriole.*

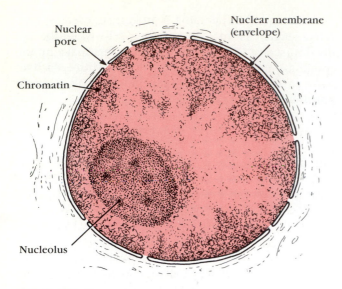

Nuclear pore — **Nuclear membrane (envelope)**

Chromatin —

Nucleolus —

FIGURE 1-11 *The nucleus.*

membrane of the envelope gives rise to and is continuous with membranes of the endoplasmic reticulum.

Distinct nuclear structures may be observed in some cells. Two commonly seen structures are the nucleolus and the condensed strands of chromatin called chromosomes, which are readily identified during cellular mitosis (see p. 15).

The *nucleolus* ("little nucleus") is a collection of dense fibers and granules forming a small spherical mass that is most visible when the cell is not in the process of mitosis (see Figure 1-11). The nucleolus is composed primarily of RNA and protein, together with smaller

amounts of DNA. These nucleic acids play key roles in the cellular synthesis of proteins. The granules of the nucleolus are precursors of ribosomes, which are the sites of protein synthesis in the cytoplasm.

Chromatin is composed of long molecules of DNA in association with protein. Chromatin fibers are too small to be seen with the light microscope. Before cell division begins, however, chromatin fibers coil and condense into compact structures that are visible under the light microscope. These visible, x-shaped structures are called *chromosomes* (Fig. 1-12). There are 46 chromosomes (23 pairs) in the human cell. The pairs of chromosomes differ from one another in size and shape.

Genes

The nucleus directs and controls the activities of the entire cell through the genes. A gene is a linear sequence of nucleotides on the DNA molecule that codes for (serves as a master mold for) the production of a single protein.[5] The sequence is divided into units of three nucleotides, each called a *triplet* or *codon*. The exact sequence of nucleotide bases (guanine, thymine, cytosine, and adenine) in each codon determines a unique code and ultimately codes for a single amino acid. The genes determine the specific code that is transcribed as RNA. The gene being transcribed is located on one of the two DNA strands, which serves as a master strand or *template* (pattern) for *messenger RNA* (mRNA) transcription. Other parts of DNA serve as templates for the formation of *transfer RNA* (tRNA) or *ribosomal RNA* (rRNA). The genetic code, transmitted to the ribosomes,

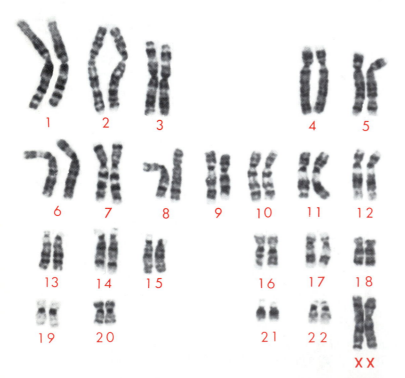

FIGURE 1-12 *Appearance of chromosomes. (Courtesy of Dr. David Ledbetter, National Institutes of Health, Bethesda, Md.)*

allows for the formation of several thousand types of proteins that are essential to the various functions of human cells (Fig. 1-13). Most proteins contain 100 to 1,000 amino acids.[5]

Protein Synthesis

Almost all of the chemical reactions associated with normal cellular function are enzyme dependent. All known enzymes are proteins, and their synthesis is controlled by nuclear DNA. Therefore, the activity of the cytoplasmic organelles is regulated either directly or indirectly by the nucleus. In addition to enzymes, nuclear DNA contains the blueprints that specify construction of other types of proteins, such as hormones and structural proteins. The synthesis of proteins occurs in two major steps, known as transcription and translation (see Figure 1-13).

Transcription occurs in the nucleus and involves DNA and mRNA. During transcription, the DNA molecule partially unwinds into two separate strands. One of the strands acts as a template on which mRNA is synthesized, while the other strand is noncoding. The genetic message carried by DNA in the form of a series of triplets is transcribed to mRNA by complementary base-pairing; thus, the formation of mRNA results in the synthesis of a molecule having a linear sequence of bases that is complementary to that of the DNA from which it was transcribed. The mRNA molecule separates from the DNA template as fast as it forms.

After synthesis, the mRNA escapes the nucleus by way of the pores in the nuclear envelope and enters the cytoplasm, where it becomes associated with ribosomes, the organelles that link amino acids into the polypeptide chains of proteins. Within the ribosome, the genetic message carried by mRNA in the form of codons is deciphered, and correct amino acids are joined in the proper sequence to form a protein molecule. This process is called *translation*, and it involves tRNA. One or more specific tRNA molecules exist for each type of amino acid. Each tRNA molecule binds itself to a specific amino acid and carries it to the site of protein synthesis in the ribosome. The tRNA molecule contains a binding site in the form of an anticodon, which recognizes and attaches to the correct codon on mRNA. Thus, as tRNA molecules bearing specific amino acids sequentially bind to mRNA

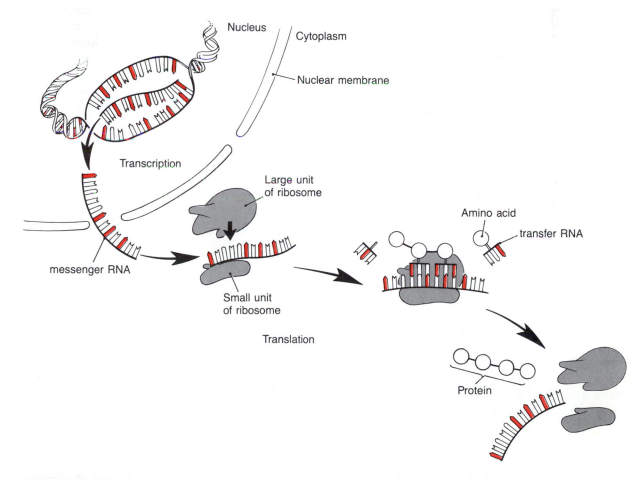

FIGURE 1-13 *Mechanism for the production of a protein through the sequencing of specific amino acids. DNA serves as the template for messenger RNA and transfer RNA, which are used in the assembly of the amino acids.*

in the ribosome, the amino acids are sequenced into a protein that is then released from the ribosome.

Once the mRNA template becomes associated with the ribosome, the process of peptide synthesis occurs rapidly, taking about 1 second for each new amino acid to be added to the peptide chain. The synthesis of a protein such as the hormone insulin (51 amino acids) takes about 1 minute. Several ribosomes may simultaneously translate a single strand of mRNA so that protein synthesis may occur more rapidly.

▼ *Reproductive Ability of Cells*

Most cells have the ability to reproduce themselves through the complex process of *mitosis*. In the adult, new cells take the place of old, worn out, or damaged cells in a rigidly defined order that maintains cellular numbers and allows for the replacement of only the needed cells. The turnover rate is billions of cells per day, but rigid controls inherently limit the number of cells to be reproduced.

Specific controls on the reproductive process produce precisely the correct quantity of cells. For example, if the erythrocyte (red blood cell) count decreases, specific stimulating factors cause the bone marrow to increase production of erythrocytes, leading ultimately to increased numbers of circulating red blood cells. After the appropriate level is reached, some factor, either diminished stimulation or an inhibitor, suppresses further production of erythrocytes (see p. 376).

REGENERATION OF CELLS

The ability of cells to reproduce themselves is called the regenerative capacity of cells. *Labile cells* regenerate frequently and have a life span that is usually measured in hours or days. Some examples of labile cells are leukocytes (white blood cells) and epithelial cells. Other cells retain the ability to regenerate or reproduce but do so only under special circumstances. These are called *stable cells*, and their life spans are measured in years or, sometimes, the entire life span of an organism. Some examples of stable cells are osteocytes of bone, parenchymal cells of the liver, and cells of the glands of the body. In the normal liver cell, for example, mitotic figures are rare, but after injury, mitoses are abundant because the liver has a remarkable ability to repair itself. The third type of cells, the *permanent cells*, live for the entire life of the organism. They include the nerve cell bodies and probably most of the muscle cells. The neuron loses its ability to undergo mitosis at about 6 months of age.[5] Myocardial muscle does not regenerate; when it dies, it is repaired by the formation of scar tissue.

REPRODUCTION OF CELLS

THE CELL CYCLE.   All human cells have a life cycle, called the cell cycle, that begins when the cell is produced by division of its parent and ends when the cell either divides to give rise to daughter cells or dies. A complete cell cycle consists of four stages, labeled G_1, S, G_2, and M (Fig. 1-14). All of the stages between mitotic divisions are called *interphase*.

The G_1 stage is the time interval after the formation of the cell that precedes replication of DNA. The S stage is the time during which DNA replication occurs. The G_2 stage is the time interval after DNA replication and before the beginning of the M stage. The M stage is that period of time in which cell division occurs. Cells not destined for an early repeat of the division cycle are commonly arrested at the G_0 stage. Stable cells can be stimulated from G_0 into G_1 with an appropriate stimulus, to provide for regeneration of lost cells.[1]

The process by which a cell divides to form two identical daughter cells is mitosis. Before a cell can undergo mitosis, its chromosomes must duplicate themselves, a process called *replication*.

Replication

Replication of DNA occurs during the S stage of interphase. During this time, the chromosomes appear to be spread out in a tangled mass known as chromatin. In replication, the two strands of the DNA molecule partially uncoil, and each serves as a template for the formation of another strand (Fig. 1-15). Each template and its

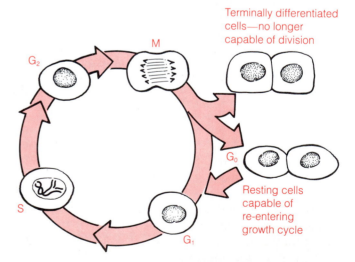

FIGURE 1-14   *The cell cycle. The cycle consists of four stages: G_1, S, G_2, and M. Cell division occurs during the M phase. In the S phase, synthesis of DNA occurs. Daughter cells may undergo differentiation and no longer be capable of division, or they may enter G_0. Cells in G_0 are mitotically inactive but may be recalled to the growth fraction under appropriate conditions. (Slauson, D.O., Cooper, B.J. Mechanisms of Disease [2nd ed.]. Baltimore: Williams & Wilkins, 1990.)*

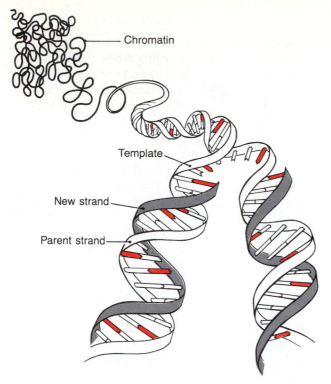

FIGURE 1-15 *Replication occurs when the two strands of DNA separate and a new strand is synthesized on each original strand. Each new molecule of DNA is identical to the original DNA molecule.*

complement then form a new DNA molecule. During mitosis, each daughter cell inherits a DNA molecule that consists of one new strand and one parental strand.

Each chromosome is furnished with a single centromere, an area that holds together the two daughter chromosomes produced when a chromosome replicates. After replication, the two identical, double-stranded molecules of DNA are called *chromatids* as long as they remain attached to each other by the centromere.

Mitosis

Mitosis is described in terms of phases through which the cell passes as it divides (Fig. 1-16). The phases are defined by the appearance of chromosomes under the light microscope and are designated (in sequence) as prophase, metaphase, anaphase, and telophase.

During *prophase*, the chromatin condenses into distinct chromosomes that are visible as pairs of chromatids joined at the *centromere*, the point of junction of the chromatin threads. In prophase, the nuclear membrane disappears, as does the nucleolus, and appears to be part of the cytoplasm. The centrioles migrate to opposite poles of the cell, and a spindle of microtubules forms between the centrioles.

During *metaphase*, the assembly of the spindle is completed and the chromosomes align in a plane mid-

way between the poles. This plane is called the *equatorial plane*. The chromosomes align at the equatorial plane because they experience an equal pull through the attached microtubules from the two poles of the spindle.

Anaphase starts with centromere division, which allows the newly divided chromosomes to move to opposite poles of the spindle. They assume a V shape as they are pulled through the cytoplasm by microtubules and filaments of the spindle apparatus.

At the beginning of *telophase*, two sets of daughter chromosomes are gathered at opposite poles. A new nuclear envelope is assembled from saccules of ER and surrounds each set of chromosomes. The chromosomes gradually unravel and disperse in the nucleus, disappearing from view. The spindle disintegrates, but the duplicated centrioles remain, and nucleoli reappear. As these events of telophase are occurring, a cleft, or cleavage furrow, forms in the plasma membrane. The cytoplasm is divided equally during anaphase or early telophase between the two newly formed daughter cells. This process is called *cytokinesis*. Complete division occurs when the furrow deepens until opposite surfaces make contact and the cell splits.

Meiosis

The process of reproduction of a new organism involves meiosis or reduction division, which is a special nuclear division of the chromosomes that produces 23 chromosomes in each sex cell rather than the 23 pairs found in all somatic cells. The sex cells, called *gametes*, are the ovum (female egg cell) and sperm (male sex cell). The union of male and female gametes is called fertilization. The resulting *zygote* contains a set of chromosomes from each parent, or a total of 23 pairs. Multiple divisions of the zygote eventually produce a new being.[5] The production of sperm is called *spermatogenesis*, and production of ova is called *oogenesis*. Fertilization and growth of the embryo and fetus are described in Chapter 5. Normal and altered reproductive function are discussed in Chapters 55 and 56.

▼ Cellular Exchange

For the cell to produce its own cytoplasm, synthesize chemicals for export, or derive energy from chemicals and convert the energy into useful work, the cell must acquire chemicals from the extracellular fluid (ECF). On the other hand, cell metabolism produces waste products which must be eliminated by the cell into the extracellular environment. Because the plasma membrane separates the intracellular fluid (ICF) from the ECF, all substances that either enter or leave the cell must pass through the plasma membrane.

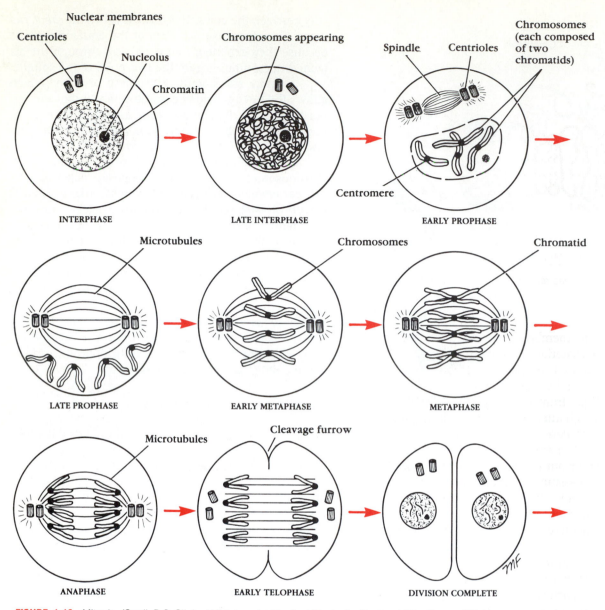

FIGURE 1-16 *Mitosis. (Snell, R.S.* Clinical Histology for Medical Students. *Boston: Little, Brown, 1984.)*

In general, the mechanisms of cellular exchange can be divided into passive and active movement across the cell membrane. Passive movement includes the processes of diffusion, osmosis, and facilitated diffusion. Active movement involves active, energy-driven and carrier-mediated transport systems as well as endocytosis and exocytosis (Fig. 1-17).

PASSIVE MOVEMENT ACROSS THE CELL MEMBRANE

Diffusion

Diffusion is defined as the net movement of a substance from a region of higher concentration to a region of lower concentration; that is, down a concentration gradient.

If the substance is equally distributed between two regions, no concentration gradient exists, and diffusion equilibrium is said to be present. The rate of net diffusion of a given substance, or the time that it takes for diffusion equilibrium to occur, is directly proportional to the concentration gradient, the cross-sectional or surface area of the diffusion pathway, and the temperature of the diffusing substance. The rate of net diffusion is determined by the amount of substance available, by kinetic motion, and by cell membrane openings through which the substance can move.[2] Additional factors include the atomic or molecular size and configuration, the ability of the diffusing solute to dissolve in lipids, and the presence or absence of an electrical charge on the diffusing solute particles.

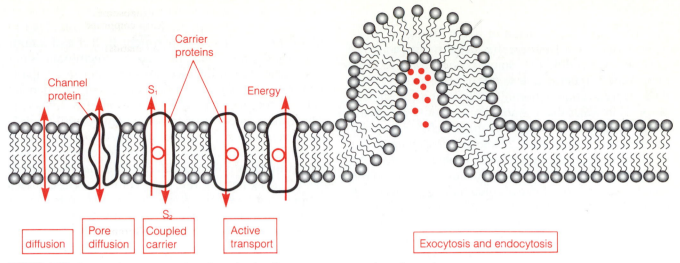

FIGURE 1-17 *Schematic representation of mechanism for transport across the cell membrane.*

The plasma membrane presents a barrier to the movement of materials in and out of the cell. Substances that diffuse through the membrane must either dissolve in the fluid structure of the plasma membrane and then diffuse from one side to the other, or they must pass through interruptions in the membrane called *channels* or *pores*. Pores are fluid-filled channels formed by proteins within the membrane. Small substances may diffuse in or out through the pores, including sodium (Na^+), potassium (K^+), calcium (Ca^{++}), chloride (Cl^-), bicarbonate (HCO_3^-), and water.[5] In general, substances with diameters greater than 8 Å have difficulty or are unable to pass through plasma membrane channels.

Uncharged particles pass through the membrane more readily than charged particles (*ions*), and negatively charged particles (*anions*) pass through more readily than do positively charged particles (*cations*). Also, molecules that have a higher degree of lipid solubility tend to diffuse through plasma membranes more readily than molecules that are less soluble in lipids. How readily an ion or molecule diffuses in or out of a cell depends on the physical and chemical properties of both the molecule itself and the plasma membrane that the molecule or ion is attempting to cross.

The movement of oxygen molecules into cells and carbon dioxide molecules out of cells is an example of the process of diffusion. Oxygen molecules are being continually consumed by metabolic processes occurring within the cell, so the concentration gradient favors diffusion of this gas into the cell. Carbon dioxide molecules are being continually produced during cellular metabolism, so the concentration gradient favors diffusion of this gas out of the cell. Other substances that diffuse through the membrane include water, nitrogen, steroids, and fat-soluble vitamins (Fig. 1-18).

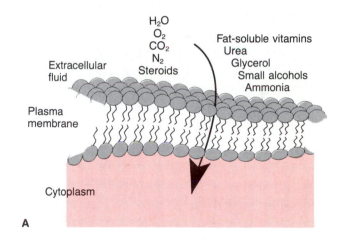

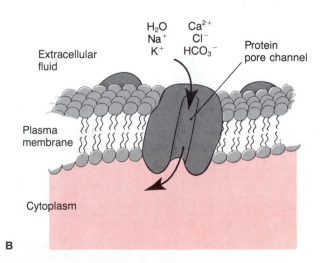

FIGURE 1-18 *Passive diffusion across the cell membrane occurs down a concentration gradient.* **A.** *Substances that can pass directly through the cell membrane.* **B.** *Substances that diffuse through a protein channel.*

Osmosis

Osmosis is the net diffusion of water through a selectively permeable membrane that separates two aqueous solutions with different solute concentrations. The membrane is impermeable to one or more of the solutes. If the concentration of nondiffusible solutes (substances dissolved in water that cannot diffuse through the membrane) is greater on one side of the membrane than the other, net diffusion of water (osmosis) occurs through the membrane toward the area of greater solute concentration until the solute:solvent ratio is equal on both sides of the membrane, or until a force of equal magnitude opposing the force created by the movement of water is applied. Water molecules diffuse from an area of greater water concentration through a selectively permeable membrane to an area of lesser water concentration.

Consider a 500-mL beaker containing 280 mL of pure water divided into two equal compartments by a selectively permeable membrane (Fig. 1-19). For pur-

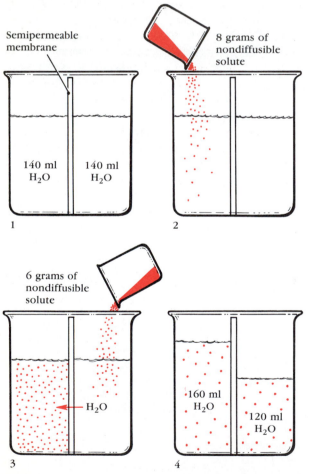

Semipermeable membrane

8 grams of nondiffusible solute

140 ml H₂O   140 ml H₂O

1   2

6 grams of nondiffusible solute

H₂O

160 ml H₂O

120 ml H₂O

3   4

FIGURE 1-19   Osmosis. **A.** A beaker of water with superimpermeable membrane separating the sides. **B.** Add 8 g of a nondiffusable substance to one side. **C.** Add 6 g of a nondiffusible substance to the other side. **D.** The water moves toward the more concentrated side and makes the concentrations equal, with more fluid on one side than the other.

poses of discussion, consider the system to be unaffected by atmospheric pressure. Compartment A contains 140 mL of water, as does compartment B. If 8 g of a nondiffusible solute, a solute to which the membrane is not permeable, is then dissolved in the water in compartment A and 6 g of nondiffusible solute is dissolved in the water in compartment B, net diffusion of water occurs from compartment B to compartment A until the solute:solvent ratios of each compartment become equal. At diffusion equilibrium, the solute:solvent ratio of compartment A is 8 g per 160 mL, and that of compartment B is 6 g per 120 mL; each compartment contains 1 g per 20 mL of fluid. A net diffusion of 20 mL water from compartment B to compartment A has occurred.

During osmosis, pressure is created on the membrane as water moves from an area of higher concentration, through the membrane, to an area of lesser concentration. This pressure is called *osmotic pressure*. The magnitude of osmotic pressure depends on the number of solute particles in the solution toward which water is moving. The greater the number of nondiffusible particles in that solution, the greater its osmotic pressure.

Fluids that contain osmotically active particles in the same concentration as that found in the plasma of blood are said to be *isotonic*. If a human erythrocyte is placed in an isotonic solution, it neither swells nor shrinks, because the net diffusion of water in or out of the cell is zero. An example of an isotonic solution is 0.9% sodium chloride in water (normal saline). Normally, the net volume of the cell remains constant. If a concentration difference for water occurs, the *water* moves, causing the cell to shrink or to swell.[2]

Fluids that contain a higher concentration of osmotically active particles than blood plasma does are termed *hypertonic fluids*. Erythrocytes that are placed in a hypertonic solution shrink and shrivel (*crenation*) because net diffusion of water out of the cells occurs. *Hypotonic solutions* contain a lower concentration of osmotically active particles than does plasma; red blood cells swell and hemolyze when placed in hypotonic solutions, because the net diffusion of water is into the cells (Fig. 1-20). In the body, osmosis is important in maintaining plasma volume, interstitial and ICF volumes, and the volumes of other fluid compartments.

Filtration

Substances, especially water, move across membranes because of pressure differences, always moving from greater to lesser pressure areas. Filtration is an important concept in the kidneys in the formation of glomerular filtrate. Larger particles remain in the capillaries owing to their size and the impermeability of the glomerular basement membrane (see pp. 621–622).

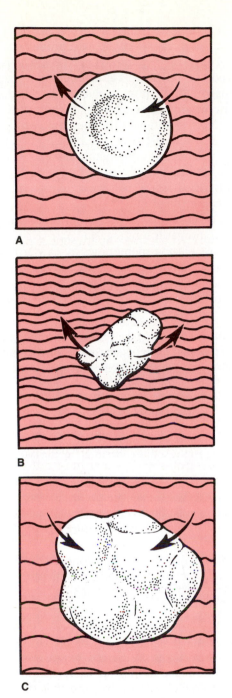

FIGURE 1-20 **A.** *Isotonic solution (cell volume unchanged).* **B.** *Hypertonic solution (cell volume decreased.* **C.** *Hypotonic solution (cell volume increased).*

Facilitated Diffusion

The process of assisted diffusion is especially important in moving glucose from the ECF to the ICF. Normally, there is a very small reserve of glucose for energy metabolism within the cell, so the cell is very dependent on the transport of glucose from the ECF. Glucose is not soluble in the lipid of the cell membrane and is too large to pass through the membrane pores. The mechanism of facili-

tated passive transport involves combining glucose with specific carrier molecules that are in the cell membrane. *Carrier systems* are composed of proteins that have receptors for specific solutes. After combining with the carrier molecule, glucose is carried into the cell by simple diffusion (Fig. 1-21). This process requires no ATP but is assisted by the pancreatic hormone insulin, which has been shown to increase the rate of glucose transport sevenfold to tenfold. Substances move only from an area of high concentration to one of low concentration (down the concentration gradient). The process is enhanced when a greater differential exists between ICF and ECF. A maximum rate for movement of solutes exists, and the mechanism can become saturated (see pp. 623–624).

ACTIVE MOVEMENT ACROSS THE CELL MEMBRANE

Active Transport

Many carrier systems transport solutes against a chemical or electrical gradient. These carrier-mediated transport systems always require the expenditure of energy and are often called "active transport" systems, or simply "pumps." All of the body's cells are capable of active transport in one way or another. For example, when a meal low in carbohydrates is ingested, cells that line the intestinal tract transport glucose out of the intestine and toward the blood, where the concentration of glucose may be much greater.

The *sodium–potassium pump* is an important example of active transport (Fig. 1-22). As mentioned previously, the ICF normally contains a much higher concentration of potassium than the ECF. Also, the ECF contains a much higher concentration of sodium (Na^+) than potassium (K^+) (see Table 1-1). These balances must be rigidly maintained for proper cellular function.

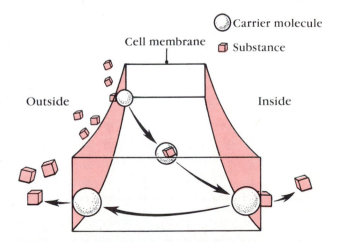

FIGURE 1-21 *Facilitated diffusion. A substance combines with a carrier molecule, which moves it to the inside of the cell and down its concentration gradient without the expenditure of energy. Each carrier molecule can carry only one specific substance.*

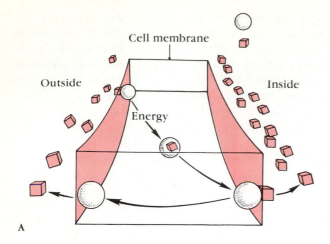

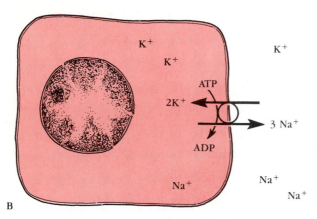

FIGURE 1-22 *Active transport. **A.** Postulated carrier system for moving substances across the cell membrane is like facilitated diffusion, except that the movement is against a concentration gradient and requires energy. **B.** Postulated mechanism for moving sodium out of the cell and potassium to the interior of the cell.*

The sodium–potassium pump transports sodium ions out of the cell, thereby preventing their accumulation inside. It also returns potassium ions to the inside of the cell. This requires direct energy from ATP.

The sodium–potassium pump prevents accumulation of sodium within the cell; by doing so, it also minimizes water influx and cellular swelling. Accumulation of sodium in ICF tends to cause osmosis of water toward the interior of the cell. The pumping of sodium ions out of the cell overcomes the continual tendency for water to enter the cell. If cellular metabolism ceases or decreases, adequate ATP to run the pump is not available, and cellular swelling begins immediately.

Carrier-Mediated Transport Systems

Although the phenomenon of carrier-mediated transport and the characteristics of transport processes have been studied for several years, the actual molecular mechanisms involved are not clear. Many carrier molecules are believed to be membrane-bound proteins (eg,

glycoprotein) that become activated (capable of picking up and transporting) when the membrane becomes energized through the breakdown of ATP. On activation of the transport protein and its attachment to the substance to be transported, the protein changes its position in the membrane in a manner that effects the transfer of the substance from one side of the membrane to the other. Evidence also indicates that the binding of some substances to receptors on the membrane causes a pore or channel to form, thereby providing a less restrictive pathway for the passive movement of materials such as ions across the membrane.[2]

Many types of solutes, such as glucose, amino acids, and various inorganic ions (eg, Na^+, Cl^-, K^+), are transported across plasma membranes by carrier molecules. Some of these transport systems are active and others are passive. Carrier-mediated transport systems often display one or more of the following characteristics:

1. *Specificity.* Carrier systems are usually specific for a particular solute. For example, the system that transports glucose will not transport other organic solutes such as amino acids.
2. *Saturation.* Many systems have a maximum rate (called the *transport maximum*, or *Tm*) at which a solute can be transported. If more solute is present than the system can handle, the system is said to be saturated and to be transporting solute at the maximum rate. Below saturation level, the rate of transport varies directly with solute concentration (ie, the higher the solute concentration, the faster the rate of transport).
3. *Competition.* If the same carrier system transports two different solutes in the same direction, the rate of transport of each is diminished by the presence of the other. In other words, the solutes compete for transport by the carrier, and some of each solute is transported at the carrier's maximum rate.
4. *Energy dependency.* Many carrier systems require energy to function. Substances (metabolic inhibitors) that interfere with energy-producing reactions of the cell often stop transport processes.
5. *Gating of protein channels.* Gating refers to the opening or closing of the channels formed by protein carriers. This opening or closing can be controlled by electrical changes in the cell membrane or by physical changes in the protein carrier molecule. *Voltage gating* occurs in response to changes in the electrical potential of the cell membrane (see pp. 21–23). *Ligand gating* occurs with a physical change in the protein molecule, which results from binding of another molecule with the protein. This molecule is called a *ligand*. The ligand can be a chemical mediator, such as acetyl COA, or a highly charged ion, such as sodium or potassium.[2]

Endocytosis and Exocytosis

Endocytosis and exocytosis are methods for bringing particles into the cell and releasing secretions to the exterior of the cell. These processes are schematically illustrated in Figure 1-7. Both are essential in carrying out the functional capabilities of specific cells. *Endocytosis* refers to the bringing in of protein and other substances through invagination of the outer cell membrane. This process occurs in the following ways.

Pinocytosis involves movement of water or material in the ECF that adheres to the outer cell membrane and stimulates invagination of the membrane. The material is encased or enclosed in a vesicle and floats into the cytoplasm. Lysosomes attach to the vesicle surface and release hydrolytic enzymes into the vesicle; the enzymes break down the material for use within the cells. A residual body may be left within the vesicle or excreted through the cell membrane to the ECF.

Phagocytosis involves the ingestion of particulate material or macromolecular substances. It often refers to the engulfment of a bacterium (see pp. 298–299).

Receptor-mediated endocytosis is the movement of substances through cell-surface receptors that stimulate the endocytotic process. Cell membranes have cell-surface receptors that pick up specific large molecules when they are found in the cell's environment. Substances termed *ligands* bind selectively to these receptors and can then be rapidly taken into the cell. In some cases, the receptor complexes escape degradation and are recycled to trap more ligand. In other cases, receptor and ligand are both degraded, which leads to a decrease in the number of surface receptors. Important compounds internalized through this process include *low-density lipoproteins*, which provide the cholesterol needed for synthesis of the cell membrane.[5] After the ligands have been taken into the cell, lysosomes attach to the vesicles and process the material.

Exocytosis has been termed *reverse pinocytosis* and is an active release of soluble products to the ECF. Secretion granules are formed, as has already been described, by the Golgi complex. The formed secretion granules move to the inner cell membrane, adhere, and cause an outpouching of the membrane. The outpouched area ruptures and releases the contents of the secretion granules into the ECF. The secretory products are vital to maintenance of the steady state of the host and include, for example, secretions necessary for digestion, glandular secretion, and neural transmission.

Both endocytosis and exocytosis require energy and are affected by the cell's ability to synthesize ATP. Both processes require enzymatic activity to enhance the rate of the reactions.

▼ *Electrical Properties of Cells*

Differences in electrical potential across the plasma membrane are characteristic of all living cells. The membrane potential exists because of unequal distribution of ions between the inner and outer surfaces of the membrane, the membrane's different permeability to various ions, and the active transport systems that maintain ionic imbalance across the membrane. The electrical charge for the inside of the cell is more negative than the outside. The *resting membrane potential* normally is about -70 to -85 mV from the inside to the outside of the cell when the cell is in the resting state. This equilibrium is attained and maintained by the sodium-potassium pump.

Some cells have the ability to respond to various types of stimuli, especially electrochemical stimuli. This response is called the cell's *excitability* and refers to the changing or altering of the electrical potential across the cell membrane. Two major types of cells, nerve and muscle, are considered to be excitable cells because they can change membrane potential, effect an action or response, and return to the resting state. The excitable tissue or cell receives a stimulus that rapidly changes its resting membrane potential. The resulting *action potential* is followed by the action of the cell, which may be a contraction, transmission of the action potential to the next cell, or another action. The cell then returns to the normal resting state, characterized by reestablishment of the resting membrane potential. Many changes occur in the cell membranes when an action potential is elicited. The following discussion of the action potential is with reference to a neuron but applies with minor variation to other excitable cells, such as skeletal and cardiac muscle cells.

When an adequate positive stimulus is applied to the neuron, a rapid and marked change occurs in the membrane potential at the point on the membrane at which the stimulus was applied. The positive stimulus increases the sodium permeability of the membrane, allowing sodium to begin entering the cell at a faster rate than it can be pumped out. As more sodium passes through the membrane, the membrane potential becomes less negative. After the membrane potential has been reduced to a critical value called the *threshold*, additional sodium channels open, increasing the membrane's sodium permeability even more and resulting in a rapid influx of sodium. The membrane potential approaches zero and then actually becomes reversed, so the inside of the membrane is positive with respect to the outside; these changes characterize *depolarization* of the membrane.

Almost immediately after sodium influx begins to depolarize the membrane, an increase in potassium diffusion out of the cell begins, and it accelerates as the movement of sodium causes the inside of the membrane to become positive. Potassium leaves the cell for the same reasons that sodium entered—favorable electrical and chemical gradients coupled with an increase in membrane permeability. As potassium efflux accelerates, further diffusion of sodium into the cell is inhibited by a decrease in sodium permeability, and the net loss of positive charges (K^+) from the inside causes the membrane potential to return to zero and then become negative once again, reestablishing the resting potential. More potassium leaves the cell than is actually required to restore the resting potential. For a short time, the inside of the membrane is more negative than it normally is at rest. This increased internal negativity is termed *hyperpolarization*. The return of the membrane potential to resting level is completed by the sodium–potassium pump, which exchanges internal sodium for external potassium, thereby restoring the normal internal:external ratios of these ions. These activities that restore the resting membrane potential after depolarization of the membrane collectively characterize the phenomenon of *repolarization*.

The action potential (membrane depolarization and repolarization) can be graphically represented as change in voltage versus time (Fig. 1-23). The duration of the action potential for a neuron is less than 0.5 msec. The action potential represents the change in membrane potential only in the region of the membrane at which an adequate positive stimulus has been applied. The entire plasma membrane does not simultaneously depolarize and then repolarize in response to an adequate stimulus.

Once an action potential has been generated, however, it spreads from one area of the membrane to another, resulting in the propagation of a nerve impulse.

A nerve impulse is a wave of depolarization followed by a wave of repolarization that travels along a nerve fiber away from the point of stimulation (Fig. 1-24). When a positive stimulus that is of sufficient strength or duration to reduce the membrane potential to threshold (sometimes called a *threshold stimulus*) is applied to the nerve fiber, the membrane depolarizes, with the inside becoming positive with respect to the outside. Adjacent areas of the membrane remain polarized (inside negative), resulting in the flow of electrical current as positive charges are attracted to adjacent negative charges. The flow of current reduces the membrane potential in adjacent areas of the membrane to threshold, allowing sodium to move in and depolarization to occur. The sequence of one area of depolarization inducing depolarization in an adjacent area results in a wave of depolarization that is propagated along the nerve fiber in a manner similar to the burning of a gunpowder fuse. As soon as the wave of depolarization passes a segment of

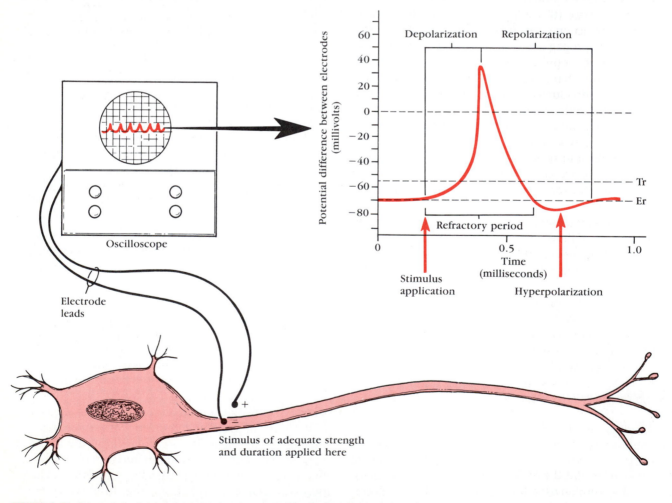

FIGURE 1-23 *Recording of an action potential. Tr, threshold potential; Er, resting potential.*

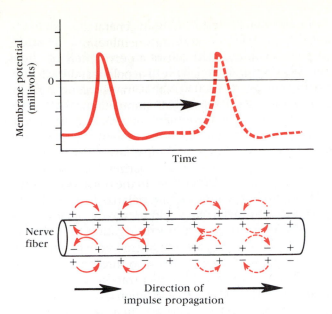

FIGURE 1-24 *Propagation of an action potential along a nonmyelinated nerve fiber.*

the fiber, that segment is repolarized and its ability to respond to another stimulus is soon restored.

If an adequate (threshold) stimulus is applied to a nerve fiber, an action potential is generated at the site of stimulus and propagated away from the site. Once generated, each impulse is conducted in an identical manner without change in magnitude or velocity. Stimuli that fail individually or collectively to reduce the membrane potential to threshold fail to generate an action potential and therefore produce no nerve impulse. In other words, weak stimuli do not generate weak impulses and strong stimuli, strong impulses. Instead, the response of a nerve fiber to a stimulus is either maximal or zero. This property is called the *all-or-none law*.

After an action potential has been generated, a minimum amount of time is required before that area of the membrane becomes capable of responding in an identical manner to a second stimulus. This minimum period is called the *refractory period*. The length of the refractory period determines the maximum number of impulses that the fiber can conduct each second. Fibers with short refractory periods can conduct impulses at a higher frequency than fibers with long refractory periods. Nerve fibers conduct impulses at a much higher rate or frequency than do myocardial muscle fibers, and their refractory periods likewise differ considerably.

▼ Cellular Movement

Many cells exhibit the ability to move. Movement may involve locomotion from one place to another, or it may involve movement of microtubules and microfilaments

within the cell. Ciliary and flagellar movements are examples of microtubular and microfilament movement. Ameboid locomotion involves movement of a cell from one location to another, and muscular contraction involves movement of muscle mass to perform work.

AMEBOID LOCOMOTION

Ameboid locomotion refers to the ability of a cell to move from one location to another in a manner similar to the way a unicellular animal, called an ameba, moves in its fluid environment. In the embryo, most of the cells exhibit ameboid motion, by which they migrate to their appropriate location. This property of ameboid movement is retained by certain defensive cells of the body, especially the leukocytes, and allows them to move from the bloodstream to the tissue spaces to contact and destroy foreign proteins[4].

Using energy (ATP) and calcium ions, the process is accomplished by the forward projection of a portion of the cell called the *pseudopodium* (Fig. 1-25). It probably depends on contraction of microfilaments in the outer portion of the cytoplasm to push out or project the pseudopodium. The remainder of the cell follows the projected area with a streaming motion. This process allows for the rapid movement of cells into an area.

MUSCULAR CONTRACTION

Approximately 50% of the body mass is skeletal, smooth, and cardiac muscle. Contraction of these muscles make possible both involuntary and voluntary movements of the body. The details of muscular contraction are described in Chapters 22, 40, and 44.

Both electrical and mechanical processes exist in muscle. Most contractions are initiated through electrical stimulation from the nerve terminals. The electrical events are followed immediately by the mechanical events in a sequential way. Electrical activation causes

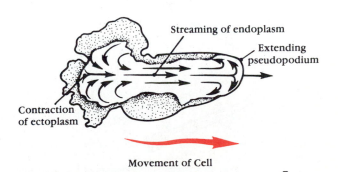

FIGURE 1-25 *Method of ameboid motion of a cell, showing contraction of ectoplasm, extended pseudopodium, and streaming of endoplasm toward the projected pseudopodium.*

depolarization, which initiates the mechanical movement of contractile proteins in relation to each other and causes a shortening of the muscle fiber. The muscle fiber is illustrated in Figure 1-26, which shows the subunits of the fiber and the appearance of two contractile proteins called *actin* and *myosin*.

Skeletal muscle has a striated appearance because of its regularly ordered proteins. These proteins make up the contractile portions of the muscle fiber. The process of skeletal muscle contraction follows a particular course. A nerve stimulation causes the release of acetylcholine at the neuromuscular junction. Acetylcholine, a chemical neurotransmitter, causes a change in muscle cell ion permeability, generating an action potential that is spread throughout the muscle cell membrane and to the

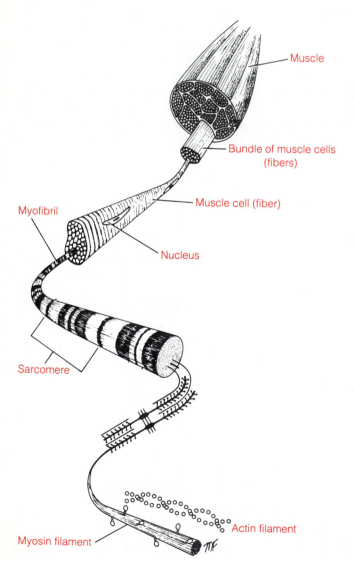

Muscle

Bundle of muscle cells (fibers)

Muscle cell (fiber)

Myofibril

Nucleus

Sarcomere

Myosin filament

Actin filament

FIGURE 1-26 *Gross to microscopic components of a skeletal muscle fiber. (Snell, R.S. Clinical Histology for Medical Students. Boston: Little, Brown, 1984.)*

T tubules that carry the stimulus to the interior of the cell. The transfer of stimulus by T tubules to the sarcoplasmic reticulum (SR) causes release of calcium from the SR. Calcium binds with the inhibitory protein *troponin*, causing troponin to interact with another protein, *tropomyosin*, which results in the uncovering of the active sites on actin, allowing for free interaction of actin with myosin. The actin filament is then pulled along the myosin filament, causing shortening of the entire sarcomere unit (Fig. 1-27). Calcium is immediately taken back up into the SR, and troponin and tropomyosin regain their normal inhibitory function. Large quantities of ATP are necessary to provide energy to pump the calcium back into the SR. During this process, sodium also leaks into the cell. The sodium pump must be activated to prevent accumulation of water in the muscle cell.

Cardiac muscle, which is also striated, follows the same general pattern for contraction but exhibits basic differences. Cardiac muscle is rapidly depolarized and contracts immediately after stimulation, but it repolarizes much more slowly than skeletal muscle. This slow repolarization apparently protects cardiac muscle from tetany, a phenomenon that may occur in skeletal muscle. Also, impulses depolarize the entire muscle mass, either atrial or ventricular, rather than individual fibers, as with skeletal muscle. This characteristic occurs because the individual cells within cardiac muscle are connected to one another by low-resistance electrical bridges (intercalated discs) that allow the electrical impulse to spread from cell to cell (see pp. 434–436).

Smooth muscle cells are smaller than skeletal muscle cells. They form two major types of muscle units, *multiunit smooth muscle* and *visceral smooth muscle*. Multiunit smooth muscle is independently innervated by nerve signals and includes the piloerector muscles of hairs (''gooseflesh''), smooth muscles of the larger blood vessels, and several muscles of the eye. Visceral smooth muscles are usually arranged in sheets, and the cell membranes contact each other so that ions can flow freely from one cell to the next. Contractions of visceral muscles are relatively slow and can be sustained for periods of up to 30 seconds. Rhythmic contractions or waves of contractions, such as intestinal peristalsis, result from the influence of nerve impulses.

▼ Cellular Organization

Although cells are the basic structural and functional units of the body, those that share a common function, such as lining a body cavity or providing for movement of the skeleton, are organized into *tissues*. In turn, tissues are organized into more complex structures known as *organs*. Organs that share a common purpose, such as the

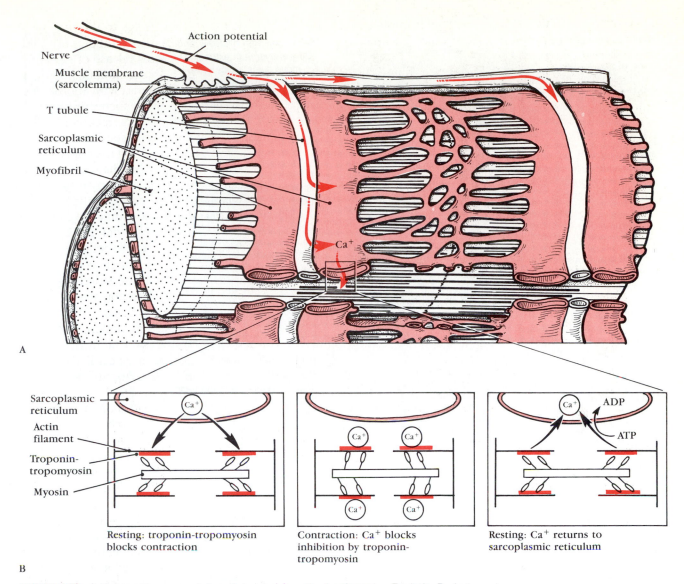

FIGURE 1-27 **A.** *Schematic representation of depolarizing stimulus through a T tubule.* **B.** *Actin and myosin filaments in the relaxed and contracted states.*

formation and excretion of urine, are grouped into *systems*. Systems work together to promote functioning of the human body. The four basic types of tissues that compose the body are the epithelial, muscular, nervous, and connective tissues.

EPITHELIAL TISSUE

Epithelial tissue provides a covering for most of the internal and external surfaces of the body. In this way, it may function as a protective barrier or it may be involved with absorption of materials, excretion of waste products, and secretion of specialized products into specific areas. Epithelial tissue is classified according to its thick-

ness (number of layers) and the shape of its cells. Fig. 1-28 illustrates different types of epithelial tissues by structure and function. It also indicates the common locations of each type of epithelial cell.

MUSCULAR TISSUE

The microstructure and functions of the muscle cells that make up muscle tissues are discussed in depth in Chapter 44. In general, muscles are classified as skeletal, cardiac, or visceral according to their appearance and function. Figure 1-29 illustrates the three types of muscle tissues and their functions.

Striated skeletal muscle provides for voluntary move-

A
Simple squamous
Flat, single layer
Lining of many areas,
  such as alveoli, glomeruli,
  gastrointestinal organs

Simple

B
Simple cuboidal
Cube-shaped cells, single layer
Lining of many ducts, especially
  in kidney and glands

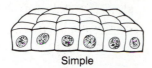
Simple

C
Stratified squamous
Several layers, cuboidal, columnar,
  and squamous
Layers of skin, linings of mucous
  membranes

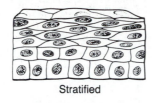
Stratified

D
Stratified cuboidal
Several layers of surface cells
Found in sweat glands,
  male urethra

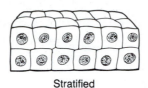
Stratified

E
Simple columnar
Single layer, columnlike
Gastrointestinal tract lining
Contains secreting goblet cells

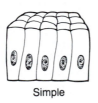
Simple

F
Columnar with microvilli and cilia
Single layer with extensions that
  move fluids along a plane
Lining of respiratory tract
  and fallopian tubes

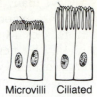
Microvilli   Ciliated

G
Stratified columnar
Layers of cells with some
  columnar, some other shapes
Contain goblet cells
Found in ducts of glands,
  male urethra, and parts of eye

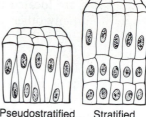
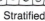
Pseudostratified   Stratified

H
Glandular
Variable layers secreting various
  products
Release products into ducts,
  such as sweat, mucus, ear
  wax, and digestive enzymes

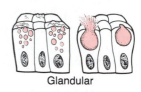
Glandular

I
Transitional
Multilayered, variable appearance
  from stratified squamous
  to cuboidal
Lining of urinary bladder, parts
  of ureters and urethra

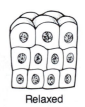
Relaxed

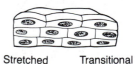
Stretched   Transitional

FIGURE 1-28 *Various types of epithelial tissues.*

ment of the body. The characteristic striated appearance results from an ordered sequence of contractile proteins which contain alternating dark and light bands. These proteins form or constitute numerous *myofibrils*, the contractile units of the muscle cell. Skeletal muscle cells are multinucleate, with the nuclei located at the periphery of the cell under the cell membrane.

Cardiac muscle forms the walls of the heart, which are the contractile portions of the organ. Its appearance is similar to that of striated skeletal muscle, except that it has a single, centrally located nucleus. Myocardial cells lie very closely approximated one to another. The importance of myocardial construction in relation to cardiac contraction is detailed on pages 433.

Smooth muscle does not exhibit the characteristic striations of skeletal or cardiac muscle, but smooth muscle cells have many fibrils that extend the length of the cell. The two major types are multiunit and visceral smooth muscles. Multiunit smooth muscles are stimulated mainly by nerve signals such as those causing contraction of blood vessels. Visceral smooth muscles are arranged in sheets or bundles, and the cell membranes contact each other through *gap junctions*, which allow the muscle to contract as a group. This type of smooth muscle is found in most of the organs of the body.[1] A single nucleus lies near the center of each cell. Smooth muscle cells are located in the viscera, blood vessels, uterus, and many other areas.

NERVOUS TISSUE

Nervous tissue is made up of neurons, the cells that conduct nerve impulses, and glial cells, which provide structural and functional support for the neurons. The typical nerve cell has a large central nucleus, multiple dendrites, and a single axon (Fig. 1-30). The dendrites carry impulses toward the cell body, and the axon carries impulses away from the cell body. The function of the neuron is described on pp. 925−930.

CONNECTIVE TISSUE

Connective tissue usually forms the framework for other cells and helps to bind together various tissues and organs. Many types of cells are included in the classifi-

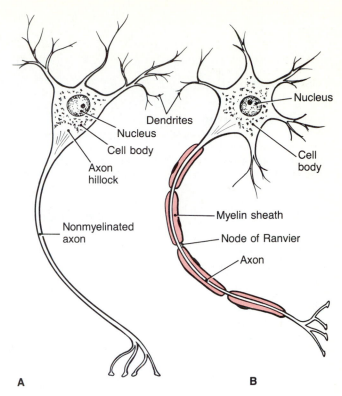

A   **B**

FIGURE 1-30 *Types of neurons.* **A.** *Example of a nonmyelinated neuron.* **B.** *Example of a neuron with its myelinated sheath.*

cation of connective tissue, and these are described in Figure 1-31. Blood cells, described in detail in Unit 6, are considered to be specialized connective tissue cells.

Bone, the hardest of the connective tissues, provides the structural framework of the body and acts as a plentiful reservoir for the minerals calcium and phosphorus. It is composed of cells, fibers, and extracellular components, which are calcified and rigid. In children, the long bones have two ends, a diaphysis and an epiphysis, separated by epiphyseal cartilage. Growth in bone length occurs as cartilage cells grow away from the shaft and are replaced by bone, resulting in an increased length of the shaft. As maturity is reached, this cartilage is entirely replaced by bone (see p. 848). Bone encloses the hematopoietic marrow, which supplies most of the blood cells of the body. *Periosteum* covers most bones and is lacking only in special areas. The principal cells of adult bone are osteocytes, which with the other bone cells—osteoblasts, osteoclasts, and osteoprogenitor cells—form and repair the bone tissue (see pp. 858−860). Bone cells adjust their number in proportion to the amount of physical stress placed on them. For example, increased deposition of collagen fibers and inorganic salts occurs in response to prolonged increase in workload. Conversely, salts are pulled from bone when stress or weight-bearing is decreased.

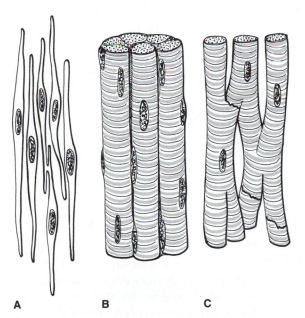

A   **B**   **C**

FIGURE 1-29 **A.** *Appearance of smooth muscle fibers.* **B.** *Striated skeletal muscle shows characteristic multiple nuclei and alternating light and dark bands* **C.** *Branched, striated, cardiac muscle fibers with a single nucleus and close approximation of cell to cell through intercalated discs.*

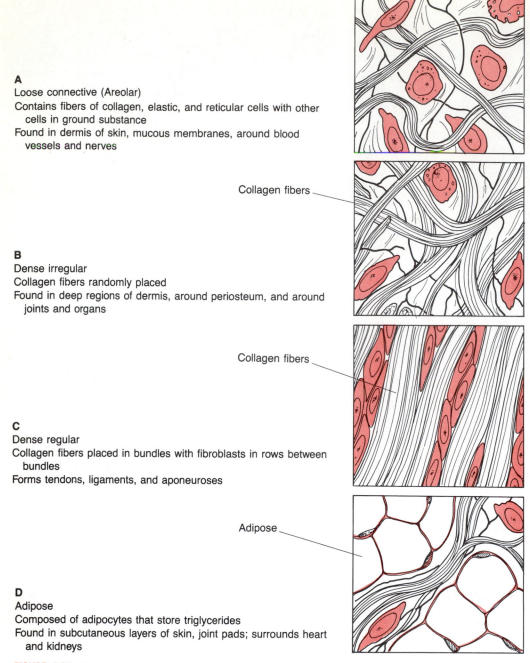

A
Loose connective (Areolar)
Contains fibers of collagen, elastic, and reticular cells with other
  cells in ground substance
Found in dermis of skin, mucous membranes, around blood
  vessels and nerves

Collagen fibers

B
Dense irregular
Collagen fibers randomly placed
Found in deep regions of dermis, around periosteum, and around
  joints and organs

Collagen fibers

C
Dense regular
Collagen fibers placed in bundles with fibroblasts in rows between
  bundles
Forms tendons, ligaments, and aponeuroses

Adipose

D
Adipose
Composed of adipocytes that store triglycerides
Found in subcutaneous layers of skin, joint pads; surrounds heart
  and kidneys

FIGURE 1-31 *Selected types of connective tissue.*

▼ *Chapter Summary*

▼ Organelles regulate the functions of the cell and the entire body (when considered in total).

▼ The cell membrane separates the intracellular from the extracellular fluid and is composed mainly of lipids and proteins.

▼ Proteins maintain cellular form and carry substances from the extracellular fluid to the intracellular fluid.

▼ The following functions are performed by specific organelles:

  ▼ Mitochondria produce energy through the production of adenosine triphosphate.

  ▼ The endoplasmic reticulum provides an area within the cell for the production of specific cellular products.

  ▼ Ribosomes produce specific proteins.

  ▼ The Golgi apparatus plays important roles in the

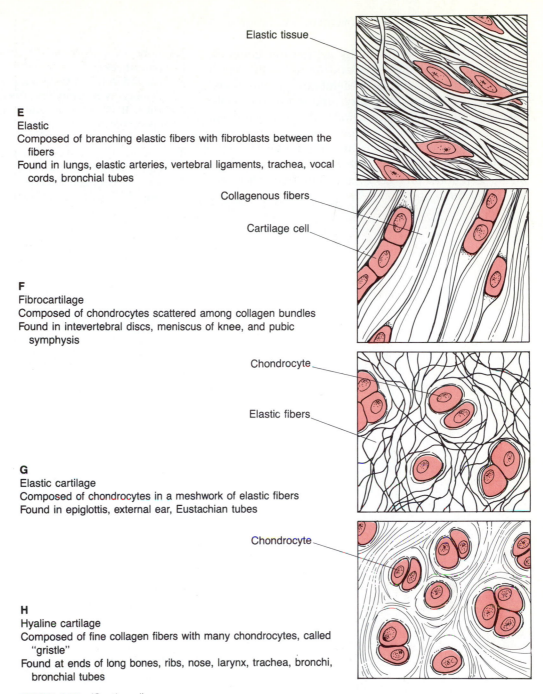

Elastic tissue

E
Elastic
Composed of branching elastic fibers with fibroblasts between the
  fibers
Found in lungs, elastic arteries, vertebral ligaments, trachea, vocal
  cords, bronchial tubes

Collagenous fibers

Cartilage cell

F
Fibrocartilage
Composed of chondrocytes scattered among collagen bundles
Found in intevertebral discs, meniscus of knee, and pubic
  symphysis

Chondrocyte

Elastic fibers

G
Elastic cartilage
Composed of chondrocytes in a meshwork of elastic fibers
Found in epiglottis, external ear, Eustachian tubes

Chondrocyte

H
Hyaline cartilage
Composed of fine collagen fibers with many chondrocytes, called
  "gristle"
Found at ends of long bones, ribs, nose, larynx, trachea, bronchi,
  bronchial tubes

FIGURE 1-31 *(Continued)*

secretory process, produces polysaccharides and lysosomes, and stores synthesized molecules.

▼ Lysosomes act as digestive enzymes that function in breaking down many substances that enter the cell.

▼ The nucleus directs and controls the activities of the cell through the genes.

▼ Cell replication depends on the cell cycle. After DNA replication, mitosis occurs when the cell divides into two genetically complete cells. The process occurs continually in some cells, according to stimulus in others, and some complex cells do not retain the capacity to divide.

▼ Cellular exchange of materials can be either passive or active, depending on the size and characteristics of the substance to be moved. Passive movement requires no expenditure of energy, and movement occurs down a concentration gradient. Active movement requires the expenditure of energy, and movement occurs against a concentration gradient.

▼   Many cells have the ability to transmit impulses. Two examples are the nerve and muscle cells, which tend to be the most excitable. Membrane potentials and refractory periods, which vary among different cells, determine the frequency of actions exhibited by the cell.

▼   Four basic types of tissues compose the body: epithelial, muscular, nervous, and connective. These tissues work together to provide the framework, movement, secretions, protection, and sensations necessary for bodily functions.

▼ *References*

1.   Cormack, D.H. *Essential Histology*. Philadelphia: J.B. Lippincott, 1993.
2.   Guyton, A.C. *Textbook of Medical Physiology* (8th ed.). Philadelphia: W.B. Saunders, 1991.
3.   Hille, B. Membranes and ions. In Patton, H.D., et al., *Textbook of Physiology* (21st ed.). Philadelphia: W.B. Saunders, 1989.
4.   Slauson, D.O., and Cooper, B.J. *Mechanisms of Disease* (2nd ed.). Baltimore: Williams & Wilkins, 1990.
5.   Tortora, G.J., and Grabowski, S.R. *Principles of Anatomy and Physiology* (7th ed.). New York: HarperCollins, 1993.

Chapter 2

Alterations in Cellular Processes

Barbara L. Bullock

▼ LEARNING OBJECTIVES

1 Define **adaptation**.
2 Describe alterations in cells that can occur because of internal and external environmental stimuli.
3 List the types of stimuli that can cause cellular alterations.
4 Differentiate between endogenous and exogenous substances.
5 Describe the abnormal intracellular accumulations that result from noxious stimulation.
6 Discuss briefly extracellular changes resulting from cellular adaptation or injury.
7 Discuss the role of free radicals in the production of cellular injury and death.
8 Discuss a clinical situation that could occur as a result of reperfusion injury.
9 Discriminate among the following pathologic cellular adaptations: atrophy, dysplasia, hypertrophy, hyperplasia, and metaplasia.
10 Differentiate between ischemia and infarction.
11 Define and describe the factors that can produce thrombosis and embolism.
12 Describe the pathologic characteristics of infarcts.
13 Specify areas in which bacterial supergrowth may occur.
14 List and describe the major types of necrosis.
15 Explain the major changes that occur after somatic death.

Barbara L. Bullock: PATHOPHYSIOLOGY: ADAPTATIONS AND ALTERATIONS IN FUNCTION, 4th ed.
© 1996 Lippincott-Raven Publishers

The life cycle of a cell exists on a continuum that includes normal activities and adaptation, injury, or lethal changes. Adaptation may be the result of normal life cycle adjustments, such as growth during puberty or the changes of pregnancy. Stressful lifestyles produce physiologic changes that may lead to adaptation or disease. Other changes occur as the result of the aging process (see Unit 2). The pathologic changes exhibited may be obvious or very difficult to detect. The cell constantly makes adjustments to a changing, hostile environment to keep the organism functioning in a normal steady state. These adaptive adjustments are necessary to ensure the survival of the organism. Adaptive changes may be temporary or permanent. The point at which an adapted cell becomes an injured cell is the point at which the cell cannot functionally keep up with the stressful environment affecting it. Injured cells exhibit alterations that may affect body function and be manifested as disease.[6]

Prevention of disease is dependent on the capacity of the affected cells to undergo self-repair and regeneration. This process of repair prevents cellular injury and death and may prevent the death of the host.

Specifically, adaptation is a return of the internal environment of the body to a normal balance after exposure to some alteration. The rigid electrolyte and water balance between the intracellular fluid and extracellular fluid must be maintained (see Chap. 10). Balance may be attained at the expense of altered intracellular metabolism and may continue for a certain period of time, after which the cell, no longer able to adapt, may undergo injurious or lethal changes.

If cells are confronted with a stimulus that alters normal cellular metabolism, they may do one or more of the following: 1) increase concentrations of normal cellular constituents; 2) accumulate abnormal substances; 3) change the cellular size or number; or 4) undergo a lethal change. These concepts are considered briefly in this chapter and delineated further in specific content areas.

▼ Stimuli That Can Cause Cellular Injury or Adaptation

Because the cell is constantly making adjustments to a changing, hostile environment, many agents potentially can cause cellular injury or adaptation. Cellular injury may lead to further injury and death of the cell, or the cell may respond to the noxious stimulation by undergoing a change that enables it to tolerate the invasion.

Stimuli that can affect the human body are categorized as physical agents, chemical agents, micro-

TABLE 2-1 *Stimuli That Can Cause Cellular Injury*

Stimuli	Injury
Physical agents	Trauma, thermal or electrical charges, irradiation
Chemical agents	Drugs, poisons, foods, toxic and irritating substances
Microorganisms	Viruses, bacteria, fungi, protozoa
Hypoxia	Shock, localized areas of inadequate blood supply, hypoxemia
Genetic defects	Inborn errors of metabolism, gross malformations
Nutritional imbalances	Protein-calorie malnutrition; excessive intake of fats, carbohydrates, and proteins
Immunologic reactions	Hypersensitivity reactions to foreign proteins, autoimmune reactions, immune deficiency

organisms, hypoxia, genetic defects, nutritional imbalances, and immunologic reactions (Table 2-1).

PHYSICAL AGENTS

Physical agents are factors such as mechanical trauma, temperature gradients, electrical stimulation, atmospheric pressure gradients, and irradiation. Physical stimuli directly damage cells, cause rupture or damage of the cell walls, and disrupt cellular reproduction. In addition to the direct damage from the physical agent, hypoxia may increase the extent of the injury.[7] Local swelling may decrease the microcirculation and produce hypoxia to the tissues.

CHEMICAL AGENTS

Chemical agents that can cause injury include both simple compounds, such as glucose, and complex agents, such as poisons. Therapeutic drugs often chemically disrupt the normal cellular balance. Chemicals produce a wide range of physiologic effects. Some chemicals directly damage the cells and cell membranes that they contact. Others may be taken into the cell and disrupt energy production, or they may be changed within the cell to form toxic metabolites.[7,8] The end result depends on the degree of disruption.

MICROORGANISMS

Microorganisms cause cellular injury in a variety of ways depending on the type of organism and the innate defenses of the human body. Some bacteria secrete exotoxins, which are injurious to the host. Others liberate endotoxins when they are destroyed. Viruses interfere with the metabolism of the host cells and cause cellular injury by releasing viral proteins toxic to the cell (see pp. 278–281).

HYPOXIA

Hypoxia is the most common cause of cellular injury and may be produced by inadequate oxygen in the blood or by decreased perfusion of blood to the tissues. The end results are disturbance of cellular metabolism and local or generalized release of lactic acid. Cellular and organ dysfunction result from lack of oxygen. This may lead to cellular, organ, and even somatic death. When cells try to adapt to the lack of oxygen, anaerobic cellular metabolism results in metabolic acidosis (see pp. 220–221).

GENETIC DEFECTS

Genetic defects can affect cellular metabolism through inborn errors of metabolism or gross malformations. The mechanisms for cellular disruption vary widely with the genetic defect but may result in intracellular accumulation of abnormal material or deficiency of substances essential for normal cell metabolism and function (see pp. 73–76).

NUTRITIONAL IMBALANCES

Nutritional imbalances produce sickness and death in more than one-half of the world's population. The imbalances include serious deficiencies of proteins and vitamins especially. Malnutrition may be primary or secondary, depending on whether it is a socioeconomic problem or is self-induced or disease-induced. No matter what the reason, nutritional deficiency is a significant cause of cellular dysfunction and death. On the other hand, excessive food intake leads to nutritional imbalances and cellular injury through the production of excessive lipids in the body. Excessive fat intake has been shown to be associated with cancer, cardiovascular diseases, and respiratory and gastrointestinal disorders.[1,9]

IMMUNOLOGIC REACTIONS

Immunologic agents can cause cellular injury, especially if hypersensitivity reactions occur, causing the release of excess histamine and other substances. The cellular response to immunologic injury is inflammation, production of scar tissue, and even tissue death. Certain structures, such as the renal nephrons, are especially susceptible to immunologic damage. Immunologic injury is discussed in more detail in Chapter 18. Immune deficiency allows opportunistic organisms to cause disease and dysfunction (see pp. 343–344).

▼ Intracellular and Extracellular Changes Resulting from Cellular Adaptation or Injury

Abnormal intracellular accumulations often result from an environmental change or an inability of the cell to process materials. Normal or abnormal substances that cannot be metabolized may accumulate in the cytoplasm. These substances may be endogenous (produced within the body) or exogenous (produced in the environment), and they may be stored by an originally normal cell. Examples of abnormal exogenous substances include carbon particles, silica, and metals that are deposited and accumulate because the cell cannot degrade them or transport them to other sites.[1,7]

Common changes in and around cells include swelling, lipid accumulation in organs, liberation of free radicals, glycogen depositions, pigmentation, calcification, and hyaline infiltration. These changes may be resolved or they may become permanent.

CELLULAR SWELLING

Hydropic cellular swelling is the initial response to disruption of cellular metabolism. It occurs most frequently with cellular hypoxia, which impairs the cell's ability to synthesize adenosine triphosphate (ATP). It results in a shift of extracellular fluid to the intracellular compartment, causing cloudy intracellular swelling with enlargement of the cell.[3,4] Ultimately, organs are affected. Cellular swelling is often reversible if sufficient oxygen is delivered to the cell and normal ATP synthesis resumes. However, as the cell swells and injury progresses, damage to the cell membrane occurs, causing a true increase in its permeability. When large molecules and enzymes leak out of (or into) the cell, severe injury or death results.[7] Continued accumulation of water in the cells often produces the appearance of small or large vacuoles of water, which may represent portions of endoplasmic reticulum (ER) that have been sequestered.[4,6]

LIPID ACCUMULATION

Lipid accumulation refers to a fatty change process that occurs in the cytoplasm of parenchymal cells of certain organs. Fat droplets accumulate in the intracellular ER and Golgi complex as a result of improper metabolism.[8] The most common location for fatty change is the liver, but the heart and kidneys also can undergo fatty change when placed under abnormal stimulation.

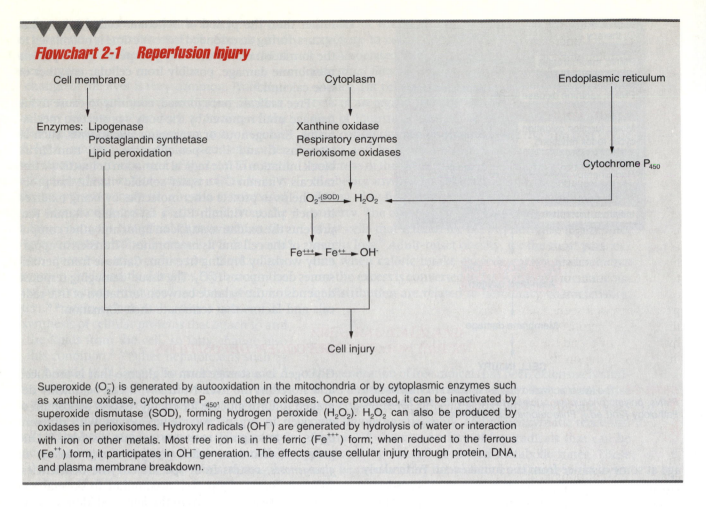

Flowchart 2-1   Reperfusion Injury

Superoxide (O_2^-) is generated by autooxidation in the mitochondria or by cytoplasmic enzymes such as xanthine oxidase, cytochrome P_{450}, and other oxidases. Once produced, it can be inactivated by superoxide dismutase (SOD), forming hydrogen peroxide (H_2O_2). H_2O_2 can also be produced by oxidases in perioxisomes. Hydroxyl radicals (OH^-) are generated by hydrolysis of water or interaction with iron or other metals. Most free iron is in the ferric (Fe^{+++}) form; when reduced to the ferrous (Fe^{++}) form, it participates in OH^- generation. The effects cause cellular injury through protein, DNA, and plasma membrane breakdown.

may be present in the brain, liver, heart, and ovaries of an elderly individual. The pigments gradually accumulate with age and apparently do not cause cellular dysfunction.[6]

Melanin is a black-brown pigment that is formed by the melanocytes of the skin. The amount of melanin imparts the degree of color to the skin. It also absorbs light and protects the skin from direct sun rays. Excessive deposition of melanin in the skin is common with Addison disease (see pp. 703–704), many skin conditions, and melanomas that arise from these cells. In the aged person, melanocyte activity is decreased and the skin becomes paler, with areas of hyperpigmentation called "liver spots" or lentigines.[4]

Hemosiderin, a derivative of hemoglobin, is a pigment that is formed from excess accumulations of stored iron. It is often formed from hemoglobin but may result from excess intake of dietary iron or impaired use of iron. One example of localized hemosiderosis is the common *bruise*, which is an accumulation of hemosiderin after the erythrocytes in the injured area are broken down by macrophages. The excess hemoglobin that is released becomes hemosiderin. The colors occur as the hemoglobin is transformed first to biliverdin (green bile), then bilirubin (red bile), and the golden-yellow hemosiderin.[1] Deposits of hemosiderin in organs and tissues, called

hemosiderosis, may occur with excess of absorbed dietary iron, impaired use of iron, or hemolytic anemia.[4] For the most part, accumulation of hemosiderin does not interfere with organ function unless it is extreme. Excessive iron storage in some organs is implicated in increased cancer risk.[6] In extreme hemosiderosis of the liver, for example, fibrosis may result.

CALCIFICATION

Normally, calcium is deposited only in the bones and teeth under the influence of various hormones. Pathologic calcification may occur in the skin, soft tissues, blood vessels, heart, and kidneys. Calcium may precipitate in areas of chronic inflammation or areas of dead or degenerating tissue.

Metastatic calcification can result from excess circulating calcium that is produced by bone reabsorption or destruction in conditions such as metastatic tumors or immobilization from fractures or spinal cord injury.[5] Sometimes, the cause of this condition is unknown. Calcium precipitates into many areas, including the kidneys, blood vessels, and connective tissue.

Calcium that precipitates into areas of unresolved healing is called *dystrophic calcification*. It may be extracellular, intracellular, or both. It often localizes in the mitochondria and propagates from there. It frequently causes organ dysfunction, as in atherosclerotic vessels or calcified cardiac valves.[2] Increased uptake of calcium into mitochondria is characteristic of injured cells.[7]

HYALINE INFILTRATION

The word *hyaline* refers to a characteristic alteration within cells or in the extracellular space that appears as a homogeneous, glassy, pink inclusion on stained histologic section. Because it does not represent a specific pattern of accumulation, different mechanisms are responsible for its formation. Intracellular hyaline changes may include excessive amounts of protein, aggregates of immunoglobulin, viral nucleoproteins, closely packed fibrils, or other substances.[4] Extracellular hyaline refers to the appearance of precipitated plasma proteins and other proteins across a membrane wall. This change is particularly well seen in and around the arterioles and the renal glomeruli. A variety of mechanisms causes the hyaline change, and the implications of this deposition differ depending on the underlying process.[1,8]

▼ Cellular Changes Caused by Injurious Stimuli

In some cases, the cell undergoes an actual change to adapt to an injurious agent. The changes often manifested are atrophy, dysplasia, hypertrophy, hyperplasia, and metaplasia and dysplasia. These adaptations are methods by which the cells stay alive and adjust workload to demand.

ATROPHY

Atrophy refers to a decrease in cell size resulting from decreased workload, loss of nerve supply, decreased blood supply, inadequate nutrition, or loss of hormonal stimulation.[4] The word implies previous normal development of the cell and cellular loss of structural components and substance (Fig. 2-3).

Physiologic atrophy occurs with aging in the parenchyma of organs and allows for survival of cells with decreased function. The cells tend to reproduce less readily. Physiologic atrophy begins in the thymus gland in early adulthood and in the uterus after menopause. Many cells in other glands and muscles also undergo atrophy with aging. These cells may develop an increase in the number of autophagic vacuoles in the cytoplasm that isolate and destroy injured organelles. The triggering mechanism for autophagia is unknown, but it may result in incompletely digested material called *residual* bodies.[1] An example of this is the lipofuscin or brownish pigment seen in the aging cell. Atrophy may progress to cellular injury and death, and the cells may be replaced with connective tissue, adipose tissue, or both.

Disuse atrophy is common after an extremity has been immobilized in a cast. The decreased workload placed on the affected muscles results in decreased size of the entire muscle. When the workload is again restored, the muscle often enlarges to its preinjury size. Atrophy

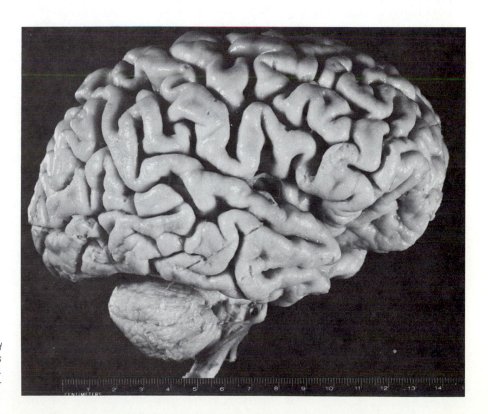

FIGURE 2-3 *Atrophy of the brain. Marked atrophy of the frontal lobes is noted in this photograph of the brain. (Widmann, F.K. Pathobiology: How Disease Happens. Boston: Little, Brown, 1978.)*

can also result from starvation, loss of nerve or endocrine stimulation, or cellular ischemia. In starvation, cellular atrophy is seen especially in skeletal muscle and in cells not vital to the survival of the organism.[6] Atrophy of a target organ of endocrine stimulation often results if the stimulating hormone for the organ hormone secretion is deficient.

Loss of nerve supply may cause muscular atrophy, such as when a spinal cord injury interrupts nervous stimulation to the muscles below the level of injury. The muscles gradually atrophy, and eventually musculature is replaced by fibrous tissue (see pp. 1044–1047). Atrophy of muscles may also be seen with chronic ischemic disease of the lower extremities. The decreased blood supply impairs the metabolism within the cell, and atrophy occurs as a protective mechanism to keep the tissue viable.

HYPERTROPHY

Hypertrophy is an increase in the size of individual cells, resulting in increased tissue mass without an increase in the number of cells. It usually represents the response of a specific organ to an increased demand for work. Hypertrophied cells increase their number of intracellular organelles, especially mitochondria. A good example of *physiologic hypertrophy* is the enlargement of muscles of athletes or weight lifters. The individual muscle cells enlarge but do not proliferate, and this provides increased strength. Physiologic hypertrophy occurs at puberty with enlargement of the sex organs (see pp. XX). Hypertrophy may also be caused by an increased functional demand such as systemic hypertension, in which the myocardium must pump under greater pressure and the size of the myocardial muscle cells increases (Fig. 2-4).

HYPERPLASIA

Hyperplasia is a common condition seen in cells that are under an increased physiologic workload or stimulation. It is defined as increase of tissue mass caused by an increase in the number of cells. Cells that undergo hyperplasia are those that are capable of dividing and thus of increasing their number. Whether hyperplasia, rather than hypertrophy, occurs depends on the regenerative capacity of the specific cell.

Physiologic hyperplasia is a normal outcome of puberty and pregnancy. *Compensatory hyperplasia* occurs in organs that are capable of regenerating lost substance. An example is regeneration of the liver after part of its substance has been destroyed. *Pathologic hyperplasia* is seen in conditions of abnormal stimulation of organs with cells that are capable of regeneration. Examples are enlargement of the thyroid gland secondary to stimulation by thyroid-stimulating hormone from the pituitary and parathyroid hyperplasia secondary to renal failure (see p. 722). Hyperplasia is induced by a known stimulus and almost always stops after the stimulus has been removed. This controlled reproduction is an important feature differentiating hyperplasia from neoplasia. There is a close relation between certain types of pathologic hyperplasia and malignancy (see pp. 54–55).

METAPLASIA

Metaplasia is a reversible change in which one type of adult cell is replaced by another type. It is probably an adaptive substitution of a cell type more suited to the hostile environment.[3] Metaplasia is commonly seen in chronic bronchitis: the normal columnar, ciliated goblet cells are replaced by stratified squamous epithelial cells. The latter cells are better suited for survival in the face of chronic, irritating smoke inhalation or environmental

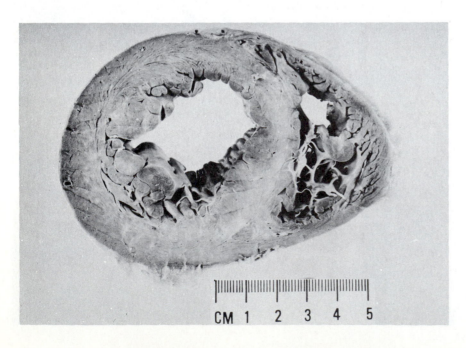

FIGURE 2-4 Hypertrophy of the myocardium (Miller, F. Peery and Miller's Pathology [3rd ed.]. Boston: Little, Brown, 1978.)

pollution. Metaplasia increases the chances of cellular survival but decreases the protective aspect of mucus secretion. Certain types of metaplasia are closely related to malignancy, which probably indicates that chronic irritation causes the initial change.

DYSPLASIA

Dysplasia refers to the appearance of cells that have undergone some atypical changes in response to chronic irritation. It is not a true adaptive process in that it serves no specific function. Dysplasia is presumably controlled reproduction of cells, but it is closely related to malignancy in that it may transform into uncontrolled, rapid reproduction.[1] The cellular changes often regress on removal of the injurious stimulus.[6] Epithelial cells are the most common types to exhibit dysplasia; changes include alterations in the size and shape of cells, causing loss of normal architectural orientation of one cell with the next. Dysplastic changes are common in the bronchi of chronic smokers and in the cervical epithelium.[1]

▼ Cellular Injury and Death

Cellular injury and death may be caused by microorganisms, by lack of oxygen, or by physical agents such as extreme temperatures, toxic chemicals, or radiation.

The mechanisms by which microorganisms cause cellular injury and death are detailed in Chapter 14. Lack of oxygen (anoxia) is the most common cause of cellular injury and death. The following conditions can produce this problem: ischemia, thrombosis, embolism, infarction, necrosis, and somatic death. The injury is reversible in some instances, or it may progress to a permanent, lethal change. Intracellular changes and their progression are detailed in the Flowchart 2-2. Physical agents often induce changes similar to those of anoxia, or they may differ depending on the agent and the tissue involved.

ISCHEMIA

Ischemia refers to a critical lack of blood supply to a localized area. It is reversible in that tissues are restored to normal function after oxygen is again supplied to them. Ischemia may precede infarction or death of the tissue, or it may occur sporadically if the oxygen need outstrips the oxygen supply. It is important to differentiate between ischemia, a clinical change, and infarction, a pathologic change. The cellular effects of ischemia have been detailed on pages 34–35 with the discussion of free radicals and reperfusion injury.

Ischemia usually occurs in the presence of atherosclerosis in the major arteries. Atherosclerosis, more fully described in Unit 7, is a lipid deposition process that

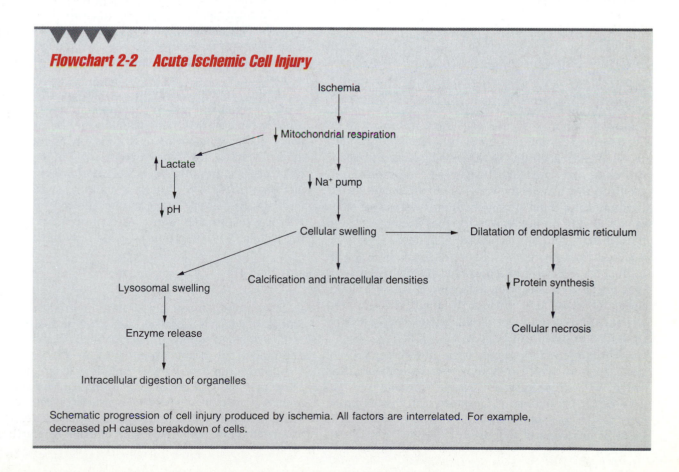

Flowchart 2-2 Acute Ischemic Cell Injury

Schematic progression of cell injury produced by ischemia. All factors are interrelated. For example, decreased pH causes breakdown of cells.

produces fibrofatty accumulations, or plaques, on the intimal layer of the artery. The medial layer of the artery may also become involved, predisposing it to atherosclerotic aneurysm formation. Atherosclerosis often gives rise to the formation of clots or thrombi on the plaque. These changes compromise blood flow through the artery, which then impairs oxygen supply to the tissues during increased need. In the later stages, the blood supply is impaired even at rest.

The classic conditions resulting from ischemia are *angina pectoris* and *intermittent claudication*. The former refers to pain from ischemia affecting the heart, and the latter refers to pain from ischemia of the extremities, usually during activity. Ischemia is often relieved by rest, and the tissues return to normal function. It may be progressive, however, and cause *ischemic infarction*, which involves cellular death from lack of blood supply or oxygen. Lack of oxygen supply to the brain, heart, and kidneys can be tolerated for only a short time; damage is irreversible. The fibroblasts of connective tissue, however, can survive much longer periods of anoxia.

Ischemia occasionally occurs after vasospasm of coronary arteries or other vessels that are unaffected by atherosclerosis. Vasospasm may be induced by many factors, including nicotine, exposure to cold, and, in some cases, stress. Vasospasm also often occurs in association with atherosclerosis.

THROMBOSIS

The word *thrombosis* refers to the formation of a clot on the intimal lining of a blood vessel. It may decrease blood flow or totally occlude the vessel. Thrombosis also may occur on the endothelial lining of the heart (*mural thrombosis*).

The most common factor in thrombosis is disruption of the endothelial lining of the blood vessels and heart. Normally, the endothelial layer is continuous from the heart throughout the vascular circuit, including the capillaries and veins. If trauma, atherosclerosis, or other factors disrupt this layer, platelets may accumulate, and the intrinsic clotting mechanism is initiated (Fig. 2-5). The body spontaneously initiates its fibrinolytic system to dissolve the clot and reopen the vessel. This may or may not be successful in reestablishing the flow of blood. Stasis of blood and increased blood viscosity also enhance coagulability of blood. Blood coagulation is described in detail in Chapter 21.

Thrombi most frequently occur in the deep veins of the legs, from which they may detach, embolize, and lodge in the pulmonary arterial circuit (see pp. 604–606). Thrombosis in an artery can disrupt blood flow to the area supplied by the vessel and cause ischemia or infarction of that area.

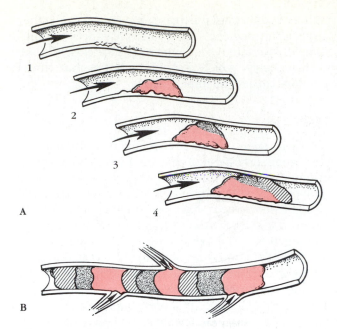

FIGURE 2-5   **A.** *stages in the development of phlebothrombosis: 1, intimal damage, sluggish circulation; 2, platelet aggregation; 3, occlusion of the lumen of the vein; 4, blood clot propagates.* **B.** *Clot propagates clot at each point of entry of the small veins.*

EMBOLISM

A thrombus may break off and become a traveling mass in the blood. This process is called *thrombotic embolization*. The most common types of emboli are derived from thrombi, but other substances such as fat, vegetations from valves, or foreign particles also may embolize. The obstruction caused by an embolus is called an *embolic occlusion*.

If the embolus arises in the venous circuit, it is carried to and trapped in the vasculature of the pulmonary capillary bed. Depending on the size of the embolus, the result may vary from clinically asymptomatic to death-producing. If the embolus arises in the left side of the heart, it may travel to any of the arteries branching off the aorta (Fig. 2-6). Arterial embolism may also occur from a larger artery, such as one affected by atherosclerosis, to a smaller artery. When it occludes the arterial tributary, it compromises blood flow to the area.

INFARCTION

Occlusion of the blood supply from an artery results in *infarction*, which is a localized area of tissue death caused by lack of blood supply. It is also termed *ischemic necrosis* and may occur in any organ or tissue.

Infarcts can have various pathologic characteristics. They may be described as *pale infarcts, hemorrhagic infarcts*, or *infarcts with bacterial supergrowth*. Pale infarcts are seen in solid tissue deprived of its arterial circulation as a result of ischemia. Red or hemorrhagic infarcts are

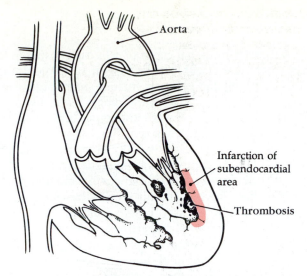

Aorta

Infarction of subendocardial area

Thrombosis

FIGURE 2-6 *Disruption of the endocardial surface, such as that after infarction affecting the subendocardial area, may lead to mural thrombosis, which may become an arterial embolus. Emboli that arise in this area are the major cause of embolic cerebrovascular accidents or strokes.*

more frequent with venous occlusion or with congested tissues. The infarcted tissue has a red appearance, owing to hemorrhage into the area, and may be poorly defined, causing difficulty in differentiation of viable from non-viable tissue.[1,3] Bacterial supergrowth is common and may be present in the area or may be brought to the area. The classification of *septic infarction* is added if there is evidence of bacterial infection in the area.[1] The lesion is converted to an abscess when it is septic and the inflammatory response is initiated. *Gangrene* is an example of infarction in which ischemic cellular death is followed by bacterial overgrowth, leading to liquefaction of the tissues. This term is frequently used to describe conditions of the extremities and the bowel.[6]

NECROSIS

The term *necrosis* refers to tissue death characterized by structural evidence of this death.[8] As cells die, the mitochondria swell, functions become disrupted, membranes rupture, and the lysosomal enzymes are released into the tissues. The nucleus undergoes specific changes that may include shrinking, fragmenting, or gradual fading. Necrosis is commonly categorized as coagulative necrosis, liquefactive necrosis, special types, and apoptosis.

Coagulative Necrosis

Coagulative necrosis usually results from lack of blood supply to an area. It is the most common pattern of necrosis. It frequently occurs as a result of infarction in organs such as the heart or kidneys, but it also may result

from chemical injury. In structured necrosis, the cellular structure and its architectural outline are preserved but the nucleus is lost; in structureless necrosis, the outline remains intact but the intracellular organelles are lost.

Caseation or *caseous necrosis* has long been described in relation to tuberculosis, but it may be present in a few other conditions. It is an example of structureless necrosis. The central area of necrosis is soft and friable and is surrounded by an area with a cheesy, crumbly appearance. The cellular architecture is destroyed. The area is walled off from the rest of the body and may become rimmed with calcium. Caseous necrosis may localize in areas of tuberculous infestation.[4]

Liquefactive Necrosis

Liquefactive necrosis most frequently occurs in brain tissue and is caused by fatal injury to the neuron. The breakdown of the neuron causes release of lysosomes and other constituents into the surrounding area. Lysosomes cause liquefaction of the cell and surrounding cells, leaving pockets of liquid, debris, and cystlike structures. Liquefactive necrosis is often described in brain infarction but also may be seen with bacterial lesions because of the release of bacterial and leukocytic enzymes. Liquefaction may occur in an area of coagulative necrosis as a secondary change.[8]

Special Types

Fat necrosis is a specific form of cellular death that occurs when lipases escape into fat storage areas. It particularly is seen in acute pancreatic necrosis and causes patchy necrosis of the pancreas and surrounding areas (see pp. 749–753). Traumatic fat necrosis, most commonly seen in the breast, gives rise to a giant cellular reaction that can resemble a carcinoma.[8]

Gangrenous necrosis is a combination of coagulative and liquefactive necroses. The term *gangrene* is applied to any black, foul-smelling area that is adjacent to living tissue. The cause of tissue death is ischemia, but bacteria and surrounding leukocytes cause liquefaction of the tissues. If the coagulative pattern is dominant, it is called *dry gangrene*; if the liquefactive process is more pronounced, it is called *wet gangrene*.[4]

Gas gangrene (myonecrosis) is a specific type of necrosis that occurs as a result of infection by bacilli of the genus *Clostridium*. Clostridia are gram-positive anaerobes that cause such conditions as tetanus, botulism, and food poisoning.[2] Gas gangrene usually occurs in large, traumatic wounds in which the organisms cause destruction of the connective tissue framework. Gas bubbles are caused by a fermentative reaction, giving a reddish-blue appearance to the involved tissues.[2] If this material reaches the bloodstream, shock and disseminated intravascular coagulation may be produced (see pp. 418–419).

Apoptosis

Apoptosis is a distinctive type of cellular death in which single or small groups of cells are deleted from their tissue of origin.[6] It can be a normal process or a programmed "suicide" process, such as that seen during embryonic development. Pathologically, the suicide process may be initiated by toxins, irradiation, or large doses of corticosteroids.[6] It is probably initiated by an endogenous endonuclease (enzyme within the cell) that becomes activated and causes destruction of the DNA and nuclear chromatin.[1]

SOMATIC DEATH

The body dies with the cessation of respiratory and cardiac function. Brain death can precede heart stoppage and is evident by irreversible coma with absent brain stem reflexes (see pp. 1024–1030). After actual bodily death occurs, the individual cells remain alive for different lengths of time. Irreversible changes then occur to cells and organs, sometimes making it difficult to determine the exact premortem pathology. Postmortem changes include rigor mortis, livor mortis, algor mortis, intravascular clotting, autolysis, and putrefaction.

Rigor mortis develops because of depletion of ATP in the muscles, beginning in the involuntary muscles; within 2 to 4 hours, it affects the voluntary muscles. The result is stiffening of the muscles, and the onset and disappearance varies among individuals. *Livor mortis* is the reddish-blue discoloration of the body that results from the gravitational pooling of blood. *Algor mortis* is the term used for the cooling of the body that occurs after death. The rate of cooling depends on the body temperature before death and the postmortem environmental temperature. *Intravascular clotting* results in clots that are not adherent to the lining of the blood vessels and heart. They may be layered in appearance, with streaks or layers of yellowish, gelatinous material. *Autolysis* refers to the digestion of tissues from released substances, such as enzymes and lysosomes. Organs may be swollen and spongy in appearance. *Putrefaction* is caused by saprophytic organisms entering the dead body, usually from the intestines. This results in a greenish discoloration of the tissues and organs, and the organisms may produce gases, leading to foamy or spongy organs.[3,8]

▼ Chapter Summary

▼   Various stimuli that confront cells can cause cellular injury or force the cells to make adjustments. Agents that can cause cellular changes include microorganisms, oxygen deprivation, and immunologic reactions.

▼   The changes that the cell undergoes depend on the cell type and the stimulus causing the changes. Common changes include cellular swelling, lipid accumulation, pigmentation, calcification, and infiltration with hyaline.

▼   The cell may produce substances that are harmful to its organelles. This is especially seen with oxygen deprivation and the production of free radicals.

▼   Cells can atrophy, hypertrophy, or undergo the changes of hyperplasia, metaplasia, or dysplasia in an attempt to adapt. Some of these changes closely relate to the changes seen when a malignant transformation occurs.

▼   Ischemia of cells is a reversible condition produced by lack of oxygen supply to the cell. Conditions that can cause ischemia include thrombosis and embolism. Ischemia may progress to an irreversible condition called infarction.

▼   Necrosis is the manifestation of cell or tissue death with a structural change in the cells. Different cells exhibit different reactions to death. The reaction may be coagulative or liquefactive. Somatic death refers to the changes that occur after the body dies.

▼ References

1. Cotran, R., Kumar, V., and Robbins, S.L. *Robbins' Pathologic Basis of Disease* (5th ed.). Philadelphia: W.B. Saunders, 1994.
2. Gilbert, D.N. Clostridial infections. In Stein, J.H., *Internal Medicine* (4th ed.). St. Louis: Mosby, 1994.
3. Golden, A. *Pathology: Understanding Human Diseases* (2nd ed.). Baltimore: Williams & Wilkins, 1985.
4. Kissane, J.M. *Anderson's Pathology* (9th ed.). St. Louis: Mosby, 1990.
5. Lemann, J. Nephrolithiasis. In Stein, J.H., *Internal Medicine* (4th ed.). St. Louis: Mosby, 1994.
6. Rubin, E., and Farber, J.L. *Pathology* (2nd ed.). Philadelphia: J.B. Lippincott, 1994.
7. Slauson, D.O., and Cooper, B.J. *Mechanisms of Disease* (2nd ed.). Baltimore: Williams & Wilkins, 1990.
8. Walter, J.B. *Pathology of Human Disease*. Philadelphia: Lea & Febiger, 1989.
9. Whitney, E., Cataldo, C., and Rolfes, S. *Understanding Normal and Clinical Nutrition* (3rd ed). St. Paul: West, 1991.

Chapter 3

Neoplasia

Barbara L. Bullock

▼ **LEARNING OBJECTIVES**

1   Relate the normal cell cycle to neoplasia.
2   Explain the difference between neoplastic and normal cells in relation to contact inhibition.
3   Relate normal cellular differentiation to neoplasia.
4   Discuss the histologic features of an anaplastic cell.
5   Define cancer at the clinical, cellular, and molecular levels.
6   Explain the morphologic differences among the subgroups of cancer.
7   Compare the characteristics of benign and malignant neoplasms.
8   Classify carcinogens and identify the neoplasms with which they are associated.
9   Explain important factors in primary tumor growth.
10   Describe the TNM classification system for staging of neoplasms.
11   Explain metastasis from invasion of the basement membrane to proliferation at a new site.
12   Describe the value of tumor markers in diagnosis and treatment of specific types of cancer.
13   Discuss the role of the immune system in the destruction of malignant cells.
14   Explain the mechanisms responsible for the development of local symptoms of neoplasms.
15   Briefly discuss paraneoplastic syndromes of the endocrine, nervous, hematologic, renal, and gastrointestinal systems.
16   Explain the anorexia–cachexia syndrome.

Cancer is the second leading cause of death in the United States. Because of the declining incidence of death from cardiovascular disease in recent years, some clinicians are predicting that cancer will predominate in the next century.[24] Despite advances in understanding of normal growth and development of cells, it is not known why cancer cells escape the normal regulations on cellular proliferation. Cancer cells generally contain the full complement of biomolecules necessary for survival, proliferation, differentiation, and expression of many functions specific to the cell type, but they lack the ability to regulate these functions.[10] The cell is constantly confronted by factors in its environment that stimulate or inhibit its activity. It responds to these factors by growth and proliferation or regression and degeneration. These responses may occur simultaneously in a cell population, or one may follow the other.[23]

As discussed in Chapters 1 and 2, the capacity to undergo mitosis is inherent in most cells. Some cells have lost their original mitotic ability and are unable to reproduce. Other cells do not reproduce unless a specific stimulus for growth occurs. Some cells reproduce constantly to replenish the cells needed for bodily functions. Every time a normal cell passes through a cycle of division, the opportunity exists for it to become cancerous. Alterations in cellular growth and proliferation may be viewed as occurring on a continuum from small, almost normal changes to grossly abnormal alterations. Hypertrophy, hyperplasia, metaplasia, and dysplasia usually are classified as controlled adaptive cellular responses (see pp. 37–39). These cellular responses are usually caused by an injurious stimulus which makes the cell vulnerable to loss of normal control of reproduction.

▼ Definitions

Neoplasia is defined as the development of an abnormal type of growth that is unresponsive to normal growth control mechanisms.[22] A *neoplasm* is a group or clump of neoplastic cells. This term is usually used synonymously with *tumor*. The term *benign neoplasia* refers to neoplastic cells that do not invade the surrounding tissue and do not metastasize. *Metastasis* is defined as the ability of the cancer cell to disseminate and establish growth in another area of the body at a distance from its origin.[14] The term *malignant neoplasia* refers to neoplastic cells that grow by invading surrounding tissue and have the ability to metastasize to receptive tissue. All malignant neoplasms are classified as cancers and then further delineated as to their tissue of origin. A tumor may be benign or malignant. Table 3-1 lists and describes terms commonly used in discussions about abnormal cellular growth. *Aberrant cellular growth* is an alteration in normal cellular growth, which usually means that the normal cell escapes the host's controls on growth and differentiation. *Anaplasia* is a term used for the loss of

TABLE 3-1 *Terms Used in Discussions of Neoplasia*

Term	Definition
Neoplasm	New growth, abnormal cellular reproduction
Aberrant cellular growth	Alteration in normal cellular growth
Tumor	A growth of neoplastic cells clustered together; may be benign or malignant
Benign	Characterized by abnormal cell division but does not metastasize or invade surrounding tissue
Malignant	Abnormal cell division with ability to invade, metastasize, and recur
Cancer	Malignant growth accompanied by abnormal cell division, invasion of surrounding tissues, and metastasis to distant sites
Carcinogenesis	Production or origination of a cancer
Carcinoma	Malignant growth originating in epithelial tissue
Sarcoma	Malignant growth originating in mesodermal tissues that form connective tissue, blood vessels, lymphatic organs
Metastasis	Ability to establish secondary tumor growth at a new location away from the primary tumor

cellular differentiation such that the cell looks less like the parent cell.

▼ Epidemiology of Cancer

Malignant neoplasms constitute more than 100 distinct disease entities. Cancer can strike at any age. It kills more children between ages 3 and 14 than any other disease.[2] The three leading death-producing cancers in men are cancer of the lung, colon and rectum, and prostate gland. For women, the most common cancers are those of the breast, lung, and colon and rectum. Even though breast cancer is much more frequently diagnosed in women than lung cancer, lung cancer became the leading cause of cancer deaths in women in 1989.[5] Advancing age increases the risk of developing cancer. The frequency rises sharply as age increases; for example, the death rate from cancer of the large intestine increases 1000-fold between ages 20 and 80. Figure 3-1 shows the 1994 estimate of cancer deaths by site and sex. Table 3-2 indicates the commonly accepted differences between benign and malignant neoplasms.

Current research indicates that almost 90% of all cancers are related to lifestyle and environmental factors.[6] These factors are briefly discussed in this section, and their mechanisms of carcinogenesis are further described on pages 54–55. Combinations of risk factors provide a higher incidence of specific cancers. The main

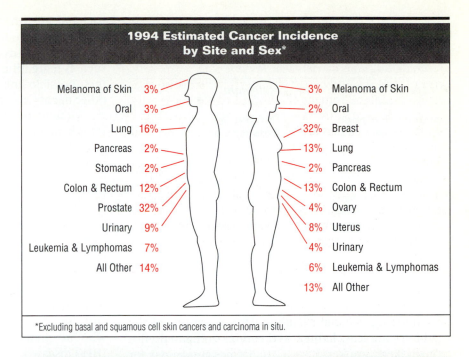

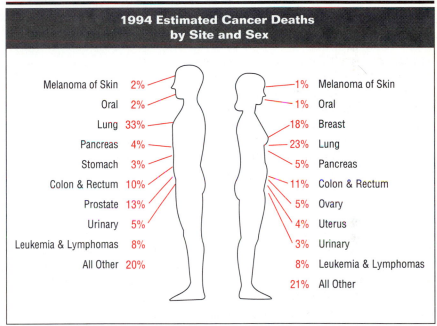

FIGURE 3-1 *1994 estimate of cancer deaths by site and sex (From Cancer Facts and Figures 1994, New York, American Cancer Society, 1993)*

risk factors for cancer include tobacco, alcohol, diet, reproductive and sexual behavior, occupation, pollution, industrial products, and medicines. Other factors not directly related to lifestyle and environment include infectious agents, endogenous hormones, and genetics.

TOBACCO

Tobacco smoke contains several carcinogenic agents. Among these are polycyclic aromatic hydrocarbons and nitrosamines. Many studies have supported the link between bronchogenic carcinoma and cigarette smoking. The duration of smoking and the number of cigarettes smoked are highly significant for cancer incidence. The studies have also documented a drop in risk over time for smokers who stop smoking.[6] Evidence also indicates a strong relation between laryngeal cancer and smoking, with smokers having 10 to 30 times the risk of nonsmokers. Pipe and cigar smokers have a similar risk. Oral cancers are related to all forms of tobacco products, and the risk is enhanced by a synergistic relation between tobacco and alcohol use, increasing the additive risk by a factor of 2.5.[6] Esophageal cancers also exhibit a synergistic relation between smoking and alcohol use.

TABLE 3-2 *A Comparison of Benign and Malignant Neoplasms*

Benign	Malignant
Similar to cell of origin	Dissimilar from cell of origin
Edges move outward smoothly (encapsulated)	Edges move outward irregularly
Compresses	Invades
Slow growth rate	Rapid to very rapid growth rate
Slight vascularity	Moderate to marked vascularity
Seldom recur after removal	Frequently recur after removal
Necrosis and ulceration unusual	Necrosis and ulceration common
Systemic effects unusual unless it is a secreting endocrine neoplasm	Systemic effects common

Smoking is a contributing factor in cancers of the bladder, pancreas, kidney, and cervix. Compared with nonsmokers, smokers have a 2 to 5 times greater risk for developing these cancers, and the risk is also related to duration of use and number of cigarettes smoked (dose-related).

ALCOHOL

As already stated, there is a synergistic relation between alcohol and tobacco smoke for cancers of the mouth, pharynx, larynx, and esophagus. Hepatic cirrhosis is a precursor lesion for hepatocellular carcinoma, and alcohol is the most common initiator for the cirrhotic process.[5,6] Breast cancer risk is increased with moderate alcohol consumption, and pancreatic carcinoma is also thought to be associated with alcohol use.[13,19]

DIET

Much of the information on dietary linkage to carcinogenesis comes from observational rather than controlled research. Fat consumption has been implicated in colorectal, breast, uterine, prostate, and ovarian cancers.[6] Numerous studies have linked the incidence of colorectal cancer to high fat and low fiber dietary intake. This is well supported by studies of other cultures in which the diet is high in fiber and the risk of colorectal cancer is very low.

Direct ingestion of aflatoxin B, a mold of the genus *Aspergillus flavus* found on corn, barley, peas, rice, soybeans, fruit, some nuts, milk, and cheddar cheese, has been linked to liver cancer in humans. Aflatoxin B has been shown to cause liver, stomach, colon, and kidney cancer in animals.[5] Chewing of betel nuts has been directly related to cancers of the oral cavity. Nitrites are food additives that are used to preserve the color of foods, to enhance its flavor, and to protect against

bacterial growth.[25] These agents can be converted to nitrosamines and may be contributors to gastric carcinomas.[25] Azo dyes were used in the past to color foods such as margarine and maraschino cherries. Because of their possible link to the production of bladder cancer, other agents are now used.

Vitamin deficiency can cause altered growth patterns in tissues. Vitamins A, C, and E may be particularly important because of their roles in epithelial growth and their antioxidant effects.

REPRODUCTIVE AND SEXUAL BEHAVIOR

Certain types of malignancies are related to sexual practices. Cervical carcinoma is linked to the age at first intercourse and the number of sexual partners. It is correlated with multiparity and is rare among women who are not sexually active or whose partners are circumcised.[20] Cancer of the penis is rare among men who are circumcised. Human immunodeficiency virus (HIV) disease is a sexually transmitted viral disease that permits cancer by decreasing immune resistance (see page 344.

OCCUPATIONAL, INDUSTRIAL, POLLUTION, OR PHARMACEUTICAL LINKS

More than 60,000 chemicals are in widespread use in the environment today. Occupational carcinogens may accounts for 4% to 6% of cancer deaths, especially among those with high rates of exposure.[6] These chemicals are sources of environmental pollution through air, soil, and water. Table 3-3 summarizes the main chemical carcinogens and their sites of action. Polycyclic aromatic hydrocarbons are present in automobile exhaust and other products of combustion, including tobacco smoke. They are also produced from animal fats in broiling meats and in smoked meat and fish.[5]

Asbestos, cadmium, chromium, and nickel are some of the substance involved in carcinogenesis. All are associated with cancer of the lung. Chromium and nickel also may cause nasal cavity tumors. Cadmium is associated with cancer of the prostate gland. Asbestos may cause cancer of the pleural cavity and gastrointestinal tract. Asbestos fibers are thought to function as promoters for other carcinogens such as cigarette smoke. Industrial compounds such as polyvinyl chloride, which is used in the manufacture of plastics, may cause angiosarcomas of the liver.

PHARMACEUTICAL AGENTS

Specific pharmaceutical agents used in the past and some used in the present have been linked to cancer causation. Arsenicals were prescribed for many years for

TABLE 3-3 *Summary of Chemical Carcinogens and Their Sites of Action*

Carcinogens	Source Examples	Sites of Action
Polycyclic aromatic hydrocarbons	Soots, tars, cigarette smoke, benzpyrene	Lips, tongue, oral cavity, head, neck, larynx, lungs, bladder
Aromatic amines	Dyes, naphthalene, 2-acetylaminofluorene	Bladder
Alkylating agents	Nitrogen mustard and mustard gas, drugs (cyclophosphamide, melphalan)	Lungs, larynx, bladder, hemopoietic system
Nitrosamines and nitrosocompounds	4-Nitrobiphenyl	
Naturally occurring products	Aflatoxin B, betel nut	Liver, oral cavity
Drugs	Griseofulvin, hycanthone, metronidazole, diethylstilbestrol	Cancers in rats, vagina, bladder, hemopoietic system

a variety of conditions and are directly related to the development of squamous and basal cell carcinomas of the skin.[6] Diethylstilbestrol, given to pregnant women 50 years ago for the prevention of miscarriage, is linked to a high incidence of adenocarcinoma of the vagina and cervix in females. Estrogen supplements are associated with a increased risk of endometrial hyperplasia and uterine cancer. Oral contraceptives and androgen therapy are linked to hepatic tumors. Antineoplastic drugs increase the risk for acute myelogenous leukemia, especially in association with radiation therapy.[6] Phenacetin users may increase the risk of renal cell carcinoma. Immunosuppressive agents increase the risk of many forms of cancer. An antifungal agent called griseofulvin, used to treat mycotic disease of the skin, has been shown to cause cancer in rats.

RADIATION

Ionizing radiation is recognized as a cause of cellular mutations. Damage to DNA can be direct or indirect. Direct damage results from interaction of the electron itself with the DNA of the cell. Indirect damage occurs when a secondary electron interacts with a water molecule, giving rise to a free radical, which then damages the DNA (see pp. 34–35). A long latent period often exists between exposure and the development of clinical disease. Firm evidence links exposure to large doses of radiation and development of leukemia. Survivors of the atomic bombings of Hiroshima and Nagasaki in the 1940s had a very high incidence of leukemia. Miners of radioactive elements have suffered a tenfold increase in lung cancer incidence.[5]

Even low doses of radiation may cause cancer in susceptible people. The frequency of breast cancer increases with small, widely spread doses of radiation, and that of thyroid cancer increases with head and neck radiography during childhood. Radiography of the fetus in utero increase its chances of developing leukemia.[6] Women undergoing fluoroscopy of the lung for tuberculosis experienced an increased incidence of breast cancer 10 years after irradiation.[6]

Ultraviolet radiation from the sun is a major cause of skin cancers. Fair-complexioned people are more likely to develop skin cancers than their darker-complexioned counterparts because of the lack of protective melanin. Skin cancers are more often seen on sun-exposed areas of the body and in elderly persons.

INFECTIOUS AGENTS

A viral etiology for the development of cancer has been investigated for many years. Viruses are thought to cause some human malignant neoplasms and have been directly associated with tumor induction in animals. Viruses implicated in human cancers are called *oncogenic viruses*; they apparently alter the genome of the infected cell, which affects the resulting offspring of the cell.[5] The two types of oncogenic viruses are DNA viruses and RNA viruses. The DNA viruses are incorporated into the genes of the host and transmitted to subsequent generations. The genes are then expressed without the usual symptoms that accompany infection. The RNA viruses, or *retroviruses*, also contribute genetic information to the host cell. These viruses use an enzyme called reverse transcriptase to develop new DNA sequences that are not attacked and destroyed by the immune system (Fig. 3-2).

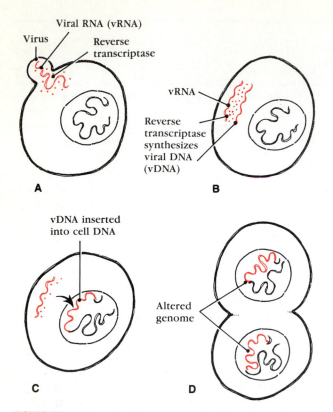

FIGURE 3-2 *Schematic showing how RNA viruses change the genome of the cell and cause replication of new cells with altered genome.* **A.** *Virus infects the cell.* **B.** *Alteration of cell RNA by virus (vRNA).* **C.** *Alteration of cell DNA.* **D.** *Duplication of the cell, with altered DNA going to the progeny.*

Some viruses associated with human malignant neoplasms are the C-type and B-type RNA viruses and certain DNA viruses (Table 3-4). Although the mechanisms are not clearly established, the C-type RNA viruses are implicated as causative agents in the development of certain types of leukemias; the B-type RNA viruses may be factors in causing breast cancer. Herpes viruses (DNA type) may be associated with cervical cancer. The Epstein-Barr virus, a DNA virus of the herpes type, has been closely associated with Burkitt lymphoma and nasopharyngeal carcinoma.[5,6,20] The hu-

man papillomaviruses have many distinct types, and the virus directly causes human warts. The connection with skin cancers, anogenital malignancy, and carcinoma of the cervix suggests the coexistence of the herpes simplex type 2 virus and papillomaviruses.[6]

The human T-cell lymphotropic virus, type 1, (HTLV−1) is a retrovirus linked to a T-cell leukemia seen in Japan, among American blacks in the southeastern USA, and among immigrants from the West Indies.[6] Hodgkin disease is an example of a number of malignancies that appear to have an infectious cause but for which no organism has been identified.

The DNA virus that causes hepatitis B is closely linked with the development of hepatocellular carcinoma.

Schistosoma haematobium is a parasite that in certain areas of Africa causes an increased incidence of bladder cancer. Liver flukes are causes of chronic liver infections that can increase the risk of cholangiocarcinoma.[6]

ENDOGENOUS HORMONES

A hormonal link is apparent in cancers of the breast, ovary, uterus, and prostate, but the exact mechanism of causation is unclear. Pregnancy is associated with a decreased risk of female cancers. The breast tissue exhibits changes with the fluctuations of hormones during the menstrual cycle. Inherited patterns of hormone production may increase the risk among family members. High levels of unopposed estrogen increase the risk of endometrial cancer. Ovarian carcinoma may be related to increased stimulation, and protection may be afforded by increased parity and by use of oral contraceptives that inhibit ovulation.[6]

Androgen excess has been an area of research in cancer of the prostate, because prostate cancer is not seen in men who have been castrated. Testosterone alone can cause prostate cancer in rats.[6]

GENETICS

A few genetically inherited disorders are directly associated with increased risk for cancer. These include autosomal recessive disorders such as ataxia-telangiectasia, which is closely associated with leukemia, lymphoma, and ovarian cancer. Autosomal dominant disorders such as neurofibromatosis are associated with increased risks of neurofibrosarcoma and acute myelocytic leukemia. Some of the X-linked recessive disorders, especially the immunodeficiency syndromes, are associated with an increased risk of leukemia and lymphoma.

More common are familial predispositions for specific types of cancer that cannot be genetically identified. Often the cancers appearing in these families are hormone-related cancers whose metabolism may be genetically determined.

TABLE 3-4 *Viruses Implicated in Malignant Neoplasia*

Virus	Associated Cancer
C-type RNA	Leukemia
B-type RNA	Breast cancer
Herpes II	Cancer of cervix
Epstein-Barr	Burkitt's lymphoma, nasopharyngeal cancers
Human papilloma virus	Cancer of cervix, anogenital cancers

▼ The Cell Cycle in Neoplasia

The cell cycle is composed of all the steps in the process of reproduction, or that period extending from one mitosis to the next. In a normal cell population, inhibitory controls slow or stop reproduction, whereas stimulating factors cause the process to proceed more rapidly. Therefore, the actual length of a cell life cycle varies. The four phases are designated G_1, S, G_2, and M, with a fifth phase, G_0, being composed of cells that have left the normal cell cycle but can be induced to reenter the cycle by specific stimuli (Fig. 3-3). The letter G is an abbreviation for "gap" and refers to the time between mitosis and synthesis (G_1) or between synthesis and mitosis (G_2). The symbol G_0 is used to describe a cell that performs all metabolic activities except for mitosis. The cell remains at this level until some stimulus, such as the death of other cells of the same cell population, triggers the beginning of G_1. A cell can remain in the G_1 phase for long periods until some key process occurs to signal its entrance into the S phase of DNA synthesis. After the S phase, the cell enters the G_2 phase, during which some residual RNA is synthesized in preparation for mitosis (M). Mitosis creates two daughter cells that have identical genetic information. The daughter cells may enter into G_1 or G_0, or they may be immediately stimulated to reproduce. Some cells are terminally differentiated and never reenter the cell cycle. These cells (eg, neurons, myocardial cells) do not become neoplastic.

The concept of the cell life cycle has helped in the basic understanding of the process a neoplastic cell goes through in its proliferation. Neoplastic cell populations ignore normal growth limitations and enter the cell cycle repeatedly at different rates. The terms growth fraction, cell cycle time, cell loss, and doubling time are used to describe these neoplastic characteristics. *Growth fraction* refers to the proportion of cells in a given cell population

undergoing cell cycle activity at any given time. Rapidly growing neoplasms have a larger number of cells in active reproduction at any given time than do slow-growing neoplasms. The *labeling index* is a measure of cells that are synthesizing DNA, or those in the S phase. This index provides a relatively simple method for estimating rates of growth of neoplastic cells.[10] The labeling index and growth fraction are the parameters that usually differentiate cancer growths from normal tissues. The actual *cell cycle time* (the time from the onset of one mitosis to the onset of the next mitotic phase) may actually be slower in cancer growths than in normal tissues. *Cell loss* refers to the number of cells lost in the process of growth. Because of the difference between the possible growth and the actual observed growth of tumors, it has been estimated that as many as 97% of the proliferated cells die spontaneously or are lost to metastasis.[20] The *doubling time* is the rate at which a neoplasm doubles its cell population. Internal cancers are not often detected before they are about the size of a cubic centimeter, which corresponds to 10^8 to 10^9 cells. The mass would have doubled at least 30 times to reach this size.[20] The actual rate of doubling varies with the tumor because of host defenses and variable death rates.

▼ Cellular Changes in Neoplasia*

CELL MEMBRANE

All cells are surrounded by a limiting membrane that constantly exists in a dynamic state (see pp. 5–6). Parts of the membrane have the capacity to redistribute and change the surface properties of the cell, which may have an effect on the cell's growth, metabolism, and behavior.[23] The outer cell membrane is the point of contact between cells. Interactions that involve the outer cell membrane have been shown to function in the control of normal cellular growth.[10] Changes in the membrane are apparent in neoplastic cells and have been implicated in the failure of the neoplastic cells to respond to normal growth-control mechanisms. They involve alterations in appropriate cell recognition, cellular adhesion, and intercellular communication. Escape from growth control could involve breakdown at any of these points.

Appropriate cell recognition is the term used for the mechanisms by which specific cells recognize one another. These mechanisms are not well understood, but they can be demonstrated by mixing cells of different types in culture media; specific cells eventually segregate themselves. Membrane enzymes and surface sugar residues are thought to contribute to recognition. Sugar-

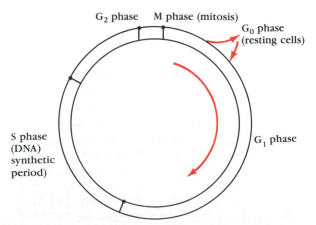

FIGURE 3-3 *The cell cycle. Interphase (G_1), DNA synthesis (S), intermediate phase (G_2), and mitosis (M) intervals are shown. The G_0 period may be entered from G_1, and reentry from G_0 to G_1 may occur.*

---

* Most of the cell changes in neoplasia relate to those seen with malignant neoplasia. Some concepts also apply to benign neoplasms. The different characteristics are discussed in a later section of this chapter.

binding enzymes, the glycosyltransferases, in the outer cell membrane may recognize sugar residues on glyco-proteins in the membrane of neighboring cells.[22] In neo-plastic cells, glycolipids are altered. Glycoproteins or glycolipids, or both, may be missing from the membrane or have an abnormal structure.[10]

Cellular adhesion is a complex process that involves the development of connections between cells.[4] Three types of connections have been described.

1. The *desmosome* is a mechanical way of holding cells together. Because it is composed of fibrous protein, it can be destroyed by a proteolytic enzyme such as trypsin.
2. The *tight junction* involves the actual fusion of two cell membranes, forming a barrier to the movement of ions and solutes from one side of the membrane to the other. It is present in areas in which sharp physical separation is needed, such as the endothelial lining of the cerebral blood vessels that form the blood-brain barrier.
3. The *gap junction*, a pore passing through the outer cell membrane, permits the movement of low-molecular-weight substances from one adjoining cell to the next.[4]

A decrease in the number of desmosomal, tight, and gap junctions often occurs in the neoplastic cell population. This causes a decrease in cellular adhesion. The communication of cells evidently is dependent on the junctions described. If cells cannot communicate in this way, the loss of contact inhibition can lead to neoplastic change. Cellular adhesion properties also include the electrical charge of the outer cell membrane. Under physiologic conditions, all mammalian cell surfaces have a negative charge, but this charge becomes more negative in neoplasia. The more aggressive the behavior of the neoplasm, the more negative the cell surface charge. This tends to push the cells away from one another.[21]

Intercellular communication is the way that cells communicate growth information. Contact-inhibition, or density-dependent growth control, is observed when normal cells are grown in culture media. The cells move around freely in the culture media until they touch one another. On contact, they adhere to one another and form parallel lines. They then grow on a single layer until they reach the edge of the culture dish, and then growth stops. The cells of a neoplasm, however, respond by continuing to divide and migrate until they are several layers deep. In other words, normal cells respond to a crowded environment, but neoplastic cells do not, because they have lost their ability either to receive or to send the necessary information to stop growth (Fig. 3-4).

Cancer cells have been described as antisocial, fairly autonomous units that do not respond to the constraints and regulatory signals imposed on normal cells.[5] It is thought that normal cellular growth is controlled by growth stimulators and growth inhibitors. Many growth factors have been described, especially polypeptide growth factors, that stimulate a variety of cell-type proliferations.[5] The lack of response to growth inhibitor influences accounts for the *uncontrolled proliferation* char-

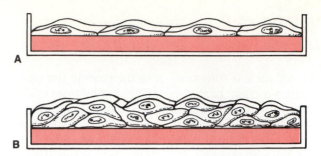

FIGURE 3-4 **A.** *Normal cells are inhibited by a crowded environment.* **B.** *Neoplastic cells continue to grow despite cell contact.*

acteristic of neoplastic cells. This lack of response allows the neoplastic growth *autonomy*. In other words, the cells reproduce through the cell cycle again and again as long as nutrients and oxygen are available. Growth control information is carried through gap junctions in many cells. With loss of gap junctions, as occurs with neoplasia, the cell may become isolated from the growth-control messengers of its normal neighboring cells as well as its own (Fig. 3-5).

NUCLEAR CHANGES IN NEOPLASIA

Just as changes occur in the outer cell membrane in neoplasia, changes occur within the cell. It is difficult to ascertain whether they are a function of the neoplasia or of the increased growth rate. All cancers are the result of some genetic changes. The genetic changes induced are inherited by all of the subsequent tumor cells formed. The genetic changes can be induced by certain substances called oncogenes. *Oncogene* is a collective term for a multiple set of growth regulatory genes that can promote the development of cancer when they are activated. Their discovery came from the study of RNA viral tumor induction.[12] Figure 3-6 illustrates mechanisms of growth promotion by an oncogene.

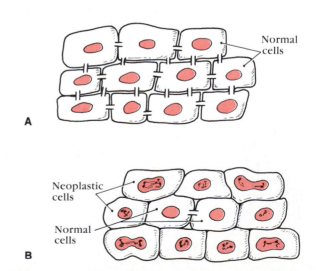

FIGURE 3-5 **A.** *Normal cells pass growth control information through the gap junctions.* **B.** *Neoplastic growth may isolate normal cells from neighboring cells.*

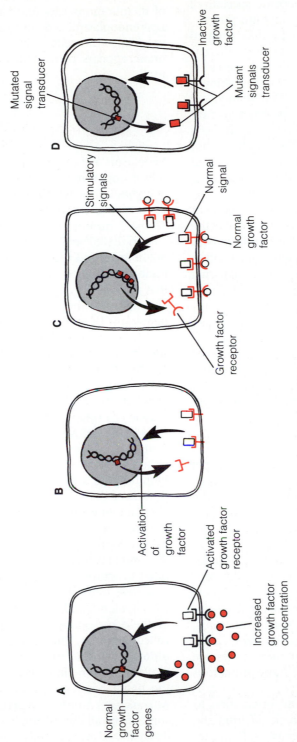

FIGURE 3-6 *Mechanisms of growth promotion by an oncogene.* **A.** *the oncogene codes for a growth factor and stimulates tumor cells.* **B.** *The growth factor receptor may be defective and constantly activated.* **C.** *An increased number of growth receptors may cause amplification of oncogene.* **D.** *Defective signal transducers may promote growth without an external trigger.*

Normal growth factor genes

Increased growth factor concentration

Activation of growth factor

Activated growth factor receptor

Growth factor receptor

Stimulatory signals

Normal signal

Normal growth factor

Mutated signal transducer

Inactive growth factor

Mutant signals transducer

A

B

C

D

DIFFERENTIATION AND ANAPLASIA

During fetal development, cells undergo changes in their physical and structural properties as they form the different tissues of the body. This process is called cellular differentiation. Differentiated cells become specialized and differ from one another physically and functionally. Nerve cells, for example, are terminally differentiated and do not undergo mitotic division. The more differentiated a cell is, the less likely it is to divide and, therefore, the less susceptible it is to malignant transformation.

The factors controlling cellular differentiation are not well understood but probably involve selective repression of genetic information. Repressor substances in the cytoplasm are apparently responsible for differentiation, with the repressor substance in one cell acting to repress one genetic characteristic, and that of another cell acting to repress a different genetic characteristic. The full set of genetic information is always present, but parts of it are repressed.[11] Cells that look and act like the cell of origin (parent cell) are called *well-differentiated cells*. All benign tumors are well differentiated, often being impossible to differentiate from the normal tissue. The cells of a malignant neoplasm are not as well differentiated as the cells of normal tissue. Neoplasms composed of cells that resemble the mature cells of the tissue of origin are called well-differentiated tumors.[5] Neoplasms composed of cells that bear little or no resemblance to the tissue of origin are called *poorly differentiated* or *undifferentiated tumors*. The lack of differentiation is called *anaplasia* and is considered a hallmark in recognizing malignant tumors.[5]

Well-differentiated cancer cells may elaborate relatively normal products of the tissue of origin, whereas poorly differentiated cancer cells may lose all specialized functional characteristics. Very anaplastic tumors may elaborate a product that is completely foreign to the tissue of origin. An example is the elaboration of a hormone like the antidiuretic hormone from the oat cell carcinoma of the lung.

Anaplasia describes the regression of a cell population from being well differentiated to being less differentiated. Anaplastic cells vary in morphology and may either resemble the tissue of origin or bear little resemblance to it.[5] The anaplastic cell usually is pleomorphic, which means that it has many shapes and sizes. Large, hyperchromatic nuclei with irregular membranes are exhibited, and they have larger and more numerous nucleoli.[5]

Less differentiated tumor cells lose orientation to one another, and tumor cells can break off from the primary tumor and metastasize to other areas. The functional efficiency of anaplastic cells correlates with the level of morphologic differentiation. Mitoses of anaplastic cells frequently are abnormal, and various chromosomal defects result. Most cells exhibit atypical and bizarre mitotic figures.[5] Few mitoses faithfully reproduce

the abnormality, and new aberrations with chromosome deletions or translocations occur.

The cytoplasmic organelles of the anaplastic cells are less numerous than those of normal cells and are abnormal in form. Pseudopodia, microfilaments, and clumps of membranous sacs and tubules usually are present. Less endoplasmic reticulum and fewer mitochondria are present, so less cellular work occurs. The nuclear membrane appears convoluted, irregular, and doubled on itself.[7]

▼ *Classification of Neoplasms*

Neoplasms are customarily classified according to their cell of origin and whether their behavior is benign or malignant. The terminology places the cell or type of tissue of origin as the first part of the name, and the suffix "-oma" (tumor) forms the last portion (Table 3-5).

Epithelial benign tumors of squamous and basal cell origin are called *papillomas*. Glandular epithelial benign tumors are called *adenomas*. Papillomas or adenomas that grow at the end of a stem or pedicle are referred to as *polyps*, and they may become malignant. Malignant neoplasms of epithelial origin are *carcinomas*. Those of glandular epithelial origin are called *adenocarcinomas*, such as adenocarcinoma of the breast.

Neoplasms of muscle cell origin are named according to muscle type, such as *leiomyoma*, which means "smooth-muscle tumor." Malignant neoplasms of muscle cell origin are *sarcomas*, an example of which is *leiomyosarcoma*. Neoplasms of glial cells of the nervous system and connective tissue cells are named in a similar manner. Neoplasms of the blood-forming cells and lymph nodes are named according to the type of blood cell affected.

Pigmented and embryonic cells also are indicated in the nomenclature of neoplasms. In normal embryological development, three layers of cells become apparent. The outer layer is the *ectoderm*, which forms the skin and other structures in the adult human. The middle layer, or *mesoderm*, forms the supporting structures of bone, muscle, fat, blood, and connective tissue. Malignant tumors of these mesodermal or mesenchymal structures are called sarcomas. The inner layer is the *endoderm*, which ultimately forms the gastrointestinal tract and other structures. Sometimes *blastoma* is used to denote that the tissue has a primitive or embryonic appearance. A *teratoma* is another embryonic-appearing tumor that comes from all three germ layers but appears as a highly disorganized array of cells. The teratoma is considered to be benign, whereas the *teratocarcinoma* is malignant. The teratocarcinoma also contains embryonal carcinoma cells, which are a population of stem cells whose proliferation is responsible for the malignancy of these tumors.[5] Neoplasms of pigmented cells are named for their

TABLE 3-5 *Classification of Common Benign and Malignant Neoplasms*

Cell	Benign	Malignant
EPITHELIAL		
Squamous	Squamous cell papilloma	Squamous cell carcinoma
Basal cell	Basal cell papilloma	Basal cell carcinoma
Glandular	Adenoma	Adenocarcinoma
Pigmented	Benign melanoma	Malignant melanoma
MUSCLE		
Smooth muscle	Leiomyoma	Leiomyosarcoma
Striated muscle	Rhabdomyoma	Rhabdomyosarcoma
NERVE		
Nerve sheath	Neurilemmoma	Neurofibrosarcoma
Glial cells	Glioma	Glioblastoma
Ganglion cells	Ganglioneuroma	Neuroblastoma
Meninges	Meningioma	Malignant meningioma
CONNECTIVE TISSUE		
Fibrous	Fibroma	Fibrosarcoma
Fatty	Lipoma	Liposarcoma
Bone	Osteoma	Osteosarcoma
Cartilage	Chondroma	Chondrosarcoma
Blood vessels	Hemangioma	Angiosarcoma
Lymph vessels	Lymphangioma	Lymphangiosarcoma
Bone marrow		Multiple myeloma
		Leukemia
		Ewing's sarcoma
LYMPHOID		Malignant lymphoma
		Lymphosarcoma
		Reticulum cell sarcoma
		Lymphatic leukemia
		Hodgkin's disease
OTHER BLOOD CELLS		
Erythrocytes		Polycythemia vera (?)
Granulocytes		Myelogenous leukemia
Monocytes	Mononucleosis (?)	Monocytic leukemia
Plasma cells		Multiple myeloma
T or B lymphocytes		Lymphocytic leukemia

cell of origin, the melanocyte. Neoplasms of embryonic cell origin also may contain bits of the germinal layers, such as hair or teeth.

▼ Benign Neoplasms

Benign neoplasms consist of cells that are similar in structure to the cells from which they are derived. The cells of benign neoplasms are more cohesive than those of malignant neoplasms. Growth occurs evenly from the center of the benign mass, usually resulting in a well-defined border. The edges move outward, smoothly pushing adjacent cells out of the way (Fig. 3-7). As this occurs, many of these tumors become encapsulated. The capsule, composed of connective tissue, separates the tumor from surrounding tissues. A benign neoplasm usually grows slowly and is limited to one area. Its blood supply is less profuse than that of a malignant neoplasm. A benign neoplasm seldom recurs after surgical removal, and seldom ulcerates, undergoes necrosis, or causes systemic problems. An exception is a secreting endocrine neoplasm, which causes symptoms resulting from excess hormone secretion.

Benign tumors produce their effects from obstruction, pressure, and secretion. A benign tumor in an

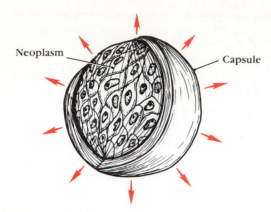

FIGURE 3-7 *Encapsulated benign neoplasm. Arrows indicate equal expansion from the center.*

BOX 3-1 ▼ Biological and Cellular Characteristics of Malignant Tumors

Pleomorphic—cells and nuclei vary in size and shape
Anaplastic—cells bear little resemblance to the parent cell. *Differentiated* cells appear much like the parent cells and growth pattern is slow; *undifferentiated* cells do not resemble parent cells and are usually rapidly growing tumors.
Abnormal mitoses—products of cell division often result in abnormal cells with a high percentage of cell death
Abnormal or no function—malignant cells rarely function like normal cells and often elaborate products not normally seen in that tissue
Nonencapsulated—tumor invades surrounding tissue rather than compressing it like benign tumors do
Metastatic—tumor has the ability to spread to other sites and establish new growth there

enclosed space such as the skull can produce serious disruption that may lead to death.[22] Intestinal obstruction may result from a benign tumor growing in that location.

▼ *Malignant Neoplasms*

Malignant neoplasms have atypical cellular structure, with abnormal nuclear divisions and chromosomes. The malignant cell loses its differentiation or resemblance to the cell of origin. The tumor cells are not cohesive, and, consequently, the pattern of growth is irregular; no capsule is formed, and distinct separation from surrounding tissues is difficult (Fig. 3-8). Malignant cells invade adjacent cells rather than pushing them aside. Tumors have varying growth rates and develop a greater blood supply than normal tissues or benign neoplasms. The hallmark of a malignant neoplasm is its ability to metastasize or spread to distant sites. Box 3-1 summarizes the biologic

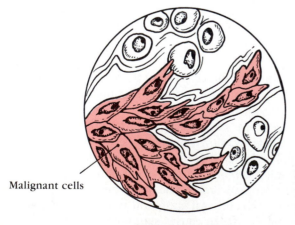

Malignant neoplasm

FIGURE 3-8 *Malignant neoplasm with irregular borders, indistinct from surrounding tissues.*

characteristics of the tumor. It frequently recurs after surgical removal and can cause systemic problems.

MECHANISMS OF CARCINOGENESIS

Cancer is revealing itself as a highly logical, coordinated process by which cells turn the usual benign life purposes to the most dangerous of ends.[1] Many areas of study have evolved to explain the nature of the different diseases that are cumulatively called cancer.

The theory of *somatic cell mutation* was formulated by Bauer in 1928. It supports the concept that genetic abnormalities can be induced by mutational carcinogenic agents and hereditary susceptibility. The proposed mutational process is progressive and involves many steps.[5]

In the 1940s, Berenblum described a two-step mutational model that involved *initiation* and *promotion*. Some factor must initiate the process. These chemical, physical, and viral factors are called carcinogens, and they induce the initial mutation. The initial mutation, called initiation, increases the sensitivity of the cell to surrounding promoters, causing the formation of a larger population of initiated cells. The *initiator* causes DNA structure alterations and mutations. The *promoter* stimulates replication of mutant cells but does not promote their mutation.[23] The process of initiation and promotion probably goes on for several cycles with subsequent mutations of initiated cells before a tumorous mass is formed.

The carcinogens were described previously as those substances that are capable of inducing neoplastic growth in susceptible persons. Carcinogens are known to increase the likelihood that exposed people will develop a neoplasm. *Cocarcinogens* increase the activity of carcinogens. *Procarcinogens* are carcinogens that must be activated or modified in the cell in order to induce cellular changes. Numerous substances have been identified as having cancer-causing abilities. These have been described on pages 44–48. It is thought that a number of steps are necessary for the expression of the fully malignant cell. The change in the first cell is a random (carcinogen-induced) mutation. Whether that cell reproduces or dies depends on a number of interrelated factors. Carcinogenesis is now being described on the basis of these interrelated mechanisms (Fig. 3-9). The carcinogenic substances must undergo molecular modification inside the cell to cause the cancer. When they are modified in such as way as to bind to the nuclear DNA, the

modification is called *activation*. In many cases, the DNA disruption is repaired and the process does not progress.

GROWTH OF THE PRIMARY MALIGNANT TUMOR

The growth rate of malignant tumors does tend to correlate with their level of differentiation. Therefore, the more undifferentiated or anaplastic a tumor, the greater is its potential for aggressive growth and dissemination.

The primary tumor usually grows for years before

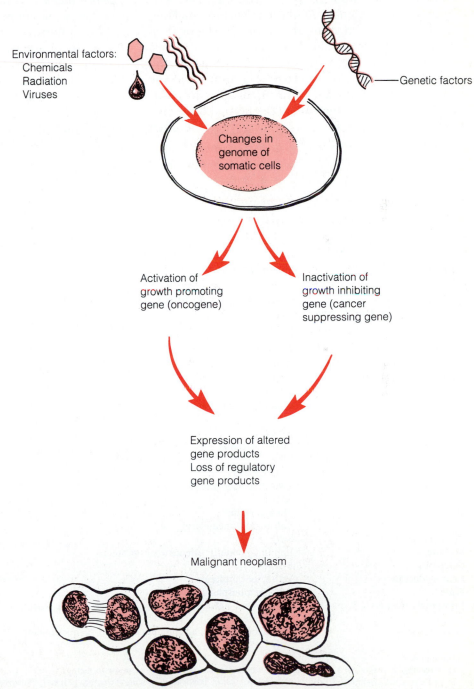

FIGURE 3-9 *Flow chart showing simplified scheme of cancer pathogenesis.*

producing a clinically overt mass.[5] It depends on the cellular reproduction of tumor cells. Each time a cell reproduces, it doubles the tumor mass, from 1 to 2 to 4 to 8, and so on. It is estimated that a typical tumor has doubled 30 times before it becomes clinically observed. A doubling of 40 times often proves to be fatal to the host.

The rate of tumor growth is affected by many factors, including blood supply, nutrition, immune responsiveness, and in some tumors, endocrine support. Studies have shown that many tumors elaborate a *tumor-angiogenesis factor* that promotes directional blood vessel growth into the tumor mass.[13,23] The increased vascularity of the malignant tumor is critical to providing nutrients and oxygen to sustain its continued growth. If a tumor outgrows its blood supply, central ischemic necrosis may occur. In a nutritionally depleted host, the tumor growth may slow because of a decrease in the supply of adequate nutrients. The tumor takes the nutrients from the host, which alters the normal body processes and produces the tumor cachexia syndrome, often called *anorexia–cachexia syndrome* (see pp. 62–63).

TUMOR MARKERS

Tumor markers are substances not normally present in the blood or not present in large quantities that may indicate that a particular type of cancer is present. The presence of these substances has not been found to be helpful except in a few cancers for several reasons: 1) by the time they are found, the markers are elevated and the disease is far advanced; 2) most are not specific for a given tumor; and 3) blood levels may be increased by various nonmalignant diseases.[3] Table 3-6 lists some examples of tumor markers. The markers used in clinical practice include 1) oncofetal proteins such as the carcinoembryonic antigen (CEA) and the alpha fetoprotein (AFP); 2) hormones such as human chorionic gonadotropin (HCG) and ectopic hormones such as adrenocorticotropic hormone (ACTH) and antidiuretic hormone (ADH); 3) immunoglobulins of abnormal type or amount; 4) tumor-associated antigens such as prostate-specific antigen (PSA); and 5) normal enzymes at elevated levels, which often reflect the involved tissue.[3]

Assays of the particular markers are used to 1) screen

TABLE 3-6 *Circulating Serum Tumor Markers*

Cancer	Tumor Markers	Recommended Use[†]
Breast	CEA,* CA 15-3, CA 549, CA M26, M 29, CA 27.29, MCA	4
Gastrointestinal (colorectal, pancreas, stomach)	CEA*	3, 4
	CA 19-9, CA 195, CA 72-4, CA 50	4
Prostate	PSA*	1(?), 3, 4
	PAP*	3, 4
Hepatocellular	AFP*	1–4
	CEA*	4
Ovary	CA 125*	3, 4
	Galactosyl transferase	4
Testicular (germ cell tumors)	AFP*	2–4
	β-hCG	2–4
	LDH,* placental-like AP* (seminoma)	3, 4
Trophoblastic	β-hCG	2–4
Lung (small cell)	NSE, CK-BB	4
Neuroblastoma	VMA,* catecholamines*	1–4
	NSE	4
Thyroid	Thyroglobulin*	1, 4
	Calcitonin* (medullary)	2, 4
Head and neck	SCC	3, 4
Myeloma	Immunoglobulins* (Bence Jones protein)	2, 3
Carcinoid	5-HIAA	2
Neuroendocrine	Variety of hormones	2
Bone	Alkaline phosphatase	2–4
Nonspecific markers	Lipid-bound sialic acid, tissue polypeptide antigen, ferritin, sialytransferase	3, 4
Liver metastases	Glycolytic enzymes, alkaline phosphatase, 5'-nucleotidase	3, 4

*FDA approved.

†1, screening; 2, diagnosis; 3, prognosis; 4, monitoring course of disease or response to therapy.

From DeVita, V.T., Hellman, S., and Rosenberg S.A., *Cancer: Principles and Practice of Oncology* [4th ed.]. Philadelphia: J.B. Lippincott, 1993.

high-risk people for the presence of cancer; 2) diagnose the exact nature of a cancer; 3) monitor the effectiveness of therapy; 4) detect recurrence of cancer; and 5) detect metastases using radioactive-labeled antibodies.[17] Because a particular substance is consistently found in the serum of people with a certain type of cancer, a measurement of that substance can be used to screen for cancer and to monitor for recurrences.[3] Chromosomal abnormalities also have been identified in certain cancers, the most consistent of which is the Philadelphia chromosome in chronic myelogenous leukemia (see pp. 399–402). The HCG hormone has been used as a marker for trophoblastic tumors and testicular and ovarian germ cell tumors. The serum levels of HCG can be used to make decisions on discontinuing and reinstituting therapy.[3, 17]

Histocompatibility antigens are being studied in neoplastic tissue, with the goal being to use a host-versus-tumor reaction to destroy the tumor or metastasis. If the immune system can recognize the tumor as foreign, immunization prepared from host tumor or from tumor cell membranes of a donor may cause the host to reject the tumor. In animal studies, these processes have been quite successful, but in humans, the response has been variable.[23] The immune system has natural defenses for tumor destruction. If the tumor cell antigen is recognized by the immune system as being foreign, it may be destroyed by T-cell cytotoxic response, by natural killer (NK) cells, by macrophage intervention, or by B cells and complement activation (see pp. 320–322). T lymphocytes and NK cells apparently contact the foreign material directly and destroy its membrane. Activated macrophages bind to and destroy neoplastic cells more readily than normal cells. In antibody reactions, the antibody apparently serves as a bridge between the effectors (eg, NK cells, macrophages, polymorphonuclear leukocytes) and target cells (tumor). If complement is involved, the final activated complement can cause the destruction of tumor cells.[1]

If the immune system is capable of destroying neoplastic tissue, how do tumor cells escape destruction? Many human tumors lack tumor-specific antigens, or the antigen is not expressed at the cell surface to be recognized as foreign. Some tumors can modulate the expression of antigen after exposure to the immune system. Immune suppression in individuals debilitated by systemic disease, irradiation, or chemotherapy predisposes them to a higher than normal frequency of later cancers, especially leukemia and lymphoma. People with cancers may have specific and nonspecific suppressor factors, which may be particularly active against T cells.[1]

▼ *Staging of Neoplasms*

Staging is an effort to describe the extent of a neoplasm in terms that are commonly understood. The purposes of staging are to determine treatment, to evaluate survival rates, to establish the relative merits of different methods of treatment, and to facilitate the exchange of information among treatment centers. The staging of cancers is based on the size of the primary tumor and the spread of tumor to regional lymph nodes or other distant areas.[5] The TNM classification varies slightly with different types of cancer but provides some general principles of staging. Box 3-2 shows an example of staging for breast cancer.

The letters used in the classification system are used to denote the following: T, the tumor or primary lesion and its extent; N, lymph nodes of the region and their condition; and M, distant metastasis.[5] Tumor in situ, or localized tumor, is abbreviated Tis. TX is used when the extent of tumor cannot be adequately assessed. Using the letter T and adding ascending numbers indicates the increasing tumor size. The spread of cancer to regional lymph nodes is indicated by N1, referring to "few," with N2 or N3 referring to many nodal metastases. The presence or absence of distant metastasis is designated by an M0 or M1. If the amount or extent of metastasis cannot be assessed, an MX may be used.

▼ *Metastasis*

The ability of a malignant neoplasm to spread to distant sites is termed *metastasis*. A clump of malignant cells, no longer attached to the original neoplasm, travels to and becomes established at a new site. The original cancer is the primary neoplasm, tumor, or site. Metastasis involves the release of many malignant cells, only some of which are able to survive the body's defense mechanisms and hostile environment.[24] Five phases are involved in metastasis: invasion, cell detachment, dissemination, arrest and establishment, and proliferation (Fig. 3-10). Table 3-7 indicates the process of metastasis from initiation to resistance to therapy.

INVASION

To invade normal adjacent cells, the malignant cells grow out from their original location into the neighboring areas. To infiltrate a body cavity or blood vessel, the malignant cells must break through the basement cell membrane. They may escape into the bloodstream through gaps between endothelial cells as rapidly growing capillary tubes penetrate the basement membrane of the capillaries.

A major structural component of the basement cell membrane is type IV collagen. It has been suggested that an enzymatic action causes dissolution of the basement membrane so that tumor cells can penetrate the membrane. There is a loss of expression of proteinase inhibitors.[15] An important enzyme in the process is collagenase type IV, which actively attaches to and dissolves type

---

BOX 3-2 ▼ *Representative Clinical Staging System for Breast Cancer*

T   Primary Tumors

TX   Primary tumor cannot be assessed
T0   No evidence of primary tumor
Tis   Carcinoma in situ: intraductal carcinoma, lobular carcinoma, or Paget's disease with no tumor
T1   Tumor 2 cm or less in its greatest dimension
     a. 0.5 cm or less in greatest dimension
     b. Larger than 0.5 cm but not larger than 1 cm in greatest dimension
     c. Larger than 1 cm but not larger than 2 cm in greatest dimension
T2   Tumor more than 2 cm but not more than 5 cm in greatest dimension
T3   Tumor more than 5 cm in its greatest dimension
T4   Tumor of any size with direct extension to chest wall or to skin (Chest wall includes ribs, intercostal muscles, and serratus anterior muscle but not pectoral muscle)
     a. Extension to chest wall
     b. Edema (including peau d'orange), ulceration of the skin of the breast, or satellite skin nodules confined to the same breast
     c. Both of the above
     d. Inflammatory carcinoma

N   Regional Lymph Nodes

NX   Regional lymph nodes cannot be assessed
N0   No regional lymph node metastases
N1   Metastasis to movable ipsilateral axillary node(s)
N2   Metastases to ipsilateral axillary nodes fixed to one another or to other structures
N3   Metastases to ipsilateral internal mammary lymph node(s)

M   Distant Metastasis

M0   No evidence of distant metastasis
M1   Distant metastases (including metastases to ipsilateral supraclavicular lymph nodes)

DeVita, V.T., Hellman, S., Rosenberg, S.A. *Cancer: Principles and Practice of Oncology* [4th ed.]. Philadelphia: J.B. Lippincott, 1993, pp. 1278–1279.

IV collagen. Damaged endothelium has high levels of collagenase IV, which may allow invasion to occur more easily.[15]

CELL DETACHMENT

After invading the neighboring tissues, body cavities, and blood vessels, malignant cells separate from the primary neoplasm and penetrate lymphatic or blood vessels. Tumor cells lack the normal property of adhesion and are easily shed into the surrounding tissues, blood, and lymph.

DISSEMINATION

The most common route that malignant cells take to distant sites from the primary neoplasm is through the lymphatic and blood vessels. Malignant cells move from lymphatic to blood vessels and vice versa. A malignant neoplasm of just a few grams may shed several million cells into the circulation each day. A large proportion of these cells die, and few possess the factors necessary for survival in the hostile, turbulent circulatory system.[18] To survive in the circulatory system and to effect arrest in the endothelium, malignant cells undergo a variety of cellular interactions that involve immunity and adherence. Some of these are described on pages 49–50.

Lymphatic Dissemination

As the tumor invades surrounding tissue, it penetrates the small lymphatic vessels. Tumor cell emboli are shed into the vessels and are trapped in the first lymph node encountered.[8] All the lymph nodes of a group may become involved with disease, or some may be skipped.[16] The lymph node often enlarges, which may be caused by a localized reaction to the tumor cells or by growth of the tumor within the node. Stimulation of the immune defense system may serve to contain the material within the node or to filter the tumor cells from the circulation, decreasing the net spread of tumor.[9]

There are numerous venous-lymphatic communications by which tumor cells can pass between the blood and lymph systems. The main communication lies at the thoracic duct, where lymphatic fluid empties directly into the venous circulation. Tumor cells brought to the venous circulation by the thoracic duct may be transported to the pulmonary capillary bed, where growth can be established, or they may break into the pulmonary veins and reach the systemic circulation.[8]

A. Primary tumor grows and invades the surrounding tissues. Cells are easily shed and can invade the basement membrane of the highly vascular tumor bed. The increased vascularity is caused by the elaboration of tumor angiogenesis factor (TAF) or by procoagulant factors.

B. The tumor cells move between the endothelial capillary junctions or penetrate the basement membrane of the capillary.

C. The shed tumor cells become arrested in a capillary bed, often liver, lungs, or brain. At this point they can penetrate the capillary wall and establish in the new environment.

D. Proliferation at the new site requires a receptive environment, with blood supply and nutrition to encourage tumor growth. Most tumor cells are killed in the process of metastasis.

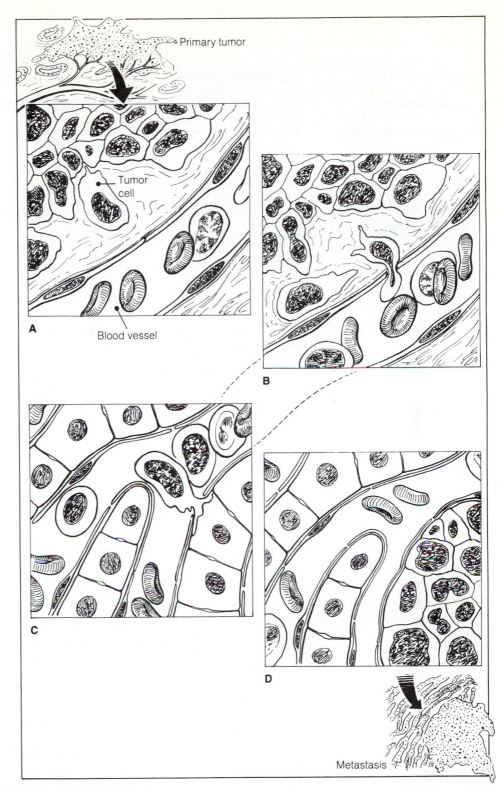

FIGURE 3-10 *Metastasis of tumor cells to nonadjacent tissues.*

TABLE 3-7 *Tumor-Host Interactions During the Metastatic Cascade*

Metastatic Cascade Event	Potential Mechanisms
1. Tumor initiation	Carcinogenic insult, oncogene activation or derepression, chromosome rearrangement
2. Promotion and progression	Karyotypic, genetic, and epigenetic instability; gene amplification; promotion of associated genes and hormones
3. Uncontrolled proliferation	Autocrine growth factors or their receptors; receptors for host hormones such as estrogen
4. Angiogenesis	Multiple angiogenesis factors including known growth factors
5. Invasion of local tissues, blood, and lymphatic vessels	Serum chemoattractants, autocrine motility factors, attachment receptors, degradative enzymes
6. Circulating tumor-cell arrest and extravasation	Tumor-cell homotypic or heterotypic aggregation
a. Adherence to endothelium	Tumor-cell interaction with fibrin, platelets, and clotting factors; adhesion to RGD-type receptors
b. Retraction of endothelium	Platelet factors, tumor-cell factors
c. Adhesion to basement membrane	Laminin receptor, thrombospondin receptor
d. Dissolution of basement membrane	Degradative proteases, type IV collagenase, heparanase, cathepsins
e. Locomotion	Autocrine motility factors; chemotaxis factors
7. Colony formation at secondary site	Receptors for local tissue growth factors; angiogenesis factors
8. Evasion of host defenses and resistance to therapy	Resistance to killing by host macrophages, natural killer cells and activated T cells; failure to express or blocking of tumor specific antigens; amplification of drug resistance genes

From DeVita, V.T., Hellman, S., and Rosenberg S.A., *Cancer: Principles and Practice of Oncology* [4th ed.]. Philadelphia: J.B. Lippincott, 1993.

Bloodstream Dissemination

Just as the tumor sheds its cells into the lymphatic system, it also can spread into the microcirculation. The spreading is facilitated if collagenase IV is present, because this enzyme dissolves the capillary basement membrane and enhances dissemination. Tumor then may grow at the site of vascular spread, or it may embolize to other parts of the body. Most tumor cells do not survive the turbulence of circulating blood. The chances for survival improve if the tumor cells aggregate with one another or with host cells, such as platelets or leukocytes.

Metastasis requires entrapment in the capillary bed or distant organs.[16] Fibrin deposits often form around the new tumor and may protect it from destruction by immune defensive cells. After the tumor is carried to the lungs, it may invade branches of the pulmonary veins and be released into the systemic circulation to travel to the brain or viscera.[8] If the tumor is shed into the portal venous system, it often ends in metastatic growth in the liver.

The *vertebral vein plexus* provides some answers regarding the odd distributions of metastases of certain tumors. This plexus of veins has no valves and communicates with all major vein systems. It can carry neoplastic cells from the primary site to odd locations. For example, cancerous cells from the prostate gland may establish in the vertebra, pelvis, and femur in the absence of evidence of other metastatic disease. Cancer of the breast may metastasize specifically to the dorsal vertebrae, as do lung cancers. Even some of the cerebral metastases may be a result of cells passing through the vertebral venous plexus.[8]

Adherence also is involved in the survival of malignant cells in the circulatory system and in their arrest in the endothelium of the capillary. Malignant cells form clumps that enter the capillary bed and adhere to endothelial cells lining the capillary, where they become entrapped or arrested. There the clump surrounds itself with fibrin, which protects it during growth.

ARREST, ESTABLISHMENT, AND PROLIFERATION

After becoming trapped in the small vessels of the arteries or veins, the aberrant clump of malignant cells must break through the vessel into the interstitial spaces to continue to grow. Cell-free spaces in the endothelial lining of the capillary appear to be induced by the malignant cells, a process that involves alterations in cellular adhesion and consequent retraction of the endothelial cells. A new environment conducive to cellular growth must be established after the malignant cells have entered the interstitial spaces.

After the clump of malignant cells, the tumor, has grown to exceed about 2 cm in diameter, it can no longer supply its nutritional needs by diffusion. Its own blood supply becomes essential for further development. The establishment of a blood supply is the factor that changes a self-contained clump of malignant cells into a rapidly growing metastatic tumor. As in primary tumor growth, the clump of metastasized cells secretes tumor-angiogenesis factor, which causes the blood vessels to send out new capillaries. These new capillaries grow toward and eventually penetrate the malignant cells, creating a blood supply through which the malignant cells receive nourishment and have their waste products removed. Establishment and proliferation of these cells also depends on the immunologic and outer cell membrane properties discussed previously. The malignant cell adjusts its environment to further its own growth. Flowchart 3-1 shows the possible outcomes of metastasis from the primary tumor.

SITES OF METASTASIS

Primary tumors have a tendency to metastasize to and grow in specific organs. Because a small tumor can release several million tumor cells a day into the bloodstream, some inevitably arrest and survive at a receptive site.[15] Patterns of metastasis apparently are determined by individual cellular characteristics and by environmental factors.[18]

Certain primary malignant neoplasms metastasize more readily to specific sites. For example, cancer of the breast metastasizes to the lungs and brain, whereas cancer of the prostate or adrenals metastasizes to the bone. The site of the metastatic neoplasm is not randomly chosen but may be based on mechanical considerations involving cellular size, pressure, vessel size, and other physical features. Also, the site of metastasis may be similar to the site that fostered the primary growth. Vascularity of the secondary site is essential, and the entrapment of the cells in a capillary network may allow for an environment conducive to secondary growth.

▼ Clinical Manifestations of Neoplasms

In their earliest stages of development, benign and malignant neoplasms are asymptomatic. The mass of cells simply is not large enough to interfere with any bodily

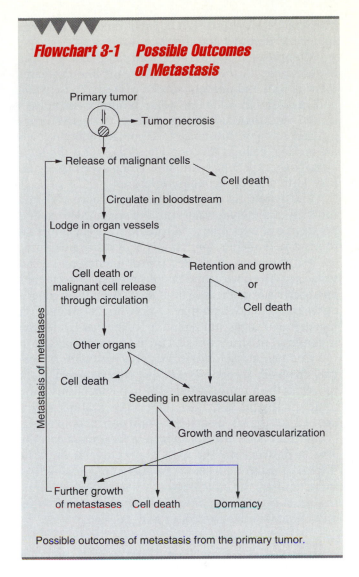

Flowchart 3-1   Possible Outcomes of Metastasis

Possible outcomes of metastasis from the primary tumor.

functions. As the tumor increases in size, local alterations in function occur. As malignant neoplasms grow and metastasize, they interfere with function at distant sites and disrupt the biochemical and nutritional balances of the body.

LOCAL MANIFESTATIONS

The nature and development of local symptomatology depends on the location of the neoplasm and on the size and distensibility of the space it occupies. A neoplasm located in the abdomen, which is large and distensible, may grow to considerable size without producing symptoms. A neoplasm the size of a pea located in the cranial vault, a rigid space controlling vital sensory and motor function, may cause major symptoms.

The mass of cells that makes up a primary or a metastatic neoplasm compresses surrounding tissues and organs and their blood supply. The resulting symptomatology is related to interference with blood supply, interference with function, and mobilization of compensatory mechanisms and immune responses.

Compression by the neoplasm interferes with the blood supply to the tissues and organs and decreases their oxygen and nutrient supply, resulting in ischemia and necrosis. In addition, waste products are not removed, and toxic substances, such as lactic acid, accumulate. As these substances accumulate, blood vessels are eroded, cellular function diminishes, and the individual may experience pain or bleeding. Necrotic tissues may form sites of secondary infection.

The symptoms produced by interference with the function of the organ vary with the organ involved and the degree of interference. A carcinoma of the lung that obstructs a bronchus, for example, may cause atelectasis, abscess formation, bronchiectasis, or pneumonitis distal to the site. The obstruction inhibits removal of secretions and bacteria from the area distal to it. The person experiences coughing, which may or may not be productive, together with signs and symptoms of infection. Infection is common in structures obstructed by a neoplasm.

Compensatory mechanisms also vary with the organ involved. Sometimes the first sign of a malignant process is the attempt by the body to compensate for the obstruction caused by the tumor. An example is increased peristalsis associated with obstruction of the bowel. This is an attempt to force a fecal mass past the area of obstruction. The mass may cause the immune system to try to rid itself of the foreign material, which may stimulate the inflammatory response, and systemic responses of increased pulse rate, elevated temperature, and elevated leukocyte count may be seen.

SYSTEMIC MANIFESTATIONS

Neoplasms have systemic as well as local effects. Systemic symptoms may be the first indication that a person has a neoplasm, or they may accompany more advanced metastatic disease. They include anorexia, nausea, weight loss, and malaise as well as signs and symptoms of anemia and infection. These signs and symptoms occur away from the primary tumor or metastasis and reflect system-wide alterations in bodily processes. The term used to describe these multiple syndromes is *paraneoplastic syndromes*. Up to 75% of all persons with a malignant neoplasm experience a paraneoplastic syndrome sometime during their illness. Significant paraneoplastic syndromes involve the endocrine, nervous, hematological, renal, and gastrointestinal systems.

Only those hormones produced by nonendocrine neoplastic tissues are considered to be paraneoplastic. Symptoms that occur as a result of endocrine paraneoplastic syndromes vary with the hormone produced. For example, all types of lung cancer can produce adrenocorticotropic hormone, causing the person to experience symptoms of Cushing syndrome—moon face, salt and

water retention, and so on. Another example is the hypercalcemia or hypocalcemia that can be caused either by production of a parathyroid hormone-like or calcitonin-like agent by ectopic neoplastic tissues. This type of paraneoplasia is sometimes found in multiple myeloma, breast, or lung cancer.[16]

Persons with malignant tumors may experience neurologic difficulties that are caused by direct effects of the neoplasm, its metastasis, or fluid and electrolyte alterations. A few neurologic symptoms are paraneoplastic, however, and may be the primary signs of cancer. The neurologic symptoms can be grouped according to the area involved: cerebral, spinal cord, or peripheral nerves. Cerebral symptoms include ataxia, dysarthria, hypotonia, abnormal reflexes, dementia, and coma. Spinal cord symptoms include muscle weakness, atrophy, spasticity, hyperreflexia, and paralysis. Peripheral nerve symptoms include sensory loss, weakness, wasting, and depressed reflexes.

Hematological alterations most frequently result from the direct effect of the malignant neoplasm, its metastasis, or response to therapeutic agents used in treatment. Paraneoplastic alterations include polycythemia, which may result from an erythropoietin-secreting tumor; disseminated intravascular coagulation, which is initiated by tumor secretions; and anemia, which may result from bone marrow suppression of erythrocytes.

Renal paraneoplastic syndromes are caused by renal obstructions from neoplastic products. Tumor antigens and immune complexes may precipitate in the glomeruli, and the end result may be renal failure.

Gastrointestinal paraneoplastic syndromes include malabsorption, liver dysfunction, and anorexia-cachexia. More than 90% of persons with advanced disease have a low serum albumin, which may result from loss of protein into the gut or poor absorption of protein from the intestines. Liver enlargement and decreased function may be associated with the hypoalbuminemia. The *anorexia-cachexia syndrome* is a common change seen in most persons with advanced malignant disease. This syndrome is manifest by loss of strength, anorexia, loss of body fat, protein loss, anemia, water and electrolyte imbalance, and major weight loss, all of which are a result of tumor-induced starvation.[25] This condition is a classic illustration of malnutrition and may manifest as starvation or kwashiorkor (see pp. 235–239). Treatment for cancer, especially chemotherapy and radiotherapy, often intensifies the anorexia-cachexia syndrome.

Generalized effects from paraneoplastic phenomena include metabolic alterations such as lactic acidosis, hyperlipidemia, amylase elevation, and muscle and joint alterations. Fever frequently occurs and, in this case, involves an unexplained temperature elevation that subsides with the destruction of the cancer but recurs with its reappearance. Tumor fever occurs with a variety of neoplasms such as Hodgkin disease, myxomas, hypernephroma, and osteogenic sarcoma.

▼ Chapter Summary

▼ Abnormal cell growth that does not respond normally to growth control mechanisms is termed neoplasia. It may be benign or malignant in nature. Benign neoplasms do not invade or metastasize to other tissues, but malignant neoplasms do.

▼ Malignant tumors or cancers are the second leading cause of death in the United States. Related factors include environmental, dietary, infectious, and smoking sources as well as genetic and familial predispositions.

▼ Neoplastic growth proliferation is considered in terms of doubling time and loss of intercellular communication signals. All malignant cells have some degree of anaplasia, which means that the cells lose resemblance to their parent cells. Well-differentiated malignant tumors have less anaplasia, usually grow slowly, and do not readily invade surrounding tissue. Undifferentiated tumors usually grow rapidly, invade, and metastasize to other locations.

▼ Neoplasms are staged or evaluated for their severity in order to determine treatment approaches and to facilitate research. Standard staging methods are being developed internationally.

▼ Metastasis of malignant neoplasms involves invasion, cell detachment, dissemination, arrest and establishment, and proliferation at a new site. Sites chosen for metastasis are very specific to individual malignancies and must be receptive to new growth.

▼ Clinical manifestations of neoplasms may be local (ie, compromising the function of the area in which they arose) or systemic (caused by paraneoplastic syndromes).

▼ References

1. Bast, R.C. Principles of cancer biology: Tumor immunology. In Devita, V.T., Hellman, S., and Rosenberg, S.A., *Cancer: Principles and Practice of Oncology* (4th ed.). Philadelphia: J.B. Lippincott, 1993.
2. *Cancer Facts and Figures 1994.* Rochester, N.Y.: American Cancer Society, 1993.
3. Capizzi, R.L. Principles of treatment of cancer. In Stein, J.H. *Internal Medicine* (4th ed.). St. Louis: Mosby, 1994.
4. Cormack, D.H. *Essential Histology.* Philadelphia: J.B. Lippincott, 1993.
5. Cotran, R.S., Kumar, V., and Robbins, S.L. *Pathologic Basis of Disease* (5th ed.). Philadelphia: W.B. Saunders, 1994.
6. Daly, M.B. Epidemiology of cancer. In Weiss, G., *Clinical Oncology.* Norwalk: Appleton & Lange, 1993.
7. DeVita, V.F., Hellman, S., and Rosenberg, S.A. *Cancer: Principles and Practice of Oncology* (4th ed.). Philadelphia: J.B. Lippincott, 1993.
8. DelRegato, J.A., Spjut, H.J., and Cox, J.D. *Ackerman and delRegato's Cancer: Diagnosis, Treatment and Prognosis* (6th ed.). St. Louis: Mosby, 1985.
9. Fidler, I.J. and Hart, I.R. Biological diversity in metastatic neoplasms: Origin and implications. *Science* 217:998, 1982.
10. Fingert, H.J., Campisi, J., and Pardee, A.B. Cell proliferation and differentiation. In Holland, J.F., et al., *Cancer Medicine* (3rd ed.). Philadelphia: Lea & Febiger. 1993.
11. Guyton, A. *Textbook of Medical Physiology* (8th ed.) Philadelphia: W.B. Saunders, 1991.
12. Klein, G. Oncogenes. In Holland, J.F., et al., *Cancer Medicine* (3rd ed.). Philadelphia: Lea & Febiger, 1993.
13. Krontiris, T.G. Molecular and cellular biology of cancer. In Stein, J.H., *Internal Medicine* (4th ed.). St. Louis: Mosby, 1994.
14. Liotta, L.A. Biochemical mechanisms of tumor cell invasion and metastases. *Prog. Clin. Biol. Res.* 256:3, 1988.
15. Liotta, L.A., Stetler-Stevenson, W.G., and Steeg, P.S. Invasion and metastasis. In Holland, J.F., et al., *Cancer Medicine* (3rd ed.). Philadelphia: Lea & Febiger, 1993.
16. Liotta, L.A. and Stetler-Stevenson, W.G. Molecular cell biology of cancer metastasis. In DeVita, V.T., Hellman, S., and Rosenberg, S.A., *Cancer: Principles and Practice of Oncology* (4th ed.). Philadelphia: J.B. Lippincott, 1993.
17. Mendelsohn, J. Principles of neoplasia. In Wilson, J.D., et al., *Harrison's Principles of Internal Medicine* (12th ed.). New York: McGraw-Hill, 1991.
18. Nicholson, G.I. Tumor metastasis. In Davies, A.J.S., and Rudland, P.S., *Medical Perspectives in Cancer Research.* Chichester, Engl.: Ellis Horwood, 1985.
19. Regan, P. Pancreatic disease. In Stein, J.H., *Internal Medicine* (4th ed.). St. Louis: Mosby, 1994.
20. Rubin, E. and Farber, J.L. *Pathology* (2nd ed.). Philadelphia: J.B. Lippincott, 1994.
21. Taussig, M.J. *Processes in Pathology and Microbiology* (2nd ed.). Boston: Blackwell, 1984.
22. Walter, J.B. *Pathology of Human Disease.* Philadelphia: Lea & Febiger, 1990.
23. Weiss, G. *Clinical Oncology.* Norwalk, Conn.: Appleton & Lange, 1993.
24. Weiss, L. *Principles of Metastasis.* Orlando, Fla.: Academia Press, 1985.
25. Whitney, E.N., Cataldo, C.B., and Rolfes, S.R. *Understanding Normal and Clinical Nutrition* (3rd ed.). St. Paul: West, 1991.

Chapter 4

Genetic Disorders

Miguel da Cunha

▼ CHAPTER OUTLINE

▼ LEARNING OBJECTIVES

1 Define the three broad types of genetic disorders.
2 Discuss briefly the chromosome set (karyotype) of the human species.
3 Differentiate between the terms homozygous and heterozygous.
4 Define **allele, genotype**, and **phenotype**.
5 Draw a Punnett square to compute the progeny of specific genotypes.
6 Describe briefly autosomal dominant inheritance patterns.
7 Describe briefly autosomal recessive inheritance patterns.
8 Describe briefly X-linked dominant inheritance patterns.
9 Describe briefly X-linked recessive inheritance patterns.
10 Explain the three types of chromosomal aberrations.
11 Compare the inheritance pattern of multifactorial disorders with the inheritance pattern of single-gene disorders and chromosomal disorders.
12 Identify at least one disease or disorder that is determined by each type of inheritance pattern.
13 Identify the biochemical defects or structural alterations associated with phenylketonuria, albinism, sickle cell disease, and Marfan syndrome.
14 Differentiate between hemoglobinopathies and thalassemias.
15 Discuss the concepts of oncogenes and tumor suppressor genes.
16 Define **teratogen** and give examples of physical and chemical teratogenic agents.

Barbara L. Bullock: PATHOPHYSIOLOGY: ADAPTATIONS AND ALTERATIONS IN FUNCTION, 4th ed.
© 1996 Lippincott-Raven Publishers

Genes control the functions of a cell by determining what proteins are synthesized within the cell. Genes are also responsible for the transmission of characteristics from one generation to the next. This chapter describes the principles of inheritance, the classification of genetic disorders, and the mechanisms by which alterations in genetic material can produce structural or functional defects. Table 4-1 presents some essential terminology for the study of genetics. A large and diverse assortment of conditions has now been recognized as genetic diseases. It is likely that the expression of any disease is influenced by the genotype of the affected person.[7]

TABLE 4-1 *Genetics Terminology*

Term	Definition
Chromosome	Microscopic structure in the cell nucleus that stores genetic information as base sequences in deoxyribonucleic acid (DNA), and whose number is constant in each species. Chromosomes are found in pairs in somatic cells (homologous chromosomes), one member of the pair being of paternal and one of maternal origin. Homologous chromosomes have identical number and arrangement of genes.
Diploid	The number of chromosomes normally present in somatic (body) cells (notation: 2n); in humans, 2n = 46.
Gene	A segment of DNA that contains genetic information necessary to control a certain function, such as the synthesis of a polypeptide (protein); that segment is often referred to as a site, or locus, on a chromosome.
Homologous	Referring to chromosomes with matching genes, or to those genes individually.
Gamete	A mature reproductive cell containing the haploid number of chromosomes. In males, the spermatozoa; in females, the ova (eggs).
Haploid	The number of chromosomes present in a gamete (notation: n); in humans, n = 23. The diploid number of chromosomes is reconstituted in the zygote on fertilization of two haploid gametes.
Gametogenesis	A series of mitotic and meiotic divisions, occurring in the gonads, that leads to formation of gametes. In males, spermatogenesis; in females, oogenesis. Reduction in the number of chromosomes (2n → n) during gametogenesis occurs in the first meiotic division (Meiosis I).
Alleles	Alternative expressions of a gene at a given locus; for example, the alleles *H* and *h* of the gene *HEXA* would determine synthesis (*H*), or no-synthesis (*h*) of the enzyme hexosaminidase A, whose absence causes Tay-Sachs disease.
Homozygous (homozygote)	An individual possessing a pair of identical alleles at a given locus on a pair of homologous chromosomes. In the above example, *HH* and *hh*.
Heterozygous (heterozygote)	An individual who has two different alleles at a given locus on a pair of homologous chromosomes. In the above example, *Hh*.
Karyotype	The chromosome constitution of an individual, usually represented by a laboratory-made display in which chromosomes are arranged by size and centromere position.
Aneuploidy	An abnormal chromosome pattern in which the total number is not a multiple of the haploid number. For example, persons with 45 or 47 chromosomes, as in Turner or Down syndrome, respectively, have an aneuploid number of chromosomes.
Trisomy	A condition characterized by a chromosome patten marked by the presence of one chromosome. For example, persons with Down syndrome (trisomy 21) carry an extra chromosome G(21), giving them a total of 47 chromosomes in somatic cells.
Monosomy	A condition characterized by a chromosome pattern marked by the absence of one chromosome. For example, women with Turner syndrome (XO females) have a missing X chromosome, giving them a total of 45 chromosomes in somatic cells.
Genotype	The basic combination of genes of an organism.
Phenotype	The measurable expression of gene function in an individual (eg, eye color, hemoglobin type).
Dominant traits	Traits for which one of a pair of alleles is necessary for expression (eg, polydactyly).
Recessive traits	Traits for which two alleles of a pair are necessary for expression (eg, cystic fibrosis).
Pedigree chart (genogram)	A schematic method for classifying genetic data.

▼ *Principles of Inheritance*

Gregor Mendel, an Austrian monk, is credited with discovering the basic principles of heredity. In 1865, Mendel presented the results of his experiments with garden peas, in which he crossed varieties with distinct characteristics and followed the progeny (offspring) of the crosses for at least two generations. Mendel proposed the idea of hereditary factors that are passed from one generation to the next, but his ideas were not accepted because the existence of chromosomes had not yet been recognized. In 1900, when chromosomes had been observed and their movements during cell division had been noted, Mendel's findings were rediscovered and accepted.

Mendel proposed two principles to describe the inheritance of characteristics in his garden peas. He concluded that the pea plant contains two inherited factors (now called alleles) for the determination of each characteristic. The principle of segregation describes the separation of these two alleles during gametogenesis, such that one half of the gametes receive one allele and the other half the other. The principle of independent assortment expresses the relationship between alleles that determine different inherited characteristics. It states that pairs of alleles segregate independently of each other. Therefore, a gamete may contain either member of one allelic pair and either member of another pair. This principle is true, provided that the alleles are not linked (eg, they are located on different chromosomes). Mendel also recognized that some alleles are dominant and are expressed whenever one copy is present, whereas other alleles are recessive and require two copies for expression.

The distribution of genetic material, as proposed by Mendel, takes place during both divisions of meiosis. Mitosis, outlined on page 15, is a type of cell division in which each of the two resulting daughter cells receives the same number of chromosomes as originally carried by the dividing mother cell. Therefore, mitosis is referred to as an equational process. This replenishment type of cell division is characteristic of somatic cells. Meiosis, one of the cell division types encountered during gametogenesis, consists of two division processes in tandem, referred to as meiosis I and II. During meiosis I, the number of chromosomes in the two resulting daughter cells is reduced to one-half of the number in the original mother cell. This is the reductional portion of meiosis. Meiosis II, which rapidly follows, is a mitosis-like (equational) division, by which each of the entering cells produces two daughter cells. In spermatogenesis, a process in which there is no cell loss, each original cell entering meiosis produces four cells at the end of the completed process. Segregation of the X and Y chromosomes during meiosis is outlined in Figure 4-1.

Studies in biochemical genetics reveal that the unit of heredity is the gene, which consists of a particular sequence of nucleotides in the deoxyribonucleic acid (DNA) of the chromosome. The sequence of nucleotides in a gene either determines the structure of a polypeptide chain or has a regulatory function in protein synthesis. The genes dictate which proteins are found in a cell, and these proteins determine the form and function of the cell. It has been estimated that humans have between 50,000 and 100,000 genes, which are arranged linearly in chromosomes. Given the different sizes of human chromosomes, it becomes obvious that the larger chromosomes carry greater number of genes than the smaller ones (Fig. 4-2). Clinically, this is illustrated by the fact that trisomies for larger chromosomes result in much more severe malformations than those for smaller groups. Trisomy 21 (Down syndrome), for example, in spite of its multiple physical and mental consequences, is still in most cases compatible with a fairly good quality of life. Trisomy 13 (Patau syndrome), however, carries significantly more severe abnormalities and shortens life span to an average of 6 to 12 months.

The karyotype (characteristic chromosome makeup) of each species defines the species chromosome number and morphology. In humans, the cell most commonly used for the study of chromosomes is the lymphocyte. To study the karyotype of an individual, cytogeneticists obtain lymphocytes from a blood sample and grow them in a nutrient medium. Colchicine is added to stop cell division in metaphase, allowing a large number of cells in the same stage of cell division to accumulate. Application of a hypotonic solution causes the cells to swell, separating the chromosomes from each other. They are

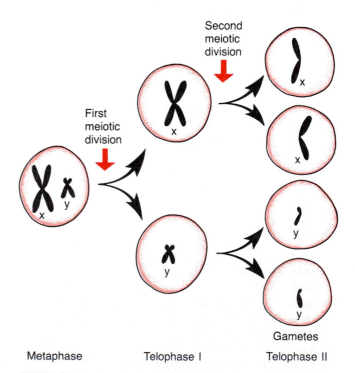

Second meiotic division

First meiotic division

Gametes

Metaphase   Telophase I   Telophase II

FIGURE 4-1 *Selected stages in the process of meiosis. These are illustrated for the XY pair of chromosomes, the sex chromosomes in the male.*

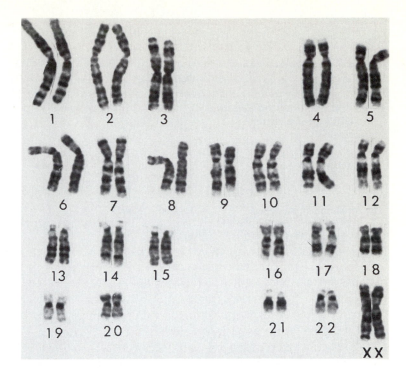

FIGURE 4-2 *Appearance of chromosomes (Courtesy of Dr. David Ledbetter, National Institutes of Health, Bethesda, Md.)*

then placed on a glass slide, stained, and photographed. The photographs are cut out, arranged into groups, and identified by number according to the length of the chromosome and position of its centromere (the constricted portion). A normal female karyotype is shown in Figure 4-2. Normal human somatic cells contain 23 pairs of chromosomes, for a total of 46. Gametes contain only one member of each chromosome pair, for a total of 23.

▼ Classification of Genetic Disorders

Genetic disorders are classified into three broad groups: single-gene, chromosome, and multifactorial. In these three groups, altered genetic material is passed from parent to offspring. Analysis of the genetics and pathophysiology of any genetic disorder first requires its categorization into one of these types. Table 4-2 shows examples of conditions that can be caused by genetic abnormalities.

Single-gene disorders result from mutation in a single gene. The mutated gene may be present on one or both chromosomes of a pair. In the former case, the matching gene on the partner (homologous) chromosome is normal. Single-gene disorders may be recognized as hereditary by analysis of pedigree, the characteristic pattern of distribution of a specific trait in a family. Table 4-3 shows examples of some of the more common single-gene disorders and their frequency.

In chromosome disorders, the defect is caused by an abnormality in chromosome number or structure. In contrast to single-gene disorders, which involve mutated genes, the structure of the genes in chromosome disorders is normal but the genes are present in multiple copies or situated on a different chromosome than is normally the case. For example, Down syndrome results from the presence of an extra chromosome 21 (trisomy 21). Chromosome disorders affect about 7 infants per 1,000 births and account for about one-half of all spontaneous first-trimester abortions.[16]

Multifactorial disorders result from a combination of small variations in genes that, when combined with environmental factors, produce serious defects. Although they do not show the distinct pedigree patterns

---

TABLE 4-2 *Common Examples of Genetic Disorders*

Disorder	Classification	Genetics
Huntington disease	Single-gene disorder	Autosomal dominant
Cystic fibrosis	Single-gene disorder	Autosomal recessive
Hypophosphatemia (vitamin D-resistant rickets)	Single-gene disorder	X-linked dominant
Hemophilia	Single-gene disorder	X-linked recessive
Down syndrome	Chromosome disorder	Trisomy 21
Turner syndrome	Chromosome disorder	45,XO
Cleft lip/palate	Multifactorial	?

TABLE 4-3 *Selected Examples of Single-Gene Disorders*

Disorder	Occurrence	Brief Description
AUTOSOMAL DOMINANT INHERITANCE		
Familial hypercholesterolemia (type II)	1:200–1:500	Deficiency in cell receptors for low-density lipoproteins, resulting in hypercholesterolemia, xanthomas, coronary heart disease
Huntington disease	1:18,000–1:25,000 (United States) 1:333,000 (United Kingdom)	Progressive neurologic disease, involuntary muscle movements, mental deterioration with memory loss, personality changes
Neurofibromatosis, type I	1:4,000–1:5,000	Disorder of neural crest–derived cells with skin and central and peripheral nervous system manifestations; café au lait spots, neurofibromas, and malignant progression are common; variable expression of manifestations
Polycystic renal disease (adult)	1:250–1:1,250	Enlarged kidneys with cysts, hematuria, proteinuria, abdominal mass; may be associated with hypertension, hepatic cysts
Tay-Sachs disease	1:3,600 (Ashkenazi Jews)	Lipid storage disease; progressive mental and motor retardation with onset at about age 6 months, deafness, blindness, convulsions, death by age 3–4 years
X-LINKED DOMINANT INHERITANCE		
Pseudohypoparathyroidism (Albright hereditary osteodystrophy)	Rare	Short stature, delayed dentition, hypocalcemia, hyperphosphatemia, mineralization of skeleton, round facies
Vitamin D-resistant rickets (familial hypophosphatemia)	1:20,000	Disorder of renal tubular phosphate transport; low serum phosphate, rickets, short stature
Polydactyly	1:100–1:300 (African-Americans) 1:630–1:3,300 (Caucasians)	Extra (supernumerary) digit on hands or feet
AUTOSOMAL RECESSIVE INHERITANCE		
Albinism (tyrosinase negative)	1:15,000–1:40,000 1:85–1:650 (Native Americans)	Melanin lacking in skin, hair, and eyes; nystagmus; photophobia; increased susceptibility to neoplasia
Cystic fibrosis	1:2,000–1:2,500 (Caucasians) 1:16,000 (African-Americans)	Abnormal exocrine gland function with pancreatic insufficiency and malabsorption, chronic pulmonary disease, excessive salt in sweat
Cystinuria	1:10,000	Defect in transport of cystine, lysine, arginine, and ornithine in intestines and renal tubules, tendency toward renal calculi
Familial dysautonomia (Riley-Day syndrome)	1:10,000–1:20,000 (Ashkenazi Jews)	Dysfunction of autonomic nervous system, sensory abnormalities, small stature, poor coordination, scoliosis, lack of tears leading to corneal ulcers
Hurler syndrome (Mucopolysaccharidosis, type I)	1–2:100,000	Mucopolysaccharide disorder; mental retardation, coarse facies, skeletal and joint deformities, deafness, dwarfism, corneal clouding, onset age 6–12 months, fatal in childhood
Phenylketonuria (PKU)	1:15,000 (United States) 1:5,000 (Scotland)	Deficiency in phenylalanine hydroxylase causing excess phenylalanine in blood and urine, mental retardation if untreated, normal development and life span with low phenylalanine diet
Sickle cell disease	1:400–1:600 (African-Americans)	Hemoglobinopathy with chronic hemolytic anemia, growth retardation, susceptibility to infection, painful crises, leg ulcers, dactylitis, priapism

(continued)

TABLE 4-3   *(continued)*

Disorder	Occurrence	Brief Description
X-LINKED RECESSIVE INHERITANCE		
Color blindness (red-green deutan)	8:100 (Caucasian males) 4–5:100 (Caucasian females) 2–4:100 (African-American males)	Normal visual acuity, defective color vision with red-green confusion
Duchenne's muscular dystrophy	1:3,000–1:5,000 males	Progressive muscle weakness, atrophy contractures, eventual respiratory insufficiency and death; 95% wheelchair-bound by 12 years of age
G6PD (glucose-6-phosphate dehydrogenase) deficiency	1:10 African-American males 1:50 African-American females	Enzyme abnormality with subtypes, manifestations involve erythrocytes because if cannot replace unstable enzyme; usually asymptomatic unless person is under stress or exposed to certain drugs or infection, which increase need for chemical-reducing power generated by action of G6PD; decreased reducing power eventually results in denaturation of hemoglobin and hemolysis
Hemophilia A	1:2,500–1;5,000 male births	Coagulation disorder caused by deficiency or defect of factor VIII
Hemophilia B	1:30,000 male births	Coagulation disorder caused by deficiency or defect of factor IX
X-linked ichthyosis	1:5,000–1:6,000 males	May be born with sheets of scales (collodion babies), dry scaling skin, corneal opacities, steroid sulfatase deficiency

of single-gene disorders, multifactorial disorders tend to cluster in families. It has been estimated that as many as 10% of the population are affected by these conditions.[7]

Another group of disorders are alterations in fetal development caused by the environment. In this case, the conditions are not hereditary, but they often involve a change in the expression of the cell's genetic material that causes a defect in the structure or function of the cell. Environmental factors such as toxic chemicals, infectious agents, and irradiation are responsible for certain congenital abnormalities. Fetal development may also be affected by an unfavorable intrauterine environment caused by maternal disease.

▼ Single-Gene Disorders

TERMINOLOGY

Transmission patterns in hereditary disorders are described in specific terms that must be defined for precise understanding. The members of a pair of matching chromosomes (those carrying genes that influence the same traits) are termed homologous chromosomes. Each gene has a specific site or locus on a specific chromosome. Genes at the same locus on a pair of homologous chromosomes are called alleles. An individual in whom both

members of a pair of alleles are the same is homozygous (a homozygote) with respect to that gene locus; if the members of a pair of alleles are different, the individual is heterozygous (a heterozygote) for that gene locus (Fig. 4-3).

Genotype is the word used to describe the genetic constitution of an individual. The measurable expression of a gene in an individual is the phenotype.

An allele that is expressed when it is present on one or both chromosomes of a pair is dominant. An allele that is expressed only if it is present on both chromosomes of a pair (with the exception of the XY pair) is

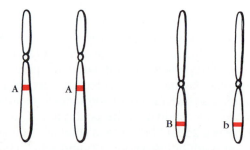

FIGURE 4-3 *Two pairs of homologous chromosomes. One pair has similar alleles at locus A. The other pair has dissimilar alleles at locus B. A person with these chromosomes would be homozygous for allele A and heterozygous for allele B.*

recessive. The terms *dominant gene* and *recessive gene* are commonly used. The trait (phenotype) that these genes determine can also be referred to as dominant or recessive. In genetic disorders, a dominant disorder is one in which the person who carries the gene (in either a heterozygous or homozygous state) is clinically affected. To be clinically affected by a recessive disorder, the individual must be homozygous for the gene. An exception is genes found on the X chromosome in a male. Because these gene loci are not matched by corresponding loci on his Y chromosome, a recessive gene on the male's X chromosome will be expressed. A disorder carried on the X chromosome is an X-linked disorder. There are no known Y-linked genetic disorders of medical interest.

PRINCIPLES OF TRANSMISSION

Phenotypes determined by single genes occur in fixed proportion in the progeny of a mating. The pedigree patterns of such traits depend on whether the gene is located on an autosomal chromosome (any chromosome other than a sex chromosome) or on the X chromosome, and on whether the gene is dominant or recessive. These factors allow four basic patterns of inheritance for single-gene traits: autosomal dominant, autosomal recessive, X-linked dominant, and X-linked recessive.

Patterns of single-gene inheritance can be exhibited in a pedigree chart, which is a schematic method for classifying data. Some symbols used in construction of a pedigree chart are shown in Figure 4-4. Gene symbols are always expressed in italics. Usually a capital letter is used to signify a dominant allele and the lower case of the same letter is used to signify the corresponding recessive allele. By this method, a genotype may be shown as *TT*, *Tt*, or *tt*, as in Figure 4-5.

An example of a phenotype determined by a single pair of autosomal alleles is the ability to taste phenylthiocarbamide (PTC). The bitter taste of the drug is detected by persons with the dominant gene but not by persons homozygous for the recessive allele. Therefore, those with the genotype *TT* (homozygous dominant) or *Tt* (heterozygous) are able to taste the drug and are classified as having a phenotype, taster. Persons with the genotype *tt* (homozygous recessive) are not able to taste the drug and are classified as phenotype, nontaster.

Figure 4-5 illustrates the use of a Punnett square to predict the genotypes and phenotypes of the progeny of a heterozygous (*Tt*) male and a *Tt* female. Mendel's law of segregation and the concept of dominance are used for this prediction. As shown in the genotypes of the offspring, there is a 25% chance that a child of this mating will be a dominant homozygote (*TT*) and a 50% chance of the child's being a heterozygote (*Tt*). Both of these genotypes produce the phenotype, taster. There is a 25% chance that the child will be a recessive homozygote (*tt*)

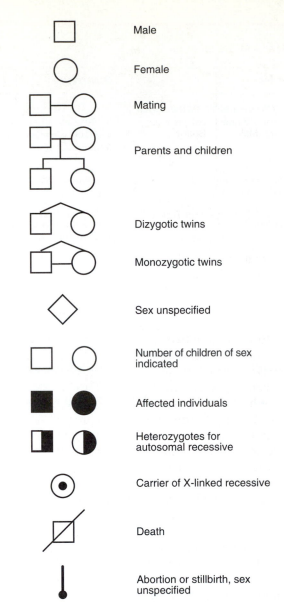

□	Male
○	Female
□—○	Mating
	Parents and children
	Dizygotic twins
	Monozygotic twins
◇	Sex unspecified
□ ○	Number of children of sex indicated
■ ●	Affected individuals
◧ ◐	Heterozygotes for autosomal recessive
⊙	Carrier of X-linked recessive
⊘	Death
⦙	Abortion or stillbirth, sex unspecified

FIGURE 4-4 *Symbols used in pedigree charts.*

and have the phenotype, nontaster. As discussed in the next section, the pattern of inheritance seen in the ability to taste PTC is typical of a dominant mode of inheritance.

Figure 4-6 illustrates all possible genotypes of offspring from matings involving a single pair of autosomal alleles. Using the same trait of PTC taster as an example, there are three possible genotypes for each male and each female (*TT*, *Tt*, and *tt*) and the different combinations of genotypes that could be found in the offspring of each mating. With respect to autosomal dominant disorders, a common clinical situation is that of a couple in which one member is affected and the other is genetically normal (eg, *Dd* × *dd*). With autosomal recessive disorders, the typical situation is that of a couple of heterozygote carriers (*Rr* × *Rr*) who seek genetic advice after producing an affected child (rr). The outcome of

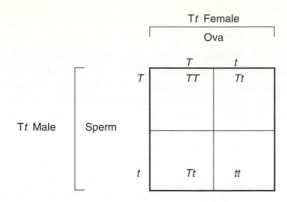

FIGURE 4-5 *Progeny of Tt and Tt mating.*

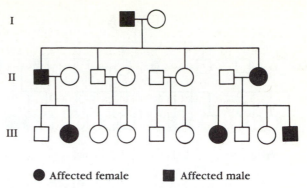

FIGURE 4-7 *Stereotypical pedigree of autosomal dominant inheritance.*

those matings and their implications are discussed in the following sections.

AUTOSOMAL DOMINANT INHERITANCE

In autosomal dominant inheritance of a genetic defect, the abnormal allele is dominant and the normal allele is recessive. According to Mendelian laws, individuals with genotypes DD and Dd express an affected phenotype, whereas the genotype dd results in a normal individual. Usually, the heterozygous person displays a more mild phenotype than the affected homozygote. For example, in achondroplastic dwarfism, the affected homozygous exhibits severe malformations, such as hydrocephalus, which usually result in severe mental retardation in addition to the physical impairment. The heterozygous person, however, usually displays the typical physical manifestations and functions well in the societal structure. For this reason, it is usually safe to assume that the affected individual in a couple is a heterozygote whose disease did not impede him or her from developing the complex societal skills that led to courtship, marriage, mating, and reproduction. In most cases, the typically observed mating is that of $Dd \times dd$ individuals. The stereotypical pedigree of this pattern is shown in Figure 4-7. If either parent is heterozygous for the autosomal dominant allele (in this case the father) and the other parent is homozygous for the normal allele, each child has a 50% risk of receiving the dominant allele and thus being affected. Each child receives a normal allele from the normal parent. Although one-half of the children will theoretically receive the dominant allele, the chances are independent in each zygote formation, and in a small sample such as a family, the ratio of normal to affected children may not be 1:1. Because the allele is autosomal and not X-linked, either sex may be affected. All affected children have an affected parent, unless the disorder results from a fresh mutation.

Characteristics of autosomal dominant inheritance are summarized as follows: 1) affected persons usually have an affected parent; 2) affected persons mating with normal persons have equal chances of producing affected and unaffected offspring; 3) unaffected children born to affected parents will have unaffected children; and 4) males and females have equal chances of being affected.

AUTOSOMAL RECESSIVE INHERITANCE

In autosomal recessive disorders, the abnormal allele is recessive, the normal allele is dominant, and, as a result, the genotypes RR and Rr both express a normal phenotype. Only affected homozygotes (rr) express the disorder. The difference between the two unaffected individuals above is that the heterozygote has a certain risk of transmitting the defective allele (r); in fact, approximately 50% of this person's gametes will carry the defective allele. Because heterozygotes are usually clinically normal but are able to transmit the disorder, they are referred to as heterozygous carriers. This accounts for the carrier state in autosomal recessive disorders. Because the dominant or normal allele masks the trait, most persons who are heterozygous for an autosomal recessive allele go undetected. If two heterozygous individuals mate (the most common pattern in autosomal recessive inheritance) and an offspring receives the recessive allele from each parent, the trait is expressed. *Consanguineous* marriage (marriage of persons who are blood relatives) may increase this probability.

If a heterozygous person mates with a homozygous normal person, each offspring receives a normal allele

Paternal genotype	Maternal genotype		
	TT	*Tt*	*tt*
TT	*TT*	*TT, Tt*	*Tt*
Tt	*TT, Tt*	*TT, Tt, tt*	*Tt, tt*
tt	*Tt*	*Tt, tt*	*tt*

FIGURE 4-6 *Parental genotypes for autosomal alleles T and t and the genotypes that could be found in progeny of the various mating pairs.*

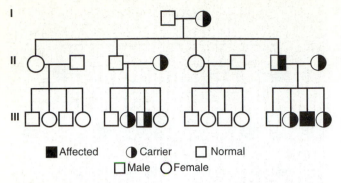

■ Affected ◑ Carrier □ Normal
□ Male ○ Female

FIGURE 4-8 *Stereotypical pedigree of autosomal recessive inheritance.*

from the normal parent and cannot express the trait. Figure 4-8 illustrates a stereotypical pedigree of autosomal recessive inheritance. In line I, a homozygous normal male mates with a heterozygous female, and each offspring receives a normal gene from the father. Fifty percent of the offspring receive the recessive allele from the heterozygous mother and are therefore carriers of the trait. Line II shows a heterozygous male mating with a heterozygous female. The progeny of this mating have a 1 in 4 risk of receiving a recessive allele from each parent and thus being affected with the trait.

Characteristics of autosomal recessive inheritance are summarized as follows: 1) the trait usually appears in siblings only, not in the parents; 2) males and females are equally likely to be affected; 3) for parents of one affected child, the recurrence risk is one in four for every subsequent birth; 4) both parents of an affected child carry the recessive allele; and 5) the parents of an affected child may be consanguineous.

SEX-LINKED INHERITANCE

Sex-linked traits are those for which the causative gene is located on one of the sex chromosomes, the X or the Y chromosome. Of the 46 chromosomes in a somatic cell, 22 pairs are autosomes, and the remaining two are sex chromosomes—XX in females, XY in males. Because the two X chromosomes in women are of equal size and homologous, they constitute a true pair. During meiosis I, homologous chromosomes pair side-by-side, allowing for exchange of genetic material (crossing over) between chromosomes of paternal and maternal origin. In males, however, the sex chromosomes are of unequal size and with different centromere positioning, and areas of homology, if they exist, are few. This leaves alleles located on the X chromosome without homologous counterparts on the Y chromosome. For this reason, males are *hemizygous* for genes located on the X chromosome, and traits determined by either dominant or recessive genes are expressed in the male.

The establishment of chromosomal sex in a male is

determined at conception by fertilization of an X-bearing ovum by a Y-bearing spermatozoon, resulting in an XY zygote. A female receives one X chromosome from each parent. Therefore, paternal genes located on the X chromosome are transmitted from father to daughter, and those on the Y chromosome from father to son.

An important function of the Y chromosome is to determine the organization of the testes in developing XY embryos. This is carried out by a complex of genes located on the Y chromosome, called the testis-determining region. As a result, all males, as well as a few phenotypically female individuals who have an XY constitution (those with testicular feminization, or androgen-insensitivity syndrome) have testes or some residual testicular tissue.

Because no genes of medical significance have been found to date on the Y chromosome, the terms *sex-linked* and *X-linked* inheritance are often (and incorrectly) used interchangeably. The discussion of sex-linked inheritance in this chapter refers to X-linked traits only.

X-Linked Dominant Inheritance

Genetic disorders caused by X-linked dominant genes are rare. The main characteristic of this inheritance pattern is that an affected male transmits the gene to all his daughters and to none of his sons. The affected female may transmit the gene to offspring of either sex (Fig. 4-9).

Characteristics of X-linked dominant inheritance are summarized as follows: 1) affected males have normal sons and affected daughters; 2) affected females (heterozygous) have a 50% risk of transmitting the abnormal gene to each daughter or son; and 3) the disorder tends to be more severe in males (hemizygous) than in females (heterozygous).

X-Linked Recessive Inheritance

Several genetic disorders associated with a recessive gene on the X chromosome have been identified. Again, the inheritance pattern of these disorders results from the morphologic differences between the X and Y chromosomes. The recessive gene located on the one X chro-

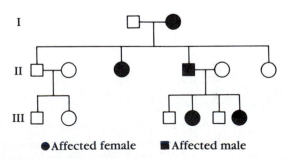

● Affected female ■ Affected male

FIGURE 4-9 *Stereotypical pedigree of X-linked dominant inheritance.*

mosome of the male is not balanced by a dominant allele on the Y chromosome and is therefore expressed. The recessive gene should be expressed in the female only if she is homozygous. Therefore, X-linked recessive disorders are rare in females. Only matings between an affected male and a carrier or affected female should result in an affected female.

Occasionally, a carrier (heterozygous) female manifests some of the signs of a recessive disorder. This is a result of the fact that, during early embryogenesis, one or the other of the X chromosomes in each of the somatic cells (cells other than the gametes) of all females degenerates, leaving only one functioning X chromosome in each cell.[4] Therefore, approximately one-half of the cells in a normal female express the genes on one of her X chromosomes, and the other half express the genes on her other X chromosome. If this "X-chromosome inactivation" is unequal, one of the X chromosomes may have a greater effect on the female's physiology than the other, resulting in the ability of a recessive gene on that chromosome to be expressed.[4]

Males affected with an X-linked recessive disorder cannot transmit the gene to their sons, but transmit it to all their daughters. An unaffected female who is heterozygous for the recessive gene transmits it to 50% of her sons and daughters. Figure 4-10 gives a stereotypical pedigree of X-linked recessive inheritance.

Characteristics of X-linked recessive inheritance are summarized as follows: 1) males are predominantly affected; 2) affected males cannot transmit the gene to sons but transmit it to all daughters; 3) sons of female carriers have a 50% risk of being affected; and 4) daughters of female carriers have a 50% risk of being carriers.

PATHOPHYSIOLOGY OF SINGLE-GENE DISORDERS

Because the genes of a cell are primarily responsible for directing the synthesis of the cell's proteins, it is not surprising that the manifestations of single-gene disorders result from alterations in protein synthesis. In many cases, the affected protein is an enzyme, part of a syn-

thetic or degradation pathway. In other instances, the altered protein is a constitutive protein (eg, hemoglobin), is part of the cell membrane (eg, a receptor of a transport protein); or is mainly supportive in function (eg, collagen). Sometimes the disorder is classified by its pattern of transmission as a single-gene defect, but its basic pathology is not known.

Altered Activity of an Enzyme in a Metabolic Pathway

Alterations in the activity of one enzyme in a metabolic pathway may have several results, including a deficiency in the end product of the pathway or the accumulation of a toxic intermediate or a toxic byproduct. These possibilities are illustrated in Figure 4-11, which shows selected pathways for the metabolism of phenylalanine and tyrosine and metabolic blocks that are responsible for three genetic disorders—albinism, alkaptonuria, and phenylketonuria.

ALTERATIONS IN AMINO ACID METABOLISM. As indicated in Figure 4-11, both phenylalanine and tyrosine are normally available from the digestion of dietary protein. Phenylalanine is also converted to tyrosine, which has many uses in the cell, one of which is to produce melanin, the pigment in skin, hair, and eyes. In *classic albinism*, a deficiency in the enzyme tyrosinase results in decreased or absent melanin production. Manifestations of this condition are listed in Table 4-3. Another single-gene disorder, *alkaptonuria*, is caused by the absence of homogentisic acid oxidase, which results in the accumulation of the pathway intermediate homogentisic acid (alkapton). Homogentisic acid is excreted in the urine and turns black in the presence of oxygen, which produces darkening of the urine. In later life, deposits of dark pigment may be noted in connective tissue and may lead to arthritis.

The most serious genetic disorder involving phenylalanine metabolism is *phenylketonuria* (PKU). In classic PKU, absence of phenylalanine hydroxylase from liver cells prevents the conversion of phenylalanine to tyrosine. Consequently, phenylalanine accumulates in the blood, and some is converted to phenylpyruvic acid, phenyllactic acid, or phenylacetic acid. These compounds are excreted in the urine, giving it a characteristic musty odor. The excess of phenylalanine and its byproducts in the blood results in various metabolic disturbances, especially alterations in nervous system development, including delayed psychomotor development, seizures, hyperactivity, and mental retardation. In addition, excess phenylalanine in the blood inhibits the activity of tyrosinase. Because this enzyme is necessary for the synthesis of melanin and catecholamines, children with PKU tend to have lighter eyes and skin than their relatives and may show a decrease in circulating epineph-

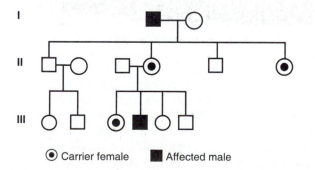

⊙ Carrier female ■ Affected male

FIGURE 4-10 *Stereotypical pedigree of X-linked recessive inheritance.*

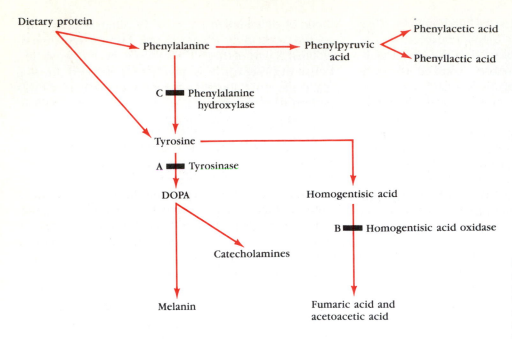

FIGURE 4-11 *Metabolism of phenylalanine and tyrosine. Arrows represent one or more chemical reactions. The indicated enzyme defects result in (A) classic albinism, (B) alkaptonuria, and (C) classic phenylketonuria (PKU). DOPA, dihydroxyphenylalanine.*

■ = Blocked reaction

rine. In the untreated infant, manifestations of PKU appear at approximately 3 to 6 months of age.

Fortunately, tests are available to detect phenylalanine or its metabolites in blood or urine. PKU screening is mandatory for newborns in most states.[4] The most commonly used test, the Guthrie bacterial-inhibition assay, which indicates phenylalanine level in the blood, is not positive until the infant has consumed enough protein to allow phenylalanine buildup. If the test is performed during the first 2 days of life, as may occur with the current trend for early hospital discharge of mother and baby, it may have to be repeated, ideally before the infant is 3 weeks old.[4] In PKU-positive infants, neurologic damage can be prevented by restriction of phenylalanine in the diet. The restrictive diet should be started as early as possible and followed until neurologic development is complete. Estimates regarding the age at which a normal diet may be allowed vary widely, from 3 years to never.[4] If a woman with PKU becomes pregnant, it is necessary for her to resume her low-phenylalanine diet to protect the fetus.[5]

With the advent of widespread neonatal PKU screening, other causes of hyperphenylalaninemia have been identified, involving closely related aspects of phenylalanine metabolism. Classic PKU accounts for approximately 90% of all cases of hyperphenylalaninemia.[5] Other causes are deficiencies of related enzymes in the liver other than phenylalanine hydroxylase. Classic PKU exhibits autosomal recessive transmission; tests are available to detect heterozygous carriers.[16]

ALTERATIONS IN CARBOHYDRATE METABOLISM. Loss of activity of enzymes in the varied pathways for carbohydrate metabolism account for many single-gene disorders. These include alterations in the metabolism of glucose, galactose, or fructose, glycogen storage diseases, and disorders involving mucopolysaccharides. In *galactosemia*, deficiency of an enzyme needed for the conversion of galactose 1-phosphate to glucose 1-phosphate leads to the accumulation of galactose and galactose 1-phosphate in tissues. This interferes with normal liver and kidney function and produces other metabolic disturbances that may result in osmotic changes in the lens of the eye and cataract development.

Glucose-6-phosphate dehydrogenase deficiency, a relatively common disorder in African-Americans, is described in Table 4-3. In *glycogen storage diseases*, various enzymes needed for the synthesis or breakdown of glycogen may be altered. The accumulation of glycogen in tissues, especially the liver, interferes with their functions. The most common glycogen storage disease is *von Gierke disease*, in which developing liver pathology produces hepatomegaly, acidosis, increased glucose and lipids in the blood, and retarded growth. *Mucopolysaccharides* are large, complex carbohydrates that form part of the extracellular matrix of connective tissue. They are constantly being turned over in the tissues and are degraded by enzymes contained in the lysosomes of a cell. A deficiency in any of the necessary lysosomal enzymes leads to the accumulation of partially degraded mucopolysaccharides within the lysosome (one type of *lysosomal storage disease*). This interferes with various activities of the cell. Manifestations of mucopolysaccharidosis, type I, or *Hurler syndrome*, are listed in Table 4-3.

DISORDERS OF SPHINGOLIPID METABOLISM. Accumulations of sphingolipids produce *lipid storage diseases* such as Gaucher disease and Tay-Sachs disease. Sphingolipids are lipids present in membranes, especially in the myelin of brain and other nervous tissue. The three classes of sphingolipids are sphingomyelins, cerebrosides, and gangliosides. Like many compounds in the body, sphingolipids are continually being turned over, and a block in their metabolism pathway can lead to their accumulation in various tissues. *Gaucher disease* is the most common lipid storage disease, exhibiting a relatively high frequency in Ashkenazi Jews (Jews of European, as opposed to Mediterranean, origin). Glucocerebrosides accumulate in reticuloendothelial cells, producing Gaucher cells, which are found most often in the spleen, lymph nodes, liver, and bone marrow. Manifestations of this disease, which has several forms, include splenomegaly, hepatomegaly, osteoporosis, anemia, tendency to bleed, and, in some forms, neurologic damage and mental retardation. In *Tay-Sachs disease*, which is also most prevalent in Ashkenazi Jews, the accumulation of one type of ganglioside in the lysosomes of neurons results in ballooning of neurons, degeneration of axons, and demyelination, producing nervous system manifestations such as those indicated in Table 4-3. At present, there is no treatment for this disease. Fortunately, screening is available to detect heterozygous carriers of this autosomal recessive disorder.

OTHER METABOLIC PATHWAY DEFECTS. Other biochemical pathways that are known to be altered by single-gene mutations include ones that involve the metabolism of purines, pyrimidines, or heme, and those that are used for the biotransformation of certain drugs. The synthesis of heme occurs by way of several precursors, called porphyrins. The *porphyrias* are disorders in which an enzyme defect leads to the accumulation and excretion of porphyrins or porphyrin precursors. Some porphyrias are hereditary, and some are caused by the toxic effect of chemicals. Of the hereditary porphyrias, four types display autosomal dominant transmission and one is autosomal recessive.

General characteristics of porphyrias include the excretion of reddish urine, photosensitization of the skin and skin eruptions, excessive hair on the face and limbs, and neurologic and psychologic manifestations. This constellation of signs and symptoms may have led to afflicted persons being called the werewolves of European folklore.

Loss or Alteration of Circulating Proteins

Other types of single-gene disorders can involve proteins that circulate in the bloodstream. Serum albumin is deficient in *analbuminemia*, producing oncotic pressure problems. Serum globulins that may be affected by single-gene mutations include complement components, α_1-antitrypsin, α_2-macroglobulin, transferrin, and various immunoglobulins (the immunoglobulins in *X-linked agammaglobulinemia* or *severe combined immunodeficiency*).[4] Clotting factor VIII, IX, or XI is absent from the blood in the *hemophilias*. Von Willebrand factor is a protein that interacts with and possibly stabilizes clotting factor VIII. It is also necessary for formation of a platelet plug. Lack of the factor occurs in *von Willebrand disease*.[1]

HEMOGLOBIN ABNORMALITIES. Disorders involving the synthesis of the protein component of hemoglobin include the *hemoglobinopathies* and the *thalassemia syndromes*. The hemoglobin molecule consists of the protein globin and four heme complexes. In adult hemoglobin, the globin component is made up of four polypeptide chains: two identical α chains and two identical β chains (see p. 374). A single-gene mutation could change the structure of the α or the β chains. Hundreds of variations in the globin chains have been identified.[1]

Sickle cell anemia results from a single-gene mutation that leads to the substitution of valine for glutamic acid at one location on the β chains of adult hemoglobin (HbA), forming HbS. The hemoglobin of a person who is homozygous for the abnormal gene contains abnormal β chains. Under low oxygen conditions, this hemoglobin tends to precipitate within erythrocytes and causes them to assume a characteristic sickle shape. These abnormal red blood cells tend to compromise blood flow to the tissues and also to lyse, resulting in anemia. A person who is homozygous for the gene is said to have *sickle cell disease*. A person who is heterozygous for the abnormal gene produces both HbS and HbA and exhibits sickling of erythrocytes only under conditions of extremely low oxygen tension. This person may never exhibit signs of sickle cell anemia and is said to have the *sickle cell trait*, rather than the disease (see pp. 383–384).

Whereas hemoglobinopathies such as sickle cell disease involve an alteration in the structure of the globin component of hemoglobin, the thalassemias result from reduced synthesis of normal hemoglobin molecules. They are classified as α- and β-thalassemias, depending on which polypeptide chain is synthesized in reduced amounts (see p. 384).

LIPOPROTEINS. Hereditary alterations in the level and function of certain lipoproteins that are normally found in the blood occur in conditions such as *familial hypercholesterolemia*, *abetalipoproteinemia*, and *familial combined hyperlipidemia*. Familial hypercholesterolemia is one of the most frequent single-gene disorders, possibly an autosomal dominant trait. Individuals who are homozygous for this gene display significant and life-threatening manifestations such as an early onset of atherosclerotic disease. Postmortem examination of children as young as 3 to 4 years of age, and of U.S. servicemen killed in the Vietnam War (average age, 19 years) has revealed early arterial changes with lipid deposition, a precursor of coronary artery disease. Cholesterol level in these individuals may be elevated from a very early age, sometimes as high as two or three times the normal amount. Homozygotes, in whom cholesterol levels can be increased fivefold to sixfold, carry a much greater risk for coronary, cerebral, and peripheral vascular atherosclerosis. Myocardial infarction from coronary atherosclerosis may occur before age 20. The genetic defect in familial hypercholesterolemia is a mutation in a gene that controls the synthesis of membrane receptors for low-density lipoprotein (LDL). Decreased receptor activity is accompanied by a loss in feedback control of cholesterol synthesis that results in increased levels of circulating cholesterol in the form of LDL. Heterozygotes for this gene have some residual receptor (and feedback) activity, but the homozygote has almost no normal LDL receptors. Various mutations in the familial hypercholesterolemia gene have been identified, increasing the complexity of this disease, but the understanding of its molecular mechanisms has led to the development of pharmacotherapeutic drugs, such as lovastatin, which lower cholesterol by augmenting the synthesis of LDL receptors.[7, 12] Lipoprotein synthesis and function are discussed in detail on pages 526–528.

Collagen Disorders

Several hereditary disorders result from abnormalities in the synthesis of collagen. This protein, which is the most abundant protein in the body, has a complex structure with several levels of organization. Thirteen different types of collagen are present in the various connective tissues of the body.[3] One example of a collagen disorder is *osteogenesis imperfecta*, which is discussed on page 854.

Another is *Marfan syndrome*, which results from an autosomal dominant gene defect or, in 15% of the cases, from a new mutation.[3] In this disorder, a defect in the structure of collagen or another connective tissue protein, elastin, is thought to be the basis for changes in skeletal, ocular, and cardiovascular tissues. Among the manifestations of Marfan syndrome are a tall, thin stature with arachnodactyly (excessively long fingers), lax ligaments that allow hyperextension of the limbs, dislocation of the optic lenses, and a tendency toward formation of dissecting aneurysms of the aorta. The stature of Abraham Lincoln and the violin virtuosity of Paganini have been attributed to Marfan syndrome.

Single-Gene Disorders in Which the Basic Defect Is Unknown

Among the disorders that appear to be transmitted as single-gene defects are several for which the basic physiologic deficiencies are not known. These include cystic fibrosis, the muscular dystrophies, and Huntington disease, all of which are mentioned briefly in Table 4-3.

Preliminary studies indicate that some manifestations of cystic fibrosis may be caused by faulty control of channels for the diffusion of chloride through cell membranes.[10] Other possible basic defects in cystic fibrosis include hypersecretion of calcium by mucous glands, increased intracellular calcium, and the production of serum glycoproteins, which inhibit the activity of cilia.[10]

Huntington disease is an autosomal dominant disorder in which symptoms do not usually appear until 35 years of age or later. By the time of diagnosis, the affected person may already have reproduced, with a 50% chance of passing this lethal trait to each of his or her offspring. There is no treatment for the disease, and progressive neurologic deterioration is inevitable. Until recently, there was no way to identify persons carrying the gene for Huntington disease before symptoms appeared. Modern techniques for DNA analysis have now shown a characteristic pattern of fragments produced when the DNA of chromosome 4 from cells of persons with the disease is cleaved by a particular enzyme, one of several *restriction enzymes*.[2, 7] Similar treatment of DNA from persons who do not carry the gene yields different fragments. This test is available for predicting which young persons will eventually develop the symptoms of Huntington disease. Use of the predictive test must be accompanied by consideration of the impact of a positive result on the person and the family.

▼ Chromosome Disorders

Chromosomal aberrations (deviations from normal) can be either numeric or structural. They can affect either autosomes or sex chromosomes, although it is rare for both to be affected simultaneously. Chromosome aberrations resulting in two or more cell lines with different chromosome numbers produce *mosaics*. In these situations, one or more of the cell lines is abnormal.

NUMERICAL ABERRATIONS

Deviations or abnormalities in chromosome number are classified in terms of loss or gain of chromosome sets. As has been discussed, the normal chromosome number in humans is 46 (23 pairs). To compare abnormalities with the normal karyotype, several terms must be defined.

Normal somatic cells, with two sets of 23 chromosomes, are said to be *diploid* (double), or 2n; gametes, with a single set of 23, are *haploid* (single), or n. A cell with an exact multiple of the haploid number is *euploid*; euploid numbers are 2n, 3n (*triploid*), or 4n (*tetraploid*). Chromosome numbers that are exact multiples of n but greater than 2n are called *polyploid*. *Aneuploid* refers to a chromosome complement that is abnormal in number but is not an exact multiple of n. An aneuploid cell may be *trisomic* (2n + 1 chromosomes) or *monosomic* (2n − 1 chromosomes). Any cell with a chromosome number that deviates from the characteristic n and 2n is *heteroploid*.

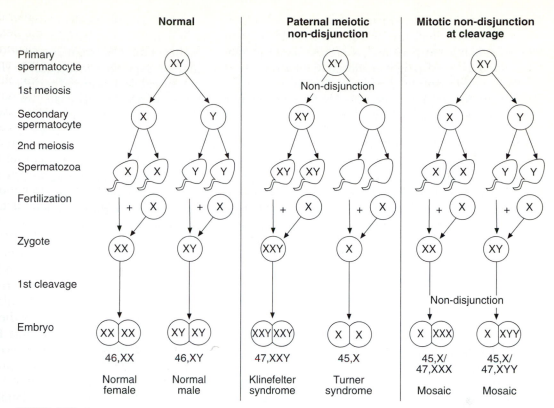

	Normal		**Paternal meiotic non-disjunction**		**Mitotic non-disjunction at cleavage**	

FIGURE 4-12 *Diagram showing mitotic non-disjunction of sex chromosomes at first meiosis and early cleavage.*

Disjunction is the normal separation and migration of chromosomes during cell division. Failure of the process, called *nondisjunction*, in a meiotic division results in one daughter cell receiving both homologous chromosomes and the other receiving neither. It is the primary cause of aneuploidy. If this deviation from the normal process occurs during the first meiotic division, one-half of the gametes will contain 22 chromosomes and one-half will contain 24. If joined with a normal gamete, a gamete produced in this manner will produce either a monosomic (2n − 1) or trisomic (2n + 1) zygote. Monosomic gametes and zygotes are much less likely to survive than their trisomic counterparts, which accounts for a much greater frequency of trisomies. Normal disjunction and nondisjunction at the first and second meiotic divisions of the ovum are illustrated in Figure 4-12. The figure also shows the union of normal sperm with gametes of varying chromosome complement. A common example of a disorder that results from an abnormality of chromosome number is *trisomy 21*, or *Down syndrome*. This disorder can result when nondisjunction of chromosome 21 occurs at meiosis, producing one gamete with an extra chromosome 21 (n + + 1 = 24) and one gamete with no chromosome 21 (n − 1 = 22). Union of the 24-chromosome gamete with a normal sperm produces a 47-chromosome zygote, or trisomy 21.

The overall incidence of Down syndrome is 1 per 700 live births. The incidence increases with increasing maternal age. Because the extra chromosome is of paternal origin in 20% to 30% of cases, the role of increased paternal age is being investigated. Presently, it is suggested that in couples in which the father is age 55 or older, the mother's age-specific risk should be doubled to estimate the couple's risk of having an infant with trisomy 21.[4]

Clinical diagnosis of trisomy 21 is often based on facial appearance. The palpebral fissures are upslanting with speckling of the edge of the iris, the nose is small, and the facial profile is flat. Figure 4-13 illustrates other manifestations of trisomy 21. The simian crease (a single

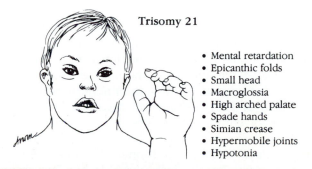

Trisomy 21

- Mental retardation
- Epicanthic folds
- Small head
- Macroglossia
- High arched palate
- Spade hands
- Simian crease
- Hypermobile joints
- Hypotonia

FIGURE 4-13 *Down syndrome phenotype. (Judge, R.D., Zuidema, G.D., and Fitzgerald, F.T. Clinical Diagnosis: A Physiologic Approach [4th ed.]. Boston: Little, Brown, 1982.)*

midpalmar fold) is found in approximately 50% of persons with Down syndrome and in approximately 5% to 10% of nonafflicted persons.[4] The presence of mental retardation is consistent in children with Down syndrome, but the degree may vary. The average intelligence quotient (IQ) is approximately 50; infrequently, values may range up to 70 or 80.

STRUCTURAL ABERRATIONS

Deviations in the normal structure of chromosomes result from the reassembling of chromosome material in an abnormal arrangement. These changes in structure may be either stable (persisting through future cell divisions) or unstable (incompatible with cell division). Stable types of structural abnormalities include the following:

1. *Deletion*, loss of a portion of a chromosome. The missing segment may be a terminal portion of the chromosome, resulting from a single break, or an internal section, resulting from two breaks.
2. *Duplication*, presence of a repeated gene or gene sequence. A deleted segment of one chromosome becomes incorporated into its homologous chromosome.
3. *Inversion*, reversal of gene order. The linear arrangement of genes on a chromosome is broken, and the order of a portion of the gene complement is reversed in the process of reattachment.
4. *Translocation*, transfer of part of one chromosome to a non-homologous chromosome. This occurs if two chromosomes break and the segments are rejoined in an abnormal arrangement.

MOSAICS

Nondisjunction occurring in cell division other than gametogenesis results in two or more cell lines with different chromosome numbers. Persons with at least two cell lines with different karyotypes are labeled mosaics. Although several different mosaics have been described, most of the cases of different cell lines involve sex chromosome constitution.

SEX CHROMOSOME ABERRATIONS

In comparison with other hereditary disorders, sex chromosome aberrations are fairly common. Of the types found in males, the incidence is about 1 in 400 births; of the types found in females, about 1 in 650 births.[4]

Most sex chromosome abnormalities are caused by numeric aberration resulting from nondisjunction during meiosis. The disorders are described by the total number of chromosomes present. A normal male is 46,XY and a normal female is 46,XX. Any variation from these values constitutes a disorder. The most common genotype with female phenotype is 45,XO (Turner syndrome), and the most common with male phenotype is 47,XXY (Klinefelter syndrome).

The overall incidence of *Turner syndrome* is 1 in 2,500 female births. The frequency at conception is higher, but 99% spontaneously abort. The diagnosis may be suggested in the newborn by the presence of redundant neck skin and peripheral lymphedema. Diagnosis can also be made later during the investigation of short stature or primary amenorrhea.

The incidence of 47,XXY (*Klinefelter syndrome*) is 1 per 1,000 males. The risk increases with increased maternal age.[4] Diagnosis is usually made during adult life as a result of the investigation of infertility. This syndrome is the most common cause of hypogonadism and infertility in men. Other manifestations include long lower extremities, sparse body hair with a female distribution, and, in approximately 50%, breast development.

▼ *Multifactorial Disorders*

Multifactorial inheritance includes the disorders in which a genetic susceptibility interacts with the appropriate environmental agents to produce a phenotype that is classified as disease. Although the word *polygenetic* is sometimes used to describe multifactorial disorders, the term more accurately describes disorders determined by a large number of genes, each with a small effect, acting additively.[7] To date, there is no method of establishing the exact effects of environmental factors or the additive effects of genes in determining the expression of a trait.[7] For this reason, multifactorial inheritance is more difficult to analyze than other types of inheritance. Multifactorial traits tend to cluster in families, but their genetic patterns are not clearly predictable, as they are with single-gene traits and chromosome disorders.

A characteristic of multifactorial inheritance is the unimodal distribution of a trait in the population. (Note the presence of only one peak in the curve in Fig. 4-14.)

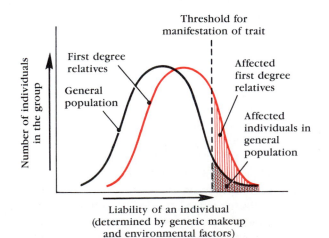

FIGURE 4-14 *Threshold model for multifactorial inheritance. First-degree relatives of the affected individual have more genetic and/or environmental factors that increase their risk of manifesting the disorder.*

Some normal characteristics such as stature and intelligence are distributed unimodally and have family patterns that are characteristic of multifactorial inheritance. The correlation among relatives with such traits is proportional to the number of genes they have in common (inherited from a common ancestral source). The more distant the relationship, the fewer genes they have in common.[7] Abnormalities that are thought to be multifactorial include congenital heart disease, congenital dislocation of the hip, neural tube defects, cleft lip, cleft palate, and atherosclerotic heart disease.

The *threshold model* of multifactorial inheritance (see Fig. 4-14) can be used to explain some of the features of the family distribution of multifactorial disorders. It is based on information collected on the frequency of the disorders in the general population and in different categories of relatives (eg, first-degree relatives such as parents, siblings, and offspring; second-degree relatives such as aunts, uncles, nieces, and nephews). Through this method of analysis, the empiric risk (recurrence risk based on experience) can be estimated. Knowledge of genetic and environmental factors in the pathogenesis of the disorder is not considered.

▼ Genetics of Cancer

The hereditary influences in cancer have been known since 1866, when the French physician Brocca described an increased frequency of breast cancer in his wife's family. Evidence has accumulated since that time leading to the following considerations:[15]

1. Large epidemiologic studies support the observations that certain tumors (especially cancer of the breast and colon, as well as the leukemias) occur more frequently within certain families, termed "cancer families."
2. Certain malignant tumors were found to be transmitted from parent to offspring. A major example is bilateral retinoblastoma, which is transmitted as an autosomal dominant trait.
3. Chromosomal studies of malignant cells have demonstrated a wide variety of chromosomal aberrations, both numerical and structural.
4. Some fixed patterns of chromosome abnormality are associated with certain tumors, with major examples being the Philadelphia translocation in chronic myelogenous leukemia and the translocation between chromosomes 8 and 14 in Burkitt lymphoma.
5. Some genetic disorders predispose to cancer development, as is the case in multiple polyposis coli and colon cancer.

The discovery of *oncogenes*, or cancer-causing genes, in the early 1970s, placed the idea of hereditary tumors in a better conceptual frame.[15] Oncogenes are natural mammalian genes which, on activation by a variety of factors, trigger malignant transformation of normal cells. Genetic studies have allowed researchers to differentiate active from inactive oncogenes and to recognize the presence of activated oncogenes in malignant cells when their inactive form is found in normal surrounding tissue. Suggested oncogene activating mechanisms included chromosomal breakage and rearrangement, as in Burkitt lymphoma, environmental agents, such as chemical carcinogens, and viral infections (see pp. 47–48).

The discovery of *tumor suppressor genes* has provided for a modern interpretation of cancer genetics. If present in normal, nonmutated states, these genes exert a negative regulation of cellular multiplication. If mutated, they permit uncontrolled cellular proliferation. An example of such genes is the *P53* gene, which is involved in the control of cell division. A wide variety of tumors exhibit mutations in *P53*.

More recently, genes have been identified that are associated with susceptibility to breast cancer (*BRCA1*) or to colon cancer (*APC*, the gene for adenomatous polyposis coli, and *HNPCC*, the gene for hereditary nonpolyposis colon cancer).[13] These genes do not appear to act as typical tumor suppressor genes. Instead, they seem to be involved in DNA repair, and errors in these genes lead to genomic instability, which then permits malignant transformation. Although extensively investigated in experimental protocols, a direct clinical application for the use of this knowledge in cancer prevention or in predicting the risk of cancer is not yet available. This new genetic tool should become available for clinical use within the very near future.

▼ Environmental Alterations in Fetal Development

The effect of environmental influences on fetal development has been a subject of increasing concern. Reasons for this include the facts that more women have entered the workplace, the level of environmental chemical exposure is increasing for all people, and birth defects caused by environmental exposure are preventable. Publicity generated by thalidomide damage in the 1960s brought the problem to the attention of the general public.

A *teratogen* is an agent that acts on the embryo or fetus, causing abnormalities in form or function. Teratogenic agents can also be referred to as fetotoxic or developmentally toxic. Exposure to these agents results in a wide spectrum of consequences, from no apparent effect to altered fetal growth, abnormal development in one or more systems, congenital anomalies, carcinogenesis, or fetal death. Whether or not the agent causes damage depends on both maternal and fetal factors, including dose of the agent (and virulence if it is a microorganism), timing of the exposure, and host susceptibility (that of both mother and fetus).

Exposure of the mother during the first 2 weeks after fertilization may not affect the fetus because implantation has not yet occurred. Exposure of the fetus during this time may result in failure to implant or another lethal event. During the first trimester, teratogenic agents are likely to produce gross structural abnormalities because organogenesis is occurring at this time. Particularly sensitive periods for different organs are illustrated in Figure 4-15. After the first trimester, only the nervous system continues to differentiate. Fetotoxic effects in the last two-thirds of gestation mainly involve interference with the size and number of cells, producing more minor structural or functional defects.[6, 11]

Teratogenic effects may be produced by chemical agents, microorganisms, radiation, or abnormalities in the maternal environment. In addition, the carcinogenic properties of such environmental agents, especially those of ionizing radiation, must be considered (see discussion of radiation effects later in this chapter). Pregnant women, or those of childbearing age, must become

aware of the risk to their offspring posed by maternal exposure to environmental and occupational agents (eg, organic solvents, lead, mercury), certain pharmacotherapeutics (eg, prescription or over-the-counter medicinal drugs), and recreational (nonmedical) drugs. Potential consequences of exposure to such agents include both teratogenic effects and postnatal withdrawal syndromes.

Exposure to organic solvents, such as vapors of gasoline, paints, aerosol sprays, and toluene-containing glues, has been implicated as a cause of low-birth-weight infants, "spontaneous" abortions, and central nervous system effects. Exposure to lead has been associated with the occurrence of stillbirths, "spontaneous" abortions, and prematurity. One of the main concerns regarding lead is its ability to cause neuropsychologic impairment in children. An ongoing Canadian study (the Motherisk Project, Toronto) has reported on 395 women, 335 of

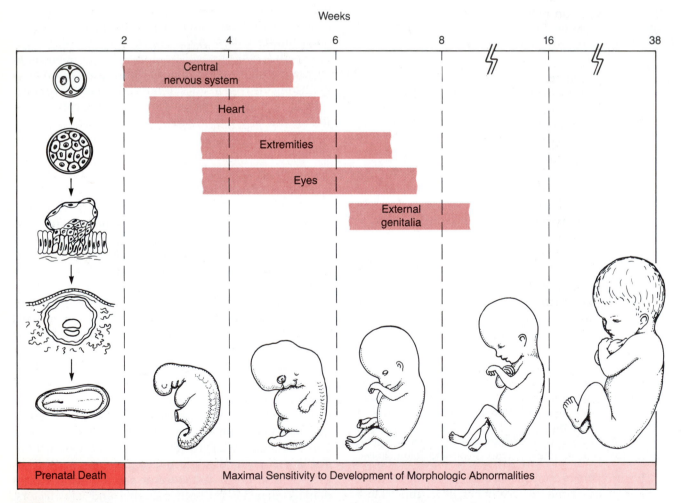

FIGURE 4-15   Sensitivity of specific organs to teratogenic agents at critical stages of human embryogenesis. Exposure to adverse influences in the preimplantation and early postimplantation stages of development (far left) leads to prenatal death. Periods of maximal sensitivity to teratogens (horizontal red bars) vary for different organ systems but overall are limited to the first 8 weeks of pregnancy. (Rubin, E., and Farber, J. Pathology [2nd ed.]. Philadelphia: J.B. Lippincott, 1994.)

them pregnant, who consulted the service for advice about risks to their present or potential pregnancies.[9] A total of 155 (45%) had been exposed to either known or suspected human teratogens. Among the chemicals used, the highest ranking (in descending order) were antidepressants, oral contraceptives, cannabinoids, antibiotics, ethanol, and cocaine.

Historically, birth defects associated with antidepressants include jejunal obstruction, ventricular septal defects (from fluoxetine), hydrocele, and congenital hip dislocation (from tricyclic antidepressants). Those associated with oral contraceptives include primarily progesterone-induced virilization of female embryos, resulting in female pseudohermaphroditism. Cannabinoids (marijuana) have not been implicated in causing birth defects in humans, but neonatal studies have shown increased tremors and startle reflexes in newborns. Tetracycline is known to cause yellow, gray-brown, or brown staining of decidual teeth and destruction of enamel in children exposed in utero. The first effects of cocaine on pregnancy were reported around 1985 and include "spontaneous" abortions, prematurity, intrauterine growth retardation, perinatal cerebral infarction, and a tenfold increase in the incidence of abruptio placentae. In addition, a withdrawal syndrome and neurobehavioral abnormalities have been described among children of cocaine-using mothers.[9]

Although the harmful effects of alcohol consumption during pregnancy have been recognized since Biblical times, it was not until 1973 that the name *fetal alcohol syndrome* was used to describe a specific constellation of abnormalities seen in the children of chronic alcoholic mothers.[14] The Fetal Alcohol Syndrome Study Group of the Research Society on Alcoholism has proposed that fetal alcohol syndrome be diagnosed by the presence of signs in each of three categories: 1) prenatal or postnatal growth retardation; 2) central nervous system involvement; and 3) characteristic facial dysmorphism.[14] The term *fetal alcohol effects* is sometimes used to describe the manifestations of fetal alcohol exposure when all of the criteria for fetal alcohol syndrome are not present.

Abundant evidence links *maternal cigarette smoking* to fetal damage. Problems include an increased spontaneous abortion rate, an increased perinatal mortality rate, an increased incidence of maternal complications such as abruptio placentae and placenta previa, decreased birth weight and size in later childhood, increased incidence of preterm delivery, and lower Apgar scores at 1 minute and 5 minutes after birth.[5] The mechanism by which cigarette smoking produces damage is not known, but it may be related to a lack of available oxygen or to toxicity of certain products of the smoke.

Microorganisms that infect a pregnant woman may damage the fetus by direct infection or by alteration of the maternal environment. Consequences of maternal infection include increased reproductive loss, prematurity, congenital malformations, and growth retardation. Fetotoxic effects can be produced by certain viruses, bacteria, fungi, and protozoa, with the majority attributable to viruses. Among these are cytomegalovirus, rubella, varicella zoster, herpes simplex types 1 and 2, and Venezuelan equine encephalitis virus. In the United States, most fetal damage is produced by members of the STORCH group of infections: syphilis (a bacterial infection), toxoplasmosis (a protozoan infection), rubella, cytomegalovirus, and herpes simplex.[6, 16]

Exposure to ionizing radiation at any time during gestation increases the risk of damage to the developing embryo or fetus, and even moderate doses can have catastrophic effects.[8] The effects depend on the age of gestation, the radiation dosage, and the dose rate (dose/time). Gestation time may be divided into three discrete phases: preimplantation (0 to 9 days), organogenesis (day 10 to 6 weeks), and the fetal period (6 weeks to term). The main radiation effects on a developing embryo or fetus are growth retardation; embryonic, fetal, or neonatal death; and congenital malformations and functional impairment such as mental retardation. During the preimplantation period, the main risk of radiation exposure is embryonic death. Animals irradiated during the early stages of development undergo severe growth retardation, but the effect is usually reversible; irradiation during the fetal period, however, results in the greatest degree of growth retardation, and it is usually permanent.

Among the Japanese survivors of the atomic explosions in the Pacific at the end of World War II, radiation-induced malformations other than central nervous system effects were rare. Microcephaly and mental retardation did occur, the former three times more often than the latter. Most cases of mental retardation were observed among persons irradiated during weeks 8 to 15 of gestation, a time that is characterized by intense cell migration in the brain.

Another effect of radiation exposure is the development of malignancies. In utero exposure to diagnostic x-rays multiplies by 1.5 to 2 times the risk of childhood malignancy during the first 10 to 15 years of life. Among the Japanese survivors who were irradiated in utero there was a significant increase in adult cancer that developed as much as four decades later.

Establishing a dose threshold for radiation is a difficult task. The consensus is that a dose of 0.1 Gy (10 rad)* given to an embryo during the sensitive period of gestation (10 days to 26 weeks) is the cutoff point, and the option of a therapeutic abortion may be considered to avoid the possibility of an anomalous child.

Advances in the treatment of chronic diseases, such

---

*The new unit of absorbed dose, the centiGray (cGy) has replaced the rad. 1cGy = 1 rad, or 1 Gray (Gy) = 100 rad.[8]

as diabetes mellitus, have resulted in an increase in the number of women with metabolic or genetic disorders who survive and become pregnant. These pregnancies are often at high risk because of the *altered maternal environment* in which the fetus must develop. Probably the hyperglycemia and ketoacidosis that accompany poorly controlled diabetes are the cause of the threefold to fourfold increase in congenital anomalies and the other problems encountered with offspring of diabetic women.

The possibility of damage to offspring of mothers with PKU has been mentioned. Other conditions in which the maternal physiology has been known to affect the fetus include hyperthermia (from fever, sauna, or hot tub), Marfan syndrome (from stress on the maternal cardiovascular system), homocystinuria, histidinemia, myotonic dystrophy, and acute intermittent porphyria.

▼ Chapter Summary

▼ The study of genetics requires understanding of the principles of inheritance. The unit of heredity is the gene, which consists of specific nucleotide sequences in the DNA of the chromosome. As was discussed in Chapter 1, the genes dictate which proteins are found in the cells, and these proteins determine the characteristics of the cell. The chromosome pattern is called the karyotype; normal human cells contain 23 pairs of chromosomes.

▼ Genetic disorders are classified into the three groups of single-gene, chromosome, and multifactorial. In all cases, the altered genetic material is passed from the parent to the offspring. Single-gene disorders are classified as autosomal dominant, X-linked dominant, autosomal recessive, and X-linked recessive. Chromosome disorders result from an abnormality in chromosome number or structure. Multifactorial disorders result from combinations of small variations that produce serious defects, especially if compounded with environmental factors. Continuing study of these disorders has produced the recognition that their incidence is very common and has been unrecognized in the past.

▼ The study of the genetics of cancer is in its infancy. That there is a hereditary influence has been recognized for a number of years, with certain types of malignancies occurring more frequently in "cancer families." Some malignancies are transmitted from parent to offspring as autosomal dominant traits. There is a predisposition to cancer development in certain individuals with genetic disorders.

▼ The period of fetal development is a sensitive period for the effect of teratogenic agents. Many different environmental agents have been shown to affect the developing fetus in ways ranging from minor to lethal. For example, the recognition of the harmful effects of

alcohol consumption during pregnancy has led to improved education of pregnant women.

CASE STUDY 4-1

Mr. and Ms. S. were both in their early forties when their first child, Jonathan, was born. Immediately after birth, the diagnosis of Down syndrome was made. Jonathan had an Apgar score of 7 and continued to have apparent cyanosis in the intensive care nursery.

1. *What factors would cause Ms. S. to be at risk for having a child with Down syndrome?*
2. *What clinical features allowed the physician to diagnose the condition immediately after birth?*
3. *What is the underlying genetic defect that produces trisomy 21? Which other defects are similar to trisomy 21?*
4. *Describe the expected growth and development pattern and potential complications for this child.*
5. *What could be the explanation for the continuing cyanosis after birth? (See also p. 493).*

See Appendix G for discussion.

▼ References

1. Babior, B.M., and Stossel, T.P. *Hematology: A Pathophysiological Approach* (3rd ed.). New York: Churchill Livingstone, 1994.
2. Bishop, C.E. DNA-based prenatal diagnosis. In Simpson, J.L., and Elias, S. (eds.), *Essentials of Prenatal Diagnosis.* New York: Churchill Livingstone, 1993.
3. Byers, P.H. Disorders of collagen biosynthesis and structure. In Scriver, C.R., Beaudet, A.L., Sly, W.S., and Valle, D. (eds.), *The Metabolic Basis of Human Diseases* (6th ed.). New York: McGraw-Hill, 1989.
4. Cohen, F.L. *Clinical Genetics in Nursing Practice.* Philadelphia: J.B. Lippincott, 1984.
5. Cotran, R., Kumar, V., and Robbins, S. *Robbins' Pathologic Basis of Disease* (5th ed.). Philadelphia: W.B. Saunders, 1994.
6. Creasy, R.K., and Resnick, R. *Maternal-Fetal Medicine* (3rd ed.). Philadelphia: W.B. Saunders, 1994.
7. Gelehrter, T.D., and Collins, F.S. *Principles of Medical Genetics.* Baltimore: Williams & Wilkins, 1990.
8. Hall, E. *Radiobiology for the Radiologist* (4th ed.). Philadelphia: J.B. Lippincott, 1994.
9. Koren, G. (ed.). *Maternal-Fetal Toxicology: A Clinician's Guide* (2nd ed.). New York: Marcel Dekker, 1994.
10. Kueppers, F. Chronic obstructive pulmonary disease. In King, R.A., Rotter, J.I., and Motulsky, A.G. (eds.). *The Genetic Basis of Common Diseases.* New York: Oxford, 1992.
11. Moore, K.L., and Persaud, T.V.N. *The Developing Human: Clinical Oriented Embryology* (5th ed.). Philadelphia: W.B. Saunders, 1993.
12. Motulsky, A.G., and Brunzell, J.D. The genetics of coronary atherosclerosis. In King, R.A., Rotter, J.I., and

Motulsky, A.G. (eds.). *The Genetic Basis of Common Diseases.* New York: Oxford, 1992.

13. Peltomaki, R., Aaltonen, L.A., Sistonen, P., et al. Genetic mapping of a locus predisposing to human colorectal cancer. *Science* 260:810–812, 1993.

14. Schardein, J.L. *Chemically Induced Birth Defects* (2nd. ed.). New York: Marcel Dekker, 1993.

15. Schimke, R.N. Cancer in families. In King, R.A., Rotter, J.I., and Motulsky, A.G. (eds.). *The Genetic Basis of Common Diseases.* New York: Oxford, 1992.

16. Simpson, J.L., and Globus, M.S. *Genetics in Obstetrics and Gynecology* (2nd ed.). Philadelphia: W.B. Saunders, 1992.

▼ *Unit Bibliography*

Babior, B.M., and Stossel, T.P. *Hematology: A Pathophysiological Approach* (3rd ed.). New York: Churchill Livingstone, 1994.

Beaudet, A.L., Scriver, C.R., Sly, W.S., et al. *Introduction to Human Biochemical and Molecular Genetics.* New York: McGraw-Hill, 1990.

Berne, R.M., and Levy, M.N. *Principles of Physiology.* St. Louis: C.V. Mosby, 1990.

Berne, R.M., and Levy, M.N. (eds.). *Physiology* (3rd ed.). St. Louis: Mosby, 1993.

Blackburn, S.T., and Loper, D.L. *Maternal, Fetal, and Neonatal Physiology.* Philadelphia: W.B. Saunders, 1992.

Brown, T.A. *Genetics: A Molecular Approach* (2nd ed.). New York: Chapman & Hall, 1993.

Cohen, F.L. *Clinical Genetics in Nursing Practice.* Philadelphia: J.B. Lippincott, 1984.

Connor, J.M., and Ferguson-Smith, M.A. *Essential Medical Genetics* (3rd ed.). Boston: Blackwell, 1991.

Cormack, D.H. *Essential Histology.* Philadelphia: J.B. Lippincott, 1993.

Cotran, R., Kumar, V., and Robbins, S. *Robbins' Pathologic Basis of Disease* (5th ed.). Philadelphia: W.B. Saunders, 1994.

Creasy, R.K., and Resnik, R. *Maternal-Fetal Medicine* (3rd ed.). Philadelphia: W.B. Saunders, 1994.

DeVita, V.T., Hellman, S., and Rosenberg, S.A. *Cancer: Principles and Practice of Oncology* (4th ed.). Philadelphia: J.B. Lippincott, 1993.

Dimmick, J.E., and Kalousek, D.K. (eds.). *Developmental Pathology of the Embryo and Fetus.* Philadelphia: J.B. Lippincott, 1992.

Ganong, W.F. *Medical Review of Physiology* (16th ed.). Norwalk: Appleton & Lange, 1993.

Govan, A.D., Macfarlane, P.S., and Callander, R. *Pathology Illustrated* (3rd ed.). New York: Churchill Livingstone, 1991.

Guyton, A. *Textbook of Medical Physiology* (8th ed.). Philadelphia: W.B. Saunders, 1991.

Holland, J.F. *Cancer Medicine* (3rd ed.). Philadelphia: Lea & Febiger, 1993.

Johnson, L. (ed.). *Essential Medical Physiology.* New York: Raven Press, 1992.

Jones, K.L. *Smith's Recognizable Patterns of Human Malformation.* (4th ed.). Philadelphia: W.B. Saunders, 1988.

Kent, T.H., and Hart, M.N. *Introduction to Human Disease* (3rd ed.). Norwalk: Appleton & Lange, 1993.

King, R.A., Rotter, J.I., and Motulsky, A.G. *The Genetic Basis of Common Diseases.* New York: Oxford, 1992.

Kissane, J.M. (ed.). *Anderson's Pathology* (9th ed.). St. Louis: Mosby, 1990.

Koren, G. (ed.). *Maternal-Fetal Toxicology: A Clinician's Guide* (2nd ed.). New York: Marcel Dekker, 1994.

Kumar, V., Cotran, R.S., and Robbins, S.L. *Basic Pathology* (5th ed.). Philadelphia: W.B. Saunders, 1992.

McKusick, V.A. *Mendelian Inheritance in Man* (10th ed.). Baltimore: Johns Hopkins, 1992.

Moffett, D., Moffett, S., and Schauf, C. *Human Physiology: Foundations and Frontiers* (2nd ed.). St. Louis: Mosby, 1993.

Moore, K.L. *Clinically Oriented Anatomy* (3rd ed.). Baltimore: William & Wilkins, 1992.

Moore, K.L., and Persaud, T.V.N. *The Developing Human: Clinically Oriented Embryology* (5th ed.). Philadelphia: W.B. Saunders, 1993.

Mulvihill, M.L. *Human Diseases: A Systemic Approach* (3rd ed.). Norwalk: Appleton & Lange, 1991.

Nora, J.J., Fraser, F.C., Bear, J., et al. *Nora and Fraser Medical Genetics: Principles and Practice* (4th ed.). Philadelphia: Lea & Febiger, 1993.

Rubin, E., and Farber, J.L. (eds.). *Pathology* (2nd ed.). Philadelphia: J.B. Lippincott, 1994.

Schardein, J.L. *Chemically Induced Birth Defects* (2nd ed.). New York: Marcel Dekker, 1993.

Scriver, A.L., Beaudet, A.L., Sly, W.S., and Valle, D. (eds.). *The Metabolic Basis of Inherited Human Diseases* (6th ed.). New York: McGraw-Hill, 1989.

Sheldon, H. *Boyd's Introduction to the Study of Disease* (11th ed.). Philadelphia: Lea & Febiger, 1992.

Simpson, J.L., and Elias, S. *Essentials of Prenatal Diagnosis.* New York: Churchill Livingstone, 1993.

Simpson, J.L, and Globus, M.S. *Genetics in Obstetrics and Gynecology* (2nd ed.). Philadelphia: W.B. Saunders, 1992.

Slauson, D.O., and Cooper, B.J. *Mechanisms of Disease* (2nd ed.). Baltimore: Williams & Wilkins, 1990.

Therman, E., and Sussman, M. *Human Chromosomes: Structure, Behavior, and Effects* (3rd ed.). New York: Springer-Verlag, 1993.

Thompson, M.W., McInnes, R.R., and Huntington, F.W. *Thompson & Thompson Genetics in Medicine* (5th ed.). Philadelphia: W.B. Saunders, 1991.

Tortora, G.J., and Grabowski, S.R. *Principles of Anatomy and Physiology* (7th ed.). New York: HarperCollins, 1993.

Underwood, J.C.E. (ed.). *General and Systemic Pathology.* New York: Churchill Livingstone, 1992.

Walter, J.B. *An Introduction to the Principles of Disease* (3rd ed.). Philadelphia: W.B. Saunders, 1992.

Walter, J.B. *Pathology of Human Disease.* Philadelphia: Lea & Febiger, 1990.

Weatherall, D.J. *The New Genetics and Clinical Practice* (3rd ed.). New York: Oxford University Press, 1991.

Weiss, G. *Clinical Oncology.* Norwalk: Appleton & Lange, 1993.

Unit 2

Development

THROUGHOUT LIFE, developmental changes affect the ability of the human body to maintain the steady state. Periods of growth are common in certain stages, and degenerative changes are dominant in others. A variety of factors affect the rate of these changes. Because of the extensive nature of this topic, no attempt has been made to deal with all aspects of development but only to present normal developmental changes and the more common susceptibilities to disease at different developmental levels.

Chapter 5, Biophysical Development of Reproduction, discusses fetal development and factors affecting labor and delivery. Further information relating to the female reproductive system may be found in Chapter 56.

Chapter 6, Biophysical Development of Children, describes physiologic changes occurring from the neonatal period through adolescence. Although it is recognized that societal and cultural factors have a great impact on development, these have been briefly discussed or omitted owing to the extensiveness of these topics.

Chapter 7, Biophysical Developmental Changes of Adults, presents a topic with a great deal of controversy and variability. Biophysically, adults do not age at the same rate. Some generalities are made, and several sociocultural concepts are discussed because of their importance. The impacts of nutrition and physical fitness are considered.

Chapter 8, Biophysical Changes of the Older Adult, deals with the theories of aging and the bodily systems affected. Older adults age at different rates and have different systemic problems, but the changes themselves seem to be an innate process. The societal and cultural impacts of an aging society are only briefly alluded to because of the extensiveness of the topic.

Chapter 9 considers the concepts of stress and sleep as they relate to different age groups. The main emphasis of this chapter is the physiology of stress and sleep and their alterations.

The reader is encouraged to use the learning objectives at the beginning of each chapter as a study guide outline for essential concepts. The unit bibliography provides general and specific resources for further study.

Chapter 5

Biophysical Development of Reproduction

Sharron P. Schlosser / Joy H. Whatley

▼ CHAPTER OUTLINE

▼ LEARNING OBJECTIVES

1   Identify the stages of fetal development and discuss the biophysical development associated with each stage.
2   Discuss the process of placenta formation.
3   Trace the circulation of blood through the placenta and fetus.
4   Relate the effects of maternal illnesses on the biophysical development of pregnancy.
5   Discuss the effects of sexually transmitted diseases and infections on the biophysical development of the pregnancy and the fetus.
6   Identify and define fetal factors that affect biophysical development.
7   Identify demographic, obstetric, miscellaneous, and medical factors that place a fetus at risk for less than optimal outcome of pregnancy.
8   Compare the normal nutritional requirements for a woman in the childbearing years with the additional requirements needed during pregnancy and lactation.
9   Discuss selected nutritional conditions that affect the biophysical development of pregnancy.
10 Discuss common agents that have a teratogenic effect on the fetus.
11 Differentiate currently used techniques and studies to assess fetal well-being.
12 Discuss the risks and benefits of currently used prenatal diagnostic screening procedures.
13 Identify and discuss the various theories regarding initiation of labor.
14 Identify and define the four stages of labor and discuss the processes occurring in each stage.
15 Examine the alterations associated with the four Ps: power, passage, passenger, and psyche; describe the adaptation problems associated with each.

Barbara L. Bullock: PATHOPHYSIOLOGY: ADAPTATIONS AND ALTERATIONS IN FUNCTION, 4th ed.
© 1996 Lippincott-Raven Publishers

The period of gestation begins with fertilization of the ovum and continues throughout development of the fetus. The duration of gestation is approximately 280 days, or 10 lunar months from the last menstrual period. Typically, the period of gestation is divided into three 3-month periods, termed *trimesters*. During this time, two processes account for the biophysical development of the fetus—*hyperplasia* and *hypertrophy*.[12] The early first trimester (first 12 weeks after conception) is characterized by hyperplasia, in which the mitotic cell division accounts for an increase in the number of cells but the size of the cells remains relatively stable. The second trimester (weeks 13 to 24) is characterized by both hyperplasia and hypertrophy. The process of hypertrophy predominates in the third trimester (week 25 to birth). During this trimester, the fetus experiences a very rapid period of growth; the number of cells does not change, but rather those cells present increase significantly in size. This chapter is concerned with prenatal development and the birth process, including factors affecting biophysical development and prenatal diagnostic studies. The genetic aspects of reproduction is discussed in Chapter 4.

▼ *Fetal Development*

STAGES

The biophysical development of the fetus is traditionally divided into three stages: the germinal period, the embryonic period, and the fetal period.

Germinal Period

The germinal period, also referred to as the period of the ovum or the period of the zygote, extends from conception through approximately the first 2 weeks. Within hours of fertilization the process of mitosis begins, usually in the outer third of the fallopian tube. Mitotic cell division continues every 10 to 12 hours throughout the zygote's journey through the fallopian tube. At this time, the mass of cells is referred to as a *morula*. After approximately 4 days in the fallopian tube, the morula reaches the uterine cavity. At this point, the cells of the morula begin to differentiate and are known as the *blastocyst* (Fig. 5-1). A fluid-filled cavity appears as the cells differentiate into two layers. The cells along the outer layer are termed the *trophoblast*; they will begin the implantation in the endometrium to form the placenta. The inner cluster of cells is termed the inner cell mass or embryoblast, and it eventually develops into the embryo.

For an additional 3 to 4 days, the blastocyst remains free within the uterine cavity, edging toward the site of implantation. As the blastocyst comes into contact with the endometrium, proteolytic enzymes from the trophoblast allow the blastocyst to virtually digest its way into the endometrium (see Fig. 5-1). This invasion of the soft and succulent endometrium erodes the maternal blood vessels in the endometrium, forming pools of maternal blood. It is here within the placenta that exchange of nutrients and waste products occurs throughout pregnancy. By approximately the 11th day, the implantation process is complete and the blastocyst appears as a slight bulge on the endometrium.

The implanting trophoblast also secretes human chorionic gonadotropin. This hormone is responsible for positive pregnancy tests and for the continued functioning of the corpus luteum and resultant production of progesterone.

Embryonic Period

The embryonic period begins with the complete implantation of the blastocyst (approximately at the end of the second week) and extends through the eighth week of prenatal development. Four major accomplishments are associated with this period of development: rapid growth, placenta formation and function, early structural development of organs, and development of a form that is recognizable as a human being.

The cells of the inner cell mass begin a rapid differentiation and are referred to as the embryonic disc. At this point, two germ layers have evolved. The primitive yolk emerges from the endoderm, and the ectoderm gives rise to the amniotic sac. By about the 16th day, the cells of the embryonic disc have further differentiated into a third primary germ layer, the mesoderm (Fig. 5-2). These three layers eventually give rise to all major fetal organs. Table 5-1 lists the structures evolving from each of the three layers. Cephalocaudal and proximodistal principles of development become evident as one explores the developing embryo. By the 22nd day, the ectoderm has folded into the neural tube, from which the brain, head, and spinal cord will develop. During this same time, two tubes form in the mesoderm; by the 22nd day, they have fused to form the fetal heart, which becomes the first functioning organ of the fetus (Fig. 5-3). Eyes, ears, nose, and mouth begin to take shape by the 22nd day. By the 26th day, arm and leg buds appear. Development continues as the elbows and knees appear and fingers and toes lose their webbing. External genitalia are evident but not distinguishable. By the end of the embryonic period, the circulation is well established. The embryo measures approximately 3 cm (1.2 inches) from crown to rump and weighs only about 2 to 4 grams.

Fetal Period

The fetal period begins with the ninth week and terminates with the birth of the fetus, at approximately 40 weeks gestation. As the embryo enters this stage of bio-

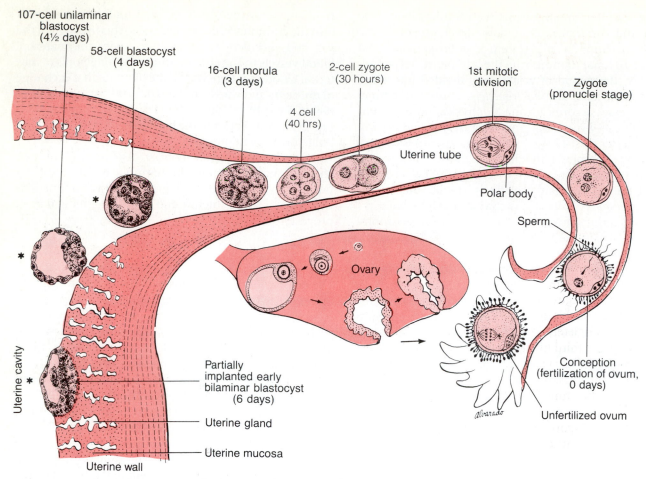

FIGURE 5-1 *Transport of the ovum into the fallopian tube and fertilization within the tube followed by cleavage (cell division) to the 8- to 16-cell stage. The product, now referred to as a morula, is delivered into the uterus, where it develops into a blastocyst and implants in the endometrium on the sixth or seventh day after fertilization. (Reeder, S.J., Martin, L.L., and Koniak, D.* Maternity Nursing *[17th ed.]. Philadelphia: J.B. Lippincott, 1992.)*

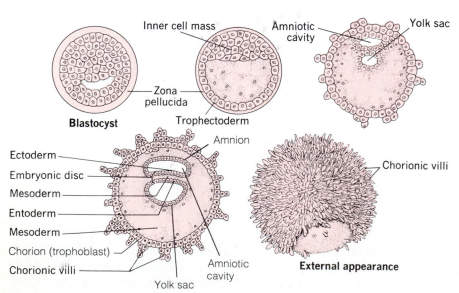

FIGURE 5-2 *Early stages of development. The cells of the blastocyst separate into a peripheral layer and an inner cell mass (top, left and center). The peripheral layer is called a blastodermic vesicle. The amniotic cavity and yolk sac are formed (top, right). The former is lined with ectoderm, the latter with entoderm. The embryonic disc and the three germ layers are shown at bottom left, together with beginning of the chorionic villi. The external appearance of the developing mass is shown at bottom right; the chorionic villi are abundant. (Reeder, S.J., Martin, L.L., and Koniak, D.* Maternity Nursing *[17th ed.]. Philadelphia: J.B. Lippincott, 1992.)*

TABLE 5-1 *Evolution of Body Organs From Primary Germ Layers*

Endoderm	Mesoderm	Ectoderm
Gastrointestinal system	Skin	Epidermis
Liver, pancreas	Bones	Hair, nails
Trachea, lungs	Muscle	Urethra
Pharynx	Heart, blood	Teeth enamel
Thyroid	Spleen	Nervous system
Tonsils	Kidneys, ureters	Mammary glands
	Ovaries, uterus	
	Testes	

physical development, the head accounts for about 50% of the overall body length, and human characteristics are evident. Bones begin to harden, muscles develop, and sex is distinguishable by the fourth lunar month. The placenta is completely formed and fetal circulation established by the third lunar month. Reflexes appear and movement becomes evident to the mother by 20 weeks' gestation. Lanugo (soft, downy hair) develops over the body by the fifth lunar month, and vernix caseosa (a cheeselike substance) appears on the skin in the sixth lunar month. Figure 5-4 illustrates the month-by-month development of the fetus.

SUPPORT STRUCTURES

Placenta

As noted, the blastocyst is covered with a layer of cells known as the trophoblast. Those trophoblasts in direct contact with the endometrium produce fingerlike projections called chorionic villi that invade and digest the endometrium (see Fig. 5-2). This invasive process results in erosion of the maternal blood vessels in the endometrium and formation of maternal lakes filled with maternal blood. The placenta is formed from the fusion of the endometrium and enlarging chorionic villi. Tiny blood vessels also form in the chorionic villi. These vessels carry fetal blood that does not mix with the maternal blood. The processes of diffusion and active transport account for the exchange of nutrients, oxygen, and waste products in the placenta after completion of its development (by the third month). The levels of estrogen and progesterone, originally produced by the corpus luteum, are now maintained by the placenta. The placenta functions as a barrier to infection, as an endocrine gland in the production of estrogen and progesterone, and as the organ of metabolic and nutrient exchange. The fetal surface of the placenta is covered with the amnion. At term (38 to 42 weeks), the placenta is a rather large organ covering almost one-half of the internal uterine wall. At this time, it measures approximately

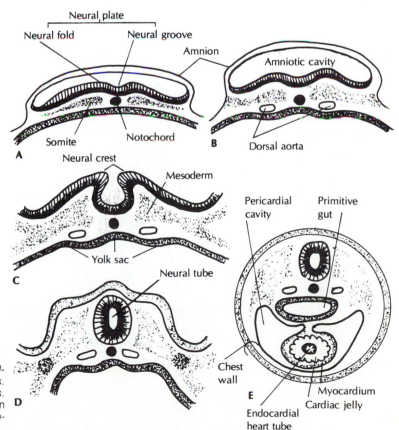

FIGURE 5-3 *Schematic representation of growth and folding of the germ layers. **A.** About 18 days. **B.** About 20 days. **C.** About 22 days. **D.** About 25 days. **E.** About 28 days. (Schuster, C.S., and Ashburn, S.S. The Process of Human Development: A Holistic Approach. Philadelphia: J.B. Lippincott, 1994.)*

Fetal Development
1st Lunar Month

The fetus is 4–5 mm in length.

Trophoblasts embed in decidua.

Chorionic villi form.

Foundations for nervous system, genitourinary system, skin, bones, and lungs are formed.

Buds of arms and legs begin to form.

Rudiments of eyes, ears, and nose appear.

4 weeks

4 weeks

2nd Lunar Month

The fetus is 27–31 mm in length and weighs 4 g.

Fetus is markedly bent.

Head is disproportionately large, owing to brain development.

Sex differentiation begins.

Centers of bone begin to ossify.

8 weeks

8 weeks

3rd Lunar Month

The fetus is 6–9 cm in length and weighs 45 g.

Fingers and toes are distinct.

Placenta is complete.

Fetal circulation is complete.

3 months

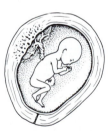

3 months

4th Lunar Month

The fetus is 12 cm in length and weighs 110 g.

Sex is differentiated.

Rudimentary kidneys secrete urine.

Heartbeat is present.

Nasal septum and palate close.

4 months

4 months

5th Lunar Month

The fetus is 19 cm in length and weighs 300 g.

Lanugo covers entire body.

Fetal movements are felt by mother.

Heart sounds are perceptible by auscultation.

5 months

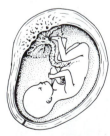

5 months

6th Lunar Month

The fetus is about 23 cm in length and weighs 630 g.

Skin appears wrinkled.

Vernix caseosa appears.

Eyebrows and fingernails develop.

6 months

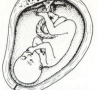

6 months

7th Lunar Month

The fetus is 27 cm in length and weighs 1100 g.

Skin is red.

Pupillary membrane disappears from eyes.

The fetus has an excellent chance of survival.

7 months

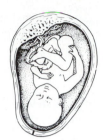

7 months

8th Lunar Month

The fetus is 28–30 cm in length and weighs 1.8 kg.

Fetus is viable.

Eyelids open.

Fingerprints are set.

Vigorous fetal movement occurs.

8 months

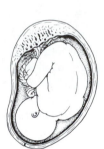

8 months

9th Lunar Month

The fetus is 32 cm in length and weighs about 2500 g.

Face and body have a loose wrinkled appearance because of subcutaneous fat deposit.

Lanugo disappears.

Amniotic fluid decreases.

9 months

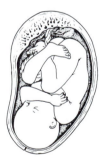

9 months

10th Lunar Month

The fetus is 36 cm in length and weighs 3000–3600 g.

Skin is smooth.

Eyes are uniformly slate colored.

Bones of skull are ossified and nearly together at sutures.

FIGURE 5-4 *Fetal development. (Adapted from Reeder, S.J., Martin, L.L., and Koniak, D. Maternity Nursing [17th ed.]. Philadelphia: J.B. Lippincott, 1992.)*

15 to 20 cm (5.9 to 7.9 inches) in diameter, 2.5 to 3.0 cm (1.0 to 1.2 inches) in thickness, and weighs about 400 to 600 grams (14 to 21 ounces).

The umbilical cord results from the elongation of the body stalk, which connects the embryo to the yolk sac. Tiny blood vessels develop and extend into the chorionic villi. As the body stalk elongates, these tiny vessels merge into the umbilical vein and two umbilical arteries. These blood vessels are surrounded by a special connective tissue referred to as Wharton's jelly. At term, the umbilical cord measures approximately 2 cm (0.8 inch) in diameter and about 55 cm (22 inches) in length.

Fetal Membranes

The chorion and the amnion are the fetal membranes that constitute the "bag of waters." Parts of the trophoblasts not directly involved with the implantation process soon begin to degenerate and form the chorion or outer lining. The amnion is a smooth membrane that evolves from the ectoderm and forms the inner lining of the bag of waters (Fig. 5-5). Amniotic fluid, ranging from 500 to 1,500 mL, is secreted by the amnion. Amniotic fluid functions to regulate temperature, aid in fetal movement, and protect the developing fetus from injury.

Yolk Sac

The yolk sac arises from the endoderm at about the eighth or ninth day after conception. It is responsible for production of red blood cells (RBCs) for about 6 weeks,

until the fetal liver is capable of this function. However, it is not responsible for the developing embryo's nutrition.

FETAL CIRCULATION

Three unique structures function during fetal development to provide sufficient blood flow for metabolic and nutrient functions of the placenta. These structures are the ductus venosus, the foramen ovale, and the ductus arteriosus. Oxygenated and nourished blood from the placenta enters the fetus through the umbilical vein. Soon after it enters the abdominal wall, the umbilical vein branches. The smaller branch enters the hepatic circulation and later empties into the inferior vena cava through the hepatic vein. The second, larger branch enters the inferior vena cava directly through the ductus venosus. Blood from the inferior vena cava empties directly into the right atrium, where it mixes with blood from the superior vena cava. The majority of this blood passes through the foramen ovale and into the left atrium, where it mixes with deoxygenated blood from the lungs. This blood is then pumped into the left ventricle and out to the fetal body through the aorta. The remaining blood in the right atrium is pumped through the tricuspid valve into the right ventricle and out the pulmonary artery. Only a small portion of this blood continues to the nonfunctioning lungs to nourish them; the remainder passes through the ductus arteriosus and enters the body circulation directly. Deoxygenated blood returns to the placenta through the umbilical arteries, where the process repeats itself (Fig. 5-6).

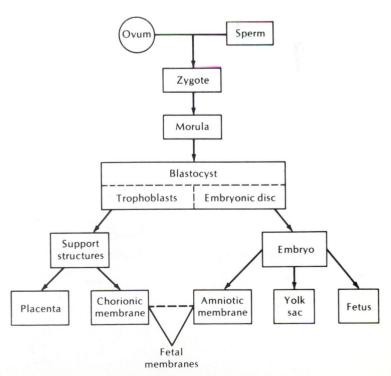

FIGURE 5-5 Origin of embryo and support structures. (Schuster, C.S., and Ashburn, S.S. The Process of Human Development: A Holistic Approach. Philadelphia: J.B. Lippincott, 1994.)

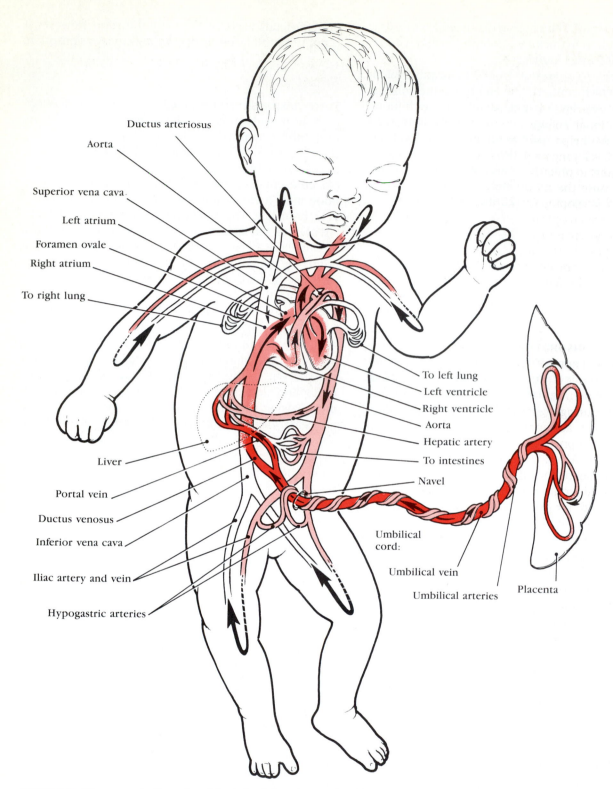

Ductus arteriosus

Aorta

Superior vena cava

Left atrium

Foramen ovale

Right atrium

To right lung

Liver

Portal vein

Ductus venosus

Inferior vena cava

Iliac artery and vein

Hypogastric arteries

To left lung

Left ventricle

Right ventricle

Aorta

Hepatic artery

To intestines

Navel

Umbilical cord:

Umbilical vein

Umbilical arteries

Placenta

FIGURE 5-6 *Diagrammatic illustration of fetal circulation. Arrows show the direction of blood flow.*

▼ Factors Affecting Biophysical Development

MATERNAL FACTORS

The event of conception activates a complex chain of events. Additional energy is needed for cell division, while hormones help to prepare body systems to accommodate the developing pregnancy and fetus. Alterations and adaptations to pregnancy involve all maternal body systems. Because the mother reacts as a total unit or system to the developing fetus, the intrauterine environment operates at an optimal level only to the degree that the maternal system is capable of adapting and adjusting to the developing fetus. Maternal illnesses and infections affect the intrauterine environment and the biophysical development of the fetus.

Illnesses

HYPERTENSIVE DISORDERS OF PREGNANCY. Hypertension occurs in approximately 10% of pregnancies. It is the second leading cause of maternal death and the major cause of perinatal mortality in the United States. Hypertension during pregnancy may lead to eclampsia, cerebral vascular accidents, cardiopulmonary insufficiency, aspiration pneumonia, or premature separation of the placenta. All of these conditions contribute to death from hypovolemic shock or disseminated intravascular coagulation. The infant is often growth-retarded, or small for gestational age, and may be born prematurely because of placental insufficiency. The infant may also suffer from hypoxia and acidosis if the mother experiences eclampsia. The only known cure for this disorder is the delivery of the fetus.[5]

There are several types of hypertension that can occur during pregnancy. To differentiate and categorize the various types of hypertensive diseases, the American College of Obstetricians and Gynecologists developed the classification system found in Box 5-1.[8]

Late or transient hypertension is the name given to hypertension that occurs only during pregnancy. It usually develops during the latter half of pregnancy, has no associated symptoms, and disappears within 10 days after delivery. Late or transient hypertension should be differentiated from *chronic hypertension*, which occurs before the 20th week of gestation and continues more than 42 days after delivery.

The term *pregnancy-induced hypertension* (*PIH*) refers to the development of proteinuria or edema, or both, in the presence of hypertension. PIH usually occurs after the 20th week of gestation. If these conditions develop in a person who already displayed hypertension before pregnancy, it is called *chronic hypertension with superimposed PIH*. Progression of PIH can cause convulsions

---

BOX 5-1 ▼ Classification of Hypertensive Disorders of Pregnancy With Diagnostic Criteria

Pregnancy-induced hypertension (PIH)
Preeclampsia: Hypertension with proteinuria, edema, or both developing after the 20th week of gestation
Mild: B/P of 140/90 or greater; *or* an increase of 30 mm Hg in the systolic or 15 mm Hg in the diastolic pressure over baseline
Severe: B/P of 160/110 or greater; proteinuria of 5 g/24 h; cerebral disturbances, pulmonary edema, or HELLP syndrome
Eclampsia: Extension of preeclampsia with tonic-clonic seizures

Chronic hypertension
Hypertension (140/90 mm Hg) before pregnancy; or discovery of hypertension before the 20th week of gestation; or continuation of hypertension indefinitely after pregnancy

Chronic hypertension with superimposed PIH
Preexisting chronic hypertension complicated by PIH
Superimposed preeclampsia
Superimposed eclampsia

Late or transient hypertension
Transient elevations of blood pressure during labor or in the early postpartum period, returning to baseline within 10 days of delivery

The American College of Obstetricians and Gynecologists. *Management of Preeclampsia.* ACOG Technical Bulletin #91. Washington, DC: ACOG, 1986.

(*eclampsia*) in the absence of associated cerebral disorders such as epilepsy.

The cause of PIH is still unknown. In the past, the disorder was referred to as toxemia because it was believed to be caused by an unknown toxin. Currently, the prevailing theory is that PIH is caused by a maternal vascular endothelial cell injury, possibly resulting from a toxin in the blood.[4] In the later stage of pregnancy, a sensitivity to the increased amount of angiotensin II, which is a vasoconstrictor, may occur. Only a small amount of angiotensin is required to elevate the blood pressure and cause vasoconstriction and decreased peripheral blood flow (see Flowchart 5-1). Diminished placental blood flow also occurs and affects fetal perfusion. The glomerular filtration rate is decreased in response to the decreased blood flow to the kidneys. The glomerular capillaries become edematous and allow protein to be excreted in the urine. This produces a decrease in the serum albumin level. Because of the decreased blood flow to the kidneys, serum levels of blood urea nitrogen (BUN), uric acid, and creatinine become elevated. Sodium is conserved, and urine output is decreased. Sodium retention increases angiotensin II sensitivity.[2]

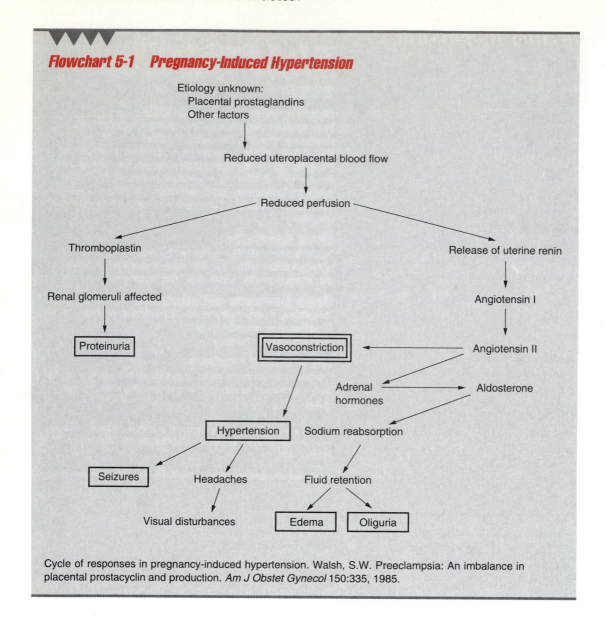

Flowchart 5-1   Pregnancy-Induced Hypertension

Etiology unknown:
    Placental prostaglandins
    Other factors

Reduced uteroplacental blood flow

Reduced perfusion

Thromboplastin

Release of uterine renin

Renal glomeruli affected

Angiotensin I

Proteinuria

Vasoconstriction

Angiotensin II

Adrenal hormones

Aldosterone

Hypertension

Sodium reabsorption

Seizures

Headaches

Fluid retention

Visual disturbances

Edema

Oliguria

Cycle of responses in pregnancy-induced hypertension. Walsh, S.W. Preeclampsia: An imbalance in placental prostacyclin and production. *Am J Obstet Gynecol* 150:335, 1985.

HELLP syndrome is a variant of PIH that can be fatal for both mother and fetus. The characteristics of HELLP are hemolysis (H), elevated liver enzymes (EL), and a low platelet count (LP). HELLP always occurs in association with PIH. However, because HELLP syndrome symptoms may be present before the symptoms of PIH, it is often misdiagnosed as disseminated intravascular coagulation, acute hepatitis, gallbladder disease, or another condition.[2] Flowchart 5-2 outlines the pathophysiology that occurs in HELLP syndrome.

DIABETES MELLITUS.   Diabetes mellitus, the inability to properly metabolize glucose, is a challenging condition during pregnancy (see also pp. 733–747). White developed a classification system for the diabetic who is pregnant[16] (Table 5-2). The National Diabetic Data Group has

also classified diabetes according to the woman's need for insulin as well as other contributing factors[4] (Box 5-2).

The maternal mortality rate for the pregnant diabetic patient has decreased in recent years. However, the pregnant patient with diabetes is still at risk for higher mortality than the general obstetric population. The increase in maternal mortality may be influenced by the increased frequency of PIH, infection, and hemorrhage. Spontaneous abortions occur more frequently because of compromised placental circulation associated with diabetic vascular complications. Polyhydramnios (excessive amniotic fluid) occurs in about 10% to 25% of pregnant diabetics owing to increased osmotic pressure, increased secretion of amniotic fluid, and diuresis from fetal hyperglycemia.

The fetal mortality rate in these cases is greater than

Flowchart 5-2   Pathophysiology of HELLP Syndrome

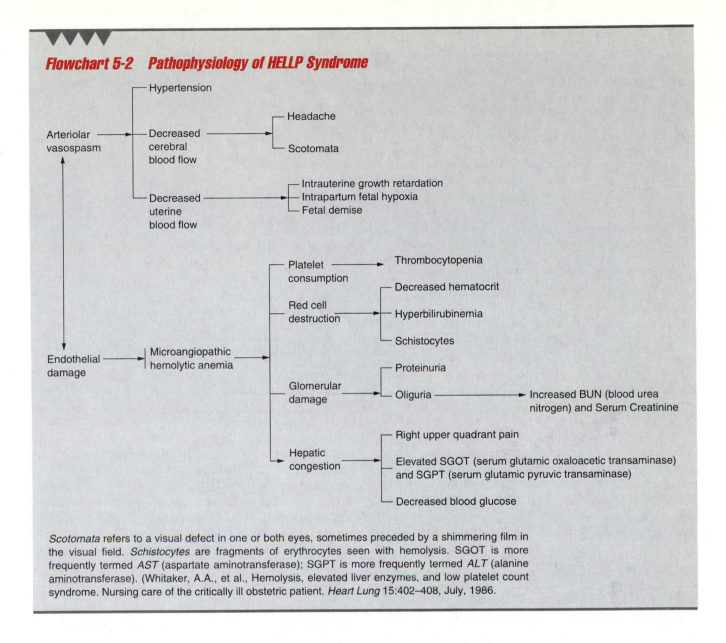

Scotomata refers to a visual defect in one or both eyes, sometimes preceded by a shimmering film in the visual field. *Schistocytes* are fragments of erythrocytes seen with hemolysis. SGOT is more frequently termed *AST* (aspartate aminotransferase); SGPT is more frequently termed *ALT* (alanine aminotransferase). (Whitaker, A.A., et al., Hemolysis, elevated liver enzymes, and low platelet count syndrome. Nursing care of the critically ill obstetric patient. *Heart Lung* 15:402–408, July, 1986.

the mortality rate for fetuses born to nondiabetic mothers. Fetal mortality may be attributed to fetal hyperglycemia and hyperinsulinemia. A previous history of stillbirth, PIH, or vascular involvement increases the frequency of intrauterine fetal death.

After delivery, there is also an increase in the rate of infant mortality among infants of diabetic mothers. Complications frequently occurring in infants of diabetic mothers include hypoglycemia, hypocalcemia, hyperbilirubinemia, and respiratory distress syndrome. Congenital abnormalities, particularly in the cardiac, renal, and central nervous systems, occur more frequently in infants of diabetic mothers. *Macrosomia* (an abnormally large body) is present in infants whose mothers are in White's classes A through C and is associated with an increased frequency of traumatic complications during

vaginal delivery. *Intrauterine growth retardation* (*IUGR*) is seen in infants whose mothers are in classes D through F, as a result of the vascular complications occurring in these groups.

Gestational diabetes mellitus, also called class A diabetes or type III gestational diabetes mellitus, is defined as carbohydrate intolerance with onset during pregnancy. Approximately 2% to 3% of pregnant women develop gestational diabetes mellitus during pregnancy.

CARDIAC DISEASE.   The increase in blood volume that occurs in pregnancy begins as early as the sixth week of gestation. The blood volume rises slowly in the first trimester, reaching a peak at about 30 to 34 weeks' gestation. A woman who is healthy and without a cardiac disorder can withstand the additional stress from

TABLE 5-2 *White's Classification of Diabetes in Pregnancy with Implications*

Class	Characteristics	Implications
A_1	Glucose intolerance diagnosed during pregnancy	Treatment with diet is adequate to maintain euglycemia Least risk of complications
A_2	Glucose intolerance diagnosed during pregnancy	Treatment requires administration of insulin in addition to diet More likelihood of fetal macrosomatia
B	Onset after age 20; duration less than 10 y No vascular disease	Some endogenous insulin secretion Characterized by insulin resistance Insulin treatment *before* pregnancy Increased risk of PIH, hypertension, fetal anomalies, and macrosomatia
C	Onset between age 10 and 20 No vascular disease	Insulin treatment *before* pregnancy Increased risk of PIH, hypertension, fetal anomalies, and macrosomatia
D	Onset before age 10; duration more than 20 y Retinopathy	Fetal growth retardation is possible Retinopathy may accelerate during pregnancy and then regress Increased risk of PIH, hypertension, fetal anomalies, or intrauterine growth retardation possible
F	Diabetic nephropathy with proteinuria	Anemia, hypertension, PIH, preterm labor common; anomalies and intrauterine growth retardation common
H	Coronary artery disease	Grave maternal and fetal risk for death

May, K.A., and Mahlmeister, L.R. *Maternal & Neonatal Nursing: Family-Centered Care* [3rd ed.]. Philadelphia: J.B. Lippincott, 1994, p. 763.

the increased blood volume. However, if there is cardiac pathology, the pregnancy may be complicated. The complications that can occur are related to the degree of disability, as categorized in the New York Heart Association functional classification of heart disease (Box 5-3).[10]

The three major types of heart disease that affect pregnancy are rheumatic heart disease, congenital anomalies, and changes in the heart resulting from hypertension. Maternal risks associated with cardiac disease are increases in the rates of spontaneous abortion and premature labor. Premature birth, respiratory acidosis, and growth retardation related to low oxygen levels in the mother are seen in infants born of mothers who suffer from cardiac disease.

ACUTE FATTY LIVER OF PREGNANCY. Acute fatty liver of pregnancy is a rare, serious perinatal complication associated with a high rate of maternal morbidity and mortality.[15] It occurs most often in the third trimester of pregnancy in nulliparas and in twin gestations.[3] Clinical manifestations of malaise, nausea, jaundice, and altered sensorium are similar to those of acute viral hepatitis, cholestasis, and severe preeclampsia.[3] Table 5-3 provides

---

BOX 5-2 ▼ National Diabetes Data Group Classification of Diabetes

Type I: Insulin-dependent diabetes
Usual onset in childhood or young adulthood
Lack of insulin production by pancreatic beta cells
Prone to ketoacidosis

Type II: Non–insulin-dependent diabetes
Usual onset after age 30
70%–80% of people with disease are obese
Have adequate insulin, but delay release or abnormal reaction in peripheral tissues

Type III: Gestational diabetes mellitus (GDM)
Onset during pregnancy
May be controlled by diet or may require insulin
Usually resolves after pregnancy

Type IV: Secondary diabetes
Develops secondary to a disease process

May, K.A., and Mahlmeister, L.R. *Maternal & Neonatal Nursing: Family-Centered Care* (3rd ed.). Philadelphia: J.B. Lipppincott, 1994, p. 760.

BOX 5-3 ▼ New York Heart Association Classification of Heart Disease

Class I	No symptoms of cardiac insufficiency on exertion; no limitations of physical activity
Class II	Symptoms felt on ordinary exertion, a slight limitation in physical activity
Class III	Symptoms felt even during limited activity
Class IV	Symptoms occurring during any physical activity, even at rest

TABLE 5-3 *Differential Diagnosis of Acute Fatty Liver of Pregnancy*

	Acute Fatty Liver of Pregnancy	Acute Viral Hepatitis	Cholestasis	Severe Preeclampsia
Trimester	Third	Variable	Third	Third
Parity	Nullipara	No association	No association	Nullipara
Clinical manifestations	Malaise, nausea, jaundice, altered sensorium	Malaise, nausea, jaundice, anorexia, altered sensorium	Pruritus, jaundice	Hypertension, edema, proteinuria, oliguria, central nervous system hyperexcitability, coagulopathy
Bilirubin	Increased	Increased	Increased	Normal or increased
Transaminases	Minimal increase	Marked increase	Minimal increase	Normal or minimal to moderate increase
Alkaline phosphatase	Normal for pregnancy	Minimal increase	Moderate increase	Normal for pregnancy
Histology	Fatty infiltration, no inflammation or necrosis	Marked inflammation and necrosis	Biliary stasis, no inflammation	Inflammation, necrosis, fibrin deposition
Perinatal mortality	Marked increase	Minimal increase	Minimal increase	Moderate increase
Maternal mortality	Marked increase	Minimal increase	No increase	Moderate increase
Recurrence in subsequent pregnancy	No	No	Yes	Yes

Clark, S.L., Cotton, D.B., Hankins, G.D.V., and Phelan, J.P. *Critical Care Obstetrics.* Cambridge MA: Blackwell Scientific, 1991, p. 489.

a comparison of acute fatty liver of pregnancy with each of these conditions. The cause is unknown, and although several theories have been proposed, none has been confirmed with clinical studies.[14]

Liver function studies, liver biopsy, coagulation studies, and computed tomography scanning may aid in the diagnosis. Treatment includes adequate oxygenation, correction of electrolyte imbalances and altered coagulation, and prompt delivery, preferably vaginal.[3, 14]

Sexually Transmitted Diseases and Infections

Sexually transmitted diseases (STDs) and infections are specific diseases or syndromes that are transmitted primarily through sexual contact (see Chapter 57). The pregnant woman, the unborn fetus, and the neonate suffer severe symptoms and complications as a result of a STD during pregnancy. More than 20 STDs have been identified, and they cause a wide variety of complications during pregnancy, such as spontaneous abortion, premature birth, IUGR, stillbirth, congenital anomalies, and neonatal death. Table 5-4 lists infections and their effects on the mother and fetus during pregnancy.

HIV infection is caused by the retrovirus human immunodeficiency virus (HIV). The pathophysiology of this disease is discussed in detail on pages 336–343. The infant born to an HIV-infected mother has an approximately 25% risk of acquiring the virus from the mother.[9] The infant is born without symptoms but shows maternal antibodies at birth. Symptoms usually occur within the first year of life. The most common signs are enlargement of the liver and spleen, lymphadenopathy, thrush, and failure to thrive. Infants frequently develop chronic bacterial infections, meningitis, pneumonia, osteomyelitis, septic arthritis, and septicemia.[5] As in the adult, the disease progresses over a period of years, to the death of the child.

FETAL FACTORS

The first 2 months of pregnancy are an especially vulnerable time in the development of the embryo. Spontaneous abortion is most likely to occur during this period, often before the woman is even aware that she is pregnant. Factors associated with spontaneous abortion include uterine anomalies, abnormal implantation, and genetic anomalies of the embryo. Genetic influences on development are discussed in Chapter 4. The fetal factors most associated with altered development are placental anomalies and multiple pregnancies.

Placental Anomalies

As discussed previously, the fertilized ovum begins its implantation process approximately 1 week after conception. Normally, this implantation occurs in the upper portion of the body of the uterus. The formation of the placenta occurs in this position and is complete by the third lunar month.

PLACENTA PREVIA. Placenta previa involves an implantation of the placenta in the lower portion of the

TABLE 5-4 *Effects of Infections During Pregnancy*

Infection	Maternal Effects	Fetal Effects
Condylomata acuminata	Vulvar warts; may require cesarean birth	None noted
Cytomegalovirus disease	Asymptomatic or mimics mononucleosis	Increase in perinatal mortality; fetal malformations
Gonorrhea	Asymptomatic or vaginal discharge; scarring of the fallopian tubes, which can affect ability to conceive	Fetal death, mental retardation, ophthalmia neonatorum
Herpes simplex type II	Vulvovaginitis	Increased perinatal mortality; fetal malformations
Influenza	Can produce critical illness if pneumonia develops	Fetal death and congenital anomalies
Hepatitis Infectious (type A) Serum (type B)	Abortion or premature labor	Fetal death, fetal deformities, congenital hepatitis
Monilial vaginitis	Thick, irritating vaginal discharge	Thrush in newborn
Poliomyelitis	More susceptible during pregnancy	Increased perinatal mortality
Rubella (German measles)	Fever and typical rash, abortion	Increased perinatal mortality and congenital defects
Rubeola (3-day measles)	Fever and typical rash, abortion	Increased perinatal mortality; congenital or neonatal infection will produce rash
Syphilis	May be asymptomatic or produce primary and secondary lesions	Fetal death, congenital syphilis
Toxoplasmosis	Asymptomatic	Increased perinatal mortality, congenital anomalies, congenital toxoplasmosis
Chlamydia	Often asymptomatic	Increased incidence of preterm labor and postnatal eye and respiratory infection
Urinary tract infection	Asymptomatic or fever, chills, dysuria, urinary frequency, and pain; abortion and premature labor	No effects unless sulfonamides are used in late pregnancy; they may cause jaundice
Varicella	Typical lesions; may precipitate shingles	Fetal death, growth retardation, and fetal malformations

Auvenshine, M.A. and Enriquez, MG. *Comprehensive Maternity Nursing: Prenatal and Women's Health.* Boston: Jones & Bartlett, 1990.

uterus (Fig. 5-7). This implantation may involve only the lower uterine segment, or it may completely cover the cervix. The most frequent symptom associated with placenta previa is painless vaginal bleeding in the third trimester of pregnancy. The threat to the fetus depends on the presence or absence of hemorrhage and the degree to which the birth canal is blocked. Conservative treatment and vaginal delivery may provide a healthy newborn if the placenta is implanted in the lower segment. However, the only way to ensure the baby's survival if there is a complete placenta previa is through cesarean delivery. Although the exact cause of placenta previa is unknown, several factors have been associated with it. These factors include advanced maternal age, increased parity, uterine scarring, multiple gestation, and enlarged placenta. Ultrasonography is especially helpful in identifying the exact location of the placenta. Risks for the fetus are also determined by the length of gestation and maturity of the fetus at the time of delivery.

ABRUPTIO PLACENTAE. Another placental anomaly associated with high risk for poor fetal outcome is abrup-

tio placenta (Fig. 5-8). In this condition, the placenta begins an abrupt premature separation from the uterine wall. The severity of the outcome depends on the amount of hemorrhage and whether or not a clot forms. Usually, an immediate delivery is essential if the fetus is to survive and develop normally. The exact cause of abruptio placentae has not been determined, but the condition is often associated with diabetes, PIH, and chronic hypertension. Increased frequency of abruptio placentae has also been associated with high parity, overdistention of the uterus, and physical injury, as well as cigarette smoking and the use of cocaine. Frequently, the woman presents with complaints of severe abdominal pain and a hard, boardlike abdomen. Fetal maturity at the time of emergency delivery greatly influences fetal outcome.

ECTOPIC PREGNANCY. Ectopic pregnancy is a third implantation anomaly. This condition involves the implantation of a fertilized ovum outside of the uterine cavity (Fig. 5-9). The most common site is the fallopian tube, where the fertilized ovum may get caught or become too

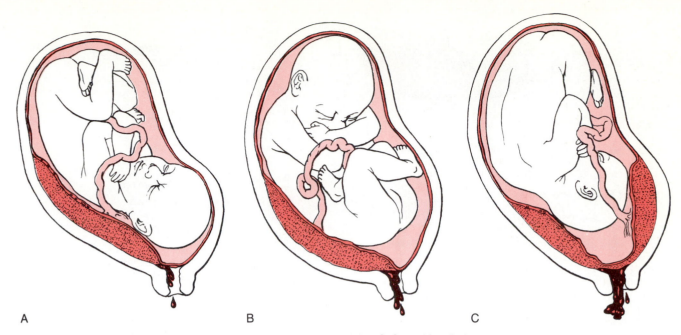

FIGURE 5-7   *Placenta previa* **A.** *Low implantation.* **B.** *Partial placenta previa.* **C.** *Central (total) placenta previa. (Reeder, S.J., Martin, L.L., and Koniak, D.* Maternity Nursing *[17th ed.]. Philadelphia: J.B. Lippincott, 1992.)*

large to proceed through the tube. The frequency of ectopic pregnancy has increased because of the increased number of women of childbearing age with a history of pelvic inflammatory disease and the use of intrauterine devices for contraception, either of which can cause scarring and alterations within the tube. Ectopic pregnancy is a life-threatening condition for the mother because of the hemorrhage and the emergency surgery associated with a ruptured ectopic pregnancy. If

this condition is diagnosed before tubal rupture, hemorrhage may be avoided and surgery scheduled for removal of the affected tube. Pregnancy tests and ultrasonography aid in the diagnosis of the presence of a fetal sac outside of the uterus.

PLACENTAL INSUFFICIENCY.   Placental insufficiency is most often associated with IUGR and may produce dysfunction of maternal-placental or fetal-placental cir-

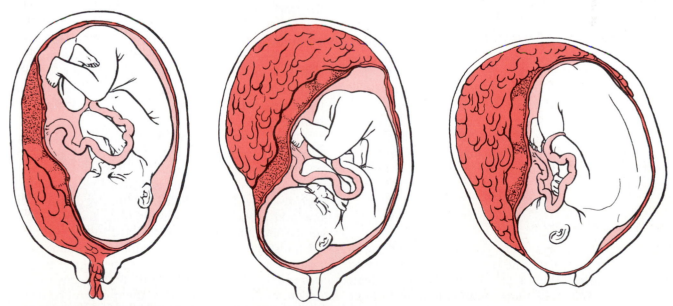

FIGURE 5-8   *Abruptio placentae of various separation sites. (Left) External hemorrhage. (Center) Internal or concealed hemorrhage. (Right) Complete separation. (Reeder, S.J., Martin, L.L., and Koniak, D.* Maternity Nursing *[17th ed.]. Philadelphia: J.B. Lippincott, 1992.)*

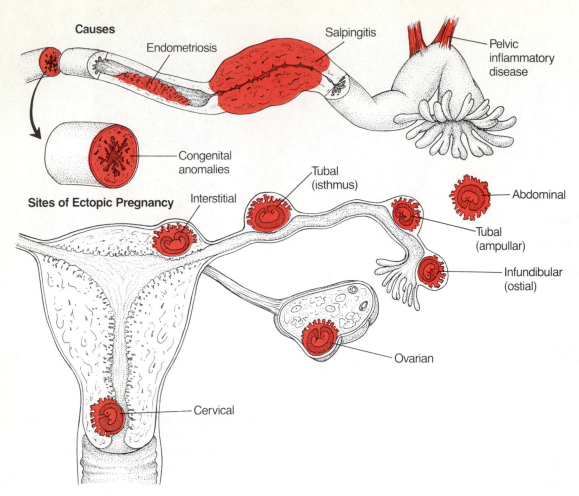

FIGURE 5-9 *Causes and sites of ectopic pregnancy. (Reeder, S.J., Martin, L.L., and Koniak, D. Maternity Nursing [17th ed.]. Philadelphia: J.B. Lippincott, 1992.)*

culation that compromises fetal nutrition and oxygenation. Occasionally, the placenta may be too small or inadequately developed to support fetal growth and development. Causes of placental insufficiency include multiple pregnancy, postmaturity, systemic diseases, hypertension, and abnormalities of the placental membranes.

Infarctions, usually found on the maternal side of the placenta, may develop if the blood supply is decreased and necrosis occurs. Infarctions appear as circular lesions ranging from dark red to yellowish white in color. Fetal risk is greatest if the infarctions occur in the central portion of the placenta and interfere with fetal circulation.

Multiple Gestations

Multiple gestations constitute yet another risk factor to fetal growth and development, and they have increased greatly because of the use of fertility drugs in the treatment of infertility. The most common form of multiple gestation is twinning. There are two major types of twins. *Monozygotic* (identical) twins occur if one ovum,

fertilized by one sperm, splits after conception. Genetically, monozygotic twins are identical. Depending on the stage of development when cleavage occurs, the twins may share an amnion or chorion, or both (Fig. 5-10). *Dizygotic* (fraternal) twins occur if two individual ova are fertilized by two separate sperm. Two placenta, two chorions, and two amnions are present (see Figure 5-10). The only similarities between dizygotic twins are those similarities associated with other siblings in the same family.

Because of the limited intrauterine space, prematurity is the most common problem associated with multiple gestation. Abnormal positioning is more frequent and may necessitate cesarean delivery. Additional high-risk conditions include hypertensive disorders, hydramnios (condition of excess amniotic fluid), and uterine dysfunction. Monozygotic twins are especially at risk for transfusion syndrome, in which one infant is well nourished and developed but the other is pale and anemic and displays evidence of intrauterine growth retardation. In monozygotic twins, the umbilical cords may also become entangled, leading to fetal demise of one twin.

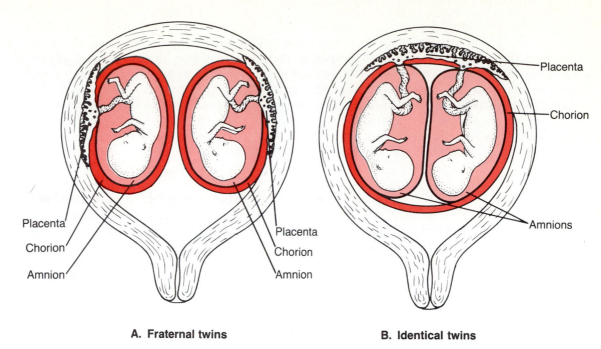

A. Fraternal twins   **B. Identical twins**

FIGURE 5-10 *Twin pregnancies.* **A.** *Fraternal twins with two placentas, two amnions, and two chorions.* **B.** *Identical twins with one placenta, one chorion, and two amnions. (Reeder, S.J., Martin, L.L., and Koniak, D.* Maternity Nursing *[17th ed.]. Philadelphia: J.B. Lippincott, 1992.)*

ENVIRONMENTAL FACTORS

Maternal Nutrition

Pregnancy is a unique developmental time. At no other stage in the life cycle does the well-being of one individual, the fetus, depend so directly on the well-being of another individual, the mother. The nutritional status of the mother is a critical determinant of her own well-being and also that of the fetus. Proper nutrition during pregnancy reduces the risks for maternal complications such as PIH and anemia, ensures adequate tissue growth, and promotes optimal infant birth weight. The recommended daily allowances for pregnant and non-pregnant women, infants, children, and adult males is found in Appendix A.

Inadequate maternal nutrition has a direct effect on fetal brain development. If maternal nutrition is insufficient, the fetal brain does not develop properly. Inadequate maternal nutrition also has a significant effect on infant birth weight. Infants with low birth weight are at risk for more frequent illnesses, hearing and vision disabilities, behavioral disorders, and learning problems than infants whose weight is within the normal range.

Several maternal conditions or factors aid in identification of women who are nutritionally at risk. Some of these conditions are 1) adolescence; 2) overweight; 3) underweight; 4) inadequate weight gain; 5) excessive weight gain; 6) anemia; 7) smoking or use of alcohol or drugs; 8) pica; 9) poor diet; and 10) medical problems such as diabetes. Several of these factors are discussed in this section.

ADOLESCENCE. The pregnant adolescent has increased nutritional needs to provide for the developing maternal musculoskeletal system. Musculoskeletal growth is not complete at puberty, and growth may continue for 1 to 2 years after puberty. The pregnant adolescent must meet her own nutritional needs as well as those required by the developing fetus. The recommended daily allowances for pregnancy and lactation are found in Appendix B.

PICA. Pica, the practice of eating nonfood substances such as laundry starch, clay, or dirt, occurs most often among pregnant African-Americans who have a family history of pica. Although this practice occurs more commonly in the southeastern United States, it is found in all geographic regions, races, and socioeconomic levels. Ingestion of pica substances may result in a less than optimal intake of essential nutrients. Iron deficiency anemia, which was once thought to cause pica, is now considered to be a result of the practice.[5] Other conditions that may occur as a result of pica include dystocia, which is pathologic or difficult labor caused by fecal impaction from clay, parasitic infection from contaminated dirt and clay, and obstruction of the small bowel resulting from excessive intake of laundry starch.[2] Some pica substances contain toxic compounds (eg, lead) that can seriously affect fetal growth and development.

IRON DEFICIENCY ANEMIA. Iron deficiency anemia during pregnancy is defined as a hemoglobin level of 11 g/dL or less during the second and third trimesters.[8] Mild anemia presents no real threat to the mother but is evidence that the maternal nutritional status is less than optimal. Iron deficiency anemia results from a decrease in hemoglobin production caused by the expenditure of iron stores. Iron stores become depleted from insufficient intake of iron, blood loss, malabsorption, or hemolysis.[8] Ferrous sulfate and vitamin C are usually given together for iron deficiency anemia since vitamin C promotes iron absorption.[8] However, these supplements should never be considered a replacement or substitute for proper nutrition.

Teratogens

A teratogen is a substance or agent that produces abnormalities in embryonic or fetal development. The most common teratogens that affect pregnancy and the fetus are tobacco, possibly caffeine, drugs including alcohol, infections, and radiation.

Maternal smoking produces low-birth-weight infants. This condition is preventable if the mother abstains from smoking during pregnancy. Approximately 32% of women are smokers at the time of conception, and 20% to 25% continue to smoke throughout pregnancy.[8] Fetal tobacco syndrome is a phrase that has been introduced to refer to the specific conditions that result from prenatal exposure to tobacco smoke.[2]

The clinical implications of caffeine use during pregnancy are not as clear as those for alcohol and tobacco. Recent research indicates that heavy caffeine users have four times the risk for having an infant with IUGR than those who abstained from the use of caffeine during pregnancy.[4]

Use of cocaine produces a vasoconstrictive effect on the smooth muscle of the uterus, which leads to premature labor that is not affected by the administration of tocolytic drugs to stop the contractions. The transfer of cocaine from mother to fetus occurs rapidly. The fetal kidney excretes cocaine and its metabolites into the amniotic fluid, and it is recycled when the fetus swallows amniotic fluid.[2]

The most serious effect of alcohol use during pregnancy occurs in fetal alcohol syndrome. In addition, fetuses of mothers who are heavy drinkers also suffer from maternal malnutrition and hypoglycemia.

▼ Prenatal Diagnostic Studies

Prenatal diagnostic studies of fetal well-being and maturity provide much-needed information regarding pregnancy status. Careful selection of tests can predict placental insufficiency, fetal anomalies, genetic abnormalities, and the ability of the fetus to survive in the existing intrauterine or extrauterine environment. Because maternal morbidity and mortality associated with modern childbearing are low, the focus of prenatal assessment of fetal well-being is to decrease fetal death and disease.

Assessment of fetal health and well-being ideally begins before conception. Those persons anticipating parenthood should prepare physically and psychologically by attaining and maintaining physical health, eating nutritiously, and avoiding substances such as drugs, alcohol, and cigarettes. Women taking prescription medications for preexisting medical conditions should confer with their physicians before conception.

RISK FACTORS

After conception has occurred, pregnancy presents a slightly greater risk of morbidity and mortality over the nonpregnant state. Factors that increase mortality and morbidity have been categorized into obstetric and preexisting medical conditions. Persons identified in either of these categories may require prenatal diagnostic studies to monitor the development of the pregnancy and fetus. Certain demographic factors are associated with increased risk during pregnancy, including maternal age younger than 15 years or older than 35 years, nonwhite race, single status, and dependency on welfare or public assistance. Obstetric risk factors include previous infertility, previous abortion, premature or low-birth-weight infant, postterm pregnancy, incompetent cervix, PIH, and multiple gestation. Miscellaneous factors that place a pregnancy at risk are related to maternal nutrition, smoking, and substance use. Medical factors that place a pregnancy at risk are anemia, heart disease, diabetes mellitus, STDs, psychiatric disorders, and any other chronic medical condition.[8]

PRENATAL DIAGNOSTIC TECHNIQUES

Several antenatal diagnostic tests are currently available to assess fetal health and well-being. Selective use of the tests provides information concerning the development of the fetus and fetal adaptation to the intrauterine environment. Table 5-5 lists diagnostic tests and their most frequent use by trimester.

Ultrasonography

Ultrasound, or sonography, is a noninvasive procedure that uses high-frequency sound waves above the highest range of hearing to provide images of the fetus, placenta, and uterus as early as 4 to 5 weeks after the last menstrual period (LMP). The first ultrasound scanning used a static B-scan method that provided two-dimensional images in cross-section. The B-scan method also provided data on tissue density and consistency. Currently, real-time ultrasound is the newest and most sophisticated form of sonography. This method provides continuous cross-section pictures of internal structures and the motion that occurs in these structures. With this method, an entire field can be scanned to show movement such as the fetal heart beating or the motion of

TABLE 5-5 *Prenatal Diagnostic Tests and Most Frequent Use by Trimester*

First Trimester, Weeks 1–13	*Second Trimester, Weeks 14–27*	*Third Trimester, Weeks 28–40*
ULTRASOUND (CROWN–RUMP LENGTH/CRL) ▼ Diagnose pregnancy ▼ Assess gestational age ▼ Identify congenital anomalies ▼ Evaluate vaginal bleeding ▼ Confirm multiple gestations ▼ Assess fetal growth ▼ Augment other prenatal tests ▼ Evaluate pelvic mass	**ULTRASOUND (BIPARIETAL DIAMETER/BPD)** ▼ Assess gestational age ▼ Confirm multiple gestations ▼ Assess fetal growth ▼ Identify structural abnormalities of fetus such as hydrocephalus ▼ Guide amniocentesis and fetoscopy procedures ▼ Determine placenta location and condition	**ULTRASOUND** ▼ Determine fetal position ▼ Estimate fetal size
DOPPLER ULTRASOUND	**DOPPLER ULTRASOUND**	**DOPPLER ULTRASOUND**
CHORIONIC VILLUS SAMPLING	**DOPPLER VELOCIMETRY**	**DOPPLER VELOCIMETRY**
	AMNIOCENTESIS (UP TO 20 WEEKS) ▼ Determine genetic make-up ▼ Determine isoimmunization (20–22 weeks)	**AMNIOCENTESIS** ▼ Determine fetal lung maturity ▼ Determine blood grouping ▼ Detect amnionitis
	α-FETOPROTEIN	**PHOSPHATYLGLYCEROL (PG)**
	ACETYLCHOLINESTERASE (ACE)	**PLACENTAL GRADING**
	PLACENTAL GRADING	**PERCUTANEOUS UMBILICAL BLOOD SAMPLING (PUBS)**
	FETOSCOPY (16–20 WEEKS)	**FETAL BIOPHYSICAL PROFILE**
	PERCUTANEOUS UMBILICAL BLOOD SAMPLING (PUBS)	

an extremity. Diagnosis of a pregnancy can be made as early as 4 to 5 weeks after the LMP through the use of static scanning. At this time, the gestational sac that is implanted in the endometrial cavity can be pictured because it is filled with fluid, is echo-free, and is surrounded by solid uterine tissue. Early diagnosis of pregnancy expedites determination of the expected date of delivery (EDD), identifies persons with risk factors, and promotes planning and referral needed for persons identified as being at high risk.

The most frequent use of ultrasound during the first trimester is to determine gestational age. Because of the rapid growth that occurs during the first trimester, EDD can be most accurately determined between 7 and 13 weeks after the LMP.[8] Through the use of real-time ultrasound, gestational age can be estimated to within 1 to 3 days by measurement of the fetal crown-rump length. After 14 weeks' gestation, the biparietal diameter, the widest transverse diameter of the fetal head, can be measured to determine gestational age. The optimal time to assess gestational age from the biparietal diameter measurement is between 16 and 20 weeks' gestation. At this time, ultrasound is accurate to within 1 week.

In addition to determination of gestational age, ultrasound is used to identify congenital anomalies, particularly in the large structures of the head and trunk. If fetal anomalies are identified, additional studies, such as amniocentesis or fetal blood sampling, are done to identify possible chromosomal disorders.

Assessment of placental condition and location is also possible because ultrasound, unlike radiography, detects soft tissue. Assessment of placental location is important, particularly in the presence of vaginal bleeding. Ectopic pregnancy can also be ruled out if an intrauterine pregnancy is identified. In cases in which there is intraabdominal pathology, such as an ovarian cyst, and examination of the abdomen is difficult, ultrasound helps to determine the presence of a pregnancy. Ultrasound can also be used to grade the placenta. Assessment of a mature placenta is based on the identification and distribution of increasing calcium deposits.[5]

Because a large number of fetuses are aborted during the first trimester, serial ultrasounds done in weekly intervals may help to authenticate fetal growth or deterioration. Several parameters of fetal growth, such as measurement of head and trunk size, soft tissue mass, general size including length and weight, and the proportions of body parts to one another should be examined to develop a growth profile.[2]

Ultrasound is also used to identify the presence of multiple gestation. Multiple gestation often produces associated risk factors such as prematurity and hypertension.

Doppler Ultrasound

Doppler ultrasound is a diagnostic technique used to assess the movement of blood in blood vessels and body organs such as the uterus and the fetal heart. Doppler ultrasound differs from conventional ultrasound because images of body structures are not provided with this method. The Doppler instrument sends out sound waves at a particular frequency which are directed at moving RBCs. The sound waves that locate and ''bounce off'' the RBCs return at a different frequency. The rate at which the RBCs move causes the change in frequency.[13]

Doppler velocimetry uses the Doppler principle to measure visual velocity waveforms. These waveforms compare the systolic and diastolic rates of blood flow. The umbilical waveform can be assessed as early as 15 weeks' gestation. It is expressed as a ratio of systolic to diastolic rate (S:D); the normal ratio is 3:1 at 28 to 30 weeks' gestation. The ratio usually decreases as pregnancy advances in response to a normal decrease in resistance in placental circulation.[8]

Chorionic Villus Sampling

Chorionic villus sampling (CVS) is used during the first trimester of pregnancy to diagnose chromosomal abnormalities and biochemical disorders. It can be performed as early as 8 weeks after the LMP. Chorionic villi are vascular extensions from the blastocyst that provide an attachment to the endometrium and result in the formation of the placenta. CVS may be performed transcervically or transabdominally. The transcervical method with direct real-time ultrasound is the more widely used procedure. Viability and gestational age are determined by ultrasound before CVS is undertaken. A gonorrhea cervical culture is also collected and analyzed before the CVS is performed. The woman must have a negative gonorrhea culture to prevent dissemination of *Neisseria* gonorrhea into the bloodstream after the test.

With ultrasound for direction, a plastic catheter is placed into the chorion and a specimen of chorionic villi is removed (Fig. 5-11). The sample is placed in a sterile culture medium and studied in a cytogenetic laboratory. Women who are Rh-negative and unsensitized to Rh-positive blood should receive anti-D globulin RhoGAM.[5]

The risks associated with CVS are similar to those after amniocentesis and may include amniotic fluid leakage, infection, intrauterine fetal death, IUGR, Rh

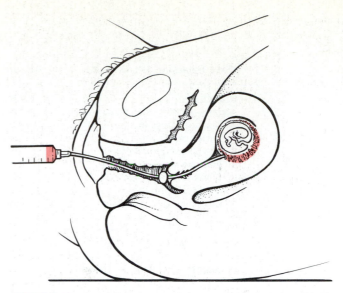

FIGURE 5-11 *Diagram of the uterus at 10 weeks gestation with biopsy catheter in position.*

isoimmunization, spontaneous abortion, septic shock, and damage to the placental membranes.[7] There is less than 1% error in interpretation of the test results. Infection can occur because the catheter is passed transvaginally, and the risk increases with the number of catheters used. Higher infection rates are noted in primigravidas because of the opposition of the cervix to passage of the catheter. In addition, there is the potential for mistakes to occur if maternal tissue is analyzed or if multiple gestation is present but unnoticed.

The greatest benefit of CVS is that the procedure can be performed during the first trimester, as opposed to amniocentesis, which cannot be done until approximately 14 to 16 weeks' gestation, after sufficient amniotic fluid is present. Because cell division occurs rapidly and the cells do not have to be grown in a laboratory, direct microscopic analysis can be done during the metaphase of mitosis. Preliminary results can then be obtained in as little as 24 to 48 hours, and these results can be verified in 5 to 10 days. First-trimester termination of pregnancy then becomes an option if an abnormality is identified. Another benefit of CVS compared with amniocentesis is that CVS uses living tissue rather than dead, sloughed epithelial cells, permitting identification of more potential disorders.

Amniocentesis

Amniocentesis is a procedure that involves the aspiration of amniotic fluid from the uterus by way of an abdominal puncture. The test can be performed in any trimester of pregnancy as long as sufficient fluid is present. If it is done in the first trimester, it is usually for genetic studies; in the second trimester, for Rh isoimmunization studies; and in the third trimester, for assessment of fetal lung maturity. Amniocentesis is preceded by ultrasound to confirm fetal viability and gestational age, locate the position of the placenta, and identify pockets of amniotic fluid. The site for needle insertion is chosen to avoid the placenta and fetus while providing an adequate amount of fluid. Approximately 20 mL of amniotic fluid is aspirated for analysis. RhoGAM is given to the Rh-negative, unsensitized mother after the procedure.

AMNIOCENTESIS FOR GENETIC STUDIES. Of the more than 5,000 single-gene disorders along with others that affect humans, more than 70 can be diagnosed by amniocentesis.[1] The test is considered a conventional part of prenatal care, especially with advanced maternal age. Most women who are age 35 years or older at the time of delivery have amniocentesis performed. At age 35, the risk for cytogenetic abnormality, most frequently trisomy 21, is one in 80, and the risks increase with advanced maternal age.

In many cases, amniocentesis can identify missing enzymes that indicate a fetal biochemical abnormality. Biochemical disorders involve lipid, amino acid, and mucopolysaccharide abnormalities; neural tube defects (NTDs); trisomy 21; hemophilia; and muscular dystrophy.[1]

Amniocentesis is also appropriate if a previous pregnancy has involved a fetus or infant with a chromosomal abnormality or NTD, or if a parent has a genetic disorder or is a known translocation carrier. One of every 500 people carries a balanced chromosomal translocation. This translocation in a parent who is phenotypically normal will produce genetic imbalance in the offspring.

Single-gene X-linked recessive disorders, such as hemophilia and muscular dystrophy, can be identified by amniocentesis through fetal sex determination. The recurrence risk for X-linked recessive transmission is 25% with each pregnancy for male fetuses. Females are carriers and are unaffected. Therefore, amniocentesis is indicated in pregnancies in which the mother is a known carrier of an X-linked disorder. Autosomal recessive single-gene disorders, such as sickle cell anemia, can also be diagnosed by amniocentesis.

α-FETOPROTEIN. The level of α-fetoprotein (AFP), which is increased in the presence of an NTD, can also be determined through amniocentesis. AFP is produced by the fetal yolk sac and liver and reaches its highest level at about 13 weeks' gestation. AFP in maternal serum reaches its highest serum peak at about 30 weeks' gestation. The protein enters the maternal serum through the placenta and the amniotic fluid through the fetal urine. The normal level of AFP at 18 weeks' gestation is 18.5 mg per milliliter of amniotic fluid. AFP levels may be increased in situations of fetal leakage, hemorrhage, or multiple pregnancy. The actual procedure of amniocentesis can also increase AFP levels; maternal serum AFP should be determined before the test, to prevent errors in interpretation of AFP. In families with an increased risk for NTDs, maternal serum AFP evaluation combined with ultrasound is recommended. If the maternal serum AFP level is increased and the sonar is normal, an amniocentesis may be necessary to make the diagnosis of a possible NTD.

ACETYLCHOLINESTERASE. The test for acetylcholinesterase is more reliable than those for AFP or maternal serum AFP to diagnose NTDs. Acetylcholinesterase is produced in the fetal central nervous system and is more fetal-specific than AFP or maternal serum AFP. Increased levels of acetylcholinesterase indicate an NTD, and decreased levels indicate recent fetal demise.

AMNIOCENTESIS FOR RH ISOIMMUNIZATION. An Rh-negative mother with an antibody titer of 1:8 or 1:16 or higher should have the first amniocentesis at approximately 24 to 25 weeks' gestation. Through amniocentesis, the quantitative amount of bilirubin is determined, indicating the degree of fetal RBC hemolysis. Depending on the severity of hemolysis, an intrauterine fetal blood transfusion of Rh-negative blood may be indicated to decrease maternal antibody formation and to correct the fetal anemia that results from hemolysis. In severe cases, fetal hydrops and fetal demise can result if intrauterine treatment is not performed.

AMNIOCENTESIS FOR FETAL LUNG MATURITY. The most frequent use of amniocentesis in the third trimester is to assess fetal lung maturity. Fetal lung maturity is measured by two phospholipids produced by fetal lung tissue, lecithin and sphingomyelin. Owing to their detergent effect, lecithin and sphingomyelin mix with amniotic fluid in the lung to promote a decreased surface tension and protect the alveoli from collapse. If both lecithin and sphingomyelin, which are expressed as a ratio (L:S), are adequate, breathing of the neonate after delivery prevents collapse of the alveoli. If the L:S ratio is inadequate, alveoli collapse and respiratory distress syndrome may develop.

An L:S ratio of 2:1 indicates two times as much lecithin as sphingomyelin and is usually an acceptable indicator of fetal lung maturity. Before 30 to 32 weeks' gestation, there is more sphingomyelin than lecithin. At about 32 weeks' gestation, lecithin and sphingomyelin are equal in amount. At 35 weeks, lecithin increases rapidly and sphingomyelin remains constant.

PHOSPHATIDYLGLYCEROL. Phosphatidylglycerol and phosphatidylinositol are two other phospholipids that are also associated with fetal lung maturity. Phosphatidylglycerol is used in conjunction with the L:S ratio. If the L:S ratio is low, a positive phosphatidylglycerol level may indicate fetal lung maturity.

Fetoscopy

Fetoscopy is a high-risk procedure used to diagnose and treat the fetus in utero. It is used in combination with ultrasound to locate the placenta and umbilical cord and to assess fetal growth. A needlescope, a flexible endoscope and needle, is inserted into the uterus through the maternal abdomen. Fetal skin tissue and samples of blood can be collected for diagnosis of genetic disorders. Intrauterine blood transfusions can be performed in cases of severe the fetal anemia that result from hemolysis when there is blood incompatibility. There is a 5% risk for spontaneous abortion after fetoscopy. Bleeding, infection, injuries to the fetus, amniotic fluid leakage, and premature birth may also occur. These risks, along with its cost and the lack of availability of the procedure in prenatal centers, have limited its present use.

Percutaneous Umbilical Blood Sampling

Percutaneous umbilical blood sampling (PUBS) is a procedure that allows direct entry to fetal circulation. The PUBS procedure produces a pure specimen of fetal blood, permitting speedy determination of fetal karotype, blood typing, antibody testing, acid-base evaluation, assessment of isoimmune hemolytic anemia, and intrauterine fetal blood transfusion.[2]

Through the use of ultrasound, the placenta and cord are located before the procedure. Needle insertion and aspiration of the fetal blood sample take place near the insertion of the cord into the placenta because less movement of the cord occurs at this location. However, maternal intervillous blood lakes are situated near the insertion of the umbilical cord and the placenta, which results in an increased chance of contamination with maternal blood. Potential complications after the PUBS procedure are chorioamnionitis, premature labor and rupture of the amniotic membranes, bleeding, and injury to the umbilical cord. Infection occurs in 1% of procedures.[2]

Through the PUBS procedure, direct assessment of fetal hemoglobin concentration is possible. Direct transfusion of RBCs to the fetus immediately corrects fetal anemia and is preferred over intraabdominal transfusion of packed RBCs, which take several weeks to be absorbed across the peritoneal membrane.[2] PUBS can be performed in an outpatient setting and has replaced fetoscopy for fetal blood sampling and transfusions.

Fetal Biophysical Profile

A fetal biophysical profile involves evaluation of five variables that are assessed by the use of real-time ultrasound. The five variables are fetal movement, fetal breathing movements, fetal tone, amniotic fluid volume, and fetal heart rate. These variables are assessed and scored by the sonographer. Each variable receives a score of 2 if it is assessed as normal and a score of 0 if it is abnormal.[1] Table 5-6 presents a list of variables and the criteria for determining the score. High scores indicate fetal well-being, and low scores indicate the need for additional testing. Indications for assessment of the fetal biophysical profile are hypertension, diabetes, postmature pregnancy, and suspected IUGR.

▼ Biophysical Factors Affecting Labor and Delivery

INITIATION OF LABOR

After approximately 266 days of being nourished and nurtured within the mother's womb, the fetus is ready for its transition to extrauterine life. The exact cause of the onset of labor has not been identified. However, various theories or a combination of theories are now being accepted as possible explanations for the initiation of labor.

Theories of Onset

HORMONAL STIMULATION. Throughout pregnancy, estrogen and progesterone play important roles in maintaining the gestation. Estrogen is believed to increase the oxytocin receptors in the uterus, and progesterone exerts a relaxing effect. Although research findings continue to be inconsistent, estrogen may increase and progesterone may decrease at or near term.[7] Oxytocin, produced by both fetus and mother, has a stimulating effect on the smooth muscle of the uterus, producing uterine contractions.

UTERINE DISTENTION THEORY. This theory is based on knowledge regarding the stretching of uterine muscle as it increases in size during pregnancy. During pregnancy, progesterone exerts a relaxing effect on the myometrium. As the pregnancy approaches term, the level of progesterone declines, allowing the overdistended uterus to begin contracting.

PROSTAGLANDIN THEORY. Prostaglandin levels are known to increase just before the onset of labor. This action may be a response to estrogen stimulation.[7] Prostaglandin exerts a stimulating effect on the smooth muscle of the myometrium, possibly leading to the onset of the contractions of labor.

Premonitory Signs

Some evidence of impending labor is noted by most women. These premonitory signs include lightening. Lightening heralds the entry of the presenting part into the pelvis. This process is accompanied by downward movement of the uterus and a release of pressure on the

TABLE 5-6 *Biophysical Profile Scoring: Technique, Interpretation, and Recommended Clinical Management*

Technique and Interpretation

Biophysical Variable	Normal (Score = 2)	Abnormal (score = 0)
Fetal breathing movement (FBM)	At least one episode of FBM of at least 30-sec duration in 30-min observation	Absent FBM or no episode of >30 sec in 30 min
Gross body movement	At least three discrete body or limb movements in 30 min (episodes of active continuous movement considered as single movement)	Two or fewer episodes of body or limb movements in 30 min
Fetal tone	At least one episode of active extension with return to flexion of fetal limb(s) or trunk; opening and closing of hand considered normal tone	Either slow extension with return to partial flexion or movement of limb in full extension, absent fetal movement
Reactive fetal heart rate (FHR)	At least two episodes of FHR acceleration of >15 bpm and of at least 15-sec duration associated with fetal movement in 30 min	Less than two episodes of acceleration of FHR or acceleration of >15 bpm in 30 min
Qualitative amniotic fluid volume (AFV)	At least one pocket of amniotic fluid that measures at least 1 cm in two perpendicular planes	Either no AF pockets or a pocket <1 cm in two perpendicular planes

Recommended Clinical Management Based on These Results

Test Score Result	Interpretation	Management
10 of 10 8 of 10 (norm fluid) 8 of 8 (NST not done)	Risk of fetal asphyxia extremely rare	Intervention only for obstetric and maternal factors; no indication for intervention for fetal disease
8 of 10 (abnorm fluid)	Probable chronic fetal compromise	Determine that there is functioning renal tissue and intact membranes; if so, deliver for fetal indications
6 of 10 (norm fluid)	Equivocal test possible fetal asphyxia	If the fetus is mature—deliver. In the immature fetus repeat test within 24 h; if <6/10, deliver
6 of 10 (abnorm fluid)	Probable fetal asphyxia	Deliver for fetal indications
4 of 10	High probability fetal asphyxia	Deliver for fetal indications
2 of 10	Almost certain fetal asphyxia	Deliver for fetal indications
0 of 10	Certain fetal asphyxia	Deliver for fetal indications

May, K.A., and Mahlmeister, L.R. *Maternal & Neonatal Nursing: Family-Centered Care* [3rd ed.]. Philadelphia: J.B. Lippincott, 1994, p. 310.

diaphragm. This movement is often accompanied by leg cramps, pelvic pressure and urinary frequency, increased vaginal secretions, and venous stasis.

BRAXTON-HICKS CONTRACTIONS. Braxton-Hicks contractions, present throughout pregnancy, become stronger and more regular and begin to produce cervical changes. These contractions sometimes become so uncomfortable that the woman goes to the hospital or physician's office for evaluation. Cervical dilatation is the most accurate way of differentiating between true and false labor.

CERVICAL CHANGES. Cervical changes are another indication of the onset of labor. Softening (ripening) of the cervix occurs as a result of Braxton-Hicks contractions. Cervical dilatation and effacement may also occur before the onset of regular contractions.

SHOW. Show is the pink-tinged secretion associated with the expulsion of the mucus plug from the cervix as it begins to dilate and efface. Labor usually begins within 24 to 48 hours of expulsion of the mucus plug. Show should be differentiated from the blood-tinged discharge associated with rupture of small vessels during vaginal examination.

RUPTURE OF THE MEMBRANES. Rupture of the membranes may precede the onset of labor or occur during the process. There is increased risk of infection with prolonged rupture of the membranes. The color of the amniotic fluid should be noted when membranes rupture; meconium-stained fluid may be associated with fetal distress. There is also risk of prolapsed cord when the membranes rupture if the presenting part is not adequately engaged in the true pelvis or if there is abnormal fetal positioning, including breech position.

STAGES OF LABOR

The process of labor and delivery has been divided into four stages. *Stage one* begins with the first regular uterine contractions and ends with complete cervical dilatation (10 cm) (Fig. 5-12). *Stage two* begins with complete dilatation and ends with expulsion of the fetus. The *third stage* of labor begins with delivery of the fetus and ends with delivery of the placenta. The *fourth stage* of labor encompasses the first hour or so after the delivery of the placenta.

First Stage

The first stage of labor is divided into three phases: latent, active, and transition. Although both physical and emotional changes are associated with each stage, only the physical changes are discussed here.

The *latent phase* begins with the first regular uterine contractions. Contractions are usually mild, lasting 15 to 20 seconds and occurring every 5 to 7 minutes. The cervix effaces and dilates up to 3 to 4 cm. The average latent phase is 8.6 hours for nulliparas and 5.3 hours for multiparas.

The *active phase* ends when cervical dilatation reaches 8 cm. It is accompanied by cervical effacement and fetal descent in the birth canal. Uterine contractions become moderate in intensity and occur every 3 to 5 minutes, lasting 35 to 40 seconds.

Transition is associated with cervical dilatation between 8 and 10 cm. Contractions occur every 2 to 3 minutes, last 60 to 90 seconds, and are moderate to severe in intensity. Transition is also associated with nausea, vomiting, diaphoresis, periods of amnesia, and increased anal pressure.

Second Stage

The second stage of labor is also referred to as the expulsion stage. In nulliparas, delivery usually occurs within 2 hours. The second stage of labor averages only 15 minutes in multiparas. As the fetus progresses through the birth canal, it undergoes a series of movements, referred to as the mechanism or movements of labor. These movements include descent, flexion, internal rotation, extension, restitution, external rotation, and expulsion. These movements are illustrated in Figure 5-13.

The mother experiences an involuntary urge to push. Intraabdominal pressure works with the uterine contractions to expel the fetus. As the presenting part begins to emerge, the perineum bulges and flattens out. The anus dilates and the labia separate. Intense rectal pressure, pain, stretching, tearing, and burning of the perineum are common sensations as the woman delivers the fetal head. On delivery of the fetal head, the mother experiences a sense of relief and decrease of pain and pressure. A small perineal incision, called an episiotomy,

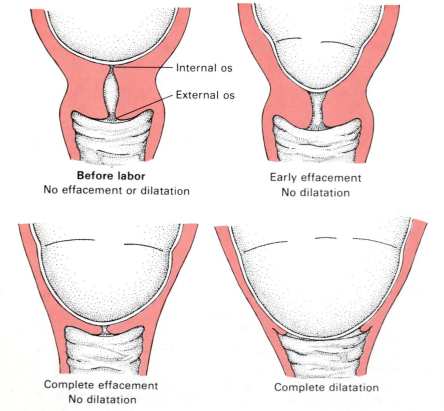

Before labor
No effacement or dilatation

— Internal os
— External os

Early effacement
No dilatation

Complete effacement
No dilatation

Complete dilatation

FIGURE 5-12 *Stages in cervical effacement and dilatation. (Reeder, S.J., Martin, L.L., and Koniak, D. Maternity Nursing [17th ed.]. Philadelphia: J.B. Lippincott, 1992.)*

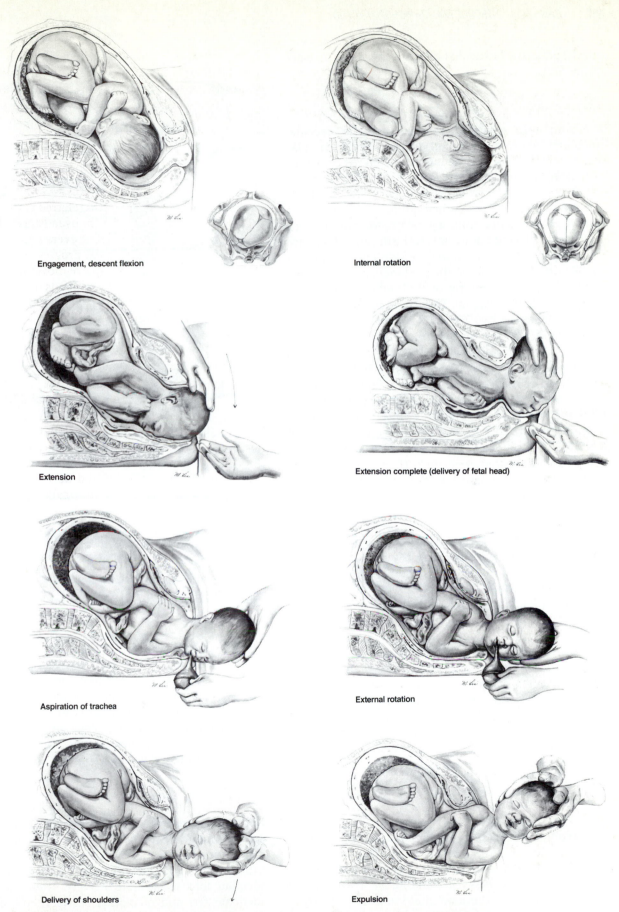

Engagement, descent flexion

Internal rotation

Extension

Extension complete (delivery of fetal head)

Aspiration of trachea

External rotation

Delivery of shoulders

Expulsion

FIGURE 5-13 *Mechanism of delivery for a vertex presentation. (Whitley, N. A Manual of Clinical Obstetrics. Philadelphia: J.B. Lippincott, 1985.)*

may be performed to avoid laceration and aid in delivery of the fetus.

Third Stage

The third stage of labor is referred to as the placental stage and involves separation and delivery of the placenta. After delivery of the infant, the uterus contracts, decreasing its size and the surface area for placental attachment. Separation of the placenta results in bleeding and the formation of a hematoma. This hematoma further enhances placental separation. Membranes separate as the placenta descends the birth canal. Evidence that the placenta has separated include a firm, globular-shaped uterus that rises in the abdomen, a sudden gush of blood, and lengthening of the umbilical cord as it protrudes from the vagina. The length of the third stage ranges from about 5 to 30 minutes. The risk for complications is increased after 30 minutes.

The most common mechanism for delivery of the placenta is Schultz's mechanism (Fig. 5-14A). Placental separation occurs first in the center and results in delivery of the fetal side first. The second mechanism for placental delivery is referred to as the Duncan mechanism (Fig. 5-14B). In this mechanism, separation occurs first along the outer edges, causing the placenta to roll and present the maternal side first. There is increased risk of retained placental parts with the Duncan mechanism.

Fourth Stage

Technically, the immediate postpartum period is not a true stage of labor. However, it is a critical period of adaptation. The uterus should remain firmly contracted, in the midline, and midway between the symphysis pubis and umbilicus. Relaxation of the uterus results in hemorrhage and even maternal death if not immediately treated by fundal massage or oxytocic drugs, or both, to control the bleeding. Although there may be a slight drop in blood pressure and slight increase in pulse immediately after delivery, vital signs should return to prelabor values very quickly. A shaking chill may be experienced in the recovery room in response to the exertion of labor, anesthesia, and sudden release of intra-abdominal pressure. The mother may also complain of thirst and hunger. A summary of the four stages of labor is found in Table 5-7.

ALTERATIONS AND ADAPTATIONS

The accomplishment of a spontaneous delivery requires the interaction of numerous factors. Problems in adaptation can occur as a result of alterations in any of the four Ps—*power, passage, passenger,* and *psyche.* Power represents the frequency, duration, and intensity of contractions, as well as the pushing effort of the woman. Passage refers to the size and type of pelvis and the ability of the

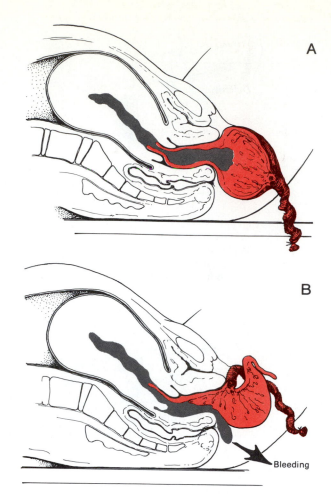

FIGURE 5-14 *Expulsion of the placenta. **A.** Schultze's mechanism. The placenta is turned inside out within the vagina and is delivered with the glistening fetal surfaces to the outside. **B.** Duncan's mechanism. The placenta is rolled up in the vagina and is delivered with the maternal surface to the outside. (Reeder, S.J., Martin, L.L., and Koniak, D.* Maternity Nursing *[17th ed.]. Philadelphia: J.B. Lippincott, 1992.)*

cervix and vagina to respond and allow passage of the fetus. Passenger is used to refer to the fetus, its head size, position, presentation, attitude, and umbilical cord. Psyche, critical in the birth process, includes the effects of anxiety, tension, and fear, which can lengthen the duration of labor and delivery. Specific problems associated with alterations in power, passage, and passenger are discussed in the following section.

Power

The timing, strength, and efficiency of uterine contractions in producing cervical dilatation and effacement are major forces in the timely descent and delivery of the fetus. Uterine contractions must be rhythmical and of adequate force to facilitate delivery. There must also be adequate rest and relaxation between contractions to allow for sufficient uteroplacental exchange. Alterations in the contraction forces occur when contractions hap-

TABLE 5-7 *Summary of Stages of Labor*

Stage	Definition	Duration	Uterine Activity	Maternal Behavior and Manifestations
First stage (dilating stage)	Period from first true labor contractions to complete cervical dilation	Varies with phase and parity		
Latent phase	Begins at true labor onset and ends with onset of active labor	Approximately 8.6 h for the nullipara and 5.3 h for the multipara	Mild, often irregular contractions 5–30 min apart, 10–30 sec duration; cervix becomes softer and thinner, 0 to 3–4 cm dilatation	Laboring woman is generally excited, alert, talkative or quiet, calm or anxious; may experience abdominal cramps, backache, rupture of membranes, pain controlled fairly well, may ambulate
Active phase	Begins with onset of active labor and ends with full dilatation	Approximately 4.6 h for the nullipara and 2.4 h for the multipara	Moderate to strong uterine contractions every 2–5 min; 30–90 sec duration, cervical dilation for nulliparas of 1.2 cm/h and for the multipara 1.5 cm/h	Laboring woman generally feels increasing discomfort, perspiring, nausea, and vomiting, flushed; experiences trembling of thighs and legs, pressure on bladder and rectum, backache, circumoral pallor, amnesia between contractions; may be more apprehensive, fear losing control, self-focused; may become irritable
Second stage (pelvic stage)	Period from complete cervical dilatation to delivery of infant	Approximately 1 h for the nullipara and 1/2 h for the multipara	Strong uterine contractions every 2–3 min, 45–90 sec duration; intraabdominal pressure is exerted	May experience decreased pain, feels pressure on rectum, bulging perineum, urge to bear down, often excited and eager, grunting sounds or expiratory vocalization
Third stage (placental stage)	Period from delivery of infant to delivery of placenta and membranes	5–30 min	Strong uterine contractions; uterus changing to globular shape; intraabdominal pressure is exerted	Focus on newborn, excited about birth, feeling of relief
Fourth stage	Period from delivery of placenta and membranes to first hour postpartum	1 h	Uterus firm at level of two fingerbreadths above umbilicus	Exploration of newborn; family integration begins; infant alert and responsive

Reeder, S.J., Martin, L.L., and Koniak, D. *Maternity Nursing*. [17th ed.]. Philadelphia: J.B. Lippincott, 1992.

pen continuously, are prolonged, or are insufficient to produce dilatation and effacement. Any of these alterations may result in dysfunctional labor and may even predispose to additional alterations such as dehydration, exhaustion, infection, and fetal compromise.

DYSFUNCTIONAL LABOR. Four labor patterns are reflective of dysfunctional labor. These are *hypertonic labor, hypotonic labor, precipitous labor,* and *prolonged labor.* The characteristics, maternal implications, and fetal or neonatal implications of each pattern are presented in Table 5-8.

PRETERM LABOR. Preterm labor refers to the onset of labor between 20 and 38 weeks' gestation. Labor before

38 weeks' gestation occurs in 5% to 10% of all pregnancies. As much as 75% of neonatal morbidity and mortality can be attributed to preterm delivery of the fetus. Even if the preterm neonate survives, long-term complications such as physical and mental handicaps may occur. Although the exact cause of preterm labor is unknown, fetal, maternal, and placental factors have been known to contribute to the onset of preterm labor. Table 5-9 reflects low-, medium-, and high-risk factors associated with preterm labor.

Early diagnosis is essential if preterm labor is to be interrupted. Contractions occurring at less than 10-minute intervals for 30 to 60 minutes and resulting in cervical dilatation and effacement are strongly suggestive of preterm labor. Conservative management—consisting

TABLE 5-8 *Comparison of Dysfunctional Labor Patterns*

Pattern	Characteristics	Maternal Implications	Fetal/Neonatal Implications
Hypertonic	Occurs in early labor (latent phase)	Exhaustion	Fetal distress
Primary uterine inertia	Occurs most often in nulli-para	Dehydration	Sepsis
	Irregular, ineffective contractions	Uterine rupture	Birth injury
	Lack of uterine relaxation between contractions	Infection of uterus	
	Little to no progress in dilatation of cervix	Vaginal lacerations if delivery is difficult	
	Failure of presenting part to descend		
Hypotonic	Occurs in active labor	Exhaustion	Fetal distress
Secondary uterine inertia	Established contraction pattern converts to one in which contractions occur less often, decrease in intensity, and decrease in duration	Dehydration	Birth injury
		Infection of uterus	
		Increased risk of postpartum hemorrhage	
Precipitous labor	Labor less than 3 h in length	Ruptured uterus	Increased risk for cerebral hemorrhage
		Lacerations	Fetal hypoxia
		No one in attendance for delivery	No immediate care to clear airway, maintain body temperature

of bed rest, increased fluids, and prenatal assessment—is instituted before tocolytic therapy begins. Increased prenatal assessment includes more frequent office visits and possibly home fetal monitoring.

Two major *tocolytics* used in current practice are ritodrine hydrochloride (Yutopar) and terbutaline sulfate (Brethine). Both medications are β-sympathomimetic agents that act on type II β-adrenergic receptors in uterine muscle, bronchioles, and the diaphragm to produce uterine relaxation, bronchodilation, vasodilation, and muscle glycogenolysis. In addition to uterine relaxation, the mother may experience hypotension and a resultant increase in heart rate. Other new drugs used in the treatment of preterm labor include calcium channel blockers and prostaglandin inhibitors.

Magnesium sulfate, a central nervous system depressant, may be administered intravenously in an attempt to control preterm labor. This drug is believed to act by blocking the function of calcium and thus inhibiting uterine contractions. Magnesium toxicity, resulting in respiratory depression and depression of the patellar reflex, is a common problem associated with its use.

POSTTERM LABOR. Postterm labor is a term used to refer to labor occurring after 42 weeks' gestation. The cause is unknown, but it has been associated with anencephaly in the fetus, administration of prostaglandin synthetase inhibitors (aspirin and ibuprofen), and low serum and urine estriol levels.

The greatest risks in postterm pregnancy are related to placental aging and a decreased transfer of oxygen and nutrients to the fetus. Amniotic fluid volume may also decrease, resulting in umbilical cord compression and fetal death. Most often, postmature neonates are pale and have dry, cracked, and peeling skin. The neonate may appear alert but distressed. Both lanugo and vernix tend to be absent. Hair and fingernails are long. Depending on the degree of oxygen deprivation to which the fetus was subjected, the amniotic fluid, umbilical cord, and skin may be meconium-stained, with a green to yellow appearance. This neonate is at increased risk for meconium aspiration, asphyxia, hypoglycemia, cold stress, and polycythemia.

After 40 weeks' gestation, it is essential that close surveillance of the fetus be instituted. This increased surveillance includes physician examinations, nonstress testing, and contraction stress testing if indicated.

CERVICAL FACTORS. One of the most common cervical conditions affecting the process of reproduction is *incompetent cervix*. Incompetent cervix refers to the condition in which the cervix is unable to support the weight of the enlarging uterus during pregnancy. Factors predisposing to incompetent cervix include cervical conizations or bi-

TABLE 5-9 *Low-, Medium-, and High-Risk Factors for Preterm Labor*

Low-Risk Factors	Medium-Risk Factors	High-Risk Factors
Any three of the following factors together equals a high-risk factor	Any two of the following factors together equals a high-risk factor	*MATERNAL FACTORS* Abdominal surgery during pregnancy Acute systemic bacterial infections Incompetent cervix
MATERNAL FACTORS Age: under 16 or over 40 y Anemia Bacteriuria Cholestasis of pregnancy Chronic renal disease Chronic cardiovascular disease Fibroid tumors Low socioeconomic factors Poor prenatal care Repeat first trimester abortions Single parent status Smoking Stature: under 5 ft tall Strenuous demanding work Weight: under 100 lbs prepregnancy weight	*MATERNAL FACTORS* Age: under 16 y Chemical abuse Cone biopsy Hyperthyroidism Narcotic addiction One second trimester abortion Poorly controlled diabetes mellitus Pyelonephritis Unexplained vaginal bleeding after 16 wk gestation Uterine anomalies *PLACENTAL FACTORS* Placenta previa	Intrauterine infections Maternal trauma Multiple gestation Pregnancy-induced hypertension Previous preterm labor Two or more second trimester abortions Untreated Cushing's disease *FETAL FACTORS* Congenital adrenal hyperplasia Fetal infections Multiple gestation Oligohydramnios Polyhydramnios
FETAL FACTORS Breech presentations after 30 wk gestation		

Holmes, J., and Magiera, L. *Maternity Nursing*. New York: Macmillan, 1987.

opsy, prior second-trimester abortion, prior difficult delivery, and exposure to diethylstilbestrol. During subsequent pregnancies, pressure from the enlarging uterus causes painless cervical dilatation. If it is detected early, McDonald's procedure can be performed and a suture placed around the cervical os (Fig. 5-15). The suture is removed at or near term, and the woman is allowed to deliver vaginally. This procedure must be repeated with each subsequent pregnancy.

An alternative procedure is the Shirodkar procedure, in which a purse-string suture is placed around the internal cervical os to maintain a closed cervix. This procedure may be performed before pregnancy occurs and is left in place, necessitating cesarean delivery in subsequent pregnancies.

Passenger

The fetus, as a passenger, must be able to accommodate and descend through the woman's pelvis. The fetal head represents the most important part of the passenger and in most deliveries is the presenting part. If size or mobility of the fetal head prevents descent through or accommodation to the pelvis, vaginal delivery is difficult or impossible.

In addition to the size and mobility of the fetal head, the position, presentation, and attitude of the fetus affect

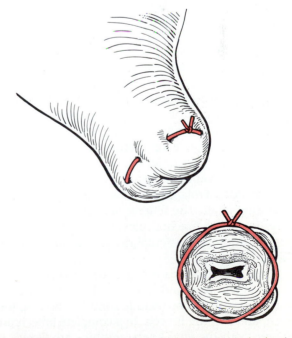

FIGURE 5-15 *A cross section of an incompetent cervix showing a cerclage suture in place. The suture is removed at term to allow cervical dilatation and delivery of the baby.*

accommodation to and descent through the pelvis. Position refers to the relation of a particular fetal point to the front, sides, or back of the maternal pelvis.

MALPOSITION. Malposition refers to any presentation other than occiput anterior, and it can influence labor and birth. An occiput posterior presentation presents a larger diameter to the maternal pelvis. This position increases pressure on the sacral nerves, causing the woman to complain of low back pain and pelvic pressure during labor.

Presentation refers to the fetal part which enters, or presents to, the maternal pelvis. Attitude is the term used to refer to the relation of fetal parts to each other. The most common presentation, cephalic, requires the least adaptation in the birth process. In the normal cephalic presentation, the occiput is the presenting part and the fetal head is completely flexed on the chest. This position allows the smallest diameter of the fetal head to present to the maternal pelvis.

MALPRESENTATIONS. Malpresentations include brow, face, breech, and shoulder presentations. Any one of the malpresentations may result in the need for a cesarean delivery. In a brow presentation, the fetal head is partially extended. This causes the largest anteroposterior (occipitomental) diameter to present to the maternal pelvis. Difficult vaginal delivery may result in cerebral and neck compression, as well as damage to the trachea and larynx. The fetus is also at risk for increased infection if labor is prolonged.

In a face presentation, the fetal head is hyperextended and the occiput may even be in contact with the fetal back. The presenting part is the face. Edema and bruising are common if a face presentation is delivered vaginally. The neonate may also suffer physical injury to the neck if the delivery is difficult. With the use of ultrasound to document the breech position and tocolytic therapy to relax the uterine muscles and prevent contractions, an attempt is sometimes made to turn the fetus to a vertex position. Important prerequisites for successful version are an adequate amount of amniotic fluid and a complete or footling breech that is not engaged at the pelvic inlet.[7]

Breech deliveries account for approximately 3% of term deliveries. Prolapsed cord is a common complication during labor. The fetus is also at risk for physical injury, including brachial plexus palsy, fractures, and spinal cord injury, if vaginal delivery is attempted and difficult.

These presentations are classified according to the attitude of the hips and knees of the fetus. The most common classifications include complete breech, frank breech, and footling breech. In a complete breech presentation, both the fetal knees and hips are flexed. The buttocks and feet present to the maternal pelvis. A frank breech is the most common breech presentation and is characterized by flexions of the fetal thighs and extension of the knees. The presenting part to the maternal pelvis is the buttocks. The footling breech is characterized by extension of knees and legs. Either one foot (single footling) or two feet (double footling) present to the maternal pelvis.

Shoulder presentation is also referred to as transverse lie. In this presentation, the fetal shoulder presents to the maternal pelvis. The acromion process of the scapula may be located either anterior or posterior and either to the woman's right or to her left side.

Any malposition or malpresentation may necessitate a cesarean delivery, depending on the size of the fetus, the maternal pelvis, and the progress of labor. Cesarean delivery is frequently indicated in shoulder, face, and some breech presentations. Prolapsed cord is most often associated with shoulder and breech presentations.

PREMATURE RUPTURE OF THE MEMBRANES. Premature rupture of the membranes refers to the spontaneous rupture of the membranes or leakage of amniotic fluid before the onset of labor. Preterm rupture occurs before 37 weeks' gestation. Predisposing factors include multiparity, incompetent cervix, maternal age greater than 35 years, low weight gain during pregnancy, and cervical damage from surgical instrumentation. Diagnosis can usually be confirmed with Nitrazine Paper, which turns dark blue in the presence of amniotic fluid, and by the presence of ferning.

Risk for the development of chorioamnionitis (infection of the chorion and amnion) is increased, especially if delivery does not occur within 24 hours of rupture. Signs of chorioamnionitis include maternal tachycardia and fever, fetal tachycardia, foul-smelling amniotic fluid, and uterine tenderness. If the membranes rupture more than 48 hours before delivery, the fetus is at increased risk for septicemia, pneumonia, and infection of the umbilical cord.

Premature rupture of the membranes early in pregnancy is more threatening because of prematurity of the fetus, possible malposition, risk of prolapsed cord, and infection. Occasionally, corticosteroids are used to increase fetal lung maturity and lessen the chance of respiratory distress syndrome in the preterm neonate.

PROLAPSED UMBILICAL CORD. A prolapsed umbilical cord is one that descends into the birth canal before the presenting part (Fig. 5-16). As a result, pressure is placed on the umbilical cord, which can interfere with fetal circulation. The progress of labor is not affected, nor is the woman's physical adaptation. However, this condition represents an obstetrical emergency for the fetus and requires immediate action.

Prolapsed umbilical cord is often associated with rupture of the membranes if the presenting part is not fully engaged in the pelvis or in cases of malpresentation.

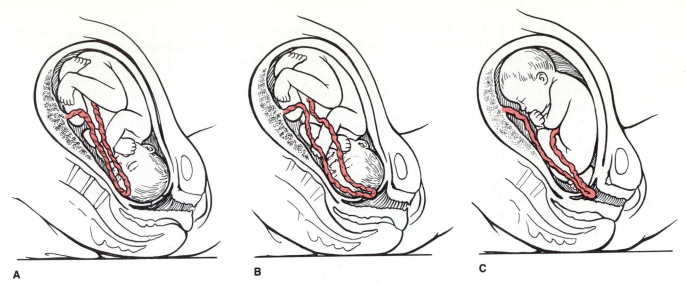

A **B** **C**

FIGURE 5-16 *Umbilical cord prolapse.* **A.** *Occult prolapse and compression of cord by fetal head.* **B.** *Forelying cord palpable in cervical os.* **C.** *Complete cord prolapse with breech presentation (Childbirth Graphics). (May, K.A., and Mahlmeister, L.R.* Comprehensive Maternity Nursing *[3rd ed.]. Philadelphia: J.B. Lippincott, 1994.)*

The umbilical cord may prolapse in varying degrees. It may protrude from the vagina, it may prolapse into the vagina but not be visible to the naked eye, or it may be compressed from pressure of the presenting part.

Evidence of cord compression can also be observed during fetal monitoring. Compression of the umbilical cord and reduction in blood flow between fetus and placenta result in variable decelerations on the monitor. Reduced blood flow leads to increased peripheral resistance and increased fetal blood pressure. This response stimulates the baroceptors in the aortic arch and carotid sinuses, which produces a slowing of the fetal heart rate.

Perinatal mortality depends on the degree of cord compression and the time between diagnosis and delivery. Knee-chest or Trendelenburg position can aid in circulation until delivery is possible. A gloved hand to provide pressure on the presenting part may also be used to relieve compression on the cord. The administration of oxygen to the mother increases the oxygen supply to the fetus.

Passage

The passage through which the fetus must pass includes not only the bony pelvis but also the cervix, vagina, and introitus. Size and shape of the pelvis are key factors in determining whether the woman can deliver the fetus vaginally. There are four classifications of pelves: gynecoid, android, anthropoid, and platypelloid (Fig. 5-17). The gynecoid pelvis is most often referred to as the

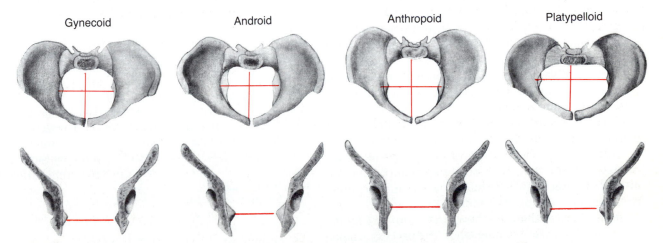

Gynecoid   Android   Anthropoid   Platypelloid

FIGURE 5-17 *Caldwell-Maloy classification of pelvic types. The typical shape of the inlet for each type is shown at the top. A line has been drawn through the widest transverse diameter, dividing the inlet into an anterior and posterior segment. The longitudinal line illustrates the anteroposterior diameter of the inlet. The typical interspinous diameter of each type is depicted at the bottom. (Reeder, S.J., Martin, L.L., and Koniak, D.* Maternity Nursing *[17th ed.]. Philadelphia: J.B. Lippincott, 1992.)*

typical female pelvis. Pelvic measurements for this type of pelvis are sufficient for the average full-term fetus.

In determining the adequacy of the pelvis for vaginal delivery, it is important to examine the sacrum, the ischial spines, and the pubic arch. A concave sacrum provides optimal capacity, but a sacrum that is flat or convex decreases pelvic capacity. A fixed sacrum may also interfere with descent of the presenting part. Sharp ischial spines decrease the transverse pelvic measurement, and a pubic arch that is narrow with a decreased angle prevents the fetal head from pivoting as it passes under the arch. Ideally, the pubic arch is wide, with at least a 90-degree angle.

In making a determination regarding the adequacy of the pelvis, the examiner must consider not only pelvic measurements but also the position and size of the fetus. Radiographic pelvimetry and computed tomography pelvimetry are useful tools in determining pelvic adequacy relative to fetal size.

▼ Chapter Summary

▼ Throughout the gestational period, fetal development encompasses three stages: the germinal, embryonic, and fetal periods. The placenta, which forms from fusion of the endometrium and enlarging chorionic villi, the fetal membranes, and the yolk sac are critical elements in the process of fetal development. Three unique structures of fetal circulation—the ductus arteriosus, the ductus venosus, and the foramen ovale—are responsible for the oxygenation and nutritional functions of the placenta.

▼ Maternal factors that affect the biophysical development of the fetus include hypertensive disorders of pregnancy, diabetes mellitus, cardiac disease, and sexually transmitted disease and infections. Maternal nutrition and teratogens also affect the development of the fetus. Fetal factors affecting the biophysical development include the following: placenta previa, abruptio placentae, ectopic pregnancy, placental insufficiency, and multiple gestation.

▼ Prenatal diagnostic studies that provide information regarding the status of the pregnancy include ultrasonography, chorionic villus sampling, amniocentesis, fetoscopy, percutaneous umbilical blood sampling, and fetal biophysical profile.

▼ After approximately 266 days within the uterus, the process of labor begins. Possible explanations for the onset of this process include hormonal stimulation, uterine distention, and prostaglandins. Braxton-Hicks contractions, cervical changes, show, and rupture of membranes are signs of impending labor. The process of labor is divided into four stages: dilatation and effacement, expulsion, placental expulsion, and recovery. The four Ps—power, passage, passenger, and psyche—represent the various alterations requiring adaptation in the delivery process. Alterations in the *power* of timing, strength, and efficiency of uterine contractions may result in dysfunctional labor, preterm labor, postterm labor, or incompetent cervix. Malposition, malpresentation, premature rupture of the membranes, and prolapsed umbilical cord are *passenger* factors that necessitate adaptation during the process of labor and delivery. *Passage* factors include alterations in the pelvis, cervix, vagina, and introitus. *Psyche* factors include the effects of anxiety, tension, and fear, which can lengthen the duration of labor and delivery.

▼ References

1. Auvenshine, M.A., and Enriquez, M.G. *Comprehensive Maternity Nursing: Prenatal and Women's Health*. Boston: Jones & Bartlett, 1990.
2. Dickason, E.J., Schult, M.O., and Silverman, B.L. *Maternal-Infant Nursing Care*. St. Louis: Mosby, 1990.
3. Duff, P. Acute fatty liver of pregnancy. In Clark, S., Cotton, D., Hankins, G., and Phelan, J. (eds.), *Critical Care Obstetrics*. Cambridge: Blackwell Scientific, 1991.
4. Fenster, L. Eskenazi, B., and Swan, S. Caffeine consumption during pregnancy and fetal growth. *Am. J. Public Health* 81:458–461, 1991.
5. Gortrie, T.M., McKinney, E.S., and Murray, S.S. *Foundations of Maternal Newborn Nursing*. Philadelphia: W.B. Saunders, 1994.
6. Khong, T., Sawyer, I., and Heryet, A. An immunohistologic study of endothelialization of uteroplacental vessels in human pregnancy. *Am. J. Obstet. Gynecol.* 167:751, 1992.
7. Martin, L.L., and Reeder, S.J. *Maternity Nursing* (17th ed.). Philadelphia: J.B. Lippincott, 1992.
8. May, K.A., and Mahlmeister, L.R. *Maternal and Neonatal Nursing: Family-Centered Care* (3rd ed.). Philadelphia: J.B. Lippincott, 1994.
9. Mendez, H., and Jule, J.E. Care of the infant born exposed to human immunodeficiency virus. *Obstet. Gynecol. Clin. North Am.* 17:637–650, 1990.
10. New York Heart Association. *Nomenclature and Criteria for Diagnosis and Diseases of the Heart and Blood Vessels* (5th ed.). New York: New York Heart Association, 1955.
11. Poole, J.H. Getting perspective on HELLP Syndrome. *Matern. Child. Nurs. J.* 13:432, 1988.
12. Schuster, C.S. Intrauterine development. In Schuster, C.S., and Ashburn, S.S. (eds.). *The Process of Human Development: A Holistic Approach*. Boston: Little, Brown, 1986.
13. Sherwen, L.N., Scoloveno, M.A., and Weingarter, C.T. *Nursing Care of the Childbearing Family*. Norwalk: Appleton & Lange, 1991.
14. Simpson, K.R., Moore, K.S., and LaMartina, M.H. Acute fatty liver of pregnancy. *J. Obstet. Gynecol. Neonatal. Nurs.* 22:213–219, 1993.
15. Watson, W.J., and Seeds, J.W. Acute fatty liver of pregnancy. *Obstet. Gynecol. Surv.* 45:585–593. 1990.
16. White, P. Classification of obstetric diabetes. *Am. J. Obstet. Gynecol.* 130:228, 1978.

Chapter 6

Biophysical Development of Children

Joy H. Whatley / Sharron P. Schlosser

▼ **CHAPTER OUTLINE**

▼ **LEARNING OBJECTIVES**

1 Discuss the respiratory, cardiovascular, thermoregulation, and hepatic adaptations of the neonate during transition from intrauterine to extrauterine life.
2 Describe the biophysical developments that occur during the neonatal period.
3 Describe the physiologic changes occurring in each body system during the various stages of childhood.
4 Identify the basic nutritional needs of children and adolescents.
5 Identify and discuss those factors that affect development in the various stages of childhood.
6 Discuss the role that accidents play in alterations and adaptations during childhood and adolescence.
7 Summarize motor and sensory development from birth throughout childhood.
8 Differentiate among the terms pubescence, puberty, and adolescence.
9 Describe the physiologic changes that occur in each body system as a response to puberty.
10 Discuss the pathophysiologic risks of obesity, anorexia nervosa, and bulimia nervosa in adolescence.
11 Describe the mechanisms involved in the pathophysiology of acne vulgaris.
12 Differentiate suicidal behavior and methods in males and in females.
13 Discuss the various chemical agents most commonly abused by adolescents and their actions and effects.
14 Discuss the physiologic and psychosocial risks associated with sexual activity during adolescence.
15 Discuss the more common menstrual disorders of adolescence.
16 Discuss the prevalence and problems associated with homosexual behavior in adolescents.

▼ *Neonate*

The neonatal period, the first 28 days of life, represents a time of dramatic anatomic and biochemical changes as the neonate adapts from intrauterine to extrauterine life. Before delivery, the fetus was dependent on the mother for oxygen, elimination, nutrition, thermoregulation, and fluid balance. In the first minute after birth, the normal newborn changes from a dependent intrauterine existence to an independent being who is capable of oxygenating, perfusing, and heating his or her own body. The vital occurrence that must follow birth is the change from respiration through the placenta to respiration through the newborn lungs.

INTRAUTERINE PULMONARY ADAPTATION

Fetal respiratory movements have been documented as early as the 13th week of gestation. These movements increase in frequency and strength as the pregnancy approaches term, or 40 weeks gestation. About 3 days before birth, the frequency decreases dramatically. Because the intrauterine oxygen needs are met by the placenta, fetal breathing movements apparently contribute very little to the oxygen needs of the fetus. It is thought that the fetal breathing movements may stimulate the synthesis, release, and distribution of surfactant.[23]

In utero, in addition to the fetal breathing movements, the fetal lungs produce fluid that helps prevent their collapse. *Surfactant*, produced by type II alveolar cells beginning at approximately 20 to 24 weeks gestation and continuing to term, increases and is part of the lung fluid as term approaches. Surfactant helps to stabilize the alveoli and decrease surface tension, preventing alveoli collapse. It also helps to establish a functioning residual capacity. Maternal health stressors, such as pregnancy-induced hypertension or heroin abuse, stimulate an increase in surfactant production. It is thought that the mother, who is stressed, produces more steroids. If the fetus needs to be removed from the intrauterine environment before term, the mother may be given steroids to enhance fetal lung maturity.

Fetal lung fluid is significant in births that involve certain presentations and in cesarean births. During vaginal delivery, the infant's chest is squeezed and then reexpands rapidly. It is thought that the thoracic compression in a vaginal delivery, along with the effect of gravity in the vertex presentation, helps to force out fetal lung fluid just before the first breath. The small amount of fetal lung fluid that remains in the lungs after birth is absorbed by the lymphatic system. The cesarean section delivery does not allow for the thoracic compression or for drainage of fluid by gravity. Therefore, the infant delivered by cesarean section or by a presentation other than vertex is at a greater risk for respiratory problems.

EXTRAUTERINE PULMONARY ADAPTATION

It is thought that several stimuli are responsible for the initiation of respiration. These stimuli are mechanical, sensory, chemical, and thermal in nature. Flowchart 6-1 outlines the interaction of stimuli in the initiation of respiration.

The mechanical forces are the thoracic compression that occurs with vaginal delivery and the change from intrauterine to extrauterine pressure subsequent to uterine contraction in labor. In addition to expelling fetal lung fluid, the thoracic compression creates a negative intrathoracic pressure that helps the lungs reexpand or "recoil," pulling in a small amount of air. When the uterus is relaxed, the intrauterine pressure is 15 cm H_2O. If the membranes are still intact, the 15 cm H_2O pressure is evenly dispersed and cannot influence the amount of pressure in the lungs. On rupture of the membranes and descent of the fetus into the lower uterine segment, uterine contractions provide up to 75 cm H_2O pressure, producing thoracic compression and expelling lung fluid.

The neonate is overstimulated during the birth process. Sensory stimuli that probably contribute to the initiation of respiration are bright lights, noise, and the sensation of weight with the addition of gravity.

Cold is a powerful thermal stimulus in the initiation of the first breath. The normal intrauterine temperature is 37°C. The delivery room may be as cold as 22°C. Extreme cooling of the infant increases the oxygen need and produces respiratory and metabolic acidosis. Chemical changes in transition occur as a result of transient asphyxia. Mild asphyxia (hypercapnia, hypoxia, and acidosis) normally occur at delivery. If chemical changes are prolonged, the respiratory center becomes depressed. Drugs given to the mother near the time of delivery can also depress the respiratory center. The normal infant

---

TABLE 6-1   *Arterial Blood Gas Values Prior to the Initial Breath Compared to Adult Values*

Substance	Values
BEFORE INITIAL BREATH	
Oxygen saturation	10%–20%
Carbon dioxide partial pressure or tension	58 mm Hg
Arterial pH	7.28
ADULT	
Oxygen saturation	96%–100%
Carbon dioxide tension	35–45 mm Hg
Arterial pH	7.35–7.45

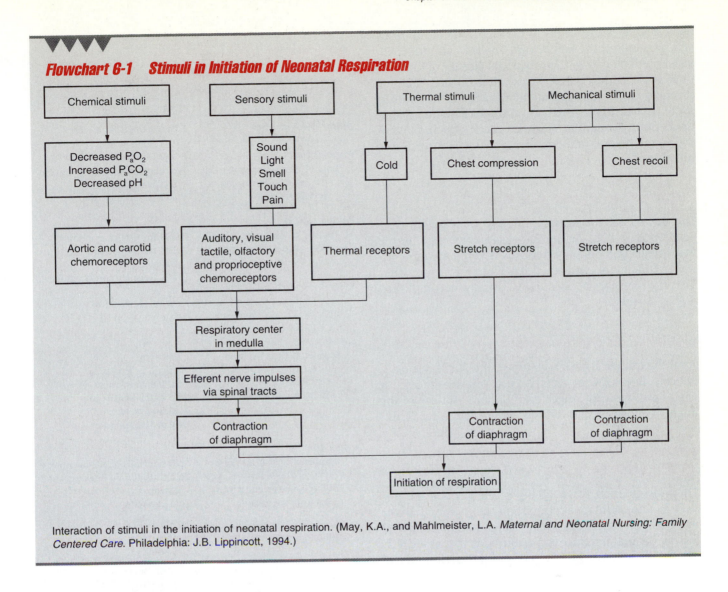

Flowchart 6-1   Stimuli in Initiation of Neonatal Respiration

Interaction of stimuli in the initiation of neonatal respiration. (May, K.A., and Mahlmeister, L.A. *Maternal and Neonatal Nursing: Family Centered Care.* Philadelphia: J.B. Lippincott, 1994.)

usually takes the first breath within 30 seconds after delivery, and a normal neonatal breathing pattern is usually established within 90 seconds.

Once established, the respirations range 30 to 60 per minute. It is not unusual for the respirations to be 80 per minute for the first few minutes after birth. Characteristics of newborn respirations are irregularity of rate, rhythm, and depth. As respirations continue, the arterial partial pressure of oxygen (Pao_2) increases, the arterial partial pressure of carbon dioxide ($Paco_2$) decreases, and blood pH approaches adult values (Table 6-1). Pulmonary blood vessels that were constricted in utero dilate in response to the increased oxygen levels, causing an increase in blood flow to the infant's lungs. The results of pulmonary transition are the following: 1) surfactant production is maintained; 2) residual volume is established; 3) physiologic acid–base balance continues; 4) blood flow to the lungs is increased; 5) vital signs are within normal limits, and 6) the infant demonstrates a pink, oxygenated color.[9]

EXTRAUTERINE CIRCULATORY ADAPTATION

The anatomic and biochemical changes that occur during conversion from fetal to adult circulation are closely related to the changes that occur in the respiratory system. These changes result from the alterations in systemic and pulmonary pressures after the initial breath, establishment of respirations, and clamping of the umbilical cord. The major cardiovascular changes that occur in response to initiation of respiration and clamping of the umbilical cord are closure of the foramen ovale, closure of the ductus arteriosus, and closure of the ductus venosus (see also pp. 489–491).

Closure of the Foramen Ovale

After the initial breath and after the clamping of the umbilical cord, a large amount of blood is returned to the heart and lungs. Pulmonary arteries dilate in response to the increased oxygen, and the pulmonary pressure is decreased. Pressure drops in the right side of the heart and increases in the left atrium. The increase in the left atrial pressure causes the functional closure of the foramen ovale within a few hours after birth. It may be several months before permanent closure of the foramen ovale occurs. Right-to-left shunting of blood may continue until permanent closure occurs, which explains the nonpathologic murmurs heard in the neonate during this time.[18]

Closure of the Ductus Arteriosus

The ductus arteriosus is sensitive to increases in oxygen concentration. As the Pao_2 levels increase after the first breath, the ductus arteriosus is stimulated to constrict. Functional closure occurs within 15 hours after delivery. Permanent closure is usually accomplished within 3 weeks.

Closure of the Ductus Venosus

After the umbilical cord is clamped, the ductus venosus, which connected fetal portal circulation with the inferior vena cava, can no longer carry blood. Fibrosis of the ductus venosus occurs within 3 to 7 days after birth.[3]

EXTRAUTERINE THERMOREGULATION ADAPTATION

Thermoregulation is the ability of the neonate to produce heat to maintain a normal body temperature. In the newborn, the balance between heat production and heat loss, or the maintenance of a stable body temperature, is possible with limited fluctuations in the environmental temperature.[3]

Newborns are prone to heat loss because of their unique anatomic characteristics and the exposure to environmental influences that occurs at delivery. Factors contributing to loss of heat are a large surface area in relation to body weight, a limited metabolic capability, and limited fat deposits. A decreased amount of adipose tissue results in decreased thermal regulation. The skin of the newborn is thin, and blood vessels lie close to the skin surface, which result in transfer of heat to the environment. The newborn is wet at delivery, and the environmental temperature in the delivery room is much lower than the intrauterine temperature.

Four specific mechanisms cause heat loss in the neonate: 1) evaporation, which is the conversion of water on the wet newborn skin to vapor; 2) convection, or the transfer of heat in response to cool air; 3) conduction, which is the transfer of heat when the infant is placed on a cool surface; and 4) radiation, or the transfer of heat from the infant to cool surfaces not in direct contact with the infant's skin. Table 6-2 outlines the major environmental factors that contribute to neonatal heat loss.

TABLE 6-2 *Environmental Factors Contributing to Neonatal Heat Loss*

Major Mechanisms	Environmental Factors
EVAPORATION Loss of heat when water on the infant's skin is converted to a vapor	Wet blankets or diapers in contact with skin Water or urine on skin
CONVECTION Transfer of heat when a flow of cool air passes over the infant's skin	Drafts from open windows Drafts from open portholes on isolette Drafts from air-conditioning ducts Flow of unheated oxygen over face
CONDUCTION Transfer of heat when the infant comes in direct contact with cooler surfaces and objects	Cold mattresses, cold sidewalls in crib or isolette Cold blankets, shirts, diapers Cold hands of caregiver Cold weight scale Cold stethoscope
RADIATION Transfer of heat from the infant to cooler surfaces and objects not in direct contact with the infant	Cold sidewalls of crib or isolette Cold outside building walls and windows Cold equipment in infant's environment

The neonate responds to heat loss through vasomotor control, thermal insulation, limited shivering, muscular activity, and nonshivering thermogenesis.[3] Vasomotor control helps to control heat loss through vasoconstriction of the blood vessels in the skin. The amount of thermal regulation in the newborn is directly related to his or her amount of white fat, which is a heat-retaining tissue. Fat accumulation begins about 32 weeks gestation; premature babies and infants with intrauterine growth retardation (IUGR) are at an increased risk for heat loss because of their inadequate thermal regulation capability. Shivering, a major mechanism of heat production in adults, is limited in the newborn. Muscular activity contributes somewhat to heat production but is not a significant source of heat. Nonshivering thermogenesis is the primary mechanism for heat production in the neonate. In response to a decrease in skin temperature, thermal receptors transmit impulses to the central nervous system (CNS). In response to stimulation of the sympathetic nervous system, norepinephrine is released by the adrenal glands and by nerve endings in a special type of adipose tissue, brown fat. Brown fat is remarkably vascular and is metabolized to produce heat. Brown fat makes up about 1.5% of total body weight and is found between the scapulae, behind the sternum, and around the neck, head, heart, great vessels, kidneys and adrenal glands.[3]

Nonshivering thermogenesis and the increase in the metabolic rate are effective mechanisms for heat production. However, they also cause increased demands for glucose and oxygen. Normal term infants counterbalance these increased demands by increasing their respiratory rate and releasing glucose that is stored in the liver. If cold stress continues or the neonate is compromised, brown fat and glucose become expended. This depletion of brown fat and glucose leads to a decrease in surfactant production and an increase in pulmonary vascular resistance. In this situation, an external heat source is essential to maintain a normal body temperature.[19]

EXTRAUTERINE HEPATIC ADAPTATION

Before birth, the placenta is responsible for the breakdown and excretion of bilirubin; after birth, the liver assumes this role. However, it is thought that the liver of the normal neonate produces inadequate amounts of glucuronosyltransferase, which is needed to change indirect or unconjugated bilirubin to direct bilirubin (see p. 809). Bilirubin is the end product of the breakdown of red blood cells (RBCs). The normal lifespan of the RBC in the neonate is only 80 to 120 days. As the RBCs become older, they become fragile and hemoglobin is split into two fragments, heme and globin. Heme is the unconjugated, indirect fraction, which is fat soluble. Direct bilirubin is water soluble and can be excreted by the kidneys. The unbound or indirect form of bilirubin can exit the vascular system and infiltrate other extravascular tissues, such as the skin or sclera, causing jaundice or icteric (yellow) skin color.

Physiologic Hyperbilirubinemia

The most frequent factors thought to contribute to physiologic jaundice are the short life span of RBCs, decreased production of liver enzymes, and increased numbers of RBCs in the neonate.[3,4] Physiologic jaundice occurs in approximately 50% of newborns, most often around 48 hours of age. Physiologic jaundice usually disappears by 1 week of age, and bilirubin levels usually do not exceed 12 mg per 100 mL. If jaundice occurs as early as 24 hours of age, it is considered pathologic, not physiologic.

Phototherapy, the process of exposing the newborn's skin to intense fluorescent light, is frequently used to treat physiologic jaundice. Phototherapy causes a structural alteration of bilirubin in the skin of the newborn by oxidizing the unconjugated, indirect bilirubin, which is fat soluble, into a water-soluble form. The water-soluble form, or direct, conjugated bilirubin, is excreted in bile, urine, and feces without going through the usual conjugation process in the liver.[29]

BIOPHYSICAL DEVELOPMENT

Normal values and variation of normal for weight, head circumference, chest circumference, temperature, pulse, respirations, and blood pressure of the normal, full-term neonate are found in Table 6-3.

▼ Infant

BIOPHYSICAL DEVELOPMENT

Biologic Growth

The period of infancy encompasses the first year after birth. The rapid, continuous growth that began at conception proceeds in a specific and orderly manner. Evidence of this rapid growth pattern can be seen in the month-by-month changes in the infant. Specific measures of height, weight, chest and head circumference, dentition, reflexes, and motor development provide evidence of these changes. A summary of average biologic growth on a month-by-month basis is found in Table 6-4. One must remember that these findings only represent the norm and that individual infants vary. Individual variation may be more evident in premature infants.

During the period of infancy, the baby grows an average of 2.5 cm (1 inch) per month during the first 6 months of life, and about 1.5 cm (0.5 inch) per month from 7 to 12 months of age. This rate of growth indicates a gain of approximately 50% of birth length during the first year of life. Although this growth occurs primarily in the trunk, the head continues to constitute a large proportion of the infant's body surface. The normal weight gain provides for the doubling of the birth weight during the first 4 to 6 months of life and tripling of the birth weight by 12 months, at which time the average weight is 9.75 kg (21.5 pounds).

Head circumference represents another area of rapid growth during infancy, indicative of brain maturation. From birth to 6 months, the head increases in size by approximately 1.5 cm per month, and from 7 to 12 months, by 0.5 cm per month. This accounts for an approximately 33% increase during the first year of life. This growth is accompanied by closure of the posterior fontanel (soft spot at the sagittal and lambdoid sutures). The anterior fontanel (soft spot at the coronal, frontal, and sagittal sutures) closes between 12 and 18 months.

Chest measurements can also indicate the overall growth of the individual infant. By the time the infant is 1 year of age, the head and chest should be about equal in size. The chest also changes in contour during this

TABLE 6-3 *Biophysical Measurements of Normal Full-Term Neonate*

Value	Average Findings	Normal Variations
Weight	3400 gm (7.5 lbs); birth weight is regained within 2 wk	2700–4000 gm (6–9 lb.); acceptable weight loss is 5%–10% of birth weight
Head circumference	33–37 cm (13–14..5 in)	Molding of head can affect head circumference
Chest circumference	31–35 cm (12.5–14 in)	2 cm less than head circumference; breast engorgement can affect chest circumference
Length	48–53 cm (19–21 in)	44–55 cm (18–22 in)
Temperature	Rectal 36.5–37°C (97.7–98.6°F) Axillary 36.5–37°C (97.7–99°F)	Environmental temperature extremes, sepsis, and altered neurologic function can contribute to hypothermia or hyperthermia
Apical pulse	120–160 beats per min (bpm)	100 bpm while sleeping, 180 bpm while crying
Respirations	40–60 breaths per min (bpm)	First hour following birth normal tachypnea, >60 bpm, and grunting, flaring, and retracting may occur
Blood pressure	71/49 mm Hg	Varies with activity level. Systolic: 60–82 mm Hg. Diastolic: 42–50 mm Hg. At 10 days of age: systolic 94–100 mm Hg; diastolic slightly increased

Values summarized from Reeder, S.J., Martin, L.L., and Koniak, D. *Maternity Nursing* (17th ed.). Philadelphia: J.B. Lippincott, 1992.

time, as the lateral diameter become larger than the anteroposterior diameter.

Dentition

The eruption of the primary teeth represents a continuation of development begun in utero. The first two deciduous (temporary) teeth erupt between 5 and 7 months of age. During the period of teething, the infant may drool, chew on hard objects, and become irritable. There is no physiologic basis for high temperature and diarrhea. If the infant refuses to eat, however, teething may be associated with low-grade fever from slight dehydration.

Neuromuscular Development

Neuromuscular development follows the general principles of cephalocaudal and proximodistal as the infant refines both gross and fine motor skills. Gross motor skills include head control, sitting, standing, and walking. Fine motor skills make use of the hands and fingers.

Head lag, noted as the neonate is pulled from a lying to a sitting position, becomes minimal by 4 months of age. Increased head control becomes evident as the infant progresses to lifting the head and chest while supporting the weight on the forearms. By 6 months of age, the infant can lift the head, chest, and abdomen and support the weight on the hands. This development facilitates rolling over. The infant can willfully roll from front to back at 5 months of age and from back to front at the age of 6 months. As the back becomes straighter and stronger, the infant develops the ability to sit by leaning forward for support at 7 months of age and unsupported at 8 months.

Before about 7 months of age, the infant is unable to support weight on the feet and legs. However, by age 9 months the infant has developed the ability to stand while holding onto furniture. The ability to crawl occurs by 10 months of age, the child takes steps while holding furniture or having hands held by 11 months of age, and walks with one hand held by 12 months of age. Walking unsupported occurs between 12 and 15 months of age.

During the first 2 to 3 months of life, grasping occurs as a reflex. Gradually, the infant progresses from a visual grasp, to palmar grasp, and finally to pincher grasp of smaller objects by 9 to 10 months of age.

Sensory Development

Sensory development involves the eyes, ears, tongue, nose, and skin. In addition to visual acuity, visual development is concerned with binocularity and stereopsis. In binocularity, the infant develops the ability to fuse

TABLE 6-4 *Biophysical Measurements of the Infant*

	1 Month	3 Months	5 Months	6 Months	7 Months	9 Months	12 Months
WEIGHT	4.4 ± 0.8 kg (10 ± 1.5 lb); gains about 680 g/mo (1.5 lb) for first 6 mo	5.7 ± 0.8 kg (12.3 ± 2 lb)	Doubles birth weight	7.4 ± 1 kg (16.5 ± 2.5 lb); gains about 340 gm/mo (0.75 lb)			10 ± 1.5 kg (22 ± 3 lb); triples birth weight
HEAD CIRCUMFERENCE	Increases 1.5 cm (0.5 in) per mo for first 6 mo			43 cm (17 in); increases 0.5 cm (0.25) in per mo for 6–12 mo	46 cm (18 in); increased by one-third since birth; head and chest measurement equal		Girl: 46 cm Boy: 47 cm
LENGTH	Approximately 53 ± 2.5 cm (21 ± 1 in); increases about 2.5 cm (1 in) per mo for first 6 mo	60 ± 2 cm (23.5 ± 1 in)					Length increases by 50% Average girl: 72 cm Average boy: 74 cm
PULSE	110–180 bpm				120–130 bpm		90–140 min
RESPIRATIONS	35 ± 10				30 ± 10		20–40/min
BLOOD PRESSURE	80/50 ± 20/10	80/50 ± 20/10		90/60 ± 28/10	96/66 ± 30/24		
DENTITION				two lower central incisors 6 ± 2 mo	upper central 7.5 ± 2 mo; lower lateral 7 ± 2 mo	upper laterals 9 ± 2 mo	6–8 deciduous teeth

Values summarized from D.B. Jackson and R.B. Saunders. *Child Health Nursing.* Philadelphia: J.B. Lippincott, 1993.

two ocular images into one cerebral image. This ability should be well developed by 4 months of age. Strabismus occurs when there is a lack of binocularity and may result in blindness if left untreated.

Stereopsis, or depth perception, is developed by 7 to 9 months of age. Throughout infancy, children display a preference for the human face. By 6 months of age, infants respond to facial expressions and react to the faces of strangers. This ability contributes to the stranger anxiety that evident by 7 or 8 months of age.

The parachute reflex develops by 7 months of age and persists indefinitely. This reflex response produces forward extension of hands and fingers when the infant, suspended in a horizontal prone position, is suddenly thrust downward.

The ability to hear is evident from birth: the neonate responds to loud noise with a startle reflex. The quieting effect of low-pitched sounds, such as the human heartbeat or a lullaby, is thought to originate from prenatal time. By 3 months of age, the infant attempts to locate sound by turning the head in the direction of the sound. The infant begins to imitate sounds at about 4 months and responds to his or her own name by 4 to 6 months of age. By the time the infant is 1 year of age, he or she can recognize the sound of words such as "no" and the names of other family members.

Smell, touch, and taste continue to develop throughout infancy. Various taste preferences are present at 7 months of age and continue to develop throughout childhood.

FACTORS AFFECTING DEVELOPMENT AND HEALTH

Sleep

The infant should begin to sleep through the night in 8- to 10-hour intervals by 3 to 4 months of age. Total sleep needs, including naps, are variable, but average 13 to 15 hours per day. Persistent night feedings, night crying, and nightmares are the most common sleep problems during infancy.

Nutrition

Adequate caloric intake is essential to support the rapid growth of infancy. As growth decreases in the first year, energy requirements decrease from 120 kcal/kg/day at birth to 100 kcal/kg/day at 1 year.[5] The primary food during infancy is milk. For breast-fed infants, the only supplements needed are iron and fluoride, and vitamin D if the mother's diet is deficient. Fluoride is a dietary supplement needed by infants who are bottle-fed. Formula intake for bottle-fed babies should not exceed 32 oz/day.[36]

There has long been a controversy about when solid food should be introduced into the infant's diet. Most authorities advocate the introduction of solid food at about 5 to 6 months of age. Several developmental factors support this time frame: 1) the gastrointestinal tract should be sufficiently mature to allow digestion of the more complex solid foods; 2) there is disappearance of the tongue thrust or extrusion reflex; 3) the infant has the ability to control the head and neck; and 4) the eruption of the primary teeth facilitates biting and chewing.

After the decision is made to introduce solid foods, new foods should be introduced one at a time and in small amounts (approximately 1 teaspoon the first time). Cereal is the first food because of its high iron content. Fruit, vegetables, and meat are then added sequentially. Egg yolk is usually introduced before egg white because of the sensitivity associated with egg white. Crackers and zwieback are finger foods recommended at about 6 months of age.

By 12 months of age, the infant usually has sufficient maturity to drink from a cup and indicates readiness for weaning. Weaning occurs gradually as the bottle is replaced one feeding at a time. Dental caries related to bottle feeding are a significant health problem associated with milk or juice bottle-feeding at bedtime. From the time primary teeth erupt, care should be taken to clean the teeth with a damp cloth.

Malnutrition, failure to thrive, and *colic* are alterations associated with nutrition. Malnutrition reflects poor or inadequate nutrition or overnutrition. Iron deficiency anemia and vitamin deficiencies are the most common examples of inadequate nutrition. Overnutrition often occurs with the introduction of solid foods if there is no decrease in milk intake. Social, cultural, and economic factors contribute to malnutrition.

Failure to thrive (FTT) is a condition associated with a weight below the third percentile when charted on a growth chart. FTT can be further classified as organic or inorganic. Organic FTT is associated with such physical conditions as heart disease, cystic fibrosis, gastroesophageal reflux, malabsorption, and endocrine or renal dysfunction. Inorganic FTT is a failure to grow in the absence of diagnosed disease. Psychosocial problems between the infant and primary caregiver, including inadequate parent–child bonding, isolation, and caregiver inadequate coping, are the basis for inorganic FTT. On occasion, a combination of physical and psychosocial problems may be present.

Colic is a common condition associated with early infancy. It occurs primarily in the first 3 to 4 months of life and is characterized by paroxysmal intestinal cramping associated with increased gas, abdominal distention, and pain. The infant exhibits loud crying accompanied by drawing of the legs up on the abdomen. Tolerance for food continues to be good, and the infant demonstrates a steady gain in weight.

Immunity and Immunizations

The immune system of the infant does not respond to environmental antigens even though the cells of the system are present. Infants are not able to localize antigens at a site of infection. Early in life, maternal antibodies provide some protection from infection, both through maternal-placental transmission and through breast-feeding. As these antibodies decline in number and effectiveness, the infant must actively produce specific antibodies to combat a wide array of infectious organisms. The infant exhibits adult levels of immunoglobulin M (IgM) by 9 months of age and approximately 40% of adult levels of immunoglobulin (IgG) by 12 months. Both T- and B-lymphocyte function gradually increase, and immunity to many antigens is attained through natural exposure and through immunizations (see pp. 318–320).

The advent of immunizations has been instrumental in decreasing mortality and morbidity from communicable diseases in children. Immunizations should include diphtheria-tetanus-pertussis (DTP), trivalent oral poliovirus (OPV), measles-mumps-rubella (MMR), *Haemophilus influenzae* B, and hepatitis B. The Committee on Infectious Diseases of the American Academy of Pediatrics and the Advisory Committee on Immunization Practices of the U.S. Public Health Service recommend that immunizations commence at 2 months of age with DTP and OPV and follow the recommended intervals. The MMR immunization is recommended at age 15 months. One conjugated vaccine for *Haemophilus influenzae* B has now been approved for initial injection at 2 months of age. Hepatitis B immunizations should begin at birth, with additional injections at 1 and 6 months after the initial injection.

ALTERATIONS AND ADAPTATIONS

Sudden Infant Death Syndrome

Sudden infant death syndrome (SIDS) is the major cause of death between 1 week and 1 year of age. It is especially devastating for the family because it involves the loss of an apparently normally developed, healthy infant. Even the postmortem examination sometimes fails to reveal the cause of death. Major characteristics associated with SIDS are summarized in Box 6-1. Although the specific cause of SIDS remains unknown, chronic hypoxia, prolonged apnea, or both may contribute to the death. Flowchart 6-2 shows some factors that may be causative in some SIDS deaths. Pulmonary edema, inflammatory changes of the upper respiratory passage, and petechial hemorrhages in the lungs and pericardium are characteristic findings on postmortem examination.

Accidents

Accidents represent another important cause of injury and death in infants, especially from 6 to 12 months of age. During this period, the infant is growing and devel-

BOX 6-1 ▼ Major Characteristics Associated with Sudden Infant Death Syndrome	
Family background	Highest in low birth weight, premature infants of adolescent mothers; underweight white males; black infants; and infants of multiple births
Siblings	No greater risk than general population when matched for maternal age and birth order
Previous health	Detailed history may show abnormalities
Age	Greatest in 1–6 mo old; peak incidence 2–4 mo
Sex	Males greater risk
Season of year	Fall and winter months
Time of day	Between midnight and 9 AM

oping rapidly. Curiosity leads to an irresistible urge to explore. This exploration involves the use of hands, legs, and the mouth and places the infant in a vulnerable position. Accidents during the first year of life commonly involve suffocation, aspiration, falls, burns, poisoning, and motor vehicle accidents. Many of the accidents can be prevented by paying special attention to the environment and using child safety restraints when traveling.

Otitis Media

Otitis media, one of the most common disease of infants and young children, frequently occurs as a complication of nasopharyngitis.[5, 36] Inflammation of the middle ear is

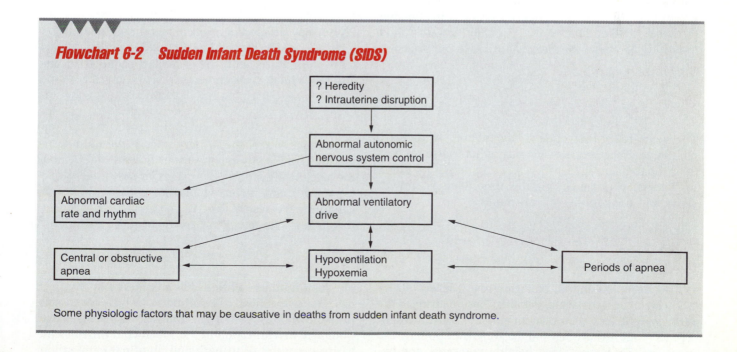

Flowchart 6-2 Sudden Infant Death Syndrome (SIDS)

Some physiologic factors that may be causative in deaths from sudden infant death syndrome.

especially common in infants and young children because they have a short, straight eustachian tube with undeveloped cartilage within it. Peak incidence for otitis media occurs between the ages of 6 months and 2 to 3 years. It is also more prevalent during winter months.

Eustachian tubes function to protect the middle ear from nasopharyngeal secretions, drain normal middle ear secretions, and equalize pressure between the middle ear and the external ear. The eustachian tubes can become obstructed from allergy, infection, enlarged adenoids, or nasopharyngeal tumors. This obstruction prevents drainage of normal secretions from the middle ear (serous otitis media). Negative middle-ear pressure occurs when air which normally escapes is absorbed. After the tube becomes fully or partially open, organisms enter the middle ear, where they multiply and produce infection. Organisms most frequently associated with otitis media are *Streptococcus pneumoniae, Haemophilus influenzae,* and *Staphylococcus aureus.* Continued or untreated otitis media can result in hearing loss from negative ear pressure, effusion in the middle ear, or damage to the tympanic membrane. Subsequently, hearing loss may lead to speech and language problems.

Although acute otitis media can be asymptomatic, classic clinical manifestations include fever, severe pain, irritability, lethargy, anorexia, vomiting, and diarrhea. Sucking and chewing increase the pain. Findings from otoscopic examination include reddened and bulging tympanic membrane and the absence of normal landmarks and light reflex.

Severe pain and fever are usually absent in serous otitis media. However, the child may experience a feeling of fullness and a popping sensation on swallowing. If air is present above the fluid, the child may experience a feeling of motion. Otoscopic examination reveals a dull, gray tympanic membrane, which may be either bulging or depressed. Landmarks are obscured. A visible fluid level may be present if there is air above the fluid.

▼ Early Childhood

The years from 1 through 5 are referred to as early childhood. These years encompass what is also referred to as the toddler (age 1 to 3 years) and preschool (age 3 to 5 years) periods. During this time, biologic growth slows and the various systems mature.

BIOPHYSICAL DEVELOPMENT

Biologic Growth

During early childhood, biologic growth levels off. By 2.5 years of age, the average toddler has quadrupled the birth weight and increased height by two-thirds. At 2 years of age, the average toddler weighs 27 pounds and measures 34 inches. This height represents approximately one-half of the predicted adult height. Increase in leg length accounts for the major gain in height of about 4 to 5 inches per year for the toddler and 2.5 inches per year for the preschooler.

The toddler gains 4 to 6 pounds per year, and the preschool child gains about 4 pounds per year. By 6 years of age, the preschool child weighs about 48 pounds and stands about 46 inches tall. Table 6-5 summarizes early childhood growth by year.

Body Proportion

During early childhood, the head continues to be relatively large in comparison to the body. By 2 years of age, the chest is larger than the head. Between 1 and 2 years, the head circumference increases about 1 inch; by 5 years, this increase is only about 0.5 inch per year.

The toddler characteristically displays a long trunk with short extremities. Immature abdominal muscles contribute to the protruding or "pot-bellied" abdomen. The typical two-year-old also displays flat feet and slightly bowed legs. The body of the preschool child begins to resemble that of an adult. The preschooler becomes taller and thinner as the lower extremities grow faster than the head, trunk, and arms. The protruding abdomen also disappears.

Dentition

The two-year-old toddler has about 16 primary teeth. By 2.5 years of age, all 20 deciduous teeth have erupted. There is very little change in dentition during the preschool years.

PHYSIOLOGIC DEVELOPMENT

Physiologic development occurs as the individual systems mature. By the end of the toddler period, all systems are mature, with the exception of the endocrine and reproductive systems.

Genitourinary System

By 2 years of age, the urinary tract of the toddler has matured sufficiently to concentrate urine. Completion of the myelinization process provides for increased sphincter control and increased bladder capacity. After the genitourinary system has attained sufficient maturity, the child is physiologically ready for toilet training.

Nervous System

The total number of brain cells is achieved by 1 year of age. However, these cells continue to increase in size, until the brain is 75% of the adult size by 3 years of age. Complete myelinization of the spinal cord provides the basis for control of urinary and intestinal elimination.

TABLE 6-5 *Biophysical Measurements of Early Childhood*

2 Years	3 Years	4 Years	5 Years
WEIGHT			
12–13 kg (27–28 lb) +2–3 kg/yr	+2–3 kg/yr	+2–3 kg/yr	+2–3 kg/yr
HEIGHT			
86–88 cm (34–36 in); about one-half adult height	+6–8 cm	+5 cm/yr	+5 cm/yr
HEAD CIRCUMFERENCE			
Slightly smaller than chest circumference	Smaller than chest by 5–7 cm		
PULSE			
110 ± 20; average 100/min	100 ± 15; average 95/min	100 ± 10; average 92/min	95 ± 15; average 90/min
RESPIRATIONS			
26–28 min	24 ± 6/min	24 ± 4/min	22 ± 3/min
BLOOD PRESSURE			
80–112 / 50–80		82–110 / 50–78	
DENTITION			
16 temporary teeth; 30 mo—full set temporary			

Values summarized from Jackson, D.B. and Saunders, R.B. *Child Health Nursing.* Philadelphia: J.B. Lippincott, 1993; Castiglia, P.T. *Child Health Care.* Philadelphia: J.B. Lippincott, 1992.

Maturation of the nervous system also accounts for the improved coordination evident during early childhood.

Gastrointestinal System

Increased stomach capacity and delayed emptying of the stomach allow the child to eat three basic meals per day with between-meal snacks. Anal sphincter control is possible as the spinal cord achieves complete myelinization.

Immune System

Continuing maturation of the immune system provides adult levels of IgG during the toddler period. Adult levels of IgM are reached toward the end of infancy. During the preschool years, the child achieves adult levels of immunoglobulin A (IgA). Development of immunoglobulins D and E continues during early childhood, but adult levels are not reached until later childhood (see p. 320).

MOTOR DEVELOPMENT

Large muscles, legs, and arms account for the most growth during early childhood, with muscles growing faster than bones. The individual in early childhood becomes a more coordinated person as hand-eye coordination and small muscle coordination improve, especially in the preschool years. The clumsy little toddler at 2 years of age who learns to ride a tricycle continues to refine the ability to run, skip, jump, and climb. The preschool child develops an ability to catch and throw a ball, but throwing is not accurate at this age. Fine motor development concentrates on the smaller muscles of the fingers. At 2 years of age, the toddler has fat fingers and incomplete myelinization. As myelinization is completed, fine motor skills improve, allowing the child to use crayons, pencils, and scissors with increasing skill.

FACTORS AFFECTING DEVELOPMENT

Nutrition

The toddler needs approximately 1,300 calories and the preschooler needs about 1,800 calories per day to maintain nutritional status and promote adequate growth. Protein intake should be about 16 and 24 g daily, respectively, for the toddler and preschooler.[5] These recommendations represent an increase during this period to provide for the rapid growth in the muscles of the body. Calcium requirements are about 800 mg per day. The child eats at least five to seven times per day.

There continues to be a great deal of controversy over the need for dietary supplements. The best guide in determining whether a child should be placed on supplements is a review of the normal dietary intake. If a child's nutritional intake is consistently below the daily recommendations, then dietary supplements are definitely indicated.

Children in early childhood should also be observed for adverse reactions to various foods and food substances. Food substances known to produce adverse reactions include sugar, artificial coloring, and various preservatives. Allergic reactions to foods may be evidenced by urticaria, itching, headache, and changes in behavior, including hyperactivity.

Accidents

Between 1 and 4 years of age, the leading cause of death is accidents. The rate of deaths from accidents is highest in this period, with the exception of adolescence. The incidence of accidents is closely related to the development occurring in the child at this time. Children in this age group exhibit tremendous curiosity about the world that surrounds them. They explore this world with their hands and mouths and display increasing control of fine motor skills. Additionally, children of this age are walking, climbing, running, and learning to ride tricycles and other motion toys. Major areas of injury include motor vehicles, drowning, burns, poisoning, falls, aspiration, and suffocation. Table 6-6 indicates the ranking of accidents by sex for children in early childhood.

Control of Bodily Functions

It is during the early childhood years that the individual gains control of bodily functions. Most children are physically mature enough to begin toilet training at about 2 years of age. However, individual variation in development and cultural practices may prevent the child from gaining control of bodily functions until 3 or 4 years of age. The absence of control of bodily function until 4 to 5 years of age indicates a need for assessment and evaluation of the individual child for enuresis and encopresis. Both of these conditions represent alterations associated with bodily function.

Enuresis is defined as involuntary voiding after the age at which bladder control should have been achieved. This involuntary voiding occurs most often at night. Primary enuresis occurs if there has never been a long, dry, symptom-free period. Secondary or acquired enuresis occurs after at least a year of dryness. This condition occurs twice as often in boys as in girls and affects 5% to 17% of children between 3 and 15 years of age who are otherwise considered normal.[36]

No one cause of enuresis has been identified. One very common factor is urinary tract infection or obstruction. An abnormal stream, including dribbling, is often indicative of a physiologic problem.[5] Enuresis has been associated with a history of bedwetting in parents, siblings, or other close relatives of affected children. A higher frequency of enuresis has been found among children of lower socioeconomic groups and in African American children. Maturational lags, characterized by frequent urination, small bladder capacity, and delayed inhibitory control, have been shown to contribute to enuresis, as has dysfunction of the reticular activating system in rapid eye movement sleep.[13] Diagnostic evaluation includes a complete history of the family and child, as well as a urinary workup. Urine cultures should be ordered to rule out an infection, and bladder capacity should be determined.

Clinical management includes use of an electronic conditioning device to alert the child and drug therapy. Imipramine (Tofranil) is frequently used to inhibit urination. Bladder training may be used in an attempt to increase bladder capacity. Withholding of fluids before bedtime and not interrupting sleep also help in achieving bladder control at night.

Encopresis is the repeated voluntary or involuntary passage of stool into clothing after the age when toilet training should have been achieved.[30] Primary, or continuous, encopresis occurs when the child has never achieved bowel control. Secondary, or discontinuous, encopresis occurs when the child has achieved bowel control before the onset of incontinence. This condition occurs more often in males than in females and affects 1.5% to 5.7% of children.[30] Encopresis is a physiologic as well as a behavioral disorder, and it is now referred to as idiopathic fecal incontinence, unless a psychiatric disorder is a direct contributing factor.[31] Emotional problems associated with encopresis include fear of parents, altered parent–child relationships, and psychosocial stress associated with life changes such as a sibling's birth or starting school.

Clinical manifestations of idiopathic fecal incontinence include a history of chronic constipation, often beginning in infancy, painful defecation, complaints of poor appetite, abdominal pain, and distention. Passage

---

TABLE 6-6 *Rankings of Accidental Deaths in Early Childhood*

Ranking	Boys	Girls
1	Motor vehicle	Motor vehicle
2	Drowning	Burns
3	Burns	Drowning
4	Suffocation	Falls
5	Falls	Suffocation

of small, hard, formed stool with diarrhea is indicative of impaction. Frequently stools are extremely large and accompanied by blood.

Diagnosis is based on a complete history and physical examination. Neurologic assessment, including deep tendon reflexes, sensory function, muscle strength, and tone of lower extremities, is suggestive of spinal cord pathology.[31] Abdominal examination reveals tenderness, masses, and organ enlargement. A kidney, ureter, and bladder flat-plate radiograph of the abdomen reveals any stool retained in the colon. Therapeutic management of ideopathic fecal incontinence includes a diet high in fiber, lubricants, cathartics, and behavior reinforcement.[31] The high-fiber diet is directed toward the prevention of constipation. Mineral oil helps soften the stool and reduce its size. The administration of cathartics aids in establishment of regularity, but most children achieve bowel control without medication in 6 to 12 months.

Hearing and Vision Problems

One of the most common handicapping disorders in the United States is hearing impairment.[36] Routine auditory screening during early childhood aids in diagnosis and prevention of speech disorders associated with hearing loss. Normal hearing function and disorders of hearing are discussed on pages 978–985. Hearing impairment in the child may be classified as conduction, sensorineural, mixed, or central auditory dysfunction. Conduction hearing losses are the most common type. They may be caused by congenital anomalies, such as ear malformation and atresia, or by acquired loss as a result of otitis media, trauma, or blockage from a foreign body. Surgical correction may be possible.

Sensorineural hearing loss in children may be caused by rubella, cytomegalovirus, meningitis, *Streptococcus pneumoniae,* hyperbilirubinemia, Down syndrome, exposure to excessive noise, or drugs such as gentamycin and chemotherapeutic agents. Head injury may also lead to a sensorineural hearing loss. Central auditory dysfunction includes birth trauma and hypoxia at birth as well as infantile autism and conversion hysteria.

Approximately 30 to 64 children per 1,000 population experience some visual impairment, even with glasses.[8] Visual impairment refers to visual loss that cannot be corrected with prescription glasses. In childhood, visual impairment can produce delays in the child's growth and development. Normal visual function and disorders of vision are described on pages 970–978.

The causes of visual impairment may be classified into four groups according to their basis in familial or genetic factors, prenatal factors, perinatal factors, or postnatal factors. Familial or genetic factors include Tay-Sachs disease, Down syndrome, galactosemia, and retinoblastoma. Prenatal factors that may lead to visual impairment in the child include syphilis, rubella, and toxoplasmosis. Visual impairment may include blindness and cataracts. Prematurity, maternal infection, and high oxygen concentrations associated with respiratory distress syndrome are among the perinatal factors producing visual impairment. Measles, mumps, rubella, chicken pox, poliomyelitis, leukemia, myasthenia gravis, juvenile rheumatoid arthritis, and trauma constitute postnatal factors responsible for visual impairment.

Visual disorders seen most often in children include errors of refraction, amblyopia, strabismus, cataracts, and glaucoma. Infections and trauma also constitute major visual alterations to which children must adapt. Specifically, errors of refraction are seen in farsightedness, nearsightedness, astigmatism, and anisometropia.

▼ Middle Childhood

The years from age 6 to 12 are referred to as middle childhood. This period is one of quiescence in biophysical development compared with the rapid growth and development noted in infancy and early childhood and the growth spurts associated with youth and adolescence. This period of physical quiescence allows for control and mastery of skills which, up until now, were unrealistic.

BIOPHYSICAL DEVELOPMENT

Biologic Growth

Biophysical growth and development proceed at a slower but steadier pace during the middle childhood years. The average gain in height during middle childhood is 2 to 3 inches per year. The school-age child gains an average of 5 to 7 pounds per year. By 12 years of age, children are approximately 58 to 59 inches tall and weigh about 86 pounds, although boys tend to be slightly shorter than girls (Table 6-7). However, wide variations occur in height and weight, indicative of the influence of genetics and nutrition on physical development. Periodic measurements of both height and weight are helpful in early diagnosis of significant deviations and are essential in to determine appropriate medication dosage.

Body Proportion

School-age children are significantly different from preschoolers and adolescents in body proportions. Arms and legs increase significantly in length. Both the brain and the bones of the head remain relatively stable, while the facial structure shows the greatest growth. As a result, the head constitutes less of the body surface (Fig. 6-1). The waist also decreases in relation to height.

TABLE 6-7 *Developmental Milestones for the School-Age Child*

Age	Physical	Motor	Social	Language	Perceptual	Cognitive
6 years	Average height 116 cm Average weight 21 kg Loses first tooth Six-year molar	Ties shoes Can use scissors Runs, jumps, climbs skips Constant activity	Increased need to socialize with same sex Egocentric	Uses every form of sentence structure Vocabulary of 2500 words Sentence length about 5 words	Knows right from left May reverse letters Can discriminate vertical, horizontal, and oblique Perceives pictures in parts or in wholes but not both	Recognizes simple words Conservation of number Defines objects by use Can group according to an attribute to form subclasses
7 years	Weight is 7 times birth weight Gains 2–3 kg/yr Grows 5–6 cm/yr	More cautious Swims Rides a bicycle Printing is smaller than 6-year-old's Activity level lower than 6-year-olds	More cooperative Same-sex play group and friend Less egocentric	Can name day, month, season Produces all language sounds	b, p, d, q confusion resolved Can copy a diamond shape	Begins to use simple logic Can group in ascending order Grasps basic idea of addition and subtraction Conservation of substance Can tell time
8 years	Average height 127 cm Average weight 25 kg	Movements more graceful Writes in cursive Can throw and hit a baseball Has symmetrical balance and can hop	Adheres to simple rules Hero worship begins Same-sex peer group	Gives precise definitions Articulation is near adult level	Can catch a ball Visual acuity is 20/20 Perceives pictures in parts and whole	Increasing memory span Interest in causal relationships Conservation of length Seriation
9–10 years	Average height 132–137 cm Average weight 27–35 kg	Good coordination Can achieve the strength and speed needed for most sports	Enjoys team competition Moves from group to best friend Hero worship intensifies	Can use language to convey thoughts and look at other's point of view	Eye-hand coordination almost perfected	Classifies objects Understands explanations Conservation of area and weight Describes characteristics of objects Can group in descending order
11–12 years	Average height 144–150 cm Average weight 35–40 kg Pubescence may begin Girls may surpass boys in height Remaining permanent teeth erupt	Refines gross and fine motor skills Can do crafts Uses tools increasingly well	Attends school primarily for peer association Peer acceptance is very important	Vocabulary of 50,000 words for reading Oral vocabulary of 7200 words	Can catch or intercept ball thrown from a distance Possible growth spurts may cause myopia	Begins abstract thinking Conservation of volume Understands relationship among time, speed, and distance

Source: P.T. Castiglia. *Child Health Care.* Philadelphia: J.B. Lippincott, 1992.

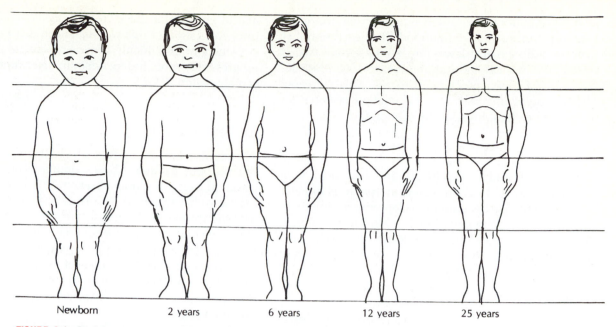

FIGURE 6-1 *Body proportions and form change as an individual progresses through the early years of the life cycle. (Schuster, C.S., and Ashburn, S.S. The Process of Human Development: A Holistic Life Span Approach [3rd ed.]. Philadelphia: J.B. Lippincott, 1992.)*

Dentition

By 5 to 6 years of age, children begin to lose baby teeth, which are replaced by permanent teeth. This process tends to occur earlier in girls than in boys. At the same time, the facial structure changes, with the jaw lengthening and the face increasing in size. By 12 to 13 years of age, all permanent teeth should have erupted, with the exception of the second and third molars.

PHYSIOLOGIC DEVELOPMENT

Musculoskeletal Changes

The steady weight gain during this period of development is caused primarily by the increase in size of the skeleton and muscles. Skeletal growth continues until the epiphyseal disks close and ossify (see p. 848). Damage to the epiphyseal disk is especially important during the middle childhood years. Injury during this time can result in premature fusion of the ossification centers and a permanent shortening of the bone. Adequate nutrition, including protein, vitamins, and minerals, is especially important to the growth of healthy bone. Kidney disease, endocrine problems, inadequate metabolism and food absorption, and interference with growth hormone production can alter bone maturation.

Muscle tone improves, and the "baby fat" of earlier years decreases as muscle mass and strength increase. Boys have more muscle cells than girls, which contributes to their greater strength. Girls tend to have more fat than muscle tissue. Increased muscle tone helps account for the improved posture during the middle years. However, increased muscle tissue and strength does not indi-cate muscle maturity. Therefore, school-age children are at increased risk for muscular injury from overuse.

Central Nervous System

Growth of the brain and head is minimal during middle childhood. Primary changes in the nervous system are evidenced in the myelinization process. The myelin sheath increases in thickness, resulting in improved conduction of nerve impulses. The effects of a maturing nervous system and improved nerve impulse conduction are seen as the clumsy child of 6 years becomes a coordinated sports participant in later childhood.

Other Systems

The maturation of the gastrointestinal system accounts for the decreased complaints of stomach ache and increased tolerance to food. Because of increased capacity and intake, the school-age child is also able to tolerate longer intervals between meals.

Middle childhood is also associated with maturation of the urinary system. Increased kidney size and function allow the child to better control elimination and adhere to a more controlled schedule.

The development of a mature immune system helps to account for the period of health associated with the school years. Tonsils and adenoids are enlarged, and this is believed to contribute to the production of antibodies when the child is exposed to various antigens. Tonsillectomies and adenoidectomies should be considered only if there is a history of frequent severe infection of the tonsils, adenoids, or middle ears, or if breathing or swallowing is impaired. The cardiovascular system continues to mature during middle childhood. The heart continues to grow, although at a slower rate. As the cardiovascular system matures, cardiac output increases, heart rate decreases, and blood pressure increases. This increased cardiac output increases the oxygenation essential for the energy expenditures of the school-age child.

MOTOR DEVELOPMENT

The years of middle childhood are associated with smoother and more coordinated motor development. Improvement of gross motor development during these years allows the school-age child to learn to ride a bicycle, jump rope, swim, and skate. Running and climbing are mastered also. Motor development during these years allows children to participate in team and individual sports because they now have the strength and skills to hit or kick a ball, throw, and catch.

Myelinization of the CNS accounts for the improvement in fine motor skills seen during the early school years. This fine motor development is evidenced as the child progresses from large printing with large pencils and crayons at age 6 to smaller writing with a regular pencil by 10 years of age. A preference for the right or left hand emerges early in the school years. Mastery of fine motor skills is also seen as school-age children learn to play musical instruments, sew, and work with models.

FACTORS AFFECTING DEVELOPMENT

Physical Fitness

Exercise is especially important to biophysical development during the middle childhood years. Physical exercise allows the child to improve muscle tone and strength as well as balance and coordination. School-age children usually display tremendous energy and need guidance in directing this energy. However, a survey of school fitness indicated that American children are not physically fit. The primary factor in the lack of fitness is the amount of time spent watching television. By the age of 18, the average child will have spent more time watching television (15,000 hours) than in school (11,000 hours).[25]

Sports participation is common for children of this age group. However, parents must be certain that the child is truly interested in the sport and that adequate protective equipment is provided. Placement of children in a sport for which they are not physically prepared or interested in may lead to problems with self-esteem or injury.

Nutrition

Overall caloric needs decrease during this period of growth and development. However, it is important that a well-balanced diet be maintained to promote growth and to prepare for the increased needs of adolescence. Implementation of this well-balanced diet becomes increasingly more difficult, however, because the child is progressively more independent in determining what is actually eaten.

Allergic Disorders

Allergic disorders in childhood include urticaria, allergic rhinitis, and asthma. These conditions are the most common cause of school absences.[10] Urticaria is a skin reaction characterized by pruritus and pale wheals. Allergic rhinitis is the most common allergic disorder affecting children.[18] Hay fever and seasonal rhinitis are terms used to refer to allergic rhinitis, which occurs with the various seasons. The release of histamine in response to inhaled irritants causes the symptoms of nasal congestion, itching, sneezing, and watery discharge in predisposed children.

It is estimated that school-age children account for approximately 2% to 5% of all asthmatics and that the condition accounts for 25% of all school absences in children younger than 17 years of age.[18] During middle childhood, asthma occurs more often in boys than in girls. However, during adolescence the incidence is about equal in boys and girls.[18]

Learning Disabilities and Attention Deficit Disorder

Learning disabilities and attention deficit disorder (ADD) represent a complex group of conditions which may not be diagnosed until the school years, when the impact is seen in the classroom. The term "learning-disabled" is applied to children of normal intelligence who exhibit disorders in understanding or using written or spoken language. Manifestations of learning disabilities vary and may include problems with the ability to listen, speak, read, write, spell, or do math.[33] Learning problems associated with visual and hearing impairment, mental retardation, emotional disorders, and motor disability are excluded from this definition. It has been estimated that 1% to 30% of school-age children exhibit some type of learning disability.[6] The condition is more common in boys than in girls and is more common in children from the lower socioeconomic levels. Reading problems, including dyslexia, represent the most common learning disability.

There is no single causative factor for learning disabilities. Problems associated with oxygen deprivation in the prenatal, perinatal, or postnatal periods, as well as complications of labor and delivery, may be contributing factors. Encephalitis, meningitis, and lead poisoning in early childhood may also contribute to the disorder.[5]

Diagnosis is based on a variety of diagnostic aids.

Physical and neurological examinations, including visual and hearing tests and serology for lead levels, aid in ruling out other causative factors. A detailed history of academic progress as well as social interactions should be obtained. Additional diagnostic aids include Pupil Rating Scale: Screening for Learning Disabilities, Conner's Teacher Questionnaire, and personal questionnaires developed by individual psychologists.

Attention deficit hyperactive disorder is the most common ADD and refers to "developmentally inappropriate degrees of inattention, impulsiveness, and hyperactivity."[2] It may also be associated with a learning disability. It has been estimated that from 1.2% to 20% of school-age children are affected by attention deficit hyperactive disorder. It occurs more frequently in upper-middle-class children and traditionally was believed to occur more often in boys than in girls.[28] More recent evidence, however, indicates that girls may be equally affected.[14]

Children with ADD have a hard time focusing on one thing for a long period of time. They are easily distracted and impulsive; they may be disorganized and prone to daydream, and they have a hard time completing tasks. These children often procrastinate, cannot plan, require extra supervision, and have trouble with details. The exact cause of ADD is unknown. A possible genetic link indicates the need for a careful family history. Oxygen deprivation in the prenatal, perinatal, or postnatal periods and complications of labor and delivery may be contributing factors. It has been suggested that food additives, caffeine, and sugar may contribute to the problem. Other research indicates that these factors may not play an important role in causation.[14]

Treatment for ADD may include medication, special education programs at school, manipulation of the environment, and behavior modification. The most common medications used to treat the condition include methylphenidate (Ritalin), amphetamine sulfate (Benzedrine), and dextroamphetamine (Dexedrine). These drugs help the child to control impulses and improve the attention span. Behavior modifications programs include reward systems, contracting, and cognitive-behavioral approaches. A structured environment and firm but reasonable limits seem to work well. Early diagnosis is the most important factor to avoid the emotional and behavioral problems and low self-esteem often associated with ADD. Diagnosis is based on criteria established by the American Psychiatric Association.[2]

▼ *Adolescence*

The period of adolescence is considered a transitional time from childhood to adulthood. During this time, rapid physical, intellectual, emotional, and social developmental changes occur. Although changes occur in all four domains and are interrelated, it is the purpose of this section to consider mainly the biophysical changes that occur during this stage of development. Alterations and adaptations specific to the adolescent are also discussed.

OVERVIEW OF GROWTH AND DEVELOPMENT STAGES

Prepuberty or pubescence is a 2- to 3-year period between childhood and adolescence. This stage of development is characterized by rapid physical growth and the appearance of secondary sex characteristics. Puberty begins in girls with menarche, which is the onset of monthly flow of bloody fluid from the uterus, called the menses. On the average in the United States, menarche occurs at 12.3 years of age. Puberty ends between ages 12 to 14 years in girls. In boys, puberty begins with the ability to produce spermatozoa and the occurrence of nocturnal emissions and ends 1 to 2 years later than with girls. The developmental stage of adolescence officially begins with the appearance of secondary sex characteristics and ends when somatic growth is complete. Adolescence is generally divided into three stages: early adolescence, ages 12 to 13; middle adolescence, ages 14 to 16; and late adolescence, ages 17 to 21. At the end of adolescence, the individual should be psychologically mature and capable of becoming a contributing, independent member of society.[5] Table 6-8 gives specific normal values related to adolescent physical development.

PHYSICAL DEVELOPMENT

Musculoskeletal System

Although all body systems undergo rapid maturation during the time of intense growth, the most noticeable change is observed in body height. The skeletal system, which doubles in mass during adolescence, grows at a faster rate than the supporting muscles. Because of this fact, the adolescent often appears to be clumsy and lacking in coordination.[5] Boys usually average an 8-inch gain in height during this growth spurt, and girls, just over 3 inches. By 18 years of age, most adolescents have attained 99% of their adult height.[5]

Lean body mass and nonlean body mass, which is primarily fat, double during puberty. The increase in skeletal mass, muscle mass, and nonlean body mass contributes significantly to the increased weight gain that occurs in adolescence. In boys, individual muscle cells increase in both number size, but in girls they increase only in size.[5] Androgen is thought to be responsible for the increased muscle mass that occurs in boys, which possibly accounts for the greater strength seen in

TABLE 6-8 *Average Biophysical Development of Young, Middle, and Late Adolescents*

Young adolescents, 12–13 Years		Middle Adolescents, 14–16 Years		Late Adolescents, 17–21 Years	
Males	Females	Males	Females	Males	Females
HEIGHT					
154–172 cm	153–167 cm	164–180 cm	155–169 cm	163–182 cm	156–170 cm
(60–68 in)	(60–66 in)	(65–71 in)	(61–66.5 in)	(64–72 in)	(61–67 in)
WEIGHT					
38–60 kg	40–60 kg	50–60 kg	42–64 kg	50–80 kg	48–72 kg
(84–132 lb)	(88–132 lb)	(110–132 lb)	(92–141 lb)	(100–176 lb)	(106–158 lb)
HEART RATE					
65 beats/min ± 10	65 beats/min ± 10	63 beats/min ± 10	66 beats/min ± 10	70 beats/min ± 10	70 beats/min ± 10
RESPIRATIONS					
19/min ± 3	19/min ± 3	17/min ± 3	17/min ± 3	17/min ± 3	17/min ± 3
BLOOD PRESSURE					
110/65 ± 10	110/60 ± 10	115/70 ± 10	115/70 ± 10	120/70 ± 10	120/70 ± 10
DENTITION					
Second molars	Second molars	—	—	Third molars	Third molars
HEARING					
Adult	Adult	Adult	Adult	Adult	Adult

Values summarized from Jackson, D.B. and Saunders, R.B. *Child Health Nursing.* Philadelphia: J.B. Lippincott, 1993.

most males. At physical maturity, girls average two times as much body fat as boys.[5]

After the appearance of secondary sex characteristics, the rate of growth declines. Ossification slows, the epiphyses of the long bones mature owing to the influence of the sex hormones, and growth of the long bones ceases.[36]

Central Nervous System

In contrast to all other body systems, the CNS does not undergo a rapid increase in growth during puberty. By 10 years of age, growth of the cerebellum, cerebrum, and brain stem is basically complete. Myelinization of the greater cerebral commissures and reticular formation of the CNS continue until middle adulthood. Adult visual abilities and normal adult hearing are attained during childhood.[5]

Respiratory System

The increase in vital capacity of the lungs corresponds with the height of the individual: the greater the height, the larger the vital capacity. As the vital capacity increases, the respiratory rate decreases in both boys and girls.[36]

Cardiovascular System

The heart doubles in size during puberty. The strength of the pumping mechanism increases.[36] This increased pumping strength causes an elevation in blood pressure. During the height of the growth period, the pulse rate may increase slightly. However, the increased body size allows stabilization of the pulse at a slower rate. Blood volume is directly correlated with weight and therefore increases more rapidly in boys. Pulse, respiration, and blood pressure values are within the adult range by 15 or 16 years of age[5] (see Table 6-8).

Gastrointestinal System

The digestive tract enlarges during adolescence. Because of the increased need for food required for growth, the size of the stomach enlarges to accommodate the additional food. Gastric acidity also increases to aid in digestion of the additional food intake.

Integumentary System

During adolescence, the sebaceous glands of the face, chest, and back become overactive and secrete increased amounts of sebum. Small pores trap the sebaceous material beneath the skin, producing a pimple or acne (see pp. 900–902).[5]

Basal Metabolic Rate

During puberty, the thyroid gland increases thyroxine secretion under the influence of the thyroid-stimulating hormone from the anterior pituitary. The increased thyroxine levels cause an increase in total body metabolism. The basal metabolic rate (BMR) increases during periods of growth, reaching a peak at puberty. The increase in BMR also causes an increase in body temperature, often causing the teenager to complain of feeling too warm. As the growth rate slows, the BMR gradually declines.

Nutritional Needs

The increased need for calories coincides with the increased rate of overall body growth and higher BMR. At the height of growth periods, girls need 2,200 calories per day and boys need 2,800 or more.[21] Protein needs correspond closely to the rate of growth. Higher proportions of proteins may be necessary in the earlier years in response to the rapid growth occurring at that time.

Adequate calcium intake is necessary for growth of bone and formation of teeth. Because of the periods of rapid skeletal growth, adolescents, particularly boys, may consume inadequate calcium. Girls on weight reduction diets may take in less than adequate calcium. Iron needs for girls vary depending on the amount of blood lost during menstruation. For replacement and maintenance, an intake of 15 mg of iron daily is recommended.[20]

PHYSIOLOGIC DEVELOPMENT

The physiologic developments of puberty are complex and poorly understood. After differentiation in the embryo, the gonads remain immature, unstimulated, and dormant until puberty. It is thought that the events of puberty are influenced by the anterior pituitary in response to stimulation from the hypothalamus. The gonadotropin-releasing hormone stimulates the anterior pituitary to produce gonadotropic hormones that, in turn, stimulate the gonads to begin functioning. The gonadotropic hormones are follicle-stimulating hormone (FSH), luteinizing hormone (LH), and luteotropic hormone or prolactin. FSH stimulates the growth of ova in girls and Leydig cells in the testes of boys. At the time that estrogen and testosterone are produced by the ovaries and testes, respectively, the adrenal cortex increases the production of androgen. The increased amounts of androgen that are produced at puberty are antagonistic to the pituitary growth hormone that is produced by the anterior pituitary (see pp. 682–684). This antagonistic effect is partially responsible for the decline in rate of body growth.

Estrogen, testosterone, and androgen are the hormones responsible for the development of the secondary sex characteristics. All persons produce both male and female hormones, and the secondary sex characteristics that appear depend on which hormone is produced in the greatest amount. The androgens produce the male characteristics, and the estrogens produce the female characteristics. The appearance of secondary sex characteristics is orderly, yet widely variable. Because there is such a wide variation in sexual maturity and development of the adolescent in comparison with chronological age, Tanner developed a system to describe and label the different stages for use in evaluating the adolescent's stage of sexual maturity.[32] Tables 6-9 and 6-10 describe the stages of sexual maturity in females and males.

ALTERATIONS AND ADAPTATIONS IN ADOLESCENCE

The developmental stage of adolescence is described as a phase of identity versus role confusion.[11] It has been identified as a time of conflict, confusion, and intense emotions. Relationships with parents change and are replaced with peer relationships. At the same time that adolescents are searching for independence from parents and authority figures, they also still maintain an element of dependence. During this developmental stage, adolescents are formalizing behavioral decisions and practices for adult life. In an effort to explore all possible boundaries and options, adolescents often participate in risk-taking behaviors. Accidents, suicides, and homicides are the leading causes of death among adoles-

TABLE 6-9 *Classification of Sexual Maturity Stages in Females*

Stage	Pubic Hair	Breasts
1	Preadolescent	Preadolescent
2	Sparse, light pigmentation, straight	Breast and papilla small mound; areola increases in diameter
3	Darker, begins to curl and increase in amount	Breast and areola enlarged
4	Coarse, curly, abundant in quantity but less than adult	Areola and papilla form secondary mound
5	Adult feminine triangle to medial surface of thighs	Mature, erect nipple, areola part of general breast contour

Adapted from Behrman, R.E. *Nelson Textbook of Pediatrics*. Philadelphia: W.B. Saunders, 1992.

TABLE 6-10 *Classification of Sexual Maturity in Males*

Stage	Pubic Hair	Penis	Testes
1	None	Preadolescent	Preadolescent
2	Scanty, long, slightly pigmented	Slight enlargement	Enlarged scrotum, pink
3	Darker pigmentation, small in amount, begins to curl	Longer	Larger
4	Resembles adult type, coarse and curly, but less in amount than adult	Larger, glans and breadth increase in size	Larger, dark pigmentation
4	Adult distribution to medial surface of thighs	Adult	Adult

Adapted from Behrman, R.E. *Nelson Textbook of Pediatrics*. Philadelphia: W.B. Saunders, 1992.

cents in the United States. Teenage drivers contribute significantly to vehicular fatalities, both their own and those of others. Drug and alcohol use are common among junior high school and high school students. Cigarette smoking, which is currently becoming more prevalent among female than male adolescents, is associated with respiratory symptoms during the teen years. Sexual activity is widespread and contributes significantly to pregnancy and sexually transmitted diseases (STDs). Other alterations and adaptations that occur in response to the physiologic and psychosocial changes of adolescence are eating disorders and acne.

Eating Disorders

Obesity, anorexia nervosa, and bulimia nervosa have increased significantly among adolescents in the last decade. They are specific syndromes that represent a disturbance in eating behavior and psychological adjustment. Left untreated, they can become life-threatening and seriously affect future development (see also pp. 240–249).

OBESITY. Obesity is thought to be caused by an increase in the number of fat cells or adipocytes that accumulate in subcutaneous tissue. It is proposed that these adipocytes are produced in infancy when the infant ingests increased calories. The potential then exists for the presence of increased weight later in life. Diagnosis of obesity is made when the weight-to-height ratio and the skinfold thickness are greater than the 95th percentile.[4] Obesity is present in 5% to 25% of children and adolescents. The risk or potential for obesity is greater for the child who has obese parents.

Many theories have been proposed as to the cause of obesity; however, there remains no definite answer. One theory is the *appestat* or *set-point theory*. This theory proposes that each person possesses an internal control system that keeps body weight stable. Through body metabolism, this set-point is maintained. If excess calo-

ries are consumed, the BMR increases to burn the additional calories. If calorie intake is reduced, the BMR decreases.[36] Another theory is the *adipose cell theory*. This theory proposes that the number and size of adipose cells is increased. Obese children may have larger adipose cells that remain large and increase in number during childhood and adolescence.[36]

Many causal and environmental factors have also been cited as contributing to childhood obesity. Examples of these are inactivity, possibly attributed to increased time watching television and playing video games, tiredness during physical activity, and avoidance of activity, leading to poor physical condition and further weight gain.[36]

ANOREXIA NERVOSA. Anorexia nervosa is a disorder of eating that involves self-induced starvation, an intense fear of fatness, dissatisfaction with body shape, and the belief that being thin and having control over body weight is essential for happiness.[17] Amenorrhea occurs in females, and males experience a decrease in sex drive. To achieve weight loss, the anorexic individual may restrict food, abuse laxatives and diuretics, self-induce vomiting, or engage in excessive exercise. Although the syndrome is labeled "anorexia," there is no loss of appetite.[5]

Anorexia nervosa affects about 1 in 200 white, adolescent females, usually from middle to upper socioeconomic classes. The most common age for problems to begin is at 12 years, with peak years at ages 13 to 14 and 17 to 18. Although less common, anorexia nervosa may occur in females until the mid-thirties and in young males.

The anorexic individual may present with a variety of complaints. Amenorrhea may occur before weight loss, although it is more common after weight loss. Nonspecific gastrointestinal symptoms are present. Hypertrophy of the parotid gland occurs, causing a chipmunk-like face. Dry skin with the texture of sandpaper, yellow discoloration of the palms of the hands, and thin scalp hair associated with lanugo-like hair over the face and body are common. Hypotension and hypothermia are late-developing symptoms. If vomiting is used as a weight control measure, enamel erosion of the teeth occurs in response to frequent exposure to the high acidity of vomitus. Left untreated, anorexia nervosa has a 15% to 21% mortality rate from starvation.[1]

The physiologic manifestations that occur in anorexia nervosa are the result of starvation. Cognitive changes that occur are loss of concentration and of general interests, mood swings, irritability, depression, apathy, and sleep disturbances. Amenorrhea, an early symptom of anorexia nervosa, is caused by a reversal of gonadotropic secretion, as seen in pubescence. Low levels of LH and FSH are associated with estrogen deficiency. The estrogen deficiency may contribute to the osteoporosis that is common in anorexia nervosa.

Some anorexic individuals have problems concentrating urine because of water deprivation. This may be caused by defective osmoregulation or vasopressin secretion. Many anorexic individuals experience abnormal thermoregulatory responses on exposure to heat or cold. Gastrointestinal symptoms are also common. Gastric emptying is delayed, and intestinal motility is decreased. This produces the complaints of bloating, constipation, and abdominal pain. Increased hepatic enzymes may indicate fatty infiltrates of the liver.

BULIMIA NERVOSA. Bulimia is the term used to explain the binge eating that occurs in this disorder. Binging is a secretive, rapid eating of large amounts of high-calorie foods. The average number of calories consumed in one binge is 5,000.[21] After binging, the individual purges through self-induced vomiting, or laxative or diuretic abuse. Binges increase in frequency and eventually become the way of meeting nutritional needs, because considerable food is absorbed in spite of the purging. The number of individuals affected with bulimia nervosa in the United States is not known. However, the frequency is apparently increasing. Like anorexia nervosa, onset of bulimia nervosa most frequently occurs in adolescent females.

The physical changes associated with anorexia nervosa may also occur with bulimia. Amenorrhea may occur, although not as commonly as in anorexia nervosa. The individual with bulimia nervosa has physical difficulties associated with repetitive purging. Swelling of the parotid glands and tooth enamel erosion may be present from the self-induced vomiting. Epigastric distress from chronic esophagitis and gastrointestinal bleeding also occur. Dilation and rupture of the esophagus can occur from binging. Some of the most serious complications of bulimia nervosa are hypokalemic alkalosis from persistent vomiting, cardiac dysrhythmia from hypokalemia, dehydration from laxative abuse, potassium depletion with cardiac arrest, and spastic colitis.

Diagnosis of bulimia nervosa is made from the following American Psychiatric Association criteria:

1. There are reoccurring episodes of binging.
2. During binging, the individual has a feeling of lack of control over eating behavior.
3. The individual regularly engages in purging behaviors, strict dieting, fasting, or excessive exercise to prevent weight gain.
4. Binge eating occurs a minimum of twice per week for at least 3 months.
5. The individual is overly concerned with body shape and weight.[2]

Acne Vulgaris

Acne vulgaris is the classic skin condition of adolescents. Between 12 and 25 years of age, approximately 85% of adolescents experience varying degrees of acne.[5] It is caused primarily by increased androgen production, which stimulates hair follicles and sebaceous gland structures on the skin of the face, neck, shoulders, and upper chest. It occurs in almost all boys and in 80% of girls.

The pathophysiology of acne vulgaris involves three mechanisms: androgens, obstruction of follicles, and bacteria. During puberty, the secretion of androgen, in addition to its role in the appearance of secondary sex characteristics, leads to increased size of sebaceous glands and increased production of sebum. If sebum is secreted into open follicles, it flows onto the skin and evaporates. In acne vulgaris, the follicles become obstructed. The ducts leading from the glands to the skin may be small and unable to handle the large amount of material produced. This causes the sebum to occlude ducts and dilate glands. Normal skin bacteria colonize sebaceous follicles, and free fatty acid is released, which irritates surrounding tissue. The whitehead or closed comedo can continue to dilate until it becomes an open comedo (blackhead), or it can rupture below the skin and spread into surrounding tissue. The skin reacts as if to a localized foreign body, responding to the comedo core and to acids from the ruptured comedos (see pp. 900–902).

Accidents and Suicide

Accidents are the leading cause of death in adolescence. Motor vehicle accidents account for the greatest number of accidental deaths and most often are associated with alcohol intoxication. In addition to intoxication, peer pressure, high energy levels, and feelings of immortality contribute to the reckless, risk-taking behavior of adolescents.[5] Adolescents are also prone to injuries from snowmobiles, minibikes, and motorcycles. Injuries may be sustained from falls, collisions, burns, or even hearing loss. Most deaths involving motorcycles result from head injuries, most of which could be prevented by using a safety helmet.[36]

Homicides are the second leading cause of death in adolescents between the ages of 15 and 19. Death usually results from knives and firearms used by non–family members.[36]

Suicide is the third leading cause of injury and death to adolescents.[36] The frequency of suicide has increased in the past decade, particularly in younger age groups.[5] Suicidal behavior affects all educational levels and all ethnic, socioeconomic, and religious groups. Adolescent males more often commit suicide, but more females admit to having difficulty with stress and depression.[22] Males choose more violent means of suicide, such as firearms, hanging, reckless behavior, and use of motor vehicles. Females choose more passive means, such as prescription and nonprescription drugs, poison ingestion, and cutting of the wrists. Impulsive suicide occurs more frequently in the adolescent age group than in any other group.

Adolescents at risk for suicidal behavior have vegetative symptoms of depression such as sleep or appetite disturbances, somatic complaints, truancy, substance abuse, sexual promiscuity, or a proneness to accidents.[12] Possible precursors or crisis events have been identified that affect an adolescent's ability to cope with life. Some of the more common events are divorce or separation; death or an extreme change in health of a family member or close friend; breakup of a romantic relationship; pregnancy, abortion, or birth of a child, and the anniversary of these events; poor personal achievement; friendship squabbles; and overachievement expectations.[22]

Advanced warning and talk of suicide usually occur in adolescents who are contemplating suicide. These warnings should be responded to. However, adolescents frequently distance themselves from help by severing important relationships and not communicating with parents, family, and friends.[12]

Substance Use

Substance use is a problem of adolescence, and the etiologic factors are related to the psychosocial development occurring at this age. Any combination of the following may be an incentive for adolescent substance abuse:

1. Emotional influences: as an attempt to increase self-esteem and self-confidence, as an emotional escape, to decrease tension and anxiety, to assert independence.
2. Physical influences: to feel relaxed, to block pain, to increase sensation, to increase energy or endurance.
3. Social influences: to be accepted in the peer group, to overcome shyness or loneliness, to escape problems.
4. Intellectual influences: to decrease boredom and mental fatigue, to improve attention span.

5. Environmental influences: because of the popular acceptance of substance use, the changing role of the family, or the influence of negative role models.[16]

Adolescents use and abuse both licit and illicit chemical substances.[35] Several chemical substances, although not identified as drugs by society, produce mild to moderate euphoric effects. Some of the more commonly abused chemical substances are caffeine, chocolate, and common analgesics. Hallucinogens, narcotics, hypnotics, and stimulants are mind-altering drugs and are available to adolescents through illegal means, the "black market." Several substances are sniffed or inhaled to produce altered sensation, including antifreeze, airplane cement, and typewriter correction fluid.[36] The abuse of cocaine by adolescents is increasing rapidly, perhaps as a result of increased availability and affordability.

The use of anabolic steroids is a major problem in professional and amateur sports. The drugs are used to enhance performance in athletic events by increasing muscular strength and size. Effects of anabolic steroids may be toxic and irreversible.[5]

ALCOHOL. Drunk driving is the leading cause of death among 15- to 24-year-olds. Students in high school seem to be drinking less alcohol, but this trend does not hold true for college-age students and young adults. Most adolescents start to drink because it seems like "grown-up" behavior, and they continue to abuse alcohol for the same reasons that adults abuse it. Alcohol is considered to be a means of escape, a way to reduce anxiety, and essential for social occasions.[21]

NICOTINE. Nicotine is physically and psychologically addicting. Long-term use of this substance contributes to respiratory diseases, cancer, and cardiovascular diseases. Approximately 70% of children and adolescents experiment with cigarettes. However, the number who become regular smokers seems to be decreasing. More female than male adolescents smoke cigarettes, but males substitute smokeless tobacco for cigarettes.[36]

Smokeless tobacco is a tobacco product that is placed in the mouth and not ignited. Examples of smokeless tobacco are snuff and chewing tobacco. Smokeless tobacco has been found to be carcinogenic. Regular use of these substances cause foul-smelling breath, periodontal disease, erosion of enamel, and loss of teeth.[36]

Adolescent Sexuality

There are 21 million adolescents in the United States between the ages of 15 and 19. Eleven million of these are sexually active.[7] By 17 years of age, 50% of adolescent females have become sexually active. More than 1.5 million adolescents admit to having had four or more sex partners.[7] The average age at first sexual experience for white males is 14.5 years.[7]

Many physical and psychosocial problems occur as the adolescent begins to physically mature and develop secondary sex characteristics. At this time, the adolescent is physically capable of procreation yet is still emotionally, socially, and intellectually too immature to handle the responsibilities and problems associated with sexual activity. The physical and psychosocial well-being of sexually active adolescents is at risk from two significant threats: STDs and unwanted pregnancy.

SEXUALLY TRANSMITTED DISEASES. STDs are occurring at epidemic proportions in the United States, with a disproportionate number of cases among adolescents. Adolescents who are sexually active are at risk for developing STDs because they tend to delay seeking medical care and do not practice safe sexual practices. The most common STDs in adolescents are gonorrhea and chlamydia.[36] Approximately 29% of persons newly diagnosed with the human immunodeficiency virus (HIV) became infected as adolescents or young adults.[5]

The major modes of HIV infection are unsafe sexual practices and substance abuse. Because both sexual activity and substance abuse are prominent behaviors in the adolescent, HIV and clinical acquired immunodeficiency syndrome (AIDS) is an enormous risk to adolescents.[7] The sexually transmitted diseases are discussed in Chapter 57. HIV infection is discussed in detail on pages 336–346.

ADOLESCENT PREGNANCY. The United States has the highest adolescent pregnancy rate of any developed country in the world.[19] Annually in the United States, 11% of the total adolescent population become pregnant. Adolescent girls give birth to 1,300 infants each day. Even with these figures, the nation's pregnancy rate stabilized in the 1980s except for those adolescents age 15 years and younger, a statistic which reflected an increase in sexual activity in this young group. Five hundred abortions are performed each day on adolescents. Forty percent to 50% of adolescents experience repeat pregnancies within 24 months of the initial pregnancy.[19] Birth control measures among adolescents are very inconsistent.

Identification of the causes of the increased incidence of adolescent pregnancy has met with limited success. Several interrelated factors contribute to the adolescent birth rates. Socioeconomic factors may play a major role. Adolescents from minority groups and lower socioeconomic groups have an increased risk for pregnancy, often begin sexual activity at an earlier age, and more frequently have illegitimate births than other adolescent girls.[3] Girls from the lower socioeconomic groups usually have lower self-esteem and limited educational achievement.

Absence of family support, especially maternal support, appears to predispose adolescents to increased risk for pregnancy. Many times the adolescent lives in a single-parent home and competes with siblings for parental attention. Often adolescents view pregnancy as the means of providing a change of direction for the future. Negative as this change may be, the young girl sees the change as a way of escaping a bad home environment, boring home town, or poor school experience, or a way of getting her boyfriend to marry her.

The extent of psychosocial risks to the pregnant adolescent depends on several factors: availability of care, family support, socioeconomic status, and developmental level of the adolescent. Adolescent childbearing results in more negative consequences than positive outcomes for the individual and society. It has been called the "syndrome of failure." Interruption or termination of education is a major contributing factor to the syndrome. Eight of 10 pregnant adolescents younger than 17 years of age do not complete high school; 4 of 10 younger than 15 years of age do not complete the eighth grade. Teen fathers are 40% less likely to graduate from high school than nonfathers. The limited education decreases job opportunities, which causes the adolescents to depend on a welfare system or have a marginal existence. The divorce rate is 72% for 14- to 17-year-olds and 46% for 18- to 19-year-olds. Children born to adolescent parents have a much higher incidence of poor school performance and impaired intellectual functioning. Adolescent pregnancy represents a cycle of repetition. Twenty-five percent of adolescent mothers and 50% of adolescent fathers were children of at least one adolescent parent.[33]

Parenting by adolescent mothers is less than optimal because of several maternal factors: insensitivity to infant behavior; harsh, impulsive physical punishment; tendency to spend less than the needed time for play and stimulation with the infant; and lack of knowledge of normal infant and child growth and development. Maternal behavior affects infant development and well-being, so these maternal characteristics are reason for concern. The extent to which the mother adapts to the infant may depend on the degree of maternal self-esteem, knowledge of growth and development, and educational and developmental status.[9]

Adolescent lifestyle, vulnerability to complications, lack of adequate prenatal care, nutritional deficiencies, and noncompliance with health regimens predispose the pregnant adolescent and fetus to less than optimal pregnancy outcomes. Adolescents receiving adequate prenatal care do not have an increased incidence of physical and medical complications compared with older women. Problems usually arise from poverty and social conditions more than from age.

Adolescents frequently have preterm labor and delivery and infants who are small for gestational age, partially as a result of low socioeconomic status, poor nutrition, lower prepregnancy weight, and delayed prenatal care. Adolescent pregnancy is also associated with pregnancy-induced hypertension.

Sexually transmitted diseases, chlamydia, and trichomoniasis, which contribute to preterm birth and infant mortality, are more common in the adolescent. Adolescents who are in the 15- to 19-year-old group have the second highest rate for gonorrhea. Infections late in pregnancy contribute to chorioamnionitis, postpartum endometritis, and neonatal septicemia.

Pregnant adolescents are at increased risk for anemia. The fetal and adolescent stages of development are the two most rapid growth periods and are associated with the greatest iron requirements. The combination of irregular eating habits with rapid growth presents an even greater risk for iron deficiency anemia.

MENSTRUAL DISORDERS. Two common problems or concerns associated with the menstrual cycle in adolescence are dysmenorrhea, and amenorrhea (see pp. 1141–1143). Two types of dysmenorrhea occur in adolescents. The most common type is primary dysmenorrhea, in which all pelvic organs are normal. In secondary dysmenorrhea, known pathology such as endometriosis or pelvic inflammatory disease exists.

Primary dysmenorrhea is thought to be caused by increased prostaglandin production. The increased levels of prostaglandins produce uterine hyperactivity and contractions. In addition to the abdominal discomfort, the young woman may also experience nausea and vomiting, pallor, and syncope. The abdominal discomfort is usually mild to severe and lasts from a few hours up to 2 days. Diagnosis of dysmenorrhea is based on a thorough history and physical examination. The physical examination should include a pelvic examination, Pap smear, and gonorrhea culture.[36]

Two types of amenorrhea occur in the adolescent: primary and secondary. Primary amenorrhea occurs when menarche is delayed past age 17 years. Secondary amenorrhea occurs when one or more menstrual cycles have occurred, followed by an absence of menses for 4 or more months. Primary and secondary amenorrhea may be caused by chromosome or endocrine disorders or by structural abnormalities. Strenuous physical activity, such as cross country running and marathon swimming, frequently produce amenorrhea. Pregnancy is the most common cause of secondary amenorrhea.

HOMOSEXUALITY. Homosexual activity is a widely publicized risk factor for AIDS and the major mode for its transmission during adolescence. Many heterosexual males admit to engaging in some homosexual activity during adolescence. Approximately 17% to 37% of adolescent males engage in at least one homosexual activity to orgasm.[24] It is estimated that 1 of 10 individuals is homosexual.

It is not known what produces a homosexual orientation. However, there are many theories. Because homosexual activity occurs in most societies, many think there is a biologic basis for the behavior.[27] Other theories suggest a genetic connection and hormonal influences.[27] Review of the literature indicates that homosexual males have normal testosterone levels and homosexual females also have testosterone levels consistent with healthy, nonlesbian females.[27] Another theory, the psychoanalytic theory, refers to homosexuality as a developmental condition related to the preoedipal and oedipal periods of development.[27] Social process theory explains homosexual behavior as a learned behavior occurring within an interpersonal setting involving family and peers.[27] Research involving 979 homosexual and 477 heterosexual males and females found that orientation to homosexuality was not statistically associated with ineffective parenting, seduction, traumatic experiences with the opposite sex, labeling, or any other theoretical environmental influence.[25]

Development of homosexual behavior occurs in four stages: sensitization, identity confusion, identity assumption, and commitment.[34] The stage of sensitization occurs before puberty. During this time, the children do not consider themselves to be homosexual but realize that they are different from their peers. Girls may feel different because they feel unfeminine, unattractive, and not interested in boys. Boys may be interested in the arts, not sports, and may often be called "sissies."[34]

During identity confusion, the adolescents begin to think that maybe they are homosexual because of their lack of heterosexual interests or their gender-atypical interests. Most homosexual (gay) males realize their sexual orientation at about 17 years of age, and homosexual (lesbian) females at about 18 years of age.[15] Most adolescents deny their feelings during the stage of identity confusion, hoping to "repair" themselves. They may assume heterosexual relationships, even to the point of pregnancy, and they may try to escape through substance abuse.[34]

During the third stage, the adolescent assumes the homosexual identity and shares it with others. Gay males assume this identity at about 20 years of age and lesbians at about 21 years.[34]

In the fourth stage, commitment to the homosexual identity is made. Internally, the person has a valid self-identity as gay or lesbian and is satisfied with that identity. Externally, this is the stage of "coming out" or disclosing the homosexual identity to society. The time that it takes for disclosure to occur varies because of the homophobia in our society. It is extremely frightening for gay or lesbian adolescents or adults to reveal their sexual identity.[26, 34]

▼ Chapter Summary

▼ In order to adapt to the extrauterine environment, the fetus must undergo major physiologic changes involving respiration, circulation, thermoregulation, and hepatic adaptations. The changes allow the infant to survive in the environment through oxygenating, perfusing, and heating his or her own body.

▼ Infancy is the period from birth through 12 months of age. It is a period of rapid growth and maturation of all body systems. Success in this period depends on nutrition, sleep, psychosocial support, and the absence of diseases.

▼ The early childhood period is the period between ages 1 and 5. Growth continues at a rapid rate but is less intense than during infancy. Body configuration changes and maturation of the body systems is essentially complete. Learning, coordination, and bodily control progress at a rapid rate, and risks for accidents increase because of children's curiosity about the world that surrounds them.

▼ Middle childhood is considered to be from ages 6 to 12. During this time, growth and development slows, and refinement of motor skills occurs with the assistance of a maturing nervous system and improved muscular strength. Learning disabilities are often diagnosed after the child starts attending school.

▼ Adolescence is the transitional time from childhood to adulthood. It is a time of rapid developmental changes that cause the individual to be physically mature enough to reproduce although still emotionally and socially immature. Unplanned pregnancy and sexually transmitted diseases are two major threats to the sexually active adolescent's well-being. Accidents, suicide, acne, and eating disorders are common threats to the physical and emotional well-being of the individual.

▼ References

1. Akridge, K. Anorexia nervosa. *J. Obstet. Gynecol. Neonatal Nurs.* 18:25, 1989.
2. American Psychiatric Association. *Diagnostic and Statistical Manual of Mental Disorders* (3rd ed.). Washington, D.C.: American Psychiatric Association, 1987.
3. Auvenshine, M.A., and Enriquez, M.G. *Comprehensive Maternity Nursing: Perinatal and Women's Health.* Boston: Jones & Bartlett, 1990.
4. Behrman, R.E., and Vaughn, V.C. (eds.). *Nelson Textbook of Pediatrics.* Philadelphia: W.B. Saunders, 1987.
5. Betz, C.L., Hunsberger, M., and Wright, S. *Family Centered Nursing Care of Children* (2nd ed.). Philadelphia: W.B. Saunders, 1994.
6. Cowell, J. Dilemmas in assessing the health status of children with learning disabilities. *J Pediatr Health Care* 4:24–31, 1990.
7. Davidson, J., and Grant, C. Growing up is hard to do . . . in the AIDS era. *Matern. Child. Nurs. J.* 13:352, 1988.
8. Davidson, P.W. Visual impairment and blindness. In Levine, M.D., Carrey, W.B., and Crocker, A.C. (eds.), *Developmental-Behavioral Pediatrics* (2nd ed.). Philadelphia: W.B. Saunders. 1992.
9. Dickason, E.J., Schultz, M.E., and Silverman, B.L. *Maternal Infant Nursing Care* (2nd ed.) St. Louis: Mosby, 1994.
10. Eggleston, P.A. Asthma. In Oski, F.A., et al. (eds.), *Principles and Practice of Pediatrics.* Philadelphia: J.B. Lippincott. 1990.
11. Erikson, E. *Childhood and Society.* New York: W.W. Norton, 1963.
12. Gemma, P.B. Coping with suicidal behavior. *Matern. Child. Nurs. J.* 14:101, 1989.
13. Gibson, L.Y. Bedwetting: A family's recurrent nightmare. *Matern. Child. Nurs. J.* 14:270, 1989.
14. Hynd, G.W., Horn, K.L., Voeller, K.K., and Marshall, R.M. Neurological basis of attention-deficit hyperactivity disorder (ADHD) *School Psychology Review* 20:174–186. 1991.
15. Janke, J. Dealing with AIDS and the adolescent population. *Nurse Pract.* 14:35, 1989.
16. Kleber, H.D. Cocaine abuse: Historical, epidemiological, and psychological perspectives. *J. Clin. Psychiatry* 49:3, 1988.
17. Krantz, M. *Child Development: Risk and Opportunity.* Belmont, CA: Wadsworth, 1994.
18. Marlow, D.R., and Redding, B.A. *Textbook of Pediatric Nursing.* Philadelphia: W.B. Saunders, 1988.
19. May, K.A., and Mahlmeister, L.R. *Comprehensive Maternity Nursing* (3rd ed.). New York: J.B. Lippincott, 1994.
20. National Research Council Committee on Dietary Allowances. *Recommended Dietary Allowances.* Washington, D.C.: National Academy of Sciences, 1980.
21. Papalia, D.E., and Olds, S.W. *Human Development.* New York: McGraw-Hill, 1992.
22. Rankin, W.W. Teenage suicide. *J. Pediatr. Nurs.* 4:130, 1989.
23. Reeder, S.J., Martin, L.L., and Koniak, D. *Maternity Nursing: Family, Newborn, and Women's Health Care* (17th ed.). Philadelphia: J.B. Lippincott, 1992.
24. Remafedi, G.J. Preventing the sexual transmission of AIDS during adolescence. *J. Adolesc. Health* 9:139, 1988.
25. Rothenberg, M.B. In my opinion . . . Role of television in shaping attitudes of children. *Child Health Care* 13:148, 1985.
26. Sanford, N.D. Providing sensitive health care to gay and lesbian youth. *Nurse Pract.* 14:30, 1989.
27. Savin-Williams, R. Theoretical perspectives accounting for adolescent homosexuality. *J. Adolesc. Health* 9:95, 1988.
28. Shaywitz, S., and Shaywitz, B. Attention deficit disorder: Current perspective. In Kavanagh, J., and Truss, T. (eds.), *Learning Disabilities: Proceedings of the National Conference.* Parkton, Md.: York Press, 1988.

29. Sherwen, L.N., Scoloveno, M.A., and Weingarten, C.T. *Nursing Care of the Childbearing Family*. Norwalk: Appleton & Lange, 1990.

30. Sprague-McRae, J.M. Encopresis: Developmental, behavioral and physiological considerations for treatment. *Pediatric Nurs* 8:229, 1990.

31. Stroh, S.E., Stern, H.P., and McCarthy, S.G. Fecal incontinence in children: A clinical update. *Matern. Child. Nurs. J.* 14:252, 1989.

32. Tanner, J.M. *Growth at Adolescence*. Oxford: Blackwell Scientific, 1962.

33. *The Law and Disabled People*. Washington, D.C.: U.S. Government Printing Office, 1980.

34. Troiden, R.R. Homosexual identity development. *J. Adolesc. Health* 9:105, 1988.

35. United States Department of Health, Education and Welfare. National Institute on Drug Abuse, 1989.

36. Wong, D. *Whaley and Wong's Essentials of Pediatric Nursing* (4th ed.). St. Louis: Mosby, 1993.

Chapter 7

Biophysical Developmental Changes of Adults

Barbara L. Bullock

▼ **LEARNING OBJECTIVES**

1 Identify the developmental tasks and conflicts characteristic of each stage of adulthood.
2 Specify physiologic changes that occur during adulthood.
3 Describe the significance of lifestyle patterns during each stage of adult development.
4 Discuss destructive lifestyles and disease processes that are commonly experienced by the adult.
5 Discuss the physiology of exercise.
6 Explain why adults are less physically fit today.
7 Describe the factors causing acute and chronic fatigue.
8 Describe the hazards of using tobacco in any form.
9 Discuss the detrimental effects of substance abuse.
10 List signs and symptoms of the most common eating disorders.
11 Discuss the relationship of sedentary lifestyles to the development of disease.

Adulthood is usually defined as the years from the early twenties to the mid-sixties, which is the largest portion of a person's life span. During this period, human beings are usually at their most productive. It is a time of job achievement and recognition, childrearing, and the establishment of values and attitudes that will be transmitted to succeeding generations. Most adults are in relatively good health; however, the prevalence of both chronic disease and fatal illness increases with age. Accidental deaths, suicides, and homicides cause a higher percentage of deaths during young adulthood, and illness and disability are more frequently seen in later adulthood.[25] Alterations to health may result from self-destructive lifestyle habits rather than from nonpreventable biologic phenomena.[24] This chapter explores adult developmental changes, lifestyle patterns, destructive lifestyles, and some of the related disease processes that are commonly experienced by the adult.

▼ Adult Development

The life cycle, or life span, begins at birth and ends at death. Chapters 5 and 6 have chronicled the developmental changes through adolescence. Chapter 8 describes changes characteristic of the older adult. Chapter 9 deals with the universal concepts of stress and sleep, which affect all periods of the life cycle. Recently, attempts have been made to identify developmental characteristics of the adulthood years. Several theorists have figured prominently in our understanding of developmental changes in the adult. Some of their research results are described briefly here.

DEVELOPMENTAL THEORISTS

Recognizing that physical and cognitive growth is mostly completed by adulthood, early developmental theorists described personality and psychosexual growth as if it ended at adolescence. Erikson was the first to suggest that development continues into adulthood. He conceptualized eight stages that encompass the life span. During each stage, individuals successfully or unsuccessfully resolve specific emotional and social conflicts before moving to the next stage.[9] Figure 7-1 shows the usual developmental tasks, as defined by Erikson, and their approximate placement along the life cycle. The developmental tasks may be resolved in a healthy or unhealthy manner, and the method of resolution is important for later stages of development to proceed smoothly.[25]

Havighurst advanced the theory by organizing information about adult development into tasks each individual needs to accomplish during certain periods of life. Like Erikson, Havighurst related the successful achievement of developmental tasks of one stage to happiness and the potential for success in later stages.[13]

Research by Gould and Levinson has resulted in developmental stages that roughly approximate certain ages. Figure 7-2 shows Levinson's life cycle transitions, especially focusing on those of early and middle adulthood. Vaillant modified Erikson's adult stages, which allows for the agreement about the nature of adult stages that is shown in Figure 7-3.

Each stage of the adult development process contains transitions or turning points that are commonly identified as maturational crises. Although maturational crises can be anticipated and prepared for, the individual experiences stress as they occur. The impact of stress depends on the overall coping ability of the person, the intensity of the stressor, and the number of stressors that occur within a particular time frame (see pp. 178–179).

YOUNG ADULTHOOD

Young adulthood usually is described as that period of time after the teenage years until approximately age 30. It is that period of early adult transition and entrance into the adult world. Neurologic development is complete by age 20. The young adult continues to refine and develop intellectual and cognitive processes. The potential for improved judgment and problem solving is influenced by the types of life experiences the individual has. Reaction times to various stimuli usually peak during young adulthood until the late twenties.

For the most part, physical development is also complete. Men may experience some physical growth after adolescence as their bodies reach the peak in muscular strength and reproductive ability. Athletic ability may reach a peak owing muscular strength and capability during the twenties.[24] Except for accidents and injury, this is normally the healthiest period of life.

The early years of this developmental stage are a time of transition from adolescence into adulthood. Young people may seem caught in both worlds as they attempt to consolidate the sense of identity that was developed during adolescence with the independence that comes from completing an education, beginning an occupation, and moving away from parental decision-making. This is the time when young people validate the perception they have of their identity as they move through new experiences. Ideally, the earlier years of adulthood are a time to try out different lifestyles, jobs, and new relationships before settling down. In addition, the young person begins the process of developing a life plan that will help set the course of his or her life.[8]

The early twenties, however, may be a period of prolonged struggle with adolescent identity issues, especially if the person must remain dependent on parents while in school, unemployed, or searching for a job. The transition may be even more difficult if the young person continues to live at home or remains financially dependent on his or her parents.

PHASES OF THE LIFE CYCLE							
	Infancy	Early childhood	Middle and late childhood	Adoles-cence	Young adulthood	Middle adulthood	Late adulthood
1	Basic trust vs. mistrust						
2		Autonomy vs. shame, doubt					
3			Initiative vs. guilt				
4				Industry vs. inferiority			
5					Identity vs. role confusion		
6						Intimacy vs. isolation	
7							Generativity vs. stagnation
8							Ego integrity vs. despair

FIGURE 7-1 *Erikson's eight stages of development. (Santrock, J.W. Adult Development and Aging. Dubuque, Iowa: W.C. Brown, 1985.)*

A major task of young adulthood is choosing and developing a career. The career decision is so important that most people feel pressure to begin the process in early adolescence and to complete it before the end of their formal education. A choice must be made, despite the fact that young people do not always have a true picture of their abilities or how well they are suited for a particular occupation. Men usually understand the role of work in their lives, but women may feel that there is conflict in their roles and expectations of them.

A second major task of young adulthood is developing the capacity for an intimate relationship. Intimacy implies a shared identity. For healthy relationships to develop, individuals must feel secure enough in their own identities to permit acceptance of the other person. The inability to form intimate relationships at this period may result in isolation and a diminished ability to deal with stress.

A major developmental task is developing a satisfying sexual pattern. Sexual activity occurs frequently in early adulthood, and there are a variety of options avail-

able to young adults.[25] The choice of sexual patterns is individual for each person.

Marriage, childbearing, and childrearing are often a part of this early adulthood transition. The demands on a couple to adequately perform the work role and successfully balance it with home responsibilities can limit the time and energy necessary to develop their own relationship. They may find themselves in conflict about money, responsibility, decision-making, and traditional or nontraditional values about male and female roles. Children add stress to the marital relationship and to career decisions for both men and women. Some couples postpone having children because of career factors.

The inability of a couple to develop and maintain the relationship itself or to cope effectively with external pressure can lead to separation and divorce. Regardless of the circumstances, divorce is an intensely stressful event. Divorce has been compared to experiencing the death of a spouse without either the comfort of formalized mourning or the social supports that accompany such an event.[12] Most divorces occur in the first 3 to 5

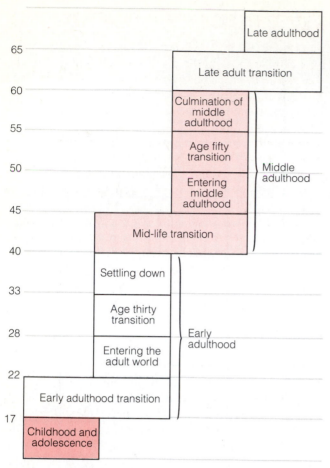

FIGURE 7-2 *Development periods in the eras of early and middle adulthood, as defined by Levinson. (Santrock, J.W. Adult Development and Aging. Dubuque, Iowa: W.C. Brown, 1985.)*

skin elasticity and a few gray hairs remind the individual that aging is occurring. These changes are a source of stress that are compounded by career pressures and family problems. Good nutrition, proper rest, and physical activity can lessen the effects of aging, but the rate of onset of signs of aging is largely determined by genetic factors. The adult developmental conflict involves increasing independence and self-reliance. Individuals are expected to be productive, contributing members of society who participate in the maintenance and continuation of social values. The major tasks include career development and parenting.

The transition to adulthood, at about age 30, may be marked by conflict between stabilizing or modifying the structure of life. The individual must decide between either "settling down" and strengthening relationships and career goals or making changes in the existing life plan before it is too late to do so.[14] Changes, especially in the area of work or relationships, may introduce considerable turmoil without providing guarantees of either success or happiness.

After the transition period, adult men focus on settling down and becoming their own persons.[14] They usually place primary importance on career advancement and productivity. Even though many men take

years after marriage and involve persons younger than 30 years of age. Separation or divorce can result in poor nutrition, inadequate or disturbed sleep, and high levels of stress.

Destructive lifestyles often have their beginning in late adolescence or early adulthood. The effect of these lifestyles may not be apparent until middle or late adulthood. Examples of destructive behaviors are cigarette smoking, excessive alcohol consumption, high fat or cholesterol dietary intake, illegal drug abuse, and risky sexual practices. These behaviors can lead to chronic lung and liver diseases, myocardial infarction, acquired immune deficiency syndrome (AIDS), neurologic dysfunction, and many other conditions. The use of illegal drugs also places individuals at high risk for accidental and homicidal death.

Adulthood

The stage of adulthood is said to include the years between the ages of 30 and 45. Although there are no major physical changes in adulthood, gradual loss of

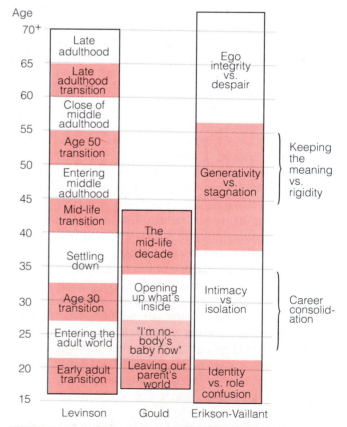

FIGURE 7-3 *A comparison of the adult stages of Levinson, Gould, and Erikson-Vaillant. (Santrock, J.W. Adult Development and Aging. Dubuque, Iowa: W.C. Brown, 1985.)*

more responsibility for childrearing than did their counterparts in previous generations, the career usually absorbs most of their energies. Women who combine work and family, on the other hand, find that they must divide their energies between the two. Career advancement often becomes more difficult for women than for men.

Whatever the occupation, there will be stress associated with it. Correlation between stress-related disorders and specific occupations is assumed, but there is definitely stress associated with all types of work. Some jobs are repetitive and monotonous, some are dangerous or physically demanding, and others may occur in a repressive or restrictive environment. Persons experience stress if their jobs make demands beyond their abilities or if work does not challenge them. Loss of employment, a common reality, causes great stress on the developing family and social relationships.

For couples who choose to have children, parenting is a major task of adulthood. For those who choose not to have children, other fulfillments must be found. Parenthood provides the couple with the opportunity to transmit personal, family, and societal values to a new generation. Some persons may feel that parenthood creates a sense of responsibility for the lives of others; for some, it limits their freedom to take risks and experiment with different roles or occupations. The traditional expectation that adulthood is the stage of life when women devote themselves exclusively to the task of mothering, raising children, and maintaining a household has been challenged by the events of the past 30 years. Yet neither remaining in the home and being a full-time mother nor combining work and parenting is fully or comfortably accepted by all segments of American society. Role conflict invariably is generated for both men and women related to career and parenting responsibilities.

Couples who have divorced may find childrearing complicated by their relationship after the divorce. Both parents may find themselves taking on roles and responsibilities previously handled by the other. Children live with one parent in most cases, with the noncustodial parent fulfilling his or her role intermittently. There may be struggles over money, discipline, privileges, time, and a variety of other concerns. Remarriage adds to the difficulty of raising children after divorce. If one or both spouses bring children to a new marriage, the task of blending the two families can seem overwhelming.

A significant number of couples want to bear children and find themselves unable to conceive. A period of significant stress begins, and self-concepts change as the couple searches for the cause of the infertility. The infertility workup itself is frustrating, time consuming, and expensive, and in the end treatment is not always successful.

At about 35 years age for women and between 40 and 45 years of age for men, the midlife crisis is viewed as another transition period. This period serves as a bridge between adulthood and middle age. It is a time when the individual determines whether the dreams of early adulthood match the realities of life. The individual begins to recognize the limits to achievement and to the time available to accomplish the plans made in early adulthood. Men worry that the opportunities for advancement are decreasing as younger workers begin to challenge their positions. Women who chose a career as young adults are forced to make a decision about having children before their "biological clock" makes the decision for them. They must also contend with the fact that the risks of complications with pregnancy and childbirth increase with age.

Other issues emerge during the midlife crisis. People begin to recognize the inevitability of aging and death. Their parents are aging and may become dependent on their children. The "sandwich" generation may be caught between responsibilities for their children and responsibilities for their parents. Decisions must be made about whether to accept and value life as it is or to make changes before middle age.

Middle Age

Intelligence, memory, and learning do not decrease in the period between ages 45 and 65 unless there are problems associated with central nervous system (CNS) functioning. There is, nevertheless, a gradual slowing of the functional capacity of all organ systems. Of particular concern is the increase of disease processes, such as cardiovascular disease and cancer.

Sexual relationships change according to physiologic changes. Women experience menopause, and men experience a plateau of sexual responsiveness (stable testosterone levels) that leads to slower response and recovery time. Adaptation to these changes maintains the capacity for satisfying sexual relationships.

If individuals have effectively resolved the internal confrontation and the need for change generated by the midlife crisis, they are able to adapt to middle age. Middle age can be a period of giving something back to society, of economic productivity, and of preparation for retirement. Without successful resolution, middle-aged persons may feel a sense of impoverishment, dissatisfaction, and boredom.

As the last child leaves home, parents may feel free to emphasize other interests in life, or they may develop feelings of loneliness and depression. How stressful this time is depends on how the couple engaged in childrearing. If childrearing has absorbed the emotional energy of the couple, they must restructure the marital relationship to again make it meaningful for them.

There is a tendency for people to become more introspective as they move through middle age. They begin to look at life in relation to the time left, not in terms of the time since birth.

▼ Physiologic Developmental Changes During Adulthood

Physiologic changes are an ongoing process. Cell death begins even during embryonic development, as does cell renewal. Over the years, there is gradual decrease in cellular function and the number of cells. Because of aging, human beings pass through stages of immaturity, maturity, and deterioration. Theories regarding the physiologic changes of aging are varied and focus on aging at the cellular level or the wearing out of biologic systems. Cells apparently gradually lose the capacity for self-repair.[24]

BIOPHYSICAL CHANGES IN YOUNG ADULTHOOD AND ADULTHOOD

The physical changes of aging have more variations among adults than among children. Aging rarely progresses uniformly throughout the bodily systems. Persons of the same age appear to be of different ages.[6] Gradual physical decline occurs in many systems of the body. The reserve in the systems accounts for continued optimal organ function.

Young adults begin to have a few physical signs of aging. The skin may develop a few wrinkles, and loss of elasticity may produce some sagging. Hair changes may include graying or balding, depending on the genetic heritage of the individual. Muscle growth continues until about the age of 39 and muscle loss begins after that. Active muscles, especially those that are routinely exercised, atrophy more slowly than sedentary muscles.

The gradual changes in the sensory system do not interfere with functioning until late adulthood. Visual acuity often declines early in adulthood, and minute perceptual changes for the colors of blues, greens, and violets occur.[6] Hearing also declines slowly and often becomes a significant problem late in life. Hearing loss may be accelerated by loud, high-pitched sounds such as those of loud rock music.[23]

Cardiopulmonary changes are insignificant in adulthood unless these systems are weakened by substance or nicotine abuse. There is normally a gradual functional loss, especially in the lungs, which is accelerated by cigarette smoking. Cocaine abuse has been shown to produce myocardial weakening and coronary artery spasm.[7, 19]

The endocrine system is affected by decreased secretion and decreased tissue receptiveness to hormone. The endocrine system affects all bodily activities, including metabolism and sexual functioning. The reproductive system is at peak function in the young adult. This is often the period of reproduction and an active sexual life. The woman's reproductive function declines rapidly after age 30, and this is evidenced by changing menstrual cycles.[19]

BIOPHYSICAL CHANGES IN MIDDLE AGE

The physical changes in the forties and fifties are also variable, but all persons show signs of aging. These signs are expressed throughout all of the body systems. The integumentary system shows wrinkling caused by collagen fiber changes. Over the life cycle, the water content of the body decreases from about 61% to 53%, and fat content increases from 14% to 30%.

The bony skeleton ceases its growth after full height has been reached. Bone mass rapidly declines after age 40 (see pp. 168–170). Calcium loss becomes pronounced during the menopausal years in women; men also lose calcium, but at a later age and at a slower rate than women do. Osteoporosis is most common in thin, white females and least common among blacks.[23] The use of calcium, Vitamin D, and estrogen supplements may decrease the rate of demineralization of the bone. Studies are supporting estrogen replacement in early menopause to decrease the rate of bone loss. Loss of height is common during the aging process. It may be caused by change in the normal 130-degree angle of the hip-femur joint to an angle of 135 degrees or greater.[19]

Muscle strength and mass are directly related to muscle use. Muscle loss is caused by decreased muscle use. Changes in collagen fibers cause a sagging or drooping of muscles, especially those of the face, breast and abdomen.[6]

Some individuals experience a gradual decline in CNS function, which may be seen as a decline in mental functioning and mood. Slower reflexes and decreased responsiveness to changes in the environment are common alterations.[19] CNS function is not often impaired, even though brain cell loss is continuous, because of the large reserve of CNS neurons. CNS changes in middle age are offset by experience and problem-solving ability.[23] Visual changes may become marked after age 40. Presbyopia from loss of elasticity in the lens of the eye causes loss of near vision (see p. 973). Hearing and smell loss may become noticeable at about age 50.

Cardiopulmonary changes are very dependent on lifestyle and genetic factors. Middle-aged individuals with high blood pressure or high cholesterol levels and those who smoke are at much higher risk for cardiopulmonary problems than those without these risk factors (see pp. 458–459). Maintaining an active lifestyle prevents loss of myocardial tone. Lung tissue becomes thicker, stiffer, and less elastic with age, but this process is markedly accelerated by smoking.[19] Repeated respiratory illnesses such as pneumonia, asthma, and bronchitis alter the lung tissue.

Genitourinary problems commonly include stress incontinence and urinary tract infections, especially in women. Stress incontinence is caused by a decrease in urethral muscle support and decreased sphincter control.[19] Some problems with incontinence can be improved by changing voiding patterns, treating urinary tract infections, or surgery.

The gastrointestinal tract exhibits a decline in gastric juice secretion, so that total daily acid production decreases.[19] Ptyalin in the saliva decreases sharply after age 40.[23] Stress and lifestyle changes may affect gastric acid production. Pancreatic enzymes may also gradually decrease between the ages of 20 and 60.[23]

The endocrine system usually exhibits no marked changes, but it is affected by stress and illness, which markedly affect the regulation of blood sugar and electrolyte balance. Middle-aged adults have an increased incidence of adult-onset diabetes mellitus, which is related to familial hereditary factors and obesity.

The reproductive system undergoes the most marked changes in middle life, especially in women. During the climacteric period in women, the ovaries cease to function and the menstrual cycle ceases, either suddenly or erratically. The menopause usually occurs in women at approximately 51 years of age but may occur earlier or later.[6, 19] The resultant estrogen deficiency and pituitary influences cause "hot flashes" and other symptoms (see pp. 1134–1136). Symptoms are aggravated by stress and family changes that may be occurring at this time. The male climacteric is a much slower process and is related to decline in testosterone production (see pp. 1110–1111). Male sexual performance declines in middle age, and impotence in males older than age 50 years is a common problem.

▼ Lifestyle Patterns Affecting Adults

NUTRITION

A significant proportion of adults in the United States have chronic diseases that are caused by nutritional imbalance. Worldwide, nutritional inadequacies are major determinants of resistance to disease and increased mortality. Nutrition is a major environmental factor in the achievement of longevity, in resistance to disease, and in the tolerance and response to stress.

Dietary needs of adults vary according to the amount of energy expended in the course of everyday living. Decreased metabolic needs without decreased intake leads to the development of excess fat, the "middle-age spread." The kinds of foods consumed by many Americans also contribute to the development of excess fat. The most common deleterious dietary practice among Americans is the disproportionate intake of dietary fats and cholesterol at the expense of complex carbohydrates and fiber.[17]

Public education is producing an improvement in the American diet. Even fast food restaurants are beginning to provide foods with less fat and cholesterol. Further education is necessary, especially for persons in poverty-stricken circumstances, to prepare low-fat, nutritious meals. The rate of obesity in the United States is very high (see pp. 240–243). Excess weight is often accompanied by elevated blood levels of cholesterol and triglycerides. These lipids are involved in producing the lesions of atherosclerosis, which may lead to coronary artery disease. Poor nutrition is also associated with hypertension, diabetes mellitus, gastrointestinal problems, renal dysfunction, and periodontal disease.

PHYSICAL FITNESS

Between the ages of 20 and 40 years, the adult begins to view life more seriously, and advancement becomes a predominant task. Major life goals are established. A positive self-image, including body image, is very important. Body image goals for most Americans are for physical beauty and fitness. However, a minority of men and women are physically fit. The reasons for this disparity include inconvenience, discouragement, fear of death, and approach-avoidance behavior. Approach-avoidance behavior is manifested when the person who initially takes part in a fitness program begins to see the program as requiring too much exertion and effort and then drops out of the program. He or she becomes torn between the need and desire for fitness and the tendency to avoid such behavior. Other reasons for not attaining physical fitness include social constraints and commitments, limited convenient access to facilities, loss of interest, declining physical ability, and breakdown of social contacts and networks.[21]

Primitive man's survival depended to a great extent on his physical prowess or efforts. Today, most persons survive through the use of intellect rather than physical abilities. In a highly technological society, there is little reason for many persons to move very much. Machines do much of the work that used to require great physical effort. Major modes of transportation have changed from walking or horseback riding, which requires physical activity, to driving a car, which requires minimal hand and foot movements. Leisure activities have changed from participation to observation. It has become almost impossible to maintain fitness through activities of daily living.

Individuals in the adulthood age group tend to exercise sporadically. This can lead to detrimental effects, because the body is put under stress for which the cardiovascular system is not conditioned. Sporadic exercising can lead to angina or even to myocardial infarction. The ideal physical fitness program must be tailored to the individual, increased gradually, and performed regularly over time to prevent unwanted effects. Recent efforts have been made to overcome one of the most often cited reasons for lack of participation in a physical fitness program, that of inconvenience. Businesses have begun to provide facilities in the workplace for physical fitness, some of which are extended to retirees. Other programs are being offered in neighborhood settings instead of in centrally located health care facilities.[8]

Adults between ages 40 and 65 begin to look at life in terms of the amount of time remaining rather than the amount of time lived since birth. Emphasis is focused on self-development, reexamination, and reevaluation. Physical changes become more dramatic, with the most common being weight gain. These changes may result in increasing stress and frustration. Selye reported research that supported regular exercise as a means to resist stress.[26] Successful aging, which can be defined as being free of pathology and long-lived, occurs when a person is moderately physically active, is a nonsmoker, has a positive outlook on life, and maintains a functional role in society.[22]

There are many advantages to remaining physically fit. The benefits of exercise include improved cardiovascular health, improved flexibility, improved skeletal and muscle strength, increased endurance, and increased respiratory capacity. In addition, increased mobility, physical and psychological stimulation, and relaxation increase the benefits of physical activity. Many studies indicate that sedentary living habits and cigarette smoking are contributing factors to the development of atherosclerosis. A positive relationship between exercise levels and lipoproteins has been identified, and it has been hypothesized that triglyceride levels can be reduced with regular, vigorous physical activity. Medical research supports the therapeutic benefits of exercise, including its effect on rehabilitation of patients with coronary heart disease. Exercise reconditions heart and skeletal muscles, decreases heart rate and blood pressure, and decreases cardiac workload. There is evidence to suggest that exercise may retard age-related declines in neuromuscular efficiency and psychomotor speed.[29]

Lack of activity leads to increases in illness and costs society billions of dollars for health care services. Research suggests that atrophy secondary to inactivity may be responsible for approximately 50% of physical decline in the elderly.[28] Physical activity may not increase the quantity of life but may increase the quality of life for the adult.[18]

Some individuals with mild arthritis have been discouraged from exercising because they are afraid of more severe arthritis. In fact, lack of physical activity accelerates joint degeneration and worsens arthritis.[2] Even with severe arthritis, low-impact aerobic exercise tends to keep the joints flexible and decrease the immobility problems associated with severe disease.

Physiology of Exercise

Exercise involves movement of muscles, which require nutrients, oxygen, and blood flow to supply and remove waste products from the metabolically active muscle. The heart and blood vessels work to provide blood flow to the muscles which delivers the substrates for energy production. The pulmonary system increases the amount of oxygen available to meet the needs of the exercising muscle. During exercise, the cardiac output may more than double, and the respiratory rate may increase threefold. Caloric expenditure in world class athletes may double as the result of 3 or 4 hours of hard training.[16]

The minimal level of energy required to sustain the body's vital functions is called the *basal metabolic rate* or BMR. It reflects the body's heat production and is determined by measuring oxygen consumption. The term MET is used to define the amount of energy needed to complete certain activities. A MET unit is a multiple of the resting metabolic rate. A MET unit of 1 is equal to the BMR. Working at 2 METs is working at twice the resting metabolism. The MET unit can also be expressed in terms of oxygen consumption per unit of body weight, with 1 MET being equal to 3.6 mL/kg/min.[16]

When a person is exercising, the body shunts blood to the skin; this not only releases heat but also provides the skin with nutrients and removes waste products.[2] Bone tissue responds to stresses placed on it; bone density and mass are increased with weight-bearing exercises such as walking and hiking.[2] When bone mass is increased in adulthood, there is a decreased incidence of osteoporosis in later life. Strengthening of muscles also prevents back problems by increasing abdominal and leg muscle strength. This prevents lordosis (an exaggerated lumbar curve) and improves the posture.[2, 16] The addition of weight training increases muscle strength and also has been shown to increase bone density. Proponents of weight training believe that it may help to prolong independence in older adults because it helps to retain the basic strength needed to carry out activities of daily life.[2] Besides the obvious physiologic benefits of exercise, physically fit adults report a generally improved feeling of well-being and a positive self-image.

Exercise is prescribed for persons with heart or vascular conditions. Gradual improvement of aerobic fitness increases the high-density cholesterol levels, which is apparently protective against atherosclerosis of the vessels. Weight loss, sodium restriction, and exercise are routinely prescribed for persons with hypertension; often, if this prescription is followed, medication is not necessary.

As the individual exercises, the heart must provide more blood flow, which it does through increases in contractility and cardiac output.[11] There is increased blood flow to the tissues through vasodilatation, and the heart rate is elevated through the activation of the sympathetic nervous system. During aerobic exercise, the blood pressure is not markedly elevated but with anaerobic exercise, such as weight lifting, there may be a significant rise in the arterial pressure.[11] Effects of exercise on the cardiovascular system and its effects on skeletal muscle are described on pages 839–840.

FATIGUE

The term fatigue refers to a loss of power or strength on exertion.[34] It has been described as a feeling of overwhelming tiredness. Fatigue can be emotionally induced if there are extreme stresses or depression in one's life. It also may result if exercise is performed to the extent that liver glycogen is depleted and glucose is not available for muscle metabolism. Therefore, fatigue may be a subjective or objective condition. The condition may be temporary, or it may occur consistently. It must be differentiated from weakness caused by muscle, neuromuscular, or organic disorders.[34]

Acute fatigue usually occurs as a result of physical exertion, and the extent of the fatigue depends on the physical condition of the person affected. It has a rapid onset and is relieved by varying periods of rest. Individuals also may complain of acute fatigue related to a particularly stressful situation.

Chronic Fatigue Syndrome

Chronic fatigue is often the outcome of chronic illnesses that limit the endurance for activity. It is also one of the main complaints of individuals who consult a physician for assistance. From the complaints of chronic fatigue, a peculiar syndrome has been identified. This is *chronic fatigue syndrome* (CFS) or, more recently, *chronic fatigue and immune dysfunction syndrome* (CFIDS), which is described as disabling fatigue, usually associated with low-grade fever, that has been present for a period of months.[30] It may be preceded by a flu-like illness that leaves the patient with muscle aches and pains, headaches, confusion, depression, sleep disruption, low-grade fever, and sometimes lymph node enlargement or pain.[27]

Chronic fatigue syndrome has been associated with infection with the fungus, *Candida albicans*; with chronic mercury poisoning from dental fillings; with anemia, hypoglycemia, or hypothyroidism; and with sleep disorders. More often, it is associated with Epstein-Barr virus infection, which is probably a result or complication of CFIDS rather than its cause. Diagnosis of CFIDS is made when there is persistent fatigue with associated symptoms lasting longer than 6 months and other significant diseases have been ruled out. Not all CFS cases can be linked with EBV, and there remains substantial disbelief as to the existence of the condition at all.[27]

Research suggests that CFIDS is caused by immune system dysfunction which is probably an overactive state. Over time or in some individuals, there is evidence of immune suppression with functional deficiencies in natural killer cells (see pp. 321–322). CFS symptoms are copious, varied, and often elusive but they comprise a syndrome that is extremely debilitating.[30] CFS sufferers have symptoms that plateau early in the illness and recur with varying degrees of severity for months to years. Victims describe "good" and "bad" days, with the good days contributing to the skepticism of others. The Centers for Disease Control has recognized CFS as a disease that forces individuals to quit work for months or years at a time. CFS is thought to represent a major threat to world health, and its victims in all countries include teachers, health care workers, clergy, flight attendants, and other individuals who have close contact with the public on a regular basis. Even though the disease does not apparently produce death, 60% to 70% of CFS victims remain significantly ill for at least 1 to 3 years. If the illness extends longer than 3 years, the chance of total recovery becomes less than 10%.[27]

Sleep problems are frequently described despite the complaint of chronic tiredness. Antidepressants or antihistamines may improve the sleep disorder component of the disease. The drug Ampligen has been shown in studies to improve the symptoms through immunomodulatory and direct antiviral effects. Whether it will become a standard treatment measure is unknown at this time.

DESTRUCTIVE LIFESTYLES

Given proper diet, exercise, rest, and the ability to cope with the stresses of adult living, adulthood should be characterized by peak physical condition and performance. However, a number of destructive lifestyle patterns place adults at risk for the development of illnesses. Cigarette smoking, substance abuse, eating disorders, and sedentary lifestyles are examples of unhealthful behaviors that often originate in response to stress and contribute to destructive lifestyle patterns.

Smoking

The controversy surrounding the use of tobacco has been evident for a long time. In 1859, Fairholt stated that "tobacco was a comfort to the poor, a luxury for the rich, and . . . united all classes in a common pleasure."[10] The modern period of cigarette manufacture began after the Civil War; however, cigarettes did not begin to be mass-manufactured until about 1890. Before that time, snuff was the tobacco form of choice in both America and Europe.

The literature is replete with evidence regarding the hazardous effects of smoking. Cigarette smoking has been found to decrease or totally paralyze the mucociliary escalator system (see p. 554). It has also been clearly implicated as a major cause of emphysema and chronic bronchitis. The risk of lung cancer increases with the number of cigarettes smoked. The male smoker is 10 times as likely to develop lung cancer as is the male nonsmoker. The American Cancer Society has estimated that 85% of lung cancer can be attributed to cigarette smoking.[3] The nicotine in cigarettes has been shown to increase the risk of heart disease.[1] Smoking has also been associated with the development of cancer of the bladder.[7] Current focus is on exposure to environmental tobacco smoke or passive smoke, which may significantly increase the risk to the nonsmoker.

Despite clear evidence that smoking cigarettes is a health hazard, people continue to smoke. It is estimated that 29% of adults in the United States are smokers, but a 0.5% decline per year is being seen.[1] In the past, smoking was an acceptable habit within society. Smoking is a learned behavior that requires practice and becomes a habit. Nicotine in cigarettes is an addictive substance, and withdrawal signs are common. These include craving for nicotine, irritability, difficulty in concentrating, and weight gain.[1] True addictive behavior is indicated when the person must have a cigarette within 30 min-utes of awakening or smokes more than 25 cigarettes per day.[1] Otherwise, smoking is a habit and may be seen as purposeful (eg, for appetite control) as well as pleasurable. Adolescents view smoking as mature behavior while rationalizing that the health hazards could never happen to them. As a result, the behavior learned at this age is carried with them into adulthood.

Substance Abuse

Many people cope with the stressors of life by the use of substances that alter their mood or perception. Most use depressants, narcotics, or stimulants (Table 7-1). A major problem with psychoactive drug use is the potential for abuse and dependence.

Abuse occurs when a person continues using a substance despite the fact that it is creating problems in major areas of his or her life. Individuals are considered

TABLE 7-1 Problems with Psychoactive Substance Use

Substance	Potential Problems
CNS DEPRESSANTS	
Alcohol	Based on alcohol blood levels, CNS depressant effects increase from sedation and anxiety relief to incoordination, slurred speech, ataxia, stupor, unconsciousness, circulatory collapse, and death. Tolerance develops. Chronic use can lead to peripheral nerve injury; polyneuritis; dementia; myocardial lesions; pancreatitis; impaired liver function; nutritional deficiencies, especially B complex; fetal alcohol syndrome. Withdrawal without treatment can progress from nausea and vomiting, tremors, restlessness, tachycardia, and hypertension to hallucinations, seizures, profound confusion, delirium, and death.
Tranquilizers	Potentiates the effect of alcohol; cross-tolerance with alcohol and sedatives; physical dependence; may accumulate in body with slow excretion by kidneys; fetal deformities. Withdrawal is similar to alcohol.
Barbiturates	Decreases cortical function; ataxia; depresses respiratory centers in medulla; shortens REM sleep; accelerates function of hepatic microsomal enzymes (decreases effectiveness and speeds tolerance); when dependence develops, even temporary abstinence leads to withdrawal symptoms. Withdrawal is similar to that for alcohol.
CNS STIMULANTS	
Amphetamines	Potentiates endogenous catecholamine activity which elevates mood and increases alertness and concentration. Intoxication produces excitation, hyperactive reflexes, hostility, aggression, convulsions. Prolonged use can lead to dysrhythmias, cerebral vascular spasm, CVA, paranoidlike state, severe abdominal pain. Physical dependency occurs. Withdrawal leads to fatigue, lethargy, depression.
Cocaine	Immediate and short-lived CNS stimulation similar to amphetamines. Chronic use is associated with multisystem problems including dysrhythmias, CVA, pulmonary edema, perforation of the nasal septum, anorexia, CNS disturbances, and sexual dysfunction. Psychologic dependence can occur.
NARCOTICS	Relieves pain and anxiety and produces a temporary euphoria. CNS depression, pupillary constriction, depressed respirations occur. I.V. abuse can lead to malnutrition, infection, contaminant toxicity, hepatitis, thromboembolic complications, and AIDS. Tolerance develops with repeated use. Withdrawal includes yawning, tearing, chills and fever, tremors, muscle spasms, and tachycardia. Withdrawal, though uncomfortable, is not life-threatening.

Adapted from Malseed, R.T., and Harrigan, G.S. *Textbook of Pharmacology and Nursing Care.* Philadelphia: J.B. Lippincott, 1989.

to be dependent on psychoactive substances if they use larger quantities than they originally intended to and they are unable to control or decrease use. In addition, much of life revolves around securing and using the substance. If individuals need to increase the amount of the substance to achieve the desired effect, they have developed tolerance to it.[15] Withdrawal is the term used for the symptoms that result from abstinence from the abused substance. Whether withdrawal occurs depends on the quantity and duration of use of the substance.[1]

ALCOHOL. Alcohol is the most frequently abused substance in the United States. Up to 90% of Americans use alcohol, but the frequency of use varies. It is estimated that 10% of male users and 3% to 5% of female users meet the criteria for the disease of alcoholism.[1] Alcoholics do not recognize the impact of alcohol on their lives or the lives of their families. The complications of alcoholism include physiologic impact on the liver and pancreas as well as psychologic and social problems (Fig. 7-4). Some of the physical complaints of the alcoholic

are sleep disorders, gastrointestinal problems, and liver complications (see p. 825). Acute, massive alcohol consumption can have damaging to lethal effects (Fig. 7-5). These may be seen in the individual who consumes massive amounts of alcohol.

Withdrawal symptoms in the alcoholic may be seen within 4 to 8 hours after the last drink. Withdrawal is marked by tremor and irritability, which progresses to agitation, hyperreflexia, and then to visual and auditory hallucinations. Seizures, disorientation, hyperadrenergism, and fever may be seen; these are the hallmarks of true delirium tremors and usually resolve within 72 hours. Delirium tremors may claim as many as 10% to 15% fatalities.[1]

OPIOIDS. Opioids—including morphine, heroin, codeine, oxycodone, and meperidine—are commonly abused drugs. The effects desired by abusers of these drugs are euphoria, sedation, and analgesia, but overdoses cause respiratory depression, coma, and death. Complications usually result from overdoses or nonsterile injection. Systemic reactions to the preparations used cause a high incidence of chronic liver disease, especially in heroin abusers. Withdrawal begins within 2 to 48 hours after the last usage. Especially with heroin, the abrupt stoppage causes rapid onset of restlessness, rhinorrhea, shivering, tachycardia, and hypertension. Treatment is aimed at suppressing many of the autonomic symptoms of withdrawal.[1]

COCAINE AND AMPHETAMINES. Cocaine is a very commonly abused drug that is usually inhaled nasally but may be smoked, ingested, or injected. Free-basing the drug with diethyl ether produces high serum concentrations and great potential for toxicity. Amphetamines are usually taken orally. Both cocaine and amphetamines produce a sense of euphoria and elation resulting from catecholamine release by the CNS. Over time, with abuse of the drugs, acute and chronic paranoid psychoses have been seen. Physical problems have to do with route of administration and include nasal perforation, rhinitis, renal failure, cerebrovascular accidents, and cor pulmonale.[1] Withdrawal is characterized by lethargy, somnolence, and depression. Craving for the effect of the drug makes it very difficult to stop this addiction.

Eating Disorders

Common eating disorders of early adulthood are *anorexia nervosa* and *bulimia nervosa* (see pp. 243–249). Anorexia nervosa usually begins in adolescence but may continue into adulthood. Bulimia is thought to occur more often in early adulthood. Although they are treated as two separate disorders, many of the behaviors overlap.

Anorexia nervosa is a potentially life-threatening

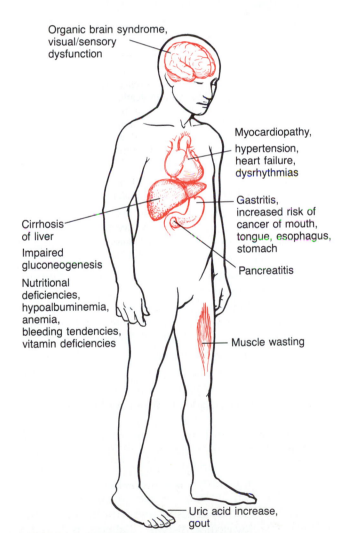

Organic brain syndrome, visual/sensory dysfunction

Myocardiopathy, hypertension, heart failure, dysrhythmias

Gastritis, increased risk of cancer of mouth, tongue, esophagus, stomach

Pancreatitis

Cirrhosis of liver

Impaired gluconeogenesis

Nutritional deficiencies, hypoalbuminemia, anemia, bleeding tendencies, vitamin deficiencies

Muscle wasting

Uric acid increase, gout

FIGURE 7-4 *Alcoholism can have damaging systemic effects.*

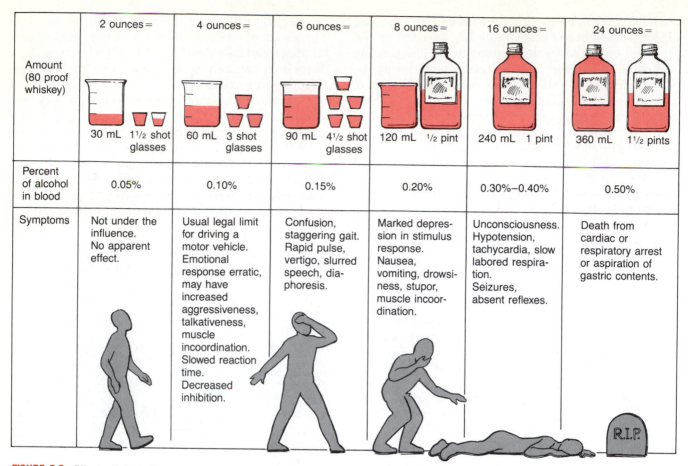

	2 ounces =	4 ounces =	6 ounces =	8 ounces =	16 ounces =	24 ounces =
Amount (80 proof whiskey)	30 mL 1½ shot glasses	60 mL 3 shot glasses	90 mL 4½ shot glasses	120 mL ½ pint	240 mL 1 pint	360 mL 1½ pints
Percent of alcohol in blood	0.05%	0.10%	0.15%	0.20%	0.30%–0.40%	0.50%
Symptoms	Not under the influence. No apparent effect.	Usual legal limit for driving a motor vehicle. Emotional response erratic, may have increased aggressiveness, talkativeness, muscle incoordination. Slowed reaction time. Decreased inhibition.	Confusion, staggering gait. Rapid pulse, vertigo, slurred speech, diaphoresis.	Marked depression in stimulus response. Nausea, vomiting, drowsiness, stupor, muscle incoordination.	Unconsciousness. Hypotension, tachycardia, slow labored respiration. Seizures, absent reflexes.	Death from cardiac or respiratory arrest or aspiration of gastric contents.

FIGURE 7-5   *Effects of alcohol ingestion on the average 68-kg (150-pound) male. Females usually react earlier to ingestion, even when body sizes are comparable. Symptoms are those generally seen.*

illness that is characterized by the loss of at least 15% of body weight, a voluntary refusal to eat, an obsessive concern about food and gaining weight, a distorted body image, and a tendency toward strenuous exercise.[5] The majority of affected persons (95%) are women. The anorexic person sees herself as fat, no matter what her weight. Often the only control she feels over her life is the control she is able to exert over food and its consumption. Therefore, it is common for the individual to deny the need for treatment and resist attempts to force weight gain.

Physical symptoms of anorexia nervosa include weight loss, an emaciated, malnourished appearance, slow pulse, and amenorrhea. Other symptoms include lanugo, brownish discoloration of the skin, hypotension, dry, lifeless hair, decreased gastric motility, and listlessness.[5] In addition, there may be anemia, lymphocytosis, leukopenia, hypocholesterolemia, hypoglycemia, and hypoproteinemia. Changes occur in the gonadotropins and ovarian hormones. Death may result from malnutrition, infection, or cardiac problems.

Bulimia is characterized by binge eating (consuming a large amount of food quickly) and purging (the process of eliminating what has been eaten by vomiting or by use of laxatives or enemas, or both). Bulimics tend to be somewhat overweight or of normal weight, but they too are concerned with the size and shape of their bodies. Unlike people with anorexia nervosa, those with bulimia are aware of the abnormality of their eating patterns but are unable to stop.

The dentist may be the first to identify bulimia from tooth enamel erosion caused by the high acid content of the vomitus. Concentrated urine, abnormal electrolytes, fever, poor skin turgor, weakness, and lethargy may occur if body fluids are depleted.[5] Abuse of syrup of ipecac can cause cumulative systemic toxicity that affects the neuromuscular, gastrointestinal, and cardiovascular systems.

Obesity is the most common nutritional problem in the United States. The nation as a whole overconsumes calories but remains undernourished because of an imbalanced diet. It has been estimated that 25% to 40% of adults older than 30 years of age are more than 20% overweight.[35] Obesity is associated with increased incidence of cardiovascular disease, diabetes, pulmonary dysfunction, and gallstones.[35] Obesity is characterized by a number of metabolic changes related to lipid metabolism. Obese individuals often have elevated serum cholesterol and triglyceride levels and lower concentrations of high-density lipoprotein; these changes increase the risk for coronary heart disease.

Sedentary Lifestyles

The current best estimate is that only about 10% to 20% of adults participate in enough exercise to provide for cardiorespiratory benefit. In one community-based study of cardiovascular disease, physical inactivity was estimated to account for as much as 23% of cardiovascular risk.[20] Recent surveys indicate that fewer than 10% of Americans older than 18 years of age meet the criteria for exercise proposed by the Centers for Disease Control as 1990 objectives for the nation, and the amount of physical activity at work and in the home has declined steadily with increasing automation and labor-saving aids.[4]

Television viewing is the most pervasive pastime in the United States today. After sleep and work, it is the nation's most time-consuming activity. The typical adult watches television almost 4 hours per day. If the television is on, activity ceases and time for exercise is reduced significantly. Owing to decreased calorie expenditure, adults who view 3 hours of television or more each day have twice the risk of obesity and an even higher risk of superobesity.[31]

An increase in physical activity, together with a decrease in total energy intake and a decrease in dietary fat, are needed to control obesity in sedentary affluent societies. Food intake is better regulated at higher levels of physical activity.

Individuals in sedentary occupations are more prone to cancer of the colon.[33] Physical activity is associated with a reduced intestinal transit time, supporting the hypothesis that the bowel mucosa has reduced exposure to potential carcinogens. In addition, physical exercise and leanness are associated with less cancer of the reproductive system in female athletes, whereas obesity is associated with increased risk for cancers of the breast and endometrium in postmenopausal women.

The adult years are an important time for education and medical care to preserve health and prevent or delay the onset of chronic disease. Despite the vast scientific, economic, and human resources devoted to health care, many of the deaths and disabilities that occur annually in the United States are premature. Cardiovascular disease, cancer, stroke, and injuries are the leading causes of adult death in this country, accounting for almost 75% of deaths annually, and they are intimately linked to preventable risk factors.[32] Many of these factors, including smoking, improper nutrition, alcohol misuse, overweight, lack of exercise, and maladaptive responses to stressful experience, can be modified by changes in personal behavior or social choices.

▼ Chapter Summary

▼ The adulthood span is considered to be from the ages of about 20 to the mid 60s, the largest portion of the person's life span. This era was largely ignored by developmental theorists until Erikson conceptualized the stages that included adulthood. Other theorists have modified and added to this concept. Basically, adulthood can be divided into young adulthood, adulthood, and middle age. Each of these time periods is variable with the individual and each have physiologic and psychologic aspects.

▼ Adulthood is the time when life style patterns affect the health of the individual. These include nutrition, physical fitness, stress, sleep, fatigue, and destructive lifestyles. Stress and sleep are considered in Chapter 9. There is a direct link between nutrition and onset of different diseases. Physical fitness also improves health and decreases onset of certain diseases. Besides dietary imbalances and sedentary behavior, smoking and substance abuse are major health damaging behaviors. The adult years are an important time for education and medical care to preserve health and prevent or delay the onset of chronic disease. Despite the various resources—scientific, economic, and human—devoted to health care, it is a disturbing fact that many deaths and disabilities that occur annually in the United States are premature. Cardiovascular disease, cancer, stroke, and injuries—the leading causes of adult death in this country, accounting for nearly 75% of deaths annually—are intimately linked to preventable risk factors.[32] Many of these factors, including smoking, improper nutrition, alcohol misuse, overweight, lack of exercise, and maladaptive responses to stressful experience, can be modified by changes in personal behavior or social choices.

▼ References

1. Bauer, R.I., Kadri, A.A., and Hunt, D.K. Substance abuse. In Stein, J. (ed.), *Internal Medicine* (4th ed.). St. Louis: Mosby, 1994.
2. Brehm, B. *Essays on Wellness.* New York: HarperCollins, 1993.
3. *Cancer Facts.* New York: American Cancer Society, 1993.
4. Centers for Disease Control. Progress toward achieving the 1990 national objectives for physical fitness and exercise. *MMWR Morb. Mortal. Wkly. Rep.* 38:449, 1989.
5. Chitty, K. Applying the nursing process for clients with eating disorders. In Wilson, H.S., and Kneisl, C.R. (eds.), *Psychiatric Nursing* (4th ed.). Menlo Park, Calif.: Addison-Wesley, 1991.
6. Clark-Stewart, A., Perlmutter, M., and Friedman, S. *Life-long Human Development.* New York: Wiley, 1988.
7. Cotran, R.S., Kumar, V., and Robbins, S.L. *Robbins' Pathologic Basis of Disease* (4th ed.). Philadelphia: W.B. Saunders, 1989.

8. Dacey, J. and Traver, J. *Human Development Across the Lifespan.* Dubuque, IA: W.C. Brown, 1991.
9. Erikson, E.H. *Childhood and Society* (2nd ed.). New York: Norton, 1963.
10. Fairholt, F. *Tobacco: Its History and Associations.* London: Chapman & Hall, 1859
11. Freeman, G.L. Cardiovascular physiology. In Stein, J. (ed.), *Internal Medicine* (4th ed.). St. Louis: Mosby, 1994.
12. Gould, R.L. *Transformations: Growth and Change in Adult Life.* New York: Simon & Schuster, 1978.
13. Havighurst, R.J. *Human Development and Education.* New York: Longman, 1972.
14. Levinson, D.J., et al. *The Seasons of a Man's Life.* New York: Ballantine, 1978.
15. Malseed, R., and Harrigan, G. *Textbook of Pharmacology and Nursing Care.* Philadelphia: J.B. Lippincott, 1989.
16. McArdle, W.D., Katch, F.I., & Katch, V.L. *Exercise Physiology* (2nd ed.). Philadelphia: Lea & Febiger, 1986.
17. McGinnis, J., and Hamburg, M. Opportunities for health promotion and disease prevention in the clinical setting. *West. J. Med.* 149:468, 1988.
18. McPherson, B. (ed.). *Sport and Aging.* Champaign, Ill.: Human Kinetics, 1986.
19. Mourad, L.A., and Ashburn, S.S. Biophysical development during middlescence. In Schuster, C.S., and Ashburn, S.S. *The Process of Human Development* (2nd ed.). Boston: Little, Brown, 1986.
20. Oberman, A. Exercise and the primary prevention of cardiovascular disease. *Am. J. Cardiol.* 55:10D, 1985.
21. Ostrow, A. *Physical Activity and the Older Adult: Psychological Perspectives.* Princeton, N.J.: Princeton Book Company, 1984.
22. Palmore, E. Predictors of successful aging. *The Gerontologist* 19:427, 1980.
23. Perlmutter, M. and Hall, E. *Adult Development and Aging.* New York: Wiley, 1985.
24. Rogers, D. *The Adult Years: An Introduction to Aging* (3rd ed.). Englewood Cliffs, N.J.: Prentice-Hall, 1986.
25. Santrock, J.W. *Adult Development and Aging.* Dubuque, Iowa: W.C. Brown, 1985.
26. Selye, H. *The Stress of Life.* New York: McGraw-Hill, 1956.
27. Shafran, S.D. The chronic fatigue syndrome. *Am. J. Med.* 90:730–739, 1991.
28. Smith, E., and Serfass, R. (eds.). *Exercise and Aging.* Hillside, N.J.: Enslow, 1981
29. Spirduso, W. Physical fitness, aging, and psychomotor speed: A review. *J. Gerontol.* 35:850, 1980.
30. Tauber, M.G. Fever of unknown origin. In Stein, J. (ed.), *Internal Medicine* (4th ed.). St. Louis: Mosby, 1994.
31. Tucker, L., and Friedman, G. Television viewing and obesity in adult males. *Am. J. Public Health* 79:516, 1989.
32. U.S. Department of Health and Human Services. *Health United States: 1986.* Publication No. (PHS) 87-1232. Hyattsville, Md.: National Center for Health Statistics, 1986.
33. Vena, J., Graham, S., Zielezny, M., Brasure, J., and Swanson, M. Occupational exercise and risk of cancer. *Am. J. Clin. Nutr.* 45(Suppl):318, 1987.
34. Vesely, D.L. Weakness. In Stein, J. (ed.), *Internal Medicine* (4th ed.). St. Louis: Mosby, 1994.
35. Weser, E., and Young, E.A. Nutrition and internal medicine. In Stein, J. (ed.), *Internal Medicine* (4th ed.). St. Louis: Mosby, 1994.

Chapter 8

Biophysical Changes of the Older Adult

Gretchen McDaniel

▼ CHAPTER OUTLINE

Biologic Theories of Aging
Early Theories of Aging
Modern Theories of Aging
  Free Radical Theory
  Waste Product Theory
  Immunologic Theory
  Cross-Link Theory
  Somatic Mutation Theory
  Genetic Aging Theory
Biophysical Effects of Aging and
  Susceptibility to Disease
General Effects
Nervous System
Cardiovascular System
  Anatomic Changes
  Physiologic Changes
  Conduction System Changes
  Arterial Changes
  Venular Changes

Diseases Related to the Aging Cardiovascular
  System
Respiratory System
  Anatomic Changes
  Functional Changes
Genitourinary System
  Anatomic Changes in the Kidneys
  Physiologic Changes in the Kidneys
  Diseases and Problems With Aging Kidneys
  Bladder Changes
  Gynecologic Changes in the Elderly Woman
  Reproductive Changes in the Elderly Man
Gastrointestinal System
  Normal Anatomic Changes
  Esophageal Changes
  Stomach Changes
  Colon Changes
  Pancreatic Changes
  Liver Changes

Musculoskeletal System
  Characteristic Changes in Anatomic Structure
    and Function
  Joint Changes
  Problems Related to Skeletal Degeneration
  Fractures and Risk of Falling
Skin and Dermal Appendages
  Changes in the Skin, Nails, and Hair
  Diseases Associated With Aging Skin
Sensory System
  Vision Changes
  Hearing Changes
  Other Sensory Changes
Aging and Cancer
Variables That Modify Biophysical Effects
  of Aging
Aging and Infection
Pharmacology and the Elderly
Chapter Summary

▼ LEARNING OBJECTIVES

1 *Discuss important research on the aging process.*
2 *Describe the biologic cellular theories of aging: free radical, waste product, immunologic, cross-linkage, somatic mutation, and genetic theories.*
3 *List the general effects of aging.*
4 *Describe the causes and effects of nervous system alterations.*
5 *Relate anatomic alterations in the cardiovascular system to the resultant physiologic changes.*
6 *Describe how the arterial changes in the elderly alter blood flow and pressure.*
7 *Discuss causes and effects of hypertension in the elderly.*
8 *Describe the physiologic result of the respiratory changes caused by aging.*
9 *Explain why elderly persons are at risk for the development of respiratory failure after stressful situations.*
10 *Compare renal function of the young adult with that of the elderly person.*
11 *List common organisms that can cause bladder infection in the elderly.*
12 *Describe the effects of lack of estrogen in postmenopausal women.*
13 *Describe the effects of hormone changes in elderly men.*
14 *Discuss briefly the many factors that cause digestive disturbances in the elderly.*
15 *Characterize the alterations in body movement that occur as a consequence of aging.*
16 *Explain the factors that lead to increased risk of bone fractures in the elderly.*
17 *List the joint changes that are common in the elderly, at what age they begin, and when they become symptomatic.*
18 *Describe the characteristic changes in skin, nails, and hair associated with aging.*
19 *Explain how sensory alterations affect adjustment in the aging process.*
20 *Describe one variable that can modify the biophysical effects of aging.*
21 *List at least two cancers that are more common in elderly persons than in the younger population.*
22 *Describe the atypical presentations of four infections to which the elderly have an increased susceptibility.*
23 *Discuss the factors associated with aging that cause alterations in drug metabolism.*

Barbara L. Bullock: PATHOPHYSIOLOGY: ADAPTATIONS AND ALTERATIONS IN FUNCTION, 4th ed.
© 1996 Lippincott-Raven Publishers

The phenomenon of aging is variable and complex in nature. It is very difficult to define what aging is or to establish the facts about the process. Much of the confusion arises from the difficulty of differentiating between normal aging and changes secondary to disease. The causes of aging have been investigated for centuries, yet no researcher has been able specifically to identify any single causative factor. Modern health care practices have resulted in an increased life expectancy in the United States. The variability of life span for humans seems to be a function of several factors: heredity, culture, race, nutrition, and environment. Total life span seems to be limited to 90 to 105 years, which supports the belief that aging is an innate process.

▼ Biologic Theories of Aging

Biology, sociology, and psychology have arrived at various explanations for the changes that occur with the aging process. Some theories have been thoroughly researched, whereas others do not enjoy the support of clinical testing or the acceptance of the medical community.

EARLY THEORIES OF AGING

Until the 19th century, most of the interest in the aging process was concerned with ways to prevent it. The ancient Egyptians tried to find the fountain of youth. Hippocrates (c. 460–377 B.C.) perceived aging as stemming from a decrease in body heat, a natural, irreversible, and unavoidable phenomenon. Galen (c. 130–201 A.D.) had a similar theory postulating that the increased coldness and dryness of aging resulted from changes in body humor. Also, Galen viewed aging as a lifelong process, as opposed to an event occurring late in the life span.[28] Leonardo da Vinci stimulated later development of theories of biologic aging through his descriptions and drawings.[9]

Theorists in the 18th and 19th centuries claimed that life was intrinsic energy which gradually decreased over time to the point of death. Darwin viewed aging as the body's inability to respond to stimuli as a result of decreased nervous and muscular tissue irritability. The predominant aging theories in the early 1990s included the "autointoxication" theory and the "wear and tear" theory.[28]

MODERN THEORIES OF AGING

To understand differences among theories of aging, it is necessary to examine the processes that take place within the aging organism. Of importance to research is the number of times cells replicate themselves.[22] Research evidence has shown that the number of times normal diploid human fibroblasts can replicate in vitro is limited. Hayflick reported, "The sum of population doublings undergone by normal fetal human fibroblasts both before and after preservation is always equal to 50 ± 10."[20] Cells isolated from older persons show progressively fewer doublings before finally stopping.

Other researchers noted that the homeostatic mechanisms that govern immunity and cellular replication decrease as a person grows older. Both cell division and ribonucleic acid (RNA) synthesis of protein slow down. There is also increasing heterogenicity of cells in terms of size, shape, and mitotic capabilities.

Common in metabolism of the older person is increased collagen cross-linkage. Cross-linkages are stable molecules that prevent deoxyribonucleic acid (DNA) strands from dividing in the normal cell reproductive cycle. Cross-linkage molecules accumulate and affect proteins in elastin and collagen, resulting in cell death. The cell death results in decreased elasticity of blood vessels and skin.[12]

This section describes biologic cellular theories of aging. No one theory answers all the questions, but each provides a clue to the aging process and certain interrelationships that do appear to exist.

Free Radical Theory

The free radical theory proposes that free radicals serve as central agents in the changes observed with aging at the tissue, cellular, and subcellular levels.[10] Free radicals are parts of molecules that have broken off or molecules that have had an electron stripped from their structure. Free radicals are normally produced in certain metabolic reactions; they are within the cellular structural system and do not diffuse freely within the cells. When they become diffusible, they damage or alter the original structure or function of other molecules by attaching themselves to them.[10]

The free radical theory has been linked to the idea of oxygen toxicity. Oxidation of proteins, fats, carbohydrates, and other elements in the body results in the formation of these free radicals.[11] Lipofuscin, a pigmented material that accumulates in some organs with aging, is associated with oxidation of unsaturated lipids. Lipofuscin is thought to have a relationship to free radicals and the aging process because of this lipid oxidation.[28] Diffusible free radical end products and compounds can cause cellular disruption. In the aging process, the number of free radical compounds appears to increase faster than body cells can repair the damage. Some scientists consider the cell membrane as the key to survival and believe that the greatest damage could be perpetrated by free radicals at this membrane level.[12]

Vitamin E is thought to protect the mitochondria from the hazards of the free radical activity. Vitamin E may function as an *antioxidant* and binding agent in the antioxidation process. This theory supports the use of antioxidants such as vitamin E in an attempt to delay cellular aging.

Free radical activity is also fostered in the body by such environmental factors as smog, byproducts of the plastics industry, gasoline, and atmospheric ozone. The human body appears to be bombarded from both external and internal sources of free radicals. If this theory is as fundamental to aging as proponents believe, careful monitoring of the environment and proper food selection should lead to better health in old age.

Waste Product Theory

The waste product theory is derived from observations of increased pigment in aging cells. The pigment, called lipofuscin, is a dark, irregular, granular inclusion within cells.[11] There is some evidence that lipofuscin occurs in cells as a result of a variety of processes such as autophagocytosis, oxidation of lipids, and copolymerization of organic molecules. It has been suggested that lipofuscin forms as an end product of free radical–induced lipid peroxidation. This suggestion provides a connection between oxygen consumption, free radicals, lipofuscin, and aging.[30] The actual effect of lipofuscin on cellular function is not known.

Immunologic Theory

The immunologic theory asserts that aging is an autoimmune process. The body's immune system fails to recognize its own cells as the cells change with age. Autoimmune responses damage or destroy cells, leading to cell death.[14] Tissue damage and increased susceptibility to infection may be caused by the presence of autoantibodies and decreased numbers of immunocompetent cells (see Chapter 16). Whether the diminished capacity for immune responses is a cause of aging is not known, but it certainly is the source of many of the disease problems of the aged, such as increased frequency of autoimmune diseases, cancers, and infections of all types.

Aging affects all parts of the immune system, but especially the T cells. A decline in T cell–dependent immune function begins at sexual maturity with the onset of involution of the thymus gland. This factor is associated with increased frequency of diseases such as cancer and autoimmune diseases. Macrophages that play a major role in protecting the body against infection do not seem to diminish in number as the body ages. The number of B cells remains elevated, but responsiveness to stimulation by antigens decreases markedly, probably because of dependence on T-cell stimulation.

Cross-Linkage Theory

The cross-linkage theory, also called the collagen theory, suggests that strong chemical reactions create strong bonds between molecular structures that are normally separate. Cross-linking produces irreparable damage to DNA and leads to cell death. Cross-linkage agents are so numerous and varied in the diet and in the environment that they are impossible to avoid.[12] Connective tissue changes are an indicator that cross-linkage has occurred. Collagen, which makes up a large part of the proteins of the body, is the substance that maintains strength, support, and structural form. As a result of the chemical action of cross-linking, aging collagens become more insoluble and rigid, resulting in inhibition of cellular permeability. Passage of nutrients, metabolites, antibodies, and gases through the blood vessel walls is inhibited. Also, the linings of the lungs and the gastrointestinal tract are affected.

Elastin, another of the fibrillar proteins present in connective tissue, is very prone to cross-linkage. It differs from collagen on the basis of its chemical composition and physical properties. Both elastin and collagen respond to cross-linkage in the same manner. Aging elastin becomes frayed, fragmented, and brittle, leading to many changes in connective tissue throughout the body. A good example of this is skin changes, such as dryness and loss of turgor, elasticity, and tone. Cross-linkage also affects cell division because cross-linkage molecules prevent division of the strands of the DNA. If only one strand is affected, no damage results. If the cross-linkage molecule attaches itself to both sides of the DNA, the cell dies because division is prevented. Such cell death has a profound effect on the elasticity of blood vessels and skin. As a result of the changes in collagen and elastin, cross-linkage is thought to be a primary cause of aging.

Somatic Mutation Theory

The somatic mutation theory asserts that spontaneous mutation occurs in DNA. This mutation occurs by hydrolysis, miscoding of enzymes, or irradiation. The mutation may be perpetuated during cellular replication if it is not corrected by repair enzymes. Mutant cells decrease the efficiency of cellular function, and thus organ function declines.[14]

Genetic Aging Theory

The genetic aging theory is based on the belief that the life span is programmed before birth into the genes in the DNA molecule. This means that a person fortunate enough to have long-lived parents or grandparents has a longer life expectancy than he or she would have had with short-lived parents. This theory is supported by genealogical studies that indicated that children whose parents died before age 60 had an average life expectancy almost 20 years shorter than that of children whose parents died at 80 years of age.[28]

▼ *Biophysical Effects of Aging and Susceptibility to Disease*

Aging leads to a gradual diminution in the functional capacity of the organ systems. In working with the elderly, it is important to distinguish between problems attributed to primary structural organ changes and secondary, reversible processes amenable to intervention.[32] Also, it must be realized that the aging process is extremely variable among different individuals. Chronologic age is a poor index of physiologic age or of performance, and advancing years are not necessarily equated with illness.

GENERAL EFFECTS

The appearance of the aging person characteristically is altered. Stature is lost, body proportions are changed, skin is dry and wrinkled, hair is thinning and gray, and there are changes in body movement characterized by slowness, stiffness, and diminished coordination and balance. The intervertebral disks become thin, as do the vertebrae themselves, leading to reduction in height. The thoracic curve of the vertebral column increases, resulting in a kyphosis. This development, along with changes in lung elasticity, results in increased anteroposterior diameter of the chest. The cervical curve increases to compensate for the thoracic curve, causing a tilting of the head. Height loss, therefore, is in the trunk. The length of the long bones is unchanged. The effect is a short trunk and long limbs, which is just the opposite of what is seen in a child (Fig. 8-1).

The total body composition is altered. Lean body mass is reduced, including fat-free body tissues such as nerves, organ parenchyma, and skeletal muscle. Increased amounts of fat are laid down in mesenteric or perinephritic areas rather than in subcutaneous fat. Decreased subcutaneous fat leads to increased skin folding.

Amounts of total body potassium, water, and intracellular fluid decrease; however, there is no change in the amount of extracellular fluid. The bone mineral mass is reduced, with increased bone porosity. Figure 8-2 shows the major changes in the body components with aging. The aggregate effect of these losses is reduced total body density.[29]

Weight changes are characteristic. In men, the average maximum weight is 172 pounds at ages 35 to 54 years. This falls to 166 pounds at ages 55 to 64. In women, the average maximum weight is 152 pounds at 55 to 64 years, 146 pounds at ages 65 to 74, and 138 pounds at ages 75 to 89 (see Appendix C). The weight of women declines less than that of men.[26]

Visible changes in movement are primarily caused by alterations in the nervous system, with diminished muscle strength and joint mobility contributing only minimally. Movement is an extremely complex activity requiring integration of many portions of the nervous system. Intact sensory information going to the brain must be coupled with integration of cortical, basal ganglionic, and cerebellar function. The extrapyramidal system is subject to early changes in function owing to diminished presence of neurotransmitters. Vascular supply to all portions of the brain is critical to coordinated function for movement. Locomotion becomes increasingly precarious with aging.

Fasting blood sugar, blood volume, serum pH, red blood cell count, and osmotic pressure are unchanged with aging in the absence of disease. The ability to respond to severe stresses is altered, however. For example, normal pH may be well maintained under normal circumstances, but should ventilatory failure or metabolic acidosis occur, the elderly person takes much longer to restore normal pH. Responses to events such as infection may be diminished or slowed. An elderly person may have an infectious illness with subnormal or normal temperature and a normal heart rate.

NERVOUS SYSTEM

The general integrative effects of aging are strongly affected by alteration in the central nervous system. Nerve impulses decrease their rate of conduction by about 10%, which may lead to ischemia, generally lower basal metabolism, and decreased temperature in nerve fibers.[6] The transmission strength of signals from the brain to the body parts decreases as a result of the dwindling number of neurons, the degenerating myelin sheath, and the formation of senile plaque with age. The signals become slightly blurred, and the threshold for arousal of an organ system may be altered. Adaptation to physiologic stressors does not occur as rapidly in the elderly as in younger persons. The increased recovery time within the autonomic system causes an organ to take longer to return to base level activity after stressful situations.

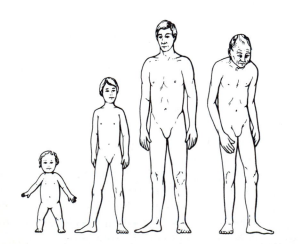

FIGURE 8-1 *Changes in body proportions through the life span.*

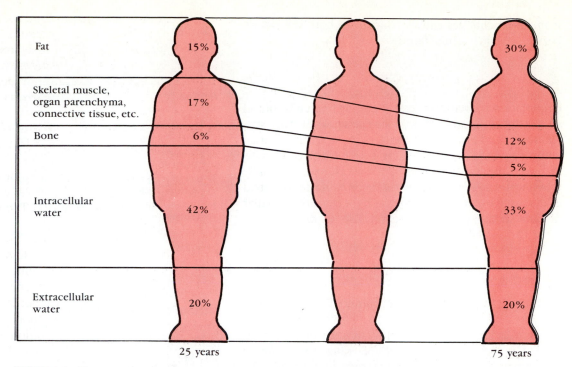

FIGURE 8-2 *Changes in major body components with the aging process.*

Substantial metabolic changes within the synaptic complexes are related to neurotransmitter production. Changes are particularly evident in Alzheimer's disease, where there is evidence of marked degeneration in the cell bodies of the cortical cholinergic nerve terminals. In normal aging, there is evidence of decreased numbers of dopaminergic neurons in the substantia nigra and noradrenergic neurons in the locus cerulens at the base of the fourth ventricle[32] (see pp. 1095–1096). Changes in neurotransmitter effects are known to be related to many brain functions associated with neuroendocrine events, such as sleep, temperature control, memory, and especially mood. Depression is associated with reduced levels of norepinephrine in the brain, a common occurrence in older persons. Despite these changes, intellectual function in the older adult seems to be sustained.

Physical changes also occur in the brain. The brain loses an average of 100 g in weight between 25 and 70 years of age.[24] In the older individual, changes occur in the cortex and in the white matter. White matter volume decreases by 11% between 70 and 90 years of age. During this period, there is a 2% to 3% decline in the number of neurons in the cortex.[24] Little loss occurs in the brainstem. Atrophy of the convolutions of the brain is common, with widening of the sulci and gyri, especially in the frontal lobe. Dilatation of the ventricles also is common. Despite these anatomic changes, there is little reduction in the total amount of DNA, nucleic acid, or protein.

The intracellular accumulation of lipofuscin pigment has been studied extensively. A major accumula-

tion of this pigment in the brain is in storage vacuoles, especially in the medulla and hippocampus, and this is quantitatively correlated with age. The amount per cell varies, but there can be enough to fill the cytoplasm and force the nucleus into an abnormal position. Although little is known about the effect of lipofuscin on cellular function, it is thought that its accumulation can hamper oxygen use.[4]

Neurofibrillary tangles frequently occur in the aging brain, but these are not exclusive to the older adult. This abnormal tissue appears to interrupt intraneuron communication. Large numbers of neurologic tangles have been found in people with neurologic disorders, such as Alzheimer's disease and senile dementia.[14]

Because of physiologic and metabolic changes in the brain and reduced oxygen consumption, less intracellular energy is produced; glucose use is diminished, and cerebral blood flow is reduced. The electroencephalogram (EEG) of the older adult remains within the normal limits of other age groups except that it is about one cycle slower. Also, physical changes contribute to degeneration of the blood-brain barrier in elderly persons, which has implications for medication administration and may help to explain acute confusional states related to medication administration.

The effects of general changes in the brain are associated with the common characteristics of aging. These include decreasing motor strength; lack of dexterity and agility; difficulties in association, retrieval, and recall; diminished memory and cognitive ability and change in affect; and, often, depression. The behavior resulting from these changes causes concern to both the elderly person and his or her family.

CARDIOVASCULAR SYSTEM

Under normal circumstances, the aging heart adapts and allows the person to maintain an average level of activity. Anatomic and physiologic changes cause reduced stroke volume and cardiac output (Table 8-1). The heart begins to have difficulty adapting to the workload, especially when unusual demands are made on it. If the workload is increased by such conditions as hypertension, valvular disease, or myocardial infarction, the result can be altered cardiac adaptation.

Anatomic Changes

Anatomic changes in the heart lead to diminished contractility and filling capacity. Loss of muscle fiber in the heart, with localized hypertrophy of individual fibers, is caused by the increased amount of collagenous material that surrounds every fiber. Thickening of the semilunar and atrioventricular valves causes increased resistance to blood flow. The end result is a heart encased in a more rigid collagen matrix, which leads to diminished contraction and decreased filling capacity of the heart chambers.

Physiologic Changes

The numerous physiologic changes that occur in the heart include alterations in the conduction system, loss of contractile efficiency, and decreased levels of circulating catecholamines. The evidence of changes in the heart differs at rest and with exercise. After 60 years of age, peripheral vascular resistance increases 1% per year.[12]

TABLE 8-2 *Cardiovascular Changes With Age (>60 y)*

Resting	Exercise
1. Decreased left ventricular stroke volume (SV)	Decreased maximum oxygen consumption
2. Decreased total cardiac output (C.O.)	Decreased maximum C.O.
3. Increased systolic blood pressure (SBP)	Increased SBP
4. Increased systemic vascular resistance (SVR)	Increased SVR
5. Decreased heart rate (HR)	Decreased maximal HR

The change in peripheral resistance, coupled with the anatomic and physiologic changes previously described, produces numerous alterations in the capacity of cardiac performance. Cardiac output decreases approximately 1% per year.[12] The heart rate increase that occurs in response to stress is less effective, and the range of optimal heart rate narrows. Mild tachycardia or bradycardia may lead to a significant deficit in blood flow in vital organs.

The combination of all these factors results in a heart that no longer has the capacity to meet all the demands that it met in earlier years (Table 8-2). Excessive fluid load, excessive workload (as in shock or hemorrhage), and insult to the heart muscle (as in ischemia or infarction) are met by a heart muscle that is less able to compensate. Output may be inadequate relative to demands, leading to many circulatory problems, such as cardiogenic shock and congestive heart failure. Even in situations of mild stress, all organs are less well perfused and therefore function less adequately.

Conduction System Changes

The changes in the conduction systems of the hearts of elderly persons are caused by alterations in the conduction system per se and by ischemia from interrupted blood supply through the coronary arteries. Disturbances of the autonomic nervous system and the local chemical (ionic) environment of the pacemaker cells may initiate dysrhythmias. The conduction impulses may be blocked as a result of increased fibrous tissue and fat in the myocardium, and by loss of fibers in the bifurcating main bundle of His and the junction of the main bundle and its left fascicles.[5] Parts of the system may become irritable and susceptible to irregular discharge. Digitalis administration is a common cause of dysrhythmias in elderly persons that can be potentiated by low serum potassium levels. A danger exists if potassium-depleting diuretics are used in association with digitalis.

TABLE 8-1 *Age-Related Changes in Heart Rate, Cardiac Output, and Blood Volume*

Age	HRm	HRr	C.I.	BV
20–40	180–190	70–75	3.0–3.7	2.7
50	175	70	2.8–3.1	2.6
60	165	65	2.6–3.6	2.6
70	155	62	2.4–3.2	2.5
80	145	59	2.4–3.2	2.4

BV, blood volume (L/m²); C.I., cardiac output indexed to surface area (cardiac index L/min/m²); HRm, heart rate maximum; HRr, heart rate resting.

Cardiac dysrhythmias contribute to poor cardiac output and may result in cardiac arrest.

Arterial Changes

Blood vessels are markedly affected by degenerative changes in aging, particularly the arteries. Basic to the problems of all arteries is the progressive stiffness caused by the cross-linkage effect on elastin and smooth muscle as the amount of collagen increases. This generalized problem in the arteries leads to increased peripheral resistance. The major arteries demonstrate these changes as follows:[25]

1. The tunica intima becomes thickened and less smooth as arteriosclerotic streaks are accumulated.
2. In the tunica media, muscle fibers are replaced by collagen or connective tissue and calcium material.
3. The ability to expand or stretch decreases owing to the changes in the intimal layers.
4. Higher blood pressures become common in the older adult because of decreased interior diameter of the arteries and diminished stretchability.
5. The aorta and its branches tend to dilate and become tortuous.

In addition, *atherosclerosis* develops. Fatty streaks in the intima have been found to be present in the first year of life. These may or may not be related to the subsequent development of atherosclerotic changes. As a person ages, the number of atheromatous plaques increases, resulting in raised areas with a central core of degenerative lipid on the tunica intima. These plaques are most numerous in the major arteries, particularly the aorta and the iliac, coronary, and carotid arteries. They also occur frequently in the renal and femoral arteries. Pathologically, they cause two problems: thrombosis and occlusion in the lumen of the artery and destruction of the tunica media leading to aneurysm. Aneurysms occur most typically in the abdominal or thoracic aorta. Arterial changes are widespread and result in diminished circulation to all organs and tissues. Of particular consequence is reduced circulation to the brain and to the kidneys. Renal plasma flow is reduced approximately 6 mL per year, from 600 mL per minute per kidney in early adulthood to 300 mL per minute per kidney by 80 years of age.[25]

Venular Changes

The thin-walled veins have valves formed from the internal layer that assist the blood to flow toward the heart, but prevent a reversal of the flow. Veins constrict and enlarge, store large quantities of blood, make the blood available when it is required by the circulation, and can actually propel blood forward.[21]

Because muscle contractions in the legs provide the upward propelling force for venous return, every time the legs are moved or the muscles are tensed, a certain amount of blood is propelled toward the heart. Varicose veins occur when the valves of the venous system are destroyed. They are common in older persons, and are usually caused by inactivity, constricting clothing, and crossing the legs at the knees. The venous stasis that occurs with varicose veins further complicates the circulatory problems.

A major vascular problem of aging is that of venous thrombosis and pulmonary emboli. Immobilization from increased time spent sitting and in bed enhances the risk of thrombosis.

Diseases Related to the Aging Cardiovascular System

Hypertension becomes substantially more common with age, even though it is not an essential aspect of aging. Approximately 40% of whites and more than 50% of African Americans older than 65 years of age have hypertension.[28] The systolic pressure gradually increases with age because of decreased aortic elasticity. The increase in diastolic pressure is less marked and results from increased resistance in the peripheral blood vessels. The diastolic pressure tends to level off in later life. Cardiac output and blood volume are also factors in the regulation of blood pressure. Blood pressure is elevated because of increased resistance to blood flow caused by arteriolar constriction. Blood pressure lowers when arteriolar relaxation reduces resistance to blood flow.

Benign essential hypertension is the most common type in persons older than 70 years of age, with more than 90% of all cases in this category.[33] Elevated pressure usually develops slowly and with little untoward effect in benign essential hypertension. Complications of hypertension account for a significant number of deaths in the United States. Hypertension contributes considerably to diseases of the cardiovascular system. It is associated with increased frequency of coronary artery disease and myocardial infarction and with hemorrhagic problems and infarcts in the brain. It is also associated with major hemorrhage from cerebral arteries and resultant strokes.

Transient cerebral ischemic attacks may occur before major strokes. These attacks are caused by arterial occlusion or hypotension. The occlusive phenomena occur most frequently in the carotid artery. The signs are hemiparesis, hemianopsia, aphasia, and loss of vision in one eye. The vertebral artery is more often involved with hypotensive states, causing the person to fall forward on the knees (without loss of consciousness), along with vertigo, vomiting, dysarthria, visual blurring, or diplopia.[8] The baroreceptors in the aorta and carotid arteries become less sensitive to pressure changes, and sudden changes in position may cause dizziness or syncope. Pressure on the carotid sinus may cause serious slowing of the heart rate and may be elicited by twisting and turning of the head.

RESPIRATORY SYSTEM

Alterations in the respiratory system in the aged impose many limitations that are not always obvious when the person is at rest but appear with exertion or stress. Under usual circumstances, older persons are capable of maintaining normal daily activities, but various changes make them more susceptible to pulmonary infections. Various consequences of the aging respiratory system are presented in Flowchart 8-1. Among aged individuals, influenza and pneumonia are the fourth leading cause of death, with bronchitis, emphysema, and asthma ranking eighth.[13]

Anatomic Changes

Loss of elasticity affects the older person's pulmonary compliance and results from increased cross-linkage in collagen and elastin fibers around the alveolar sacs. Pressure builds up within the alveolar sacs during inspiration, some of which tends to be retained during expiration, and finally results in an increased residual air volume. In addition, there is a decrease in the quantity of air that can be taken in during normal breathing.

Changes in the costal cartilage result in a diminution of chest wall compliance, which is further complicated by skeletal deformities of the thorax and postural changes such as stooped shoulders. In the older adult, the changes in the muscular system lead to a decline in the strength of muscles that assist respiration. Degeneration of the intervertebral disks of the thoracic spine result in increased anteroposterior diameter of the chest and a chest wall that is less compliant during respiration.

The end result of the loss of elasticity, muscle weakness, and changes in the structure of the chest is difficulty in expiration of air. Results of pulmonary function studies are altered by this reduced capacity to empty the lungs. Total lung capacity is changed little, but vital capacity is gradually and progressively reduced. The forced expiratory volume and maximum breathing capacity are both reduced, and the residual volume and functional residual capacity of the lungs are increased (Fig. 8-3). The residual volume increases 50% between the ages of 30 and 90. The maximum breathing capacity is diminished by 60% between ages 20 and 80.[19] Actual air flow is reduced 20% to 50% throughout the adult years.

Functional Changes

The main functional respiratory problems in the elderly person without pulmonary disease are reduced ventilation of all alveoli, especially at the bases of the lungs, and

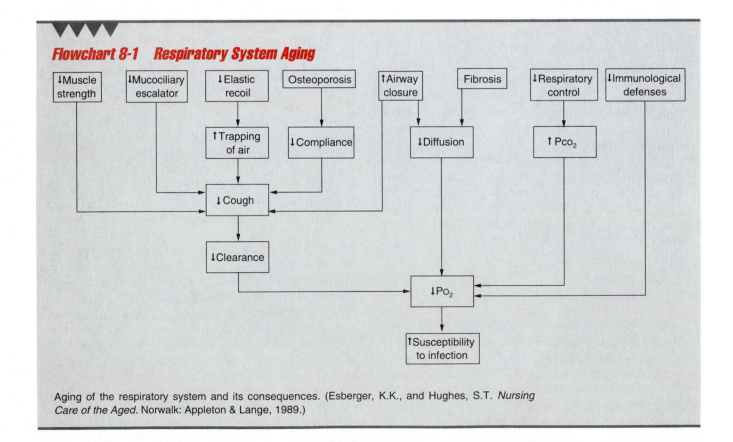

Flowchart 8-1 Respiratory System Aging

Aging of the respiratory system and its consequences. (Esberger, K.K., and Hughes, S.T. *Nursing Care of the Aged.* Norwalk: Appleton & Lange, 1989.)

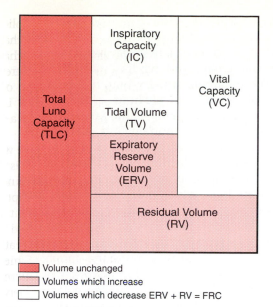

Volume unchanged
Volumes which increase
Volumes which decrease ERV + RV = FRC

FIGURE 8-3 *Changes in lung volume with aging. TLC does not change with aging. As the amount of trapped air increases, the amount of air that is moved by breathing is decreased. (Adapted from Esberger, K.K., and Hughes, S.T. Nursing Care of the Aging. Norwalk: Appleton & Lange, 1989.)*

reduced oxygen partial pressure in the arterial blood. The partial pressure of arterial oxygen (Pao_2) declines with age, averaging 75 mm Hg in the seventh decade. The partial pressure of carbon dioxide ($Paco_2$), however, remains the same unless disease is superimposed on the diminished ventilation; this constancy is probably a result of the higher rate of diffusion of carbon dioxide. With the structural and mechanical changes that have been described, the bases of the lungs are ventilated less and less. The part of the lungs that is well perfused is the part of the lungs not being ventilated. Blood must be shunted to the ventilated upper portions of the lungs. The redistribution of blood is usually insufficient to compensate, and the Pao_2 falls. The condition becomes worse when the elderly person lies down, and nocturnal hypoxemia may be a major cause of confusion.

Functional deficits may not impair function under baseline conditions or with minimal physical exertion. However, changes in the capacity to increase the work of breathing, resulting from structural changes that reduce the maximum breathing capacity, put the elderly person at risk for respiratory infections. The need to increase oxygen intake rapidly or to blow off carbon dioxide rapidly because of acidemia may cause decompensation and rapid respiratory failure in an elderly person with no respiratory disease per se. Sudden increases in physical activity or sudden psychologic stress may overwhelm a respiratory system that handles moderate stress well.

An elderly person with little previous difficulty may develop respiratory failure rather rapidly after stress such as surgery, excessive exercise, a sudden rise in

environmental pollution (eg, in smog crises), or infection (eg, pneumonia). The assumption must be made that all elderly individuals are at risk for respiratory failure. Respiratory failure is evidenced by a diminishing Pao_2 and a rising $Paco_2$ associated with a drop in arterial pH.

Potential causes of respiratory failure are surgery, the use of depressant drugs, lung infections, bed rest, pulmonary edema caused by circulatory problems, and pulmonary embolism. Pulmonary embolism occurs frequently in elderly patients who are immobilized because of bone fractures or other conditions requiring bed rest. Any acute condition such as trauma, burns, or myocardial infarction in the elderly may be complicated by respiratory failure. The potential of unrecognized pulmonary changes, particularly those caused by environmental effects, is present in all persons older than age 40.

In addition to functional changes, which are normal alterations with aging, most persons in modern industrialized society have lung changes caused by chronic environmental pollution. Inhalants such as smoke, various industrial end products, and the end products of combustion of petrochemicals have a profound effect on respiratory function. They cause decreased ciliary action, increased mucus production, and deposition of foreign materials in the functional alveoli and in intercellular spaces. These pollutants have two main effects: they increase the obstructive component in lung function, and they decrease the compliance of the lung tissue through deposits of foreign material that increase its stiffness. The latter effect is common among miners and industrial workers who constantly inhale coal dust or asbestos.

GENITOURINARY SYSTEM

Genitourinary problems in older adults are common conditions that many of these individuals are reluctant to discuss. In addition to causing embarrassment, they are bothersome and are frequently thought of as a sign of growing old. Renal dysfunctions are potentially life-threatening and become more so because of delay in detection and treatment.

Anatomic Changes in the Kidneys

The urinary tract undergoes many changes with age. The kidneys are affected by involutional processes, and normal age-related changes occur in renal vascular anatomy and function independent of disease. The nephrons begin to degenerate and disappear by the seventh month in utero. The normal young adult has approximately 800,000 to 1 million nephrons in each kidney.[21] These gradually degenerate, and their number is reduced by one-third to one-half by the seventh decade.[19] Changes

TABLE 8-3 *Changes in Kidney Size, Volume, and Filtering Surface Across the Life Span*

	At Birth	Young Adult	Over 65 Years	Percentage Loss
Kidney mass (g)	50	270	185	31
Kidney volume (mL)	20	250	200	20
Filtering surface area (m²)	0.02	1.6	0.9	43

in kidney size, volume, and filtering surface over the life span are shown in Table 8-3.[20]

In addition to the loss of nephrons, there is some degeneration of the remaining nephrons. The degeneration starts as a sclerosis or scarring of the glomeruli, followed by atrophy of the afferent arterioles. The glomeruli, deep in the cortex of the kidney, retain one capillary that enlarges and acts as a shunt between the afferent and efferent arterioles. The compensation that does occur results from enlargement of the remaining nephrons. Despite enlargement of the nephrons, the net weight of each kidney decreases by about 20% to 30%, and this occurs primarily in the cortex.[12]

Physiologic Changes in the Kidneys

Because of the loss of nephrons or functional units of the kidneys, a decline in function is to be expected with age. The kidneys do not concentrate urine as well because of the loss of nephrons. Under normal circumstances, however, the kidneys are capable of maintaining acid-base balance.

The renal filtration rate decreases about 6% per decade. As general arteriosclerosis occurs throughout the body, the arterioles in the kidneys are also affected. The result is that some of the blood is diverted to other parts of the body and does not pass through the glomerular filtration system. Gradual decreases in renal blood flow and glomerular filtration rate are related to decreases in cardiac output, renal mass, and filtering surface of the kidneys.[28]

The physiologic alterations result in slower renal adaptation to excess acid or alkaline loads in the elderly. Even minor stress can cause disruption in kidney function, and aged kidneys have difficulty in restabilizing.

Diseases and Problems With Aging Kidneys

Renal function in the elderly may be compromised by one or more of the following: inadequate fluid intake, fluid loss from vomiting or diarrhea, shock due to hem-

orrhage, acute or chronic cardiac failure, septicemia caused by gram-negative bacteria, and injudicious use of diuretics.[15] Any one of these may result in renal ischemia and acute renal shutdown if not promptly corrected.

The minimum urinary output should be 400 mL daily. Output of 20 mL per hour or less may herald acute renal failure. Acute renal failure frequently arises in the elderly and carries a mortality rate of 80% in persons 70 years of age and older. The dangers of acute renal failure include fluid overloading, which leads to congestive heart failure and pulmonary edema, and rising serum potassium level, which may cause cardiac arrest.

Diseases of the kidneys, regardless of the cause, create long-term problems. In addition to the various pathologic events associated with such diseases, the elderly person also must adapt to the normal changes of aging. The most frequent chronic kidney disease in the elderly is pyelonephritis. Other physiologic conditions that can lead to kidney dysfunction include hypertension, sodium and water retention, marked sodium or water loss, retention of potassium, and loss of serum protein. The greatest concern is inability of the kidneys to handle changing concentrations of hydrogen ion. The responses to increased hydrogen ion concentration are slowed and diminished, leading to metabolic acidosis.

Several antibiotics often used to treat infections in elderly persons are nephrotoxic, including tetracycline, cephaloridine, and gentamycin. Occasionally, penicillin also has this effect. It is not uncommon for an elderly person who has sepsis from an infection to develop acute renal failure after treatment with one of these antibiotics. It is difficult to ascertain under such circumstances whether renal failure is caused by the antibiotic or by the shock associated with the infection.

Bladder Changes

Two of the most common and bothersome problems elderly persons encounter are nocturnal frequency of micturition and urinary incontinence. Among changes that contribute to these problems are loss of muscle tone, which results in relaxation of the perineal muscles in the female, prostatic hypertrophy in the male, bladder diverticuli, sphincter relaxation, and altered bladder reflexes (Fig. 8-4). Frequently, bladder capacity is reduced. Incomplete emptying of the bladder predisposes the elderly person to residual urine and infection.

Escherichia coli is the most frequent cause of bladder infection in women, whereas *Proteus* species are the most common in men.[11] Bladder infections can result from poor hygienic practices or from anything that impedes urinary flow, such as neoplasms, strictures, or a clogged indwelling catheter. Urine may become alkaline in the presence of an infection, leading to the formation of small inorganic salt calculi. Gross or microscopic hematuria may occur with urinary tract infections (see p. 634).

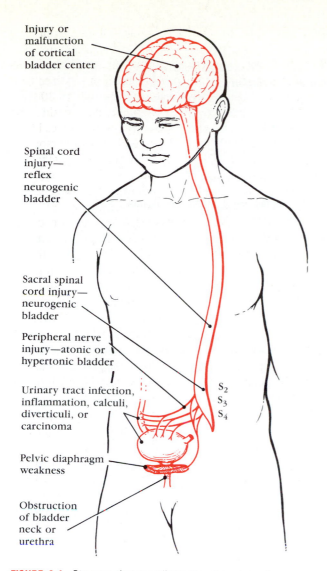

Injury or
malfunction
of cortical
bladder center

Spinal cord
injury—
reflex
neurogenic
bladder

Sacral spinal
cord injury—
neurogenic
bladder

Peripheral nerve
injury—atonic or
hypertonic bladder

Urinary tract infection,
inflammation, calculi,
diverticuli, or
carcinoma

Pelvic diaphragm
weakness

Obstruction
of bladder
neck or
urethra

S_2
S_3
S_4

FIGURE 8-4 *Stresses that contribute to urinary incontinence.*

Gynecologic Changes in the Elderly Woman

In the elderly woman, objective gynecologic findings are directly related to the effects of estrogen deprivation. General atrophy occurs in the reproductive system, causing a reduction in the size of the uterus and cervix, thinning of the vaginal walls, changes in mucous secretions, and greater friability and susceptibility of vaginal tissue to irritation and infection. Because of diminished secretions, the vagina loses the normal flora that create its protective acid environment. Atrophic changes result in a vulva that is pallid and has a loss of subcutaneous fat accompanied by a flattening and folding of the labia. Breast tissue thins and sags as a result of replacement of atrophying glandular tissue with fat.

Reproductive Changes in the Elderly Man

Physiologic changes in the elderly man are also caused by lowered hormone production but occur much more gradually than in the female. The testes undergo cellular change with no significant change in size. Fat content increases in testicular cells, and the number of cells decreases. The number of sperm ejaculated decreases by up to 50% by 90 years of age. Sperm change in size and shape and lose their fertilization ability.[3] Androgen production begins to decline at age 30 years and continues to decline until age 90.

Most elderly men have some benign prostatic hyperplasia, which is considered to be a normal aging change. The changes result in a prostate that is more fibrous and has irregular thickening. The frequency of prostatic cancer also increases with age (see pp. 648–649).

GASTROINTESTINAL SYSTEM

Normal Anatomic Changes

The gastrointestinal system is the site of many diseases in the elderly, ranging from simple dyspepsia to carcinoma. Contributing to the prevalence of these conditions are many normal features of aging (Table 8-4). The grinding surfaces of the molars have worn down, and many elderly persons have lost most or all of their teeth. With the loss of chewing ability, they may eat only soft food, thereby developing gum and digestive problems. Altered taste sensation, caused by a decline in the number of taste buds, fosters a poor appetite, and this can result in malnutrition.

Esophageal Changes

Changes in esophageal motility begin to occur with aging. Degenerative changes in the smooth muscle that lines the lower two-thirds of the esophagus result in delayed esophageal emptying, dilatation of the esophagus, and an increase in nonpropulsive contractions.[1, 6] Obstructive phenomena can occur as a result of tumors, rings, or strictures.

The risk of hiatal hernia in persons older than age 50 may be as high as 40% to 60%. Small hiatal hernias are so common that they are frequently considered a normal finding on radiography.[34] Difficulty in swallowing is one of the primary symptoms. Hiatal hernias can mimic pulmonary distress and angina; therefore, radiography should be performed to verify the diagnosis.

Stomach Changes

It is thought that the stomach mucosa becomes thinner; however, in some studies have indicated that gastric mucosa remains normal in individuals up to 80 or 90 years of age.[1] It is generally thought that gastric acid secretion is decreased with age. Pernicious anemia is common in the elderly because vitamin B_{12} is dependent on the gastric intrinsic factor for its absorption (see

TABLE 8-4 *Gastrointestinal Changes of Aging*

Change	Complication or Association
Loss of teeth	Poor intake, large bolus
Loss of tongue papilla, taste, and smell	Poor appetite, weight loss
Reduced salivary ptyalin	Slight reduced carbohydrate digestion
Reduced esophageal peristalsis	Delayed emptying, presbyesophagus
Irregular nonperistalitic esophageal waves	Delayed emptying, presbyesophagus
Poor relaxation of esophageal sphincter	Delayed emptying, presbyesophagus
Hiatal hernia	Esophagitis, bleeding
Thinned gastric mucosa and muscularis; decreased gastrin, gastric acid, pepsin, and intrinsic factor	Atrophic gastritis, iron deficiency anemia, pernicious anemia, ulcer, carcinoma
Decreased colonic muscle tone; decreased colonic motor function	Constipation
Diverticulosis	Diverticulitis
Reduced liver weight and blood flow	None
Decreased inducible enzymes of the liver	Altered drug metabolism
Reduced serum albumin	Weakness, weight loss
Increased globulin	None
Cholelithiasis	Cholecystitis

O'Hara-Devereaux, M., Andous, L.H., Scott, C.D. (eds.). *Eldercare: A Practical Guide to Clinical Geriatrics.* New York: Grune & Stratton, 1981, p. 100.

pp. 785–786). Gastric motility and gastric emptying appear to decrease with age.

Colon Changes

Constipation is one of the most frequent complaints of the elderly population. In a large percentage, constipation is caused by cultural eating patterns, decreased exercise, decreased gastric motility, low fluid intake, and the ingestion of drugs such as antihypertensives and sedatives. Constipation in elderly persons is compounded by the abuse of purgatives, laxatives, and enemas, which are employed to resolve constipation-thus creating a vicious cycle.

Diseases of the colon that are common in the elderly include diverticulosis, diverticulitis, polyposis, and cancer of the colon (see Chapter 41). Diverticulosis is considered to be a disease of aging, with the majority of diverticuli arising in the sigmoid colon. Most of these diseases are asymptomatic, but occult blood in the stool is common, especially with colon cancer.

Pancreatic Changes

The changes in the pancreas with age are associated with pancreatic ductal epithelial hyperplasia and intralobular fibrosis.[1] On rare occasions, this fibrosis may lead to atrophy. The volume of pancreatic secretions declines and enzyme output diminishes with advanced age. However, the importance of these changes in causing dysfunction or nutritional impairment has not been thoroughly researched.[1]

Liver Changes

There is a decrease in liver size and hepatic blood flow with advancing age. Hepatocytes tend to be larger and have increased nuclear DNA. A brown, atrophied appearance of the liver is seen in older persons as a result of deposited lipofuscin granules in hepatocytes. However, this trait has also been found in younger individuals who have cachexia or malnutrition.[1] Hepatic parenchymal fibrosis may be present, but it has no apparent functional significance.

MUSCULOSKELETAL SYSTEM

One of the most visible characteristics of aging is the change in posture and patterns of movement (Fig. 8-5). Successful portrayal of an old person by an actor nearly always includes certain features of body movement, such as stooped posture, muscular rigidity, slow movement, and lack of coordination and stability. Alterations in neuromuscular function result from the combined effect of changes in the muscles, the peripheral motor neurons, the myoneural synapses, and the central nervous system. Diet, heredity, and hormonal balances also are influences on the musculoskeletal system.

Characteristic Changes in Anatomic Structure and Function

General wasting of skeletal muscles occurs because of loss of muscle fibers. Muscle strength, endurance, and agility are affected by the decrease in muscle mass. All

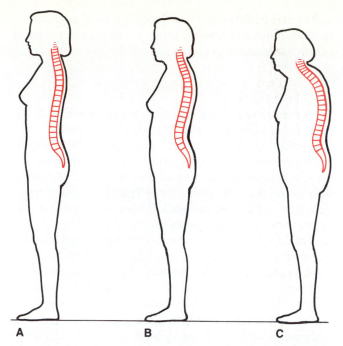

FIGURE 8-5 *Posture changes occur gradually as aging occurs.* **A.** *Early to middle adulthood, spine is straight.* **B.** *Middle age to early aging with early osteoporosis changes weakening the vertebrae.* **C.** *Late aging changes may show a height loss of 10 cm or more.*

Joint Changes

Joint changes in the elderly include erosion of the cartilagenous surfaces of the joints, degenerative changes of the soft tissues in the joints, and calcification and ossification of the ligaments, especially those around the vertebrae. The name given to the degenerative processes of the joints is *osteoarthritis*. Once again, it is difficult to determine how much of this process is normal aging because it is present in all persons to some degree. It may begin at 20 years of age, and by age 50 radiologic changes may be present.[19]

The cartilage of the joints loses elasticity, becomes dull and opaque, and then softens and frays, denuding the underlying bone. The underlying bone develops a proliferation of fibroblasts, and new bone is formed. At the joint margins, extensive proliferation produces bony outgrowths or spurs. If spurs project into the joint, they can cause considerable pain and limitation of motion. Pieces of cartilage and bone may break off to form loose bodies in the joint that require surgical removal.

Changes in joints are probably the result of long-term trauma. Alterations resulting from osteoarthritis are easily seen in the fingers with the development of Heberden's and Bouchard's nodes (Fig. 8-6). Overgrowth of the bone margins on the fingers, which occurs most often in women, may be unsightly but is usually

muscle activity in the elderly is affected by the degree of oxygen supply and its alterations, which are related to reduced circulatory and respiratory function. The peripheral motor neurons also have some decrease in protein synthesis, with thickening at the myoneural junction and decrease in acetylcholine levels.

The general decrease in movement, coupled with muscle stiffness and slowness, particularly in initiating movement, is attributable primarily to prolongation of contraction time, latency period, and relaxation period of motor units, as well as changes in the extrapyramidal system. A resting tremor may also be present. These changes are considered normal. If the extrapyramidal function becomes severely impaired, Parkinson syndrome, chorea, or dystonia of various types may appear.

In addition to the wasting of skeletal muscles, loss of minerals causes the bones to become more brittle. The amount of trabecular bone begins to decrease in the midthirties. By 90 years of age, women have lost 43% of trabecular bone, and men lose 27% by 80 years of age. Cortical (compact) bone loss begins to occur in the mid-forties in women and in the fifties in men. This bone loss results in a change in cortical-trabecular bone ratio, from 55:45 at age 15 years to 70:30 by age 85.[28] Reduction in height results from hip and knee flexion, kyphosis of the dorsal spine, and shortening of the vertebral column.

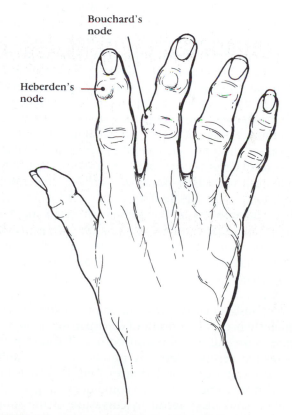

FIGURE 8-6 *Heberden's and Bouchard's nodes in an elderly individual. Note the lateral deviation of the third and ring fingers.*

not painful. If bone overgrowth occurs about the hip, the femoral head may become trapped, painful, and immobile. Hip replacement surgery may be required. The cartilaginous disks that exist between the vertebrae undergo the same pathologic changes that take place in the other joints. The degenerative changes are contributed to by the predisposing factors of aging, extensive involvement in physical activities leading to injury, excessive use of the joint, and obesity. These pathologic changes are accompanied by pain and limitation of motion.

Problems Related to Skeletal Degeneration

Osteoporosis is basically caused by an increase of bone absorption over bone formation. This primarily affects trabecular bone and also the cortices of long bones. The outer surfaces of long bones continue to grow slowly throughout life, but with osteoporosis, the inner surfaces are reabsorbed at a slightly faster rate. The end result is a long bone that is slightly longer in external diameter but with thinner walls and with markedly diminished trabecular bone in its ends. Vertebral bodies, which have a larger percentage of trabecular bone, are severely affected by this process.[2]

In osteoporosis, there is evidence of decreased calcium absorption from the gastrointestinal tract. Also, the disease has some relation with gonad deficiency, because its frequency is greatly increased in postmenopausal women. Immobilization and lack of weight-bearing on the skeletal system causes osteoporosis at any age. Also, elevated levels of cortisone, either exogenous or endogenous, cause the condition. Regardless of the underlying pathologic process, osteoporosis occurs to a degree in all elderly persons but is much more marked in women.

Of primary concern in osteoporosis is the tendency for bone fracture, most frequently of the vertebrae and the femurs. Studies of elderly persons show that 34% of fractures of the femur are caused by accidents.[3] Twenty-five percent occur because of a "drop attack," which is a sudden fall caused by postural instability that results from changes in the hindbrain and cerebellum. The person suddenly falls to the ground without warning or with a momentary vertigo. Among 384 persons evaluated in one study, the most frequent cause of falls was tripping, followed by loss of balance and drop attack.[3] Forty-three percent of the total sample had neurologic disease.

Kyphosis, or curvature of the spine, in older persons frequently occurs as a result of osteoporosis of the vertebrae. Vertebral atrophy also occurs. Because of the progressive degeneration, the number of cells diminishes, the water content decreases, and the tissues lose turgor and become friable. The combined changes in the vertebrae and disks result in curvature of the spine. Kyphosis causes decreased respiratory capacity of the chest wall and other conditions related to impingement on various spinal nerves as a result of the narrowed disks

and vertebral changes. These problems most often occur in the lumbar and cervical spine. Compression fractures of the spine are also common.[27]

Fractures and Risk of Falling

In the aged individual, there is an increased risk for falling and bone fractures. This may be related to cerebral vascular disease, which often causes difficulty in locomotion in elderly persons. Arteriosclerosis of the carotid and vertebral arteries that results in ischemia may cause transient paralysis or lightheadedness, poor balance, and falling episodes. If such events occur, the person becomes anxious and tense about moving, and coordination is reduced even further. Older persons who fear falling tend to take fewer and fewer risks; the result is increased immobility. Individuals who have had cerebrovascular accidents tend to have hemiparesis or hemiplegia. Those who recover from such episodes tend to have some motor disability that creates difficulty in walking, postural changes in both sitting and standing, residual spasticity, and footdrop. These factors increase the risk for falling. Injury from falling is a major problem for the elderly. Fractures of the hip and wrist are frequent, as is head injury. The fractures are often the result of decreased bone strength related to osteoporosis. Hospitalization and surgical procedures for fractures carry multiple risks.

SKIN AND DERMAL APPENDAGES
Changes in the Skin, Nails, and Hair

Next to alterations in the musculoskeletal system, changes in the integument are the most obvious signs of aging. With loss of elasticity, wrinkles, lines, and drooping eyelids occur. Exposed areas, such as the hands, develop age spots or excessive skin pigmentation. The skin becomes dry, thin, fragile, and prone to injury. Nails become dry and brittle. Toenails become susceptible to fungal infection and appear thickened; there is a lifting of the nail plates. The rate of change is very individual and is dependent on such factors as nutrition, genetics, emotions, and environment. Typical changes that occur in the skin are depicted in Figure 8-7.

Numerous problems occur because of the changes in the skin. The loss of water, which is the basis for many problems in the elderly, results from atrophy of all skin layers, with diminished vascularity and decreased elasticity. Lack of water leads to pruritis and decubitus ulcers. Lesions such as tumors, warts, and keratoses may arise with no pain; however, lesions such as herpes zoster are often very painful. Sebaceous and sweat glands become less active and contribute to dry skin.

Another inevitable change is the loss of hair pigment, or graying; its onset and degree may vary greatly. There is also generalized thinning of the hair, con-

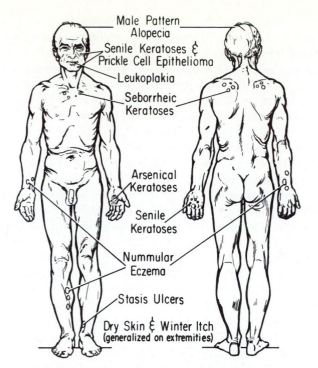

FIGURE 8-7 *Typical skin changes with aging. (Sauer, G.C. Manual of Skin Diseases [6th ed.]. Philadelphia: J.B. Lippincott, 1991.)*

tributed to by a decrease in the density of hair follicles. In older females, the hair appears finer and more sparse; some axillary and pubic hair is lost. Often, an increase in facial hair is noted because of decreased estrogen production after menopause. Older males frequently have hair growth in ears and nares, and the eyebrows grow more bushy. Men are more susceptible to alopecia than women, with genetics playing a part in the degree and rapidity of balding.

Diseases Associated With Aging Skin

The skin often reflects other disease conditions such as liver or cardiac disease. Relatively minor skin problems, such as overgrowths of epidermal tissue, cause cosmetic problems but rarely need surgical excision. *Senile telangiectasias*, small scarlet growths scattered over the skin, increase in number after middle age. *Hyperkeratotic warts*, raised brown or black epidermal overgrowths, also develop in increased numbers with age. These two types of lesions, together with others that occur less frequently, have no clinical significance and do not require removal unless irritated by clothing or jewelry. Cancers of the skin are very common, especially in fair-skinned individuals or in sun-damaged skin (see pp. 909–911).

SENSORY SYSTEM

Few persons escape sensory deficits as they age. They become more vulnerable to injury, more isolated from society, and less able to care for their personal needs as these deficits occur. Deficits are greatest in sight, hearing,

taste, smell, and touch, and they interfere with the ability to communicate.

Vision Changes

With age, changes take place in both the structural and functional aspects of the eyes. Eyelids become thinner and wrinkled, and skinfolds result from loss of orbital fat, leading to proptosis. Inversion or eversion of the lids is common, and the conjunctivae are thinner and more fragile.

Arcus senilis, a bluish gray ring, may surround the corneal limbus and be visible against the darker pigments of the eye. Arcus senilis is a harmless change and does not affect visual acuity. Light brown patches may occur in the irides, changing their appearance but not their ability to regulate pupil size. The lenses may develop changes that cause vision problems such as loss of elasticity or presbyopia (see p. 976).

Cataracts may develop because of loss of soluble proteins and subsequent loss of lens transparency. The cloudy, hazy lens results in visual loss. Reduced transmission of light causes distant objects to become hazy. Surgical excision may become necessary if the cataracts become too dense.

Glaucoma is another major eye problem that affects the aged. Glaucoma accounts for about 10% of all blindness in the United States.[13] Intraocular pressure rises rapidly in acute glaucoma and slowly in chronic glaucoma. Peripheral vision and night vision are both affected. The decline in peripheral vision may occur slowly and interferes with driving ability. Medications and surgery are now available to treat glaucoma. Early treatment is essential because the blindness that results is irreversible.

Hearing Changes

With aging, changes may develop in the functional ability of the ears as well as their external appearance. Population studies indicate that hearing gradually deteriorates beginning in the third decade of life.[16] The external ears undergo very little change other than some slight elongation of the lobes. Cerumen decreases in amount but contains a greater amount of keratin, which easily becomes impacted and difficult to remove. Impacted cerumen can block sound waves and cause temporary hearing loss until it is removed.

Sclerosis or atrophy of the tympanic membrane affects the middle ear, usually by reducing the number of high-frequency sound waves reaching the inner ear. Loss of cells at the base of the cochlea leads to retrocochlear loss of efficiency. The ability to hear high-frequency sounds is reduced first, followed by loss of ability to hear lower frequencies. The term used to describe progressive hearing loss in the aged is *presbycusis*. This bilaterally symmetric perceptive hearing loss starts at about the fourth decade, but the effects are usually not noticeable at their outset.

Exposure to excessive noise, recurrent otitis media in younger years, trauma to the ears, and certain drugs contribute to hearing loss. Persons living or working in highly industrialized areas experience more hearing loss than those in nonindustrial areas.

Other Sensory Changes

The aging process does not have as dramatic an effect on taste, smell, and touch as it does on vision and hearing, but these senses are also reduced. There is an obvious decrease in ability to taste sweet and salty flavors, owing to a decrease in the number of taste buds. Diet becomes an important factor because the aging person tends to eat more sweets and to salt food more heavily. The sweets lead to obesity and increased dental problems, and the salt may aggravate existing hypertension. Olfactory function may diminish, resulting in inability to smell, which also interferes with appetite. It also can present a hazard in the case of fire or smoke.

A decrease in tactile sensation may be manifested by difficulty in discriminating between different temperatures. Older persons tend to burn themselves because of this change. Minor injuries occur as a result of occasional unawareness of pain or pressure.

VARIABLES THAT MODIFY BIOPHYSICAL EFFECTS OF AGING

In 1958, a group of gerontologists began a comprehensive and ambitious longitudinal study on aging known as the Baltimore Longitudinal Study of Aging (BLSA). After almost 40 years of investigation, the BLSA researchers believe that the changes of aging are not limited to a single cause. It was found in a number of tests that older people performed as well as younger people, that aging did not always result in gradual loss of intellectual functions, and that in some cases lifestyle modification improved test performance.[23] These results are part of the emerging body of evidence that suggests that the effects of the changes thought to normally occur with aging can be modified by lifestyle and environmental variables. An active versus a sedentary lifestyle is preferred. Physical activity reduces the rate at which aerobic capacity is lost. Moderate weight-bearing activity is beneficial in increasing bone mass.[17] Dietary modifications, such as adopting a low-cholesterol diet, can influence the occurrence of some age-associated diseases. Discontinuation of cigarette smoking can also decrease the occurrence of disease in the elderly.

AGING AND CANCER

Cancer is a serious problem, regardless of age. Because cancers are multifaceted diseases whose prevalence often increases with age, a brief discussion of cancer and aging is presented here. Even though the prevalence of cancer is higher in older persons, certain types are diagnosed less frequently in this age group, including cervical cancer and sarcoma. Several factors are associated with cancer, although the exact cause is unknown. Constant irritation from smoking a pipe can cause oral cancers, chewing tobacco can result in cancer of the mouth, and smoking cigarettes can lead to carcinoma of the lung. The percentage of lung cancer was once highest in men, but the disease is increasing in women because of the increased number of women who smoke.

Environmental factors such as air pollution, food additives, asbestos, and certain chemicals are carcinogenic. According to the National Research Council, evidence indicates that most common cancers are influenced by diet, although there are no precise estimations of the impact of foods on cancer. Chemical carcinogens produce different effects at different periods of life. Chemical carcinogenesis occurs most readily in the aged. The assumption is that there is either an accumulated effect on the DNA of the cell or an accumulated risk for a cell to become malignant.

The majority of persons with carcinoma of the colon are in the older age group. This cancer is usually very slow-growing and remains localized for a long time. Early surgical removal is beneficial.

Cancer of the prostate is the most common tumor of men older than 85 years of age.[19] The disease is known to metastasize to the pelvis, vertebrae, and other bony sites, as well as to the brain. Breast cancer is common in elderly women and is often discovered during examination for other conditions.

Chronic lymphocytic leukemia, lymphosarcoma, and myeloma are malignancies with a high incidence in the elderly population. Hodgkin disease tends to run a rapid course in the aged, but malignancies of the lung, oral cavity, larynx, and gastrointestinal tract seem to have a similar prognosis in young and old.

AGING AND INFECTIONS

Both nosocomial and community-acquired infections are more common in the elderly (Fig. 8-8). Predisposing factors include a decline in immune competence, chronic illness, diminished organ reserves, development of resistant organisms, alteration in natural barriers, inadequate nutrition, and diminished sensory perception. In the immune system, T lymphocytes are reduced and neutrophils become less efficient with advanced age, thereby decreasing the elderly person's ability to fight infectious diseases. Also, the fever response to infectious disease may be blunted or absent; this factor increases the morbidity and mortality associated with infections in the elderly population.[18]

Elderly persons are especially susceptible to respiratory, urinary tract, and skin infections because of the systemic changes discussed previously. Also, the presentation of infections in the elderly may be somewhat atypical, compared with those in younger adults. A summary of atypical presentations of pneumonia, tuberculosis, urinary tract infections, and skin infections is presented in Table 8-5.

▼ Pharmacology and the Elderly

Aged persons use one-third of all prescribed drugs used in this country. Most take several drugs and also use over-the-counter agents frequently.[31] All drugs can pose risks to elderly persons and can decrease their mental, physical, and functional status.[26] Nutritional status may be impaired by long-term use of certain drugs.

The elderly are the least able to tolerate injudicious use of drugs because many physiologic changes make them respond to medication in more variable ways than do younger adults. These physiologic changes result in a system that is less able to distribute, metabolize, and excrete drugs. The liver, kidneys, and heart are most involved with drug excretion and metabolism. Because they have lost some of their efficiency, compounds may accumulate and cause toxicity. The cumulative effects of trauma, prior illnesses, accidents, and disabilities further reduce the aging person's ability to handle drugs.

Pharmacokinetic factors (those related to drug disposition in the body) have been studied in relation to absorption in the gastrointestinal tract, which would theoretically be reduced in elderly as a result of changes in intestinal mucosa, blood flow, and motility. However, there is not yet convincing evidence that alterations in

TABLE 8-5	Atypical Presentations of Common Infections in Elderly Persons
Pneumonia	Blunted fever response; decreased evidence of consolidation in 30% of patients; confusion, disorientation, and changes in behavior are common presenting signs and symptoms.
Tuberculosis	Cough, weight loss, and weakness may be subtle symptoms and may be attributed to other chronic diseases; chest pain, hemoptysis, and night sweats are seen in later stages of disease.
Skin infections	Decreased inflammatory response may delay diagnosis; peripheral vascular disease will decrease erythema, warmth, and swelling, which are commonly used to determine infection.
Urinary tract infections	Blunted fever response; anorexia, nausea, vomiting, and abdominal pain; confusion and change in behavior; increased incidence of asymptomatic bacteriuria.

Adapted from Fraser, D. *Patient Assessment: Infection in the elderly*. J. Gerontol. Nurs. 19:5, 1993.

absorption actually occur.[7] With age, the total body composition changes, resulting in a higher percentage of fat tissue and less lean tissue and water. The disposition of drugs that are selectively used in different tissues is affected. Also, body size decreases, so the concentration of a drug in the body is higher with standard dosages. Plasma binding by albumin in the elderly decreases 20%. Drugs that are normally plasma-focused are therefore increased in concentration in the tissues.

Metabolism of drugs by the liver is diminished in the elderly by poor circulation to the liver, by a reduction in the hepatic mass, and by the possible decrease in hepatic enzymes. Any disease of the liver aggravates this situation considerably. Some of the most common drugs metabolized by the liver that have increased half-life in the elderly are the antidepressants diazepam (Valium) and chlordiazepoxide (Librium).

Another problem is reduced excretion caused by diminished renal function. Renal reserve is markedly reduced as people age, and the ability to excrete drugs is also markedly reduced. Drug action in the elderly is also altered by changes in tissue responses. There may be an increased threshold to a drug's actions. There may be a decrease in the number of receptive sites for the drug, coupled with a decrease in the necessary enzymes. A summary of alterations in the pharmacokinetic variables in the elderly is presented in Table 8-6.

Listed high among drugs that can be dangerous to the elderly are antibiotics, such as tetracyclines and gentamycin. Antibiotics are excreted by the kidneys, and reduced kidney function can lead to toxic accumulation of the agents. Mental disturbances, gastrointestinal side

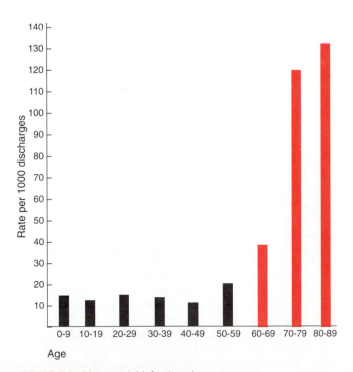

FIGURE 8-8 *Nosocomial infections by age group.*

TABLE 8-6 *Alteration of Pharmacokinetic Values in the Elderly*

Factor	Altered Physiology	Clinical Importance
Absorption	Elevated gastric pH Reduced gastrointestinal blood flow Possible changed number of absorbing cells Possible altered gastrointestinal motility	Studies have not supported any loss of absorptive ability
Distribution	Decreased total body water Decreased lean body tissue mass per kg body weight Increased body fat	Higher concentration of drugs distributed in body fluids Possible longer duration of action of fat-soluble drugs
Protein binding	Decreased serum albumin concentrations	Increased unbound plasma concentrations of highly protein-bound drugs
Metabolism	Decreased hepatic blood flow; decreased hepatic mass; possible decreased enzyme activity	Decreased hepatic clearance
Elimination	Decreased glomerular filtration rate Decreased renal plasma flow Altered tubular function	Decreased renal clearance of drugs and metabolites

effects, and rashes are some toxic effects.[7] If diuretics, which cause potassium loss, are given in combination with digoxin, the danger of dysrhythmias is greatly increased. The effect of digitalis on the conduction system is enhanced by low serum potassium levels. Many of the antihypertensive agents have diverse side effects, but they all possess the ability to cause hypotension. Orthostatic hypotension can lead to falls and fractures. Elderly persons should be warned of this possibility, and if they are taking antihypertensives they should be cautioned not to rise too rapidly from a supine or sitting position.

The elderly person does not display the toxic effects of digoxin, such as gastrointestinal and ocular symptoms, that usually arise in younger adults. This makes digoxin one of the drugs that places the older individual at grave risk. Digoxin blood levels are not always a good guide to toxicity; the elderly person more commonly exhibits electrocardiographic changes and confusion. Toxic blood levels may not be seen, but the effects may be present.

Many elderly persons develop nutritional problems from long-term use of medications such as laxatives. Mineral oil can interfere with absorption of nutrients and vitamins in the intestinal tract, and its use should be discouraged.

▼ Chapter Summary

▼ The causes of aging are not specifically known. Biologic cellular theories provide some insight into the changes seen, but all of the theories support the known concepts that there is a decreased function in all of the organ systems. The exact age at which each change occurs, but the pattern of change exists.

▼ Systemic changes are seen in the nervous system, the musculoskeletal system, the cardiopulmonary system, the genitourinary system, the gastrointestinal system, the sensory system, and the skin. These contribute to alterations, especially in emotional responses, in gait, and in responses to stressful situations.

▼ Elderly individuals are much more susceptible to developing cancer, and certain types of malignancies are more common among the elderly. Infections, especially opportunistic infections, are more common in the elderly because of the progressive immune suppression seen with aging.

▼ Elderly individuals tend to have more chronic diseases than the younger population and therefore take more prescription drugs than younger individuals. All drugs pose risks to elderly persons and can affect their mental, physical, and functional abilities. The systemic changes of age make elderly persons less able to distribute, metabolize, and excrete drugs.

▼ References

1. Altman, D.F. Changes in gastrointestinal, pancreatic, biliary, and hepatic function with aging. *Gastroenterol. Clin. North. Am.* 19:227, 1990.
2. Barzel, U. Common metabolic disorders of the skeleton in aging. In Reichel, W. (ed.), *Clinical Aspects of Aging* (3rd ed.). Baltimore: Williams & Wilkins, 1989.
3. Birren, J.E., and Schaie, K.W. (eds.). *Handbook of the Psychology of Aging* (3rd ed.). San Diego: Academic Press, 1990.
4. Burggraf, V., and Donlon, B. Assessing the elderly. *Am. J. Nurs.* 85:976, 1985.
5. Caird, F., Dall, J., and Williams, B. The cardiovascular system. In Brockehurst, J.C. (ed.), *Textbook of Geriatric*

Medicine and Gerontology (4th ed.). New York: Churchill Livingstone, 1992.

6. Carnevali, D.L., and Patrick, M. *Nursing Management for the Elderly* (3rd ed.). Philadelphia: J.B. Lippincott, 1993.

7. Carruthers, S. Pharmacokinetics. In Rossman, I. (ed.), *Clinical Geriatrics* (3rd ed.). Philadelphia: J.B. Lippincott, 1986.

8. Carter, A. The neurologic aspects of aging. In Rossman, I. (ed.), *Clinical Geriatrics* (3rd ed.). Philadelphia: J.B. Lippincott, 1986.

9. Clark, K. *Leonardi da Vinci*. London: Cambridge University Press, 1939.

10. Cotran, R. Cell injury and Adaptation. In Robbins, S.L., and Kumar, V. (eds.), *Pathologic Basis of Disease* (5th ed.). Philadelphia: W.B. Saunders, 1994.

11. Davies, I. Biology of aging-Theories of aging. In Brockehurst, J.C. (ed.), *Textbook of Geriatric Medicine and Gerontology* (4th ed.). New York: Churchill Livingstone, 1992.

12. Ebersole, P., and Hess, P. *Toward Healthy Aging: Human Needs and Nursing Response* (4th ed.). St. Louis: Mosby, 1994.

13. Eliopoulos, C. *Gerontological Nursing* (3rd ed.). Philadelphia: J.B. Lippincott, 1993.

14. Esberger, K.K., and Hughes, S.T. *Nursing Care of the Aged*. Norwalk: Appleton & Lange, 1989.

15. Faubert, P., Shapiro, W., Porush, J., and Kahn, A. Medical renal disease in the aged. In Reichel, W. (ed.), *Clinical Aspects of Aging* (3rd ed.). Baltimore: Williams & Wilkins, 1989.

16. Fisch, L. Special senses-DThe aging auditory system. In Brockehurst, J.C. (ed.), *Textbook of Geriatric Medicine and Gerontology* (4th ed.). New York: Churchill Livingstone, 1992.

17. Frantz, R., and Ferrell-Torry, A. Physical impairments in the elderly populations. *Nurs. Clin. North. Am.* 28:363, 1993.

18. Fraser, D. Patient assessment: Infection in the elderly. *J. Gerontol. Nurs.* 19:5, 1993.

19. Gioiella, E., and Bevil, C. *Nursing Care of the Aging Client: Promoting Healthy Adaptation*. Norwalk: Appleton-Century-Crofts, 1985.

20. Goldman, R. Aging of the excretory system. In Finch, C., and Schneider, E. (eds.), *Handbook of the Biology of Aging* (2nd ed.). New York: Van Nostrand Reinhold, 1985.

21. Guyton, A.C. *Textbook of Medical Physiology* (8th ed.). Philadelphia: W.B. Saunders, 1991.

22. Hayflick, L. Current theories of biological aging. *Fed. Proc.* 34:9, 1975.

23. Hayflick, L. *How and Why We Age*. New York: Ballantine. 1994.

24. Hubbard, B.M., and Squier, M. The physical aging of the neuromuscular system. In Tallis, R. (ed.), *The Clinical Neurology of Old Age*. New York: John Wiley & Sons, 1989.

25. Kohn, R. Heart and cardiovascular system. In Finch, C., and Schneider, E. (eds.), *Handbook of the Biology of Aging* (3rd ed.). New York: Van Nostrand Reinhold, 1990.

26. Lamy, P.P. Drugs and the elderly: A new look. *Fam. Community Health* 5:34, 1982.

27. Malasanos, L., et al. *Health Assessment* (4th ed.). St. Louis: Mosby, 1990.

28. Matteson, M.A., and McConnell, E.S. *Gerontological Nursing: Concepts and Practice*. Philadelphia: W.B. Saunders, 1988.

29. Rossman, I. Anatomic and body composition changes with aging. In Finch, C., and Schneider, E. (eds.), *Handbook of the Biology of Aging* (2nd ed.). New York: Van Nostrand Reinhold, 1985.

30. Sohal, R., and Allen, R. Relationship between metabolic rate, free radicals, differentiation and aging: A unified theory. In Woodhead, A., Blachett, A., and Hollaender, A. (eds.), *Molecular Biology of Aging*. New York: Plenum Press, 1985.

31. Vestal, R.D., and Cusack, B.J. Pharmacology of aging. In Schneider, E.L., and Rowe, J.W. (eds.), *Handbook of the Biology of Aging* (3rd ed.). San Diego: Academic Press, 1990.

32. Walker, M. The physiology of normal aging: Implications for nursing management of critically compromised adults. In Fulmer, T., and Walker, M. (eds.) *Critical Care Nursing of the Elderly*. New York: Springer, 1992.

33. Williams, G.H., and Braunwald, E. Hypertensive vascular disease. In Braunwald, E., et al., *Harrison's Principles of Internal Medicine* (12th ed.). New York: McGraw-Hill, 1991.

34. Winsberg, F. Roentgenographic aspects of aging. In Rossman, I. (ed.), *Clinical Geriatrics* (3rd ed.). Philadelphia: J.B. Lippincott, 1986.

Chapter 9

Concepts of Stress and Sleep

Barbara L. Bullock

▼ **LEARNING OBJECTIVES**

1 Describe the general adaptation syndrome according to Selye's studies.
2 Explain the chemical and hormonal mediators important in the stress response.
3 Differentiate between the general and local adaptation syndromes.
4 Describe the three physiologic mechanisms that respond to stress stimulation.
5 Discuss the relation between stress and disease.
6. Describe the effects of stress on the immune system.
7 Identify the effects of stress on target organs and systems of the body.
8 Describe the physiology of sleep.
9 Discuss the importance of sleep as a basic human need on which the physical and emotional health of an individual depends.
10 Explain the major characteristics of each stage of sleep.
11 Identify common sleep pattern disturbances.
12 Discuss the relation of the circadian rhythm to the sleep cycle.
13 Describe the changes of aging as they relate to the sleep cycle.

Barbara L. Bullock: PATHOPHYSIOLOGY: ADAPTATIONS AND ALTERATIONS IN FUNCTION, 4th ed.
© 1996 Lippincott-Raven Publishers

▼ *Stress*

All persons experience certain amounts of stress during each stage of the development process. *Stress* has been defined as the nonspecific response of the body to any demand placed on it.[23] Stress-producing factors are called *stressors*; these may be physiological or psychological, or both. Reactions to stressors may be adaptive or maladaptive. The stressors may be pleasant or unpleasant, and they may evoke many different emotional or psychologic responses while eliciting similar physiologic reactions. Closely associated with stress is the concept of *emotions*. This concept includes a wide range of behaviors, expressed feelings, and changes in body states.[21] Emotions often elicit the stress response, which can be viewed as a physiologic response to the emotion that encompasses the reported feelings. Stressors may be actual physical threats or perceived threats. They also may be the emotional side of joys or sorrows that elicit a physiologic response.

THEORIES OF EMOTION

Several theories have attempted to explain the relation between emotions and visceral activity. Three prominent theories are the James-Lange theory, the Cannon-Bard theory, and Schachter's cognitive theory. These are briefly described here, and the reader is referred to the bibliography for further reading.

The James-Lange theory suggests that strong emotions and activation of the skeletal muscle and autonomic nervous system are inseparable factors. An example of this is the emotion of fear, which is a reaction to some sort of stimulus with results perceived as an emotion.[21] This theory emphasizes peripheral physiologic events, the vasomotor response, in emotions.

The Cannon-Bard theory focuses on the brain and emotion, especially cerebral integration of emotional experience (stressor) and emotional response (stress). This theory emphasizes that some emotions are an emergency response of the sympathetic nervous system (SNS) to a sudden, threatening condition.[21] These emotions provoke a nonspecific response of increased heart rate, glucose mobilization, and other SNS responses.[23]

Schachter's cognitive theory suggests that individuals interpret visceral activation in terms of the specific stimulus, the surrounding situation, and their cognitive states. This allows for differences among individuals that are molded by experience. An emotional state results from the interaction of physiologic stimulation, activation, and interpretation.[21]

Studies linking emotion to physiologic responses have discovered that even if the physiologic receptors are blocked, the emotional response to a stimulus is not reduced. Other studies have demonstrated a specific pattern of autonomic arousal for each different emotion.[21]

The study of emotional responses is in its infancy, but the relation of stimulus to physiologic response is intriguing. The linkage of emotion to the stress response was extensively studied during and after World War II, when it was observed that one-third of American casualties had sustained no physical injury but were victims of fear, exertion, sleep deprivation, death of colleagues, and exposure to heat, cold, and noise.[27]

The ability to cope successfully with emotions directly affects the health status of the individual at any age. Many health problems are related to inability to handle the stresses of everyday living. Because stress is a great threat to health during the life span, it is important to understand the body's responses to stress. Although there are many ways to explain the physiology of stress, the concept of the systems theory provides a logical means for describing this phenomenon.

SYSTEMS THEORY

Systems theory is one of the older models for organizing and examining relations among units. It describes closed systems as those that do not interact or exchange energy with their environments. The sciences of physics and physical chemistry are limited to the examination of closed systems. Conversely, open systems do exchange matter, energy, and information with their environments.[26] A relative state of balance or dynamic equilibrium, called the *steady state*, is achieved. Human beings, as open, physiologic organisms, use relations among their component parts to achieve this state. The steady state is said to exist when the composition of the system is constant despite continuous exchange of components of the system. The three fundamental qualities of open systems are structure, process, and function. *Structure* refers to the arrangement of all defined elements at a given time. *Process* is the transformation of matter, energy, and information between the system and the environment. *Function* relates to the unique manner that each open system uses to achieve its required end.[16]

A feedback scheme is used to describe the fundamental qualities of open systems. In the human, this means that if a factor becomes excessive or inadequate in the body, alterations in function are initiated to decrease or increase that factor in an attempt to bring it into normal range. The processes used in this scheme include input, throughput, output, and feedback. Input is the energy, matter, or information absorbed by the system. Throughput is the transformation of this energy into useful information, matter, or energy that is used by the system. The excess information, matter, or energy is discharged to the environment in a process called output.

Feedback is the process of self-regulation by which open systems determine and control the amount of input and output of the system. The two types of feedback in the human body are *negative* and *positive feedback*. Negative feedback refers to a process of returning to a state of equilibrium, and positive feedback indicates movement away from equilibrium. Negative feedback indicates a return to normal balance, whereas positive feedback, unchecked, produces illness and finally death. In the human body, negative feedback can be readily illustrated by many functions. Flowchart 9-1 illustrates the feedback system used to maintain the balance of thyroid hormones. Loss of hormonal control, for example, causes disease states because the body produces either too many hormones or not enough, which alters the metabolic processes.

THE STRESS RESPONSE

The individual, as a system, encounters physiologic, psychosocial, environmental, and other stressors (Flowchart 9-2). These stressors may produce adaptive coping responses, or they may result in physical changes that become pathophysiologic. The study of the effects of

stress on the human body was pioneered by Selye. He studied the nonspecific response of the body to a demand and noted differences in individual abilities to withstand the same demands. He defined stress as a specific syndrome that is nonspecifically induced. He also defined stressors as tension-producing stimuli that potentially can cause disequilibrium.[22] The perceived significance of the stressor is important and varies among individuals.

Psychologic and physiologic stressors both elicit a response that includes enlargement of the adrenal cortex, atrophy of the thymus gland, and SNS activation. A pattern including fatigue, loss of appetite, joint pains, gastric upset, and other nonspecific complaints comprises the syndrome which Selye called "the syndrome of just being sick." Later, he termed this condition the *general adaptation syndrome*, or the GAS.[23] The GAS may be elicited by a variety of stimuli or stressors and may be of a physiologic, psychogenic, sociocultural, or environmental nature. The GAS is divided into three stages: alarm reaction, resistance, and exhaustion (Flowchart 9-3).

In the *alarm* stage, a stressor causes an initial activation of the defensive abilities of the body.[2] The hypothalamus is activated, releasing corticotropin-releasing factor, which stimulates the adenohypophysis to release adrenocorticotropic hormone (ACTH). Glucocorticoids are then released. The so-called *fight-or-flight* mechanisms is activated mainly through the SNS, which releases two catecholamines, *norepinephrine* and *epinephrine*. The physiologic action of these hormones causes vasodilation in the heart and skeletal muscles. These hormones also cause vasoconstriction in the skin, viscera, and kidneys, increased blood pressure, and increased rate and force of cardiac contractions. All of these physiologic actions prepare the body for an assault.

In the stage of *resistance*, levels of corticosteroids, thyroid hormones, glucagon, and aldosterone are increased. These is a reduction in the alarm reactions. The adrenal cortex enlarges and becomes hyperactive. A hypermetabolic state exists, increasing blood sugar for available energy and stabilizing the inflammatory response. The immune system becomes depressed. There is depression of T cells and B cells and atrophy of the thymus gland, which leads to a depression of the primary antigen-antibody response. This immune suppression is probably caused by the effect of excess ACTH and circulating glucocorticoids. The end result, immunologically, is suppression and atrophy of all immune tissues (see p. 336). If infection is present, this suppression causes delayed clearing of the organisms and delayed healing. This stage is not always beneficial, especially if it persists for a period of time.

If stage 3, *exhaustion*, occurs, resistance to the stressor is depleted and death ultimately occurs (see Flowchart 9-3). Exhaustion is frequently caused by the

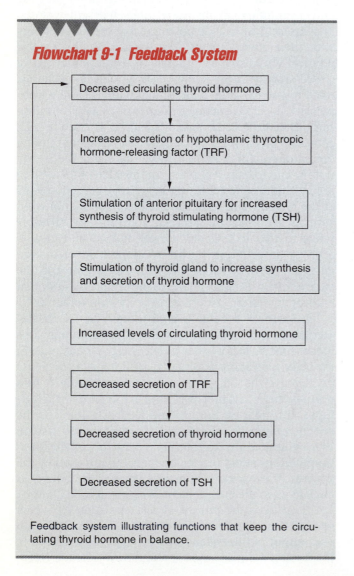

Flowchart 9-1 Feedback System

Decreased circulating thyroid hormone

Increased secretion of hypothalamic thyrotropic hormone-releasing factor (TRF)

Stimulation of anterior pituitary for increased synthesis of thyroid stimulating hormone (TSH)

Stimulation of thyroid gland to increase synthesis and secretion of thyroid hormone

Increased levels of circulating thyroid hormone

Decreased secretion of TRF

Decreased secretion of thyroid hormone

Decreased secretion of TSH

Feedback system illustrating functions that keep the circulating thyroid hormone in balance.

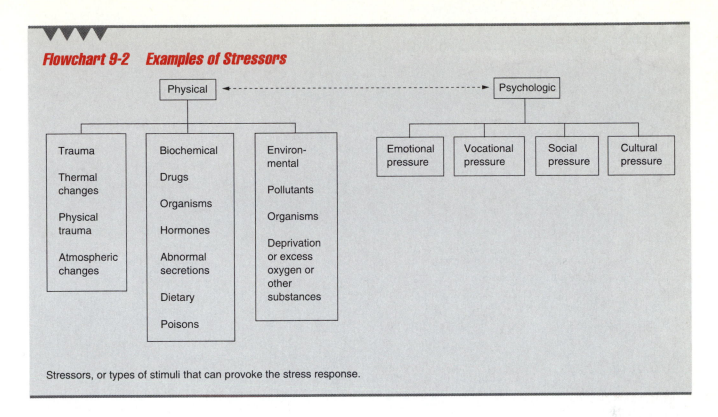

Flowchart 9-2   Examples of Stressors

Stressors, or types of stimuli that can provoke the stress response.

lack of immunologic defense and is considered to be an immunodeficiency secondary to stress. Selye proposed that exhaustion is a correct term for aging, a wearing down of the human body from lifelong stress.[23] This conclusion is not supported in some of the recent literature but provides one way to explain the aging process (see p. 159).

Individuals differ in their reactions to stressors. Response to the same stressor can also vary from one day to the next in the same person. Some types of stress are positive; positive stress is called *eustress*. These sources are associated with some sort of control over the outcome and include such stressors as getting married, buying a house, and travel. Negative stress is termed *distress* and reflects situations over which one has little control, including sickness, death, and divorce.[3] As discussed in a later section, the perception of stress has important implications for health, and it has been shown that the hormonal changes in response to eustress are less harmful than those of distress.[3] The emotions of anger, hostility, and distrust are particularly damaging to health.

Localized reaction to stressors is called the *local adaptation syndrome* (LAS); it is well illustrated by the process of inflammation. The usual outcome of inflammation is localization and destruction of the foreign substance that triggered the process.[19] The LAS assumes the same general pattern as the GAS, with an acute phase followed by a resistance phase and then exhaustion. Exhaustion of the LAS causes breakdown of the localizing mechanism and spread of the process, ultimately leading to a generalized response.

ADAPTATION

Adaptation is defined as adjustment of an organism to a changing environment. It refers to adjustments that are made as a result of stimulation or change, with the end result of modifying the original situation. An adaptive response is a type of negative feedback that maintains the organism in the steady state. Physiologic adaptation refers to the adjustments made by the organs and systems in response to stress or physiologic disruption. This response is often called *compensation* for abnormal stimuli. *Maladaptation* is disruptive. It moves toward positive feedback, a disordering of the physiologic response. This positive feedback can be considered a vicious cycle: if not interrupted, it can become disruptive to the individual.

Physiologic responses to stressors comprise three separate and interactive mechanisms: neurologic, endocrine, and immunologic. These mechanisms may promote adaptation to the stressor. Long-term application of stressors ultimately causes end-organ dysfunction through these same mechanisms.[2]

Neurologic Mechanisms

Both the voluntary and the autonomic divisions of the nervous system are reactive to stress. The voluntary system is mediated through the cerebral cortex, which is responsive to the stress stimulus. The cerebral cortex directs the muscles to move to avoid danger and effects the flight response. The combination of vasodilation in the skeletal muscle and the voluntary flight response

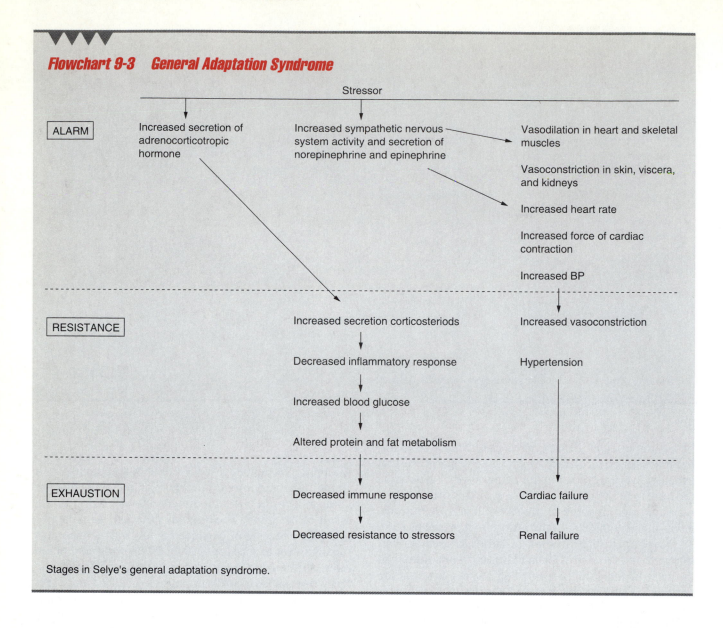

Flowchart 9-3   General Adaptation Syndrome

Stages in Selye's general adaptation syndrome.

are sometimes termed the *musculoskeletal response* to a stressor.

The autonomic nervous system is involuntary and is regulated through the hypothalamus. In the stress response, stimulation of the SNS occurs. Two hormones, epinephrine and norepinephrine, which are classified as *catecholamines*, are important factors in the stress response. Both are synthesized in the adrenal medulla and released when the SNS is activated. Norepinephrine is also synthesized and secreted at adrenergic (sympathetic) nerve terminals throughout the body and is directly released when the SNS is stimulated. Epinephrine is excreted rapidly in the urine after being biotransformed in the liver. Norepinephrine, liberated at the axon endings, is actively taken up, restored, or biotransformed.

The primary action of epinephrine is to increase the rate and force of cardiac contraction. It is secreted as part of the stress response from the SNS stimulation of the adrenal medulla. Epinephrine is a potent stimulus for glycogenolysis in the liver, which leads to an increased blood glucose level.[9] In addition to accelerating the degradation of glycogen, epinephrine diverts blood from the viscera to the skeletal muscles. Its action provides the fuel and the circulatory effort necessary to meet an increased need.

Norepinephrine is secreted in small quantities in the flight-or-fight response and in acute physical or mental stress. Studies have shown a constant increase in norepinephrine levels in individuals under chronic, unremitting stress. Norepinephrine exerts its primary control over the arterioles, leading to intense vasoconstriction and increased systemic vascular resistance, which causes increased blood pressure and increased cardiac workload (afterload). The vasoconstriction to the gut and reduced blood flow to the gastric mucosa is implicated in

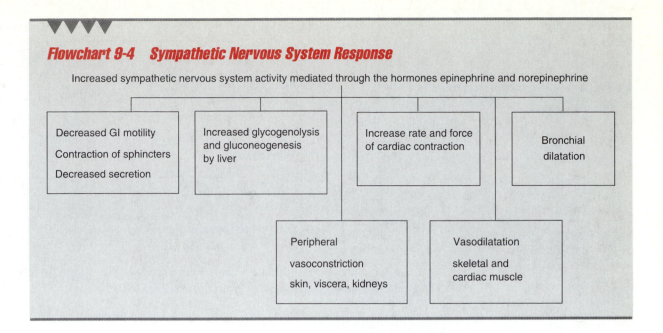

Flowchart 9-4   Sympathetic Nervous System Response

Increased sympathetic nervous system activity mediated through the hormones epinephrine and norepinephrine

Decreased GI motility Contraction of sphincters Decreased secretion	Increased glycogenolysis and gluconeogenesis by liver	Increase rate and force of cardiac contraction	Bronchial dilatation

Peripheral vasoconstriction skin, viscera, kidneys

Vasodilatation skeletal and cardiac muscle

the development of stress ulcers. Flowchart 9-4 illustrates the sympathetic response to stress as it is mediated through epinephrine and norepinephrine.

In addition to the above effects, epinephrine and norepinephrine are responsible for bronchial dilatation, increased respiratory rate, inhibition of the activity of the gastrointestinal tract, and pupillary dilation. Elevated levels of these hormones may be related to the development of hyperlipidemia and stress-induced cardiovascular disease.

Endocrine Mechanisms

The endocrine hormones are increased in the stress response through hypothalamic stimulation of the pituitary, leading to stimulation of target organ secretion. This relation is illustrated in Flowchart 9-5. Stimulation of the pituitary can increase secretion of ACTH, antidiuretic hormone (ADH), thyroid-stimulating hormone, and others. Secretion of aldosterone from the adrenal cortex is also increased.

The target organs of ACTH are the adrenal glands. Stimulation from this hormone causes an increased synthesis of the glucocorticoids, especially cortisol, cortisone, and small amounts of hydrocortisone. These substances increase serum glucose and alter the metabolism of carbohydrates, fats, and proteins. Gluconeogenesis, glycogenolysis, protein catabolism, and lipolysis are increased. The result is that more fuel is made available for energy.

In individuals who are awake in the day and sleep at night, the glucocorticoids are thought to be synchronized by light. Their concentration in blood and urine decreases during sleep and rises to their highest levels in the early morning.[9] This pattern of glucocorticoid secretion follows a particular pattern called the *circadian rhythm*. The early-morning high levels drop at about 10 AM, increase slightly again about 2 PM, then gradually decline until 10 PM (Fig. 9-1). Disruptions in circadian rhythm are often produced by stress, which especially disturbs the rhythmic patterns involving blood glucose, leukocytes, and temperature regulation.[2] Alterations in the circadian rhythm have been shown to increase with the duration of the stress.[2] Changes in circadian rhythm may relate to illness in that phase relationships seem to be consistent in particular maladies. For example, persons with peptic ulcer disease frequently have increased gastric acid secretion causing pain in the late night or early morning hours. Low blood levels of glucocorticoids increase the sensitivity to sounds, tastes, and smells. Continued high blood levels of the glucocorticoids produce suppression of the immune system.

The stress response increases the secretion of thyroid-stimulating hormone from the anterior pituitary, which leads to increased synthesis and secretion of the thyroid hormones and an increased basal metabolic rate. The effects of this increase are small and not well coordinated with other effects of stress.[6] The thyroid hormone, thyroxine, apparently makes the body more responsive to the effects of epinephrine and may be the major effector of prolonged stress.

Variable secretion of ADH from the posterior pituitary occurs in stressful situations. Certain types of stress and stress behaviors decrease the production of ADH, resulting in a diuresis. Other types of stress increase ADH production, which promotes water retention. The stimuli arise from a higher center than the hypothalamus but

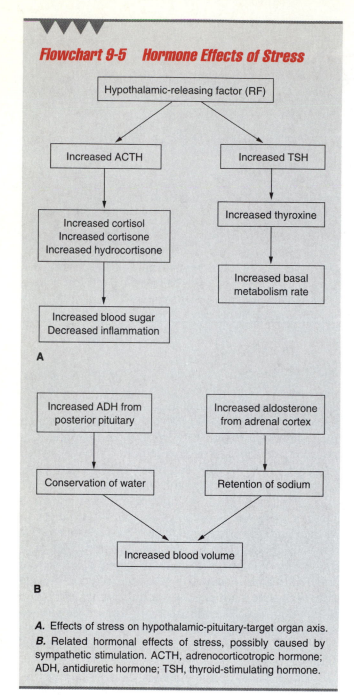

Flowchart 9-5   Hormone Effects of Stress

Hypothalamic-releasing factor (RF)

Increased ACTH → Increased cortisol / Increased cortisone / Increased hydrocortisone → Increased blood sugar / Decreased inflammation

A

Increased TSH → Increased thyroxine → Increased basal metabolism rate

Increased ADH from posterior pituitary → Conservation of water

Increased aldosterone from adrenal cortex → Retention of sodium

Increased blood volume

B

A. Effects of stress on hypothalamic-pituitary-target organ axis.
B. Related hormonal effects of stress, possibly caused by sympathetic stimulation. ACTH, adrenocorticotropic hormone; ADH, antidiuretic hormone; TSH, thyroid-stimulating hormone.

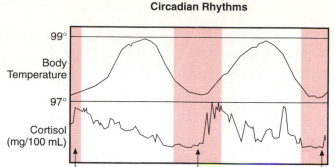

Circadian Rhythms

Body Temperature — 99° — 97°
Cortisol (mg/100 mL)
Sleep

FIGURE 9-1 *Circadian rhythms showing correlation of cortisol secretion and temperature changes in a 24-hour period.*

functions in sodium and water retention and in potassium excretion (see p. 699).

Immunologic Mechanisms

Stress, especially chronic, unremitting stress, apparently lowers the body's defenses, a response at least partly caused by increased production of corticosteroids (Flowchart 9-6). Corticosteroids suppress the inflammatory response by affecting lymphocytes and granulocytes. The B cells are depressed, and the high glucocorticoid levels reduce the production of immunoglobulins by the B cells. Sleep deprivation has been reported to caused diminished ability to destroy bacteria, presumably by suppression of granulocytic cells.[11] The T-cell response and, sometimes, the number of T cells, are affected by various forms of stress, such as death of a spouse, excessive exercise, and taking tests.[3, 11] Acceleration of normal thymic atrophy in the adult has been

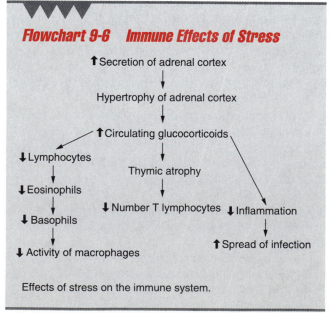

Flowchart 9-6   Immune Effects of Stress

↑ Secretion of adrenal cortex

Hypertrophy of adrenal cortex

↑ Circulating glucocorticoids

↓ Lymphocytes
↓ Eosinophils
↓ Basophils
↓ Activity of macrophages

Thymic atrophy
↓ Number T lymphocytes

↓ Inflammation
↑ Spread of infection

Effects of stress on the immune system.

act on the hypothalamus to cause the secretion or lack of secretion of ADH.[2] Examples of conditions that increase ADH include hypovolemia, anesthesia, and postsurgical stress. Decreased ADH is caused by alcohol ingestion, hypothermia, certain drugs, and other stressors (see pp. 684–685).

An increased level of aldosterone is often present in the stress response and may, like the elevated level of ADH, be a response to hemodynamic alterations or occur when there is associated renin release. Aldosterone

observed during periods of stress. The immune suppression that occurs after overwhelming insult to the body may be lifesaving in that it prevents a body-wide, inflammatory response, but the end result of suppression may be delayed healing and decreased resistance to infections.

STRESS AND DISEASE

Many studies have been conducted in an attempt to relate stress effects to actual disease development. Psychologic and physical stressors have been studied to correlate personality traits, genetic predisposition, and environmental, emotional, occupational, and social factors with specific disease. Ill health is manifested by the bodily symptoms of hyperventilation, functional bowel, musculoskeletal syndromes, and sleep disturbances.[27] These syndromes are strongly associated with anxiety, distress, and depressed moods and are closely linked to stressful experiences.[27] Ill health syndromes may also terminate in disease, but the exact link is not totally understood. The ill health is linked closely with life situations, especially uncontrollable and undesirable life experiences.[5]

A maladaptive response of the body to stressors increases the risk of disease development. It is commonly accepted that psychophysiologic arousal can cause specific end-organ pathology in certain individuals. The chronicity of the arousal state and hyperstimulation of the end organ are necessary factors in the production of pathology.[14] Genetic predisposition to a certain disease and organ susceptibility can be influenced by physical or emotional stress, or both.

Genetic Predisposition

Stressors of sufficient strength or intensity can cause an alteration in normal functioning of the body. If one has a genetic or hereditary susceptibility to the stressors, the alteration may be manifested as disease. Genetic susceptibility refers to myriad conditions that "run in the family" and seem to make the individual react in a particular way to certain stressors. A common example is an exaggerated allergic response that predisposes members of families to react to specific pollens. When the pollen count is seasonally high, these persons suffer different types of allergic responses. In this example, the stressor is the pollen count, but the response is heightened by a hyperactive, hereditary immune reaction (see p. 349).

Many other diseases seem to be familial, and development of actual disease may or may not require additional stressors to trigger the process. One example is the onset of a stroke (cerebrovascular accident) in an individual with a strong family history of stroke who also is obese, has high cholesterol levels from a high-fat diet, and smokes cigarettes.

Organ Susceptibility

Organs of different individuals are not equally resistant to stressors. Some persons under stress conditions may develop cardiovascular disorders, others may develop peptic ulcers under the same conditions, and still others may suffer migraine headaches or other maladies. The "weak organ" theory suggests that certain organs have increased susceptibility in certain individuals.[29] Why the heart is the target organ in some persons and the stomach is targeted in others is not known.

STRESS-INDUCED DISEASES

Selye referred to the production of disease as maladaptation and categorized stress-induced diseases as indicated in Box 9-1.[23] The stress connections of cardiovascular, immune deficiency, digestive diseases, cancer, and other conditions is explored in the following section.

Cardiovascular Disease

For many years it has been recognized that stress is important in the development of coronary artery disease. It can be in the form of emotional, occupational, societal, cultural, hereditary, or physical stress.

Major studies of the relations between high-fat diets, stressful living situations, and personality have led to some theories concerning coronary artery disease. Individuals who have hypercholesterolemia have a greater risk of developing atherosclerotic heart disease than those with normal cholesterol levels. The production and relations of various types of cholesterol are explored in Chapter 27. In some cases, hypercholesterolemia "runs in the family," in some cases it is diet-induced, and in some cases its cause is a mystery. During stressful periods, the serum cholesterol has been shown to rise,

BOX 9-1 ▼ Selye's Classification of Stress-Induced Diseases

1. Hypertension
2. Heart and blood vessel disease
3. Kidney disease
4. Eclampsia
5. Arthritis
6. Skin and eye inflammation
7. Infections
8. Allergic and hypersensitivity diseases
9. Nervous and mental diseases
10. Sexual derangements
11. Digestive diseases
12. Metabolic diseases
13. Cancer
14. Diseases of resistance

perhaps because of lipolysis induced by the increased levels of circulating catecholamines.

Studies also link serum lipid levels and personality patterns. Stress-induced lipemia is considered to be the principal mechanism for stress-related atherosclerosis. Stress may induce coronary artery vasospasm, which can cause myocardial injury. Emotional stress, especially anger, can precipitate anginal pain and aggravate heart problems.[2] Life stressors, such as bereavement or loss of employment, are significant risk factors for myocardial ischemia and infarction.[27]

Many facets of current lifestyles in the United States have been studied. One area of study is the commonly observed personality pattern in which the individual feels a loss of control over his or her occupation or social environment. One study identified a behavior pattern consistent with hypertension and heart attack. It includes competitiveness in work, fast work pace, time pressure, and inability to relax at work or play. This personality pattern apparently offers the greatest risk for the development of symptomatic coronary artery disease even after the other risk factors are taken into account.[28]

Immune Deficiency

The decreased immune response after exposure to stressful situations appears to be caused by increased secretion of glucocorticoids from the adrenal cortex. The major effect is suppression of T lymphocytes, which, in turn, decreases the cell-mediated immune response. Both T and B lymphocytes are affected by glucocorticoid release, but the lymphopenia (decreased numbers of lymphocytes) is caused by redistribution rather than by actual loss of T cells. Physiologically or psychologically stressful events precipitate a decrease in lymphocytes and other leukocytes.[2]

The administration of glucocorticoids in conditions of hypersensitivity or exaggerated response has long been shown to be beneficial. This is especially true in such conditions as rheumatoid arthritis, acute asthmatic attacks, and specific types of malignancy, especially leukemia. Conversely, the stress-induced response of decreased immunity can be very detrimental in conditions such as cancer. Often an individual who was declared "cured" of cancer undergoes relapse after an acute stressful situation, such as the death of a loved one. The stress-induced depression of the immune system may allow for an increased rate of malignant growth (see p. 60).

Digestive Diseases

The relation between stress and peptic ulcers has been studied for many years. Three types of stress-induced ulcer disease are briefly described here and in more detail on pages 785–790.

Overwhelming stress frequently leads to the development of stress ulcers. These may be related to gastric mucosal ischemia and gastric acid secretion. The ischemia is a result of vasoconstriction by the circulating catecholamines. The mechanism for the related gastric acid secretion is not entirely understood but may be a result of cerebral stimulation of the dorsal motor nucleus of the vagus nerve. Hypersecretion has been demonstrated clearly only in the development of Cushing ulcers, which are associated with brain lesions. Stress ulcers are very frequent in individuals who experience overwhelming conditions such as shock due to trauma, surgery, burns, or infections.

An increased rate of gastric secretions between meals has been demonstrated in persons who have duodenal ulcers; those with gastric ulcers often have normal or decreased secretion of hydrochloric acid. It would appear that duodenal ulcers result from a chronic increase in gastric acid secretion and affect the duodenum before the alkalinizing secretions can buffer the acid. Gastric ulcers seem to be related to gastritis and to decreased resistance of the gastric mucosa.

Stress has been indicated in many other digestive conditions, including such diverse ones as constipation, diarrhea, ulcerative colitis, and Crohn's disease. Personality and stress factors in ulcerative colitis and regional enteritis have been studied extensively, leading to much additional knowledge of the very complex pathogenesis of these disorders. Anger and anxiety may precipitate or exacerbate ulcerative colitis symptoms.[2]

Cancer

Specific stressors are linked with cancer causation. These carcinogens are discussed on pages 45–48. Numerous studies have linked psychosocial attitudes with development and progression of cancer. The findings vary, but depression, isolation, introverted personality, and feelings of hopelessness tend to support development of the disease.

The relation between stress and cancer may be that depression of the immunologic response by the stress allows cancer to be initiated.[11] Local exposure to carcinogen stressors may result in tumorigenesis. Stress can be viewed as having a twofold influence on malignancy: it increases the production of abnormal cells, and it decreases the capability of the body to destroy these cells.[22] All individuals are exposed daily to a host of potential carcinogens, and resistance is multifactorial, including physiologic and behavioral responses and attitudes.[20]

Other System Effects of Stress

The skin is a target organ for stress reactivity, and when stress occurs, the vessels constrict and peripheral blood flow decreases. Some of the vasospastic conditions, such as Raynaud phenomenon, are partly stress-induced.

Other stress-related disorders include eczema, urticaria, psoriasis, and acne.[2]

The musculoskeletal system exhibits stress effects by chronically tensed muscle, producing the common syndromes of backache, headache, and colon spasms.[27] Arthritis, especially rheumatoid arthritis, is aggravated by high degrees of stress, and symptoms may be exacerbated at these times.

The respiratory system participates in the acute stress reaction by hyperventilation. Stress may be exhibited also by heightened allergic sinusitis and episodes of bronchial asthma. Onset of acute ashmatic attacks may occur with sleeplessness, worry, and grief.[2]

▼ *Sleep*

Sleep is an essential component in maintaining the physiologic balance for all humans. The amount of sleep needed varies among individuals. Sleep is a basic human need on which the physical and emotional health of an individual depends.

FUNCTIONS OF SLEEP

The function of sleep is primarily to allow the body to restore itself and prepare for the next day. The heart and respiratory rate decrease during sleep, thus preserving respiratory and cardiac function. During sleep, the body conserves energy by lowering the basal metabolic rate. Epithelial and specialized cells are also repaired and revitalized during sleep.

The function of dreaming is unknown, but it is thought that some memory and problem-solving aspects are related to this function. Studies of dream content suggest that in the early stage they are oriented toward reality but in the second half of sleep the sequence of events and content become more emotionally intense and bizarre.[21] Nightmares are long, frightening dreams that awaken the sleeper; night terrors are characterized by arousal from deep sleep, often with screaming, and then amnesia as to the cause of the arousal.

Several factors can alter the quantity and quality of an individual's sleep in various ways throughout the lifetime. These factors have been identified as physical illness, sleep schedule variations, emotional stress, exercise and fatigue, weight loss and weight gain patterns, environmental factors, a person's lifestyle, and various drugs and substances. Almost everyone has at some time had difficulty in some part of the sleep cycle.

SLEEP PATTERNS

The normal human sleep-wake cycle covers a 25-hour period. Normally, its onset occurs with a decrease in activity and lasts from 7 to 9 hours.[24] There is variability in sleep needs, with some individuals requiring only 4 to 5 hours a night and others requiring 11 to 12 hours.

The pattern of an individual's sleep can be identified in a sleep lab. A sleep lab is set up to look like a bedroom. The individual is attached to leads for the recording of an electroencephalogram (EEG), which measures brain activity; an electrocardiogram (ECG), which measures electrical impulses of the heart; an electromyogram (EMG), which measures muscle tone; and an electrooculogram (EOG), which measures eye movement. These provide information on the physiology of sleep. The individual's oxygen concentration and blood pressure are also monitored. During the sleep process, the technician records sleep activity observed or heard through a microphone and video camera. A comprehensive graphic recording of the vital functions and measurements is produced during the sleep period.

PHYSIOLOGY OF SLEEP

Sleep and wakefulness physiology is a very complex phenomenon associated with many neurochemical transmitters and various areas of the brain. The coordinating mechanisms either activate or suppress the center in the brain that controls sleep. The reticular activating system (RAS), located in the upper brain stem area, contains certain cells that maintain a person's state of being awake and alert. The catecholamine-releasing neurons that release dopamine may be the cause of wakefulness. Spontaneous activity in the RAS excites the cerebral cortex and the peripheral nervous system. The feedback from these areas to the RAS tends to sustain the wakefulness state.[8, 9] It is thought that the neurons in the RAS fatigue and are susceptible to inhibition by sleep-producing chemicals. During sleep, the feedback system is tremendously slowed or inhibited, and activity in the RAS is very low.[25]

Sleep may be the result of the release of serotonin or other mediators from special cells in the raphe nuclei of the pons and medulla. Serotonin may play a role in synthesis of a hypnogenic factor that directly causes sleep.

Sleep is composed of a set of physiologic processes involving a sequence of states within the central nervous system.[10] Each sequence can be readily identified with an EEG, EMG, and EOG by the various levels of activity that are measured. Two distinct phases of sleep have been identified by these instruments. They are active or rapid eye movement (REM) sleep and quiet or non-REM sleep.[4]

As the individual falls asleep, he or she enters non-REM sleep, which is characterized by four progressive stages. Non-REM sleep is recognized by snoring, slow regular respiration, absence of body movement, and slow regular brain activity. Each stage of non-REM sleep is progressively deeper. At the end of stage 4, individuals enter stage 3, then stage 2, then finally REM sleep (Table

TABLE 9-1 *Characteristics of NREM Sleep*

Stage	Characteristics
I	Is transitional stage between wakefulness and sleep
	The person is in a relaxed state but still somewhat aware of the surroundings.
	Involuntary muscle jerking may occur and waken the person.
	The stage normally lasts only for minutes.
	The person can be aroused easily.
	Constitutes only about 5% of total sleep.
II	The person falls into a stage of sleep.
	The person can be aroused with relative ease.
	Constitutes 50% to 55% of sleep.
III	The depth of sleep increases and arousal becomes increasingly difficult.
	Composes about 10% of sleep.
IV	The person reaches the greatest depth of sleep, which is called *delta sleep.*
	Arousal from sleep is difficult.
	Physiologic changes in the body include the following:
	Slow brain waves are recorded on an EEG.
	Pulse and respiratory rates decrease.
	Blood pressure decreases.
	Muscles are relaxed.
	Metabolism slows and the body temperature is low.
	Constitutes about 10% of sleep.

(Source: C. Taylor, C. Lillis, P. LeMone. *Fundamentals of Nursing* [2nd ed] Philadelphia; JB Lippincott, 1993)

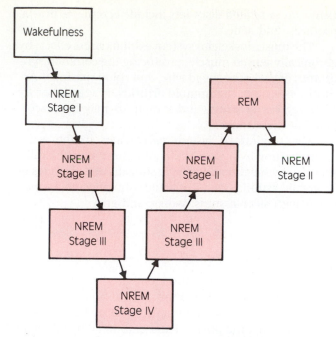

FIGURE 9-2 *A single normal sleep cycle. In the normal nocturnal pattern, the shaded cycle is repeated four or five times. Periods of REM sleep generally increase in duration, and periods of deep sleep (stage IV) progressively decrease as morning approaches. (Taylor, C. Lillis, C., and LeMone, P. Fundamentals of Nursing: The Art and Science of Nursing Care [2nd ed.] Philadelphia: J.B. Lippincott, 1993.)*

9-1). REM sleep is characterized by irregular respirations, absence of snoring, rapid eye movement, and twitching of the face and fingers. It usually takes about 90 minutes for an individual to reach REM sleep. Each person is different, but a typical night's sleep consists of four to six sleep cycles, each beginning with stage 1 and progressing through REM sleep (Fig. 9-2).

EFFECTS OF AGING ON THE SLEEP CYCLE

The characteristics of the sleep-wake cycle and the percentage of time spent in the various stages of sleep change over a person's life cycle.[21] Infants apparently have the highest amount of REM sleep. Young adults (20–40 years of age) spend 50% of their sleep time in stage 2, 25% in REM, 10% in stage 3, 10% in stage 4, and 5% in stage 1.[15]

Total sleep time and the total nightly amounts of sleep are age-dependent. Usually sleep time is greatest in infancy and gradually decreases in childhood. The total sleep time stabilizes in adulthood until it starts to decrease with old age. In addition, the number of awakenings that occur during sleep tends to increase after 40 years of age. Most of these awakenings occur during REM sleep.[15] Figure 9-3 illustrates a typical pattern of sleep in an elderly person.

SLEEP PATTERN DISTURBANCES

Sleep pattern disturbances most often fall into four basic groups: disorders of initiation and maintenance of sleep; disorders of excessive somnolence; disorders of the sleep-wake schedule; and dysfunctions associated with sleep, sleep stages, or partial arousals (Box 9-2). Individuals may have one or more type of sleep pattern disturbance, and these can be either acute or chronic. Acute episodes are not usually a problem because of their short duration. However, chronic disturbances usually require intervention.

Disorders of Initiating and Maintaining Sleep (DIMS)

These problems can be caused by multiple factors, both internal and external. Several aspects of an individual's sleep environment can alter sleep patterns. Examples are noise, uncomfortable beds, and sick children. Internal factors such as stress, pain, and ingested chemicals can alter sleep patterns.

Inability to sleep, or insomnia, may be exhibited by difficulty falling asleep, recurrent awakenings, or early-morning awakening without being able to return to sleep.[13] It causes a high level of frustration in the affected individual and is described as the feeling of being tired

Children

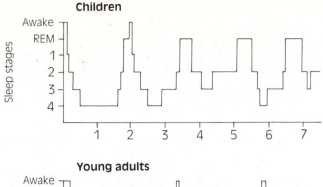

Young adults

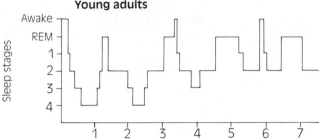

Elderly

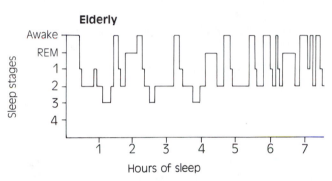

Hours of sleep

FIGURE 9-3 *A comparison of developmental differences in NREM and REM cycles during nocturnal sleep for children, young adults, and elderly people. (Taylor, C. Lillis, C., and LeMone, P.* Fundamentals of Nursing: The Art and Science of Nursing Care *[2nd ed.] Philadelphia: J.B. Lippincott, 1993.)*

from not getting enough sleep. It may indicate a pathologic disorder, or it may be psychologic in origin. Examples of pathologic disorders are pain, obstructive uropathy, endocrine disorders such as hyperthyroidism, and congestive heart failure. Musculoskeletal disorders, such as arthritis, often interfere with sleep patterns. Psychological disorders include anxiety, obsessive worrying, and depression.[1] A sleep log helps to document factors that may be causing the problem, and it is critical to review life situations and drug use, especially caffeine or alcohol use.

Disorders of Excessive Somnolence (DOES)

DOES is defined as the tendency of an individual to fall asleep whenever he or she becomes sedentary.[13] Excessive daytime sleepiness may indicate either sleep apnea or narcolepsy. Sleep apnea may result from obstruction of the airway or changes in the pacemaker respiratory neurons in the brain stem.[21] There may be chronically

reduced performance and inattention to tasks. Individuals may cite blackouts, forgetfulness, poor concentration, and amnesia.[13]

Intrinsic sleep disorders include obstructive apnea, which occurs with progressive relaxation of the muscles of the chest, diaphragm, and throat and causes airway obstruction for as long as 30 seconds.[7] The individual still attempts to breathe, because the chest and abdomen continue to move. Each breath gets stronger until the obstruction is relieved. This condition most frequently occurs in the morbidly obese individual.

Defects in the brain's respiratory center, which paces respiration, are involved in central apnea. The impulse to breathe temporarily fails, and air flow and chest wall movement cease. Central apnea may be the cause of crib death (sudden infant death syndrome, or SIDS) in infants and is related to immaturity of the respiratory neurons. DOES may also be associated with head injury or brain tumors or lesions.

BOX 9-2 ▼ A Classification of Sleep Disorders

1. Disorders of initiating and maintaining sleep (insomnia)
   Ordinary, uncomplicated insomnia
     Transient
     Persistent
   Drug-related
     Use of stimulants
     Withdrawal of depressants
     Chronic alcoholism
   Associated with psychiatric disorders
   Associated with sleep-induced respiratory impairment
   Sleep apnea
2. Disorders of excessive somnolence
   Narcolepsy
   Associated with psychiatric problems
   Associated with psychiatric disorders
   Drug-related
   Associated with sleep-induced respiratory impairment
3. Disorders of sleep-waking schedule
   Transient
     Time zone change by airplane flight
     Work shift, especially night work
   Persistent
     Irregular rhythm
4. Dysfunctions associated with sleep, sleep stages, or partial arousals
   Sleepwalking (somnambulism)
   Sleep enuresis (bed-wetting)
   Sleep terror
   Nightmares
   Sleep-related seizures
   Teeth grinding
   Sleep-related activation of cardiac and gastrointestinal symptoms

Source: M.R. Rosenzweig and A.L. Leiman, *Physiological Psychology* (2nd ed.). New York: Random House, 1989.

Narcolepsy is a condition in which the individual complains of excessive daytime sleepiness. There is also an abnormality in REM sleep.[21] During the day, the individual may suddenly fall asleep, and REM sleep can occur within 15 minutes. Sleep attacks can occur at any time and may be caused by brain stem dysfunction that involves failure of a waking mechanism to suppress the brain stem centers controlling REM sleep.

Depressive disorders cause a variety of sleep disorders, from difficulty falling asleep to extended sleep periods. Analysis of sleep character shows marked decreases in stage 3 and stage 4 sleep, with increases in stage 1 and stage 2 and frequent, vigorous REM sleep. This may be caused by neurotransmitter imbalance, and measures of sleep are used as a prognostic tool in the treatment of depression.[21]

Disorders of the Sleep–Wake Schedule

When people work the evening or night shift or travel by air across numerous times zones, the sleep–wake cycles are disrupted. Irregular patterns characterize the sleep, and frequently the sleep cycles are shortened. The inconsistent schedules result in "desynchronization" of body rhythms as they adjust at different rates to schedule changes. Internally, it disrupts the timing of metabolic and behavioral activities in the body. Concentration is impaired, digestion is altered, and sleeping is difficult.[12] The problem then becomes chronic fatigue, which occurs gradually and may result in the patient's feeling run down, depressed, and generally lacking in energy.[12]

If the individual works the night shift, sleeping must be done during the daylight hours, and the sleep pattern is disrupted. The circadian rhythm is apparently controlled by a cluster of neurons in the hypothalamus called the suprachiasmatic nucleus. This area takes its cues from light in the environment, which is monitored by the retina of the eye. It responds by sending messages to other parts of the body that influence the circadian rhythm.[17, 18] Treatment can be effected by using light therapy to alter the biorhythms or by regulating the sleep environment to simulate the night cycle during the daylight hours.

Dysfunctions Associated With Sleep, Sleep Stages, or Partial Arousals

These dysfunctions are grouped under the term *parasomnias*, and they include such diverse sleep disturbances as sleepwalking (somnambulism), night terrors, and bedwetting.[24] These conditions are occasional problems in adults and seem to occur mainly in stage 2 and stage 4 sleep. Certain illnesses, such as peptic ulcer disease and cardiovascular disease, seem to be aggravated during the normal, intense REM sleep periods. Symptoms such as chest pain or epigastric distress may occur during this time, and arousal from sleep may result.[1]

CASE STUDY 9-1

Mr. Jim Lord is a 43-year-old ex-football player who has gained 150 pounds since college football days. He comes to the clinic with complaint of constant sleepiness and "nodding off" during any sedentary periods such as watching television or even at his desk at work. He weighs 385 pounds with a large, protuberant abdomen. Vital signs are within normal limits except that it is noted that accessory muscles are used in the breathing process. Mr. Lord's wife complains that he snores loudly, especially at night in bed and awakens her with his restlessness.

1. *What type of sleep disorder is probably occurring with Mr. Lord? What clinical manifestations lead you to this diagnosis?*
2. *What are methods that could be used to diagnose this condition?*
3. *Explain the pathophysiology of the sleep disorder described. What alterations in the REM/nonREM pattern might be seen?*
4. *Compare this sleep disorder with others in the sleep disorder classifcation.*

See Appendix G for discussion.

▼ Chapter Summary

▼ Human emotions are closely linked to physiologic responses involving autonomic nervous system activities. Coping with emotional stress directly affects the health status of the individual, and different organs may be the targets of disease resulting from failure to cope.

▼ The systems theory has been used for many years to describe relations among units. The open system of the body achieves the a steady state and maintains adequate function through a negative feedback process that causes the functioning to balance the system.

▼ The pioneer of stress response research was Selye, who described the effects of stress on the human body, which he called the general adaptation syndrome. This syndrome comprises alarm reactions as well as the stages of resistance and exhaustion. In the study of the stress response, maladaptation to stressors can be seen as a basis of disease. Certain stress-induced diseases are well known, and many have to do with depression of the immunologic response.

▼ Sleep is essential to maintain the physiologic balance in all human functioning. Sleep patterns have been identified, and these vary with the age of the individual. Proper rest depends on a balance of the various stages of sleep. Sleep pattern disturbances are described in four categories: disorders of initiation and maintenance of sleep, disorders of excessive somnolence, disorders of the sleep-wake schedule, and dysfunctions associated with sleep, sleep stages, or partial arousals.

▼ *References*

1. Aldrich, M.S. Cardinal manifestations of sleep disorders. In Kryger, M.H., Roth, T., and Dement, W.C., *Principles and Practice of Sleep Medicine* (2nd ed.). Philadelphia: W.B. Saunders, 1994.

2. Asterita, M. *The Physiology of Stress*. New York: Human Sciences Press, 1985.

3. Brehm, B.A. *Essays on Wellness*. New York: Harper Collins, 1993.

4. Carskadon, M.A., and Dement, W.C. Normal human sleep: An overview. In Kryger, M.H., Roth, T., and Dement, W.C., *Principles and Practice of Sleep Medicine* (2nd ed.). Philadelphia: W.B. Saunders, 1994.

5. De La Torre, B. Psychoendocrinologic mechanisms of life stress. *Stress Med.* 10:107–114. 1994.

6. Dunn, A.J., and Kramaarcy, N.R. Neurochemical responses in stress: Relationships between the hypothalamic-pituitary-adrenal and catecholamine systems. In Iverson, L.L., and Iverson, S.D., *Drugs, Neurotransmitters, and Behavior*. New York: Plenum Press, 1984.

7. Fierman, J. Disordered sleep. *Emerg. Med.* 17:160, 1985.

8. Gaillard, J.M., Nicholson, A.N., and Pascoe, P.A. Neurotransmitter systems. In Kryger, M.H., Roth, T., and Dement, W.C. *Principles and Practice of Sleep Medicine* (2nd ed.). Philadelphia: W.B. Saunders, 1994.

9. Guyton, A.C. *Textbook of Medical Physiology* (8th ed.). Philadelphia: W.B. Saunders, 1991.

10. Hoch, C., and Reynolds, C. Sleep disturbances and what to do about them. *Geriat. Nurs.* 7:24, 1986.

11. Irwin, J., and Anisman, H. Stress and pathology: Immunological and central nervous system interactions. In Cooper, C.I., *Psychosocial Stress and Cancer*. New York: Wiley, 1984.

12. Klein, M. *The Shift Worker's Handbook*. Lincoln, NE: SynchroTech, 1991.

13. Matheson, J.K. Sleep and its disorders. In Stein, J., *Internal Medicine* (4th ed.). St. Louis: Mosby, 1994.

14. Meerson, F.Z. *Adaptation, Stress and Prophylaxis*. New York: Springer-Verlag, 1984.

15. Mendelson, W., Gillin, J. and Wyatt, R. *Human Sleep and Its Disorders*. New York: Plenum Press, 1977.

16. Miller, J. Living systems: Basic concepts. In Gray, W., et al., *General Systems Theory and Psychiatry*. Boston: Little, Brown, 1969.

17. Montplaisir, J., and Godbout, R. *Sleep and Biological Rhythms: Basic Mechanisms and Applications to Psychiatry*. New York: Oxford University Press, 1990.

18. Rae, S. Bright light, big therapy. *Modern Maturity* 37:1, 1994.

19. Roitt, I., Brostoff, J., and Male, D. *Immunology* (2nd ed.). Philadelphia: J.B. Lippincott, 1989.

20. Rosch, P.J. Stress and cancer. In Cooper, C.I., *Psychosocial Stress and Cancer*. New York: Wiley, 1984.

21. Rozenzweig, M.R., and Leiman, A.I. *Physiological Psychology* (2nd ed.). New York: Random House, 1989.

22. Selye, H. Stress, cancer, and the mind. In Day, S.B., *Cancer, Stress and Death*. New York: Plenum Press, 1968.

23. Selye, H. *The Stress of Life*. New York: McGraw-Hill, 1956.

24. Smith, P.L. Approach to the patient with sleep disorders. In Kelley, W.N., *Textbook of Internal Medicine*. Philadelphia: J.B. Lippincott, 1989.

25. Tortora, G. and Grabowski, S. *Principles of Anatomy and Physiology* (7th ed.). New York: HarperCollins, 1993.

26. Von Bertalanffy, I. *General Systems Theory: Foundations, Development and Applications*. New York: Brazillier, 1986.

27. Weiner, H. *Perturbing the Organism*. Chicago: The University of Chicago Press, 1992.

28. Wheatley, D. *Stress and the Heart*. New York: Raven Press, 1977.

29. Wolff, H.G. *Stress and Disease* (2nd ed.). Springfield, Ill.: Charles C. Thomas, 1968.

▼ *Unit Bibliography*

American Psychiatric Association. *Diagnostic and Statistical Manual of Mental Disorders* (3rd ed.). Washington, D.C.: American Psychiatric Association, 1987.

Asterita, M. *The Physiology of Stress*. New York: Human Sciences Press, 1985.

Belsky, J. *The Psychology of Aging*. Monterey, Calif.: Brooks/Cole, 1984.

Beregi, E. *Centenarians in Hungary: A Sociomedical and Demographic Study*. New York: Karger, 1990.

Biancuzzo, M. Six myths of maternal posture during labor. *Matern. Child. Nurs. J.* 18:264–269. 1993.

Binstock, R.H., and George, L.K. *Handbook of Aging and the Social Sciences*. San Diego: Academic Press, 1990.

Birren, J.E., and Schaie, K.W. *Handbook of the Psychology of Aging* (3rd ed.). San Diego: Academic Press, 1990.

Bliss-Holtz, J. Determination of thermoregulatory state in full-term infants. *Nurs. Res.* 42:204–207, 1993.

Brouillard-Pierce, C. Indications for induction of labor. *Matern. Child. Nurs. J. Suppl.* 14S-22S, 1993.

Campinha-Bacote, J., and Bragg, E.J. Chemical assessment in maternity care. *Matern Child Nurs J* 18:24–28, 1993.

Cosner, K.R., and deJong, E. Physiologic second-stage labor. *Matern. Child. Nurs. J.* 18:38–43. 1993.

Crumley, F.E. Substance abuse and adolescent suicidal behavior. *JAMA* 263:3051, 1990.

Dacey, J. and Travers, J. *Human Development Across the Lifespan*. Dubuque, IA: W.C. Brown, 1991.

Ebersole, P., and Hess, P. *Toward Healthy Aging* (4th ed.). St. Louis: Mosby, 1994.

Erikson, E. *Childhood and Society*. New York: W.W. Norton, 1963.

Fleming, B.W., Munton, M.T., Clarke, B.A., & Strauss, S.S. Assessing and promoting positive parenting in adolescent mothers. *Matern. Child. Nurs. J.* 18:32–37. 1993.

Gebauer, C.L., and Lowe, N.K. The biophysical profile: Antepartal assessment of fetal well-being. *J. Obstet. Gynecol. Neonatal Nurs.* 22:115–124. 1993.

Gormly, A.V., and Brodzinsky, D.M. *Lifespan Human Development* (4th ed.). New York: Holt, Rinehart & Winston, 1989.

Hazzard, W.R. (ed.) Geriatrics. In Kelley, W.N. (ed.), *Textbook of Internal Medicine* (2nd ed.) Philadelphia: J.B. Lippincott, 1992.

Henker, B., and Whalen, C.K. Hyperactivity and attention deficits. *Am. Psychol.* 44:216, 1989.

Homer, P., and Holstein, M. *A Good Old Age?* New York: Simon & Schuster, 1990.

Kain, C., Reilly, N., and Schultz, E. The older adult: A comparative assessment. *Nurs. Clin. North. Am.* 25:833, 1990.

Kleber, H.D. Cocaine abuse: Historical, epidemiological, and psychological perspectives. *J. Clin. Psychiatry* 49:3, 1988.

Krantz, M. *Child Development: Risk and Opportunity*. Belmont, CA: Wadsworth, 1994.

Lancaster, E. Tuberculosis comeback: Impact on long-term care facilities. *J. Gerontol. Nurs.* 19:16, 1993.

LeFrancois, G.R. *Of Children: An Introduction to Child Development* (6th ed.). Belmont, Calif.: Wadsworth, 1989.

Markides, K.S., and Cooper, C.L. *Aging, Stress and Health*. New York: Wiley, 1989.

Matti, L.K., and Caspersen, V.M. Prevalence of drug use among pregnant women in a rural area. *J. Obstet. Gynecol. Neonatal Nurs.* 22:510–514, 1993.

Moore, M.M. Recurrent teenage pregnancy: Making it less desirable. *Matern. Child. Nurs. J.* 14:104, 1989.

Muscari, M.E. Effective nursing strategies for adolescents with anorexia nervosa and bulimia nervosa. *Pediatr. Nurs.* 14:475, 1988.

Ott, M.J., and Jackson, P.L. Precocious puberty: Identifying early sexual development. *Nurse Pract.* 14:21, 1989.

Papke, K.R. Management of preterm labor and prevention of premature delivery. *Adv. Clin. Nurs. Res.* 28:279–288.

Papalia, D.E., and Olds, S.W. *Human Development*. New York: McGraw-Hill, 1992.

Patterson, E.T., Douglas, A.B., Patterson, P.M., and Bradle, J.B. Symptoms of preterm labor and self-diagnostic confusion. *Nurs. Res.* 41:367–372.

Perlmutter, M. *Adult Development and Aging*. New York: Wiley, 1985.

Peterson, M. Physical aspects of aging: Is there such a thing as "normal"? *Geriatrics* 49:45, 1994.

Pfeffer, C.R. *The Suicidal Child*. New York: Guilford Press, 1986.

Reber, A.M. *Nutrition and Aging* (2nd ed.). Denton, Tx.: Center for Studies in Aging, 1988.

Roebothan, B., and Chandra, R. Relationship between nutritional status and immune function of elderly people. *Age Ageing* 23:49, 1994.

Rogers, D. *The Adult Years: An Introduction to Aging* (3rd ed.). Englewood Cliffs, N.J.: Prentice-Hall, 1986.

Rosenzweig, M.R., and Leiman, A.L. *Physiological Psychology* (2nd ed.). New York: Random House, 1989.

Santrock, J.W. *Adult Development and Aging*. Dubuque, Iowa: W.C. Brown, 1985.

Santrock, J.W. *Children* (2nd ed.). Dubuque, Iowa: W.C. Brown, 1990.

Schrader, B.D., Heverly, M.A., and Rappaport, J. Temperament, behavior problems, and learning skills in very low birth weight preschoolers. *Res. Nurs. Health* 13:27, 1990.

Schuster, C.S., and Ashburn, S.S. (eds.). *The Process of Human Development: A Holistic Life Span Approach* (2nd ed.). Boston: Little, Brown, 1986.

Selye, H. *The Physiology and Pathology of Exposure to Stress*. Montreal: Acta, 1950.

Selye, H. *Stress Without Distress*. Philadelphia: J.B. Lippincott, 1974.

Selye, H. *Selye's Guide to Stress Research*. New York: Van Nostrand Reinhold, 1983.

Shaffer, D.R. *Developmental Psychology: Childhood and Adolescence* (2nd ed.). Pacific Grove, Calif.: Brooks/Cole, 1989.

Simpson, J. Elderly people at risk of falling: The role of muscle weakness. *Physiotherapy* 79:831, 1993.

Simpson, K.R., Moore, K.S., and LaMartina, M.H. Acute fatty liver of pregnancy. *J. Obstet. Gynecol. Neonatal Nurs.* 22:213–219, 1993.

Starn, J., Patterson, K., Bemis, G., Castro, O., and Bemis, P. Can we encourage pregnant substance abusers to seek prenatal care? *Matern. Child. Nurs. J.* 18:148–152. 1993.

Stephens, M.A. *Stress and Coping in Later Life Families*. New York: Hemisphere, 1990.

Surratt, N. Severe preeclampsia: Implications for critical-care obstetric nursing. *J. Obstet. Gynecol. Neonatal Nurs.* 22:500–507, 1993.

Tappen, R., and Beckerman, A. A vulnerable population: Multiproblem older adults in acute care. *J. Gerontol. Nurs.* 19:38, 1993.

Thomas, L.E. *Research on Adulthood and Aging*. Albany: State University of New York, 1989.

Vander Zanden, J.W. *Human Development* (4th ed.). New York: Alfred A. Knopf, 1989.

Williams, M., Wallhagen, M., and Dowling G. Urinary retention in hospitalized elderly women. *J. Gerontol. Nurs.* 19:7, 1993.

Fluid, Electrolyte, Acid-Base, Nutritional Balance, and Shock

FLUID, ELECTROLYTE, and acid–base balance is achieved through the complex cooperation of various systems of the body. Continual movement and exchange of water results in a regulated balance between plasma, interstitial fluid, and intracellular fluid. Nutritional balance participates in promoting homeostasis through nutrient utilization. Because the subject encompasses many other systems, the intent of this unit is to provide the basis for further exploration in the specific systems of the body.

Chapter 10 summarizes water and electrolyte balance and explores the major alterations that can occur with disease states. The functions of the major electrolytes are detailed. Edema refers to a shift of fluid volume between compartments caused by protein deficiency and pressure alterations. Specific reference to electrolyte and water regulation is found in many other areas of the text.

Chapter 11 deals with the basic concepts of the regulation of acid-base balance and how alterations in the balance can result. Respiratory alterations are described in greater detail in Unit 8, and the metabolic alterations are specifically explored in Unit 9. Other systems that function in the regulation of hydrogen ion concentration are noted in Units 6, 7, 10, 11, and 14.

Chapter 12 covers the principles of nutrition and alterations in nutritional balance. Activities of vitamins and minerals are also discussed. Chapter 13 explores the underlying mechanisms for the production of the altered hemodynamic state called shock. Alterations in cardiac output are also detailed in Unit 7. Because the shock state affects other organs and systems, this content is also found in the specific chapters that describe those effects.

The reader is encouraged to use the learning objectives as a study guide outline; the bibliography listed at the end of the unit can aid in further investigation of the topic.

Chapter 10

Normal and Altered Fluid and Electrolyte Balance

Barbara L. Bullock

▼ **CHAPTER OUTLINE**

▼ **LEARNING OBJECTIVES**

1 Describe the mechanisms by which water and sodium balance is normally regulated.
2 List the normal serum concentrations of the major electrolytes and plasma proteins.
3 Describe the relations between the intracellular and extracellular compartments in terms of fluid and electrolyte composition.
4 Describe in detail the normal fluid dynamics at the capillary line.
5 Define the terms **hydrostatic pressure, oncotic pressure, colloid osmotic pressure**, and **outward and inward forces** as they relate to capillary fluid dynamics.
6 Describe briefly the role of the lymphatic system in controlling extravascular fluid volume.
7 Describe the role of sodium in controlling osmotic pressure in the extracellular fluid.
8 Explain the probable effects of atrial natriuretic peptide on fluid volume and sodium regulation.
9 Differentiate the clinical effects of hypernatremia from those of hyponatremia.
10 Define **dilutional hyponatremia**.
11 Discuss how the syndrome of inappropriate antidiuretic hormone can cause hyponatremia.
12 Describe the function of potassium in the body.
13 Distinguish between the pathophysiologic changes resulting from hypokalemia and those caused by hyperkalemia.
14 Discuss the numerous functions of calcium in the body.
15 Describe the physiologic effects of hypocalcemia and hypercalcemia.
16 List the functions of phosphate in the body.
17 Explain the relations between calcium and phosphates in body functions.
18 Explain how hypochloremia is related to metabolic alkalosis.
19 Describe the effects of magnesium on the body.
20 Discuss the five pathologic mechanisms that can produce edema and their relations to each other.
21 Differentiate pitting from nonpitting edema.

Barbara L. Bullock: PATHOPHYSIOLOGY: ADAPTATIONS AND ALTERATIONS IN FUNCTION, 4th ed.
© 1996 Lippincott-Raven Publishers

The volume and composition of body fluids must remain constant to support life. Continual movement and exchange of water and electrolytes occur and are regulated by the body to compensate for wide variations in intake and output. Table 10-1 lists the normal laboratory values for the electrolytes and water. Measured values may reflect environmental changes or disease states. The protein composition of plasma plays a major role in regulation of fluid movement at the capillary line.

TABLE 10-1 *Normal Laboratory Values for Electrolytes and Water*

WATER	
Serum osmolality	285–295 mOsm/kg
	285–295 mmol/kg (SI units)
Urine osmolality	50–1,200 mOsm/kg
	50–1,200 mmol/kg (SI units)
SODIUM	
Serum sodium	136–145 mEq/L
	136–145 mmol/L (SI units)
Urine sodium	40–220 mEq/L/24 hr
	40–220 mmol/L/24 hr (SI units)
POTASSIUM	
Serum Potassium	3.5–5.0 mEq/L
	3.5–5.0 mmol/L (SI units)
Urine Potassium	25–120 mEq/L/24 hr
	25–120 mmol/L/24 hr (SI units)
CALCIUM	
Serum Calcium	Total: 9.0–10.5 mg/dL
	2.25–2.75 mmol/L (SI units)
	Ionized: 4.5–5.6 mg/dL
	1.05–1.30 mmol/L (SI units)
Urine Calcium	100–300 mg/24 hr
	2.5–7.5 mmol/24 hr (SI units)
PHOSPHATE	
Serum Phosphate	2.5–4.5 mg/dL, 1.7–2.6 mEq/L
	0.78–1.52 mmol/L (SI units)
Tubular Reabsorption	Ratio of creatinine clearance to phosphate clearance
Phosphate	Detects hyperparathyroidism, increased levels 82%–95% on normal diet
CHLORIDE	
Serum Chloride	90–110 mEq/L
	98–106 mmol/L (SI units)
Urine Chloride	110–250 mEq/L
	110–250 mmol/day (SI units)
MAGNESIUM	
Serum Magnesium	1.8–3.0 mg/dL, 1.5–2.5 mEq/L
	0.65–1.05 mmol/L (SI units)
Urine Magnesium	6.0–10.0 mEq/24 hr
	3.0–5.0 mmol/24 hr

▼ *Regulation of Water and Sodium Balance*

WATER

Water balance refers to an equilibrium maintained between intake and output. Water, a necessary solvent, is used in many metabolic processes of the body and carries waste products for excretion through the urine, skin, lungs, and feces. Water cushions, protects, lubricates, insulates, and provides structure for and resilience to the skin.

Water accounts for approximately 60% of body weight in the adult. This amount normally decreases with age and is affected by other components of body composition (Fig. 10-1). The lean individual has a greater percentage of body water than the obese person, because fat cells contain less water than muscle cells. The amount of water intake necessary to maintain life in the adult is about 1,500 mL per day. Water intake, although intermittent, is usually higher than necessary, with an average total of 2,000 mL per day. Water is ingested in liquids and in foods and is also produced by oxidation of foodstuffs. It is directly conserved by the antidiuretic hormone (ADH) and indirectly conserved by aldosterone.

The composition of the body fluids is regulated by the kidneys, gastrointestinal tract, nervous system, and lungs, with input from the heart and glands. Hormones, especially aldosterone and ADH, regulate the composition of plasma and other fluid compartments.

The intake of water must be balanced by output. The kidneys rid the body of excess water. Obligatory urinary output to eliminate waste and maintain minimal renal function is 300 to 500 mL per 24 hours. The volume of urinary excretion can be increased tremendously, and usually totals approximately 1,500 mL per 24 hours. Water is also lost through the lungs (300 mL/24 h), skin (500 mL/24 h), and feces (200 mL/24 h). This loss is termed insensible loss. In the adult, body water gains and losses are balanced at a total of approximately 2,600 mL per 24 hours (Table 10-2).[5]

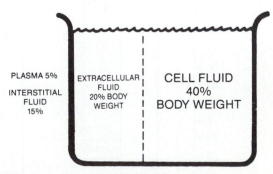

FIGURE 10-1 *Total body fluid, 60% body weight. (Metheny, N.M. Fluid and Electrolyte Balance: Nursing Considerations. Philadelphia: J.B. Lippincott, 1991.)*

TABLE 10-2 *Average Intake and Output in an Adult for a 24-Hour Period*

Intake		Output	
Oral liquids	1300 mL	Urine	1500 mL
Water in food	1000 mL	Stool	200 mL
Water produced by metabolism	300 mL	*INSENSIBLE:*	
Total	2600 mL	Lungs	300 mL
		Skin	600 mL
		Total	2600 mL

Metheny, N.M. *Fluid and Electrolyte Balance: Nursing Considerations* [2nd ed.]. Philadelphia: J.B. Lippincott, 1992.

Water imbalance can occur as a result of excess or depletion of body fluids. It is closely associated with changes in sodium concentration. Body water loss is aggravated by elevated body temperature, diarrhea, vomiting, and other excessive depletion such as occurs through kidneys, skin, lungs, and the gastrointestinal tract. Water excess is often caused by sodium retention, but it may occur with excess ADH secretion or excessive ingestion of water.

Water accounts for the *osmotic pressure* in the tissues and cells of the body. Osmotic pressure is actually determined by the movement or draw of water through a selectively permeable membrane toward an area of greater solute concentration (see p. 187). To determine the osmotic pressure of a solute, the osmolality of the solution must be determined. Osmolality is defined as the number of osmoles (Osm) of a substance contained within a kilogram of water; an osmole is the number of molecules in one gram molecular weight of undissociated solute.[6] A solution with 1 Osm in each kilogram of water has an osmolality of 1 Osm/kg, and a solution with an osmolality of 1 milliosmole (mOsm) per kilogram contains .001 Osm/kg of solute.[6] Normal serum osmolality is 285 to 295 mOsm/kg. Electrolytes, primarily sodium, determine serum osmolality, and serum osmolality can easily be estimated by doubling the serum sodium value (see Table 10-1). An elevated osmolality is indicative of either excessive solutes, especially sodium, or inadequate fluid volume.[17]

FLUID BALANCE IN BODY COMPARTMENTS

Fluids are maintained in strict volume and concentration in each of the three compartments: 1) extracellular intravascular (plasma); 2) extracellular extravascular (interstitial fluids); and 3) intracellular fluids (ICF). Figure 10-2 shows the relations of fluid balance and composi-

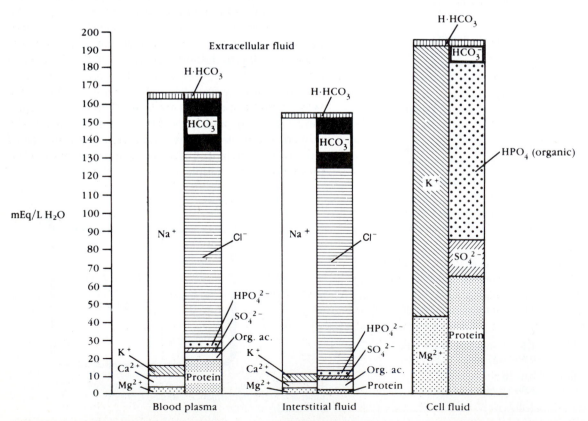

FIGURE 10-2 *Electrolyte composition of the body fluid compartments.*

tion among these three compartments. In normal distribution, about 70% of body fluid is intracellular, and the rest is extracellular in the form of interstitial fluid, plasma, and secretion or excretion fluids. The relations of cations, anions, and volumes must be maintained rigidly to preserve life. Interstitial fluids and plasma basically contain the same electrolyte composition, but plasma contains a large amount of protein. The composition of intracellular electrolytes is quite different from that of extracellular electrolytes, but the number of charges (cations and anions) is basically equal in the compartments (see Figure 10-2). To maintain life, fluid containing oxygen and nutrients from the blood is filtered into the interstitial spaces and carried to the ICF, and excess carbon dioxide and other cellular waste products are returned to the bloodstream to be circulated and excreted by the lungs and kidneys. The process requires the constant movement and exchange of fluids and gases.

Thirst

Thirst, defined as the conscious desire for water, is the principal regulator of water intake. It is usually first expressed when the osmolality of plasma reaches about 295 mOsm/kg.[14] Osmoreceptors located in the thirst center in the hypothalamus are sensitive to changes in the osmolality of extracellular fluids (ECFs). As osmolality increases, the cells shrink and the sensation of thirst is experienced as a result of dehydration. This stimulates thirst through the following mechanisms:

1. Decreased renal perfusion stimulates the release of renin, which eventually leads to the production of angiotensin II (see p. 698). Angiotensin II stimulates the hypothalamus to release neural substrates that are responsible for generating the sensation of thirst.[7]
2. Osmoreceptors in the hypothalamus detect elevations in osmotic pressure and activate nervous pathways that result in the thirst sensation.
3. Thirst may be induced by local dryness of the mouth in true hyperosmolar states, or it may occur to relieve the unpleasant dry sensation that results from reduced salivation.

Thirst may result from depleted circulatory volume due to hemorrhage or from decreased cardiac output secondary to pump failure. The sensation may be diminished or unrecognized in elderly and confused individuals and in individuals with decreased levels of consciousness, resulting in inadequate fluid consumption.

Generally, the thirst sensation prompts the individual to consume water, thereby correcting the hypovolemia or state of increased osmolality. After the thirst sensation has been satisfied, intake of fluid ceases. Excessive intake of water that is unrelated to thirst usually has a psychogenic basis. Obsessive preoccupation with and indulgence in excessive water intake can lead to fluid volume overload, decreased serum osmolality, and decreased serum osmotic pressure.

RENAL REGULATION

The kidneys regulate the volume and electrolyte concentration of body fluids. ECF is filtered through the renal glomeruli. Selective reabsorption and excretion of water and solutes occurs in the renal tubules (see pp. 623–627). Glomerular filtration rate and renal perfusion, reflective of cardiac output, determine the rate of this process. Hypovolemic states result in reduced urinary output, which reflects the body's attempt to conserve or retain fluid volume. The mechanism by which this occurs is related to decreased renal perfusion. Underperfused kidneys release renin, which converts first to angiotensin I and then to angiotensin II. The latter hormone stimulates the release of aldosterone from the adrenal cortex. The action of aldosterone is to facilitate renal reabsorption of sodium and water, thus increasing circulating fluid volume.[9]

ANTIDIURETIC HORMONE

ADH is formed in the hypothalamus and stored in the neurohypophysis of the posterior pituitary. The area of ADH storage and release may overlap with the thirst center, which accounts for the integration of thirst and ADH release.[6] The major stimuli for ADH secretion are increased osmolality and decreased volume of ECF. Secretion may also occur with the stress of trauma, surgery, pain, and some anesthetics and drugs. The hormone increases reabsorption of water at the collecting ducts, thereby conserving water to correct the osmolality and restore the volume of ECF (Fig. 10-3).

Also called vasopressin, ADH has a minor vasoconstrictive effect on the arterioles that can increase blood pressure. A significant decrease in ADH secretion secondary to lesions or trauma of the hypophyseal tract results in diabetes insipidus, which is characterized by a massive increase in urinary output. Blood volume depletion does not result in diabetes insipidus as long as the thirst mechanism remains intact. Increased secretion of ADH, stimulated by pituitary hypersecretion or by extrapituitary tumors, results in a marked decrease in serum osmolality, an increase in blood volume, and a decrease in urinary output. This is known as the syndrome of inappropriate ADH secretion (SIADH) (see pp. 691–692).

ALDOSTERONE

Aldosterone, a hormone secreted by the adrenal gland, acts on the renal tubules to increase the sodium uptake. The increased sodium retention causes an increase in water retention (see Figure 10-3). The amount of water retention is directly related to the amount of sodium retained. Aldosterone release is stimulated by changes in potassium concentration, by serum sodium concentrations, and by the renin-angiotensin system (see p. 698). Normally, the rate or amount of aldosterone secretion is

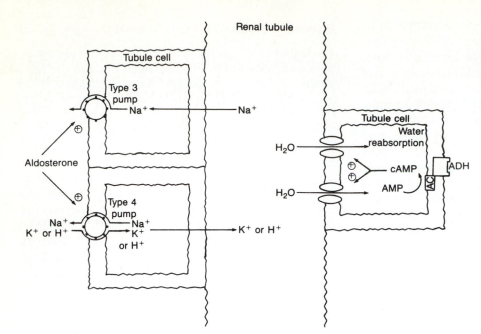

FIGURE 10-3 *Location and influence of aldosterone and antidiuretic hormone (ADH) receptors. Aldosterone stimulates sodium pumps and exchange pumps in the serosal membranes of renal tubule cells, creating a gradient that draws sodium out of the renal tubule and pushes potassium and hydrogen into the tubule. ADH activates an adenylate cyclase-linked receptor on the serosal membrane of tubule cells that initiates formation of cyclic adenosine monophosphate (cAMP), which promotes aggregation of proteins in the luminal membrane that serve as water channels. (Swonger, A.K., and Matejski, M.P. Nursing Pharmacology Philadelphia: J.B. Lippincott, 1991.)*

closely regulated by the potassium concentration, and it is very effective in controlling hyperkalemia.[7]

PROSTAGLANDINS

The prostaglandins are naturally occurring fatty acids that are present in many of the tissues of the body and function in the inflammatory response, blood pressure control, uterine contractions, and gastrointestinal motility. In the kidneys, renal prostaglandins cause vasodilation and, in most cases, promote sodium excretion by inhibiting the response of the renal distal tubules to ADH. Prostaglandin-mediated renal vasodilation protects the kidneys from ischemia when levels of vasoconstrictors, such as angiotensin II and norepinephrine, increase.[23] Sodium retention may result when endogenous prostaglandin production is decreased.

GLUCOCORTICOIDS

The glucocorticoids, secreted by the adrenal cortex, exert weak activity that promotes the reabsorption of sodium and water. This increases blood volume and sodium retention. Therefore, alterations in glucocorticoid levels cause alterations in the blood volume balance.

ATRIAL NATRIURETIC PEPTIDE (ANP)

ANP, first identified in 1981, is a 28-amino acid peptide released from myocytes in the coronary sinuses of the atria in response to increased atrial stretch. Although ANP is released on a continual basis in healthy persons, its release is accelerated by any condition that results in increased atrial stretch, especially fluid volume excess.

Research is being done to determine the physiologic function of this hormone in the body.[8,19] It has been shown in laboratory studies to have the following effects: 1) increases the kidneys' ability to excrete both water and sodium; 2) improves glomerular filtration rate and hence increases sodium filtration by dilatation of the afferent and efferent arterioles[4]; 3) inhibits the reabsorption of sodium by the collecting ducts; 4) inhibits renin secretion by the juxtaglomerular apparatus, thereby preventing release of aldosterone from the adrenal cortex; and 5) inhibits release of ADH.[4,22] Circulating levels of ANP are elevated in congestive heart failure, renal insufficiency, and cirrhosis and have been shown to be low or normal in volume depletion and in the nephrotic syndrome.

▼ Movement of Fluids at the Capillary Line

The capillaries are formed of endothelium, which is permeable to all of the solutes and water of the plasma. It is impermeable to the large molecules and cells in the plasma. Substances move through the gaps or spaces in the endothelial cells, and some substances, such as carbon dioxide, oxygen, and small solutes, move through the endothelial membrane as well. The process occurs by diffusion, so that near-equilibrium exists at the capillary line: the amount of fluid leaving the capillary nearly equals the amount reabsorbed. This dynamic equilibrium is called *Starling's law of the capillaries.*[24] The equilibrium occurs mostly through a balance achieved between the hydrostatic pressure of the blood and the colloid osmotic pressure within the capillaries.

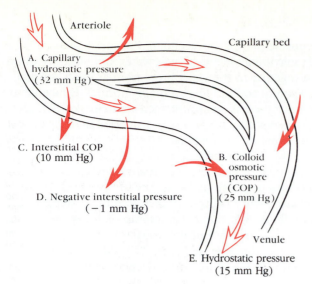

FIGURE 10-4 *Fluid dynamics at the capillary line.* **A.** *Capillary hydrostatic pressure is higher at the arteriolar end and tends to push fluid out.* **B.** *Colloid osmotic pressure (COP) generated by the plasma proteins maintains a constant inward pull or force.* **C.** *Interstitial COP is an outward force.* **D.** *Negative interstitial pressure is an outward force.* **E.** *Venular hydrostatic pressure is lower than the COP that is maintained in the vessel, which provides an inward force.*

Blood entering the capillary comes in at a *hydrostatic pressure* that is generated by the heart. This hydrostatic pressure varies in the different systemic arterioles, but it is always higher at the arteriolar end of the capillary than at the venular end (Fig. 10-4). As fluid filters out of the capillary into the tissue spaces, the hydrostatic pressure decreases. The high pressure exerted at the arteriolar end of the capillary has been called a simple *outward force,* or pushing force, which moves fluid from the vessel to the interstitial spaces. The average hydrostatic pressure at the arteriolar end is 32 mm Hg, and it drops to 15 mm Hg at the venous end.[6] This hydrostatic pressure provides the main outward force, but it is enhanced by a negative

interstitial pressure and the interstitial fluid colloid osmotic pressure, as shown in Figure 10-4.

The interstitial fluid colloid osmotic pressure results from plasma proteins that are leaked into the interstitial spaces and that exert a colloid, or water-pulling, effect. The pressure exerted by the plasma proteins, the *colloid osmotic* or *oncotic pressure (COP),* is an osmotic pulling or *inward force* that draws water toward it. Because the plasma proteins cannot move into the interstitial area, they exert their colloidal effect by drawing water back into the vessel. The average COP is 25 mm Hg, a pressure that remains constant across the capillary.

Note in Figure 10-4 that at the arteriolar end of a schematic capillary the hydrostatic pressure exceeds the COP by about 7 mm Hg, causing fluid movement to the interstitial area. At the venous end, the hydrostatic pressure has dropped to 15 mm Hg and is now lower than the COP, which causes movement of fluid back into the capillary. The COP in the capillaries is mainly generated by albumin, because it is the most abundant of the plasma proteins. Table 10-3 lists the relative concentrations of plasma proteins.

Although the amount of fluid filtered out of the vessel almost equals that reabsorbed, a larger amount is filtered into the tissue spaces than is reabsorbed. Also, small amounts of protein escape into the tissue spaces during the process of fluid movement and cannot be reabsorbed by the blood vessels. These excesses of fluid and protein are absorbed by the *lymphatic system* and returned through lymphatic channels to the blood. The lymphatic system provides the only means to return plasma proteins in the tissues to the bloodstream.[6]

Edema does not normally occur until there is an increase of 17 mm Hg in the gradient favoring filtration, or the outward force.[6] This is because the lymph channels can increase the amount of fluid carried and thus compensate for increased fluid escaping into the tissue spaces. Edema does result if there is significant alteration

TABLE 10-3 *Concentration and Function of Major Plasma Proteins*

Proteins	Concentration	Functions
TOTAL PLASMA PROTEINS	6.0–8.0 g/dL	Synthesized by liver; maintain blood osmotic pressure; function in acid-base balance and coagulation; provide substrate for structure and energy and for transport of drugs and hormones.
ALBUMIN	3.2–4.5 g/dL (50%–65% of total)	Most abundant; main protein in production of osmotic pressure; maintains blood volume; transports stored hormones; participates in binding drugs and in acid-base balance.
GLOBULIN	2.3–3.5 g/dL (30%–45% of total)	Antibodies in form of immunoglobulins; provide for humoral immunity; transport iron, fats, and other substances.
FIBRINOGEN	150–400 mg/dL	Essential function in blood coagulation.

in the balance of the inward (COP) and outward (hydrostatic) forces.

▼ Water-Sodium Deficits and Excesses

Water and sodium imbalances are categorized as *volume* or *osmolar*. Volume, or isotonic, imbalances occur when sodium and water increase or decrease together in the same ratio that is normally found in the ECFs. Osmolar imbalances result when there is an alteration in the normal relation of water to solutes in the ECFs. The serum sodium level is the best indicator of osmolality of blood because it is the most abundant solute in the vascular space.[14]

HYPOVOLEMIA

Hypovolemia, or extracellular volume depletion, is an isotonic imbalance in which water and electrolytes are lost together in the same proportion as exists normally. The serum sodium level remains normal. Hypovolemia occurs if there is an abrupt decrease in intake of fluids or if the extracellular volume is decreased because of such conditions as hemorrhage, diarrhea, vomiting, burns, excessive diaphoresis, draining wounds, ascites, or severe uncontrolled diabetes mellitus. Hypovolemia results in a decrease in the size of the extracellular space and circulatory collapse, which eventually depletes cellular fluid. Signs and symptoms of hypovolemia are related to the cause of the imbalance (Table 10-4). Regardless of the cause of the fluid volume loss, the volume depletion is quite advanced by the time symptoms are

---

TABLE 10-4 *Water and Sodium Excess and Deficit*

Normal Function	Source and Cause of Imbalance	Clinical Manifestations
WATER		
Removes waste products, provides fluid medium for blood and tissues; lubricates, insulates, cushions, protects body. Composes approximately 60% of body weight or about 40 L. Forty percent is intracellular; 20% is extracellular. Average intake is 2,000 mL/day. Normal water balance (serum osmolality) is regulated by antidiuretic hormone (ADH), atrial natriuretic peptide (ANP), and aldosterone.	Normal value: 280–295 mOsm/kg Gain and loss usually equal. Loss stimulates thirst and decreases renal output. Excess intake decreases thirst and increases urine output.	
	Hypervolemia: excess extracellular fluid volume. May be caused by conditions such as excessive administration of isotonic solution; renal, liver, cardiac diseases; hyperaldosteronism.	Weight gain, distended abdomen, venous engorgement, hypertension, edema, dyspnea. Urine osmolarity <200 mOsm/L. Could indicate renal impairment if it continues after fluid restriction.
	Hypovolemia: extracellular fluid volume depletion. Loss of fluid through conditions such as burns, hemorrhage, diarrhea, vomiting, diaphoresis, diabetes mellitus, hypoaldosteronism.	Thirst, dry mucous membranes, poor skin turgor, shock, may occur with increased blood sugar in diabetes mellitus.
SODIUM		
Regulates serum osmolality by maintaining osmotic pressure. Water and sodium balance are highly correlated. Functions in neuromuscular and muscular excitability; functions in acid-base balance and enzyme systems. Supplied by dietary intake; excreted mainly by kidneys, under influence of aldosterone primarily ANP and ADH secondarily.	Normal value: 135–145 mEq/L	
	Hypernatremia (>145 mEq/L): caused by excess loss of water over sodium, excess intake, hyperalimentation, renal insufficiency. Decreased ADH or decreased aldosterone.	Cellular shrinking caused by increased extracellular osmolality leads to central nervous system irritability, tachycardia, hypotension, thirst, oliguria, anuria.
	Hyponatremia (<130 mEq/L): excess water in relation to sodium caused by hypotonic fluid administration, some diuretics, dilutional from congestive heart failure, cirrhosis, syndrome of inappropriate ADH secretion. Classified as isotonic, hypertonic, or hypotonic.	Cellular swelling caused by decreased extracellular osmolality leads to cerebral edema, headache, stupor, coma; peripheral edema, polyuria, decreased thirst, nausea, vomiting.

manifested, owing to the fact that interstitial fluid and, to a lesser extent, ICF move to the intravascular spaces to maintain circulation.

HYPERVOLEMIA

Hypervolemia, or extracellular volume excess, is an isotonic imbalance in which water and electrolytes are gained together in the same proportion as exists normally in the ECF. The serum sodium level remains normal. Hypervolemia may result from excessive administration of isotonic solutions or of adrenal glucocorticoid hormones. This imbalance also may occur in disease states such as chronic renal failure, liver disease, congestive heart failure, malnutrition, and hyperaldosteronism if homeostatic mechanisms for fluid and electrolyte balance are impaired. Hypervolemia results in expansion of the extracellular space and circulatory overload. Signs and symptoms reflect the overload (see Table 10-4).

▼ Sodium

Sodium is the major cation of the ECF. It regulates the osmotic pressure of the ECF and markedly affects the osmotic pressure of ICF. Sodium intake comes from the diet; requirements for body needs vary according to age and size. Adolescents need between 900 and 2,700 mg of sodium daily. Adults can maintain sodium balance with less than 500 mg per day. One teaspoon of salt contains approximately 2 g of sodium. The average daily intake in the United States is 2.3 to 6.9 g.[26]

Sodium is also an essential component in neuromuscular excitability and is responsible for depolarization of the cell membranes of excitable cells. It participates in acid-base balance by combining with the bicarbonate radical. Sodium exists in combination with various anions, especially chloride and bicarbonate. Sodium concentration is directly regulated by aldosterone and indirectly by ADH, ANP, and the glucocorticoids.

HYPONATREMIA

Deficits of serum sodium result either from actual loss of sodium from body fluids or from excessive gains in extracellular water that dilute the sodium concentration. This imbalance may be caused by inadequate sodium intake, diuretic therapy, adrenal insufficiency, and administration of hypotonic solutions to replace fluid lost through diaphoresis, vomiting, or gastrointestinal suctioning. Conditions that may result in water gain include psychogenic polydipsia, inadequate excretion of water secondary to renal disease or brain lesions, and administration of hypotonic solutions after surgical procedures or trauma.[18] The cells become swollen as water moves

from ECF to ICF to compensate for the solute deficit. The neuromuscular system is particularly sensitive to this imbalance (see Table 10-4).

Hyponatremic disorders are commonly classified as *isotonic*, *hypertonic*, and *hypotonic* states, depending on the serum osmolality. Isotonic hyponatremia occurs with the infusion of isotonic solutions that are sodium-free and dilute the ECF. The hyponatremia is gradually transformed from isotonic to hypotonic as the glucose in the isotonic solutions is oxidized.[25] Hypertonic hyponatremia occurs with very high glucose states, which pull water from the cells (eg, in diabetic ketoacidosis). If the initial volume is normal, each 100 mg/dL increase of blood glucose decreases the serum sodium by 1.6 mEq/L.[16]

The term hypotonic hyponatremia refers to a hypo-osmolar plasma associated with decreased serum sodium. The degree of hyponatremia may not reflect total body sodium. An example is hypervolemic hypotonic hyponatremia which, as its name implies, refers to water intoxication such as that which can occur with an excess secretion of ADH (the syndrome of inappropriate ADH secretion). The hyponatremic individual has clinical manifestations of weight gain, edema, hypoalbuminemia, hypertension, and, sometimes, increased intracranial pressure.[16] The hypervolemic individual may have *dilutional hyponatremia*, which means that water has been reabsorbed in excess proportion to sodium. With water restriction and administration of diuretics, the serum sodium may be restored to normal.[11]

The person with hypovolemic hyponatremic clinical syndrome may show signs of dehydration with a decreased urine output and signs of vascular collapse. This clinical condition may be treated with intravenous saline to correct the sodium deficit. In hyponatremia, it is critical to recognize the source of the problem, because the treatment could be lifesaving or life-threatening to the affected individual.

HYPERNATREMIA

Serum sodium excess results from decreased intake or increased output of water. Overingestion of sodium may also cause this imbalance. Conditions that may lead to hypernatremia include impaired thirst sensation, dysphagia, profuse diaphoresis, watery diarrhea, polyuria due to diabetes insipidus, excessive water loss from the lungs, and excessive administration of hypertonic solutions. Cells shrink and dehydration occurs as water moves from the ICF to the ECF to compensate for the solute excess. Brain cells are very sensitive to this imbalance (see Table 10-4).

Hypernatremia may be associated with normal, decreased, or increased serum volume. Normal volume hypernatremia is most commonly seen in persons who have inadequate water intake and are pulling intracellular water intravascularly. The goal of therapy is aimed at repletion of total body water lost. Hypovolemic hypernatremia indicates a marked loss of fluids, with water being lost at a greater rate than sodium. The symptoms of dehydration are often profound, and restoration of volume is a priority. Hypervolemic hypernatremia is often iatrogenic, as when large amounts of sodium bicarbonate are administered for metabolic acidosis.

▼ Potassium

Potassium is normally concentrated in the ICF. It directly affects the excitability of nerves and muscles and contributes to the intracellular osmotic pressure (Table 10-5). Secretions and excretions contain large amounts of potassium. The source of potassium is the diet, which normally provides much more than is needed by the body. Urine potassium concentration varies, providing an efficient mechanism for the excretion of excess potassium to maintain the narrow range of normal serum concentrations.

Potassium moves into the cell during the formation of new tissues, the anabolic phase. During tissue breakdown, the catabolic phase, potassium leaves the cell. Potassium does not move into cells if there is a deficit of oxygen, glucose, or insulin.

The human body very effectively excretes potassium but has little mechanism for renal conservation. Potassium deficit occurs in 2 to 3 days if there is no intake. This deficit is enhanced by conditions such as surgery that increase anabolic needs. Anything that increases the

excretion of potassium, such as use of diuretics, may also cause the depletion.

The major route for the loss of potassium is the kidneys, but some loss can occur through gastrointestinal secretions or the skin. In the kidneys, the final excretion of potassium is under the control of aldosterone at the distal tubules. At this point, hydrogen, potassium, and sodium tend to compete with each other for excretion. Sodium is usually preferred for absorption in the presence of aldosterone. If the plasma hydrogen ion concentration is elevated above normal, the tubules preferentially tend to excrete hydrogen and conserve potassium, which leads to the hyperkalemia often seen in association with acidosis. The reverse is true in alkalosis: If the hydrogen concentration is low, potassium is preferentially excreted and hydrogen is conserved, thus causing the hypokalemia associated with alkalosis (see pp. 221–222).

HYPOKALEMIA

A serum deficit of potassium may be caused by any of the following: lack of intake; use of potassium-depleting diuretics; major gastrointestinal surgical procedures, especially with nasogastric suctioning and incomplete replacement; excessive gastrointestinal secretions; hyperaldosteronism; malnutrition; and trauma or burns (see Table 10-5).

Hypokalemia affects every system. In the gastrointestinal system, anorexia, nausea, vomiting, and paralytic ileus may occur. In the muscles, flaccidity and weakness may be exhibited and may lead to respiratory muscle weakness and arrest. Cardiac dysrhythmias are

---

TABLE 10-5 *Potassium Excess and Deficit*

Normal Function	Source and Cause of Imbalance	Clinical Manifestations
Regulates osmolality of ICF; functions in neuromuscular excitability and in acid-base balance. Important to rate and force of cardiac contractility. Dominant cation in ICF.	Normal value: 3.5–5mEq/L Supplied by diet, excreted by kidney, about 40 mEq/day. Some loss of K^+ in sweat and stool. Loss is regulated by aldosterone; no mechanism for conservation.	
	Hyperkalemia (levels >5.0 mEq/L): renal failure, cellular damage, metabolic acidosis. Excessive K^+ intake; drugs: β-adrenergic blockers, captopril, cyclosporine, heparin.	Depression of cardiac conductivity. Peaked T waves and widened QRS complex on ECG, muscle cramping, nausea, diarrhea; seen with metabolic acidosis.
	Hypokalemia (levels <3.5 mEq/L): gastrointestinal loss, lack of dietary intake, vomiting, metabolic alkalosis, surgical loss. Drugs: K^+-depleting diuretics, steroids, amphotericin.	Muscle cramping, fatigue, weakness, increased cardiac irritability, U waves on ECG, dysrhythmias, vomiting, paralytic ileus, decreased ability of kidney to concentrate urine.

common and the electrocardiogram (ECG) may show the presence of a U wave that was not previously present (Fig. 10-5). Ventricular tachycardia and cardiac arrest may occur if the levels are very low. Central nervous system depression and decreased deep tendon reflexes also may be noted. Hypokalemia causes decreased ability of renal tubules to concentrate waste, leading to increased water loss.

Hypokalemia causes an increased sensitivity to digitalis and may precipitate the effects of digitalis toxicity in persons taking a preparation of the drug. Hypokalemia enhances automaticity and may precipitate ventricular fibrillation in the heart.

HYPERKALEMIA

Excess potassium is usually secondary to temporary or permanent kidney dysfunction (see Table 10-5). It frequently occurs in association with renal failure. It also may be present transiently (with normal renal function) after major tissue trauma or after the rapid transfusion of stored bank blood. As blood is stored, the red blood cells begin to break down and release their potassium into the surrounding fluid. A unit of blood 1 day old has approximately 7 mEq of potassium per liter, but a unit that is 21

days old has 23 mEq per liter.[13] Certain drugs or excessive potassium intake can also cause hyperkalemia. Pseudohyperkalemia results if blood samples are allowed to hemolyze.[13]

Hyperkalemia mainly affects the cardiovascular system. A decreased membrane potential causes a decrease in the intensity of the action potential, resulting in a dilated, flaccid heart. Various kinds of conduction defects may be noted together with ectopic dysrhythmias. The ECG shows a shortened PR interval, tall peaked T waves, a short QT interval, and widening of the QRS complex (see Figure 10-5). In the gastrointestinal system, nausea, vomiting, and diarrhea are common. Initial irritability of the skeletal muscles gives way to weakness and flaccid paralysis. Digital numbness and tingling may be described.

▼ *Calcium*

Calcium is present in the body in the form of calcium salts and as ionized and protein-bound calcium. Ninety-nine percent is in the bones and teeth in the crystalline form, which gives hardness to these structures. Of the 1% that is circulating, approximately 40% is bound to plasma proteins, especially albumin. The serum albu-

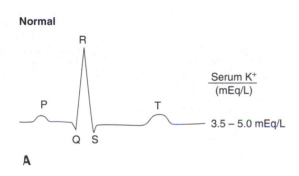

Normal

Serum K+ (mEq/L)

3.5 – 5.0 mEq/L

A

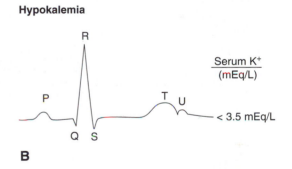

Hypokalemia

Serum K+ (mEq/L)

< 3.5 mEq/L

B

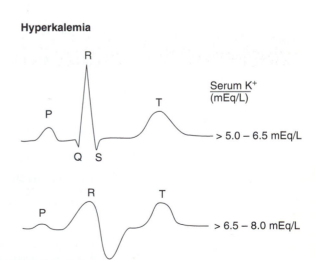

Hyperkalemia

Serum K+ (mEq/L)

> 5.0 – 6.5 mEq/L

> 6.5 – 8.0 mEq/L

C

FIGURE 10-5 **A.** *Electrocardiagram with potassium range.* **B.** *In hypokalemia, the T wave become flatter, and the U wave is seen.* **C.** *In hyperkalemia below 6.5 mEq/L, the T wave becomes tall and peaked; above 6.5 mEq/L, the QRS becomes widened and the T wave large and rounded. The P wave flattens and the PR interval increases. When the potassium level is >8.0 mEq/L, cardiac arrest is imminent.*

min is the major circulating calcium-binding protein. If its value is normal, 50% of the calcium is in the free ionized form. If the serum albumin is low, the ionized calcium level is greater than 50%, and the hypercalcemia is greater than that indicated by total serum calcium.[3] The ionized form of calcium is the active portion, and it functions in membrane integrity, coagulation, and muscle contraction, and in the electrophysiology of the excitable cells (Table 10-6).

Calcium can be released from its bound form, especially in the presence of a decreased serum pH. The reaction, simply stated, is a reversible equation:

$$Ca^{++} \text{ (protein-bound} + H^+) \leftrightarrow Ca^{++} \text{ (ionized)} + H^+ \text{ (protein complex)}$$

The reaction is driven toward the right in acidosis, causing an increase in ionized serum calcium. In alkalosis, the reaction is driven more toward the left, which can cause hypocalcemia. This is the method used by the body plasma proteins to buffer hydrogen ion (see pp. 221–222).[21] Calcium concentration in the blood is under the influence of *parathyroid hormone* (PTH) and *calcitonin*. PTH is released by the parathyroid glands when the extracellular level of ionized calcium is decreased (see p. 711). Calcitonin enhances the deposition (uptake) of calcium into bone if increased calcium levels are present, and it inhibits bone reabsorption. Calcitonin is produced by C cells in the thyroid gland. It functions to reduce serum calcium and phosphate levels but may have more important roles in bone development in the fetus.[12]

Calcium stabilizes the cell membrane and blocks sodium transport into the cell. Because of this, decreased calcium levels increase the excitability of cells, and increased levels decrease excitability.

Vitamin D affects calcium absorption as well as bone deposition and reabsorption. Vitamin D is produced in the skin through the action of ultraviolet light and is present also in most American diets. It is changed by the liver to 25-hydroxycholecalciferol by hydroxylation and is further metabolized by the kidneys with the aid of PTH to form the most active type, 1,25-dihydroxycholecalciferol (see pp. 720–723). This substance is important in enhancing calcium uptake from the gastrointestinal tract and functions with PTH in bone reabsorption.[6, 12, 21]

RELATION OF CALCIUM TO PHOSPHATE

Phosphate is an anion that is also regulated by PTH and activated vitamin D. Normally, the aggregate concentration of calcium and phosphate is constant: if the calcium level increases, the phosphate level decreases. Calcium joins with phosphate to form calcium phosphate ($CaHPO_4$). If an excessive amount of $CaHPO_4$ is formed, it is not ionizable, and hypocalcemia results.

HYPOCALCEMIA

If calcium levels decrease, the blocking effect of calcium on sodium also decreases. As a result, depolarization of excitable cells occurs more readily as sodium moves in.

TABLE 10-6 *Calcium Excess and Deficit*

Normal Function	Source and Cause of Imbalance	Clinical Manifestations
Most calcium is stored in skeleton and teeth; provides a large reservoir for serum levels. Ionized Ca^{++} used to control muscular contraction, cardiac function, nerve impulses, and blood clotting.	Normal value: 9.0–10 mg/dL. Ionized: 4.5–5.6 mg/dL. Fifty percent ionized, 50% protein bound. In acidosis, ionized Ca^{++} rises because of loss from protein. In alkalosis, levels are lowered owing to protein gain.	Because of reservoir balance, is usually maintained even at expense of bones or teeth.
	Hypercalcemia (>10.5 mg/dL): immobility, hyperparathyroidism, blood or bone malignancies, excess vitamin D, renal insufficiency. Drugs: thiazide diuretics, lithium, theophylline, chemotherapy agents.	Muscle weakness from decreased neuromuscular excitability, CNS depression, stupor, coma; ECG may show shortened QT. If caused by bone loss, may have increased risk of fractures.
	Hypocalcemia (<8.5 mg/dL): hypoparathyroidism or surgical removal of parathyroid gland; insufficient vitamin D, dietary lack of calcium, hypoalbuminemia. Drugs: loop diuretics, anticonvulsants, citrate-buffered blood, phosphates, alcohol abuse, calcitonin, cisplatin, gentamycin.	Increased neuromuscular excitability. Trousseau and Chvostek signs, skeletal muscle cramps, tetany, laryngospams, asphyxia, death.

Therefore, if the calcium levels are low, increased central nervous system excitability and muscle spasms occur. Convulsions and tetany may be the result (see Table 10-6).

Hypocalcemia may be associated with decreased activation of vitamin D, which often results from renal or liver disease. Pancreatitis may cause decreased serum calcium owing to the release of pancreatic lipase, which combines with fatty acids and calcium. Blood transfusions may cause hypocalcemia as calcium binds with the citrate used in the blood preparation, thus removing ionizable calcium from the blood.[12] Hyperphosphatemia, hypoalbuminemia, parathyroid disease, administration of agents such as adrenocorticotropic hormone or glucagon, surgical removal of the parathyroid glands, gastrointestinal tract disease, and neoplastic conditions may all be associated with hypocalcemia. Functional hypoparathyroidism and hypocalcemia can be caused by hypermagnesemia and may be produced if magnesium is used to control premature labor.[3]

The results of hypocalcemia are spasms and tetany, increased gastrointestinal motility, cardiovascular problems, and osteoporosis. Muscle tetany is both common and dangerous, especially if it involves laryngeal spasm.[3] The Trousseau sign of hypocalcemia is elicited if, when a blood pressure cuff is inflated on an extremity for 1 to 3 minutes, a contraction of the fingers occurs. The Chvostek sign is elicited if tapping of the facial nerve at the temple results in a twitch on that side of the face. Cardiac problems include decreased cardiac contractility and, occasionally, symptoms of heart failure. The cardiac action potential changes are seen on the ECG by prolongation of the ST segment and resultant QT interval prolongation (Fig. 10-6B).[2, 16, 17]

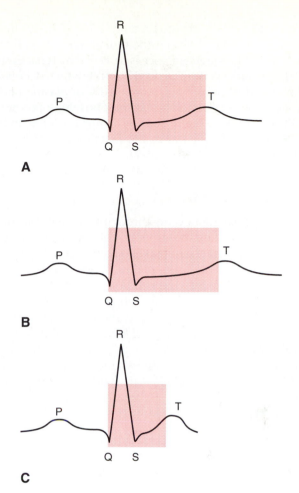

FIGURE 10-6   *A. Normal electrocardiogram tracing. **B.** Prolongation of the QT interval in hypocalcemia may increase risk of dysrhythmias or heart block and may be associated with poor contractility. **C.** Shortening of QT in hypercalcemia may cause severe dysrhythmias that may result from increased cardiac irritability.*

HYPERCALCEMIA

Excessive levels of calcium increase the blocking effect on sodium in the skeletal muscles. This leads to decreased excitability of both muscles and nerves, eventually contributing to flaccidity (see Table 10-6). Hypercalcemia is associated with decreased phosphate levels. The major cause is hyperparathyroidism, which produces increased PTH, increasing calcium uptake from the bones into the circulating blood. Thiazide diuretics also can cause increased PTH levels and hypercalcemia.[2] Some malignant tumors secrete PTH-like substances that function similarly to true PTH. Other malignant tumors, such as multiple myeloma and breast cancer, cause osteolytic lesions that can result in the release of calcium into the bloodstream and hypercalcemia. Excessive ingestion of vitamin D may cause the condition owing to increased absorption of calcium from the gut. Immobilization may cause loss of bone substance and increased levels of serum calcium.

Hypercalcemia causes skeletal muscle weakness, anorexia, nausea and vomiting, constipation, weight loss, and increased excretion of calcium in the urine. The increased circulating calcium may be deposited anywhere, but the kidneys are most vulnerable. Calcium deposition may result in kidney stones. Increased amounts may also be deposited in the arteries and cardiac valves. Central nervous system changes may include depression, bizarre behavior, and memory impairment. Acute hypercalcemia in persons on hemodialysis for renal failure can present symptoms suggestive of dementia.[1] Cardiac effects include shortening of the QT interval on the ECG with virtually no ST segment (see Figure 10-6C).[17]

▼ Phosphate

Phosphate functions with calcium to support bone formation. Most phosphate comes from dietary intake of dairy products, meat, and eggs.[26] Phosphate is the primary intracellular anion. It assists with energy transfer within the cells.[13] Approximately 85% of body phosphate is in the bones, and the remaining 15% is intracellular.[21] Phosphate balance is achieved by renal excretion; this process is influenced by PTH, which decreases absorption of phosphate. About 10% of plasma phosphate is protein-bound.[27] Plasma phosphate promotes acid-base balance of the body by acting as a buffer in the ECF. It also participates in the metabolism of glucose, fats, and proteins (Table 10-7).

HYPOPHOSPHATEMIA

Hypophosphatemia occurs through three mechanisms: decreased intestinal absorption, enhanced urinary excretion, and enhanced uptake to bone (see Table 10-7). It occurs in alcoholism, malnutrition, diabetic ketoacidosis, and hyperthyroidism. A deficit may also result from antacid use, because aluminum hydroxide, aluminum carbonate, and calcium carbonate combine with phosphate to promote loss of phosphate through the feces. Common symptoms include anorexia, dizziness, paresthesias, muscle weakness, and vague neurologic symptoms. In the alcoholic, the syndrome may appear like delirium tremens.[27] Hypercalciuria is often seen, and kidney stones may result. Extreme imbalances are characterized by hematologic abnormalities, muscle breakdown, irritability, stupor, encephalopathies, seizures, and coma.

HYPERPHOSPHATEMIA

Hyperphosphatemia can occur in renal failure or if PTH levels are decreased. It also may be seen with excess oral intake or abuse of phosphate-containing laxatives (see Table 10-7). Transfusion of stored blood and skeletal muscle breakdown may cause increased serum levels. Because calcium is inversely related to phosphate, the clinical manifestations of hyperphosphatemia resemble those of hypocalcemia.

▼ Chloride

The chloride ion is the major anion of ECF (Table 10-8). The amount of chloride in the fluid closely parallels the sodium content. Chloride is a component of hydrochloric acid in the stomach. It also serves an essential role in the transport of excess carbon dioxide by red blood cells (see p. 375). Chloride moves into the cells by passive transport.

Chloride depletion (hypochloremia) especially results from loss of gastrointestinal secretions, such as that occurring from vomiting, excessive diarrhea, and nasogastric suctioning. Diuretic therapy commonly causes hypochloremia together with hyponatremia, but urinary loss of chloride may be greater than loss of sodium. Metabolic alkalosis results as bicarbonate is conserved to maintain cation-anion balance. The clinical manifestations of hypochloremia are usually related to the associated metabolic alkalosis (see p. 221).

Hyperchloremia is often associated with hypernatremia, especially in dehydration and renal problems. It can lead to weakness, lethargy, and Kussmaul breathing.

▼ Magnesium

Magnesium is found mostly within the cells and in the bones (Table 10-9). This cation activates a number of intracellular enzyme systems and is required for protein

---

TABLE 10-7 *Phosphate Excess and Deficit*

Normal Function	Source and Cause of Imbalance	Clinical Manifestations
Essential for generation of bony tissue. Functions in metabolism of glucose and lipids for energy. Works in ICF acid–base balance.	Normal value: 3.0–4.5 mg/dL 85 percent stored in bones. Supplied in diet. Inverse relation with calcium.	
	Hyperphosphatemia (>4.5 mg/dL): most frequently seen in kidney failure, hypoparathyroidism, hypocalcemia, excessive alkali ingestion, blood hemolysis.	Symptoms like those of hypocalcemia. May develop dysrhythmias and tetany.
	Hypophosphatemia (<3.0 mg/dL): hypoparathyroidism, diabetic coma due to carbohydrate metabolism, alcohol withdrawal, hyperalimentation.	Anorexia, weakness, bone pain, muscle weakness, osteomalacia, tremors, hyporeflexia, confusion, seizures, coma, bleeding disorders.

TABLE 10-8 *Chloride Excess and Deficit*

Normal Function	Source and Cause of Imbalance	Clinical Manifestations
Predominant ECF anion; exists mainly with sodium as NaCL or with hydrogen as HCL. Affects osmotic pressure with Na. Follows Na loss and gain and acid-base balance. Essential in gastric acid.	Normal value: 98–106 mEq/L Mainly ingested as salt. Chloride rises in acidosis as bicarbonate drops. It decreases in alkalosis as bicarbonate increases. Excreted with cations through kidneys and gastrointestinal tract.	
	Hyperchloremia (>110 mEq/L): dehydration, Cushing syndrome, hyperventilation, anemia, cardiac failure, some kidney problems.	Weakness, lethargy, deep rapid breathing.
	Hypochloremia (<80 mEq/L): vomiting, diarrhea, burns, diabetic ketoacidosis, fever, acute infections, diuretics.	Hyperexcitability of CNS, signs like hyponatremia.

and nucleic acid synthesis. Magnesium is particularly essential in promoting neuromuscular integrity.[13] Magnesium is mainly regulated by renal excretion. Most magnesium is reabsorbed, but hypernatremia and hypercalcemia can decrease its reabsorption.[10]

HYPOMAGNESEMIA

The most common cause of decreased serum magnesium is excessive ingestion of alcohol. Other causes include malnutrition, diabetes mellitus, liver failure, and poor intestinal absorption. The clinical manifestations include cardiovascular dysrhythmias, increased neuromuscular irritability, paresthesias, tetany, and convulsions. Some of these are caused by refractory hypocalcemia or hypokalemia, and such conditions respond only to magnesium therapy.[10] Hypokalemia is common in association with hypomagnesemia owing to increased renal excretion of potassium when the magnesium level is low.

TABLE 10-9 *Magnesium Excess and Deficit*

Normal Function	Source and Cause of Imbalance	Clinical Manifestations
Regulates neuromuscular irritability; essential in blood coagulation. Activates many enzymes in carbohydrate and protein metabolism. Essential in absorption of calcium from gut and in calcium metabolism.	Normal value: 1.5–2.5 mEq/L Closely related to calcium levels. Also associated with potassium levels.	
	Hypermagnesemia (>2.5 mEq/L): renal failure, leukemia, severe dehydration. May be elevated with excessive taking of magnesium drugs.	Sedative effect, drowsiness, lethargy, flushing, respiratory depression, nausea, vomiting, slurred speech, bradycardia, hypotension.
	Hypomagnesemia (<1.5 mEq/L): malabsorption, cirrhosis, alcoholism, protein-calorie malnutrition, bowel resection, diarrhea, dehydration. Treatment in diabetic coma with insulin may decrease serum Mg. Drugs that will cause decrease: loop diuretics, aminoglycosides, and cisplatinum.	Muscle tremors, tetany, hypocalcemia, hyperactive reflexes, anorexia, nausea and vomiting, ventricular irritability.

HYPERMAGNESEMIA

This condition is rare but may occur in individuals with renal failure, especially if they ingest magnesium-containing antacids.[13] It also may occur as a result of therapy for toxemia of pregnancy or premature labor.[10] Clinical manifestations begin at a level of 4 mEq/L or greater and include lethargy, coma, cardiac dysrhythmias, respiratory failure, and death. Because dialysis in persons with chronic renal failure does not remove magnesium well, these individuals should be restricted from ingesting magnesium-containing medications.

▼ Edema

The word *edema* refers to the expansion or accumulation of interstitial fluid volume. It may be localized or generalized, pitting or nonpitting, depending on its cause. Edema is usually thought of as accumulation of excess fluid in the skin; however, the mechanism causing skin edema also can cause fluid shifts in other vulnerable areas of the body. These fluid shifts are sometimes termed *third-space shifts* and include ascites, pleural or pericardial effusions, and pulmonary edema.[13] Table 10-10 summarizes the etiologic mechanisms that may lead to the formation of edema and fluid shifts. Five

---

TABLE 10-10 *Etiologic Mechanisms for the Formation of Edema*

Etiologic Mechanisms	Types of Edema
Increased capillary pressure	Congestive heart failure Phlebothrombosis Cirrhosis of the liver with portal hypertension
Vasodilatation	Inflammation Allergic reactions Burns (direct vascular injury)
Decreased colloid osmotic pressure	Liver failure Protein malnutrition Nephrosis Burns
Lymphatic obstruction	Surgical removal of lymph structures Inflammation or malignant involvement of lymph nodes and vessels Filariasis
Sodium/body water excess	Congestive heart failure Renal failure Aldosteronism Excess sodium intake

---

interrelated mechanisms are commonly described: decreased COP; increased capillary hydrostatic pressure; increased capillary permeability; lymphatic obstruction; and sodium and body water excess.[6] Some forms of edema result from more than one mechanism.

DECREASED COLLOID OSMOTIC PRESSURE

If the plasma proteins are depleted in the blood, the inward forces are decreased, allowing the filtration effect to favor movement into the tissues. This leads to accumulation of fluid in the tissues with a decreased central volume of plasma. The kidneys respond to the decreased circulating volume by activating the renin-angiotensin-aldosterone system, which results in additional reabsorption of sodium and water. Intravascular volume increases temporarily. However, because the plasma protein deficit has not been corrected, the COP (ie, the inward force) remains low in proportion to capillary hydrostatic pressure. Consequently, intravascular fluid moves into the tissues, worsening the edema and the circulatory status.

Hypoproteinemia causes decreased COP and may result from malnutrition, neoplastic wasting, liver failure, or protein loss through burns, kidneys, or the gastrointestinal tract. Albumin is the primary protein affected because it is the most abundant and also because its molecules are rather small and can pass through damaged capillary endothelium or glomeruli. Loss of protein into the tissues causes decreased reabsorption of tissue fluids and edema. This is a positive feedback response, because as the central blood volume becomes depleted, the kidneys conserve more sodium and water and additional edema is formed (see Flowchart 10-1). This response can be terminated by restoring intravascular protein levels, which increases the intravascular COP and subsequently decreases the volume of edema.

The accumulation of ascitic fluid in cirrhosis of the liver is related partly to hypoproteinemia from decreased hepatic production of albumin and partly to increased hydrostatic pressure created by portal hypertension (see pp. 820–822).

INCREASED CAPILLARY HYDROSTATIC PRESSURE

The most common cause of increased capillary pressure is congestive heart failure in which increased systemic venous pressure is combined with increased blood volume. These manifestations are characteristic of failure of the right ventricle, or right-sided heart failure. Left-sided heart failure can also lead to an increase in pulmonary capillary pressure. If the pressure exceeds 25 mm Hg, pulmonary edema can occur (see pp. 502–505).

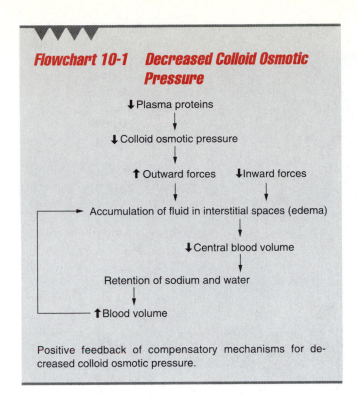

Flowchart 10-1   Decreased Colloid Osmotic Pressure

↓ Plasma proteins

↓ Colloid osmotic pressure

↑ Outward forces   ↓Inward forces

Accumulation of fluid in interstitial spaces (edema)

↓Central blood volume

Retention of sodium and water

↑Blood volume

Positive feedback of compensatory mechanisms for decreased colloid osmotic pressure.

Other causes of increased hydrostatic pressure include renal failure with increased total blood volume, increased gravitational forces from standing for long periods of time, impaired venous circulation, and hepatic obstruction. Venous obstruction usually produces localized rather than generalized edema because only one vein or group of veins is affected.

INCREASED CAPILLARY PERMEABILITY

Direct damage to blood vessels, such as with trauma and burns, may cause increased permeability of the endothelial junctions. Localized edema may occur in response to an allergen, such as a bee sting. In certain individuals, this allergen may precipitate an anaphylactic response with widespread edema initiated by the histamine type of reaction. Inflammation causes hyperemia and vasodilation, which lead to accumulation of fluids, proteins, and cells in an affected area. This results in edematous swelling (exudation) of the affected localized area (see p. 349).

OBSTRUCTION OF THE LYMPHATICS

The most common cause of lymphatic obstruction is the surgical removal of a group of lymph nodes and vessels to prevent the spread of malignancy. Radiation therapy, trauma, malignant metastasis, and inflammation may

also lead to localized lymphatic obstruction. *Filariasis*, a rare parasitic infection of the lymph vessels, can cause widespread obstruction of the vessels. Lymphatic obstruction leads to retention of excess fluid and plasma proteins in the interstitial fluid. As proteins accumulate in the interstitial spaces, more water moves into the area. The edema is usually localized.

SODIUM AND BODY WATER EXCESS

With congestive heart failure, cardiac output is decreased as the force of contraction decreases. To compensate, increased amounts of aldosterone cause the retention of sodium and water. Plasma volume increases, as does venous intravascular capillary pressure. The failing heart is unable to pump this increased venous return, and fluid is forced into the interstitial space (see p. 509). Hypervolemia also can occur with renal insufficiency and renal failure. The kidneys cannot adequately excrete the solute load and hypervolemia results.

TYPES OF EDEMA

Pitting edema refers to the displacement of interstitial water by finger pressure on the skin, which leaves a pitted depression. After the pressure is removed, it often takes several minutes for the depression to be resolved. Pitting edema often appears in dependent sites, such as the sacrum of a bedridden individual. Similarly, gravitational hydrostatic pressure increases the accumulation of fluid in the legs and feet of an upright individual.

Nonpitting edema may be seen in areas of loose skin folds such as the periorbital spaces of the face. Nonpitting edema may occur after venous thrombosis, especially of the superficial veins. Persistent edema leads to trophic changes in the skin. These changes may progress to stasis dermatitis and ulcers that heal very slowly (see pp. 537–538). Nonpitting, brawny edema is also associated with thick, hardened skin and color changes. It occurs when serum proteins become trapped and coagulated in the tissue spaces. Figure 10-7 shows some different causes of edema and the mechanisms that may produce them.

DISTRIBUTION OF EDEMA

The distribution of edema can give clues as to its cause. If it is localized in one extremity, it is probably caused by venous or lymphatic obstruction. Edema resulting from hypoproteinemia is generalized but is especially pronounced in the eyelids and face in the morning, due to the recumbent position assumed at night and the aid of

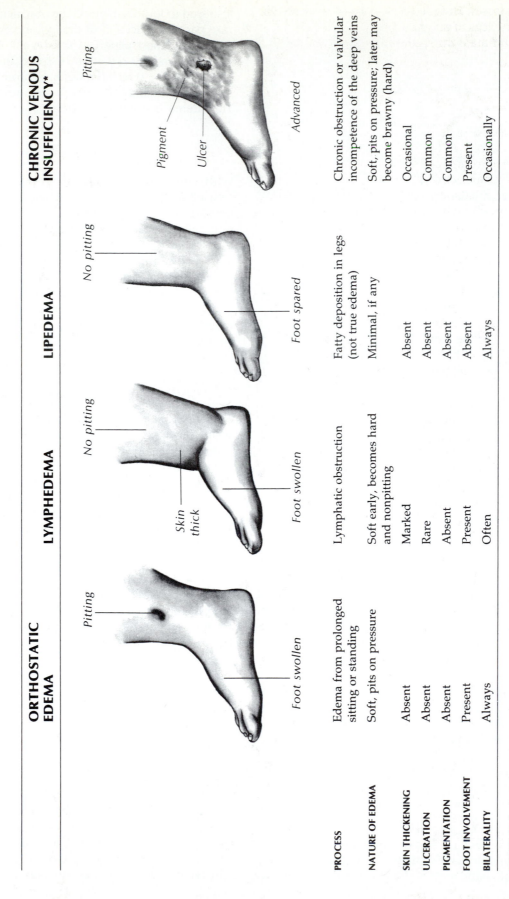

	ORTHOSTATIC EDEMA	LYMPHEDEMA	LIPEDEMA	CHRONIC VENOUS INSUFFICIENCY*
PROCESS	Edema from prolonged sitting or standing	Lymphatic obstruction	Fatty deposition in legs (not true edema)	Chronic obstruction or valvular incompetence of the deep veins
NATURE OF EDEMA	Soft, pits on pressure	Soft early, becomes hard and nonpitting	Minimal, if any	Soft, pits on pressure; later may become brawny (hard)
SKIN THICKENING	Absent	Marked	Absent	Occasional
ULCERATION	Absent	Rare	Absent	Common
PIGMENTATION	Absent	Absent	Absent	Common
FOOT INVOLVEMENT	Present	Present	Absent	Present
BILATERALITY	Always	Often	Always	Occasionally

FIGURE 10-7 *Some peripheral causes of edema. (Bates, B. A Guide to Physical Examination [6th ed.]. Philadelphia: J.B. Lippincott, 1995.)*

gravitational forces. The edema of heart failure is usually greatest in the legs of an ambulatory individual, and it tends to accumulate throughout the day.[20]

▼ Chapter Summary

▼ A rigid balance of fluid and electrolytes is essential to maintain the health of the individual. There are many complex mechanisms to rigidly maintain intracellular and extracellular electrolyte levels, and these in turn influence water balance. Water balance is intricately involved with sodium balance. Hypovolemia and hypervolemia may involve water imbalance alone or with sodium imbalance. If the sodium levels are affected, so are the transport mechanisms across the cell membrane. Thirst and renal and hormonal mechanisms function to maintain water and sodium balance.

▼ Plasma proteins are essential in maintenance of the vascular and extravascular fluid compartments. Their balance regulates the movement of fluid from the capillaries to the interstitial spaces and cells, and the movement from the interstitial spaces and cells back into the vascular system.

▼ Potassium balance is essential to normal nerve and muscle excitability. The range of normal is very narrow, with the bulk of the electrolyte being concentrated in the intracellular fluid. Potassium is poorly conserved by the kidney and is easily lost even when other electrolytes are conserved. Therefore, hypokalemia is probably the most common electrolyte disturbance seen in the clinical area. Hyperkalemia is less common, especially if the kidneys are functioning well.

▼ Most calcium and phosphate is found in the bones and teeth, and their balance is under the influence of the parathyroid hormone and other hormones. Serum calcium is carefully preserved by the body; its level is critical because low calcium levels can produce tetany, laryngeal spasm, and other severe problems. Hypercalcemia is often associated with decreased phosphate levels. Deposition of calcium throughout the body can lead to organ dysfunction.

▼ Magnesium is just now being appreciated for the cardiac problems that it can cause. It is often seen in association with hypokalemia. Hypomagnesemia is much more common than hypermagnesemia.

▼ Edema is a condition that results when there is expansion of interstitial fluid volume. The cause of edema varies, and its mechanism may cause fluid shifts in other areas of the body. The five mechanisms that cause edema are decreased COP, increased capillary hydrostatic pressure, increased capillary permeability, lymphatic obstruction, and sodium and body water excess.

▼ References

1. Benabe, J.E., and Martinez-Maldonado, M. Disorders of calcium metabolism. In Maxwell, M.H., Kleeman, C.R., and Narins, R.G. (eds.), *Clinical Disorders of Fluid and Electrolyte Metabolism* (4th ed.). New York: McGraw-Hill, 1987.
2. Bilezikian, J.P. Hypercalcemia. In Stein, J.H., *Internal Medicine* (4th ed.). St. Louis: Mosby, 1994.
3. Bilezikian, J.P. Hypocalcemia. In Stein, J.H., *Internal Medicine* (4th ed.). St. Louis: Mosby, 1994.
4. Birney, M.H., and Penney, D.G. Atrial natriuretic peptide: A hormone with implications. *Heart Lung* 19:174, 1990.
5. Epstein, M. Disorders of sodium balance. In Stein, J.H., *Internal Medicine* (4th ed.). St. Louis: Mosby, 1994.
6. Guyton, A.C. *Textbook of Medical Physiology* (8th ed.). Philadelphia: W.B. Saunders, 1990.
7. Hollenberg, N.K., and Dzau, V.J. The renin-angiotensin system. In Maxwell, M.H., Kleeman, C.R., and Narins, R.G. (eds.), *Clinical Disorders of Fluid and Electrolyte Metabolism* (4th ed.). New York: McGraw-Hill, 1987.
8. Humes, H.D., and Cox, M. Principles of the renal regulation of fluid and electrolytes. In Kelley, W.N., *Textbook of Internal Medicine*. Philadelphia: J.B. Lippincott, 1989.
9. Kikeri, D., and Mitch, W.E. The heart and kidney disease. In Schlant, R.C., and Alexander, R.W., *The Heart, Arteries and Veins* (8th ed.). New York: McGraw-Hill, 1994.
10. Kobrin, S. Disorders of magnesium homeostasis. In Stein, J.H., *Internal Medicine* (4th ed.). St.Louis: Mosby, 1994.
11. Kokko, J.P. Diuretics. In Schlant, R.C., and Alexander, R.W., *The Heart, Arteries and Veins* (8th ed.). New York: McGraw-Hill, 1994.
12. Marx, S.J., and Bourdeau, J.E. Calcium metabolism. In Maxwell, M.H., Kleeman, C.R., and Narins, R.G. (eds.), *Clinical Disorders of Fluid and Electrolyte Metabolism* (4th ed.). New York: McGraw-Hill, 1987.
13. Metheny, N.M. *Fluid and Electrolyte Balance* (2nd ed.). Philadelphia: J.B. Lippincott, 1992.
14. Morrison, G., and Singer, I. Hyperosmolal states. In Maxwell, M.H., Kleeman, C.R., and Narins, R.G. (eds.), *Clinical Disorders of Fluid and Electrolyte Metabolism* (4th ed.). New York: McGraw-Hill, 1987.
15. Narins, R.G., and Krishna, G.G. Disorders of water balance. In Stein, J.H., *Internal Medicine* (4th ed.). St. Louis: Mosby, 1994.
16. Mundy, G.R. Malignant diseases and the skeleton. In Stein, J.H., *Internal Medicine* (4th ed.). St. Louis: Mosby, 1994.
17. Rardon, D.R., and Fisch, C. Electrolytes and the heart. In Hurst, J.W., et al., *The Heart* (7th ed.). New York: McGraw-Hill, 1990.
18. Reineck, H.J., and Stein, J.H. Sodium metabolism. In Maxwell, M.H., Kleeman, C.R., and Narins, R.G. (eds.), *Clinical Disorders of Fluid and Electrolyte Metabolism* (4th ed.). New York: McGraw-Hill, 1987.
19. Schlant, R.C., and Sonnenblick, E.H. Normal physiology of the cardiovascular system. In Schlant, R.C., and Alexander, R.W., *The Heart, Arteries and Veins* (8th ed.). New York: McGraw-Hill, 1994.

20. Schlant, R.C., and Sonnenblick, E.H. Pathophysiology of heart failure. In Schlant, R.C., and Alexander, R.W., *The Heart, Arteries, and Veins* (8th ed.) New York: McGraw-Hill, 1994.

21. Schrier, R.W. *Renal and Electrolyte Disorders* (3rd ed.). Boston: Little, Brown, 1986.

22. Stanton, B.A., and Koeppen, B.M. Control of body fluid volume and osmolality. In Berne, R.M., and Levy, M.N. (eds.), *Principles of Physiology*. St. Louis: Mosby, 1990.

23. Stein, J.H., and Bakris, G.L. Principles of renal physiology. In Stein, J.H., *Internal Medicine* (4th ed.). St. Louis: Mosby, 1994.

24. Tortora, G.J., and Grabowski, S.R. *Principles of Anatomy and Physiology* (7th ed.). New York: Harper-Collins, 1993.

25. Weisberg, L., Szerlip, H.M., Davidson, R.L., and Cox, M. Approach to the patient with altered sodium and water homeostasis. In Kelley, W.N., *Textbook of Internal Medicine*. Philadelphia: J.B. Lippincott, 1989.

26. Whitney, E.N., Cataldo, C.B., and Rolfes, S.R. *Understanding Normal and Clinical Nutrition* (3rd ed.). St. Paul: West, 1991.

27. Ziyadeh, F.N. Disorders of phosphate homeostasis. In Stein, J.H., *Internal Medicine* (4th ed.). St. Louis: Mosby. 1994.

Chapter 11

Normal and Altered Acid–Base Balance

Barbara Bullock

▼ **LEARNING OBJECTIVES**

1 List the normal values of the blood gases and pH of the different body fluids.
2 Differentiate between volatile and nonvolatile acids.
3 Describe the major buffer systems.
4 Describe specifically how the carbonic acid–bicarbonate system is affected by the respiratory and renal systems.
5 Explain how the kidneys maintain a constant hydrogen ion concentration in the plasma.
6 Describe the activity of hemoglobin as a protein buffer.
7 Differentiate between acidosis and alkalosis on the basis of physiologic disruption.
8 Compare respiratory acidosis and metabolic acidosis with respect to pathophysiology and compensatory mechanisms.
9 Define the term ''anion gap'' and relate it to an acid–base abnormality.
10 Differentiate the etiology of respiratory and metabolic alkalosis.
11 Describe the clinical manifestations of respiratory and metabolic acidosis and alkalosis.

▼ *Normal Acid–Base Balance*

All living cells of the human body are surrounded by a fluid environment called extracellular fluid (ECF). The chemical composition of the ECF is regulated within narrow limits that provide an optimal environment for maintaining normal cell function. The most precisely regulated ion concentration in ECF is that of the hydrogen ion, normally ranging from 37 to 43 nEq/L. A nanoequivalent (nEq) is 10^{-9}, or 0.000000001 equivalent, a very small measurement; the abbreviation saves writing a lot of zeros.[10] The ionic concentration can also be expressed as nmol/L, which has the same meaning. Deviation from normal hydrogen ion concentration can upset normal reactions of cellular metabolism by altering the effectiveness of enzymes, hormones, and other chemical regulators of cell function. It can also affect the normal distribution of other ions (such as sodium and potassium) between the intracellular fluids and the ECFs, thereby disturbing a variety of cell and tissue ion-dependent functions, such as conduction, contraction, and secretion. Therefore, normal ECF hydrogen ion concentration is essential for normal body functions. The concentration is determined by the types and amounts of acids and bases present, and its regulation is commonly called acid–base balance.

Some hydrogen ions are ingested in foods, but most are produced as a result of metabolism of glucose, fatty acids, and amino acids.

FUNDAMENTAL CONCEPTS

An electrolyte is a substance that *dissociates* and forms ions when mixed with water; the process is called *ionization*. It is composed of *cations* (positively charged electrolytes, such as sodium), and *anions* (negatively charged electrolytes, such as chloride). Ionic solutions readily conduct electric current, hence the term *electrolyte*.

An *acid* is any electrolyte that ionizes in water and forms hydrogen ions and anions. An acid is a *hydrogen ion donor* and thus elevates the hydrogen ion concentration of the solution to which it is added. The strength of an acid is determined by its degree of ionization in water. Strong acids completely ionize in water and readily liberate hydrogen ions. Hydrochloric acid (HCl) is a strong acid because 99.9% of the HCl molecules ionize in pure water. Weak acids partly ionize in water and therefore do not liberate hydrogen ions as readily as strong acids. The acidity of the solution depends on how much the acid dissociates.

A *base* is any substance that can bind hydrogen ions. An *alkali* is a substance that contains a base. A strong base binds hydrogen ions readily. Hydroxides such as sodium hydroxide (NaOH) contain the hydroxyl (OH) ion, a strong base. A weak base binds hydrogen ions less

readily. Sodium bicarbonate is a weak alkali containing the bicarbonate ion, a weak base. When *sodium bicarbonate* ($NaHCO_3$) is added to water, it completely dissociates. A small percentage of the resulting bicarbonate ions binds hydrogen ions and forms carbonic acid ($HCO_3^- + H^+ \rightleftharpoons H_2CO_3$).

Because a base is a hydrogen ion acceptor, the addition of a base to a solution containing hydrogen ions lowers the hydrogen ion concentration; the opposite occurs when an acid is added.

PH AND HYDROGEN ION

The pH is simply a negative logarithm of hydrogen ions (H^+) in a solution. This system was developed by Sorensen in the early 1900s to simplify the annotation of the number. One liter of water contains 0.0000001 g of hydrogen ions. This figure is equal to $1/10^7$, as shown by the following equation:

$$0.0000001 = 1/10,000,000$$
$$= 1/(10 \times 10 \times 10 \times 10 \times 10 \times 10 \times 10)$$
$$= 10^7 = 10^{-7}$$

This simplified formula denotes the negative notation of a pH of 7 for neutral water. For any given solution, the numeric value of pH decreases as the hydrogen ion concentration increases. Therefore, because water is neutral at a pH of 7, when hydrogen ions are added to it, the solution becomes more acidic. The greater the hydrogen ion concentration, the more acidic the solution and the more the pH number falls. Acidic solutions range in pH between 0 and 7. Alkalotic or basic solutions, conversely, have less hydrogen ion concentration and range in pH between 7 and 14. The smaller the hydrogen ion concentration, the more alkaline the solution. Box 11-1 shows the approximate pH compositions of body fluids. Note that the relationship between the pH and the hydrogen ion figures is logarithmic rather than linear. This

---

BOX 11-1 ▼ pH Values of Certain Body Fluids

Gastric juice	1.2–3.0
Vaginal fluid	3.5–4.5
Urine	4.6–8.0
Saliva	6.4–6.9
Blood (arterial)	7.35–7.45
Semen	7.20–7.60
Cerebrospinal fluid	7.4
Pancreatic juice	7.1–8.2
Bile	7.6–8.6

means that an increase or decrease of one pH unit represents a 10-fold change in hydrogen ion concentration.[3]

In the fluids of the human body, the acceptable pH range is 7.35 to 7.45. Normal blood gas values are indicated in Table 11-1. Levels below 7.35 indicate a state of acidosis, whereas levels above 7.45 indicate alkalosis. When the hydrogen ion concentration is in the normal range of 40 nEq(nmol)/L, the pH is 7.40.

The broadest range of hydrogen ion concentration in ECFs compatible with mammalian life is 16 to 125 nEq/L, corresponding to a pH range of approximately 7.8 to 6.8. Cells of the human body usually function normally when the pH of ECF (interstitial fluids and plasma) remains constant at about 7.40. Alterations in plasma H^+ concentration alter the functioning of many enzyme and hormone systems; for example, acidosis depresses the function of epinephrine. H^+ concentration also affects neurologic functioning and the distribution of other ions. Acidosis depresses nervous system functioning, leading to coma, whereas alkalosis causes hyperexcitability, which may lead to convulsions.

In the processes of cellular metabolism, acid is continually being formed. The excess hydrogen produced must be eliminated from the body to maintain a steady

TABLE 11-1 *Arterial Blood Gases*

Term	Normal Value	Definition—Implications
pH	7.35–7.45	Reflects H^+ concentration; acidity increases as H^+ concentration increases (pH value decreases as acidity increases) pH < 7.35 (acidosis) pH > 7.45 (alkalosis)
Pa_{CO_2}	35–45 mm Hg	Partial pressure of CO_2 in arterial blood When < 35 mmHg, hypocapnia is said to be present (respiratory alkalosis) When >45 mmHg, hypercapnia is said to be present (respiratory acidosis)
Pa_{O_2}	80–100 mm Hg (decreases with age)	Partial pressure of O_2 in arterial blood Any reading above 80 mm Hg (on room air) is considered acceptable In adults younger than 60 yr (on room air) <80 mmHg indicates mild hypoxemia <60 mmHg indicates moderate hypoxemia <40 mmHg indicates severe hypoxemia Somewhat lower levels are accepted as normal in aged persons because there is some loss of ventilatory function with advanced age
Standard HCO_3	22–26 mEq/L	HCO_3 concentration in plasma of blood that has been equilibrated at a Pa_{CO_2} of 40 mm Hg and with O_2 to fully saturate the hemoglobin
Base excess	$-2 \rightarrow +2$ mEq/L	Reflects metabolic (nonrespiratory) body disturbances, which may be primary or compensatory in nature Always negative in metabolic acidosis (deficit of alkali or excess of fixed acids) Always positive in metabolic alkalosis (excess of alkali or deficit of fixed acids) Arrived at by multiplying the deviation of standard HCO_3 from normal by a factor of 1.2, which represents the buffer action of red blood cells

(Source: Metheny, N. M. *Fluid and Electrolyte Balance: Nursing Considerations* [2nd ed.]. Philadelphia: J.B. Lippincott, 1992).

state. The acids formed are often described as 1) *volatile* acids that are excretable by the lungs and 2) *nonvolatile* acids that are excreted by the kidney.

METABOLISM: VOLATILE AND NONVOLATILE ACIDS

Volatile Acids

A volatile acid is defined as an acid that can be excreted from the body as a gas. Either the acid itself or a chemical product of the acid can be converted to a gas and excreted. Carbonic acid, produced by the hydration of carbon dioxide in body fluids, is the only volatile acid in the body. The formation can be expressed in the following equation:

$$CO_2 + H_2O \; \underset{\text{(carbonic anhydrase)}}{\rightleftarrows} \; H_2CO_3$$

Note that the enzyme carbonic anhydrase is necessary to accelerate the reaction. A normal adult produces about 300 L of carbon dioxide per day from metabolic reactions, which results in the production of a large amount of carbonic acid. Normally, the lungs excrete carbon dioxide as rapidly as cell metabolism produces it by increasing the rate and depth of breathing. In this way, carbonic acid is not allowed to accumulate in the body and alter the pH of the ECF.

Nonvolatile Acids

A nonvolatile acid, also called a *fixed acid*, cannot be eliminated by the lungs and must be excreted by the kidneys. All metabolic acids present in body fluids except carbonic acid are classified as nonvolatile and include sulfuric acid, phosphoric acid, lactic acid, ketoacids (acetoacetic acid, β-hydroxybutyric acid), and smaller amounts of other inorganic and organic acids.

To some extent, fixed acids are neutralized by fixed bases in our diet. Fruits and vegetables contain such alkaline substances as potassium citrate. In a typical American diet, however, metabolic breakdown of foodstuffs, especially proteins, leads to an excess of fixed acids (about 50 to 100 mEq/day), and these acids must be eliminated by the kidneys to maintain a normal pH of the ECF. Research does not support that diets can produce a more acidic or basic urine on their own merit, because much has to do with individual metabolism.[11]

REGULATION OF BODY FLUID PH

As previously stated, ECF pH is normally maintained between 7.35 and 7.45. This occurs through three main mechanisms: 1) buffer systems, 2) exhalation of carbon dioxide, and 3) kidney excretion of hydrogen.[10]

Buffer Systems

Buffers include weak acids and the salt of that acid, which functions as a weak base. The most important buffers in the body fluids consist of weak acids plus the salts of their conjugate bases, together referred to as acid–base buffer pairs. In ECF fluids, the salts are primarily sodium salts, and in the intracellular fluids they are primarily potassium salts. They act within a fraction of a second for immediate defense against either increases or decreases in hydrogen ion concentration. Buffers minimize changes in pH by taking up hydrogen ions when acids are added to body fluids or by releasing hydrogen ions when the pH of body fluids becomes too high. The function of buffers is to convert strong acids, which would strongly decrease overall pH, into weak acids, which have a minimal effect on pH. Buffers also convert strong bases, which strongly increase overall pH, into weak bases, which have a minimal effect on pH. When acid or base is added to ECF, approximately half of the added ions eventually diffuse into cells, where they are buffered. These ions or others that affect acid–base balance are exchanged across the cell membrane for intracellular ions or are accompanied into cells by ions of opposite charge. For example, if an acid is added to ECF, some of the hydrogen is buffered chemically within the ECF. Some is also diffused across cell membranes into cells. Because the hydrogen ion is positively charged, it must either be exchanged across the cell membrane for another cation, such as Na^+ or K^+, or be accompanied into the cell by an anion, such as Cl^-. Although both processes occur, the movement of cations out of the cell is quantitatively more important. In metabolic acidosis, for example, extracellular potassium levels, as measured in blood plasma, are frequently elevated as intracellular stores are depleted to allow intracellular buffering of hydrogen ions. Often, in metabolic acidosis, plasma chloride is also reduced.

CARBONIC ACID–BICARBONATE SYSTEM. This system buffers volatile and nonvolatile acids in the interstitial fluid and in plasma. The bicarbonate ion can act as a weak base and the carbonic acid can act as a weak acid, so the system can compensate for either excess or deficit hydrogen ion.[10]

The carbonic acid–bicarbonate system is the most important extracellular buffer, because it can be regulated by both the lungs and the kidneys. Normally, the carbonic acid (H_2CO_3) to bicarbonate (HCO_3^-) ratio is maintained at approximately 1:20 (Fig. 11-1). This ratio keeps the pH at approximately 7.40. The actual content required to maintain this balance is 1.2 mEq/L of H_2CO_3 to 24 mEq/L of HCO_3^-. As long as the ratio of 1:20 is maintained, the pH will also be stabilized. If, for example, a retention of carbon dioxide and a reciprocal compensatory retention of bicarbonate occurs, the amounts

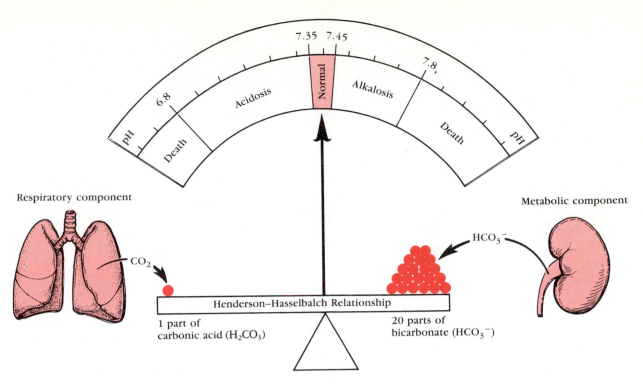

FIGURE 11-1 *Mechanisms for the defense against changes in body fluid pH.*

might be 2.0 mEq/L of H_2CO_3 and 40 mEq/L of HCO_3^-, which would still maintain the ratio (2:40 instead of 1:20), and the pH would remain 7.40.[9] The respiratory system works very rapidly in the excretion or retention of CO_2, whereas the renal system functions much more slowly to retain or excrete HCO_3^-, as is discussed in the subsequent sections.

PHOSPHATE BUFFER SYSTEM. This system acts in almost the same way as the carbonic acid–bicarbonate system except that sodium salts of dihydrogen phosphate ($H_2PO_4^-$) and sodium monohydrogen phosphate (HPO_4^-) ions are used. The dihydrogen phosphate acts as a weak acid and can buffer strong bases, whereas the monohydrogen phosphate ions acts as the weak base and can buffer strong acids.[9] Phosphate is highest in the intracellular fluid, so this buffer system is most active in the intracellular fluid. It also acts to buffer acids in the urine by combining Na_2HPO_4 with a strong acid such as HCl to form sodium chloride (NaCl) and sodium dihydrogen phosphate (NaH_2PO_4), a weak acid.[10] This is a mechanism for acidification of the urine and decreasing plasma acidity.

PROTEIN BUFFER SYSTEM. The most plentiful buffer in body cells and plasma is the protein buffer system. All proteins can act as acidic and basic buffers. Hemoglobin buffers carbonic acid by causing the carbonic acid, formed from the union of carbon dioxide and water, to dissociate into hydrogen ions and bicarbonate ions. At the time that carbon dioxide is moving into the cell, the oxygen from the hemoglobin is released to the tissue. The reduced hemoglobin combines with the hydrogen ion, which decreases its acidity and provides a mechanism for carrying the acid back to the lungs. Once in the lungs, hydrogen again attaches to the bicarbonate ions and dissociates into carbon dioxide and water. The carbon dioxide gas readily diffuses out through the alveoli as new oxygen is being picked up (Fig. 11-2). Seven of the 20 amino acids have side chains that can release or bind hydrogen.[10] Their activity may be seen in both acidosis and alkalosis by releasing hydrogen or binding it when necessary.

Exhalation of Carbon Dioxide

The respiratory system plays an important role in acid–base balance by controlling the partial pressure of carbon dioxide (P_{CO_2}) in arterial blood. As excess carbon dioxide is formed during cellular processes, most of it is picked up by the red blood cells and carried to the lungs.

Carbon dioxide reacts with body water to form carbonic acid, which then dissociates into hydrogen ion and bicarbonate ion, as the following reaction sequence indicates:

$$CO_2 + H_2O \underset{\text{hydration}}{\overset{\text{dehydration}}{\rightleftarrows}} H_2CO_3 \underset{\text{dissociation}}{\overset{\text{association}}{\rightleftarrows}} H^+ + HCO_3^-$$

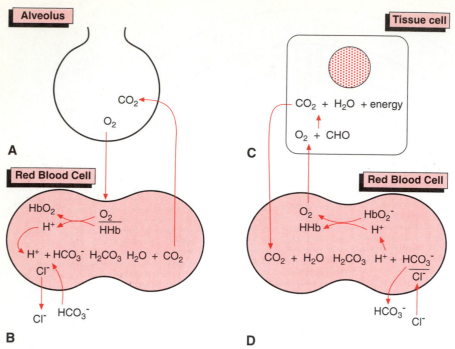

FIGURE 11-2 **A.** *Alveolus exchanges O_2 and CO_2 with* **B.** *Red blood cell (RBC), which adds O_2 to hemoglobin (Hb) and releases CO_2 to be blown off in alveolus.* **C.** *Tissue cell takes up O_2 and gives off CO_2 to* **D.** *RBC which carries CO_2 as HHb and HCO_3^-, which can be donated to the plasma when the pH of the plasma is decreased.*

These reactions are readily reversible. The hydration of dissolved carbon dioxide to form carbonic acid and the dehydration of carbonic acid to form carbon dioxide and water are slow reactions if uncatalyzed. The enzyme carbonic anhydrase, present in red blood cells, renal tubular cells, and other cells speeds up these reactions. The dissociation of carbonic acid to hydrogen ion and bicarbonate ion, or the reaction in the opposite direction, occurs virtually instantaneously. As long as the rate at which carbon dioxide is being eliminated from the body by the lungs equals the rate at which carbon dioxide is produced, no net change in the hydrogen ion concentration of that reaction will occur.

An increase in carbon dioxide tension results in the liberation of hydrogen ions; thus, the pH decreases. If alveolar ventilation is decreased, metabolically produced carbon dioxide accumulates in the blood, carbonic acid concentration rises, and blood pH falls.

A decrease in carbon dioxide tension results in less free hydrogen ions and, consequently, a more alkaline pH. If ventilation is stimulated so that elimination of carbon dioxide temporarily exceeds its production, the blood P_{CO_2} moves to a lower level and alkaline blood pH results. Thus, changes in alveolar ventilation profoundly influence blood pH.

Alveolar ventilation is normally adjusted so that pH changes in the arterial blood are kept to a minimum. Increases of hydrogen ion concentration in body fluid (decreased pH), specifically in arterial blood and cerebrospinal fluid, result in a reflex increase in respiratory rate and depth. This respiratory response acts to blow off more carbon dioxide. The result is that the hydrogen ion concentration is decreased toward normal. Excess carbonic acid in the blood (due to failure to eliminate carbon dioxide adequately) is a powerful stimulus to ventilation. The increase in ventilation serves to diminish the retention of carbon dioxide and thereby minimizes the accumulation of carbonic acid in the blood. The ventilatory response also is reactive to acidosis from other acids. Fixed, nonvolatile acids cause a marked increase in ventilation rate and depth.

Decreases of body fluid hydrogen ion concentration (increased pH) depress respiratory activity. This allows carbon dioxide to build up in the blood. Consequently, more hydrogen ions are made available, minimizing the alkaline shift in pH. A decrease in respiration due to an alkaline pH is usually not as dramatic as the increase seen due to acidosis. The decreased ventilation produces *hypercapnia* (high serum carbon dioxide), which is a powerful stimulus to ventilation in persons with healthy lungs. Hypoxia becomes a stimulus to respiration when the partial pressure of arterial oxygen (Pa_{O_2}) falls to 60 mm Hg or less (see pp. 559–561).

The respiratory system normally changes its activity to minimize shifts in pH. Respiratory activity responds rapidly to acid–base stresses and shifts blood pH toward normal in minutes. A person who is hypoventilating begins to accumulate carbon dioxide rapidly and, as a reflex, increases the rate and depth of breathing to restore the blood pH. Conversely, respiratory rate is slowed when the pH elevates which causes the pH to approach normal. An increase in alveolar ventilation of two times normal can increase the pH of blood 0.23 pH units. Conversely, depressing ventilation to one fourth of normal decreases the pH by 0.4 pH units.[3, 10]

Kidney Excretion of Hydrogen

The major role of the kidneys in maintaining acid–base balance is to conserve circulating stores of bicarbonate and to excrete hydrogen ions. The kidneys maintain ECF pH by 1) increasing urinary excretion of hydrogen ions and conserving plasma bicarbonate when the blood is too acidic and 2) increasing urinary excretion of bicarbonate and decreasing urinary excretion of hydrogen ions when the blood is too alkaline.

Renal mechanisms for hydrogen ion regulation are slower (taking hours or days) than are chemical buffer or respiratory mechanisms. Renal compensation for acid–base disturbances can be complete, however, because the kidneys actually excrete hydrogen ions and eliminate them from body fluids.[4] The respiratory mechanisms described above cannot eliminate tissue-generated metabolic hydrogen ions from the body.

Renal control of acid–base balance involves three processes that occur simultaneously along the length of the nephron: 1) reabsorption of filtered bicarbonate, 2) excretion of titratable acid, and 3) excretion of ammonia. All three mechanisms involve secretion of hydrogen ions into the urine and return of bicarbonate to the plasma.

Quantitatively, the *reabsorption of filtered bicarbonate* is the most important process in renal acid–base regulation. Approximately 4500 mEq of $NaHCO_3$ are filtered each day. Normally, all but 1 or 2 mEq of $NaHCO_3$ are reabsorbed into the plasma.

Figure 11-3 illustrates the cellular mechanisms involved in the reabsorption of filtered bicarbonate. Carbon dioxide in the tubular epithelial cell reacts with intracellular water to form carbonic acid. The reaction is catalyzed by the enzyme *carbonic anhydrase*. Carbonic acid dissociates to form hydrogen ions and bicarbonate ions. The hydrogen ions are actively secreted by the luminal cell membrane into the urine in exchange for sodium ions. The bicarbonate ion moves passively across the peritubular membrane into the blood, accompanying the actively reabsorbed sodium ion. In urine, hydrogen ions react with bicarbonate ions to form carbonic acid, which then dissociates into carbon dioxide and water. Water is either reabsorbed osmotically or eliminated in the urine, depending on the body's water balance. Both blood and urine carbon dioxide are in equilibrium with carbon dioxide in tubular cells and provide the main impetus for cellular generation of bicarbonate.

The kidneys also excrete hydrogen ions in the form of *titratable acids*, which consist mostly of dihydrogen phosphate ($H_2PO_4^-$) formed when hydrogen in the tu-

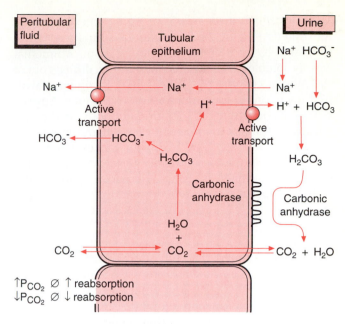

FIGURE 11-3   *Reabsorption of filtered bicarbonate.*

bular fluid combines with monohydrogen phosphate (HPO_4^-). For each hydrogen ion excreted in the form of titratable acid, an equivalent quantity of $NaHCO_3$ is added to the blood (Fig. 11-4). Adults normally produce 1 to 2 mEq/kg/day of fixed, nonvolatile acid, probably due to the high-protein diet consumed by meat-eating people.[5, 7] Approximately 40 mEq of hydrogen ions are excreted per day in combination with *ammonia*. If a chronic acid load is imposed on the body, the production and excretion of ammonia may increase more than 10-fold over several days.

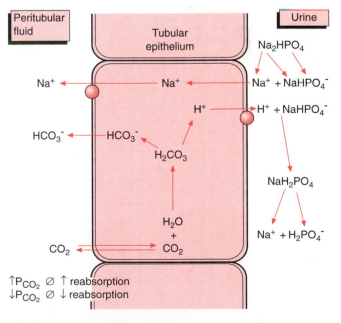

FIGURE 11-4   *Production of titratable acid.*

The cellular mechanisms of ammonia excretion are illustrated in Figure 11-5. Ammonia is produced in the tubular cells from amino acid metabolism. Ammonia, readily soluble in the luminal membrane, diffuses out of the tubular cell into the urine, where it combines with hydrogen ions to form ammonium (NH_4) ions. Ammonium ions penetrate cell membranes poorly, so they are effectively trapped in urine and excreted in combination with chloride.[3] For each hydrogen ion excreted with ammonia, an equivalent quantity of $NaHCO_3$ is added to the blood. Normally, the kidneys produce up to 40 mEq of HCO_3^- per day from NH_4 formation.[4]

Integration of Defense Mechanisms

As previously noted, the body mechanisms for defense against changes in fluid pH consist of buffer systems, respiratory mechanisms, and renal mechanisms. All of the mechanisms function simultaneously to maintain pH within normal limits, but they do not function independently of one another.

The pH of arterial blood is within normal limits (7.35 to 7.45) when the bicarbonate to carbonic acid ratio is 20:1 (see Figure 11-1).

The carbonic acid concentration in plasma is very small and cannot be measured directly. It is proportional to the concentration of dissolved carbon dioxide, so P_{CO_2} is often used to calculate H_2CO_3 levels. Note that it is the ratio of bicarbonate to P_{CO_2} that determines pH, rather than the absolute amounts of bicarbonate and carbon dioxide. Plasma bicarbonate is controlled by the kidneys, whereas arterial P_{CO_2} is controlled by the lungs. Thus, the effectiveness with which buffers operate depends on efficient respiratory and renal mechanisms to maintain

---

BOX 11-2 ▼ Henderson–Hasselbalch Equation to Determine pH, HCO_3^-, or H_2CO_3

$$pH = pK + \log \frac{[HCO_3^-]}{[H_2CO_3]}$$

pK = dissociation constant for CO_2 in water, normally 6.1
HCO_3^- = bicarbonate, usually calculated from direct measure of pH and Pa_{CO_2}
H_2CO_3 = carbonic acid, which can be calculated by multiplying $0.03 \times Pa_{CO_2}$. 0.03 is the constant for the solubility of CO_2 in plasma at 37°C.
Example: Pa_{CO_2} 40
        HCO_3 24

$$pH = 6.1 + \log \frac{[HCO_3^-]}{[H_2CO_3]}$$

$$pH = 6.1 + \log \frac{24}{40 \times 0.03}$$

$$pH = 6.1 + \log \frac{24}{1.2} \left(\frac{20}{1} \right)$$

$$pH = 6.1 + 1.3 = 7.40$$

---

proper buffer ratios. The lungs and kidneys, therefore, are sometimes referred to as physiologic buffers.

▼ Altered Acid–Base Balance

Because the hydrogen ion concentration of blood ultimately affects the hydrogen ion concentration of all body fluids and because blood is readily accessible for chemical analysis, arterial blood is used as a representative body fluid in assessing acid–base balance.

Clinical evaluation of the acid–base status of a person involves the determination of arterial blood pH, P_{CO_2}, and HCO_3^- (see Table 11-1). Usually, pH and P_{CO_2} are measured and HCO_3^- is determined from a nomogram based on the Henderson-Hasselbalch equation (Box 11-2). Sometimes, instead of determining HCO_3^- from the Henderson-Hasselbalch relationship, total carbon dioxide content of arterial plasma is measured.[2] This is the sum of plasma bicarbonate plus dissolved carbon dioxide plus carbonic acid. It is measured by acidifying the plasma sample to remove all the carbon dioxide. In a normal sample of plasma, 95% of the total carbon dioxide is bicarbonate. Also included in the arterial blood gas readings are oxygen content and hemoglobin saturation with oxygen.

ACIDOSIS AND ALKALOSIS

Acidosis in the body fluids refers to an elevation of the H^+ concentration above normal or a decrease in the HCO_3^- below normal, resulting in a decrease in the pH of the body fluids to below 7.35. The source of the excess hydrogen ion or altered H_2CO_3:HCO_3^- ratio can be respiratory (volatile) or metabolic (nonrespiratory or nonvolatile). *Acidemia* is defined as an acidic condition of the

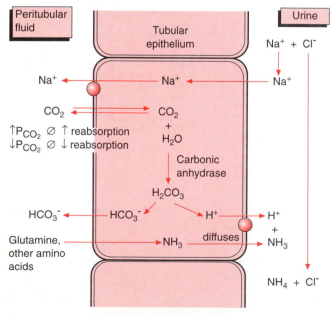

FIGURE 11-5 *Excretion of ammonia.*

Peritubular fluid

Tubular epithelium

Urine

$Na^+ + Cl^-$

Na^+ → Na^+ ← Na^+

CO_2 ← CO_2
    +
    H_2O

↑P_{CO_2} ∅ ↑ reabsorption
↓P_{CO_2} ∅ ↓ reabsorption

Carbonic anhydrase

H_2CO_3

HCO_3^- ← HCO_3^- → H^+ → H^+
    +
    NH_3

Glutamine, other amino acids → NH_3 diffuses → NH_3

$NH_4 + Cl^-$

blood signified by an arterial pH value less than 7.35. The physiologic processes causing the acidemia are defined as *acidosis* (ie, a condition of becoming acidic).[5]

Alkalosis refers to a decrease in the H$^+$ concentration of the body fluids or an excess of the HCO$_3^-$, thus increasing pH of the body fluids to above 7.45. The source of the depletion of hydrogen ion is either elimination of carbon dioxide (hyperventilation) or a metabolic excess of primary base bicarbonate. *Alkalemia* is defined as an alkaline condition of the blood signified by arterial pH greater than 7.45. The physiologic processes causing the alkalemia define the term *alkalosis* (ie, a condition of becoming alkalotic).[5] Table 11-2 summarizes some factors that may cause acidosis and alkalosis. Table 11-3 details the physiologic effects of the pH change that occur regardless of whether the change has resulted from respiratory or metabolic alterations.

Disturbances of acid–base balance may arise from respiratory or metabolic causes. The four primary types of acid–base disturbances are 1) respiratory acidosis, 2) respiratory alkalosis, 3) metabolic acidosis, and 4) metabolic alkalosis.

ETIOLOGY AND CLINICAL MANIFESTATIONS OF ACIDOSIS AND ALKALOSIS

Respiratory Acidosis

Respiratory acidosis is caused by failure of the respiratory system to remove carbon dioxide from body fluids as fast as it is produced in the tissues. Essentially, any

condition that impairs or interferes with breathing can result in respiratory acidosis. Impairment of breathing leads to an increase in arterial Pco_2 above 45 mm Hg, with a corresponding decrease in pH value to 7.35 or less. The pathophysiology of respiratory acidosis is summarized in Flowchart 11-1.

Causes of respiratory acidosis include obstructive and restrictive lung disease, interference with movements of the thoracic cage (eg, poliomyelitis), decreased activity of the respiratory center (due to brain trauma, hemorrhage, narcotics, anesthetics, etc.), and neuromuscular disease (such as myasthenia gravis, Guillain-Barré syndrome) (see Table 11-2).

Persons with severe respiratory acidosis usually show signs and symptoms of respiratory insufficiency, such as cyanosis; rapid, shallow breathing; and disorientation. Acute respiratory acidosis can produce *carbon dioxide narcosis*, with symptoms of headache, blurred vision, fatigue, and weakness. Prolonged acidosis may produce severe central nervous system symptoms, including increased intracranial pressure and permanent damage.[5] When the pH falls below 7.10, dysrhythmias and peripheral vasodilatation may cause severe hypotension.

Respiratory Alkalosis

Respiratory alkalosis is caused by the loss of carbon dioxide from the lungs at a faster rate than it is produced in the tissues. This leads to a decrease in arterial Pco_2 below 35 mm Hg, with a pH greater than 7.45. The

TABLE 11-2 *Disturbances of Acid–Base Balance*

Arterial Blood pH	Primary Abnormality	Indicator of Primary Abnormality	Examples of Causative Factors	Compensatory Mechanisms
Alkalemia pH > 7.45	Respiratory alkalosis	Decreased PCO$_2$ < 35 mm Hg	Hypoxia, anxiety, pulmonary embolus, pregnancy, other causes of hyperventilation	Kidneys retain hydrogen ions and excrete bicarbonate
	Metabolic alkalosis	Increased HCO$_3^-$ > 26 mEq/L	Treatment with diuretics and hormones that augment renal excretion of H$^+$, K$^+$, and Cl$^-$; fluid loss from stomach by vomiting or nasogastric suction; Cushing's disease, aldosteronism, excessive ingestion of alkali	Alveolar ventilation decreases, more CO$_2$ is retained. Kidneys increase H$^+$ retention and excrete bicarbonate
Acidemia pH < 7.35	Respiratory acidosis	Increased PCO$_2$ > 45 mm Hg	Obstructive lung disease, depression of respiratory center by drugs or disease, other causes of hypoventilation	Kidneys increase H$^+$ excretion and bicarbonate retention
	Metabolic acidosis	Decreased HCO$_3^-$ < 22 mEq/L	Diarrhea (loss of HCO$_3^-$), diabetic acidosis, lactic acidosis, renal failure, aspirin poisoning, treatment with ammonium chloride	Alveolar ventilation increases, more CO$_2$ is eliminated; kidneys increase H$^+$ excretion and bicarbonate retention

TABLE 11-3 *Physiologic Effects of pH Change*

	Alkalemia	Acidemia
Cardiovascular	↑ Dysrhythmias (multifocal AT, PVCs) ↓ Cerebral blood flow	Systemic vasodilation Resistance to vasoconstrictors Pulmonary vasoconstriction ↓ Venous capacitance Myocardial depression ↑ Risk of ventricular fibrillation Conduction defects

Metabolic	↓ O_2 delivery (Bohr effect)
	↑ Phosphofructokinase activity
	↑ Glycolysis
	↑ Lactate and pyruvate production
		Acute
		  ↑ Calcium solubility
		  ↑ Serum phosphate
		  ↑ Serum potassium (only if mineral acid or hyperosmolar state)
		  ↑ O_2 delivery (Bohr effect)
		Chronic
		  Loss of bone to buffering (metabolic acidosis)
		  Loss of muscle protein

Central nervous system	*Metabolic pH shifts* Little effect on CSF pH after acute or chronic changes	*Respiratory pH shifts* ↑ Pco_2 induces CSF acidosis, CNS depression and coma ↓ Pco_2 induces CSF alkalosis ↑ Seizure activity

AT: atrial tachycardia; PVC: premature ventricular contractions; CSF: cerebrospinal fluid; CNS: central nervous system.
(Source: Stein, J. (ed.). *Internal Medicine* [4th ed.]. St Louis: C.V. Mosby, 1994).

pathophysiology of respiratory alkalosis is summarized in Flowchart 11-2.

Any condition resulting in excessive loss of carbon dioxide due to alveolar hyperventilation will cause respiratory alkalosis. Respiratory alkalosis is easily produced by voluntary overbreathing. Other causes include high altitude, anxiety, fever, meningitis, aspirin poisoning, pneumonia, pulmonary embolus, and other factors that increase respiratory center activity (see Table 11-2). Symptoms of respiratory alkalosis are related to nervous system irritability and include light-headedness, altered consciousness, various paresthesias, cramps, and carpopedal spasm from clinical hypocalcemia (see pp. 723–724).[5]

Metabolic Acidosis

Metabolic acidosis results from either an abnormal accumulation of fixed acids or loss of base. The arterial blood pH falls below 7.35, and the plasma bicarbonate is usually decreased below 22 mEq/L. The pathophysiology is summarized in Flowchart 11-3.

Metabolic acidosis may result from the systemic accumulation of either hydrochloric or nonhydrochloric acids.[1] The determination of the cause is aided by determining the anion gap (see pp. 224–226). Among its multiple causes are kidney failure, in which the kidneys are unable to replenish bicarbonate stores used for buffering strong acids produced by metabolism. In diabetes mellitus, keto acid production due to incomplete oxidation of fats may lead to a severe metabolic acidosis. Anaerobic metabolism of glucose during strenuous exercise or circulatory shock may lead to lactic acidosis. Excessive administration of chloride can cause an excessive loss of HCO_3^- and metabolic acidosis. Loss of pancreatic bicarbonate from the intestine during chronic diarrhea or bilious vomiting produces metabolic acidosis, often with serious consequences in children. Acid-producing overdoses include acetylsalicylic acid, ethylene glycol, methyl alcohol, and paraldehyde (see Table 11-2).

Symptoms of severe metabolic acidosis include deep, rapid respiration (Kussmaul's breathing), disorientation, and coma. Clinical manifestations of metabolic acidosis depend on the pH level. Arterial pH of less than 7.10 can produce severe ventricular dysrhythmias and reduction of cardiac contractility. Production of lactic acidosis may occur with associated hypotension.[8] Lethargy and coma can develop, but neurologic symptoms are less prominent in metabolic acidosis than in respiratory acidosis, because the central nervous system is more sensitive to carbon dioxide changes than to pH shifts.

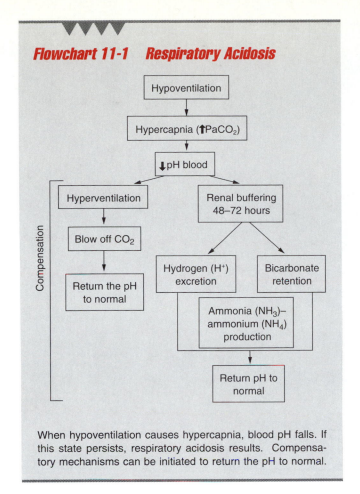

Flowchart 11-1 Respiratory Acidosis

When hypoventilation causes hypercapnia, blood pH falls. If this state persists, respiratory acidosis results. Compensatory mechanisms can be initiated to return the pH to normal.

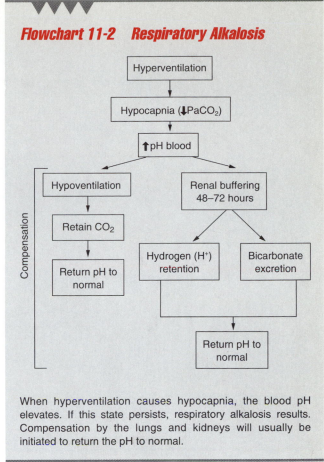

Flowchart 11-2 Respiratory Alkalosis

When hyperventilation causes hypocapnia, the blood pH elevates. If this state persists, respiratory alkalosis results. Compensation by the lungs and kidneys will usually be initiated to return the pH to normal.

The chronic acidosis of renal failure retards bone growth and causes a variety of bone disturbances, probably due to buffering of acidosis by bone calcium.[6]

The anion gap, discussed later in this chapter, is commonly used in the differential diagnosis of metabolic acidosis. Conditions with a low or normal anion gap and those with an increased gap are noted in Table 11-4.

Metabolic Alkalosis

Metabolic alkalosis results from either a loss of hydrogen ions or addition of base to body fluids. It is defined as a disorder that results in primary, not secondary, increase in plasma HCO_3^-.[1] The plasma bicarbonate increases to above 26 mEq/L, and the arterial blood pH increases above 7.45. Secondary increase in plasma HCO_3^- is often seen with chronic respiratory acidosis as a compensation to keep the pH at or about normal levels (see pp. 600–601). The pathophysiology of metabolic alkalosis is summarized in Flowchart 11-4.

One cause of metabolic alkalosis is ingestion of excessive amounts of base (eg, $NaHCO_3$, or baking soda) to treat stomach ulcers and indigestion. Administration of $NaHCO_3$ in a cardiac arrest situation can produce a "post code" metabolic alkalosis. Another cause is vomiting of gastric contents in which HCl is lost from the body. This is called *hypochloremic metabolic alkalosis* and results from loss of hydrogen (increased pH) and chloride (causing renal retention of bicarbonate, HCO_3^-). Endocrine disorders (eg, Cushing's disease) and treatment with certain types of drugs (eg, thiazide) may augment renal excretion of H^+, K^+, and Cl^- and lead to metabolic alkalosis (see Table 11-2). Clinical manifestations of metabolic alkalosis include apathy, mental confusion, shallow breathing, spastic muscles, weakness, muscle cramps, and dizziness. Some of the clinical features are associated with hypokalemia or hypocalcemia. Neurologic symptoms include paresthesia and light-headedness.[5]

EFFECTS OF PH CHANGES ON POTASSIUM, CALCIUM, AND MAGNESIUM BALANCE

Integrated into the direct effects of acidosis and alkalosis on the physiologic process are their compounding effects on potassium and calcium balance. Other electrolytes, such as magnesium and phosphate, are also affected, but

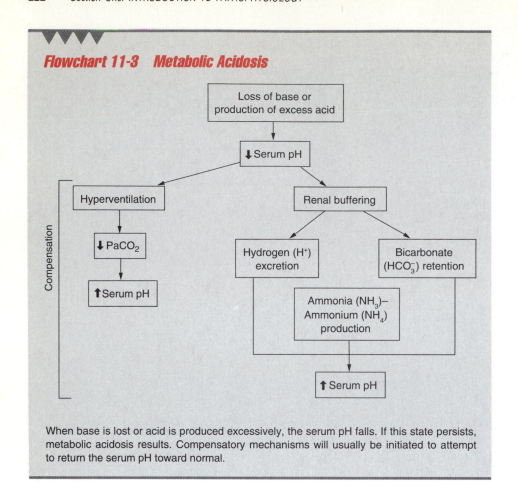

Flowchart 11-3   Metabolic Acidosis

When base is lost or acid is produced excessively, the serum pH falls. If this state persists, metabolic acidosis results. Compensatory mechanisms will usually be initiated to attempt to return the serum pH toward normal.

the systemic effects of potassium and calcium imbalances can be life threatening.

Hydrogen is preferentially excreted or retained over other cations by the renal system to maintain the blood pH. When the arterial pH falls, the excess H^+ is excreted through the kidneys. It cannot be excreted unless a cation is retained. Potassium is the cation usually retained, thus hyperkalemia develops in acidosis. Potassium may also shift out of intracellular fluid because more than 50% of the excess H^+ is buffered intracellularly. The K^+ and small amounts of Na^+ leave the cell to maintain electroneutrality.[1] The reverse is true with alkalosis. The kidney retains H^+ to normalize the blood pH, and K^+ is wasted. The intracellular hydrogen is donated to the ECF, and K^+ is retained intracellularly. Thus, hyperkalemia is associated with acidosis, and hypokalemia is associated with alkalosis (see also p. 200–201). Severe symptoms, such as cardiac dysrhythmias and coma, can result.

Changes in the arterial pH affect the ionized calcium levels in blood. The calcium in an alkalotic serum binds with serum proteins, producing the clinical effect of hypocalcemia.[12] The result can be hypocalcemia, tetany, spasm, and dysrhythmias (see p. 202–203). In an acidic environment, more calcium may be released from the plasma proteins, and ionized calcium levels may rise

transiently. The effect is not so pronounced as that seen with alkalemia.

Serum magnesium levels also may change in response to the pH levels. Hypomagnesemia is often seen in acidosis. Symptoms include weakness, mental depression, and tetany similar to that of hypocalcemia.

COMPENSATION AND CORRECTION

The two ways for an abnormal pH of arterial plasma to be returned toward normal are compensation and correction. In correction, the primary cause of the acid–base disturbance is repaired. For example, if respiratory acidosis is caused by partial blockage of the respiratory tree, removal or reduction of the obstruction improves ventilation and allows blood pH to return toward normal. Correction of an acid–base disturbance is the primary aim of persons concerned with the delivery of health care to affected individuals.

In compensation, the system or systems not responsible for causing the acid–base disturbance make physiologic adjustments to return blood pH toward normal. For example, in respiratory acidosis (high P_{CO_2}), the kidneys compensate by increasing the return of bicarbonate to the blood to return the $HCO_3^-:H_2CO_3$ ratio to normal. All processes of compensation are directed at

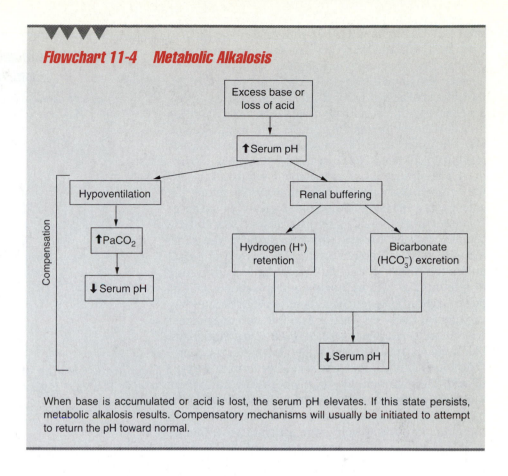

Flowchart 11-4   Metabolic Alkalosis

When base is accumulated or acid is lost, the serum pH elevates. If this state persists, metabolic alkalosis results. Compensatory mechanisms will usually be initiated to attempt to return the pH toward normal.

returning the bicarbonate to carbonic acid ratio to 20:1 and restoring the normal pH of arterial plasma.

The kidneys compensate for respiratory acidosis (high Pco_2) by elevating the plasma bicarbonate above 26 mEq/L. The kidneys compensate for respiratory alkalosis (low Pco_2) by lowering the plasma bicarbonate

---

TABLE 11-4   *Causes of Metabolic Acidosis Classified as High Anion Gap or Normal Anion Gap*

High Anion Gap (Gain of Unmeasured Anions)	Normal Anion Gap
Diabetic ketoacidosis	Diarrhea
Starvational ketoacidosis	Biliary or pancreatic fistulas
Alcoholic ketoacidosis	Excessive administration of isotonic saline or ammonium chloride
Lactic acidosis	
Renal failure	Ureteroenterostomies
Poisonings:	Renal tubular acidosis
Salicylate	Acetazolamide (Diamox)
Ethylene glycol	
Methyl alcohol	

(Source: Metheny, N. M. *Fluid and Electrolyte Balance: Nursing Considerations* [2nd ed.]. Philadelphia: J.B. Lippincott, 1992).

below 22 mEq/L. Similar compensations are made by the kidneys in nonrenal causes of metabolic acidosis and alkalosis.

The respiratory system attempts to compensate for metabolic acidosis (low HCO_3^-) by lowering the arterial Pco_2 below 35 mm Hg through hyperventilation. It attempts to compensate for metabolic alkalosis by elevating the arterial Pco_2 above 45 mm Hg through hypoventilation.

The effectiveness of the compensations depends on the amount of disruption occurring from the underlying disorder and the body's ability to make changes. Life-threatening disorders are not effectively compensated for by renal mechanisms, but they may respond quickly to respiratory compensations.

Major disturbances of acid–base balance are rarely completely compensated. Arterial pH is returned toward normal during compensation, but rarely to normal. Therefore, the arterial pH indicates whether a process of acidosis or alkalosis is present. The arterial blood Pco_2 and the plasma bicarbonate concentration indicate which process, respiratory or metabolic, is responsible for the abnormal pH and which process is compensatory.

For example, the following blood gas data indicate an acid–base abnormality: pH = 7.22; Pco_2 = 30 mm Hg; HCO_3^- = 12 mEq/L. To interpret the data, one must look at the pH to see if there is acidemia or alkalemia. In this case, the arterial pH is below normal range (7.35 to 7.45) and indicates acidemia. The body does not overcompensate, so the pH is reflective of the cause. The plasma P_{CO_2} and bicarbonate are then examined for indications of acidosis and alkalosis. Here, the bicarbonate concentration is below normal range (22 to 28 mEq/L) and indicates metabolic acidosis. The arterial P_{CO_2} is below normal range (35 to 45 mm Hg) and indicates respiratory alkalosis. Because there is acidemia, the primary disturbance is one of metabolic acidosis, whereas the compensatory process is respiratory. Therefore, the data suggest partially compensated metabolic acidosis.

Sometimes two primary disturbances of acid–base balance may be present simultaneously in the same individual. For example, a person with severely impaired pulmonary function may have respiratory acidosis due to retention of carbon dioxide and metabolic acidosis due to lactic acid production caused by inadequate oxygenation of the blood. In this example, severe acidemia will be seen. Examples of acid–base disturbances and blood values are shown in Table 11-2. Table 11-5 presents blood gases in such a way as to determine the type of acid–base abnormality that is occurring and where there is compensation for the abnormality. Note that the pH and HCO_3 changes in metabolic abnormalities go in the same direction, whereas the pH and Pa_{CO_2} changes

go in the opposite directions in respiratory abnormalities. Box 11-3 gives examples of each of these concepts with some reflective numbers.

BOX 11-3 ▼ Examples of Acid–Base Abnormalities

1. Metabolic acidosis, with partial respiratory compensation.
   pH 7.24 ↓
   Pa_{CO_2} 28 ↓
   HCO_3^- 12 ↓
2. Metabolic alkalosis with partial respiratory compensation.
   pH 7.58 ↑
   Pa_{CO_2} 50 ↑
   HCO_3^- 37 ↑
3. Respiratory acidosis, uncompensated.
   pH 7.22 ↓
   Pa_{CO_2} 56 ↑
   HCO_3^- 26 N
4. Respiratory alkalosis, uncompensated.
   pH 7.5 ↑
   Pa_{CO_2} 28 ↓
   HCO_3^- 22 N

▼ The Anion Gap

Preliminary assessment of arterial P_{CO_2}, HCO_3^-, and pH is helpful in determining which, if any, of the four major types of acid–base disturbances is present. Other measurements, computations, and tests are performed to confirm the preliminary diagnosis and establish the exact cause of the disturbance. The anion gap is commonly used in the differential diagnosis of metabolic acidosis. The number of milliequivalents per liter of cations in plasma is normally balanced by an equal number of milliequivalents per liter of anions: $Na^+ + K^+ + Mg^{++} + Ca^{++} +$ other cations $= Cl^- + HCO_3^- + HPO_4^{--} + SO_4^{--} +$ plasma proteins$^-$ + other anions. Only the concentrations of Na^+, K^+, Cl^-, and HCO_3^- are measured routinely; Mg^{++}, Ca^{++}, and other cations are considered unmeasured cations (UC); and HPO_4^{--}, SO_4^{--}, plasma proteins$^-$, and other anions are considered unmeasured anions (UA).

According to the principle of electroneutrality, plasma ionic balance can be expressed in the form of an equation between cations and anions: $[Na^+] + [K^+] + [UC] = [Cl^-] + [HCO_3^-] + [UA]$.

If the equation is rearranged so that measured ions are on one side and unmeasured ions are on the other side, the result is $([Na^+] + [K^+]) - ([Cl^-] + [HCO_3^-]) = 16 \pm 4$ mEq/L.

Notice that K^+ is included in determining the anion gap. Because plasma K^+ is small compared with Na^+, Cl^-, and HCO_3^-, it is sometimes excluded from anion

---

TABLE 11-5 *Directions of Acid–Base Abnormalities and Compensations*

Imbalance	pH	HCO₃	Pa$_{CO_2}$	Base Excess
METABOLIC ACIDOSIS				
Uncompensated	↓	↓	N	↓
Partially compensated	↓	↓	↓	↓
Fully compensated	N	↓	↓	↓
METABOLIC ALKALOSIS				
Uncompensated	↑	↑	N	↑
Partially compensated	↑	↑	↑	↑
Fully compensated	N	↑	↑	↑
RESPIRATORY ACIDOSIS				
Uncompensated	↓	N	↑	N
Partially compensated	↓	↑	↑	↑
Fully compensated	N	↑	↑	↑
RESPIRATORY ALKALOSIS				
Uncompensated	↑	N	↓	N
Partially compensated	↑	↓	↓	↓
Fully compensated	N	↓	↓	↓

N: normal.

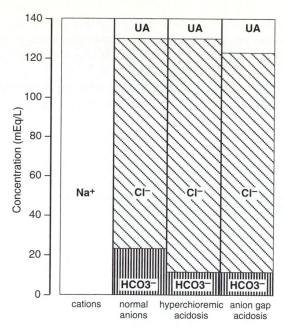

FIGURE 11-6 *The difference between cations, mainly sodium (Na +), and anions, mainly bicarbonate (HCO_3^-) and chloride (Cl^-), is the anion gap which consists of the unmeasured anions (UA^-). In hyperchloremic acidosis, the HCO_3^- is decreased and replaced by Cl^-. In anion gap acidosis, the UA^- anions increase (see text).*

gap computations, in which case the normal value for the anion gap becomes 12 ± 4 mEq/L. In other words, it is normal for the measured Na^+ to exceed the sum of Cl^- and HCO_3 by 12 ± 4 mEq/L when the plasma K is not calculated.[1,5] In metabolic acidosis, the anion gap may be normal, increased, or decreased, depending on the etiology (see Table 11-4).

A normal anion gap in metabolic acidosis occurs in such conditions as diarrhea, ammonium chloride ingestion, and renal dysfunction. A high anion gap may be present with accumulation of organic acids, such as ketoacids and lactic acids, as well as certain drugs and poisons. A normal gap is maintained by increasing chloride ions so that the sum of the HCO_3^- and Cl^- remains constant. This situation is often called *hyperchloremic acidosis*. A high anion gap occurs when the sum of HCO_3^- and Cl^- decreases due to the accumulation of other acids (Fig. 11-6).

In clinical practice, the initial determination of high-anion-gap acidosis versus normal-anion-gap acidosis leads to distinct laboratory investigations.[1] Flowchart 11-5 shows the laboratory tests that can be used to differentiate causative factors in high-anion-gap acidosis. Normal-anion-gap acidosis is further delineated by a

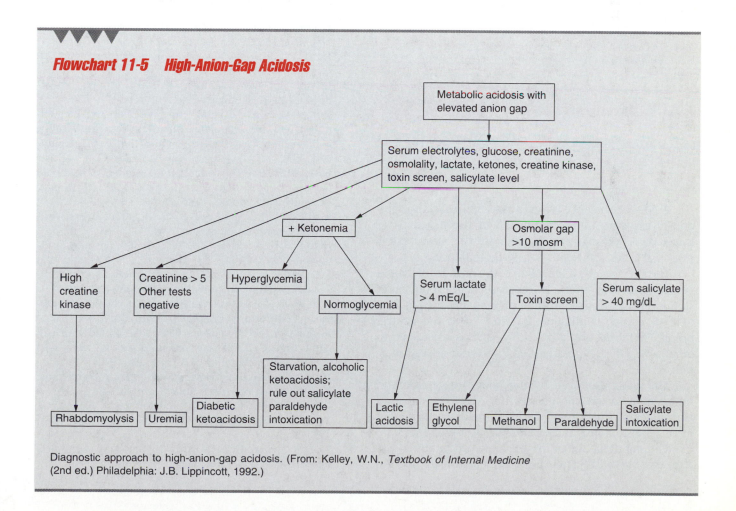

Flowchart 11-5   High-Anion-Gap Acidosis

Diagnostic approach to high-anion-gap acidosis. (From: Kelley, W.N., *Textbook of Internal Medicine* (2nd ed.) Philadelphia: J.B. Lippincott, 1992.)

history and physical examination as well as by HCO_3^- and K^+ studies. Diarrhea is the most common cause of normal-anion-gap acidosis, and there is often associated hypokalemia. Persons receiving hyperalimentation intravenous fluids with HCl or those with renal tubular acidosis may have a hyperkalemic/hyperchloremic metabolic acidosis.[1]

CASE STUDY 11-1

Ms. Ella James is an 85-year-old widow who was brought to the emergency room because of acute onset of weakness, confusion, muscle cramps, and dizziness. She has had a long history of gastrointestinal complaints and has ingested baking soda for indigestion. Her daughter reports many instances that Ms. James took at least two tablespoons of baking soda for "indigestion." On this admission her blood gases were: pH, 7.62; Pco_2, 48; Po_2, 78; HCO_3^-, 36. Other significant laboratory results include: Na^+, 152 mEq/L; K^+, 2.8 mEq/L, CO_2, 38.

1. *What is the acid-base abnormality seen in this situation? Is there any compensation seen?*
2. *Compare the pathophysiology of this acid-base abnormality with other types of acid-base abnormalities.*
3. *What is the explanation for the abnormalities seen in the sodium and potassium levels?*
4. *Discuss the clinical manifestations in relation to the degree of abnormality seen.*
5. *What measures should be instituted to prevent recurrence of this acid-base abnormality?*

See Appendix G for discussion.

▼ Chapter Summary

▼ Acid–base balance is rigidly maintained by the body and is essential in promoting all of the functions of the body. The lungs and kidneys are the main organs responsible for the regulation of the balance.

▼ The pH is simply a reflection of the number of hydrogen ions in a solution. In the case of the body, that solution is the plasma. Normal pH is maintained at 7.35 to 7.45, which is alkaline, because 7.0 is the neutral point. Therefore, any point below 7.35 is considered to be acidotic, whereas greater than 7.45 is considered alkalotic.

▼ The acids produced by the body are volatile and nonvolatile. A volatile gas, carbon dioxide is mainly eliminated by the lungs. Nonvolatile acids are those that must be exchanged and eliminated by the kidneys.

▼ The maintenance of the pH depends on buffer systems that chemically increase or decrease the pH into the normal range. The rate and depth of respiration and the retention or excretion of hydrogen by the kidneys also affect the pH. The carbonic acid/bicarbonate ratio accounts for this pH range and is 1:20.

▼ Four imbalances of acid–base balance are respiratory acidosis, respiratory alkalosis, metabolic acidosis, and metabolic alkalosis.

▼ Alterations in the pH have specific and detrimental effects on the body along with specific symptoms. Each imbalance is specifically compensated, with the rapidity of the compensatory mechanism varying depending on the imbalance. Acid–base imbalances also affect the balance of potassium, calcium, and magnesium.

▼ The anion gap is a helpful method for determining the type of acid–base disturbance present. Normal anion gap is 16 ± 4 mEq/L when potassium is included in the calculation. A normal gap may be seen in the presence of acidosis when the chloride increases to fill the gap. High-anion-gap acidosis is seen with excess production of organic acids.

▼ References

1. Breyer, M.D., and Jacobson, H.R. Approach to the patient with metabolic acidosis or alkalosis. In W.N. Kelley (ed.), *Textbook of Internal Medicine* (2nd ed.). Philadelphia: J.B. Lippincott, 1992.
2. Fischbach, F. *A Manual of Laboratory and Diagnostic Tests* (4th ed.). Philadelphia: J.B. Lippincott, 1992.
3. Guyton, A. *Textbook of Medical Physiology* (8th ed.). Philadelphia: W.B. Saunders, 1991.
4. Humes, H.D., and Cox, M. Principles of the renal regulation of fluid and electrolytes. In W.N. Kelley (ed.), *Textbook of Internal Medicine* (2nd ed.). Philadelphia: J.B. Lippincott, 1992.
5. Laski, M.E., and Kurtzman, N.A. Disorders of acid-base balance. In J.H. Stein (ed.), *Internal Medicine* (4th ed.). St. Louis: C.V. Mosby, 1994.
6. Metheny, N.M. *Fluid and Electrolyte Balance* (2nd ed.). Philadelphia: J.B. Lippincott, 1992.
7. Narins, R.G. Acid-base disorders: Definitions and introductory concepts. In M.H. Maxwell, C.R. Kleeman, and R.G. Narins (eds.), *Clinical Disorders of Fluid and Electrolyte Metabolism* (4th ed.). New York: McGraw-Hill, 1987.
8. Rice, V. Acid-base derangements in the patient with cardiac arrest. *Focus on Critical Care* 14(6):53, 1987.
9. Shoemaker, W.C. Fluids and electrolytes in the acutely ill adult. In W.C. Shoemaker (ed.), *Textbook of Critical Care* (3rd ed.). Philadelphia: W.B. Saunders, 1994.
10. Tortora, G., and Grabowski, S.R. *Principles of Anatomy and Physiology* (7th ed.). New York: Harper-Collins, 1993.
11. Whitney, E.N., Cataldo, C.B., and Rolfes, S.R. *Understanding Normal and Clinical Nutrition* (3rd ed.). St. Paul: West, 1991.
12. Zaloga, G.P., and Chernow, B. Hypocalcemia in critical illness. *JAMA* 256:1924, 1986.

Chapter 12

Normal and Altered Nutritional Balance

Roberta H. Anding

▼ CHAPTER OUTLINE

▼ LEARNING OBJECTIVES

1 Discuss the nutritional terms **macronutrients** and **micronutrients**.
2 Discuss the mechanisms by which carbohydrates are used in the body for energy production.
3 Identify foods high in dietary fiber and their benefit in the diet.
4 List at least three alternate sources of sucrose.
5 Identify essential and nonessential amino acids.
6 Discuss the functions of protein in the body.
7 Describe the importance of nitrogen balance.
8 List the main functions of fat.
9 Compare saturated, monosaturated, and polyunsaturated fats as to structure and function.
10 List the functions and sources of water-soluble and fat-soluble vitamins.
11 Compare deficiency and toxicity with water-soluble and fat-soluble vitamins.
12 Discuss the functions of the essential trace minerals.
13 Describe protein calorie malnutrition, including its components, marasmus and kwashiorkor.
14 Discuss insulin/glucagon changes in starvation.
15 Define **ketoadaptation** and the risks involved with its failure.
16 Compare hypertrophic and hyperplastic obesity.
17 Discuss the multifaceted process of weight control.
18 Explain the risks of android versus gynoid obesity.
19 Compare anorexia nervosa and bulimia regarding etiology, manifestations, and nutritional imbalances produced.
20 List the physiologic effects of vomiting and laxative and diuretic abuse.
21 Describe the diagnostic clues to the problems of anorexia nervosa and bulimia.

Nutritional balance is a major factor in promoting health and preventing disease. Balance can be altered by excessive or deficient quantities of essential nutrients. Vitamins, minerals, carbohydrates, proteins, and fats all provide these essential nutrients. This chapter presents an overview of the macronutrients, the micronutrients, and the effects of an imbalance of each. Macronutrients include carbohydrates, proteins, and lipids. Micronutrients include the vitamins and particular trace minerals. Other minerals and water balance are discussed in Chapter 10. Water is essential for the absorption of nutrients and elimination of wastes from the body. Further discussion of nutrition is found in Unit 11, especially in relation to absorption and nutrient production. Alterations of nutritional balance affect all of the body processes and are discussed throughout the book.

▼ *Macronutrients*

CARBOHYDRATES

Carbohydrates function to supply the body with energy. The simpler forms of carbohydrates, called simple sugars, are monosaccharides and disaccharides. Monosaccharides contain one sugar unit; disaccharides contain two (Fig. 12-1). The more complex carbohydrates are classified as starches, or polysaccharides. They are also sources of dietary fiber. Polysaccharides contain 20 or more sugar units (monosaccharide molecules). Oligosaccharides are intermediate carbohydrates containing 3 to 10 sugar units. Glycogen, also referred to as animal starch, is the storage form of carbohydrate and is stored in liver and muscle.

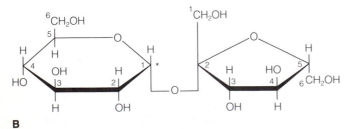

A.

B.

FIGURE 12-1 *A. Structure of monosaccharide glucose.* **B.** *Structure of disaccharide sucrose. (Redrawn from: Luke, B. Principles of Nutrition and Diet Therapy. Boston: Little, Brown, 1984.)*

TABLE 12-1 *Forms of Carbohydrates and Food Sources*

Type of Carbohydrate	Food Sources
MONOSACCHARIDES	
Glucose	Breakdown of product (complex carbohydrates)
Fructose	Fruits, honey, corn syrup
DISACCHARIDES	
Maltose	Grains
Lactose	Milk, milk products, filler in nondairy products
Sucrose	Sugar, honey, maple syrup
OLIGOSACCHARIDES	Dried beans, peas (carbohydrate used in enteral medical nutrition products)
POLYSACCHARIDES	Breads, grains, starches

In the United States, carbohydrates supply 45% of energy, with one-half coming from simple sugars and one-half from complex carbohydrates. Dietary goals for Americans include decreasing the amount of simple sugars and increasing the amount of complex carbohydrate intake. Table 12-1 lists forms of carbohydrate and food sources.

Functions

Dietary carbohydrate yields four calories per gram (kcal/g), whereas dextrose administered intravenously yields 3.4 kcal/g. A 5% dextrose solution has 5 g of dextrose per 100 mL of intravenous solution, which means that a liter bottle of this solution contains 170 kcal.[82] Certain tissues of the body, particularly the brain and red blood cells, rely on glucose as a preferred energy source. In the absence of adequate carbohydrate, *gluconeogenesis* ensues to synthesize glucose from noncarbohydrate sources, primarily protein. Most gluconeogenesis occurs in the liver (see pp. 806–807). To spare protein, the daily consumption of 100 g of carbohydrate is necessary. The provision of adequate carbohydrate will also prevent ketosis, which results from fat breakdown.

Dietary Fiber

Complex carbohydrates are also sources of dietary fiber. Dietary fiber refers to the foodstuffs that remain undigested as they enter the large intestine. Certain fibers, the water-soluble forms, are digested or fermented by the bacteria in the large intestine. Fiber, therefore, cannot always be defined as the undigested portion of carbohydrate-containing foods. Current intake of fiber in the United States averages 10 to 13 g/day.[49] Recommended goals for dietary fiber range from 20 to 40 g/day.[80]

Proposed benefits of adequate fiber intake include decreased risk of problems, such as colon cancer, diverticular disease, constipation, and hemorrhoids. Dietary fiber may also be used as an adjunct to the treatment of gastrointestinal (GI) disorders, diabetes, and coronary artery disease. Classification of fiber is based on its solubility, which determines its physiologic function. Table 12-2 lists the type, function, and representative food sources of dietary fiber and amounts of water-soluble/insoluble fiber.

Increasing dietary fiber should be done gradually to minimize GI discomfort. It requires a concomitant in-

crease in fluid, especially water, to maintain GI motility. Increased dietary fiber in elderly individuals may create problems due to decreased ability to increase fluid intake and chronic ingestion of constipating medications. These factors may lead to fecal impactions, which are often difficult to recognize clinically. Intake of large amounts of fiber also is associated with the development of *bezoars*, an accumulation of fiber in the stomach, and may cause a decreased absorption of minerals, particularly divalent calcium, zinc, and iron.[70]

Alternate Sweeteners

To reduce simple sugar consumption and as an adjunct to weight control, Americans have increased consumption of alternatives to sucrose. Sweeteners can be classi-

TABLE 12-2 *Major Types of Fiber: Their Sources and Physiologic Effects*

Water-Soluble Fibers	Sources
PHYSIOLOGIC EFFECTS Slow gastric emptying and intestinal transit time / Lower serum cholesterol levels / Delay glucose absorption, which helps improve glucose tolerance in diabetics	
GUMS	Oat bran and oatmeal / Dried peas and beans
PECTIN	Apples, citrus fruits, strawberries / Dried peas / Squash, cauliflower, cabbage, carrots, potatoes

Water-Insoluble Fibers	Sources
PHYSIOLOGIC EFFECTS Absorb water to increase fecal bulk / Reduce pressure within the colon / Decrease intestinal transit time / Have little effect on serum cholesterol or glucose	
HEMICELLULOSE	Wheat bran and whole grains and cereals
CELLULOSE	Whole-wheat flour and wheat bran / Vegetables: cabbage, peas, green beans, wax beans, broccoli, brussel sprouts, root vegetables / Apples
LIGNIN	Cereals and wheat bran / Mature vegetables / Pears, strawberries / Eggplant, green beans

(Dudek, S. G. *Nutrition Handbook for Nursing Practice* [2nd ed.]. Philadelphia: J.B. Lippincott, 1993.)

TABLE 12-3 *Alternate Sweeteners and Their Relative Sweetening Power Compared With Sucrose*

Caloric	Noncaloric
Fructose 1.0–1.8 ×	Aspartame* 180–200 ×
Sugar Alcohols 0.5 ×	Cyclamate
Sorbitol	Acesulfame 200 ×
Mannitol	Saccharin 375 ×

* Although aspartame is a dipeptide (protein), it is used as a carbohydrate alternative.

(Adapted from *Diabetes Care* 11(2):174–82, 1988.)

fied as caloric and noncaloric. Table 12-3 lists sweeteners and their relative sweetening power as compared with sucrose.

FRUCTOSE. Fructose is a naturally occurring carbohydrate found in fruit and honey. It has a slow postprandial rise in blood glucose compared with sucrose. Excessive consumption of fructose is linked with hypertriglyceridemia.[57]

SORBITOL AND MANNITOL. Sorbitol and mannitol are sugar alcohols that contain 4 kcal/g. Slow absorption from the GI tract causes intestinal gas and osmotic diarrhea. Children are particularly sensitive to the laxative effects of sorbitol.

ASPARTAME. Aspartame is a chemical compound of phenylalanine and aspartic acid. Although technically noncaloric, it is extremely sweet, and very small amounts are required to achieve desired sweetness. Safety issues concerning aspartame include the following:

1. There are nonspecific side effects, including headache, nausea, and dizziness.[12]
2. Methanol production forms momentarily as a by-product of aspartame metabolism. Methanol is oxidized to formal-dehyde and then to carbon dioxide. The amounts generated are below a harmful level.[82]
3. Aspartame can alter neurotransmitters in the brain. High levels of aspartame increase the level of phenylalanine and its metabolic product, tyrosine, in experimental animals. Tyrosine is essential in the production of epinephrine and norepinephrine as well as thyroxine and melanin. Consumption of a high carbohydrate meal exacerbates these effects while blocking the increase in tryptophan and serotonin normally seen after a high carbohydrate meal.[88]
4. Aspartame use is contraindicated in persons with phenylketonuria (PKU). PKU results when there is a deficiency of phenylalanine hydroxylase, an enzyme that converts phenylalanine to tyrosine.

The Food and Drug Administration (FDA) has set an acceptable daily intake for aspartame at 50 mg/kg. This is equivalent to approximately 14 soft drinks per day or 71 packets of Equal.

CYCLAMATES. Cyclamates were banned by the FDA in 1970 after animal studies indicated a potential cancer risk as well as testicular atrophy and chromosomal damage. Further review has failed to establish cyclamates as carcinogenic.[23, 82]

Derangement of Carbohydrate Metabolism

Alterations of carbohydrate usage can be caused by defects in absorption, metabolism, or storage. Table 12-4 lists representative defects of carbohydrate metabolism and the cause. These defects are discussed in greater detail in other sections of this text.

PROTEIN

The recommended dietary allowance for protein is 0.8 g/kg of ideal body weight for healthy individuals. The average intake of protein in the United States is 75 to 110 g or approximately 1.5 times the needed amount. Protein must be consumed daily because there is no storage or reserve of protein in the body. All protein in the body is functional. Any loss of body protein represents a loss of physiologic function.

TABLE 12-4 *Defects of Carbohydrate Metabolism*

Disease State	Type of Defect	Clinical Presentation
Diabetes mellitus	Metabolic defect in insulin secretion or use	Hyperglycemia
Lactose intolerance	Absorption deficiency of lactose	Diarrhea, gas, cramps, bloating
Glycogen storage	Storage deficiency of glucose 6-phosphatase deficiency (von Gierke's disease)	Hepatomegaly, severe hypoglycemia, hyperlipidemia

Amino acids are the building blocks of protein. The key component of the molecule is the amine group, which is the nitrogen component. Twenty amino acids are required by the body, of which nine are essential, indicating dietary need. Eleven amino acids are synthesized by the liver. Table 12-5 lists the essential and nonessential amino acids.

Protein metabolism/catabolism is controlled by the liver, and excretion of the end products of protein metabolism (urea nitrogen and creatinine) is dependent on the kidneys.

Dietary protein can be classified as complete (high biologic value) or incomplete (low biologic value). Complete proteins contain all the essential amino acids in proper proportion, indicating the ability to perform physiologically the functions of protein. Incomplete proteins alone cannot function as proteins and are deaminated. Deamination is the process of removing the amine group and converting the remaining carbon skeleton (keto analogue) to glucose or ketones. Complimentary proteins, or mutual supplementation, result from the combining of two plant proteins that are deficient in one or more essential amino acids, thereby improving overall protein quality. Box 12-1 list examples of complimentary proteins.

Functions

The primary function of protein is to build and repair tissue in healthy individuals. Protein requirements are greatest during periods of rapid growth and development. Table 12-6 lists the recommended dietary allowances of protein.

The blood proteins, albumin and globulin, are

BOX 12-1 ▼ Examples of Complementary Proteins

Rice and beans
Croutons and split pea soup
Tortilla and beans
Corn bread and chili beans
Chick peas and tahini (sesame seed paste)
Tofu and sesame seeds

hydrophilic molecules that contribute to blood oncotic pressure and thereby function in fluid balance and blood pressure (see pp. 206–207). Deficiencies of protein can eventually cause leaking of fluid into the extracellular spaces with resulting edema. Proteins regulate acid–base balance through their buffering capabilities. Proteins function in the transport of nutrients and the enzymatic reactions of metabolism. Proteins also function

TABLE 12-5 Amino Acids

Essential	Nonessential
Histidine	Alanine
Isoleucine	Arginine
Leucine	Asparagine
Lysine	Aspartic acid
Methionine	Cystine (cysteine)
Phenylalanine	Glutamic acid
Threonine	Glutamine
Tryptophan	Glycine
Valine	Hydroxyproline
	Hydroxylysine
	Proline
	Serine
	Tyrosine

(Dudek, S. G. *Nutrition Handbook for Nursing Practice* [2nd ed.]. Philadelphia: J.B. Lippincott, 1993.)

TABLE 12-6 Recommended Dietary Allowances of Protein

Category	Age (years) or Condition	Weight (kg)	RDA (g/kg)*	RDA (g/day)
Both sexes	0–0.5	6	2.2	13
	0.5–1	9	1.6	14
	1–3	13	1.2	16
	4–6	20	1.1	24
	7–10	28	1.0	28
Males	11–14	45	1.0	45
	15–18	66	0.9	59
	19–24	72	0.8	58
	25–50	79	0.8	63
	51+	77	0.8	63
Females	11–14	46	1.0	46
	15–18	55	0.8	44
	19–24	58	0.8	46
	25–50	63	0.8	50
	51+	65	0.8	50
Pregnancy	1st trimester			+10
	2nd trimester			+10
	3rd trimester			+10
Lactation	1st 6 months			+15
	2nd 6 months			+12

* Amino acid score of typical U.S. diet is 100 for all age groups, except young infants. Digestibility is equal to reference proteins. Values have been rounded upward to 0.1 g/kg.

(Dudek, S. G. *Nutrition Handbook for Nursing Practice* [2nd ed.]. Philadelphia: J.B. Lippincott, 1993.)

TABLE 12-7 *Alterations in Protein Requirements in Selected Disease States*

Disease	Protein Requirements
Renal disease	
Early renal failure (serum creatinine 2–6 mg/mL)	0.6 g/kg (75% human biologic value)
Advanced renal failure	0.3 g/kg
Dialysis—hemo	1.0–1.2
peritoneal	1.2–1.5
Nephrotic syndrome	0.6 g plus urinary losses
Neoplastic disease	1.5–2.5 g/kg
Liver disease	
Hepatic encephalopathy	50 g/d with increased amounts of branched chain amino acids
Cirrhosis with encephalopathy	Decreased aromatic amino acids 0.8 gm–1.0 g/kg
Trauma	1.0–1.5 g/kg
Sepsis	1.5–2.0 g/kg

in clotting, connective tissue, and visual pigments. As an energy source, protein yields 4 kcal/g.

Alterations in Protein Requirements

Disease processes, through their effect on absorption, metabolism, or excretion, affect protein requirements. Decreased protein tolerance may also occur. Table 12-7 lists various disease states and protein requirements or

restrictions. Altering the amount and type of amino acids may compensate for the inability of the body to metabolize the substrate. The branch chain amino acids, *valine*, *isoleucine*, and *leucine*, may be preferred amino acids in liver disease and trauma because they help to decrease muscle proteolysis.

NITROGEN BALANCE. Nitrogen balance (NB), or equilibrium, is the amount of protein required to allow for normal physiologic functioning. NB studies are useful in determining the amount of protein required to remain in nitrogen homeostasis (ie, to achieve or maintain a positive NB). NB can be calculated as follows: NB = (protein intake in grams × 0.16) − (24-hour urine urea nitrogen in grams + 3 g). The extra 3 g of urea nitrogen added to the equation is that amount normally lost in fecal material. Figure 12-2 summarizes the concept of nitrogen equilibrium and those factors that can produce a positive or negative balance.

LIPIDS

Fats are the most concentrated source of energy, supplying 9 kcal/g. Excessive saturated fat consumption is highly correlated with atherosclerosis and cancer incidence. A national dietary goal is to decrease saturated fat to about 10% of total dietary intake, balancing the total fat intake with polyunsaturated and monounsaturated fats.

Functions

The average fat intake in the United States is 38%. The physiologic requirement for essential fatty acids is 4% of total calories. The main functions of fat are 1) as a caloric

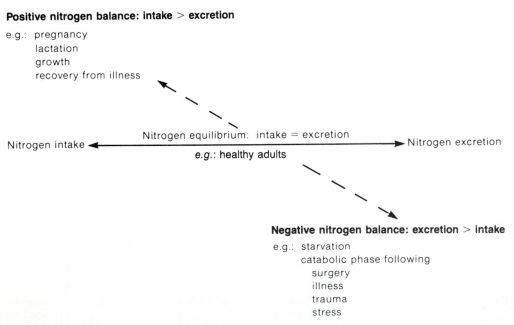

Positive nitrogen balance: intake > excretion

e.g.: pregnancy
    lactation
    growth
    recovery from illness

Nitrogen intake ←   Nitrogen equilibrium: intake = excretion   → Nitrogen excretion
e.g.: healthy adults

Negative nitrogen balance: excretion > intake

e.g.: starvation
    catabolic phase following
      surgery
      illness
      trauma
      stress

FIGURE 12-2 *States of nitrogen balance. (From : Dudek, S.J. Nutrition Handbook for Nursing Practice [2nd ed.]. Philadelphia: J.B. Lippincott, 1993.)*

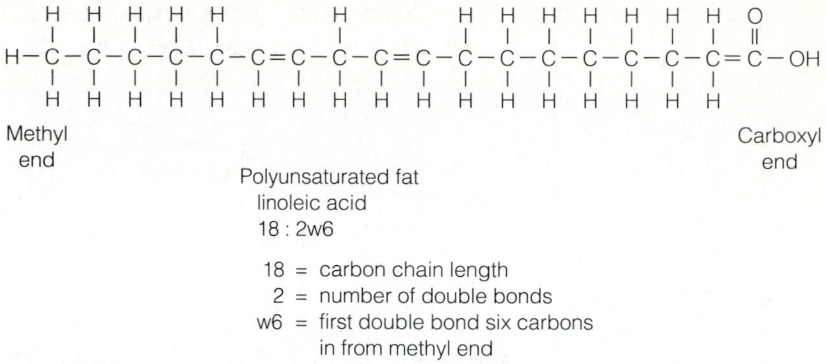

FIGURE 12-3 *Structure of a fatty acid.*

source; 2) to provide satiety; 3) to insulate the body; 4) to transport fat-soluble vitamins; 5) to form prostaglandin (eicosanoid) by essential fatty acids; and 6) to provide substrate for hormones, including cholecalciferol and estrogen.

Families of Fatty Acids

Fatty acids are carbon chains of varying lengths with a carboxyl or acid group at one end and a methyl group at the other. Figure 12-3 illustrates the structure of a fatty acid.

A fatty acid is saturated if all the bonds between carbon atoms are single bonds. Saturated fats solidify at room temperature and can be of animal or plant origin. Saturated fats are the most atherogenic (atherosclerosis-causing) family of fatty acids. Table 12-8 lists common food sources of saturated fat and cholesterol.

Monounsaturated fats are those containing a single double bond. Dietary sources include olive oil, peanut oil, and canola (rapeseed) oil. Monounsaturated fats lower serum cholesterol.[31]

Polyunsaturated fats are long chain fatty acids (≥ 18 carbons in the chain). Essential fatty acids, linoleic (omega-6), and alpha linolenic (omega-3) acids must be consumed in the diet. The physiologic function of these essential fatty acids is in the phospholipid layer in the cell wall and as precursors to the eicosanoids, prostaglandins, prostacyclins, thromboxanes, and leukotrienes. These compounds are integral to such vital body functions as regulation of blood pressure, blood clotting platelet aggregation, the immune response, inflammation, and the initiation of labor. Modification of dietary lipids can affect physiologic function. Flowchart 12-1 illustrates the process of eicosanoid production from dietary precursors.

In polyunsaturated fats, the position of the first double bond determines the eicosanoids synthesized. If the first double bond is located at the third carbon atom from the methyl end, it is an omega-3 polyunsaturated fat. If the first double bond is located at the sixth carbon atom from the methyl end, it is an omega-6 fatty acid. A summary of the difference in physiologic effects is found in Table 12-9. Dietary sources of omega-6 fatty acids are corn, safflower, and sunflower oils. Dietary sources of omega-3 fatty acids are soybean oil, canola oil, and cold-water fish. Polyunsaturated fats have been shown to have a hypocholesterolemic effect.[48]

Greenland Eskimos have approximately one-tenth the risk of heart attacks as compared with Danish people.[2] Although both populations consume high-fat diets, Eskimos eat primarily cold-water fish and Danes eat saturated fat. Fish oils decrease platelet aggregation and prolong bleeding time. The cholesterol-lowering effect of fish oils is slight through the reduction of very low-density lipoproteins, a primary carrier of triglycerides. When consuming a mixed diet, most individuals ingest a greater amount of omega-6 fatty acids. However, omega-6 and omega-3 fats compete for the enzymes responsible for desaturation and elongation to their respective metabolites. Affinity of the substrate for the enzyme increases with increasing number of double bonds, indicating that omega-3 fatty acids can prevent the conversion of the omega-6 fatty acids to their metabolically active end products.

TABLE 12-8 *Common Food Sources of Cholesterol and Saturated Fat*

Food	Cholesterol (mg)	Saturated Fat (g)
Ground beef (27% fat), 3 oz	80	7.0
Lean ground beef (15% fat), 3 oz	50	5.0
Chicken—white meat (no skin), 3 oz	70	1.0
Cheese, most varieties, 1 oz	30	5.0
Whole milk, 1 c	33	5.0
Skim milk, 1 c	trace	0.3
Butter, 1 T	30	7.0
Corn oil margarine, 1 T	0	2.0
Canola oil, 1 T	0	1.0
Corn oil, 1 T	0	1.8
Coconut oil, 1 T	0	12.0

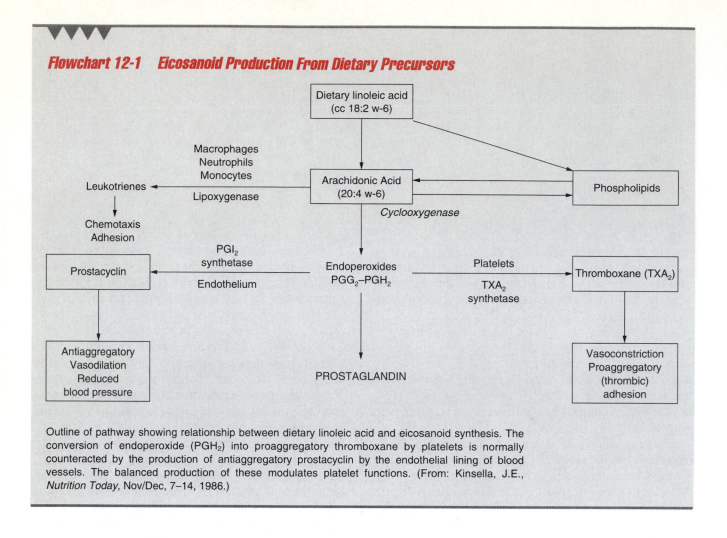

Flowchart 12-1 Eicosanoid Production From Dietary Precursors

Outline of pathway showing relationship between dietary linoleic acid and eicosanoid synthesis. The conversion of endoperoxide (PGH_2) into proaggregatory thromboxane by platelets is normally counteracted by the production of antiaggregatory prostacyclin by the endothelial lining of blood vessels. The balanced production of these modulates platelet functions. (From: Kinsella, J.E., *Nutrition Today*, Nov/Dec, 7–14, 1986.)

Fatty Acid Metabolism

The metabolism of fatty acids is, in part, determined by the length of the carbon chain. Dietary fats are mostly made up of triglycerides: three fatty acid chains of varying lengths esterified to a glycerol backbone. Long-chain triglycerides are hydrolyzed in the intestinal lumen by pancreatic lipase to monoglycerides and free fatty acids (FFAs). Poorly soluble in water, bile salts enhance solubility through miceller formation (see p. 809). Micelles are transported passively across the intestinal cell wall where re-esterification occurs. Chylomicrons are the transport vehicle for re-esterified triglyceride. Chylomicrons are released into the lymphatic system, then to

TABLE 12-9 *Effects of Products Made from Omega-3 and Omega-6 Fatty Acids in Man*

Site of Synthesis	Omega-6 (Linoleic Acid)	Omega-3 (EPA, DHA)
Cells lining blood vessels	Form prostaglandin I_2, which inhibits blood clotting	Form prostaglandin I_3, which inhibits blood clotting
Platelets* in the blood	Form thromboxane A_2, which is a strong promoter of blood clotting	Form thromboxane A_3, which is a very weak promoter of blood clotting

The net result is that omega-3 fatty acids reduce the tendency for blood to clot.
  * Platelike fragments in the bloodstream that contribute to blood clotting.
  Wardlaw, G. M., and Insel, P. M. St. Louis, Toronto, Boston: Times Mirror/Mosby, 1990.

venous circulation. Lipoprotein lipase cleaves the triglyceride into FFAs and monoglyceride. In the fed state, monoglycerides and FFAs are stored in the adipose cell. In the fasting state, muscle mitochondria oxidize FFAs for energy or the liver releases the fatty acids as very low-density lipoproteins. The transport of long-chain fats across mitochondrial membranes is dependent on *carnitine*, which acts as a carrier substance.

Medium-chain triglycerides (MCTs) have 8 to 10 carbon chains and do not require bile for emulsification or pancreatic lipase for hydrolysis. Absorption of these triglycerides is intact, and degradation into FFAs occurs through intracellular lipase. Albumin carries FFAs into portal circulation, then to the liver for oxidation. Rapid metabolism of MCTs occurs as carnitine is not needed for transport into the cell. In diseases affecting fat digestion or absorption, MCT oil can be a valuable caloric source. MCT oil does not provide essential fatty acids.

Cholesterol is a sterol found in animal products only. There is no required intake for cholesterol, because humans can synthesize cholesterol when dietary supply is inadequate. The richest dietary sources include liver, egg yolk, whole milk, whole-milk cheese, beef, and pork. Physiologic functions of cholesterol include its role in forming many hormones, in keeping the cell membrane insoluble in water, and in forming bile salts. It is unnecessary to consume cholesterol per se, because the liver efficiently produces it from saturated fat in the diet (see pp. 807–808).

▼ Micronutrients

The micronutrients include the water-soluble and fat-soluble vitamins as well as minerals. Some of the minerals (electrolytes) are discussed in Chapter 10, and other necessary trace minerals are covered in this section. A basis for understanding the functions is presented in this chapter with application of materials throughout specific sections. See Appendix D for the recommended daily allowances for different age groups as determined by the National Research Council of the Food and Nutritional Board, National Academy of Sciences.

WATER-SOLUBLE VITAMINS

Vitamins are organic compounds needed for metabolism of foodstuffs. Vitamins provide no energy but facilitate energy-yielding chemical reactions. The B vitamins and vitamin C are water soluble and are not stored in appreciable amounts. Megadoses defined at 10 times recommended dietary allowance are taken by some individuals, and toxicity may develop.

Disease states can significantly increase the need for water-soluble vitamins. Table 12-10 summarizes function, food sources, conditions caused by deficiency, signs and symptoms of the deficiency, factors influencing or increasing requirements, and toxicity signs and symptoms.

FAT-SOLUBLE VITAMINS

The fat-soluble vitamins are A, D, E, and K and are absorbed together with dietary fat. They are readily stored in fatty tissues and are more likely than water-soluble vitamins to cause a toxic reaction. Toxicity symptoms may occur at levels as low as 10 times the recommended dietary allowance. Deficiency states may be encountered in persons with steatorrhea, or fat malabsorption. However, because stores of these vitamins exist, the development of deficiency symptoms occurs over a period of time. Table 12-11 lists the fat-soluble vitamins, chemical name, function, food sources, diseases caused by deficiency, clinical signs and symptoms of deficiency, conditions that influence requirements, and toxicity.

TRACE MINERALS

Minerals are inorganic compounds that are vital in human nutrition and cell function. Minerals function in a variety of metabolic roles, including enzyme cofactors, hormones, nerve conduction, and structural components. Bioavailability refers to the amount of mineral absorbed and used by the body. Various factors influence the bioavailability of a particular mineral, such as binding effect, fiber, and the physiologic need.[13] Minerals are necessary in a variety of body functions, including acid–base balance, osmotic pressure, cell membrane permeability, enzyme system activation, and nerve and muscle responsiveness. The activities of the minerals are discussed in the respective sections of the text. The important trace minerals are summarized in Table 12-12. The functions, food sources, disease states, factors influencing requirements, signs and symptoms, and toxicity are presented in this table. Appendix D presents recommended dietary allowances (RDAs) for vitamins and minerals.

▼ Malnutrition

Malnutrition is defined as an inadequate intake of macronutrients, vitamins, or minerals that impairs the physiologic functioning of the body. It may be the result of inadequate intake or due to increased requirements. The incidence of malnutrition has been estimated to affect 50% of hospitalized patients.[82]

Protein calorie malnutrition (PCM) is a continuum with *marasmus* (starvation or semi-starvation) at one end and *kwashiorkor* (protein deficiency, also known as hypoalbuminemic malnutrition) at the other (Fig. 12-4). Protein calorie malnutrition, as seen in the hospital, is generally classified into three categories:

(text continues on page 239)

TABLE 12-10 *Functions and Alterations in Water-Soluble Vitamins*

Vitamin	Function	Food Sources	Deficiency	Factors Influencing Requirements	Signs and Symptoms	Toxicity
Thiamine	Metabolism through oxidative reaction	Pork, whole grains, organ meats	Beriberi, chronic alcoholism	Alcoholism, fever, infection, hyperthyroidism, burns, trauma, chronic antacid use	Anorexia, fatigue, peripheral neuropathy, footdrop, cardiomegaly, depression	Nausea and vomiting
Riboflavin	Coenzyme flavin, mononucleotide, citric acid, beta-oxidation	Milk, dairy products	Cheilosis, ariboflavinosis	Thyroid dysfunction, burns, trauma, diabetes, alcoholism, oral contraceptives, tricyclic antidepressants	Seborrheic dermatitis, scrotal dermatitis, growth failure, photophobia	None known
Niacin	Coenzyme NAD, NADPH, formation of ATP, oxidation/reduction, reactions, immune competence	Mushrooms, enriched grain products, tuna, chicken, can be synthesized from dietary tryptophan	Pellegra	Alcohol, thyroid disorders, neoplasia, isoniazid for TB, burns	Diarrhea, dermatitis, dementia, weakness, fatigue	In large amounts, nicotinic acid functions as a vasodilator; nausea, vomiting, hypocholesterolemic effect
Pyridoxine (B₆)	Coenzyme form, pyridoxical phosphate, transamination of amino acids, synthesis of hemoglobin, neurotransmitter synthesis	Meat, fish, poultry, bananas, cantaloupe, broccoli	Irritability, depression	Uremia, burns, advancing age, neoplastic disease, medication, liver disease, uremia, isoniazid, hydralazine, high-protein diets, asthma, degenerative diseases	Stomatitis, glossitis, cheilosis, anemia (after prolonged deficiency)	Irreversible nerve damage, ataxia
Folic acid	One carbon transfer reaction, synthesis of RBC, nucleotides, RNA, DNA, proteins	Orange juice, liver, green leafy vegetables	Megaloblastic anemia/ macrocytic anemia	Fevers, burns, alcoholism, ileal disease, inflammatory bowel disease, gluten-induced enteropathy, gastrectomies, periods of increased growth, medications, methotrexates, common deficiency in elderly and in adolescent females	Smooth, sore tongue; dementia; diarrhea; weight loss	May mask B₁₂ deficiency
B₁₂	Coenzyme transfer of methyl (CH₃) groups, synthesis of nucleic acids and choline, RBC formation	Animal protein	Megaloblastic anemia, pernicious anemia	Vegetarian; gastrectomy; ileal resection, gastric bypass surgery; intestinal parasites; medications, such as neomycin, potassium chloride	Loss of appetite, weight loss, glossitis, leukopenia, thrombocytopenia, tingling in extremities, dementia	None known
Ascorbic acid (vitamin C)	Collagen formation, cartilage formation, synthesis of bile, acts as a reducing agent, wound healing	Green peppers, citrus fruit, strawberries, broccoli, cabbage	Scurvy	Cigarette smoking, alcoholism, use of oral contraceptives, cancer, surgery, burns	Capillary fragility, hemorrhagic disorders, fatigue, anorexia, muscle pain, gingivitis	Diarrhea, nausea, excess converted to oxalate and forms kidney stones, interferes with urine glucose tests, rebound scurvy

NAD: nicotinamide adenine dinucleotide; NADPH: nicotinamide adenine dinucleotide phosphate; ATP: adenosine triphosphate; TB: tuberculosis; RBC: red blood cells.

TABLE 12-11 *Functions and Alterations in Fat-Soluble Vitamins*

Vitamin	Function	Food Sources	Deficiency	Factors Influencing Requirements	Signs and Symptoms	Toxicity
Vitamin A (retinoids) beta carotene (precursor)	Visual adaptation, adrenal hormone biosynthesis, mucopolysaccharide and glycoprotein synthesis, maintenance of epithelial structure, wound healing, immunocompetence	Whole milk, butter, carrots	Xerophthalmia	Preterm infants, gastrointestinal dysfunction, respiratory ailments, burns, trauma	Night blindness, keratinization of epithelial cells, diarrhea	Nausea, vomiting, alopecia, hypercalcemia, long bone tenderness (pregnant women and persons with chronic renal disease may be more susceptible)
Vitamin D cholecalciferol, synthesized via ultraviolet light	Absorption of calcium and phosphorus, calcium reabsorption from kidney, removal of calcium and phosphorus from bone, immunoregulatory	Milk, dairy products	Rickets, osteomalacia	Tropical sprue, regional enteritis, pancreatic insufficiency, gastric resection, jejunoileal bypass, chronic renal failure, hypoparathyroidism, medications (anticonvulsants, cimetidine, isoniazid), total parenteral nutrition	Bone pain, increased serum alkaline phosphatase, decreased serum calcium levels, bone demineralization	Nausea, vomiting, anorexia, headache, diarrhea, confusion, calcification of soft tissue
Vitamin E (tocopherols)	Antioxidant, cell membrane integrity, immunoregulatory	Vegetable oil	Hemolytic anemia	Increased intake of polyunsaturated fats, steatorrhea, protein calorie malnutrition, infancy, cystic fibrosis, short-bowel syndrome, respiratory distress syndrome, retrolental fibroplasia, bronchopulmonary dysplasia, smoking	Increased platelet aggregation, neurologic abnormalities, decreased serum creatinine, excessive creatinuria	Nausea, headache, antagonist to vitamin K
Vitamin K (phylloquinone) diet (menaquinone) gut flora	Clotting factors	Greens, broccoli, cauliflower	Hemorrhagic disease	Stage of life cycle (newborn, elderly), renal failure, ulcerative colitis, chronic pancreatitis, biliary dysfunction, medications (antibiotics, coumadin, cholestyramine)	Prolonged bleeding times	With prescription menadione, jaundice, anemia

TABLE 12-12 *Functions and Alterations in Trace Minerals*

Mineral	Function	Food Sources	Deficiency	Factors Influencing Requirements	Signs and Symptoms	Toxicity
Zinc	Ligand in albumin, nucleotides, thymus integrity, cellular immunity, sexual maturation	Oysters, wheat germ, crab, shrimp, red meat	Growth retardation, delayed secondary sex characteristics	Trauma, burns, surgery, inflammatory bowel, short-bowel syndrome, increased intake of fiber, recovery from malnutrition, total parenteral nutrition	Hair loss, skin inflammation, poor wound healing, decreased taste	Decreased use of copper, iron; decrease in HDL cholesterol; diarrhea; nausea and vomiting; immunosuppresion
Copper	Component of enzymes of iron metabolism, cross-binding of collagen, myelination of nerves	Meat, liver, cocoa, legumes, nuts, affected by soil conditions	Rare, induced by copper; free total parenteral nutrition; microcytic hypochromic anemia; increased serum cholesterol levels	Short-bowel syndrome, chronic diarrhea, Crohn's disease, celiac disease, burns, antacids, high zinc intake	Skeletal demineralization, impaired glucose tolerance, hair depigmentation	Vomiting
Selenium	Antioxidant, glutathione, peroxidase	Fish, organ meats, eggs, shellfish	Muscle pain, muscle wasting, heart disease	AIDS, cystic fibrosis, cancer	Growth retardation, muscle pain/weakness, cardiomyopathy	Narrow range of essentiality to toxicity; nausea, vomiting; death
Iron	Essential component of hemoglobin, respiratory oxidation, enzyme cofactor, hydroxylation of lysine and proline	Heme: liver, lean red meat, oysters; nonheme: green leafy vegetables	Hypochromic, microcytic anemia	Vegetarianism; running; periods of rapid growth; bioavailability decreased with tannins, calcium carbonate, magnesium oxide, zinc/copper, oxalate	Shortness of breath, impaired motor development, spoon-shaped nails (koilonychia), increased susceptibility to infection	Excess unbound iron, promotes bacterial/fungal growth, hemochromatosis

HDL: high-density lipoprotein; AIDS: acquired immunodeficiency syndrome.

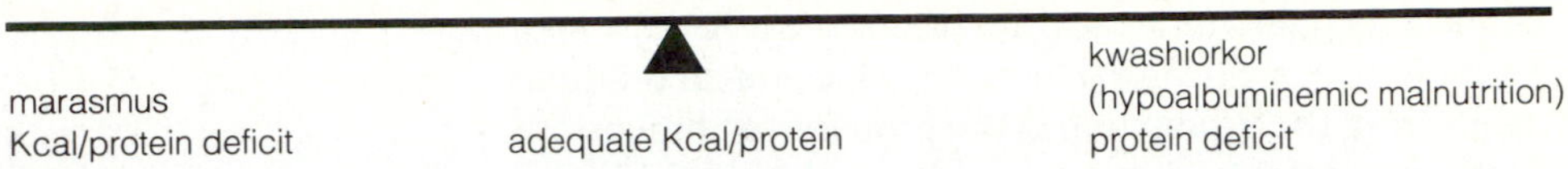

FIGURE 12-4 *The continuum of marasmus and kwashiorkor. Balance requires adequat Kcal and protein. Alteration in either will tip the delicate balance.*

1. *Marasmus*. This is semi-starvation caused by poor intake or poverty, where fat and muscle provide most of the calories required. It is characterized by a reduction of body weight but a preservation of serum proteins and immune competence unless it is very severe. The maintenance of serum proteins is at the expense of somatic (muscle) and visceral (organ) protein.

2. *Kwashiorkor*. Kwashiorkor means "the disease that the first child gets when the second one comes" and is typically seen in underdeveloped countries where children are weaned from the breast to a protein-poor gruel. The pathogenesis of kwashiorkor is evidenced by a low ratio of protein to calories as well as a "flaky paint" dermatitis and hair changes.[66] *Hypoalbuminemic malnutrition*, or hospital-based kwashiorkor, develops in persons who have the stress of injury or infection with poor intake or inappropriate nutrition support. There is a generalized protein loss with increasing impairment of visceral function, evidenced by a decrease in immunocompetence and hypoalbuminemia. This condition is also known as *stressed starvation*.

3. *Combined malnutrition*. This third and most serious form of macronutrient malnutrition is commonly seen in the elderly or in persons with chronic disease. The stress of illness or trauma is superimposed on a marasmic individual. This person needs early nutritional intervention to increase survival rate.

CALORIE RESERVES IN STARVATION

During starvation, physiologic sources of calories include glycogen, somatic and visceral protein, and fat. In the early hours of a fast, glycogen serves as the primary energy source. Metabolism favors glucose homeostasis to support tissues dependent on glucose as a sole energy source, such as the brain, nerves, red blood cells, and renal medulla. During the initial stage of starvation, a fall in arterial blood glucose levels causes a decrease in *insulin*, which is a major anabolic hormone. As insulin levels fall, the levels of the counterregulatory or catabolic hormones increase. The major catabolic hormone involved in the process is *glucagon*. The decrease in the insulin-to-glucagon ratio stimulates glycogenolysis and the release of hepatic glucose. Glycogenolysis is the major source of glucose for approximately 24 hours. Gluconeogenesis from protein serves as the major source of glucose after the initial stage of starvation. Urinary excretion of nitrogen (from protein catabolism) increases as losses of 12 g of nitrogen per day become common. As the fast continues, the decreased level of insulin allows lipolysis and the release of FFAs, oxidation of fatty acids, and synthesis of ketones. The brain cannot use FFAs

because fatty acids do not cross the blood–brain barrier. Ketones and ketoacids can cross the blood–brain barrier and serve as alternative energy sources for the brain, a major consumer of glucose. This process is known as *ketoadaptation*. The rate of protein breakdown is slowed, and urinary nitrogen losses become approximately 3 to 5 g per day. Serum proteins (also known as the proteins of homeostasis) are preserved until the individual is close to death and fat reserves are exhausted. At this point, gluconeogenesis increases, nitrogen excretion increases, and death is likely.

Concomitantly, a decrease in metabolic rate reduces the caloric need of the body and slows the rate of deterioration. A decrease in voluntary work and loss of lean body mass from metabolically active organs such as the pancreas and gut may also contribute to a decrease in metabolic activity. Cardiac workload decreases, and bradycardia lowers the basal metabolic rate.

NUTRITIONAL/METABOLIC CONSEQUENCES OF STRESS

Hypoalbuminemic malnutrition, or stressed starvation, has a profound and significantly different effect on body composition, protein use, and organ function when compared with marasmus. Neuroendocrine control mechanisms are altered and mediate changes in nutritional status. Increases in catecholamines as well as increased levels of glucagon increase the blood glucose level. This is often referred to as "stress diabetes." The hyperglycemia does stimulate insulin release, but insulin resistance, coupled with increases in glucagon levels, allows hyperglycemia to persist. Gluconeogenesis is accentuated, and losses of protein continue at a greater rate than with simple starvation alone. In this hypermetabolic state, there is an increase in lipolysis, but there is a marked decline in ketone production, possibly due to adequate levels of circulating insulin. This failure to ketoadapt has the greatest clinical implications for the individual who is obese. Often viewed as having ample calorie reserves, the major calorie source in stressed starvation is protein and not fat. Therefore, an obese person may not be perceived at nutritional risk based on physical size rather than on the degree of stress. In clinical nutrition, the provision of intravenous dextrose prevents ketoadaptation. When dextrose is given, nutritional support, including adequate protein, should begin as soon as possible.

Skeletal muscle is catabolized to gain access to the

branched-chain amino acids, which serve as energy substrates through gluconeogenesis. Hepatic protein synthesis shifts from the production of the proteins of homeostasis (albumin, transferrin, prealbumin, and retinol-binding protein) to the production of acute phase reactants, such as interleukin-1, ceruloplasmin, and clotting factors, thereby contributing to hypoalbuminemia. Alterations in the serum levels of the proteins of homeostasis can be used to assess the degree of nutritional depletion (Table 12-13). Stress can decrease the serum albumin levels as much as 0.5 g/dL, even in the absence of systemic pathology.[20, 82] Hypoalbuminemia has deleterious effects on wound healing and makes nutritional repletion difficult. Box 12-2 summarizes the effects of hypoproteinemia.

Hypermetabolism is a hallmark of stress, and this causes caloric and protein requirements to increase. Factors influencing caloric and protein requirements include the type of stress, such as infection, fractures, trauma, fever, and respiratory support. To promote anabolism, 150 kcal should be provided for each gram of nitrogen given. An alternative formula allows 35 kcal/kg.[20] Alterations in plasma levels of branched-chain amino acids, glutamine, and arginine may indicate unique roles for these amino acids in the critically ill.[16, 69]

▼ Disorders of Weight Management

OBESITY

Obesity is the most common nutritional disorder in the United States. Although weight reduction promotions are a multimillion dollar industry, Americans are becoming more obese than ever. Although calorie intake has decreased by 10% in the last century, the frequency of obesity has doubled during that time span. Since 1975, obesity in children ages 6 to 11 years has increased by 54% and by 39% in the 12- to 17-year-old group. It has been estimated that 40% of children who are obese at age 7 years will be obese adults.[55] Thirty-four million Americans are obese, and 13 million more are severely obese.[78]

Definition

Obesity is generally defined as being 20% above ideal body weight (IBW) and severely obese as 40% above IBW. A quick estimation of IBW can be performed as shown in Box 12-3. Resting metabolic (energy) expenditure is defined as the amount of calories the body uses at rest for involuntary metabolic activities in the nonfasting state. It is influenced by a variety of factors. Resting energy expenditure decreases with age, starvation, inactivity, and loss of lean body mass. Lean body mass is lost during dieting. It is increased by fever, physiologic stress,

TABLE 12-13 *Relationship Between Nutritional Depletion and Serum Proteins*

Indicator	Normal	Degree of Depletion		
		Mild	*Moderate*	*Severe*
Albumin (g/dl)	3.5–5.5	2.8–3.4	2.1–2.7	<2.1
Transferrin (mg/dl)	180–260	150–200	100–149	<100
Prealbumin (mcg/dl)	200–300	10–15	5–9	<5
Retinol-binding protein[a] (mcg/dl)	40–50	—	—	—

Note: To convert albumin (g/100 ml) to international standard units (nmol/L), multiply by 37.06. To convert transferrin (mg/100 ml) to standard international units (g/L), multiply by 0.01.

[a] Levels of <3 mg/100 ml suggest compromised protein status. The actual degree of depletion (mild, moderate, and severe) has not been defined.

Adapted from Whitney, E. N., Cataldo, C. B., and Rolfes, S. R. *Understanding Normal and Clinical Nutrition* (3rd ed.). St Paul: West, 1991.

and physical activity. In most individuals, the resting energy expenditure accounts for about 75% of the total daily energy expenditure. Voluntary physical activity accounts for the remaining 25%. Although many formulas and techniques exist for the calculation of resting energy expenditure, it may be estimated by using the individual's IBW × 10. (Appendix E shows recom-

---

BOX 12-2 ▼ Effects of Hypoproteinemia

1. Decreased wound tensile strength
2. Poor wound healing
3. Decreased blood volume
4. Decreased bone marrow activity—anemia, leukopenia
5. Decreased coagulation mechanisms
6. Increased atrophy of spleen, lymph tissue
7. Decreased antibody production
8. Decreased cell-mediated immunity—resistance to infection
9. Decreased resistance of liver to toxic agents
10. Decreased urine output and water retention
11. Decreased pulmonary function and ventilation
    Atrophy of respiratory muscles
    Retained secretions
    Decreased albumin—interstitial edema
    Decreased serum buffering capacity
12. Increased tendency to develop decubitus ulcers
13. Diarrhea

Adapted from A. Barrocas, G. L. Webb, W. R. Webb, and C. M. St. Romain, *Hypoproteinemia in Nutritional Considerations in the Critically Ill* 75(7):849, 1982.

mended energy intakes in the United States.) Body mass index, also known as Quetelet's index, can also be used in defining obesity.[26] A body mass index of 30 kg/m^2 can be categorized as obese. (See Appendix E for the body mass index).

Types of Cellular Obesity

Hypertrophic obesity is characterized by an increase in the size of the existing adipocyte, or fat cell. Hypertrophy is present in all obesity, and 80% to 90% of adult onset obesity is hypertrophic. Hyperplastic obesity is defined as an increase in the number of fat cells available to be filled. Hyperplasia occurs primarily during periods of rapid growth, such as infancy and adolescence, and is often called "juvenile-onset" obesity. Weight loss and weight maintenance are more difficult to achieve in hyperplastic obesity.[9]

Regulation of Body Weight

In most individuals, body weight is maintained within a narrow range over time by short- and long-term regulation. Short-term regulation refers to the onset of eating on a meal-to-meal basis and is largely dependent on appetite. Long-term regulation refers to the modulation of intake and output so that body weight is maintained within a range.[79] It is a multifaceted process influenced by genetics, thermogenesis, hormones, enzymatic activity, and activity level.

APPETITE CONTROL. Appetite is regulated internally by the hypothalamus. The lateral hypothalamus, or *hunger center*, initiates food consumption after receiving clues, such as hypoglycemia, indicating macronutrient depletion. The ventromedial hypothalamus, or *satiety center*, monitors rising nutrient levels and signals the termination of hunger.[33] Many physiologic clues are directed to the hypothalamus. The gut releases brain–gut peptides, including cholecystokinin and bombesin, throughout the process of eating, signaling satiety.[29] Increasing nutrient levels in the blood, rising blood glucose levels, and tryptophan also cue satiety.[8] Tryptophan, an amino acid precursor to serotonin, is a powerful regulator of carbohydrate intake.[27] Norepinephrine release by the sympathetic nervous system stimulates hunger, and epinephrine and dopamine inhibit hunger. Obesity may, in part, be due to a defect in the stimulation and inhibition of the sympathetic nervous system.[7, 60]

External factors, such as the type, appearance, and smell of food; the social impetus to eat; and environmental stressors also increase or decrease food intake. Control of appetite through internal and external manipulations is essential in controlling obesity.[5]

GENETIC INFLUENCES. Obesity is highly familial. Adoption studies have demonstrated positive correlations between parents and their biologic children and little or no correlation in body weight between adoptees and their adoptive parents.[63, 73] An estimated 25% of all obesity is linked to genetic factors.[9]

A "thrifty gene" theory has been proposed as one possible expression of obesity. A thrifty metabolism is described as having high metabolic efficiency, meaning that a higher proportion of excess calories is stored as fat, better equipping the individual to withstand starvation, or dieting.[24] When overfed, lean individuals gain a higher proportion of lean body mass. The amount of lean body mass is a major determinant of basal metabolic rate.[25]

BROWN ADIPOSE TISSUE. Brown adipose tissue is a richly innervated, highly vascular tissue possessing metabolic activity through its mitochondria. This tissue has a high capacity for heat production and is involved in thermogenesis. Most fat in the human body does not possess metabolic activity, functioning instead as a storage depot. During periods of overconsumption, often called "luxus consumption," brown adipose tissue may be involved in the increased rate of heat production seen in lean individuals.[38] Brown adipose tissue is controlled by the sympathetic nervous system. Under conditions of overconsumption, failure to stimulate brown adipose tissue results in the storage of excess calories as fat rather than in their release as heat.[38] An estimated 50 g of brown adipose tissue could increase energy turnover by 10% to 15%.[71] Research is focusing on pharmacologic agents that can activate brown fat.[38]

Another facet of thermogenesis is the thermic effect of food- or diet-induced thermogenesis. When food is eaten, the basal metabolic rate rises, and calorie expenditure can be 10% to 15% of the meal. The thermic effect of food is blunted in formerly obese individuals and may contribute to the regaining of lost weight.[38]

SET-POINT THEORY. The set-point theory of obesity implies that body weight, like body temperature, is regulated at a physiologically, possibly genetically, predetermined level. Obesity can be defined in this context as a regulation at an elevated set point.[45] In normal starvation, a decrease in metabolic rate accompanies restricted intake. Obese individuals decrease metabolic rate accordingly but exhibit minimum weight loss, indicating a physiologic process that appears to be defending the current weight.[44] Interventions in individuals with regulated body weight at a higher level may prove disappointing to client and practitioner alike.[86] Methods to alter set point are not proven to work.

ENZYME ACTIVITY: CONTROL OF LIPOLYSIS. Lipoprotein lipase is the enzyme that facilitates the removal of lipids from the blood. Lipoprotein lipase hydrolyzes triglyceride into FFAs and glycerol. The FFAs enter the fat cell and are reesterified. Lipoprotein lipase activity increases during periods of weight gain in all individuals. However, after weight reduction in the obese, lipoprotein lipase activity remains elevated and may contribute to the rapid regaining of weight often seen after dieting attempts.[21]

Adenyl cyclase also stimulates lipolysis, but within the cell. It increases FFA concentration. This, in turn, decreases hepatic clearance of insulin.[59] The activity of adenyl cyclase is greater in abdominal depots than in gluteal fat and may contribute to the health risks associated with obesity by hyperinsulinemia.

UNIQUE ROLE OF INSULIN. The major health risks of obesity, such as cardiovascular disease, hypertension, noninsulin dependent diabetes mellitus, and cancer, are generally ascribed to obesity. Excess body weight, or increasing body mass index, has been the major determinant of risk. However, upper body obesity, known as android obesity, is now considered a better predictor of risk, especially cardiovascular risk, than body weight alone.[42] Lower body obesity, or *gynoid* obesity, is an overall health risk but is not seen as a risk factor. Figure 12-5 provides a nomogram for calculating the waist-to-hip ratio used in determining upper body versus lower body obesity. Table 12-14 compares the general features of android versus gynoid obesity.

Obesity is often accompanied by an increase in beta-cell secretion, peripheral resistance to insulin, and resultant hyperinsulinemia. Hyperinsulinemia may precede the development of obesity and be a cause rather than a

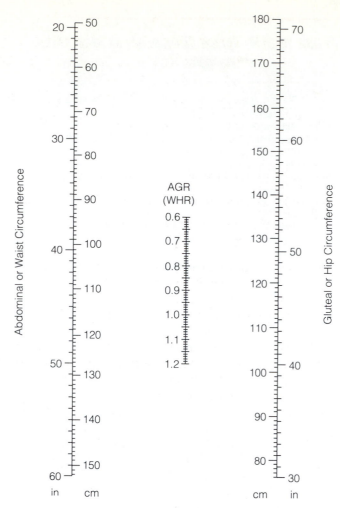

FIGURE 12-5 *The abdominal (waist) and gluteal (hips) ratio (AGR) can be determined by placing a straight edge between the column for waist circumference and reading the ratio from the point where this straight edge crosses the AGR, or waist-hips ratio (WHR), line. The waist or abdominal circumference is the smallest circumference below the rib cage and above the umbilicus, and the hips or gluteal circumference is the largest circumference at the posterior extension of the buttocks. (From: Bray, G.A., and Gray, D.S. Obesity, Part I: Pathogenesis. West. J. Med. 149:429, 1988.)*

consequence. Hyperinsulinemia is responsible for the "deadly quartet": upper body obesity, glucose intolerance, hypertriglyceridemia, and hypertension.[43] Research over the last decade has focused on the link between android obesity and hyperinsulinemia and the increased risk of diabetes, hypertriglyceridemia, lowered high density lipoprotein (HDL) levels, hypertension, and coronary artery disease.[3, 22, 50, 53, 67, 72, 77] The proposed mechanism is dependent on the evidence suggesting that abdominal fat is more metabolically active than peripheral or gluteal fat. Increases in adenyl cyclase in the cell and lipoprotein lipase in the blood allow an increase in FFA concentration, which decreases hepatic clearance of insulin. This coupled with a positive energy balance and increasing levels of plasma-free testosterone (android) yields a cascade effect, with hyperinsulinemia

TABLE 12-14 *Terms for the Two Different Distributions of Body Fat*

Android	Gynoid
Upper body	Lower body
Apple	Pear
Abdominal	Visceral, gluteal, femoral
Central	Peripheral
Subscapular skinfold thickness >25	Subscapular skinfold thickness <25
Waist-to-hip girth ratio >0.85	Waist-to-hip girth ratio <0.85

as the end result (Flowchart 12-2). Therefore, many of the generalized overall health risks of obesity may be attributed to hyperinsulinemia.[47]

Management of upper-body obesity may differ from conventional treatment of obesity. Diet therapy for obese individuals usually consists of a traditional high-carbohydrate, low-fat diet. However, persons with upper-body obesity, hyperinsulinemia, and hypertension may require lower carbohydrate and higher unsaturated fat diets, because a high-carbohydrate diet may exacerbate hyperinsulinemia.[59] Hypertensive, hyperinsulinemic persons should be treated cautiously with diuretics and beta blockers, because these medications can worsen glucose tolerance.[19]

Inactivity

Inactivity, or lack of exercise, contributes to the development and maintenance of obesity. Television watching has been positively correlated with the development of obesity in children. The prevalence of obesity increases 2% per each hour of daily television viewing.[18] Although obese individuals use more calories per any given activity, most obese individuals choose to be less active compared with their lean counterparts.

Benefits of exercise for obese individuals include an increase in metabolically active lean body mass, decrease in hunger, increase in basal metabolic rate, and decrease in insulin levels. Cardiovascular endurance improves, and HDL cholesterol levels may rise with exercise. Exercise should be strongly encouraged as an adjunct to weight control.

Besides exercise, traditional management of obesity includes weight-loss diets and behavior modification. Other options include surgery for severe obesity and pharmacologic interventions.

Complications of Obesity

Multiple medical and psychologic complications have been related to obesity. It has been associated with increased risk for diabetes mellitus, hypertension, stroke, heart and respiratory failure, liver and kidney problems, arthritis, thromboembolism, GI disorders, and even reproductive dysfunction (Fig. 12-6).

ANOREXIA NERVOSA

Definition and Incidence

Anorexia nervosa is an eating disorder considered to be a psychologic disorder with physiologic manifestations. It is characterized by 1) a relentless pursuit of thinness that does not diminish as weight loss progresses; 2) disturbed body image; and 3) amenorrhea. To the affected individual, the eating pattern and weight loss are not viewed as

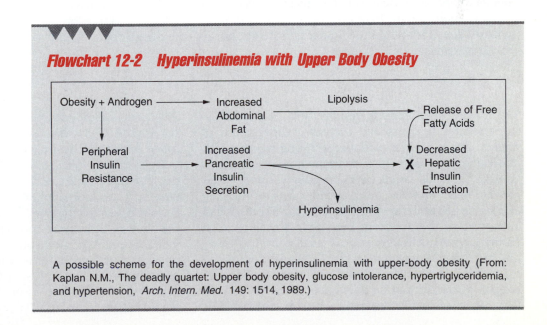

Flowchart 12-2   Hyperinsulinemia with Upper Body Obesity

A possible scheme for the development of hyperinsulinemia with upper-body obesity (From: Kaplan N.M., The deadly quartet: Upper body obesity, glucose intolerance, hypertriglyceridemia, and hypertension, *Arch. Intern. Med.* 149: 1514, 1989.)

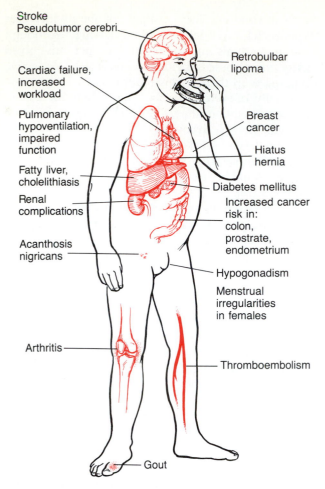

Stroke
Pseudotumor cerebri

Retrobulbar
lipoma

Cardiac failure,
increased
workload

Pulmonary
hypoventilation,
impaired
function

Breast
cancer

Hiatus
hernia

Fatty liver,
cholelithiasis

Diabetes mellitus

Renal
complications

Increased cancer
risk in:
colon,
prostrate,
endometrium

Acanthosis
nigricans

Hypogonadism

Menstrual
irregularities
in females

Arthritis

Thromboembolism

Gout

FIGURE 12-6 *Complications associated with obesity.*

BOX 12-4 ▼ *Diagnostic Criteria for Anorexia Nervosa*

▼ Refusal to maintain body weight over a minimal normal weight for age and height, eg, weight loss leading to maintenance of body weight 15% below that expected; or failure to make expected weight gain during period of growth, leading to body weight 15% below that expected

▼ Intense fear of gaining weight or becoming fat, even though underweight

▼ Disturbance in the way in which one's body weight, size, or shape is experienced, eg, the person claims to "feel fat" even when emaciated, believes that one area of the body is "too fat" even when obviously underweight

▼ In females, absence of at least three consecutive menstrual cycles when otherwise expected to occur (primary or secondary amenorrhea) (A woman is considered to have amenorrhea if her periods occur only following hormone, eg, estrogen, administration)

American Psychiatric Association. *Diagnostic and Statistical Manual of Mental Disorders III-R*. Washington, D.C.: American Psychiatric Association, 1987.

abnormal. Although anorexia has been recognized since the Middle Ages, the psychogenesis of the disorder has changed in modern times. Currently, weight control is seen as a form of self-control. The disorder affects primarily women, and the frequency of anorexia is approximately 1% to 3% in the United States.[37] The diagnostic criteria are presented in Box 12-4.

Etiology

The etiology of anorexia is multifactorial. Societal pressures toward thinness and increased expectations of women are possible explanations. Young women with anorexia are usually from enmeshed, or overly close, families.[46] Family conflicts go unresolved and feelings are repressed. Mothers are often viewed as overbearing and fathers as underinvolved. Hence, the anorectic can be viewed as the symptom bearer for a dysfunctional family. Persons with anorexia are usually overachievers and are thought of as the "perfect little girl." Although many women in our culture are preoccupied with weight, anorectics can be differentiated on the basis of their sense of ineffectiveness, lack of personal fulfill-

ment, interpersonal distress, and fear of maturity.[37] Female athletes are subjected to weight expectations and are more prone to develop eating disorders.

Behavioral disturbances seen in anorectics mimic those exhibited in persons undergoing simple starvation. In landmark research, Keys described a "starvation syndrome" in which healthy young male volunteers were put on restrictive diets for several months. Subjects in this study developed a preoccupation with food and food preparation as well as elaborate food rituals. Cognitively, the men experienced difficulty with decision making and decreased alertness. Socially, the subjects withdrew from group activities and became isolated and depressed and experienced a decrease in sex drive.[46] These biologic effects of starvation are also seen in anorectics. This underscores the importance of weight loss in the development of symptoms seen in anorexia.

Medical Complications

The medical complications of anorexia are dependent on the variant of the disease manifested. Clinically, two major variants exist: "restrictors," who control weight through caloric restriction alone, and "bulimic anorectics," who alternate calorie restriction with binging and purging.[54] An estimated 30% to 50% of anorectics use various purging behaviors.[75] Medical complications are most severe in bulimic anorectics.[34] The mortality rate for both variants of the disorder are as high as 20%.[36] The physical signs and symptoms associated with anorexia are summarized in Box 12-5. (Figure 12-7 illustrates the complications that are associated with both types of anorexia.)

BOX 12-5 ▼ Physical, Mental, and Behavioral Signs and Symptoms of Anorexia

Physical Symptoms
▼ Extreme weight loss and muscle wasting (anorexics may lose 25% of their body weight over a period of months); bulimics experience weight fluctuations, but may appear normal weight
▼ Arrested sexual development, amenorrhea
▼ Dry, yellow skin related to the release of carotenes as fat stores are burned for energy
▼ Loss of hair or change in hair texture
▼ Pain on touch
▼ Hypotension, bradycardia
▼ Anemia
▼ Constipation
▼ Severe sleep disturbances, insomnia
▼ Dental caries and periodontal disease

Mental and Behavioral Symptoms
▼ Bizarre eating habits, refusal to eat
▼ Feelings of failure, low self-esteem, social isolation
▼ Perfectionist, overachiever
▼ Preoccupation with food, dieting, and death
▼ Intense fear of becoming fat that does not lessen with weight loss
▼ Distorted body image and denial of eating disorder
▼ Frantic pursuit of exercise
▼ Frequent weighing
▼ Use of laxatives, diuretics, emetics, and diet pills
▼ Manipulative behavior

(Dudek, S. G. *Nutrition Handbook for Nursing Practice* [2nd ed.]. Philadelphia: J.B. Lippincott, 1993.)

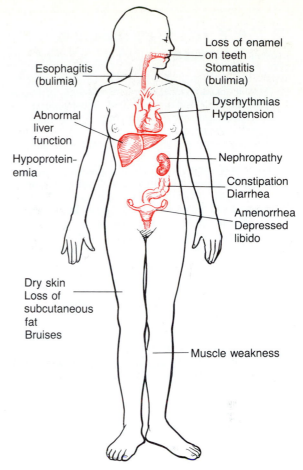

FIGURE 12-7 Complications associated with both types of anorexia nervosa.

RESTRICTORS: COMPLICATIONS OF SEMISTARVATION. Cardiac abnormalities account for most deaths associated with anorexia. Reductions in cardiac muscle mass, decrease in cardiac chamber size, and alterations in myocardial contractility have been documented.[30] Clinical presentation includes hypotension, sinus bradycardia, and abnormal exercise tolerance.[68] Overzealous nutritional repletion may precipitate congestive heart failure. Refeeding edema is associated with an increase in intracellular and extracellular volume and heart failure. Decreased basal metabolic rate and subnormal body temperature are associated features of starvation. Consequently, resting caloric expenditure can decrease to approximately half normal.[76] This is a compensatory mechanism to preserve physiologic functioning, although at a lowered rate. Therefore, refeeding chronically starved individuals requires a conservative intake of calories at approximately 75% of basal requirements.[14] Clinicians faced with a cachectic client often begin parenteral dextrose solutions either alone or as part of a total parenteral nutrition program. These solutions cause an increase in

insulin production by the beta cell. Increasing levels of insulin force phosphate into the cell, resulting in hypophosphatemia. Phosphate participates in many enzymatic reactions as either adenosine triphosphate or 2,3-diphosphoglycerate. Profound muscular weakness and progressive encephalopathy, coma, and death may develop. Hematologic disturbances associated with hypophosphatemia include hemolytic anemia and impaired leukocyte and thrombocyte function. Although the ideal form of nutritional repletion needs to be delineated for anorectics, care should be given to not increase feeding too rapidly and to monitor electrolyte disturbances. Recommended weight gain per day should not exceed one-quarter to one-half pound per day.[14]

METABOLIC DISTRUBANCES. Metabolic findings in anorexia are similar to those seen in starvation (Box 12-6). Restrictors normally experience a "fixed hypoglycemia" secondary to ketoadaptation and adequate glucogenic substrates. As weight loss progresses to a critical point, fat reserves are exhausted and gluconeogenic precursors

BOX 12-6 ▼ Laboratory Findings in Anorexia Nervosa

Chemical/Metabolic

Normal results on most laboratory tests early in process

Elevated BUN levels, secondary to dehydration; decreased glomerular filtration rate

Hypercarotenemia

Elevated serum cholesterol levels (early; may decrease later)

Decreased transferrin, associated anemia (usually normal protein and albumin-globulin ratio); low complement, fibrinogen, and prealbumin

Elevated serum lactic dehydrogenase and alkaline phosphatase (possibly related to growth)

Depressed phosphorus level (a late and ominous sign); depressed magnesium and calcium levels (calcium may be elevated)

Possible depression of plasma-zinc, urinary zinc, and urinary copper levels

Fixed hypoglycemia, possible hypoglycemic coma

Negative nitrogen balance

Elevated uric acid

Endocrine

Low leutinizing hormone (LH); low or pseudo-normal follicle-stimulating hormone (FSH); deficiency of gonadotropin-releasing hormone (GnRH); normal prolactin; low testosterone in men and low estradiol in women

Elevated circulating cortisol (normal production; does not suppress with dexamethasone)

Low normal fasting glucose (increased insulin binding by red blood cells and growth hormone deficiency reported)

Low normal thyroxine (T_4); reduced triiodothyronine (T_3); elevated reverse T_3; normal TSH

Possible elevation of parathyroid hormone (PTH) secondary to hypomagnesemia with resultant hypercalcemia

Elevated resting growth hormone levels

Hematologic

Leukopenia with relative lymphocytoses (bone marrow hypoplasia), absolute lymphopenia

Thrombocytopenia

Very low erythrocyte sedimentation rate, almost always

Anemia late (especially with rehydration)

Adapted from Comerci, G. D. Medical complications of anorexia nervosa and bulimia nervosa. *Med. Clin. N. Am.* 74(5):1293, 1990.

---

body fat contributes to amenorrhea. Lack of estrogen, cortisol excess, and malnutrition are central to the pathogenesis of the bone disease exhibited in women with the disorder. In most women, the onset of the disorder occurs before peak bone mass is achieved (approximately age 24). Therefore, the prolonged duration of amenorrhea increases the severity of osteopenia.[4] Increased exercise may increase the risk of pathologic fractures. Osteonecrosis and femoral head collapse have also been reported.[81]

GI DISORDERS. GI disorders are often presented as a reason to eliminate certain foods from the diet. Nausea, epigastric pain, bloating, flatus, and early satiety are common complaints in anorexia. Gastric emptying time is often delayed but is secondary to decrease in food intake and subsequent malnutrition. As gradual refeeding commences, emptying time improves and normalization occurs while body mass index is still subnormal.[74]

NEUROPATHY. Chronic malnutrition contributes to the development of peripheral neuropathy. Compression neuropathies may also develop due to excessive loss of supportive subcutaneous tissue.[52]

BULIMIA

Definition and Incidence

Bulimia, meaning "ox hunger," is a disorder of weight maintenance characterized by a preoccupation with weight, an increased interest in dieting, and ultimate control of weight through caloric restriction alternating with binge eating and purging. Purging is generally accomplished through vomiting, laxative abuse, and/or diuretic abuse. Other purgatives include syrup of ipecac, milk in the lactose intolerant, sorbitol, and a decrease in insulin in insulin-dependent diabetics.[61] Actual incidence of bulimia is controversial, but estimates are that 4% to 10% of adolescents and young women are affected.[89] It is a disorder almost exclusively confined to women. Affected males are generally those who pursue interests or careers in which body image and weight are of paramount importance, such as wrestlers, jockeys, and dancers. Most of the women are from the upper socioeconomic classes. The age of onset is generally in the late teens. A bulimic episode is considered an "out-of-control" experience, and the food consumed is deemed excessive. The average calories consumed during a binge are 500 to 10,000. Foods chosen are high in calories, nondietetic, and easily consumed. Unlike anorectics, affected persons are aware that the eating habits are abnormal but are unable to stop.[62] Shame and secrecy accompany this disorder and prevent appropriate diagnosis and treatment. Box 12-7 lists the diagnostic criteria for bulimia.

---

are diminished. Profound hypoglycemia and hypoglycemic coma may develop. Hence, severe hypoglycemia represents a grave prognosis, and prompt medical treatment is warranted.[64] Elevation in uric acid may be present and also can serve as an index of severity. Strenuous exercise, starvation, alcohol consumption, and thiazide diuretics contribute to hyperuricemia.[32]

ENDOCRINE ABNORMALITIES. Hypogonadism is a characteristic feature of anorexia, and loss of needed

BOX 12-7 ▼ Diagnostic Criteria for Bulimia Nervosa

▼ Recurrent episodes of binge eating (rapid consumption of a large amount of food in a discrete period of time)

▼ A feeling of lack of control over eating behavior during the eating binges

▼ Engagement in either self-induced vomiting, use of laxatives or diuretics, strict dieting or fasting, or vigorous exercise to prevent weight gain

▼ A minimum average of two binge eating episodes a week for at least 3 months

▼ Persistent overconcern with body shape and weight

American Psychiatric Association, *Diagnostic and Statistical Manual of Mental Disorders III-R*. Washington, D.C.: American Psychiatric Association, 1987.

Etiology

The psychogenesis of bulimia is complex. Bulimia is considered a "disorder of maturation" and usually occurs at a time of separation from home or loved ones. It signals difficulty in making the transition from adolescence to young adulthood.[85] As with anorexia, increased societal expectations of women, difficulty in defining the female role, and a desire for thinness are central to the development of the disorder. Family or individual history is often significant for affective disorders, such as depression.[51] Childhood sexual abuse, once considered more common in bulimic women than in the general population, is present approximately 30% of the time, similar to the incidence in the general population.[10, 15] As opposed to the anorectic's family, families of bulimic women often exhibit overt conflict and less cohesion. Bulimic women sense greater neglect and rejection. Mothers are disengaged or distant from their daughters. Daughters, in turn, feel anxious and disorganized.[87]

Dieting initiates the disorder; however, the maintenance of the disorder is attributed to the new role binging and purging takes on. The rapid consumption of large amounts of food followed by purging functions to reduce anxiety. Therefore, anxiety reduction contributes to the continuance of the bulimic behavior.[87]

Medical Complications

Medical complications are common and may produce lasting effects or even death. Some of the more common complications are discussed below.

ELECTROLYTE ABNORMALITIES: EFFECTS OF LAXATIVES, DIURETICS, AND VOMITING. Electrolyte disturbances are a common manifestation in bulimic anorec-

tics and bulimics and are dependent on the purgative method used.

Hypokalemia is a common and dangerous electrolyte disturbance. Continual vomiting and laxative and diuretic abuse precipitate hypokalemia, because 80% of body potassium is excreted in the urine and 20% in the feces.[17]

Other causative factors in the development of hypokalemia include decreased plasma volume, metabolic alkalosis, and coexisting magnesium deficiency.[35] Chronic laxative abuse may produce nephropathy and a urine concentration deficit. The resultant polyuria and hypovolemia result in hyperaldosteronism and the development of edema.[84]

Chronic laxative abuse affects GI and renal functioning and, therefore, affects the development of electrolyte abnormalities. GI effects include atrophy of smooth muscle, progressive loss of innervation, and decrease in colonic neurons. Cathartic colon, a permanent alteration in bowel function, may result in severe constipation as well as GI bleeding. Anemia, steatorrhea, and protein-losing enteropathy may be present. Effects on the renal system include dehydration and sodium loss. Hyponatremia stimulates the renin aldosterone system, resulting in sodium and fluid retention and hypokalemia. Abrupt cessation of laxatives promotes secondary hyperaldosteronism, and peripheral edema results. Weaning from laxatives prevents rapid weight gain, reduces anxiety, and decreases the likelihood of returning to laxatives.[83] Diarrhea from laxative abuse causes electrolyte abnormalities but does not cause a significant malabsorption of calories. Ingestion of 50 laxative tablets results in a calorie loss of only 12%, indicating that 88% of the calories from the binge have been absorbed. Therefore, laxative abuse is an ineffective method of weight control.[6, 58]

Acid–base disturbances occur in bulimia secondary to the purgative method used. Metabolic alkalosis is the most common. Loss of hydrogen ions in vomiting and in diuretic abuse leads to an increase in plasma bicarbonate, contributing to alkalosis. Metabolic acidosis can occur during the starvation or restricting phase, in which ketoacids are being used as a primary energy source. Additionally, laxative abuse causes a profound bicarbonate loss and leads to metabolic acidosis. Flowchart 12-3 illustrates the electrolyte/acid–base abnormalities seen in eating disorders. The physical signs and symptoms associated with bulimia are summarized in Box 12-8.

ENDOCRINE ABNORMALITIES. The endocrine disturbances in bulimia are not clearly defined or understood. Endocrine dysfunction exists and may be related to poor nutritional intake or starvation during the restricting phase.[56] Menstrual and ovulatory disturbances occur in normal-weight bulimics, and the etiology is unknown.[11]

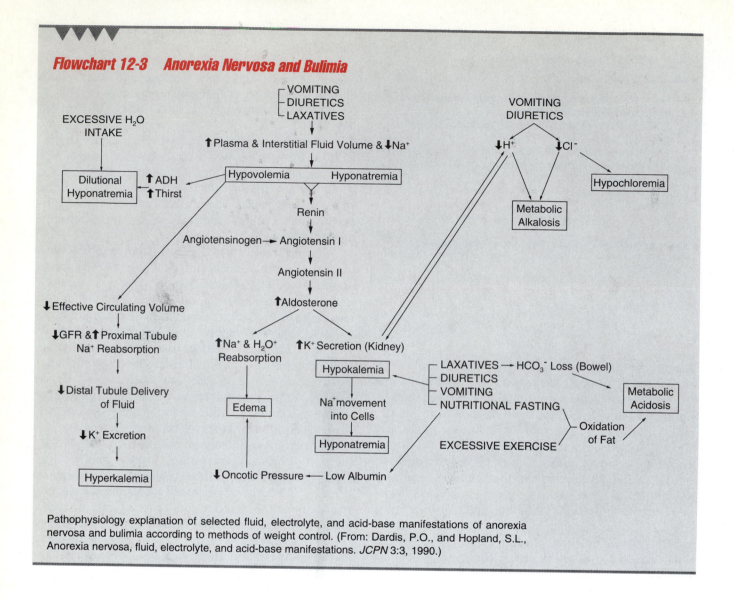

Flowchart 12-3   Anorexia Nervosa and Bulimia

Pathophysiology explanation of selected fluid, electrolyte, and acid-base manifestations of anorexia nervosa and bulimia according to methods of weight control. (From: Dardis, P.O., and Hopland, S.L., Anorexia nervosa, fluid, electrolyte, and acid-base manifestations. *JCPN* 3:3, 1990.)

UPPER GI DISORDERS. Dysphagia may develop in bulimics secondary to a poor or absent pharyngeal gag reflex and increased duration of dry swallow. The defect in swallowing may be attributed to desensitization from prolonged vomiting as well as being a learned response.[65] Bulimics often have increased stomach capacity due to repeated binging, but gastric emptying time may be increased or normal.[28,41] Gastric rupture and esophageal tears are the most severe form of upper GI disorders.

ORAL DISORDERS. In bulimic anorectics and bulimics who vomit, enamel erosion is the most common oral disorder. Other oral abnormalities include dentin hypersensitivity, caries, xerostomia, parotid gland enlargement, and periodontal disease. The low pH of vomitus is the major cause. Postvomiting rinsing with tap water may contribute to oral disease, because it reduces the buffering capacity of saliva.[1] Due to the secretive nature

of bulimia, oral disorders may provide the first diagnostic clue to health professionals, particularly the dental hygienist and dentist.

DERMATOLOGIC COMPLAINTS. Bulimics often exhibit a fine dry rash on the hands secondary to dehydration. Calluses on the knuckles may be present when the fingers are used for vomiting.

NUTRITIONAL DEFICIENCIES OF ANOREXIA NERVOSA AND BULIMIA

The nutritional deficiencies exhibited in persons with eating disorders are many and varied. Chronic protein deficiency, hypoalbuminemia, and negative nitrogen balance are seen in anorectics and bulimics.[39] Vitamin deficiencies, especially water-soluble vitamins, can be evidenced by angular stomatitis, mucosal ulcers, and

BOX 12-8 ▼ Physical Symptoms and Signs in Bulimia Nervosa

Presenting Physical Symptoms
Weight may be normal, overweight, or underweight
Complaints of bloating, diarrhea, swelling
Hyperactivity (mental and motor); exceptions common
Constant or extreme thirst and increased urination (hypokalemic nephropathy-hypovolemia)
May present with depression, anxiety, despair, and suicidal ideation

Physical Signs
Usually well groomed and good hygiene; definite exceptions, especially patients with a severe character disorder or chronic addictive conditions
Usually normal weight or mild to moderate obesity (exception: food restrictors or anorexia nervosa patients with associated bulimia, vomiting, purging)
Generalized or localized edema at lower extremities (compensatory renal retention of sodium and water, ie, hypovolemia with secondary hyperaldosteronism or pseudo-Bartter's syndrome)
Physical findings of extreme weight loss (self-starvation) if bulimia, vomiting, and purging are complications of anorexia nervosa or food restriction
Loss of scalp hair, skin changes of anorexia nervosa
Amenorrhea, effects of estrogen deficiency
Hypothermia
Swelling of parotid and other salivary glands, hyperamylasemia
Dental enamel dysplasia and discoloration due to gastric juices (vomiting)
Bruises and lacerations of palate and posterior pharynx; lesions of fingernails, fingers, and dorsum of hand(s) (due to self-induced vomiting)
Pyorrhea and other gum disorders
Diminished reflexes, muscle weakness, paralysis, and, infrequently, peripheral neuropathy with muscle weakness and paralysis
Muscle cramping (with induced hypoxia or positive Trousseau's sign)
Signs of hypokalemia (cardiac dysrhythmias, hypotension, decreased cardiac output, weak pulse, poor-quality heart sounds, abdominal distention, ileus, acute gastric dilatation, myopathy, shortness of breath, depression, and mental clouding)
Cardiomyopathy secondary to ipecac poisoning

Modified from Comerci, G. D. Medical complications of anorexia nervosa and bulimia nervosa. *Med. Clin. N. Am.* 74(5):1293, 1990.

hair loss.[34] Zinc and copper deficiency is commonly seen in restrictors and bulimics and may impair appetite regulation. Deficiency of zinc results in altered taste acuity, altered taste sensitivity, and impairment in the sense of smell.

Zinc deficiency may contribute to the chronicity of eating disorders. It develops secondary to poor intake, impaired absorption, and the consumption of low-zinc foods during a binge.[40]

CASE STUDY 12-1

Mr. Wainwright is a 5'10", 185-lb. construction worker. He was admitted to the hospital after a fall from a scaffolding. He sustained a broken femur, radius, and two broken ribs and has internal bleeding. On day 10 of a complicated hospitalization, his albumin level is 2.0 g/dL and his weight is 162 lb. He has been maintained on D_5W as his only caloric source, and he has received only clear liquids orally.

1. *What form of malnutrition does Mr. W have?*
2. *Describe the pathophysiologic consequences of this form of malnutrition.*
3. *What degree of protein depletion is indicated in the above data?*
4. *Compare the clinical manifestations of this form of malnutrition with other forms of malnutrition.*
5. *When nutritional support is initiated, what serum protein is the most sensitive marker of repletion? What nutritional support should be used to restore Mr. W's nutritional status?*

See Appendix G for discussion.

▼ Chapter Summary

▼ The macronutrients required to sustain life are carbohydrates, proteins, and fats, which are used for energy production and anabolic processes. The dietary supply of these nutrients provides the resources for plasma proteins, defensive cells, and the enzymatic reactions of metabolism. Fat intake is essential for energy resources, insulation, hormone substrate, and other essential functions.

▼ The micronutrients include the water- and fat-soluble vitamins as well as the minerals that are essential in cell function. Each micronutrient has a specific function and is made available through the diet.

▼ Malnutrition is a condition of inadequate intake of macronutrients or micronutrients. Protein–calorie malnutrition is common in hospitalized patients. Malnutrition may affect only protein stores ("kwashiorkor") or may be caused by poor intake and is termed "marasmus." During starvation, the basal metabolic demands of the body are decreased to conserve energy. The stress of illness increases the need for nutrients, and these may not be provided in the diet or intravenous fluids.

▼ Obesity is the most common nutritional disorder in the United States. It is a growing problem among children and adults alike. Causes of obesity are multiple and include excessive intake and genetic influences. Other theories are being investigated, including the type of adipose tissue, the set-point theory, and the control of lipolysis. Obesity is also closely related to lack of exercise and level of fitness.

▼ Anorexia nervosa and bulimia are considered to have a psychological basis. The etiology of these conditions varies, but the result is an imposed nutritional deficiency that may be manifested by semistarvation or major pathologic disruptions.

▼ *References*

1. Altshuler, B.D., Dechow, P.C., Waller, P.A., and Hardy, B.W. An investigation of the oral pathologies occurring in bulimia nervosa. *Intl. J. Eating Disorders* 9:191, 1990.
2. Bang, H.O., et al. The composition of the Eskimo food in northwestern Greenland. *Am. J. Clin. Nutr.* 33:2657, 1980.
3. Baumgartner, R.M., Roche, A.F., Chumlea, W.C., Survogel, R.M., and Gevech, C.J. Fatness and fat patterns: Associations with plasma lipids and blood pressures in adults, 18 to 57 years of age. *Am. J. Epidemiol.* 126:614, 1987.
4. Biller, B.M.K. Mechanism of osteoporosis in adult and adolescent women with anorexia nervosa. *J. Clin. Endocrinol. Metab.* 68:548, 1989.
5. Blundell, J.E. Appetite disturbance and the problems of overweight. *Drugs* (39 Suppl.) 3:1, 190.
6. Bo-Linn, G.W., et al. Purging and caloric absorption in bulimic patients and normal women. *Ann. Intern. Med.* 99:14, 1983.
7. Bray, G.A., York, D.A., and Fisher, J.S. Experimental obesity: A homeostatic failure due to defective nutrient stimulation of the sympathetic nervous system. *Vitamins and Hormones* 45:1, 1989.
8. Bray, G.A. Obesity. In M.L. Brown (ed.), *Present Knowledge in Nutrition* (6th ed.). Washington, D.C.: Internal Life Sciences Institute, Nutrition Foundation, 1990.
9. Bray, G.A., and Gray, D.S. Obesity Part I: Pathogenesis. *West. J. Med.* 149:429, 1988.
10. Bulik, C.M., Sullivan, P.F., and Rorty, M. Childhood sexual abuse in women with bulimia. *J. Clin. Psychol.* 50(12):460, 1989.
11. Cantopher, T., Evans, C., Lacey, J.H., and Pearce, J.M. Menstrual and ovulatory disturbances in bulimia. *Br. Med. J.* 297:836, 1988.
12. Centers for Disease Control, Division of Nutrition, Center for Health Promotion and Education. Evaluation of consumer complaints related to aspartame use. *Morbid. Mortal. Weekly Rep.* 33:605, 1990.
13. Clydesdale, F.M. The relevance of mineral chemistry to bioavailability. *Nutr. Today* pp. 23–27, March/April 1989.
14. Comerci, G.D. Medical complications of anorexia nervosa and bulimia. *Med. Clin. N. Am.* 74(5):1293, 1990.
15. Conners, M.E., and Morse, W. Sexual abuse and eating disorders. *Int. J. Eat. Disord.* 13:1, 1993.
16. Daly, J.M., et al. Immune and metabolic effects of arginine in the surgical patient. *Ann. Surg.* 208:512, 1988.
17. Dardis, P.O., and Hofland, S.L. Anorexia nervosa: Fluid and electrolyte and acid base manifestations. *J. Child Adolesc. Psychol. Mental Health Nurs.* 3(3):85, 1990.
18. Dietz, L., and Gortmaker, S.L. Do we fatten our children at the television set? Obesity and television in children and adolescents. *Pediatrics* 75:807, 1985.
19. Dornhorst, A., Powell, S.H., and Pensky, J. Aggravation by propranolol of hyperglycemic effect of hydrochlorothiazide in type II diabetics without alteration of insulin secretion. *Hypertension* 11:244, 1985.
20. Doweiko, J.P., and Nompleggi, D.J. The role of albumin in human physiology and pathophysiology, Part III: Albumin and disease states. *JPEN* 15(4):476, 1991.
21. Elliot, D.L., et al. Obesity: Pathophysiology and practical management. *J. Gen. Int. Med.* 2:188, 1987.
22. Ferrarinini, E., et al. Insulin resistance in essential hypertension. *N. Engl. J. Med.* 317:350, 1987.
23. Food and Drug Administration. *Cancer Assessment Committee Report*. Washington, D.C.: U.S. Government Printing Office, FDA Docket No. 82F-0320, 1984.
24. Forbes, G.B. Do obese individuals gain weight more easily than nonobese individuals? *Am. J. Clin. Nutr.* 52:224, 1990.
25. Forbes, G.B. Lean body mass–body fat interrelationships in humans. *Nutr. Rev.* 45:225, 1987.
26. Ganrow, J.S., and Webster, J. Quetelet's index (W/H²) as a measure of fatness. *Int. J. Obesity* 9:147, 1985.
27. Garattini, S., et al. Progress in assessing the role of serotonin in the control of food intake. *Clin. Neuropharmacol.* 2(Suppl. 1):8, 1988.
28. Geliebter, A., Melton, P.M., Roberts, D., McCray, R.S., Gage, D., and Haskim, S.A. The stomach's role in appetite regulation in bulimia. *Ann. N. Y. Acad. Sci.* 575:512, 1989.
29. Gibbs, J., and Smith, G.P. Satiety: The role of peptides from the stomach and the intestine. *Fed. Proc.* 45:1391, 1986.
30. Gottdiener, J.S., Gross, H.A., Henry, W.L., Borer, J.S., and Ebert, M.H. Effects of self induced starvation on cardiac size and function in anorexia nervosa. *Circulation* 58:425, 1978.
31. Grundy, S. Monounsaturated fatty acids, plasma cholesterol and coronary heart disease. *Am. J. Clin. Nutr.* 45:1168, 1987.
32. Gupta, M.A., and Kavanaugh-Danelon, D. Elevated serum uric acid in eating disorders: A possible index of strenuous physical activity and starvation. *Int. J. Eating Disorders* 8:463, 1989.
33. Guyton, A. *Textbook of Medical Physiology* (8th ed.) Philadelphia: W.B. Saunders, 1991.
34. Hall, R.C.W., and Beresford, T.P. Medical complications of anorexia and bulimia. *Psychol. Med.* 7:165, 1989.
35. Hall, R.C., et al. Refractory hypokalemia secondary to hypomagnesemia in eating disorders patients. *Psychosomatics* 29(4):435, 1988.
36. Halmi, K. Anorexia nervosa: Demographic and clinical features in 94 cases. *Psychol. Med.* 36:18, 1974.
37. Herzog, D.B., and Copeland, P.M. Eating disorders. *N. Engl. J. Med.* 315:295, 1985.
38. Himms-Hajen, J. Brown adipose tissue thermogenesis and obesity. *Prog. Lipid Res.* 28:67, 1989.
39. Hooker, C., and Hall, R.C.W. Nutritional assessment of patients with anorexia and bulimia: Clinical and laboratory findings. *Psychol. Med.* 7(3):27, 1989.
40. Humphries, L., Vivian, B., Stuart, M., and McClain, C.J.

Zinc deficiency and eating disorders. *J. Clin. Psychol.* 50: 456, 1989.

41. Hutson, W.R., and Wald, A. Gastric emptying time in patients with bulimia nervosa. *Am. J. Gastroenterol.* 85:41, 1990.
42. Jointhorp, B. Obesity and adipose distribution as risk factors for the development of disease: A review. *Infusionstherapie* 17:24, 1990.
43. Kaplan, N.M. The deadly quartet: Upper body obesity, glucose intolerance, hypertriglyceridemia and hypertension. *Arch. Intern. Med.* 149:1514, 1989.
44. Keesey, R.E. The body weight set point: What can you tell your patients? *Postgrad. Med.* 83:114, 1988.
45. Keesey, R.E. A set point theory of obesity. In K.D. Brownell and J.P. Foreyt (eds.), *Handbook of Eating Disorders: Physiology, Psychology and Treatment of Obesity, Anorexia and Bulimia.* New York: Basic Books, 1986.
46. Keys, A., et al. *The Biology of Human Starvation.* Minneapolis: University of Minnesota Press, 1950.
47. Kissebah, A.H., Freedman, D.S., and Peiris, A.N. Health risk of obesity. *Med. Clin. N. Am.* 73:111, 1989.
48. Lands, W.E.M. Renewed questions about polyunsaturated fats. *Nutr. Rev.* 44:189, 1986.
49. Lanza, E., et al. Dietary fiber intake in the U.S. population. *Am. J. Clin. Nutr.* 46:790, 1987.
50. Lavaroni, I., et al. Risk factors for coronary artery disease in healthy persons with hyperinsulinemia and normal glucose tolerance. *N. Engl. J. Med.* 320:702, 1989.
51. Levy, A.B., Dixon, K.N., and Stern, S. How are depression and bulimia related? *Am. J. Psychol.* 146:162, 1989.
52. MacKenzie, J.R., La Ban, N.M., and Sacheyfio, A.H. The prevalence of peripheral neuropathy in patients with anorexia nervosa. *Arch. Phys. Med. Rehabil.* 70(12):827, 1989.
53. Maicardi, V., Camellini, L., Bellodi, G., Coscelli, C., and Ferramini, E. Evidence for an association of high blood pressure and hyperinsulinemia in obese man. *J. Clin. Endocrin. Metab.* 62:1302, 1986.
54. Mitchell, J.E. Medical complications of anorexia and bulimia. *Psychol. Med.* 1(3):229, 1984.
55. Morgan, B.L.G. Obesity. *Nutr. Health* 8:1, 1988.
56. Newman, M.M., and Halmi, K.A. The endocrinology of anorexia nervosa and bulimia nervosa. *Endocrinol. Metab. Clin. N. Am.* 17(1):195, 1988.
57. Nikkila, E.A., and Kekki, M. Effects of dietary fructose and sucrose on plasma triglyceride metabolism in patients with endogenous hypertriglyceridemia. *Acta. Med. Scand. Suppl.* 542:221, 1972.
58. Oster, J.R., Materson, B.J., and Rogers, A.I. Laxative abuse syndrome. *Am. J. Gastroenterol.* 74:451, 1980.
59. Peiris, A.N., Mueller, R.A., Smith, G.A., Struve, M.F., and Kissebah, A.H. Relationship of androgenic activity to splanchic insulin metabolism and peripheral glucose utilization in premenopausal women. *J. Clin. Endocrinol. Metab.* 64:162, 1986.
60. Peterson, H.R., et al. Body fat and the activity of the autonomic nervous system. *N. Engl. J. Med.* 318:1077, 1988.
61. Peveler, R.C., Fairburn, C.G., Boller, I. and Dunger, P. Eating disorders in adolescents with IDDM: A controlled study. *Diabetes Care* 15: 1356, 1992.
62. Pope, H.G., et al. Anorexia and bulimia among 300 female suburban shoppers. *Am. J. Psychol.* 141:292, 1984.
63. Price, R.A., and Stunkard, A.J. Comingling analysis of obesity in twins. *Hum. Hered.* 39:121, 1989.
64. Rich, L.M., Caine, M.R., Findling, J.W., and Shaker, J.L. Hypoglycemic coma in anorexia nervosa. Case report and review of the literature. *Arch. Intern. Med.* 150(4):894, 1990.
65. Roberts, M.W., et al. Dysphagia in bulimia nervosa. *Dysphagia* 4(2):106, 1989.
66. Rossow, J.E. Kwashiorkor in North America. *Am. J. Nutr.* 49:58, 1989.
67. Saad, M.F., Knowler, W.C., Pettitt, D.J., Nelson, R.G., Mott, D.M., and Bennett, P.H. Sequential changes in serum insulin concentration during development of non insulin dependent diabetes. *Lancet* 1:1356, 1989.
68. Schochen, D.D., Holloway, J.D., and Powers, P. Weight loss and the heart: Effects of anorexia nervosa and starvation. *Arch. Intern. Med.* 149:877, 1989.
69. Souba, W.W., Smith, R.J., and Wilmore, D.W. Glutamine metabolism by the intestinal tract. *JPEN* 9:608, 1985.
70. Stevens, J., et al. Comparison of the effects of psyllium and wheat bran on gastrointestinal transit time and stool characteristics. *J. Am. Diet. Assoc.* 88:323, 1988.
71. Stock, M.J. Thermogenesis and brown fat: Relevance to human obesity. *Infusionstherapie* 16:282, 1989.
72. Stout, R.W. Insulin and atheroma: 20 year perspective. *Diabetes Care* 13:631, 1990.
73. Stunkard, A.J., Foch, T.T., and Hrubec, Z. A twin study of human obesity. *JAMA* 256:51, 1986.
74. Szmukler, G.I., Young, G.P., Lichtenstein, M., and Andrew, J.T. A serial study of gastric emptying time in anorexia nervosa and bulimia. *Aust. N. Z. J. Med.* 20(3):220, 1990.
75. Vaisman, N., Corey, M., Rossie, M.F., et al. Changes in body composition during refeeding in patients with anorexia nervosa. *J. Pediatr.* 113(5):925, 1988.
76. Vaisman, N., et al. Energy expenditure and body composition in patients with anorexia nervosa. *J. Pediatr.* 113(5): 919, 1988.
77. Van Gaal, L.F., Vansant, G.A., and De Leeuw, I.H. Upper body obesity and the risk for atherosclerosis. *J. Am. Coll. Nutr.* 8:504, 1989.
78. Van Itallie, T.B. Health implications of overweight and obesity in the United States. *Ann. Intern. Med.* 103:983, 1985.
79. Vaselli, J.R., and Maggio, C.A. Mechanism of appetite and body-weight regulation. In F.T. Frankle and M.U. Yang (eds.), *Obesity and Weight Control.* Rockville, Md.: Aspen, 1988.
80. Vinik, A.I., and Jenkins, D.J.A. Dietary fiber in the management of diabetes. *Diabetes Care* 11:160, 1988.
81. Warren, M.P., et al. Femoral head collapse associated with anorexia nervosa in a 20 year old ballet dancer. *Clin. Orthop.* 251:171, 1990.
82. Whitney, E.N., Cataldo, C.B., and Rolfes, S.R. *Understanding Normal and Clinical Nutrition* (3rd ed.). St. Paul: West Publishing Co., 1991.
83. Willard, S.G., Winstead, D.K., Anding, R., and Dudley, P.

Laxative detoxification in bulimia nervosa. In W.G. Johnson (ed.), *Advances in Eating Disorders* (Vol. 2). Greenwich, Conn.: JAI Press, 1989.

84. Wolff, H.P., Vecsei, P., Kruch, R., et al. Psychiatric disturbance leading to potassium depletion, sodium depletion, raised plasma renin concentration and secondary hyper-aldosteronism. *Lancet* 1:257, 1968.

85. Wooley, S.C., and Kearney-Cooke, A. Intensive treatment of bulimia and body image disturbance. In K.D. Brownell and J. Foreyt (eds.), *Handbook of Eating Disorders*. New York: Basic Books, 1986.

86. Wooley, S.C., and Wooley, O.W. Should obesity be treated at all? In A.J. Stunkard and E. Stellar (eds.), *Eating and Its Disorders*. New York: Raven Press, 1984.

87. Yates, A. Current perspectives on eating disorders: I. History, psychological and biological aspects. *J. Am. Acad. Child Adolesc. Psychol.* 28:813, 1989.

88. Yokogoshi, H., Roberts, C.H., Caballero, B., and Wurtman, R.J. Effects of aspartame and glucose administration on brain and plasma levels of large neutral amino acids and brain 5- hydroxyindoles. *Am. J. Clin. Nutr.* 40:1, 1984.

89. Zuckerman, D., et al. Prevalence of bulimia among college students. *Am. J. Pub. Health* 76:1135, 1986.

Shock

Barbara L. Bullock

▼ **LEARNING OBJECTIVES**

1 *Discuss the physiologic mechanisms responsible for maintaining normal tissue perfusion.*
2 *Discuss compensatory responses to the shock state.*
3 *Describe the stages of shock.*
4 *List causes, indicators, and consequences of irreversible shock.*
5 *Identify the etiologies of shock relative to their designated classifications.*
6 *Differentiate among the pathologic processes associated with each classification of shock.*
7 *List and explain the basis for symptoms associated with each classification of shock.*
8 *Define* **toxic shock syndrome**.
9 *Explain the basis for the development of the complications of shock.*
10 *Describe multiple organ dysfunction syndrome.*

Barbara L. Bullock: PATHOPHYSIOLOGY: ADAPTATIONS AND ALTERATIONS IN FUNCTION, 4th ed.
© 1996 Lippincott-Raven Publishers

The occurrence of the shock state represents the most severe complication of a variety of diseases. It is a complex problem that causes multiorgan effects, and the etiology does not begin and end with a single pathophysiologic alteration. The interactions, including compensatory mechanisms, cause changes in volume, flow, and oxygen transport regardless of the initiating event. These changes are the main factors that lead to survival or circulatory failure and death.[19] Therapy can alter the interactions; however, it should address not only the primary insult but also the systemic effects of the insult. The physiology of tissue perfusion that underlies normal metabolism is reviewed in the first part of this chapter as a basis for understanding the alterations that occur when that balance is disturbed.

▼ Maintenance of Tissue Perfusion

Any discussion of the state of shock must be preceded by an overview of the physiologic mechanisms that maintain and regulate normal blood pressure (BP). Basically, blood pressure is the product of cardiac output (CO) times total peripheral resistance (TPR) and can be expressed by the equation $BP = CO \times TPR$. Any condition or derangement that increases or decreases either CO or TPR may raise or lower BP accordingly. Normally, alterations in BP due to an increase or decrease in either CO or TPR are transient and momentary in healthy persons. Because there is an inverse relationship between CO and TPR, an increase or decrease in one component prompts an opposite response in the other so that BP remains constant. For example, if CO decreases, TPR automatically increases and BP returns toward normal. The physiologic mechanisms responsible for activating this inverse relationship and maintaining BP are mostly generated by autonomic nervous system responses (see pp. 454–455).

CARDIAC OUTPUT

Cardiac output is defined as the volume or load of blood ejected by the left ventricle each minute. In the average-sized adult, this volume is approximately 5 liters. It is usually slightly less in females due primarily to lower body weight, size, or both. Cardiac output, although relatively consistent in most individuals, is not an absolute or constant value, because it may be influenced directly or indirectly by many factors. Cardiac output is the product of stroke volume (SV) times heart rate (HR) $(CO = SV \times HR)$. SV is that quantity of blood ejected by each ventricle with each cardiac contraction. It is determined or influenced by such factors as the volume (preload) and compliance, contractility, and afterload of the ventricles.[1] The relationship is shown in Flowchart 13-1.

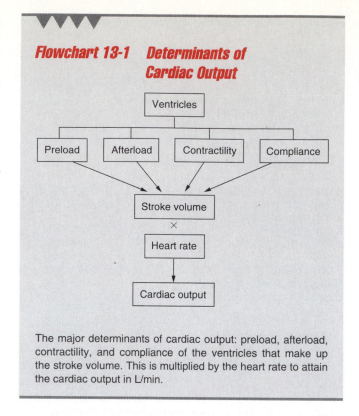

Flowchart 13-1 Determinants of Cardiac Output

The major determinants of cardiac output: preload, afterload, contractility, and compliance of the ventricles that make up the stroke volume. This is multiplied by the heart rate to attain the cardiac output in L/min.

Circulating blood volume with an adequate venous return plays an important role in determining stroke volume. Conditions that alter either atrial pressure, ventricular function, or venous return affect stroke volume and, consequently, cardiac output. If stroke volume increases or decreases, an automatic opposite response in heart rate serves to maintain constant cardiac output. For example, a decrease in venous return results in a decreased stroke volume, but cardiac output remains constant due to an increase in heart rate.

The second determinant of cardiac output is heart rate. Heart rate is mediated by autonomic nervous system (parasympathetic and sympathetic) influence on the sinoatrial node. This node is influenced by the parasympathetic system to decrease its rate, whereas sympathetic innervation increases it.

TOTAL PERIPHERAL RESISTANCE

Total peripheral resistance is determined primarily by the diameter of the arteries. Total peripheral resistance is also termed systemic vascular resistance. Resistance is high in vessels with small diameters (vasoconstriction) and low in vessels with larger diameters (vasodilation). Therefore, systemic blood pressure is increased when vessels are constricted and decreased when vessels are dilated. Like heart rate, blood vessel diameter and hence resistance, is influenced by the autonomic nervous system. Sympathetic stimulation results in vasoconstriction, whereas parasympathetic stimulation results in vasodilation.

AUTONOMIC RESPONSE

The influence of the autonomic nervous system on peripheral resistance and heart rate plays a critical role in regulating blood pressure. The effects of autonomic nervous system innervation arise from two areas in the medulla of the brain stem: the cardiac center and the vasomotor center. Both centers respond promptly to autonomic innervation through stimulation by the sympathetic branch or inhibition by the parasympathetic branch.

Sympathetic nervous system stimulation of the cardiac center results in acceleration of heart rate, whereas parasympathetic nervous system stimulation results in deceleration of heart rate. Sympathetic nervous system stimulation of the vasomotor center produces vasoconstriction and an increase in total peripheral resistance. Parasympathetic nervous system stimulation of the vasomotor center produces vasodilation and a decrease in total peripheral resistance (see pp. 436–438).

The structures responsible for instigating autonomic activity are the baroreceptors located in the aortic arch and carotid sinuses. The baroreceptors are sensitive to changes in the degree of stretch or tension in the walls of these major arteries. Decreased stretch or tension is indicative of low cardiac output and/or decreased peripheral vascular resistance consistent with low blood pressure. Conversely, increased stretch or tension indicates elevated cardiac output and/or increased peripheral vascular resistance consistent with high blood pressure. Marked decrease in stretch in the arterial wall prompts a reflex at the baroreceptors, resulting in sympathetic stimulation of the cardiac center, which then causes acceleration of heart rate, increased cardiac output, and simultaneous stimulation of the vasomotor center, which, in turn, increases peripheral resistance. The net effect is an elevation in blood pressure.[9] Increased stretch in the arterial wall causes the baroreceptors to respond by stimulating the parasympathetic nervous system and elicits a decelerating effect from the cardiac center, resulting in a decreased heart rate and cardiac output. A concomitant decrease in total peripheral resistance through inhibition of vasomotor center activity results. The overall effect is a reduction in blood pressure.

INTRAVASCULAR FLUID VOLUME

Without sufficient quantities of circulating intravascular volume, autonomic nervous system innervation would be ineffective in executing normal physiologic functions related to blood pressure control. Physiologically, adequate circulating fluid volume ensures adequate venous return, which, with other factors such as ventricular function and heart rate being normal, ensures adequate cardiac output. Increases or decreases in circulating fluid volume can either raise or lower blood pressure accordingly.

An additional component in the fluid volume influence over blood pressure is the process of autoregulation. Autoregulation is the mechanism whereby blood vessels either constrict or dilate in response to respective increases or decreases in oxygen stimulation and/or intravascular volume.[22] This constriction or dilatation is called a myogenic response.[8] In the case of increased volume and pressure, autoregulation results in vasoconstriction to normalize or equilibrate acceptable blood flow to tissues and organs. Vasoconstriction in peripheral vessels increases total peripheral resistance and systemic blood pressure.

Low or inadequate fluid volume and pressure induce autoregulative vasodilation to increase the amount of blood flow to tissues and organs. Vasodilation reduces total peripheral resistance, thereby lowering blood pressure. Another explanation for autoregulation is that as volume and pressure increase or decrease, an accumulation of metabolites may be present. These *vasoactive factors* include vasodilators, such as *endothelium-derived relaxation factor* and lactic acid, and vasoconstrictors, such as *thromboxane* A_2 and *superoxide radicals*.[22]

Intravascular fluid volume is determined greatly by the body's sodium content, which is regulated by the thirst mechanism, aldosterone, and antidiuretic hormone. All of these depend on an intact renal function.

HORMONES

The hormones responsible for blood pressure regulation are the catecholamines (epinephrine and norepinephrine), renin-angiotensin-aldosterone (RAA), and antidiuretic hormone. Each regulates blood pressure through different, but equally effective, mechanisms.

Catecholamines

The catecholamines, epinephrine and norepinephrine, released by the adrenal medulla as well as by various adrenergic terminals located throughout the body, are categorized as short-term, immediate determinants of blood pressure. Epinephrine increases the rate and strength of cardiac contractions. In instances of hypotension, epinephrine secretion elevates the blood pressure mainly by this mechanism. The role of norepinephrine in restoring and maintaining blood pressure is related mainly to its vasoconstrictive effects and elevated total peripheral resistance. Both epinephrine and norepinephrine are released into the circulation through stimulation of autonomic adrenergic sympathetic nervous system influence on the adrenal medulla and various other sympathetic terminals located throughout the body.

Renin-Angiotensin-Aldosterone (RAA) System

The role of the RAA system in blood pressure restoration is shown in Flowchart 13-2. This system is prompted into action by the effects of hypotensive episodes on renal perfusion. Low or decreased renal perfusion stimulates the juxtaglomerular apparatus in the kidney to release renin. Renin has little or no direct effect on blood pressure, but it acts on angiotensin, a plasma protein, to produce angiotensin I, which is then converted in the lungs to angiotensin II. Angiotensin II has two profound effects on blood pressure restoration. First, it is a very potent vasoconstrictor and, as such, produces a generalized increase in total peripheral resistance, thereby elevating blood pressure. Second, angiotensin II stimulates the hypothalamus to induce thirst and prompts the release of aldosterone from the adrenal cortex. Aldosterone increases the reabsorption of sodium from the distal tubules and collecting ducts. Increased sodium reabsorption causes a concomitant reabsorption of water. These mechanisms raise blood pressure by elevating intravascular fluid volume.

Antidiuretic Hormone

Antidiuretic hormone (ADH), also called *vasopressin*, is secreted by the posterior pituitary in response to hyperosmolality, water deficit, or low blood volume. Hyperosmolality (especially due to hypernatremia) and water deficit conditions are detected by osmoreceptors located in the supraoptic nuclei of the hypothalamus. These structures, in turn, stimulate pituitary release of ADH. The action of the hormone is that of water conservation. It is accomplished by a mechanism that stimulates the collecting ducts of nephrons to increase reabsorption of water. Increased plasma water dilutes or offsets the hyperosmolar condition and corrects the water deficit. It also raises intravascular volume, augments venous return, improves cardiac output, and thereby raises blood pressure.

Secretion of ADH is enhanced by low blood volume, which causes decreased stretch on the baroreceptors in the carotid sinus and aortic arch. This stimulates the secretion of ADH. In addition to its water conservation action, ADH also produces a vasoconstrictive effect on arterioles, ultimately raising blood pressure.[12]

▼ Shock—An Overview

Shock is defined as a condition of profound hemodynamic and metabolic disturbance due to inadequate blood flow and oxygen delivery to the capillaries and tissues of the body.[17,21] It is typically manifested by hy-

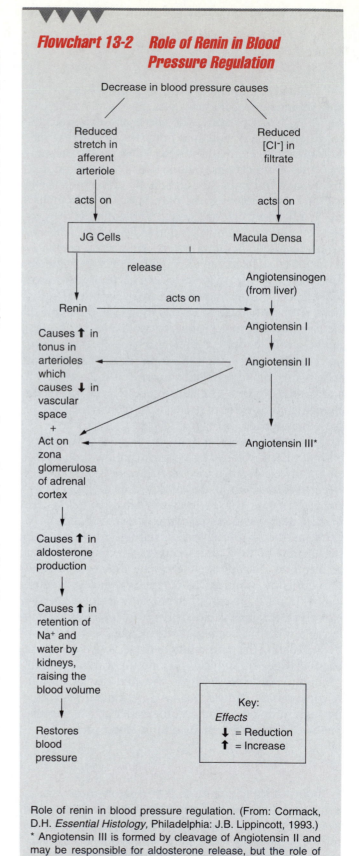

Flowchart 13-2   Role of Renin in Blood Pressure Regulation

Role of renin in blood pressure regulation. (From: Cormack, D.H. *Essential Histology*, Philadelphia: J.B. Lippincott, 1993.)
* Angiotensin III is formed by cleavage of Angiotensin II and may be responsible for aldosterone release, but the role of this substance in unclear.

potension; tachycardia; oliguria; cool, moist skin; restlessness; and altered levels of consciousness. It usually is induced by such conditions as hemorrhage, heart failure, sepsis, and neurologic damage.

Regardless of its etiology or pathologic basis, every form of shock is characterized by compromised or inadequate tissue and organ perfusion. Flowchart 13-3 shows the pathogenesis of shock. In effect, a discrepancy exists between the tissues' need for oxygen and various nutrients and the actual supply of those elements. The ultimate result of this discrepancy is multisystem deterioration and related loss of function. Table 13-1 presents the general etiologic classification of circulatory shock.

Compromised tissue and organ perfusion characteristic of shock is caused by *low cardiac output* or *reduced tissue perfusion pressure* or both. Every type of shock can easily be grouped with or related to one or sometimes both of these categories.

▼ *Stages of Shock*

There are essentially three stages of the shock state. Various authors refer to them by different names: initial, progressive, and final;[8] nonprogressive, progressive, and irreversible;[9] early, tissue hypoperfusion, and cell and organ injury;[5] and compensated, decompensated, and irreversible shock.[5] Despite the variation in nomenclature, persons experiencing shock progress through fairly distinguishable phases ranging from compensation to var-

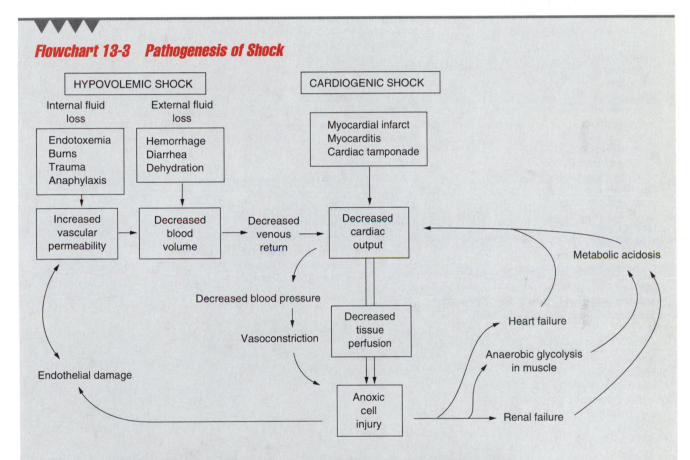

Flowchart 13-3   Pathogenesis of Shock

This flowchart shows the integration of many factors in the progression of shock. Shock is initiated by one of two principal events: pump failure or "cardiogenic shock," and loss of circulatory volume, or "hypovolemic shock." Hypovolemic shock follows internal fluid loss, such as that in endotoxemia, burns, trauma, and anaphylaxis, or external fluid loss, such as that caused by hemorrhage, diarrhea, and dehydration. The effects of both events is decreased cardiac output and decreased tissue perfusion. The resulting cell injury prompts several vicious circles. Metabolic acidosis (renal failure, anaerobic glycolysis) and heart failure lead to further decline in cardiac output. Endothelial damage increased vascular permeability and decreases effective blood volume, reducing venous return and decreasing cardiac output. (Source: Rubin, E., and Farber, J. *Pathology* [2nd ed.]. Philadelphia: J.B. Lippincott, 1994.)

TABLE 13-1 General Etiologic Classification of Circulatory Shock

Reduction of Intravascular Volume (Hypovolemic Shock)

Loss of blood volume—Hemorrhage
External loss
  Trauma
  Gastrointestinal bleeding
  Severe hemoptysis
Internal or sequestered blood loss
  Hemothorax
  Hemoperitoneum
  Retroperitoneal hemorrhage
  Ruptured aortic aneurysm
  Fractures
Loss of plasma volume
Loss of protein-rich body fluids
  Burns
  Desquamated-exudative lesions
Dehydration
  Gastrointestinal loss
    Vomiting
    Diarrhea
  Renal loss
    Diabetic ketoacidosis
    Hyperosmolar nonketotic diabetes
    Diabetes insipidus
    Adrenal insufficiency
    High-urine-output renal failure
    Overly aggressive diuretic therapy
  Cutaneous loss
    Nonreplaced perspiration or insensible loss
  Internal or sequestered loss
    Peritonitis
    Pancreatitis
    Budd-Chiari syndrome
    Bowel ischemia and infarction

Increased Vascular Capacitance (Vasogenic, Veno-Vasodilatory Shock, Distributive Shock)

Neurogenic
Spinal cord injury
Cerebral damage
Severe dysautonomia
Toxic, Humoral
Septicemia
Endotoxemia
Anaphylaxis
Drugs
Anesthesia
Sympatholytics
Adrenergic blockers
Veno-vasodilators
Barbiturates
Narcotics

Failure of the Heart as a Pump (Cardiogenic Shock)

Impaired Systolic Performance
Myocardial injury or depression
  Myocardial ischemia-infarction
  Myocarditis
  Cardiomyopathy
  Drugs (eg, doxorubicin, cocaine)
  Septic shock
  Acidosis
Misdirected systolic ejection
  Papillary muscle or chordal rupture
  Ruptured ventricular septum or free wall
Cardiac dysrhythmias
  Marked bradycardia or tachycardia
  Ventricular fibrillation
Inadequate Ventricular Diastolic Filling
Extracardiac or extravascular compression
  Pericardial tamponade
  Tension pneumothorax
  Positive-pressure ventilation
Obstruction to blood flow
  Pulmonary embolization
  Cardiac tumors (eg, myxoma)
Valvular Incompetence or Malfunction
Acute severe aortic or mitral valvular
  regurgitation
Obstruction or incompetency of prosthetic heart
  valve

Miscellaneous Causative Factors

Microcirculatory Injury and/or Obstruction
Thrombotic thrombocytopenic purpura
Disseminated intravascular coagulation
Anaphylaxis
Septic shock
Trauma
Tissue and Cell Membrane Injury
Septic shock
Pancreatitis
Prolonged hypoxia or shock

From W. N. Kelley et al., *Textbook of Internal Medicine* (2nd ed.). Philadelphia: J.B. Lippincott, 1992.

TABLE 13-2 *Clinical Picture Exhibited According to Degree of Shock*

	Compensated (Nonprogressive)	Decompensated (Progressive)	Irreversible
Sensorium	Oriented to time, place, person	Remains oriented; words slurred	Disoriented to comatose
Pulse	Rate increased; Quality full to decreased	Rate very high; Quality decreased and variable	Rate over 150; Quality weak, thready, difficult to feel
Blood pressure	Normal to low (10–20% decrease but may be slightly increased as compensatory mechanism)	Decreased 40–50 mm Hg below normal (20–40% decrease)	Systolic less than 80; Diastolic may not be heard
Urinary output	35–50 mL/h	20–35 mL/h	Less than 20 mL/h
Color	Pale	Pale	Mottled
Capillary refill	Circulation return slightly slowed; 3–5 sec	Circulation return slowed; 5–10 sec	Circulation return very slow; >10 sec
Blood gases	pH normal	pH below 7.35	pH very low; 7.0–7.2

ious states or degrees of decompensation. Table 13-2 shows the differences in the clinical picture according to the degree of shock.

COMPENSATED (NONPROGRESSIVE) SHOCK

Compensated shock represents the initial or early phase during which, in response to the initial insult, several physiologic compensatory mechanisms are activated. Frequently, when these mechanisms are fully operational, they may compensate for the shock state, depending on the extent of the insult.

During this early phase, cardiac output, total peripheral resistance, or both are decreased as a consequence of the initial insult, regardless of its origin or nature. These decreases result in decreased stretch or tension in the walls of major arteries. Baroreceptors situated in these arterial walls, specifically in the aortic arch and carotid sinuses, detect the reduced stretch and activate the autonomic nervous system response.

The sympathetic branch of the autonomic nervous system responds to baroreceptor innervation by instigating two processes. Sympathetic activity stimulates the cardiac center to increase heart rate by inhibiting vagal tone, which increases cardiac output. It simultaneously stimulates the vasomotor center to increase total peripheral resistance through vasoconstriction. Both of these responses represent an effort to raise blood pressure and improve or restore adequate tissue and organ perfusion. They are usually operational within several seconds to minutes.

Another compensatory mechanism set into motion in this early stage of shock is activation of the RAA system. Renin, released in response to low renal perfusion, triggers the eventual production of angiotensin II. Angiotensin II exerts its effects on blood pressure by vasoconstriction and by both stimulation of the thirst mechanism and release of aldosterone from the adrenal cortex. The vasoconstrictive effect raises blood pressure by increasing total peripheral resistance, and the other effects do so by increasing circulating intravascular fluid volume. The RAA system is fully activated about 20 minutes after the initial stimulus, so its action follows that of the sympathetic nervous system.

In response to the decreased blood pressure, vasopressin (ADH) is released. Its primary action is on the kidneys to promote water conservation and on the systemic arterioles to cause arteriolar vasoconstriction. Both of these actions tend to elevate blood pressure.

Symptoms that predominate in this initial stage are directly related to the compensatory activities described above. The individual is usually awake and alert but somewhat anxious. Heart rate is elevated with low to normal blood pressure. The skin is usually pale, moist, and cool. Pupillary dilatation from sympathetic nervous system stimulation may be evident. The hematocrit level becomes depressed when the condition is due to hemorrhage, because interstitial fluid is absorbed into the blood vessel and dilutes the blood. Respirations may be shallow, and the rate is increased in response to inadequate tissue oxygen delivery. Urinary output is slightly reduced, and the person usually complains of thirst. Bowel sounds may be hypoactive, related to compensatory vasoconstriction and reduced blood delivery to the intestines. Muscle weakness and hyporeactive reflexes may be present.

The shock state usually resolves within several hours, as long as the initiating event is not overwhelming and compensatory mechanisms are intact and functional.[22] Otherwise, shock progresses to a more advanced stage in which compensatory mechanisms become virtually incapable of restoring blood pressure.

DECOMPENSATED (PROGRESSIVE) SHOCK

Decompensated shock represents a condition in which compensatory responses fail to restore blood pressure and tissue perfusion. In addition, the deleterious effects of prolonged tissue and organ hypoperfusion with resultant ischemic deterioration begin to compound the worsening clinical picture. During this stage, the potentially devastating complications of shock usually begin to develop.

In the decompensated stage, the effects of ischemia on organs generating compensatory responses become evident. Exhaustion of compensation results. The medullary vasomotor center reacts to decreased perfusion and oxygen deprivation by ceasing activity, thereby causing even lower blood pressure due to generalized vasodilatation.[22] Similarly, the myocardium, subjected to inadequate coronary artery perfusion and increased work in efforts to sustain cardiac output, begins to deteriorate and is unable to generate adequate cardiac out-

put. Flowchart 13-4 shows the effect of shock on contractility. Despite the underlying mechanism causing the alteration, myocardial depression results.[3] Additional factors responsible for myocardial ineffectiveness are related to the influence of lactic acid and the myocardial depressant factor. Lactic acid is produced in the myocardium and in tissues throughout the body as a by-product of anaerobic glycogenesis consistent with stages of oxygen deprivation. It can greatly suppress myocardial contractility. The myocardial depressant factor is thought to exert a potent negative inotropic effect (see p. 512). It is released by the pancreas, which suffers from compromised splanchnic organ circulation consistent with shock states.[5] Eventually, myocardial contractility is impaired and stroke volume declines. The shock state, especially septic shock, may cause the release of *tumor necrosis factor*, which decreases myocardial contractility.[1]

Renal integrity is compromised relatively early in this stage of shock. The kidneys are sensitive to low perfusion pressure and respond quickly to reduced glomerular filtration by activating the RAA system. The kidneys, like the gastrointestinal system, skin, and splanchnic organs, are targeted as nonessential organs and are further compromised by selective vasoconstriction induced by sympathetic activity. The more essential organs, the heart and brain, are not affected by sympathetic vasoconstriction. Renal effects of the shock state and this vasoconstriction are seen in the form of acute tubular necrosis secondary to ischemia and prompt acute renal failure (see pp. 658–662).

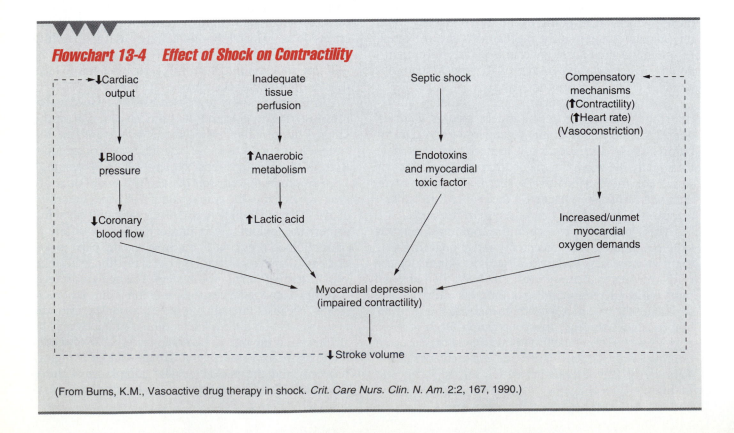

Flowchart 13-4   Effect of Shock on Contractility

(From Burns, K.M., Vasoactive drug therapy in shock. *Crit. Care Nurs. Clin. N. Am.* 2:2, 167, 1990.)

Hypoperfusion, ischemia, and selective vasoconstriction also affect other organs. Lung tissue undergoes ischemic deterioration, resulting in adult respiratory distress syndrome, or shock lung (see pp. 587–589). The ischemic gastrointestinal tract undergoes necrotic changes and releases endotoxins, which are vasodilating substances that further compound shock. Liver function deteriorates, and the liver becomes incapable of performing metabolic or biotransformation functions.[4]

Late in this decompensated stage, hypoxia leads to increased blood capillary permeability. The resultant loss of blood plasma components into the tissues decreases circulating blood volume, which increases interstitial hypoxia.[22]

Symptoms associated with the decompensated stage of shock are related to organ failure and the development of complications. Levels of consciousness and orientation decrease. Bradycardia and hypotension progress, urine output ceases, pulmonary and peripheral edema develop, and tachypnea with dyspnea becomes prominent. Abdominal distention and paralytic ileus are common. The person appears critically ill, with cold, diaphoretic, ashen skin. The arterial pH becomes acidotic due to lactic acid accumulation. Recovery at this point depends on the underlying condition and rapid, effective therapeutic management.

IRREVERSIBLE SHOCK

Irreversible shock denotes the final progression and is basically the point at which the person becomes refractory or unresponsive to all forms of therapeutic management. There is progressive decrease in cardiac output and blood pressure together with increased severity of the metabolic acidosis. Ischemic cell death occurs and is manifested by renal, heart, pulmonary, and brain dysfunction.[5] Progressive renal and heart failure, manifestations of respiratory difficulties, and coma mark the ultimate outcome of the condition. Survival is virtually impossible. Flowchart 13-5 summarizes the different types of feedback that promote the progression of shock.

Flowchart 13-5   Progressive Shock

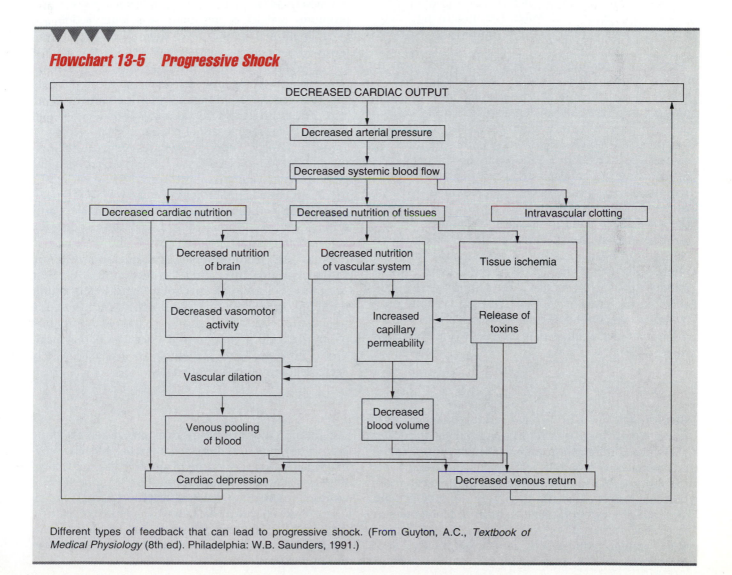

Different types of feedback that can lead to progressive shock. (From Guyton, A.C., *Textbook of Medical Physiology* (8th ed). Philadelphia: W.B. Saunders, 1991.)

▼ *Classifications of Shock*

Shock can be classified by etiology or associated physiologic impairment. For example, hypovolemic shock is caused by loss of intravascular volume, cardiogenic shock is the result of cardiac decompensation, and distributive shock results from internal fluid loss or redistribution. Hypovolemic shock refers to volume depleting conditions, such as hemorrhage, burns, dehydration, and trauma. Cardiogenic shock includes pump failure and decreased venous return, referring to insufficient quantity of blood entering the heart. Distributive (vasogenic) shock involves conditions that result in a maldistribution of blood volume, such as nervous system failure, septicemia, and anaphylaxis.

HYPOVOLEMIC SHOCK

Hypovolemic shock, or that shock state resulting from loss of circulating fluid volume, may result from any condition that significantly depletes normal volumes of whole blood, plasma, or water. The underlying pathology, regardless of the exact type of fluid loss, is related to actual circulatory fluid pressure/volume deficits. Decreased circulating fluid volume decreases venous return, which reduces cardiac output and, therefore, lowers blood pressure. Consequently, lowered blood pressure impedes tissue and organ perfusion and oxygen delivery. This leads to ischemia, necrosis, organ malfunction, and shock. Compensatory mechanisms are activated to adjust for the reduced tissue and organ perfusion. These mechanisms, discussed previously, include sympathetic nervous system stimulation to increase cardiac rate and total peripheral resistance, activation of the RAA system, and increased secretion of ADH.

These mechanisms, working together, effectuate an elevation in blood pressure. If treatment to correct or remove the underlying cause of fluid volume loss is initiated, the shock remains in the nonprogressive stage and crisis is averted or resolved. If the fluid volume loss is overwhelming or therapeutic measures are ineffective, this initial stage of shock may progress to the irreversible stage.

Hemorrhage

Hemorrhagic shock occurs as a result of massive loss of whole blood. Some conditions that produce drastic loss of blood include gastrointestinal bleeding, postoperative hemorrhage, hemophilia, childbirth, and trauma. For the shock state to ensue, blood loss must be extensive. Minimal loss of blood, up to 10% of the total volume, does not produce noticeable changes in blood pressure or cardiac output. Blood loss of up to 45% of the total blood volume reduces both cardiac output and blood pressure to zero.[9] Symptoms depend on the actual volume of blood lost and whether the loss was sudden or gradual.

In addition to the compensatory mechanisms, certain humoral substances are released in hemorrhage in an attempt to restore the steady state. In shock due to abrupt hemorrhage, adrenocorticotropic hormone is increased, which, in turn, increases glucocorticoid levels. The *glucocorticoids* maintain capillary integrity and combat the effects of the mediators of the inflammatory response. Erythropoietin levels rise and stimulate bone marrow to produce red blood cells. Circulating volume of *2-3,diphosphoglycerate*, a substance that interacts with hemoglobin to promote the release of oxygen, increases. This increases the liberation of oxygen, thereby reducing the effects of the tissue and organ hypoxia characteristic of shock.[13] The *prostaglandins*-DPGE$_2$, PG$_{12}$, PGF$_2$-alpha, and PGA$_2$—play a mixed role in hemorrhagic shock, exerting beneficial and detrimental effects. Both PGE$_2$ and PG$_{12}$ dilate liver and renal vessels, thereby improving perfusion to these organs; PGF$_2$-alpha and PGA$_2$ constrict blood vessels. PG$_{12}$ retards aggregation of platelets, whereas PGA$_2$ exerts the opposite effect and actually promotes platelet aggregation. This latter action has been implicated in the development of disseminated intravascular coagulation (see pp. 418–419).

In addition to these humoral agents released in hemorrhagic shock, other substances released in response to cellular deterioration can perpetuate the shock state. For example, lysosomal enzymes extend cellular damage, depress myocardial contractility, and constrict coronary vessels. The kinins depress myocardial contractility, promote vasodilation, and, together with histamine, make capillaries more permeable, contributing to fluid volume loss. Serotonin causes potent arteriolar constriction and thus impedes microcirculation. Lactic acid, generated by anaerobic metabolism, depresses myocardial contractility. Endotoxins are released in response to gastrointestinal ischemia and result in vasodilation and myocardial depression.[4] All of these substances—lysosomal enzymes, kinins, histamine, serotonin, lactic acid, and endotoxins—are released in response to cellular damage and are normal by-products of injured cells. Their overall effect in hemorrhagic shock, however, is to perpetuate the vicious cycle of decreased perfusion and hypoxia.

Dehydration

Dehydration shock results from extensive and profound loss of body fluid. Conditions that classically cause dehydration are profuse sweating; extensive gastrointestinal fluid loss related to diarrhea, vomiting, or upper gastrointestinal suctioning; diabetes insipidus; ascites; the diuretic phase of acute renal failure; diabetic ketoacidosis; Addison's disease; hypoaldosteronism; lack of adequate fluid volume intake; osmotic diuresis; and injudicious use of diuretics.

Dehydration must be severe to produce a shock state, because fluid shifts from the interstitial spaces and intracellular compartments to maintain intravascular volume. Simple or moderate dehydration does not produce symptomatology consistent with shock, because fluid moves along a pressure gradient from tissue spaces to the intravascular space. Fluid volume in the vascular compartment is maintained at the expense of the tissues. Once fluid volume loss becomes severe, however, the transfer of water is not sufficient to maintain intravascular volume, and the shock state ensues.

The mechanisms involved in producing shock from dehydration are similar to those that produce shock with hemorrhage. Fluid lost from the body diminishes vascular volume, which reduces venous return. Cardiac output decreases, blood pressure falls, and tissue and organ perfusion declines. Physiologic adaptive mechanisms are activated in an attempt to restore blood pressure, fluid volume, and, ultimately, perfusion. Fluid replacement and treatment of the underlying cause often can rapidly restore the blood pressure.

Burns

Burns, especially third-degree burns, often cause hypovolemic shock. The mechanism by which this type of shock occurs is related not so much to fluid loss as to loss of plasma proteins through the burn surface. Loss of plasma proteins significantly decreases colloidal osmotic pressure. In an effort to restore colloidal and hydrostatic pressure equilibrium, water leaves the vascular space and enters the interstitium. Consequently, intravascular volume decreases, venous return decreases, cardiac output is inadequate, and blood pressure falls.

Shock secondary to burns also may be caused by associated hemorrhage and sepsis. Burn surfaces promote platelet aggregation and activation of factor XII, which leads to localized intravascular clot formation. These localized clots can impair microcirculation, resulting in tissue ischemia and necrosis, and can consume factors of coagulation, causing disseminated intravascular coagulation. Sepsis can result from extensive burns because of loss or destruction of the body's natural barrier, the skin, to bacterial invasion. In addition, burned surfaces release toxins into systemic circulation that can injure intestinal capillaries, thereby releasing intestinal bacteria and endotoxins into systemic circulation. The mechanisms of septic shock are discussed on pages 265–266.

Trauma

Trauma, in the forms of crushing injuries to muscles and bones, gunshot wounds, and penetration of blood vessels, the viscera, or other vital organs by knives or sharp instruments, produces the shock state primarily through extensive and sudden blood loss. An astounding amount of blood lost internally due to trauma can be concealed in tissue, organs, and "third spaces" for variable lengths of time before symptoms of shock are manifested. For example, the thigh muscle can hold up to 1,000 mL of blood resulting from a fractured femur or a tear in a femoral vessel without a noticeable increase in thigh diameter.[8] Loss of 1 liter of whole blood represents a significant hemorrhage, especially if it goes undetected and uncorrected. Because of the massive blood loss usually associated with extensive trauma, traumatic shock is almost identical to hemorrhagic shock in terms of pathologic mechanisms and adaptive responses.

Another aspect of trauma is that loss of plasma, even without overt blood loss, often occurs.[19] Loss of plasma alone from capillary damage can lead to hypovolemia extensive enough to produce shock. Similarly, release of endotoxin and intestinal bacteria due to injury or ischemia to the gastrointestinal tract results in septic shock, which compounds the trauma-induced shock.

CARDIOGENIC SHOCK

That shock state that is directly attributable to impaired or compromised cardiac output is referred to as cardiogenic shock. Two categories of conditions can induce shock of cardiac origin: *pump failure*, which is the inability of the heart to contract effectively, and *decreased venous return*, which is the inability of sufficient quantities of blood to enter the heart.

Pump Failure

Pump failure shock is always directly attributable to heart failure, which most often results from massive myocardial infarction. Other conditions causing cardiogenic shock from pump failure include the myocardiopathies, drug toxicity, and dysrhythmias (see Table 13-1). The mechanism by which myocardial infarction causes pump failure is related to extensive myocardial damage that results in greatly diminished cardiac output. The predominant and prevailing defect accounting for low cardiac output is impaired myocardial contractility with loss of functional myocardium (see Chapter 25). Pump failure results when nearly half of the myocardial tissue is nonfunctional.

Decreased Venous Return

Decreased venous return is a category of cardiogenic shock that is not caused by inadequate circulating volume but by actual impedance of blood flow into the heart. It results from such conditions as cardiac tamponade, acute pericardial effusion, and mediastinal shifts that squeeze or compress the heart to such an extent that venous inflow is impaired.[12] Decreased venous return always results in decreased cardiac output and, hence, lowered blood pressure with impaired tissue and organ perfusion.

Progression of Cardiogenic Shock

In response to low cardiac output, regardless of the cause, compensatory mechanisms are activated for the purpose of improving or restoring tissue perfusion by increasing blood pressure through acceleration of heart rate and elevation of total peripheral resistance. The decreases in stroke volume, cardiac output, and perfusion brought about by impaired myocardial contractility are compounded and worsened by the autonomic sympathetic responses intended to improve them. The autonomic response increases heart rate, thus increasing oxygen demand and decreasing diastolic filling time, both of which further compromise an impaired myocardium. In addition, autonomically mediated vasoconstriction increases afterload, forcing the failing myocardium to work even harder in its attempt to sustain adequate cardiac output. Selective vasoconstriction shunts blood away from organs, such as the kidneys, skin, and splanchnic organs, and toward the heart and brain, resulting in additional reduction of tissue and organ perfusion. Eventually, these selectively deprived organs experience and demonstrate the effects of inadequate perfusion. Flowchart 13-3 depicts the pattern of cardiogenic shock development.

Left ventricular filling pressure and cardiac index obtained through use of a flow-directed, balloon-tipped pulmonary artery (Swan-Ganz) catheter are universal values for determining not only the extent of cardiac decompensation, but also the prognosis for survival in cardiogenic shock. Generally, persons with high left ventricular end-diastolic pressure or pulmonary artery end-diastolic pressure (greater than 15 mm Hg) and/or low cardiac index (less than 2 L/min/m^2) have statistically higher rates of mortality (see pp. 505–511). The higher the left ventricular or pulmonary artery end-diastolic pressure and the lower the cardiac index, the greater the likelihood of death from cardiogenic shock.[1, 5]

In addition to pressure values recorded from the Swan-Ganz catheter, other signs indicative of cardiogenic shock include varying degrees of pulmonary edema; hypotension; decompensation, such as oliguria/anuria; ascites; cold and diaphoretic skin with pallor; decreased or altered sensorium; and abdominal distention with hypoactive or absent bowel sounds. Bradycardia and hypotension denote advanced stages of shock and usually indicate that sympathetic compensatory activity has failed and that survival is unlikely.

Early recognition and prompt treatment of conditions that result in cardiogenic shock may preclude its development. This is true especially in cardiogenic shock secondary to venous inflow impedance. If the shock state is related to acute myocardial infarction, however, prompt treatment may or may not alter the eventual outcome, depending on the extensiveness of the infarct.

DISTRIBUTIVE SHOCK

The shock state that develops as a consequence of profound and massive vasodilatation as opposed to hypovolemia or cardiac dysfunction is referred to as low-resistance, or distributive, shock. The term "distributive shock" is used because central blood volume is redistributed to peripheral vascular beds, especially venous beds.[12] The primary defect is a marked increase in vascular capacity or vasodilatation relative to the amount of circulating blood volume. Blood volume per se is not reduced, but rather the circulatory capacity to accommodate that volume is increased. Categories of conditions that result in extensive vasodilatation or increased vascular capacity are *vasomotor center depression, sepsis,* and *anaphylaxis.*

Regardless of the initiating event or insult, the sequence of pathologic events that culminates in distributive shock is uniform and consistent. Profound arteriolar dilatation and vasodilatation related to the vasomotor center depression, sepsis, or anaphylaxis lead to a relaxation or reduction of total peripheral resistance. Reduced total peripheral resistance results in a decrease in the volume of blood returning to the heart. This is related to blood vessel size or diameter and velocity or force of blood flow. The smaller the vessel, the brisker is the blood flow through it. Similarly, the larger the vessel diameter, the less forceful, more sluggish, and slower is the blood flow through it. Dilated vessels are unable to generate sufficient force or pressure to propel blood adequately. Hence, in vasodilatation, venous return to the heart is reduced. The consequence of diminished venous return is decreased filling pressures in the chambers of the heart, with subsequent diminution of heart muscle fiber stretch or tension, which lowers stroke volume. The consequence of reduced stroke volume is impaired perfusion of tissues and organs, which deprives them of needed oxygen and nutrients. This sets the stage for the vicious cycle of positive-feedback, shock-related pathology. The general pathogenesis of distributive shock is displayed in Flowchart 13-6.

The vasodilatation that promotes or leads to the shock state interferes with or impairs tissue and organ perfusion for a variable time before the actual development of shock. Thus, the onset of shock actually compounds and worsens the existing perfusion deficit. In addition, compensatory mechanisms instituted to restore blood pressure and, hence, tissue perfusion are hampered and even offset by the underlying disease process, which is either vasomotor failure or potent vasodilator substances.

One of the major compensatory mechanisms activated in the shock state, the sympathetic vasomotor

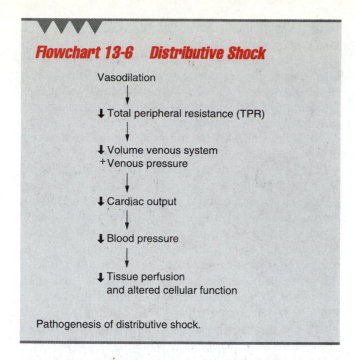

Flowchart 13-6   Distributive Shock

Vasodilation

↓ Total peripheral resistance (TPR)

↓ Volume venous system
+ Venous pressure

↓ Cardiac output

↓ Blood pressure

↓ Tissue perfusion
and altered cellular function

Pathogenesis of distributive shock.

stimulation, may be futile and ineffective owing to the nature of the primary defect. As long as the initiating vasodilatatory event prevails, vasomotor response is unable to contribute to the restoration of blood pressure and tissue perfusion.

Pure symptoms of distributive shock are difficult to distinguish from those of the primary condition due to the predominant feature of vasodilatation. Therefore, some overlap or dual causation of symptoms is unavoidable. Symptoms include hypotension; tachycardia; cool, moist-to-diaphoretic skin; fever; oliguria; hypoactive bowel sounds; increased hematocrit level; anxiety; and tachypnea.

Neurogenic Shock (Vasomotor Center Depression)

Neurogenic shock, also known as spinal shock, is the result of loss of vasomotor tone that induces generalized arteriolar and venous dilatation. This leads to hypotension, with pooling of blood in storage or capacitance vessels and splanchnic organ capillaries. Vasomotor tone is controlled and mediated by the vasomotor center in the medulla and the sympathetic fibers extending down the spinal cord to peripheral blood vessels, respectively. Thus, any conditions that depress medullary function or spinal cord integrity and innervation can precipitate neurogenic shock. One example of such a condition is head injury that directly or indirectly adversely affects the medullary area of the brain stem. Indirect injury results from cerebral edema, with increased intracranial pressure that accompanies head trauma or ischemia of the brain. Other instances that may promote neurogenic

shock from medullary brain stem depression are deep general anesthesia and drug overdose, especially barbiturates, opiates, and tranquilizers.[5,9] Spinal cord injury and high spinal anesthesia may also induce neurogenic shock or profound vasomotor failure because of interference with or interruption of sympathetic pathways to blood vessels, which blocks vasoconstrictive responses and promotes vasodilatation. Syncopal episodes, or fainting, are considered to be a mild form of neurogenic shock that is relatively transient and inconsequential.

Septic Shock

Septic shock is defined as a severe and profound condition of generalized vascular collapse secondary to a systemic infection commonly caused by a gram-negative organism. The development of the shock state due to infection is believed to be related to the release of endotoxin from the bacterial cell wall. For this reason, septic shock is commonly referred to as *endotoxin shock* or simply *toxic shock*. Toxic shock is usually caused by gram-negative organisms but also may be caused by viruses, fungi, or gram-positive bacilli. Gram-positive bacteria produce toxins on the surface of their cell walls, called exotoxins. Shock produced by these organisms is called *exotoxic shock*.[11] Table 13-3 summarizes the most frequently occurring gram-negative bacteremias and their sites of origin.

Endotoxin, a lipopolysaccharide made up of the layers of the bacterial cell wall, is capable of interacting with and influencing the activity of other cells and plasma proteins throughout the body. The net symptomatic effects of endotoxin activity include fever, abnormal clotting, hypotension, and elevated complement levels. In addition to being released by bacteria in sys-

TABLE 13-3 Sites of Origin of Hospital-Acquired Bloodstream Infections

Organism	Contaminating Sites
1. *Staphylococcus aureus* (methicillin-resistant)	Skin, wounds, IV lines, urinary tract
2. *Enterococci*	Urinary tract, feces, wounds
3. *Escherichia coli*	Feces, urinary tract, peritonitis
4. *Proteus mirabilis*	Urinary tract
5. *Acinetobacter* sp.	IV lines
6. *Klebsiella/Serratia/ Enterobacter* sp.	Lungs, IV lines, urinary tract, wounds
7. *Pseudomonas* sp.	Lungs, wounds, IV lines, urinary tract
8. *Bacteroides* sp.	Decubiti, wounds, abscesses
9. *Candida* sp.	Oral, skin, mucous membranes
10. *Aspergillus* sp.	Lungs, sinuses

temic circulation, endotoxin is released from necrotic bowel.[5, 14]

The release of endotoxin by the bacterial cell wall initiates the process by which septic shock develops. Endotoxin is liberated from gram-negative bacteria through phagocytic activity of the macrophage system. If the bacterial infection is relatively minor, endotoxin is eventually neutralized and rendered harmless by the cells of the mononuclear phagocyte system.[20] In more extreme infections, the release of greater quantities of endotoxin virtually overwhelms the defensive system, thereby allowing endotoxin activity to prevail and the shock state to develop. The lipopolysaccharide binds to a specific protein, which with a specific receptor site on the macrophages causes them to secrete large amounts of tumor necrosis factor. The development of a sudden shocklike state may be a direct result of tumor necrosis factor.[17] Tumor necrosis factor and interleukin-1 are major *monokines* (released by macrophages) that cause the vascular permeability. The term monokine has been replaced by the term *cytokine*, because it has been shown that many cells can release vasoactive mediators.[5] Cytokines are initially beneficial in shock, because they mobilize body nutrients stores for energy. If the shock state is protracted, however, these substances can lead to metabolic deterioration through muscle tissue catabolism, depletion of carbohydrate stores, and ineffective use of fat for energy.[5, 23] The macrophage system also activates other shock-mediating substances, such as complement, coagulation factors, and prostaglandins. Many of these factors work together to produce capillary damage, which causes the leakage of plasma that produces marked fluid volume loss. The inevitable consequence of this plasma loss is a circulating fluid volume deficit with resultant hypotension. This capillary insult is also the basis for the development of adult respiratory distress syndrome in septic shock.[15]

The overall systemic effects of septic shock are shown in Figure 13-1. The process is initiated by some form of infectious agent that enters the body and overwhelms normal defenses to foreign invasion. As a consequence of host defense activity, mediators of such shock are liberated. The collective effects of these mediators are vasodilatation, capillary endothelial cell damage, platelet aggregation with microemboli formation, myocardial depression, and impaired myocardial contractility. The alterations in peripheral venules and arterioles as well as those of myocardial function impair tissue and organ perfusion, resulting in lactic acidemia. Lactic acidemia further depresses myocardial contractility, total peripheral resistance, and the vital organ functions. Death ensues predictably unless this chain of events is interrupted.[14, 19]

Three identifiable patterns of response or states are associated with septic shock. The first state, referred to as the *hyperdynamic state*, presents the familiar picture of

acute infection with chills, fever, and warm, dry, flushed skin (hence, the synonymous term "pink shock"). Tachycardia, tachypnea with respiratory alkalosis, and little alteration of blood pressure occur in the early stage. Blood pressure is relatively normal, because cardiac output remains high, despite early widespread vasodilatation and the beginning stage of increased capillary permeability induced by endotoxin-stimulated release of vasoactive substances. The predominant physiologic feature of the hyperdynamic state is high cardiac output, which is attributable to an intact and functional compensatory sympathetic response to decreased peripheral resistance.[9] The second or intermediate state in septic shock is called *normodynamic* and represents a transitional period between the first and third states. It is that pattern or state during which the effects of endotoxin liberation begin to become manifested by signs and symptoms such as hypotension, oliguria, cool skin, and thirst.[15] Tachycardia persists in an attempt to restore blood pressure and tissue perfusion. Therapy involves treatment of the underlying cause with specific antibiotics and restoration of the blood pressure to permit tissue perfusion.

The final state is called *hypodynamic* and can be equated with the irreversible stage of hemorrhagic shock. The affected person is obviously acutely ill and moribund, with cold, clammy, diaphoretic skin, anuria, severe hypotension, tachycardia, and tachypnea. Metabolic acidosis from increased tissue catabolism and lactic acidosis is usual. Effects of myocardial depression are evidenced by pulmonary edema and low cardiac output. Once septic shock has progressed to this state, survival is doubtful and therapeutic measures are usually futile.

A special condition called *toxic shock syndrome* may produce septic shock. It also may be a relatively mild condition that resolves with treatment. Toxic shock syndrome is highly correlated with the use of tampons in menstruating women (50% to 70% of cases).[2, 18] The causative organism, *Staphylococcus aureus*, is absorbed and releases a large amount of pyogenic exotoxin, called toxic shock syndrome toxin.[1, 7] Signs and symptoms of infections include fever, nausea and vomiting, diarrhea, peritoneal irritation, conjunctivitis, hypotension, renal dysfunction, headache, hypocalcemia, diffuse erythroderma, and desquamation of the palms and soles of the feet.[6] Circulatory collapse and death are rare.

Anaphylactic Shock

Anaphylactic shock, or anaphylaxis, is the most drastic, acutely developing, and rapidly progressing form of shock. Onset often occurs within seconds, and profound peripheral vascular collapse may become well established in only a few minutes. Without immediate treatment, irreversible shock develops promptly and death occurs in about an hour. This form of the shock state is

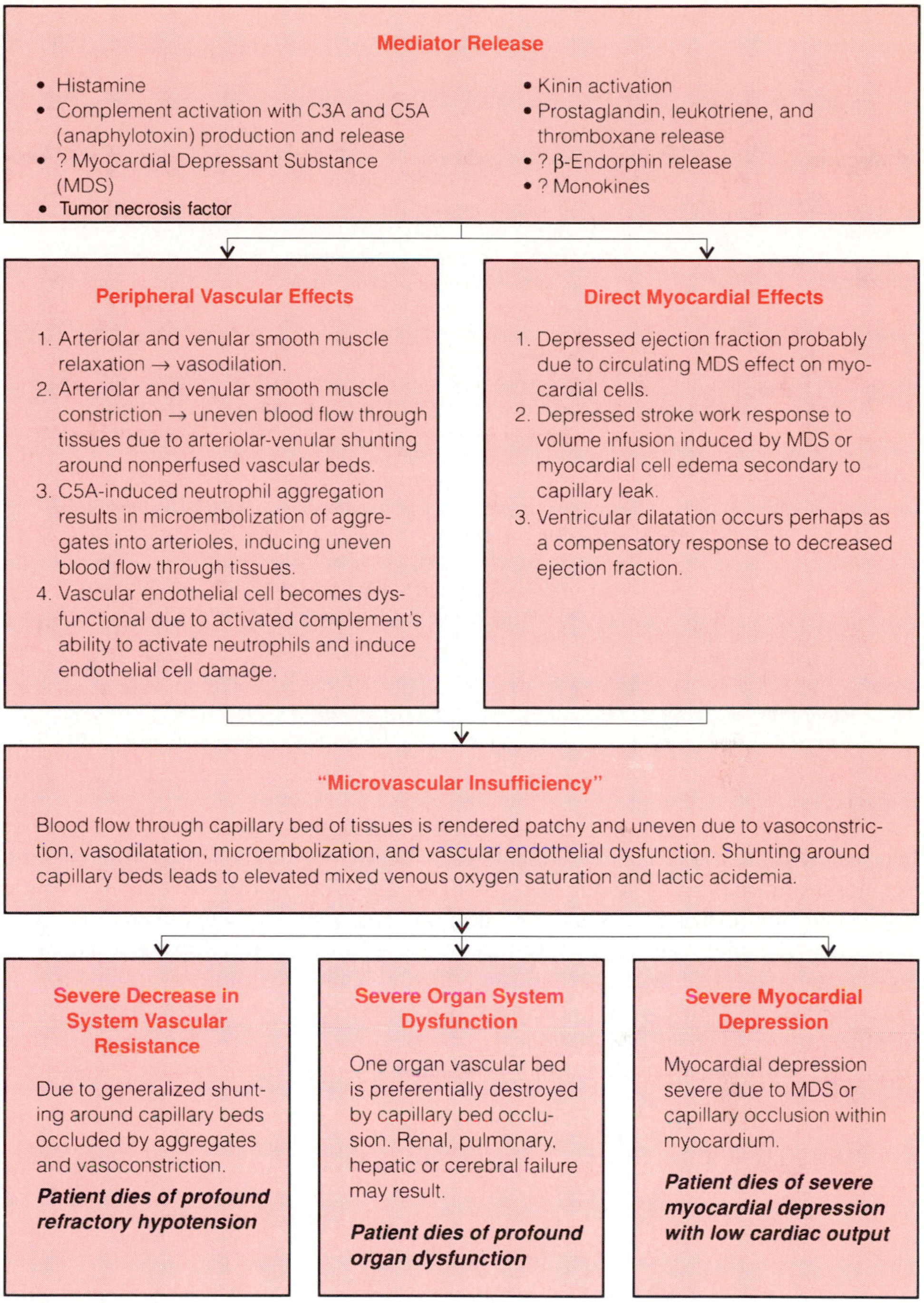

Mediator Release

- Histamine
- Complement activation with C3A and C5A (anaphylotoxin) production and release
- ? Myocardial Depressant Substance (MDS)
- Tumor necrosis factor

- Kinin activation
- Prostaglandin, leukotriene, and thromboxane release
- ? β-Endorphin release
- ? Monokines

Peripheral Vascular Effects

1. Arteriolar and venular smooth muscle relaxation → vasodilation.
2. Arteriolar and venular smooth muscle constriction → uneven blood flow through tissues due to arteriolar-venular shunting around nonperfused vascular beds.
3. C5A-induced neutrophil aggregation results in microembolization of aggregates into arterioles, inducing uneven blood flow through tissues.
4. Vascular endothelial cell becomes dysfunctional due to activated complement's ability to activate neutrophils and induce endothelial cell damage.

Direct Myocardial Effects

1. Depressed ejection fraction probably due to circulating MDS effect on myocardial cells.
2. Depressed stroke work response to volume infusion induced by MDS or myocardial cell edema secondary to capillary leak.
3. Ventricular dilatation occurs perhaps as a compensatory response to decreased ejection fraction.

"Microvascular Insufficiency"

Blood flow through capillary bed of tissues is rendered patchy and uneven due to vasoconstriction, vasodilatation, microembolization, and vascular endothelial dysfunction. Shunting around capillary beds leads to elevated mixed venous oxygen saturation and lactic acidemia.

Severe Decrease in System Vascular Resistance

Due to generalized shunting around capillary beds occluded by aggregates and vasoconstriction.

Patient dies of profound refractory hypotension

Severe Organ System Dysfunction

One organ vascular bed is preferentially destroyed by capillary bed occlusion. Renal, pulmonary, hepatic or cerebral failure may result.

Patient dies of profound organ dysfunction

Severe Myocardial Depression

Myocardial depression severe due to MDS or capillary occlusion within myocardium.

Patient dies of severe myocardial depression with low cardiac output

FIGURE 13-1 *Sequential steps in the pathogenesis of septic shock in patients who die. Surviving patients would have the sequential steps interrupted at some stage before the last three mechanisms of the patient death (bottom three boxes). (Modified from: Parrillo, J.E., and Ayres, S.M. Major Issues in Critical Care Medicine. Baltimore: Williams and Wilkins, 1984.)*

induced by an antigen–antibody reaction that occurs when an antigen to which the individual had previously been sensitized enters the body. Anaphylaxis rarely occurs on initial exposure to an antigen. Antigens known to precipitate anaphylaxis are therapeutic drugs (ie, antibiotics, anesthetics, and contrast media, particularly those containing iodine) and foreign protein, such as that found in blood products and snake and insect venom (Table 13-4).[10]

Anaphylaxis, or type I hypersensitivity reaction, is brought about or initiated by the action of immunoglobulin E (IgE) (see p. XX). An antibody present in serum, IgE binds to mast cells and basophils when stimulated by exposure to a specific antigen. On a second or repeat exposure, the antigen adheres to the mast cell or the basophil, resulting in the release of substances that mediate shock.[5, 10] These substances, which include histamine, bradykinin, leukotrienes, and prostaglandins, mediate shock by different mechanisms and produce most of the overt symptomatology associated with anaphylactic shock (Fig. 13-2).

Histamine dilates blood vessels, constricts respira-

TABLE 13-4 *Agents Commonly Implicated in Anaphylactic and Anaphylactoid Reactions*

Antibiotics	Penicillin and penicillin analogues, cephalosporins, tetracyclines, erythromycin, streptomycin
Nonsteroidal antiinflammatory agents	Salicylates, aminopyrine
Narcotic analgesics	Morphine, codeine, meprobamate
Other drugs	Protamine, chlorpropamide, parenteral iron, iodides, thiazide diuretics
Local anesthetics	Procaine, lidocaine, cocaine
General anesthetics	Thiopental
Anesthetic adjuncts	Succinylcholine, tubocurarine
Blood products and antisera	Red blood cell, white blood cell, and platelet transfusions, gamma globulin, rabies, tetanus, diphtheria antitoxin, snake and spider antivenom
Diagnostic agents	Iodinated radiocontrast agents
Foods	Eggs, milk, nuts, legumes (peanuts, soybeans, kidney beans), fish, shellfish
Venoms	Bees, wasps, hornets, snakes, spiders, jellyfish
Hormones	Insulin, corticotropin, pituitary extract
Enzymes and other biologicals	Acetylcysteine, pancreatic enzyme supplements
Extracts of potential allergens used in desensitization	Pollen, food, venoms

W. C. Shoemaker et al. *Textbook of Critical Care* (3rd ed.). Philadelphia: W.B. Saunders, 1995.

tory smooth muscle, and increases vascular permeability. Bradykinin also causes vasodilatation and makes capillaries more permeable but has little or no effect on respiratory smooth muscle. The leukotrienes C_4, D_4, and E_4 (formerly called SRS-A, or slow-reacting substances of anaphylaxis) constrict bronchial smooth muscle and increase venule permeability.[5] The prostaglandins exert a variety of effects depending on their type. They increase, decrease, or do not influence vascular permeability, blood vessel size, or respiratory smooth muscle. The mechanism by which antigen–antibody reactions induce shock is directly related to the effects of the substances liberated at the outset of the reaction. Specifically, the shock state develops as a consequence of hypotension from profound vasodilatation and low cardiac output secondary to central fluid volume deficits due to increased capillary permeability and peripheral pooling of blood. Compensatory mechanisms are not capable of reversing or re-

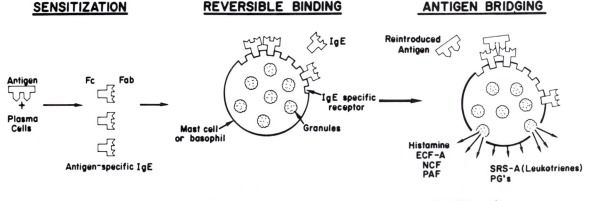

FIGURE 13-2 *The sequence of events leading to mediator release. During the initial exposure to antigen (sensitization) antigen-specific IgE is synthesized by plasma cells. The Fc portion of the IgE molecules then reversibly binds to receptors on mast cells or basophils. When antigen is subsequently reintroduced, two cell-bound IgE molecules are linked by a divalent antigen molecule (antigen-bridging). This initiates a series of biochemical events leading to primary mediator release. (From: Shoemaker, W.C. Textbook of Critical Care (3rd ed.). Philadelphia: W.B. Saunders, 1995).*

tarding the progression of this form of shock because the initial shock-producing insult develops rapidly and acutely.

In addition to overwhelming hypotension and tissue and organ ischemia, anaphylactic shock is often characterized by severe laryngeal spasm, edema, and bronchoconstriction. These pathologic developments compound the shock state by adding further hypoxemia to the overall pattern of response. Hypoxemia perpetuates the cycle of anaerobic metabolism and lactic acid production.

Signs and symptoms of anaphylaxis include profound hypotension, tachycardia, urticaria, pruritus, fever, dyspnea with hoarseness or stridor with wheezing, oliguria, cool and moist skin with pallor, cyanosis, and anxiety. The individual has a recent history of contact with a known allergen or an antigen capable of inducing the anaphylactic reaction. Respiratory complications, such as stridor and inspiratory wheezing, may precede respiratory arrest. Immediate treatment with epinephrine administered intravenously can have dramatic and often lifesaving effects.

▼ *Complications of Shock*

Complications that are directly caused by the shock state are devastating and often fatal. These complications stem from and are produced by the pathologic processes inherent in shock. The pathology is often seen in a number of organs (Fig. 13-3). The three most common processes that induce severe complications are vasodilatation with inadequate tissue and organ perfusion, damage to the capillary endothelial lining, and activation of clotting factors. Complications of these processes include lactic acidosis, adult respiratory distress syndrome, disseminated intravascular coagulation, and organ necrosis.

LACTIC ACIDOSIS

The basis for lactic acidosis in shock is the relentless production of lactic acid related to continual hypoxia of tissues from impaired perfusion. Hypoperfusion to tissues deprives them of oxygen. Cells are unable to metabolize nutrients appropriately without oxygen. In the absence of sufficient oxygen, cells are forced to metabolize nutrients anaerobically, which invariably results in the production of lactic acid.

Lactic acid exerts two major effects on the body. It depresses myocardial contractility, which interferes with cardiac output, further reducing the already compromised perfusion and oxygenation of tissue. This establishes a cycle of further compromised tissue perfusion. The second untoward effect of lactic acid production is that it contributes acid to the body, leading to metabolic acidosis and further impairment of cellular metabolic function.

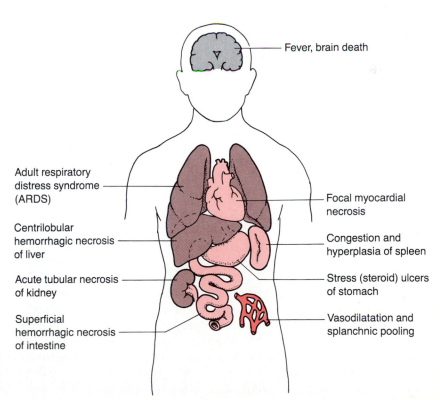

FIGURE 13-3 *Complications of shock. (Source: Rubin, E., and Farber, J. Pathology [2nd ed.). Philadelphia: J.B. Lippincott, 1994.)*

ADULT RESPIRATORY DISTRESS SYNDROME

Adult respiratory distress syndrome develops secondary to shock because of at least two processes associated with the shock state. Pulmonary ischemia from hypoperfusion and aggregation of platelets in pulmonary capillaries significantly damage the endothelial lining of the pulmonary capillaries, causing them to lose selective permeability. Consequently, water, electrolytes, red blood cells, and plasma proteins are extravasated into the interstitium of the lungs. This greatly impedes pulmonary compliance. Later, these fluids and blood components penetrate the alveoli, leading to frank pulmonary edema, further reduction in compliance, bronchospasm, atelectasis, and, ultimately, significant hypoxemia (see pp. 587–589).[5]

DISSEMINATED INTRAVASCULAR COAGULATION

Disseminated intravascular coagulation is a complex coagulopathy that occurs rather frequently among persons who are acutely ill, especially those who have experienced some form of shock. The bases for the development of disseminated intravascular coagulation are abnormal platelet aggregation and activation of factors of clotting, both of which are prominent features of shock. In response to the platelets and clotting factors, generalized coagulation occurs in the microcirculation and impedes capillary flow. In addition, the clotting process consumes fibrin, platelets, and other factors of clotting and initiates fibrinolysis. Active fibrinolysis produces and releases fibrin degradation products, which are the end products of fibrin, fibrinogen, and plasmin lysis. The presence of these fibrin degradation products plus the consumption of platelets and other clotting factors interrupts subsequent coagulation and leads to widespread bleeding.[5]

Symptoms of microcirculation (capillary) coagulation are present, including cool skin with mottling and cyanotic nail beds and concomitant signs of profuse bleeding, especially from puncture sites, incisions, and the gastrointestinal tract. The overall picture of disseminated intravascular coagulation is one of a vicious cycle of coagulation and anticoagulation (see pp. 418–419).

ORGAN ISCHEMIA AND NECROSIS

Organ ischemia with resultant necrosis and loss of function are the inevitable consequences of shock, particularly if the condition is protracted or progresses to the irreversible stage. Organ ischemia occurs secondary to shock as a consequence of hypotension, selective vasoconstriction of sympathetic activity, platelet aggregation with microcirculation clotting, and capillary endothelial damage. Organ systems that undergo the most pronounced damage are the heart, brain, kidneys, liver, and lungs. Necrotic lesions secondary to the shock state have been identified in liver, myocardial, renal, and lung tissue with resultant dysfunction or complete loss of function.[5, 19]

CASE STUDY 13-1

Joey Green, an 18-year-old college freshman, was involved in a one-car motor vehicle accident at 1:00 AM on a Saturday morning. He received multiple superficial lacerations along with a fracture of three ribs on the left side. He was admitted with a blood pressure of 70/48, pulse of 148, and respirations of 36. Examination revealed abdominal tenderness and diminished breath sounds on the left side. He was alert and oriented, but pale and perspiring profusely. After initial stabilization, a Swan-Ganz catheter was placed which showed a pulmonary artery pressure of 20/8 and a pulmonary capillary wedge pressure of 2. His central venous pressure was 1 mm Hg.

1. *What type of shock is Joey exhibiting? From the clinical picture described, explain the source of the shock.*
2. *Explain the pathophysiology of this form of shock and compare it with other types.*
3. *What is the significance of the Swan-Ganz catheter readings?*
4. *What would the expected course of treatment be for this type of shock?*

See Appendix G for discussion.

▼ Multiple Organ Dysfunction Syndrome

The term multiple organ system failure, or multiple organ dysfunction syndrome (MODS), refers to a progressive loss of function in two or more organs following a major bodily insult.[6] The precipitating factors include a variety of diseases and mechanisms that usually precipitate shock and organ hypoxia (Box 13-1). The most common association with MODS occurs when it follows sepsis and/or septic shock. Circulating mediators damage vital organs, whose function is disrupted. The effects of MODS are illustrated in Flowchart 13-7.

The pathogenesis of other causes besides sepsis is unclear. MODS is the major cause of death in shock survivors and seems to be related to the number of organ systems involved. It can affect anyone who has undergone a major body insult and usually begins with pulmonary failure manifested by adult respiratory distress syndrome. This is followed rapidly by acute renal failure. Cardiovascular effects may be the result of septic mediators or shock-induced myocardial depression. Gastrointestinal and liver dysfunction are manifested by ileus and altered liver function tests. Central nervous system deficits appear and are closely related to the magnitude of the shock state. The onset of immune deficiency markedly depletes the host's ability to withstand opportunistic organisms. The syndrome of disseminated intravascular coagulation markedly decreases the chance for survival, because it further damages oxygen-depleted tissues and organs.

The clinical signs of MODS are variable but usually begin with the respiratory abnormalities of adult respiratory distress syndrome, which precipitate further hypoxia to all tissues. Early signs of extrapulmonary MODS include confusion, decreased urine output, evidence of gastrointestinal bleeding, thrombocytopenia,

altered coagulation studies, glucose intolerance, and worsening of a previously stable shock picture.[16]

The critical action to prevent death is to ascertain and treat the underlying etiology; to prevent and/or treat superinfection; and to exclude other etiologies of organ dysfunction, such as nephrotoxicity from antibiotics.[16] The incidence of MODS in intensive care units has increased, probably due to more efficient treatment of the major insult that precipitated the syndrome. The mortality rates for MODS depend on the number of organs affected and the degree of disruption. Mortality figures of up to 90% have been described.

▼ Chapter Summary

▼ The shock state results from a major disruption of the mechanism of tissue perfusion. It is caused by many different diseases or trauma and leads to multiorgan effects. Tissue perfusion is maintained by a cooperative effort of cardiac output and vascular supply. This requires the combined effects of total peripheral resistance, autonomic nervous system actions, intravascular fluid volume, hormones (catecholamines and sodium/water retaining hormones), and the ability to pump blood to all areas of the vascular tree.

▼ Shock is a profound hemodynamic and metabolic disturbance that results when the tissues of the body are not properly perfused. It results from fluid volume deficit, vascular volume deficit, and inadequacy of the circulatory pump. Shock occurs in stages from compensated to noncompensated to irreversible.

▼ Hypovolemic shock may result from anything that decreases circulating volume of blood or plasma. The source of the loss must be determined and corrected to prevent the progression of the circulatory collapse. Cardiogenic shock results from impairment of the pumping mechanism of the heart. The compensatory mechanisms of the body function like those for hypovolemia, which is detrimental to the functioning of the heart. Distributive shock develops as a consequence of vasodilatation caused by different mechanisms. These mechanisms may be vasomotor center depression, anaphylaxis, or sepsis. The underlying mechanism must be treated to remove the source of the vasodilatation.

▼ The shock state produces many serious complications that are often the cause of the patient's death. Lactic acidosis produced from anaerobic metabolism in the cells produces a metabolic disruption to the body tissues. Other common complications affect the lungs and the coagulation system. Organ ischemia and necrosis produce loss of organ function.

▼ Closely associated with this organ function disruption is MODS, with its progressive loss of function in two or more organs. MODS has a very high mortality rate unless the underlying problem can be treated.

Flowchart 13-7   Multiple Organ Dysfunction Syndrome (MODS)

Development of multiple organ dysfunction syndrome.

Chapter 14

Infectious Agents

Barbara L. Bullock

▼ **CHAPTER OUTLINE**

▼ **LEARNING OBJECTIVES**

1 Describe the major defense mechanisms of the host.
2 List the major characteristics of each type of infectious agent.
3 Explain how infectious agents are classified.
4 Describe the modes of viral infection and how viruses multiply.
5 Describe at least six viral infections, differentiating DNA and RNA viruses, incubation periods, mode of transmission, and clinical effects.
6 Define chlamydiae in terms of their importance in disease causation.
7 Describe the pathologic effects of the rickettsial organism in spotted and typhus fevers.
8 Discuss the role of toxins produced by bacterial organisms.
9 Describe at least six gram-positive and gram-negative bacterial infections in terms of pathogenesis and clinical effects.
10 List three major classifications of fungi that are infectious to humans and describe the relationships among them.
11 Explain how protozoa move and reproduce.
12 Briefly describe three infections that may result from protozoa.
13 Categorize the types of helminths and describe how each can cause pathology in humans.

Barbara L. Bullock: PATHOPHYSIOLOGY: ADAPTATIONS AND ALTERATIONS IN FUNCTION, 4th ed.
© 1996 Lippincott-Raven Publishers

Infectious diseases are produced by living organisms: viruses, chlamydia, rickettsia, bacteria, fungi, protozoa, and helminths. These diseases have been present in enormous numbers and have caused epidemics by their contagiousness. Although developments in nutrition, insect control, immunization, sanitation, and drug therapy have decreased the mortality and morbidity of infectious diseases, microbial infections have not been eliminated.[13] Microbes have developed mutant strains that are resistant to once-effective antimicrobial therapy. Infectious diseases still occur in great numbers and often are fatal to very young or elderly, debilitated victims. People in less developed countries have a much greater risk of contracting and dying of infectious diseases than do those in industrialized countries.[13]

▼ Host–Parasite Relationships

The occurrence of infectious diseases depends on many factors, including the virulence of the organism, the number of invading organisms, the defense mechanisms of the body, and the relationship with the normal human flora. Infectious organisms characteristically cause infection in one organ system. This propensity is called *tissue tropism*, which is determined by specific biochemical substances on the surface of the organism complemented by receptors on the target organ.[3]

VIRULENCE

Virulence is the ability of the infecting organism to cause disease, requiring a receptive host in which it can settle and multiply. The mechanisms by which an organism can cause disease require epithelial attachment, penetration into tissues, production of toxins, and the ability to cause alterations in the genome of the new host.[6,8] Some organisms are highly virulent in most normal hosts, which means that in most individuals they will cause disease.[17] The number of invading organisms must be sufficient to overwhelm the defenses of the host. In some cases, the organism is not naturally virulent but the host has a decreased ability to resist the infection. When an infection results under this circumstance, it is called an *opportunistic infection*. This term refers to the organism that is normally *nonpathogenic* but *pathogenic* when the immune defense of the host is compromised.[17] The importance of opportunistic infections has been underscored by the emergence of many unusual infections in people infected with the human immunodeficiency virus that causes acquired immune deficiency syndrome (see p. 343).

The emergence of opportunistic infections has also been enhanced by the medical therapeutics administered to combat disease. These treatment measures can impair the ability of the host to withstand infection, allowing organisms that normally reside on the surfaces of the body to gain access and cause disease. The amount of immune compromise and the elements of the immune system compromised are key factors in the severity of the disease manifestations. Many disease conditions and even emotional stress can suppress the immune response and leave the individual vulnerable to disease.

DEFENSE MECHANISMS OF THE BODY

The defense mechanisms of the human body reside on the external and internal surfaces and include physical, chemical, and immune barriers. Whether the organism can cause disease largely depends on the success or failure of these mechanisms and barriers to provide adequate defense. The main physical external barrier to infection is the skin, an intact epidermis being almost impervious to infection. The mucous membranes lining various organs also remove organisms by secreting mucus, which provides a washing effect and prevents organisms from adhering to membranes. Chemical secretions, such as hydrochloric acid in the stomach and the normally acidic pH urine, contribute to the sterile environment in the organs. The immune system targets pathogens for destruction. When organisms gain access to the body, lymphocytes recognize and destroy them, often without producing disease manifestations. The competence of the immune system, therefore, plays a major role in the outcome of infectious disease (see Chapter 16).

The defense mechanisms can be grouped into physical or chemical characteristics, immune factors, and nature of the host (Table 14-1). Clinically apparent infec-

---

TABLE 14-1 *Defense Mechanisms of the Body*

Mechanism	Characteristics of Defense
Physical	Intact epidermis Mucus-secreting membranes Mucus blanket movement in respiratory tract Connective tissue
Chemical	Hydrochloric acid in stomach Acid pH of urine Lysozyme enzyme present in many secretions Resident flora in mouth, on skin, in large intestine
Immune	Specific antigen–antibody reactions Immunoglobin A Inflammatory response
Host factors	Age Sex Genetic susceptibilities Nutritional balance Stress—physiologic or emotional Presence of other diseases

tions occur when the defense mechanisms have not been sufficient to hold the growth of the organism in check. The pathogenesis of infection depends on the capability of the specific organism and its ability to bypass or inactivate the defense mechanisms of the body. Manifestations of infections can be ascribed to injury, dysfunction, destruction of host cells, and alterations in the immune response. Once actual infection is established, it often causes nonspecific signs and symptoms that characteristically include fever, chills, muscle pain, lymph node enlargement, and variable elevation in the white blood cell count. Each microorganism is distinct and has its own means of invasion and reproduction. The major classifications of living organisms are described in this chapter. The effects of the resultant diseases are also described in the chapters relating to specific organs and systems.

Infections may produce illness, as described earlier, or they may be inapparent or *subclinical*, in which state they are so mild that signs and symptoms are not seen. A particular form of subclinical infection is the *carrier state*, in which the person remains a reservoir of infection and retains the ability to infect others.[17] Another important form of infection is *latent infection*, in which bouts of disease occur, interrupted by periods of no disease manifestation or infectivity. Herpes viral infections are common latent infections that can be reactivated by stress, other infections, or other factors.[13]

All infectious organisms are communicable (transmissible) from one member of the same species to another. The modes of transmission vary and depend on the source, quantity of organisms, transit survival, and a susceptible new host.[17]

The human organism can contact and combat a multitude of potential pathogens in the environment. This is evidenced by the state of relative disease freedom in most people. This active defense is maintained through the complex immune system, which demonstrates a high degree of selectivity for organisms. The defensive ability of this system is affected by age, genetic factors, psychological factors, and environmental and nutritional factors.

NORMAL HUMAN FLORA

Many infections arise from normal flora of the host due to change in parasite virulence or change in host resistance. When the normal barriers to infections are broken, such as in hospital settings with invasive procedures, there is a much greater risk of normal flora causing infection. Infections that are caused by the hospital or other medical setting are called *iatrogenic infections*, which would not occur if the individual had not been placed in the environment or been subjected to a particular procedure. When this is compounded by a decrease in host resistance, such as the stress of surgery or a reaction to antibiotic therapy, organisms normally under control will proliferate rapidly and become pathologic. If the normal microbes in an area are known, then the source and significance of microorganisms isolated from a clinical infection also become known.[14]

The organisms that are indigenous to specific areas vary. Table 14-2 categorizes the sites and the organisms that normally reside in those sites.

▼ *Viruses*

Viruses are the smallest infectious agents known. They are not complete cells in themselves and essentially exist as parasites on living cells. These organisms use the biochemical products of other living cells to replicate.

STRUCTURE, REPRODUCTION, AND PATHOGENESIS

Viruses vary in size, appearance, and behavior. They are classified as either DNA or RNA viruses, according to their genetic material. Many contain nucleic acid, which is protected by a closed protein shell called the *capsid*. Some are surrounded by a lipid envelope.

Mature virus particles are called *virions* and contain a core of nucleic acid of either DNA or RNA.[4] Viruses appear to be species- and organ-specific and can replicate only in permissive or receptive cells. Some viruses enter a receptive cell by being enveloped (endocytosis), and some fuse with the cellular membrane, after which the process of multiplication can begin.

The structure of the virus has been studied with the electron microscope and is described according to its appearance. The complete infective particle is called a *virion*. The *capsid* is the protein coat, which is made up of protein subunits called *capsomeres*. The viral nucleic acid and the capsid are called the *nucleocapsid*.[4] Complex virions may contain additional layers, or envelopes. Figure 14-1 illustrates the different forms of viruses and their component parts. The protein covering of the virus is type specific. The surface structure is responsible for attachment to particular cell receptors. Infection depends on the compatibility of the viral surface with the host cell receptors and the ability of viral nucleic acid to use the host cell to manufacture viral products. All viruses are similar in their method of attachment to the specific receptors on the host cell membrane, the so-called "lock-and-key" attachment. Some have amino acids that are similar to the actively transported substances in the cell membrane of the host. Viruses can fool the cell, attach themselves to receptor sites on the host cell, and block the movement of normally transported materials.

Viruses affect and infect specific cells. Some B lymphocytes, for example, carry receptors for the Epstein-Barr virus, whereas cells in the tracheal lining have receptors for the influenza virus. Viruses produce specific diseases that involve specific tissues, but their modes of

TABLE 14-2 *Microorganisms Commonly Found on the Body*

Site Affected	Organism	Site Affected	Organism
Skin	*Staphylococcus epidermidis*	Large intestine	Gram-negative bacilli
	Staphylococcus aureus		*Escherichia coli*
	Propionibacterium acnes (anaerobic corynebacteria)		Enterobacteriaceae
	Lactobacilli		*Klebsiella* sp.
	Clostridium perfringens		*Enterobacter* sp.
	Acinetobacter calcoaceticus		*Candida albicans*
	Aerobic corynebacteria		*Bacteroides fragilis*
Nose/Nasopharynx	*Haemophilus parainfluenzae*		*B. melaninogenicus*
	Staphylococcus aureus		*B. oralis*
	Staphylococcus epidermidis		*Fusobacterium nucleatum*
	Aerobic corynebacteria		*F. necrophorum*
Mouth/Oropharynx	*Staphylococcus aureus*		Gram-positive bacilli
	Staphylococcus epidermidis		Lactobacilli
	Aerobic corynebacteria		*Eubacterium limosum*
	Alpha- and nonhemolytic streptococci		*Bifidobacterium bifidum*
	Streptococcus mutans		Gram-positive cocci
	S. milleri		*Staphylococcus aureus*
	S. mitis		Enterococci
	S. sanguis		Peptostreptococci
	S. salivarius	Genitourinary tract	*Lactobacillus*
	Branhamella catarrhalis	Vagina	*Bacteroides*
	Anaerobic micrococci		Peptostreptococci
	Veillonella alcalescens		Aerobic corynebacteria
	Enterobacteriaceae		*Staphylococcus epidermidis*
Small intestine	*Candida albicans*		Enterococci
			Candida albicans
			Trichomonas vaginalis

Note: Not all organisms are found in every individual. These organisms are common in sites listed. Other sites are usually sterile.

transmission and diseases produced are numerous. Cells respond to viral infection in different ways. There may be no apparent cellular change, because viral DNA may adopt a symbiotic relationship with the host cell. Conversely, cellular pathologic effects, such as death or virus-induced hyperplasia, may occur. Cytopathic effects are common and include aggregation of host cells into clusters with shrinkage, lysis, and fusion of the cells. The effects differ and are influenced by the effects of the virus on cellular synthesis of macromolecules; alteration in cellular organelles, such as the lysosomes; and changes in the host cell membrane. Figure 14-2 shows a generalized viral life cycle including the courses the infection may take.

Although no one virus is typical, the replication and transmission of this organism have been assessed extensively by studying the bacteriophage (virus that attacks bacteria). The genetic material of the bacteriophage is enclosed in an angular head or protein-containing capsid. The hollow head contains the viral genetic material and connects with a hollow cylinder of protein surrounded by protein contractile fibers. The contractile fibers coil around the cylinder like a spring. At the end of the tail, the fibers and an enzyme are important in attaching the virion to the host cell (Fig. 14-3).

Viral multiplication usually occurs in several steps. The first step is recognition and attachment (adsorption) of the virus to the host cell. The mechanism varies with the type of virus. The second step is penetration or injection of viral DNA into the cell. Replication follows through nucleic acid synthesis and assembly into new virus particles. At a certain point, these virus particles are released from the cell into the extracellular environment (Fig. 14-4).[2] The formed particles can survive outside the host cell for variable periods of time, often until a new susceptible host cell can be found.

Each type of virus infects the host cell uniquely. The resulting signs and symptoms of the viral disease reflect the manner in which the virus has affected the host.[18] Some viruses are *endogenous* and can remain latent within the host for years, only to be later reactivated (Fig. 14-5). Examples of this type are herpes zoster and genital herpes. In most cases, the disease results from exposure to an *exogenous virus*, either through direct contact with another infected host or through indirect transmission, such as by means of contaminated water or shellfish.[4]

Viral infections stimulate the immune system's antibody production. Neutralizing antibodies are formed during viremia, but the main host defense is through cell-mediated immunity (see pp. 326–327).[13] The initial

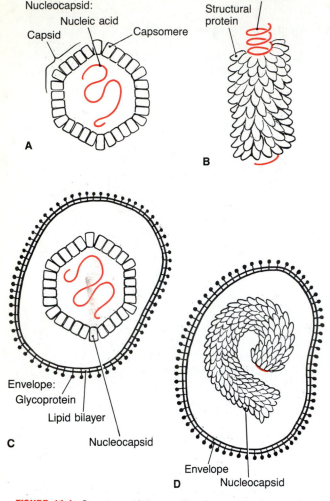

FIGURE 14-1 *Structures of viruses. The morphology varies by shape and presence or absence of an envelope.* **A.** *and* **B.** *represent two forms of naked or nonenveloped viruses.* **C.** *and* **D.** *represent two types of enveloped viruses that are highly variable in shape (pleomorphic) because the membrane is not rigid. These are more complex viruses.*

initiate a rapid reproductive cycle, the more virulent the virus. Activation or induction causes the latent viruses to become active and reprograms the cell for viral reproduction. It has been suggested that activation may be initiated by cold temperatures, carcinogens, or materials in food, air, or water. Each virus responds to a specific induction mechanism. Sometimes a few cells with viruses within them escape induction, so that not all affected cells are lysed. In this way the host cell carries viral DNA as part of its own DNA, and the virus can remain latent in the host tissues throughout the life of the cell.

Viral infections produce many diseases, including hepatitis, meningoencephalitis, pneumonia, rhinitis, skin diseases, and numerous other disorders that affect almost every body system. Research is being conducted on many other disease conditions, such as multiple sclerosis, diabetes mellitus, and cancer, in the hopes of finding a viral connection.[8, 13] Identification of viral infections can be made by cell culture during the prodromal and early acute stages of disease. Later identification of certain types of viruses can be made by complement-fixing antibodies, which elevate and remain elevated for a period of time following the disease. A high titer of complement-fixing antibody to a specific virus is suggestive of recent contact with that virus.[15] The polymerase chain reaction is a new test that can amplify a single DNA

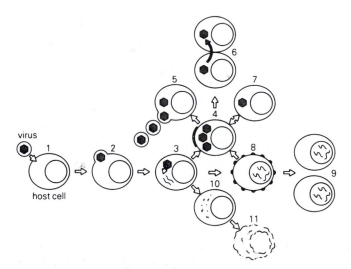

FIGURE 14-2 *A generalized viral life cycle. The virion becomes absorbed by its receptors to a host cell (1). The virus then penetrates the cell and becomes uncoated (2 and 3). Infection may take several courses, depending on the viral species. Some viruses replicate their components, which then assemble in the host cell (4) and are released by budding from the cell membrane (5). Alternatively, the virus can spread by cell-to-cell contact (6), without being released. Viruses also remain dormant within cells, to be reactivated at a later date (7). Some viruses are capable of inserting their genetic material into the host genome, where they remain latent (8). The cell subsequently may become productive (4) or, in certain circumstances, can undergo neoplastic transformation (9). Some virus infections may be absorptive (10), either because the host cell is nonpermissive for infection or because the virus is defective. Both abortive infections and productive infections can lead to cell death (11). (From I. Roitt, J. Brostoff, and D. Male,* Immunology *[2nd ed.]. Philadelphia: J.B. Lippincott, 1989.)*

response to viral infestation usually is by the mononuclear cells, the monocytes and lymphocytes. At the site of entry of viruses into the body, the immunocompetent (antigen-specific) cells accumulate and initiate the inflammatory process. Macrophages often attach to the virus and enhance T- and B-cell interaction. Exposure to viral agents initially causes the synthesis of specific IgM antibodies, which is followed after about 10 days by the synthesis of IgG antibodies. When the virion is sufficiently coated with antibody, it is rendered noninfectious. The specific T lymphocytes provide for long-term immunity. Viruses and other substances stimulate the production of *interferon*, a family of antiviral proteins that inhibits viral spread from cell to cell.[5]

After attachment, an *eclipse* stage may be entered, during which viral DNA becomes part of the host chromosome and remains *latent*. The greater the capability to

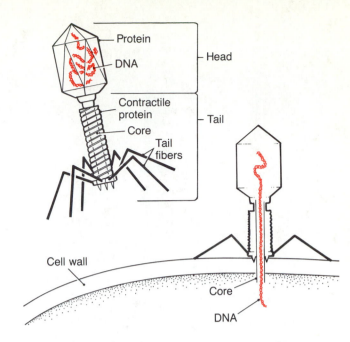

FIGURE 14-3 *A bacteriophage is a virus that attacks bacteria. It has been used to study viral activity. The bacteriophage is composed of DNA, protein, a hollow core, and tail fibers. It attaches to the cell wall of a* E. coli *bacteria and injects its DNA through the bacterial cell wall.*

molecule, which yields a detectable signal, especially for viral diseases. The polymerase chain reaction technique has been used to detect hepatitis B virus in chronic hepatitis and human immunodeficiency virus and especially for typing of the genital human papillomavirus as well as other viruses.[15]

Although there are multitudes of types of viruses, most of them can be classified into DNA or RNA structural viruses. Table 14-3 presents this classification, listing the common disease-producing groups, their modes of transmission, and the resulting symptomatology.

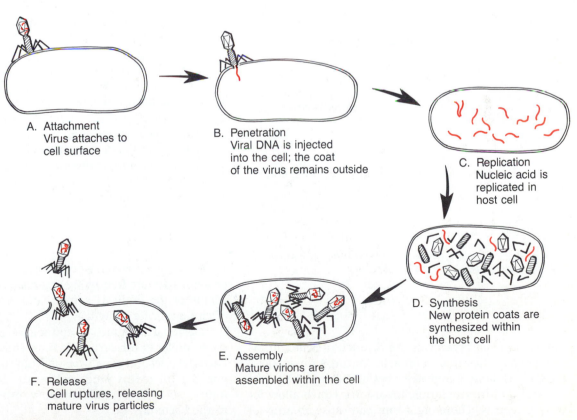

A. Attachment
Virus attaches to
cell surface

B. Penetration
Viral DNA is injected
into the cell; the coat
of the virus remains outside

C. Replication
Nucleic acid is
replicated in
host cell

D. Synthesis
New protein coats are
synthesized within
the host cell

E. Assembly
Mature virions are
assembled within the cell

F. Release
Cell ruptures, releasing
mature virus particles

FIGURE 14-4 *Steps in replication cycle of a virus.*

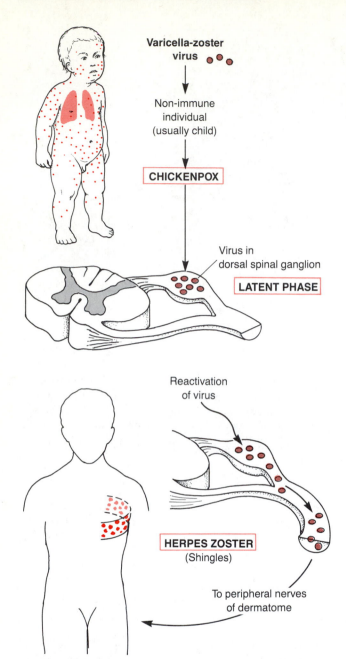

FIGURE 14-5 *Varicella (chickenpox). Varicella-zoster virus (VZV) in droplets is inhaled by a nonimmune person (usually a child) and initially causes a "silent" infection of the nasopharynx. This progresses to viremia, seeding of fixed macrophages, and dissemination of VZV to skin and viscera. The VZV resides in a dorsal spinal ganglion, where it remains dormant for many years. Herpes zoster. Latent VZV is reactivated and spreads from ganglia along the sensory dermatomes. (Adapted from: Rubin, E. and Farber, J.L.* Pathology *[2nd ed.]. Philadelphia: J.B. Lippincott, 1994.)*

▼ Chlamydia

The chlamydial organisms are distinct, obligate, intracellular parasites that cannot be cultured on artificial media.[10] Chlamydiae possess both DNA and RNA and cell walls with cytoplasmic inclusions, which allow for their diagnosis. These organisms can cause an array of diseases, and the most common sexually transmitted disease in developed countries is caused by *Chlamydia trachomatis*. The *C. psittaci* or *C. pneumoniae* can cause an acute flulike illness that may progress to pneumonia.[13] Trachoma is caused by a subtype of *C trachomatis* and causes conjunctivitis as well as urethritis, cervicitis, proctitis, and salpingitis. Lymphogranuloma venereum is venereally transmitted as a subtype of *C. trachomatis* and produces lymphadenopathy in the inguinal areas in males and in the pelvic and perirectal lymph nodes in females.[13]

▼ Rickettsia

Rickettsia, once thought to be related to viruses because of their small size, are obligate, parasitic organisms. They possess all of the features of bacteria except that they can multiply only within certain cells of susceptible hosts.[12] Their normal reservoir most often is the arthropods, especially ticks, mites, lice, and fleas, in which they multiply without causing disease. Most rickettsial diseases are transmitted to humans through the bite or feces of the infected arthropod. An exception to this is Q fever, which probably is spread from person to person by respiratory droplets. The classification of rickettsia is based on the clinical features and epidemiologic aspects of the diseases they cause. The organisms are classified into the 1) spotted fever group; 2) typhus group; and 3) others, including Q fever.

All rickettsial diseases cause fever, and most cause a rash that is the result of rickettsial multiplication in the endothelial cells of the small blood vessels. The cells become swollen and necrotic, leading to the vascular lesions noted on or through the skin. Aggregations of lymphocytes, granulocytes, and macrophages accumulate in the small vessels of the brain, heart, and other organs.

Laboratory tests demonstrate the presence of rickettsial antigen and antibodies. Broad-spectrum antibiotics, such as tetracycline, suppress the growth of rickettsia, but full recovery requires an intact immune system that can develop antibodies against the organism.[20]

The most common diseases resulting from rickettsial infection include Rocky Mountain spotted fever and the typhus fevers (Table 14-4).

▼ Bacteria

Unlike viruses, bacteria do not require living cells for growth. They are free-living organisms that use the nutrients of the body as a food source and a favorable environment for growth.

Bacteria can attach to epithelial tissue and, like viruses, prefer to infect specific sites. Pathogenic effects of bacterial infection usually result from substances such as enzymes or toxins produced by the bacteria or from injury caused by the inflammatory response of the body to the bacteria.

(text continues on page 287)

TABLE 14-3 *Common Viruses That Cause Pathologic Effects in Humans*

Type	Nucleic Acid Present	Incubation Period	Epidemiology	Clinical Manifestations
Herpesviruses Varicella (chicken pox)	DNA	10–21 days	Highly contagious through respiratory droplets	Fever, disseminated vesicular eruption profuse on trunk and on oral mucosa; increased risk in immunosuppressed people
Zoster (shingles)	DNA	Variable		Follows chickenpox—may occur years after a primary attack; spreads down peripheral nerves of skin; active ganglionitis causes burning or dull pain; vesicles follow nerve fibers
Herpes simplex Type 1	DNA	2–12 days	Skin contact (oral)	Fever, vesicular eruption of mucous membranes, conjunctivitis, oral lesions (fever blisters); encephalitis occasionally results when virus ascends to central nervous system; manifestations more severe in immunosuppressed people
Type 2	DNA	5–14 days	Skin contact (genital); attack rate with sexual contact 1 : 3; through small mucosal cracks	Genital vesicles, fever, burning, urinary urgency in males; dysuria, vulvar burning, dyspareunia in females
Epstein-Barr	DNA	30–50 days	Respiratory droplet, transfusion	Sore throat, lymphadenopathy, splenomegaly, supraorbital edema; causative agent of infectious mononucleosis; virus has been isolated from Burkitt's lymphoma
Cytomegalovirus	DNA	?20–50 days	Saliva, urine, feces, semen, transplacental, transfusion	Vary with age of onset: *Congenital*: failure to thrive, jaundice, respiratory distress; may be fatal *Postnatal*: infection may cause anemia, hepatomegaly, lymphocytosis *Adult form*: fever, lymphocytosis, Guillain-Barré syndrome *Immunosuppressed people*: interstitial pneumonia, hepatitis, increased frequency of rejection of transplanted organs
Vaccinia	DNA	About 2 wk after vaccination	Inoculation for smallpox	Probably hybrid of variola or cowpox virus; may cause widespread eczematous reaction or encephalomyelitis that causes death in 30%–40% of patients

(continued)

TABLE 14-3 *(continued)*

Type	Nucleic Acid Present	Incubation Period	Epidemiology	Clinical Manifestations
Adenovirus (many strains identified)	DNA	5–10 days	High frequency in children and military recruits; respiratory aerosol or droplet	Febrile pharyngitis; headache, regional lymphadenopathy, nasal obstruction and discharge, conjunctivitis, *pneumonia*
Papovavirus (warts—many types)	DNA	1–20 months	Skin contact, contact with contaminated secretions; sexually transmitted	Solid, rounded tumors with horny projections 1–2 cm in size; often asymptomatic unless located on area of irritation; often found on hands, neck, shins, forearms, genital area
Molluscum contagiosum	DNA	1–25 weeks	Sexual/nonsexual skin contact	3–5 mm, firm, smooth lesions, usually on genitalia, asymptomatic
Picornavirus—coxsackie viruses A & B (many strains)	RNA	2–5 days	Fecal-oral contact; insects may be passive vectors	Depend on type; acute myocarditis, fever, muscle and pleuritic pain, vesicular lesions on soft palate and tonsils, pharyngitis; associated with many systemic problems
Coronavirus	RNA	3 days	Respiratory droplet	Common cold, rhinitis, pneumonia, bronchitis
Rhinovirus (many strains)	RNA	1–2 days	Respiratory droplet	Common cold; fever, cough, croup, and pneumonia may develop in children; sore throat, nasal congestion, and nasal discharge without fever common in adults
Morbillivirus	RNA	3–5 days	Respiratory droplet	Measles rash follows exposure usually associated with rhinorrhea, rash disseminates bodywide
Poliovirus	RNA	2–5 days	Fecal-oral contact	Undifferentiated febrile illness may spread to involve anterior horn cells of spinal cord and motor nuclei of cranial nerves; causes various muscle paralyses, hemiplegia, paraplegia; bladder and respiratory muscle dysfunction; poliovaccines can prevent disease
Orthomyxovirus—influenza A, B, and C	RNA	18–36 hours, up to 7 days	Epidemic, new strains evolve frequently; transmitted by infected respiratory secretions	Respiratory symptoms, cough, headache, muscle pain, fever, chills, sneezing, nasal discharge, prostration common; symptoms among strains similar

(continued)

TABLE 14-3   *(continued)*

Type	Nucleic Acid Present	Incubation Period	Epidemiology	Clinical Manifestations
Paramyxovirus	RNA	15–21 days	Very communicable in crowded conditions; transmitted by upper respiratory tract secretions	Painful enlargement of salivary glands; orchitis occurs in 20%–35% postpubertal males; small percentage develop meningitis or may affect other glands
Rhabdovirus—rabies	RNA	Variable; average 2–6 wk in humans	Animal bite of nonimmunized domestic dogs or cats, or of wild animals such as skunks, foxes, raccoons, bats, wolves	Virus introduced through mucous membranes or epidermis; replicates in striated muscle and then spreads up peripheral nerve bundles to central nervous system; passes to all organs but major effects on CNS; acute encephalitis, brain stem dysfunction and death; rapidly fatal if not treated; hydrophobia (excessive salivation) characteristic
Arbovirus—four groups cause CNS disease	RNA	4–14 days	Mosquito bite transmits to humans; can multiply in horses, birds, bats, snakes, insects	Age-related; younger people often have high fever and convulsions; headache, fever, drowsiness, confusion, disorientation; some manifest mainly by lethargy, "sleeping sickness"; muscle weakness; residual effects range from none to convulsions; speech difficulties
Hepatitis A	RNA similar to picornaviruses	15–45 days	Fecal-oral enhanced by poor hygiene, overcrowding, contaminated food, water; sexual; percutaneous	Onset acute, most frequent in young people; causes anorexia, malaise, and other symptoms followed by jaundice; dark urine, clay-colored stools; recovery usually complete
Hepatitis C	RNA	60–160 days	Parenteral; possible fecal-oral	Clinical course variable; debilitation and liver dysfunction not infrequent, chronic hepatitis
Hepatitis B	DNA-type	45–160 days	Percutaneous, sexual, fecal-oral	Chronic active hepatitis may occur; jaundice, liver dysfunction may progress to liver failure; recovery slow
Delta virus	RNA	28–180 days	Blood, homosexual contact	People susceptible to hepatitis B or HBV carriers can be infected; clinical picture like HBV; may progress to chronic hepatitis
Hepatitis E	RNA	14–56 days	Fecal-oral; contaminated water	Chronic active hepatitis, cirrhosis, chronic carrier, like Hepatitis B

(continued)

TABLE 14-3 *(continued)*

Type	Nucleic Acid Present	Incubation Period	Epidemiology	Clinical Manifestations
Human immuno-deficiency virus	RNA retrovirus	Not known	Homosexual or heterosexual contact; parenteral transmission; perinatal transmission	May be dormant; may cause clinical AIDS; immunodeficiency affects resistance to cytomegalovirus and Epstein-Barr virus with high percentage affected; pneumonia caused by *Pneumocystis carinii*; series of opportunistic infections; Kaposi's sarcoma; swollen lymph glands, fatigue, weight loss; clinical AIDS usually results in death

CNS: central nervous system; AIDS: acquired immunodeficiency syndrome.

TABLE 14-4 *Common Rickettsia That Cause Pathologic Effects in Humans*

Rickettsia	Morphology	Epidemiology	Clinical Effects
Spotted fevers (*Rickettsia rickettsii*; Rocky Mountain spotted fever)	Small organism, stains purple; usually gram-negative cell wall antigen; elaborates endotoxinlike substance	Multiply in nucleus and cytoplasm of infected cells of ticks and mammals; commonly occurs in Western hemisphere; transmitted by bite of infected tick or through skin abrasions contacting tick feces or tissue juices; incubation 3–12 days	Swelling and degeneration of endothelial cells, vascular damage, myocarditis, pneumonitis; peripheral vascular collapse may cause death; impairment of hepatic function and consumption coagulopathy may occur; severe headache, muscle pain, fever for 15–20 days; characteristic rash begins as small discrete, nonfixed pink lesions on wrists, ankles, forearms, etc., becomes petechial; mortality 7%–10%
Typhus fevers (*R. prowazekii*; epidemic typhus)	Small, gram-negative organism; always multiplies within cytoplasm of cells	Inhalation of dried louse feces; louse feces often rubbed into broken skin as with scratching of bite; incubation approximately 1 wk	Intense headache; continuous pyrexia for 2 wk; macular rash in axilla spreads to extremities, becomes petechial; peripheral vascular collapse as with Rocky Mountain spotted fever
R. typhi (endemic typhus)	Similar to *R. prowazekii*	Transmitted by fleas, widespread in U.S., especially southeastern and Gulf Coast states	Headache, fever, chills; fever up to 12 days; rash generalized, dull red macular, over thorax and abdomen; prognosis good with or without treatment
Q fever (*C. burnetti*)	Appearance similar to other rickettsiae	Inhalation of infected dust, of ticks on body and lice feces; sheep, goats, cows often affected; incubation 2–4 wk; present throughout the world	Fever, headache, weakness, interstitial pneumonitis, dry cough, chest pain; hepatitis and endocarditis may follow; rash not characteristic
Trench fever (*R. quintana*)	Appearance like other rickettsiae	Transmitted by body louse feces into broken skin; found in Europe, Africa, North America; incubation usually 1–4 wk	Headache, fever, malaise, pain, tenderness, splenomegaly, macular rash common; recovery usually rapid
Scrub typhus (*R. tsutsugamushi*)	Appearance like other rickettsiae	Transmitted by chigger bite, especially in Asia, northern Australia	Fever, usually undiagnosed. Rash and eschar rarely seen

Bacteria are classified in many ways. They may be gram-positive or gram-negative, depending on the chemical composition of their cell walls and their absorption of staining dye. *Gram-positive bacteria* stain purple because their cell walls resist decolorization by acetone alcohol. *Gram-negative bacteria* are first decolorized and then stained with a red dye to make them stand out.

Bacteria also are classified by their morphology. Spherical bacteria are *cocci*; rod-shaped are *bacilli*; and spiral are *spirochetes*. They can be pyogenic (pus producing), granulomatous, aerobic, or anaerobic. Organisms such as *Mycobacterium tuberculosis* elicit a granulomatous inflammatory response that involves a chronic inflammatory process with a nodule of granulation tissue and actively growing fibroblasts and capillary buds (see pp. 575–576).

PATHOGENESIS

All bacteria are capable of localizing in specific organs and often produce acute inflammatory reactions. The degree of tissue damage depends on the number of bacteria present, the virulence of the organisms, the site of infestation, and the resistance of the host to the organism. The bacteria must resist engulfment by the defensive neutrophil cell. Some organisms elaborate toxins that kill or depress the phagocytic cell; others develop resistant strains to escape recognition. Some of these organisms are *facultative intracellular bacteria* that counteract the defensive phagocyte after being interiorized. In this way, latent foci can be reactivated years after the initial infection.[13] The most common example of this is tuberculosis. Table 14-5 presents a classification of some of the more common bacteria that affect humans. The list is necessarily incomplete because there are thousands of bacterial organisms.

The virulence of bacteria is enhanced by the elaboration of endotoxins and exotoxins. *Endotoxins* are produced by many gram-negative organisms and, when released, are pyrogenic and confer antigenic specificity to the toxin.[13] These enhance chemotaxis, and some activate complement by the alternate pathway (see pp. 300–301). *Exotoxins* usually are produced by gram-positive bacteria. These toxins have specific effects on target organs; for example, elaboration of diphtherial toxin causes the formation of a thick membrane on the respiratory structures and toxic effects on the heart and nervous system. *Coagulase*, an enzyme produced by many staphylococcal organisms, can initiate the coagulation sequence and produce coagulation in various areas. Coagulase also may cause the deposition of fibrin on the surface of staphylococci that may inhibit the ability of defensive phagocytes to destroy the bacteria. It is thought that the presence of coagulase is largely responsible for the virulence of *Staphylococcus aureus*.[16]

▼ *Fungi*

There are 50,000 to 100,000 different species of fungi. Of these, about 180 have been shown to have the capacity to cause disease.[19] Disease-producing fungal or mycotic organisms are divided into three groups, according to the part of the body they infect. *Systemic* or *deep mycoses* affect the internal organs or viscera. The pathogens involved can attack major systems and organs and may cause death. *Subcutaneous mycoses* infect the skin, subcutaneous tissue, fascia, and bone. Infection usually occurs from direct contamination with fungal spores or mycelia (mycelia are filamentous parts of fungi) fragments that enter wounds or broken areas of the skin. *Superficial mycoses* involve only the epidermis, hair, and nails. The principal habitat of the organisms is mammalian skin.[13]

Unlike bacteria, most pathogenic fungi produce no extracellular toxic substances. Their pathogenicity is probably a result of the hypersensitivity that is produced to their antigenic components or metabolites. The structure of pathogenic fungi is similar to that of other fungi. Long branching filaments called *hyphae* are produced, which may divide into a chain of cells by forming walls or septa. As hyphae grow and branch, they form a mesh of growth called a *mycelium*. Fungi reproduce sexually by spores when there is fusion or asexually by nuclei when there is no fusion.[18] Saprophytic fungi that grow in the soil usually cause a systemic mycosis. The infection is transmitted from the soil or the droppings of fowl to humans through the inhalation of spores. Most deep mycoses are caused by free-living organisms and are limited to certain geographic locations.[1] The severity of the disease depends on the degree of hypersensitivity of the host. The usual pathologic lesion is a chronic inflammatory granuloma that can produce abscess and necrosis.

An important funguslike organism is *Pneumocystis carinii*, which was formerly classified as a protozoan. It has been identified in immune-compromised individuals and is the most common, severe, life-threatening infection among persons infected with the human immunodeficiency virus.[9] The clinical picture includes fever, cough, chest tightness, and diffuse interstitial infiltration of the lungs. It is usually fatal if not treated, and even after treatment with pentamidine, relapses are common.

Saprophytic fungi in the soil or on vegetation also can cause subcutaneous mycotic infection. This infection is opportunistic in that it occurs by direct implantation through a crack or sore on the skin. As with the systemic mycoses, necrotic granulomatous lesions of any area may occur.

The superficial mycoses may represent allergic reactions to fungi. These organisms do not invade deeper tissues or become disseminated.

(text continues on page 291)

TABLE 14-5 Bacteria That Cause Pathologic Effects in Humans

Bacteria	Gram Stain	Morphology	Epidemiology	Clinical Effects
Pseudomonas aeruginosa	Gram-negative	Motile rod; greenish yellow pigment formed; saprophytic but can establish infection and invade when host resistance is decreased	Commonly present on skin and mucous membranes; often attacks debilitated, immunosuppressed, burned, premature, or elderly people; transmitted by contact, especially to urinary tract, lungs, or damaged skin	Purulent drainage from wounds; characteristic greenish mucous from site of infection; bacteremia carries a 75% mortality; high fever, confusion, chills followed by circulatory collapse and sometimes leukopenia
Proteus	Gram-negative	Active motile rod; hydrolyzes urea; actively decomposes protein	Commonly present in decaying matter, soil, water, and human intestine; affects skin, urinary tract, ears, and other areas secondarily in susceptible people	Localized purulent infections may spread and cause bacteremia, symptoms of bacteremia; usually sensitive to penicillin therapy
Enterobacter, Klebsiella	Gram-negative	Short, plump, nonmotile rods; type-specific capsular antigens	Urinary tract and respiratory infections; especially pneumonia; often found in immunosuppressed, alcoholics, or people with diabetes mellitus	Symptoms of pneumonitis; productive cough, weakness, anemia; may resemble TB; responds well to aminoglycoside therapy
Shigella	Gram-negative	Nonmotile rods; aerobic or nearly anaerobic	GI tract resident; transmitted through fecal-oral route, or through contaminated food, water, swimming pools; common in countries where sanitation is poor; incubation usually less than 48 h	Fever, colicky abdominal pain, diarrhea; liquid, greenish stools may contain various amounts of blood; dehydration may result
Escherichia coli	Gram-negative	Non–spore-forming rods; different strains characterized by their antigens	Normal inhabitant of colon; may spread to urinary tract directly or through bloodstream; opportunistic organism in debilitated people	Accounts for more than 75% of urinary tract infections; abscesses may form on any area; bacteremia characterized by fever, chills, dyspnea; may develop endotoxic shock
Salmonella S. typhi (typhoid fever)	Gram-negative	Motile; type identified by specific antigens	Ingestion of contaminated foods, water, or milk; transmitted through fecal contamination of foodstuffs; totally transmitted by human carriers; incubation period about 10 days	Rare in U.S.; onset of fever, chills, abdominal pain, and distention; rash of small macules on upper abdomen and thorax; without treatment often causes intestinal bleeding and perforation
Other Salmonella organisms	Gram-negative	Varies with type	Food contamination; disease onset within hours of food ingestion	Enteritis, massive vomiting, diarrhea, dehydration, fever; antibiotic treatment normally not helpful
Haemophilus H. influenzae	Gram-negative	Small, pleomorphic nonmotile, aerobic non–spore-forming	Respiratory transmission, especially to very young and aged	Nasopharyngitis may be epidemic, especially in impoverished and rural populations; often outbreaks during winter months may develop into pneumonia, ear infections, rarely meningitis

(continued)

TABLE 14-5 *(continued)*

Bacteria	Gram Stain	Morphology	Epidemiology	Clinical Effects
H. pertussis (Bordetella pertussis)	Gram-negative	Small, aerobic, slow-growing	Respiratory droplets; very contagious; incubation about 1 wk	"Whooping cough"; characterized by catarrhal stage followed by paroxysmal cough and laryngeal stridor; without immunization, epidemics occur; immunization or disease does not provide lifelong immunity
H. ducrey (Chancroid)	Gram-negative	Small, anaerobic, slow-growing	Sexual contact; increased incidence in males	Chancroid, painful genital ulcer, diagnosed by Gram's stain
Staphylococcus	Gram-positive	Spherical, grapelike clusters or organisms on solid media		
S. aureus	Gram-positive	Coagulase positive; remains viable on surfaces of furniture or clothing	Commonly resides on skin and mucosal surfaces; invades skin through hair follicles, thence to bloodstream; occasionally through urinary or respiratory tract	Most common cause of *skin infections*, furuncles, boils, and carbuncles; may have localized lymphadenopathy; impetigo results from exfoliative toxin from a form of *S. aureus*; *pneumonia* more common in hospitalized patients; causes fever, tachycardia with localized areas of pneumonia; also may cause empyema; *bacteremia* may produce fever, tachycardia with abscess throughout the body; often fatal, nearly 50% mortality; *acute osteomyelitis* commonly caused by this organism; may result from skin or bloodborne infection or from open or closed trauma of affected bone; high fever and bone pain; may cause much osseous destruction; usually responds well to antimicrobials; urinary tract infections most frequently result from contamination of indwelling catheter, ascends to kidneys from bladder
Streptococci	Gram-positive	Spherical, anaerobe non-motile, non–spore-forming		
Group A, *S. pyogenes* (at least 60 subtypes), B hemolytic	Gram-positive		Respiratory droplet	Streptococcal *pharyngitis* very common in crowded living situations, greatest frequency ages 5–15 yr; fever, extremely painful and inflamed pharynx, tonsils, uvula; *scarlet fever* may result when a specific strain of *Streptococcus* A produces a toxin causing rash, diffuse erythema, with petechiae on soft palate, scarlet "strawberry" tongue in early stages; later tongue becomes beefy in appearance, called "raspberry" tongue; desquamation of skin occurs up to 3–4 wk after the disease; may occur before rheumatic fever; *rheumatic fever* may follow acute streptococcal infection and apparently is immune reaction to organism; acute *glomerulonephritis* also may follow streptococcal infection; *erysipelas*, an acute infection of the skin and subcutaneous tissue from *S. pyogenes*, causes malaise, itching, erythema that spreads rapidly with edema and encrustation; localized skin lesions, cellulitis, and pneumonia may also result

(continued)

TABLE 14-5 (continued)

Bacteria	Gram Stain	Morphology	Epidemiology	Clinical Effects
Group B, *S. agalactiae*	Gram-positive		Frequently colonize in the female genital tract, throat, and rectum; may be transmitted to susceptible person directly or by respiratory contact	May occur in puerperium to cause septicemia, pulmonary involvement, and meningitis in newborns
S. pneumoniae (pneumococcus)	Gram-positive	Diplococcal form, lancet-shaped	Transmitted by respiratory tract droplet; rapidly progressive once established	Preceded by "cold" or "sinus" complaints; fever, chills, pleuritic pain, cough productive of rusty sputum; hypoxia occurs with infiltration of lung tissue; progresses to atelectasis in one or more lobes; responds well to antibiotic therapy
Neisseria N. *meningitides*	Gram-negative	Single cocci, grows well in media with small amount of oxygen	Resides in nasopharynx of carriers, spreads through respiratory droplets; transmitted by bloodstream to meninges	*Meningococcemia* begins with cough, headache, sore throat followed by high fever and sometimes manifestations of endotoxic shock; *meningitis* evidenced by presence of meningococcus in cerebrospinal fluid and neurologic symptoms
N. *gonorrhoeae* (gonorrhea)	Gram-negative	Diplococcus	Humans only natural hosts; transmitted almost solely through sexual intercourse; incubation period usually less than 1 wk	Men develop dysuria, urethral discharge; because of penicillin treatment, complications are rare; women have dysuria, vaginal discharge, abnormal menstrual bleeding, Bartholin's gland may be involved; pelvic inflammatory disease may result
Corynebacterium diphtheriae (diphtheria)	Gram-positive	Nonmotile rod, club-shaped; elaborates exotoxin	Most frequently transmitted through respiratory tract but may be transmitted by skin, genitalia; incubation 1 day to 1 wk	Respiratory effect on pharynx, larynx, and trachea; formation of thick, leathery membrane on these structures, causing respiratory obstruction; exotoxin effects: heart, causing myocarditis; nervous system, causing peripheral neuritis, motor denervation; peripheral vascular collapse occurs in late stages; without antitoxin protection, mortality about 35% with 90% of those having laryngeal involvement
Clostridium tetani (tetanus)	Gram-positive	Anaerobic, motile rod, spore-bearing; exotoxin production	Found in soil and intestinal tract of humans and some animals; puncture or laceration of skin usual mode of entry; incubation variable, usually about 14 days	Exotoxin attacks CNS, causing muscle rigidity and spasms; pain and stiffness of jaw early symptoms; *lockjaw* refers to inability to open jaw; laryngospasm may lead to hypoxia; overall mortality 40%–60%

(continued)

TABLE 14-5   *(continued)*

Bacteria	Gram Stain	Morphology	Epidemiology	Clinical Effects

Mycobacterium
  M. tuberculosis
  (tuberculosis)
		Aerobic, acid-fast; resists decolorization with acid or acid alcohol; curved, spindle-shaped	Respiratory droplet; reinfection or activation of dormant infection; incubation 4–8 wk if not walled off	*Primary TB*: usually lung involvement, macrophages wall off viable organisms; these may be seen on radiograph as rims of calcification; *clinical TB*: fever, pleurisy, night sweats, cough, weight loss; can spread to bone or cause liquefaction and cavitation of lung

M. leprae		Hansen's bacillus; acid-fast rod	Prolonged exposure, especially familial; skin or nasal mucosa may be portal of entrance; incubation about 3–5 yr; little immunity has been demonstrated; endemic regions: tropical countries and few states in U.S.	Destructive lesions of skin, peripheral nerves, upper respiratory passages, testes, hands, and feet; treatment may be curative
Treponema pallidum (syphilis)		Spiraled organism, with fibrile, 3 at each end, contractile elements for motility	Almost always transmitted by sexual contact; incubation averages 3 wk	Organism can penetrate any mucous membrane, enters blood and lymphatics; primary lesion of site of infection heals; secondary effects are lymphadenopathy, rash, arterial inflammation; tertiary syphilis involves CNS changes, dementia, inflammatory changes of aorta, etc.

Table 14-6 summarizes some of the common human fungal infections. The reaction to these organisms often depends on host resistance and nutritional balance. Systemic fungal infections are more commonly seen in people who have a depressed immune resistance.

▼ *Protozoa*

Protozoa are complex, unicellular organisms that may be spherical, spindle-shaped, spiral, or cup-shaped.[18] Many absorb fluids through the cell membrane, and all possess the ability to move from place to place. Pathogenesis caused by protozoa often occurs in the gastrointestinal tract, genitourinary tract, and circulatory system. Table 14-7 summarizes several common protozoal diseases in humans.

The protozoa may be divided into four groups, or *subphyla*. The *flagellates* (Mastigophora) have flagella, or undulating membranes. They are considered to be some of the more primitive protozoa. This group includes members of *Giardia*, *Trichomonas*, and *Enteromonas* genera, which infect the intestinal or genitourinary tract.[7] Other flagellates, such as *Leishmania*, tend to be localized to skin, tissue, or mucous membranes. *Trypanosoma* organisms cause a systemic disease that is often fatal.[8] *Trichomonas vaginalis*, a common protozoal infection in women, is discussed on page 1169.

Typical ameboid characteristics are seen in the subphylum Sarcodina. Species of the genera *Entamoeba*, *Endolimax*, and *Iodamoeba* are representative of this group.

Organisms in the Sporozoa subphylum have a definite life cycle that usually involves two different hosts, one of which often is an arthropod and the other a vertebrate. *Plasmodium*, genus of the malaria parasites, is representative of this group.

Together with the Sporozoa, organisms in the subphylum Ciliata are the most complex of the protozoa. These organisms have cilia distributed in rows or patches, and the shape of the organism varies according to the amount of material it has ingested.[7] *Balantidium coli* is the only representative that is pathogenic to humans. It is a rare cause of infection, with only a few cases having been recorded.

The motility of the protozoa is accomplished by pseudopod or by the action of flagella or cilia. In *pseudopod* movement, characteristic of many ameboid cells,

TABLE 14-6 *Common Fungi That Cause Pathologic Effects in Humans*

Fungus	Morphology	Epidemiology	Clinical Effects
Superficial dermato-phytoses: tinea pedis (athlete's foot), tinea capitis (scalp ringworm), tinea corporis (body ringworm)	Branching hyphae on microscopic examination; found on keratinized portion of skin, nail plate, and hair	Contact with fungus through skin; maceration or poor hygiene favor acquisition	Fissuring of toe webs, itching, irritation, areas of alopecia, and scaling; circumscribed lesion with round borders of inflammation leads to designation of *ringworm*; treatment curative
Systemic candidiasis (C. albicans)	Small, yeastlike cells; blastospores with budding; forms clusters of round growths on cornmeal agar	Contact with normal flora of mouth, stool, vagina; may be superficial or systemic in susceptible immunosuppressed people	*Oral* lesions: white plaques on mouth and tongue, may cause fissures and open sores; *urinary tract infection* after broad-spectrum antibiotic therapy or in person with diabetes mellitus; *vaginal* discharge may be profuse and irritating; *Candida* in serum may cause disseminated abscesses
Coccidioidomycoses (C. immitis)	Yeastlike cells; no budding is formed; divided into multiple small cells	Soil saprophyte in southern U.S., Mexico, South America; infection occurs with inhalation of arthrospores; symptoms begin 10–14 days after inhalation	*Primary form*: respiratory infection causes flulike symptoms, sometimes pneumonia; pleural effusion may occur; *progressive form*: dissemination to regional lymph nodes, skin, meninges, etc. may occur, especially with immunosuppressed, other than Caucasian; fever, cough, chest pain, pulmonary coin lesion
Histoplasmosis (H. capsulatum)	Dimorphic fungus; forms cottony white growth on glucose agar	Grows as mold, prefers moist soil; airborne exposure by cleaning chicken coops, working with soil	Cough, fever, weight loss, hilar adenopathy; progressive fibrosis of mediastinal structures; difficult to diagnose; treatment with amphotericin B may or may not be helpful; ultimate prognosis poor for disseminated type
Blastomyosis (B. dermatitidis)	Dimorphic fungus; budding, round, yeastlike cells	Majority of cases in southeast, central and mid-Atlantic U.S.; infection acquired by inhalation of fungus, reservoir unknown; incubation may be about 4 wk	Fever, cough, weight loss, chest pain, pneumonia, large skin lesions; responds well to treatment with amphotericin B
Cryptococcosis (C. neoformans)	Yeastlike, budding	Infection through inhalation in lungs, often opportunistic with immunosuppressed people (AIDS, lymphoma, etc.); fungus excreted in pigeon droppings	More common in males; pulmonary infection causes chest pain, cough, infiltrates; meningoencephalitis causes headache, dementia, confusion, cranial nerve palsies, cerebral edema, and death 2 wk to several years after diagnosis
Pneumocystis carini	Fungus-like cysts with dark bodies	Mainly confined to immunosuppressed individuals, especially AIDS. Transmitted through respiratory droplets	Fever, nonproductive cough, shortness of breath, pneumonitis, progressive to pneumonia (PCP), often fatal
Aspergillosis (Aspergillus fumigatis)	Molds, in colonies, smoky gray color	Opportunistic with immunosuppressed individuals, especially neutropenic individuals	Allergic bronchopulmonary asthmatic response, focal consolidation, lobar pneumonia

TABLE 14-7 *Common Protozoa That Cause Pathologic Effects in Humans*

Protozoa	Morphology	Epidemiology	Clinical Effects
Amebiasis (*Entamoeba histolytica*)	Motile trophozoite usually seen in active disease; cysts form usual means of disease transmission; anaerobic	Cysts transmitted from human feces; contaminated food, poor personal hygiene	Chronic, mild diarrhea to fulminant dysentery; stools may contain mucus and blood, may persist for months or years; numerous trophozoites found in stools; fever, abdominal cramps, and hepatomegaly common
Malaria (*Plasmodium vivax, Plasmodium ovale, Plasmodium malariae, Plasmodium falciparum*)	Asexual phase passed in human body; multiple in liver, called *exoerythrocytic* cycle; then enter RBCs and multiply, *trophozoite* stage; as RBCs hemolyze, segments called *merozoites* released into blood	Transmitted by bite of infected female *Anopheles* mosquito; incubation period varies with type of organism from 10 days–7 wk	Anemia due to loss of RBCs; hemolyzing process with release of parasites cause chills and fever; immunologic mechanisms cause normal as well as infected RBC hemolysis; debilitation progressive; hepatitis complications may cause permanent damage
Toxoplasmosis (*Toxoplasma gondii*)	Intracellular protozoa exist in trophozoites; cysts and oocysts form; trophozoites invade all cells; cysts often take the form of transmission; oocysts transmitted through cycle by cat; form not seen in humans	Transplacental transfusion or fecal-oral cysts; may be in lamb or pork	Focal areas of necrosis, especially of eye, but may cause CNS or disseminated effects; lymphadenopathy common in immunosuppressed people; CNS involvement leads to high mortality; may infect fetus of affected mother
Giardiasis (*Giardia lamblia*)	Flagellated protozoan in upper small intestine; both tropozoite and cyst stages; cyst can remain viable in cold or tepid water 1–3 months	Water spread in U.S.; found in persons with achlorhydria, genetic susceptibility, Type A blood	Subtotal villous atrophy of small intestine. Inflammatory infiltrate. Incubation period 1–3 weeks, acute diarrheal period, nausea, anorexia, may last 1–2 months; chronic illness occurs rarely

the projection is actively pressed forward and is rapidly followed by the rest of the organism. The movement usually is directional, toward a specific focus. *Flagella* are whiplike projections that cause rapid movement of the organism from place to place. *Cilia* are shorter and more delicate and cover the entire outer surface of the organism. The synchronous action of these structures allows the organism to move rapidly.[11]

Reproduction may be sexual or asexual, depending on the species. The sexual cycle, when it occurs, takes place in the definitive host, whereas the asexual cycle takes place in the intermediate host.[18] Protozoa capable of sexual reproduction are called *gametes*, and those capable of asexual reproduction are called *zygotes*. Protozoa can also form cysts, which means that they can surround themselves with a resistant membrane. This prevents destruction and allows them to live for a long time.

▼ Helminths

The word *helminth* means worm and usually refers to pathogenic worms, many of which are parasitic. The common intestinal helminths are divided into three general groups: 1) *nematodes*, or roundworms; 2) *trematodes*, or flukes; and 3) *cestodes*, or tapeworms. Helminths are complex organisms in both their structure and their life cycle. Many spend part of their developmental life in several locations and in various hosts, such as fish, hogs, rats, snails, and humans. Their eggs, or larvae, often are eliminated in the feces or urine of humans and may be found in the feces on microscopic examination. The mode of infection for helminths is mainly through fecal–oral transmission or through broken skin.

Table 14-8 summarizes some common diseases caused by helminths. These conditions, although rarely fatal, are an important cause of disability worldwide.

TABLE 14-8 *Common Helminths That Cause Pathologic Effects in Humans*

Helminths	Morphology	Epidemiology	Clinical Effects
Schistosomiasis: *S. mansoni, S. haematobium, S. japonicum*	Blood flukes grow and mature in portal venous system; may attain 1–2 cm in length; life span 4–30 yr	Eggs of worm pair excreted in feces or urine of humans hatch miracidia that penetrate a specific snail host and transform into infective larvae; these penetrate human skin and are carried to rest finally in portal venous circulation; worldwide distribution	Usually asymptomatic; may cause dermatitis at focus of entry; cause mild fever and malaise; acute fever begins 1–2 mo after exposure, often associated with lymphadenopathy and hepatomegaly, eosinophil levels markedly elevated; mucosa of bowel may become ulcerative and ova may be recovered from stool specimens. *S. haematobium* causes hematuria with involvement of kidneys, ureters, bladder, and seminal vesicles
Cestodes (tapeworms; *Taenia saginata* [beef], *Taenia solium* [pork], *Hymenolepis nana* [dwarf], *Dypylidium caninum* [dog])	Segmented ribbon-shaped hermaphroditic worms; absorb food through their surface; attach to host intestinal mucosa by sucking cups; length varies with species from 1 cm–10 m	Transmitted when raw or poorly cooked beef or pork eaten; other types may be transmitted by fecal-oral route, man to man or dog to man; usually matures in adult intestines	Weight loss, hunger, epigastric discomfort; in *T. solium*, encysted larvae may deposit in muscles, eyes, and brain; leads to eosinophilia, weakness, muscle pain; anemia may result from tapeworm competition for nutrition
Nematodes	Elongated, cylindric, unsegmented organisms form a few millimeters to a meter in length; life span 1–2 mo–10 yr		
Trichinosis (*Trichinella spiralis*)		Encysted larvae of *T. spiralis* ingested in poorly cooked pork or bear meat; larvae released in intestinal mucosa; multiply, and new larvae migrate into vascular channels throughout body; lodge in skeletal muscle, become encysted and grow for 5–10 yr	Severe inflammation of muscles in major infestation of muscle; may begin with diarrhea and fever; muscle pain, conjunctivitis, and rash may develop; eosinophilia common; neurotoxic symptoms and myocarditis may be seen
Trichuris trichiura	Embryonated eggs in soil; worms develop in small intestine; cylindrical shape	Common in southeastern U.S. and in tropical/subtropical areas	Often asymptomatic; may have abdominal pain, diarrhea, weight loss
Enterobiasis (pinworm, threadworm; *Enterobius vermicularis*)	Female 10 mm, male 3 mm; live attached to mucosa of bowel; female deposits eggs on perianal skin at night, then dies	Fecal-oral transmission, transfer of eggs from anus to mouth; contamination of bed linens, remains viable 2–3 wk; common infection in humans	Pruritus of anal and genital region common, especially at night; bladder infection or other foci relatively rare; simultaneous treatment of entire families and group essential
Hookworm (*Ancylostoma duodenale, Necator americanus*)	Four prominent hooklike teeth attach worm to upper part of small intestine; adults about 1 cm in length	Affects about 700 million persons worldwide; greatest incidence in Africa, Asia, tropical Americas; transmitted by invasion of exposed skin by larvae, migrates through lungs and resides in GI tract; excretion of larvae in fecal material perpetuates cycle	Iron deficiency anemia and hypoalbuminemia result from chronic intestinal blood loss; most infections asymptomatic but may have GI distress or ulcerlike pain; eosinophilia common

▼ *Chapter Summary*

▼   Infectious diseases are produced by living organisms of different types and cause their disabilities through different mechanisms. These diseases are common and often are fatal to the very young and the very old.

▼   Whether an organism will cause disease depends on the virulence of the organism and the resistance of the host. The defense mechanisms of the body include physical, chemical, and immune barriers.

▼   Viruses are the smallest of the infectious agents and exist as parasites on the living cells. They are classified as DNA or RNA viruses according to their manner of infectivity. Viruses affect only specific cells on which they attach, then penetrate and multiply. At a certain point the viral particles are released to the surrounding environment to find other target cells.

▼   Chlamydial organisms are similar to viruses in that they are intracellular parasites. These organisms cause many of the sexually transmitted diseases.

▼   Rickettsia are small organisms that are like bacteria except that they can multiply only within certain susceptible cells. They are transmitted to humans through the bite or feces of an infected arthropod and produce disease with a variable clinical picture.

▼   Bacteria are free-living organisms that are classified according to their morphology and toxin-secreting characteristics. They can localize on specific organs and often produce an inflammatory reaction. The severity of the infection depends on the organ or tissue affected and the host's ability to mount an immune response.

▼   Fungi are common organisms, and most of them do not cause disease in humans. The mechanism by which they produce disease is probably a result of a hypersensitivity reaction to their components or metabolites. Most diseases caused by fungi are superficial unless the host's immune system is depleted.

▼   Protozoa are complex organisms that can move from place to place through pseudopods or flagella or cilia. Protozoa can form cysts that are resistant to the attempts by the body to destroy them.

▼   Helminths are the pathogenic worms that are usually parasitic to humans and animals. They are usually transmitted through fecal–oral ingestion or through broken skin.

▼ *References*

1. Bennett, J.E. Fungal infections. In J. Wilson et al. (eds.),, *Harrison's Principles of Internal Medicine* (12th ed.). New York: McGraw-Hill, 1991.
2. Brock, T.D., and Madigan, M.T. *Biology of Microorganisms* (5th ed.). Englewood Cliffs, N.J.: Prentice-Hall, 1988.
3. Denson, P., Weinbaum, D.L., and Mandell, G.L. Host defense against infection: The roles of antibody, complement, and phagocytic cells. In J.H. Stein (ed.), *Internal Medicine* (4th ed.). St. Louis: C.V. Mosby, 1994.
4. Fields, B.N. The biology of viruses. In J. Wilson et al. (eds.), *Harrison's Principles of Internal Medicine* (12th ed.). New York: McGraw-Hill, 1991.
5. Herold, B.C., and Spear, P.G. Virus-host interactions. In S.T. Shulman, J.P. Phair, and H.M. Sommers (eds.), *The Biologic and Clinical Basis of Infectious Diseases* (4th ed.) Philadelphia: W.B. Saunders, 1992.
6. Istorico-Sanders, L.J. Gram-negative bacteremia and the sepsis syndrome. In J.H. Stein (ed.), *Internal Medicine* (4th ed.). St. Louis: C.V. Mosby, 1994.
7. Klaas, J. Parasites. In B.J. Howard (ed.), *Clinical and Pathogenic Microbiology*. St. Louis: C.V. Mosby, 1987.
8. Merlin, T.L., Gibson, D.W., and Connor, D.H. Infections and parasitic diseases. In E. Rubin and J. Farber (eds.), *Pathology* (2nd ed.). Philadelphia: J.B. Lippincott, 1994.
9. Murphy, R. Infection in the compromised host. In S.T. Shulman, J.P. Phair, and H.M. Sommers (eds.), *The Biologic and Clinical Basis of Infectious Diseases* (4th ed.). Philadelphia: W.B. Saunders, 1992.
10. Murphy, R. Sexually transmitted diseases. In S.T. Shulman, J.P. Phair, and H.M. Sommers (eds.), *The Biologic and Clinical Basis of Infectious Diseases* (4th ed.). Philadelphia: W.B. Saunders, 1992.
11. Plorde, J.J. Trichomonas and other protozoan infections. In J. Wilson et al. (eds.), *Harrison's Principles of Internal Medicine* (12th ed.). New York: McGraw-Hill, 1991.
12. Rubin, S.J. Viruses, chlamydiae, and rickettsiae. In B.J. Howard (ed.), *Clinical and Pathogenic Microbiology*, St. Louis: C.V. Mosby, 1987.
13. Samuelson, J., and von Lichtenberg, F. Infectious diseases. In R.S. Cotran, V. Kumar, and L.S. Robbins (eds.), *Robbins' Pathologic Basis of Disease* (5th ed.). Philadelphia: W.B. Saunders, 1994.
14. Sommers, H.M., and Shulman, S.T. The indigenous microbiota of the human host. In S.T. Shulman, J.P. Phair, and H.M. Sommers (eds.), *The Biologic and Clinical Basis of Infectious Diseases* (4th ed.). Philadelphia: W.B. Saunders, 1992.
15. Shulman, S.T., Sommers, H.M., and Sharon, N. Laboratory diagnosis of infections. In S.T. Shulman, J.P. Phair, and H.M. Sommers (eds.), *The Biologic and Clinical Basis of Infectious Diseases* (4th ed.). Philadelphia: W.B. Saunders, 1992.
16. Shulman, S.T. Staphylococci, staphylococcal disease, and toxic shock syndrome. In S.T. Shulman, J.P. Phair, and H.M. Sommers (eds.), *The Biologic and Clinical Basis of Infectious Diseases* (4th ed.). Philadelphia: W.B. Saunders, 1992.
17. Shulman, S.T., and Phair, J.P. Host-bacteria interactions. In S.T. Shulman, J.P. Phair, and H.M. Sommers (eds.), *The Biologic and Clinical Basis of Infectious Diseases* (4th ed.). Philadelphia: W.B. Saunders, 1992.
18. Smith, A.L. *Principles of Microbiology* (10th ed.). St. Louis: C.V. Mosby, 1985.
19. Tilton, R.C., and McGinnis, M.R. Fungi and actinomycetes. In B.H. Howard (ed.), *Clinical and Pathogenic Microbiology*. St. Louis: C.V. Mosby, 1987.
20. Woodward, T.E. Rickettsial diseases. In J. Wilson et al. (eds.), *Harrison's Principles of Internal Medicine* (12th ed.). New York: McGraw-Hill, 1991.

Chapter *15*

Inflammation and Resolution of Inflammation

Barbara L. Bullock

▼ CHAPTER OUTLINE

▼ LEARNING OBJECTIVES

1 Define and describe different types of mechanical and physical wounds.
2 Describe the vascular and cellular phases of acute inflammation.
3 Define **chemotaxis** and **chemotactic gradient**.
4 Explain leukocyte response in inflammation.
5 Draw or describe phagocytosis.
6 Describe the functions of the major mediators of the inflammatory system.
7 Draw the classic and alternate pathways for complement activation.
8 Differentiate chronic inflammation from acute inflammation.
9 Describe the reasons for the effects of inflammation, including fever, leukocytosis, lymphadenopathy, lymphangitis, lymphadenitis, and neutropenia.
10 Briefly explain the process of simple resolution in inflammation.
11 Explain why regeneration occurs in some tissues and not in others.
12 Describe the process of repair by scar tissue.
13 Differentiate between healing by first intention and healing by second intention.
14 Describe exuberant granuloma and keloid scar formation.
15 Define **contracture**, **stenosis**, **constriction**, **adhesion**, **dehiscence**, and **evisceration**.

Barbara L. Bullock: PATHOPHYSIOLOGY: ADAPTATIONS AND ALTERATIONS IN FUNCTION, 4th ed.
© 1996 Lippincott-Raven Publishers

In the process of living, injury to the body tissues and organs inevitably occurs. Healing and repair of these tissues and organs must proceed for life to be maintained. Wound healing and inflammation are part of many disease processes and are modified or altered by many environmental and individual factors. Healing normally is preceded by inflammation, which provides a cellular environment conducive to healing.

Injury normally is prevented by the body's host defense system, which includes both physical and chemical barriers (Box 15-1). The inflammatory response, which includes white blood cells and their chemical mediators, provides a mechanism for ridding the body of microorganisms and decreasing their injury potential.[7]

A *wound* is a break or interruption of the continuity of a tissue caused by *mechanical* or *physical* means (Table 15-1). A mechanical wound is caused by some kind of trauma that damages the tissues. Physical wounds may result from organisms, chemical or thermal agents, or death of tissues or organs. Each type of wound results in inflammation, which is the reaction of the body to tissue injury.

Inflammation usually is a beneficial response to invasion by microbial agents or to tissue injury. It normally proceeds on a continuum from the inflammatory phase to the healing phase. Inflammation can be defined as a tissue reaction to injury that characteristically involves vascular and cellular responses working together to destroy substances recognized as being foreign to the body. The tissue is then restored to its previous state or repaired in such a way that the tissue or organ can retain viability. The process of inflammation is closely related to the process of immunity (see Chapter 16).

Healing ideally involves the return of tissue to its previous state. Tissue regeneration also participates in the healing process. If the injured area cannot be bridged by tissue regeneration, scar tissue may be formed.

Inflammatory states may be classified as *acute* or *chronic*. Acute inflammation involves the vascular and cellular changes that characterize the process. Chronic inflammation follows a persistent, self-perpetuating course, with the source of the inflammation being unresolved. The most common causes of inflammation are 1) infection from microorganisms in the tissues; 2) physical trauma, often with the release of free blood in the tissues; 3) chemical, irradiation, mechanical, or thermal injury, causing direct irritation to the tissues; and 4) immune reactions, causing tissue-damaging hypersensitivity responses.

▼ *Acute Inflammation*

VASCULAR PHASE

When injury occurs, large amounts of strong chemical substances are released in the tissue. These substances create a "chemical wall" called a *chemotactic gradient*, which provides a source toward which fluids and cells begin to move. The first reaction to injury is a neural reflex that causes vasoconstriction, which initially decreases the blood flow. It is rapidly followed by arteriolar and venular dilatation, the hyperemic response, which allows fluids to cross from the capillaries into the tissue spaces. The increased permeability allows protein-rich fluid high in fibrinogen to move into the area of high chemical concentration. This fluid may dilute the injurious chemicals and bring complement, antibodies, and other chemotactic substances to the area. The leakage of fluid allows for a collection of extravascular fluid and edema in the area. The plasma proteins leaked into the tissues provide an osmotic gradient, or pull, that brings more water in from the plasma (Fig. 15-1**A**).

CELLULAR PHASE

The components of the fluid exudation cause a characteristic response by the leukocytes commonly described as margination and pavementing, directional emigration, aggregation, recognition, and phagocytosis. These leukocyte activities provide for the elimination of the foreign material from the tissues. Leukocyte properties are discussed in detail in Chapter 20.

Margination, Pavementing, and Adherence

Margination refers to the movement of granulocytes and monocytes toward the endothelial lining of the vessel. Because of the increased capillary permeability that

---

BOX 15-1 ▼ *Mechanisms of Host Defense*

Physical and chemical barriers
    Morphologic integrity of skin, mucous membranes
    Sphincters
    Epiglottis
    Normal secretory and excretory flow
    Endogenous microbial flora
    Gastric acidity
Inflammatory response
    Circulating phagocytes
    Complement
    Other humoral mediators (bradykinins, fibrinolytic systems, acid cascade)
Reticuloendothelial system
    Tissue phagocytes
Immune response
    T lymphocytes and their soluble products
    B lymphocytes and immunoglobulins

Wilson, J. D., et al. *Harrison's Principles of Internal Medicine* (12th ed.). New York: McGraw-Hill, 1991.

TABLE 15-1 *Types of Mechanical and Physical Wounds*

Wound	Definition
MECHANICAL	
Incision	Caused by cutting instrument; wound edges are in close proximity, aligned
Contusion	Caused by blunt instrument, usually disrupting skin or organ surface; causes hemorrhage or ecchymosis of affected tissue
Abrasion	Caused by rubbing or scraping of epidermal layers of skin or mucous membranes
Laceration	Caused by tissue tearing, with blunt or irregular instrument; tissue nonaligned with loose flaps of tissue
Puncture	Caused by piercing of tissue or organ with a pointed instrument accidentally, such as with a nail, or intentionally, such as a venipuncture
Projectile or penetrating	Caused by foreign body entering tissues at high velocity; fragments of foreign missile may scatter to various tissues and organs
Avulsion	Caused by tearing of a structure from its normal anatomic position; damage to vessels, nerves, and other structures may be associated
PHYSICAL	
Microbial agents	Living organisms may affect skin, mucous membranes, organs, and bloodstream; secrete exotoxins; or release endotoxins or affect other cells
Chemical agents	Agents toxic to specific cells include pharmaceutic agents, substances released from cellular necrosis, acids, alcohols, metals, and others
Thermal agents	High or low temperatures can produce wounds of various thicknesses; these in turn may lead to cellular necrosis
Irradiation	Ultraviolet light or radiation exposure affects epithelial or mucous membranes; large doses of whole-body radiation cause changes in CNS, blood-forming system, and GI system

CNS: central nervous system; GI: gastrointestinal

results from the initial injury, the movement of blood is slowed. The polymorphonuclear leukocytes (PMNs), mostly neutrophils, drop to the side of the capillary to form a layer close to the endothelial lining. This layer assumes a particular appearance called *pavementing* (Figure 15-1**B**). The platelets and a few red blood cells may join the PMNs on the endothelial lining. The endothelial cells normally repel passing blood cells, but the changes that occur during inflammation appear to inhibit this property. *Adherence* of inflammatory cells to the endothelial lining is a critical aspect in the recruitment of these cells to the sites of tissue injury.[8] This adherence is effected by glycoproteins, called adhesion molecules. These contribute to the migration and function of the leukocytes in the inflammatory response.[8] The PMNs then move into the tissue spaces and adhere to the surface of the microorganism.[10]

Emigration

White blood cells move to the area of injury by emigration. Neutrophils move by ameboid motion toward the chemotactic signal (chemical gradient) by projecting a pseudopodium into the gap between two endothelial cells. This active process is followed by the cytoplasm streaming toward the projected extension (Figure 15-1**C**).[3] The entire leukocyte then arrives in the tissue spaces. The first leukocytes on the scene are neutrophils. Monocytes (macrophages) and lymphocytes arrive later. Red blood cells may passively leak into the tissues along with the PMNs or because of hydrostatic pressure changes.

Directional orientation for the movement of the PMNs is through chemotaxis. *Chemotaxis* is the directional movement of ameboid cells along a concentration gradient composed of substances such as bacterial toxins, products of tissue breakdown, activated complement factors, and other factors. The gradient provides a directional force that draws phagocytic cells to the area (Figure 15-1**D**).

Recognition and Phagocytosis

Phagocytosis is a highly specific process that requires recognition of the foreign particle by the phagocyte before actual attack and engulfment can take place. The

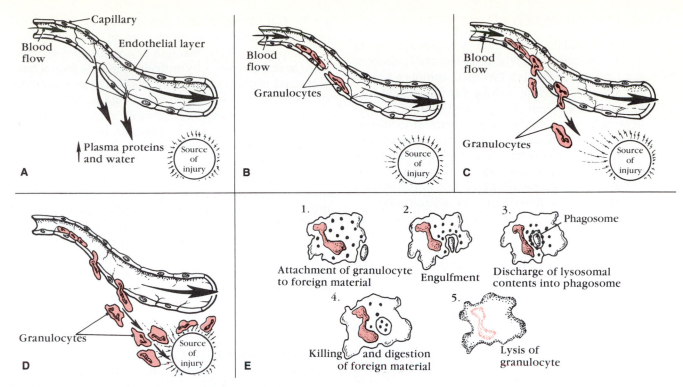

FIGURE 15-1 *Acute inflammation. **A.** Vascular phase. Increased permeability of endothelial junctions allows the movement of plasma proteins into interstitial spaces, pulling water into the area and leading to edema. This increased permeability is induced by chemical mediators given off by the foreign agent or by the cells' reaction. It occurs immediately after the injury and primarily affects the venulae. **B.** Cellular phase. Granulocytes marginate to the wall of the blood vessel. This also is probably a response to the chemical messengers. As groups stick to the endothelium, a pavementing pattern is seen. The leukocyte then begins to move by ameboid action toward the endothelial junctions. **C.** Emigration. Granulocytes move by ameboid action through the endothelial gaps toward the chemotactic source. **D.** Chemotaxis. Large numbers of granulocytes accumulate in the area of injury. **E.** Phagocytosis engulfs and destroys foreign material. Many granulocytes also are destroyed and may release their lytic enzymes into surrounding tissues.*

major phagocytes are neutrophils and macrophages. Neutrophils usually require the foreign material to be coated with a substance called *opsonin*. Opsonins include immunoglobulins, especially IgG, and the opsonic fragment of C3 (see p. 301).[3] Once the foreign particles are recognized, their receptors are attached by the leukocyte, and phagocytosis occurs. Macrophages also may respond to opsonized or other foreign material.

Phagocytosis involves the engulfment of foreign material. The cytoplasm of the phagocyte flows around the foreign particle and ingests it. Cytoplasmic lysosomes attach to the ingested particle and release hydrolytic enzymes into it, which often kill the microorganisms or dissolve foreign proteins (Figure 15-1**E**). In the process, the phagocyte often dies and releases its proteolytic enzymes into the surrounding tissue, causing injury to surrounding cells and resulting in the digestion of the cell membrane of the phagocyte.

Accumulations of large numbers of phagocytes in the area of inflammation lead to pus accumulation and, eventually, the destruction and removal of foreign mate-

rial. Phagocytosis localizes or walls off foreign material, preventing the spread of the process to other areas.

Phagocytosis is an energy-dependent process and stimulates the production of hydrogen peroxide within the lysosomes of the phagocyte. The pH of the lysosome drops to about 4.0, which enhances the action of the hydrolytic enzymes.[3] The quantities of hydrogen peroxide produced are insufficient to induce a bactericidal effect, but they increase in the presence of myeloperoxidase and a halide ion. Myeloperoxidase is present in the granules of the neutrophils.[9] Superoxide, formed during oxidative metabolism, is a lethal oxidant that results in bacterial killing in a process called the *respiratory oxidative burst*.[10] These and other tissue-injuring by-products have been called free radicals, which function in bacterial killing and in tissue-damaging reactions.

Some organisms are virulent and resistant to destruction by the phagocytes. The toxins of the organisms may destroy the phagocytes. Other organisms, such as the tuberculosis bacillus, are engulfed, but not destroyed, by macrophages and live within the cell for years.[3]

MEDIATORS OF INFLAMMATION

Many mediators of the inflammatory system are responsible for the effectiveness of the response and limitations of tissue damage. General factors that promote a beneficial inflammatory reaction include adequate blood supply, good nutrition, youth, and general health. This section deals with some of the major chemical mediators known to play an important role in promoting inflammation. Research has disclosed complicated interplay among the various mediators and a cooperative system with enhancers and depressors to the response. Box 15-2 indicates the most likely mediators in inflammation.

Complement

The complement system has been identified as a major mediator of the inflammatory response. It is essential in promoting the acute inflammatory reaction elicited by bacteria, some viruses, and immune complex disease.[6,10] The system contains about 20 distinct proteins and their cleavage products. Complement components normally are present in the blood in the form of inactive proteins called *zymogens*.[6] These are sequentially activated, with each component activating the next in the series (Fig.

BOX 15-2 ▼ *Most Likely Mediators in Inflammation*

Vasodilation
  Prostaglandins
  Histamine
  Serotonin
Increased vascular permeability
  Vasoactive amines
  C3a and C5a (through liberating amines)
  Bradykinin
  Leukotrienes C, D, E
Chemotaxis
  C5a
  Leukotriene B$_4$
  Other chemotactic lipids
  Bacterial products
Fever
  Endogenous pyrogen
  Prostaglandins
Pain
  Prostaglandins
  Bradykinin
Tissue damage
  Neutrophil and macrophage lysosomal enzymes
  Oxygen-derived free radicals
  Growth factors
  Platelet-activating factors (PAF)
  C8-C9

Adapted from Cotran, R., Kumar, V., and Robbins, S. L. *Robbins Pathologic Basis of Disease* (5th ed.). Philadelphia: W.B. Saunders, 1994. Reprinted by permission.

15-2). The complement system enhances chemotaxis, increases vascular permeability, and, in the final conversion, causes cell lysis. Fixation or activation of complement at the C1 level is by antigen–antibody interaction. This *classic pathway* continues a reaction pattern until the C8 and C9 enzymes are activated (see p. 325).

The *alternate pathway* is initiated by cleavage or activation of the C3 portion by plasmin, trypsin, bacterial proteases, and other enzymes found in the tissues. The C5 fragment also can be activated by many of these same substances. These pathways may be important mediators of the inflammatory process to clear agents that have little immunologic specificity, such as some bacterial products and proteases present in normal tissue.[6]

The inflammatory process is greatly diminished in the absence of complement enzymes. Deficiency of C3 especially causes a depression of the response and poor clearing of infection (see p. 335).[4]

Autocoids (Arachidonic Acid Metabolites)

Prostaglandins and related substances belong to a group of so-called autocoids or local, short-range mediators that exert their effects locally and are rapidly broken down. These substances can be synthesized by most connective tissue, blood, and parenchymal cells. Through a complex conversion process, another group of active substances, called *leukotrienes*, is formed. Some of these substances (previously called slow-reacting substances of anaphylaxis, or SRS-A) are potent mediators of smooth-muscle contraction and increased chemotaxis (Fig. 15-3).[8,9] During cell injury, phospholipids become available for conversion to prostaglandins. Other mediators of inflammation, such as bradykinin, also have been shown to stimulate prostaglandin synthesis. Some of the prostaglandins function as vasodilators by enhancing vascular permeability. This leads to edema, with increased concentrations of these substances in the fluids and exudates of inflammatory reactions. The mechanism by which prostaglandins increase fever is not known, but local production is thought to affect the hypothalamus, which then transmits the information to the vasomotor system, resulting in stimulation of the sympathetic nervous system (see p. 304).

Kinins

Substances called kinins can cause vasodilation. *Bradykinin*, a small polypeptide, is activated by the enzyme *kallikrein*. Kallikrein, present in the body fluids in an inactive form, can be activated by a decreased pH of body fluids, changes in temperature, contact with abnormal surfaces, and especially by activation of the Hageman factor (factor XII) of the clotting system.

The Hageman factor may be activated by endotoxins, cartilage contact, and contact with basement membrane tissue. When it comes in contact with plasma

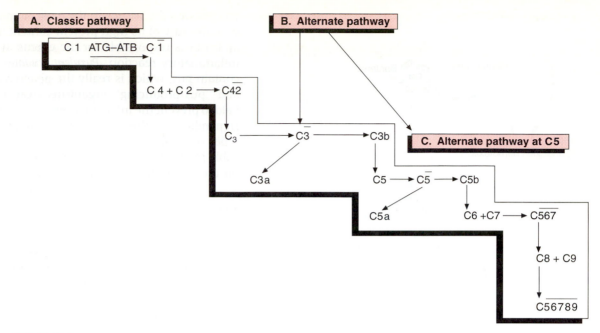

FIGURE 15-2 *Complement activation.* **A.** *Classic pathway activated by ATG-ATB reaction.* **B.** *Alternate pathway at C3 activated by endotoxins, trypsin, plasmin, and tissue proteases.* **C.** *Alternate pathway at C5 activated by trypsin, bacterial proteases, and macrophages. C3a increases vascular permeability; anaphylatoxin causes liberation of histamine from mast cells and platelets; C3b is an opsonic factor; C5a increases chemotaxis and vascular permeability; C567 complex is chemotactic; C89 causes breakdown of cell membrane (cell lysis).*

kallikrein, it can generate bradykinin, which is a powerful vasodilator. Bradykinin is inactivated by kininases, which render it biologically inactive.[8]

Coagulation System

Factor XII, the Hageman factor, activated by surface-active agents, causes the activation of the coagulation proteins as well as conversion of prekallikrein to kallikrein (Flowchart 15-1).[3,8] Complement also works in the coagulation system through activation of the Hageman factor. The process is not fully understood but may be an underlying factor in causing disseminated intravascular coagulation (see pp. 418–419).[6] Plasminogen may be activated to plasmin in the process that lyses fibrin clots and also activates the alternate pathway of complement. Several factors in this system lead to increased vascular permeability.

Histamine and Serotonin

In the immediate postinjury phase, histamine and serotonins are the major mediators of increased vascular permeability. Histamine is present mostly in mast cells, basophils, and platelets. Many agents promote its release from tissue, including mast cell and IgE reactions, C3 and C5a fragments, trauma, heat, and lysosomes of neutrophils.[3] The release is due to increased vascular permeability and histamine-releasing factors.

Some serotonin is present in the platelets, but the major source of this amine is the mucosal layer of the gastrointestinal tract. It is not present in mast cells of humans. Release from platelets occurs when platelet aggregation is stimulated.

Lymphokines

Lymphokines are released from T lymphocytes during immunologic reactions (see p. 321). This group of vasoactive substances plays a major role in immunologic reactions and also induces chemotaxis for neutrophils (PMNs) and macrophages.

Neutrophils

The lysosomes of neutrophils contain potent proteins and proteases that can activate the alternate pathway for complement, release kininlike substance, and release cationic proteins, all of which increase vascular permeability.[3,4] As the neutrophils die and release their products into the surrounding tissue, chemotaxis and vasodilation are enhanced.

EXUDATES

In the process of inflammation, different types of exudates are formed, the analysis of which may offer clues to the nature of the process. An exudate is fluid or matter collecting in a cavity or tissue space. The simplest exudate, the *serous* exudate, is the protein-rich fluid that

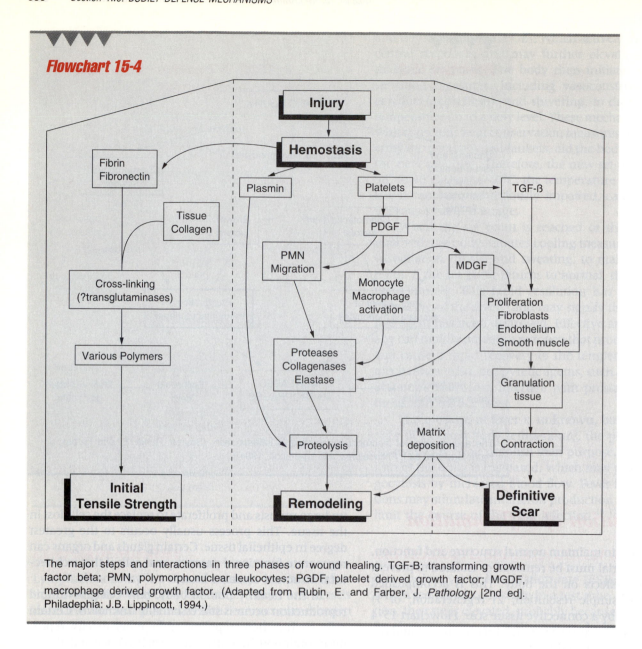

Flowchart 15-4

The major steps and interactions in three phases of wound healing. TGF-B; transforming growth factor beta; PMN, polymorphonuclear leukocytes; PGDF, platelet derived growth factor; MGDF, macrophage derived growth factor. (Adapted from Rubin, E. and Farber, J. *Pathology* [2nd ed]. Philadephia: J.B. Lippincott, 1994.)

Cells may be classified according to reproductive capability. Differences in reproductive ability cause these cells to react differently during wound healing. All of the *labile* cells undergo complete regeneration by the proliferation of reserve cells. *Stable* cells regenerate if they are stimulated to do so. For example, bone injury causes fibroblasts to differentiate into osteoblasts and osteocytes. Studies of muscle regeneration have shown that smooth muscle shows little regenerative ability, whereas voluntary muscle may partially regenerate if conditions are optimal.[5] Synovial cells in the tendons may be reformed under optimal healing conditions. *Permanent* cells do not regenerate, so their death requires replacement by scar tissue.

If tissue cells are to regenerate, they must preserve 1) part of the original structure, and 2) the architectural framework of the injured tissue.

REPAIR BY SCAR

Repair by scar occurs when dead tissue cells are replaced by viable cells that are of a different type than the original cells. The new cells form granulation tissue, which later matures to fibrous scar tissue.

Wound healing begins with inflammation. There is no distinct line between the time when inflammation ends and healing begins. Healing follows several typical steps or stages. The first stage requires a cleanup of cellular debris, organisms, or clot, which is carried out mostly by macrophages and a few neutrophils. Replacement of necrotic material, clot, or exudate by granulation tissue is called *organization*. *Granulation tissue* is proliferative connective tissue that is highly vascularized. The gradual laying down of *collagen* by these connective tissue cells eventually causes a dense fibrous scar to form.[5] Collagen is the main component that provides strength to healing wounds.[3,4] The scar begins as collagen bridges the defect and provides the initial strength to a wound. Epithelialization also occurs from the wound margins across the surface of the wound (Fig. 15-4).

As granulation tissue forms, it is very vascular and bleeds readily. As the scar forms, it tends to mold to the shape of the surrounding tissue and increases in tensile strength by compressing the collagen. In the early weeks, the scar is red because of the many blood vessels infiltrating it. The new vessels originate by a budding or sprouting process called *angiogenesis*, or *neovascularization*. The new vessels are leaky and allow fluid and protein to pass through them into the extravascular spaces. This leakiness accounts for long-term edema after the acute inflammation has subsided. The red scar color fades as vessels become smaller, until the scar assumes a white, fibrous appearance. Wound remodeling occurs throughout healing. Contraction, or shortening, is effective in pulling the wound edges closer together in the early stages of scar formation.

Cicatrization denotes formation of mature scar tissue. It has been described as less vascular, pale, and contracting scar tissue. The *cicatrix* denotes the scar, which has less elasticity than most normal tissue.

Healing by First Intention

First-intention healing refers to scar tissue that is laid down across a clean wound whose edges are in close apposition. The edges are sealed together by a blood clot, which dries to protect and seal the wound. The best example of this is a clean surgical wound closed by sutures (Fig. 15-5).

An acute inflammatory reaction occurs within the first 24 hours, with neutrophilic infiltration of the area. By the 3rd day, macrophages have moved in to clear up cellular debris, and fibroblasts begin to synthesize collagen on the margins of the incision.[1] By the 5th day, the collagen fibrils begin to bridge the defect. Maximum vascularization occurs at this time. Collagen continues to accumulate to form a firm, tough scar, progressively increasing in strength until about the 21st day.[1] Epithelialization across the superficial layers restores a smooth contour. The scar initially is bright red from the extensive vascularization, but it fades to a thin white line as vascularity decreases. Wound contraction occurs in all major scars, and this pulls the margins closer together.[1]

Healing by Second Intention

Second-intention healing parallels first-intention healing, except that it occurs in larger wounds in which large sections of tissue have been lost or in wounds compli-

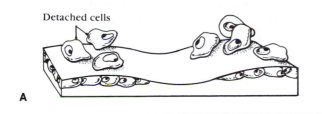

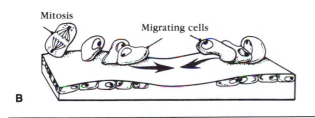

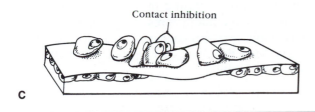

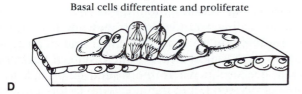

FIGURE 15-4 *Epithelialization of a wound.* **A.** *With injury, epidermal cells detach from basement membrane and enlarge.* **B.** *Undifferentiated basal cells migrate toward center of wound defect.* **C.** *Contact inhibition occurs when migrating cells meet in the center and touch.* **D.** *Basal cells proliferate to restore epidermis.*

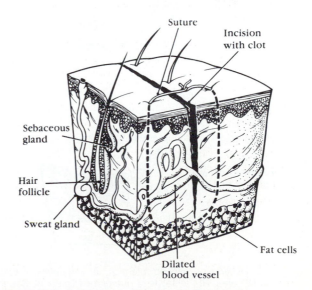

FIGURE 15-5 *Initial stage of healing by first intention.*

cated by infection. Much more time is necessary to remove the necrotic debris and infection from this type of wound. The inflammatory reaction is more extensive with the larger wound surface and occurs over a longer period. Large amounts of granulation tissue must be formed. The wound must granulate from its margins and base, with collagen gradually filling the defect. Epithelialization across the granulation tissue occurs to provide a smooth surface. Wound contraction results, mostly caused by fibroblast contraction that tends to pull the wound edges closer together (Fig. 15-6).

Healing by second intention is similar to healing by first intention, except that more cellular debris must be cleared, much more granulation tissue is formed, and a large, often deforming scar results. This type of healing is required in third-degree burns, deep skin ulcerations, and infected and other large wounds. Structures normally found in the scarred area cannot be replaced, so hair follicles, sweat glands, and melanin-producing cells are lost.

Because healing by second intention requires much more time than first intention, nutritional needs to promote the healing process are accelerated. Large amounts of collagen must be synthesized, and this requires protein availability. These wounds often become contaminated and heal over the surface only to open up again due to infectious processes smoldering below the surface. A wound must heal from the base upward, and large wounds are often opened surgically and packed to allow for granulation tissue to form at the base of the wound.

SUMMARY OF THE OUTCOMES OF THE HEALING RESPONSE

The principles of wound healing affect all tissues of the body. The response of individual tissues to injury and the amount of injury determine the type of healing that occurs. Some tissues regenerate freely (labile cells), others regenerate only under specific circumstances (stable cells), and other tissues do not retain the capacity to regenerate (permanent cells). In the first group, regeneration without scarring can occur easily, in the second group, regeneration may occur, while in the third group, the injured tissue must be replaced by scar tissue to repair the defect. In all cases, if the defect is large, the result will be scar formation. The presence of large amounts of exudate may produce a defect large enough to require scarring. Also, if the framework of a tissue is destroyed, scarring usually results.

FACTORS THAT DELAY WOUND HEALING

Many factors affect the body's ability to heal a wound. Oxygen deficiencies, malnutrition, and electrolyte imbalances are examples of conditions that can markedly affect the efficiency of the normal defense mechanisms. Immune suppression and clotting deficiencies also can disturb the primary closure of a wound surface. The effects of systemic bodily stress from injury or illness produce immune suppression, resulting in delayed healing. Table 15-3 lists local and general factors that can delay wound healing.

ABERRANT HEALING

Aberrant means deviating from the normal, typical, or usual. In healing wounds, deviations from the normal may cause complications, deformity, and decreased function of the injured tissue. The results of aberrant healing depend on where the wound is located, the degree of deviation, and the modifying factors present in the patient. Aberrant healing results from an abnormality in healing mechanisms that leads to formation of excess scar tissue, contracture, constrictions, or adhesions.

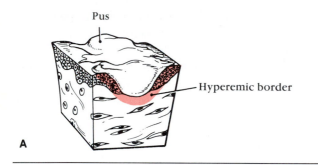

Pus

Hyperemic border

A

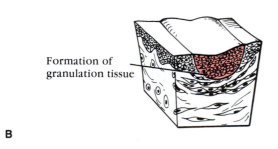

Formation of granulation tissue

B

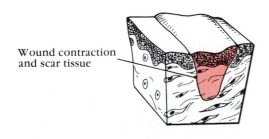

Wound contraction and scar tissue

C

FIGURE 15-6 *Healing by second intention.* **A.** *Hyperemic border around infected area.* **B.** *Formation of granulation tissue.* **C.** *Wound contraction and scar tissue.*

TABLE 15-3 *Factors that Delay Wound Healing*

General Factors	Local Factors
Age	Devitalized tissue
Nutrition status	Tissue damage at time of injury
Vitamin deficiencies—particularly of A, D, C, K, thiamine, riboflavin, and pantothenic acid	Tissue destruction by dessication before closure
Protein depletion	Cellular injury from use of excessively strong antiseptics
Fluid-electrolyte balance	Compromised tissue converted to an avascular state, such as by excessively restrictive dressings or an underlying expanding hematoma
Dehydration, edematous conditions, or both	Seroma or hematoma, which provide excellent conditions for bacterial growth
Medication, such as immunosuppressives, glucocorticoids, and anticoagulants	Bacterial infection
Diseases, such as diabetes mellitus, hemophilia, and other disease states in which nutrition, fluid-electrolyte imbalance, or methods of treatment compromise the normal progression of wound healing	Retained foreign body, including buried suture material
	Failure to close a dead space
	Closure under tension
	Improper approximation of wound edges

From Barnes, H. V. *Clinical Medicine.* Chicago: Yearbook, 1988:103.

Exuberant Granulations and Keloids

Exuberant granulations, or "proud flesh," occurs when excessive accumulation of scar tissue is present. They may vary in size from small to very large protrusions of granulation tissue that block the epithelialization of the wound. Once removed, they do not return. Keloids are excessive, bulging, tumorous scars that extend beyond the confines of the original wound and seldom regress.[2] They can result with any wound but occur most often around the face, neck, and shoulders.

Keloid formation probably results from abnormalities in collagen synthesis and degradation. Inadequate lysis of collagen by *collagenase* may be the main defect, or elevated levels of propylhydroxylase, necessary for collagen formation, may contribute to the excess scar formation. Research has demonstrated that in contrast to normal fibroblasts, keloid fibroblasts synthesize collagen rapidly, possibly because of excessive histamine in the area. Keloid formation also may be a type of autoimmunity in people with elevated levels of serum immunoglobulins.[2] Dark-skinned people develop keloids more frequently than do light-skinned people. Persons younger than age 30 also have a propensity for development of these abnormalities. Keloids tend to recur after removal.

Contracture

Wound contraction is a normal part of healing and involves migration of wound margins toward the center. Some wounds continue to contract after closure, and a disfiguring scar or disability results. The ability of a wound to close depends in part on the flexibility of the surrounding skin. The ability of skin to stretch on the scalp and tibial area is limited, especially if little subcutaneous tissue is present. Contractures may interfere with joint mobility or with other body movements, such as breathing and head movement. They can occur in any area, in skin, and in subcutaneous tissue as well as after bone fractures and tendon, muscle, or nerve injuries.

Dehiscence and Evisceration

Dehiscence is the surface disruption that results in the bursting open of a previously closed wound. This can occur as a result of interruption of primary or secondary healing. Dehiscence occurs when the strength of the collagen framework is not adequate to hold against the forces imposed on the wound. Poor collagen synthesis often is related to poor circulation.

Evisceration refers to the internal organs moving through a dehiscence. This most frequently occurs with the abdominal organs, but others also may eviscerate.

Stenosis and Constriction

If scar tissue forms in and around tubular areas, such as the ureter or esophagus, a stricture may develop, leading to narrowing or obstruction of an opening. Scar tissue contracts normally, and in tubular structures this may form a stricture. Excessive scarring may occur around an incision line due to inflammation.

Adhesions

When serous or mucous membrane surfaces are inflamed, the exudate may cause scar tissue to bind or adhere to adjacent surfaces. Adhesions commonly occur in the peritoneal cavity between loops of bowel or abdominal viscera, especially after abdominal surgical procedures. Partial or complete intestinal obstruction can result from the fibrinous bands extending from organ to organ or from organ to peritoneal wall. Adhesions also frequently develop after pleuritis, causing dense fibrous pleural adhesions that obliterate the pleural space and restrict respiratory excursion.

CASE STUDY 15-1

Sally Smith is an obese, white, diabetic female who underwent a cholecystectomy seven days ago. She had an incision that measured 3 inches and was secured with staples. The staples were removed and the wound margins immediately opened revealing an open area filled with white, purulent material. The wound margins were red and the base of the wound appeared to be closed with no apparent dehiscence.

1. *Describe the phases of wound healing.*
2. *What type of healing or nonhealing is described in the above example?*
3. *What factors are necessary, in this case, to promote healing? What are early indications that the healing process is occurring?*
4. *What are factors, in this case, that may delay wound healing?*
5. *Plan an appropriate treatment for this situation.*

See Appendix G for discussion.

▼ Chapter Summary

▼ Inflammation is the body's response to injury. It is usually beneficial because it rids the body of abnormal stimuli so that normal functioning of that tissue can resume.

▼ In acute inflammation, a vascular phase results in vasodilatation after the initial neural reaction of vasoconstriction. In the cellular phase, the leukocytes, mainly neutrophils, move toward the abnormal stimulus. After recognition through opsonin covering, phagocytosis of the antigen occurs.

▼ Many mediators of inflammation determine the effectiveness of the inflammatory response. Complement, a series of sequentially activated protein mediators, is essential in promoting the inflammatory response. The mediators work effectively together in most inflammatory responses to assist in the destruction of the foreign agent. The debris left from the battleground is cleared by macrophages and neutrophils. Sometimes the effects of the mediators damage normal tissue surrounding the foreign agent.

▼ When the acute inflammatory process cannot be cleared, a chronically inflamed area is infiltrated by mononuclear leukocytes, and persistent signs of inflammation may be present.

▼ The inflammatory process causes local and systemic effects of heat, pain, redness, swelling, lymphadenopathy, fever, elevated ESR, and, usually, leukocytosis.

▼ Resolution of inflammation may be through simple neutralization and destruction of the foreign agent. It may require regeneration of the tissue destroyed, or if the defect is large, the cells may be replaced by scar tissue.

▼ Scar tissue is made of collagen by infiltrating connective tissue cells. Small defects are repaired by first-intention healing, whereas large defects require healing by second intention. These terms refer mainly to the amount of scar tissue laid down.

▼ Many factors affect the ability of the body to heal a wound, including the nature of the foreign agent, the nutritional status of the individual, and oxygen supply. Immune deficiency and clotting deficiencies may also delay healing.

▼ Healing also may progress abnormally, causing exuberant granulations, contractures, dehiscence, evisceration, adhesions, and stenosis of various areas.

▼ References

1. Barnes, H.V., et al. *Clinical Medicine*. Chicago: Yearbook, 1988.
2. Cohen, I.K., and Diegelmann, R.F. The biology of keloid and hypertrophic scar and influence of corticosteroids. *Clin. Plast. Surg.* 4:2, 1977.
3. Cotran, R., Kumar, V., and Robbins, S.L. *Robbin's Pathologic Basis of Disease* (5th ed.). Philadelphia: W.B. Saunders, 1994.
4. Guyton, A. *Textbook of Medical Physiology* (8th ed.). Philadelphia: W.B. Saunders, 1991.
5. Kissane, J.M. *Anderson's Pathology* (9th ed.). St. Louis: C.V. Mosby, 1990.
6. Laurell, A.B. The complement system. In L.A. Hanson and H. Wigzell (eds.), *Immunology*. London: Butterworth, 1985.
7. Masur, H., and Fauci, A.S. Infections in the compromised host. In J.D. Wilson et al. (eds.), *Harrison's Principles of Internal Medicine* (12th ed.). New York: McGraw-Hill, 1991.
8. Rubin, E., and Farber, J.L. *Pathology* (2nd ed.). Philadelphia: J.B. Lippincott, 1994.
9. Slauson, D.O., and Cooper, B.J. *Mechanisms of Disease* (2nd ed.). Baltimore: Williams & Wilkins, 1990.
10. Tortora, G.J., and Grabowski, S.R. *Principles of Anatomy and Physiology* (7th ed.). New York: Harper-Collins, 1993.
11. Walter, J.B. *Pathology of Human Disease*. Philadelphia: Lea & Febiger, 1989.

▼ *Unit Bibliography*

Balk, R.A., and Bone, R.C. The septic syndrome: Definition and clinical implications. *Crit. Care Clin.* 5:1, 1989.

Benenson, A.S. *Control of Communicable Diseases in Man* (14th ed.). Washington, D.C.: American Public Health Association, 1985.

Cormack, D.H. *Essential Histology*. Philadelphia: J.B. Lippincott, 1993.

Cotran, R.S., Kumar, V., and Robbins, S.L. *Robbins' Pathologic Basis of Disease* (5th ed.). Philadelphia: W.B. Saunders, 1994.

Dineen, P., and Hildick-Smith, G. *The Surgical Wound*. Philadelphia: Lea & Febiger, 1981.

DuPont, H.L. (ed.). Infectious diseases. In W.N. Kelley (ed.), *Textbook of Internal Medicine* (2nd ed.). Philadelphia: J.B. Lippincott, 1992.

Fox, R.A. *Immunology and Infection in the Elderly*. Edinburgh: Churchill Livingston, 1984.

Gantz, N.M., et al. *Manual of Clinical Problems in Infectious Disease* (2nd ed.). Boston: Little, Brown, 1986.

Govan, A.D.T., Macfarlane, P.S., and Callander, R. *Pathology Illustrated* (3rd ed.). New York: Churchill Livingstone, 1991.

Guyton, A. *Textbook of Medical Physiology* (8th ed.). Philadelphia: W.B. Saunders, 1991.

Kissane, J.M. *Anderson's Pathology* (9th ed.). St. Louis: C.V. Mosby, 1990.

LiVolsi, V.A., et al. *Pathology* (2nd ed.). Media, Pa.: Harwal, 1989.

Lynch, J.M. Helping patients through the recurring nightmare of herpes. *Nursing82* 12:52, 1982.

Morello, J.A., Mizer, H.E., and Wilson, M.E. *Microbiology in Patient Care*. New York: Macmillan, 1984.

Roitt, I., Brostoff, J., and Male, D. *Immunology* (3rd ed.). St. Louis: C.V. Mosby, 1993.

Roitt, I., Brostoff, J., Male, D.K., and Gray, A. *Case Studies in Immunology*. St. Louis: C.V. Mosby. 1994.

Rubin, E., and Farber, J. *Pathology* (2nd ed.). Philadelphia: J.B. Lippincott, 1994.

Schaechter, M., Medoff, G., and Eisenstein, B.I. *Mechanisms of Microbial Disease* (2nd ed.). Baltimore: Williams and Wilkins, 1993.

Segreti, J. Nosocomial infections and secondary infections in sepsis. *Crit. Care Clin.* 5:172, 1989.

Shulman, S.T., Phair, J.P., and Sommers, H.M. *The Biologic and Clinical Basis of Infectious Diseases* (4th ed.). Philadelphia: W.B. Saunders. 1992.

Smith, A.M. *Principles of Microbiology* (10th ed.). St. Louis: C.V. Mosby, 1985.

Standler, N., and Klionsky, B. *Cases in Pathology: A Clinical Approach for Students*. New York: Churchill Livingstone. 1992.

Stroud, M., Swindell, B., and Bernard, G.R. Cellular and humoral mediators of sepsis syndrome. *Crit. Care Nurs. Clin. North Am.* 2:2, 1990.

Taylor, D.L. Wound healing: Physiology, signs, and symptoms. *Nursing83* 13:44, 1983.

Walter, J.B. *Pathology*. Philadelphia: W.B. Saunders, 1990.

Wilson, J.D., et al. *Harrison's Principles of Internal Medicine* (12th ed.). New York: McGraw-Hill, 1991.

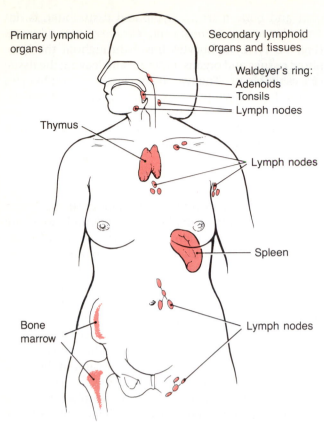

FIGURE 16-1 *Illustration of major lymphoid organs and tissues. The thymus gland processes and matures T lymphocytes, and the bone marrow produces and matures B lymphocytes. The lymph nodes and tissues drain and filter much of the tissue spaces. The lymphoid cells in the spleen trap antigens.*

The node consists of a stroma in which different types of free cells are held in place by reticular and collagen fibers. The lymph sinusoid is a thin-walled vessel through which lymph flows. The lymph sinus in the subcapsular space is like a hollow space that conducts the lymphatic flow.[3] Basically, lymph nodes serve as a series of in-line filters, so that all lymph in the lymph vessels is filtered by at least one node. Lymph nodes receive lymph from an afferent lymphatic vessel, and the lymph then passes through the cortical, paracortical, and medullary regions. Many lymphocytes and macrophages reside in these areas.

Thymus

The thymus gland, a primary lymphoid organ, is located in the mediastinal area (see Figure 16-1). It processes lymphocytes, and rapid production of lymphocytes occurs in this region from the early years of life until puberty. In the medullary area, lymphocytes appear to become more differentiated, after which they enter the circulation. Many of the cells, called thymocytes, that are produced by the thymus die in the gland.[20] The thymus and other lymphatic tissues undergo marked changes in size in relation to age (Fig. 16-3). The thymus weighs about 22 g at birth, grows rapidly in children, and reaches maximum size at puberty (about 35 g), after which it gradually begins the process of involution, beginning in the cortical zone and progressing to the medullary area.[20] The gland never completely disappears, but in elderly people, it is a collection of reticular fibers, some lymphocytes, and connective tissue.

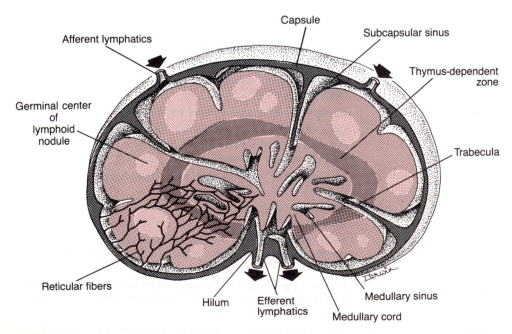

FIGURE 16-2 *Basic organization of a lymph node. (Source: Cormack, D.H. Essential Histology. Philadelphia: J.B. Lippincott, 1993.)*

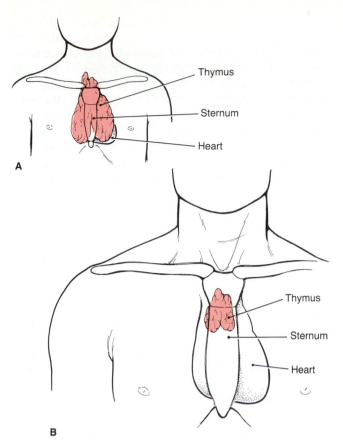

FIGURE 16-3 *A. Large, active thymus gland in childhood.* **B.** *Atrophy and fat infiltration in adulthood.*

cytes and plasma cells that can be seen with the naked eye throughout the parenchyma of the spleen are called the *white pulp*. These cells function in the process of immunity.

Mucosa-Associated Lymphoid Tissue

Aggregates of lymphoid tissue are found in many organs, especially those of the gastrointestinal, respiratory, and urogenital tracts. These systems normally are the main portals of entry for microorganisms.[16] Therefore, the presence of lymphoid tissue can, through secretory IgA and other immune factors, prevent entry of these microorganisms into the body. The tonsils are aggregations of lymphoid tissue and are named according to their location (Fig. 16-5). Those of the mouth and pharynx are called *palatine, lingual,* and *pharyngeal*. They are composed of lymphoid tissue and many lymphocytes. In the intestinal area, *Peyer's patches* are accumulations of lymphoid tissue, as is the vermiform appendix.

▼ Cells of the Immune System

Mononuclear and polymorphonuclear leukocytes are involved in the immune response. Mononuclear T and B lymphocytes are considered to be the only *immunocompetent cells*. They provide for specificity, or recognition,

Lymphocyte maturation is regulated by transformation of lymphocyte precursor cells into antigen-specific lymphocytes. This process occurs in the cortical and medullary areas under the influence of the *thymic hormones*. A group of hormones that affect cell activities has been identified, but not all of their effects are known. These hormones appear to be necessary to cause the differentiation of the stem cell precursor received from the bone marrow into mature T cells.[20]

Spleen

The spleen is the largest lymphatic organ. It can function as a reservoir for blood in two areas, the venous sinuses and the pulp (Fig. 16-4). As the spleen enlarges, the quantity of red blood cells within its *red pulp* (so called because of its dark red tissue that is rich in blood) also can increase. One of the main functions of the spleen is to process the red blood cells that squeeze through its pores. Red blood cells that are nearing the end of their life span often break down here (see p. 377). The macrophages in the splenic tissue clear the cellular debris and process hemoglobin.

Many phagocyte cells, especially macrophages, line the pulp and sinuses of the spleen. Groups of lympho-

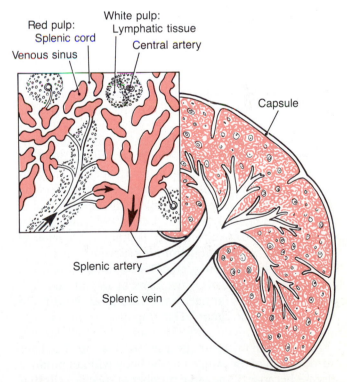

FIGURE 16-4 *Organization of lymphoid tissue in spleen. Note venous sinuses in red pulp.*

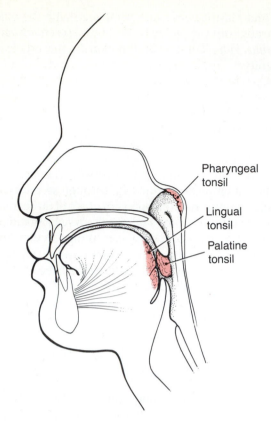

FIGURE 16-5 *Appearance and location of the tonsils.*

of specific antigens by specific lymphocytes. An *antigen* is a substance recognized by the immunocompetent cells as being foreign, against which an immune reaction is initiated.

Polymorphonuclear leukocytes are *nonspecific cells* that interact with the lymphocytes and antigen to produce an inflammatory reaction (see pp. 298–299). Phagocytic macrophages also play an important role in the immune response, in that macrophages can be used to process antigen.

The interaction among B cells, T cells, and macrophages with antigen provides the basis for the development of immunity. The cell- or tissue-specific antigens provoke specialized cells (immunocytes) that protect the human organism from microorganisms, foreign tissue, and diseases caused by altered cells, especially tumor cells. This protective function is known as *immune surveillance*.[2, 11, 24] Through immune surveillance, the *immune response* may be triggered. The immune response is a complex sequence of events set off by the introduction of a foreign agent (antigen) and usually ends with the elimination of the agent.[8] This response requires recognition of the antigen with the appropriate cellular and humoral mechanism to effect its elimination. The later introduction of the antigen to the body will not produce disease because of the large number of specific cells that recognize it and ultimately destroy it. This is *immunity*. The remainder of this chapter elucidates this process.

B LYMPHOCYTES

The B lymphocytes are responsible for *humoral-* or *immunoglobulin*-mediated immunity. These cells originate in the bone marrow and mature either there or in some other portion of the system. They are capable of proliferating and differentiating into *plasma cells* and *memory cells* when exposed to antigen. Plasma cells secrete large quantities of specific immunoglobulin. Memory cells are a method of stockpiling a specific clone of B cells so that immediate production of the specific immunoglobulins results when the cells are exposed to a particular antigen.

Immunoglobulin secreted by plasma cells is called *antibody*. Antibody has exquisite specificity for antigen, so that within the many classes of antibody are molecules that recognize only their specific antigen.[19] The specificity resides in a portion of the molecule that has binding affinity for antigen. Some lymphoblasts are formed by activation of a clone of specific B lymphocytes. These form numbers of new B lymphocytes that are similar to the original clone. The net effect is to increase the population of specific B cells for a specific antigen.[17] These B cells circulate throughout the lymphoid tissue and are available to combat antigen whenever it is encountered. An expanded clone causes a rapid response when new contact occurs.[12] These are the methods for fighting infection through the primary and secondary immune response described on pages 324–327.

The basic unit of every immunoglobulin molecule is a symmetric arrangement of four polypeptide chains. Two of the polypeptide chains, called *heavy chains (H)*, are identical and have a greater molecular weight than the two *light chains (L)*. These heavy and light chains are kept together as a symmetric four-chain molecule (H_2L_2).[10] The chains are held together by disulfide bonds. Figure 16-6 shows a representative model of an immunoglobulin. The Fab (fragment, antigen-binding) portion is the *variable* portion, and the Fc (fragment, crystallizable) portion is the *constant* portion of the immunoglobulin class. The constant portion almost

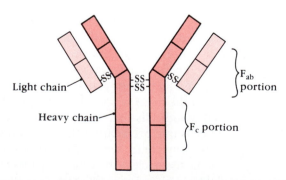

FIGURE 16-6 *Schematic appearance of an immunoglobulin showing two light and two heavy polypeptide chains. The constant portion, or Fc, accounts for the biologic activity, and the variable portion, or Fab, provides for the binding of specific antigen. SS: disulfide bonds.*

certainly directs the biologic activity of the antibody and perhaps the distribution or location of the immunoglobulin within the body.[22] The variable portion provides individual specificity for binding antigen and varies among immunoglobulin molecules.

Five major classes of immunoglobulins have been identified: IgG, IgM, IgA, IgE, and IgD. The classification depends on the structure of the heavy-chain portion of the molecule.[22] Table 16-2 lists the main properties of each major classification. The ability of the antibody to combine with a specific antigen resides in the Fab portion of the molecule, whereas the biologic properties that determine how the antigen is destroyed or rendered harmless are found in the Fc portion of the molecule.

IgM

Often called the macroglobulin (because it is the largest), IgM is the first immunoglobulin produced during an immune response. It is made up of five units held together by a short peptide chain called the J chain. It makes up about 10% of normal immunoglobulins.[10, 22]

IgM (in association with IgD) is efficient in agglutinating antigen as well as in lysing cell walls. It is present in high concentrations in the bloodstream and also early in the course of an infection. It can react efficiently with bacteria and viruses. The level of IgM normally decreases in about a week as the IgG response increases.[10] IgM activates (fixes) complement and has five binding sites for antigen.

IgG

IgG makes up about 75% of the antibodies in plasma. During the secondary response, it is the major immunoglobulin to be synthesized. This antibody freely diffuses into the extravascular spaces to interact with antigen. The amount of IgG synthesized is closely related to the amount of *antigenic* stimulation presented to the host. In prenatal life, it diffuses across the placental barrier to provide the fetus with passive immune protection until the infant can produce an adequate immune defense. Various subtypes of IgG exist, each with slightly different biologic characteristics.[10] It has been shown to

TABLE 16-2 *Immunoglobulin Classification*

Characteristic	Immunoglobulin				
	IgG	*IgA*	*IgM*	*IgD*	*IgE*
Serum concentration (mg/dL)	1000	200	120	3	0.05
Molecular weight	150,000	160,000 (serum) 400,000 (secretory)	900,000	180,000	190,000
Serum half-life (days)	23	6	5	3	2
Binds to mast cells	−	−	−	−	+
Fixes complement	+ +	−	+ + +	−	−
Antiviral activity	+	+ + +	+	?	?
Antibacterial lysis	+	+	+ + +	?	?
Total (%)	75–80	10–15	6	1	0.002
Crosses placenta	+	−	−	−	−
Function	Major antibody formed in secondary response; most common antibody in response to infection; long-lived	External secretions and surfaces, saliva, tears, mucus, bile, colostrum; protective function in preventing entry of microorganisms through portals of entry	First antibody formed in primary response; mediates cytotoxic responses; can produce antigen–antibody complexes that precipitate	Not known; found with IgM on surface of B cells	Reaginic antibody binds to mast cells and basophils; causes allergic symptoms through attaching to mast cells and release of histamine and other substances

−: negative; +: positive; + +: active; + + +: highly active.

Summarized from Cormack, D. *Essential Histology*. Philadelphia: J.B. Lippincott, 1993; Roitt, I., Brostoff, J., and Male, D. *Immunology*. St. Louis: C.V. Mosby. 1993; Stites, D. P., and Terr, A. I. *Basic Human Immunology* (8th ed.). Norwalk, Conn.: Appleton & Lange, 1994.

carry the major burden in neutralizing bacterial toxins partly through its ability to fix complement. This property functions in accelerating phagocytosis.

IgA

Most IgA is in the form of *secretory* IgA in the external body secretions, such as saliva, sweat, tears, mucus, bile, and colostrum. It provides a defense against pathogens on exposed surfaces, especially those entering the respiratory and gastrointestinal tracts. More than 85% of plasma cells in the intestinal area produce IgA. Secretory IgA is derived from specific plasma cells. A *secretory component* is synthesized by exposed epithelial cells. These two factors interact to form specific defense against bacterial and viral antigens. The first exposure causes increased amounts of secretory IgA and secretory component to be formed, so that on second exposure, the body surfaces are defended by specific antibody when exposed to specific antigen.[5] Antibodies to IgA may inhibit the adherence of pathogens to mucosal cells. The structure of the IgA molecule appears to facilitate its transport into the external secretions.

IgD

IgD is present in plasma and readily broken down (half-life in plasma, 2 to 8 days). Its exact function is unknown, but its presence on lymphocyte surfaces together with IgM suggests that it may be the receptor that binds antigens to the cell surface. Its levels are elevated in chronic infections, but it has no apparent affinity for particular antigens.[10]

IgE

IgE is called the reaginic antibody because it is involved in immediate hypersensitivity reactions. Concentrations normally are low in the serum, and the antibody apparently remains firmly fixed on the tissue surfaces, probably bound to mast cells. Contact with an antigen triggers the release of the mast cell granules. The released vasoactive amines cause the signs and symptoms of allergy and anaphylaxis (see pp. 349–352). High serum levels of IgE occur in allergy-prone people and in those infected with certain parasites, especially helminths.[10]

FORMATION OF SPECIFIC ANTIBODIES

To be specific, an antigen and an antibody must fit together precisely, the way the right key fits into a lock (Fig. 16-7). The antigen-binding, or variable, region of the antibody binds others of similar structure. A person is confronted every day with many different antigens, both environmental and synthetic, against which the body must provide defense. Figure 16-8 shows how this

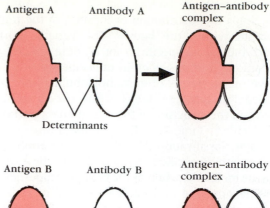

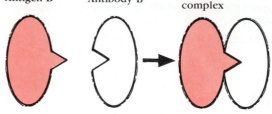

FIGURE 16-7 *Highly schematic appearance of specificity of antibody for antigen, the so-called lock-and-key response. The determinants on the surface of the antigen and antibody provide for recognition of antigen by antibody (ATG-ATB interaction).*

might work when the antibody is confronted with two microbes and responds to one.

Each immunoglobulin molecule has a *constant region* and a *variable region*. The constant region is similar in molecules of each class of immunoglobulin. The variable region must be able to bind many different antigens and provides for specificity. Several theories have been proposed to try to explain immunoglobulin specificity. One of these, the *clonal-selection theory*, proposes that each lymphocyte contains all the genetic information necessary to produce all possible antibodies. Thus the gene for specific antibody is activated by contact with the antigen, and large amounts of the antibody are formed.[17] The binding of antigen stimulates the small number of B cells that recognize it to proliferate, producing sufficient cells to mount an immune response.[10] The clonal-selection model assumes that large amounts of antigenic stimulation trigger the immunocompetent lymphocyte to divide and make large amounts of specific antibody.[10] When the B cell first encounters its specific antigen, it may become either a *memory cell* or a *plasma cell*.

T LYMPHOCYTES

The long-lived T lymphocytes account for about 70% to 80% of the blood lymphocytes. Their life span ranges from a few months to the duration of a person's life, and they account for long-term immunity. The T lymphocytes are thought to originate from stem cells in the bone marrow but are matured in the thymus gland, thus they are sometimes called *thymocytes*. The process proceeds from stem cell to prothymocyte to immature thymocyte to the mature, immunocompetent T lympho-

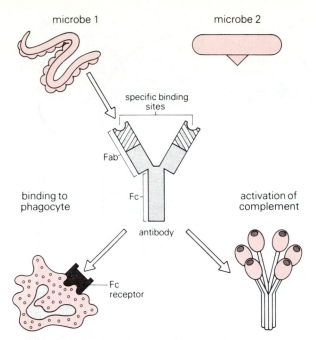

FIGURE 16-8 *Antibody—a flexible adaptor. When a microorganism lacks the inherent ability to activate complement or bind to phagocytes, the body provides a class of flexible adaptor molecules with a series of different shapes that can attach to the surface of different microbes. These flexible adaptor molecules are antibodies, and the body can make several million antibodies that are able to recognize a wide variety of infectious agents. Thus the antibody shown binds microbe 1 but not microbe 2, by its "antigen-binding portion" (Fab), while the Fc portion (which may activate complement) binds to Fc receptors on host tissue cells, particularly phagocytes (Source: Roitt, I.M., Brostoff, J., and Male, D.K. Immunology [2nd ed.]. Philadelphia: J.B. Lippincott, 1989.)*

cyte.[20] These cells develop distinctive receptors on their cell surfaces, which differentiate their functions from those of B cells. The T lymphocytes proliferate rapidly in the thymus and produce large numbers of antigen-specific cells.

The T lymphocytes leave the thymus to enter special regions called thymus-dependent zones, mainly in the paracortical region of the lymph nodes and part of the white pulp of the spleen. They may remain in the lymphoid tissue, enter the blood circulation, or enter the extravascular spaces to encounter antigens that correspond to the membrane receptors on their surfaces. If a T cell encounters its specific antigen, it divides and proliferates to form a clone of T cells that can destroy the antigen. The T lymphocyte can be functionally divided into three subgroups: killer, helper, and suppressor cells.

T lymphocytes recognize antigen in the form of peptide fragments that are bound to molecules of the *major histocompatibility complex* (MHC).[14] MHCs are antigen fragments presented on the surface of cells.[17] The T-cell receptor for antigen recognizes these antigenic peptides that are bound to MHC molecules.[14] The result is that individual T lymphocytes respond only to a specific combination of antigen and MHC.

Major Histocompatibility Complex

The mature T lymphocyte can recognize the MHC. A lack of reaction to *self*-MHC proteins is acquired, whereas a strong reaction to *nonself* or foreign proteins is developed. The T cell becomes a major defender against infected host cells or nonself cells such as transplanted tissue.[17]

All nucleated cells contain histocompatibility antigens that are genetically determined and expressed on their membranes. The MHC genes are critical in initiating and regulating immunity.[6] The MHC is found in the HLA (human leukocyte antigen) on chromosome 6. These HLA antigens are so named because they were first seen on the leukocyte population. The products of the MHC are expressed on the cell surface of nucleated cells, which are part of the genetic makeup of the individual.[14, 17, 18] The T lymphocyte recognizes, as noted above, the MHC peptides that are foreign through the use of its T-cell receptors.

Killer Cells

Killer T lymphocytes (cytotoxic T cells) bind to the surface of the invading cell, disrupt its membrane, and kill it by altering its intracellular environment. Killer T cells secrete cytotoxic proteins onto the target cell and "murder" the target or foreign cell.[14] The toxic proteins, often called *lymphokines* (which is a general term for chemotactic substances that signal immune cells), include perforin (cytolysin) and granzymes (a family of complement-like proteases).[14] The substances may be *chemotactic,* establishing a chemical gradient that helps to bring leukocytes and other substances into the area. The cytotoxic cells can stimulate the target cell to commit suicide, a mechanism called *apoptosis.* The mechanisms used by the cells are not well understood but involve fragmentation of the DNA and disintegration of the cell.[21] After killing, the activated cytotoxic T cell moves on with the ability to kill again.[14]

Cytolytic T lymphocytes directly kill cells and are essential in killing virally infected cells. They accomplish this by binding to virally infected host cells and secreting cytotoxic substances into the host cytoplasm. This kills the cells and stops the spread of viral particles.[13] These cells are also active in the destruction of some of the parasitic organisms. The recognition mechanism of the T cells must be tightly controlled to discriminate between self and nonself, because they recognize the membrane proteins of the host cell rather than free antigen. Therefore, cytolytic T lymphocytes are the chief mechanisms to react to and reject foreign tissue.[14, 18] The lymphokines secreted draw macrophages to the area and stimulate the production of interferon, which may function to suppress the spread of viruses from cell to cell (Fig. 16-9). Interferon made through recombinant technology has

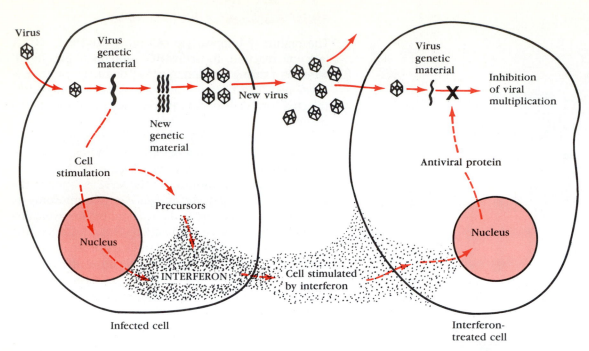

FIGURE 16-9 *Schematic representation of interferon activity (From: Bellanti, J.A.* Immunology III. *Philadelphia: W.B. Saunders, 1985.)*

been effective in the treatment of certain leukemias, chronic hepatitis, and life-threatening rabies.[13]

Helper T Cells

Helper T cells stimulate B lymphocytes to differentiate into antibody producers. A message from antigen-sensitized T lymphocytes also induces sensitized B cells to divide and mature into plasma cells, which begin to synthesize and secrete immunoglobulins. The synthesis of IgM seems to be the least dependent on T cell activity, whereas the IgA response is the most dependent. Another group of helper T cells interacts with the mononuclear phagocytes with the result of enhancing the destruction of pathogens.[17]

Suppressor T Cells

Suppressor T cells reduce the humoral response. The production of immunoglobulins against a particular antigen can be reduced or abolished in the presence of these cells. The mechanism of action may be to control the production of immunoglobulins either by regulating the proliferation of B cells or by inhibiting the activity of helper T cells.

Figure 16-10 shows the comparative formation and differentiation of T and B lymphocytes.

NATURAL KILLER CELLS

Some cells cannot be classified as T or B lymphocytes because they lack the surface markers that are characteristic of these cells. Morphologically, these cells are mainly large granular lymphocytes and account for up to 15% of blood lymphocytes. Natural killer (NK) cells are functionally identified through their abilities to kill virus-infected cells, tumor cells, and targets coated with IgG antibody.[15] The ability to kill (lyse) target cells is called *natural killer activity* or *antibody-dependent cellular cytotoxicity*, depending on the specific activity of the cell. NK cells also may release interferon or other cytokines and may be important in the regulation of immune response and hemopoiesis.[15] As can be readily seen, the functions of NK cells overlap with those of other leukocytes.

MACROPHAGES

Macrophages are the mature cells of the *mononuclear phagocyte system* or monocyte–macrophage system that function in phagocytosis of antigen and in processing and presenting antigen to specific lymphocytes.[15, 20] They are mature forms of blood monocytes and migrate into the different tissues of the body and function as phagocytes. Tissue macrophages make up a network of phagocytic cells throughout the body. These have special names in different areas, for example, Kupffer's cells in the liver, alveolar macrophages in the lungs, peritoneal macrophages in the peritoneal cavity, and histiocytes in the connective tissue. In the central nervous system, the special cells of the neuroglia classification called *microglia* can undergo changes and develop the property of phagocytosis during pathologic states. Figure 16-11 shows these different monocytes and macrophages.

Macrophages serve an essential function in removing foreign and devitalized material from the body. They

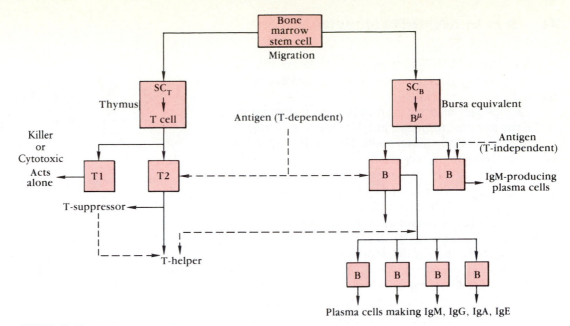

FIGURE 16-10 *Schematic appearance of T and B lymphocyte maturation. Both T and B lymphocytes arise from the bone marrow stem cell (SC) and migrate to the thymus gland (T cell) or to an unknown area (B cell), where they mature to immunocompetent cells. The T cells may act in cooperation with B cells or alone. Some antigens can stimulate B cells.*

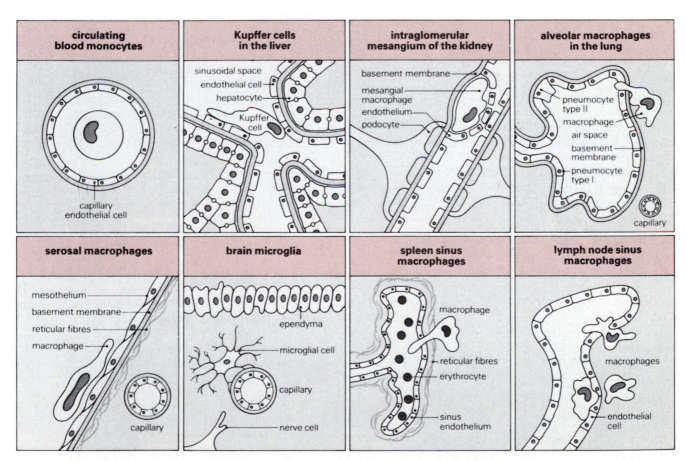

FIGURE 16-11 *Mononuclear phagocyte system. The cells of this system include circulating blood monocytes and dispersed phagocytes in connective tissue or fixed to the endothelial layer of the blood capillaries that in the liver are known as Kupffer cells. Endothelium-fixed phagocytes include the intraglomerular mesangial cells in the kidney. Alveolar and serosal macrophages are examples of "wandering" macrophages, whereas brain microglia are cells that enter the brain around the time of birth and differentiate into fixed tissue cells. (From: Roitt, I., Brostoff, J., and Male, D. Immunology [2nd ed.]. Philadelphia: J.B. Lippincott, 1989.)*

are active at a site of injury during wound healing and in removing microorganisms, cellular debris, and necrotic material.

Macrophages also have an important cooperative role in the immune response, but their method of functioning is not entirely understood. These cells trap and process antigens to present them to lymphocytes. They may play a secondary or accessory role in promoting lymphocytic activity and may function as an intermediary between specific T cells and specific B cells.[9]

The macrophage moves by ameboid motion toward a chemical concentration of soluble substances released into its environment by antigens or by lymphocytes. This is called movement toward a *chemotactic gradient*, or signal, that is elicited by soluble substances such as lymphokines (see p. 321). The monocyte migration inhibition factor and the macrophage-activating factor, which, respectively, tend to retain the macrophage in an area and increase its phagocytic activity, are especially important cytokines. The release of these cytokines results from activation of the macrophage by organisms and in association with lymphocytes and/or NK cells.[21]

ANTIGEN, IMMUNOGEN, OR HAPTEN RECOGNITION

An *antigen* is a molecule that can detect immune response when introduced into the body. When an antigen stimulates an immune response, it is said to have *immunogenicity*.[1,8] It then stimulates the immune response, denoting an active production of antibodies or sensitized cells. Most antigens and immunogens are proteins, but other large molecules, such as polysaccharides and nucleoproteins, also may function in this way.

Several characteristics appear to determine whether a molecule can stimulate an immune response, and these include such aspects as size, foreignness, shape, and solubility. Some molecules become antigenic only when they are combined with a carrier. Called *haptens*, these substances fail to elicit an immune response because they are small. These molecules cannot serve as complete antigens until they are combined with protein carriers (Fig. 16-12). An example is the contact allergens, which probably attach to proteins of the skin and stimulate the proliferation of a T-cell population sensitized to the substance. Later, exposure to the allergen leads to a more rapid reaction. Other examples include drugs, dust particles, dandruff, industrial chemicals, and poisons.[12]

▼ *Types of Immunity*

HUMORAL IMMUNITY

Humoral immunity refers to immunity effected by antibody synthesis or the production of specific immunoglobulin that coats the antigen and targets it for

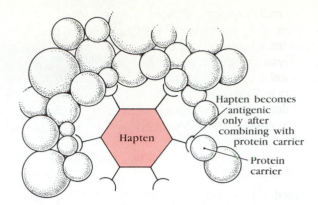

FIGURE 16-12 *Some molecules become antigenic only after they have combined with a carrier, usually a protein. These molecules, called "haptens," when combined with a carrier are fully antigenic.*

destruction by polymorphonuclear neutrophils. The interaction of antigen with antibody activates the classic pathway of the complement system (see p. 300).

Most antigens are recognized by T helper cells, which promote the activation of specific B cells. These B cells are "turned on" by either direct T-cell interaction or T-cell secretions. In some cases, a macrophage serves as an intermediary between the T and B cells. The B cell then divides and differentiates into a plasma cell that secretes specific immunoglobulin to target the antigen for destruction. Antigen recognition by a T or B cell often is enhanced by macrophage interaction, which processes the antigen and presents it to the appropriate cell (Fig. 16-13).

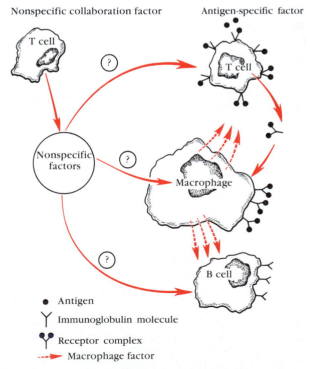

FIGURE 16-13 *The macrophage often enhances antigen recognition and probably serves as an intermediary between T and B cells.*

Certain antigens, designated as *thymus-independent antigens*, elicit strong B-cell responses without T-cell interaction. Examples include *Escherichia coli*, pneumococcal polysaccharide, dextrans, and other large polymers.[7] Humoral immunity often is described in terms of the *primary* and *secondary* immune responses. This terminology refers to the time lapse between the introduction of antigen and the humoral or immunoglobulin response.

Primary Response

The first time a particular antigen enters the body, a characteristic pattern of antibody production is induced. As the antigen binds to specific B cells, activation occurs and causes the cells to proliferate and differentiate into specialized antibody-producing plasma cells. After about 6 days, antibodies specific to the antigen can be measured in the blood. This *lag* or *latent* phase is the time during which activation of T and B lymphocytes is occurring.[8] The first antibodies or immunoglobulins to be produced in measurable quantities usually are IgMs. These are produced in large quantities, with levels increasing up to 14 days and then gradually declining in production to little IgM production after a few weeks.[3] After the initial IgM elevation, IgG immunoglobulins appear at about day 10, peak at several weeks, and maintain high levels much longer. During the course of the primary immune response, the immunoglobulins improve in their ability to bind the inducing antigen. The mechanisms responsible for this change are not known, but it is likely that firmer binding occurs because of greater precision in matching surface receptors. IgG is considered the highest-affinity antibody that binds antigenic groupings firmly.[4, 12] A *steady-state phase* is eventually reached, during which antibody synthesis and degradation are about equal. Then a *declining phase* occurs, when the synthesis of new antibody decreases. Figure 16-14 shows primary and secondary immune responses to the same antigen.

Secondary Response

The secondary response differs from the primary response in that the production of specific antibodies for the antigen begins almost immediately. More antibody is produced, and specific immunoglobulin is produced early and in large amounts.

The secondary response is called the memory response because the immune system responds much faster to a second exposure to a particular antigen. Both T and B memory cells are involved, because in the primary response, lymphocytes proliferate and differentiate into T and B memory cells. If the antigen is introduced into the host a second time, these cells begin immediate production of antibodies of a higher binding capacity than in the primary response. Small amounts of antigen

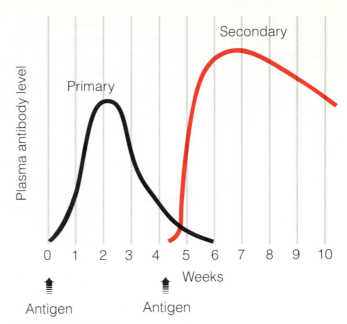

FIGURE 16-14 *Primary and secondary immune response by antibody to the same antigen.*

stimulate a highly specific response with the specific antibody.[8]

Complement Activation

Complement is a system of at least 18 proteins and their fragments that circulate as functionally inactive molecules. They can interact with one another in a sequential activation cascade. They are designated by numbers, with nine numbers indicating the major molecules and symbols or names indicating the components (see p. 300).

The *classic pathway* for the activation of complement involves binding the first component, C1, with a portion of the immunoglobulin molecule. This begins the cascade of complement activation, which is essential in promoting the inflammatory process. Figure 15-2 on page 301 shows the major pathway of activation and the end result of the process. The system promotes inflammation by increasing vascular permeability, chemotaxis, and phagocytosis and, finally, causes lysis of the foreign cell. Activation of complement also promotes opsonization of target material. Opsonization occurs with the fixation of complement proteins to antigen particles.[23] This sets the stage for phagocytosis by neutrophils or macrophages. Complement activation (fixation) is the result of complement-fixing antibody, especially IgG. The results of the components of the cascade cause some damage to normal tissue around the foreign tissue, and in some cases, this process can be damaging to the host. In most cases, an antigen–antibody reaction is required for the activation of complement. The *alternate complement activation* described on page 300 results in no immunologic memory, because there is no antigen–antibody reaction. The complement factors participate in inflammation with the result of destroying foreign material along with some normal tissue.

CELL-MEDIATED IMMUNITY

Cell-mediated immunity, caused by T-lymphocyte activity, is mediated through contact between T cells and antigen, with subsequent destruction of the antigen.[1] The T lymphocyte recognizes antigen by receptors on the surface of the T cell. Destruction may occur through the release of soluble chemical compounds directly into the target cell membrane or through the secretion of the lymphokines discussed earlier (see Flowchart 16-1). Direct contact with an antigen is often called *killer activity*.

Killer activity is mediated through a group of cytotoxic T cells that function in the destruction of cells with identified surface antigens. The specific recognition is through the lock-and-key approach described earlier. The killer T lymphocyte may directly destroy the antigen by binding to the cell and producing a break in its membrane. This results in disruption of the intracellular osmotic environment and the death of the cell. The activated killer cell also may release cytotoxic substances directly into the target cell.

The activated T lymphocytes release lymphokines, which affect other lymphocytes by enhancing or suppressing their activity. These cells also may create a chemotactic gradient that causes macrophages to accumulate in the area. The activation of a very few antigen-specific T cells leads to a reaction that involves a large number of mononuclear cells that destroy the antigen.[1] The specific antigen involved may be foreign tissue (transplant reactions), intracellular parasites (such as viruses or mycobacteria), soluble protein, or penetrating chemicals. The chemotactic gradient also attracts eosinophils, basophils, and neutrophils to the area.

Cell-mediated immunity, often termed *delayed hypersensitivity* because the response usually takes days, involves the direct intervention of T cells in a response without a corresponding humoral immunity. It results in the accumulation of macrophages around the small blood vessels, resulting in destruction of vessels. This may lead to minor vascular lesions—for example, the wheal-and-flare response—or it may result in major destruction and massive necrosis. The antigen initially may react with a few specific T cells in the area and produce the chemotactic response as well as macrophage-inhibiting factor, which tends to keep macrophages in the area. The response seems to be dose related in that the greater the amount of antigen present, the greater the development of sensitized T lymphocytes. The end result is cytolysis of the antigenic cell. This mechanism, which involves the T cells and associated macrophages, is responsible for rejecting transplanted organs and, in this process, is called *cell-mediated lymphocytolysis*.[18] The *tuberculin reaction* is a good clinical example, in that people infected with *Mycobacterium tuberculosis* develop a wheal-and-flare response when injected intradermally with a lysate of tuberculin material.[1]

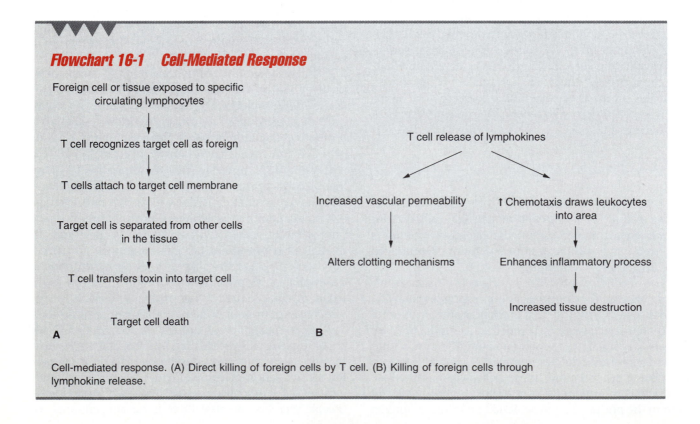

Flowchart 16-1   Cell-Mediated Response

Foreign cell or tissue exposed to specific circulating lymphocytes

↓

T cell recognizes target cell as foreign

↓

T cells attach to target cell membrane

↓

Target cell is separated from other cells in the tissue

↓

T cell transfers toxin into target cell

↓

Target cell death

A

T cell release of lymphokines

Increased vascular permeability   ↑ Chemotaxis draws leukocytes into area

↓   ↓

Alters clotting mechanisms   Enhances inflammatory process

↓

Increased tissue destruction

B

Cell-mediated response. (A) Direct killing of foreign cells by T cell. (B) Killing of foreign cells through lymphokine release.

The T cells function in *immunosurveillance* to detect cells in the host that have foreign antigens on their surface. They can be thought of as defensive cells that patrol the blood and tissue spaces. This self-protective function prevents the transplantation of tissue from one person to another unless the antigens on the surface of the cells in the tissue are similar enough for the host tissue to accept the transplanted tissue as self.

▼ Summary of the Process of Immunity

As previously described, the term *immunity* refers to all of the mechanisms used by the body to prevent foreign material from causing harm to the body.[1] The agents may be microorganisms or other environmental factors.

TABLE 16-3 *Immunizing Preparations (Vaccines and Antisera) Useful in Humans*

Vaccines	Type of Vaccine
BACTERIAL	
Anthrax	Alum-precipitated antigen from culture filtrate
Cholera	Killed *Vibrio cholerae*
Haemophilus influenzae	Type b polysaccharide
Meningococcal meningitis	Polysaccharide, group A, C, Y, W135 of *Neisseria meningitidis*
Pertussis	Killed *Bordetella pertussis*
Plague	Killed *Yersinia pestis* (attenuated strain in some parts of the world)
Pneumococcal infection	Polysaccharide (capsule) of 23 serotypes of *Streptococcus pneumoniae*
Tetanus	Toxoid
Tuberculosis	Attenuated live bacille Calmette-Guérin (BCG)
Typhoid	Killed *Salmonella typhi* (attenuated)
Botulism	Toxoid, limited use in research workers
Brucellosis	Attenuated live *Brucella abortus* strain 19 (limited use in humans outside the United States)
RICKETTSIAL	
Typhus fever	Formalin-inactivated *Rickettsia prowazekii* (attenuated, live; shows promise)
Rocky Mountain spotted fever	Inactivated *Rickettsia rickettsii*
VIRAL	
Hepatitis B	Inactivated HB surface antigen
Influenza	Inactivated; whole or "split" virus
Measles	Attenuated
Mumps	Attenuated
Polio	Attenuated or inactivated
Rabies	Inactivated
Rubella	Attenuated
Varicella	Attenuated
ANTISERA	
Botulism	Human immune globulin; equine immune globulin
Diphtheria	Equine immune serum
Hepatitis A	Pooled human serum globulin (ISG)
Hepatitis B	Specific anti-HB (HBIB) or ISG
Hypogammaglobulinemia	Pooled human ISG
Measles	Pooled human ISG
Rabies	Human immune globulin, RIG, equine immune serum
$Rh_{o(D)}$	Immune (human) globulin vs. $Rh_{o(D)}$ factor
Tetanus	Human immune globulin (TIG)
Vaccinia	Vaccinia immune globulin
Varicella zoster	Zoster immune globulin (VZIG)
Antilymphocyte serum	Equine
Black widow spider	Equine antivenin
Coral snake bite	Equine antivenin
Crotalid snake bite	Polyvalent equine antiserum

Benjamin, E. and Leskowitz, S. *Immunology: A Short Course.* New York: Alan R. Liss, 1988.

Innate immunity refers to those factors a person is born with to prevent disease. These factors, broadly speaking, can be physical barriers, such as skin or mucous membranes. Chemical barriers also work cooperatively to decrease microorganism invasion. The internal factors include the cells of the mononuclear phagocyte system and leukocyte secretions.

Acquired immunity refers to passive and active immune processes. In early neonatal life, some of the mother's immunity, passed through the placenta prenatally, continues to protect the infant from disease. This *passive immunity* protects the neonate only for the first few months of life. *Active acquired immunity* involves the response mounted by the person's own immune system. It requires all of the factors described earlier. Scientists have discovered the process of inducing acquired immunity through *vaccination*. The resultant individual response can be induced against microorganisms and their products as well as against thousands of natural and synthetic compounds. The vaccine prepared uses the least amount of antigenic material to provide the maximum human response and, thus, protection from disease. People are vaccinated against antigens that are threatening to them in the environment in which they live. Table 16-3 lists the main immunizing preparations that are useful in humans.

▼ Chapter Summary

▼ The immune system is a highly complex, integrated system that directs the protection of the body from foreign invasion. The system is highly specific and distinguishes foreignness from self, a concept called the development of self-tolerance.

▼ The actions of the immune system are effected through lymphoid organs, tissues, and cells. The lymphoid organs are the lymph nodes, spleen, thymus, and mucosa-associated lymphoid tissue. The cells of the immune system are the specific T and B lymphocytes, which are closely related to the nonspecific macrophages and polymorphonuclear leukocytes. Functionally, these organs and cells work together to provide protection against disease.

▼ B lymphocytes are responsible for humoral- or immunoglobulin-mediated immunity. These cells produce antibody, which is immunoglobulin and is found in five major classes: IgM, IgG, IgA, IgD, and IgE. When the B cell first encounters its specific antigen, it makes a plasma cell and a memory cell, which function on the second encounter with the antigen.

▼ T lymphocytes are the long-lived cells that account for long-term immunity. They originate in the bone marrow but are processed and matured in the thymus gland. The T lymphocyte can recognize MHC proteins, which means that it can react strongly with foreign MHC proteins (such as incompatible blood transfusions).

▼ T lymphocytes may be killer cells that function alone in the destruction of a target antigen, or they may work with the B lymphocyte as helper cells. Some T cells reduce the humoral response and are called suppressor cells.

▼ Macrophages and other cells work in the immune reaction in processing and presenting antigen to the T lymphocyte and also remove foreign and devitalized material from the body. The process of immunity requires the process of inflammation and depends on the activation of complement to destroy foreign material.

▼ The immune response may be T lymphocyte plus B lymphocyte with complement and neutrophils. It may involve T lymphocyte alone, which destroys the target cells and usually requires the assistance of the macrophage.

▼ Passive immunity results when antibodies are given to the individual without the active development of individual immunity, such as with transplacental transfer of antibodies to the fetus.

▼ Acquired immunity always requires the cooperative effect of sufficient specific immune cells to protect the body from many organisms in the environment.

▼ References

1. Benjamini, E., and Leskowitz, S. *Immunology: A Short Course.* New York: Alan R. Liss, 1988.
2. Beverly, P. Tumour immunology. In I. Roitt, J. Brostoff, and D. Male (eds.), *Immunology* (3rd ed.) St. Louis: C.V. Mosby. 1993.
3. Cormack, D.H. *Essential Histology.* Philadelphia: J.B. Lippincott, 1993.
4. Cotran, R.S., Kumar, V., and Robbins, S.L. *Robbins' Pathologic Basis of Disease* (5th ed.). Philadelphia: W.B. Saunders, 1994.
5. Ganong, W.F. *Review of Medical Physiology* (15th ed.). Los Altos, Calif.: Lange, 1991.
6. Goodman, J.W. Antigen presentation and the major histocompatibility complex. In D.P. Stities, A.I. Terr, and T.G. Parslow (eds.), *Basic and Clinical Immunology* (8th ed.). Norwalk, Conn.: Appleton & Lange, 1994.
7. Goodman, J.W. Immunogens & antigens. In D.P. Stites, A.I. Terr, and T.G. Parslow (eds.), *Basic and Clinical Immunology* (8th ed.). Norwalk, Conn.: Appleton & Lange, 1994.
8. Goodman, J.W. The immune response. In D.P. Stites, A.I. Terr, and T.G. Parslow (eds.), *Basic and Clinical Immunology* (8th ed.). Norwalk, Conn.: Appleton & Lange, 1994.
9. Goodman, J.W. The immune response. In D.P. Stites and A.I. Terr (eds.), *Basic Human Immunology.* Norwalk, Conn.: Appleton & Lange, 1994.
10. Goodman, J.W., and Parslow, T.G. Immunoglobulin proteins. In D.P. Stites, A.I. Terr, and T.G. Parslow (eds.), *Basic and Clinical Immunology* (8th ed.). Norwalk, Conn.: Appleton & Lange, 1994.
11. Greenberg, P.D. Mechanisms of tumor immunology. In D.P. Stites, A.I. Terr, and T.G. Parslow (eds.), *Basic and*

Clinical Immunology (8th ed.). Norwalk, Conn.: Appleton & Lange, 1994.

12. Guyton, A.C. *Textbook of Medical Physiology* (8th ed.). Philadelphia: W.B. Saunders, 1991.

13. Herold, B.C. Virus-host interactions. In S.T. Shulman, J.P. Phair, and H.M. Sommers (eds.), *The Biologic and Clinical Basis of Infectious Diseases* (4th ed.). Philadelphia: W.B. Saunders, 1992.

14. Imboden, J.B. T lymphocytes and natural killer cells. In D.P. Stites, A.I. Terr, and T.G. Parslow (eds.), *Basic and Clinical Immunology* (8th ed.). Norwalk, Conn.: Appleton & Lange, 1994.

15. Lydyard, P., and Grossi, C. Cells involved in immune responses. In I. Roitt, J. Brostoff, and D. Male (eds.), *Immunology* (3rd ed.). St. Louis: C.V. Mosby. 1993.

16. Lydard, P., and Grossi, C. The lymphoid system. In I.M. Roitt, J. Brostoff, and D.K. Male (eds.), *Immunology* (3rd ed.). St. Louis: C.V. Mosby, 1993.

17. Male, D., and Roitt, I. Introduction to the immune system. In I. Roitt, J. Brostoff, and D.K. Male (eds.), *Immunology* (3rd ed.). St. Louis: C.V. Mosby, 1993.

18. Marrack, P., and Kapplar, J. The T cell and its receptor. *Sci. Am.* 254:32, 1986.

19. Owen, M., and Steward, M. Antigen recognition. In I. Roitt, J. Brostoff, and D.K. Male (eds.), *Immunology* (3rd. ed.). St. Louis: C.V. Mosby, 1993.

20. Parslow, T.G. Lymphocytes and lymphoid tissue. In D.P. Stites, A.I. Terr, and T.G. Parslow (eds.), *Basic and Clinical Immunology* (8th ed.). Norwalk, Conn: Appleton & Lange, 1994.

21. Rook, G. Cell-mediated immune reactions. In I. Roitt, J. Brostoff, and D.K. Male (eds.), *Immunology* (3rd ed.). St. Louis: C.V. Mosby, 1993.

22. Turner, M., and Owen, M. Antigen receptor molecules. In I. Roitt, J. Brostoff, and D.K. Male (eds.), *Immunology* (3rd ed.). St. Louis: C.V. Mosby, 1993.

23. Walport, M. Complement. In I. Roitt, J. Brostoff, and D.K. Male (eds.), *Immunology* (3rd ed.). St. Louis: C.V. Mosby, 1993.

24. Ziegler, J.L. Cancer in the immunocompromised host. In D.P. Stites, A.I. Terr, and T.G. Parslow (eds.), *Basic and Clinical Immunology* (8th ed.). Norwalk, Conn.: Appleton & Lange, 1994.

Chapter 17

Immunodeficiency and Human Immunodeficiency Virus Disease

Miguel da Cunha

▼ CHAPTER OUTLINE

▼ LEARNING OBJECTIVES

1 *Differentiate between primary and secondary immunodeficiency.*
2 *Differentiate between cell-mediated and humoral immunodeficiency.*
3 *Describe severe combined immunodeficiency.*
4 *Characterize the age of onset of signs and symptoms in the major primary immune deficiencies described.*
5 *Explain the different symptoms that can occur according to the types of cells affected.*
6 *Briefly describe complement abnormalities and how these affect the immune response.*
7 *List at least six disorders that can cause secondary immunodeficiency.*
8 *Specify how stress alters the immune response.*
9 *List several immunosuppressive agents, giving benefits and drawbacks of their use.*
10 *List three causes of malnutrition or protein depletion and explain how these can disrupt the immune response.*
11 *Describe human immunodeficiency virus (HIV) disease and acquired immunodeficiency syndrome.*
12 *Explain the changes in outlook for people with HIV infection.*
13 *Discuss how opportunistic diseases become a serious threat in immunodeficiency.*

Barbara L. Bullock: PATHOPHYSIOLOGY: ADAPTATIONS AND ALTERATIONS IN FUNCTION, 4th ed.
© 1996 Lippincott-Raven Publishers

▼ *Immunodeficiency Syndromes*

The primary function of the immune system is to distinguish "self" from "nonself" antigens. Once that recognition takes place, a multifaceted immune response will be mounted against antigens perceived as "nonself" in an effort to inactivate them and render them harmless to the host. However, in the process of performing its normal function as a protective device, the immune system may cause detrimental effects to the host. Such is the case of rejection of a graft that would have enhanced the host's quality of life or increased life span. Pathologic alterations of immune function are traditionally grouped as 1) hypersensitivity reactions in which small immunogenic stimuli generate exaggerated immune responses; 2) autoimmune diseases in which the ability to distinguish self from nonself is lost; and 3) immunodeficiency syndromes in which the ability to mount an efficient immune response is impaired or nonexistent. The reactions in categories 1 and 2 are discussed in detail in

---

TABLE 17-1 *Selected Causes of Secondary Immunodeficiency and Their Consequences to Normal Immune Response*

Disease States	Consequences
Diabetes mellitus	Depressed chemotaxis/phagocytosis Depressed T-cell functions
Disseminated tuberculosis	Depressed T-cell functions
Malignancies	Depressed B- and T-cell functions
Malnutrition	Depressed phagocytosis Depressed T-cell functions Depressed B-cell functions
Uremia	Depressed T-cell functions Decreased macrophage activation/phagocytosis
Viral infections (including human immunodeficiency virus)	Depressed B- and T-cell functions Decreased macrophage activation/phagocytosis

Iatrogenic Causes	Consequences
Corticosteroid therapy	Depressed B- and T-cell functions Depressed macrophage activation/phagocytosis
Immunosuppressive therapy (including radiotherapy)	Depressed multiplication/activation of T- and B-cells Depressed macrophage activation/phagocytosis
Splenectomy	Depressed humoral immunity

Chapter 18. This chapter addresses immunodeficiency of various causes.

From an etiologic viewpoint, immunodeficiency syndromes can be classified as primary or secondary. *Primary* or *congenital immunodeficiency syndromes* result mostly from genetically determined abnormalities that impair cell-mediated and/or humoral responses. *Secondary* or *acquired immunodeficiency syndromes* are conditions that develop as consequences of disease states (eg, malignancies, malnutrition, viral infections) or result from medical treatment (especially with immunosuppressive drugs) (Table 17-1). From a pathogenesis viewpoint, immunodeficiencies may be classified according to the component of immune response involved, such as 1) B-cell, or antibody-mediated, immunity; 2) T-cell–mediated immunity; 3) immunity mediated by the action of phagocytic cells; and 4) immunity associated with the activation of complement.[30]

The hallmark of immunodeficiencies is an increased susceptibility to infections. The nature of the infection depends on which component (and consequently, function) of the immune system is involved. For example, B-cell mediated (humoral) deficiencies predispose to infections with pyogenic bacteria, whereas T-cell deficiencies increase the susceptibility to bacterial, fungal, and viral infections (Table 17-2). In addition, immunodeficiency syndromes may predispose to cancers (such as HIV-related lymphomas) and to autoimmune disease. It is important to remember, however, that immunodeficiency syndromes are extremely heterogeneous entities, because various components of the immune system may be compromised.

▼ *Primary Immunodeficiency*

A primary defect in the immune system results from the failure of an essential part of the immune system to develop. The defect can occur at any point during the development of the immune system and may involve organ or cellular defects. Many types of primary immunodeficiency states have been described according to the cell type affected and the developmental stage of the cellular system (Table 17-3). The more common disorders are described below.

B-CELL (HUMORAL) IMMUNODEFICIENCIES

Several pathophysiologic defects in the immune system result in abnormal immunoglobulin synthesis or a deficiency of immunoglobulins. These can affect production of all of the immunoglobulins or of only specific classes. Antibody deficiency is suspected in people with persistent, recurrent, severe, or unusual infections. Different types of deficiencies can arise at any age (Table 17-4).

TABLE 17-2 *Common Pathogens in Immunodeficiency Disorders*

Defective Element	Common Microorganisms
T-cell deficiencies	Bacteria: Intracellular: *Mycobacterium tuberculosis*, *Listeria monocytogenes* Extracellular: salmonella, legionella, nocardia Fungi: Candida, histoplasma, cryptococcus, aspergillus Viruses: Cytomegalovirus, herpes simplex, herpes zoster Protozoa: Pneumocystis, toxoplasma, cryptosporidium
B-cell dysfunction	
Hypogammaglobulinemia	Pyogenic extracellular bacteria
IgA deficiency	Bacteria infecting sinuses, lungs; *Giardia lamblia*; hepatitis viruses
Splenectomy	*Streptococcus pneumoniae*, salmonella
Phagocytic/bactericidal deficiency	Many staphylococci and streptococci, *Haemophilus influenzae*, candida
Complement deficiencies	
C3	*Streptococcus pneumoniae*
C5-C9	*Neisseria* species

From Widmann, F. K. *An Introduction to Clinical Immunology*, pg. 180. Philadelphia: F.A. Davis, 1989. (Used with permission.)

TABLE 17-3 *Examples of Primary Immunodeficiency Disorders Affecting T- and B-Cell Lines*

Congenital B-Cell (Humoral) Deficiencies

DISEASE	FUNCTIONAL DEFICIENCIES
X-linked agammaglobulinemia	All Ig isotypes decreased; reduced B cells
Selective IgA deficiency	Decreased serum IgA1 and IgA2; normal B cells
Selective IgG subclass deficiency	Decrease in one or more IgG subclasses
Transient hypogammaglobulinemia of infancy	IgG and IgA decreased; detectable bacterial antibodies; normal B cells
Common variable immunodeficiency	Variable decreases in multiple IgG isotypes; normal or decreased B cells

Congenital T-Cell and Combined Immunodeficiencies

DISEASE	FUNCTIONAL DEFICIENCIES
DiGeorge syndrome	Decreased T cells; normal B cells; normal or decreased serum Ig
X-linked SCID	Markedly decreased T cells; reduced serum Ig
Ataxia-telangiectasia	Decreased T cells; normal B cells; variable reduction in IgA, IgE, and IgG subclasses

SCID: severe combined immunodeficiency disease.

Adapted from Abbas, A. K., Lichtman, A. H., and Pober, J. S. *Cellular and molecular immunology* (2nd ed.). Philadelphia: W.B. Saunders, 1994.

TABLE 17-4   *Age of Onset of Selected Primary Immunodeficiency Disorders*

Usual Age Group	Immunodeficiency Disorder
Earliest infancy	Reticular dysgenesis* SCID† DiGeorge syndrome*
2–6 months	Infantile hypogammaglobulinemia‡
6–24 months	Transient hypogammaglobulinemia of infancy‡ Wiscott-Aldrich Syndrome (bleeding may occur earlier)*
Childhood	Ataxia-telangiectasia† (ataxia may occur earlier) IgA deficiency (symptomatic)‡
Adolescence or adulthood	Deficiencies of complement Common variable immune-deficiency‡

Adapted from Widmann, F. K. *An introduction to clinical immunology.* Philadelphia: F.A. Davis, 1989.
   SCID: severe combined immunodeficiency disease.
   * Disorders of T-cell (cell-mediated) immunity.
   † Combined B-cell and T-cell immunodeficiencies
   ‡ Disorders of B-cell (humoral) immunity

The most common primary B-cell deficiencies are X-linked agammaglobulinemia, variable immunodeficiency, and IgA deficiency.

X-Linked Agammaglobulinemia

A defect in the maturation of stem cells into B cells occurs in X-linked hypogammaglobulinemia (Bruton-type agammaglobulinemia). This congenital disease first appears in male infants at about age 5 to 6 months, when the maternally transmitted level of antibodies has decreased. The B cells are virtually absent from the blood, and the basic defect seems to be failure of B cells to mature.[38]

Levels of immunoglobulins IgM, IgG, and IgA are low. Antigens are not cleared well from the body, causing infants with this condition to be extremely susceptible to bacterial infections, especially those caused by *Staphylococcus aureus, Streptococcus pyogenes, Haemophilus influenzae,* and pneumococci. The result is a high frequency of respiratory, sinus, and throat infections.[1]

The cellular immune system remains competent. Allograft rejection and the ability to resist viral, fungal, and parasitic infections are apparently normal. Autoimmune disease occurs frequently, especially rheumatoid arthritis and systemic lupus erythematosus.[7]

Variable Immunodeficiency

Variable immunodeficiency may be seen in various forms, with the common feature being hypogamma-globulinemia, usually of all antibody classes but sometimes of only IgG. These conditions may be congenital or acquired; in the latter case, they may be seen along with malnutrition or immunosuppressant chemotherapy. Variable immunodeficiency can manifest as a B-cell defect in which antigen is recognized and B cells proliferate but do not differentiate into plasma cells. In some cases, autoantibodies are directed at the T and B cells, which cause a general immunodeficiency disorder. It may be associated with T-helper cell suppression or the presence of activated T-suppressor cells.[24] Autoimmune diseases and cancer occur with high frequency, but the main problem is the inability to clear infectious diseases from the body.[1, 24]

IgA Deficiency

Selective IgA deficiency, which occurs in apparently healthy people who may have normal serum levels of the other immunoglobulins, is the most common immunodeficiency disorder (occurring in 1 of every 600 persons). Affected persons lack IgA in serum and external secretions. The disease has a hereditary basis.[15]

The presence of normal numbers of B cells with IgA expressed on their surface suggests failure in the synthesis and release of IgA rather than the absence of IgA B lymphocytes. The defect appears to be in differentiation of IgA B lymphocytes, perhaps because of hyperactivity of IgA suppressor cells that prevents the differentiation. A defect in the helper cells specific for IgA synthesis also may be present.[10] Acquired IgA deficiency may occur in persons treated with phenytoin and penicillamine.

The most common symptoms relate to those surfaces that normally are covered with mucosal secretions. Infections of the sinuses and respiratory tract are common. Related gastrointestinal problems include ulcerative colitis, pernicious anemia, and malabsorption states. About 50% of people with IgA deficiency also have some atopic disease.[15] The prevalence of autoimmune diseases, such as systemic lupus erythematosus and rheumatoid arthritis, is markedly increased, and the diagnosis can be supported by the presence of anti-IgA antibodies.[6] A high frequency of cancer cases in the respiratory and gastrointestinal tracts and lymphoid system has been reported.

The reason for this increased susceptibility to atopic disease, autoimmune disease, and cancer is unknown, but one theory is that IgA normally interacts with many antigens on the mucosal surfaces and prevents their entry into the body.[15] A deficiency of IgA would allow the body to be exposed to more antigens than it can combat successfully. Because of increased antigenic stimulation, more antigen can react with IgE and produce allergic manifestations. Increased risk of production of antibody that will cross react with a self-antigen increases the risk of autoimmune disease. Chronic irritation and inflammation caused by the large amount of antigen could predispose the exposed tissue to malignant transformation.

T-CELL (CELL-MEDIATED) IMMUNODEFICIENCIES

Primary deficiencies in T-cell function have been recognized for many years. However, immunodeficiencies of T-cell function will affect other cells of the immune system, due to the regulatory action of some T lymphocytes (helper/inducer T cells and suppressor T cells). Consequently, selective T-cell immunodeficiencies are rare, because they often result in secondary B-cell (humoral) dysfunction. Primary T-cell deficiencies are those that occur initially as a result of impairment in T-cell maturation, the most common example being primary thymic hypoplasia, or DiGeorge syndrome.

DiGeorge Syndrome

This selective T-cell deficiency is due to a developmental malformation of the 3rd and 4th pharyngeal pouches that may result in congenital hypoplasia or complete absence of the thymus and parathyroids, abnormalities of the great vessels, and facial deformities. The degree of severity varies among individuals. In some cases, the primary (initial) defect has been associated with maternal ethanol consumption. In others, it has demonstrated an autosomal dominant pattern of inheritance, suggesting a genetic etiology.[1] The complete DiGeorge syndrome is characterized by the presence of all the anomalies above, so that the child will present with deficient cell-mediated immunity (due to agenesis or hypoplasia of the thymus); abnormal calcium homeostasis, often expressed by muscle twitching or tetany (a result of agenesis or hypoplasia of the parathyroid glands); facial malformations, such as low-set ears and slanted eyes; and malformations of the great vessels.[3]

From a morphologic viewpoint, the disease is characterized by the absence or severe reduction of circulating T lymphocytes, and the resulting defective cell-mediated immunity is manifested by an increased susceptibility to infections with viruses, fungi, intracellular bacteria, and protozoa. Because such parasites often survive and multiply within cells, their successful eradication depends on the presence of an intact T-cell function. In many cases the disease is severe and potentially fatal in early childhood. However, T-cell function tends to improve with age and is often normal by age 5 years, either because of the presence of some residual thymic tissue or because other structures assume the function of that missing site of T-cell maturation. In refractory cases, the disease can be corrected by transplantation of fetal thymic tissue, or bone marrow grafting.[1]

SEVERE COMBINED IMMUNODEFICIENCY DISEASE

Severe combined immunodeficiency disease is thought to arise from a deficiency of the stem cell population that forms the lymphocytes. It is manifested by T- and B-cell deficiency associated with a hypoplastic thymus. A tremendous decrease in the number and maturity of lymphocytes provides for little, if any, immune response to antigen. The loss of T cells usually is greater than that of B cells, and T-cell immaturity may be manifested by failure to differentiate to a mature form on antigen stimulation.[19] The two mechanisms for the development of severe combined immunodeficiency disease are 1) a defect in stem cell population and 2) abnormal differentiation of T cells because of abnormalities in the thymus gland.[24] The result is deficiency of both humoral and cell-mediated responses.

Stem cell deficiency severely depresses a person's ability to mount any type of immune response. The thymus remains small and embryonic, resembling that of a 6- to 8-week-old fetus.[15] The few lymphocytes present are not activated by antigen. Few B cells are present, so all classes of immunoglobulins are depressed, resulting in lack of production of specific antibodies.

An infant with this condition is affected from birth and is unable to cope with a germ-laden environment. Such children are vulnerable to all forms of infections, and many die within the first year of life. The initial problem in early infancy is failure to thrive, which is followed in the first few weeks of life by serious infections, such as pneumonia and infectious diarrhea. Any type of infection may develop, and none responds well to treatment. If severe combined immunodeficiency disease is suspected within hours of birth, the child may be placed in a germ-free environment, with a later attempt to perform bone marrow transplantation.

In some cases, full immunologic ability can be attained if *graft-versus-host disease* does not limit the success. This disorder occurs when immunocompetent cells are transplanted to recipients who lack the usual immune defense. The normal cells react against those of the recipient. Involvement of the skin, liver, and intestinal mucosa is most common (Fig. 17-1). Graft-versus-host disease can be ameliorated by close matching of bone marrow for transplantation and, in some cases, pretreating bone marrow cells.[31]

PHAGOCYTIC CELL DEFICIENCIES

Deficiencies in the phagocytic cell system results in increased susceptibility to bacterial infections, with little or no increase in viral or fungal diseases. Because of the high frequency of bacterial infections, antibiotic therapy is a major consideration in the management of phagocyte deficiencies.[6] A classic example of such disorders is

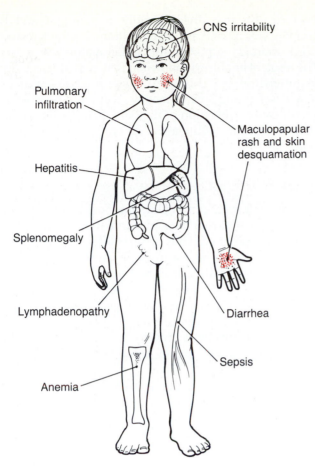

FIGURE 17-1   *Major clinical features of the graft-versus-host disease (GVHD).*

TABLE 17-5   *Complement Protein Deficiencies and Their Clinical Consequences*

Protein	Associated Diseases/Pathology
C1q, C1r, C1S	Systemic lupus erythematosus Recurrent pyogenic infections
C2	Systemic lupus erythematosus Vasculitis Glomerulonephritis Recurrent pyogenic infections
C3	Immune complex disease Glomerulonephritis Recurrent pyogenic infections
C4	Glomerulonephritis Systemic lupus erythematosus
C5, C6, C7, C8	Disseminated neisserial infections
C9	None
Properdin, factor D	Neisserial infections Other pyogenic infections

Adapted from Abbas, A. K., Lichtman, A. H., and Pober, J. S. *Cellular and molecular immunology* (2nd ed.). Philadelphia: W.B. Saunders, 1994.

Chédiak-Higashi disease, which is characterized by albinism, extreme sensitivity to light, and frequent bacterial infections. The most frequent cellular change in Chédiak-Higashi disease is the presence of abnormally large granules within phagocytic cells (mostly neutrophils). These changes appear to decrease the cells' ability to internally destroy phagocytized bacteria, although their phagocytic ability remains intact. Eventually the neutrophils will become overloaded and undergo lysis, and the bacteria will be released unharmed to continue the infectious process.

COMPLEMENT ABNORMALITIES

Complement factors are necessary to promote the inflammatory process. Complement deficiency has been detected in an increased number of persons with autoimmune disease (Table 17-5). Various symptoms occur, depending on the complement factor that is deficient.

Deficiency of complement inhibitors also can result in allergic reactions; the most frequent is hereditary angioedema, caused by a genetic deficiency of C1 esterase inhibitor. This produces uncontrolled activation of the complement system, causing angioedema in the skin, larynx, and gastrointestinal and genitourinary tracts.[1]

Deficiencies of complements 2 and 3 (C2 and C3) are fairly common. Deficiency of C2 is transmitted as an autosomal dominant trait, and people with this condition have a high frequency of systemic lupus erythematosus and other connective tissue disorders.[1,37]

Deficiency of C3 results in impairment of the inflammatory response and difficulty in clearing pyogenic and gram-negative infection. The deficiency can be inherited or acquired. The substance is used faster than it can be made in major systemic infections or in a nutritionally depleted host.[31]

▼ *Secondary Immunodeficiency*

MULTIFACTORIAL SECONDARY IMMUNODEFICIENCY

Secondary immunodeficiency states result from the loss of a previously effective immune system. They include any disorder that exhibits loss of immunocompetence as a result of another condition. A broad classification includes immunodeficiency secondary to stress, aging, immunosuppressive drugs, systemic infection, cancer, malnutrition, renal diseases, and radiation therapy. These conditions may lead to a loss of immunoglobulins, inadequate synthesis of immunoglobulins, loss of specific lymphocytes responsible for cell-mediated immunity, loss of phagocytic inflammatory cells, or a combination of these. Even though decreased effectiveness of the immune system frequently is not life-threatening, it often results in decreased ability of the organisms to mount an inflammatory or immune response. Therefore, susceptibility to infection by bacteria, viruses, fungi, or all three is increased. In some cases, the loss of immunocompetence causes enough alteration in host resistance to increase morbidity and mortality.

Effects of Stress

Stress response has been the target of much research with respect to how it disrupts the physiologic functioning of the body. Stress appears to alter the immune response through neural interruption from the hypothalamus, which ultimately decreases the functioning of the thymus through secretion of glucocorticoids. Glucocorticoid hormones mainly diminish the inflammatory response by suppressing macrophages, decreasing the number of white blood cells, and causing regression of lymphatic tissue. This can enhance the spread of infection (see p. 184).

Effects of Aging

Immune system changes with aging have been studied extensively. Some studies have related aging changes to immune system deterioration. Most studies of immune system cell numbers show little change over the life span.[31] The activities of T cells may change because of an increased number of immature T cells in the blood. As a person ages, thymic hormone levels decrease, which may cause a decline in cell-mediated immunity.[1] When the T cells are less functional, the ability of B cells to mount specific antibody responses decreases. In an older person, there is an increase in the production of autoantibodies and apparently nonfunctional monoclonal immunoglobulin proteins.[1] The results of immune system dysfunction include 1) a decrease in the ability to control infections; 2) possibly a decrease in immune surveillance, which leads to an increased risk of cancer; and 3) possibly an increase in autoimmune diseases related to increased autoantibody production.[7, 24, 30]

Effects of Immunosuppression

Immunosuppression usually refers to the pharmacologic suppression of the immune system. Drugs have been used extensively to decrease the rejection phenomenon in transplanted tissue, the rate of growth of malignant tumors, and the inflammation involved with autoimmune disorders. Agents used to achieve these effects are cytotoxic drugs, such as methotrexate, and corticosteroids, such as hydrocortisone. The cytotoxic drugs are toxic to cells that divide rapidly, including T and B lymphocytes as well as polymorphonuclear leukocytes. Corticosteroids suppress the inflammatory response. The result of immunosuppression is increased sensitivity to the environmental antigens. Superimposed infections may develop and spread readily. Many pharmacologic agents cause depression of the bone marrow formation of leukocytes and thus affect all types of white blood cells.[38]

Effects of Other Conditions

Systemic infection can deplete the host defense to the point at which further antigen stimulation may result in decreased resistance. Thus host resistance is decreased, and opportunistic organisms may cause serious problems. Cancer usually causes malnutrition as a result of protein wasting. Decreased synthesis of lymphocytes results. Immunodeficiency caused by B lymphoproliferative disorders, such as chronic lymphocytic leukemia and multiple myeloma, results in impairment of the antibody responses, causing secondary infections with pyogenic bacteria.

Radiation therapy, usually instituted against cancer, affects rapidly proliferating cells and results in a decrease in all of the cells of the inflammatory response, including the T and B lymphocytes. Opportunistic infections, especially those caused by gram-negative bacteria, viruses, and fungi, occur more frequently.[38]

Renal disease probably causes most of its immunosuppressive effects from proteinuria leading to hypoproteinemia or from acid–base disruptions that can affect the formation of lymphocytes, especially T cells. Many pathologic processes of the kidneys are treated with corticosteroids, and immunosuppression may result from drug therapy.

▼ Human Immunodeficiency Virus (HIV) Disease and Acquired Immunodeficiency Syndrome

HISTORICAL CONSIDERATIONS

Acquired immunodeficiency syndrome (AIDS) was first recognized as a new disease in 1981, when the Centers for Disease Control and Prevention received reports of small clusters of *Pneumocystis carinii* pneumonia (PCP) and Kaposi sarcoma (KS) occurring among young, otherwise healthy male homosexuals. Although they were known diseases, PCP and KS had not affected that target population before 1981. PCP had been restricted mainly to young malnourished children, and KS was found in elderly men of Mediterranean ancestry. Immunosuppressed persons had been shown to have both PCP and KS. This new clinical entity was originally termed "gay-related immunodeficiency." In 1982, the term AIDS was adopted, because new cases of this disease were reported among various groups outside the gay community, namely, recipients of blood products (eg, freeze-dried factor VIII concentrate for hemophilia A) and injecting-drug users. Such horizontal transmission through sexual activity and blood-to-blood contact as well as reports of vertical transmission from infected women to their offspring raised the possibility of an infectious etiology. In 1983, researchers led by Dr. Luc Montagnier of the Institut Pasteur in Paris reported the discovery of the virus that causes AIDS. It was determined to be a retrovirus (RNA-containing) initially named lymphadenopathy virus and now termed human immunodeficiency virus type 1 (HIV-1). In 1986, a group of investigators led by Kanki discovered in West Africa another retrovirus related to HIV-1 whose infection also resulted in an acquired immunodeficiency.[17] Formerly called human T-lymphotropic virus type IV (HTLV-4), this second "AIDS virus" is now called HIV-2. HIV-2 is found primarily in countries in West Africa (Guinea-Bissau, Ivory Coast, Senegal) and in France, Germany, Portugal, Canada, Cuba, and Brazil. Although HIV-2 appears to have existed in West Africa longer than HIV-1, fewer cases of AIDS have been reported in West Africa than in Central and East Africa. A recent account of a study from 1985 to 1993 in Senegal reported that HIV-2 is less virulent than HIV-1 by showing that 5 years after seroconversion, one third of women infected with HIV-1 had developed AIDS symptoms, whereas none of the women infected with HIV-2 were symptomatic. That study also revealed that the rate of developing abnormal CD4 + cell counts was lower for HIV-2 infections.[22] Differences in viral load may be responsible for the low rate of HIV-2 transmission, because it has been shown that the amount of virus carried by HIV-2–infected persons remains fairly low until the immunodeficiency is severe.[11] Because HIV-2 prevalence in the United States is quite low, the current discussion addresses only HIV-1, which is hereafter referred to simply as HIV.

The awareness that HIV was a blood-borne virus prompted the development of tests to screen donated blood for the presence of HIV antibodies, which would reveal a previously infected donor. A commonly used screening antibody test, the enzyme-linked immunosorbent assay (ELISA) was approved for general clinical use in 1985. A confirmatory antibody test, the Western blot was licensed by the Food and Drug Administration in kit form in 1987.

It took 9 years, from the first recognition in 1981, for the total cumulative number of AIDS cases to reach 100,000. The second 100,000 cases were reached in 1991, which gives AIDS a doubling time of approximately 2 years. This figure, added to the fact that AIDS is sexually transmitted, has made this disease one of the major public health issues in the world. Many countries have mobilized extensive resources to curtail the spread of AIDS through testing and public education, but much remains to be done to control this epidemic.[29]

MODES OF HIV TRANSMISSION

Three modes of transmission of HIV have been identified since the beginnings of the epidemic: 1) through unprotected sexual activity, which means without the use of adequate barriers; 2) through blood-to-blood contact; and 3) through vertical transmission (Box 17-1).

Sexual Activity

Most cases of HIV reported in the United States (57%) occurred through male-to-male sexual activity, reflecting a high virus load in seminal fluid. This finding is confirmed by cases of heterosexual transmission, of which the vast majority of cases involves man-to-woman transmission. Although it is easy to conceptualize how the virus may be acquired by the recipient of infected semen, the portal of HIV entry into the circulation in male-to-female transmission has not been clearly determined, especially in the case of nonforceful, well-lubricated vaginal penetration.[4] Female-to-male spread may be achieved through virus-containing vaginal fluids, cervical mucus, or menstrual blood, but the portal of entry in the male, likewise, has not yet been conclusively identified. However, data on transmission of hepatitis B virus and HIV among homosexual males suggest that transurethral exposure is an important transmission method.[18]

BOX 17-1 ▼ *Modes of HIV Transmission*

Unprotected Sexual Activity
▼ Vaginal intercourse
▼ Anal intercourse
▼ Oral intercourse (?)

Blood-To-Blood Contact
▼ Needle sharing among injected-drug users
▼ Transfusion of HIV-infected blood and blood products
▼ Occupational exposure to HIV-infected body fluids among health care workers

Vertical Transmission (Maternal-To-Offspring)
▼ Transplacental transmission
▼ Intrapartum transmission
▼ Postpartum transmission via breast-feeding (?)

HIV: human immunodeficiency virus.
   (?) Questionable due to other concomitant modes or activities (see text).

The recipient of unprotected anal or vaginal intercourse carries the highest risk of HIV infection, followed by the inserter in these two activities, respectively.[26] The efficiency of a latex barrier, such as latex condoms (as opposed to "skin," or natural membrane, condoms), in reducing the rate of sexually transmitted diseases, including HIV infection, has been documented. In a study of 343 female sex partners of HIV-infected men, the annual seroconversion rate for couples who never or not always used condoms was respectively 6% and 10%, compared with 1% among those who always used this protective device.[27] Transmission of HIV through oral sex remains questionable; although biologically possible, due to portals of entry through the oral cavity, systematic studies have not been conducted due to the difficulty in identifying study populations who practice this form of sexual activity exclusively. It must be noted that it is the sexual activity practiced, and not the gender or sexual orientation of the participants, that determines the risk factors in sexual transmission of HIV. In the reporting of HIV statistics, therefore, the phrase "groups at risk" is being increasingly replaced by the phrase "activities at risk."

Blood-to-Blood Contact

Blood-to-blood contact accounts for the transmission of HIV among injecting-drug users (formerly referred to as intravenous-drug users) through the sharing of hypodermic needles and devices; among the recipients of blood products, including clotting factors; and, rarely, among health care workers through occupational infection from HIV-positive patients.

The incidence of HIV infection in injecting-drug users, their sex partners, and their offspring has increased significantly in recent years, with a disproportionate number of cases among African-American and Hispanic populations. A now classic study of 452 persons enrolled in a methadone-treatment program revealed an overall HIV seroprevalence of 40%, with 49% in African Americans (who account for 12% of the general U.S. population), 42% in Hispanics (who account for 7%), and 17% in non-Hispanic whites.[28]

The rate of HIV infection among hemophiliacs averages 55% and is a function of frequency of clotting factors infusion, which indicates that severe hemophiliacs are at increased risk. The risk was much greater before 1985 and has been virtually eliminated with the development of viral-inactivation measures and donor antibody testing.[13] Likewise, HIV infection through blood transfusions has declined after 1985, because all units of donated blood since that time are antibody tested. However, because there is a window of time between infection and seroconversion, blood units can test antibody-negative but actually be virus-positive. The current risk of HIV transmission from screened blood is in the range of 1 in 38,000 to 1 in 153,000 units

of donated blood, a risk which increases in areas of high HIV prevalence.[5]

The incidence of HIV infection by occupational exposure among health care workers is relatively small (less than 0.3% seroconversion), given their extensive contact with HIV-infected persons and/or their body fluids.[8, 21]

Vertical Transmission

Vertical transmission from an HIV-positive woman may occur through prenatal (during gestation), intrapartal (during labor and delivery), or postpartal (through breast-feeding) exposure. Reported rates of transmission of HIV from pregnant women to their offspring range from 25% to 35%.[23] Because the virus can cross the placenta, variation in transmission rates appears to be related to the maternal virus load. Women who become pregnant soon after infection have a lower transmission risk than those who conceive many months or years after infection. Those who have previously given birth to HIV-positive children also have an increased risk of transmitting it again. In intrapartum transmission, infants delivered by cesarean section have a lower rate of HIV infection than do babies delivered vaginally. Transmission through breast milk has been challenged, because nipple fissures during lactation are common, and transmission through blood cannot be ruled out.

EPIDEMIOLOGIC TRENDS

"The changing face of AIDS" is a metaphor often used to expressed the evolution of epidemiologic trends in HIV disease in the United States. The first wave of persons with AIDS was represented by homosexual/bisexual men infected through sexual activity. This was followed by a second wave of injecting-drug users who acquired the virus through the sharing of contaminated needles. Traditionally heterosexual injecting-drug users, in turn, proceeded to infect their sex partners through unprotected sexual activity. The United States has now witnessed the emergence of the fourth wave, the offspring of those women who were infected through intravenous drug use or through sexual activity with an infected injecting-drug user.

A decrease in the number of cases among homosexual/bisexual men was first noted in 1991.[33] Overall, the proportion of cases attributed to male-to-male contact has decreased from 67% in 1985 to 46% in 1993.[35] This trend is probably due to intensive educational efforts directed at that community, resulting in stricter adherence to safer sex practices and reduction in number of sex partners. However, most reported cases of AIDS in the United States (57%) continues to occur among gay/bisexual men. Although the number of cases among gay/bisexual men continued to decrease, the proportion of cases attributed to injecting-drug users among women and heterosexual men increased from 17% in 1985 to 28% in 1993. In 1993 alone, AIDS cases attributed to heterosexual contact increased 130% over 1992. Of those, 42% were contacts with an injecting-drug user, and 50% represented contacts with an HIV-infected partner whose risk was unreported or unknown. As with other sexually transmitted diseases, women are at greater risk of acquiring HIV through heterosexual contact. In 1993, 4% of men and 37% of women with AIDS were reported as having HIV infection associated with heterosexual transmission. Because almost 90% of pediatric AIDS cases result from perinatal transmission from an infected mother, it is not surprising to see a proportionally large increase in perinatal transmission.[35]

HIV-related mortality also presents a sobering picture. In 1992, HIV disease became the leading cause of death for men age 25 to 44 years, and the fourth leading cause of death for women within the same age bracket.[34] In the absence of curative therapies for HIV infection, strategies aimed at decreasing the spread of this disease must have an educational focus. Risk-reduction efforts directed at women in reproductive age groups will have the double benefit of decreasing infection risk for themselves and for their offspring.

NATURAL HISTORY AND IMMUNOLOGIC ASPECTS

HIV belongs to the HTLV and to the *lentivirus* (lentus is Latin for slow) family of nononcogenic, cytopathic retroviruses. Other lentiviruses found in nonhuman animals share some morphologic and pathogenic properties with HIV. They all cause slow, progressive wasting disorders, including neurologic degeneration, that are often fatal. Retroviruses, or RNA-containing viruses, were identified several decades ago as oncogenic, or cancer-causing, viruses. In 1971, Howard Temin and David Baltimore identified an enzyme present in retroviruses that allowed them to integrate their genetic information into the genome of the host cells by reversing the process of DNA to RNA transcription. Appropriately, that enzyme was termed *reverse transcriptase*. The HIV virion (free virus particle) is approximately 100 nm in diameter and consists of a central core surrounded by a lipid envelope (Fig. 17-2). The core consists of the RNA genome and several viral proteins, which include p24, p18, and reverse transcriptase. Viral proteins are encoded by specific RNA-contained viral genes, while other genes control viral replication functions. From the lipid membrane protrude glycoprotein molecules, gp120 and gp41.[9]

HIV and Its Target Cells

After appropriate exposure to an HIV-infected body fluid, viral particles gain access to the host's blood circulation and lymphatic structures. At these sites, and eventually at various other organs, HIV initiates the infective

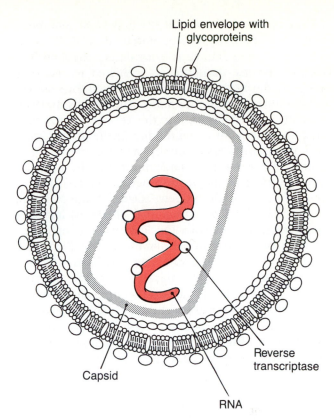

FIGURE 17-2 *Structure of human immune deficiency virus type 1 (HIV-1). The internal core structure consists of the viral genome (two identical RNA strands) and reverse transcriptase molecules surrounded by various core capsid proteins (p24, p18). The virus membrane consists of a lipid envelope from which protrude molecules of glycoproteins (gp41 and gp120).*

process through the binding of one of its envelope glycoproteins, gp120, to specific receptor sites present on the surface of a variety of cells. The preferred binding site is a glycoprotein receptor termed CD4. Among the cells that display CD4 receptors (CD4+ cells), helper/inducer T lymphocytes (or T4 cells) and monocytes—macrophages are the primary targets of HIV. Other targets include various antigen-presenting cells, such as Langerhans cells in the skin and mucous membrane, dendritic cells in lymph nodes and peripheral blood, and microglial cells in the central nervous system. Despite HIV's preference for CD4 cells, studies in vitro have identified a variety of cells that do not display detectable CD4 molecules (CD4− cells) but that can be infected by HIV.[9] These include some central nervous system cells (such as neurons, glial cells, astrocytes, and endothelial cells), muscle cells, colorectal cells, B cells, and bone marrow progenitor cells. The entry and proliferation of HIV in CD4− cells in vitro, however, is inefficient and not yet understood. HIV infection of cells not known to be CD4+ has also been documented in vivo, including cells of the colon, rectum, duodenum, cervix, retina, and brain. These studies indicate that mechanisms other than CD4 affinity may be involved in HIV infection.

After the binding of viral gp120 with an appropriate cellular receptor, the HIV membrane fuses with the cell membrane, and the virus core enters the host cell. Through reverse transcriptase–mediated reverse transcription, the incoming viral RNA controls the synthesis of viral DNA and viral proteins. This results in 1) the integration of viral DNA into the host cell's genome in the form of a latent provirion and 2) the production of new viral particles. Eventually, as a long-term consequence of viral infection, large numbers of host cells are killed, possibly by apoptosis (programmed cell death), a form of "physiologic cellular suicide" induced by the viral gp120.[14, 20] The cumulative effects of increased numbers of viruses with the loss of T4 lymphocytes result in progressive impairment of cell-mediated and humoral immunity, which renders the host vulnerable to the opportunistic diseases that are the hallmark of HIV infection. The production of host cells with integrated progeny virus ensures the availability of viruses for future infection, because these progeny viral genomes are activated into infective particles by undetermined factors.

T4 Cell Loss as a Predictor of Disease Progression

In the intact immune system, the regulatory effects of helper/inducer T cells are modulated by the action of suppressor T cells (T8 cells). For example, T4 cells stimulate blast proliferation of antigen-activated B cells, thus they indirectly stimulate the production of antibodies by the resulting plasma cells. Conversely, T8 cells inhibit B-cell blast proliferation and therefore suppress antibody production. The balance between the two effects is achieved through a T4/T8 ratio of approximately 2:1. This signifies in an intact immune system the tendency toward stimulation and not inhibition of antibody production. The T4/T8 ratio is an important predictor of disease progression in HIV disease. When the ideal ratio of 2:1 falls to approximately 1:1, it reflects a reduction in T4 numbers and is indicative of significant immune suppression. Ratios below 0.5:1 signal the onset of impending opportunistic diseases. Reduction in total T4 cell count is also prognostic of immune dysfunction. When the normal count (650 to 1,200 cells/mm^3) drops to 500 cells/mm^3, significant impairment of immune function is expected. A reduction to 200 or fewer cells/mm^3 indicates impending opportunistic disease and is an AIDS-defining condition.[32] Although T4 cell count is the most reliable indicator of disease progression, the clinician should not be surprised to encounter HIV-infected persons with markedly reduced counts (sometimes in the range of 10 to 100 cells/mm^3) exhibiting no signs or symptoms of immune dysfunction for long periods of time. This discrepancy between decreased T4 cell counts and a relative disease-free state suggests that some other cell of the immune system may play a more significant role as a predictor of disease progression. Until such cells can be identified and better studied, reduction in T4 cell counts will provide clinicians with a guideline in determining when to institute antiretroviral therapy. On the basis of clinical trials with available agents, treatment with single agents should be initiated when the T4 count has fallen below 500 cells/mm^3 and combination therapy be given when the T4 count has fallen to 300 cells/mm^3 or when the person become symptomatic. In addition, prophylactic measures to delay the onset of pneumocystic pneumonia, the most common opportunistic disease, usually is added at the level of 200 or fewer cells per cubic millimeter.

Decrease in cell-mediated and humoral immunity that result from loss of T cells will eventually cause a severe, overall immune dysfunction which also includes 1) the production of nonspecific immunoglobulins (including IgM hyperimmunoglobulinemia, which is common in pediatric cases); and 2) impaired macrophage and natural killer cell function, resulting in decreased cancer immunosurveillance ability. The ensuing opportunistic infections and malignancies are characteristic of advanced HIV infection.

CLINICAL SPECTRUM OF HIV DISEASE

Most AIDS researchers agree that the clinical course and pathologic changes that follow a successful HIV infection represent a continuum of disease progression. On this continuum, AIDS is the terminal event. These clinicians espouse the belief that HIV + Time = AIDS. However, a fraction of infected individuals have remained disease-free for as long as 12 years after exposure.[34] The existence of such nonprogressors (so called "long-term survivors") raises the question of whether HIV infection is invariably fatal or whether these survivors are perhaps protected by unidentified defense mechanisms. AIDS researchers have changed much of their focus from the causation of AIDS to what protects some infected individuals from developing AIDS. The most recent data on nonprogressors reveal that these individuals may exhibit HIV-specific humoral and cellular immune responses that might contribute to control of viral replications, as demonstrated by the finding that CD8+ cells (suppressor T cells) from such persons strongly inhibit the growth of HIV in culture. Another explanation is the presence of attenuated forms of the virus that may have defective replication mechanisms. Both of these characteristics are markedly different from those of most HIV-infected persons (Dr. David Ho, personal communication, October 6, 1994).

Once an appropriate exposure to HIV occurs, predictable phases of disease progression result (Box 17-2). An appropriate exposure to HIV refers to that which results in infection.

BOX 17-2 ▼ *Clinical Spectrum of HIV Disease (1993 CDC Classification)*

A. Clinical Category A
1. Acute retroviral syndrome
   a. Negative antibody test.
   b. Acute influenza-like symptomatology occurring 2–4 weeks after infection. Rash may occur.
2. Asymptomatic infection (asymptomatic "carriers")
   a. Positive antibody test (2 ELISAs + 1 WB).
   b. No disease process.
3. Persistent generalized lymphadenopathy
   a. Positive antibody test (2 ELISAs + 1 WB)
   b. Lymphadenopathy (>1 cm diameter at 2 or more extrainguinal sites for more than 3 months)

B. Clinical Category B
1. Usually a positive antibody test (2 ELISAs + 1 WB)
2. Examples of conditions (partial list):
   Oropharyngeal candidiasis (oral thrush)
   Vulvovaginal candidiasis, persistent, frequent, or poorly responsive to treatment
   Cervical dysplasia (moderate to severe), or cervical carcinoma in situ
   Constitutional symptoms, such as fever (38.5°C) or diarrhea lasting >1 month
   Oral hairy leukoplakia
   Herpes zoster (shingles) involving at least 2 distinct episodes or more than one dermatome
   Pelvic inflammatory disease, particularly if complicated by tubo-ovarian abscess
   Peripheral neuropathy

C. Clinical Category C (AIDS-Defining)
1. Usually a positive antibody test (2 ELISAs + 1 WB).
2. AIDS-defining diseases are (complete list):
   a. Opportunistic infections:
   Pneumocystis carinii pneumonia

Candidiasis of bronchi, trachea, or lungs
Esophageal candidiasis
Cytomegalovirus (CMV) disease (other than liver, spleen, or nodes)
CMV retinitis (with loss of vision)
Herpes simplex: chronic ulcers (>1 month), herpetic bronchitis, pneumonitis, esophagitis
Myocobacterium avium complex or *M. kansaii*, disseminated or extrapulmonary
Mycobacterium tuberculosis, any site
Mycobacterium sp. any site
Recurrent pneumonia
Toxoplasmosis of the brain
Salmonella septicemia
Coccidiodomycosis, disseminated or extrapulmonary
Cryptococcosis, extrapulmonary
Cryptosporidiosis, chronic intestinal (>1 month)
Histoplasmosis, disseminated or extrapulmonary
Isosporiasis, chronic intestinal (>1 month)
   b. Malignancies
   Kaposi's sarcoma
   Invasive cervical cancer
   Lymphomas: primary lymphoma of brain, Burkitt's lymphoma, immunoblastic lymphoma
   c. Neurologic disease:
   HIV-related encephalopathy
   Progressive multifocal leukoencephalopathy
   d. HIV wasting syndrome

D. T4 Lymphocyte Categories
1. Category 1: ≥500 cells/mm³
2. Category 2: 200–499 cells/mm³
3. Category 3 (AIDS-defining): <200 cells/mm³

CDC: Centers for Disease Control and Prevention; HIV: human immunodeficiency virus; AIDS: acquired immunodeficiency syndrome; ELISA: enzyme-linked immunosorbent assay; WB: Western blot.
Adapted from U.S. Centers for Disease Control and Prevention. 1993 revised classification system for HIV infection and expanded surveillance case definition for AIDS among adolescents and adults. *MMWR* 41 (No. RR-17):1, 1992.

Acute Retroviral Syndrome

Within 3 weeks after exposure, approximately 90% of all infected persons develop a transient mononucleosis-like symptoms complex. This complex is termed *acute (primary) HIV infection*, or *acute retroviral syndrome*. Although fever, pharyngitis, headache, malaise, and a diffuse skin rash may be the most frequently reported findings, other clinical manifestations may include arthralgias, lymphadenopathy, gastrointestinal symptoms, and photophobia. The cutaneous manifestations usually present as a diffuse roseola-like eruption occurring mainly on the trunk and limbs. This temporary and self-limiting illness usually subsides within 1 to 2 weeks, and the infected person returns to an asymptomatic status.[36] Acute retro-

viral syndrome probably represents an attempt by the immune system to control the infection in its early stages. With virus multiplication progressing unopposed, seroconversion usually occurs within 6 to 12 weeks after infection. This seroconversion time represents the time it takes for HIV-infected asymptomatic persons to yield positive results on antibody tests such as the ELISA and the Western blot. In a few discrete populations, seroconversion times of up to 3 years or more have been reported, but these are rare.[16] Once seroconversion occurs, most persons will continue to test HIV antibody–positive. The lack of detectable antibodies may occur during a time called the "seroconversion window," during which a virally infected individual will have a negative result on an antibody test. For this reason, it is imperative that tests with negative results be repeated at determined intervals to confirm the absence of HIV infection (Flowchart 17-1).

Asymptomatic HIV Disease

After the resolution of acute retroviral syndrome, infected persons regain an asymptomatic state and may remain relative healthy for a long time. The term *asymptomatic* refers to the absence of clinical manifestations that can be directly attributed to the HIV infection. In some cases, a few nonspecific manifestations, such as headache and lymphadenopathy, may be seen in this otherwise asymptomatic phase. The presence of lymphadenopathy resulting in lymph nodes with diameters greater than 1 cm and occurring at two or more extra-inguinal sites for more than 3 months is termed *persistent generalized lymphadenopathy*. Despite the absence of clinical findings in the majority of cases, such laboratory abnormalities as anemia, neutropenia, and thrombocytopenia may occur. Although these changes are not specific to HIV disease, they are often present in advanced stages of infection. The most HIV-specific change seen during this phase is a steady decline in T-helper cells, corresponding at times to annual losses of 40 to 80 cells/mm^3. In the absence of any symptomatology, infected persons can only be identified by a positive HIV-antibody test result. It must be noted that viral proliferation continues throughout this phase and that antibodies produced against HIV are unable to inactivate the virus.

Therefore, asymptomatic persons who test HIV antibody–positive must be considered virus-positive and capable of transmitting the virus through sexual activity or blood sharing. Despite the inaccuracy of the terminology, persons in this phase are commonly termed HIV-positive carriers, signifying persons who are asymptomatic but who carry the virus in their blood. The median duration of the asymptomatic phase, as limited by the diagnosis of HIV-related disease process, has been reported to be as long as 12 years, which is called the incubation time.

Early Symptomatic HIV Disease

Formerly termed AIDS-related complex, early symptomatic disease is usually precipitated by a progressive loss of T-helper cells, which results from long-standing infection. The depression of immune function facilitates the development of conditions that are relatively rare among immunocompetent persons. These include opportunistic infections caused by various microorganisms, such as viruses (eg, varicella-zoster virus), fungi (eg, *Candida albicans*), and protozoa (eg, toxoplasmosis) as well as a variety of conditions such as fever, night sweats, chronic diarrhea, fatigue, headache, hairy leukoplakia, idiopathic thrombocytopenic purpura, pelvic inflammatory disease, peripheral neuropathy, and cervical dysplasia. The severity of these manifestations range from minor to life-threatening.

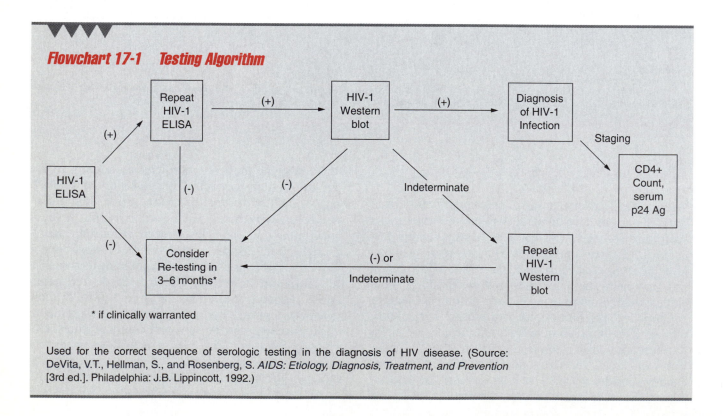

Flowchart 17-1 Testing Algorithm

* if clinically warranted

Used for the correct sequence of serologic testing in the diagnosis of HIV disease. (Source: DeVita, V.T., Hellman, S., and Rosenberg, S. *AIDS: Etiology, Diagnosis, Treatment, and Prevention* [3rd ed.]. Philadelphia: J.B. Lippincott, 1992.)

Late Symptomatic Disease (AIDS)

With the total T-helper cell count reaching below 200 cells/mm^3, the symptomatic HIV-infected person is now vulnerable to a series of more severe disease processes and opportunistic diseases which are *AIDS defining*. These include opportunistic infections caused by protozoa (eg, *Toxoplasma gondii, Cryptosporidium, Isospora belli*), viruses (eg, herpes simplex virus, varicella-zoster virus, cytomegalovirus), bacteria (*Mycobacterium tuberculosis, M. avium* complex, *Nocardia* species, *Listeria monocytogenes, Salmonella* species), and fungi (eg, *Pneumocystis carinii, Candida albicans, Cryptococcus neoformans, Coccidioides immitis*). Other AIDS-defining illnesses include malignancies (eg, Kaposi sarcoma, primary lymphoma of the brain, invasive cervical carcinoma), neurologic disorders (eg, HIV-related encephalopathy, progressive multifocal leukoencephalopathy), and HIV wasting syndrome. Although some of the opportunistic infections can be avoided or managed with adequate prophylactic or therapeutic intervention, their underlying cause is severe immune dysfunction. Even if controlling *Pneumocystis* pneumonia spares many lives, a T-helper cell count below 50 cells/mm^3 greatly increases the risk of death.[36]

CLINICAL CLASSIFICATION

In January, 1993, the Centers for Disease Control and Prevention adopted a new classification system for HIV infection based on three clinical categories (Categories A, B, and C) and three T-cell categories (Categories 1, 2, and 3) (Table 17-6).[32]

Clinical category A includes persons with acute retroviral syndrome, *persistent generalized lymphadenopathy*, and symptomatic disease. Category B is defined as symptomatic conditions in an HIV-infected adolescent/adult that are not included among conditions listed in Clinical category A or C. For classification purposes, Category B conditions take precedence over those in Category A. Clinical category C includes the clinical conditions that are AIDS-defining. For classification purposes, once a Category C condition has occurred, the person remains in that category.

T-cell category 1 is represented by persons who have a T-helper cell count greater than 500 cells/mm^3. T-cell category 2 reflects a count between 200 and 499 cells/mm^3. T-cell category 3 constitutes those persons with a T-helper cell count below 200/mm^3 (AIDS-defining).

REPRESENTATIVE OPPORTUNISTIC DISEASES IN HIV INFECTION

Pneumocystis carinii *Pneumonia*

A disease rarely seen before the emergence of the HIV epidemic in the 1980s, PCP is the most common and life-threatening disease in HIV infection. PCP is caused by a funguslike organism, formerly classified as a protozoan, which results in a pattern of interstitial pulmonary consolidation similar to that seen in fungal pneumonias.

TABLE 17-6 *1993 Revised Classification System for HIV Infection and Expanded AIDS Surveillance Case Definition for Adolescents and Adults**

	Clinical categories		
CD4$^+$ T-Cell Categories	*(A)* Asymptomatic, Acute (Primary) HIV or PGL[†]	*(B)* Symptomatic, not (A) or (C) Conditions[†]	*(C)* AIDS-Indicator Conditions[†]
(1) ≥500/mm^3	A1	B1	C1
(2) 200–499/mm^3	A2	B2	C2
(3) <200/mm^3 AIDS-indicator T-cell count	A3	B3	C3

HIV: human immunodeficiency virus; AIDS: acquired immunodeficiency syndrome; PDL: persistent generalized lymphadenopathy.

  * The shaded cells illustrate the expanded AIDS surveillance case definition. Persons with AIDS-indicator conditions (Category C) as well as those with CD4 + T-lymphocyte counts <200/mm³. (Categories A3 or B3) are reportable as AIDS cases in the United States and Territories, effective January 1, 1993.

  † See text for discussion.

  From the U.S. Centers for Disease Control and Prevention. 1993 revised classification system for HIV infection and expanded surveillance case definition for AIDS among adolescents and adults. *MMWR* 41 (No. RR-17):1, 1992.

Research supports the belief that infection with *P. carinii* occurs during early life, and the microorganism is kept in check by an intact immune system until immunosuppression occurs. In this sense, PCP as seen in HIV-infected adults represents a reactivation of a preexisting infection. HIV-infected persons at highest risk for developing PCP include those with a baseline T4 cell count of 200 or fewer cells/mm^3, those with thrush and fever, and those who have previously had an episode of PCP. Manifestations of PCP include a persistent, nonproductive cough; progressive shortness of breath; tachypnea; and fever.

Toxoplasmosis

The second most common neurologic disease in AIDS, toxoplasmosis is an infection caused by a protozoan, *Toxoplasma gondii*, whose definitive host is the domestic cat. Humans usually acquire the microorganism by ingesting its oocysts (ova) excreted in cat feces or cysts present in inadequately cooked meats. Infection with *T. gondii* is the most common cause of focal encephalitis in HIV-infected persons. Immunologic evidence for the presence of *T. gondii* can be found in a least 50% of the adult U.S. population, which again suggests that the disease seen in HIV-infected persons is a reactivation of previous infection. Clinical manifestations of toxoplasmosis include headache, fever, hemiparesis, seizures, ataxia, aphasia, altered mental states, confusion, dizziness, and coma.

Chronic Cryptosporidiosis

This disease is caused by a variety of species of the genus *Cryptosporidium*, a coccidian protozoan traditionally found in farm animals and recently in humans. Sources of infection include infected humans and contaminated food or water. Fecal–oral transmission is the presumed mode of transmission. In persons with AIDS, this infection causes a persistent, voluminous watery diarrhea, resulting in massive fluid loss and weight loss. Spread to other organs, such as the lung and gallbladder, has been reported.

Isosporiasis

An enteric infection with coccidian protozoan, *Isospora belli* produces symptoms similar to those of cryptosporidiosis. Although rare in the United States, it has been reported in increasing numbers among immigrants from the Caribbean and Africa.

Recurrent Pneumonias

Included in the AIDS-defining category in 1993 are bacterial or viral pneumonias occurring at the rate of two or more episodes per year.

Tuberculosis

Infection with *Mycobacterium tuberculosis* (TB) at pulmonary or extrapulmonary sites has also been included among Category C diseases. Mycobacterial tuberculosis may be the presenting illness in HIV-infected individuals, especially among injecting-drug users. TB has been an increasing concern due to its communicability and increased prevalence. In addition, some strains of *M. tuberculosis* have become resistant to traditionally efficient therapeutic agents. Clinical manifestations include persistent cough, fever, night sweats, fatigue, and weight loss (see pp. 575–576).

Mycobacterium avium *Complex*

Infection with *Mycobacterium avium*, or *M. kansasii*, results in a type of tuberculosis found in 20% to 40% of persons with advanced HIV disease. The hallmark of this infection is extensive extrapulmonary involvement. The gastrointestinal tract is usually the site of entry, and dissemination to the bone marrow, lymph nodes, and liver is common. Clinical manifestations include fever, anorexia, night sweats, malaise, weight loss, and weakness. Cough, headache, diarrhea, and abdominal pain are other symptoms of this infection.

Malignancies

Various forms of cancer have been included in Category C disease. *Kaposi sarcoma* (KS), an angiosarcoma, is significantly prevalent (26%) among HIV-infected gay and bisexual men, but for an unknown reason, it has remained rare in other HIV-infected groups. This epidemic form of KS has characteristics different from the other major KS type found in elderly men of Mediterranean ancestry. The epidemic form is more aggressive and has a higher metastatic potential.

Invasive carcinoma of the cervix in HIV-infected women has become an AIDS-defining condition in the 1993 classification. Other gynecologic manifestations, such as abnormal vaginal cytologic results, can also occur in early symptomatic HIV disease. By including these disorders of the female reproductive system, this classification emphasizes the risk to women of AIDS. The most common malignancy in HIV-infected children is a B-cell non-Hodgkins lymphoma.

Neurologic Disease

HIV-related encephalopathy, including AIDS dementia complex, and progressive multifocal leukoencephalopathy (PML) are central nervous system consequences of HIV infection that have different etiologies. PML and some encephalopathies result from opportunistic infections, with PML being caused by a papovavirus, whereas AIDS dementia complex most likely results from HIV infection of brain cells, such as the microglial cells and neurons. Additionally, peripheral neuropathies may result from opportunistic infections or from direct HIV effect. AIDS dementia complex is a subcortical degeneration similar to that of Huntington disease that results in cognitive, motor, and behavioral changes.

HIV Wasting Syndrome

First identified in sub-Saharan African countries and described under the term "slim disease," this syndrome was later associated with HIV infection. HIV wasting syndrome is defined as a weight loss of more than 10% of a person's body mass within 6 months and with the absence of any attempts at losing weight. The precise cause or pathogenesis of this syndrome is unknown, but it probably represents an entity similar to the anorexia/cachexia syndrome seen in cancer patients, which is refractory to weight-gaining measures. It is often associated with massive and persistent diarrhea.

TREATMENT APPROACHES

Because the major clinical manifestations of HIV infection result from opportunistic diseases secondary to immunosuppression, specific curative or palliative treatments are indicated for each individual disorder. For example, fungal infections, such as those caused by *Cryptococcus neoformans*, can be successfully controlled by antifungal agents, such as ketoconazole or amphotericin. Pneumocystis pneumonia is the presenting disease in approximately 60% of all cases of HIV infection and until recently accounted for 75% to 80% of all deaths. However, intravenous and aerosolized administration of pentamidine has produced remarkable results in the prophylaxis and treatment of PCP. Management of KS is still not greatly successful in controlling tumor growth or metastasis. Treatment approaches for KS include chemotherapy with vinblastine, immunotherapy with interferon, and palliative radiation therapy.

Total management of HIV infection will need to be approached on a three-prong basis: 1) prophylactic vaccination of uninfected individuals; 2) treatment of infected persons with antiretroviral agents; and 3) administration of immune modulators or biologic response modifiers. A new concept in vaccine development has been introduced with the AIDS epidemic, that of a therapeutic vaccine in addition to the traditional prophylactic vaccine approach. A prophylactic or preventive vaccine stimulates the immune system of a person still uninfected to produce antibodies that would protect the individual from infection on future exposures to the virus. For persons who are already HIV-infected, a therapeutic vaccine could be used. This type would stimulate the immune system to effectively destroy HIV already present in the host's body. Most vaccines being developed belong to this second group.

The development of an effective vaccine has been hindered by various obstacles. First, variability of the viral genome exists due to the high HIV mutation rate. Second, infected persons produce anti-HIV antibodies that are inefficient in neutralizing the virus. Third there is a lack of adequate animal models to use for testing. Until recently, only the chimpanzee could be used, but in the early 1990s, an HIV-sensitive ring-tailed macaque in Southeast Asia and a recently developed HIV-sensitive mouse have been discovered. Fourth, definitive evidence of vaccine safety has been unavailable, because genetically engineered vaccines must not contain any traces of infectious fragments of the virus. Fifth, demonstration of efficacy is unavailable, because success in animal models may not transpose to clinical success.

Treatment approaches for infected persons will vary according to the disease progression. In early stages, when the immune system is not so severely compromised and opportunistic diseases are absent, treatment could be restricted to antiretroviral agents to prevent HIV replication and disease progression. In later stages, the presence of severe immunosuppression and opportunistic diseases will require the combination of antiretrovirals and immune modulators. Immune modulators studied thus far have been proven unsuccessful. These include replacement methods, such as lymphocyte transfer and bone marrow transplant, and the use of biologic-response modifiers, such as interleukin-2 and other cytokines. However, the U.S. National Institutes of Health is sponsoring trials that combine antiretrovirals with alpha-interferon, and preliminary data appear encouraging.

At the time of the current writing, the most promising approach is the development of new antiretrovirals. Of all pharmaceuticals used in the treatment of AIDS-related illness, only four are antiretrovirals: zidovudine (AZT), didanosine (dideoxyinosine, or ddI), zalcitabine (dideoxycytidine, or ddC), and stavudine (d4T). All four drugs act by blocking reverse transcription and consequently arresting intracellular viral replications. Therefore, these agents are only active against intracellular virus particles and not free circulating viruses. Consequently, these drugs need to be taken for life and therefore must have manageable side effects. The oldest and perhaps the most successful is AZT, whose use has significantly reduced the signs and symptoms of infection and extended the life span of symptomatic persons.[25] One disadvantage of AZT is that persons who have received the drug for longer than 18 to 33 months develop a tolerance, and the drug ceases to be effective. This means that the sooner the treatment is instituted, the sooner it must be discontinued. The development of the other three similar drugs has now allowed for replacement once tolerance to AZT is reached.[2] The most significant side effect of AZT is bone marrow suppression, with approximately 50% of patients developing anemia and becoming transfusion dependent. Concurrent administration of erythropoietin significantly increases red blood cell production.[12]

The existence of different side effects among the antiretrovirals represents an enormous advantage in the development of multiple drug protocols, which is the essence of modern treatment approaches to various diseases. Among the side effects of ddI, the most significant are pancreatitis and a painful peripheral neuropathy. Those of ddC include fever, rash, oral ulcerations, and peripheral neuropathy. The side effects of d4T include peripheral neuropathy and, in advanced disease, pancreatitis. Despite some overlap, researchers are encouraged in initiating sequential or multidrug regimens. If this approach proves to be successful in preventing asymptomatic HIV-positive persons from developing dis-

ease processes, HIV disease may be managed as a chronic illness, much like controlled diabetes mellitus.

▼ Chapter Summary

▼ Immunodeficiency syndromes may be classified as primary and secondary. Primary immunodeficiency syndrome results from impairment of the cell-mediated or humoral response due to a genetic deficiency. Secondary immunodeficiency syndrome results from the impairment of a previously intact immune system. The major problem with all types of immunodeficiency syndromes is a marked susceptibility to infections, an increased predisposition to cancers, and an increased incidence of autoimmune disease.

▼ Developmental immunodeficiencies include B-cell immunodeficiency, which can affect any or all components of the humoral response, T-cell immunodeficiency, or both. Associated developmental deficiencies include deficiencies of the phagocytic cells or complement abnormalities.

▼ Secondary immunodeficiencies have multiple causes, including stress, aging, immunosuppressive drugs, systemic infection, and cancer. Major illness almost always affects immune competence.

▼ The worldwide epidemic of HIV disease and AIDS is the result of a specific retrovirus that attacks the T-helper population and renders the individual virtually immunodeficient. This virus is spread through sexual contact, through blood contamination, and from mother to offspring. The disease was first described among the male homosexual population, but the incidence is rapidly increasing among the heterosexual population, especially among injecting-drug users. Clinically, the individual is often asymptomatic for varying periods of time after the primary HIV infection, which often causes a flulike illness. Most of the symptomatic HIV disease is due to opportunistic infections. *Pneumocystis carinii* pneumonia is the most common cause of death. Many other opportunistic infections, malignancies, and neurologic manifestations are seen in the progression of this disease. Despite progress in treatment and vaccination research, the outcome of the disease is universally fatal.

CASE STUDY 17-1

Cindy Ham is a 28-year-old divorced female with an 8-year-old daughter. Since her divorce 5 years ago, she has dated casually but has not been sexually active. Ms. Ham reported that her husband was her only sex partner. She is now a graduate student who presented to the Student Health Service with a severe vaginal yeast infection which has been refractory to short-term treatment with antifungal vaginal treatment. Physician examination revealed mild lymphadenopathy of the cervical chains and pelvic examination was positive for a whitish discharge and vaginal and vulvar inflammation consistent with yeast infection. *Candida sp.* was confirmed by wet mount preparation and blood was drawn for HIV screening. During a follow-up visit, Ms. Ham was informed that her HIV antibody tests (2 ELISAs and a confirmatory Western Blot) were positive. When questioned about any other HIV-related manifestations, Ms. Ham was unsure about having experienced acute retroviral syndrome symptoms, but acknowledged an episode of "sore throat with swollen lymph nodes in her neck sometime in the past." Ms. Ham believes that she acquired the virus from her husband, who reportedly had had various sexual relationships during the times they were separated. Laboratory tests indicate a T4 cell count of 360/mm³. A repeat count showed 300 cells/mm³. Ms. Ham's daughter was tested for HIV and the results were negative. Treatment with zidovudine (AZT) was initiated and psychosocial intervention with counseling was begun.

1. *Why did Ms. Ham's persistent yeast infection alert the medical team to the possibility of HIV infection?*
2. *If Ms. Ham was infected by her husband several years ago, how did she remain healthy for such a long time?*
3. *If Ms. Ham was a blood donor and had been routinely tested for HIV antibody, how long after infection would she become positive?*
4. *What is the significance of acute retroviral syndrome (ARS)?*
5. *Considering the modes of transmission of HIV, why is Ms. Ham's disease probably caused by her ex-husband?*
6. *What is the significance of the T4 count?*
7. *What is the mode of action of antiretrovirals such as zidovudine (AZT)? What are its limitations and side effects?*
8. *Considering the prognosis of HIV infection, what psychosocial interventions would be recommended?*

See Appendix G for discussion.

▼ References

1. Abbas, A.K., Lichtman, A.H., and Pober, J.S. *Cellular and Molecular Immunology* (2nd ed.). Philadelphia: W.B. Saunders, 1994.
2. Abrams, D.I., Goldman, A.I., Launer, C., et al. A comparative trial of didanosine or zalcitabine after treatment with zidovudine in patients with human immunodeficiency virus infection. *N. Engl. J. Med.* 330: 657, 1994.
3. Ammann, A.J., and Hong, R. Disorders of the T-cell sys-

tem. In Stiehm, E.R. (ed.) *Immunologic Disorders in Infants and Children* (3rd ed.). Philadelphia: W.B. Saunders, 1989.

4. Alexander, N.J. Sexual transmission of human immunodeficiency virus: Virus entry into the male and female genital tract. *Fertil. Steril.* 54:1, 1990.
5. Alter, H.J. Epstein, J.S., Swenson, S.G., et al. Prevalence of human immunodeficiency virus type 1 p24 antigen in U.S. blood donors—an assessment of the efficacy of testing in donor screening.*N. Engl. J. Med.* 323: 1312, 1990.
6. Barrett, J.T. *Medical Immunology: Text and Review*. Philadelphia: F.A. Davis, 1991.
7. Benjamin, E., and Leskowitz, S. *Immunology: A Short Course* (2nd ed.). New York: Wiley-Liss, 1994.
8. Chamberland, M.E., Peterson, L.R., Munn, V.P. et al. Human immunodeficiency virus infection among health workers who donate blood. *Ann. Intern Med.* 121: 269, 1994.
9. Connor, R.I. and Ho, D.D. Etiology of AIDS: Biology of human retroviruses. In V.T. DeVita, S.Hellman, and S.A. Rosenberg (eds.), *AIDS: Etiology, Diagnosis, Treatment, and Prevention* (3rd ed.). Philadelphia: J.B. Lippincott, 1992.
10. Cotran, R.S., Kumar, V., and Robbins, S.L. *Robbins Pathologic Basis of Disease* (5th ed.). Philadelphia: W.B. Saunders, 1994.
11. De Cock, K.M., Adjordolo, G., Ekpini, E., et al. Epidemiology and transmission of HIV-2—why there is no HIV-2 pandemic. *JAMA* 270: 2083, 1993.
12. Fischl, M.A., Galpin, J.E., Levine, J.D., et al. Recombinant human erythropoietin for patients with AIDS treated with zidovudine. *N. Engl. J. Med.* 322: 1488, 1990.
13. Goedert, J.J., Kessler, C.M., Aledort, L.M., et al. A prospective study of human immunodeficiency virus type 1 infection and the development of AIDS in subjects with hemophilia. *N. Engl. J. Med.* 321: 1141, 1989.
14. Gougeon, M.L., and Montagnier, L. Apoptosis in AIDS. *Science* 260: 1269, 1993.
15. Hong, R., and Ammann, A.J. Disorders of the IgA system. In Stiehm, E.R. (ed.) *Immunologic Disorders in Infants and Children* (3rd ed.) Philadelphia: W.B. Saunders, 1989.
16. Imagawa, D.T., Lee, M.H., Wolinsky, S.M., et al. Human immunodeficiency virus type 1 infection in homosexual men who remain seronegative for prolonged periods. *N. Engl. J. Med.* 320: 1458, 1989.
17. Kanki, P.J. West African human retroviruses related to HTLV-III, *AIDS* 1: 141, 1987.
18. Kingsley, L.A., Rinaldo, C.R., Lyter, D.W., et al. Sexual transmission efficiency of hepatitis B virus and human immunodeficiency virus among homosexual men. *JAMA*, 264: 230, 1990.
19. Kissane, J.M. (ed.) *Anderson's Pathology* (9th ed.). St. Louis: C.V. Mosby, 1990.
20. Koga, Y., Sasaki, M., Nakamura, K., et al. Intracellular distribution of the envelope glycoprotein of human immunodeficiency virus and its role in the production of cytopathic effects in CD4+ and CD4—human cell lines. *Virology.* 64: 4661, 1990.
21. Marcus, R., Kay, K., and Mann, J. Transmission of human immunodeficiency virus in health care settings worldwide. *Bulletin of the World Health Organization*, No. 67, pp. 577–582, 1989.
22. Marlink, R., Kanki, P., Thior, I., et al. Reduced rate of disease development after HIV-2 infection as compared to HIV-1, *Science* 265: 1587, 1994.
23. Mofenson, L.M., and Wolinski, S.M. Current insights regarding vertical transmission. In P.A. Pizzo and C.M. Wilfert (eds.), *Pediatric AIDS: The Challenge of HIV Infection in Infants, Children, and Adolescents* (2nd ed.). Baltimore: William and Wilkins, 1994.
24. Mudge-Grout, C.L. *Immunologic Disorders*. St. Louis: Mosby Year Book, 1992.
25. Osmond, D., Charlebois, E., Lang, W., Shiboski, S., and Moss, A. Changes in AIDS survival time in two San Francisco cohorts of homosexual men, 1983 to 1993. *JAMA* 271: 1083, 1994.
26. Peterman, T.A., Cates, W., and Wasserbeit, J.N. Prevention of the sexual transmission of HIV. In V.T. DeVita, S. Hellman, and S.A. Rosenberg (eds.), *AIDS: Etiology, Diagnosis, Treatment, and Prevention* (3rd ed.). Philadelphia: J.B. Lippincott, 1992.
27. Saracco, A., Musicco, M., Nicolosi, A. et al. Man-to-woman sexual transmission of HIV: longitudinal study of 343 steady partners of infected men. *J. Acquir. Immun. Defic. Syndr.* 6:497, 1993.
28. Schoenbaum, E.E., Hartel, D., Selwyn, P.A., et al. Risk factors for human immunodeficiency virus infection in intravenous drug users. *N. Engl. J. Med.* 321: 874, 1989.
29. Sepulveda, J., Fineberg, H., and Mann, J. (eds.). *AIDS Prevention Through Education: A World View*. New York: Oxford University Press, 1992.
30. Stiehm, E.R., General considerations. In Stiehm, E.R., (ed.) *Immunologic Disorders in Infants and Children* (3rd ed.). Philadelphia: W.B. Saunders, 1989.
31. Stites, D.P., Terr, A.I., and Parslow, T.G. (eds.). *Basic and Clinical Immunology* (8th ed.). Norwalk: Appleton and Lange, 1994.
32. U.S. Centers for Disease Control and Prevention. 1993 revised classification system for HIV infection and expanded surveillance case definition for AIDS among adolescents and adults. *MMWR* 41 (No. RR-17): 1, 1992.
33. U.S. Centers for Disease Control and Prevention. Update: acquired immunodeficiency syndrome—United States, 1992. *MMWR* 42: 547, 1993.
34. U.S. Centers for Disease control and Preventions. Update: mortality attributable to HIV infection among persons aged 25–44 years—United States, 1991 and 1992. *MMWR* 42: 869, 1993.
35. U.S. Centers for Disease Control and Prevention. Heterosexually acquired AIDS—United States, 1993. *MMWR* 43: 155, 1994.
36. Volberding, P. A. Clinical spectrum of HIV disease. In V.T. DeVita, S. Hellman, and S.A. Rosenberg (eds.). *AIDS: Etiology, Diagnosis, Treatment, and Prevention* (3rd ed.). Philadelphia: J.B. Lippincott, 1992.
37. Whaley, K., and Lemercier, C. The complement system. In E. Sim (ed.). *The Natural Immune System: Humoral Factors*. New York: Oxford University Press, 1993.
38. Widman, F.K. *An Introduction to Clinical Immunology*. Philadelphia: F.A. Davis, 1989.

Hypersensitivity and Autoimmune Reactions

Barbara L. Bullock

▼ **CHAPTER OUTLINE**

▼ **LEARNING OBJECTIVES**

1 Describe the types of hypersensitivity reactions according to underlying pathophysiologic mechanisms and how they are manifested as disease.
2 Differentiate between anaphylaxis and atopy.
3 Identify the mechanisms of red blood cell destruction seen with cytotoxic hypersensitivity reactions.
4 Describe the results of hemolysis with respect to transfusion reactions, erythroblastosis fetalis, and warm and cold antibody diseases.
5 Describe the development of Goodpasture's syndrome as a result of cytotoxic hypersensitivity.
6 Explain the underlying pathophysiology of immune complex disease.
7 Describe the mechanisms that occur in serum sickness and the Arthus reaction.
8 Describe the relation of hypersensitivity reactions and autoimmune disorders.
9 Describe the pathophysiologic mechanisms by which delayed hypersensitivity can result.
10 Identify the histology of contact dermatitis.
11 Describe transplant graft rejection using the transplanted kidney as an example.
12 Differentiate conditions that are organ-specific and nonorgan-specific that probably result from the mechanisms of autoimmunity.
13 Name the main clinical finding that supports diagnosis of the autoimmune phenomena.
14 Describe systemic lupus erythematosus in terms of pathology and resultant clinical effects.
15 Describe the basis for classifying rheumatoid arthritis as an autoimmune disease.
16 Explain the pathophysiologic results of rheumatoid arthritis on the joints and on other body systems.
17 Describe the syndrome of scleroderma.

Tissue-damaging immune disorders have been classified in various ways to clarify their pathophysiologic basis. Four mechanisms of immunologically mediated disorders have been described according to the manner in which tissue injury occurs.[5] Some of these conditions also may be classified as autoimmune reactions.

The classic term for immunologic tissue-damaging reactions is *hypersensitivity reactions*, which refers to an exaggerated response of the immune system to an antigen. The antigen that elicits the response is called an *allergen*. Allergens produce different responses, depending on a person's genetic predisposition for an exaggerated response. In some cases, the antigen that produces the response is unknown.

▼ Classifications of Tissue Injury Caused by Hypersensitivity

The types of hypersensitivity reactions are described in this section according to the underlying pathophysiologic mechanisms and how they manifest themselves in different diseases (Table 18-1). Figure 18-1 shows a summary diagram of the four types of hypersensitivity reactions.

TYPE I: IMMEDIATE HYPERSENSITIVITY: ANAPHYLAXIS OR ATOPY

Anaphylaxis refers to an acute reaction usually associated with a wheal-and-flare type of skin reaction and vasodilation that may precipitate circulatory shock. Atopy, which results from the same mechanism, recurs chronically in responses that depend on the antigen, frequency of contact, route of contact, and sensitivity of the organ system to the antigen.

Atopy is the most common of the immediate hypersensitivity reactions. These reactions, commonly called *allergies*, occur in organs that are exposed to environmental antigens. Thus, the skin, respiratory tract, and gastrointestinal system are especially affected. Many types of antigens or allergens can initiate the hypersensitivity state in susceptible people. The most common of these are environmental allergens, such as pollens, dander, foods, insect bites, and certain household cleaning agents. Drug sensitivity reactions can effect the same response. Other disease states that are classified in this group include hay fever, urticaria (hives), asthma, and atopic eczema. Susceptibility to allergy is determined by genetic factors and by other factors that allow for exposure to the allergen.[22]

Pathophysiologically, the immune response is activated when antigen binds to IgE antibodies attached to the surface of mast cells. Mast cells are present in profusion in connective tissue, skin, and mucous membranes. The reaction proceeds when the IgE molecule specific for a particular antigen becomes cross-linked on the surface of the mast cell and triggers the release of intracellular granules. These granules contain large quantities of histamine and other chemotactic substances, especially mediators from arachidonic acid and platelet-activating factor (see pp. 300–301). Histamine is probably the most potent mediator. It constricts smooth muscle and causes microvascular peripheral vasodilation along with an increase in vascular permeability, resulting in local vascular congestion and

TABLE 18-1 *Classification of Hypersensitivity States*

Type	Cause	Responsible Cell or Antibody	Immune Mechanism	Examples of Disease States
I—Immediate hypersensitivity (anaphylaxis, atopy)	Foreign protein (antigen)	IgE	IgE attaches to surface of mast cell and specific antigen, triggers release of intracellular granules from mast cells	Hay fever, allergies, hives, anaphylactic shock
II—Cytotoxic hypersensitivity	Foreign protein (antigen)	IgG or IgM	Antibody reacts with antigen, activates complement, causes cytolysis or phagocytosis	Transfusion, hemolytic drug reactions, erythroblastosis fetalis, hemolytic anemia, vascular purpura, Goodpasture's syndrome
III—Immune complex disease	Foreign protein (antigen) Endogenous antigens	IgG, IgM, IgA	Antigen–antibody complexes precipitate in tissue, activate complement, cause inflammatory reaction	Rheumatoid arthritis, systemic lupus erythematosus, serum sickness, glomerulonephritis
IV—Delayed/cell-mediated	Foreign protein, cell, or tissue	T lymphocytes	Sensitized T cell reacts with specific antigen to induce inflammatory process by direct cell action or by activity of lymphokines	Contact dermatitis, transplant graft reaction, granulomatous diseases

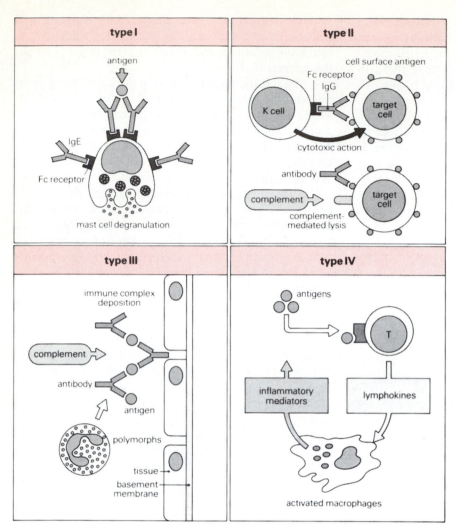

FIGURE 18-1 *Summary diagram of the four types of hypersensitivity reactions. Type I. Mast cells bind IgE by way of their F_c receptors. On encountering antigen, the IgE becomes cross-linked, inducing degranulation and release of mediators. Type II. Antibody is directed against antigens on a person's own cells (target cell). This may lead to cytotoxic action by K (killer) cells or complement-mediated lysis. Type III. Immune complexes are deposited in the tissue. Complement is activated, and polymorphs are attracted to the site of deposition, causing local damage. Type IV. Antigen-sensitized T cells release lymphokines after a secondary contact with the same antigen. Lymphokines induce inflammatory reactions and activate and attract macrophages, which release mediators. (From Roitt, I., Brostoff, J., and Male, D., Immunology [3rd ed.] Philadelphia: J.B. Lippincott, 1989.)*

edema.[15] The constriction of smooth muscle in the bronchioles accounts for the bronchiolar constriction often associated with the allergic reaction (Fig. 18-2).

Testing for a reaction to a particular allergen may be performed with a needle prick to the skin. Sensitivity to the allergen on the needle is exhibited by a rapid wheal-and-flare reaction. Systemic reactions are usually avoided because the amount of allergen used is very small.[22] A provocation test also may be performed in which the allergen is applied to the mucous membrane of the eyes or nose, or a skin patch test for contact dermatitis may be used. Elimination diet testing with foods suspected to be causative of the symptoms is frequently used, but the diagnosis of allergies is often erroneous due to the subjective nature of the procedure.[22]

Anaphylaxis and Anaphylactic Shock

Anaphylaxis is defined as an antigen-specific allergic hypersensitivity reaction of the body to a foreign protein or a drug. It is mediated primarily by IgE interaction with mast cells. Anaphylactic shock occurs when the reaction becomes systemic and thus a life-threatening event. The reaction results in a subject who has been previously sensitized to the antigen. The antigen–antibody reaction occurs on the mast cells in the connective tissue and around small blood vessels. It causes the mast cells to release histamine and other mediators, which results in contraction of smooth muscle and increased vascular permeability. This causes bronchospasm and the loss of intravascular fluid into the tissue spaces in some cases. Edema follows and is particularly noticeable around the eyes. This edema, called *angioneurotic edema* or *angioedema*, may appear in the skin or mucous membranes. Laryngeal edema associated with bronchospasm often causes acute dyspnea and air hunger.[18]

Hives, or urticaria, may appear on any skin surface as cutaneous localized swellings. These are sudden, generalized eruptions of papules or wheals, and intense itching is exhibited.

Fluid shift from increased vascular permeability may be significant enough to result in decreased blood pressure and shock. Signs and symptoms of anaphylactic shock include acute anxiety, pruritus, urticaria, angioedema,

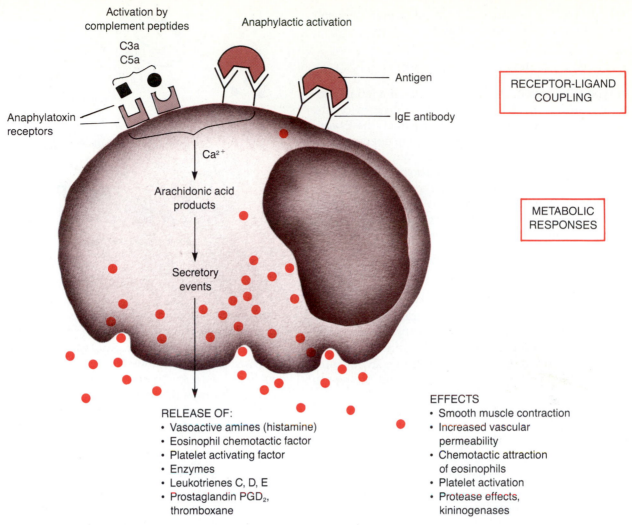

FIGURE 18-2 *Type I hypersensitivity. Activation of the mast cell and the potent inflammatory mediators released or synthesized by the cell. (Source: Rubin, E., and Farber, J.L. Pathology [2nd ed.]. Philadelphia: J.B. Lippincott, 1994.)*

dyspnea, hypoxia, and hypotension.[18] Some people experience vascular collapse without signs of respiratory distress.

Bronchial Asthma

Atopic allergy may cause bronchial asthma, frequently induced by the inhalation of environmental antigens (see pp. 592–595). The mechanism for bronchial asthma, like atopy, may result from interaction of antigen with specific IgE antibodies. The inflammation produces mucosal edema, increased secretion of mucus, and bronchospasm, all of which cause narrowing of the airways and increased airway resistance. The early signs and symptoms of asthma are dyspnea and wheezing. Repeated attacks result in hypertrophy of the smooth muscle, which can exaggerate bronchoconstriction and increase the severity of each subsequent attack. Bacterial or viral infections may precipitate asthmatic attacks.

Atopic Eczema

Atopic eczema is an acute or chronic, noncontagious inflammatory condition that may occur after contact with irritants to which a person has a specific sensitivity.In some cases, it results from a cell-mediated reaction (as described on pages 356–357 with the type IV reactions), and in others, it is mediated by IgE, with liberation of chemotactic mediators into dermal areas. It often is associated with respiratory allergy.[19]

Atopic eczema causes urticaria and angioedema. Urticaria involves the superficial capillaries, and angioedema involves the capillaries of the deeper skin layers. The wheals of urticaria have well-defined margins, erythema, and vesicles filled with clear fluid. Pruritus frequently is severe. Angioedema causes nonpitting swelling of localized areas of the skin.[6] This skin reaction to an allergen is often associated with respiratory hypersensitivity, especially hay fever or other type of allergy. Drug reactions may result in the same dermatologic manifestations, probably caused by the same mechanisms.

TYPE II: CYTOTOXIC HYPERSENSITIVITY

In type II hypersensitivity response, a circulating antibody, usually an IgG, reacts with an antigen on the surface of a cell. Because people normally have antibodies to antigen of the ABO blood group not present on their own membranes, the antigen may be a normal component of the membrane.[12] It also may be a foreign antigen, such as a pharmacologic agent, that adheres to the surface of the host's own cells. Antibodies produced to the host's own red blood cells may produce an autoimmune hemolytic anemia. The cell is destroyed by the reaction on its surface either by phagocytosis or lysis. The effect on the host depends on the number and types of cells destroyed.

Examples of this hypersensitivity response include hemolytic reactions, such as autoimmune hemolytic anemia, erythroblastosis fetalis, and specific target cell destruction, as exemplified by Goodpasture's syndrome. These are briefly discussed following a review of some of the general pathophysiologic features of the type II response.

The pathophysiology of type II hypersensitivity usually involves the activation of complement and resultant destruction of red blood cells or specific target cells. Opsonic coating of target cells with IgG antibody sets the stage for effector cells to destroy the target cells.[12] Specific IgG or IgM activation of complement results from complement activation through C89 (Fig. 18-3). Red blood cell destruction may be triggered by IgG opsonization and the attachment of lymphocytes or macrophages to the cell surface.[6]

Hemolytic Reactions

Examples of reactions that destroy red blood cells are transfusion reactions, erythroblastosis fetalis, autoimmune hemolytic anemia, and drug-induced hemolysis. The reaction of host antibody with the surface antigens on the red blood cells of an incompatible donor results in hemolysis. The surface antigens that make up the ABO and Rh systems are common sources of incompatibility (see pp. 376–377).

Transfusion reactions may result in hemolysis of donor red blood cells with the liberation of large quantities of hemoglobin into the plasma. Some of the hemoglobin is broken down into unconjugated bilirubin. If the amount of free hemoglobin is greater than 100 mg/dL of plasma, the excess diffuses into the tissue or through the renal glomeruli into the renal tubules. Precipitation of large amounts of hemoglobin in the renal tubular fluid forms sharp needles in the acid urine, which can cause tubular damage and obstruction.[8] Precipitation in the tubules of the shells of red blood cells also frequently

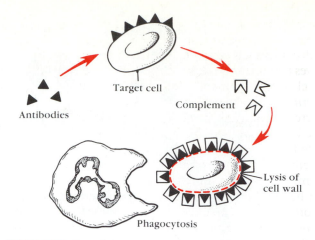

FIGURE 18-3 *Type II hypersensitivity response. The target cell is covered with antibody that activates complement and sets the stage for phagocytosis.*

contributes to tubular damage and renal failure. Transfusion reactions may also increase the risk of renal failure by causing circulatory shock, renal vasoconstriction, and decreased renal blood flow. The antigenic nature of mismatched blood transfusions depends on the type and Rh factor of the donor blood. For example, people with type A blood possess anti-B antibodies. Therefore, the incompatible blood is coated with antibodies, usually of the IgM class. This causes agglutination of the donor cells, and lysis rapidly follows.[4] Signs and symptoms of a transfusion reaction include chills, fever, low back pain, hypotension, tachycardia, anxiety, hyperkalemia, nausea and vomiting, red- or port wine–colored urine, and, occasionally, urticaria. These may progress to shock and irreversible renal failure.

Erythroblastosis fetalis may result if a mother without Rh antigens carries a child with Rh antigens, or if mother and fetus have ABO incompatibility. A mother who lacks Rh antigens on her red blood cells (Rh-negative) can be sensitized to the Rh antigen carried on the cells of the fetus by mixing her red blood cells with fetal red blood cells. If the woman again becomes pregnant with a fetus that has Rh antigens, her anti-Rh antibodies may cross the placenta and enter the fetal circulation. The result is destruction of fetal red blood cells through a hemolytic reaction. More commonly, *ABO blood group incompatibility* causes the free passage of antibodies from the mother through the placenta to the fetus.[3,6] Blood types interact in different ways, but the result is attachment and hemolysis of fetal red blood cells by maternal antibodies.[3] Hemolysis of fetal red blood cells results in severe *anemia*, which may lead to heart failure. Also, the release of high concentrations of bilirubin from hemoglobin may result in brain damage, called *kernicterus*, as unconjugated bilirubin passes across the still permeable blood–brain barrier, causing edematous swelling of brain parenchyma. The mechanism by which unconjugated bilirubin crosses the blood–brain barrier is not clearly understood. The barrier apparently is more permeable in neonates and premature infants.[6] Hyperbilirubinemia is common in an affected infant who survives for more than several days. This increased bilirubin level usually is manifested as jaundice and is termed *icterus gravis*. The red blood cell activity in bone marrow increases, and extramedullary hematopoiesis begins in the liver, spleen, and perhaps other organs to compensate for lost red blood cells. The risk of erythroblastosis fetalis in subsequent pregnancies can be reduced by administering anti-Rh antibodies to the mother within 72 hours after the birth of the first Rh-positive infant. More difficult to predict is ABO erythroblastosis, but the condition can be monitored if both parents are aware of their blood incompatibility.

Two types of hemolytic anemias with a probable autoimmune basis are *warm antibody disease* and *cold antibody disease*. Warm antibody disease is called *autoimmune hemolytic anemia* and usually is due to IgG antibody that attacks the host's own red blood cells. The disease can be life-threatening, depending on the amount of hemolysis. The red blood cells develop a limited life span, and the resulting anemia can be severe. Autoimmune hemolytic disease may develop for no known reason, or it may be associated with other autoimmune diseases, cancer, or systemic infection.[6] Cold antibody disease results when an autoantibody, usually IgM, binds to erythrocytes at temperatures below 31°C. These temperatures may be reached in the fingers or toes during very cold weather. The red blood cells thus coated with cold antibodies reenter the general circulation, activate complement, and hemolyze the red blood cells. These hemolytic attacks occur only after exposure to cold and tend to be self-limiting. The major diagnostic criterion for hemolytic anemia is the Coombs' antiglobulin test. In this test, agglutination of red blood cells occurs when immunoglobulins are attached to the red blood cell membranes.[6]

Drug-induced hemolysis may result from drug–antibody complexes that bind passively to red blood cells and initiate the complement reaction. Other drugs may act as haptens and bind to a red blood cell carrier. Antibody is formed and induces hemolysis of the red blood cells. Some drugs produce changes in the surface antigens of the red blood cells, resulting in antibody production against the host's own erythrocytes. Most drug-induced hemolytic reactions stop once use of the drug is discontinued. Table 18-2 indicates some of the drugs that have been implicated in producing immune hemolytic anemias.

Specific Target Cell Destruction

The best illustration of specific target cell hypersensitivity reaction is *Goodpasture's syndrome*, which is a rapidly occurring condition characterized by the development of *antiglomerular basement membrane antibodies*.

TABLE 18-2 *Classification of Immune Hemolytic Anemias*

AUTOIMMUNE HEMOLYTIC ANEMIAS
A. Warm-antibody types
1. Idiopathic warm autoimmune hemolytic anemia
2. Secondary warm autoimmune hemolytic anemias
a. Systemic lupus erythematosus and other autoimmune disorders
b. Chronic lymphocytic leukemia, lymphomas, etc.
c. Hepatitis and other viral infections
B. Cold-antibody types
1. Idiopathic cold agglutinin syndrome
2. Secondary cold agglutinin syndrome
a. *Mycoplasma pneumoniae* infection, infectious mononucleosis and other viral infections
b. Chronic lymphocytic leukemia, lymphomas, etc.
3. Paroxysmal cold hemoglobinuria
a. Idiopathic
b. Syphilis, viral infections

DRUG-INDUCED IMMUNE HEMOLYTIC ANEMIAS
1. Drug absorption mechanism
2. Membrane modification mechanism
3. Immune complex mechanism

PARTIAL LIST OF DRUGS:

Aminosalicylic acid (PAS)	Methyldopa
Antihistamines	Penicillin
Cephalothin	Pyramidon
Chlorinated hydrocarbons	Quinidine
Chlorpromazine	Quinine
Dipyrone	Rifampin
Insulin	Stibophen
Isoniazid	Sulfonamides
Levodopa	Sulfonylureas
Mefenamic acid	Tetracyclines
Melphalan	

ALLOANTIBODY-INDUCED IMMUNE HEMOLYTIC ANEMIAS
A. Hemolytic transfusion reactions
B. Hemolytic disease of the newborn
C. Allograft-associated anemias

Stites, D. P., Terr, A. J., Parslow, T. G. *Basic and Clinical Immunology* (8th ed.). Norwalk, Conn.: Appleton-Lange, 1994.

These antibodies are directed at the glomerular basement membrane of the kidneys as well as the basement membrane of the pulmonary alveoli. The initiator is unknown, but the condition is associated with influenza and the inhalation of hydrocarbons.[7] It may rapidly progress to death because of the destruction of the basement membranes, which frequently leads to hemoptysis or uremia. Improvement in prognosis has been reported with use of plasmapheresis to remove antiglomerular basement membrane antibodies along with high-dose corticosteroids and cytotoxic therapy.[7] Both pulmonary and glomerular improvement have been seen.

Other examples of specific target cell destruction

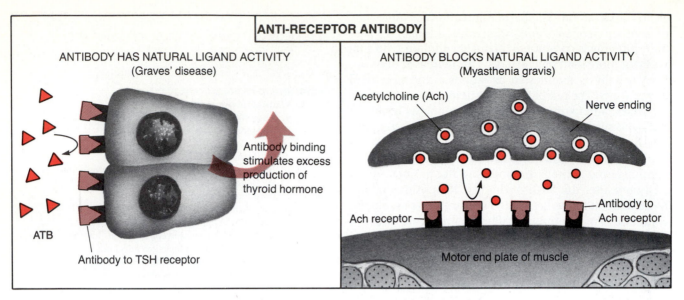

FIGURE 18-4   *Type II hypersensitivity. Noncytotoxic antireceptor antibodies in Graves' disease and myasthenia gravis. The binding of the antibody to the TSH receptor in Graves' disease results in hyperthyroidism, whereas the inhibition of synaptic transmission in myasthenia gravis leads to profound muscle weakness. (Source: Rubin, E., and Farber, J.L. Pathology [2nd ed.]. Philadelphia: J.B. Lippincott, 1994.)*

include the autoimmune diseases of myasthenia gravis and Graves' disease. These conditions are discussed further on pages 1087 and 714, respectively. Figure 18-4 illustrates how the anti-receptor antibodies function to cause the effects of these conditions.

Type III: Immune Complex Disease

Immune complex disease results in the formation of antigen–antibody complexes that activate a variety of serum factors, especially complement.[6] This results in precipitation of complexes in vulnerable areas, leading to inflammation as a consequence of complement activation. The end result is an intravascular, synovial, endocardial, and other membrane inflammatory process that affects the vulnerable organs (Fig. 18-5). Each person apparently has some unique vulnerability in target organs.

Antigen–antibody complexes may be present in the plasma without causing disease manifestations. If the complexes are not removed by the mononuclear phagocyte system, they may lodge in the tissue, where they initiate an inflammatory reaction that leads to tissue destruction. The complexes frequently are small, and their size seems to determine whether they will be cleared and whether they can lodge at a place where significant damage can occur. The antigen–antibody complexes that remain in solution cause reactions when they circulate through the body and lodge in the tissue and small vessels.[21] Increased vascular permeability allows the complexes to be deposited in the extravascular spaces. Deposition also appears to be greater at points of high pressure, high flow, and turbulence.[9] Once precipitated, the immune complexes initiate the inflammatory process by activating complement and releasing vasoactive substances from the defense cells (Flowchart 18-1). Complement activation can be initiated through either the classic or the alternative pathway, depending on which immunoglobulin class is involved.[9] Box 18-1 summarizes the pathogenesis of inflammatory lesions in type III reactions.

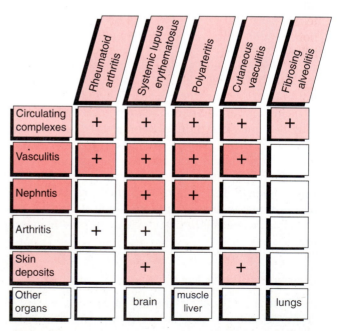

	Rheumatoid arthritis	Systemic lupus erythematosus	Polyarteritis	Cutaneous vasculitis	Fibrosing alveolitis
Circulating complexes	+	+	+	+	+
Vasculitis	+	+	+	+	
Nephritis		+	+		
Arthritis	+	+			
Skin deposits		+		+	
Other organs		brain	muscle liver		lungs

FIGURE 18-5   *Immune complex deposits and their clinical effect.*

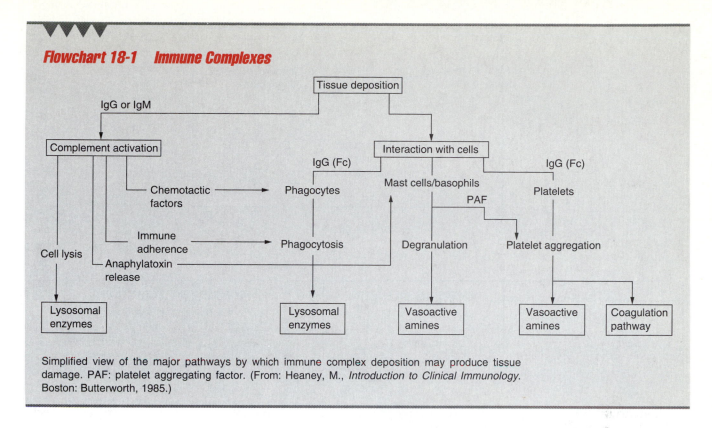

Flowchart 18-1 Immune Complexes

Simplified view of the major pathways by which immune complex deposition may produce tissue damage. PAF: platelet aggregating factor. (From: Heaney, M., *Introduction to Clinical Immunology*. Boston: Butterworth, 1985.)

Serum Sickness

Serum sickness results from injection of large doses of foreign material and can cause various types of arthritis, glomerulonephritis, and vasculitis. Antigen–antibody complexes form in the bloodstream and precipitate into vulnerable areas. First reported after passive immunization with horse serum (equine tetanus antitoxin), which contains at least 30 antigens, serum sickness can cause an acute reaction or a chronic condition. Vaccines, protein-based drugs, and beestings may cause this condition. It may occur rarely as an allergic reaction to penicillin, sulfonamides, and cephalosporins.[21]

BOX 18-1 ▼ Pathogenesis of Type III Reactions

1. Antigen (endogenous or exogenous)–antibody complexes form
2. Localization of complexes in vessels, often in joint areas
3. Activation of complement inflammatory pathway
4. Chemotaxis for cells and exudate
5. Inflammation with swelling, heat, and pain in joints and tissues
6. Infiltration of area with polymorphonuclear leukocytes and macrophages
7. Tissue damage and destruction
8. Continuing inflammation and fibrin deposition
9. Scarring and collagen deposition; may cause joint or tissue deformity

If the antigen concentration is greater than the antibody concentrations, the resulting antigen-antibody complexes tend to be small and remain in solution for as long as 15 days after initial injection. Immune complexes are deposited throughout the vasculature of the body; complement is activated, and neutrophils and macrophages move into the area in response to chemotactic signals. Phagocytosis of the immune complexes begins with the release of lysosomal enzymes into the area, which causes acute vasculitis with destruction of the elastic lamina of the arteries. Once phagocytosis of the immune complexes is complete, the inflammatory process decreases, leaving some scarring of the blood vessel walls.[6]

Renal glomerular deposits of complexes occur even when the immune complex concentrations are not high, probably because of the efficient filtering action of the kidneys. The complexes form characteristic deposits in the glomerular walls that activate complement and lead to destruction of glomerular tissue. Increased permeability of the glomerular basement membrane often produces hematuria and proteinuria. Figure 18-6 shows the process of vasculitis and glomerulonephritis that can result.

Arthus Reaction

Another type III disorder, the Arthus reaction, involves inflammation and cellular death at the site of injection of antigen into a previously sensitized person. Pathologically, it causes acute, localized edema with tissue inflammation and little vasculitis.[15] Antibody precipita-

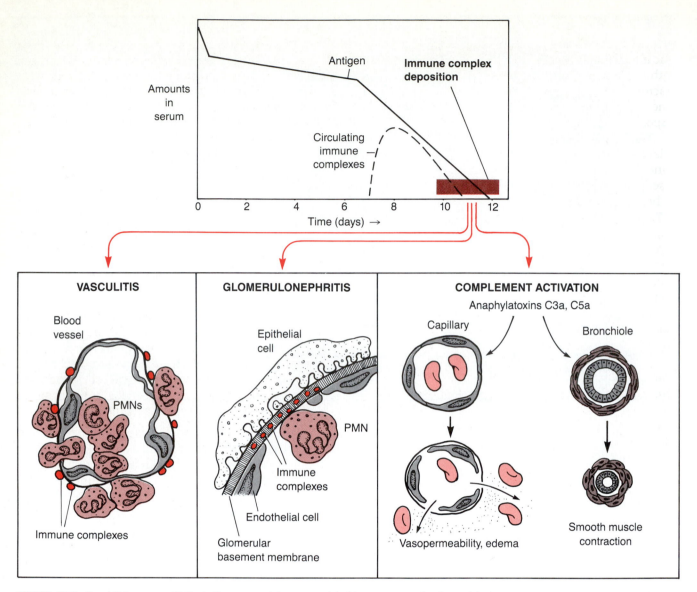

FIGURE 18-6 *Type III hypersensitivity. In the serum sickness model of immune complex tissue injury, antibody is produced against a circulating antigen, and immune complexes form in the blood. These complexes deposit in tissues such as blood vessels and glomeruli and, augmented by complement activation, induce tissue injury or dysfunctional responses. (Source: Rubin, E., and Farber, J.L.* Pathology *[2nd ed.]. Philadelphia: J.B. Lippincott, 1994.)*

tion and complement activation cause all of the effects of inflammation, with activation of the complement fragments through C89, which destroys antigen and surrounding tissue.

Hypersensitive pneumonitis may be an Arthus reaction from the inhalation of antigenic materials from molds, plants, or animals.[9] This reaction is primarily due to IgG response, but some relation with the type IV hypersensitivity reaction has been described.[6,9,20]

Other Type III Conditions

Many of the common autoimmune conditions are classified as immune complex disorders. The mechanism for inflammation and damage is the precipitation of immune complexes into vulnerable areas. Immune complex disorders are dynamic, everchanging processes that are manifested in the tissues in which they become lodged. Systemic lupus erythematosus (SLE), rheumatoid arthritis, and some types of glomerulonephritis are examples. SLE and rheumatoid arthritis are discussed more fully on pages 359–362. Glomerulonephritis is described in detail on pages 636–642.

TYPE IV: CELL-MEDIATED HYPERSENSITIVITY

Type IV response is the result of specifically sensitized T lymphocytes without the participation of antibodies. Activation causes a delayed-type response.

Delayed Hypersensitivity

Delayed hypersensitivity responses are due to the specific interaction of T cells with antigen. The T cells react with the antigen and release lymphokines that draw macrophages into the area. Macrophages release monokines. These substances enhance the inflammatory response that destroys the foreign material (Fig. 18-7).

The tuberculin response is the best example of the delayed hypersensitivity response and is used to determine whether a person has been sensitized to the disease. Reddening and induration of the site begin within 12 hours of injection of tuberculin and reach a peak in 24 to 72 hours.[2] It is mainly a dermal reaction. The positive response occurs because of the persistent presence of mycobacterium organisms that the macrophages are unable to destroy. Delayed hypersensitivity responses usually are caused by infectious agents, such as mycobacteria, protozoa, and fungi. These organisms present a chronic antigenic stimulus, and the T lymphocytes and macrophages react, sometimes conferring protective immunity against later exposure.

Exposure to the chemicals in poison ivy is another example of the delayed hypersensitivity response. Even though the chemicals are not proteins, they bind to cell membrane proteins and are recognized by antigen-specific lymphocytes.[15] The effect reaches greatest intensity 24 to 48 hours after exposure.

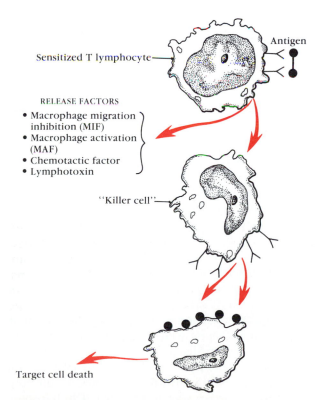

FIGURE 18-7 *Type IV cell-mediated hypersensitivity. The T lymphocyte contacts the foreign material, and through direct intervention or secretion of substances toxic to the foreign material, it destroys the foreign protein.*

Granulomatous Hypersensitivity Response

Granulomatous hypersensitivity response is the most important form of delayed hypersensitivity because it results in the formation of granulomas in different areas of the body. The epithelioid cell is the characteristic morphologic feature and appears as a large, flattened cell that may be derived from activated macrophages. Sometimes the formation of multinucleate giant cells occurs.[2] The granuloma may be surrounded by fibrosis, and necrotic material may be contained within it.

Precise classification of diseases that manifest delayed hypersensitivity with or without granuloma formation is difficult. A wide variety of chronic diseases are included, most of which are related to infectious agents. Table 18-3 describes the common chronic diseases together with etiology, pathology, and clinical manifestations.

Contact Dermatitis

A common allergic skin reaction, contact dermatitis seems to be a T-cell response with a delayed reaction. It occurs on contact with certain common household chemicals, cosmetics, and plant toxins. These may alter the normal skin protein so that it becomes antigenic, or they may act as haptens that combine with proteins in the skin.[2]

The area of contact becomes red and indurated, and vesicles begin to appear. This type of dermatitis is mainly confined to the epidermis. Lymphocytes and macrophages infiltrate the area and react against the epidermal cells. Sterile, protein-rich fluid fills the blebs. If the blebs are opened, the antigen may be spread to a new area. The affected cells are destroyed, slough off, and are replaced by the regeneration of new cells.

CASE STUDY 18-1

Julie Edwards, a 37-year-old woman, was working in her yard when she received a sting on the right wrist from a yellow-jacket wasp. Several minutes later she complained of a itching sensation and cramping abdominal pain. She then became acutely short of breath with wheezing. A patchy erythema radiating from the area of the sting was noted along with swollen eyelids and lips. A neighbor took her to an emergency center where she became very faint. Vital signs were: blood pressure, 60/34; pulse, 156; respirations, 40. Epinephrine 1/1000 was immediately administered intravenously along with 100 mg of hydrocortisone. Within minutes, an improvement in the respiratory rate was noted and blood pressure increased to 100/70 with a pulse rate of 112.

1. *What type of hypersensitivity response is described above?*
2. *Explain the pathophysiologic mechanism involved in producing the clinical picture.*
3. *What is the rationale for the treatment given?*
4. *How could this reaction be prevented? What should Mrs. Edwards be taught to prevent this occurrence?*

See Appendix G for discussion.

TABLE 18-3 *Examples of Granulomatous Inflammations*

Disease	Cause	Tissue Reaction
BACTERIAL		
Tuberculosis	*Mycobacterium tuberculosis*	*Noncaseating tubercle* (*granuloma prototype*): a focus of epithelioid cells, rimmed by fibroblasts, lymphocytes, histiocytes, occasional Langhans' giant cell; *caseating tubercle*: central amorphous granular debris, loss of all cellular detail; acid-fast bacilli
Leprosy	*Mycobacterium leprae*	Acid-fast bacilli in macrophages; granulomas and epithelioid types
Syphilis	*Treponema pallidum*	*Gumma*: Microscopic to grossly visible lesion, enclosing wall of histiocytes; plasma cell infiltrate; center cells are necrotic without loss of cellular outline
Cat-scratch disease	*Gram-negative bacillus*	Rounded or stellate granuloma containing central granular debris and recognizable neutrophils; giant cells uncommon
PARASITIC		
Schistosomiasis	*Schistosoma mansoni, S. haematobium, S. japonicum*	Egg emboli; eosinophils
FUNGAL	*Cryptococcus neoformans*	Organism is yeast-like, sometimes budding; 5 to 10 μm; large, clear capsule
	Coccidioides immitis	Organism appears as spherical (30–80 μm) cyst containing endospores of 3 to 5 μm each
INORGANIC METALS AND DUST		
Silicosis, berylliosis		Lung involvement; fibrosis
UNKNOWN		
Sarcoidosis		*Noncaseating granuloma*: giant cells (Langhans' and foreign-body types); asteroids in giant cells; occasional Schaumann's body (concentric calcific concretion); no organisms

From Cotran, R., Kumar, V., and Robbins, S. L. *Robbins Pathologic Basis of Disease* (5th ed.). Philadelphia: W.B. Saunders, 1994.

TRANSPLANT OR GRAFT REJECTION

Rejection of tissue and transplanted organs involves several of the hypersensitivity responses. Targeting of transplanted organs depends on whether the *histocompatibility antigens* are similar enough between the donor and the recipient to prevent activation of the rejection phenomenon. The surface antigens on cells distinguish them from cells of other people and from the cells of other organs. These are the self-proteins to which a person develops tolerance. Identical twins have identical histocompatibility antigens, so that organs or tissue can be transplanted from one to the other with ease. Donor and recipient tissues are matched; the closer the match, the more likely the transplantation will be successful.[10]

Rejection is a complex reaction that involves both cell-mediated and humoral responses. It is defined as the process by which the immune system of the host recognizes, develops sensitivity to, and attempts to eliminate the antigenic differences of the donor organ.[10] Cytolytic T lymphocytes may either attack grafted tissue directly or secrete chemotactic lymphokines that enhance the activity of macrophages in tissue destruction. Humoral responses may be due to circulating antibodies that were formed during previous exposure to the antigen. After transplantation, the lymphocytes become sensitized as they pass through the donor site. When antibody is involved, it appears to target the vasculature of the graft, especially the graft site.[6, 10]

The rejection phenomenon of a transplanted kidney has been studied extensively. It appears to involve both humoral and cell-mediated hypersensitivity. The sensitized lymphocytes interact with the graft proteins and release mediators that attract macrophages and polymorphonuclear leukocytes to the area. The lysosomal enzymes released by these cells cause endothelial destruction, especially of the blood vessels, that leads to decreased glomerular filtration rate and renal failure.

The T lymphocytes are directly cytotoxic to the donor cells. They also may activate B lymphocytes to form antibodies and immune complexes that activate complement and further damage the vascular endothelium.

The process may be acute or chronic. The more adequately matched the donor and recipient, the less acute the reaction. Also, recipients are given immunosuppressive drugs that delay the rejection. Chronic changes usually affect the vasculature and lead to organ ischemia and eventual failure.

Graft rejection is common, and most cadaver grafts are rejected within 5 years. Long-term survival of grafts has not been achieved except in twin or closely matched human leukocyte antigen transplants. Adequate immunosuppression has been helpful in prolonging graft survival.[6, 10]

▼ *Autoimmunity*

The study of autoimmunity has been spurred by the discovery of antibodies directed toward specific cells in certain people. Many people demonstrate serum autoantibodies but show no evidence of disease. This is especially true in the elderly, and much research related to the loss of self-tolerance with aging is being conducted. Even people who have suffered myocardial infarction may exhibit myocardial autoantibodies but experience no further myocardial disruption. In diabetes mellitus, autoantibodies to the islet cells of the pancreas often are demonstrated, which leads to the theory that some forms of diabetes mellitus may be a result of an autoimmune attack on these cells.[14]

A wide spectrum of autoimmune responses has been divided clinically into non-organ-specific and organ-specific diseases.[14] Figure 18-8 indicates the spectrum of common organ-specific and non-organ-specific diseases. Many of these are described in other sections of the book. The relations of destructive autoimmune reactions are clearly demonstrated in myasthenia gravis, Graves' disease, rheumatoid arthritis, SLE, and others (Table 18-4). SLE, rheumatoid arthritis, and scleroderma are considered in further detail in the section below and in Chapter 45. The possibility of autoimmunity as a causative factor has been speculated in conditions as diverse as multiple sclerosis, hepatitis, and cancer. Autoantibodies, however, have not been consistently demonstrated in cancer. The appearance of *autoantibodies* and the symptomatology of a disease lend support for an autoimmune classification.

Observations of autoimmune phenomena have resulted in the following generalizations:

1. Specific autoimmune phenomena occur with greater frequency in certain families, which suggests a genetic disorder related to a fundamental disorder of thymic immune control.

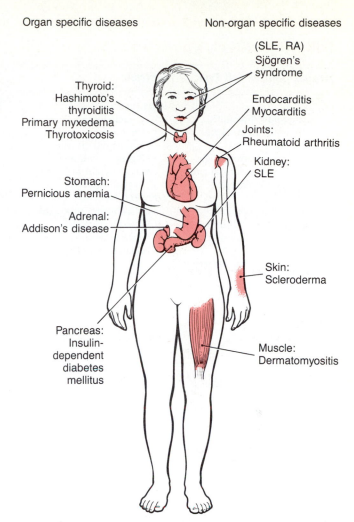

FIGURE 18-8 *Autoimmune diseases have been classified as organ specific and non-organ-specific. Organ-specific diseases only affect certain organs. Non-organ-specific diseases can target multiple organs or have system wide effects.*

2. Autoimmune diseases are more common in females than in males, which indicates a relation between the sex hormones and the immune response.
3. Elderly people have a greater prevalence of autoantibodies, which may be the result of genetic errors because of the immune system's wearing out through the aging process.
4. Viruses may play a role in the occurrence of autoimmunity because of their ability to disrupt the immune system at any one of several levels.
5. Sequestered tissue (tissue and protein not normally in contact with T and B cells) may be exposed to these cells through disease or disruption.
6. Tissue self-antigen is altered by disease or injury, so that the host no longer recognizes it as self.[6, 14, 17]

SYSTEMIC LUPUS ERYTHEMATOSUS

SLE is a multisystem, chronic, remitting and relapsing, rheumatic disease that may assume several forms. The disease is found with the greatest frequency in women 20 to 40 years of age. It is much more common and more

TABLE 18-4 *Autoimmune Diseases*

Single Organ or Cell Type	Systemic
PROBABLE	**PROBABLE**
Hashimoto's thyroiditis	Systemic lupus
Autoimmune hemolytic	erythematosus
anemia	Rheumatoid arthritis
Autoimmune atrophic gas-	Sjögren's syndrome
tritis of pernicious anemia	Reiter's syndrome
Autoimmune encepha-	
lomyelitis	**POSSIBLE**
Autoimmune orchitis	Inflammatory myopathies
Goodpasture's syndrome*	Systemic sclerosis
Autoimmune thrombocyto-	(scleroderma)
penia	Polyarteritis nodosa
Insulin-dependent diabetes	
mellitus	
Myasthenia gravis	
Graves' disease	
POSSIBLE	
Primary biliary cirrhosis	
Chronic active hepatitis	
Ulcerative colitis	
Membranous glomerulone-	
phritis	

*Target is basement membrane of glomeruli and alveolar walls.
From Cotron, R., Kumar, V., and Robbins, S. *Robbins Pathologic Basis of Disease* (5th ed.). Philadelphia: W.B. Saunders, 1994.

severe in African American women, with a reported incidence of 1 in 245.[6]

Pathologically, widespread degeneration of connective tissue occurs, especially in the heart, glomeruli, blood vessels, skin, spleen, and retroperitoneal tissue. Skin changes include atrophy, dermal edema, and fibrinoid infiltration. The renal glomeruli characteristically demonstrate fibrinoid changes, necrosis with scarring, and deposits of immunoglobulin and complement in the basement membrane.[11] Antinuclear antibody is found in the serum of 80% to 100% of persons with SLE. The antinuclear antibody may represent antibodies to DNA, to nucleoproteins, or to other nuclear components. The lupus erythematosus cell is present in about 76% of affected people. It is basically a mature polymorphonuclear leukocyte that has engulfed nuclear material. These cells may be clustered around masses of nuclear material and are then called lupus erythematosus rosettes.[6] The lupus erythematosus cell is the result of targeting by antinuclear antibodies.

The American Rheumatism Association issued a list of 14 criteria indicative of SLE. If the person exhibits four or more of these, the diagnosis is probable (Table 18-5).

Stiffness and pain in the hands, feet, or large joints are common complaints. The joints appear red, warm, and tender but do not exhibit the deformities of rheumatoid arthritis. The exposed skin shows signs of a patchy atrophy. An erythematous rash frequently occurs in a butterfly pattern over the nose and cheeks. The dermis becomes edematous and infiltrated by lymphocytes, plasma cells, and histiocytes with an underlying small-vessel vasculitis.[13]

Renal involvement, a serious complication, results from the precipitation of immune complexes in the renal glomeruli. The complexes on the endothelial side of the basement membrane cause inflammatory lesions, thickened basement membrane, tubular atrophy, and interstitial spaces filled with lymphocytes and plasma cells.[6] The course of renal involvement is characterized by remissions and exacerbations ranging in severity from mild proteinuria to massive hematuria and proteinuria, resulting in total renal failure.[13]

Systemic problems, including fever, fatigue, anorexia, and weight loss, are common. Cardiopulmonary effects include pericarditis and pleural effusions and pneumonitis. Raynaud's phenomenon is observed in approximately one-third of affected persons (see p. 534).[13] Neurologic manifestations are often nonspecific and include headache, organic brain syndrome, and seizures. Besides antibody demonstration, hematologic abnormalities include hemolytic anemia, thrombocytopenia, and leukopenia, which result from direct cytoxicity to the hematologic cells.[13]

The prognosis for SLE depends on the degree of effect on target organs. The 10-year survival rate has improved from 50% to 90% with the advent of dialysis, the use of glucocorticoids, and renal transplantation.[13]

RHEUMATOID ARTHRITIS

Rheumatoid arthritis is a chronic, systemic, inflammatory disease that specifically affects the small joints of the hands and feet in its early stages and involves the larger joints in later stages. It occurs throughout the world and affects 1% to 2% of the population, with a more common incidence in women between the ages of 25 and 55.[23] It is nonsuppurative but results in the destruction of cartilage and joints. It also may produce lesions of the heart valves, pericardium, myocardium, and pleura.[11]

The pathophysiologic manifestations of rheumatoid arthritis appear to result from the development of antibody against IgG. These antibodies, called *rheumatoid factor (RF)*, belong to the IgM, IgG, and IgA classes.[6] The RF is present in 85% to 90% of persons with rheumatoid arthritis and may be stimulated by a self-antigen, an antigen in the synovial cavity, or an infectious antigen. The RF continues to interact with IgG even in the absence of any specific antigen.[1] Chronic antigenic stimulation, such as occurs in chronic respiratory infections, causes the production and destruction of large amounts of antibody. The RF-IgG complexes are present in the

TABLE 18-5 *Clinical Features of Systemic Lupus Erythematosus*

Organ System	ARA Criteria for Classification of SLE	Other Features
Constitutional		Fever, malaise, anorexia, weight loss
Cutaneous	1. Malar rash	Alopecia
	2. Discoid rash	Raynaud's phenomenon
	3. Photosensitivity	Other rashes: subacute cutaneous LE, urticaria, bullous lesions
	4. Oral/nasopharyngeal ulcers	Vasculitis
		Panniculitis (lupus profundus)
Musculoskeletal	5. Nonerosive arthritis	Arthralgia/myalgia
		Myositis
		Ligamentous laxity
		Avascular necrosis of bone
Cardiopulmonary	6. Pleuritis	Pleural effusions
	Pericarditis	Myocarditis
		Pneumonitis
		Verrucous endocarditis (Libman-Sacks syndrome)
		Interstitial fibrosis
		Pulmonary hypertension
Renal	7. Proteinuria (>500 mg/dL)	Nephrotic syndrome
	Urinary cellular casts	Renal insufficiency
		Renal failure
Neurologic	8. Psychosis	Organic brain syndrome
	Seizure	Cranial neuropathies
		Peripheral neuropathies
		Cerebellar signs
Gastrointestinal		Serositis
		Ascites
		Vasculitis (bleeding/perforation)
		Pancreatitis
		Elevated levels of liver enzymes
Hematologic	9. Hemolytic anemia	Anemia of chronic disease
	Leukopenia (<4000/mL)	Lupus anticoagulant
	Lymphopenia (<1500/mL)	Thrombosis
	Thrombocytopenia (<100,000/mL)	Splenomegaly
		Lymphadenopathy
Other systems		Sicca complex
		Conjunctivitis/episcleritis
Laboratory	10. Antinuclear antibody	Lupus band test on skin biopsy
	11. Anti-dsDNA	Anticardiolipin antibody
	Anti-Sm	Lupus anticoagulant
	False-positive VDRL	Hypocomplementemia
	LE preparation	

dsDNA: double-stranded DNA; VDRL: Venereal Disease Research Laboratory test; ARA: American Rheumatism Association; SLE: systemic lupus erythematosus.

From Kelley, W. N. *Textbook of Internal Medicine* (2nd ed.). Philadelphia: J.B. Lippincott, 1992.

rheumatoid lesions and apparently activate complement or prostaglandins or other substances that promote the inflammatory response (Flowchart 18-2).

Acute attacks of rheumatoid arthritis occur as the RF-IgG complexes precipitate in the synovial fluid. Complement is activated and attracts polymorphonuc-

lear leukocytes, whose main function appears to be phagocytosis of the complexes. The lysosomal enzymes released by these cells intensify the inflammatory reaction and increase destruction of the articular cartilage. Granulation tissue and inflammatory cells form a mass of tissue called *pannus* that erodes the articular cartilage.

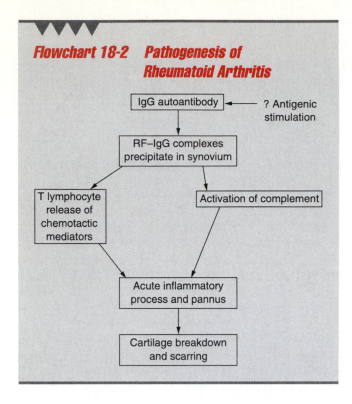

Flowchart 18-2   Pathogenesis of Rheumatoid Arthritis

The joint space is destroyed, and the resultant scarring may completely immobilize the joint or cause bleeding and thrombosis in the area.

Rheumatoid subcutaneous nodules often are seen and are described as firm, nontender oval masses up to 2 cm in diameter. These are present on the forearms and sometimes the Achilles tendons or are attached to underlying periosteum or tendons.

Other systems also are affected. A necrotizing arteritis may lead to thrombosis of small arteries. Fibrinous pericarditis, cardiomyopathy, and valvular lesions may affect the heart. Pleuritis and interstitial fibrosis may affect the lungs. The rheumatoid nodules may occur on bone, and other effects are seen in the nervous system and the eyes.[1]

The signs and symptoms of rheumatoid arthritis are due to both systemic and local inflammatory lesions. Fatigue, weakness, joint stiffness, and vague arthralgias are early symptoms. The person complains of morning stiffness, which gradually improves after rising. Joints in the hands or feet may be inflamed and swollen; these symptoms tend to spread symmetrically, so that the corresponding joints on the contralateral extremity become involved. Systemic symptoms are variable and rarely cause significant problems.[23] The joint and systemic manifestations are summarized in Box 18-2.

Laboratory values, besides the positive RF, include a normochromic or hypochromic anemia, mild leukocytosis with eosinophilia, and elevated erythrocyte sedimentation rate. Synovial fluid shows exudation with polymorphonuclear leukocytes, and the fluid appears turbid.[23]

The course of rheumatoid arthritis is variable, with remissions and exacerbations. Some people have a relatively benign disease, whereas others experience disease progression to severe deformity and total disability.

SCLERODERMA

Scleroderma, also called systemic sclerosis, is a relatively uncommon condition that involves thickening and fibrosis of the skin together with vascular, organ, and immunologic derangements. It affects about four times as many women as men, with the highest onset occurring between ages 50 and 60 years.[6] The disease appears to follow a more severe course in African American women.[6] Different forms of the disease exist, but the initial onset usually is marked by Raynaud's phenomenon. The condition may be more prevalent than is thought because of missed diagnosis.

The initial skin changes of edema may be accompanied by arthralgia or morning stiffness. This is followed by skin thickening that results from accumulation of collagen in the dermis.[16] The skin changes are continuous, causing taut restrictions over the joints, the thoracic cavity, and even the face. The serum antinuclear antibody is positive in 90% of persons with systemic sclerosis, and other antibodies may be demonstrated. As the disease progresses, organ changes occur. Patchy fibrosis of the myocardium may result from intermittent myocardial ischemia. Pulmonary changes are varied and may include interstitial inflammatory fibrosis and vascular injury.[6] Progressive renal insufficiency and marked hypertension result from renovascular changes. The gastrointestinal changes are varied and include esophageal reflux, malabsorption, intussusception, and volvulus. Endocrine changes include hypothyroidism and repro-

---

BOX 18-2 ▼ Joint and Systemic Manifestations of Rheumatoid Arthritis

Subcutaneous nodules—firm, freely movable at joint points, such as knuckles and elbows

Morning stiffness—lasts at least 1 hour, then improves

Arthritis—bilateral involvement, usually of same joint areas. Hand joints usually affected and swollen. Usually at least three joint areas involved

Serum rheumatoid factor positive—autoantibody that is seen with systemic autoimmune diseases, positive in nearly all cases of rheumatoid arthritis

Inflammation—persistence of synovitis leads to disability from destruction of cartilage, bone, and tendons. Contractures are common, usually flexion

Peripheral nerve entrapment—causes carpal tunnel syndrome. Paresthesias, pain, burning, muscle wasting, and weakness are present

Vasculitis of small arteries—causes pericardial, cardiac, and pulmonary lesions. Digital necrosis is common

Scleritis—results from loss of normal fluid in the film of the eye

ductive disorders.[16] In some cases, affected persons are said to have the CREST syndrome, which is a more limited form that may develop visceral changes much later in the course of the disease, if at all. The CREST syndrome refers to the manifestations of *c*alcinosis (calcium deposits in various body tissues), *R*aynaud's phenomenon, *e*sophageal dysmotility, *s*clerodactyly (the fixed semiflexed fingers with tightened skin), and *t*elangiectasia (permanent dilatation of the capillaries in various areas of the body).[6]

Morbidity and mortality depend on the degree of organ involvement, and a 60% overall 5-year survival rate is reported in systemic sclerosis.[16]

▼ Chapter Summary

▼ Hypersensitivity reactions are tissue-damaging, immune-mediated disorders. They are usually classified as type I, anaphylaxis or atopy; type II, cytotoxic hypersensitivity; type III, immune complex; and type IV, cell-mediated hypersensitivity. Autoimmune reactions usually fall in the type II and type III reactions.

▼ Type I reactions involve a hypersensitivity response to an environmental antigen. It is IgE mediated and involves release of mast cell mediators, which can result in hives or anaphylactic shock. Bronchial asthma and atopic eczema are forms of this reaction.

▼ Type II reactions occur when a circulating antibody, usually IgG, reacts with a cell surface antigen. The product of this reaction is either hemolysis or target cell destruction. A common and potentially fatal type II reaction is the transfusion reaction to the surface antigens on the red blood cell.

▼ Type III reactions involve the formation and precipitation of immune complexes into vulnerable areas, usually the small vessels. There is a resulting vasculitis and inflammation of the area affected. Many type III disorders are those described as the classic, systemic autoimmune disorders.

▼ The type IV reaction involves the sensitized T lymphocyte without the participation of antibodies. Usually, the response is delayed and the severity of the reaction depends on the initial antigenic stimulation. Certain contact dermatitis reactions are type IV, as are some of the hypersensitivity responses to organisms.

▼ The study of autoimmunity requires the understanding of an excessive, self-targeted immune response. Many different conditions are thought to have an underlying autoimmune basis, which means the loss of self-tolerance and self-tissue destruction.

▼ Autoimmune responses have been categorized as organ-specific and nonorgan-specific. Most of the organ-specific responses are described in other areas of the text. The common nonorgan-specific responses of SLE, rheumatoid arthritis, and scleroderma are detailed in this chapter.

▼ References

1. Ball, G.V., and Koopman, W.J. Rheumatoid arthritis. In W.N. Kelley (ed.), *Textbook of Internal Medicine* (2nd ed.). Philadelphia: J.B. Lippincott, 1992.

2. Barnetson, R., and Gawkrodger, D. Hypersensitivity type IV. In I. Roitt, J. Brostoff, and D. Male (eds.), *Immunology* (3rd ed.). St. Louis: C.V. Mosby, 1993.

3. Beckerman, K.P. Reproduction & the immune system. In D.P. Stites, A.I. Terr, and T.G. Parslow (eds.), *Basic and Clinical Immunology* (8th ed.). Norwalk, Conn.: Appleton & Lange, 1994.

4. Bellanti, J.A. *Immunology III.* Philadelphia: W.B. Saunders, 1985.

5. Brostoff, J., and Hall, T. Hypersensitivity type I. In I.Roitt, J. Brostoff, and D. Male (eds.), *Immunology* (3rd ed.). St. Louis: C.V. Mosby, 1993.

6. Cotran, R.S., Kumar, V., and Robbins, S.L. *Robbins' Pathologic Basis of Disease* (5th ed.). Philadelphia: W.B. Saunders, 1994.

7. Fulmer, J.D. Interstitial lung disease. In J. Stein (ed.), *Internal Medicine* (4th ed.) St. Louis: C.V. Mosby, 1994.

8. Govan, A.D.T., Macfarlane, P.S., and Callander, R. Genitourinary system. In *Pathology Illustrated.* New York: Churchill Livingstone, 1991.

9. Hay, F. Hypersensitivity—Type III. In I.Roitt, J. Brostoff, and D. Male (eds.), *Immunology* (3rd ed.) St. Louis: C.V. Mosby, 1993.

10. Hutchinson, I. Transplantation and rejection. In I. Roitt, J. Brostoff, and D. Male (eds.), *Immunology* (3rd ed.) St. Louis: C.V. Mosby, 1993.

11. Kissane, J.M. *Anderson's Pathology* (9th ed.). St. Louis: C.V. Mosby, 1990.

12. Male, D. Hypersensitivity—Type II. In I. Roitt, J. Brostoff, and D. Male (eds.), *Immunology* (3rd ed.). St. Louis: C.V. Mosby, 1993.

13. McGuire, J.L., and Lambert, R.E. Lupus erythematosus. In W.N. Kelley (ed.), *Textbook of Internal Medicine* (2nd ed.) Philadelphia: J.B. Lippincott, 1992.

14. Roitt, I. Autoimmunity and autoimmune disease. *Immunology* (3rd ed.). St. Louis: C.V. Mosby, 1993.

15. Rubin, E., and Farber, J.L. *Pathology* (2nd ed.). Philadelphia: J.B. Lippincott, 1994.

16. Seibold, J.R. Scleroderma. In W.N. Kelley (ed.), *Textbook of Internal Medicine* (2nd ed.). Philadelphia: J.B. Lippincott, 1992.

17. Steinberg, A.D. Mechanisms of disordered immune regulation. In D.P. Stites, A.I. Terr, and T.G. Parslow (eds.), *Basic and Clinical Immunology* (8th ed.). Norwalk, Conn.: Appleton & Lange, 1994.

18. Terr, A.I. Anaphylaxis and urticaria. In D.P. Stites, A.I. Terr, and T.G. Parslow, *Basic and Clinical Immunology* (8th ed.). Norwalk, Conn.: Appleton & Lange, 1994.

19. Terr, A.I. The atopic diseases. In D.P. Stites, A.I. Terr, and T.G. Parslow (ed.), *Basic and Clinical Immunology* (8th ed.). Norwalk, Conn.: Appleton & Lange, 1994.

20. Terr, A.I. Cell-mediated hypersensitivity diseases. In D.P. Stites, A.I. Terr, and T.G. Parslow (ed.), *Basic and Clinical Immunology* (8th ed.). Norwalk, Conn.: Appleton & Lange, 1994.

21. Terr, A.I. Immune-complex allergic diseases. In D.P. Stites, A.I. Terr, and T.G. Parslow (ed.), *Basic and Clinical Immu-*

Chapter 19

Normal and Altered Erythrocyte Function

Barbara L. Bullock

▼ LEARNING OBJECTIVES

1 Describe the composition of whole blood.
2 Discuss the primary functions of blood.
3 Explain the stem cell theory.
4 Diagram the process for the development of erythrocytes.
5 Explain the structure and function of hemoglobin.
6 Explain the factors that influence erythropoiesis.
7 Explain blood typing and how transfusion reactions can occur.
8 Describe the process of red blood cell destruction.
9 Differentiate between physiologic erythrocytosis and polycythemia.
10 Discuss the neoplastic process involved in polycythemia vera.
11 List and differentiate the morphologic characteristics of the different types of anemia.
12 Explain how aplastic anemia can develop.
13 List and describe the cause and result of the hemolytic anemias.
14 Describe the precipitating cause of and environment that produces sickle cell anemia.
15 Explain why iron deficiency anemia is common in children and young women.
16 Explain the relation of intrinsic factor deficiency to the development of pernicious anemia.
17 Differentiate the causes of pernicious anemia and folic acid anemia.
18 Briefly explain why posthemorrhagic anemia may not occur immediately after an acute hemorrhage.
19 Discuss the anemias associated with chronic disease.
20 Briefly describe the laboratory findings and diagnostic tests that are helpful in diagnosing disorders of red blood cells.

Barbara L. Bullock: PATHOPHYSIOLOGY: ADAPTATIONS AND ALTERATIONS IN FUNCTION, 4th ed.
© 1996 Lippincott-Raven Publishers

All living cells require materials to survive and to perform functions that are necessary to maintain life. Blood and interstitial fluid provide the means by which essential substances are delivered to the cells and materials not needed are removed from the cells. Transportation of cellular and humoral messages by the blood helps to integrate physiologic processes, thus enabling the body to function as a unified whole.

Since ancient times, there has been much interest in and curiosity about blood and its relation to life. Blood was known to be essential to human existence; loss of large amounts became associated with loss of life. The first description of red blood cells (RBCs) came with the discovery of the microscope by Leeuwenhoek (1632–1723). He examined the blood and described the red corpuscles.[30] Sophisticated and advanced technology now makes it possible to examine and describe blood components and their functions in minute detail.

▼ General Physical Characteristics of Blood

The primary roles of blood in general are to integrate body functions and to meet the needs of specific tissues. This is accomplished through transportation, regulation, and protection mechanisms.[22] Blood transports oxygen, nutrients, waste products, and hormones from one place to another. Regulation is accomplished through buffers in the blood, plasma proteins, and heat transport, such as muscle-generated temperature. The protection function of the blood includes antibodies and phagocytes to protect against disease as well as factors that participate in hemostasis.

Blood consists of a clear yellow fluid called *plasma*, in which cells and many other substances are suspended. Proteins are the major solutes in plasma and consist primarily of albumins, globulins, and fibrinogen. The composition of plasma is similar to that of interstitial fluid, except that it has a much higher protein concentration. This higher concentration of proteins in the blood maintains the intravascular volume by the exertion of colloid osmotic pressure. In addition to holding water in the intravascular spaces, plasma proteins bind such substances as lipids and such metals as iron, contribute to viscosity of blood, and participate in the coagulation of blood. They also are important in regulating acid–base balance.

The total blood volume is divided into two main categories: plasma and cells. Ninety-nine percent of the cells are RBCs. Table 19-1 summarizes the main substances present in blood.

The blood volume is the sum of volumes of plasma and formed elements of blood in the vascular system. It can be calculated from either plasma volume or cell volume, which, in the healthy man, average 45 mL/kg and 30 mL/kg body weight, respectively.[17] If the average man weighs 75 kg, the total blood volume (including plasma and cell volume) will be about 5,500 to 6,000 mL, or about 8% of total body weight.[22] The variation of normal blood volumes is indicated in Box 19-1. Although numerous factors affect blood volume, it remains relatively stable in the healthy person. Several compensatory mechanisms contribute to this stability; for example, decreased RBC volume is followed by increased plasma volume, thereby returning total blood volume to its normal level. In this situation, the total blood volume may be normal, but the ratio of plasma to cells is altered. Capillary dynamics and renal mechanisms play major roles in maintaining plasma volume.

General physical characteristics of the blood are summarized in Table 19-2. Oxygenated arterial blood is bright red, changing to dark red or crimson when oxygen is lost and carbon dioxide is added. The pH is regulated within the narrow limits of 7.35 to 7.45 (see pp. 212–214). The relatively high viscosity of blood is primarily due to the suspension of cells and plasma components, which causes it to flow more slowly than water.

The circulation of blood provides for maintenance of a consistent (homeostatic) state in individual body cells. The constituency of blood rapidly and continuously changes, but the overall concentration of substances remains relatively constant. This constancy in the environment of individual body cells is essential for life.

▼ Hematopoiesis

BONE MARROW

In the adult, the bone marrow produces all of the blood cells and platelets. At birth, *red marrow* is present in all bone marrow cavities, and blood cells are formed there as well as in the liver and spleen.[26] In children, blood cells are produced in the marrow of all bones. By age 20 to 25 years, red marrow is present in the cranial bones, vertebrae, sternum, ribs, clavicles, scapulae, pelvis, and proximal ends of the femora and humeri (Fig. 19-1). The other marrow areas become inactive and infiltrated with fat and are called *yellow marrow*. In the aged person, red marrow begins to leave the cranial bones and lower vertebrae.[16] The blood supply to the marrow comes from large-lumina, thin-walled arteries that branch into a network of capillaries to become a bed of sinusoids. Between the sinuses lies the hematopoietic tissue in which blood cells are formed. The new cells enter the sinuses through small openings in the walls. Blood cells gain access to the sinusoids at a critical moment in their maturation phase, and maturation is completed in the circulatory system and tissues.[26] Loss of integrity of the sinus walls or increased need may allow the release of immature cells into the circulation.

TABLE 19-1 *Main Substances Present in Blood*

Acetoacetate	0.3–2.0 mg/dL	G6PD screen, qualitative	Negative
Acid phosphatase	0–0.8 U/mL	Haptoglobin	100–300 mg/dL
Acid phophatase, prostatic	2.5–12.0 IU/L	Hemoglobin A_2	0%–4% of total Hb
Albumin	3.0–5.5 g/dL	Hemoglobin F	0%–2% of total Hb
Aldolase	1–6 IU/L	Immunoglobulin, quantitation	
Alkaline phosphatase		IgG	600–1800 mg/dL
15–20 years	40–200 IU/L	IgA	70–400 mg/dL
20–101 years	35–125 IU/L	IgM	
Alpha-1 antitrypsin	200–500 mg/dL	Male	30–350 mg/dL
ALT	0–40 IU/L	Female	30–375 mg/dL
Ammonia	11–35 μmol/L	IgD and IgE	minimal
Amylase, serum	2–20 U/L	Insulin, fasting	6–20 μU/mL
Anion gap	8–12 mEq/L (mmol/L)	Iron-binding capacity	250–400 μg/dL
Ascorbic acid	0.4–1.5 mg/dL	Iron, total, serum	40–150 μg/dL
AST	5–40 IU/L	Lactic acid	0.6–1.8 mEq/L
Bilirubin		LDH, serum	20–220 IU/L
Total	0.2–1.2 mg/dL	Leucine aminopeptidase (LAP)	30–55 IU/L
Direct	0–0.4 mg/dL	Lipase	4–24 IU/L
Calcium, serum	8.7–10.6 mg/dL	Magnesium, serum	1.5–2.5 mEq/L
Carbon dioxide, total	18–30 mEq/L (mmol/L)	5′-Nucleotidase	0.3–3.2 Bodansky units
Carcinoembryonic antigen,	<2.5 μg/L	Osmolality, serum	278–305 mOsm/kg serum water
serum		Phenylalanine	3 mg/dL
Carotene (carotenoids)	50–300 μg/dL	Phosphorus, inorganic, serum	2.0–4.3 mg/dL
C3 complement	55–120 mg/dL	Potassium, plasma	3.1–4.3 mEq/L
C4 complement	15–51 mg/dL	Potassium, serum	3.5–5.2 mEq/L
Ceruloplasmin	15–60 mg/dL	Protein, total, serum	
Chloride, serum	95–105 mEq/L (mmol)	2–55 years	5.0–8.0 g/dL
Cholesterol, total	100–180 mg/dL	55–101 years	6.0–8.3 g/dL
Copper	100–200 μg/dL	Sodium, serum	135–145 mEq/L
Creatine kinase, total	20–200 IU/L	Sulfate	0.5–1.5 mg/dL
		T_3 uptake	25%–45%
Creatinine, serum		T_4	4–11 μg/dL
Female adult	0.5–1.3 mg/dL	Triglycerides	20–180 mg/dL
Male adult	0.7–1.5 mg/dL	Urea nitrogen, serum	
Folate, serum	1.9–14.0 ng/mL	2–65 years	5–22 mg/dL
Gamma glutamyl		Male	10–38 mg/dL
transpeptidase		Female	8–26 mg/dL
Male	12–38 IU/L	Uric acid	
Female	9–31 IU/L	10–59 years	
Gastrin	150 pg/mL	Male	2.5–9.0 mg/dL
Glucose, serum (fasting)	70–115 mg/dL	Female	2.0–8.0 mg/dL
Glucose-6-phosphate	5–10 IU/g Hb		
dehydrogenase			

Hematopoiesis (the normal formation of blood cells in the bone marrow) is a dynamic, constant process, with rapid turnover of blood cells and a constant need for new cells. Bone marrow can meet the body's changing needs for various types and numbers of cells. It maintains a reserve supply of cells for stressful and unexpected situations that create an increased demand. Normally, the ratio of white blood cell precursors to RBC precursors is between 2:1 and 4.5:1.[26]

STEM CELL THEORY

Most of the formed elements of the blood have a limited life span. Erythrocytes live an average of 120 days. Granulocytes circulate in the blood for an average of 6 hours and then move into the tissues, where they may live for several days.[15] Other cells, such as macrophages and lymphocytes, may live months or years. When cells are lost through use or age, they must be continually replaced through a rigidly controlled process.

The origin of cells that develop into mature erythrocytes, leukocytes, and platelets has been investigated for many years. The *stem cell theory* helps to explain the various stages of cell differentiation in the bone marrow. The cellular elements finally present in blood are the more differentiated and mature cells. The pluripotential stem cells transform to committed precursors and finally differentiate (mature) into recognizable precursors of mature cells (Fig. 19-2). Stem cells can be *pluripotent*, from which any type of blood cell can form,

BOX 19-1 ▼ *Variations of Normal Blood Volumes*

A wide variation in normal blood volumes exists because of the following factors:

1. *Weight*. Because fatty tissue contains little water, the total blood volume correlates more closely with lean body mass than with total body weight.
2. *Sex*. Because women usually have a higher ratio of fat tissue to lean tissue, the blood volume per kilogram for them usually is lower than that for men.
3. *Pregnancy*. Total blood volume gradually rises as a pregnancy progresses, with the greatest increase occurring primarily in plasma volume.
4. *Posture or position*. Volume tends to increase when a person is in bed for a period of time and decreases when he or she assumes the erect position. The variation in blood volume may result from alterations in capillary pressure that lead to changes in glomerular filtration.
5. *Age*. Percentage of blood volume is higher in the newborn and decreases with increasing age.
6. *Nutrition*. Lack of nutrients may cause a decrease in RBCs or plasma formation, thus decreasing the total blood volume.
7. *Environmental temperature*. The volume of blood increases when the environmental temperature is increased.
8. *Altitude*. At high altitudes, the environmental oxygen pressure is greatly decreased, and a greater number of RBCs are produced for oxygen transport.

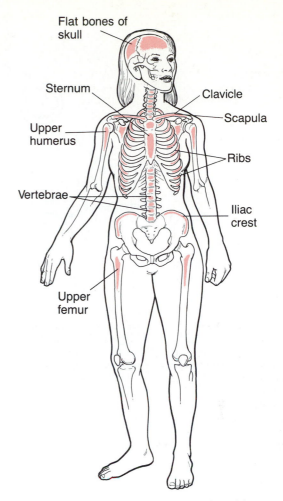

FIGURE 19-1 *Sources of red bone marrow in the adult.*

or *unipotent*, from which only one type of cell develops.[17] The appearance of these cells cannot be distinguished by ordinary microscopic techniques.

Stem cells have the morphologic appearance of small mononuclear cells that resemble lymphocytes. They are grouped in pools or compartments that can

TABLE 19-2 *Physical Characteristics of Blood*

Characteristic	Normal	Example of Alterations
Color	Arterial: bright red Venous: dark red or crimson	Anemia
pH	Arterial: 7.35–7.45 Venous: 7.31–7.41	Decrease in acidosis; increases in alkalosis
Specific gravity	Plasma: 1.026 RBC: 1.093	
Viscosity	3.5–4.5 times that of water	Increases in polycythemia; decreases in anemia
Volume	5000 mL (70-kg male) About 3 L in plasma 2 L blood cells	Decreases in dehydration Increase in pregnancy

maintain themselves and produce cells that can become committed to a certain line of blood cells. The committed stem cells group into colony-forming units (CFUs). Colony-forming units that are designated to form erythrocytes are termed CFU-E, those that form granulocytes and monocytes have the designation CFU-GM, and those forming megakaryocytes are termed CFU-M.[17]

Complex feedback loops of humoral regulation of hematopoiesis are beginning to be recognized. Colony-stimulating and -inhibiting factors are important in regulating the proliferation and differentiation of blood cells.[8] As noted in Figure 19-2, the stem cell becomes committed to the lymphoid or trilineage myeloid stem cell lines. From that point, further changes determine the ultimate cell formed. The stem cell maintains the property of self-renewal. Pools of pluripotent or uncommitted cells must be present, because once the cell line becomes differentiated (eg, proerythroblast), the cells are in active cell division and cannot self-replicate.[8] The pool apparently can recover if injured but not lethally damaged, which works in favor of chemotherapeutic agents that damage differentiated cells but may not affect the stem cells.[1] RBC formation is the most well under-

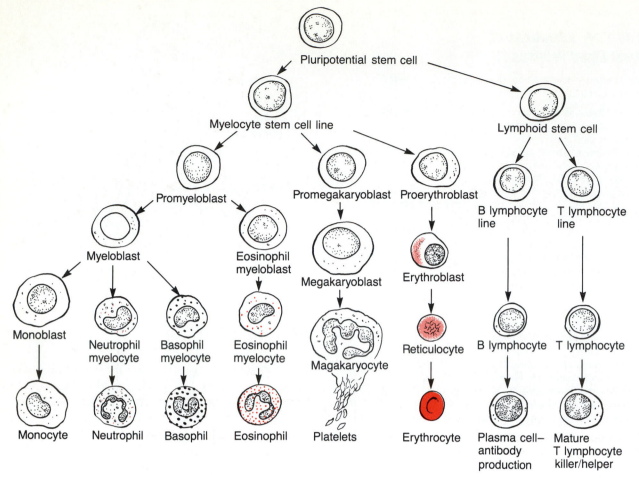

FIGURE 19-2 *Differentiation of hematopoietic blood cells.*

stood of hematopoietic cell formation and differentiation. The reader is referred to Chapters 16, 20, and 21 for discussions of the other blood cells.

SPLEEN

The spleen is a large, highly vascular organ with elements of the lymphoid and mononuclear phagocyte systems. It is located in the left upper abdominal cavity, directly beneath the diaphragm, above the left kidney, and behind the fundus of the stomach (Fig. 19-3). The spleen is covered by peritoneum and held in position by the peritoneal folds. It has a connective tissue capsule from which trabeculae (supporting strands) extend inside the organ and form a framework. Splenic pulp is present in the small spaces of this framework.

The major areas of the spleen are the *red pulp*, the *white pulp*, and the *venous sinuses*. As can be seen in Figure 19-4, a small splenic artery penetrates into the splenic pulp and terminates in highly porous capillaries. Cells move from these capillaries into the red pulp and then gradually squeeze through the trabecular network, eventually ending up in the venous sinuses.[8, 17] This

exposure of cells to phagocytic cells gives a large surface area to get rid of unwanted debris in the blood. Old RBCs, bacteria, platelets, or parasites, for example, can be removed from the circulation and destroyed. The destruction of old and imperfect RBCs sometimes is referred to as "culling." Reticulocytes and many platelets are stored in the spleen. Much of the spleen contains white pulp, which consists of a large number of phagocytic and immunocompetent cells. The cells also line the venous sinuses to cleanse the blood. Splenic enlargement is seen in some infectious conditions in the same manner as is seen with lymph node enlargement.

Blood is brought to the spleen by the splenic artery, which divides into several branches before entering the concave side of the spleen. The small arteries divide into smaller vessels and finally to arterioles and capillaries. After passing through the substance of the spleen just described, the capillaries empty into thin-walled veins that terminate in the splenic vein, which itself terminates in the portal vein.[7]

The spleen is not a muscular organ, but dilatation of vessels within it can cause it to store several hundred milliliters of blood and release this blood into the circulation with vascular constriction.[17]

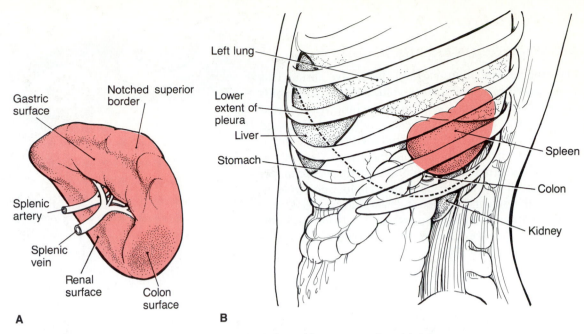

FIGURE 19-3   *Spleen.* **A.** *Structure and position.* **B.** *Relationship to surrounding structures.*

Although the spleen is not necessary for survival, it is involved in four important functions: 1) production of lymphocytes in the white pulp; 2) destruction of erythrocytes in the red pulp; 3) filtration and trapping of foreign particles in both areas, destroying bacteria and viruses; and 4) storage of blood.[8] In fetal life, the spleen is active in hematopoiesis, a function that mostly ends at or before birth. The normal adult spleen holds about 150 to 200 mL of blood, but because of its structure, the spleen often enlarges with increased volume when the systemic venous pressure becomes elevated, such as with right-sided heart failure.

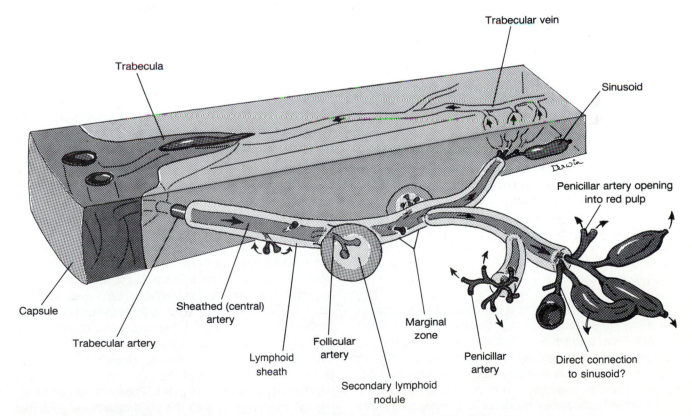

FIGURE 19-4   *Basic organization of the spleen, showing its various blood vessels and associated white pulp. (Source: Cormack, D.H. Essential Histology. Philadelphia: J.B. Lippincott, 1993.)*

▼ *Erythropoiesis*

DESCRIPTION OF ERYTHROCYTES

Erythrocytes are nonnucleated, biconcave disks. This shape provides a large surface-volume ratio that permits distortion of the cells without stretching their membrane. RBCs can traverse very small capillaries, and normal RBCs adapt to the sinusoids of the spleen, escaping without being trapped and destroyed. The unique shape of erythrocytes also is conducive to gas exchange. The membrane of the RBC is made of lipids and proteins, making it resilient, flexible, and water-insoluble. Erythrocytes contain hemoglobin, which binds loosely with oxygen and carbon dioxide to carry essential gases to and away from the tissues.

DEVELOPMENT OF ERYTHROCYTES

Erythrocytes are formed in the blood islands of the yolk sacs during the first several weeks of gestation. During the second trimester of pregnancy, fetal RBCs are produced in the liver, spleen, and lymph nodes. After birth, the bone marrow becomes the principal site of RBC production. After adolescence, the red marrow of the membranous bones, especially the pelvic bone, sternum, ribs, and vertebrae, take over the major erythropoietic function. This marrow cell pool provides a constant supply of peripheral RBCs.

The mature RBC is the end result of several divisions and differentiations before reaching the final stage of maturity (Fig. 19-5). During maturation, the nucleus decreases in size until it disappears, the total size of the cell shrinks, the amount of ribonucleic acid lessens, and hemoglobin synthesis increases. Hemoglobin reaches a concentration of 34% of cell volume. The reticulocyte stage is the final stage before the mature erythrocyte is formed. The reticulocyte contains remnants of the Golgi apparatus and other organelles. It normally remains in the marrow about 1 day and then in the bloodstream 1 day before becoming a mature erythrocyte. Normally, only 1% to 2% of the erythrocytes in the blood are in the form of reticulocytes.[7]

HEMOGLOBIN

The protein hemoglobin is a conjugated, oxygen-carrying red pigment with a molecular weight of about 64,500. The synthesis of hemoglobin begins in the erythroblast and continues through the normoblast stage. Small amounts of hemoglobin are formed for a day or so by the reticulocytes. Two parallel processes are involved in hemoglobin synthesis: the formation of the porphyrin structure (heme) that contains iron and the

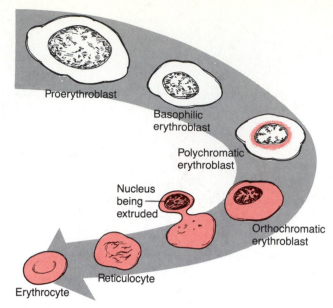

FIGURE 19-5 *Development of red blood cell. Proerythroblast stage is the first stage following the erythroid colony forming unit (CFU-E), which is a cell with a very large nucleus. The basophilic erythroblast stage is when hemoglobin synthesis begins. The polychromatic erythroblast, or normoblast stage, is the last stage of DNA synthesis and cell division. Hemoglobin synthesis continues. The orthochromatic erythroblast stage shows the shrinking and autolysis of the nucleus. The remains of the nucleus are extruded from the cell. In the reticulocyte stage, the cell does not have a nucleus and enters the circulation, where it becomes a mature erythrocyte. The erythrocyte is a disk-shaped, pliable cell that can move in tight spaces to pick up or release oxygen.*

formation of the polypeptide chains that make up globin (Fig. 19-6). *Heme* is a large disk that contains iron and porphyrin, a nitrogen-containing organic compound.[19] The adult hemoglobin molecule (HbA) is composed of a globin (made of two alpha and two beta large polypeptide chains) with four heme (iron porphyrin) complexes. The structure of hemoglobin changes in the last 3 months of gestation from primarily fetal hemoglobin (HbF) to HbA. In certain congenital hemolytic anemias, the HbF persists, which, along with globin chain synthesis imbalance, provides the basis for the pathophysiology of these disorders (see pp. 381–383).[9] One iron atom is present for each heme molecule. Each of the four iron atoms of the molecule combines reversibly with an atom of oxygen, forming oxyhemoglobin. When oxygen concentration is high, as in the lungs, oxygen combines with hemoglobin, but when the concentration is lower, as in the tissues, oxygen is released. In the lungs, about 95% of hemoglobin becomes saturated with oxygen. The high density of hemoglobin in each RBC allows a large amount of oxygen to be transported. The disk shape of the erythrocytes provides a large surface area per unit mass of hemoglobin, enhancing gas exchange in both the pulmonary and systemic capillary system.

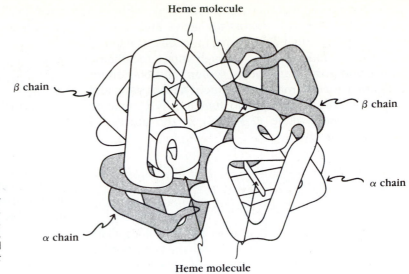

Heme molecule

β chain

β chain

α chain

α chain

Heme molecule

FIGURE 19-6 *Structure of the hemoglobin molecule. The hemoglobin molecule is made up of four polypeptide chains. Two identical chains are called A chains, and the other two identical chains are called B chains. Each chain encloses a heme molecule. (From: Schmid, G. The Chemical Basis of Life, General, Organic, and Biological Chemistry for the Health Science.* Boston: Little, Brown, 1982.)

SUBSTANCES NEEDED FOR ERYTHROPOIESIS

Several substances are essential for the proper formation of RBCs and hemoglobin. Among these are amino acids, iron, copper, pyridoxine, cobalt, vitamin B_{12}, and folic acid. Iron is essential for the production of heme, and about 65% of body iron is present in hemoglobin. The total amount of iron in the body equals about 4 g, with 15% to 30% of this amount being stored as *ferritin*, primarily in the liver. Ferritin (storage iron) is formed from a combination of iron with a protein called *apoferritin*.[17] It is readily available for hemoglobin synthesis when needed through the aid of a beta-globulin called *transferrin*. Transferrin has specific binding capabilities that facilitate the transfer of iron across the membranes of immature erythrocytes. Transferrin also carries the iron released from worn-out erythrocytes to the bone marrow, where it is reused for hemoglobin synthesis. The presence of reduced ferrous iron allows the formation of hemoglobin, which is capable of binding and releasing oxygen normally. Oxidized ferric iron, however, results in the formation of *methemoglobin*, which cannot carry oxygen. Certain drugs, such as nitrates, phenacetin, sulfonamides, and lidocaine, may cause the production of excess ferric iron.[2]

Daily losses of iron are replaced by dietary intake or transferred to apoferritin to make ferritin. Iron is absorbed mostly in the duodenum by an active process that apparently continues until all of the transferrin is saturated. When transferrin can accept no more iron, absorption of iron almost entirely ceases in the duodenum. Conversely, if the stores are depleted, larger amounts of iron are absorbed. The result is a feedback mechanism that keeps a stable level of iron for hemoglobin synthesis.[16] Lack in the diet or poor absorption of iron leads to iron deficiency anemia (see pp. 385–386).

Vitamin B_{12} (cyanocobalamin) is essential for the synthesis of deoxyribonucleic acid (DNA) molecules in the forming RBCs. This large molecule does not easily penetrate the mucosa of the gastrointestinal tract, but must be bound to a glycoprotein known as the *intrinsic factor* for its absorption. The intrinsic factor is secreted by the parietal cells of the gastric mucosa and binds to vitamin B_{12} to protect it from the digestive enzymes. After absorption from the gastrointestinal tract, vitamin B_{12} is stored in the liver and is available for the production of new erythrocytes. Long-standing lack of B_{12} leads to maturation-failure anemia (pernicious anemia) (see pp. 384–385).

Folic acid (pteroylglutamic acid) also is necessary for the synthesis of DNA and promotes RBC maturation. Lack of folic acid causes folic acid anemia, a type of maturation-failure anemia that readily responds to dietary replacement.

Copper is a catalyst in the formation of hemoglobin and in this way helps to make RBCs.[29] Cobalt is a mineral in the vitamin B_{12} molecule so that its deficiency will lead to the same type of maturation-failure anemia as that seen with lack of the intrinsic factor.

ENERGY PRODUCTION IN ERYTHROCYTES

Mature erythrocytes cannot synthesize nucleic acids, complex carbohydrates, lipids, or proteins because they do not have a nucleus or other intracellular organelles. Because there are no mitochondria for oxidative metabolism, the energy of mature RBCs is generated from the metabolism of glucose by the anaerobic pathway. The RBCs carry about 280 million hemoglobin molecules, and this is available oxygen transport space. Because their energy is produced anaerobically, RBCs do not use any of the oxygen that they transport.[28] Even without a nucleus, the RBC is metabolically active and requires energy to provide for the following functions: 1) maintenance of osmotic stability through intact membrane pumps and active transport of sodium and potassium; 2) maintenance of iron in the reduced ferrous state; and 3) modulation of hemoglobin function by generating 2,3-diphosphoglycerate (2,3-DPG) in the process of generating energy.

FUNCTION OF RED BLOOD CELLS IN OXYGEN AND CARBON DIOXIDE TRANSPORT

Most of the oxygen that crosses the alveolocapillary membrane to the blood combines with the heme portion of hemoglobin. This combination is in a loose bond called *oxyhemoglobin*. Hemoglobin saturation with oxygen usually is 95% in arterial blood, and oxygen is rapidly released when it reaches the tissues, which have an oxygen pressure (P_{O_2}) of about 40 mm Hg. In normal venous blood, the P_{O_2} is about 40 mm Hg, with a hemoglobin saturation of about 70% (see pp. 559–560).[17]

As stated before, hemoglobin becomes nearly saturated with oxygen as it passes through the lungs. This oxygen is unloaded at the tissue level to meet cellular needs. The affinity of hemoglobin for oxygen is affected by hydrogen ion concentration, carbon dioxide levels, and the amount of 2,3-DPG. Increased levels of any of these causes a decreased affinity for oxygen and more effective oxygen unloading to the tissues. This could be viewed as a compensatory mechanism for tissue oxygenation. Elevated levels of 2,3-DPG have been seen with some chronic hypoxic states. The presence of excess DPG also decreases the ability of hemoglobin to combine with oxygen in the lungs. Conversely, if the 2,3-DPG levels are decreased or hydrogen and carbon dioxide levels are lowered, there may be a defect in oxygen unloading.[17]

Transport of carbon dioxide from the tissues of RBCs occurs in two major ways: 1) in combination with hemoglobin as carbaminohemoglobin (20–25%); and 2) in the dissolved form of bicarbonate (70%). When carbon dioxide is released from the tissue cell, it diffuses into the RBC and combines with water, with carbonic anhydrase as the catalyst, to form carbonic acid. Carbonic acid (H_2CO_3) almost immediately dissociates into free hydrogen and bicarbonate ions. Free hydrogen attaches to hemoglobin because it is a powerful acid–base buffer, and bicarbonate is free to diffuse into the plasma or attach to a positive ion within the RBC. When bicarbonate diffuses into the plasma, it usually is replaced by chloride in the *chloride shift*. This is made possible by a bicarbonate–chloride carrier protein that rapidly moves these ions in opposite directions. The end result is a greater amount of chloride in venous RBCs than in arterial cells, and CO_2 is carried from the tissue cells as bicarbonate ions in the plasma.[17, 28]

FACTORS THAT INFLUENCE ERYTHROPOIESIS

The normal life span of adult RBCs is 120 days. Old RBCs are continuously destroyed, and new ones are regenerated daily for replacement. There normally is little variation in the rate of destruction and production, so that the total RBC mass in the body remains relatively constant. Erythropoiesis is stimulated by a decrease in the P_{O_2} of arterial blood. If the number of RBCs decreases, the bone marrow is stimulated to produce more erythrocytes. Oxygen delivery may decrease due to anemia or hypoxia of any cause, and there is usually stimulation of the bone marrow by erythropoietin to produce more RBCs. Chronic hypoxemia, such as with chronic lung disease, produces an increase in the number of circulating RBCs (polycythemia).

Erythropoietin hormone stimulates the bone marrow to produce increased numbers of RBCs through conversion of certain stem cells to proerythroblasts. These stem cells are derived from pluripotent stem cells but are more sensitive to erythropoietin than are other stem cells. These cells are referred to as erythropoietin-responsive cells, which are part of a fast cycling system for RBC production. These cells also mature faster than other precursor cells.[15, 28] Erythropoietin principally comes from renal glomerular epithelial cells, but some may be released from liver epithelium. The usual stimulus for erythropoietin secretion is hypoxia, but androgens and possibly other hormones have an effect on its secretion. The androgen connection accounts for the higher RBC count in men than in women.[15] A negative feedback system is established, with hypoxemia being a stimulus for erythropoietin and resulting in increased production of RBCs (Fig. 19-7). The hypoxic stimulus is relieved, so that both the stimulus for erythropoietin synthesis and the rate of erythropoiesis decrease.

ANTIGENIC PROPERTIES OF ERYTHROCYTES

More than 300 RBC antigens have been identified, the molecular structure of which is determined by genes at various chromosomal loci.[16] Because distinct RBC antigenic properties are genetically determined, the antigens and antibodies are almost never precisely the same among individuals. The antigens in the blood of one person may react with plasma or cells of another, especially during or after a blood transfusion. The antibody to the RBC antigen attaches to the antigenic sites and may cause hemolysis or agglutination of the RBCs.

Blood is classified into different groups and typed according to the antigens present on the red cell mem-

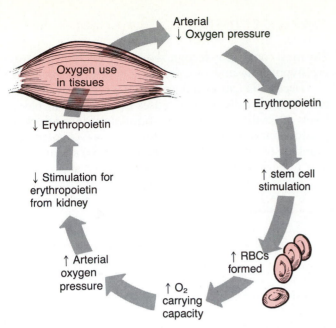

FIGURE 19-7 *Feedback mechanism for maintaining red blood cell population.*

brane. The term *blood group* refers to any well-defined system of RBC antigens; 21 systems are recognized.[11] The term *blood type* refers to identification of the antigens to determine a person's blood group. The antigens most commonly present on RBC membranes are antigens A, B, and Rh. These make up the ABO system of antigens and the Rh system (Table 19-3). A person may inherit neither of these antigens (type O) or one (A or B) or both (A and B). Type O blood is referred to as the universal donor because it lacks A or B antigens. Type AB blood, referred to as the universal recipient, contains neither anti-A nor anti-B antibodies. Either may contain other antigens that can account for a blood transfusion reaction.

The Rh type is determined by the presence or absence of particular antigens on the RBC. Type Rh negative refers to the absence of these antigens, and Rh positive refers to the presence of these antigens. There are six types of Rh factors: C, D, E, c, d, and e. The most common is D, which, when present, accounts for the Rh + (positive) designation. Blood that does not have the D antigen is called Rh − (negative). The other factors are considered in blood transfusion reactions. Eighty-five percent of whites and 95% of African Americans in the United States are Rh + .[9, 17] Types A and B surface antigens are called *agglutinogens*, and plasma antibodies that can cause agglutination are called *agglutinins*. Antibodies to the agglutinogens are almost always present if the agglutinogen is not present on a person's RBCs.[10] For example, anti-A agglutinins are present in the plasma of someone who does not have a type A agglutinogen.

DESTRUCTION OF ERYTHROCYTES

When RBCs are released into the circulation from bone marrow, they have a limited life span of about 120 days. The metabolism of glucose begins to fail in the aging erythrocytes, causing a gradual decrease in the amount of available adenosine triphosphate (ATP). Without an adequate supply of ATP, the cells are no longer able to maintain functions that are essential for life. The fragile cell membrane may rupture when passing through a tight spot in the circulation, such as the spleen, or it may be taken up by macrophages in the spleen, liver, or bone marrow. After lysis of the RBC, hemoglobin is reduced, releasing iron, which is then recycled. After the iron is removed, the remainder of the components in the heme molecule are converted to bilirubin. Bilirubin is taken to the liver to be conjugated with glucuronide (see p. 809).

A few RBCs undergo intravascular destruction. When the RBC membrane is damaged, hemoglobin moves out of the cells and quickly becomes bound with a plasma globulin called *haptoglobin*. The resulting complex prevents renal excretion of hemoglobin. The complex is then taken up by phagocytic cells in the liver and processed. When the amount of hemoglobin presented for uptake exceeds renal absorptive capacity, free hemoglobin and methemoglobin appear in the urine.[9] The membranous remains of RBCs are called "ghosts" when they are present in blood samples.

▼ Polycythemia

No general agreement has been reached regarding the use of the term *erythrocytosis* versus the term *polycythemia*. The term polycythemia is the more commonly used term for an increase above normal of circulating RBCs.[13] Erythrocytosis is a term used more frequently now for conditions of *absolute* or *secondary polycythemia*, in which there is an actual increase in total RBC mass. Erythrocytosis denotes an increase in RBCs secondary to

TABLE 19-3 *Blood Groups*

Percentage of Population	Type	
44	O:	neither antigen A nor B
43	A:	antigen A on RBC; no anti-A antibodies; contains anti-B antibodies
9	B:	antigen B on RBC; no anti-B antibodies; contains anti-A antibodies
4	AB:	both antigen A and antigen B on RBC; no anti-A; no anti-B antibodies in plasma
85	D	RH +
15	NoD	RH −

a known stimulus, whereas *polycythemia vera* refers to a primary myeloproliferative disorder.

Relative polycythemia, or *spurious polycythemia,* occurs when, through plasma loss, the concentration of RBCs becomes greater than normal in the circulating blood.[13] The term *myeloproliferative disorders* includes a large group of syndromes whose common denominator is the ability to proliferate hematopoietic elements. Table 19-4 lists the classifications and causes of polycythemia along with pertinent laboratory features.

ERYTHROCYTOSIS

The most commonly recognized causes of erythrocytosis are hypoxemia and overproduction of erythropoietin.

Hypoxemia causes a decrease in oxygen availability to the tissue cells, which causes an increase in blood levels of erythropoietin. This stimulates the marrow to produce more RBCs and causes a release of increased numbers of reticulocytes. In the process of acclimatization to high altitudes which have a low atmospheric

---

TABLE 19-4 *Causes of Polycythemia*

Clinical Pathophysiologic Mechanisms	Salient Laboratory Features
Normal RBC mass (spurious polycythemia)	Normal measured (^{51}Cr) red blood cell mass
Acute: hemoconcentration (eg, dehydration)	Decreased plasma volume
Chronic: Spurious or relative	
(stress; Gaisböck's syndrome)	
Increased RBC mass (absolute polycythemia)	Increased measured (^{51}Cr) red blood cell mass
Neonatal: physiologic	
Familial: altered hemoglobin structure or	Decreased P_{50} of whole blood
function	Left shift in oxygen dissociation curve
Decreased 2,3-diphosphoglycerate (DPG)	Decreased P_{50} of whole blood
DPG mutase deficiency	
Hereditary high adenosine triphosphate	
Autonomous erythropoietin production	Increased erythropoietin
Acquired	
Primary: polycythemia vera	Splenomegaly
	Increased platelets and white blood cells
	Increased vitamin B_{12} and B_{12}-binding proteins
Secondary to decreased arterial oxygen	Arterial oxygen saturation tension below 92%
High altitudes	
Pulmonary diseases with hypoventilation	Pao$_2$ below 65 mm Hg
Cardiovascular shunts	
Secondary to decreased oxygen-carrying	Direct measurement:
capacity	Carboxyhemoglobin
Elevated carboxyhemoglobin	
("smoker's polycythemia")	
Methemoglobinemia	Methemoglobin
Secondary to decrease oxygen delivery	Decreased P_{50} of whole blood
Hemoglobin with altered structure or func-	Left shift in oxygen dissociation curve
tion: high oxygen affinity for hemoglobin	
(see Familial)	
Secondary to aberrant (inappropriate)	Increased erythropoietin
erythropoietin production	
Renal: renal artery stenosis, systemic dis-	
ease, renal cell carcinoma, transplant	
rejection	
Liver: hepatoma	
Uterus: leiomyoma	
Adrenal: pheochromocytoma	
Secondary to blood transfusion	
("blood doping")	
Secondary to administration of erythropoietin	
Secondary to other hormones	Hormone assays
Cushing's syndrome	
Androgens	

(Source: Kelley, W. N. *Textbook of Internal Medicine* [2nd ed.] Philadelphia: J.B. Lippincott, 1992)

oxygen level, physiologic erythrocytosis occurs. The plasma volume reduces, RBC volume slowly rises, and total hemoglobin increases, resulting in an increase in total blood volume. Hypoxemia often is noted in patients with pulmonic disease, and many of those affected have an associated erythrocytosis. Heavy smokers often have an increased hematocrit level, which is probably due to either an increase in RBC mass or a decrease in plasma volume or both. This probably results from the high carbon monoxide levels in cigarette smoke that displace oxygen from the hemoglobin and reduce oxygen content.

Overproduction of erythropoietin results when there is inappropriate, excessive production of erythropoietin. This condition has been associated with renal disease, malignant tumors, or conditions in which there is a disturbance of renal blood flow. Secondary polycythemia is always related to elevated levels of circulating erythropoietin, and the bone marrow remains normal without proliferation of the leukocytes. As stated above, this proliferation of erythropoietin may represent a normal renal response to tissue hypoxia, or it may result from production of erythropoietin from an outside or uncontrolled source.[12]

The pathogenesis of chronic spurious polycythemia is not known, but a condition of chronic plasma depletion is present.[12] This condition has been seen with hypertensive individuals, often males. Smoking and high blood pressure have been considered to cause the volume depletion, and treatment of any vascular insufficiency through phlebotomy may be considered.[12]

POLYCYTHEMIA VERA

Polycythemia vera is a myeloproliferative disorder in which there is increased production of all the formed elements (RBCs, granulocytes, and platelets) of blood. The cause of this condition is unknown. Polycythemia vera must be differentiated from polycythemia secondary to excessive erythropoietin secretion. It is associated with normal or lower-than-normal levels of serum and excreted erythropoietin.[9] The condition is relatively rare, occurring slightly more frequently in men than in women and between ages 50 and 70.[14]

The abnormal proliferation often initially involves both white and red elements of the marrow. Thrombocytosis and erythrocytosis may be much greater than normal values. Evidence supports the belief that the disease is a neoplastic disorder that stimulates abnormal erythropoietin-hypersensitive stem cells while suppressing normal stem cells.[14]

The results of the proliferating cellular elements are increases in RBC count, blood viscosity, and blood volume. The liver and spleen become congested and packed with RBCs. The thick blood causes stasis and thrombosis in many areas, which may lead to infarction in any area. Vascular thrombosis mainly results from associated

elevated platelet levels.[5] The course of the disease may change, resulting in aplastic, fibrotic, or even leukemic bone marrow.[9] The polycythemia may be gradually replaced by an anemia. The cause of anemia or leukemic change may be related to the effects of the chemotherapy used to treat the disease.[1] A terminal acute myeloblastic leukemia is seen to result in patients treated with chlorambucil or marrow irradiation.[9]

The clinical onset of polycythemia vera is insidious. Most symptoms appear to be related to the increased blood volume, increased blood viscosity, and changes in cerebral blood flow. Light-headedness, visual disturbances, headaches, and vertigo may be described. Ruddy cyanosis of the face usually is apparent. Pruritus is a common complaint, possibly caused by histamine release from the basophils.[18] Increased cardiac work may be manifested by eventual congestive heart failure. Thrombophlebitis and thrombosis of digital arteries, accompanied by gangrene, may occur. Associated laboratory values are increased hematocrit, hemoglobin, RBC mass, basophils, eosinophils, neutrophils, thrombocytes, leukocyte alkaline phosphatase, serum B_{12} and B_{12}-binding protein, and uric acid. The RBC count may be 7 to 9 million/μL or higher, and the total blood volume is elevated.

▼ Anemias

The term anemia refers to a condition in which there is a decrease in hemoglobin concentration, the number of circulating RBCs, or the volume of packed cells (hematocrit) compared with normal values. Anemias usually are categorized according to cause or morphology (Table 19-5). To diagnose the type of anemia present, one must determine the underlying mechanism of the disease. Almost all anemias can be divided into two kinds: 1) those caused by impaired RBC formation and 2) those caused by excessive loss or destruction of RBCs.[19] The reticulocyte count is of primary importance in diagnosis, as are the size, shape, color, and hemoglobin content of RBCs as determined on blood smear. Morphologic characteristics of RBCs usually are used in the classification of anemias. The terms used include the following:

1. *Normocytic/normochromic*: Normal size and color of RBCs imparted from hemoglobin concentration
2. *Microcytic/hypochromic*: Decreased size and color of RBCs caused by inadequate hemoglobin concentrations
3. *Macrocytic*: Large size of RBCs
4. *Anisocytosis*: Variations in RBC size
5. *Poikilocytosis*: Variations in RBC shape

Alterations in RBC size or hemoglobin content are common in anemias related to deficiencies of iron, folate, or vitamin B_{12}. The shape of the cells gives valuable clues in diagnosis of inherited membrane abnor-

TABLE 19-5 *Classification of Anemias*

Type	Morphologic Characteristics	Causes
Aplastic	Normocytic, normochromic RBCs, depletion of leukocytes and platelets	Drug toxicity Genetic failure Radiation Chemicals Infections
Hemolytic	Normocytic, normochromic, increased number of reticulocytes	Mechanical injury RBC antigen–antibody reaction Complement binding Chemical reactions Hereditary membrane defects
Macrocytic or megaloblastic; pernicious or folic acid	Macrocytic with variation in size (anisocytosis), shape (poikilocytosis) of RBCs	Inadequate diet Lack of intrinsic factor for pernicious anemia Impaired absorption
Microcytic; iron deficiency; chronic blood loss	Microcytic; hypochromic	Inadequate diet Blood loss, chronic Increased need
Posthemorrhagic; acute hemorrhage	Normocytic, normochromic, increased number of reticulocytes within 48–72 h	Loss of blood leading to hemodilution from interstitial fluid within 48–72 h Internal or external hemorrhage, leading to blood volume depletion

malities, hemolytic anemias, and hemoglobinopathies. In addition, the blood smear provides information regarding RBC inclusions. Increased stimulus for erythrocyte production is indicated by an increased number of reticulocytes or normoblasts in the peripheral blood.

APLASTIC ANEMIA

Aplastic anemia occurs as a result of reduced bone marrow function and causes a drop in levels of all blood elements. The number of pleuripotent stem cells appears to decrease, and the blood-forming cells are not formed or matured. A severe anemia results, with the formed RBCs sometimes appearing morphologically as slightly macrocytic. The cells also may be normocytic and normochromic.

The cause of aplastic anemia is poorly understood, and in more than one-half of cases, it is unknown.[10] Genetic failure of bone marrow development or injury to stem cells may prohibit the cells' reproduction and differentiation. Physical agents, such as whole-body irradiation, have been implicated. Chemical agents that may cause aplastic anemia include cytotoxic drugs used for treatment of malignant disease; antimicrobial agents, such as chloramphenicol; anticonvulsants; and antiinflammatory drugs. Aplastic anemia also may occur as a sequelae to systemic infections. Box 19-2 lists some of the factors that can cause aplastic anemia.

A routine blood examination and marrow aspiration and biopsy provide essential information regarding bone marrow function. The marrow is hypocellular or, in rare cases, hypercellular. Marrow biopsy reveals large areas of fat with clusters of lymphocytes, reticular cells, and plasma cells. Uptake of iron by the marrow is decreased, and serum iron is increased. Smears most frequently show normocytic, normochromic RBCs that are profoundly decreased in number.[9]

The onset of symptoms is variable and usually gradual. Symptoms often are associated with the progressive anemia and concomitant decrease in oxygen transport. Weakness, dyspnea, headaches, and syncope are common. Symptoms resulting from associated leukopenia (decreased white blood cells) include decreased immunologic defense and recurrent infections. The associated thrombocytopenia (decreased platelets) is variable, with bleeding tendencies ranging from formation of small petechiae to severe bleeding.

Bone marrow transplantation may be a treatment option for the younger person with refractory aplastic anemia if a compatible family donor is available. Blood components may be replaced by blood transfusions to allow time for bone marrow to recover in cases of transient marrow failure. Therapy with drugs and other chemical agents should be discontinued until recovery of the bone marrow begins. Splenectomy may be indicated if active hemolysis is associated.

The prognosis of aplastic anemia varies, depending on the causative agent. Gradual recovery of hematopoiesis can occur once the agent is discontinued. Severe, progressive anemia is a poor prognostic sign, with infec-

(Source: Kelley, W. N. *Textbook of Internal Medicine* [2nd ed.]. Philadelphia: J.B. Lippincott, 1992).

BOX 19-2 ▼ Causes of Aplastic Anemia

Congenital

Acquired
Drugs
Chemotherapeutic drugs
Antiinflammatory
　Phenylbutazone
　Indocin
　Gold
Antibiotics
　Chloramphenicol
　Sulfonamide
Sulfonylurea
　Chlorpropamide
　Tolbutamide
Antiseizure
　Phenytoin
　Trimethadione
Quinacrine

Toxins
Benzene
Toluene (glue) and trinitrotoluene
Arsenic
Insecticides
Paint thinner
Lacquers
Infections
Hepatitis non-A, non-B
Mononucleosis
Radiation
Immune suppression
Pregnancy

Hereditary spherocytosis is an inherited autosomal dominant condition that results in a molecular defect on the RBC membrane.[26] The RBCs are spheric and are prematurely destroyed in the spleen. The cells rapidly hemolyze in a hypotonic solution.[16,25]

Clinical signs depend on the amount of hemolysis present and can include jaundice, splenomegaly, and signs of anemia. The splenic enlargement is characteristic and is a key determinant in clinical expression.[19] Crises in hereditary spherocytosis are related to associated problems, such as infections, especially parvovirus, and gallstones.[20]

Acquired immune hemolytic anemia results from destruction of the RBCs by the immune system. It is diagnosed by the Coombs' test. A *positive direct Coombs' test* means that a plasma protein, usually IgG or complement, has become fixed to the surface of an RBC. The type involving IgG is associated with lymphoma, systemic lupus erythematosis, and drug reactions, or it may

tion and hemorrhage being the most frequent causes of death.

Red Blood Cell Aplasia

Pure RBC aplasia is much less common than aplastic anemia. It is characterized by severe normocytic, normochromic anemia with no reticulocyte response.[10] It may be congenital, immunologically mediated, drug-induced, or preleukemic, or it can occur after a viral infection. RBC aplasia frequently is secondary to end-stage renal failure (see p. 665).

HEMOLYTIC ANEMIA

The life span of the RBC may be shortened by intrinsic or extrinsic factors that adversely affect the cell; the shortening may be compensated for by an increase in erythrocyte production. Hemolytic anemias can be classified in numerous ways. Categories often overlap, and no classification seems to be satisfactory. A classification of hemolytic anemias by mechanism of RBC injury is found in Box 19-3, which indicates the wide diversity of causative conditions. The more common diseases are discussed in greater detail below.

Abnormalities of the Red Cell Membrane and Metabolic Deficiencies

These inherited and acquired disorders of the RBC membrane include such conditions as hereditary spherocytosis, acquired immune hemolytic anemia, and glucose-6-phosphate dehydrogenase deficiency.

BOX 19-3 ▼ Classification of Hemolytic Anemias by Mechanism of Red Blood Cell Injury

Abnormalities of Membrane and Shape
Hereditary
　Spherocytosis
　Elliptocytosis
　Stomatocytosis
Acquired
　Immune hemolytic anemia (spherocytes)
　Anemia of liver disease (acanthocytes, stomatocytes, target cells)
　Anemia of uremia (echinocytes)
　Exotoxinemia (spherocytes)
　Membrane sensitivity to complement—paroxysmal nocturnal hemoglobinuria

Metabolic Deficiencies
Hexose-monophosphate shunt enzyme deficiencies
Glycolytic pathway enzyme deficiencies
Purine and pyrimidine pathway enzyme deficiencies

Hemoglobinopathies
Disorders of hemoglobin structure
　Sickling disorders
　Hemoglobin C, D, and E disorders
　Unstable hemoglobins
Disorders of hemoglobin synthesis
　Thalassemias: α-, β- and related disorders

Physical Red Blood Cell Injury
Fragmentation hemolytic anemias
　Microangiopathic
　Heart valve hemolysis
Thermal and chemical hemolysis
Red blood cell parasitization (malaria, babesiosis)

(Source: Kelley, W. N. *Textbook of Internal Medicine* [2nd ed.]. Philadelphia: J.B. Lippincott, 1992).

be idiopathic.[24] Some people with this type of disease have an antibody against a specific antigen on their own RBCs.

The IgG-related Coombs' test agglutination of RBCs sometimes is called *warm antibody disease*, because antibody-coated cells adhere to macrophages in the spleen and precipitate RBC destruction at 37°C. Cold antibody disease is mediated through the IgM antibodies, which, at temperatures below 30°C, trigger the complement sequence that destroys RBC membranes, leading to loss of hemoglobin.[26] Most cold antibody disease is idiopathic, but it has been described with some of the myeloproliferative disorders. Hemolysis is localized to those body parts exposed to cold temperatures.[9]

The *indirect Coombs' test* uses normal RBCs exposed first to the suspected serum and then crossed with the Coombs' serum, which induces agglutination of RBCs if anti-RBC antibodies are present in the suspected serum. It often is used as a screening test to detect the presence of antibodies, especially in cross-matching blood for transfusions. Both direct and indirect Coombs' tests may be positive, especially in relation to drugs such as penicillin, quinidine, quinine, and methyldopa.[23] The signs and symptoms of anemia, hemolysis, and fever often are temporal and remit after the drug is withdrawn.

Blood transfusion reactions are a good example of secondary defects of the red cell membrane. These reactions are immunologically mediated and directed at the antigens in the transfused blood that are deemed foreign. Flowchart 19-1 shows the process and the results of the immune attack. Major hemolysis usually results from incompatibilities of the ABO system or, occasionally, the Rh factor.[16] Other hemolytic reactions may be directed toward any of the other RBC antigens. Hemolysis usually occurs intravascularly, but it also may occur in extravascular spaces. Symptoms of the reaction usually involve the sudden onset of restlessness, anxiety, fever, chills, flushing, chest or back pain, nausea, vomiting, and then early onset of disseminated intravascular coagulation, renal failure, and shock. Laboratory tests show hemoglobinemia, elevated bilirubin, and often a positive direct Coombs' test.[16] Early identification of the reaction and stopping further blood transfusion may be lifesaving. Table 19-6 indicates factors to consider in differential diagnosis of acute transfusion reactions.

Glucose-6-phosphate dehydrogenase deficiency is a deficiency of this X-linked RBC enzyme. It occurs in 13% of African American males, and 25% of African American females are carriers. Levels of the enzyme reflect the susceptibility of the carrier to hemolysis. One in four

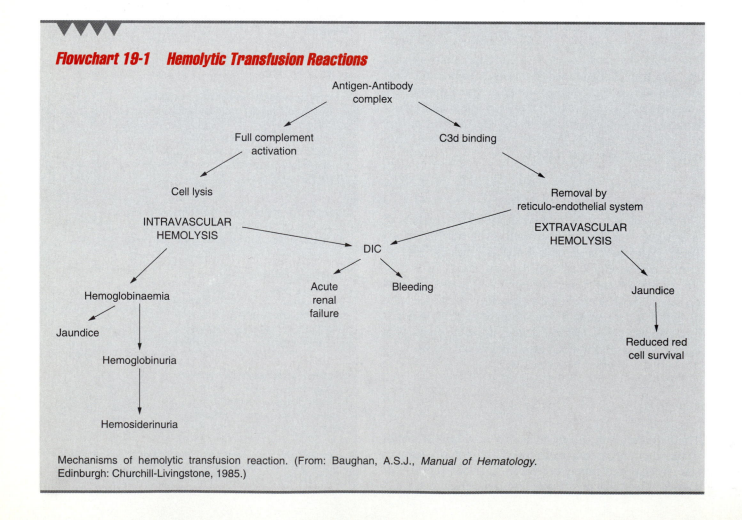

Flowchart 19-1 Hemolytic Transfusion Reactions

Mechanisms of hemolytic transfusion reaction. (From: Baughan, A.S.J., *Manual of Hematology.* Edinburgh: Churchill-Livingstone, 1985.)

TABLE 19-6 *Differential Diagnosis of Acute Transfusion Reactions*

Clinical Feature	Possible Diagnosis
Fever and chills	Major hemolytic transfusion reaction
	Reaction to foreign HLA antigens on transfused white blood cells and platelets
	Contaminated blood
Dyspnea	Fluid overload
	Major hemolytic transfusion reaction
	Contaminated blood
	Air embolism
	Anaphylactic reaction due to transfusion of IgA-containing plasma to IgA-deficient recipient with anti-IgA
	Pulmonary leukoagglutinin
Bleeding	Disseminated intravascular coagulation due to major hemolytic transfusion reaction or contaminated blood
	Thrombocytopenia due to massive transfusion of packed red blood cells
	Washout of coagulation factors due to massive transfusion of packed red blood cells
Arrhythmia	Circulatory overload
	Hyperkalemia
	Hypothermia
	Hypocalcemia
	Major hemolytic transfusion reaction
	Contaminated blood
	Air embolism
Hypotension	Major hemolytic transfusion reaction
	Contaminated blood
	Anaphylaxis due to IgA deficiency
Hemoglobinuria	Major hemolytic transfusion reaction
	Excessive infusion pressure through small-bore needle
	Overheating with blood warmer
	Contaminated blood

(Source: Kelley, W. N. *Textbook of Internal Medicine* [2nd ed.] Philadelphia: J.B. Lippincott, 1992)

carriers is subject to hemolysis. Oxidant drugs, such as sulfonamides and primaquine, may precipitate the development of hemolysis in susceptible people. Conditions that may precipitate an acute hemolytic episode include viral or bacterial infections and diabetic ketoacidosis. Two main variants of the disease have been described, with profound hemolytic anemia occurring in affected African blacks and people of Mediterranean descent. Once the infection is controlled or the triggering drug discontinued, recovery usually occurs.[16, 26]

Hemoglobinopathies

Hemoglobinopathies are inherited disorders that are characterized by structural variations of hemoglobin. Two related genetic disorders are described as *sickle syndromes: sickle cell trait* and *sickle cell anemia*. These syndromes occur almost exclusively in blacks and are demonstrated by the curved shape of the RBCs when they are exposed to decreased oxygen tension. About 10% of blacks carry HbS on the hemoglobin molecule and about 0.2% exhibit the actual disease.[9] The designation HbS is given when there is substitution of an amino acid (valine) for the normal glutamic acid. The sickle cell trait is carried by heterozygous individuals; sickle cell anemia occurs when an individual is homozygous.

The altered amino acid sequence alters the solubility of hemoglobin. At low blood pH and with decreased oxygen tension, the HbS precipitates out of solution, and the cells become sickle-shaped and then become stuck in the small vessels.[3] After vascular obstruction, there is hemolysis of the RBCs. Symptoms depend on the number of hemolyzed and sickled RBCs.

Most people with the sickle cell trait have no symptoms unless they suffer a hypoxic episode, during which some hemolysis and anemia may be noted. Because the sickle cell trait is heterozygous, RBCs require very low oxygen tension to precipitate the characteristic sickling effect, and overall RBC life span usually is not affected.

Sickle cell anemia causes symptoms beginning at about 6 months of age. The hemoglobin, HbS, when deoxygenated, distorts the RBC into a sickle or holly-leaf shape. Small blood vessels become blocked by aggregates of these sickle cells, and the blood supply to all parts of the body may be compromised. The damaged RBCs are trapped in the spleen, and the entire organ eventually may become infarcted.

Infections or hypertonic plasma greatly increase the chances of sickling. As the RBCs obstruct blood flow to the tissues, further deoxygenation and more sickling occurs. The characteristic shape usually returns to normal when oxygen again becomes available.

Hemolysis occurs when RBCs assume the sickle form, and average RBC survival time becomes 10 to 15 days. Bilirubin is released from the hemoglobin during hemolysis, and jaundice may become evident when increased conjugated and unconjugated bilirubin accumulates in the plasma.

The bone marrow often becomes hyperplastic, with evidence of increased erythropoiesis. Reticulocytes and even normoblasts may be released into the circulating blood.

Signs and symptoms of sickle cell anemia vary in severity from sickle crisis in acute hemolysis to impairment of growth and maturity. Because of increased susceptibility to infections, especially those caused by pneumococci, repeated episodes of painful crisis occur. These result from microinfarcts from the vasoocclusive phenomenon.[9] Anemia usually is severe, with most of the hemolysis occurring in the extravascular spaces. Chronic leg ulcers, attacks of abdominal pain, and neurologic complications of sudden onset are common. Joint pains may mimic osteomyelitis, and joint effusions are frequent. Any organ may be permanently impaired. Flowchart 19-2 summarizes the pathogenesis of sickle cell anemia. Severe renal impairment may lead to frank renal failure. The prognosis for sickle cell anemia is improving, and with proper oxygenation and hydration, more persons are surviving to adulthood.

Thalassemias are intrinsic, congenital disorders that result from defects in the synthesis of hemoglobin and cause a hypochromic, microcytic anemia. They are classified as *major* and *minor*, according to the features of the disease. Defects of both beta and alpha chains are known, and many forms have been diagnosed according to the number of these defects. Disease involving defects of beta-chain synthesis occurs most frequently in inhabitants of the Mediterranean areas, Central Africa, Asia, the South Pacific, and parts of India. Defects in alpha-chain synthesis are most frequent among southern Asians. The effects vary markedly, depending on whether the disorders are heterozygous or homozygous.[26]

Thalassemia major is homozygous and exhibits ineffective erythropoiesis and peripheral hemolysis, which stimulates enlargement of the red marrow to increase RBC formation. Sometimes the liver also becomes involved in erythropoiesis, resulting in hepatomegaly. Clinical manifestations include profound anemia, wasting, jaundice, hepatomegaly, and characteristic ''chipmunk'' facies. Typical expansion of the bone marrow leads to thin cortical bone, causing enlargement of the bones of the face and jaws. The long bones become vulnerable to fracture. Growth retardation is common, as are marked splenomegaly and hepatomegaly. Death may occur early in fetal life, and the condition is diagnosed with severe hemolytic anemia along with hypochromic, microcytic RBCs.[2, 26] A less severe form of the disease may permit the homozygote to survive to adulthood, and transfusion therapy has diminished some of the effects.[26]

Thalassemia minor is a heterozygous disorder that may be diagnosed in studies of persons having chronic, asymptomatic, mild anemia. It is diagnosed by blood smear and must be differentiated from iron deficiency anemia.[26]

Direct Physical Trauma

Direct physical trauma to RBCs can induce hemolytic anemias. External trauma from blows, as may be inflicted in the martial arts, usually is self-limiting. Turbulent blood flow also can cause trauma to the RBCs. Trauma to circulating RBCs has been reported from prolonged exercise, artificial cardiac valves, extracorporeal circulation devices, and conditions in which fibrin deposited in the microvasculature causes fragmentation of RBCs. The results include mild to severe hemolysis and bilirubinemia. The degree of hemolysis is related to the severity of the symptomatology; for example, artificial cardiac valves may be replaced if significant hemolysis is noted.

MATURATION-FAILURE ANEMIA

Megaloblastic anemias refer to those that demonstrate large, immature, poorly functional erythrocytes. The two most common causes are vitamin B_{12} deficiency and folate deficiency. Other conditions, such as drug-induced suppression and inborn errors, also may produce this type of anemia (Box 19-4).

Pernicious Anemia

Vitamin B_{12} deficiency usually results from malabsorption of the vitamin because of a deficiency of the intrinsic factor that protects the vitamin so that it can be absorbed in the ileum (see p. 767). Pernicious anemia, which results from this deficiency, occurs most frequently in people older than age 60 who have fair complexions and a family history of the disease.

Flowchart 19-2   Pathophysiology of Sickle Cell Anemia

```
Arterial pO2          →    Capillary Venous pO2
oxy Hb S                   deoxy Hb S
(soluble)                  (polymerized)
                                 ↓
Stiff, viscous        ←    Membrane changes
sickled cell               Ca++ influx, K+ leakage
     ↓                           ↓
Capillary venule          Shortened red cell
occlusion                 survival
                          (hemolytic anemia)
     ↓                           ↓
Micronfarction            Anemia
Ischemic tissue pain      Jaundice
Ischemic organ malfunction Gallstones
Autoinfarction of spleen  Leg ulcers
```

Pathophysiology of sickle cell anemia. The diagram summarizes the pathogenesis of the dual stigmata of sickle cell disease, hemolytic anemia, and vasoocclusive crises. (Adapted from: Kelly, W.N. [ed.]. *Textbook of Internal Medicine* [2nd ed.] Philadephia: J.B. Lippincott, 1992.)

The onset of symptoms usually is insidious but may be hastened by conditions such as infection. Persons with pernicious anemia do not secrete hydrochloric acid (on gastric analysis) even after parenteral stimulation with histamine. Many of the signs and symptoms of pernicious anemia are common to any of the anemic states. Anorexia, fatigue, shortness of breath, and irritability are common. Soreness of the tongue characteristically occurs early in the illness and progressively worsens. The soreness is quickly relieved after adequate vitamin B_{12} treatment. Symmetric numbness and tingling of the toes and fingers occur in 10% of these people, and this may indicate early neurologic disease. Ataxia and loss of vibration sense also may be noted. Neurologic symptoms may not entirely remit after treatment.

Folic Acid Anemia

A deficiency of folic acid produces anemia with characteristics similar to those of pernicious anemia. The two conditions cannot be distinguished morphologically. The RBCs are large (megaloblastic) with fragile membranes. A definite dietary deficiency can be demonstrated, and the anemia develops 1 to 2 months after a continued dietary deficiency. Folic acid anemia is common in alcoholism and chronic malnutrition. Increased frequency during pregnancy relates also to poor nutrition.[4] It usually responds well to oral dietary replacement unless malabsorption is a problem.

IRON DEFICIENCY ANEMIA

Iron deficiency anemia is characterized by deficient hemoglobin synthesis caused by a lack of iron. With severe deficiency, the RBCs become *microcytic* and *hypochromic* because of low concentrations of hemoglobin. This is the most common type of anemia, and it occurs in all geographic locations and in all age groups.[19] The main causes of iron deficiency are increased loss, as in chronic or acute bleeding, and decreased dietary intake. The blood lost during menstruation accounts for a high frequency of iron deficiency in women. Iron deficiency is common among preschool children, presumably because of increased dietary need and poor dietary supply.[6]

Because iron is absorbed mostly in the duodenum and its ionization and absorption are enhanced by gastric hydrochloric acid, iron deficiency anemia may accompany pernicious anemia or gastrectomy. Also, malabsorption syndromes impair absorption of iron along with other nutrients.

Laboratory values reflect decreased levels of serum iron and apoferritin (iron-binding protein produced by the liver) in the early stages. Normal serum iron levels range from 60 to 190 µg/dL or 13 to 31 mol/L (SI units), but 20% of affected adults have normal iron indices.[23]

Vitamin B_{12} normally binds chemically with the intrinsic factor that promotes its absorption. In certain conditions, such as atrophy of the gastric mucosal cells, lack of secretion of the intrinsic factor leads to malabsorption of vitamin B_{12}. Normal erythrocyte maturation is dependent on adequate amounts of vitamin B_{12} for the synthesis of DNA molecules. Without B_{12}, a *macrocytic* or *megaloblastic anemia* results, with marked anisocytosis (variation in RBC size) and poikilocytosis (variation in RBC shape). Ineffective erythropoiesis and increased erythroblast destruction result in hyperbilirubinemia. Although the most pronounced changes arise in the RBCs, mild neutropenia and thrombocytopenia also may occur.

Anemia, characterized by microcytic and variably sized hypochromic RBCs, is a relatively late manifestation.[23]

Clinical manifestations are nonspecific, and their onset is insidious. Fatigue, tachycardia, irritability, and pallor with epithelial abnormalities, such as sore tongue or stomatitis, may occur. Thinning or spooning of the nails (koilonychia) occasionally is encountered (Fig. 19-8). Pica may be striking, with affected people craving dirt, starch, or ice.[6,21] Late manifestations may include cardiac murmurs, congestive heart failure, loss of hair, and pearly sclera.

POSTHEMORRHAGIC ANEMIA

Posthemorrhagic anemia may occur after acute or chronic blood loss, although chronic blood loss usually results in iron deficiency anemia. Plasma and RBCs are both lost during a hemorrhage, so laboratory values may reveal a normal hemoglobin level and RBC count immediately after a hemorrhage. The dominant clinical picture is that of hypovolemia and shock.

Blood volume is restored by the movement of fluid from the interstitial spaces into the capillaries, causing dilution of the remaining RBCs (dilutional anemia) with a maximum effect in 48 to 72 hours. This dilute blood carries too few RBCs to efficiently oxygenate the tissues. Anemia of a normocytic and normochromic type becomes apparent. The bone marrow is stimulated to produce increased numbers of RBCs, but this process requires a period of time that varies according to the amount of blood lost. Within 7 days, the reticulocyte count can be elevated to 15%.[26] In acute massive bleeding, this compensatory effect may not occur in time to be lifesaving without transfusions of whole blood.

ANEMIAS ASSOCIATED WITH CHRONIC DISEASE

Anemias of chronic disease are those which exhibit a mild-to moderate decrease in hemoglobin concentration. There is a decrease in the proliferation of RBCs and a shortened RBC survival.[27] This very common anemia is associated with various types of infections, autoimmune diseases, neoplastic diseases, and inflammatory disorders (Box 19-5). The reticulocyte count is less than 2%, and the RBC morphology is normochromic and normocytic.

This condition has an insidious onset; the symptoms

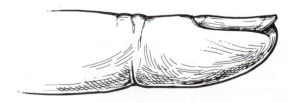

FIGURE 19-8 *Spoon-shaped nails in iron deficiency anemia.*

BOX 19-5 ▼ **Some Causes of Anemia from Chronic Disease**

Superimposed Infections
  Acute bacterial, viral, or fungal
Chronic Infections
  Osteomyelitis
  Tuberculosis
  Chronic fungal diseases
  Chronic bladder and kidney infection
  Chronic hepatitis
Chronic Inflammatory Disorders
  Systemic lupus erythematosus
  Collagen vascular diseases
  Rheumatoid arthritis
  Osteoarthritis
Malnutrition
  Cirrhosis of the liver
  Pancreatitis
  Dietary inadequacy
Malignancy
  Any metastatic carcinoma or sarcoma
  Any hematologic malignancy

---

are vague, with pallor and fatigue, and they must be differentiated from iron deficiency anemia.[21] Treatment is aimed at control of the underlying disease process.

CASE STUDY 19-1

Millie Pallor, 44-year-old woman, was seen by her family physician because she was feeling worn-out and unable to carry out activities of daily living. She indicated that her menstrual periods were very heavy, lasting 8 to 9 days and occurring every 21 days. She also reported that she had been dieting to lose 20 pounds. Examination revealed a thin, pale woman with spooning of the nails and thin, lifeless hair.

1. *What is the most probable diagnosis for this woman? What laboratory test would be used and what would confirm the diagnosis suspected?*
2. *Compare the pathophysiology, clinical picture, and laboratory features of the different types of anemias.*
3. *What treatment would be effective in this form of anemia? What teaching should be used to prevent recurrence of this clinical picture?*

See Appendix G for discussion.

▼ Laboratory and Diagnostic Tests

HEMATOLOGIC STUDIES

Examination of the blood provides valuable information in the diagnosis and treatment of blood disorders. Normal hematologic values, summarized in Table 19-7, are based on the examination of statistically significant

Levels may be decreased in anemia or circulatory over-load and are increased in polycythemia.

Red Blood Cells

Erythrocytes are the mature circulating RBCs whose primary function is to transport oxygen and carbon dioxide. Increases and decreases in RBC counts usually vary in the same direction as the hemoglobin, as previously mentioned.

Packed Cell Volume or Hematocrit

The packed cell volume is the ratio of packed cells to total volume in a sample that has been centrifuged. The packed cell volume is used to determine RBC indices, calculate blood volume and total RBC mass, and roughly measure the concentration of RBCs.[23] Levels increase in conditions associated with hemoconcentration (burns, shock, and trauma), hypovolemia, and polycythemia. The hematocrit level decreases in hypervolemic states (cardiac failure, overhydration with intravenous fluid), hemorrhage, and hemolysis.

Erythrocyte Sedimentation Rate

Blood is a suspension of formed elements in plasma; therefore, when it is mixed with an anticoagulant and stands, the heavier RBCs sink to the bottom. The rate at which the RBCs settle is a function of fibrinogen and globulin. These proteins enhance clumping of erythrocytes, thus increasing the rate at which the cells fall. Other factors that affect the rate are alterations in the positive charge of plasma, the ratio of plasma protein fractions to each other, and changes in the erythrocyte surface.

The erythrocyte sedimentation rate is a nonspecific test, butbecause the sedimentation rate is increased in many inflammatory conditions, it can serve in the differential diagnosis in such conditions as acute myocardial infarction, angina pectoris, rheumatoid arthritis, and osteoarthritis. A moderately increased erythrocyte sedimentation rate often is noted in patients older than age 60.

Mean Corpuscular Volume

The mean corpuscular volume measures the volume and size of each RBC. The mean corpuscular volume increases in megaloblastic anemias (large cells) and decreases in iron deficiency (small cells).[23]

Mean Corpuscular Hemoglobin

The mean corpuscular hemoglobin gives the amount of hemoglobin by weight in the average RBC. Macrocytic cells with a large volume of hemoglobin show increased

---

TABLE 19-7 *Normal Hematologic Values*

RED BLOOD CELLS

Infant, 1 month	3.3–5.3 mL/mm^3
Child, 1 year	3.8–4.8 mL/mm^3
Child, 6–10 years	4.1–5.2 mL/mm^3
Adult	
Female	3.8–5.1 mL/mm^3
Male	4.3–5.7 mL/mm^3
Adult >65 years	3.8–5.8 mL/mm^3

HEMOGLOBIN

Infant, first day	14–20 g/dL
Child, 1 year	10–14 g/dL
Child, 6–10 years	11–15 g/dL
Adult	
Female	12–16 (1.86–2.48 nmol/L)
Male	13.5–17.5 (2.09–2.71 nmol/L)
Adult >65 years	11.7–17

VOLUME PACKED RBC (HEMATOCRIT)

Infant, first day	50%–62% (0.50–0.62 volume fraction)
Child, 1 year	32%–40% (0.3–0.4)
Child, 6–10 years	33%–43% (0.33–0.43)
Adult	
Female	37%–47% (0.37–0.47)
Male	40%–54% (0.40–0.54)
Adult >65 years	35%–50% (0.35–0.50)

ERYTHROCYTE SEDIMENTATION RATE (WESTERGREN METHOD)

Female	0–20 mm/h
Male	0–13 mm/h
Children	0–10 mm/h

MEAN CORPUSCULAR VOLUME

Female and male	87–103 μm^3

MEAN CORPUSCULAR HEMOGLOBIN

Female and male	26–34 pg/cell or 0.40–0.53 fmol/cell

MEAN CORPUSCULAR HEMOGLOBIN CONCENTRATION (MCHC)

Female and male	31–37 g/dL (41.81–57.1 mmol/Hgb/L)

RETICULOCYTE COUNT

Male	0.5%–1.5% of erythrocytes
Female	0.5%–2.5% of erythrocytes

Values summarized from: Fischbach, F. A *Manual of Laboratory and Diagnostic Tests* [4th ed.] Philadelphia: J.B. Lippincott, 1992.

---

numbers of healthy people. They vary with age, environment, sex, genetics, and physiologic state. The most important erythrocyte studies are discussed below.

Hemoglobin

The primary function of hemoglobin is to carry oxygen in the form of oxyhemoglobin; therefore, the oxygen-combining capacity of blood is directly proportional to the hemoglobin concentration. The hemoglobin level varies significantly with sex and age (see Box 19-5).

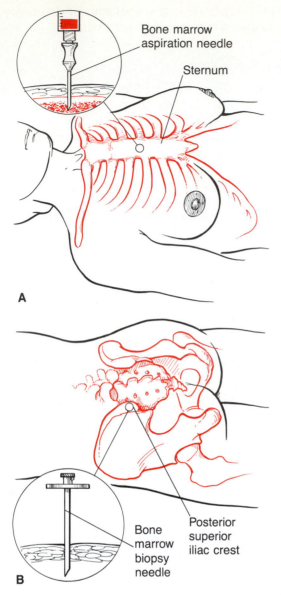

Bone marrow
aspiration needle

Sternum

A

Bone
marrow
biopsy
needle

Posterior
superior
iliac crest

B

FIGURE 19-9 *Technique and sites available for bone marrow aspiration for biopsy.*

levels, as in macrocytic anemia. Levels of mean corpuscular hemoglobin are decreased in conditions related to hemoglobin deficiency, as in iron deficiency anemia.

Mean Cell Hemoglobin Concentration

The mean cell hemoglobin concentration gives the average percentage of hemoglobin saturation or concentration of hemoglobin in the average red cell. Decreased levels occur in hemoglobin deficiency.

Reticulocyte Count

The reticulocyte is a young, nonnucleated cell of the erythrocyte line. An elevated reticulocyte count is indicative of increased bone marrow activity, with early release of increased numbers of reticulocytes, as in hemolytic anemias.

Bone Marrow Studies

Bone marrow may be obtained for examination by aspiration or biopsy. Data obtained from bone marrow examination are useful in the diagnosis, progression, and prognosis of blood disorders. Figure 19-9 shows a method for obtaining bone marrow contents for examination.

DIAGNOSTIC TEST

Schilling Test

This test measures the absorption of vitamin B_{12}. Radioactive B_{12} is administered orally, and a 24-hour urine collection is begun. The presence of radioactivity in the urine indicates gastrointestinal absorption of vitamin B_{12}. Above 8% excretion of the radioactive dose is normal. This test is used in the diagnosis of pernicious anemia.

▼ Chapter Summary

▼ Blood is composed of formed elements and plasma. The formed elements include all of the blood cells, and the plasma consists of water, electrolytes, and plasma proteins. The bone marrow produces the blood cells and platelets with the active hematopoietic areas being red marrow.

▼ Blood cells have a limited life span and are replenished constantly through specific stimuli. The process of blood cell replacement involves the stem cell, which become committed to the cell line and finally produces the appropriate cell.

▼ Erythropoiesis is the developmental process to produce erythrocytes, a process that requires erythropoietin. In this process, hemoglobin is formed, which has the ability to carry oxygen and carbon dioxide in normal cellular respiration. Many substances are essential in the formation of erythrocytes and hemoglobin, without which anemias may result.

▼ Erythrocytes are active metabolic cells that have no nucleus and live for approximately 120 days. They have specific antigenic properties, which become the basis for blood typing before transfusion.

▼ Polycythemia is a condition of increased erythrocytes in the circulating blood. This response may be physiologic or pathologic, depending on its response to hypoxia and erythropoietin.

▼ Anemia refers to a condition of inadequate hemoglobin, circulating RBCs, or volume of RBCs in comparison to normal. Anemias are classified according to their morphologic characteristics. Categories include aplastic, hemolytic, maturation failure, posthemorrhagic, and those associated with chronic disease.

▼ Underlying mechanisms causing anemias are complex and varied. Many environmental agents can cause anemia, especially drugs and toxic substances. The cause of the anemia is sometimes unknown. Hematologic studies are performed to provide information for the diagnosis and treatment of blood disorders.

▼ References

1. Baserga, R. Principles of molecular cell biology of cancer: The cell cycle. In V.T. DeVita, S. Hellman, and S.A. Rosenberg (eds.), *Cancer: Principles and Practice of Oncology* (4th ed.). Philadelphia: J.B. Lippincott, 1994.
2. Benz, E.J. Hemoglobinopathies: Genetics, pathophysiology, and clinical features. In W.N. Kelley et al. (eds.), *Textbook of Internal Medicine* (2nd ed.) Philadelphia: J.B. Lippincott, 1992.
3. Benz, E.J. Structure, function, and synthesis of hemoglobins. In W.N. Kelley et al. (eds.), *Textbook of Internal Medicine* (2nd ed.). Philadelphia: J.B. Lippincott, 1992
4. Carmel, R. Nutritional biochemistry of megaloblastic anemias. In W.N. Kelley et al. (eds.), *Textbook of Internal Medicine* (2nd ed.) Philadelphia: J.B. Lippincott, 1992.
5. Castle, W.B. The polycythemias. In W.S. Beck (ed.), *Hematology* (4th ed.). Cambridge, Mass.: MIT Press, 1985.
6. Cook, J.D. Iron metabolism and ferrokinetics. In W.N. Kelley et al. (eds.), *Textbook of Internal Medicine* (2nd ed.). Philadelphia: J.B. Lippincott, 1992.
7. Cormack, D.H. *Essential Histology*. Philadelphia: J.B. Lippincott, 1993.
8. Cormack, D.H. *Ham's Histology* (9th ed.). Philadelphia: J.B. Lippincott, 1987.
9. Cotran, R.S., Kumar, V., and Robbins, S.L. *Robbins' Pathologic Basis of Disease* (5th ed.). Philadelphia: W.B. Saunders, 1994.
10. Deisseroth, A.B., and Wallerstein, R.O. Approach to the patient with bone marrow failure. In W.N. Kelley et al. (eds.), *Textbook of Internal Medicine* (2nd ed.). Philadelphia: J.B. Lippincott, 1992.
11. Deisseroth, A.B., and Wallerstein, R.O. Blood groups, tissue typing, and transfusions of blood products. In W.N. Kelley et al. (eds.), *Textbook of Internal Medicine* (2nd ed.). Philadelphia: J.B. Lippincott, 1992.
12. Dessypris, E.N. Abnormal hematocrit. In J.H. Stein (ed.), *Internal Medicine* (4th ed.) St. Louis: C.V. Mosby, 1994.
13. Frenkel, E.P., and Fleishman, R.A. Approach to the management of polycythemia. In W.N. Kelley et al. (eds.), *Textbook of Internal Medicine* (2nd ed.) Philadelphia: J.B. Lippincott, 1992.
14. Frenkel, E.P., and Fleishman, R.A. Polycythemia vera. In W.N. Kelley et al. (eds.). *Textbook of Internal Medicine* (2nd ed.) Philadelphia: J.B. Lippincott, 1992.
15. Ganong, W.F. *Review of Medical Physiology* (15th ed.). Los Altos, Calif.: Lange, 1991.
16. Giblett, E.R. Blood groups and blood transfusion. In J. Wilson et al. (eds.), *Harrison's Principles of Internal Medicine* (12th ed.). New York: McGraw-Hill, 1991.
17. Guyton, A. *Textbook of Medical Physiology* (8th ed.). Philadelphia: W.B. Saunders, 1991.
18. Hutton, J.L. The leukemias and polycythemia vera. In J.H. Stein (ed.), *Internal Medicine* (4th ed.). St. Louis: C.V. Mosby, 1994.
19. Jandle, J.A. *Blood: Textbook of Hematology*. Boston: Little, Brown, 1987.
20. Lessin, L.S., and Palek, J. Hemolytic anemias due to intracorpuscular abnormalities. In W.N. Kelley et al. (eds.), *Textbook of Internal Medicine* (2nd ed.). Philadelphia: J.B. Lippincott, 1992.
21. Lipschitz, D.A. Iron deficiency anemia, the anemia of chronic disease, sideroblastic anemia, and iron overload. In J.H. Stein (ed.), *Internal Medicine* (4th ed.). St. Louis: C.V. Mosby, 1994.
22. Memmler, R.L., Cohen, B.J., and Wood, D.L. *The Human Body In Health and Disease* (7th ed.). Philadelphia: J.B. Lippincott, 1992.
23. Pagana, K.D., and Pagana, T.J. *Mosby's Diagnostic and Laboratory Text Reference*. St. Louis: C.V. Mosby, 1992.
24. Petz, L.D. Hemolytic anemias due to acquired abnormalities of the red blood cell membrane. In W.N. Kelley et al. (eds.), *Textbook of Internal Medicine* (2nd ed.). Philadelphia: J.B. Lippincott, 1992.
25. Roodman, G.D. Hemolytic anemia. In J.H. Stein (ed.), *Internal Medicine* (4th ed.). St. Louis: C.V. Mosby, 1994.
26. Rubin, E., and Farber, J.L. *Pathology* (2nd ed.). Philadelphia: J.B. Lippincott, 1994.
27. Siegel, R.S., and Lessin, L.S. Anemias associated with chronic disease. In W.N. Kelley et al. (eds.), *Textbook of Internal Medicine* (2nd ed.). Philadelphia: J.B. Lippincott, 1992.
28. Tortora, G., and Grabowski, S.R. *Principles of Anatomy and Physiology* (7th ed.). New York: Harper Collins, 1993.
29. Whitney, E.N., Cataldo, C.B, and Rolfes, S.R. *Understanding Normal and Clinical Nutrition* (3rd ed.). St. Paul: West Publishing Co., 1991.
30. Wintrobe, M.M. *Blood, Pure and Eloquent*. New York: McGraw-Hill, 1980.

Chapter **20**

Normal and Altered Leukocyte Function

Barbara L. Bullock

▼ **LEARNING OBJECTIVES**

1 List and describe the five types of leukocytes.
2 Differentiate leukocytes on the basis of morphology and function.
3 Describe the differential white count and list the relative proportion of each cell type.
4 Describe phagocytosis and discuss its significance with respect to the destruction of microorganisms.
5 Compare the average life span of the five types of leukocytes.
6 Explain locomotion, diapedesis, degranulation, killing, chemotaxis, and opsonization.
7 Explain the function of the mononuclear phagocyte (macrophage) system.
8 Describe the characteristics of a myeloproliferative disorder.
9 Differentiate between malignant and nonmalignant disorders in leukocytes.
10 Explain the basis of classification of leukemias.
11 Differentiate between acute and chronic leukemia.
12 Differentiate generally between reactive lymphadenopathies and malignant lymphomas.
13 Differentiate Hodgkin's disease and other lymphomas on the basis of laboratory findings.
14 Explain the significance of Sternberg–Reed cells with respect to Hodgkin's disease.
15 Discuss the clinical features and pathologic alterations in multiple myeloma.

Barbara L. Bullock: PATHOPHYSIOLOGY: ADAPTATIONS AND ALTERATIONS IN FUNCTION, 4th ed.
© 1996 Lippincott-Raven Publishers

Leukocytes, larger and less numerous than erythrocytes, play a key role in the defense mechanisms of the body. As the name implies, leukocytes are almost white (the Greek *leukos* means "white"). Examination of a centrifuged tube of whole blood reveals a fuzzy gray-white layer between the packed red blood cells and the clear yellow plasma. This white layer, called the *buffy coat*, contains leukocytes and platelets.

The most important function of the leukocytes is to defend the body against invasion by foreign organisms and to produce, transport, and distribute defensive elements, such as antibodies or other factors, that are necessary for the immune response. The various types of leukocytes work together in an integrated system. Each type performs different functions in the defense mechanisms, and all functions are necessary for a total integrated and effective defense.

▼ Normal Leukocyte Function

CHARACTERISTICS OF LEUKOCYTES

There normally are about 5,000 to 10,000 leukocytes per microliter, or 5 to 10^9 per liter of adult human blood.[7] Of these, *granulocytes* (polymorphonuclear leukocytes, or polys) make up the largest portion of the total number, about 65%. The *agranulocytes* compose the remaining 35%. Granulocytes have large granules and horseshoe-shaped nuclei that differentiate and become multilobed, with two to five distinct lobes connected by thin strands. The background cytoplasm stains blue to pink with Wright's stain, which enhances their morphologic identification (Table 20-1). Granulocytes are subdivided into three cell types: neutrophils, eosinophils, and basophils. The *neutrophils* are the most numerous, making up 50% to 70% of the total white blood cell (WBC) count. They have small, fine, light pink or lilac acidophilic granules when stained and a segmented, irregularly lobed, purple nucleus.

Eosinophils constitute about 1% to 5% of the normal WBC count. They have large, round granules that contain red-staining basic mucopolysaccharides and multilobed purple-blue nuclei.[3]

Like eosinophils, *basophils* constitute a small percentage of the WBCs, ranging from 0% to 1% of the total count. The coarse, basophilic blue granules often conceal the segmented nucleus. The content of these granules includes histamine, heparin, and acid mucopolysaccharides.[3]

Lymphocytes and monocytes are the remaining WBC types normally present in peripheral blood. They were termed *agranulocytes* because they were originally thought to have no granules. Their granules are very small and stain quite differently than the large granules

of granulocytes. Lymphocytes and monocytes also are called mononuclear leukocytes, because unlike the granulocytes, they do not have a multilobed nucleus.

Lymphocytes are cells with large, round, deep-staining nuclei and very little cytoplasm. The cytoplasm is slightly basophilic and stains pale blue. They make up about 20% to 40% of the total WBC count.

The *monocyte* is a large mononuclear leukocyte with a prominent, multishaped nucleus that sometimes is kidney-shaped. The chromatin in the nucleus looks like lace, with small particles linked together by fine strands. Chromatin is less clumped than in the mature granulocyte or lymphocyte. The gray-blue cytoplasm is filled with many fine lysosomes that stain pink with Wright's stain. Monocytes constitute about 1% to 6% of the total WBC count. Figure 20-1 shows the different types of WBCs.

TABLE 20-1 *Staining Characteristics of Leukocytes*

Leukocyte	Cytoplasm	Cytoplasmic Granules	Nucleus
Neutrophil	Blue to pink	Lilac	Purple-blue
Eosinophil	Blue to pink	Red	Purple-blue
Basophil	Blue to pink	Blue-black	Purple-blue
Lymphocyte	Pale blue		Dark blue
Monocyte	Gray-blue	Pink	Blue lighter than lymphocytes

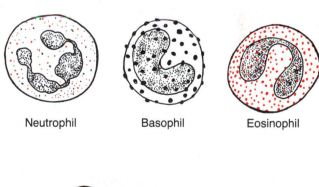

Neutrophil   Basophil   Eosinophil

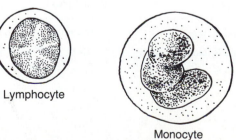

Lymphocyte   Monocyte

FIGURE 20-1 *Appearance of different types of leukocytes.*

DIFFERENTIAL WHITE BLOOD CELL COUNT

The WBC count is determined by counting cells in a diluted blood sample. The count is important as a diagnostic tool in identifying diseases that alter these cells. Significant increases or decreases of the count are known as *quantitative alterations*. Significant functional abnormalities of the cells are called *qualitative alterations*.

Each of the leukocytes has a specific function in the body's defense system. An attack by a foreign agent often elicits a response by a certain type of leukocyte. For example, a pyogenic bacterial infection may elicit an increase in neutrophils, or a parasitic infection might elicit an increase in eosinophils. Therefore, an increase or decrease in the normal percentage of leukocytes may have significant diagnostic value. The relative proportion of leukocyte cell types is called the *differential count*.

The differential count is determined on a smear of blood one cell layer thick. This layer is stained with a polychrome solution that contains both basic and acidic dyes, usually Wright's stain. The leukocyte cellular structure absorbs the dye differentially and permits evaluation not only of the relative proportions of the WBCs, but also of cellular elements and platelets. Differentials may be counted manually or electronically (Table 20-2).

Normal differential WBC proportions vary with age. The neutrophils, for example, are significantly increased at birth, but fall below the normal adult level by 2 weeks of age. Lymphocytes, more prevalent at birth and in early childhood, decrease in numbers until adult levels are reached (Table 20-3).

An *absolute count* of a particular leukocyte often is necessary for diagnosis. This can be obtained by using a special diluting fluid that lyses the erythrocytes and either lyses or does not stain the other WBCs present. The specific leukocyte can then be counted without including the other cells.

TABLE 20-3 Leukocyte Differential Count in Peripheral Blood

TOTAL WHITE BLOOD CELL COUNT	
Adult/child >2 years	5,000–10,000/mm^3
Child <2 years	6,200–17,000/mm^3
SEGMENTED NEUTROPHILS	
Adult/child >2 years	3,000–7,000/mm^3 (50–70% of total)
Child <2 years	2,400–4,000/mm^3 (25–35% of total)
BAND NEUTROPHILS	
Adult/child >2 years	500 ± 100/mm^3 (<8%)
Child <2 years	800 ± 200/mm^3 (<8.5%)
EOSINOPHILS	
Adult/child >2 years	50–250/mm^3 (1–4%)
Child <2 years	200 ± 50/mm^3 (2–4%)
BASOPHILS	
Adult/child >2 years	40 ± 101 mm^3 (0.5–1%)
Child <2 years	50 ± 10/mm^3 (0.5–1%)
LYMPHOCYTES	
Adult/child >2 years	1,000–4,000/mm^3 (20–40%)
Child <2 years	7,000 ± 2,000/mm^3 (60 ± 15%)
MONOCYTES	
Adult/child >2 years	100–600/mm^3 (2–6%)
Child <2 years	700 ± 200/mm^3 (3.5–8%)

TABLE 20-2 Normal Differential Count of Leukocytes

Leukocytes	Count (%)
Neutrophils, segmented	50–70
Neutrophils, bands or stabs	0–5
Eosinophils	1–4
Basophils	0–1
Lymphocytes	20–40
Monocytes	1–6

GENESIS OF LEUKOCYTES

The multipotential or uncommitted stem cells in bone marrow are essentially responsible for blood cell and platelet formation. They differentiate into unipotential, or committed, stem cells that ultimately become WBCs, platelets, and erythrocytes (see Figure 19-2).

Neutrophils, basophils, and eosinophils are formed in the bone marrow and can be stored there until needed. If the need is greater than the supply, immature forms may be released into the bloodstream.

Granulocytes and monocytes are thought to be derived from a common committed stem cell. The promonocyte also is formed and differentiated in bone marrow and is released into the circulation as amonocyte. The monocyte can leave the blood for the tissues, where it enlarges and is transformed or matured into a lysosome-filled *macrophage*. The macrophage is much larger than the monocyte, which is important for the phagocytosis of large particles and debris. Granulocytes and monocytes have phagocytic properties.

Lymphocytes are thought to be formed from the pluripotent stem cell that becomes committed to the lymphocyte line (see Chapter 16). Unlike granulocytes and monocytes, most lymphocytes are differentiated not in the bone marrow, but in the lymphoid tissue, thymus, or spleen. Only large and small lymphocytes and plasma cells can be identified by morphology. Identification of B and T lymphocytes involves such laboratory techniques as cell marker studies and cytochemistry. Differentiation of the B and T lymphocytes in the lymphoid tissue is an important aspect of the immunologic response.

LIFE SPAN OF WHITE BLOOD CELLS

The life span of WBCs in the circulating blood usually is short. The average half-life of a neutrophil is about 6 hours.[10] During a serious infection, neutrophils often live 2 hours or less, until they are used or destroyed.

Granulocytes mature in the bone marrow. After myelocytes (precursors of granulocytes) stop dividing, maturing granulocytes accumulate as a reserve in the bone marrow. There is normally about a 5-day supply of granulocytes in this reserve. Once the granulocytes leave the marrow, they spend an average of 12 hours in the circulation and about 2 to 3 days in the tissues before they are destroyed.

Monocytes spend less time in the bone marrow pool than granulocytes. The life span of the monocyte in the circulation is about 36 hours, or about three times as long as that of granulocytes.[3] After the monocyte has been transformed into a mobile or fixed macrophage in the tissues, its life is long, ranging from months to years.

The life span of the lymphocytes varies tremendously. A small population of extremely long-lived cells may survive for many years. These cells are necessary for maintaining immunologic memory and have the special ability to reenter cell division through specific stimulation by an antigen. Most T lymphocytes of the peripheral lymphatic tissue recirculate about every 10 hours.[19] They follow a path from the blood to the lymphatic tissue, through the lymphatic channels, and back to the blood through the thoracic duct. The survival rate of T lymphocytes ranges from a few days to months and years. In general, most T lymphocytes have slow replacement rates and a long survival time.

The B lymphocytes are largely noncirculating. They remain mainly in the lymphoid tissue and can differentiate under appropriate stimulation into plasma cells. Mature plasma cells, which can secrete specific antibodies, have a survival rate of about 2 to 3 days (see p. 318). Table 20-4 summarizes the life span of the various WBCs.

PROPERTIES OF LEUKOCYTES
Functional Classification

The properties of leukocytes can be best understood by separating them into two major functional groups: *phagocytes* and *immunocytes*. As discussed in the previous section, immunocytes and phagocytes are thought to be derived from a common stem cell in the bone marrow. The immunocytes, or lymphocytes, probably undergo a differentiation phase outside the bone marrow. Phagocytes mature in the bone marrow and are released as mature granulocytes and monocytes into the circulation. Granulocytes and monocytes are classified as phagocytes. Monocytes must enter the tissues and differentiate into macrophages to exhibit the property of phagocytosis.

TABLE 20-4 *Life Span of White Blood Cells*

Cell Type	In Circulating Blood	Tissue Life
Granulocytes	6–8 h; time shortened in acute infection	2–3 days
Monocytes	Short transit time, often less than 36 h	Months or years as tissue macrophages
T lymphocytes	Remain in the blood a few hours but recirculate about every 10 h	Varies from a few days to years
B lymphocytes	Few circulate	Most remain in lymphoid tissue; when they become secreting plasma cells, they survive 2–3 days
Platelets	Most circulate; are totally replaced every 10 days	

Phagocytosis

The most important property of the phagocytes (granulocytes and macrophages) is phagocytosis. Phagocytosis is a process similar to that by which an ameba ingests and digests its nourishment. The phagocyte can change its shape by sending out processes from its protoplasm. Microorganisms, old cells, or foreign particles can then be enveloped or engulfed in a vacuole, or *phagosome*, formed by the fusing of the processes of protoplasm. Associated with ingestion of the foreign or devitalized material are rapid increase in cellular energy and the generation of hydrogen peroxide (Fig. 20-2).

Degranulation

Phagocytosis involves not only ingestion of a microorganism or particle, but also digestion or destruction of this foreign body. After the material has become engulfed in the phagosome, degranulation occurs. This process involves lysosomes (granules) fusing with the internal membrane of the phagosome and emptying their contents into its vacuole. The biochemical events of this morphologic phenomenon are not understood completely. The granules contain hydrolytic enzymes that cause the dissolution of the phagosome contents and, eventually, lysis of the phagocyte itself.

Killing

Killing is the process by which the microorganism contained within the membrane-bound phagosome dies. Most of the hydrolytic enzymes contained in the granules serve a digestive function and are not directly involved in killing.[10] What actually kills the microorganism is peroxidation of hydrogen peroxide, which, in the presence of iodide, destroys the microbial membrane. Most bacteria can be killed by this process. Some organisms, such as acid-fast bacilli that cause tuberculosis and leprosy, are able to survive inside the phagocyte.

Dissolution is complex and involves integrated action of many hydrolytic enzymes. The phagocyte, as well as the foreign invader, often is lysed by its own enzymes and becomes part of the degradation products (see Figure 20-2).

The degradation products that remain after phagocytosis usually intensify the inflammatory process to varying degrees. The released lysosomal enzymes of degranulation or toxins released by the bacteria may damage the surrounding tissues. Degradation products

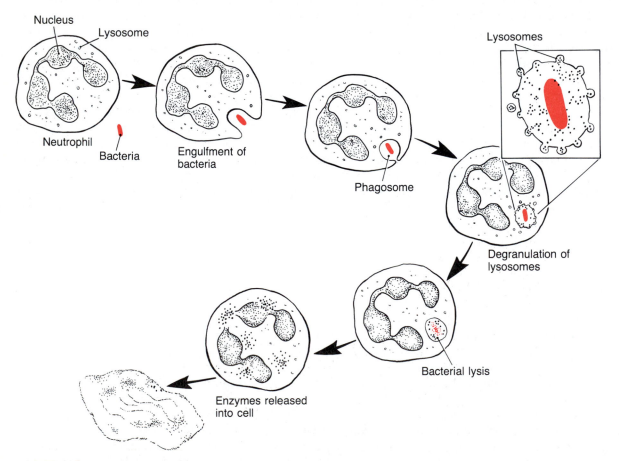

FIGURE 20-2 Phagocytosis of bacteria.

include thromboplastic products that lead to vascular clotting.

Phagocytosis is promoted by other factors, such as temperature and electrical charge. Elevated body temperatures or increased heat at the site of infection enhances phagocytosis. Fever during an infection may serve as a protective mechanism within limits. The electrical charge on antigen surfaces also may enhance phagocytosis, because the charge on dead or foreign particles is different from that on living tissues and is considered to be a dominant factor in specificity.[18]

Increased glucose metabolism and cellular oxygen consumption are needed for phagocytosis because increased energy is necessary for the production of large amounts of hydrogen peroxide used to kill bacteria.[21] Energy in the form of adenosine triphosphate is supplied by glycolysis in the WBC itself.

Diapedesis

Phagocytes can accumulate at the site of invasion or injury. Like the ameba, they form pseudopod-like processes that allow them to move through avenues of the body. Granulocytes and monocytes can leave the circulation and enter tissue by a process called diapedesis. Diapedesis refers to the ability of the phagocyte to slip through the walls of the capillary vessel by ameboid motion. A small portion of the phagocyte slides through at a time until the entire cells leaves the circulation. Diapedesis allows phagocytes to accumulate at the invasion site (see pp. 298–299).

Chemotaxis

The phagocytes must be able to find the site of a bacterial invasion or recognize that infection has taken place. Specific phagocytes break down and digest necrotic material. Chemical substances, called chemotactic agents or mediators, are released from the infected or necrotic tissues and provide a signal for the leukocytes to move toward the source of the chemotactic agent. This process, called chemotaxis, is dependent on a concentration gradient. A greater concentration of the chemical causes more leukocytes to move toward the source. Other chemotactic agents include the complement system, plasminogen, the fibrinolytic system, kallikrein (the kinin system), and substances released from the phagocytes (see pp. 300–301).

Pinocytosis

Pinocytosis, "cell drinking," is the cellular engulfment by the phagocyte of tiny particles included in a droplet of fluid. It differs from phagocytosis in that in phagocytosis the membrane sends out processes to grasp a relatively large particle using a biochemical mechanism similar to muscle action. In pinocytosis, macrophages ingest and break down molecules, such as protein molecules in suspension.[16]

Recognition of the Particle

Before a phagocyte can ingest a bacterium or particle, it must recognize the particle. Recognition of the foreign invader is achieved through mediation in one of two ways: opsonization and surface properties.[4]

Opsonization of the antigenic surface is necessary for the phagocyte to attach to the antigen. Opsonization is mediated by activation of the complement protein system or by specific antibodies. Activation of complement results in attachment of C3b to the surface of the particle, which, with specific antibody, allows it to be recognized and phagocytosed by the leukocyte (see p. 299).[4]

Some particles have special *surface properties* that cause them to adhere to the phagocyte and subsequently undergo phagocytosis. These physiochemical properties allow the particle to adhere to the cell membrane of the phagocyte while pseudopodia surround and engulf the particle. This type of phagocytosis is seen in the early phases of an illness and is most effective with tightly packed leukocytes. The exact mechanism of attachment of the phagocyte to the antigen before antibody formation, complement activation, or cell devitalization is unknown.

FUNCTION OF PHAGOCYTES

The functions of granulocytes and monocyte–macrophages overlap, but in general, granulocytes are the first line of defense against microbe invasion; neutrophils are adept at recognizing, ingesting, and killing pyogenic bacteria; and monocyte–macrophages are important in the final removal or cellular cleanup of debris after phagocytosis and cell lysis.

Monocyte–macrophages can ingest bigger particles and larger amounts of debris because of their larger size. Inert materials as large as wood or steel fragments can be engulfed by macrophages and removed from the site of inflammation. If a particle is very large, multinucleated foreign-body *giant cells* may be produced. The characteristic foreign-body giant cell may represent fusion of several macrophages.

Macrophages not only provide the final removal of microorganisms, but also clear the body of its own aged and damaged cells. Some macrophages possess the ability to break down and recycle old red blood cells (RBCs). Certain tissue macrophages break down hemoglobin, leaving products that can be recycled into new hemoglobin. Macrophages of the liver, spleen, and bone marrow can return the released iron to transferrin to be transported to the erythroid marrow for RBC synthesis. Phagocytes contain antibacterial substances, peroxidase, and lysosomal enzymes necessary for phagocytosis and other activities. Macrophages are thought to participate in killing tumor cells that have been processed by the lymphocytes. Monocytes and granulocytes also interact with other biologically active substances, such as complement.

For the phagocytes to accomplish their defensive purpose, the following must occur: 1) they must accumulate in sufficient numbers at the right place; 2) they must attach to the foreign material or agent; 3) they must envelop or engulf the agent; and 4) they must dispose of the debris.[4, 10] Alterations in any of these functions results in defective phagocytosis, which then results in a defective defensive response.

FUNCTION OF BASOPHILS AND EOSINOPHILS

The precise function of basophils and eosinophils is not well understood, but it is known that these cells participate in inflammatory and allergic reactions.

Basophils contain histamine, heparin, and small quantities of bradykinin and serotonin. They are present in small numbers in the blood and in larger numbers in the connective tissue and pericapillary areas. Their function seems to be largely to prevent clotting in the microcirculation and to cause some of the signs and symptoms of allergic reactions.[9] People with allergies often have elevated levels of immunoglobulin E (IgE). Receptor sites for IgE have been found on the basophils. When these receptor sites are attacked, histamine and other substances are released that increase chemotaxis and also enhance the allergic response (see pp. 349–350). The number of basophils increases in some of the myeloproliferative diseases, such as polycythemia vera.

Eosinophils weakly exhibit phagocytosis and chemotaxis.[23] They are present in large numbers in the mucosa of the intestinal tract and of the lungs. Because of this, they probably help to detoxify foreign proteins. The circulating level of eosinophils is increased in people with allergies, perhaps as a result of the cells removing and digesting the antigen–antibody complex. Eosinophilia is associated with worm infestation or parasitic infections. In trichinosis, the numbers of eosinophils can increase 25% to 50%.

MONONUCLEAR PHAGOCYTE SYSTEM

The mononuclear phagocyte system is the large system of stationary and mobile macrophages. It was formerly called the reticuloendothelial system, but the term "mononuclear phagocyte system" is a more descriptive term for the functional capabilities of this system. Important in the body's defense, it is considered to be more a functional than an anatomic system. It includes all the fixed and mobile phagocytic cells in the liver, spleen,

lymph nodes, and gastrointestinal tract. Fixed macrophages in these organs seem to exist in dynamic equilibrium with mobile macrophages. All tissue macrophages, including the Kupffer's cells of the liver and alveolar macrophages in the lungs, originate from the mobile circulating macrophages.[18] This system is important in preventing the spread of infection and removing cellular debris and products of metabolic degradation. Many of the metabolic products are conserved and recycled.

FUNCTION OF IMMUNOCYTES

Unlike monocytes and granulocytes, lymphocytes do not possess phagocytic capabilities, but protect the body against specific antigens. This specific immunity, discussed in Chapter 16, is integrated with other general immune responses. The lymphocytes move freely from the blood to the lymphoid tissues. They seem to patrol the tissue spaces for foreign material.

▼ Nonmalignant White Blood Cell Disorders

QUANTITATIVE ALTERATIONS OF GRANULOCYTES

Quantitative alterations of granulocytes result from several conditions that cause a significant increase or decrease in the number of leukocytes. This usually is measured by calculating the total number of leukocytes in blood. Each cell type is then considered and counted individually to identify the causative condition. Physiologic leukocytosis (increase in the number of leukocytes above 10,000/L) can be caused by exercise, emotional stress, menstruation, sunlight, cold, and anesthesia. During pregnancy, the number of polymorphonuclear leukocytes increases consistently. This increase is even more exaggerated during labor and the first postpartum week. The newborn also has increased leukocyte levels.

Neutrophils

A physiologic shift in the number of neutrophils can be influenced by several conditions. Table 20-5 lists principal causes of neutrophilia and neutropenia. *Neutrophilic leukocytosis (neutrophilia)* is defined as an absolute neutrophil count greater than 7,500/μL blood. The *leukemoid reaction* refers to persistent neutrophilia of 30,000 to 50,000/μL, which usually result from an acute infection but may be mistakenly diagnosed as a leukemia. The neutrophils in this reaction appear more mature than myelocytes and have large blue cytoplasmic inclusions, unlike those of leukemic origin.[20] A *shift to the left* occurs with increases in the number of nonsegmented neutrophils in circulating blood. When increased numbers

TABLE 20-5 Principal Causes of Neutrophilia and Neutropenia

NEUTROPENIA	NEUTROPHILIC LEUKOCYTOSIS
Decreased production	Infections (primarily
Irradiation	bacterial)
Drug-induced (acute,	Immunologic–inflammatory
chronic)	Rheumatoid arthritis
Viral infections	Rheumatic fever
Congenital	Vasculitis
Cyclic	Tissue necrosis
Ineffective production	Infarction
Megaloblastic anemia	Trauma
Myelodysplastic syndrome	Burns
Increased destruction	Neoplasia
Isoimmune neonatal	Hemorrhage
Autoimmune	Hemolysis
Idiopathic	Metabolic disorders
Drug-induced	Acidosis
Felty's syndrome	Uremia
Systemic lupus	Gout
erythematosus	Endocrinologic disorders
Complement activation–	Thyroid storm
induced dialysis	Glucocorticoids
Splenic sequestration	Pregnancy
Increased margination	Toxins
	Physical stimuli
	Cold
	Heat
	Stress
	Emotional stress
	Hereditary neutrophilia

From Rubin, E., and Farber, J. L. *Pathology* (2nd ed.). Philadelphia: J.B. Lippincott, 1994.

of neutrophils are released in an inflammatory process, some may be in immature forms called *bands* or *stabs*, which have a short life span. An increased number of these cells in the peripheral blood often is a good indicator of an inflammatory process, especially an acute bacterial infection.[7] A leftward shift usually indicates an acute infectious process. When it returns to normal mature cells, the infection often is seen to be subsiding.[4] Neutrophilic leukocytosis occurs in such pathologic conditions as acute pyogenic infections, cancer, hemorrhage, hemolysis, tissue necrosis, and metabolic chemical toxic poisonings.

Neutrophilic leukopenia (neutropenia) occurs when the absolute neutrophil count is less than 2,500/μL of blood.[13] Irradiation, anaphylactic shock, and systemic lupus erythematosus are some of the causes of this decrease. Chemical agents that affect the hematopoietic system cause a decrease in the neutrophils. Antithyroid drugs, phenothiazines, and chemotherapeutic agents are only a few of the many drugs that can cause neutropenia (see Table 20-5). Nonpyogenic bacterial, viral,

and rickettsial infections can cause a decrease in the neutrophil count. Any overwhelming bacterial infection may lead to a neutrophilic leukopenia, because the vast numbers of cells used to fight the infections is much greater than the reserve supply.[24] The body's reserve ability to form neutrophils is exhausted, and the neutrophil count falls.

Eosinophils

Eosinophilic leukocytosis (eosinophilia) is defined as an absolute eosinophil count that exceeds 500/μL of blood and often is associated with allergy and parasitic infections.[7] The increase with allergic conditions is believed to be due to the tissue reactions associated with allergy-released products that specifically increase the production of eosinophils in the bone marrow. Eosinophilic leukocytosis also occurs in response to parasitic infection. This is probably the most common cause of extremely large numbers of eosinophils. The mechanism by which the parasitic infections cause the increased count is unknown. Eosinophilic leukocytosis also can be caused by pulmonary disorders, skin diseases, and cancer.[1]

Eosinophilic leukopenia (eosinopenia) occurs when the absolute eosinophil count is less than 50/μL of blood.[7] The decrease may be due to severe infection, shock, or adrenocortical stimulation. Peripheral blood eosinophils are sensitive to adrenocortical hormones and may be reduced or absent in stress, with Cushing's disease, or in patients being treated with corticosteroids.[7] There is no reported adverse effect of eosinopenia.[8]

Basophils

Basophilic leukocytosis (basophilia) is defined as an absolute basophil count exceeding 50 to 100/μL of blood.[7] This usually is greater than 2% of the WBC differential and is associated with myeloproliferative disorders, chronic granulocytic leukemia, and, occasionally, ulcerative colitis and certain skin diseases.[17]

Basophilic leukopenia (basopenia) occurs when the absolute basophil count is less than 20/μL of blood.[7] It often is associated with suppression of other granulocytes in drug-induced suppression as well as severe infection, shock, and adrenocortical stimulation.

QUALITATIVE ALTERATIONS OF GRANULOCYTES

When granulocytes display defective physical and chemical functions, they are said to have qualitative abnormalities. Decreased resistance to infection may occur even when there is a normal granulocyte count.[20] Most of the defective functions are related to phagocytosis. The defects may be in phagocyte locomotion or in the phagocyte itself, such as that in *lazy leukocyte syndrome*, which can be seen with an intrinsic abnormality of leukocytes, such as in diabetes mellitus.[4] There may be deficient chemotaxis and related complement abnormalities. The latter are associated with collagen vascular disorders and, occasionally, bacterial infections. Some drugs, such as aspirin, corticosteroids, colchicine, and phenylbutazone, can cause dysfunction of the phagocyte.[8]

Ethanol causes a significant decrease in leukocyte migration and chemotaxis during acute intoxication. Chemotaxis also can be decreased by the use of some antibiotics, such as gentamicin, in therapeutic doses.[4, 17] *Granulomatous diseases* are rare qualitative defects of the granulocytes, especially neutrophils, that result in defective bactericidal activity. In chronic granulomatous disease, there is an inherited X-linked absence of neutrophil and monocyte oxidative metabolism. The enzymes are necessary for the actual killing of bacteria, without which leukocytes are unable to oxidize or destroy certain bacteria.[20] The disease results in severe recurrent infections of the skin, lymph nodes, lungs, liver, and bones with catalase-positive microorganisms (those that destroy their own hydrogen peroxide).[20]

Several qualitative abnormalities of the granulocytes are inherited. Altered nuclear structure and appearance, excessive granulation of the cytoplasm, and hypersegmentation of neutrophils may occur. These alterations may affect phagocytosis or may have no clinical implications.

MONOCYTE ABNORMALITIES

Monocytosis infers an absolute monocyte count greater than 750/μL in children and 500 to 600/μL in adults.[7] This disorder arises in nonpyogenic bacterial infections, such as active tuberculosis, subacute bacterial endocarditis, syphilis, and brucellosis. It is associated with chronic inflammatory disorders, viral infections, and chronic ulcerative colitis.[17]

Monocytopenia refers to a decrease in the blood monocyte counts and it often is associated with other causes of leukopenia. It frequently is secondary to acute stress reactions or glucocorticoid administration. Overwhelming infections and immunosuppressive agents decrease the monocyte count.

LYMPHOCYTIC DISORDERS

Lymphocytosis must be defined according to a person's developmental stage. The absolute lymphocyte count from birth to age 3 years is 9,000/μL of blood. From 4 to 12 years, it is 7,000/μL, and in adults, it is 4,000/μL.[24] Viral disorders that produce lymphocytosis include mumps, rubella, rubeola, hepatitis, and varicella. Lymphocytosis also occurs in pertussis and chronic lymphocytic leukemia. Numbers of atypical lymphocytes are increased in infectious mononucleosis, cytomegalic inclusion disease, and toxoplasmosis.

Lymphopenia is defined as an absolute lymphocyte count of less than 1,400/μL in the child and less than 1,000/μL in the adult.[24] This condition may be caused by such factors as stress, adrenocortical stimulation, alkylating agents, and irradiation. It is associated with Hodgkin's disease, lymphosarcoma, terminal uremia, and acute tuberculosis.

Infectious Mononucleosis

A disease that often strikes young adults, infectious mononucleosis is characterized by cervical lymphadenopathy, fever, sore throat, and splenomegaly. Exudative tonsillitis is common.

The designation "mononucleosis" is misleading, because the proliferating cells present in the lymph nodes, spleen, tonsils, and other organs are atypical lymphocytes, not monocytes. Serology shows an increase in lymphocytes, with 10% to 20% of these being abnormal.

Mononucleosis is caused by the Epstein-Barr virus (EBV). The EBV is transmitted primarily through oral secretions. Blood and sexual transmission can occur, but the incidence is uncommon.[22] This is the same herpesvirus that causes the malignant Burkitt's lymphoma that occurs in some areas in Africa. If cultured infectious mononucleosis lymphocytes are transplanted into immunosuppressed animals, a malignant lymphoproliferative disorder results. Genetically determined defects in the immune response may be the key to this cancer.[4]

EBV subclinically infects from 90% to 100% of the world's population usually by age 5.[26] Large epidemiologic studies have shown that only people without antibodies against EBV are at risk for developing infectious mononucleosis. The active disease is associated with the brief appearance of IgM antibodies against EBV. The IgM antibody increase represents a primary response and indicates recent exposure to the virus.

In the United States, infectious mononucleosis particularly affects the adolescent and young adult age groups. By adulthood, nearly 100% of the population have EBV antibodies.[26]

Hematologic changes are characteristic of mononucleosis. At first, there may be a mild leukopenia, but by the 2nd week, the WBC count reaches 15,000 to 30,000/μL of blood. Atypical lymphocytes, up to 20% of the total, are seen circulating in the peripheral blood in the 2nd through the 4th weeks.[26] The atypical lymphocytes may take one of several forms, but the most common picture includes nuclear chromatin that is finely divided or clumped. The nucleolus usually is absent, and vacuoles often are present in the cytoplasm. If atypical lymphocytes are present in large numbers, the disease may hematologically resemble acute leukemia or Hodgkin's disease, but the combination of fever, pharyngitis, lymphadenopathy, and antibody tests usually make the differential.[26]

EBV induces an increase in antibody formation by the B lymphocytes. The presence of this antibody forms the basis for laboratory diagnostic testing. The heterophil antibody titer and MonoSpot tests are used for differential diagnosis. No correlation has been noted between the levels of EBV or antibody titer and severity of the disease.[5, 26]

Symptoms of infectious mononucleosis disappear before the abnormal hematologic findings do. Clinical characteristics include profound fatigue, fever, malaise, sore throat, and weakness. Splenomegaly is characteristically seen, and hepatic dysfunction may be present. Complications are infrequent but may be seen in the immune suppressed individual. These include hemolytic anemia, splenic rupture, encephalitis, hepatitis, and pulmonary complications and death.[26] Avoidance of contact sports and increased rest usually are prescribed for 6 to 8 weeks after diagnosis. Gradual recovery is the rule and usually occurs in 2 to 4 weeks with no residual effects. Immunity to reinfection is established after having the disease, and recurrent mononucleosis is rare.[26] However, because EBV is a herpesvirus, it can persist as a latent infection, during which time asymptomatic reactivation occurs in apparently healthy young adults and provides a mechanism for the infection of those without antibodies. Persons having an impaired cell-mediated response to viral infection may develop severe or even fatal lymphoproliferative complications. This has especially been seen in persons infected with human immunodeficiency virus and in several genetic deficiency syndromes.[5, 26]

Lymphadenopathy

Lymphadenopathies are characterized by enlarged lymph nodes. The nodes may be tender or nontender and movable or fixed. Nodes involved by lymphomas or leukemias tend to be large, firm, and movable, whereas those of metastatic spread of cancer tend to be adherent to surrounding structures. In acute infections, the nodes usually are asymmetric with associated redness and edema. Localized lymphadenopathy usually indicates drainage of an inflammation that may be due to infection, neoplasm, or early lymphoma. Generalized lymphadenopathy infrequently is caused by infection in the adult, more often being caused by a malignant or nonmalignant process.

Lymphadenopathies show individual pathologic features, depending on the causative agent. Suppurative lymphadenitis is characterized by neutrophils in the sinusoids of the lymph nodes.

These nodes serve as filtration units for the regions infected by pyogenic bacteria. Lymph node enlargement may be due to reactive follicular hyperplasia of non-specific origin. There usually is hyperplasia of follicular center cells, which may be due to stimulation of B cells in viral diseases, syphilis, or autoimmune diseases, such as rheumatoid arthritis or systemic lupus erythematosus.

▼ Malignant White Blood Cell Disorders

LEUKEMIA

Leukemia is the name of a group of malignant diseases characterized by both qualitative and quantitative alterations in circulating leukocytes. It is associated with diffuse abnormal growth of leukocyte precursors in the bone marrow. The word *leukemia* is derived from the Greek *leukos* and *aima*, meaning "white" and "blood," referring to the abnormal increase in leukocytes. This uncontrolled increase eventually leads to anemia, infection, thrombocytopenia, and, in some cases, death.

Classification

Classification of leukemia usually is based on 1) *the course and duration of the illness* and 2) *the abnormal type of cells and tissue involved*. The course of the illness has been subclassified into acute and chronic.

Acute leukemia affects approximately 5 persons per 100,000 in the United States each year.[12] It is associated with rapid onset, a massive number of immature leukocytes, rapidly progressive anemia, severe thrombocytopenia, high fever, infective lesions of the mouth and throat, bleeding into vital areas, accumulation of leukocytes in vital organs, and severe infection. Laboratory studies usually show some degree of anemia and thrombocytopenia. Most advanced laboratory methods can now identify the cell type that causes acute leukemia, but a small percentage of cases cannot be classified, except that the predominant cell is an undifferentiated stem cell (Table 20-6). Demonstration of leukemic cells in the peripheral blood cannot always be relied on. Open surgical biopsy of the bone marrow usually demonstrates the abnormal cells.

Chronic leukemia constitutes 35% to 50% of all cases of leukemia.[4] The onset of this disease is characterized by gradual onset and leukocytes that are more mature. This disease mostly strikes adults and the elderly. The clinical course progresses more slowly than that of acute leukemia. Laboratory analysis usually reveals a well-differentiated leukemic cell that can be classified as lymphocytic or granulocytic (Table 20-7).

Leukemia is further classified by the type of tissue and abnormal cell involved. Three broad categories based on tissue origin are 1) *myeloid*, which includes the granulocytes (neutrophils, eosinophils, or basophils); 2) *monocytic*; and 3) *lymphocytic*. If abnormal proliferation of

TABLE 20-6 *French-American-British Classification of Acute Leukemia*

FAB Type	Morphology	Histochemistry
L1	Small blasts with scant cytoplasm and little variation from cell to cell, round nucleus with a single small nucleolus	PAS-positive; peroxidase-negative; acid phosphatase- and naphthyl esterase-positive if T-ALL
L2*	Larger cells with more abundant cytoplasm than L1; significant variation from cell to cell; irregularly shaped nucleus, often with multiple nucleoli	Same as L1
L3	Large cells with strongly basophilic cytoplasm that may be vacuolated; fine chromatin in a round nucleus; multiple nucleoli, often basophilic	PAS- and peroxidase-negative; vacuoles usually oil red O-positive
M0	Acute myelocytic leukemia—no cytoplasmic granules by light microscopy. Monoclonal antibodies demonstrate at least one myeloid antigen on cell surface.	Sudan black and peroxidase-negative. The latter can be identified by monoclonal antibody.
M1	Acute myelocytic leukemia—undifferentiated cells with only occasional cytoplasmic granules; some promyelocytes are seen	Occasional peroxidase-positive granules
M2	Acute myelocytic leukemia—granulated blasts predominate; monocytoid cells may be present in small number; differentiation beyond the promyelocyte stage is clearly evident; Auer rods may be seen	Strongly peroxidase-positive
M3	Acute promyelocytic leukemia—hypergranular promyelocytes predominate; the cells have large basophilic and eosinophilic granules	Strongly peroxidase-positive
M4	Acute myelomonocytic leukemia—both monocyte and granulocytic precursors are found; serum lysozyme is elevated	Strongly peroxidase-positive; may have punctate PAS-positive cells
M4E	Acute myelomonocytic leukemia—same as M4, but young eosinophils with small eosinophilic granules and large, basophilic primary granules constitute up to 30% or more of marrow cells. Serum lysozyme is elevated	Same as M4
M5A	Acute monoblastic leukemia—large monoblasts with abundant, relatively agranular cytoplasm that may be vacuolated and basophilic; more common in children. Serum lysozyme is elevated	May be peroxidase- and PAS-positive; nonspecific esterase stains are strongly positive
M5B	Acute monocytic leukemia—the predominant cell has a characteristic twisted, indented, or folded nucleus; more common in adults. Serum lysozyme is elevated	Same as M5A
M6	Erythroleukemia—megaloblastoid red blood cell precursors predominate, but myeloid blasts are also seen, multinucleated red blood cell precursors are common	The red blood cell precursors are PAS-positive, and ringed sideroblasts are seen with iron stains
M7	Megakaryocytic leukemia—variable morphology; megakaryocytic features may not be seen with light microscopy. This rare entity is usually identified with monoclonal antibodies to platelet antigens	Variable; platelet peroxidase can be demonstrated by electron microscopy

FAB: French-American-British; ALL: acute lymphocytic leukemia; PAS: periodic acid-Schiff.
   *L2 is the most frequent morphology in adult ALL.
   From Kelley, W. N. (ed.). *Textbook of Internal Medicine* (2nd ed.). Philadelphia: J.B. Lippincott, 1992.

granular leukocytes or their precursors is found in the blood or bone marrow, the leukemia may be called granulocytic, myelocytic, or myelogenous. With abnormal proliferation of lymphocytes or monocytes, the disease is called lymphocytic or monocytic, respectively.

If the majority of cells are immature, the suffix "blastic" is used instead of "cytic." For example, lymphoblastic, myeloblastic, or monoblastic indicates immaturity of leukocytes.

Classification of the chronic leukemias has not been a diagnostic problem, because there are usually enough mature leukocytes with abnormal mitotic figures which

TABLE 20-7 *Chronic Leukemias*

Type	Description
Chronic myeloid leukemia	Chromosome marker, Ph_1 (Philadelphia) characteristic in 90% of cases. Granulocyte precursors dominate cell line. Marked elevation of leukocyte count usually >100,000 cells/mm³. Thrombocytosis common. Marked lack of alkaline phosphatase in granulocytes. Accelerated phase may terminate in "blast" crisis, which appears like acute leukemia. Median survival 3–4 years.
Chronic lymphocytic leukemia	Various chromosomal abnormalities common (especially trisomy 12). Similar to small lymphatic lymphoma. B-cell neoplasm with long-lived nonfunctional B lymphocytes that infiltrate the bone marrow. Total leukocyte count may be 200,000 cells/mm³. Hypogammaglobulinemia common with increased susceptibility to bacterial infections. Course variable with median survival of 4–6 years.
Hairy cell leukemia	Chronic B-cell leukemia. Cells have fine, hairlike projections. Splenic, liver, and bone marrow with massive splenomegaly infiltration common; leukocytosis uncommon. Course is variable with remissions and possible cure.

Summarized from Cotran, R., Kumar, V., and Robbins, S. L. *Robbins' Pathologic Basis of Disease* (5th ed.). Philadelphia: W.B. Saunders, 1994.

allow for a diagnosis of a specific type of leukemia. Diagnosis and classification of acute leukemia present a greater challenge. Because of cellular immaturity, it is sometimes difficult to identify the cell type. Research and technologic advances have led to a more sophisticated identification and classification system that includes the use of cell marker studies, cell secretory activity, and cytochemistry as well as morphology and response to therapy.

Many factors are thought to influence the development of leukemia. These can be divided into three groups: 1) genetic factors; 2) acquired diseases; and 3) chemical and physical agents.

Genetic factors present in an identical twin pose a great risk if the other twin has leukemia. Siblings of a person with leukemia and people with Down's syndrome also are at significant risk for developing leukemia. Several chromosomal abnormalities have been associated with the onset of leukemia. The Philadelphia (Ph) chromosome, a translocation between chromosome 9 and chromosome 22, is associated with chronic granulocytic leukemia.[11] Acute and chronic leukemias often show abnormalities of many chromosomes.[14]

Acquired diseases with some increased risk for leukemia include myelofibrosis, polycythemia vera, and sideroblastic refractory anemia. Multiple myeloma and Hodgkin's disease also represent increased risk for development of the disease. The risk may be related to the underlying disease or to the treatment with chemotherapeutic agents or irradiation.

Physical and chemical agents that pose significant risk include irradiation and long-term exposure to benzene. Some risk also may be associated with the chemotherapeutic agent chloramphenicol and alkylating agents. Viral causation of leukemia in humans has been studied extensively, particularly because it has been noted in lower animals. Induction of leukemic changes in tissue cultures of human cells by RNA viruses supports the possibility of viral transmission of certain forms of leukemia.[12] The human T-cell leukemia virus, a retrovirus, has been isolated from cells of persons with adult T-cell leukemia, an aggressive cancer composed of mature T-lymphoid cells.[12] The disease is found particularly in southwestern Japan, parts of the Caribbean, and central Africa.[2]

Clinical Manifestations

Table 20-8 summarizes the clinical manifestations for the acute and chronic leukemias. Pathologic alterations caused by the disease processes create characteristic signs and symptoms.

Acute lymphocytic leukemia (ALL) usually occurs abruptly, with fever, fatigue, bleeding, signs of bone marrow dysfunction, and bone pain. Anemia is almost always present in persons with ALL.[25] The WBC count varies, usually between 10,000 and 30,000 cells/L with a platelet count of less than 100,000 cells/L.[25] The bone marrow is crowded with lymphoblasts that may be morphologically indistinguishable from myeloblasts. Infiltration of the lymph nodes, spleen, and liver is characteristic.[4]

Acute myeloblastic or *myelocytic leukemia (AML)* also arises abruptly, with symptoms similar to those of ALL. Due to the variability of the diagnostic characteristics, the terms *acute nonlymphocytic leukemia* and *acute undifferentiated leukemia* are being used to classify this form of leukemia.[12, 25] Laboratory studies may help to differentiate the cellular causation. The organ infiltration with AML is not as prominent as with ALL. Hemorrhages, small vascular occlusions, and disseminated intravascu-

TABLE 20-8 *Clinical Manifestations of Leukemia*

Anemia	Common due to replacement of erythrocytic bone marrow with leukemic elements. Causes pallor. May be profound with acute leukemia.
Fever	May be associated with infection, or the cause may be unknown.
Weight loss	Anorexia from leukemia, chemotherapy, or radiotherapy. Taste alterations are common.
Fatigue	Common and may or may not be related to degree of anemia.
Bleeding	Nosebleeds, ecchymosis, and petechiae are common in acute leukemia, usually due to depressed platelet formation. Disseminated intravascular coagulation is caused by abnormal products of leukemic infiltration, especially with acute leukemias.
Bone marrow dysfunction	Leukemic bone marrow suppression of granulocytes causes decreased resistance to infection. Chemotherapy also causes suppression. Infections are usually present, with upper respiratory tract infections or flulike illness. Infection often causes death.
Lymph node infiltration and splenic enlargement	Lymphadenopathy is common due to leukemic infiltration of lymph nodes. Splenic enlargement results from infiltration of the spleen with leukemic cells.

lar coagulation (DIC) commonly occur. Anemia is characteristic, but an elevated WBC count above 100,000/μL occurs in only about 20% of cases.[4]

Chronic myelocytic leukemia accounts for 15% to 20% of cases and may be discovered on routine physical examination, especially with evidence of an enlarged spleen.[4] In about 90% of cases, the Ph_1 chromosome can be demonstrated. This chromosome represents a translocation of part of chromosome 9 to chromosome 22.[20] This chromosomal aberration also is occasionally seen in ALL. Early signs are fatigability, weakness, weight loss, and anorexia. Bleeding, anemia, and infection are late manifestations. The WBC count is very high, from 50,000 to 500,000/μL.[11] After about 3 years, approximately 50% of people affected enter an accelerated phase which is characterized by a process like acute leukemia.[2]

Chronic lymphocytic leukemia is a long-term disease, usually of elderly people and especially among Western peoples.[6] It is characterized by generalized lymphadenopathy and often is otherwise asymptomatic. Anemia, fatigue, and night sweats may be described. The lymphocyte count is usually greater than 15,000/μL. The leukemia cells are small and mature looking but nonfunctional. The course and progression of the disease are variable, with median survival of 4 to 10 years.[1]

Hairy cell leukemia is a rare form that produces distinctive cells with hairlike projections. The origins of the cells are not known, but they are thought to be of B-lymphocyte lineage.[6] The disease occurs mainly in elderly men, with splenomegaly, hepatomegaly, and bone marrow failure resulting in *pancytopenia*. With appropriate chemotherapy, remissions and even a possible cure have been seen in at least 50% of affected persons.[2, 4]

Infection caused by marrow failure and granulocytopenia is the most common cause of fatality in all types of leukemia. It may appear in any organ or area and may be manifested by fever, chills, inflammation, and weakness. Bleeding of the skin, gingivae, or viscera often occurs because of thrombocytopenia. DIC caused by reduced platelets and coagulation factors may cause significant hemorrhage (see pp. 418–419). DIC is probably triggered by proteolytic enzymes or factors released by the leukemic cells that activate the clotting process.

Reduced appetite and hypermetabolism result in weight loss, weakness, fatigue, and pallor associated with anemia. The progression varies with the specific disease process. Calcium and magnesium abnormalities can be seen in serologic laboratory tests.

Leukemic infiltration of the meninges, central nervous system, and cranial nerves results in such clinical manifestations as headache, visual disturbances, nausea, and vomiting. Bone infiltration leads to bone tenderness and pain. Hepatosplenomegaly and infiltration of other viscera are manifested by abdominal tenderness and anorexia. Lymphadenopathy and neoplastic masses are due to local infiltration.

Disease Progression

Chemotherapy has markedly increased the survival rates for acute leukemias. Untreated ALL usually is fatal within 3 months. Studies show that more than 60% of children who receive chemotherapy are alive after 5 years.[4] AML has a poorer record, even with treatment, with average survival of 1 to 2 years.

The chronic leukemias have a variable course that can be controlled by oral alkylating agents or irradiation. Progressive anemia and susceptibility to infection are hazards, and chronic myelocytic leukemia may terminate by transforming into AML.

CASE STUDY 20-1

Mr. Gary Johns, a 65-year-old man, was admitted for chemotherapy following the diagnosis of chronic myelogenous leukemia. He had white blood cell count of 250,000/mm³ with most of the cells being mature granulocytes. Examination revealed marked splenomegaly, anemia, and temperature of 100.8°F. Mr. Johns reported a weight loss of 32 pounds during the past 6 months and upper abdominal tenderness along with nonspecific arthalgias.

1. *Describe the pathophysiology of chronic myelogenous leukemia (CML). Compare it with the other forms of leukemia.*
2. *What is the clinical marker that is characteristic of CML?*
3. *Why does anemia, bleeding, and opportunistic infection occur with CML? What types of infections might be seen in this individual?*
4. *Describe the clinical picture that results form the accelerated phase of the disease.*
5. *What is the purpose of chemotherapy in CML? What is a common side effect of this therapy?*

See Appendix G for discussion.

MALIGNANT LYMPHOMAS

Malignant lymphomas are the seventh most common causes of death from cancer in the United States.[15] The incidence of these tumors is increasing each year, which may be a result of their association with acquired immunodeficiency syndrome.[15] The etiology of malignant lymphomas includes heredity, environmental carcinogen exposure, immunosuppression, and viral and oncogenic exposure.

Lymphomas are solid neoplasms that contain cells of lymphoreticular origin. These tumors should be considered tumors of the immune system, because their principal cellular component is the lymphocyte.[15] *Lymphoreticular organs* include the lymph nodes, spleen, bone marrow, thymus, liver, and submucosa of the gastrointestinal and respiratory tracts.

Pathologically, lymphadenopathy is characteristic, with eventual involvement of the liver, spleen, and viscera. Diffusely diseased nodes are gray, with capsular infiltration occurring later in the process. The enlarged nodes may become adherent to one another and to surrounding organs and tissues.[4]

Classification

The classification of malignant lymphomas usually is based on the predominant cell type and its degree of differentiation. The disease may be further divided into nodular and diffuse types, depending on the predominant pattern of cell arrangement. Table 20-9 indicates the cellular origins and sites of disease of malignant lymphomas. With more specific antiserums, the lymphocyte origin of B cells, T cells, and monocytes can be delineated.

Diffuse lymphomas are more invasive than the nodular lymphomas. The more undifferentiated the cell, the more aggressive the tumor becomes. As with leukemia, most persons with lymphomas develop immunodeficiencies that are followed by infection. A common staging classification for lymphomas is used; the later the stage, the greater the involvement and the worse the prognosis (Table 20-10).

Hodgkin's Disease

Hodgkin's disease is a malignant lymphoma that occurs in various distinct forms. It is slightly more common in men than in women and in whites than in blacks.[20] The incidence is greater between age 20 and 30 years and again after age 50.[20] Multiple factors, like with other malignant lymphomas, are linked to its development. These factors include oncogenic exposure, viruses (especially EBV of infectious mononucleosis), genetic factors, and immunodeficiency. It is characterized by proliferation of a tumor with normal tissue, reactive lymphocytes, plasma cells, and a scattering of the characteristic malignant cells, called *Reed–Sternberg* cells. Infiltration of the nodes with eosinophils and plasma cells occurs, and this is associated with necrosis and fibrosis.

The histologic criteria in Hodgkin's disease are similar to those in non-Hodgkin's lymphomas. The Reed–Sternberg cell, which is a multinucleated, odd-looking giant cell with a prominent nucleolus, must be present to confirm the diagnosis.[4, 20] Hodgkin's disease appears to involve a defect in the B or T lymphocytes, and the total lymphocyte count is depressed. Infection often causes major complications.

Hodgkin's disease has been classified into four types: 1) lymphocyte predominant, in which there is diffuse replacement by lymphocytes; 2) mixed type, which includes several distinct cell patterns, both lymphocytic and histiocytic; 3) lymphocyte depletion, with a predominant pattern of large malignant cells; and 4) nodular sclerosing, which has extensive scarring.[4]

Staging of Hodgkin's disease is usually through the Ann Arbor staging classification (see Table 20-10). Bone marrow examination and examination of the spleen for pathology after splenectomy often are the bases for staging. As with other lymphomas, the later the stage, the poorer the prognosis.

Common clinical manifestations of Hodgkin's disease are enlarged, palpable lymph nodes, fever, weight loss, and loss of energy. Node enlargement may cause

TABLE 20-9 *Comparative Classification of Lymphomas*

International Working (Survival)	1974 (Modified 1979) Lukes-Collins (Morphologic-Immunologic)	1966 (Modified 1976) Rappaport (Morphologic–Cell Size)
LOW GRADE		
Small lymphocytic		
Consistent with chronic lymphocytic leukemia	Diffuse small lymphocytic	Diffuse well-differentiated lymphocytic
Plasmacytoid	Plasmacytoid lymphocytic	Well-differentiated lymphocytic with plasmacytoid differentiation
Follicular, predominantly small cleaved cell	Follicular small cleaved	Nodular poorly differentiated lymphocytic
	Follicular and diffuse small cleaved	Nodular and diffuse poorly differentiated lymphocytic
Follicular, mixed small cleaved and large cell	Follicular small cleaved and large cell	Nodular mixed lymphocytic-histiocytic
	Follicular and diffuse small cleaved and large cell	Nodular and diffuse, mixed lymphocytic-histiocytic
INTERMEDIATE GRADE		
Follicular, predominantly large cell	Follicular, large cell	Nodular histiocytic
	Follicular and diffuse large cell	Nodular and diffuse histiocytic
Diffuse small cleaved cell	Diffuse small cleaved	Diffuse poorly differentiated lymphocytic
Diffuse mixed small and large cell	Diffuse mixed small cleaved and large cell	Diffuse poorly differentiated lymphocytic-histiocytic
Diffuse large cell		
Cleaved cell	Diffuse large cleaved	Diffuse mixed lymphocytic-histiocytic or histiocytic
Noncleaved cell	Diffuse large noncleaved	Diffuse histiocytic
HIGH GRADE		
Large cell immunoblastic	Immunoblastic sarcoma	Diffuse histiocytic
Plasmacytoid	B-cell type	
Clear cell	T-cell type	
Polymorphous	B- or T-cell type	
Epithelioid cell component	T-cell type	
Lymphoblastic	Lymphoblastic, diffuse	Diffuse lymphoblastic
Convoluted	Convoluted	
Nonconvoluted		
Small noncleaved cell	Small noncleaved	Diffuse undifferentiated
Burkitt's	Burkitt's	Burkitt's
Follicular areas	Burkitt's-like	Non-Burkitt's

From Rubin, E., and Farber, J. L. *Pathology* (2nd ed.). Philadelphia: J.B. Lippincott, 1994.

compression on the spinal cord or other organs. The tumor may invade the vasculature or the lung parenchyma.

Anemia and immunodeficiency with lymphocytopenia occur in the later stages. Biopsy may be needed to demonstrate Reed–Sternberg cells.[4] Immunodeficiency, exacerbated by chemotherapy, leads to ineffective control of microbial invasion, especially fungal and protozoal. Infection is a common complication of both the disease and the tumor.

Treatment with chemotherapy and radiation therapy has markedly improved the prognosis for Hodgkin's disease, with a 90% to 100% remission reported.

MULTIPLE MYELOMA

Multiple myeloma, or *plasma cell myeloma*, is a malignant neoplasm of plasma cells that damages the bone marrow and skeletal structure. The aberrant myeloma cells arise

TABLE 20-10 *Staging Classification Systems for Lymphomas*

National Cancer Institute Modified Staging for Intermediate- and High-Grade Lymphomas		Ann Arbor Staging Classification for Hodgkin's Disease	
Stage	Characteristics	Stage	Characteristics
I	Localized nodal or extranodal disease (Ann Arbor state I or IE)	I	Involvement of a single lymph node region (I) or a single extralymphatic organ or site (IE)
II	Two or more nodal sites of disease or a localized extranodal site plus draining nodes with none of the following: performance status ≤ 70, B symptoms, any mass > 10 cm in diameter (particularly gastrointestinal), serum lactate dehydrogenase > 500, three or more extranodal sites of disease	II	Involvement of two or more lymph node regions on the same side of the diaphragm (II) or localized involvement of an extralymphatic organ or site (IIE)
III	Stage II plus any poor prognostic features	III	Involvement of lymph node regions on both sides of the diaphragm (III) or localized involvement of an extralymphatic organ or site (IIIE) or spleen (IIIS) or both (IIISE)
		IV	Diffuse or disseminated involvement of one or more extralymphatic organs with or without associated lymph node involvement. The organ(s) involved should be identified by a symbol: A, asymptomatic; B, fever, sweats, weight loss > 10% of body weight.

From DeVita, V. (ed.). *Cancer: Principles and Practice of Oncology* (4th ed.). Philadelphia: J.B. Lippincott, 1993.

from a single clone of plasma cells that are B cell–derived and secrete anomalous circulating immunoglobulins, also called *paraproteins*. Based on the paraprotein, multiple myeloma can be categorized as follows: 1) as IgG, IgA, IgD, IgE, and IgM types; 2) as "light chain disease"; 3) as biclonal, in which two distinct paraproteins are secreted; or 4) as a nonsecretory myeloma.[20]

Laboratory examination of the bone marrow shows proliferation of both mature and immature plasma cells, with about 20% or more having multinucleated forms. These cells often completely replace the bone marrow. Serum protein electrophoresis and immunoelectrophoresis are abnormal. Bence Jones proteinemia and proteinuria, which are proliferations of light chains of immunoglobulin molecules, are present in about 50% of affected people. A higher frequency of renal failure correlates with the amount of protein found in the urine, because the excreted light chains are thought to be toxic to the renal tubules.[3] About 1% of the affected plasma cells do not secrete antibodies.

The malignant neoplasm that arises in bone usually does not metastasize outside bone. The destructive lesions erode the bone and cause punched-out lytic lesions observable radiographically (Fig. 20-3). These lesions can be visualized in any bone but are most frequent in the vertebral column, ribs, skull, pelvis, femurs, clavicles, and scapulae.[20] The bones can become so fragile

that simple movements can cause fractures. Pathologic fractures usually occur, because the lesions seem to affect the weight-bearing regions.

Calcium metabolism often is abnormal, causing some persons to have elevated serum calcium levels. There often is a normocytic, normochromic anemia, with variable depression of WBC and platelet counts.

Bone or back pain is the most common symptom. Pallor and weakness caused by secondary anemia may occur.

In some cases, myeloma nephrosis occurs because of the infiltration and precipitation of the light chains (Bence Jones protein) in the distal tubules as the urine is concentrated. The laminated, crystalline casts in the distal tubules damage the kidney cells and obstruct the tubules. Pathologic interstitial inflammation and fibrosis further impair kidney function, leading to uremia.

Anemia, thrombocytopenia that leads to bleeding, and neutropenia resulting in infection are common results of the disorder. Vascular insufficiency may occur in the peripheral areas and apparently is related to increased blood viscosity caused by high levels of circulating immunoglobulins. Survival statistics remain poor and largely depend on the person's response to the chemotherapeutic regimen, with 2 to 3 years as the norm.[4] In about 10% of cases, the disease progresses very slowly, taking many years to run its course.

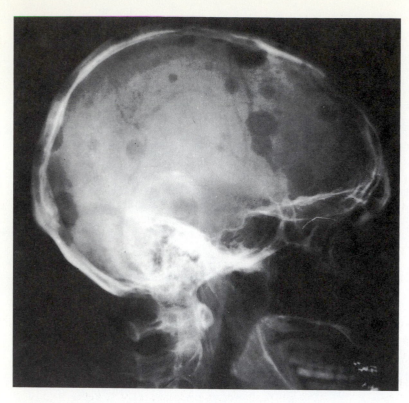

FIGURE 20-3 *Multiple myeloma. A radiograph of the skull shows numerous "punched-out" radiolucent areas. (Source: Rubin, E., and Farber, J.L. Pathology [2nd ed.]. Philadelphia: J.B. Lippincott, 1994.)*

▼ *Chapter Summary*

▼ The normal range of leukocytes per microliter of blood is between 5,000 and 10,000. Granulocytes (eosinophils, basophils, and neutrophils) and agranulocytes (lymphocytes and monocytes) compose leukocytes and can be classified as phagocytes and immunocytes. The leukocytes can be classified as phagocytes and immunocytes. WBCs have a finite life span. Neutrophils live days or hours, whereas lymphocytes may live for years. Granulocytes mature in the bone marrow and usually are delivered into the blood in their mature forms.

▼ The main purpose of the WBCs is to isolate, recognize, and kill foreign material. A major process in this action is phagocytosis, in which bacteria are killed and the effect of the organism is deleted from the body. The neutrophil and macrophage (mature monocyte) are the main phagocytes of the body. The basophils and eosinophils participate in inflammation and allergic reactions. The lymphocytes are the immunocytes discussed in Chapter 16.

▼ Nonmalignant WBC disorders include those conditions with an increase or decrease in the count of specific leukocytes or alterations in the ability of these leukocytes to perform their functions. Increased counts are especially seen in infections, whereas decreased counts occur in response to chemotherapeutic agents and exhaustion of the cellular response to infection.

▼ Malignant WBC disorders include leukemias and lymphomas. Leukemias are classified according to their cell morphology as either acute or chronic leukemia. They can be further described based on the cells affected as either lymphocytic or myelocytic.

▼ Leukemias and lymphomas are increasingly being seen in the immunosuppressed population. Lymphomas are sometimes categorized as Hodgkin's and non-Hodgkin's lymphomas, depending on their cell type and the clinical course of the disease. Treatment for Hodgkin's lymphoma has been successful, whereas the other forms have less favorable outcomes.

▼ Multiple myeloma is a malignant disease of plasma cells derived from a certain population of B cells. This disease tends to cause destructive lesions of the bones; it metastasizes outside the bones. Treatment results for this disease are very discouraging.

▼ *References*

1. Canellos, G.P. Chronic leukemias. In W.N. Kelley et al. (ed.), *Textbook of Internal Medicine* (2nd ed.). Philadelphia: J.B. Lippincott, 1992.
2. Champlin, R., and Golde, D.W. The leukemias. In J. Wilson et al. (eds.), *Harrison's Principles of Internal Medicine* (12th ed.). New York: McGraw-Hill, 1991.
3. Cormack, D.H. *Ham's Histology* (9th ed.). Philadelphia: J.B. Lippincott, 1987.
4. Cotran, R.S., Kumar, V., and Robbins, S.L. *Robbins' Pathologic Basis of Disease* (5th ed.). Philadelphia: W.B. Saunders, 1994.
5. Crowe, S. Virus infections of the immune system. In D.P.

Stites, A.I. Terr, and T.G. Parslow (eds.), *Basic and Clinical Immunology* (8th ed.). Norwalk, Conn.: Appleton-Lange. 1994.

6. Deissorth, A.B. et al. Chronic leukemias. In V.T. DeVita, S. Hellman, and S.A. Rosenberg (eds.), *Cancer: Principles and Practice of Oncology* (4th ed.). Philadelphia: J.B. Lippincott, 1993.

7. Fischbach, F. *A Manual of Laboratory and Diagnostic Tests* (4th ed.). Philadelphia: J.B. Lippincott, 1992.

8. Gallin, J. Disorders of phagocytic cells. In J. Wilson et al. (eds.), *Harrison's Principles of Internal Medicine* (12th ed.). New York: McGraw-Hill, 1991.

9. Goodman, J.W. Immunogens and antigens. In D.P. Stites, A.I. Terr, and T.G. Parslow (eds.), *Basic and Clinical Immunology* (8th ed.). Norwalk, Conn.: Appleton-Lange, 1994.

10. Guyton, A.C. *Textbook of Medical Physiology* (8th ed.). Philadelphia: W.B. Saunders, 1991

11. Hutton, J.J. The leukemias and polycythemia vera. In J.H. Stein (ed.), *Internal Medicine* (4th ed.). St. Louis: C.V. Mosby. 1994.

12. Keating, M.J., Estey, E., and Kantarjian, H. Acute leukemia. In V.T. DeVita, S. Hellman, and S.A. Rosenberg (eds.), *Cancer: Principles and Practice of Oncology* (4th ed.). Philadelphia: J.B. Lippincott, 1993.

13. Kee, J.L. *Handbook of Laboratory and Diagnostic Tests* (2nd ed.). Norwalk, Conn.: Appleton and Lange, 1994.

14. Krontiris, T.G. Molecular and cellular biology of cancer. In J.H. Stein (ed.), *Internal Medicine* (4th ed.). St. Louis: C.V. Mosby, 1994.

15. Longo, D.L., et al. Lymphocytic lymphomas. In V.T. DeVita, S. Hellman, and S.A. Rosenberg (eds.), *Cancer: Principles and Practice of Oncology* (4th ed.). Philadelphia: J.B. Lippincott, 1993.

16. Memmler, R.L., Cohen, B.J., and Wood, D.L. *The Human Body in Health and Disease* (7th ed.). Philadelphia: J.B. Lippincott, 1992.

17. Pagana, K.D., and Pagana, T.J. *Mosby's Diagnostic and Laboratory Text Reference*. St. Louis: C.V. Mosby. 1992.

18. Parslow, T.G. The phagocytes: neutrophils and macrophages. In D.P. Stites, A.I. Terr, and T.G. Parslow (eds.), *Basic and Clinical Immunology* (8th ed.) Norwalk, Conn: Appleton-Lange. 1994.

19. Roitt, I., Brostoff, J., and Male, D. *Immunology*. Philadelphia: J.B. Lippincott, 1994.

20. Rubin, E., and Farber, J.L. *Pathology* (2nd ed.). Philadelphia: J.B. Lippincott, 1994.

21. Spitznagel, J.K. Constitutive defenses of the body. In M. Schaechter, G. Medoff, and B.I. Eisenstein (eds.), *Mechanisms of Microbial Disease* (2nd ed.). Baltimore: Williams and Wilkins. 1993.

22. Straus, S.E. Herpes simplex virus and its relatives. In M. Schaechter, G. Medoff, and B.I. Eisenstein. *Mechanisms of Microbial Disease* (2nd ed.). Baltimore: Williams and Wilkins, 1993.

23. Terr, A.I. Inflammation. In D.P. Stites, A.I. Terr, and T.G. Parslow (eds.), *Basic and Clinical Immunology* (8th ed.). Norwalk, Conn: Appleton-Lange, 1994.

24. Wallach, I. *Interpretation of Diagnostic Tests* (4th ed.). Boston: Little, Brown, 1986.

25. Wiernik, P. Acute leukemias. In W.N. Kelley (ed.), *Textbook of Internal Medicine* (2nd ed.). Philadelphia: J.B. Lippincott, 1992.

26. Yungbluth, M. Infectious mononucleosis and viral infections of the upper respiratory tract. In S.T. Shulman, J.P. Phair, and H.M. Sommers (ed.), *The Biologic and Clinical Basis of Infectious Diseases* (4th ed.). Philadelphia: W.B. Saunders, 1992.

Chapter 21

Normal and Altered Coagulation

Barbara L. Bullock

▼ CHAPTER OUTLINE

▼ LEARNING OBJECTIVES

1 Define **hemostasis** and list the four major events included in this process.
2 Explain the role of vasoconstriction in hemostasis and the mechanism of stimulation.
3 Describe the function of the platelets and explain their role in the hemostatic process.
4 Describe the sequence of events in the coagulation process.
5 Describe briefly the essential clotting factors, where they are formed, and how they act.
6 Explain the common pathway of blood coagulation.
7 Differentiate between the intrinsic pathway and the extrinsic pathway in prothrombin activation.
8 Diagram the interrelationships of the major components involved in hemostasis.
9 Describe the composition of the blood clot.
10 Explain the action of the fibrinolytic system.
11 List several factors normally present in the blood that inhibit clotting.
12 Differentiate factors that enhance coagulation and those that inhibit coagulation in normal blood.
13 Explain the basis of common laboratory tests used to determine coagulation problems.
14 Explain briefly the role of liver function with respect to normal coagulation.
15 Differentiate the factor deficiencies that cause the various types of hemophilia.
16 Explain how uncontrolled bleeding occurs in disseminated intravascular coagulation.
17 Differentiate between thrombocytosis and thrombocytopenia, and list some causative conditions for each.
18 Describe some platelet disorders that are associated with hypercoagulability.

Barbara L. Bullock: PATHOPHYSIOLOGY: ADAPTATIONS AND ALTERATIONS IN FUNCTION, 4th ed.
© 1996 J.B. Lippincott-Raven Publishers

Coagulation is an essential, protective part of hemostasis that prevents blood loss when a vessel is damaged. Hemostasis refers to the arrest of bleeding. Coagulation is the ability of blood to change from a fluid to a semisolid mass. It involves the conversion of fibrinogen, a soluble macromolecule composed of three polypeptide chains, to fibrin monomers by action of the proteolytic enzyme thrombin. Polymerization (the process of combining a number of small molecules) of the monomers follows and spontaneously bonds fibrin monomers together. A fibrin-stabilizing factor acts on fibrin to cause cross-linkage bonding, which forms an insoluble, threadlike mesh on which a clot forms. This mechanism for clot initiation and formation involves a series of sequential cascadelike reactions that involve several factors in the blood and injured tissues.

▼ Characteristics and Physiology of Platelets

Platelets (also called thrombocytes) are fragments of megakaryocytes formed in the bone marrow and released into the circulation. The normal platelet concentration in the blood is about 150,000 to 400,000.[1, 11] These cell fragments are essential for normal hemostasis and clotting. They also participate in other processes, such as inflammation and fibroblast proliferation.[4]

Platelets lack a nucleus and are functionally active in the circulation for 8 to 12 days, at which time they are eliminated from the circulating blood, mostly by the macrophages in the spleen.[9] At any given time, one-third of the platelets are not circulating and are mostly seen to congregate in the red pulp of the spleen.[4] Platelets are continually being formed in the bone marrow to maintain normal levels in the body. A decrease in their number causes a marked increase in the potential for bleeding and is seen in a variety of clinical situations.

The cell membrane has on its surface a coat of glycoproteins that prevents its adherence to normal endothelium and allows it to adhere to damaged surfaces (see below). The membrane contains phospholipids with platelet factor III, which is important in the blood clotting process.[9] Within the cytoplasm of the platelets are found dense granules that contain active factors, which include actin and myosin, adenosine triphosphate and adenosine diphosphate, prostaglandins, serotonin, fibrin-stabilizing factor, and a growth factor that helps to repair damaged vascular walls.[9] The residual endoplasmic reticulum and Golgi's apparatus synthesize enzymes and store calcium ions.[9]

▼ Hemostasis

Hemostasis, the arrest of bleeding or circulation of the blood, is often divided into four main events: 1) vasoconstriction; 2) formation of a hemostatic platelet plug;

3) blood coagulation; and 4) clot formation. The interaction of all four events is essential for normal hemostasis. The general dynamic interaction of these events is illustrated in Figure 21-1.

VASOCONSTRICTION

Vasoconstriction is the result of many events that occur during an injury. Immediately after the wall of a vessel is injured, contraction of the vessel decreases the flow of blood in and out of the vessel. This contraction is due mainly to nervous reflexes and local myogenic spasms.[5] Nervous reflexes are probably initiated by pain impulses created by the tissue or vascular trauma. Local myogenic spasm is initiated by direct damage to the vascular wall and by the release of serotonin from platelets.

The greater the portion of vessel traumatized, the greater the degree of spasm. A sharply cut vessel bleeds longer than a crushed one.[5] A clean cut by a sharp razor blade, for example, bleeds longer than a scrape or jagged cut.

HEMOSTATIC PLATELET PLUG FORMATION

When a blood vessel is damaged, the endothelial lining is disrupted, exposing the underlying collagen. When platelets are exposed to collagen or other foreign surfaces, such as antigen–antibody complexes, thrombin, proteolytic enzymes, endotoxins, or viruses, they undergo a dynamic change in their appearance. They begin to swell and form irregular shapes with processes protruding from their surfaces. They become sticky and adhere to the collagen and basement membrane of the vessel. In this process of *platelet adhesion*, they become activated and liberate the contents of their granules.[15] The platelets release adenosine diphosphate, which attracts other platelets and aids in platelet adhesion and aggregation. Adenosine diphosphate also is released from disrupted red blood cells and damaged tissue. Enzymes released from the platelets cause the formation of thromboxane A (a type of prostaglandin) in the plasma.[5] Both adenosine diphosphate and thromboxane A activate nearby platelets that stick to the original platelets, thereby creating a cycle of platelet activation. The gathering of the platelets is called *platelet aggregation*, and eventually a platelet plug results, which causes the damaged endothelial vessel wall to adhere to the collagen fibers (Fig. 21-2).[9, 15] This plug is loose and arrests circulation only if the tear in the vessel is small. Later, a tight plug is formed by fibrin threads that result from the process of coagulation. Hundreds of minute ruptures occur in the capillaries each day. The platelet plug is important because it can stop bleeding completely if the damage is small. A significant decrease in the number of platelets can lead to small hemorrhagic areas under the

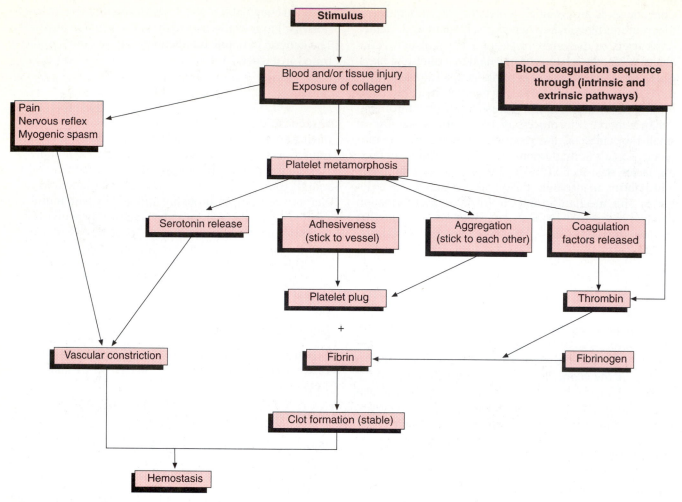

FIGURE 21-1 *Hemostatic mechanisms.*

skin and in the internal tissue.[9] Usually, the plugging mechanism seals the tear in the vessel rather than occluding the lumen.

▼ General Mechanism of Blood Coagulation

After initial hemostasis, as described above, the sequential activation of the factors for blood coagulation takes place. The interaction of these factors causes the formation of the solid clot, which ensures the prevention of blood loss in the case of a vascular tear. As will be noted, clotting within the vascular system or on damaged endothelium of the heart can occur, and this process often causes major circulatory problems.

Three basic reactions constitute the sequential pathway for blood coagulation: 1) a prothrombin activator is formed by the intrinsic or extrinsic pathway in response to tissue or endothelial damage; 2) prothrombin activator catalyzes the conversion of prothrombin to throm-

bin; and 3) thrombin catalyzes the conversion of soluble fibrinogen to solid fibrin polymer threads. These fibrin threads form the meshwork on which plasma, blood cells, and platelets aggregate to make the clot (Fig. 21-3). Before these three reactions can occur, other responses must take place. A group of reactants called clotting factors begin the process that terminates in the formation of the blood clot.

CLOTTING FACTORS

The clotting factors are a series of plasma proteins that are generally inactive forms of proteolytic enzymes. Table 21-1 summarizes these factors and indicates the international nomenclature used for each. The enzymatic proteolytic actions cause successive reactions of the clotting process in a cascadelike sequence. One activated factor is important for the activation of the next factor. The sequentially derived product of one reaction supplies the essential protease necessary for the next reaction. A low level or lack of even one of these inactive

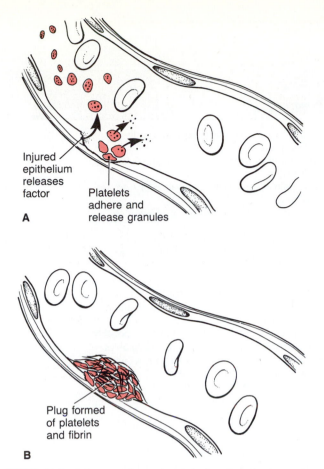

A

B

FIGURE 21-2 **A.** *Damaged vessel endothelium is a stimulus to circulating platelets, causing platelet adhesion. Platelets release mediators.* **B.** *Platelet aggregation results.*

proteolytic enzymes can lead to abnormal bleeding and hemorrhage.[5]

Fibrinogen, prothrombin, and factors VII, IX, and X are essential procoagulation factors. Fibrinogen (factor I) is synthesized in the liver at a rate that usually corresponds to the rate of use or need. The levels of fibrinogen may be increased by adrenocorticotropic hormone, growth hormone, endotoxin, pregnancy, and occlusive arterial disease. Prothrombin (factor II) and factors VII, IX, and X are also synthesized exclusively in the liver by a process that requires vitamin K. Lack of vitamin K can result from liver disease and intestinal malabsorption.[9]

FORMATION OF THE PROTHROMBIN ACTIVATOR

The coagulation process begins with the formation of the prothrombin activator, a substance or complex of substances. The mechanism is initiated by trauma to the tissues or blood, contact of the blood with damaged endothelial cells, collagen, or other substances outside the blood vessel endothelium. This injury or contact leads to the formation of the prothrombin activator, which then leads to the conversion of prothrombin to thrombin.

The prothrombin activator is formed in one of two ways: 1) through the extrinsic pathway, initiated by trauma to the vessel wall or tissues outside the vessel; or 2) through the intrinsic pathway, which begins with trauma to blood components and thus alters the platelets and factor XII.

Interplay of the intrinsic and extrinsic systems is needed for normal clotting. Deficiency of a single protein in one of these pathways may lead to a clotting disorder. The intrinsic and extrinsic pathways converge on a final common pathway, leading to the formation of a fibrin clot (see Figure 21-3). Each precursor protein is important in the clotting process because it is necessary for the activation of the next.

The clotting process occurs by a cascade of activation of one clotting factor after another. The activated form of one factor sequentially catalyzes the activation of the next in cascade fashion, leading to clot formation (Flowchart 21-1).

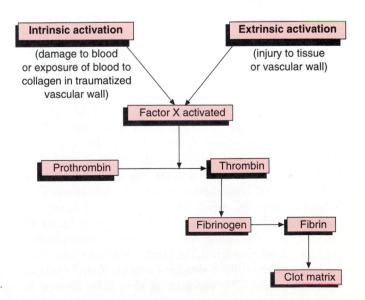

FIGURE 21-3 *Common pathway of blood coagulation.*

TABLE 21-1 *Blood Coagulation Factors*

Factor (International Nomenclature)	Common Synonyms	Remarks
I	Fibrinogen	Soluble macromolecule, synthesized in liver, fibrin precursor
II	Prothrombin	Synthesized in liver, vitamin K required for formation
III	Tissue thromboplastin; thrombokinase	Phospholipid; involved in activation of extrinsic pathway
IV	Calcium	Involved in several complexes of coagulation process
V	Proaccelerin; labile factor; Ac-globulin; Ac-G	Synthesized in liver; modifier protein, not enzyme; required in prothrombin activator complex
(VI)	Obsolete term	Same as factor V
VII	Proconvertin; stable factor; serum prothrombin conversion accelerator	Part of enzyme complex in extrinsic pathway; synthesized in the liver; vitamin K required for formation
VIII	Antihemophilic globulin (AHG); antihemophilic factor (AHF); antihemophilic factor A	Required for intrinsic pathway function; possibly synthesized in liver, spleen, RES, or kidneys
IX	Plasma thromboplastin component (PTC); Christmas factor; antihemophilic factor B	Synthesized in liver; requires vitamin K; needed for intrinsic pathway function
X	Stuart-Prower factor; Stuart factor	Synthesized in the liver; requires vitamin K, needed for both intrinsic and extrinsic pathways
XI	Plasma thromboplastin antecedent (PTA); anti-hemophilic factor C	Substrate in intrinsic activator enzymatic complex; needed for intrinsic system activation, area of synthesis unknown
XII	Hageman factor; contact factor; antihemophilic factor D	Involved in first step of activation of intrinsic system; area of synthesis unknown
XIII	Fibrin stabilizing factor (FSF); fibrinase	Causes amide cross-linkage fibrin; stabilizes clot formation, synthesized by platelets and possibly other proteins, may be activated by liver

INTRINSIC PATHWAY

The intrinsic pathway for the initiation of coagulation is through activation of components already present in the blood. This mechanism for initiating clotting begins within the vessel and occurs more slowly (it usually requires several minutes) than the extrinsic pathway.[15] When the blood comes into contact with collagen or damaged endothelium, an intrinsic activator–enzymatic complex is formed. An important part of this complex is the Hageman factor (activated factor XII), a proteolytic enzyme. This complex enzymatically activates factor XI. Sequential events continue in cascade fashion. Activated factor XI enzymatically activates factor IX. Factor IX forms factor X activation complex, which consists of activated factor IX, factor VIII, calcium, and phospholipids. Activated factor X then combines with factor V, calcium, and phospholipids to form the prothrombin activator. Within seconds, the prothrombin activator initiates the proteolytic cleavage of prothrombin bonds to form thrombin. The amount of thrombin formed is closely related to the amount of prothrombin activator present. Once thrombin is formed, the final clotting process is set in motion.

If factor VIII or the platelets are not at an adequate level, activation of factor X is impaired. Decreased factor VIII is the major problem in classic hemophilia, and decreased platelets result in bleeding disorders, such as thrombocytopenia (see pp. 420–421). All of the clotting factors are essential to the normal coagulation sequence.

EXTRINSIC PATHWAY

The extrinsic pathway for coagulation is triggered by factors not normally present in the blood, such as substances released from damaged tissues or other foreign materials. Because it has fewer steps than the intrinsic pathway, it occurs rapidly, often within seconds.[15] When the blood comes in contact with a traumatized vascular wall or extravascular tissue, substances called tissue factor and tissue phospholipids are released. Tissue factor is

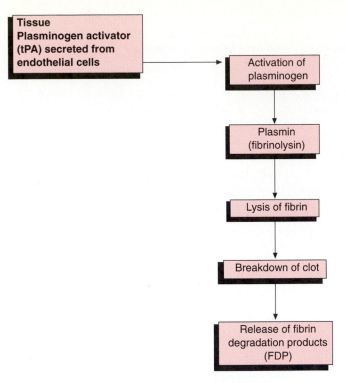

FIGURE 21-4 *The presence of fibrin causes the release of tPA which activates plasminogen, a circulating plasma protein, to plasmin which is the same as fibrinolysin. Plasmin breaks down fibrin causing the breakdown of clot and release of FDPs, also called fibrin split products (FSP).*

a proteolytic enzyme with cleavage ability, and tissue phospholipids are mainly those of the cell membrane.

The tissue factor plus factor VII, calcium, and phospholipids form a complex. This complex acts enzymatically on factor X to form activated factor X. Activated factor X then becomes part of the prothrombin activator complex, which enzymatically converts prothrombin to thrombin. Thrombin, in turn, enzymatically converts fibrinogen to fibrin.

FINAL COMMON PATHWAY TO CLOT FORMATION

With the activation of factor X and formation of the prothrombin activator complex, the final common pathway for clot formation begins (see Figure 21-3). Prothrombin activator complex causes the conversion of prothrombin to thrombin. Thrombin, in turn, enzymatically converts fibrinogen to fibrin. These reactions constitute the final coagulation pathway for both the intrinsic and extrinsic systems. The rate of the blood coagulation reaction is generally related to the amount of prothrombin activator formed and the degree of activation of factor X. If either is inhibited or stopped because of the absence of a clotting factor or other reasons, the coagulation process becomes altered and excess bleeding results.

CLOT FORMATION

Blood coagulation occurs faster with severe trauma to the vascular wall than with minor trauma. The general sequence of physical events takes place in a comparatively short time. After the vessel is severed, the platelets aggregate and fibrin appears. A fibrin clot can form in as little as 15 seconds up to 6 minutes. Clot retraction follows and may take 30 to 60 minutes. After the clot is formed, it either dissolves or organizes into a fibrous mass.

Blood Clot Composition

The blood clot is composed of a meshwork of polymerized fibrin threads that have become attached to blood cells, platelets, and plasma products. The fibrin threads adhere to the damaged vessel surface, holding the clot in place and preventing blood loss. The meshwork is produced by spontaneous aggregation of fibrin monomer to form polymer threads. Fibrin-stabilizing factor (factor XIII) acts on the fibrin to form covalent cross-links. This stabilizes the clot and makes it resistant to dissolution.[15]

Clot Retraction

The contractile physiology of the platelet response is critical in clot retraction. Failure of a clot to retract often indicates a decrease in the number of platelets. The platelets entrapped in the clot continue to release fibrin-stabilizing factor. Stronger bonding of the fibrin threads occurs and causes the threads to contract. Clot retraction pulls the edges of a broken vessel closer together, which allows the vascular wall to mend. After contraction is completed, blood serum, which includes plasma and the clotting factors, is expressed from the clot.

▼ Lysis of Blood Clots

Plasmin, or *fibrinolysin*, a proteolytic enzyme that resembles trypsin, is formed from inactive circulating plasminogen by the action of thrombin, which stimulates the production of *tissue-type plasminogen activator*.[7] It digests fibrin threads and causes lysis of the clot along with destruction of blood clotting factors. Large amounts of the inactive enzyme plasminogen are incorporated into the clot and activated by vascular endothelial factors, such as thrombin, activated factor XII, and lysosomal enzymes in damaged tissue (Fig. 21-4).[9] Bacterial organisms, especially streptococci, produce activators. In the case of the streptococcus organism, the activator is *streptokinase*, which has been used therapeutically to dissolve clots. Plasmin largely mediates the fibrinolytic system. This built-in, self-destructing system for clots breaks

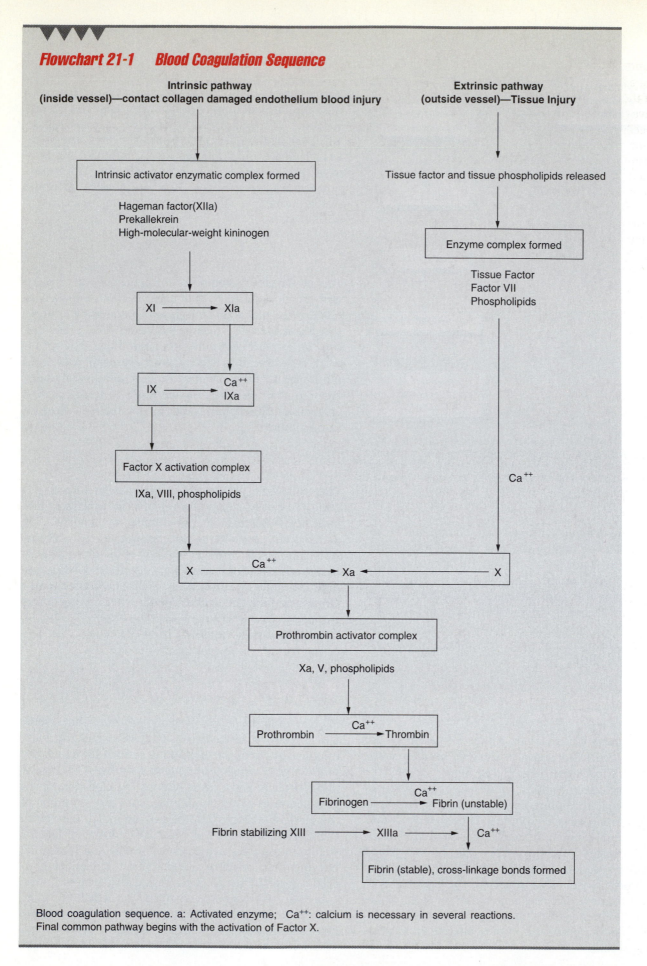

Flowchart 21-1   Blood Coagulation Sequence

Intrinsic pathway
(inside vessel)—contact collagen damaged endothelium blood injury

Extrinsic pathway
(outside vessel)—Tissue Injury

Intrinsic activator enzymatic complex formed

Tissue factor and tissue phospholipids released

Hageman factor(XIIa)
Prekallekrein
High-molecular-weight kininogen

Enzyme complex formed

Tissue Factor
Factor VII
Phospholipids

XI ⟶ XIa

IX ⟶ Ca^{++}
IXa

Factor X activation complex

IXa, VIII, phospholipids

Ca^{++}

X ⟶ Ca^{++} ⟶ Xa ⟵ X

Prothrombin activator complex

Xa, V, phospholipids

Prothrombin ⟶ Ca^{++} ⟶ Thrombin

Fibrinogen ⟶ Ca^{++} ⟶ Fibrin (unstable)

Fibrin stabilizing XIII ⟶ XIIIa ⟶ Ca^{++}

Fibrin (stable), cross-linkage bonds formed

Blood coagulation sequence. a: Activated enzyme; Ca^{++}: calcium is necessary in several reactions.
Final common pathway begins with the activation of Factor X.

down and limits excessive clot formation. Plasmin is self-limiting and localizes the fibrinolytic activity to the region of the resolving clot. Inhibitors of plasmin prevent excessive proteolytic action.

Specific substances, such as alpha$_2$-antiplasmin and alpha$_2$-macroglobulin, inhibit plasmin action. Alpha$_2$-antiplasmin binds to fibrin by factor XIII during clot formation, so that the rate of fibrinolysis depends on a balance of amounts of plasminogen, plasminogen activators, and antiplasmins within the clot.[7] The fibrinolytic system breaks down the clot so that healing can occur. Intravascularly, it ensures patency of the vascular system. The degradation products produced from fibrinolysis are called fibrinogen degradation products, which inhibit the formation of thrombin and limit the formation of the clot. A balance between the formation of thrombin and plasmin must be present for normal coagulation and clot dissolution to occur.

▼ Anticoagulation Factors in Normal Blood

Anticoagulants inhibit coagulation and are important in keeping the blood fluid. An anticoagulant can be considered as any factor that prevents blood clotting. Factors that aid in the prevention of clotting include the smooth endothelial lining of the vessel, rapid blood flow through an area, negatively charged proteins on the endothelial surface, and anticoagulant substances in the blood.

A smooth endothelium and a monomolecular layer of negatively charged proteins adsorbed on the endothelium are essential for maintaining the fluidity of blood.[9] Rapid blood flow dilutes the factors that promote coagulation, thus preventing initiation of the clotting process. An intact, smooth endothelium prevents contact activation of the intrinsic pathway, and the layer of negatively charged proteins repels clotting factors and platelets that might stick to the vessel wall.

Several plasma proteins can dampen the activity of proteolytic enzymes generated in the coagulation and fibrinolytic systems. These include antiplasmin, activated protein C inhibitor, antithrombin III, and alpha$_2$-macroglobulin.[9] These plasma proteins localize coagulation action at the site of injury and prevent propagation of the coagulation effect throughout the vascular system.

The most powerful anticoagulants in the blood are those that remove the excess thrombin formed during coagulation. These are *fibrin threads* and *antithrombin III*. During clot formation, 85% to 90% of thrombin becomes adsorbed to fibrin threads.[9] This adsorption effectively stops the action of thrombin on fibrinogen. Excess thrombin not adsorbed combines with the plasma protein antithrombin III, which blocks the effect of thrombin on fibrinogen and inactivates the thrombin.

Heparin, a potent anticoagulant, is present in the granules of the circulating basophils and the tissue mast cells. Its concentration in blood is very slight. Heparin acts as an anticoagulant mainly by inhibiting factor IX, factor X, and thrombin. It reacts with factors in both the intrinsic and extrinsic pathways.

▼ Laboratory Tests for Coagulation Problems

CLOTTING OR COAGULATION TIME

One of the oldest tests for normal coagulation is based on the amount of time drawn blood takes to clot. This can be done simply by observing the clotting time in a test tube. Increased clotting time indicates that a problem exists, but normal clotting time does not rule out a hemostatic abnormality (Table 21-2).

Causes of prolonged clotting time include deficiencies of any factor in the intrinsic clotting system or in the common pathway, fibrinogen deficiency, and excessively rapid fibrinolysis. This test has long been used for persons receiving heparin therapy but is now being replaced by the partial thromboplastin time (PTT), which is a more sensitive measurement of the coagulation factors.

PROTHROMBIN TIME

In the test for prothrombin time (PT), animal tissue extract and calcium are added to freshly drawn and separated citrated plasma. The time the mixture takes to clot is given in seconds (see Table 21-2). The tissue extract bypasses the intrinsic clotting system so that only factors VII, X, and V; prothrombin; and fibrinogen affect the test. The PT is often reported as a percentage of normal activity, which is a way of expressing the activity of factors in comparison to a normal control subject. Normal is always considered to be 100%. If the individual measures at 20%, only about one-fifth of normal clotting activity exists. A person having faster clotting activity than the control subject can have greater than 100% activity. An *increased* PT refers to a longer time for clotting to occur, with clotting ability being less than normal. A *decreased* PT refers to the reverse. Deficiencies of factors XII, XI, IX, and VIII do not affect the PT.

The PT is often used to monitor the effects of the coumarin anticoagulants. Coumarin depresses the synthesis of factors VII, IX, X, and prothrombin.

PARTIAL THROMBOPLASTIN TIME

Partial thromboplastin time is a relatively simple test for mild to moderate deficiencies of intrinsic clotting factors (see Table 21-2). It is useful for detecting many types of bleeding disorders due to decreased amounts of factors

TABLE 21-2 *Normal Blood Coagulation Values*

Test	Normal Values	Significance of Altered Values
Clotting or coagulation time	6–17 min (glass tube) 19–60 min (siliconized tube)	Prolonged in deficiency of all clotting factors except VIII and VII; used for heparin therapy control
Prothrombin time	10–14 sec	Prolonged in deficiency of factors I, II, V, VII, and X; inadequate vitamin K in diet; extrinsic pathway
Partial thromboplastin time (PTT)	30–45 sec	Prolonged by deficiency in factors I, II, V, VIII, IX, X, XI, and XII; intrinsic pathway; best single screening test; APTT most commonly used
Activated partial thromboplastin time (APTT)	16–23 sec	
Platelet count	150,000–300,000/μL	Increased in malignancy, myeloproliferative disease, iron deficiency anemia, collagen disorders, cirrhosis of the liver, thrombocytosis; decreased in thrombocytopenia, laboratory artifact, red blood cell count above 6.5 mil/mm³
Bleeding time	2.5–9 min (Ivy method) 8 min (Duke method)	Prolonged in thrombocytopenia, drug-induced with aspirin, indomethacin, phenylbutazone, myeloproliferative diseases; normal in hemophilia A and B, hypoprothrombinemia, hypofibrinogenemia
Clot retraction	Begins: 30–60 min Complete: 12–24 h	Prolonged in thrombocytopenia, thrombasthenia (oxygen release deficit)

Values summarized from Fishbach, F. A Manual of Laboratory and Diagnostic Tests (4th ed.). Philadelphia: J.B. Lippincott, 1992.

composing the intrinsic system. It is a general test that is used to monitor heparin therapy. Chemicals are often added to achieve an activated PTT (aPTT). The resulting clotting time is accelerated.

The PTT increases (becomes longer) both in hereditary factor deficiencies and in acquired conditions, such as disseminated intravascular coagulation (DIC). Therapeutic heparin is used to keep the PTT at 1.5 to 2.5 times the normal level. This therapy may be used in persons who have hypercoagulable blood as discussed on pages 421–422.[2] Deficiencies of all the factors prolong the PTT, with the exception of factor VII. A person with a factor VII deficiency has a normal PTT and a prolonged PT. Partial thromboplastin time can be used to demonstrate circulating anticoagulants in plasma. If test plasma mixed with normal plasma has a longer PTT than normal plasma alone, it indicates that something in the test plasma has inhibited coagulation.

TESTS FOR SPECIFIC DEFICIENCIES

Specific coagulation factor assays are special tests that can determine the absence of specific clotting factors. Any of the other specific factors can be tested. Small amounts of blood are added to samples of plasma known to be deficient in a particular factor. If, for example, the added plasma corrects the PTT to normal for plasma

known to be deficient in a particular factor, then that factor is not deficient in the sample. The process is repeated until the tested plasma does not correct the PTT. This identifies the missing factor in the plasma of the individual being tested. Several special tests for coagulation factors are based on this laboratory method.

PLATELET COUNT

One of the most common laboratory tests, the complete blood count, usually includes the platelet count (see Table 21-2). Platelets are difficult to count because of their inherent tendency to clump, adhere to the vessel, and aggregate. Electronic means of counting them offer the greatest accuracy.

Thrombocytosis (increased number of platelets) may occur in association with certain malignancies and with polycythemia vera. Thrombocytopenia (decreased number of platelets) may be secondary to many conditions, or it may be idiopathic (see p. 420).

BLEEDING TIME

Measurement of *bleeding time* is achieved through an incision made either on the earlobe (Duke's method) or on the inner surface of the forearm (Ivy's method). The time needed for active bleeding from the clean, superficial wound to stop is called the bleeding time (see Table 21-2). The variables involved are vascular contractility and platelet aggregation.

Secondary bleeding time can be measured by noting how long it takes for bleeding to cease after a scab is removed. Secondary bleeding time is prolonged in persons with deficiencies of factors in the intrinsic pathway or factor XIII, the fibrin-stabilizing factor.

CLOT RETRACTION

Measuring the clot retraction time consists of observing the time in which a clot retracts and expresses serum and the degree of retraction. Whole blood is left in a test tube at 37°C. Clot retraction normally begins in about 30 minutes; by 4 hours, a well-defined clot is surrounded by clear serum. Complete retraction requires about 12 to 24 hours if measured at room temperature. The norm is 50% to 100% in 2 hours.[6] If platelet function or number is decreased, clot retraction is impaired.

▼ Alterations in Blood Coagulation

Deficiency of any of the clotting factors or platelets can result in a defect or impairment of blood coagulation. This impairment may result from genetic deficiencies of clotting factors or suppression or consumption of the major clotting components. Coagulation does not occur as an isolated, independent event but continually interacts with other mechanisms of the body, such as the inflammatory process. Alterations in the process can result in injury, hemorrhage, or death.

SINGLE COAGULATION FACTOR DEFICIENCIES

Single coagulation factor deficiencies are usually hereditary. The most common deficiencies are of factor VIII, IX, and XI. All cause bleeding that may involve any of the soft tissues or the joints.

Hemophilia

The term hemophilia loosely defines several different hereditary deficiencies of coagulation factors of the intrinsic pathway. The most common cause of this coagulation disorder is a deficiency in factor VIII, accounting for about 83% to 85% of cases of hemophilia.[5] Usually, factor VIII is produced, but it is abnormal and does not promote coagulation.

The classic factor VIII deficiency is genetically transmitted through a sex-linked recessive gene. It affects males almost exclusively. Females are usually asymp-

tomatic carriers but in rare cases may manifest the disease.[1] This type of hemophilia is called *classic hemophilia* or *hemophilia A*. It is characterized by spontaneous or traumatic subcutaneous and intramuscular hemorrhages. Hematuria and bleeding from the mouth, gums, lips, and tongue are common manifestations. Repeated joint hemorrhages cause extreme pain and deformity. The severity of the bleeding depends on the coagulation factor levels with borderline factor VIII (0.05 μ/mL with a normal range of 0.5 to 2.0 μ/mL, causing problems only with posttraumatic or postsurgical bleeding). Levels below 0.02 μ per mL result in spontaneous bleeding episodes.[1] Transfusion of normal factor VIII or fresh plasma briefly relieves the bleeding tendency.

Von Willebrand disease is characterized by a quantitative and qualitative deficiency of factor VIII. Because of this deficiency, adhesion of platelets to the injury-exposed collagen is impaired. This condition produces a prolonged bleeding time with a mild to moderate bleeding disorder. Epistaxis, gastrointestinal bleeding, and menorrhagia are common.[1, 6, 12] Von Willebrand factor is one of the products of factor VIII. This condition, usually of autosomal dominant basis, has been shown to be associated with some of the autoimmune and lymphoproliferative conditions.

Factor IX deficiency, called *hemophilia B* or *Christmas disease*, is sex-linked, recessive, and accounts for about 10% to 15% of cases of hemophilia. Clinically, it is indistinguishable from factor VIII hemophilia and requires laboratory differentiation.[1] Bleeding tends to be severe, with crippling joint deformities. This condition is sometimes seen in association with severe protein-wasting glomerulopathies.[5]

Factor XI deficiency, called *hemophilia C* or *Rosenthal's disease*, is a mild bleeding disorder manifested by bruising, epistaxis, and menorrhagia. It is transmitted as an autosomal recessive trait and accounts for about 2% of hemophiliacs. The mildness of this disease is thought to be due to activation of factor XI through other mechanisms.[12]

VITAMIN K DEFICIENCY

Many disorders can lead to deficiencies of several coagulation factors. One example is fat-soluble vitamin K, which is required for the synthesis of factors II, VII, IX, and X. These vitamin K–dependent factors can be monitored by PT. Deficiencies of vitamin K may result from several conditions. A newborn normally is deficient in vitamin K due to an immature liver and lack of intestinal bacteria that are important for the synthesis of the vitamin. The newborn is often given injections of vitamin K to help prevent any possible bleeding disorder that might occur.

Obstructive liver disease and malabsorption disorders can also cause a deficiency in vitamin K. Obstructive liver disease blocks the flow of bile necessary for the absorption of fat-soluble vitamins, and malabsorption disorders do not allow enough vitamin K to be absorbed into the circulation.[13]

Coumarin anticoagulants are competitive inhibitors of vitamin K. Vitamin K can be injected as an antidote in case of excessive bleeding or possible hemorrhage due to overdose of these drugs.

LIVER DISEASE

Coagulation disorders and platelet dysfunction are present in persons with significant liver disease. The liver is essential for the synthesis of the coagulation proteins and for the removal of activated coagulation products from the circulation. Liver disease may produce platelet dysfunction and thrombocytopenia. Any form of severe liver dysfunction, such as that produced from hepatitis, shock state, poisoning, or acute alcohol-induced dysfunction, can produce abnormal coagulation.[5, 13] The abnormal coagulation results from the following: 1) reduced coagulation factor synthesis; 2) failure to remove activated products; 3) impaired clearance of the fibrinolytic enzymes; and 4) accompanying DIC.[1]

MASSIVE TRANSFUSION SYNDROME

A large volume of blood administered over a short time causes a decrease in circulating coagulation factors and platelets. Bank blood is usually deficient in factor V, factor VIII, and platelets.[8] It also is collected into bags that contain citric acid, which prevents clotting. If multiple units of blood are administered, a generalized bleeding disorder may occur.[1]

DISSEMINATED INTRAVASCULAR COAGULATION/CONSUMPTIVE COAGULOPATHY

Disseminated intravascular coagulation involves both bleeding and clotting. It occurs as a complication of several clinical conditions that trigger senseless activation of the clotting factors within the circulating blood.[13] The consumption of clotting factors and platelets result in a serious hemorrhagic condition that is accompanied by ischemic changes resulting from microvascular thrombosis.[13] It may occur secondary to a major, often life-threatening, condition or, rarely, be a subclinical disorder noted only on laboratory examination.[1, 13] The process begins with activation of the sequence causing coagulation. This hypercoagulable state produces thrombosis, especially in the small vessels.[8] Widespread coagulation activation leads to consumption of clotting factors, such as platelets and fibrin. Secondary activation of the fibrinolytic system then occurs. Table 21-3 indicates some of the diverse factors that can initiate the coagulation sequence. Persons who develop DIC are of-

TABLE 21-3 *Etiology of Disseminated Intravascular Coagulation*

Causative Agent or Condition	Probable Massive Coagulation Stimulus
Infection	
Gram-negative bacteria	Endotoxemia; endothelial damage
Gram-positive bacteria	Fulminating sepsis; endothelial damage
Rickettsia rickettsii (Rocky Mountain spotted fever)	Parasitization of endothelial cells; rupture walls of small vessels
Plasmodium falciparum (falciparum malaria)	Injury to red blood cells and platelets; possible antigen–antibody reaction
Complications of pregnancy	
Amniotic fluid embolism	Circulating thromboplastins absorbed
Saline abortion	
Hydatidiform mole	
Puerperal sepsis	Vascular damage
Toxemia	
Large hemangiomas	Turbulence of blood, stasis Endothelial damage
Disseminated carcinoma	Circulating tissue thromboplastins from malignant tissue
Hemolytic transfusion reaction anaphylaxis, hemolytic-uremic syndrome	Antigen–antibody reactions
Tissue damage	
Massive trauma	Thromboplastins released
Heat stroke	
Extensive burns	
Snake bites	
Extracorporeal circulation	Blood injury

ten critically ill as a result of the underlying disease. The DIC often develops insidiously, and widespread bleeding becomes the initial sign.

The clotting sequence is triggered either by endothelial damage that activates the intrinsic coagulation cascade or by release of thromboplastic substances. The resultant clotting causes occlusion of a large proportion of the small peripheral blood vessels. The clotting sequence activates the fibrinolytic system and thus causes diffuse fibrinolysis. The conversion of plasminogen to plasmin in the fibrinolytic system inhibits the proteolysis of fibrinogen by thrombin and may inhibit platelet aggregation. Fibrin degradation (split) products are formed by the lysis of plasmin, fibrinogen, and fibrin. These end products form a complex with the fibrin monomer, which prevents the laying down of the fibrin thread and platelet aggregation. Therefore, despite widespread clotting, the major problem is bleeding (Fig. 21-5).

Uncontrolled bleeding occurs because of consumption of the clotting factors. Normal hemostasis is pre-

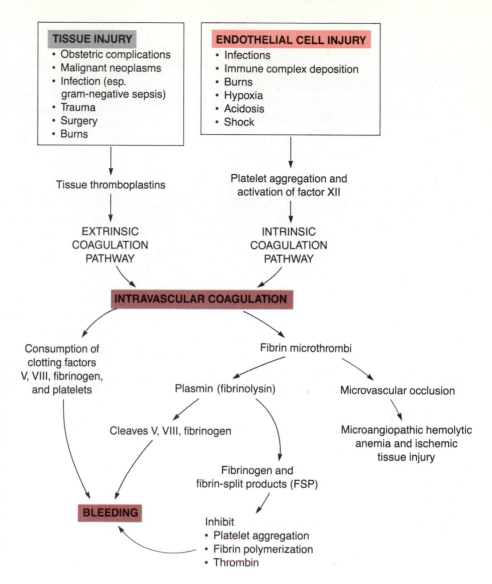

FIGURE 21-5 *The pathophysiology of disseminated intravascular coagulation (DIC). The syndrome of DIC is precipitated either by tissue injury, with release of tissue thromboplastin and activation of the extrinsic coagulation pathway, or by endothelial cell injury, with activation of the intrinsic coagulation pathway. Intravascular coagulation is induced by either one or both mechanisms. Clinically, there is bleeding from multiple sites and microvascular occlusions or thromboses with secondary microangiopathic hemolytic anemia and ischemic tissue injury. (Source: E. Rubin and J. Farber, Pathology [2nd ed.]. Philadelphia: J.B. Lippincott, 1994)*

vented, so varying degrees of ecchymoses, petechiae, and bleeding from any opening may occur. The onset may be acute, such as that after acute obstetric emergencies, or it may gradually develop, as with disseminated cancers. Bleeding problems usually predominate, and venipuncture sites or incisions may bleed profusely.

Acrocyanosis often occurs in the digits and is manifest as cold, mottled fingers and toes. Hypoxemia may cause dyspnea, cyanosis, and air hunger. Neurologic or renal symptoms may result from microthrombi that occlude the small vessels.

Laboratory tests that are helpful include the PT, PTT, fibrinogen level, and platelet count. Both the PT and PTT are prolonged, whereas fibrinogen and platelet levels are depressed. Levels of fibrin split or degradation products are elevated.

Treatment of DIC involves anticoagulation with heparin to interrupt the coagulation process followed by replacement of the clotting factors and platelets to pre-

vent further bleeding.[13] It is most important to treat the underlying disease process to decrease the stimulus for the coagulopathy.

PRIMARY FIBRINOLYSIS

Primary fibrinolysis results when massive amounts of plasminogen activator are released into the system. The activator, such as streptokinase, may be administered therapeutically to dissolve pulmonary emboli. Plasminogen activators can also be released by activator-rich neoplastic tissue, such as prostatic carcinoma. Severe anoxia, shock, or surgical procedures may also precipitate their release.

Disseminated intravascular coagulation and primary fibrinolysis reactions are similar. Both are associated with increased fibrinolytic activity, but primary fibrinolysis results in increased amounts of plasminogen activator in the plasma. In DIC, it is a secondary response to a hypercoagulable state. In primary fibrinolysis, there is a marked increase in bleeding potential at any vulnerable site, such as the mucous membranes, gastrointestinal system, and intracerebral areas.

ANTIBODY ANTICOAGULANTS

Antibodies to various coagulation factors have been observed in many disease states. About 10% of persons treated for hemophilia A develop an antifactor antibody to factor VIII.[1] Antibodies to paraproteins in persons with multiple myelomas and antibodies to multiple coagulation factors in persons with systemic lupus erythematosus are other examples of antibodies that act as circulating anticoagulants. The development of antibodies to coagulation factors results in an increased risk of hemorrhage.

▼ Platelet Disorders

THROMBOCYTOPENIA

This quantitative platelet disorder involves the presence of a very small number of platelets in the circulatory system. If the platelet count falls below 50,000, there is a potential for hemorrhage associated with trauma, such as surgery or accidents. A platelet count of about 20,000 is associated with petechiae, ecchymoses, and sometimes bleeding from mucous membranes. With a count below 5,000, a great risk exists for fatal hemorrhage through the intestinal tract or central nervous system.[3]

An abnormal decrease in the number of platelets may occur in several disorders, such as defective platelet production, increased platelet destruction, sequestration of platelets, and loss of platelets from the system. The two major types of thrombocytopenia are idiopathic thrombocytopenic purpura and secondary thrombocytopenia. Table 21-4 classifies causes of thrombocytopenia by mechanism. Figure 21-6 illustrates the evaluation of thrombocytopenia to determine the cause.

Idiopathic thrombocytopenia purpura is apparently an autoimmune condition that causes an increased rate of destruction of platelets. The result is either acute destruction of platelets, which often follows a viral infection, or chronic idiopathic thrombocytopenic purpura, which may be associated with another autoimmune disease, such as autoimmune hemolytic anemia.[11] The pathogenesis appears to involve the production of autoantibodies directed against the platelets. Clinical manifestations include diffuse petechiae, ecchymosis, epistaxis, hemorrhages into the soft tissues, melena, and hematuria.

TABLE 21-4 *Classification of the Thrombocytopenias*

Type of Disorder	Etiology
DECREASED PRODUCTION	
Hypoproliferation	Toxic agents, especially drug toxicity; radiation, infection; constitutional factors (Fanconi's anemia, etc.); idiopathic aplastic anemia; paroxysmal nocturnal hemoglobinuria; myelophthisis (tumor, fibrosis, etc.)
Infective thrombopoiesis	Megaloblastic anemia; Di Guglielmo's syndrome; familial thrombocytopenia
ABNORMAL DISTRIBUTION	Congestive splenomegaly; myeloid metaplasia, lymphoma
DILUTIONAL LOSS	Massive blood transfusion
DYSFUNCTION	
Drug-induced	Drugs that cause platelet dysfunction include aspirin, nonsteroidal antiinflammatory drugs, alcohol, antihistamines, tricyclic antidepressants, phenothiazines
Systemic disease	Renal disease; liver disease; myeloproliferative diseases; hereditary protein disorders; leukemia and myelodysplasia, multiple myeloma
ABNORMAL DESTRUCTION	
Consumption	Disseminated intravascular coagulation, vasculitis; thrombotic thrombocytopenia (TTP)
Immune mechanism	Idiopathic thrombocytopenic purpura (ITP); drug-induced thrombocytopenia; chronic lymphocytic leukemia, lymphoma, lupus erythematosus, neonatal thrombocytopenia; posttransfusion purpura
Direct trauma	Cardiopulmonary bypass, hemodialysis, continuous arteriovenous or veno-venous hemofiltration (CAVH, CVVH)

Adapted from W. S. Beck, *Hematology* (4th ed.). Cambridge, MA: MIT Press, 1985 and D. L. Barnard, *Clinical Hematology*. Oxford: Heinemann Med., 1989.

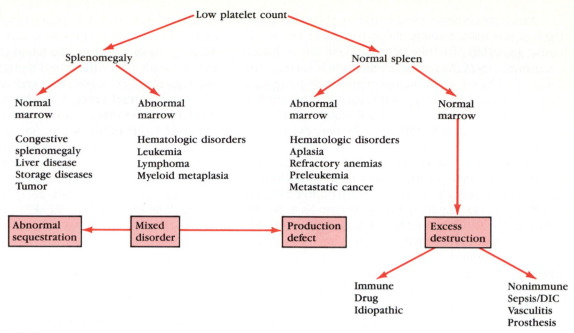

FIGURE 21-6 *A schematic approach to the clinical evaluation of thrombocytopenia. (Source: W.S. Beck, Hematology [4th ed.] Cambridge, Mass: MIT Press, 1985)*

Secondary thrombocytopenia commonly occurs in association with drug hypersensitivity, viral infections, and some of the autoimmune conditions. Some of the drugs that may induce secondary thrombocytopenia are chlorothiazide derivatives, gold thiomalate, diphenyl-hydantoin, acetaminophen, quinidine, heparin, sulfonamides, chloramphenicol, antimetabolites, and antihistamines.[14] Platelet destruction results from antibodies that target the platelets for destruction. *Heparin-induced thrombocytopenia* may be mild or severe. Aggregates of platelets may precipitate in small vessels; thus, the condition often is termed "white clot syndrome." Mild thrombocytopenia often is characterized by venous and arterial thromboses.[13] Loss of circulating platelets causes increased risk of bleeding.

PLATELET FUNCTION DISORDERS

Platelet function disorders include alterations that have a prolonged bleeding time with a normal platelet count in most instances. The disorders are due to a variety of defects of platelet function, such as in platelet adhesion in von Willebrand disease, or in platelet aggregation, as in thrombasthenia, a congenital disorder.

These platelet disorders can also be acquired. Drugs such as aspirin may impair the aggregation of platelets. In uremia, a dialyzable factor is formed that inhibits platelet aggregation.

THROMBOCYTOSIS

Thrombocytosis (thrombocythemia) is an increased number of platelets in the peripheral blood. Counts of 400,000 to 1,000,000/μL are usually asymptomatic, but counts greater than 1,000,000/μL may result in thrombosis or bleeding when the excessive numbers of platelets are dysfunctional.[3] Physiologic thrombocytosis occurs in response to infection, trauma, and other conditions. It almost always occurs after splenectomy, when platelets are circulated in the blood because they can no longer pool in the spleen.

Idiopathic thrombocythemia refers to a sustained platelet count of greater than 800,000/μL. The condition is generally regarded as one of the myeloproliferative disorders due to its responsiveness to chemotherapy. It occurs with splenic enlargement and may be associated with other myeloproliferative disorders, such as chronic myelogenous leukemia and polycythemia vera.[2] Affected individuals often exhibit peripheral thrombosis and episodes of spontaneous bleeding.

HYPERCOAGULATION

Hypercoagulation may involve accelerated rates of coagulation, hyperviscosity, and increased platelet activity or antithrombin III deficiency. The term refers to an increased propensity of the blood to clot. The condition has been seen in association with atherosclerosis, blood stasis, hemangiomas, and certain myeloproliferative diseases.

Thrombotic thrombocytopenic purpura, a rare disorder, is characterized by thrombocytopenia, anemia, neurologic deficits, and renal failure. Endothelial cell damage may be the activator in the disorder, with an immune vasculitis affecting the endothelial cells. Platelet adhesion and aggregation lead to obstruction of the vessel and ischemia of the surrounding tissues.[5]

Blood stasis in the small vessels is enhanced when the blood is more viscous. Polycythemia increases viscosity and affects the rate of blood flow. An increased number of any of the formed elements may increase the viscosity of blood. Giant hemangiomas may precipitate massive blood turbulence, with stasis in the affected vascular bed. There is an increased platelet and fibrinogen turnover, and coagulation in and around the hemangioma is common.

Hyperfunction of platelets in the absence of thrombocytosis has been postulated as a mechanism for various diseases. It is theorized that strokes and transient ischemic attacks in younger persons who have no evidence of arterial abnormalities or degenerative changes could be the result of hyperfunction of the platelets. Platelet clumping in small vessels may result in alterations of blood supply.[10, 14]

Platelet activation and release of thromboxane A_2 may lead to coronary artery spasm, ischemia, and infarction. Platelet function in these cases can be examined by laboratory means for increased sensitivity to aggregating agents and increased release of thromboxane A_2 and other platelet factors.

Antithrombin III deficiency is an inherited familial disorder that results in thrombosis. The antithrombin III inactivates most of the active proteases involved in thrombin formation. A modest decrease in this inhibitor allows the proteases to remain active longer, which results in the rapid formation of thrombi.[10] Antithrombin III deficiency can also occur as an acquired disorder and is associated with liver disease or DIC. Oral contraceptives and heparin also reduce antithrombin III levels.

The myeloproliferative diseases may elaborate clotting factors, which initiate the coagulation sequence. Usually, the coagulation pattern results in activation of the fibrinolytic system and a DIC-like syndrome.

▼ Chapter Summary

▼ Blood coagulation depends on two major processes. The first is hemostasis, which is the arrest of bleeding and which usually requires vasoconstriction and formation of a platelet plug. Part of the hemostatic process is blood coagulation and formation of a clot. This requires an intricate, sequential activation of the clotting factors, which finally results in the laying down of fibrin, which traps red blood cells and other cells to make the clot.

▼ The intrinsic pathway of blood coagulation occurs when there is disruption of the endothelial lining and the stimulus for coagulation occurs. It requires the activation of many clotting factors and proceeds very slowly. This pathway is often one of a disease state and produces abnormal clotting in vessels.

▼ The extrinsic pathway of blood coagulation is initiated when there is injury to a vessel and tissue thromboplastin is activated. It is a rapid cascade of coagulation and produces a clot in a tissue that is disrupted from injury, such as a wound. The blood clot is composed of fibrin threads that adhere to a damaged vessel surface and trap blood cells, platelets, and plasma products.

▼ Once a clot is formed, it sets the tissue up for repair. It then must be lysed and removed so that repair can proceed. Lysis results from the activation of plasminogen, a plasma protein, to plasmin, which is a proteolytic enzyme that digests threads of fibrin and destroys many of the blood clotting factors.

▼ Blood coagulation tests are routinely performed and include clotting time, PT, PTT, and platelet count. Many of these specifically determine clotting factor deficiencies.

▼ Blood coagulation defects can be produced by genetic deficiencies or suppression or consumption of the clotting factors. Hemophilia is an example of a group of genetic deficiencies that produces a bleeding diathesis. Disseminated intravascular coagulation is an example of consumptive coagulopathy that begins with abnormal clotting that uses up the clotting factors, resulting in bleeding. Platelet disorders cause bleeding, because they are necessary to stem the initial flow of blood with the platelet plug.

▼ Hypercoagulation is a common problem that is seen when there is increased blood viscosity, abnormal initiation of coagulation, or a decrease in the anticoagulant factors. Stasis of blood tends to promote coagulation, especially in the deep veins of the legs and pelvis.

▼ References

1. Barnard, D.L. *Clinical Haematology*. Oxford: Heinemann Medical, 1989.
2. Bunn, P.A., and Ridgway, E.C. Paraneoplastic syndromes. In V.T. DeVita, S. Hellman, and S.A. Rosenberg (eds.), *Cancer: Principles and Practice of Oncology* (4th ed.). Philadelphia: J.B. Lippincott, 1993.
3. Chanarin, I. *Laboratory Haematology: An Account of Laboratory Techniques*. Edinburgh: Churchill-Livingstone, 1989.
4. Cormack, D.H. *Essential Histology*. Philadelphia: J.B. Lippincott, 1993.
5. Cotran, R.S., Kumar, V., and Robbins, S.L. *Robbins' Pathologic Basis of Disease* (5th ed.). Philadelphia: W.B. Saunders, 1994.
6. Fischbach, F. *A Manual of Laboratory and Diagnostic Tests* (4th ed.). Philadelphia: J.B. Lippincott. 1992.
7. George, J.N., and Kolodziej, M.A. Hemostasis and fibrinolysis. In J.H. Stein (ed.), *Internal Medicine* (4th ed.). St. Louis: C.V. Mosby, 1994.
8. Gralnick, H.R. Acquired disorders of blood coagulation. In W.N. Kelley (ed.), *Textbook of Internal Medicine* (2nd ed.). Philadelphia: J.B. Lippincott, 1992.
9. Guyton, A.C. *Textbook of Medical Physiology* (8th ed.). Philadelphia: W.B. Saunders, 1991.
10. Hoak, J.C. Disorders associated with thrombosis. In W.N.

Kelley (ed.). *Textbook of Internal Medicine* (2nd ed.). Philadelphia: J.B. Lippincott, 1992.

11. Kelton, J.G. Abnormalities of platelet and vascular function. In W.N. Kelley (ed.), *Textbook of Internal Medicine* (2nd ed.). Philadelphia: J.B. Lippincott, 1992.
12. Rick, M.E., and Gralnick, H.R. Inherited disorders of blood coagulation. In W.N. Kelley (ed.), *Textbook of Internal Medicine* (2nd ed.). Philadelphia: J.B. Lippincott, 1992.
13. Rubin, E., and Farber, J.L. *Pathology* (2nd ed.). Philadelphia: J.B. Lippincott, 1994.
14. Shattil, S.J. Disorders of platelet function. In W.N. Kelley (ed.), *Textbook of Internal Medicine* (2nd ed.). Philadelphia: J.B. Lippincott, 1992.
15. Tortora, G.J., and Grabowski, S.R. *Principles of Anatomy and Physiology* (7th ed.). New York: Harper-Collins, 1993.

▼ *Unit Bibliography*

Babior, B.M. *Hematology: A Pathophysiologic Approach* (3rd ed.). New York: Churchill-Livingstone, 1994.

Back, R.R. Initiation of coagulation by tissue factor. *CRC: Critical Reviews in Biochemistry* 23(4):339, 1988.

Baker, W.F. Clinical aspects of disseminated intravascular coagulation: A clinician's point of view. *Semin. Thromb. Hemost.* 15(1):1, 1989.

Barnard, D.L. *Clinical Haematology*. Oxford: Heineman Medical, 1989.

Begeman, H., and Rastetter, J. *Atlas of Clinical Hematology* (4th ed.). Berlin: Springer-Verlag, 1989.

Besa, E.C. *Hematology*. Baltimore: Williams & Wilkins. 1992.

Brown, B. *Hematology: Principles and Procedures* (6th ed.). Philadelphia: Lea & Febiger, 1993.

Carr, M.E. Disseminated intravascular coagulation: Pathogenesis, diagnosis, and therapy. *J. Emerg. Med.* 5(4):311, 1987.

Chanarin, I. *Laboratory Haematology: An Account of Laboratory Techniques*. Edinburgh: Churchill-Livingstone, 1989.

Cotran, R.S., Kumar, V., and Robbins, S.L. *Robbins' Pathologic Basis of Disease* (5th ed.). Philadelphia: W.B. Saunders, 1994.

Cozzolino, F., Torcia, M., and Miliani, A. Potential role of interleukin 1 as the trigger for diffuse intravascular coagulation in acute nonlymphoblastic leukemia. *Am. J. Med.* 84(2):240, 1988.

Eastham, R.D. *Clinical Hematology* (7th ed.). Boston: Butterworth, 1992.

Fischbach, F. *A Manual of Laboratory and Diagnostic Tests* (4th ed.). Philadelphia: J.B. Lippincott, 1992.

Ganong, W.F. *Review of Medical Physiology* (16th ed.). Los Altos, Calif.: Appleton & Lange, 1993.

Govan, A.D.T., Macfarlane, P.S., and Callander, P. *Pathology Illustrated* (3rd ed.). New York: Churchill-Livingstone, 1991.

Guyton, A. *Textbook of Medical Physiology* (8th ed.). Philadelphia: W.B. Saunders, 1991.

Harmening, D.M. *Clinical Hematology and Fundamentals of Hemostasis* (2nd ed.). Philadelphia: F.A. Davis, 1992.

Hauptman, J.G., Hassouda, H.I., Bell, T.G., Penner, J.A., and Amerson, T.E. Efficacy of antithrombin III in endotoxin-induced disseminated intravascular coagulation. *Circulatory Shock* 25(2):111, 1988.

Hoffbrand, A.V. *Essential Hematology* (3rd ed.). Oxford: Blackwell Scientific, 1993.

Isselbacher, K.J. *Harrison's Principles of Internal Medicine* (13th ed.). New York: McGraw-Hill, 1994.

Kelley, W., et al. *Textbook of Internal Medicine* (2nd ed.). Philadelphia: J.B. Lippincott, 1992.

Kissane, J.M. *Anderson's Pathology* (9th ed.). St. Louis: C.V. Mosby, 1990.

Lotspeich-Steininger, C.A. *Clinical Hematology*. Philadelphia: J.B. Lippincott, 1992.

Markad, V.N., and Moore, R.B. *Sickle Cell Disease: Pathophysiology, Diagnosis, and Management*. Westport, Conn.: Praeger, 1992.

Mazza, J. *Manual of Clinical Hematology*. Boston: Little, Brown, 1988.

McDonald, G.A., Paul, J., and Cruickshank, B. *Atlas of Haematology* (5th ed.). Edinburgh: Churchill-Livingstone, 1988.

Muller-Berghaus, G. Pathophysiologic and biochemical events in disseminated intravascular coagulation: Dysregulation of procoagulant and anticoagulant pathways. *Semin. Thromb. Hemost.* 15(1):58, 1989.

Pagana, K.D., and Pagana, T.J. *Mosby's Diagnostic and Laboratory Test Reference*. St. Louis: C.V. Mosby, 1992.

Rubin, E., and Farber, J.L. *Pathology* (2nd ed.). Philadelphia: J.B. Lippincott, 1994.

Spivak, J.L., and Eichner, E.R. *The Fundamentals of Clinical Hematology* (3rd ed.). Baltimore: John Hopkins, 1993.

Turgeon, M.L. *Clinical Hematology: Theory and Procedures*. Boston: Little, Brown, 1988.

Williams, J.W., et al. *Hematology* (4th ed.). New York: McGraw-Hill, 1990.

Wilson, J., et al. *Harrison's Principles of Internal Medicine* (12th ed.). New York: McGraw-Hill, 1991.

Wintrobe, M.M. (ed.). *Wintrobe's Clinical Haematology* (9th ed). Philadelphia: Lea & Febiger, 1993.

Chapter 22

Normal Circulatory Dynamics

Barbara L. Bullock

▼ LEARNING OBJECTIVES

1 Locate the major structures of the heart, including the chambers, valves, and vessels.
2 Locate the origin and branches of the right and left coronary arteries.
3 Structurally differentiate a myocardial muscle cell and a skeletal muscle cell.
4 Compare skeletal and cardiac muscle contraction.
5 Describe clearly the properties of the heart: automaticity, rhythmicity, excitability, and conductivity.
6 Define **diastolic depolarization** in the sinoatrial node and the reason it is considered to be the pacemaker of the heart.
7 Discuss the descending order of pacemakers in the conduction system of the heart.
8 Relate the events of the cardiac cycle to the waveforms seen on an electrocardiogram tracing.
9 Using examples of different types of dysrhythmias, discuss the concepts of automaticity and reentry.
10 Describe the four interrelated factors of cardiac contraction: preload, afterload, contractility, and heart rate.
11 Define ventricular compliance and give examples of conditions that can alter this property.
12 Describe the events of the cardiac cycle.
13 Relate the normal pressures and oxygen saturations in the chambers of the heart and in the vessels to the physiology of circulation.
14 Describe the factors responsible for generating heart sounds and the sounds that are produced.
15 Explain sympathetic and parasympathetic influences on the heart.
16 Locate and define the functions of the chemoreceptors and baroreceptors.
17 Discuss the structure and related function of the arteries and veins.
18 Locate the arteries and veins beginning with the aorta and terminating in the vena cavae.
19 Describe the structure and function of the lymphatic system.
20 Describe briefly the generation of Korotkoff's sounds.
21 Describe pulse pressure and mean arterial blood pressure.
22 Describe the four direct determinants of blood pressure.

Barbara L. Bullock: PATHOPHYSIOLOGY: ADAPTATIONS AND ALTERATIONS IN FUNCTION, 4th ed.
© 1996 J.B. Lippincott-Raven Publishers

Understanding the dynamics of normal cardiac contraction provides the basis for understanding the effects of alterations of structures within the heart, myocardial muscle, and vessels. The first part of this chapter is devoted to normal cardiac anatomy and physiology; the second part deals with the dynamics of circulation.

▼ *Anatomy of the Heart*

The heart is a double pump that pumps its blood to the lungs and to the systemic arteries. It provides for oxygenation and nutrition of all of the tissues of the body.

The heart is composed of four pumping chambers: the right and left atria and the right and left ventricles. The right atrium and ventricle receive blood from the systemic veins and pump it to the lungs through the pulmonary artery. The left atrium and ventricle pump blood received from the pulmonary veins to the systemic arteries through the aorta. Figure 22-1 shows the general anatomy of the heart and blood vessels.

ATRIA

The *right atrium* is a low-pressure, thin-walled chamber that receives blood from the superior and inferior vena cava and from the veins draining the heart. The *left atrium* is slightly smaller than the right and receives blood from the four pulmonary veins that carry oxygenated blood from the lungs back to the heart.

The atrial walls are composed of three layers: 1) epicardium, a thin outer layer that is continuous with the outer layer of the ventricles; 2) myocardium, the middle or muscular layer of the atria, discontinuous with that of the ventricles; and 3) endocardium, a thin, continuous inner layer that covers the inner surface of the atria, valves, ventricles, and vessels entering and leaving the heart. The muscular layer of the atria is much thinner than that in the ventricles and accounts for the lower pressures maintained in these chambers. The atria serve mostly as storage reservoirs and as conductive passageways for the movement of blood to the ventricles.

Dividing the right atrium from the left atrium is the membranous atrial septum, a separation that prevents the communication of blood between the atria. This septum houses the fossa ovalis, which is the remains of the fetal foramen ovale (see pp. 489–491).

VENTRICLES

Like the atria, the ventricular walls are composed of three layers: epicardium, myocardium, and endocardium (Fig. 22-2). The right ventricle has been described as looking like a bellows, with a myocardial layer that is thicker than that in the atrial walls but thinner than that of the left ventricle. The left ventricle is more circular

Atria: Low pressure chambers and reservoirs. Serve as separate pump from ventricles.

Ventricles: High pressure chambers; generate pressure sufficient to sustain arterial pressure of 120/80 mm Hg. Left ventricular pressure 120/0-10; right ventricular pressure 25/0-5. Aortic pressure 120/80.

Atrioventricular valves: Attached to papillary muscles by chordae tendineae which prevent valvular eversion into the atria during ventricular contraction.

Semilunar valves: Aortic and pulmonic valves lie between the ventricles and the exiting arteries; prevent the backflow of blood from the arteries into the ventricles when the ventricles relax.

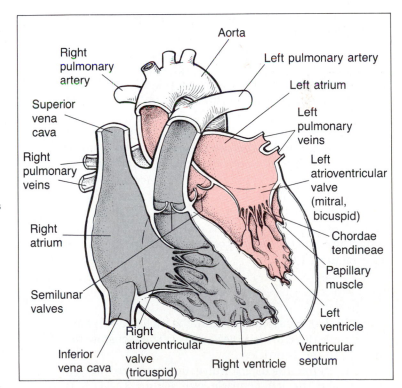

FIGURE 22-1 *Internal anatomy of the heart.*

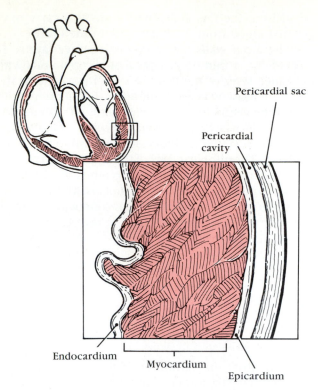

FIGURE 22-2 *Cross-section showing the layers of the ventricles. Note the thin endocardial layer in relation to the thick myocardium.*

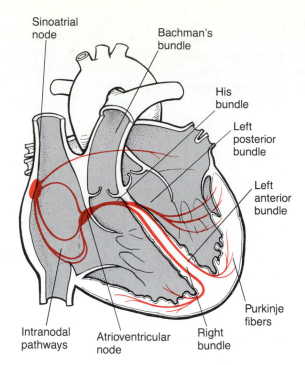

FIGURE 22-3 *Location of pathways for the conduction system of the heart.*

than the right. Its myocardial muscle layer is much thicker than that in the right ventricle, which allows it to achieve the high pressures required for systemic arterial circulation.

Separating the ventricles is the ventricular septum, a thick muscular structure that becomes membranous as it nears the atrioventricular valves (see Figure 22-1). This septum contains the branches of the conduction tissue for the transmission of an impulse (Fig. 22-3). It also provides an important fulcrum during contraction of the ventricles.

The inner surface of the ventricles contains areas of raised muscle bundles that are undercut by open spaces. These muscle bundles are called the *trabeculae carneae*. The papillary muscles project from the trabeculated surface, giving rise to two groups of papillary muscles in the left ventricle and three groups in the right. These muscles give off strong fibrous strands called *chordae tendineae*, which attach to the margins of the atrioventricular valves (see Figure 22-1).

ATRIOVENTRICULAR VALVES

The mitral, or bicuspid, valve and the tricuspid valve are called the atrioventricular (AV) valves. They separate the atria from the ventricles.

The mitral (bicuspid) valve lies between the left atrium and the left ventricle (see Figure 22-1). It is composed of two leaflets of fibroelastic tissue that

slightly overlap each other when the valve is closed (Fig. 22-4). The margins of the valve are attached to the fibrous chordae tendineae.

The tricuspid valve is composed of three leaflets and lies between the right atrium and the right ventricle. The leaflets, also composed of fibrous tissue, are thinner than

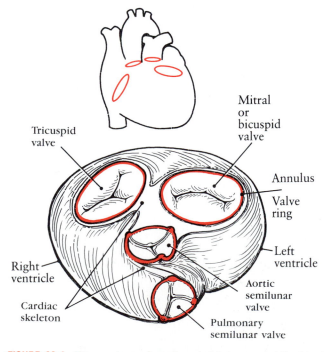

FIGURE 22-4 *Fibrous rings of cardiac skeleton surround the heart valves as viewed from above. Valves are in the closed position.*

those of the mitral valve. These are also attached to chordae tendineae that project from the right ventricular papillary muscles (see Figure 22-1). The annulus (valve ring) that surrounds each valve is flexible and distorts its shape during ventricular contraction.

SEMILUNAR VALVES

The aortic and pulmonary valves are called semilunar valves because their cusps are cuplike in appearance (Fig. 22-5). Each of the valves contains three cusps whose margins meet when the valves are closed. The valve cusps meet when they are filled with blood during the diastolic or resting phase of the cardiac cycle (see pp. 445–446). Two coronary arteries, the right and left coronary arteries, arise from the aortic sinuses of Valsalva. These sinuses are pouchlike dilatations of the valve cusps. The coronary ostia (openings) are located in the upper one-third of the aortic coronary cusps (Fig. 22-6). In about 50% of hearts, a third coronary artery called the *conus artery* arises from a separate ostium in the right sinus of Valsalva.[16]

The aortic and pulmonic valves are similar in structure except that the aortic valve is composed of slightly thicker fibrous cusps than the pulmonary valve. Both valves are supported by strong fibrous tissue or valve rings.

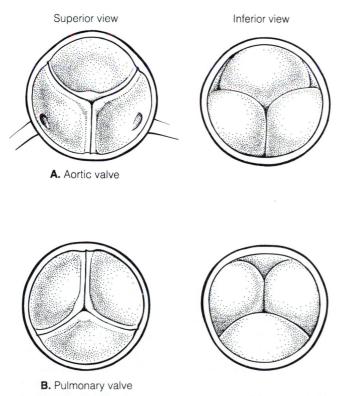

FIGURE 22-5 **A.** *Aortic valve in closed position viewed from above and below.* **B.** *Pulmonic valve in closed position viewed from above and below.*

FIBROUS CARDIAC SKELETON

Holding the main structures of the heart together is the fibrous cardiac skeleton. It provides a firm anchor for the attaching of the the atrial and ventricular muscles and the valvular tissue.[16] It is composed of compact fibroelastic tissue around the valves (see Figure 22-4). It is continuous with the membranous portion of the ventricular septum and provides support for the right coronary and noncoronary aortic cusps.[16]

VEINS

The superior and inferior venae cavae bring the systemic venous blood back to the heart. After passing through the systemic vascular (capillary) bed, the blood passes through venules, small veins, larger veins, and, finally, the inferior and superior venae cavae (see Figure 22-1). Figure 22-7 shows the larger veins of the body.

The pulmonary veins, usually four, carry oxygenated blood from the lungs back to the left atrium. These bring the entire output of the right ventricle back to the left side of the heart to be circulated.

Systemic veins are distensible, thin-walled structures that can hold large volumes of blood. For this reason, veins are often called *capacitance vessels*. The larger veins have valves that permit blood flow in one direction, that is, back toward the heart (Fig. 22-8).

ARTERIES

The two major arteries leading from the heart are the pulmonary artery and the aorta. The pulmonary artery leads from the right ventricle to the lungs. It branches into smaller and smaller vessels that finally become the pulmonary capillary bed, where oxygen and carbon dioxide exchange occurs. The pulmonary capillaries then become venules and finally the four pulmonary veins described above.

The aorta is the main systemic artery and carries oxygenated blood to all of the tissues of the body. It gives off branches that become smaller and smaller, terminating finally in systemic arterioles and capillaries, where exchange for oxygen and nutrition takes place. Figure 22-9 shows the main branches of the arteries of the body. Arteries are less numerous than veins and have thicker walls.

The aorta and pulmonary arteries are composed of three layers: tunica intima (endothelial layer or coat); tunica media (muscular layer); and tunica externa (outer, adventitial coat). These provide the structure necessary for the higher pressures generated in the arteries.

CORONARY ARTERIES

Two main coronary arteries arise from the sinuses of Valsalva of the aortic valve. The *right coronary artery* arises from the right coronary sinus, and the *left coronary*

Coronary arteries arise from 2 of the pouchlike dilations at the base of the aorta called the sinuses of Valsalva.

Right coronary artery (RCA): most frequently supplies the sinoatrial (55% of hearts) and atrioventricular (90%) nodes, right ventricle (RV), posterior septum and posterior left ventricle (LV). It turns downward in the posterior interventricular groove and is called the posterior descending coronary artery.

Left coronary artery (LCA): divides into the left anterior descending (LAD) and circumflex arteries. The LAD gives off 1–4 diagonal arteries which supply the LV wall. The LAD supplies the anterior LV and the apex of the heart. The circumflex artery supplies part of the anterior and lateral LV.

Veins of the heart: blood is returned from the heart muscle through the thebesian veins (which drain the septa and ventricular walls directly into the heart chambers) the small cardiac vein, middle cardiac vein, and great cardiac vein which drain into the coronary sinus and thence into the right atrium. Anterior cardiac veins enter the right atrium directly.

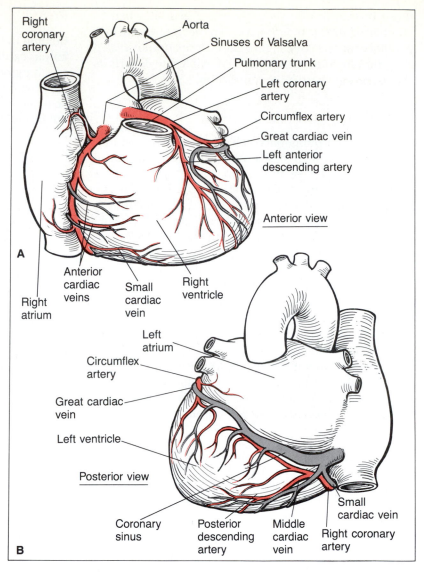

FIGURE 22-6 *Coronary arteries and veins. **A.** Anterior view; **B.** posterior view.*

artery arises from the left coronary sinus (see Figure 22-6). The right coronary artery usually arises as a singular vessel from the right coronary ostium, but two vessels may arise from this position. This second vessel, if present, is called the *conus artery*. When a single coronary artery arises on the right side, the conus artery is the first branch off the right main coronary artery.[16] The right coronary artery travels in the AV groove (sulcus) and turns downward in the posterior surface to the posterior interventricular sulcus. Smaller arterial vessels branch off the main artery. In about 55% of human hearts, the right coronary artery supplies blood to the sinoatrial (SA) node, and in about 90% it supplies the AV node. In some hearts, the right coronary artery supplies the posterior surface of the right and left ventricles and the posterior interventricular septum. It may extend to supply part of the lateral and apical surfaces of the heart. A variation in the amount of myocardial tissue supplied by

the right coronary artery accounts for the difference in myocardial disease when the right coronary artery is diseased.

The left main coronary artery arises from a single ostium in the left coronary sinus. It travels in the AV sulcus to the left for a few millimeters to a few centimeters and then divides or bifurcates into the left anterior descending coronary artery and the left circumflex. At the point of the bifurcation, other branches called *diagonal arteries* may branch off. The diagonal arteries, one to four in number, supply the anterior surface of the left ventricle. The left anterior descending coronary artery descends in the anterior interventricular sulcus and supplies blood to the anterior left ventricle, the anterior interventricular septum, and the apex of the heart. The circumflex artery comes off the main left coronary artery at a sharp angle and travels in the left AV sulcus to the posterolateral surface of the left ventricle. Its branches

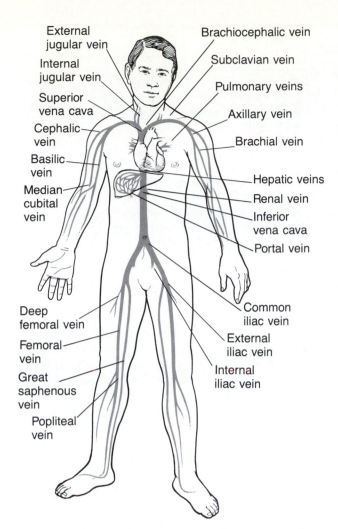

External jugular vein

Internal jugular vein

Superior vena cava

Cephalic vein

Basilic vein

Median cubital vein

Brachiocephalic vein

Subclavian vein

Pulmonary veins

Axillary vein

Brachial vein

Hepatic veins

Renal vein

Inferior vena cava

Portal vein

Deep femoral vein

Femoral vein

Great saphenous vein

Popliteal vein

Common iliac vein

External iliac vein

Internal iliac vein

FIGURE 22-7 *Some of the systemic veins of the body.*

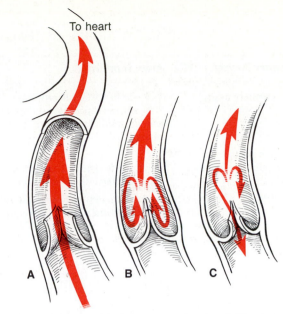

To heart

A   B   C

FIGURE 22-8 *Valves of the larger systemic veins. **A.** Blood can move forward through the valves to the heart. **B.** and **C.** Valves distend with blood and close to prevent backflow, which causes perpetual movement of blood toward the heart. Blood moves from higher pressure to the lower pressure produced by the negative intrathoracic pressure and low pressure in the right atrium.*

supply blood to the lateral left ventricle and various amounts of posterior wall. In a small percentage of persons, the circumflex is dominant and supplies the entire left ventricle and interventricular septum.[16] The circumflex also supplies the SA node in approximately 45% of persons and usually supplies blood to the left atrium. Table 22-1 summarizes the normal blood supply to the myocardium and variations that may occur.

The coronary arteries divide into smaller and smaller branches that penetrate deep into the myocardial muscle. These form a network of capillaries that supply the myocardial cells. Numerous functional and nonfunctional anastomoses exist between the coronary vessels. These have been shown to enlarge when the flow in one arterial branch is decreased. Enlargement of anastomoses can improve blood flow to myocardial segments, thus providing collateral circulation. The endocardial layer is the only portion of the heart that receives oxygen and nutrients from the blood that circulates within the chambers. The rest of the heart receives its oxygen and nutrients from branches of the coronary arteries.

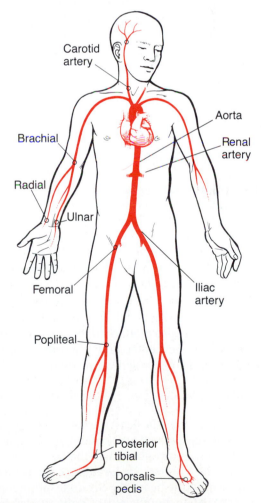

Carotid artery

Brachial

Radial

Ulnar

Femoral

Popliteal

Aorta

Renal artery

Iliac artery

Posterior tibial

Dorsalis pedis

FIGURE 22-9 *Major systemic arteries of the body. The circles represent points at which the pulse can be palpated.*

TABLE 22-1   *Normal Blood Supply to Myocardium*

Coronary Artery	Area Supplied	Variations
Right coronary artery	SA node in 55% of hearts; AV node in 90% of hearts; posterior surface of right and left ventricles; posterior interventricular system	Dominant when supplies lateral and apical left ventricle
Left main coronary artery		
Left anterior descending	Anterior left ventricle; apex of heart; anterior interventricular septum	In 5–10% of hearts supplies AV node; anterolateral left ventricle
Circumflex	SA node in 45% of hearts; left atrium; posterior lateral surface left ventricle	In 5–10% of hearts supplies AV node; dominant where supplies entire left ventricle; interventricular septum

SA: sinoatrial; AV: atrioventricular.

CORONARY VEINS

The coronary veins provide for drainage of the myocardium and empty into the right atrium. They consist of the coronary sinus and its branches, the anterior right ventricular veins, and the thebesian veins (see Figure 22-6). Most drainage from the left ventricle is received by the coronary sinus and its branches. The coronary sinus is basically an extension of the great coronary vein. The anterior cardiac veins drain the right ventricle and usually empty directly into the right atrium. The remaining venous blood empties into the heart through the small thebesian veins. These are tiny venous outlets draining directly into the right atrium and ventricles.[16]

PERICARDIUM

The heart is surrounded by a fibrous sac called the parietal pericardium, an inner layer of which is in contact with the outside of the heart. This layer is called the visceral pericardium or the epicardium (see Figure 22-2). Between the two layers there is normally about 10 to 50 mL of clear fluid, an ultrafiltrate of blood plasma, which allows for free movement of the heart within the sac.[16] The fibrous layer is attached to the sternum and the diaphragm by ligaments, and this keeps the heart in a normal position. It also is attached to the great vessels at the area where they enter and leave the heart. The pericardium limits distension of the heart.

CONDUCTION SYSTEM

Normal contraction of the heart is initiated by specialized conductive tissues, which are actually myocardial muscle cells with fewer myofibrils than the other myocardial cells. Figure 22-3 shows the location of the conductive structures within the heart: the SA node, atrial internodal tracts, AV node, bundle of His, right and left bundle branches, and terminal or Purkinje network.

The SA node is a small mass of cells located near the entrance of the superior vena cava into the right atrium. It normally serves as the pacemaker of the heart because of its ability to generate an impulse through automatic diastolic depolarization (see pp. 436–437).

The atrial internodal tracts extend from the SA node and are difficult to distinguish from the surrounding cardiac muscle. The pathways are designated as the *anterior, middle,* and *posterior internodal tracts.*[16] The electrical impulse generated by the SA node travels rapidly along these tracts to merge at the AV node. Bachmann's bundle (the anterior internodal tract) conducts the impulse to the left atrium. The remaining tracts travel through the right atrium.

The AV node and bundle of His form an interconnecting structure between the atria and ventricles that functionally joins the two units. The AV node lies in the right atrium at the juncture of the atrial septum. It is composed of dense fibrous tissue that continues into the bundle of His. The AV node along with the bundle of His pathway is the only functional connection between the atrial and ventricular muscles. The slow conduction in the AV node may be partly due to the unspecialized structure of its cells. The bundle of His directly connects with the AV node and crosses into the membranous portion of the ventricular septum. It is composed of fibrous tissue with a few myofibrils and terminates in the bifurcation of the common bundle into the right and left bundle branches.[16]

The right and left bundle branches travel down the interventricular septum to terminate in the Purkinje network. The right bundle branch descends superficially in the endocardium of the right ventricular septum. It divides into numerous branches that penetrate the walls of the right ventricle. The left bundle fans into two main *fascicles—the posterior and anterior—*which travel in the left interventricular septum for varying distances. The posterior fascicle sends its branches to the lateral and posterior wall and papillary muscle. The anterior fascicle primarily goes to the anterior and lateral wall of the left ventricle.[16] The fascicular branches subdivide into smaller and smaller subbranches and terminate in the Purkinje network.

The Purkinje network is composed primarily of Purkinje cells that have few myofibrils and are joined end to end by intercalated disks that aid in the property of accelerated conduction of the impulse (see Myocardial Cellular Structure below). A Purkinje fiber is composed of many Purkinje cells in a series. These fibers lie in the deepest layer of the myocardium and supply the papillary muscles and apical parts of the ventricles. Thus, the apical portion of the ventricles contracts before the basal parts, facilitating the excitation of the right and left ventricles.[1]

MYOCARDIAL CELLULAR STRUCTURE

Cardiac muscle cells are similar to skeletal muscle cells in many ways, but have some fundamental differences. Cardiac muscle cells have a single central nucleus, whereas skeletal cells have peripheral nuclei. The muscle cells are closely approximated so that impulses generated in one myocardial cell can be passed easily to the next.

The myofibril is the contractile unit of the myocardial muscle cell. Its action occurs through the movement of actin on myosin in the sarcomere unit. The thin actin filament also contains two inhibitory proteins, *tropomyosin* and *troponin*. The activity of these proteins in muscle contraction is described in detail on pages 836–838. The myocardial muscle cell has a poorly developed sarcoplasmic reticulum (SR) but a highly developed transverse tubular system. This tubular system probably contributes to the intracellular release of calcium.[7] The cardiac cell also contains a large number of mitochondria that have been shown to store calcium. Glycogen and lipid are also stored within the cells.

Cardiac muscle cells are close to one another. The end of one cell very closely approximates the next. The junctions of the cells consist of intercalated disks, which form a tight connection and allow impulses to pass rapidly from one cell to the next (Fig. 22-10). The myocardial cellular structure allows the entire myocardial unit to contract when one cell is stimulated to threshold level. The heart behaves as a *syncytium*; that is, if one cell is stimulated, the entire unit contracts (see below).

▼ *Physiology of the Heart*

The physiology of the heart is considered in terms of the electrical and mechanical activities of the myocardial muscle. The cellular aspects are briefly outlined to provide

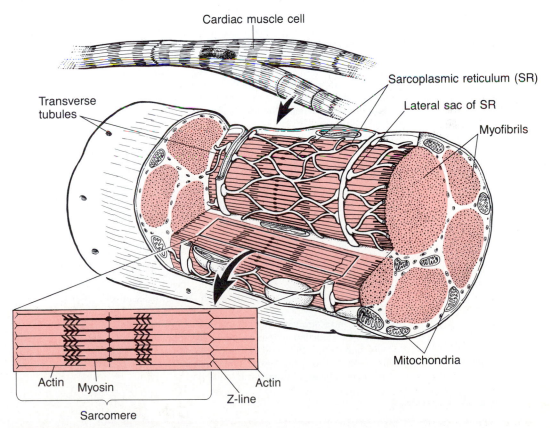

FIGURE 22-10 *Structure of a cardiac muscle cell.*

greater understanding of the process. Table 22-2 provides some definitions of terms used in cardiac physiology.

CONTRACTION OF CARDIAC MUSCLE

Cardiac contraction occurs in much the same way as skeletal muscle contraction, except that the muscle functions as a syncytium. This means that if one cardiac muscle cell is stimulated to threshold and contracts, the impulse spreads to all of the muscle cells and the entire unit contracts. The two separate syncytial units in the myocardium, atrial and ventricular, are functionally joined by the AV node and the bundle of His.

The mechanism for contraction is similar to that described in Chapter 44. The action potential generated causes the release of calcium from the SR into the sarcoplasm. Calcium binds with the inhibitory proteins troponin and tropomyosin, allowing actin to slide on myosin. Actin and myosin are the contractile proteins that make up the sarcomere units of the myocardial muscle cell. The calcium ion apparently has two major roles in excitation–contraction: as the trigger substance or initiator and as the regulator of contraction.[11] When the action potential is initiated, there is a rapid influx of sodium. As the action potential travels down the extensive T tubular system, it comes close to the terminal cisternae of the SR. The SR releases large amounts of free calcium that bind with troponin, thus inhibiting both troponin and tropomyosin. Energy for the contraction is obtained from adenosine triphosphate (ATP), which is split by an adenosine triphosphatase (ATPase) site on the myosin filament when it interacts with actin.[11]

The amount of calcium available to inhibit troponin is directly related to the rate and amount of myocardial tension developed.[13] The T tubules possess a large number of voltage-dependent calcium channels. The amount of calcium that flows across the sarcolemma through these channels largely determines the amount of calcium released by the SR.[7] It is also possible that competition between sodium and calcium for binding sites affects myocardial contractility. Calcium must be returned to the SR through a continually active calcium

---

TABLE 22-2 *Definitions of Cardiac Physiology Terms*

Term	Definition
Cardiac action potential	A rapid sequence of changes in the electrical potential across the cell membrane resulting in systole and diastole
Syncytium	A cardiac property; if one cardiac muscle fiber is stimulated to threshold, the entire myocardial unit will contract
Inotropic state	Referring to contractility; (+) inotropic refers to increased contractility; (−) inotropic refers to decreased contractility
Chronotropic state	Refers to heart rate; (+) chronotropic refers to tachycardia; (−) chronotropic refers to bradycardia
Absolute refractory period	The period in the cardiac cycle during which the cell will not respond to a second stimulus regardless of the strength of the stimulus
Relative refractory period	The period in the cardiac cycle during which the cell will respond to a strong stimulus; main cause of ectopic beats
Automaticity	The spontaneous property of depolarizing and generating an action potential; enhanced automaticity increases irritability of conduction outside SA node
Rhythmicity	Regular, rhythmic generation of an action potential
Excitability	Ability of a cell to respond to stimulation from an adjacent cardiac muscle cell
Conductivity	Ability of muscle cell to transmit action potential from one cell to adjacent cell
Preload	Volume related; degree of myocardial muscle length prior to contraction
Afterload	Pressure related; resistance against which the ventricles must pump
Contractility	Force of contraction generated by myocardial muscle
His-Purkinje system	Portion of conduction system including AV node, bundle of His, bundle branches, and Purkinje network
Cardiac work	The amount of oxygen consumption required for cardiac contractions; includes intramyocardial tension

SA: sinoatrial; AV: atrioventricular.

pump that decreases the level of free calcium. A decreased level of calcium in the sarcoplasmic fluid restores the inhibition of actin and myosin by the troponin–tropomyosin complex.[6] The sarcomere unit then returns to the resting position. Figure 22-11 summarizes the process of excitation–contraction and actin–myosin relaxation.

In recent years, *calcium channel blockers* have been developed to close or partially close the calcium channels and, thus, decrease the myocardial tension. As described on pages 444–445, the contractility or force of cardiac contraction is called its *inotropic state*. An increased ($^+$) inotropism refers to increased force of contraction and energy use within the muscle fibers. In ischemic heart disease or hypertrophic cardiomyopathy, the result of decreased available calcium is a decrease in cardiac work, thereby causing a negative ($^-$) inotropic state. The result is decreasing blood pressure and cardiac ischemia. The results of these pharmacologic agents could be detrimental if the inotropic state were not sustained to adequately maintain the blood pressure. The explanation of how some of the antidysrhythmic agents work is thought to relate to the blocking of *sodium channels*. This has led to classification of antidysrhythmic drugs according to their membrane/channel action.[10]

Action Potential

When the myocardial muscle cell is at rest, the resting membrane potential is approximately -85 to -95 mV. When an action potential occurs, it changes the membrane potential from a negative to a slightly positive value. The action potential in cardiac muscle remains in plateau longer than in other excitable cells, which allows for a longer contraction in cardiac muscle. After the action potential, contraction occurs and is followed by repolarization and a return to the resting state. As noted in Figure 22-12, these changes in potential and state of cardiac muscle can be described in terms of discrete phases: phase 0 denotes depolarization; phase 1 indicates complete depolarization and contraction; phase 2 is a plateau phase of maximum cardiac contraction; phase 3 is the period of repolarization; and phase 4 indicates the myocardium at rest.

Re-stimulation during phases 1 and 2 does not cause the muscle to contract again. This is called the refractory period and occurs in both atrial and ventricular muscle. The *absolute refractory period* is the time during which the membrane is completely depolarized and/or contracting, when no stimulus can cause it to respond or contract again. The *relative refractory period* (phase 3) occurs when

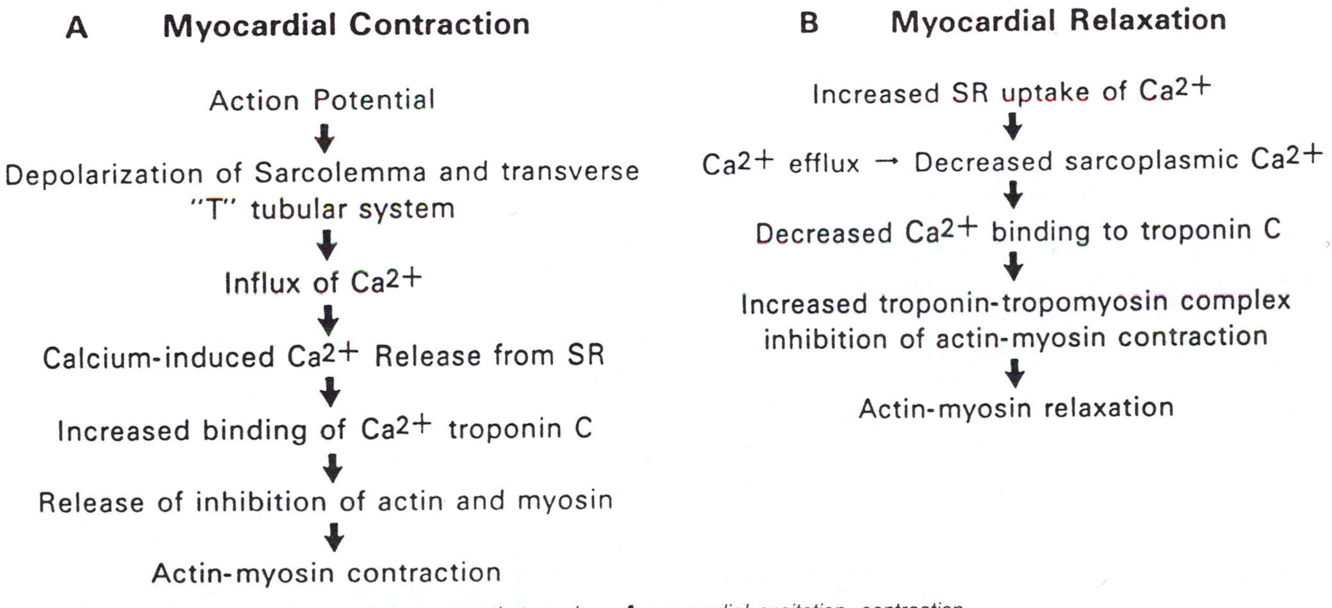

A   Myocardial Contraction

Action Potential
↓
Depolarization of Sarcolemma and transverse "T" tubular system
↓
Influx of Ca2+
↓
Calcium-induced Ca2+ Release from SR
↓
Increased binding of Ca2+ troponin C
↓
Release of inhibition of actin and myosin
↓
Actin-myosin contraction

B   Myocardial Relaxation

Increased SR uptake of Ca2+
↓
Ca2+ efflux → Decreased sarcoplasmic Ca2+
↓
Decreased Ca2+ binding to troponin C
↓
Increased troponin-tropomyosin complex inhibition of actin-myosin contraction
↓
Actin-myosin relaxation

FIGURE 22-11 *Schematic diagram of the events that produce **A** myocardial excitation–contraction coupling and **B** myocardial relaxation. With depolarization of the cardiac cell membranes (sarcolemma and transverse T system), the Na+ channels open, followed by the Ca++ channels. The initial transsarcolemmal influx of Ca++ triggers the release of Ca++ from the sarcoplasmic reticulum (SR). Ca++ in higher concentration then binds to troponin C. This produces conformational changes in whole troponin (troponin 1–troponin C–troponin T complex) that relieves a troponin 1 interaction with actin, thereby allowing tropomyosin to roll back into the grooves of the F-actin superhelix and allowing the interaction of actin and myosin to produce a contraction. The transsarcolemmal Ca++ current has both a faster and a slower component. Possibly, the former acts to trigger the release of Ca++ current from the SR, whereas the latter may cause the SR to accumulate calcium. Ca++ influx may also occur by the Na+Ca++ exchanger. Relaxation is initiated by an unknown stimulus that produces the active uptake of Ca++ by the SR Ca++ binding to troponin C and relaxation. During relaxation, Ca++ efflux may occur both by Ca++ ATPase and by an Na+Ca++ exchanger. (Source: R.C. Schlant and R.W. Alexander (eds.). Hurst's The Heart [8th ed.] New York: McGraw-Hill, 1994)*

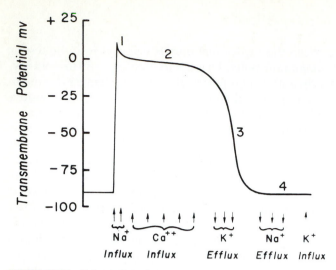

FIGURE 22-12 *Schematic action potential of human ventricular myocardium together with probable electrolyte movements. The initial phase O spike and overshoot is related to a sudden influx of Na+. This is followed by a slower, maintained influx of Ca++ during the plateau phase 2. The phase of Ca++ efflux is not well defined for human ventricular myocardium, but presumably it occurs during phase 4. (Source: R.C. Schlant and R.W. Alexander (eds.) Hurst's The Heart [8th ed.] New York: McGraw-Hill, 1994)*

the muscle membrane is repolarizing, and a strong stimulus will cause it to contract.[2]

METABOLISM OF CARDIAC MUSCLE

Cardiac muscle requires constant production of ATP. Little ATP is stored in cardiac muscle, so oxygen and nutrients for energy production must be constantly supplied. Most ATP is produced in the numerous myocardial mitochondria using fatty acids and other nutrients, especially lactate and glucose. If one substance is not available, cardiac muscle can efficiently use the other.

The amount of ATP normally produced is equivalent to the work needed to pump incoming blood into the arteries with sufficient pressure to maintain vital body functions. *Myocardial work* is generated by the ventricular wall tension during systole and diastole. The wall tension generated during systole creates the pressure to eject blood into the arteries. Cardiac work is often expressed in terms of *myocardial oxygen consumption*. The amount of oxygen consumed is closely related to the amount of stress developed in the ventricular wall. The major factors that affect oxygen consumption include the amount of myocardial muscle mass, the contractile or inotropic state, heart rate, and intramyocardial tension generated.[11] The oxygen supply for this work is delivered in the blood from the coronary arteries alone. Increased oxygen is needed in stressful situations because of enhanced contractility and tachycardia, which is induced by the catecholamines, especially epinephrine. The myocardial muscle takes up a large amount of

the oxygen delivered to it from the coronary arteries. Oxygen extraction of up to 70% leaves little oxygen reserve. Increased systemic energy needs can be met only by increasing the heart rate and respiratory rate to increase oxygen delivery (Fig. 22-13).

AUTOMATICITY

The spontaneous property of generating an action potential by the conduction tissue is called *automaticity*. This occurs through a slow, sliding depolarization that creeps toward threshold. When the threshold level is reached, spontaneous depolarization occurs. The action potential usually arises in the SA node, where an inward leakage phenomenon allows sodium to drift into the cell. Self-initiation of the action potential (diastolic depolarization) then occurs. All parts of the conduction system retain the property of automaticity but do so at inherently different rates. Figure 22-14A shows that this phenomenon normally occurs because of an unstable membrane potential, with gradual, slow depolarization at the end of the cycle (phase 4). The rate of depolarization in phase 4 is more rapid in the SA node, thus it fires more frequently. These SA node impulses dominate other automatic regions simply because they are formed with greater frequency (see Figure 22-14B). The term *enhanced automaticity* usually refers to increased irritability of cells of the conduction tissue outside the SA node.

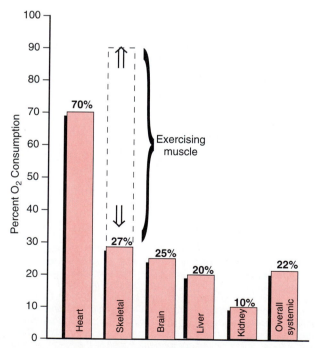

FIGURE 22-13 *Normally the brain extracts 25% of the oxygen delivered to it. The liver, kidney and systemic cells take 10 to 20%. The skeletal muscle oxygen extraction depends upon whether it is relaxed or exercising. The heart normally extracts 70 to 75% of oxygen delivered to it.*

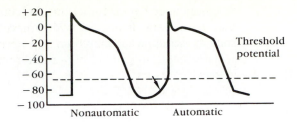

A

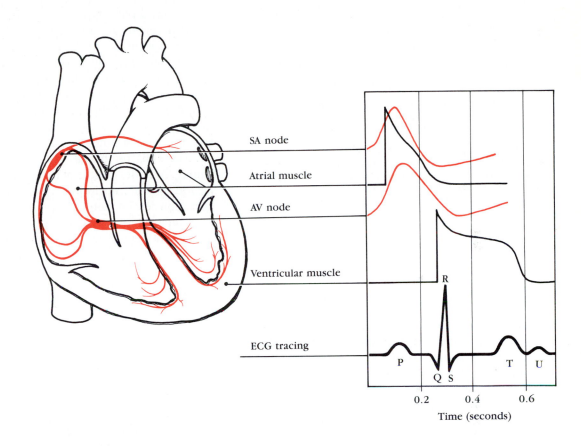

B

FIGURE 22-14 **A.** *The nonautomatic cell depolarizes with a stimulus of adequate strength. The automatic cell depolarizes at regular intervals through increased permeability to sodium.* **B.** *Various areas of the conduction system depolarize through automatic and nonautomatic mechanisms.*

Pharmaceutical agents, hypoxemia, and injury are some of the factors that can alter the threshold for myocardial response. Table 22-3 lists factors that enhance and depress automaticity. Some drugs, for example, raise the threshold for generation of the action potential and thus decrease the rate of diastolic depolarization. This is especially effective if ectopic impulses are causing ventricular dysrhythmias (see pp. 442–444).

Parasympathetic influences through the vagus nerve slow the rate of diastolic depolarization and decrease the rate of SA node automaticity. Sympathetic influences increase the automaticity and the rate of diastolic depolarization.

RHYTHMICITY

Rhythmicity is an important property of the conduction tissue that is characteristic of all of the potential pacemakers of the heart. It refers to the rhythmic or regular generation of an action potential. The leakage phenomenon described above remains regular, allowing for the same amount of time from one depolarization to the next. Therefore, the action potential discharges regularly. Rhythmicity also may be affected by the sympathetic nervous system (SNS) and the parasympathetic nervous system (PSNS). A cyclic increase and decrease in cardiac rate due to respiratory influences on the vagus

TABLE 22-3 *Factors That Enhance and Depress Automaticity*

Enhancing Factors	Depressing Factors
Sympathetic nervous system stimulation	Parasympathetic nervous system stimulation
Fever	Vagotonia
Pain	Hyperkalemia
Anxiety	Drugs
High-output states	
Hyperthyroidism	
Anemia	
AV fistula	
Congestive heart failure	
Hypoxia	
High metabolic rates	
Toxic states	
Exercise	
Drugs	
Vagolytics (atropine)	
Sympathomimetics (epinephrine, norepinephrine)	
Catecholamines	
Hypokalemia	
Acid–base imbalance	
Trauma	

AV: arteriovenous.

nerve results in an increased cardiac rate on inspiration and a decreased rate on expiration in certain persons. Rhythmicity may be interrupted by enhanced automaticity of influences, such as nervous system stimulation, electrolyte imbalances, or pharmaceutical agents.

EXCITABILITY

Excitability refers to the ability of the cell to respond to stimulation. In the heart, there are fast and slow conductors. The fast conductors include atrial and ventricular muscle cells and the Purkinje fibers, whereas the slow responses are those in the SA and AV nodes. Different cardiac muscle fibers have been shown to have both fast and slow channels. The word *excitability* denotes the ability of the muscle cell to respond to an impulse in an adjacent muscle cell.[12]

CONDUCTIVITY

Impulse transmission in cardiac muscle is affected mostly by the structure of the intramyocardial cells, which allows the current to flow easily from one cell to the next. Therefore, threshold current from one cell rapidly passes to and depolarizes the adjacent cell. Conductivity is effected through the intercalated disks, or the tight junctions between the myocardial muscle cells. It may be slowed or altered with intracellular damage, such as ischemia or infarction.

ELECTRICAL EVENTS OF THE CARDIAC CYCLE

As stated above, the cardiac cycle is initiated through specialized conduction tissue. These pacemaker cells spontaneously depolarize in a rhythmic fashion. The critical threshold is gradually reached; spontaneous depolarization occurs and is followed by repolarization.

The pacemaker of the heart is the sinus (SA) node, because spontaneous depolarization occurs more frequently here than in the other potential pacers. This depolarization supersedes the discharge of the other potential pacers. During normal pacemaking activity, the sinus node impulse suppresses the His–Purkinje system, which could be potential pacemakers.[1]

The cells of the His–Purkinje system (which includes AV node, bundle of His, and branches) are depolarized by the sinus impulse before their diastolic depolarization reaches threshold.[1] The conduction tissue has been referred to as a cascade of potential pacers that fire at different rates and can take over pacemaker function if the more rapid pacemaker is not operational.[8] Figure 22-15 shows the approximate potential rates of the inherent cardiac pacemakers.

Excitation of cardiac muscle normally follows a strict sequential pattern. The sinus node begins the excitation. This is due to the less negative resting membrane potential (-55 to -60 mV) in the sinus node than in the other cardiac muscle fibers and to increased membrane permeability to sodium. The impulse or action potential occurs and sends the excitation wave through the internodal pathways, causing depolarization of the atrial muscle and excitation of the AV node. At the AV node, the impulse is slowed as it passes through the dense fibrous tissue. This allows time for the atria to complete contraction before the depolarization wave is sent to the ventricles. The impulse is then sent down the bundle of His and the bundle branches to the Purkinje network, which causes rapid depolarization and contraction of the ventricles.

The Electrocardiogram

The electrocardiogram (ECG) graphically depicts the electrical events of the cardiac cycle. The waveforms produced are of 1) the electrical activity (action potential) generated as electrical impulses spread through the conduction system and 2) the recovery of myocardial cells after depolarization. Table 22-4 defines terms relating to normal electrophysiology and cardiac dysrhythmias. Figure 22-16 shows the appearance of the ECG in

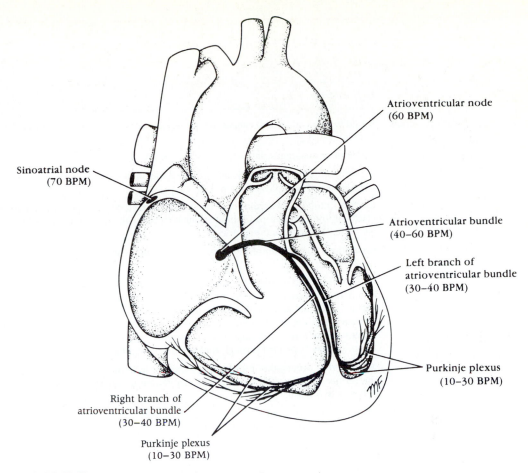

Sinoatrial node
(70 BPM)

Atrioventricular node
(60 BPM)

Atrioventricular bundle
(40–60 BPM)

Left branch of
atrioventricular bundle
(30–40 BPM)

Purkinje plexus
(10–30 BPM)

Right branch of
atrioventricular bundle
(30–40 BPM)

Purkinje plexus
(10–30 BPM)

FIGURE 22-15 *Approximate rates of inherent cardiac pacemakers.*

relation to electrical activities. This activity creates an electrical field that is distributed to the body surfaces. For example, SA node depolarization is inscribed as the P wave. The PR interval is the time it takes for the impulse to traverse the AV node. As the impulse travels down the bundle of His, the QRS complex is formed. Finally, the T wave represents repolarization. Figure 22-17 shows the activities occurring in the heart depicted by the ECG tracing. Because the myocardium is depolarized from endocardium to epicardium, an electrode placed on the epicardial surface normally shows a positive inscription. If a large amount of muscle mass is depolarized, a large inscription is formed (Fig. 22-18). Smaller muscle masses inscribe smaller R waves.

The electrical impulses are sensed by positive and negative electrodes placed in various locations on the body surface. One positive and one negative electrode make a lead. Leads record the magnitude, direction, and surface potential of impulses generated by cardiac cells. Electrical impulses moving toward a positive electrode produce a predominantly positive deflection of the QRS complex (R wave), whereas impulses traveling away from a positive electrode produce predominantly negatively deflected QRS (QS) complexes (Fig. 22-19).

The two types of leads are bipolar and unipolar. Bipolar leads were first identified by Einthoven as a triangular lead system composed of a positive and a negative electrode placed at equal distances from the heart. The electrodes are placed on the left arm, right arm, and left leg and are termed *limb leads* (see Figure 22-16). In lead I, the positive electrode is on the left arm with the negative on the right. In lead II, the negative electrode is on the right arm with the positive on the left leg. In lead III, the positive electrode is on the left leg with the negative on the left arm. The bipolar leads view the heart from the frontal plane, gathering data from the superior, inferior, right, and left surfaces.

The unipolar leads consist of the augmented limb leads and the precordial chest (V) leads. The augmented limb leads are so called because the electrical voltage is so small that it must be amplified to be seen. These leads look at the frontal plane of the heart. A positive electrode is placed on either the left arm (aVL), right arm (aVR), or left leg (aVF), with a common reference point at the heart (see Figure 22-16).

Precordial leads provide six views (V_1 through V_6) of electrical activity of the heart on the horizontal plane (Fig. 22-20). Due to the position of the electrodes in the

TABLE 22-4 *Terms Relating to Normal Electrophysiology and Cardiac Dysrhythmias*

Term	Definition
Absolute refractory period	Period where cardiac cell cannot accept any stimulus, regardless of intensity, to initiate an impulse
Accessory pathway	An extra or analogous pathway bypassing the AV node
Action potential	A change in electrical activity along the cell membrane initiating an impulse; each cardiac cell has five phases: 0, 1, 2, 3, and 4
Automaticity	Electrical property of cardiac cells that permits spontaneous depolarization generating an electrical impulse; groups of these automatic cells make up the heart's primary pacemakers: SA node, AV node, and ventricles
Circus movement	Continuous stimulation of the myocardium through conduction pathways within the myocardium
Conduction	Flow of electrical impulses through the cardiac conduction system. Normal conduction occurs in this way from the SA node to the ventricles
Aberrant conduction	Impulses that are abnormally conducted through the ventricles due to a delay in the refractory period in the bundle branches; seen on the ECG as a change in QRS morphology
Antegrade conduction	Impulses flow forward through the conduction system
Retrograde conduction	Impulses flow backward through the conduction system
Compensatory pause	A pause that occurs after a premature complex; a premature beat that does not interrupt the cardiac cycle is a full compensatory pause and is equal to twice the R to R interval between two normal beats
Reentry	Phenomenon where an impulse returns to reexcite a previously stimulated region of the myocardium through a pathway; usually the impulse is sinus or ectopic in origin and occurs in an area of slowed conduction with unequal response time in the myocardium
Rhythm	
Active rhythm	A rhythm stimulated by a premature ectopic focus that maintains a rate faster than a normal pacemaker and assumes control of cardiac rhythm regardless of the underlying rhythm
Ectopic rhythm	Impulses that originate outside of the SA node due to the inability of the SA node to generate an impulse
Normal sinus rhythm	A series of impulses generated by the SA node and conducted through the conduction system in a normal fashion
Passive rhythm	Impulses generated by a lower pacemaker when the primary pacemakers slow or fail; also termed as escape rhythm

AV: atrioventricular; SA: sinoatrial; ECG: electrocardiogram.

precordial area, these leads are particularly useful in detecting atrial and ventricular activity and chamber hypertrophy and in providing a mirror image of posterior heart activity. The electrodes are placed in specific locations on the anterior chest wall, and each gives specific important information that can be supportive of different diagnoses, particularly myocardial ischemia or infarction (see p. 464). Referring to Figure 22-20, one can note that most of the electrical impulses move away from the electrode in V_1, producing a small, positive R wave and a deep, negative S wave. Due to the placement of the V_2 through V_6 electrodes and the flow of the electrical forces, the R wave appears to grow, becoming more positive and reaching maximum height in V_4. This is known as *R wave progression on the precordium* and is characteristic of normal ECGs. The R waves in V_5 and V_6 then become somewhat smaller.

The 12-lead ECG is composed of the six limb and six precordial leads, giving a comprehensive view of the heart in two dimensions. Figure 22-21 illustrates normal results of a 12-lead ECG. It is useful in diagnosing acute and nonacute myocardial infarction, atrial and ventricular hypertrophy, and congenital defects. It can also detect the dysrhythmias associated with acute or chronic heart disease. In the diagnosis of acute myocardial infarction, the 12-lead ECG assesses anatomic areas or surfaces of the heart perfused by the right and left coronary arteries. Patterns reflecting ischemia, injury, and necrosis can be detected by examining these areas.

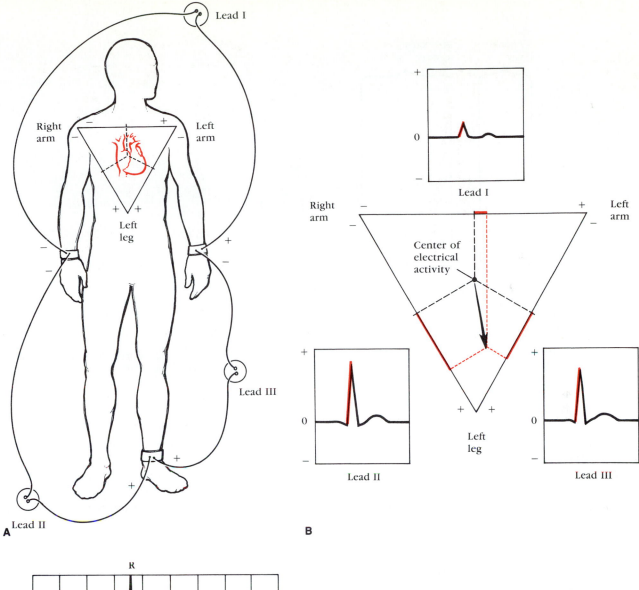

FIGURE 22-16 **A.** *The standard electrocardiographic (ECG) leads with their attachments to the body.* **B.** *ECG tracings recorded with leads I, II, and III.* **C.** *The normal ECG from lead II. Each small square represents 0.04 seconds on the horizontal plane. Measurements are made of time required for impulses to pass through different portions of the conduction system. The P wave indicates SA node initiation of the impulse. The QRS indicates ventricular depolarization, and the T wave reflects ventricular repolarization.*

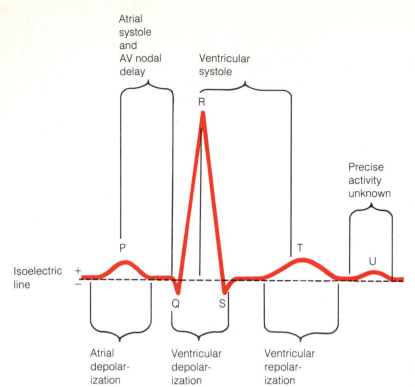

Atrial systole and AV nodal delay

Ventricular systole

Precise activity unknown

Isoelectric line

Atrial depolarization

Ventricular depolarization

Ventricular repolarization

FIGURE 22-17 *Correlation of mechanical and electrical activity within the heart.*

Cardiac Dysrhythmias

An alteration in the normal rhythm of the cardiac cycle is often labeled a dysrhythmia, arrhythmia, or ectopic rhythm. The term most widely accepted is dysrhythmia. A *dysrhythmia* is defined as an abnormality of the formation or conduction of an electrical impulse that causes an alteration in heart rate or regularity. A dysrhythmia occurs when some factor alters the normal action poten-

tial of the heart. The two primary mechanisms that initiate alterations in normal cardiac rhythm are *abnormal automaticity* and *reentry phenomena*. Automaticity may be enhanced or depressed. In enhanced automaticity, the rate of pacemaker discharge is increased, whereas in depressed automaticity there is a decreased rate of discharge. Reentry develops when an impulse has the ability to reexcite tissue previously depolarized through anatomic or functional circuits.[10] The rate of

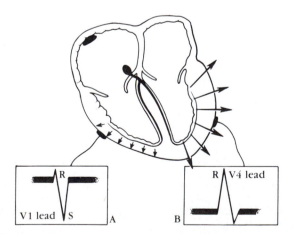

FIGURE 22-18 **A.** *As the depolarization wave spreads from endocardium to epicardium in the right ventricle, the small muscle produces a small positive wave in V_1 (the right ventricular lead of the 12-lead electrocardiogram). The deep S wave reflects left ventricular depolarization, which is seen as moving away from the V_1 lead position.* **B.** *Endocardial to epicardial depolarization produces a tall R wave in V_4 because of the thick muscle mass of the left ventricle.*

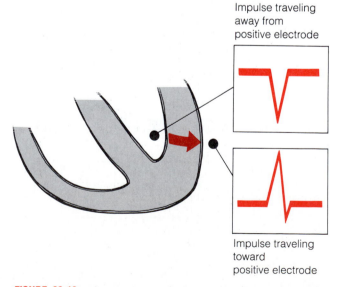

Impulse traveling away from positive electrode

Impulse traveling toward positive electrode

FIGURE 22-19 *Appearance of QRS complex relative to cardiac placement of a positive electrode.*

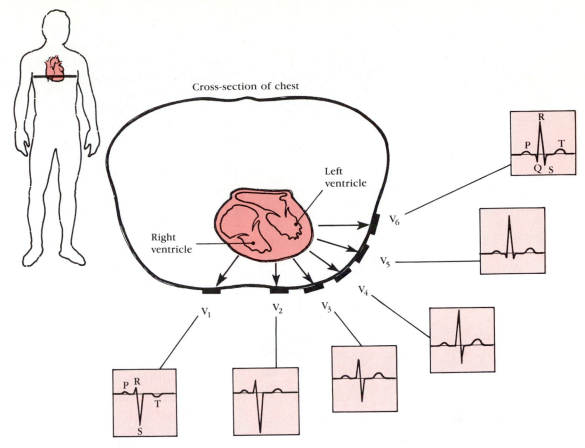

FIGURE 22-20 *Appearance of QRS complexes in precordial leads of a 12-lead electrocardiogram.*

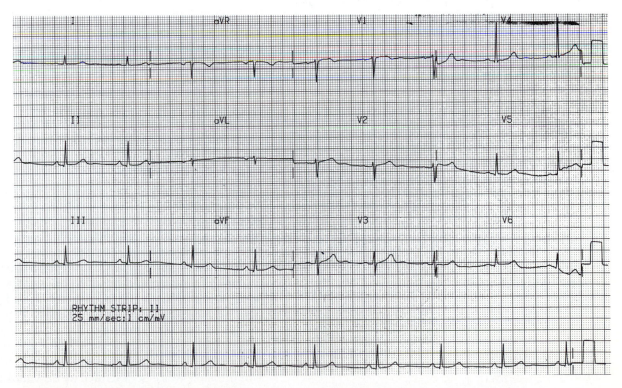

FIGURE 22-21 *Normal 12-lead electrocardiogram.*

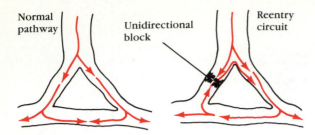

FIGURE 22-22 *Mechanism of reentry. In the reentry circuit, a unidirectional block permits the impulse to reenter the tissue and set up a circus movement. (Source: B.H. Yee, and S.I. Zorb, Cardiac Critical Care Nursing. Boston: Little, Brown, 1986)*

impulse conduction and the length of the refractory period influence the presence of reentry phenomena. Figure 22-22 illustrates how the impulses may enter the circuit and generate recurrent dysrhythmias. Continuous excitement of the myocardium by normal or abnormal paths is described as a *circus movement* or *reentrant excitation*.[10]

Alterations in cardiac rhythms can result from many etiologies (Table 22-5). The most common include disease or injury to the cardiac muscle, structures, or conduction system; systemic diseases; drug intoxication; electrolyte imbalances; and exercise.[10] Hypokalemia in association with stimulation from catecholamines is a potent cause of dysrhythmias, especially ventricular reentry circuits.[9]

Dysrhythmias are clinically significant as indicators of underlying heart disease, or they may produce life-threatening electrical events with catastrophic hemodynamic results. Dysrhythmias may be present with or without clinical signs or symptoms and in persons with and without advanced cardiac disease. Clinical symp-

TABLE 22-5 *Etiologies of Dysrhythmias*

Etiology	Examples
Underlying cardiac disease	Coronary artery disease; cardiomyopathies; valvular lesions; congenital defects; rheumatic heart disease
Acute myocardial infarction	
Systemic/metabolic diseases	Diabetes; hypertension; pulmonary disorders; hyperthyroidism; anemia
Electrolyte imbalance	
Anesthesia	
Drug intoxication	Digitalis
	Other prescription and illegal drugs
Central nervous system disorders	
Psychoneurogenic disorders	
Exercise	

toms in the person with a normal heart are usually not noted unless the heart rate exceeds 180 beats/minute or slows to below 40 beats/minute.[15] The hemodynamic effects of dysrhythmias vary depending on the heart rate and rhythm and on whether there is significant underlying heart disease.

The classification of common cardiac dysrhythmias is provided in Appendix F. The criteria for diagnosis, symptoms presented, and treatment are briefly covered. Further reference material for the comprehensive study of cardiac dysrhythmias are provided in the unit bibliography.

MECHANICAL EVENTS OF THE CARDIAC CYCLE

The mechanical events of cardiac contraction are regulated by the following interrelated factors: 1) preload; 2) afterload; 3) contractility; and 4) heart rate.[11]

Preload

This term refers to the degree of stretch (myocardial muscle length) before contraction. Preload is provided by the venous return and refers to the volume that causes a degree of stretch in the ventricles. Increased preload is responded to by an inherent increase in the force of the cardiac contraction within certain limits. This concept was described by Starling in 1918, who noted that the energy of contraction is related to the length of the muscle fiber.[9] Prior to Starling's observations, Frank had studied the concept with frog atria and ventricles. Wiggers then demonstrated that the diastolic volume increase resulted in increased magnitude of response in dogs. The general principle is often referred to as the *Frank–Starling law of the heart* but probably should be called the *Frank-Straub-Wiggers-Starling principle* to recognize those who studied this important physiologic property. A commonly used word for this property is *compliance*, which is the ratio of ventricular volume change to ventricular diastolic pressure change. Decreased compliance means increased stiffness; a compliant chamber can accept volume without an elevation in pressure.[11] Ischemia of cardiac muscle causes a decrease in compliance, whereas a normally functioning ventricle can increase volume without a significant increase of pressure, such as during exercise stress.

In Frank–Starling's law, the increased fiber length is related to increased volume of blood, which causes the initial stretch. When the fiber is stretched, it responds with an increased force of contraction. This has been related to the all-or-nothing law of the heart, which means that despite the strength of stimulus applied, cardiac muscle responds either to its fullest or not at all. This principle was first described by Bowditch in 1871.[11] In the normal, compliant ventricle, changes of volume can be accommodated quite readily. Ventricular compliance refers to the ability of the ventricle to accept more diastolic volume. Normally, right ventricular output equals that of the left, even though the stroke volumes between the chambers may vary slightly. Respiratory excursion, for example, may cause a temporary increase in right ventricular output. However, when the ventricle receives this increased volume, it increases its output to balance the minute cardiac output. Ischemia, pericardial restriction, and hypertrophy are examples of factors that can affect this compliance by limiting venous inflow or limiting the contractility that normally would occur. Increased ventricular distensibility without effective contraction may be present in heart failure (Fig. 22-23). End-diastolic volume and preload can be determined by a variety of factors. Intravascular blood volume depletion decreases preload, while overload of intravascular volume increases. Decreased efficiency or cardiac contractility, such as with heart failure, increases preload. Body position can greatly influence it because blood tends to pool in dependent parts of the body. Loss of effective negative intrapleural pressure can cause a significant decrease in preload.[2]

Afterload

This factor refers to the resistance that is normally maintained by the aortic and pulmonary valves, the condition and tone of the aorta, and the resistance offered by the systemic and pulmonary arterioles. Afterload is the net force per unit cross-sectional area across the myocardial

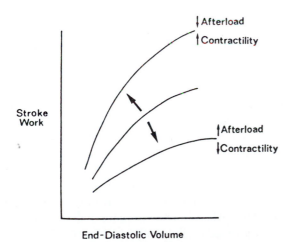

FIGURE 22-23 *Ventricular function curves with stroke work plotted as a function of the left ventricular end-diastolic volume. Each of these curves represents the effect of preload (end-diastolic volume) on cardiac performance (stroke work) at a given afterload and contractile state. An increase in contractility or a decrease in afterload shifts the curve upward and to the left, such that the stroke work is greater for a given preload. A decrease in contractility or an increase in afterload shifts the curve downward and to the right such that the stroke work is less for a given preload. (Source: W.N. Kelley, (ed.). Textbook of Internal Medicine [2nd ed.]. Philadelphia: J.B. Lippincott, 1992)*

wall during ejection. It is estimated by using Laplace's law, which is figured as follows: Wall stress = PR/2h, where P = intracavitary pressure, R = radius of curvature, and h = wall thickness.[13] It is determined primarily by aortic impedance, which is mainly determined by systemic vascular resistance. Because wall stress is difficult to measure, the mean arterial pressure or left ventricular systolic pressure is used to approximate afterload.[13] Increased blood viscosity and added preload also contribute to afterload. Pathologic states, such as hypertension and aortic stenosis, significantly increase afterload. As afterload increases, so does cardiac work and oxygen consumption.

Greater muscle mass is required to maintain cardiac output against chronic increased resistance. Over time, the ventricular muscle mass increases, leading to cardiac hypertrophy.

Contractility

Contractility refers to the force of contraction generated by the myocardial muscle. This may be expressed in terms of the *inotropic state*, which is referred to as positive (+) if the force of contraction is increased and negative (−) if the force of contraction is decreased. This factor is influenced by both preload and afterload, but it may occur independently of these influences. The SNS, through the influence of catecholamines, causes an increase in cardiac rate and force of contraction. Also, by increasing the recoil of ventricular muscle on diastole, diastolic ventricular pressure is decreased. This allows for greater filling, greater fiber stretch, and, therefore, a stronger contraction.[16] Contractility is difficult to measure independent of preload or afterload changes.[11, 14]

Heart Rate

Stress in any form stimulates the SNS, which leads to an increased cardiac rate. This increased rate leads to increases in cardiac output and ventricular contractility. Rate changes are often called the *chronotropic effect*, with a positive effect referring to an increased rate and a negative effect referring to a decreased rate. Alteration in heart rate is a significant factor in changes of cardiac output. The cardiac output equals the stroke volume multiplied by the heart rate and is measured in liters per minute. Table 22-6 lists some terms and normal values related to the cardiac cycle.

PHASES OF THE CARDIAC CYCLE

The two major phases of cardiac activity are called *systole* and *diastole*. Systole refers to contraction and diastole refers to relaxation. The events of the cardiac cycle from the atria through the ventricles relating systole and diastole are discussed in this section. Important definitions are presented in Table 22-6.

TABLE 22-6 Terms Used to Define the Cardiac Cycle

Term	Definition
Cardiac output	Amount of blood pumped from heart/minute; cardiac output = stroke volume × heart rate; normal = 4–8 L/min
Cardiac index	Cardiac output indexed to square meters of body surface area; normal = 2.5–4.0 L/min/m²
Stroke volume	Amount of blood ejected from each ventricle beat; this is not all of the blood in each ventricle, but about 60–75% of the volume, and is called the *ejection fraction*
End-diastolic volume	Amount of blood in the ventricle just before systole
Ejection fraction	Ratio of stroke volume to end-diastolic volume. Measure of left ventricular function; normal = 67 ± 9%
Isovolumic contraction	Period of ventricular pressure rise prior to opening of semilunar valves
Ejection	Period when ventricular pressure exceeds arterial pressure, and blood is ejected from heart
Incisura	Inscription of a pressure recording that occurs when aortic valve closes; caused by a momentary reversal of pressures between aorta and left ventricle
Isovolumic relaxation	Rapid drop of pressure in ventricles toward diastolic pressure. Occurs prior to opening of atrioventricular valves and ventricular filling
Systole	Contraction of the heart
Diastole	Relaxation of the heart

Atrial Filling and Contraction

As the atria receive blood from the incoming veins, blood accumulates in these structures until ventricular pressures fall below atrial pressures. As the atrial pressure rises, the flow of blood passively opens the AV valves and blood flows into the ventricles. Approximately 70% of blood flow from the atria to the ventricles occurs passively. Atrial contraction, which follows atrial depolarization from the SA pathways, provides the "atrial kick" to move the remaining atrial blood into the ventricles.

Ventricular Filling and Contraction

Rapid ventricular filling occurs after the AV valves open. Blood moves into the ventricles passively and then actively in response to the atrial kick. Ventricular depolar-ization and contraction occur from the conduction pathways and Purkinje activation of the muscle. Ventricular systole occurs in discrete phases:

1. Ventricular pressure begins to rise, causing increased tension around the AV valve structures and closure of the mitral and tricuspid valves. This is called the *isovolumetric contraction period* and occupies the time between onset of ventricular contraction and opening of the semilunar valves. It is associated with the first heart sound.[11]
2. Blood is ejected from the ventricles when the pressure in the ventricles exceeds the diastolic pressures maintained in the aorta and the pulmonary artery. This increased pressure opens the semilunar valves, and blood flows into the arteries. This period is termed *rapid ventricular ejection*.
3. After ejection of the stroke volume, the pressure in the ventricles begins to fall. At a certain point, the pressure falls below the arterial diastolic pressure, and the semilunar valves close. The second heart sound occurs at this time. On a pressure tracing, closure of the aortic valve is indicated by the *incisura* or *aortic dicrotic notch*. The *isovolumetric relaxation phase* occurs as pressure continues to descend in the ventricles toward the low diastolic pressure. This lasts until the pressure in the ventricles falls below the atrial pressure, when rapid ventricular filling begins again. Figure 22-24 summarizes the events of the cardiac cycle.

The mechanical events occur at the same time in both the right and left sides of the heart. Figure 22-25 shows some significant differences between the chambers in terms of pressures and oxygen saturations. One can see that left-sided pressures exceed right-sided pressures. Although both arteries maintain a diastolic pressure, the aortic pressure is much higher than the pulmonic. The diastolic pressure in both ventricles is normally very low, nearing zero.

Heart Sounds

Two major distinct sounds are produced in the normal heart: S_1, often called the mitral sound, and S_2, which occurs with the closure of the semilunar valves. The S_1 occurs when the ventricles begin contraction or during cardiac systole. It has always been attributed to closure of the AV valves but may or may not be a component of the sound. The S_1 is probably produced by the acceleration and deceleration of blood with tensing of the valve structures and cardiac vibrations.[12] Normally, this sound is best heard in the fifth intercostal space in the midclavicular line. This location is illustrated in Figure 22-26.

The second heart sound is mainly due to closure of the semilunar valves. It has two components: the aortic and pulmonary closure sounds. During the inspiratory phase of respiration, there is an increase in venous return to the right side of the heart, which increases the volume in the right ventricle, thereby increasing ejection time. The pulmonary valve closes slightly after the aortic valve, producing a physiologic splitting sound. This split is more obvious in young persons and during hyper-

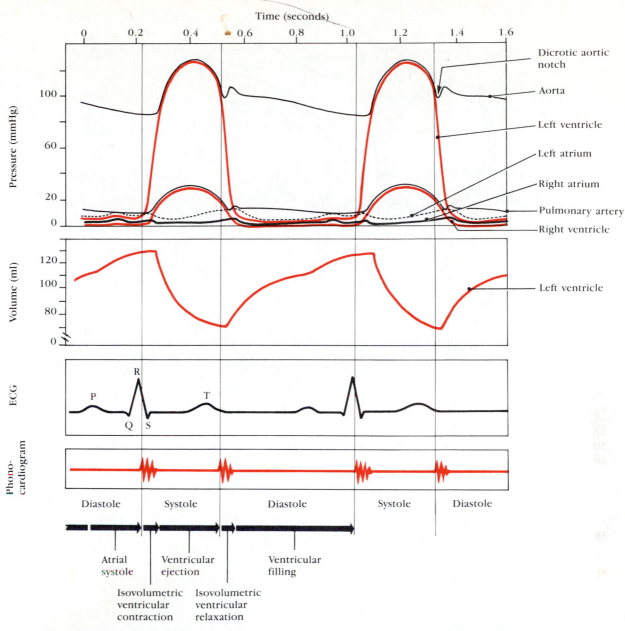

FIGURE 22-24 *Events of the cardiac cycle indicating changes in volume and pressure related to the electrocardiogram and heart sounds.*

ventilation. This sound is best heard in the aortic and pulmonic areas at the second intercostal spaces (see Figure 22-26). Figure 22-27 illustrates the splitting of the second heart sound on inspiration.

The third heart sound, S_3 (ventricular gallop), may be normally heard in young children but is usually pathologic in adults. When heard, it occurs after the S_2. It results from tensing of the chordae and AV ring during the end of the rapid filling phase.[12] It is most frequently heard when there is a dilated ventricle or volume overload, especially with heart failure.

The fourth heart sound, S_4 (atrial gallop), occurs with increased ventricular pressure during atrial contraction. It is heard immediately before S_1 and may be associated with hypertension or decreased ventricular compliance. Both S_3 and S_4 are best heard at the apex with the bell portion of the stethoscope.

Other sounds may be heard with pathology of the heart and its valves. All of the heart sounds are phonetically illustrated in Figure 22-28 and further described in Chapters 24, 25, and 26.

Figure 22-24 summarizes the relationship of S_1 (systole) and S_2 (diastole) to cardiac events. Also shown are the periods of the cardiac cycle as related to the ECG.

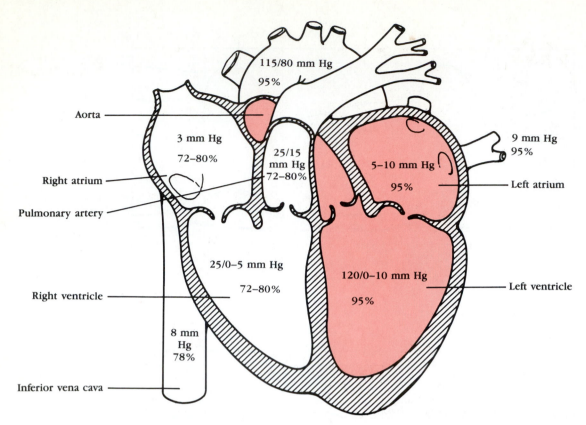

FIGURE 22-25 Normal pressures and oxygen saturations in the great vessels and cardiac chambers.

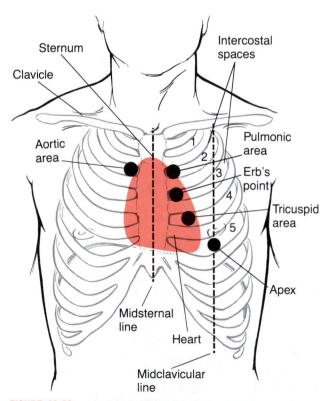

FIGURE 22-26 Locations of the auscultatory points for the various heart sounds. Note that the mitral sound is heard directly over the point of maximal impulse (PMI), which is also the apex of the heart, normally at about the midclavicular line.

CARDIAC RESERVE

As with other organs and systems of the body, the heart has a reserve. It has the capacity to regulate its cardiac output to meet the demands of the body. It can increase blood flow fivefold to sixfold during exercise.[11] The mechanisms used are interrelated and result in adequate cardiac output for metabolic needs. The mechanisms of cardiac reserve include change in pulse rate and stroke volume, increased oxygen extraction, redistribution of blood flow, anaerobic metabolism, and cardiac dilatation and hypertrophy.

Heart rate increase enhances the cardiac output

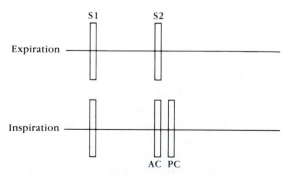

FIGURE 22-27 Illustration of splitting of the second heart sound on inspiration. Note that aortic closure (AC) occurs first; pulmonic closure (PC) follows. On inspiration, two separate sounds may be heard.

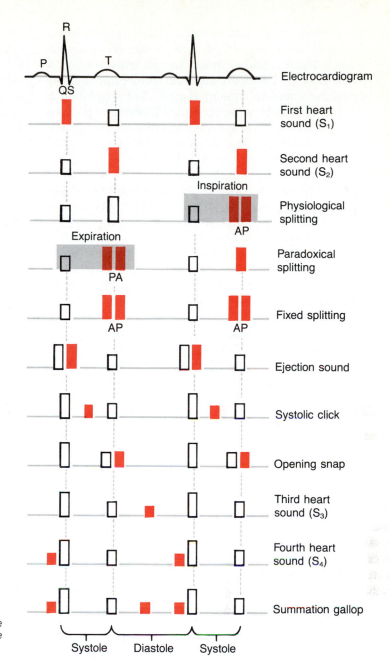

FIGURE 22-28 *Illustration of the heart sounds related to the electrocardiogram. Some normal and pathologic sounds are illustrated.*

within certain physiologic limits. Increasing the rate of contraction and maintaining the stroke volume will increase the minute cardiac output. It is mainly mediated by a decrease in the vagal tone and to some extent by increasing sympathetic stimulation (see below).

Stroke volume is the amount of blood ejected per ventricle per beat. In the normal person, this amount is related to the person's size, fitness level, and age. A good indicator of the ability of the heart to maintain contractility is the relationship between the end diastolic volume and the stroke volume. This is called the *ejection fraction* and normally is about 60% to 75%.[10] In other words, if the ventricle receives 100 mL of blood during a cardiac cycle, it should pump out 60 to 75 mL with each

beat. In the normal heart, increased return of blood to the heart is responded to by maintaining or increasing the ejection fraction through the Frank–Starling principle described earlier. A decrease in ejection fraction is the hallmark of ventricular failure, because the ventricle is unable to pump effectively (see p. 498).

In many of the systemic tissues, more oxygen can be extracted from the blood to increase tissue oxygenation when it is needed. The heart already extracts about 70% to 75% of its supplied oxygen, so this mechanism is of less use to the heart than to the systemic tissues.[11]

Systemically, the redistribution of cardiac output helps to maintain vital tissue perfusion in increased demand situations. This results in maintaining blood flow to the brain, heart, and tissues acutely requiring blood flow and decreasing blood flow to the less essential areas.[11] The two main mechanisms for redistribution of blood flow in the heart are local autoregulation and autonomic nervous system control. Autoregulation is the mechanism by which coronary blood flow remains constant and involves a myogenic, arteriolar vasodilatation and local chemical regulation through metabolic vasodilator substances, especially carbon dioxide, hydrogen, potassium, and prostaglandins. The autonomic nervous system increases or decreases heart rate either through sympathetic or parasympathetic nervous system activation (see below).

Anaerobic metabolism is a reserve mechanism that may be used during exercise. In the heart muscle, when oxygen supply is limited, the rate of glucose uptake is increased and lactate is produced. This mechanism for contraction is inefficient and cannot be sustained for long periods.[9]

Cardiac dilatation and hypertrophy are compensatory mechanisms for overload situations. Temporary dilatation results in the Frank-Starling principle of enhanced contractility, but when dilatation remains it is a classic sign of heart failure. Hypertrophy results mainly when there is a consistent increase in the work that the heart must perform. The most frequent cause is hypertension, in which there is consistent increase in afterload and the individual cardiac muscle cells enlarge to sustain the constant increase in pressure that must be maintained.

AUTONOMIC INFLUENCES ON CARDIAC ACTIVITY

The autonomic nervous system, through the sympathetic and parasympathetic nervous systems, provides an external influence on myocardial contractility and rate. The cardiovascular center in the medulla receives input from other areas of the brain and relays messages throughout the body. In the heart, this involves adjusting the heart rate and contractility to the demands of the body. The autonomic nervous system has an enhancing or restraining effect on the inherent pacemaker system and can alter the automaticity of abnormal pacemaker systems.

Sympathetic Nervous System

Fibers from the SNS are present in the atrial wall, ventricles, and SA and AV nodes. When stimulated, these cardioaccelerator fibers release norepinephrine, which stimulates beta-1 receptors to increase the rate of depolarization and impulse transmission through the conduction tissue. Increased sympathetic tone increases cardiac rate and the contractility of myocardial muscle. The increased contractility is due to enhanced calcium entry through the myocardial muscle calcium channels.[2] The predominant effect of SNS stimulation is usually on the

sinus node and causes a sinus tachycardia such as that seen in response to exercise or fear. Stimulation of the SNS also can increase the irritability of myocardial muscle cells, causing abnormal or early depolarization, such as with premature atrial or ventricular contractions. These are usually referred to as *ectopic foci* because they are outside the SA node.

The effects of the SNS on the coronary arteries are somewhat more complex. Norepinephrine has been shown to cause coronary artery vasoconstriction and causes increased oxygen extraction by the myocardial cell. Some persons have a hyperactive response to norepinephrine and exhibit coronary artery vasospasms during stressful situations. Ischemia results and causes the liberation of metabolites that, in turn, can cause vasodilation. Epinephrine, most of which is released from the adrenal glands, has a secondary dilating action on the coronary arteries. Prostaglandins, a group of chemically related substances, may be stimulated secondarily in the stress response. They are synthesized by the myocardial cells and arteries and usually dilate the coronary arteries.[6]

Normally, autoregulation of coronary blood flow appears to counteract the effects of neural stimulation. When SNS stimulation induces coronary vasoconstriction, coronary autoregulation usually overrides the mechanism and ischemia is prevented.[3]

Parasympathetic Nervous System

The PSNS is mediated through the chemical transmitter acetylcholine, which is released from vagal fibers (see pp. 951–954). The major effect of vagal stimulation is on the SA node, atrial muscle, and AV node. The result of stimulation is a restraining influence on the conduction tissue, with only a slight decrease in ventricular contractility. Vagal stimulation slows the heart rate by restraining the rate of diastolic depolarization in the conduction tissue. A balance exists between SNS and PSNS stimulation of the heart, but the predominant system appears to be the PSNS, as evidenced by the resting heart rate, which is usually lower than the inherent automatic SA pacing rate.[2]

BARORECEPTORS

Baroreceptors are pressure-sensitive structures present mostly in the carotid sinus and the aortic arch (Fig. 22-29). Decreased systolic blood pressure causes a reflex sympathetic response with increased pulse, increased contractility, and vasoconstriction. Increased pressure stimulates stretch receptors and causes a reflex vagal response, which results in decreased heart rate and passive vasodilation in the systemic arterioles. The ability of the aortic and carotid sinus reflexes to alter heart rate and blood pressure is called *Marey's law of the heart.*[2] There is also a reflex, called the Bainbridge reflex, for increased venous pressure located in the right atrium

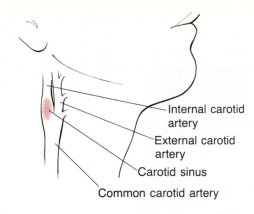

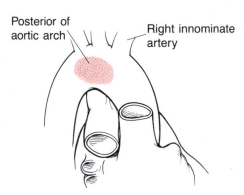

FIGURE 22-29 *Location of baroreceptors in (**A**) the carotid sinus area and (**B**) the aortic arch area.*

and venae cavae. When this pressure is increased, impulses are sent to the medulla, and the SNS is stimulated to increase the rate and force of the cardiac contraction.[2]

CHEMORECEPTORS

The major chemoreceptor of the body is the medulla oblongata, but special receptors are also located in the carotid and aortic bodies. Chemical changes in the blood, especially of pH and carbon dioxide and oxygen levels, alter cardiac activity. A decreased pH or P_{O_2} level causes a reflex sympathetic discharge that results in tachycardia, vasoconstriction, and increased myocardial contractility. A decreased P_{CO_2} and increased pH level serve to reduce the vasoconstrictor effect, leading to passive vasodilatation.[13]

▼ Anatomy of the Arteries, Capillaries, Veins, and Lymphatics

ARTERIES

The arteries are composed of three layers: tunica intima, tunica media, and tunica externa or adventitia (Fig. 22-30). The layers contain variable amounts of collagen and muscle fibers according to the type of artery. Ba-

sically, however, the outer coat supports or gives shape to the vessel, the middle or muscular coat regulates the diameter of the vessels, and the inner coat provides a smooth passageway for blood flow. The large arteries are called *elastic vessels* because they can stretch or increase their diameter to receive the stroke volume of the heart and then contract or resume their original shape, which pushes the blood forward. The *nutrient arteries* are branches of the elastic vessels; they supply oxygen and nutrients to the organs and tissues. The smallest branch of an artery is the *arteriole*, which leads into the capillary bed. The arteriole offers varying degrees of resistance to circulating blood by constricting or dilating its diameter. This mechanism regulates the volume and pressure in the artery and the capillary bed.

Blood pressure changes as blood courses down the arteries, being highest in the aorta and lowest in the capillary system (Fig. 22-31). Vasoconstriction causes increased diastolic pressure (because of increased peripheral or systemic vascular resistance; PVR or SVR) and decreased capillary pressure. Vasodilatation causes decreased diastolic pressure (decreased PVR or SVR) and increased capillary pressure. The terminal portion of the arteriole contains precapillary sphincters that constrict and relax with autonomic stimulation or with local changes in temperature, pH, and oxygen levels.

CAPILLARY NETWORK

A network of tiny blood vessels provides the microcirculation through which materials enter or leave the circulating blood. A capillary consists of a single layer of endothelial cells. These cells are lined up in such a way to allow for the exchange of fluids, dissolved gases, and small molecules.[8] Large molecules, such as the plasma proteins, are held back in the capillaries and provide osmotic pressure. Capillary pressures differ in different organs and systems (see Figure 22-31).

VEINS

The smallest veins are the venules, which receive their blood from the capillaries. These vessels have very thin walls through which some nutrients and oxygen may leave and waste products may enter. Capillaries and venules are often called *exchange vessels*. Venules join together to form the veins. Many more veins than arteries are formed. These vessels contain approximately 75% of circulating blood volume at any one time. Because they have the capability to stretch and hold blood, they are called *capacitance vessels*. The larger veins have valves that are endothelial flaps or folds interspersed along the inner surface of the veins (see Figure 22-8). These valves prevent the backflow of blood and are numerous in the lower extremities, especially in skeletal muscle areas.

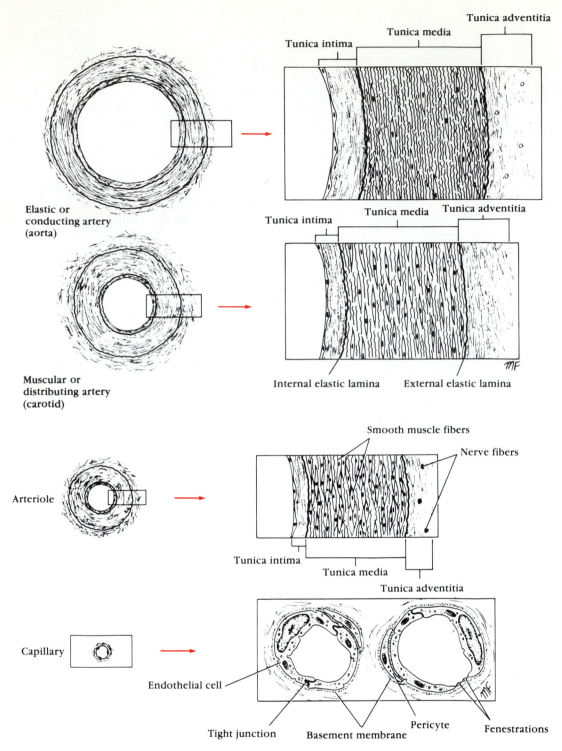

FIGURE 22-30   *Layers of the aorta, artery, arterioles, and capillary.*

Figure 22-7 illustrates the major veins of the body. These vary somewhat in anatomic position.

LYMPH VESSELS

Lymph vessels begin as blind-ended capillaries. They connect the lymph nodes and provide a secondary circulatory system. Approximately 2 liters of fluid are left in the interstitial spaces every day. This diffuses into the lymph capillaries. The lymph vessels effectively remove any excess plasma proteins that have leaked into the interstitial area.

The movement of lymph through the large lymphatic vessels occurs because of arterial pulsations and muscle movement. Backflow is prevented by the lymphatic vessel valves. Lymph flow in the thoracic duct is approx-

Arteries

Vasculature has thicker, more muscular walls, high pressure resistance circuit. Elastic property of the larger arteries permits distention to accommodate blood ejected from the left ventricle recoiling to propel blood forward. As blood moves to the periphery, arteries subdivide to become arterioles which can dilate or constrict in response to autonomic nervous system control. Dilatation decreases resistance to flow; constriction increases resistance thus decreasing and increasing the diastolic pressure maintained within the arterial circuit.

Capillaries

Large bed of single-layer walled vessels. Oxygen and nutrients are delivered to the tissues and carbon dioxide and wastes are picked up. Exchange is dependent on hydrostatic and oncotic pressures produced by actual generative forces from the heart and plasma proteins respectively.

Veins

Small veins called venules receive and collect blood from the capillaries and empty into veins. Veins have greater distensibility than arteries and lower pressures, thus this is called a capacitance system. Venous valves within the veins help to maintain a forward flow of blood toward the heart.

Pulmonary Circulation

The vasculature has thinner walls, greater distensibility, less resistance to blood flow. Pressure is 1/5 of systemic pressure. Primary function: takes up oxygen and gives off carbon dioxide.

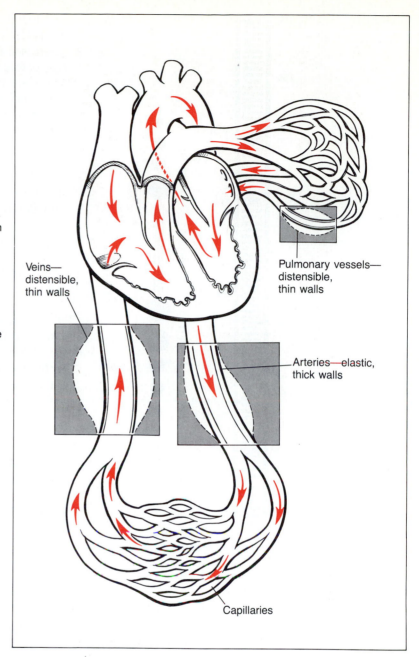

Veins— distensible, thin walls

Pulmonary vessels— distensible, thin walls

Arteries—elastic, thick walls

Capillaries

FIGURE 22-31 *Blood flow through the systemic and pulmonary vasculature circuit.*

imately 1.3 mL/kg of body weight per hour.[5] If the lymphatic circulation is decreased or blocked, *lymphedema* (edema of high protein content) occurs.

▼ Factors Controlling Arterial Pressure and Circulation

ARTERIAL BLOOD PRESSURE

Arterial blood pressure is determined by cardiac output and resistance to blood flow. The highest pressure is the *systolic pressure*, which is achieved by the contracting left ventricle in the ejection of its stroke volume. The *diastolic pressure*, maintained or stored as potential energy in the aorta during diastole, permits a continuous forward flow of blood. The difference between the systolic and diastolic pressures is the *pulse pressure*. The *mean arterial pressure* is the average pressure maintained in the aorta. It can be calculated by adding one-third of the pulse pressure to the diastolic pressure.

The sounds described in auscultating blood pressure are called *Korotkoff's sounds* (Fig. 22-32). They are generated after a cuff is placed around an extremity and pressure sufficient to occlude the blood flow is applied. As the cuff pressure is released, the beating sounds begin when the pressure falls below the systolic blood pressure. As the cuff pressure is continually released, the

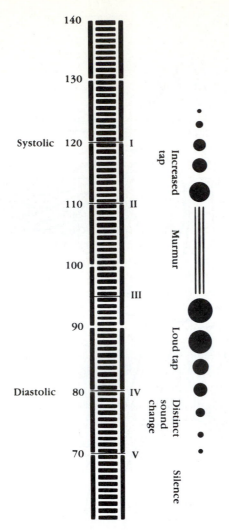

FIGURE 22-32 *Korotkoff sounds. (Source: B. Dossey, C. Guzzetta, and C. Kenner. Critical Care Nursing: Body, Mind, Spirit [3rd ed.] Philadelphia: J.B. Lippincott, 1992)*

sounds become muffled and disappear at the point of diastolic pressure. It is generally appreciated that an error of 8 to 10 mm Hg (systolic pressure underestimated by 4 to 5 mm Hg and diastolic pressure overestimated by the same amount) occurs with this indirect measurement.[5] The sounds are basically produced by turbulence of blood flow through the constricted segment. Flow of blood in an unconstricted artery is silent.

PULSE PRESSURE

The pulse pressure is the difference between the systolic and diastolic pressures and normally is about 50 mm Hg.[5] Changes are affected by changes in the systolic or diastolic level. High systolic and low diastolic pressures increase or widen the pulse pressure. Low systolic and high diastolic pressures decrease or narrow the pulse pressure. Either component can be altered with a net effect of pulse pressure alteration.

Increased pulse pressure is usually the result of increased stroke volume, decreased peripheral volume, or decreased PVR. These factors might occur during exercise or fever, with aortic insufficiency, or sometimes with atherosclerosis. A narrowed pulse pressure can occur with increased PVR, decreased cardiac output, hypovolemia, or other conditions.

DIRECT AND INDIRECT DETERMINANTS OF BLOOD PRESSURE

Contraction of the left ventricle moves its stroke volume into the aorta. The left ventricle pumps against the elastic resistance of the aortic wall, the resistance offered by the arterioles, and the residual volume in the aorta. Therefore, direct determinants of arterial blood pressure include cardiac output, vascular resistance, aortic impedance (resistance to flow), and diastolic arterial volume.[4] Indirect determinants of blood pressure include the activity of the autonomic nervous system and the renin-angiotensin-aldosterone system (see p. 520).

Variations of blood pressure occur with normal daily activities. It can be affected by such factors as the posture of the body, muscular activity, emotions, and use of tobacco, coffee, and vasoactive drugs.

Cardiac Output

The amount of blood ejected from the heart is partly determined by the length of end-diastolic fibers. Changes in stroke volume vary in healthy persons, and increased ventricular volume at the end of diastole will, of itself, produce a stronger ventricular contraction. If an individual is hypovolemic, the decreased end-diastolic fiber length leads to a decrease in the force of ventricular contraction and, subsequently, a decrease in cardiac output and blood pressure.

Vascular Resistance

Vascular resistance is often called *peripheral vascular resistance* (PVR) or *systemic vascular resistance* (SVR) and refers to the impedance offered to blood flow by the arterioles. The major factor that determines resistance to blood flow from a major artery is the caliber or radius of the arteriole. Constriction of the arterioles increases the resistance against which the heart has to pump and raises the blood pressure. Dilatation of the arterioles decreases the impedance offered and decreases blood pressure. Stimulation of the sympathetic nerves causes vasoconstriction, a mechanism that is important in blood pressure elevations with exercise or fear. Humoral mechanisms can cause an increased or decreased PVR. Prostaglandins, renin, kinins, and many other substances are being studied in relation to their regulation of PVR.

The control of blood flow by the tissues is called *autoregulation* and probably occurs with selective opening and closing of capillary sphincters. Hyperemia occurs when the channels are open and cause increased amounts of blood flow to an area.

Aortic Impedance

Aortic impedance is offered by the elastic aortic wall and the aortic valve. The aortic valve normally remains closed until the pressure in the left ventricle exceeds the pressure maintained in the aorta. After this occurs, the valve opens and the ventricle must pump against the resistance offered by the elastic aortic wall. When elasticity increases, such as with aging, more aortic impedance is offered to the left ventricle. Also, with narrowing of the aortic valve, impedance requires an increased ventricular force to eject its contents.

Diastolic Arterial Volume

The amount of blood remaining in the aorta on diastole is related to all of the factors mentioned in the previous paragraphs. If cardiac output is increased and PVR is also elevated, increased amounts of blood remain in the arterial circuit during diastole. This usually increases the diastolic pressure and the resistance against which the ventricle has to pump. If cardiac output is increased and PVR is decreased, the "run-off" decreases the diastolic volume and volume resistance against which the heart is pumping.

▼ Factors Affecting the Venous Circulation

Blood in the veins does not normally pulsate as it does in arteries. Movement of blood through the systemic veins is due to pressure differences; skeletal, thoracic, and visceral muscle pressures; and valves that prevent the backflow of blood. Pulsations may be seen in the jugular veins; these reflect the activity of the right atrium and right ventricle. Abnormalities in venous circulation can result from many conditions, such as fluid overloading, venous insufficiency, and constrictive pericarditis.

▼ Chapter Summary

▼ The heart is a double pump that sends blood to the lungs to be oxygenated and also to the systemic circulation, where it provides oxygen and nutrition for the entire body. The intricate anatomy provides the means for the forward movement of blood.

▼ The muscle of the heart is composed of three layers: epicardium, myocardium, and endocardium. The right ventricle has a much thinner myocardium than the left, and the two ventricles are separated by a thick interventricular septum. Between the atria and ventricles are the atrioventricular valves and between the ventricles and the arteries are the semilunar valves. The coronary arteries arise from the sinuses of Valsalva of the aortic valve and provide blood to nourish the myocardium.

▼ The conduction system provides the stimulus for cardiac contraction; it is an inherent mechanism that does not depend on central nervous stimulation for its basic rate. Myocardial muscle cells lie very close to one another, which allows a stimulus to pass rapidly from one muscle cell to the next. Cardiac contraction occurs much in the same way as skeletal muscle contraction except the entire muscle contracts as a group.

▼ Cardiac muscle exhibits the properties of automaticity, rhythmicity, excitability, and conductivity. The cardiac cycle is described in terms of electrical and mechanical events. The electrical events are carried out through the specialized conduction tissue. These can be recorded by electrocardiographic tracings, and alterations in the tracings indicate abnormalities in the conduction circuit. The mechanical events follow the electrical and are regulated by preload, afterload, contractility, and heart rate.

▼ The phases of the cardiac cycle include atrial filling and contraction and ventricular filling and contraction. These phases produce the heart sounds, and alterations in the sound can indicate pathology.

▼ The autonomic nervous system has an accelerating (sympathetic) and decelerating (parasympathetic) effect on cardiac rate. The baroreceptors and chemoreceptors in the carotid sinus and aortic arch cause a reflex response to increase the sympathetic or parasympathetic response.

▼ The cardiac output is carried to the arteries, where the systemic blood pressure is relayed. The capillaries receive the blood at much less pressure and provide exchange of gases and nutrients to the tissues. The blood pressure is affected by blood volume, cardiac contractility, systemic vascular resistance, and heart rate.

▼ References

1. Biggers, J.T. The electrical activity of the heart. In R.C. Schlant, R.W. Alexander, et al. (eds.), *Hurst's: The Heart* (8th ed.). New York: McGraw-Hill, 1994.
2. Cheitlin, M.D., Sokolow, M., and McIlroy, M.B. *Clinical Cardiology* (6th ed.). Norwalk, Conn.: Appleton-Lange, 1993.
3. Factor, S.M. Pathophysiology of myocardial ischemia. In R.C. Schlant, R.W. Alexander, et al. (eds.), *Hurst's: The Heart* (8th ed.). New York: McGraw-Hill, 1994.
4. Frohlich, E.D. Pathophysiology of systemic arterial hypertension. In R.C. Schlant, R.W. Alexander, et al. (eds.), *Hurst's: The Heart* (8th ed.). New York: McGraw-Hill, 1994.

5. Ganong, W.F. *Review of Medical Physiology* (15th ed.). Norwalk, Conn.: Appleton & Lange, 1991.

6. Guyton, A.C. *Textbook of Medical Physiology* (8th ed.). Philadelphia: W.B. Saunders, 1991.

7. Hathaway, D.R., and Watanabe, A.M. Biochemical basis for cardiac and vascular smooth muscle contraction. In W.N. Kelley (ed.), *Textbook of Internal Medicine* (2nd ed.). Philadelphia: J.B. Lippincott, 1992.

8. Little, R.C. *Physiology of the Heart and Circulation* (3rd ed.). Chicago: Yearbook, 1985.

9. Opie, L.H. *The Heart: Physiology and Metabolism* (2nd ed.). New York: Raven Press, 1991.

10. Rosen, M.R. Principles of cardiac electrophysiology. In W.N. Kelley (ed.), *Textbook of Internal Medicine* (2nd ed.). Philadelphia: J.B. Lippincott, 1992.

11. Schlant, R.C., and Sonnenblick, E.H. Normal physiology of the cardiovascular system. In R.C. Schlant, R.W. Alexander, et al. (eds.), *Hurst's: The Heart* (8th ed.). New York: McGraw-Hill, 1994.

12. Shaver, J.A., and Salerni, R. Auscultation of the heart. In R.C. Schlant, R.W. Alexander, et al. (eds.), *Hurst's: The Heart* (8th ed.). New York: McGraw-Hill, 1994.

13. Tortora, G.J., and Grabowski, S.R. *Principles of Anatomy and Physiology* (7th ed.) New York: Harper Collins, 1993.

14. Vatner, S.F., and Cox, D.A. Circulatory function and control. In W.N. Kelley (ed.), *Textbook of Internal Medicine* (2nd ed.). Philadelphia: J.B. Lippincott, 1992.

15. Waldo, A.L., and Witt, A.L. Mechanisms of cardiac arrhythmias and conduction disturbances. In R.C. Schlant, R.W. Alexander, et al. (eds.), *Hurst's : The Heart* (8th ed.). New York: McGraw-Hill, 1994.

16. Waller, B.F., and Schlant, R.C. Anatomy of the heart. In R.C. Schlant, R.W. Alexander, et al. (eds.), *Hurst's: The Heart* (8th ed.). New York: McGraw-Hill, 1994.

Chapter 23

Coronary Artery Disease

Barbara L. Bullock

▼ CHAPTER OUTLINE

▼ LEARNING OBJECTIVES

1 Describe the following diagnostic procedures: coronary arteriogram, thallium scan, exercise electrocardiogram, multigated blood pool scan, cardiac catheterization, and echocardiography.
2 Differentiate the pathologic and clinical manifestations of myocardial ischemia and infarction.
3 Describe the development of an atherosclerotic plaque in a coronary artery.
4 Identify the most common sites of coronary artery lesions.
5 Discuss the risk factors for coronary atherogenesis.
6 Describe the process of healing after a myocardial infarction.
7 List and explain the significance of the characteristic electrocardiogram changes of angina and myocardial infarction.
8 Describe briefly why heart pain occurs and why it radiates to other areas.
9 Explain how myocardial ischemia and infarction impair myocardial contractility.
10 Differentiate the significant changes of each of the cardiac enzymes.
11 Describe at least four common complications of myocardial infarction.

Barbara L. Bullock: PATHOPHYSIOLOGY: ADAPTATIONS AND ALTERATIONS IN FUNCTION, 4th ed.
© 1996 J.B. Lippincott-Raven Publishers

▼ Coronary Artery Disease: Ischemic Heart Disease

Cardiovascular disease is the leading cause of death and disability in the United States. One of every three men and one of every 10 women can expect to develop cardiovascular disease before age 60 years.[12] Overall, cardiovascular disease mortality has declined by 39% from a peak in the 1960s. The death rate in the United States has been falling at a rate of 2% to 3% per year, mainly due to declining mortality from cardiovascular disease.[12] Improved cardiovascular disease mortality figures may reflect widespread application of cardiopulmonary resuscitation, better medical control of emergencies, control of hypertension, lower cholesterol diets, or numerous other factors.[1] Coronary heart disease, a term used interchangeably with the term *coronary artery disease* (CAD), causes about 800,000 new heart attacks and about 450,000 recurrent heart attacks each year. Men have a higher incidence than women and at an earlier age.[11] Despite the encouraging decline in mortality, coronary heart disease is the leading cause of death in American adults, causing more than one-fourth of deaths in persons over age 35 years. More than half of these deaths are sudden out-of-hospital fatalities.[11]

Coronary artery disease is almost totally caused by atherosclerosis of the coronary arteries, a finding that has led to widespread research into the cause of atherosclerosis. There are numerous theories of the pathogenesis of atherosclerosis. Most agree that it begins early in life and progresses over decades (see pp. 526–530). Many factors probably interact to accelerate the atherogenic process. These have been identified as risk factors in epidemiologic studies, because they seem to reflect an increase in the probability of a person developing coronary atherosclerosis but do not predict the severity or extent of an atherosclerotic lesion.[13]

RISK FACTORS

The probability of developing CAD is determined by certain risk factors. These have been labeled as risk factors that cannot be altered and those that can be changed by lifestyle changes. Table 23-1 lists the major risk factors and these are described below.

Alterable Risk Factors

Diet is a main factor in the development of CAD. In the United States, the consumption of a high-fat, high-carbohydrate diet was standard in most households until the 1970s, when education in decreasing fat in the diet was begun. Despite educational efforts, the American diet remains higher in fat than in most other nations of the world. This American diet has resulted in generally high serum plasma cholesterol levels. Coronary risk is

TABLE 23-1 *Risk Factors for Coronary Artery Disease*

Alterable	*Unalterable*
Diet	Age
Smoking	Sex
Hypertension	Race
Stress	Genetic heritage
Sedentary living	
Diabetes mellitus	
Alcohol	

directly related to serum cholesterol: the higher the plasma cholesterol, the greater the risk.[13] Those who have plasma cholesterol levels below 160 mg/dL have less than half the risk of myocardial infarction (MI) than those with levels of 250 mg/dL. Foods high in saturated fat content are readily used by the liver to make cholesterol. Table 23-2 lists the various forms and risks of serum cholesterol levels (see also p. 526 and p. 807). The low-density lipoprotein (LDL) form of cholesterol is associated with an increased risk of CAD, whereas the high-density lipoprotein (HDL) form tends to exert a protective effect in preventing CAD. Factors such as exercise, age (children and premenopausal women), and diet cause increases in HDL levels and apparently decrease the risk of CAD.[13] The current recommendation of the National Cholesterol Education Program is to restrict total fat intake to 30% or less of total calories. Widespread public education has led many convenience food vendors to offer foods with a decreased fat content. The changing diet may be a major factor in the declining mortality figures for CAD. A small percentage of cases of hyperlipidemia are due to a hereditary disorder. These cases should be diagnosed at an early age and can be treated with diet restrictions and lipid-lowering drugs.

Cigarette smoking has been labeled the single most preventable cause of premature death in the United States.[12] Evidence indicates that the risk of CAD decreases after quitting, so that after 1 year the risk is similar to that of nonsmokers.[12] Risk of cerebrovascular accident is also decreased after quitting, perhaps due to decreased fibrinogen levels, which are usually elevated in smokers. Smoking is addictive and probably synergistic to other risk factors. It decreases HDL and increases LDL cholesterol and alters oxygen transport in the myocardium.[13] Because of the oxygen uptake problem, smokers have a much increased risk of cardiac dysrhythmias and sudden death.[12] Overall, smoking has declined from 50% to 31% among men and 32% to 27% among women over the past 20 years, which probably also has contributed to the declining mortality from CAD.[12]

Hypertension, described in Chapter 26, is a significant risk factor for CAD that can be decreased with antihyper-

TABLE 23-2 *Serum Cholesterol and CAD Risks*

Types of Lipids	Source	Functions and CAD Risks
Chylomicron	80–95% triglyceride (TG)	Low risk, little association with CAD; largest lipoprotein, transports triglycerides to fat and muscle and liver
Very low density lipoprotein (VLDL)	45–65% TG 25% cholesterol	Synthesized by liver, primarily transports triglycerides to tissue capillaries and fat and muscle cells
Low density lipoprotein (LDL)	70% cholesterol	Major cholesterol transport; uptake of LDL in arteries can result in the development of atherosclerosis; high levels seen with familial hyperlipoproteinemias, smokers, diabetics; often elevated in obese individuals
High density lipoprotein (HDL)	25% cholesterol	Carrier that removes cholesterol from tissues and transports it to the liver for catabolism and excretion; levels are increased in premenopausal women, athletes, moderate alcohol drinkers

Source: K. D. Pagana and T. J. Pagana. *Mosby's Diagnostic and Laboratory Test Reference.* St. Louis: Mosby Year Book, 1992.

tensive drugs, diet, and exercise. The risk of CAD is related to the elevation of the systolic pressure, especially in men over age 50 years and in the elderly population.[12, 13]

Stress or behavioral factors have always been thought to be correlated with an increased incidence of CAD. The type A behavior pattern, characterized by competitiveness, impatience, aggressiveness, and time urgency, has yet to be convincingly documented as causative in CAD.[12] Stressful life events, job problems, limited social support, and lifestyle changes have all been associated with increased CAD, although the mechanism is unknown. These psychosocial factors may also be associated with other risk factors, such as diet and smoking.

Sedentary living has been implicated in increased CAD risk, with some of the newer studies suggesting decreased risk with regular, moderate, or vigorous physical activity.[12] Controlled studies are difficult to attain, but all of the correlates of moderate exercise with its attendant psychological and physical improvement seem to have a positive effect on decreasing CAD. Cardiac rehabilitation programs have been shown to improve psychologic and physical well being of persons with CAD and may affect survival after an acute cardiac event.[21]

Diabetes mellitus causes alteration in carbohydrate and fat metabolism and increases the frequency of coronary and other atherosclerotic diseases. The mechanism of atherogenesis is poorly understood and the evidence is inconclusive as to whether elevated concentrations of serum lipoproteins occur in persons who have adequate control of their disease.[17] Keeping the body weight and blood sugar levels under control may decrease the rate of onset of CAD.

Although alcohol has not been shown to cause an increase in serum cholesterol, it is positively correlated with high blood pressure. Some studies have shown that one to two drinks per day can increase serum HDL levels. The danger in recommending this as medical therapy is that alcohol consumption is correlated with increased smoking behavior, alcoholism, obesity, and other systemic problems.[3, 13]

Unalterable Risk Factors

Increased age is associated with an increased incidence of CAD. All forms of atherosclerotic disease become more common with increased age.

Sex differences favor an increased incidence in men at an earlier age. Female hormones may be protective, but if the woman is diabetic, is a cigarette smoker, or takes oral contraceptives, her incidence increases. As men and women become elderly, the frequency of CAD becomes nearly equal.

Racial differences have been studied with little conclusive evidence of differences when the other risk factors are ruled out. Blacks have an equal incidence of CAD but a higher incidence of hypertension, whereas Asians have a somewhat lower incidence, presumably due to diet.[4]

Genetic heritage is a strong factor in the development of CAD. History taking in the young person suffering from acute MI will often reveal a close family member with early CAD. Despite controlling the other risk factors, the risk is definitely increased when heart disease "runs in the family." Persons with a family history of premature CAD (before age 55 years) in first-degree relatives have two to five times the risk of those without this history.[12] This risk is further increased with the presence of other risk factors in the individual and in the family.

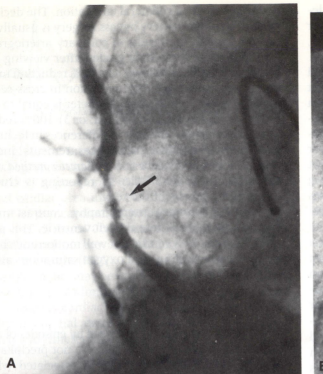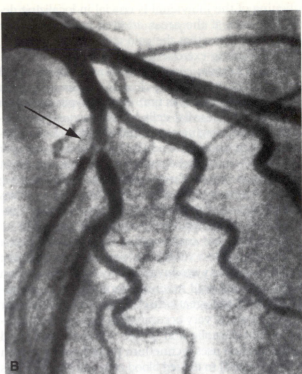

FIGURE 23-5 Coronary arteriogram. (**A**) Stenosis involving mid-right coronary artery (RCA); (**B**) Concentric stenosis of circumflex artery. (From Hudak, C.M., and Gallo, B. Critical Care Nursing: A Holistic Approach, 6th ed. Philadelphia: J.B. Lippincott, 1994.)

induced angina, but the pain may occur at night or after less and less activity during the day. The attacks usually last longer than in earlier episodes. An impending MI is often heralded by the increasing severity of anginal attacks. The ECG often shows continual signs of ischemia and injury.

ISCHEMIC MYOCARDIAL DYSFUNCTION (STUNNED MYOCARDIUM)

The term "stunned myocardium" refers to the persistent mechanical dysfunction of the ventricle due to ischemia. This type of ischemic injury is not sufficient to produce an MI, but the myocardium demonstrates significant contractile abnormalities.[6] This condition has been described in association with angina, postthrombolytic therapy, and postpercutaneous coronary angioplasty and following cardiopulmonary artery bypass. The actual pathogenesis is unknown, but it may be associated with depression of adenosine triphosphate levels, perhaps due to inadequate oxygen for formation. Other postulated mechanisms include damage caused by oxygen free radicals or abnormal calcium transport.[6] The oxygen free radicals are a product of reperfusion and induce ventricular dysfunction by an unknown mechanism, possibly peroxidation of unsaturated fatty acids of intracellular organelles.[16] This condition responds well to inotropic agents such as dobutamine or dopamine. It has been clinically noted that if the stunned heart is

allowed to rest with the use of an intraaortic balloon pump or supported with an inotropic drug, it often will regain contractility and be able to support an adequate blood pressure within several days.

▼ Myocardial Infarction

PATHOPHYSIOLOGY

Myocardial infarction, or ischemic necrosis of the myocardium, results from prolonged ischemia to the myocardium with irreversible cell damage and muscle death. The time between onset of ischemia and myocardial muscle death is approximately 20 to 40 minutes, although this varies with the vessel that is occluded and the amount of collateral circulation that has developed.[16] The resulting size of the infarct depends on 1) the extent, severity, and duration of the ischemic episode; 2) the amount of collateral circulation; and 3) the metabolic needs of the myocardium at the time of the event.[4] Myocardial infarction almost always occurs in the left ventricle and often significantly depresses left ventricular function. The larger the infarcted area, the greater the loss of contractility. Functionally, MI causes the following: 1) reduced contractility with abnormal wall motion; 2) altered left ventricular compliance; 3) reduced stroke volume; 4) reduced ejection fraction; and 5) elevated left ventricular end-diastolic pressure.[3]

Alterations in function depend not only on the size

TABLE 23-4 *Arterial Myocardial Lesion and Area of Infarction*

Coronary Artery Affected	Percentage of Cases	Areas of Infarction
Left anterior descending	40–50	Anterior left ventricle apex anterior interventricular septum
Right coronary artery	30–40	Inferior/posterior wall of left ventricle; posterior interventricular septum; right ventricle
Left circumflex	15–20	Lateral wall of left ventricle

Summarized from R. S. Cotran, V. Kumar, and S. L. Robbins, *Robbins' Pathologic Basis of Disease* (5th ed.). Philadelphia: W.B. Saunders, 1994.

but also on the location of an infarct. An anterior left ventricular infarct often results from occlusion of the left anterior descending coronary artery. Posterior left ventricular infarcts often arise from right coronary artery obstruction, whereas lateral wall infarcts usually arise from circumflex artery obstruction. Table 23-4 lists the

coronary artery affected, the areas of resulting infarction, and the percentage of infarcts that result from the lesions. This distribution varies because of individual differences in coronary artery supply. The infarct is also described in terms of where it occurs on the myocardial surface. The *transmural infarct* extends from endocardium to epicardium. The *subendocardial* type is located on the endocardial surface, extending varying distances into the myocardial muscle. *Intramural infarction* is often seen in patchy areas of the myocardium and is usually associated with longstanding angina pectoris. These terms have been largely replaced by the terms Q wave infarction and non-Q-wave infarction, which reflect the ECG appearance of Q waves in association with the clinical picture of MI. In the pathogenesis, the initiating events are coronary occlusion, but the Q-wave infarction usually results from sustained coronary occlusion and extensive necrosis, whereas the non-Q-wave type may have early spontaneous reperfusion for at least a part of the affected area.[16]

All acute MIs have a central area of necrosis or infarction that is surrounded by an area of injury; the area of injury is surrounded by a ring of ischemia (Fig. 23-6). The amount of myocardial dysfunction that re-

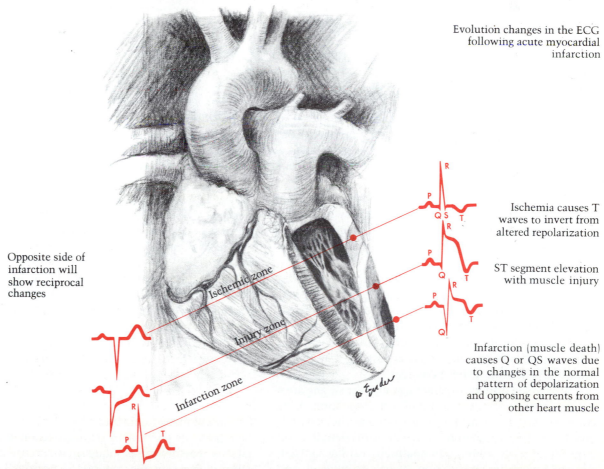

Evolution changes in the ECG following acute myocardial infarction

Ischemia causes T waves to invert from altered repolarization

ST segment elevation with muscle injury

Infarction (muscle death) causes Q or QS waves due to changes in the normal pattern of depolarization and opposing currents from other heart muscle

Opposite side of infarction will show reciprocal changes

Ischemic zone
Injury zone
Infarction zone

FIGURE 23-6 *The effects of cardiac ischemia, injury, and infarction. (Source: B.M. Dossey, C.E. Guzzetta, and C.V. Kenner, Critical Care Nursing: Body, Mind, Spirit [3rd ed.] Philadelphia, J.B. Lippincott, 1992)*

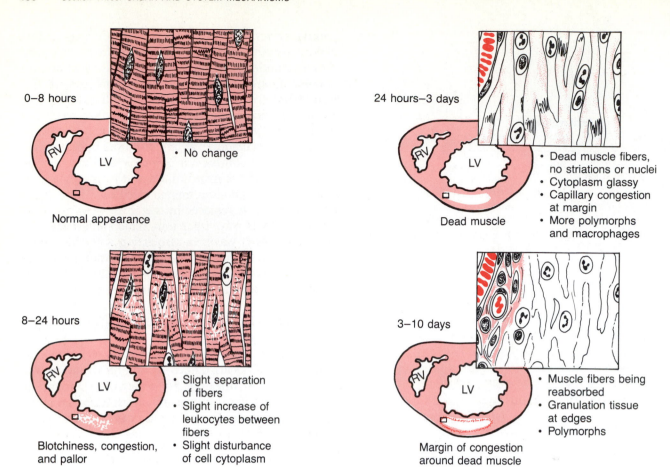

0–8 hours

RV / LV

Normal appearance

- No change

8–24 hours

RV / LV

Blotchiness, congestion, and pallor

- Slight separation of fibers
- Slight increase of leukocytes between fibers
- Slight disturbance of cell cytoplasm

24 hours–3 days

RV / LV

Dead muscle

- Dead muscle fibers, no striations or nuclei
- Cytoplasm glassy
- Capillary congestion at margin
- More polymorphs and macrophages

3–10 days

RV / LV

Margin of congestion around dead muscle

- Muscle fibers being reabsorbed
- Granulation tissue at edges
- Polymorphs

FIGURE 23-7 *Pathologic appearance of myocardial infarction over time.*

sults depends not only on the size of the necrotic lesion, but also on the amount of injury and ischemia in the area. Each area emits characteristic ECG patterns that help to localize and determine the extent of the infarct on a 12-lead ECG.

When myocardial muscle cells die, they liberate the intramyocardial cellular enzymes. These enzymes can be used to date an infarct and partially to judge its severity.[14] The significance of these enzymes is discussed with the diagnostic tests on page 467.

Because the affected myocardial muscle does not regenerate after an infarction, healing requires the formation of scar tissue that replaces the necrotic myocardial muscle. This involves a series of morphologic changes ranging from no apparent cellular change in the first 6 hours to total replacement by scar tissue. Figure 23-7 outlines these changes.

Scar tissue inhibits contractility, and the significance of this depends on the amount of scar tissue formed. As contractility falls, heart failure ensues and the body begins to use the compensatory mechanisms described on page 502 in an attempt to maintain cardiac output. Arteriolar vascular constriction, heart rate increase, and renal retention of sodium and water all help to regulate cardiac output. Ventricular dilatation is commonly seen. If a large amount of ventricular myocardium is lost, contractility may be greatly compromised, and cardiogenic shock may ensue.

Right ventricular infarction may occur with occlusion of the right coronary artery. When infarcts affect the posterior wall of the left ventricle and the posterior interventricular septum, they extend to the right ventricular wall in 15% to 30% of cases.[4] The central venous pressure may be elevated markedly if acute right ventricular failure develops. Low right ventricular output causing shock often responds well to vigorous fluid therapy but poorly to vasodilators. Infusions raise both right and left ventricular filling pressures.[16] The diagnosis of right ventricular infarction is difficult but may be established by right-sided ECG leads and echocardiographic studies.

CLINICAL MANIFESTATIONS

The clinical manifestations of MI depend on the severity of the infarct, the previous physical condition of the individual, and whether earlier infarcts have occurred. They may reflect changes in the autonomic nervous system. The location of the infarct may affect symptoms, including

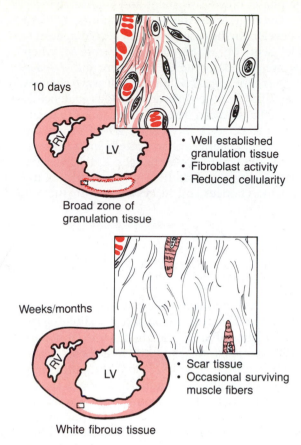

- Well established granulation tissue
- Fibroblast activity
- Reduced cellularity

Broad zone of granulation tissue

- Scar tissue
- Occasional surviving muscle fibers

White fibrous tissue

FIGURE 23-7 *(continued)*

occurs with the onset of myocardial necrosis. The erythrocyte sedimentation rate increases in the early period after MI and generally indicates an inflammatory process. Cardiac enzyme levels elevate because of cellular damage. Cardiac enzymes, normally present in myocardial muscle, are available in abnormally large amounts in the blood as a result of cellular death. These enzymes include creatinine phosphokinase, serum glutamic oxaloacetic transaminase or aspartate transaminase, and lactic dehydrogenase (Fig. 23-9). Their values elevate and return to normal in a characteristic pattern after an MI (Table 23-5). Because the enzymes are present in other tissues, coexisting disease can produce misleading enzyme elevations. Isoenzymes provide more specific accuracy. The isoenzyme creatinine phosphokinase—MB is usually considered diagnostic of MI, especially in the presence of increased levels of lactic dehydrogenase₁.

Myocardial infarction imaging, discussed on pp. 462–463, has proved to be a sensitive indicator of acute myocardial damage. The technetium pyrophosphate combines with calcium in the damaged myocardial cells and shows up on a scan as a hot spot. Also, the multigated blood pool scan is used to calculate end-diastolic volume, end-systolic volume, ejection fraction, and stroke volume. These values are beneficial in evaluating the effects of infarction on myocardial function.

magnitude and location of pain. The manifestations can range from sudden death due to dysrhythmias or ventricular rupture to no symptoms whatsoever. Acute, substernal, radiating chest pain is often described. Areas of radiation follow nerve channels described on pages 1017–1018. Diaphoresis, dyspnea, nausea and vomiting, extreme anxiety, and any type of dysrhythmia may be noted (Fig. 23-8). Often the clinical features reveal associated complications (see pp. 469–471).

Diagnosis of MI is made on physical examination as well as with specific diagnostic tests. Absence of typical symptoms cause approximately 23% of MIs to go unrecognized.[16] Of these atypical symptoms, respiratory difficulties, nausea, vomiting, and epigastric pain are common. The response of most individuals is to deny the possibility that an MI is occurring, so that atypical symptoms are either ignored or attributed to another cause.

DIAGNOSTIC TESTS

Laboratory Studies

Laboratory studies are very helpful in the diagnosis of acute MI. The complete blood count often reveals an elevated leukocyte count, which rises with the fever that

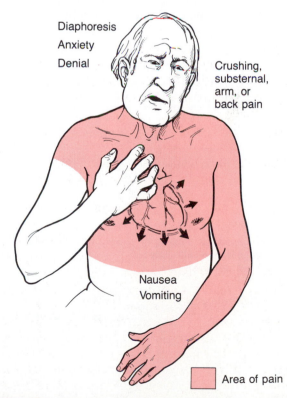

Diaphoresis
Anxiety
Denial

Crushing, substernal, arm, or back pain

Nausea Vomiting

Area of pain

FIGURE 23-8 *Clinical picture of myocardial infarction. Some or all of the signs and symptoms may be present.*

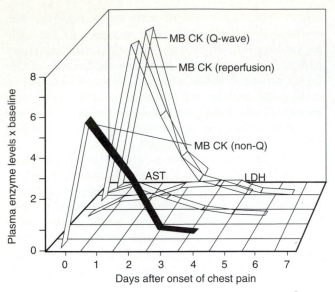

FIGURE 23-9 *Typical changes in myocardial enzymes following myocardial infarction. MB CK (non-Q) peaks earlier than MB CK Q-wave). MB CK following reperfusion peaks slightly earlier than MB CK (Q-wave). The AST (formerly called SGOT) peaks at 12 to 48 hours. The LDH peaks in 3 to 5 days. (see Text)*

Electrocardiographic Changes of Myocardial Infarction

Electrocardiographic changes of acute MI consist of pronounced Q waves and ST elevation. These changes are reflected in the leads overlying the area of injury, so that the infarction can be generally localized by the ECG. In the acute phase, only ST segment and T wave changes are seen. Over the following 36 to 48 hours, Q wave changes develop. In the early phase, the ECG diagnosis is "probable" acute MI, which changes to acute MI when Q waves are added to the ST segment and T wave changes. Over time, the ST segment and T wave changes return to normal, but the Q wave persists as evidence of an old infarction and can be used to localize the defect throughout the person's life. Figure 23-10 shows the characteristic ECG changes of an acute inferior MI relative to ST segment and T wave changes. A deep Q wave has formed as shown in lead III. This is evidence of the MI with acute changes still in evidence with the S-T segment elevation.

Bedside Measurement of Pulmonary Artery Pressures and Cardiac Output

Bedside techniques to measure pulmonary artery pressures and cardiac output are invaluable in evaluating left ventricular function after MI. Insertion of the pulmonary artery balloon-tipped thermodilution catheter intravenously through the right heart into the pulmonary artery allows for continuous monitoring of pulmonary artery pressures. When the balloon on the catheter is inflated, the pressure monitored is called the pulmonary artery wedge pressure. It reflects left ventricular function. The catheter also permits periodic calculations of cardiac output. An MI that results in significant alteration of left ventricular contractility leads to increased

---

TABLE 23-5 Serum Enzyme Changes in Myocardial Infarction

Enzyme	Elevates	Peaks	Period of Elevation	Site of Formation
CPK (creatinine phosphokinase)	4–8 h	12–36 h	72 h	
Isoenzymes				
CPK I (BB)	0	0	0	Produced mostly by brain
CPK II (MB)	4–8 h	12–36 h	72 h	Produced mostly by heart
CPK III (MM)	0	0	0	Produced mostly by skeletal muscle
SGOT (serum glutamic oxaloacetic transaminase); **also called aspartate aminotransferase (AST)**	6–12 h	36–48 h	4–6 d	Mostly heart, liver, muscles, erythrocytes
LDH (lactic dehydrogenase)	12–24 h	24–96 h	8–14 d	Heart, liver, muscles, erythrocytes
Isoenzymes LDH1	12–24 h	24–96 h	8–14 d	Produced mostly by heart and erythrocytes
LDH2	0	0	0	Produced mostly by mononuclear phagocyte system
LDH3	0	0	0	Produced mostly by lungs and tissues
LDH4	0	0	0	Produced by placenta, kidneys, pancreas
LDH5	0	0	0	Produced by liver and skeletal muscle

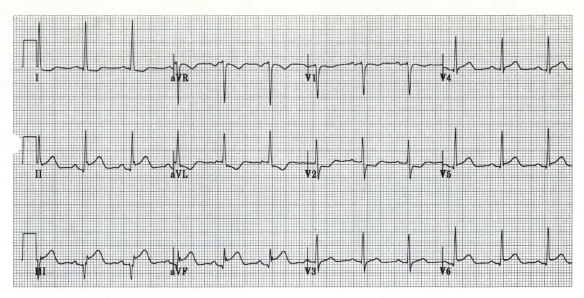

FIGURE 23-10 *Acute changes seen in inferior myocardial infarction. Note S-T segment elevation in leads II, III, and aVF. Deep Q wave is evident in lead III.*

left ventricular end-diastolic pressure. This is reflected as increased pulmonary artery wedge pressure and decreased cardiac output.

CASE STUDY 23-1

Mr. Charles Dow, a 43 year old, white business executive, was brought to the emergency room of a local hospital following successful resuscitation of collapse and ventricular fibrillation by advanced cardiac life support measures at his home. His wife indicated that he had in recent weeks complained of "tightness" in his chest following activity and eating. Mr. Dow is approximately 5'10" and weighs 265 pounds. He has a history of smoking 1 pack per day and is trying to quit. His serum cholesterol is 342 mg/% with an HDL of 65 mg/%. He recently was laid off from his job. Laboratory data include a CPK of 1620 with elevation in CPK II (MB) to 32%. Twelve-lead ECG changes revealed the following data: frequent PVCs, ST segment elevation in leads V2-V5.

1. *What are the risk factors identified for Mr. Dow?*
2. *What is the probable diagnosis for Mr. Dow's signs and symptoms?*
3. *Explain the pathophysiology of the diagnosis selected.*
4. *What is the significance of the laboratory and ECG data in terms of time of disease onset?*
5. *What is the probable cause of the collapse and ventricular fibrillation suffered by this patient?*
6. *What is the explanation for the chest tightness described by the patient?*
7. *Describe a therapeutic plan for treating Mr. Dow and helping him to prevent future recurrences of this problem.*

See Appendix G for discussion.

COMPLICATIONS OF MYOCARDIAL INFARCTION

Dysrhythmias

The most common complication (90%) of acute MI is a disturbance in cardiac rhythm. Myocardial infarction itself produces numerous predisposing factors to account for this high frequency, including 1) tissue ischemia; 2) hypoxemia; 3) sympathetic and parasympathetic nervous system influences; 4) lactic acidosis; 5) hemodynamic abnormalities; 6) drug toxicity; and 7) electrolyte imbalance. The basic mechanisms for cardiac rhythm abnormalities are abnormal *automaticity*, abnormal *conduction*, or both (see pp. 438–444). The most common dysrhythmias associated with MI are listed in Table 23-6. Dysrhythmias may cause a decline in cardiac output, an increase in cardiac irritability, and further compromise of myocardial perfusion. The most common cause of death outside of the hospital in persons with MI is probably ventricular fibrillation.

Congestive Heart Failure and Cardiogenic Shock

[handwritten: Stroke Volume - Amt of blood pumped w/@ Contraction]

Congestive heart failure is a state of circulatory congestion produced by myocardial dysfunction. Myocardial infarction compromises myocardial function by reducing contractility and producing abnormal wall motion. As the ability of the ventricle to empty becomes less effective, stroke volume falls and residual volume increases. The fall in stroke volume elicits compensatory mechanisms to maintain cardiac output (see p. 502).

Cardiogenic shock results from profound left ventricular failure, usually from a massive MI. This pump failure

TABLE 23-6 *Common Dysrhythmias After Myocardial Infarction*

Type of Dysrhythmia	Examples
Ventricular	Premature ventricular contractions (PVCs) Ventricular tachycardia Ventricular fibrillation
Atrial	Premature atrial contractions Atrial flutter Atrial fibrillation
Conduction defects	Bundle branch block, right or left Second-degree heart block Third-degree or complete heart block
Sinus	Sinus tachycardia Sinus bradycardia Sinus dysrhythmia

shock follows MI in 10% to 15% of cases; mortality is approximately 80%.[4] The Forrester classification of heart failure after acute MI is helpful in determining prognosis and treatment (Table 23-7).[22]

Thromboembolism

Mural thrombi are common in postmortem examinations of persons who die of MI. In a study of 924 persons who died of acute MI, 44% had mural thrombi attached to the endocardium.[4] These thrombi are usually associated with large infarcts and, therefore, probably occur more frequently in nonsurvivors than in survivors. Mural thrombi adhere to the endocardium overlying an infarcted area. Fragments, however, can produce systemic arterial embolization. Autopsy studies reveal that 10% of persons who

die of MI also have arterial emboli to the brain, kidneys, spleen, or mesentery.[4, 18]

Almost all pulmonary emboli originate in the veins of the lower extremities. Bed rest and heart failure predispose a person to venous thrombosis and pulmonary embolism. Both occur in persons with acute MI. When prolonged bed rest was standard therapy for all cases of MI, the rate of pulmonary embolus was 20%. With early mobilization and widespread use of prophylactic anticoagulation therapy, however, pulmonary embolus has become a rare cause of death as a complication of MI.

Pericarditis

This syndrome associated with MI was first described by Dressler and is often called Dressler's syndrome. It usually occurs after a transmural infarction but may follow cardiac surgery.[18] It is less common than in previous years due to the discontinuation of treatment of MI with anticoagulation.[18] A pericardial friction rub occurs in about 10% to 20% of persons after transmural infarction. Pericarditis is usually transient, appearing in the first week after infarction. The chest pain of acute pericarditis develops suddenly and is severe and constant over the anterior chest. The pain worsens with inspiration and is usually associated with tachycardia, low-grade fever, and a transient, triphasic, pericardial friction rub.[20]

Myocardial Rupture

Rupture of the free wall of the left ventricle accounts for 10% of deaths in the hospital due to acute MI.[18] It causes immediate cardiac tamponade and death. Cardiac tamponade causes restriction to the filling of the heart and an immediate decline in blood pressure (Fig. 23-11). Rupture of the interventricular septum is less common, occurs with extensive myocardial damage, and produces a ventricular septal defect.[16] Rupture of the papillary muscle is an un-

TABLE 23-7 *A Clinical Classification of Heart Failure After Acute Myocardial Infarction*

Class	Description	Outcome	PCWP	CI
I	No pulmonary congestion; no hypoperfusion	1–3% mortality	≤18	>2.2
II	Pulmonary congestion; no hypoperfusion	9–11% mortality	>18	>2.2
III	Peripheral hypoperfusion without congestion	18–23% mortality	≤18	≤2.2
IV	Both hypoperfusion and pulmonary congestion	51–60% mortality	>18	≤2.2

PCWP: pulmonary capillary wedge pressure; CI: cardiac index.
Summarized from: R. Roberts, D. Morris, C. M. Pratt, and R. W. Alexander. Pathophysiology, recognition, and treatment of acute myocardial infarction and its complications. In R. C. Schlant and R. W. Alexander. *Hurst's The Heart* [8th ed.]. New York: McGraw-Hill, 1994.

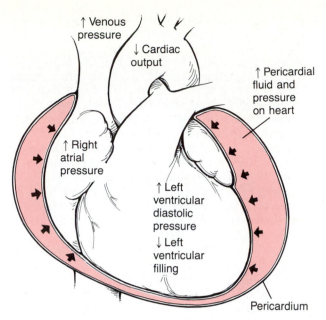

FIGURE 23-11 *Cardiac tamponade. This condition may be due to rupture of the myocardium after infarction or it may be seen with trauma to the heart or hemorrhagic pericarditis.*

common complication of MI and is more common with right coronary artery occlusions.[16] It results when there is necrosis and rupture of the papillary muscle, which causes the release of the chordae tendineae and immediate onset of mitral regurgitation. The rupture of the posteromedial papillary muscle follows infarction related to right coronary artery occlusion (Fig. 23-12). Sudden, severe onset of

mitral regurgitation is usually followed by symptoms of heart failure.

Ventricular Aneurysm

This event is a late complication of MI that involves thinning, ballooning, and hypokinesis of the left ventricular wall after a transmural infarction. The aneurysm often creates a paroxysmal motion of the ventricular wall, with ballooning out of the aneurysmal segment on ventricular contraction (Fig. 23-13). The dysfunctional area often becomes filled with necrotic debris and clot and sometimes is rimmed by a calcium ring. The debris or clot may fragment and travel into the systemic arterial circulation.[16] Occasionally, these aneurysms rupture, causing tamponade and death, but usually the problems that result are due to declining ventricular contractility or embolization. The end result of embolization relates to sudden interruption of blood supply to any systemic artery (see pp. 529–536).

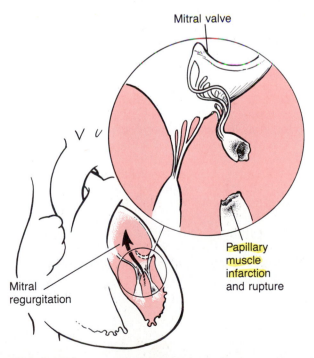

FIGURE 23-12 *Production of acute picture of mitral regurgitation due to papillary muscle infarction and rupture.*

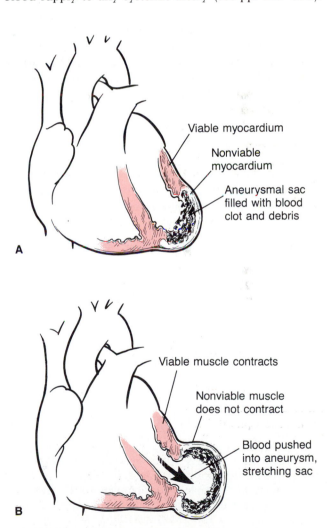

FIGURE 23-13 *Appearance of the ventricular aneurysm. A. When the myocardium is relaxed, the aneurysm remains as an aneurysmal sac, usually located at the apex of the heart. B. When the myocardium contracts, blood is pushed into the sac, causing it to bulge. This also decreases cardiac output.*

▼ *Chapter Summary*

▼   Coronary artery disease is the most common cause of death in the United States and is related to the American lifestyle (alterable risk factors) and to unalterable risk factors of aging, male gender, and genetic predisposition.

▼   Coronary artery disease is mainly due to the development of atherosclerosis in the coronary arteries or their branches. The luminal arterial narrowing is gradual in most cases and may first cause myocardial ischemia with the symptoms of angina pectoris. Ischemia is totally reversible, and between episodes of ischemia the heart muscle functions normally.

▼   Diagnostic tests for CAD include the ECG, cardiac enzymes, myocardial imaging, and cardiac catheterization.

▼   Myocardial infarction refers to the irreversible cell damage usually produced by ischemia that lasts more than 40 minutes. The clinical manifestations depend on the amount of damage that is done to the myocardial pumping mechanism. Because myocardium does not regenerate, healing requires the formation of scar tissue in the infarcted area. Scar tissue does not contract and actually impairs contractility. The cardiac enzymes are released and are very helpful in establishing the diagnosis. The ECG changes reflect the location and acuteness of the infarct. Hemodynamic monitoring gives information on the contractility of the left ventricle.

▼   Complications of myocardial infarction are common, especially the dysrhythmias (premature ventricular contractions, ventricular tachycardia, and ventricular fibrillation). Other complications include congestive heart failure, thromboembolism, pericarditis, myocardial rupture, and ventricular aneurysm.

▼ *References*

1. American Heart Association. *Facts and Figures.* Dallas, TX: American Heart Association. 1994.
2. Chatterjee, K. Ischemic heart disease. In J.H. Stein, *Internal Medicine* (4th ed.) St. Louis: C.V. Mosby, 1994.
3. Cheitlin, M.D., Sokolow, M. and McIlroy, M.B. *Clinical Cardiology* (6th ed.). Norwalk, Conn: Appleton-Lange, 1993.
4. Cotran, R.S., Kumar, V., and Robbins, S.L. *Robbins' Pathologic Basis of Disease* (4th ed.). Philadelphia: W.B. Saunders, 1989.
5. Davies, M.J. The pathology of coronary atherosclerosis. In R.C. Schlant and R.W. Alexander (eds.), *Hurst's The Heart* (8th ed.). New York: McGraw-Hill, 1994.
6. Factor, S.M. Pathophysiology of myocardial ischemia. In R.C. Schlant and R.W. Alexander (eds.), *Hurst's The Heart* (8th ed.). New York: McGraw-Hill, 1994.
7. Fletcher, G.F., and Schlant, R.C. The exercise test. In R.C. Schlant and R.W. Alexander (eds.), *Hurst's The Heart* (8th ed.). New York: McGraw-Hill, 1994.
8. Franch, R.H., King, S.B., and Douglas, J.S. Techniques of cardiac catheterization including coronary arteriography. In R.C. Schlant, R.W. Alexander, et al. (eds.), *Hurst's The Heart* (8th ed.). New York: McGraw-Hill, 1994.
9. Guyton, A.C. *Textbook of Medical Physiology* (8th ed.). Philadelphia: W.B. Saunders, 1991.
10. Johnson, L.L., and Pohost, G.M. Nuclear cardiology. In R.C. Schlant, R.W. Alexander, et al. (eds.), *Hurst's The Heart* (8th ed.). New York: McGraw-Hill, 1994.
11. Kannel, W.B., and Thorn, T.J. Incidence, prevalence, and mortality of cardiovascular diseases. In R.C. Schlant, R.W. Alexander, et al. (eds.), *Hurst's The Heart* (8th ed.). New York: McGraw-Hill, 1994.
12. Oberman, A. Epidemiology and prevention of cardiovascular disease. In W.N. Kelley (ed.), *Textbook of Internal Medicine* (2nd ed.). Philadelphia: J.B. Lippincott, 1992.
13. Rackley, C.E., and Schlant, R.C. Prevention of coronary artery disease. In R.C. Schlant, R.W. Alexander, et al. (eds.), *Hurst's The Heart* (8th ed). New York: McGraw-Hill, 1994.
14. Roberts, R. Acute myocardial infarction. In W.N. Kelley (ed.), *Textbook of Internal Medicine* (2nd ed.). Philadelphia: J.B. Lippincott, 1992.
15. Roberts, R. Ischemic heart disease. In W.N. Kelley (ed.), *Textbook of Internal Medicine* (2nd ed.). Philadelphia: J.B. Lippincott, 1992.
16. Roberts, R., Morris, D., Pratt, C.M., and Alexander, R.W. Pathophysiology, recognition, and treatment of acute myocardial infarction and its complications. In R.C. Schlant, R.W. Alexander, et al. (eds.), *Hurst's The Heart* (8th ed.). New York: McGraw-Hill, 1994.
17. Ross, R. Factors influencing atherogenesis. In R.C. Schlant, R.W. Alexander, et al. (eds.), *Hurst's The Heart* (8th ed.). New York: McGraw-Hill, 1994.
18. Rubin, E., and Farber, J.L. *Pathology* (2nd ed.). Philadelphia: J.B. Lippincott, 1994.
19. Schlant, R.C., and Alexander, R.W. Diagnosis and management of chronic ischemic heart disease. In R.C. Schlant, R.W. Alexander, et al. (eds.), *Hurst's The Heart* (8th ed.). New York: McGraw-Hill, 1994.
20. Shabetai, R. Diseases of the pericardium. In R.C. Schlant, R.W. Alexander, et al. (eds.), *Hurst's The Heart* (8th ed.). New York: McGraw-Hill, 1994.
21. Wenger, N.K. Rehabilitation of the patient with coronary disease. In R.C. Schlant, R.W. Alexander, et al. (eds.), *Hurst's The Heart* (8th ed.). New York: McGraw-Hill, 1994.
22. Zimmerman, J.E., and Knaus, W.A. Outcome prediction in adult intensive care. In W.C. Shoemaker et al. (eds.), *Textbook of Critical Care*. Philadelphia: W.B. Saunders, 1989.

Chapter 24

Alterations in Specific Structures in the Heart

Barbara L. Bullock

▼ CHAPTER OUTLINE

▼ LEARNING OBJECTIVES

1 Relate the pathophysiologic consequences of acute rheumatic fever to chronic valvular disease.
2 State the major pathophysiology and compensatory mechanisms that are used in mitral stenosis, mitral insufficiency, mitral valve prolapse, aortic stenosis, and aortic regurgitation.
3 Describe the clinical manifestations of mitral stenosis, mitral insufficiency, mitral valve prolapse, aortic stenosis, and aortic regurgitation.
4 Describe how pulmonary hypertension can develop from mitral stenosis and from congenital heart defects.
5 Describe briefly the major characteristics of cardiac murmurs produced by valvular defects.
6 Identify the pathophysiologic alterations in and clinical manifestations of infective endocarditis.
7 State the pathophysiologic alterations in and clinical manifestations of pericarditis.
8 Describe the embryologic events leading to cardiac development.
9 Differentiate the consequences of left-to-right and right-to-left shunts.
10 Identify the pathophysiologic results of patent ductus arteriosus, atrial and ventricular septal defects, tetralogy of Fallot, transposition of the great vessels, and coarctation of the aorta.

Barbara L. Bullock: PATHOPHYSIOLOGY: ADAPTATIONS AND ALTERATIONS IN FUNCTION, 4th ed.
© 1996 J.B. Lippincott-Raven Publishers

▼ Valvular Disease

Valvular disease refers to a condition, such as stenosis or insufficiency, that may interfere with valve functions and the flow of blood through the heart. In valvular stenosis, the valve orifice (opening) narrows and the valve leaflets (cusps) become fused together in such a way that the valve cannot open freely. This narrowing of the opening causes obstruction of blood flow. As a result, the chamber behind the affected valve must build up more pressure to overcome resistance. The muscle fibers in that chamber must thicken to do more work to push the blood through the narrowed opening. Gradually, the muscle hypertrophies in response to the added workload. With valvular insufficiency (regurgitation), the valve cannot close completely. The incomplete closure usually results from scarring and retraction of the valve leaflets. As a result, blood is permitted to flow backward (retrograde) through the opening. The heart chamber, which receives the additional retrograde flow, is then forced to pump the added regurgitant volume together with the volume being received. As a response to the increased volume present in the chamber behind the regurgitant valve, the muscle fibers lengthen or stretch. This dilatation of muscle fiber increases the surface area to accommodate the additional volume. Both hypertrophy and dilatation are compensatory mechanisms that occur in the presence of specific valvular defects.

When stenosis and regurgitation occur simultaneously, the defect is called a mixed lesion and usually is a feature of advanced disease. In the clinical setting, the lesions are classified in terms of the predominant mechanical load that is placed on the heart. This leads to the classification of valvular defects. Stenosis can be predominant, or "pure," as can regurgitation, or the lesions can be mixed. In addition to having a mixed lesion on one valve, there may be disease on another valve at the same time. This is known as combined valvular disease, which may present a rather complex clinical picture depending on the number of valves involved and the types of lesions.[1]

DIAGNOSTIC TESTS

Chest Radiography

The chest radiograph (roentgenogram) is used to recognize abnormalities in cardiac size and to identify certain valvular lesions that cause cardiac failure. Chronic valvular disease may show calcification on the valve cusps or leaflets. The chest x-ray is nonspecific in terms of which cardiac valve is affected. The cardiac silhouette enlarges, for example, in the presence of aortic regurgitation (insufficiency) because of the dilatation of the chamber and hypertrophy of the muscle. Cardiac failure as a sequela of mitral stenosis, for example, can be seen on chest films as accumulation of fluid in the interlobular spaces of the lung, the result of blood damming back into the pulmonary area.

Electrocardiography

The electrocardiograph (ECG), which records the electrical current produced by the excitable cells of the myocardium, is useful in diagnosing atrial, ventricular, or biventricular hypertrophy related to valvular disease. Chamber hypertrophy usually causes an increase in amplitude of the P wave or the QRS complex, and characteristic ST and T wave changes may develop.

The ECG can also be useful for evaluating acute pericarditis (see p. 487). The ST segments may be elevated or depressed in many leads; T wave inversion may or may not accompany these changes. In addition, if pericardial effusion is present, there may be low voltage in both the QRS complex and T wave in all leads.

Echocardiography

Echocardiography uses sound waves to identify intracardiac structures based on the principle of sonic reflection.[5] When a sound wave passes through a medium such as blood, it is reflected backward (echoed) when it comes in contact with a medium of different density or elasticity, such as the muscle of the heart. Intracardiac structures have different densities, which are referred to as interfaces. In echocardiography, an ultrasound wave (beam) is transmitted from the transducer to the cardiac interfaces. These waves are reflected back to the transducer as an echo. The sonic energy is then transformed into electrical energy that can be displayed in graphic form (Fig. 24-1). The recording depends on the transducer's angle and on the intracardiac structures that lie within the beam's pathway.[5]

Used as a noninvasive tool at the bedside, echocardiography assesses valvular motion and pumping action of the heart and measures cardiac chamber size. Because it assesses valvular motion, the echocardiogram can be used to diagnose such valvular abnormalities as stenosis, regurgitation, mitral valve prolapse, and ruptured chordae tendineae. Fluid inside the pericardial membrane (pericardial effusion) can also be detected. In addition, echocardiography is useful in the assessment of abnormal thickening of the ventricular walls and septum or abnormal dilatation of the cardiac chambers.

Cardiac Catheterization

Cardiac catheterization is an invasive diagnostic procedure that can yield important information regarding the chambers of the heart. A catheter is passed either to the right or left side of the heart; pressure and oxygen are recorded throughout the process. Left heart catheteriza-

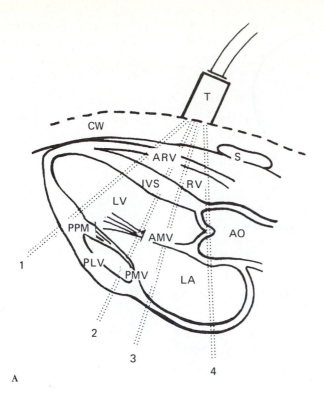

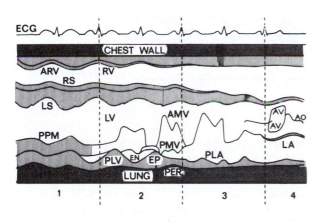

FIGURE 24-1 **A.** *Schematic representation of the course of the ultrasonic beam to achieve the echo represented in* **B.** *CW: chest wall; T: transducer; S: sternum; ARV: anterior right ventricular wall; RV: right ventricle; IVS: interventricular septum; LV: left ventricle; PPM: posterior papillary muscle; AMV: anterior mitral valve leaflet; AO: aorta; PLV: posterior left ventricular wall; PMV: posterior mitral valve leaflet; LA: left atrium.* **B.** *Schematic representation of an echocardiogram from the four transducer positions. RS: right side of interventricular septum; LS: left side of interventricular septum; EN: endocardium; EP: epicardium; PER: pericardium; PLA: posterior left atrial wall; AV: aortic valve cusps. (Reprinted with permission for H. Feigenbaum Clinical application of echocardiography. Prog. Cardiovasc Dis 14:531, 1972, Grune and Stratton, Inc., Publishers.)*

tion assesses the function of the left ventricle and aorta and the mitral and aortic valves. Right heart catheterization assesses the function of the right atrium and ventricle and the tricuspid and pulmonic valves.

In right heart catheterization, the catheter is normally inserted into the antecubital or saphenous vein and guided sequentially into the right atrium, right ventricle, pulmonary artery, and pulmonary arterial wedge position. With left heart catheterization, the catheter is inserted into the femoral or brachial artery and is advanced retrograde through the aorta into the left ventricle. Another method of insertion is the transseptal approach. This is accomplished by inserting a long curved needle through a catheter positioned in the right atrium to puncture the intact interatrial septum. This approach is not commonly used but may be employed when mitral disease is suspected.[7]

Once a catheter is in place in either the left or right heart, the chambers may be visualized through injection of a radiopaque substance (dye) through the catheter into the specific chamber under investigation. This is known as cardiac angiography. During the injection of the dye, abnormalities in valvular motion, such as stenosis or regurgitation, may be detected.

Cardiac catheterization is also useful in determining pressure differences between chambers, as in valvular stenosis, in which a pressure gradient may be present. This procedure helps to assess the severity of the disease process and to determine whether surgical intervention is necessary. Quantitative measurements of volumes, pressures, ejection fraction, and cardiac output are recorded. Because it is invasive, the procedure has inherent risks. Right heart catheterization is rarely associated with morbidity or mortality. However, left heart catheterization can produce serious complications, including cardiac perforation, major dysrhythmias, hypotension, hemorrhage, vascular thrombosis, acute myocardial infarction (MI), and cerebral embolism as well as death.[7]

ACUTE RHEUMATIC FEVER: A MAJOR CAUSE OF VALVULAR DISEASE

Rheumatic fever is an inflammatory disease that occurs in susceptible persons after untreated pharyngeal infection with group A beta-hemolytic streptococcus. It appears to be an individual immune reaction to the streptococcal organism. The production of streptococcal antigenic response may activate cytotoxic T cells, which may cross-react with certain cardiac structures and cause acute inflammation of the heart (Fig. 24-2).[14] The disease causes inflammation of the joints, heart, skin, and nervous system.[9] The attack rate of rheumatic fever is 1% to 3% in persons with untreated streptococcal sore throat. Effective treatment with penicillin virtually eliminates the disease. The most common age of onset is 9 to 11 years, and frequency is greatest in areas of crowded,

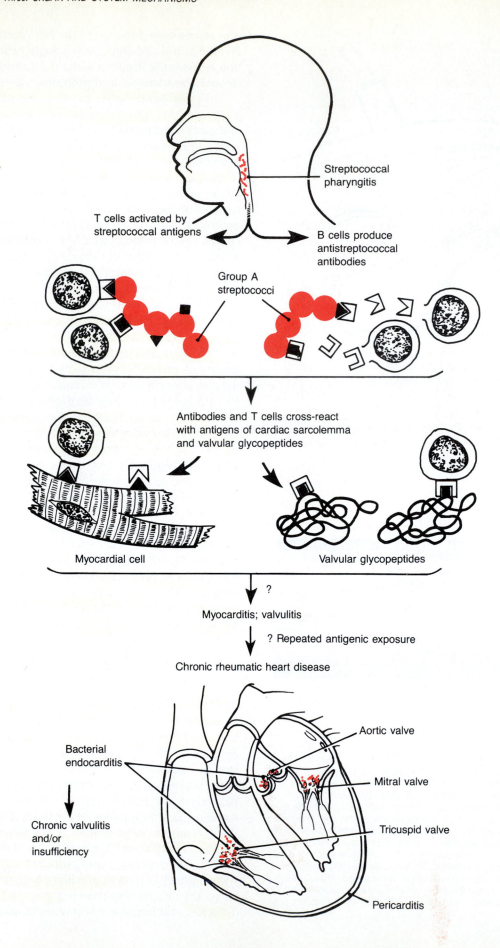

Streptococcal pharyngitis

T cells activated by streptococcal antigens

B cells produce antistreptococcal antibodies

Group A streptococci

Antibodies and T cells cross-react with antigens of cardiac sarcolemma and valvular glycopeptides

Myocardial cell

Valvular glycopeptides

?

Myocarditis; valvulitis

? Repeated antigenic exposure

Chronic rheumatic heart disease

Bacterial endocarditis

Chronic valvulitis and/or insufficiency

Aortic valve

Mitral valve

Tricuspid valve

Pericarditis

◄ **FIGURE 24-2** *Etiologic factors in rheumatic heart disease. The upper portion illustrates the initiating beta-hemolytic streptococcal infection of the throat, which introduces the streptococcal antigens into the body and may also activate cytotoxic T cells. These antigens lead to the production of anticardiac antigens, including those from the myocyte sarcolemma and from the glycoproteins of the valves. This may be the mechanism for the production of the acute inflammation of the heart in acute rheumatic fever that involves all cardiac layers (endocarditis, myocarditis, and pericarditis). This inflammation becomes apparent after a latent period of 2 to 3 weeks. The insult may progress to chronic stenosis or insufficiency of the valves. These lesions involve the mitral, aortic, tricuspid, and pulmonary valves, in that order of frequency. (Adapted from: E. Rubin and J.L. Farber Pathology [2nd ed]. Philadelphia: J.B. Lippincott, 1994)*

substandard living conditions.[14] Recurrent attacks of rheumatic fever are common in susceptible untreated persons and carry a greater risk of valvular disease with each recurrence.

Pathophysiology

The joints are affected with an exudative synovitis with associated subcutaneous nodules. A characteristic acute carditis is noted with the diagnostic lesion, the *Aschoff's body*, present in the myocardium. *Verrucae*, which are small, warty vegetations produced by fibrin or ground substance, appear on the valve leaflets. These apparently cause inflammation and exudation, leading to inter-adherence of the leaflets. These also may develop in a line on the chordae tendineae and produce scarring and shortening of these structures over a long time (Fig. 24-3).[3]

During the acute phase of rheumatic fever, the valves and endocardial surface are inflamed and edematous. Nervous system involvement is manifested by Syden-ham's chorea, which is rapid, jerky, involuntary movements of the arms and legs, and emotional instability.[3,9] No diagnostic central nervous system lesion has been found to explain this manifestation.

Clinical Manifestations

Onset of the disease may be acute or subacute. The acute form causes migratory polyarthritis, which refers to joint inflammation that moves from joint to joint. Subcutaneous nodules appear over the extensor surfaces of joints, such as the wrist or elbows.[9] Low-grade and intermittent fever is characteristic, but in severe pericarditis or myocarditis it may be as high as 102°F (39°C).[1] Tachycardia out of proportion to the level of the fever may be associated with mitral or aortic murmurs, cardiac enlargement, and congestive heart failure. Chorea is uncommon and may begin up to 3 months after the streptococcal infection.

Erythema marginatum may be noted and is described as a pink, erythematous rash on the trunk and extremities. It often appears in concentric circles that fade and enlarge in minutes to hours. Rheumatic arteritis, pneumonitis, and pleuritis are other relatively rare manifestations of the disease.

Chronic rheumatic carditis may occur and run a fatal course over a few months. Fortunately, it is rare, and cardiac involvement is subsequently expressed through valvular defects, often years after the initial disease.

Laboratory tests are not diagnostic, but the anti-

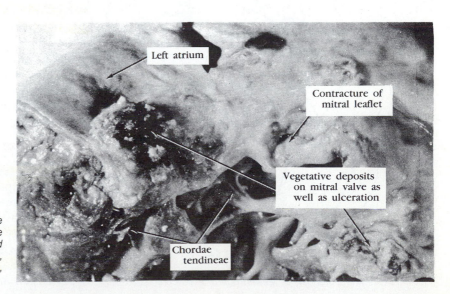

FIGURE 24-3 *Mitral valve viewed from above showing vegetative deposits, ulceration of valve leaflets, and fusion of commissures. (Reprinted from J. Kernicki, B. Bullock, and J. Matthews, Cardiovascular Nursing. New York: G.P. Putnam, 1971)*

streptolysin-O titer is increased after streptococcal infection. The erythrocyte sedimentation rate is increased, indicating an inflammatory process. Most cases of rheumatic fever abate within 12 weeks. The onset in later years of valvular dysfunction is hard to predict, but treatment of later streptococcal infections, which prevents rheumatic fever, has led to few reported cases of valvular stenosis or regurgitation in the United States. Significant numbers of cases still are reported from the Middle East, Southeast Asia, and developing countries.[3]

MITRAL STENOSIS

Stenosis of the mitral valve causes impairment of blood flow from the left atrium to the left ventricle (Fig. 24-4). The impairment is due to an abnormality in the structure of the valve leaflets that prevents the valve from opening completely in diastole. The most common cause of mitral stenosis is scarring after rheumatic endocarditis. Unusual causes are congenital mitral stenosis, atrial myxoma, mitral calcification, and atrial thrombi.[8]

Pathophysiology and Compensatory Mechanisms

The basic alteration in mitral stenosis is decreased blood flow from the left atrium to the left ventricle. As a result of the rheumatic process, the commissures (junctional areas between the leaflets) become fibrous and fused, the chordae become shortened, and the valve becomes funnel shaped. As the valve becomes more stenotic, the leaflets thicken with scar tissue and become calcified at the valve ring and at the leaflet margins. There are rarely any symptoms until the mitral valve orifice decreases in

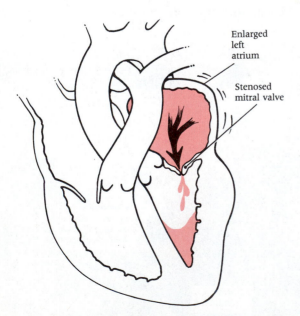

FIGURE 24-4 *Mitral stenosis as viewed during atrial contraction.*

size from the normal 4 to 6 cm to 1 to 2 cm.[8] As the orifice further decreases in size, pulmonary symptoms appear. Mitral valve orifice (opening) size correlates relatively well with symptoms. Because the size usually decreases very gradually over years, symptoms are often first noted in the fourth or fifth decade of life.

In the normal heart, there is no functional pressure gradient between the left atrium and left ventricle in diastole. A pressure gradient is the difference in pressure in two chambers when the valve dividing them is open. In mitral stenosis, the gradient is determined by the size of the mitral valve orifice and the flow across the valve. The flow is determined by the duration of diastole (during which filling occurs) and by cardiac output.[8] The stenotic mitral valve does not permit increases in blood flow, thus left atrial pressure must increase to discharge its contents into the left ventricle. Because of the constant increase in left atrial volume and pressure, the left atrium dilates and hypertrophies. As the atrium size increases, the risk of developing various atrial dysrhythmias also increases. Atrial fibrillation commonly develops, further compromising the blood flow to the ventricle because of ineffective atrial contraction. Constant increased pressure and volume in the left atrium cause an increase in pressure in the pulmonary veins and capillary bed. If the pressure in the pulmonary capillaries becomes greater than the plasma oncotic pressure, fluid passes into the interstitial spaces. Lymphatic circulation increases at least fourfold to keep the interstitial fluid drained and to prevent alveolar pulmonary edema. Fluid in the alveoli is a late manifestation of mitral stenosis.

Chronic elevation of left atrial pressure causes the onset of pulmonary hypertension. Pulmonary hypertension results from chronic elevation of pulmonary capillary pressure. This excessive pulmonary pressure can rise to nearly systemic values, causing an increased pressure load against which the right ventricle must pump. Chronic pulmonary edema (congestion) in the interstitial spaces occurs, and right ventricular failure is the result (see pp. 502–506). Early in the course of the disease, even in the presence of pulmonary hypertension, the right ventricular function may remain normal.[8] As decompensation begins, the classic manifestations of mitral stenosis are seen, including pulmonary congestion and all the signs of right heart failure.

Clinical Manifestations

Dyspnea as a result of pulmonary congestion is the most common symptom. Dyspnea is increased by any condition that increases heart rate, such as exercise, stress, fever, or atrial fibrillation with a rapid ventricular response. Paroxysmal nocturnal dyspnea may be reported by persons with some degree of right heart failure. Fatigue is also common and is related to both pulmonary hypertension and right ventricular failure. Hemoptysis may occur as a result of pulmonary venous hypertension and, in rare cases, may be massive when there is rupture of a bronchial vein.[1] Palpitations may be reported, especially in the presence of atrial fibrillation. Palpation of the precordium may reveal a parasternal lift with the development of right ventricular hypertrophy.[1] Auscultation reveals 1) a loud first heart sound; 2) an opening snap; and 3) a diastolic rumble (Fig. 24-5). The loud first heart sound is due to closure of the mitral valve apparatus when it remains deep in the left ventricle at the time of contraction. Changes in leaflet mobility also contribute to the production of the loud first heart sound. The opening snap heard on auscultation is thought to result from the sudden snapping of fused commissures of the valve into the ventricle. It also may be due to calcification of the valve leaflets. The diastolic rumble of mitral stenosis is a loud, long murmur that begins just after the opening snap and has a decrescendo pattern. It results from the movement of the valve leaflets toward the closed position in mid-diastole, despite the continuing blood flow across the mitral valve produced by the pressure gradient.[1,8]

Diagnostic Tests

The appearance of the cardiac silhouette in mitral stenosis on chest film is characteristic. In the posteroanterior view, the left heart border is straightened, the pulmonary artery is enlarged, and there is a double density due to left atrial enlargement. In the lateral view, the enlarged left atrium and right ventricle are seen. Kerley's B lines represent edema in the lobular septa, and these are noted as horizontal lines at the lung bases at their outer edges, where the pulmonary venous and arterial pressures are highest.[1,17]

The ECG characteristically shows a broad, notched P wave in lead II. This probably reflects atrial enlargement. Many persons with mitral stenosis develop atrial fibrillation. As pulmonary hypertension develops, right ventricular hypertrophy may be noted.[17]

Loss of posterior leaflet movement, left atrial enlargement, changes suggestive of pulmonary hypertension, and right ventricular enlargement may be seen on the echocardiogram. If mitral stenosis is complicated by the presence of mitral valve incompetence, left ventricular enlargement is also noted on the echocardiogram.[8] Direct measurements of a gradient across the mitral valve cannot be made by conventional means but can be assessed by simultaneous measurement of the pulmonary artery wedge and left ventricular diastolic pressure (see p. 510). Correlation of the pressure gradient with cardiac output, heart rate, and diastolic filling time provides the examiner with data to calculate the mitral valve area.[1]

Course and Complications

The uninterrupted course of mitral stenosis is long and progresses toward total disability and death. Atrial fibrillation adds an additional burden to the already compromised hemodynamics. Systemic emboli complicate the course of mitral stenosis and relate to onset of atrial fibrillation. Pulmonary hypertension develops after long exposure to high pulmonary pressures. It is associated with permanent vascular changes and the development of right heart failure. Fatigue is a major complaint and is often associated with peripheral edema, ascites, liver enlargement, and an enlarged right ventricle.

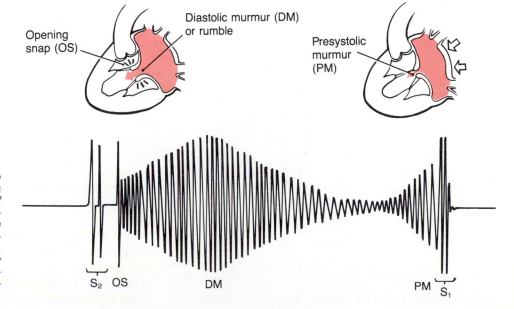

FIGURE 24-5 *The diastolic rumble characteristic of mitral stenosis is produced due to the obstruction of blood flow from left atrium to left ventricle. The stiff valve produces an opening snap (OS). The murmur intensity decreases in mid-diastole. Atrial contraction increases flow across the stiff valve, causing a presystolic increase in the murmur intensity.*

MITRAL REGURGITATION OR INSUFFICIENCY

Mitral regurgitation is described as the backflow of blood from the left ventricle across the mitral valve to the left atrium during ventricular systole. Regurgitation occurs when the mitral valve fails to close completely. The most common causes of mitral regurgitation are mitral valve prolapse, coronary artery disease, and rheumatic valve disease. Less common conditions include connective tissue disease, papillary muscle dysfunction, and infective endocarditis.[8]

Pathophysiology and Compensatory Mechanisms

The pathophysiology of mitral insufficiency depends on the underlying cause. Displacement of the leaflets of the mitral valve in mitral valve prolapse prevents closure of the valve and allows blood flow back into the left atrium (see p. 481). Rupture of the papillary muscles after MI can produce a sudden, marked mitral insufficiency. The same rheumatic processes that lead to mitral stenosis contribute to the production of mitral regurgitation. When changes in the valve leaflets and chordae cause the leaflets to stay in a closed position, stenosis results. When the changes cause the valve to stay in the open position, regurgitation results. The scarring and retraction of the mitral leaflets extend from one leaflet to another, crossing one or more commissures.

In mitral regurgitation, cardiac output is divided into regurgitant and systemic flows (Fig. 24-6). The

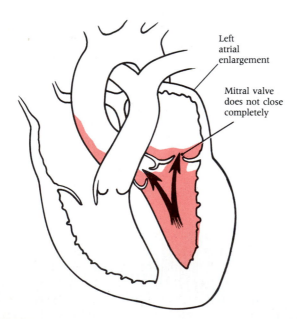

Left atrial enlargement

Mitral valve does not close completely

FIGURE 24-6 *Stroke volume in mitral insufficiency is divided into regurgitant and systemic flows. The greater the degree of mitral insufficiency, the more regurgitance there will be. The left atrium gradually dilates unless the onset of insufficiency is sudden.*

amount of regurgitant flow is determined by the degree of mitral valve incompetence and the resistance to flow through the aortic valve. Regurgitant flow increases proportionately to mitral valve orifice size. Any factor that increases resistance at the aortic valve, such as aortic stenosis, decreases systemic flow and increases regurgitant flow.

The left ventricle responds to the increased volume from the left atrium with dilatation and hypertrophy, so sufficient systemic cardiac output is maintained.[17] The regurgitant volume entering the left atrium gradually increases, and the left atrium gradually dilates, to accommodate the increased volume. As a result of left atrial enlargement, the valve annulus stretches and displaces the posterior leaflet of the mitral valve, which leads to further mitral regurgitation. As mitral regurgitation progresses, contractility of the left ventricle decreases, leading to a decrease in systemic flow and onset of left ventricular failure.

In acute mitral insufficiency, the left atrial compliance and distensibility are unable to deal with the sudden pressure overload, and the pressure rises rapidly in the left atrium and is quickly transmitted to the pulmonary capillary bed. The result is the rapid onset of acute fulminating pulmonary edema and rapid decompensation.

Clinical Manifestations

Many people with mitral regurgitation have no symptoms for several years, but acute onset causes symptoms immediately. When symptoms do appear, dyspnea and fatigue are common, due to a decreased cardiac output and increased pulmonary venous pressure. Other common symptoms include orthopnea, paroxysmal nocturnal dyspnea, and palpitations. Acute mitral regurgitation from a condition such as papillary muscle rupture post-MI causes the sudden onset of pulmonary congestion and pulmonary edema, which results in death in the absence of emergent surgical treatment.[17]

The person with mitral regurgitation usually can better tolerate the onset of atrial fibrillation than one who has mitral stenosis. Atrial fibrillation occurs in about 75% of persons with chronic mitral regurgitation.

The person's general appearance is normal, but signs of congestive heart failure may develop when the problem has been present for a long time. In chronic mitral regurgitation, the apex impulse is often displaced laterally and is larger than normal. This finding is related to left ventricular dilatation. The systolic murmur characteristic of mitral regurgitation is almost always present.[1] The murmur is loud, high pitched, holosystolic (of constant intensity throughout systole), and heard best at the apex (Fig. 24-7). The murmur may radiate to the axilla or back. The first heart sound is usually diminished in mitral regurgitation. A third heart sound that is associ-

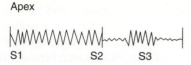

Apex

S1   S2   S3

FIGURE 24-7 *Holosystolic mitral regurgitation murmur, no opening snap. Note the usual presence of an S3.*

ated with the rapid phase of ventricular filling may also be present. If present, the third heart sound indicates some degree of cardiac decompensation.

Diagnostic Tests

Left atrial and ventricular enlargement are frequent findings on chest films in persons who have mitral regurgitation. As in mitral stenosis, the left atrium may be greatly enlarged. Pulmonary venous changes may be noted on chest films, but their occurrence is less frequent than in mitral stenosis.[8] The usual ECG findings of chronic mitral regurgitation are atrial and ventricular hypertrophy. Atrial fibrillation is common. Right ventricular hypertrophy is less common in mitral regurgitation than in mitral stenosis.[8]

Cardiac catheterization provides data to describe the amount of mitral regurgitation and the pumping ability of the left ventricle. The amount of mitral regurgitation can be measured quantitatively during catheterization. The ejection fraction is measured and is useful in determining the pumping ability of the left ventricle. Cardiac output is usually decreased in symptomatic individuals.

Echocardiographic studies are helpful in identifying left atrial and left ventricular enlargement and can be used with the echo Doppler technique to provide an estimate of the severity of the regurgitation.[8] Wall motion abnormalities and abnormalities of the papillary muscles and chordae tendineae can be assessed rapidly, and this may be very helpful in acute mitral regurgitation.

MIXED MITRAL STENOSIS AND REGURGITATION

A mitral valve that has both fused commissures and structures that fail to close properly exhibits a mixture of mitral stenosis and regurgitation. Most mixed mitral lesions are rheumatic in origin. The course of these mixed lesions depends on which one is predominant. If the degree of stenosis is greater than the degree of incompetence, there is a smaller amount of backflow of blood across the mitral valve during systole and a smaller amount of forward flow of blood across the valve in diastole. If incompetence is greater than stenosis, there is more backflow of blood across the valve in systole and more forward flow of blood across the valve in diastole.[1]

Dyspnea is the most common symptom and may be of acute onset when atrial fibrillation ensues. Palpitations are also common and are frequently related to rapid atrial dysrhythmias. The heart is usually enlarged. The first heart sound may be loud, and there may be an opening snap. Often, a third heart sound is present in addition to, or instead of, the opening snap. The characteristic pansystolic murmur of mitral regurgitation and the diastolic murmurs of mitral stenosis are usually present.[1] Pulmonary congestion in mixed stenosis and regurgitation may lead to pulmonary edema, especially with the onset of atrial fibrillation.

MITRAL VALVE PROLAPSE

Mitral valve prolapse, also called Barlow syndrome, floppy mitral valve syndrome, and systolic click–murmur syndrome, is a common condition, occurring in 5% to 7% of the adult population.[17] It is caused by posterior displacement of the posterior cusp of the mitral valve and is probably a congenital abnormality of the valve tissues in which the large posterior leaflet bulges back into the left atrium during systole.[1] It may occur as an autosomal dominant disorder, as part of the connective tissue abnormality called Marfan's syndrome, or in normal individuals.[12] As the ballooning of the leaflet into the left atrium continues, the chordae and papillary muscles become stressed. Contraction of the papillary muscles decreases and mitral regurgitation occurs. The amount of this regurgitation is usually hemodynamically insignificant but may produce symptoms. More frequently, the symptoms produced are the result of an atrial dysrhythmia.

Most persons with mitral valve prolapse are free of symptoms. For this reason, it is commonly diagnosed during a routine physical examination. A nonanginal, nonexertional type of chest pain may be present with palpitations, fatigue, and dyspnea.

Mitral valve prolapse is most commonly diagnosed in women in the second to fourth decade of life.[12] A familial tendency toward development of the condition may be seen. Auscultation at the apex reveals a late systolic murmur that is a crescendo, loud, and musical. The murmur may be preceded by one or more clicks in systole.

A normal cardiac shadow is usually evident on radiographs. The ECG often reveals several dysrhythmias, especially sinus dysrhythmias, atrial fibrillation, premature ventricular contractions, and ventricular tachycardia. Other ECG changes include ST-T wave abnormalities and prolongation of the QT interval. The echocardiogram is useful in diagnosis and helps to determine the presence and amount of insufficiency.

Complications are rare but may include bacterial endocarditis or acute mitral insufficiency from chordae rupturing or stretching.

AORTIC STENOSIS

Aortic stenosis involves obstruction to outflow of blood from the left ventricle to the aorta; the obstruction may lie at the level of the valve, above the valve, or below the valve. Supravalvular lesions are almost always congenital and may be associated with other defects in physically underdeveloped children.[1] Subvalvular and valvular stenosis may be congenital or acquired.[12] Subvalvular stenosis may be due to a subvalvular ring that interferes with valve function or a fibromuscular thickening involving the interventricular septum.[1] Among the acquired causes of aortic stenosis are rheumatic heart disease, degenerative calcific disease of the elderly, and subacute bacterial endocarditis that increases the stenosis produced from another defect.[13] Hypertrophic obstructive cardiomyopathy may cause an obstruction to outflow, producing a different clinical picture (see p. XX).[1] The most common cause in those under age 30 years is a congenital stenotic aortic valve or subaortic valve. In persons ages 30 to 70 years, rheumatic heart disease may be present, but calcification of a congenital bicuspid valve is more often the cause. In persons over age 70, the degenerative calcific type is predominant.[13]

Pathophysiology and Compensatory Mechanisms

Significant narrowing of the valve orifice leads to a decrease in blood flow from the left ventricle to the aorta. The obstruction of outflow from the left ventricle leads also to strain or pressure load on the left ventricle that occurs as the left ventricle tries to push blood through the narrowed opening (Fig. 24-8). This resistance to ejection is reflected by an increase in pressure in the left ventricle to force more blood through the stenotic valve during systole.

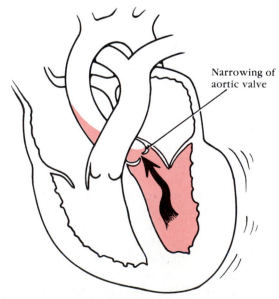

Narrowing of aortic valve

FIGURE 24-8 View of aortic stenosis during systole.

A systolic pressure gradient develops between the left ventricle and aorta and is called an *aortic valve gradient*. These hemodynamic consequences are not manifested until the valve orifice, which is normally 2.6 to 3.5 cm^2, has narrowed to approximately one-third of normal. The left ventricle is capable of compensating for increasing pressure demands through myocardial hypertrophy. This mechanism allows for increasing systolic pressures to maintain an adequate systemic blood pressure. The increased muscle mass requires increased oxygen supply that may or may not be supplied by the coronary arteries. If the stenosis becomes increasingly severe, the persistent pressure overload (strain) leads to myocardial failure. Hypertrophy is a long-term compensatory mechanism that maintains systolic blood pressure at or slightly below normal levels.

Clinical Manifestations

The classic clinical manifestations that accompany severe aortic stenosis are chest pain, syncope, and heart failure. Sudden death has been reported in 5% of persons with severe aortic stenosis.[12] Chest pain and syncope are related to reduced cardiac output, increased perfusion needs, and decreased perfusion of the coronary arteries and brain. Congestive heart failure results from the inability of the left ventricle to keep pace with the demands placed on it. Once heart failure ensues, the course of the condition is rapidly debilitating.

Chest pain is usually manifested after physical exertion as a result of inability of the heart to increase coronary blood flow.[1] This type of angina can occur in up to 70% of persons with severe aortic stenosis.[13]

Syncopal episodes and "gray outs," or periods of confusion associated with severe aortic stenosis, are dangerous signs. Without surgical intervention, the prognosis is poor.

The chronic strain imposed on the left ventricle eventually leads to heart failure and may terminate in pulmonary edema. Left ventricular failure is the cause of death in over one-half of persons who have severe stenosis.

Auscultation may reveal a paradoxic splitting of the second heart sound, which is due to aortic valve closure following that of the pulmonic valve. In addition, a diamond-shaped (crescendo–decrescendo) systolic ejection murmur begins after the first heart sound; increases in intensity, reaching a plateau toward the middle of the ejection period; and fades progressively, ending just before the aortic valve closes (Fig. 24-9). An ejection click may also occur during systole as the calcified stiff valve leaflets try to open.

Diagnostic Tests

A chest film may show apical bulging if hypertrophy is present. Calcification of the valve ring may be seen. In

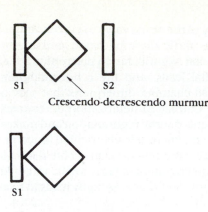

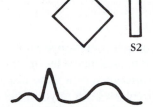

FIGURE 24-9 *Diagrammatic depiction of a crescendo-decrescendo murmur. Note the relationship of the sound to the electrocardiogram recording below. The examiner should concentrate on each component: The S1 is followed by a sound of increasing intensity that stops just before S2.*

the presence of left ventricular failure, pulmonary vascular enlargement may be noted.

Electrocardiographic abnormalities include left ventricular hypertrophy and strain. Left ventricular hypertrophy produces changes in the amplitude of the QRS complex and ST segment displacement (strain pattern) in the precordial leads particularly.[13] Conduction system disturbances, such as heart block, may be manifested.

The echocardiogram is useful in assessing valve structure and motion as well as in providing information regarding ventricular function. Changes in the thickness, calcification, and mobility of the aortic valve can be recorded, and ventricular wall thickness can be evaluated.

Cardiac catheterization is useful in determining the systolic gradient across the valve as well as the valve orifice size. The gradient may be as much as 100 mm Hg, which means, for example, that to attain a systemic systolic pressure of 100 mm Hg, the left ventricle must attain a systolic pressure of 200 mm Hg.

AORTIC REGURGITATION, INSUFFICIENCY, OR INCOMPETENCE

Aortic regurgitation is incomplete closure of the aortic valve. It can occur as a chronic or acute lesion. Causes of chronic lesions include rheumatic fever, syphilis, hypertension, connective tissue disorders, and atherosclerosis.[13] The acute lesion can result from a dissecting aneurysm of the aorta, infectious endocarditis, and, occasionally, rheumatic fever.[12]

Pathophysiology and Compensatory Mechanisms

The pathologic process in aortic regurgitation differs with each cause. For example, with rheumatic aortic insufficiency, fibrosis and unequal contracture of the leaflets lead to malalignment of the leaflets.[13] Perforation or destruction of one or more of the leaflets with infectious endocarditis may occur. In syphilitic aortic regurgitation, dilatation of the ascending aorta stretches the individual leaflets, rendering them too short to close completely during diastole. Dissecting aortic aneurysm dilates the valve ring and prevents aortic closure.[13]

The hemodynamic alterations of aortic insufficiency depend on the etiology of the process, the size of the leak, the diastolic pressure gradient across the valve, and the duration of diastole.[13] During systole, blood is ejected out of the left ventricle through the aortic valve and into the aorta, but some of it flows back into the ventricle during diastole when the pressure in the aorta exceeds that in the left ventricle. Similarly, during diastole, blood flows into the ventricle from the left atrium (Fig. 24-10). The left ventricle then becomes volume-overloaded by receiving the blood from the left atrium and that blood flowing back through the regurgitant valve. An increase in the left ventricular end-diastolic volume results.

If the increase in end-diastolic volume in the left ventricle occurs chronically, then the left ventricle gradually dilates as a compensatory mechanism, that is, the myocardial fibers stretch to increase the surface area to accommodate this extra volume. This dilatation permits the left ventricle to eject a larger stroke volume (Frank–Starling's law) to maintain the cardiac output.

Longstanding hypertrophy is associated in this case with dilatation and often results in myocardial fibrosis,

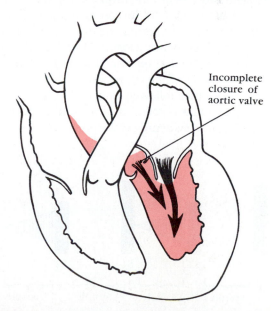

FIGURE 24-10 *View of aortic insufficiency during early ventricular diastole.*

Incomplete closure of aortic valve

so that cardiac muscle cells become unable to resume their normal shape after surgical replacement of the diseased valve has been performed. As a result, left ventricle failure and acute pulmonary edema often ensue.

In *acute aortic regurgitation*, the time factor does not permit the compensatory mechanisms to develop. The volume overload in this case is so sudden that acute dilatation occurs, and the left ventricle cannot maintain stroke volume and cardiac output. In acute aortic regurgitation, there is a sudden increase in the left ventricular end-diastolic pressure. This is reflected to the pulmonary capillary bed, causing pulmonary edema. Death often rapidly ensues unless heroic measures are instituted.

Clinical Manifestations

In chronic aortic insufficiency with the compensatory mechanisms functioning, symptoms may not develop for many years. Palpitations may be described by the affected person especially when lying on the left side. A prominent apical impulse and an observable left ventricular lift on the precordium are often noted.[1] The onset of heart failure is indicated by increasing fatigue, dyspnea, chest pain, orthopnea, paroxysmal nocturnal dyspnea, and pulmonary edema.

Auscultatory findings depend on the severity of the regurgitation. In mild regurgitation, a decrescendo diastolic murmur begins shortly after S_2 and ends before S_1 (Fig. 24-11). With moderate regurgitation, there may be another type of murmur, called an *Austin Flint murmur*, which is a diastolic rumble heard at the apex. It is caused by premature closure of the mitral valve during rapid filling of the ventricles and corresponds to the severity of aortic regurgitation.

The diastolic murmur of acute aortic regurgitation differs from those heard in chronic aortic regurgitation. The diastolic murmur can be cooing or coarsely vibrating. The first heart sound may be diminished or absent because of the premature closure of the mitral valve.[13]

In severe regurgitation, the amplitude of the pulse increases markedly when it is palpated. This is noted as a sudden sharp pulse followed by a rapid collapse of the diastolic pulse and is referred to as a *water-hammer* or *Corrigan's pulse*. A widening of the pulse pressure reflects

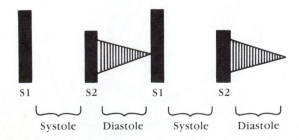

FIGURE 24-11 *Diastolic murmur of aortic regurgitation.*

inability of the aortic valve to exert its influence to maintain the aortic diastolic blood pressure.[12,13] The ECG reflects left ventricular hypertrophy, especially in the precordial leads, and the echocardiogram reflects the increased chamber dimensions that may occur in later stages.[5] Cardiac catheterization documents the severity and extent of aortic regurgitation and makes quantitative measurements of left ventricular function.

Once symptoms develop in both the acute and chronic forms, deterioration is fairly swift, and, if left untreated, the severe condition eventually leads to heart failure and death.

MIXED AORTIC STENOSIS AND REGURGITATION

When aortic stenosis and regurgitation are both present, the condition is referred to as a mixed lesion. It has been reported that most persons with aortic valve disease have mixed lesions. This involves both myocardial hypertrophy and dilatation, and the clinical features of both conditions may be present. Either stenosis or regurgitation usually predominates over the other hemodynamically.

▼ Infective Endocarditis

Infective endocarditis affects the lining of the heart and is caused by an invading microorganism. The causative agents include bacteria, fungi, rickettsiae, and, rarely, viruses and parasites.[1] Infective endocarditis has been described by a variety of terms, including 1) subacute bacterial endocarditis; 2) acute bacterial endocarditis; 3) prosthetic valve endocarditis; and 4) native valve endocarditis.[4] Although there is considerable overlap among the clinical pictures of endocarditis, the terms *subacute bacterial endocarditis* and *acute bacterial endocarditis* are useful in describing the clinical picture of these conditions. Table 24-1 provides a comparison of acute and subacute bacterial endocarditis.

The epidemiology of acute bacterial endocarditis and subacute bacterial endocarditis includes congenital heart disease, rheumatic fever, mitral valve prolapse, prosthetic valves, bacteremia or sepsis from other types of organisms, intravenous drug abuse, and degenerative changes in the cardiac valves. The frequency of the offending organisms is noted in Table 24-2 as related to susceptible individuals. Some precipitating factors for disease onset are contaminated needle usage in intravenous drug abusers and dental work or endoscopic procedures in persons with previously damaged cardiac valves.

The invading organism of subacute bacterial endocarditis is usually of low virulence, and the process can develop gradually over weeks or months.[4] The disease

TABLE 24-1 *Comparison of Acute and Subacute Bacterial Endocarditis*

Characteristic	Acute	Subacute
Duration of clinical symptoms	<6 weeks	>6 weeks
Most common organisms	*Staphylococcus aureus*, β-streptococci	α-Streptococci
Virulence of organism	Highly virulent	Less virulent
Condition of valves	Usually previously normal	Usually previously damaged
	Perforations common	Perforations rare

From E. Rubin & J. L. Farber. *Pathology* [2nd ed.]. Philadelphia: J.B. Lippincott, 1994.

usually affects an already damaged heart, such as one with congenital or rheumatic heart disease. The most common causative organism is the alpha-streptococcus, or *Streptococcus viridans*.

Acute bacterial endocarditis often occurs in persons with a normal heart but can affect persons with damaged hearts. Because the organism is of high virulence, the process usually progresses very rapidly and causes significant valvular damage. The most common causative organism is *Staphylococcus aureus*. The tricuspid or pul-

monary valves are affected in more than 50% of cases of acute bacterial endocarditis in intravenous drug abusers, but the aortic and mitral valves may also be affected.[4]

The organisms traveling in the bloodstream attach to the endocardial lining of a normal heart or to the defective area of an abnormal heart.[2] After attaching themselves, the organisms become enmeshed in deposits of fibrin and platelets, with vegetations occurring on the leaflets of the valves. These vegetations vary in size, shape, and color and may become quite friable depend-

TABLE 24-2 *Frequency of Various Organisms Causing Infective Endocarditis**

Organism	NVE, %	IV Drug Abusers, %	Early PVE, %	Late PVE, %
Streptococci	65	15	5	35
Viridans, alpha-hemolytic	35	5	<5	25
Streptococcus bovis (group D)	15	<5	<5	<5
S. faecalis (group D)	10	8	<5	<5
Other streptococci	<5	<5	<5	<5
Staphylococci	25	50	50	30
Coagulase-positive	23	50	20	10
Coagulase-negative	<5	<5	30	20
Gram-negative aerobic bacilli	<5	5	20	10
Fungi	<5	5	10	5
Miscellaneous bacteria	<5	5	5	5
Diphtheroids, propionibacteria	<1	<5	5	<5
Other anaerobes	<1	<1	<1	<1
Rickettsia	<1	<1	<1	<1
Chlamydia	<1	<1	<1	<1
Polymicrobial infection	<1	5	5	5
Culture-negative endocarditis	5–10	<5	<5	<5

NVE: native valve endocarditis; PVE, prosthetic valve endocarditis.
*These are representative figures collated from the literature; wide local variations in frequency are to be expected.
From R. C. Schlant and R. W. Alexander (eds.). *Hurst's The Heart* [8th ed.]. New York: McGraw-Hill, 1994.

ing on the invading organisms (see Fig. 24-3).[14] Acute bacterial endocarditis often produces large friable vegetations that embolize and produce embolic abscesses; subacute bacterial endocarditis produces smaller vegetations that also embolize and lodge in the microcirculation and spleen. The vegetations produced by the infectious process settle on the cardiac valves and invade the leaflets. These vegetations prevent normal alignment of the cusps and may, therefore, cause incomplete closure or regurgitation, leading to cardiac murmurs. The murmurs produced correspond to the affected valve. For example, with mitral insufficiency, a systolic murmur results, and with aortic insufficiency, the murmur is an early diastolic murmur.

If the vegetations grow and infiltrate the downstream side of the valve, small fragments may break off as blood is pushed through the valve orifice. These fragments, usually located on the left side of the heart, may embolize to the cerebral and systemic circulations. In addition, heart failure may ensue with severe hemodynamic alterations that occur from severe valvular regurgitation.[4]

The clinical manifestations of infective endocarditis include fever, hematuria, splenomegaly, petechiae, Osler's nodes, and anemia. Cardiac murmurs are common. The fever and its related symptomatology are dependent on the type of infection. With acute bacterial endocarditis, the fever has a rapid onset, with spikes to high elevations that are accompanied by shaking chills.[4] In subacute bacterial endocarditis, the fever is usually low grade, intermittent with elevations, and without chills. In addition, complaints of weakness, fatigue, night sweats, anorexia, and arthralgias and exhibition of splenomegaly are common. In both types of infective endocarditis, there may be Osler's nodes, which are painful, tender, red, subcutaneous nodules in the pads of the fingers; Janeway lesions, which are flat, small, irregular, nontender red spots on the palms and soles; and Roth's spots, which are retinal hemorrhages that have a white or yellow center surrounded by a red irregular halo.[3,4]

The diagnosis of infective endocarditis is based on positive blood cultures, which are present in most cases. The positive blood cultures and the cardiac valvular disruption confirm the diagnosis. In addition, a normocytic, normochromic anemia and an elevated sedimentation rate may be noted. Many cases of subacute bacterial endocarditis are probably not diagnosed at the time of infection. If acute bacterial endocarditis is not treated, the clinical course is rapid and often fatal. Treatment is aimed at identifying the causative microorganism followed by antibiotic therapy strong enough to penetrate the vegetation and reach the microorganism and kill it. The prognosis depends on the offending organism and the stage at which it is treated.[14] Table 24-3 summarizes the major clinical manifestations and diagnostic features of bacterial endocarditis.

TABLE 24-3   *Summary of the Major Clinical Manifestations of Infective Endocarditis*

Manifestation	History	Examination	Investigations
Systemic infection	Fever, chills, rigors, sweats, malaise, weakness, lethargy, delirium, headache, anorexia, weight loss, backache, arthralgia, myalgia Portal of entry: oropharynx, skin, urinary tract, drug addiction, nosocomial bacteremia	Fever, pallor, weight loss, asthenia, splenomegaly	Anemia, leukocytosis (variable), raised erythrocyte sedimentation rate, blood culture, results positive, abnormal cerebrospinal fluid
Intravascular lesion	Dyspnea, chest pain, focal weakness, stroke, abdominal pain, cold and painful extremities	Murmurs, signs of cardiac failure, petechiae (skin, eye, mucosae), Roth's spots, Osler's nodes, Janeway lesions, splinter hemorrhages, stroke, mycotic aneurysm, ischemia or infarction of viscera or extremities	Blood in urine, chest roentgenogram, echocardiography, arteriography, liver-spleen scan, lung scan, brain scan, CT scan, histology, culture of emboli
Immunologic reactions	Arthralgia, myalgia, tenosynovitis	Arthritis, signs of uremia, vascular phenomena, finger clubbing	Proteinuria, hematuria, casts, uremia, acidosis, polyclonal increases in gamma globulins, rheumatoid factor, decreased complement, immune complexes in serum, antistaphylococcal teichoic acid antibodies

CT: computed tomography.
From R. C. Schlant and R. W. Alexander (eds.). *Hurst's The Heart* [8th ed.]. New York: McGraw-Hill, 1994.

CASE STUDY 24-1

Jenny Jones is an 18-year-old white female who has been living "on the streets" with friends for the past 8 months. She is a known drug abuser who is brought into the emergency room with sudden onset of high fever, shaking chills, and complaints of difficulty breathing. Examination shows a thin-to-emaciated young woman with splenomegaly, petechiae all over the skin surfaces, and a loud systolic and diastolic murmur with a gallop rhythm. There are rales in the bases of the lungs and her pulse is 146 with a respiratory rate of 32.

1. *What is the probable diagnosis for Ms. Jones?*
2. *Describe clearly the basis on which you made the diagnosis. What definitive laboratory analysis is used to determine the diagnosis? Include risk factors and clinical manifestations in your assessment.*
3. *Outline the pathophysiology of the condition, including causative organisms and the target structure of these organisms.*
4. *Considering the clinical manifestations, what is the prognosis?*
5. *What is the appropriate treatment for this condition? What are preventative steps to avoid recurrence of this condition?*

See Appendix G for discussion.

▼ Pericarditis

The pericardium is the fibrous sac surrounding the heart that protects the heart and secretes a lubricant for cardiac movement. It also prevents dilatation of the chambers of the heart during exercise and hypervolemia and maintains the heart in a fixed position. In addition, it provides a barrier to infections from the lungs and pleural cavities.

Pericarditis is an inflammation of the pericardium that may be secondary to many conditions, including open heart surgery (the leading cause), MI, viral or bacterial infections, anticoagulants, or trauma.[15] Generalized conditions, such as uremia, systemic lupus, and rheumatoid arthritis, or malignancies, such as lung or breast cancer or lymphoma, also may involve the pericardium.[1]

ACUTE PERICARDITIS

In acute pericarditis, serous, serofibrinous, or purulent exudates form on the epicardial and pericardial surfaces.[3] The nature of the exudates depends on the underlying cause. The volume of the exudates also varies. Small volumes usually do not encroach on cardiac function, but larger volumes restrict cardiac input and produce a cardiac tamponade, which is described below.

Some of the clinical manifestations include fever, pain, pericardial friction rub, ECG changes, pericardial effusion with cardiac tamponade, and a paradoxic pulse. The pain can be described as severe, sharp, and aching. It is usually precordial or substernal, and it may radiate to the left or right shoulder, arms, and elbows. Occasionally, pain may spread to the jaw, throat, and ears. It may be intensified by deep breathing, sneezing, coughing, moving, or changing position. The pain may be relieved when the person sits up and leans forward. Acute pericarditis is often confused with the pain of myocardial ischemia, and this may lead to misdiagnosis.[1]

In addition to pain, one of the most important physical signs of pericarditis is a friction rub that is heard best at the apex and at the lower left sternal border. It is an intermittent, transitory sound that imitates the sound of sandpaper rubbing together. This loud, "to and fro," leathery sound may disappear one day and reappear the next.

Acute pericarditis can produce the following changes on the ECG: 1) ST elevation occurs in two or three standard limb leads and precordial leads V_2 through V_6; 2) reciprocal depressions occur in aVR and V_1; and 3) several days to weeks after the early stage, the ST segments return to normal and the T waves invert. Low voltage is characteristic and no Q waves develop; this helps to distinguish acute pericarditis from an acute MI.

Pericardial Effusion, Hemopericardium, and Purulent Pericarditis

Pericardial effusion may develop in cases of acute pericarditis. This is fluid that accumulates between the pericardium and myocardium. Pericardial effusion refers to a collection of noninflammatory fluids in the pericardial sac. This fluid may be serous, serosanguineous, chylous, or, rarely, of other compositions, such as cholesterol.[3] Serous effusions are seen in congestive heart failure and hypoproteinemia, such as that caused by liver failure. Serosanguineous effusions result from blunt chest trauma, especially postcardiopulmonary resuscitation. Chylous effusions contain lipid droplets, which are seen especially with conditions causing lymphatic obstruction.[3] Hemopericardium refers to accumulation of blood in the pericardial sac. Purulent pericarditis with pus or inflammatory exudate is not considered to be an effusion, but large volumes of bacterial, mycotic, or parasite-laden fluid can accumulate and produce a reddened, granular inflammatory reaction.[3] If the fluid accumulates rapidly, it can cause cardiac compression (see Figure 23-11). With pericardial effusion, the heart sounds are faint, and apical impulse may disappear. The chest film shows enlargement of the cardiac silhouette. The heart may appear as a "water bottle" configuration (Fig. 24-12). The echocardiogram detects the presence of pericardial fluid.

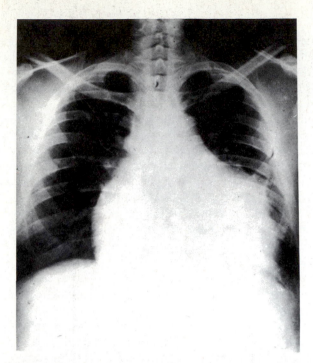

FIGURE 24-12 *Chest film of an individual with a large pericardial effusion that resulted in pericardial tamponade. (Source: Dossey, B., Guzzetta, C., and Kenner, C., Critical Care Nursing: Body, Mind, Spirit [3rd ed]. Philadelphia: J.B. Lippincott, 1992)*

CHRONIC CONSTRICTIVE PERICARDITIS

Chronic constrictive pericarditis results from the healing of acute pericarditis and formation of granular tissue that gradually contracts to form a firm scar surrounding the heart. This scar causes constriction of the heart and, therefore, interferes with filling of the ventricles. This complication is similar to the physiologic abnormality that results from cardiac tamponade, except that it develops slowly over weeks to months.

Clinical manifestations of chronic constrictive pericarditis are weakness, fatigue, weight loss, anorexia, and edema. Individuals may complain of abdominal discomfort due to systemic venous congestion. This discomfort is caused by hepatic congestion and swelling of the abdomen. A characteristic sign of constrictive pericarditis is jugular neck vein distention, which is indicative of elevated venous pressure.

The echocardiogram may show pericardial thickening and paradoxic septal motion in constrictive pericarditis. The echocardiogram also shows that the left ventricular wall moves distinctly outward in early diastole, after which there is little or no change.[15] The chest film may be diagnostic when calcification appears in the pericardium.

Cardiac Tamponade

When fluid accumulates rapidly or in an amount large enough to impair cardiac function, the condition is referred to as cardiac tamponade. The amount of fluid that can cause tamponade varies according to the rate of fluid accumulation. In rapid accumulation of fluid, 250 mL may produce significant obstruction. When an effusion develops slowly, 1,000 mL or more may accumulate before significant symptoms develop. As fluid collects in the pericardium, the pressure rises in the pericardial cavity to a level equal to the pressures in the heart during diastole. The first structures to be compressed are the right atrium and ventricle, because they have the lowest diastolic pressures. This compression causes increased venous pressure with decreased right atrial filling. Jugular venous distension and systemic venous congestion with edema and hepatomegaly result. There is also a decrease in diastolic filling of the ventricles, which leads to decreases in stroke volume and cardiac output. This can be a life-threatening complication of pericarditis, and death may result from circulatory collapse.[1]

A characteristic sign of cardiac tamponade is *pulsus paradoxus*. This is a large inspiratory reduction in arterial pressure that can be heard with a stethoscope. In pulsus paradoxus, the systolic blood pressure drops more than 10 mm Hg during inspiration. If the tamponade is severe, pulsus paradoxus may be palpated as a weakness or disappearance in the arterial pressure during inspiration.

▼ Congenital Heart Disease

Congenital cardiovascular disease is an abnormality of structure or function of the heart, circulatory system, or both. The abnormalities usually result from an alteration or failure of development of a structure within the heart. The condition causes a shunting or obstructive defect or both. A cardiovascular shunt refers to blood flow through an abnormal communication between the chambers of the heart or between the pulmonary and systemic circulations. An obstructive defect causes increased intraventricular or interatrial pressures.

The frequency of congenital cardiovascular malformations is difficult to determine, because many are asymptomatic and not diagnosed in infancy. Prolapses of the bicuspid aortic and mitral valves are common asymptomatic congenital defects. Approximately 0.9% of live births are complicated by a cardiovascular malformation.[11]

The etiology of congenital heart disease is variable and appears to result from multifactorial interactions between genetic and environmental systems. A causative factor usually cannot be identified. Some environmental insults include viral infection (especially rubella) in the first 8 weeks of pregnancy and drug and alcohol abuse. Maternal lupus erythematosus has been implicated as a major risk factor. Hereditary factors may be involved in such conditions as atrial septal defect, patent ductus arteriosus, and coarctation of the aorta. Some lesions are more prevalent in females (atrial septal defect, patent ductus arteriosus) and some in males (coarctation of the aorta, congenital aortic stenosis). Extracardiac anomalies occur in approximately 25% of infants who have significant cardiac anomalies.[6] Preterm infants often have persistence of the ductus arteriosus, a structure that normally closes at birth. Stillborn infants have a very high frequency of complex cardiac anomalies.

EMBRYOLOGY

To understand the congenital heart defects, one must understand the development of the heart. The heart develops from a straight cardiac tube, which appears in the first month of gestation. This forms a primitive atrium and ventricle, followed rapidly by a large truncus arteriosus. The tube doubles over on itself during the second month of gestation to form two parallel pumping systems, each having two chambers and a great artery (the truncus arteriosus). As a consequence of this doubling, the heart begins to situate in the left side of the chest. An *endocardial cushion* develops within the common chamber and is the first of the structures to divide the chambers of the heart. From the endocardial cushion, the mitral and tricuspid orifices develop (Fig. 24-13). The large truncus divides into the aorta and pulmonary ar-

teries. Rotation of the truncus coils the aortopulmonary septum and creates the normal spiral relationship between the aorta and pulmonary artery. The truncus arteriosus is connected to the dorsal aorta by six pairs of aortic arches that appear and disappear at different times during the formation of the heart and vessels. Abnormalities of the regression of the arch system in a number of sites can produce a wide variety of arch abnormalities. Partitioning of the heart is accomplished by septa that form actively and passively.[16] The major septa of the heart are formed between the 27th and 37th days of development.[10]

In addition to formation of heart and vessel structures, changes occur in the fetal circulation that enable the newborn to survive in the extrauterine environment. During fetal growth, the placenta performs the duties of respiration, excretion, and nourishment for the fetus. There are three essential structures: the *ductus venosus*, a vessel that connects the umbilical vein to the inferior vena cava; the *foramen ovale*, an opening in the interatrial septum; and the *ductus arteriosus*, a vessel that joins the main pulmonary artery and the distal aortic arch.

During fetal life, the blood passes from the placenta along the umbilical vein through the ductus venosus and into the inferior vena cava, where it is mixed with venous

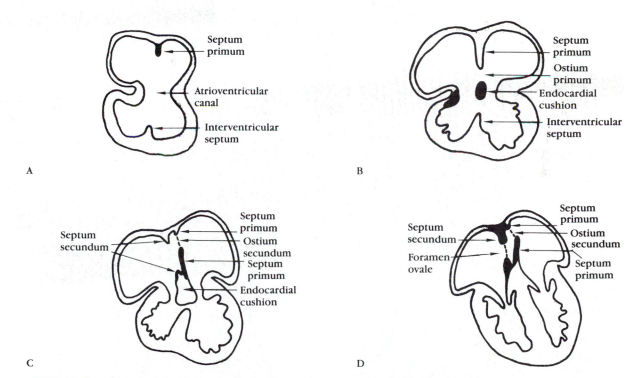

FIGURE 24-13 *Schematic illustration of the embryologic development of the atrial septum.* **A.** *Septum primum beginning to divide the fetal single atrium.* **B.** *Development of the endocardial cushion that will form a portion of the atrioventricular valves.* **C.** *Two septi, the septum primum and the osteium secundum, basically divide the atria into two chambers.* **D.** *The septum secundum forms as an incomplete structure, and the septum primum remains as a flap valve. Right-to-left flow of blood in fetal circulation keeps this foramen ovale open. When the flow of blood changes to a left-to-right shunt, the flap valve over the foramen ovale closes, anatomically dividing the chambers. (Reprinted from J. Kernicki, B. Bullock, and J. Matthews, Cardiovascular Nursing. New York: G.P. Putnam, 1971)*

return from the lower extremities. It enters the right atrium and is mainly channeled through the foramen ovale, a one-way valve, into the left atrium, where it is channeled to the rest of the body to provide oxygen and nutrients to all of the tissues. Blood flow from the head and upper extremities returns to the superior vena cava, is channeled into the right ventricle, and is pumped out of the pulmonary artery. Because of the nonfunctioning, nonexpanded lungs, the resistance to blood flow into the lungs is higher, and blood shunts through the ductus arteriosus into the descending aorta (Fig. 24-14). Because of the resistance of the lungs, the pressures in the

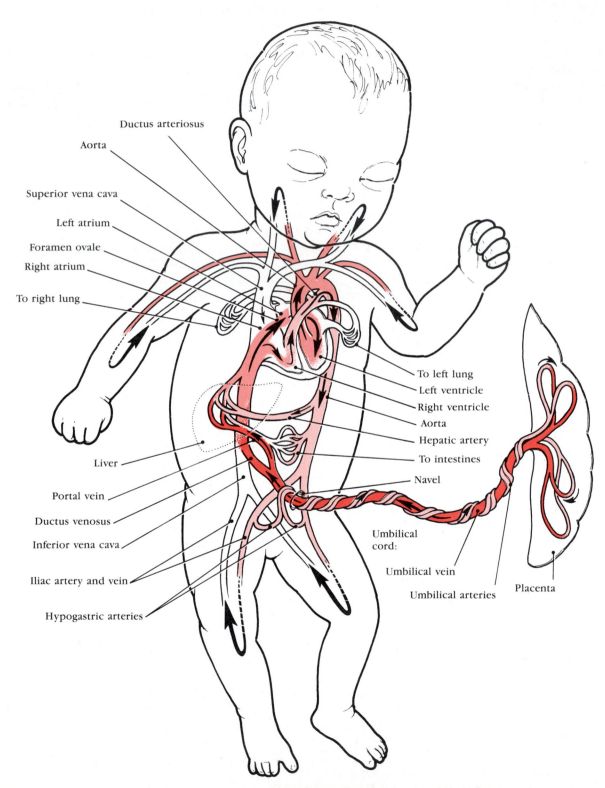

FIGURE 24-14 *Diagrammatic illustration of fetal circulation. Arrows show the direction of blood flow.*

right ventricle and those in the right atrium are elevated, causing a right-to-left shunt of blood across the foramen ovale into the left atrium.

Birth changes are as follows: the infant cries and expands its lungs, the resistance in the pulmonary circulation decreases, and the pressure lowers in the right side of the heart. With dilatation of the pulmonary vessels and lowered pulmonary arterial pressure, the flow is diminished through the ductus arteriosus, and it gradually closes, usually becoming a thin ligament-like structure within 6 to 8 weeks after birth. Clamping the umbilical cord leads to clotting of blood in the umbilical vein and ductus venosus; the latter occludes within 1 to 5 days to become a ligament also. The increased systemic resistance created with clamping of the umbilical arteries is transmitted to the left atrium. This, in conjunction with increased venous return from the lungs, causes the pressure in that chamber to exceed right atrial pressure, thus tending to create a left-to-right flow through the foramen ovale. The foramen ovale acts as a one-way valve, and the tendency toward reversal of flow causes the flap of the valve to close. Closure is followed by gradual, permanent obliteration of the opening by fibrous adherence of the flap to the interatrial septum within 6 to 8 months.

CONSEQUENCES OF CONGENITAL HEART DISEASE

Left-to-Right Shunt

Because blood flows along the path of least resistance from higher to lower pressures, most congenital defects having an abnormal communication between chambers or vessels end up with a left-to-right shunt. A portion of blood returned to the left heart is diverted back into the pulmonary circuit before it can reach the systemic capillaries. This often causes increased volume in the right heart and, subsequently, in the pulmonary circuit. Most atrial septal defects and ventricular septal defects as well as patent ductus arteriosus result in a left-to-right shunt. The result is pulmonary overloading, and eventually, pulmonary hypertension and congestion.

Pulmonary hypertension results from increased pressure in the pulmonary vascular bed, usually produced by a large left-to-right shunt. The pulmonary vasculature begins to undergo changes that eventually destroy the ability of the pulmonary arterioles to deliver blood to the pulmonary capillaries.[11] The amount of pulmonary resistance can be estimated from data obtained at cardiac catheterization. Significant pulmonary hypertension indicates permanent damage and a poor prognosis. Prevention of pulmonary overloading early in life through surgical correction or palliation must be instituted to prevent this dread complication. The systemic circulation also may become impaired if the shunt is large. The result may be right ventricular failure due to the continual volume and pressure that the right ventricle is required to pump.

Right-to-Left Shunt

This type of shunt occurs when desaturated, systemic venous blood is diverted to the left side of the heart without passing through the capillaries of the lungs. For this condition to occur, there must be a communication from the right heart to the left heart, and the pressures in the right heart must exceed those of the left. The common signs and symptoms include cyanosis, polycythemia, clubbing, squatting, and failure to thrive. When cyanosis is present, the shunt is large, with about one-third of the arterial hemoglobin being unsaturated. Polycythemia is the normal reaction of the body to the lack of oxygen. The kidneys release erythropoietin, which stimulates the release of more red blood cells. The increased numbers of red blood cells increase blood viscosity. Clubbing also occurs with long-term polycythemia and cyanosis. The ends of the phalanges become bulbous and the nails curved. The cause of clubbing may be dilatation and engorgement of the local capillaries in an attempt to gain oxygen. The child may assume a squatting position, which may be a way of centralizing the available oxygen. Failure to thrive and growth retardation may be related to tissue hypoxia and poor nutrient absorption.

Congestive Heart Failure

One child in five with any type of congenital heart defect will develop congestive heart failure.[11] It often develops early in life in the severe defects with significant shunting. In small atrial septal defects or ventricular septal defects, congestive heart failure, if seen, develops after years of pulmonary hypertension from the left-to-right shunt. In infants, congestive heart failure may be fulminant or insidious and may be associated with respiratory tract infections. It is manifested by difficulty breathing and rapid, grunting respirations.[11] Symptoms of right heart failure are less common and are usually seen in association with pulmonary hypertension or cyanosis.

PATENT DUCTUS ARTERIOSUS

When the embryonic patent ductus arteriosus (PDA) fails to close after birth, it persists as a shunt between the pulmonary artery and the aorta. It often occurs as an isolated defect and is the second most common congenital defect in infants and children.[11] The PDA often does not manifest in the early postnatal days, but within about 2 weeks the blood flow through the ductus from the aorta to the pulmonary artery first produces a systolic and then a continuous machinery-like murmur, indicating a constant flow of blood through the shunt.

The result of this condition is increased volume and pressure in the pulmonary system, basically short-circuiting one-fourth to three-fourths of left ventricular output. The signs and symptoms depend on the volume of the shunt and often are absent. The condition is usually discovered on routine physical examination when the murmur is detected. Other symptoms include pulmonary congestion and manifestations of heart failure.

ATRIAL SEPTAL DEFECTS

Congenital atrial septal defects are very common and result from failure of the atrial septum to close. There are various forms: *ostium primum, persistent atrioventricular communis*, and *ostium secundum*. Figure 24-14 shows the embryologic development of the atrial septum. Figure 24-15 shows the location of the common types of atrial septal defects.

Clinical manifestations depend on the size of the defect and the volume of shunted blood. Most atrial septal defects are asymptomatic, but right ventricular hypertrophy, frequent respiratory infections, feeding difficulties, dyspnea, fatigability, and growth retardation may develop with larger defects.

VENTRICULAR SEPTAL DEFECTS

Ventricular septal defects are considered to be the most common congenital heart lesions and account for 8% to 20% of congenital heart disease. The ventricular septum

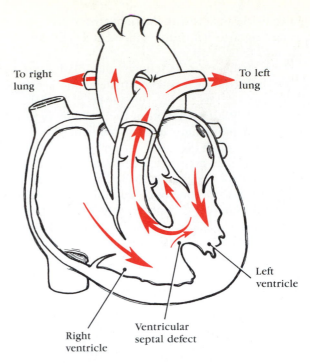

FIGURE 24-16   *Blood flow in a ventricular septal defect.*

grows in a cephalad (headward) fashion and fuses at the endocardial cushion. It begins as a muscular septum with a membranous portion at the point of closure (see Figure 24-13).[10] The shunt of blood in a ventricular septal defect is almost always left-to-right, from the high pressure in the left ventricle to the low pressure in the right ventricle (Fig. 24-16). The shunt produces a holosystolic murmur of a high grade, often creating a palpable thrill on the chest wall. In a large shunt, there is significant overloading of the right ventricle and pulmonary circulation. In the small defect, the shunt of blood is much smaller and may be occluded during part of ventricular systole by the contraction of the muscular septum.

The clinical manifestations of ventricular septal defects depend on the amount of pulmonary overloading and right ventricular strain. In some cases (as many as 30%), the defect apparently closes spontaneously, and a preexisting murmur then disappears.[1] Pulmonary hypertension and right ventricular failure are signs of poor prognosis without surgical intervention. The defect may progress to a cyanotic condition if the right ventricular pressures become high enough to reverse the shunt to right-to-left. The term *Eisenmenger's syndrome* is used to describe pulmonary hypertension that results in a reversed shunt. It accounts for about 7% of adult congenital heart disease, more commonly in women than in men.[1] It can be seen in any of the defects in which there is a reversal of shunt to a bidirectional or right-to-left shunt, but it most commonly is seen with ventricular septal defect.[1]

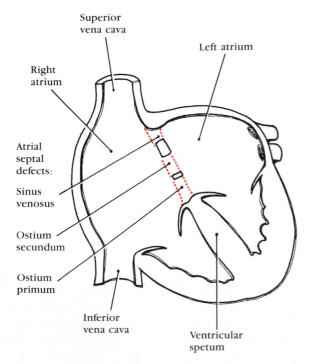

FIGURE 24-15   *Location of the common types of atrial septal defects.*

TETRALOGY OF FALLOT

This condition was first described by Fallot in 1888. It is the primary cause of cyanotic heart disease and is more common in males than in females. It involves the combination of pulmonary stenosis, ventricular septal defect, dextroposition of the aortic root, and hypertrophy of the right ventricle (Fig. 24-17). The degree of pulmonary stenosis is responsible for the volume and direction of the shunt. It increases right ventricular pressure, causing shunting of blood from the right ventricle to the left through the ventricular septal defect. Pulmonary stenosis also decreases pulmonary blood flow and the available blood for oxygenation. Direct pumping of blood to the aorta from the right ventricle causes direct access of venous blood to the systemic circulation.

Cyanosis may be severe and deepens during exertion, pulmonary infection, and dyspnea. Clubbing of the fingers also depends on the degree of cyanosis. The oxygen saturation in the arterial system may be 80% or lower, whereas venous oxygen saturation may be below 60% (normal, 75% to 80%). Polycythemia is compensatory and causes increased blood volume and elevated hematocrit levels. Cerebral anoxia may cause periods of dizziness and convulsions. Squatting is often a habitual response. Stunting of growth is characteristic when there is severe cyanosis. Complications of the condition include cerebral embolism, subacute bacterial endocarditis, and brain damage from hypoxia.

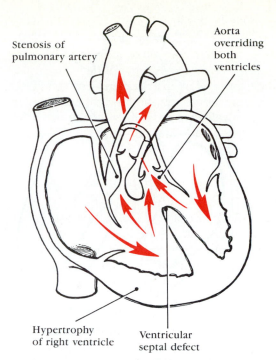

FIGURE 24-17   *Blood flow in tetralogy of Fallot.*

be severe or minimal to absent; it is intensified with exertion. Dyspnea is common, and congestive heart failure frequently occurs in early infancy. Death within the first year is common without surgical intervention.

TRANSPOSITION OF THE GREAT VESSELS

In the fourth week of gestation, the common truncus arteriosus is divided into the pulmonary artery and the aorta. The two vessels rotate so that the pulmonary artery lies anteriorly and in the right ventricle and the aorta arises posteriorly and in the left ventricle, thus providing for normal blood flow. In transposition, this rotation does not occur; the aorta arises anteriorly from the right ventricle and the pulmonary artery arises posteriorly from the left ventricle. Blood is pumped from the right ventricle through the aorta to the systemic system and returns through the cavae to the right atrium. Blood from the left ventricle passes through the pulmonary artery to the lungs and returns through the pulmonary veins to the left atrium (Fig. 24-18). These two closed circuits are obviously incompatible with life.

Other defects usually associated with this condition include atrial septal defects, ventricular septal defects, and enlarged bronchial arteries to carry blood from the aorta to the lungs. In some cases, the ductus arteriosus remains patent and the foramen ovale remains open due to the increase in right atrial pressure. The clinical manifestations depend on the amount of intermixing of blood from the associated life-sustaining defects. Cyanosis may

COARCTATION OF THE AORTA

The aortic arch develops between the fifth and seventh weeks of gestation. The area of the aorta near the ductus arteriosus may develop improperly, leaving a restricted

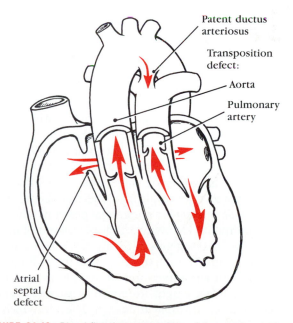

FIGURE 24-18   *Blood flow in transposition of the great vessels.*

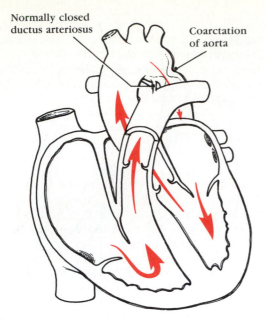

Normally closed
ductus arteriosus

Coarctation
of aorta

FIGURE 24-19 Postductal coarctation of the aorta.

lumen proximal to, at, or distal to the insertion of the ductus.[10,11] Postductal coarctation obstructs blood flow beyond the left subclavian artery, so that the blood pressure in the upper extremities is much higher than in the lower extremities (Fig. 24-19). No cyanosis is evident, because the ductus closes at birth. The symptoms result from high blood pressure and decreased circulation to the lower extremities. Headaches, dizziness, epistaxis, and intermittent claudication, coolness, or pallor in the lower extremities may be noted. Preductal or ductal coarctation usually results in persistent patency of the ductus, with blood shunting from the pulmonary artery to the aorta. The result is cyanosis of the lower extremities. In either case, congestive heart failure may result, especially after 5 years of age.[11]

OTHER DEFECTS

Less common congenital heart defects include *total anomalous pulmonary venous connection*, with the pulmonary veins connected to the right atrium; *truncus arteriosus*, in which the embryonic truncus fails to divide into the aorta and pulmonary arteries; and *endocardial cushion defect*, in which the valves and septa fail to form adequately and may result in a one-chambered heart. *Ebstein's malformation* is a congenital defect in which the basic abnormality is downward displacement of the tricuspid valve, making part of the right ventricle a part of the right atrium. This decreases output to the lungs and increases right atrial pressures. If there is an associated atrial septal defect, a right-to-left shunt causes a cyanotic clinical picture.[1] *Tricuspid atresia* is a defect in which the tricuspid valve does not form or there is no right ventri-

cle. A hypoplastic pulmonary artery may be present and a patent ductus arteriosus must be present to sustain life. The right atrium is enlarged and the left ventricle is hypertrophied. *Isolated pulmonic stenosis* is a relatively common congenital anomaly and produces symptoms when it is severe. *Bicuspid aortic valve* refers to development of the aortic valve with only two cusps. This defect is very common and usually asymptomatic. *Mitral valve prolapse*, discussed on page 481, results when the posterior leaflet of the mitral valve is abnormally large and inferiorly placed. It causes abnormal cardiac hemodynamics, which can include mitral insufficiency and various cardiac dysrhythmias. This condition is very common, especially in women, and is frequently asymptomatic.

▼ Chapter Summary

▼ Valvular disease is any abnormality of the cardiac valve that interferes with cardiac function. Valvular defects are described as stenotic or regurgitant or mixed lesions. The mitral, aortic, tricuspid, or pulmonic valves may be affected. The mitral and aortic are the most commonly diseased valves and may be damaged by rheumatic carditis or infective endocarditis or through papillary muscle defect. The valve may be genetically malformed.

▼ Acute rheumatic fever is an inflammatory disease that affects susceptible persons who are untreated after a streptococcal sore throat. The disease usually runs a relatively minor course, but repeated infections cause damage to the valves. Rheumatic heart disease is decreasing in incidence in the United States, but still is seen in significant incidence throughout the world.

▼ Mitral stenosis causes impairment of blood flow from the left atrium to the left ventricle, which increases left atrial and pulmonary pressures as the disease progresses. Clinical manifestations include weakness, fatigue, palpitations, and dyspnea. Symptoms of pulmonary congestion and right heart failure are common.

▼ Mitral insufficiency results when the valve does not close properly. Sudden onset, such as after papillary muscle rupture, causes rapid decompensation. Gradual decompensation occurs when there is a small regurgitant flow. Symptoms may be appear gradually and are often much like mitral stenosis. Atrial fibrillation is a complicating dysrhythmia of either condition.

▼ Aortic stenosis causes an obstruction to blood flow from the left ventricle to the aorta. The left ventricle hypertrophies in order to empty its contents. Systemic blood pressure may decrease, and the coronary arteries may not receive adequate blood to supply the hypertrophied cardiac muscle. The classic symptoms are chest pain, syncope, and heart failure. Sudden death is a relatively common complication.

▼ Aortic insufficiency refers to incomplete closure of

the aortic valve, in which some of the blood pumped out goes back into the left ventricle on diastole. Sudden-onset aortic insufficiency causes major alterations in the hemodynamics and onset of congestive heart failure.

▼ Endocarditis is usually caused by an invading microorganism, which may be a bacterium, fungus, rickettsiae, or, rarely, another organisms. The major classifications of endocarditis are subacute bacterial endocarditis, which often occurs on a defective valve, and acute bacterial endocarditis, which usually occurs in a healthy heart. The clinical manifestations include fever, splenomegaly, and anemia along with the production of valvular insufficiency.

▼ Pericarditis refers to an inflammation of the pericardial sac that can be seen secondary to infectious processes or due to systemic diseases. Pericardial effusion may cause restriction in cardiac function, a condition called cardiac tamponade. Pericarditis may also cause restriction of cardiac inflow due to fibrosis of the pericardium.

▼ Congenital heart disease is a defect of cardiac structure that occurs due to failure of proper development of a portion of the heart. There may be associated shunts within the heart causing a left-to-right or right-to-left shunt. Congestive heart failure is a frequent complication. The common defects are patent ductus arteriosus, atrial septal defects, ventricular septal defects, tetralogy of Fallot, transposition of the great vessels, and coarctation of the aorta. Other less common defects also can result from these developmental problems. Each defect produces its own set of hemodynamic problems.

▼ References

1. Cheitlin, M.D., Sokolow, M., and McIlroy, M.B. *Clinical Cardiology* (6th ed.). Norwalk, Conn: Appleton-Lange, 1993.
2. Cobbs, C.G., and Douglas, J.I. Approach to endocarditis, intravascular infections, pericarditis, and myocarditis. In W.N. Kelley (ed.), *Textbook of Internal Medicine* (2nd ed.). Philadelphia: J.B. Lippincott, 1992.
3. Cotran, R.S., Kumar, V., and Robbins, S.L. *Robbins' Pathologic Basis of Disease* (5th ed.). Philadelphia: W.B. Saunders, 1994.
4. Durack, D.T. Infective and noninfective endocarditis. In R.C. Schlant, R.W. Alexander, et al. (eds.), *Hurst's The Heart* (8th ed.). New York: McGraw-Hill, 1994.
5. Felner, J.M., and Martin, R.P. The echocardiogram. In R.C. Schlant, R.W. Alexander, et al. (eds.), *Hurst's The Heart* (8th ed.). New York: McGraw-Hill, 1994.
6. Fink, B.W. *Congenital Heart Disease: A Deductive Approach to Its Diagnosis* (2nd ed.). Chicago: Yearbook, 1985.
7. Franch, R.H., King, S.B., and Douglas, J.S. Techniques of cardiac catheterization including coronary arteriography. In R.C. Schlant, R.W. Alexander, et al. (eds.), *Hurst's The Heart* (8th ed.). New York: McGraw-Hill, 1994.
8. Gaash, W.H., O'Rourke, R.A., Cohn, L.H. and Rackley, C.E. Mitral valve disease. In R.C. Schlant, R.W. Alexander, et al. (eds), *Hurst's The Heart* (8th ed.) New York: McGraw-Hill, 1994.
9. Kaplan, E.L. Acute rheumatic fever. In R.C. Schlant, R.W. Alexander, et al. (eds.), *Hurst's The Heart* (8th ed.). New York: McGraw-Hill, 1994.
10. Langman, J. *Medical Embryology: Human Development—Normal and Abnormal* (2nd ed.). Baltimore: Williams & Wilkins, 1969.
11. Nugent, E.W., Plauth, W.H., Edwards, J.E., and Williams, W.H. The pathology, pathophysiology, recognition, and treatment of congenital heart disease. In R.C. Schlant, R.W. Alexander, et al. (eds.), *Hurst's The Heart* (8th ed.). New York: McGraw-Hill, 1994.
12. Rahimtoola, S.H. Valvular heart disease. In J.Stein et al. (eds.), *Internal Medicine* (4th ed.). St. Louis: C.V. Mosby, 1994.
13. Rapaport, E., Rackley, C.E., and Cohn, L.H. Aortic valvular disease. In R.C. Schlant, R.W. Alexander, et al. (eds.) *Hurst's The Heart* (8th ed.). New York: McGraw-Hill, 1994.
14. Rubin, E., and Farber J.L. *Pathology* (2nd ed.). Philadelphia: J.B. Lippincott, 1994.
15. Shabetai, R. Diseases of the pericardium. In R.C. Schlant, R.W. Alexander, et al. (eds.), *Hurst's The Heart* (8th ed.). New York: McGraw-Hill, 1994.
16. Von Mierop, L.H.S., and Kutsche, L.M. Embryology of the heart. In R.C. Schlant, R.W. Alexander, et al. (eds.). *Hurst's The Heart* (8th ed.). New York: McGraw-Hill, 1994.
17. Weiss, J.L. Valvular heart disease. In W.N. Kelley et al. (ed.), *Textbook of Internal Medicine* (2nd ed.). Philadelphia: J.B. Lippincott, 1992.

Chapter 25

Compromised Pumping Ability of the Heart

Barbara L. Bullock

▼ **CHAPTER OUTLINE**

▼ **LEARNING OBJECTIVES**

1 Differentiate between cardiac and circulatory failure.
2 Describe preload and afterload as a result of cardiac failure.
3 Discuss compensatory mechanisms of cardiac failure.
4 Describe cause and effect of dilatation of the heart chambers.
5 List the underlying factors that can precipitate heart failure.
6 Compare the pathophysiology of right and left heart failure.
7 Describe the basis for the clinical manifestations of left heart failure.
8 Describe the basis for the clinical manifestations of right heart failure.
9 Discuss radiologic changes in right and left heart failure.
10 Identify the purposes of the Swan-Ganz catheter in monitoring congestive heart failure.
11 Identify blood tests used to aid in the diagnosis of congestive heart failure.
12 Discuss pathophysiology of cardiogenic shock.
13 Identify clinical signs and symptoms of cardiogenic shock.
14 Define **primary** and **secondary cardiomyopathy**.
15 Describe congestive, restrictive, and hypertrophic cardiomyopathies.
16 Briefly discuss the clinical picture of myocarditis depending on the causative condition.

Barbara L. Bullock: PATHOPHYSIOLOGY: ADAPTATIONS AND ALTERATIONS IN FUNCTION, 4th ed.
© 1996 J.B. Lippincott-Raven Publishers

▼ Heart Failure

DEFINITIONS

Heart or *cardiac failure* refers to a constellation of signs and symptoms that result from the heart's inability to pump enough blood to meet the body's metabolic demands. The pump itself is impaired and unable to supply adequate blood to meet the cellular needs. Cardiac failure is one type of circulatory failure, a term that also includes hypoperfusion resulting from extra cardiac conditions, such as hypovolemia, peripheral vasodilatation, and inadequate oxygenation of hemoglobin. *Circulatory congestion* may result from cardiac or noncardiac causes. Cardiac causes of circulatory congestion are called *congestive heart failure* (CHF) and are described below. Noncardiac causes include conditions of increased blood volume, such as those that result from salt retention and those that primarily result from decreased peripheral resistance, such as arteriovenous fistulas and severe anemia.[14]

The clinical result of heart failure can lead to circulatory congestion, which causes circulatory overload. This is a clinical syndrome characterized by abnormal retention of sodium and water resulting from renal compensation for decreased cardiac output. Circulatory overload is enhanced by the resulting excess blood volume and increased venous return.

CAUSES OF HEART FAILURE

The causes of heart failure are varied and include intrinsic myocardial disease, malformation or injury, and secondary abnormalities (Table 25-1). Myocardial failure is often the cause of death in terminal illness of noncardiac etiology.

The causes can be further grouped into the mechanisms that produce the symptoms of heart failure. These may be classified as those that produce excessive workload for the heart; those with loss or impairment of contractile units; and those with restriction of ventricular filling.[17] Box 25-1 lists conditions that typify responses in each category.

BOX 25-1 ▼ *General Causes of Chronic Congestive Heart Failure* *

Excessive Workload

Pressure overload: Systemic hypertension, aortic stenosis, pulmonary hypertension secondary to mitral stenosis (RV)

Volume overload: mitral regurgitation, aortic regurgitation, ventricular septal defect, atrial septal defect (RV), the "high output" failures (arteriovenous fistula, anemia, thyrotoxicosis, beriberi)

Loss or Impairment of Contractile Units

Myocardial infarction (ischemic heart disease)

Congestive cardiomyopathy
  Idiopathic
  Toxic; alcohol, doxorubicin, cobalt
  Infectious: viral, trypanosomiasis

Restriction of Ventricular Filling

Hypertrophic cardiomyopathy

Restrictive cardiomyopathy: Amyloidosis, hemochromatosis

Extrinsic cardiac: Constrictive pericarditis, pericardial tamponade

Intracardiac: Mitral stenosis

RV: effect on the right ventricle.

* The diseases listed are examples that typify a class. The list is not exhaustive.

(From W. N. Kelley, *Textbook of Internal Medicine* [2nd ed.]. Philadelphia: J.B. Lippincott, 1992.)

TABLE 25-1 *Intrinsic and Secondary Causes of Heart Failure*

Intrinsic*	Secondary
Cardiomyopathy	Chronic obstructive lung disease
Myocardial infarction	Pulmonary embolism
Myocarditis	Anemia
Ischemic heart disease	Thyrotoxicosis
Congenital heart defects	Systemic hypertension
Pericarditis/cardiac tamponade	Arteriovenous shunts
Aortic/mitral valve defects	Blood volume excess
	Metabolic/respiratory acidosis
	Drug toxicity
	Cardiac dysrhythmias
	Metabolic diseases

* Intrinsic refers to myocardial, endocardial, and pericardial disease, and congenital malformations that increase ventricular volume load and ischemia or infarction of the ventricular myocardium.

PATHOPHYSIOLOGY OF HEART FAILURE

The onset of heart failure may be acute or insidious. It is often associated with systolic or diastolic overloading and with myocardial weakness. As the physiologic stress on the heart muscle reaches a critical level, the contractility of the muscle is reduced and cardiac output declines, but venous input to the ventricles remains the same or increases. The systemic responses to the decreasing cardiac output are predictable and include 1) reflex increase in sympathetic activity; 2) release of renin from the juxtaglomerular cells of the kidneys; 3) anaerobic metabolism by affected cells; and 4) increased extraction of oxygen by the peripheral cells. The responses of the heart to increased volume of blood in the ventricles are also predictable and include short-term and long-term mechanisms.

In *acute* or *short-term mechanisms*, as the end-diastolic fiber length increases, the ventricular muscle responds with dilatation and an increased force of contraction (Frank–Starling law of the heart; see pp. 444–445). In *long-term mechanisms*, ventricular hypertrophy increases the ability of the heart muscle to contract and push its volume into the circulation. The pathology of the predisposing condition determines whether heart failure is acute or insidious in onset, because compensation often occurs for long periods before the clinical manifestations of heart failure develop. An example of long-term compensation is that which results from the excessive workload of systemic hypertension (see p. 519). Because the ventricles must pump against increased pressure (increased afterload), the ventricular myocardium hypertrophies, the heart pumps with more force, and the heart rate is often elevated. These mechanisms may maintain normal cardiac output for years before the onset of failure. Symptoms of CHF signal that the pump can no longer keep up with cellular demands. Gradually, the manifestations of heart failure become apparent.

An example of acute onset of heart failure is an extensive myocardial infarction (MI), which causes direct impairment of cardiac contractility, a sudden decrease in cardiac output, and insufficient available time for the development of hypertrophy (see p. XX). The end result may be cardiogenic shock and/or pulmonary edema, which is described in detail later in this chapter.

Sympathetic Response to Heart Failure

A decrease in cardiac output results in decreased blood pressure, which causes a reflex stimulation of the sympathetic nervous system (SNS). The SNS causes an increase in the rate and force of contraction of the ventricles through the conduction system and through an increase in ventricular irritability. It also results in vasoconstriction of the arterioles throughout the body.

The SNS activity is mediated through two hormones—epinephrine and norepinephrine (see pp. 953–955). These increase the rate and force of cardiac contractions and function in systemic arteriolar vasoconstriction. Myocardial synthesis of norepinephrine is impaired, but an associated inhibition of the cardiac parasympathetic activity still produces an increased heart rate and contractility.[14] The plasma epinephrine levels become elevated, which also leads to increased heart rate.[13]

Renin-Angiotensin-Aldosterone (RAA) System

When blood pressure decreases, the decline is perceived by the renal juxtaglomerular cells, which release renin. Renin acts on angiotensinogen, a plasma protein pro-

duced by the liver, to form angiotensin I. Angiotensin I is converted to angiotensin II by an enzyme present mostly in the lungs (Fig. 25-1). Angiotensin II is a potent vasoconstrictor that constricts renal arterioles, stimulates the thirst center in the brain, and stimulates the secretion of aldosterone by the adrenal glands.[6] These actions cause vasoconstriction, which leads to increased blood pressure and expansion of the blood volume through the aldosterone effect of sodium preservation. The RAA system constantly functions to maintain fluid volume and blood pressure. The end product, angiotensin II, is rapidly destroyed by angiotensinase, a term used for a number of different blood and tissue enzymes.[6]

In persons with heart failure, this system increases cardiac preload and afterload through fluid volume retention (aldosterone effect) and vasoconstriction (angiotensin II effect). Increasing the workload on a heart that is already failing is a temporary mechanism to improve the stroke volume, but it is at the ultimate expense of the ability of the heart to compensate.

Myocardial Oxygen Needs and Oxygen Extraction from the Red Blood Cells

Myocardial oxygen needs in heart failure may be increased due to increased stress on the myocardial muscle, as with hypertension, increased heart rate, or ventricular enlargement.[11] The available oxygen and oxygen needs partially determine the ability of the heart to compensate for the problem producing the heart failure.

Oxygen extraction from the red blood cells to the tissues increases when the circulation is inadequate and perfusion is diminished. Normally, about 30% of oxygen is extracted from red blood cells by the peripheral tissue, but greater amounts can be extracted during periods of poor perfusion. Unfortunately, this mechanism is not very useful to the myocardial tissue in heart failure, because myocardial muscle normally extracts 70% to 75% of the oxygen it receives.[6]

Atrial Natriuretic Peptide or Factor (ANP or ANF)

The concentration of this substance is increased in heart failure, and its action is to promote diuresis through the suppression of aldosterone, renin, and arginine vasopressin. Atrial natriuretic peptide is made and stored in cells of the atria and is released with atrial distension. The purpose of this substance in heart failure is unclear, and the action is probably overwhelmed by the other factors that tend to promote sodium and water retention and vasoconstriction.[14]

Frank–Starling Law of the Heart

When the heart is not pumping all of its contents out, increased amounts of blood are left within the organ. This residual volume increases diastolic fiber length. The

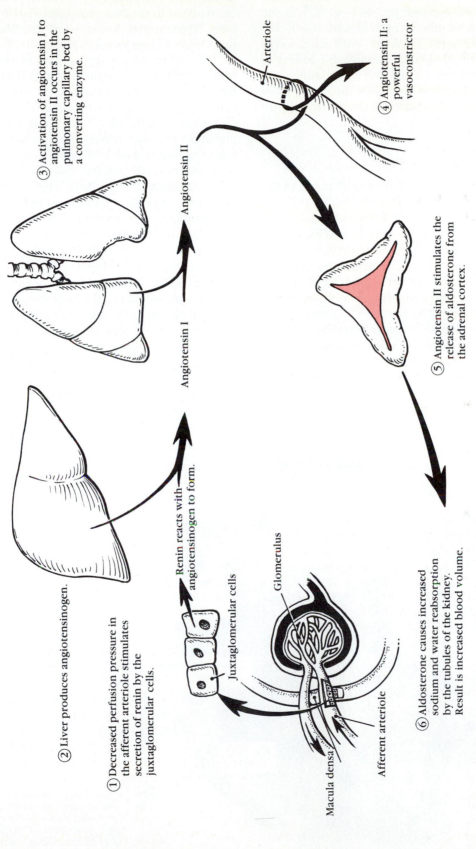

③ Activation of angiotensin I to angiotensin II occurs in the pulmonary capillary bed by a converting enzyme.

Arteriole

④ Angiotensin II: a powerful vasoconstrictor

Angiotensin II

Angiotensin I

② Liver produces angiotensinogen.

⑤ Angiotensin II stimulates the release of aldosterone from the adrenal cortex.

① Decreased perfusion pressure in the afferent arteriole stimulates the secretion of renin by the juxtaglomerular cells.

Renin reacts with angiotensinogen to form.

Glomerulus

Juxtaglomerular cells

⑥ Aldosterone causes increased sodium and water reabsorption by the tubules of the kidney. Result is increased blood volume.

Macula densa

Afferent arteriole

FIGURE 25-1 *The renin-angiotensin-aldosterone system.*

inherent compensatory mechanism is an increase in the force of recoil, so that the heart responds with increased stroke work and volume (see pp. 444–445).[17] In the failing heart, diastolic fiber length is continually increased, causing the heart to enlarge. With activation of the RAA system, blood volume is increased, adding to this diastolic preload (see Figure 25-1). The chronically dilated ventricle become less able to use the Frank–Starling mechanism to compensate for the increased preload.[14]

Hypertrophy of the Myocardium

When increased stress is placed on any chamber of the heart, hypertrophy can result. This physiologic myocardial response is caused by chronically increased workload. The individual myocardial muscle cells increase in size but not in number. Hypertrophy probably results when the wall tension of the chamber must continuously increase on systole to eject the contents of the chamber. Ventricular hypertrophy is more common than atrial hypertrophy and provides for compensatory adaptation to a chronically increased workload.

Hypertrophy may be classified as *concentric* or *eccentric*. Concentric hypertrophy reveals a thickened ventricular wall without apparent enlargement of the heart.[14] This often occurs with aortic stenosis and sometimes with systemic hypertension. Eccentric hypertrophy exhibits a proportionate increase in the wall size and diameter of the ventricle.[4, 14] This type of hypertrophy often occurs in conditions associated with increased preload. Hypertrophy maintains or increases contractility until heart failure ensues (Fig. 25-2).

The stimulus for myocardial hypertrophy is unknown, but it is thought that increased systolic wall tension with increased afterload causes synthesis of sarcomeres parallel to existing sarcomeres in the case of concentric hypertrophy.[14] The compensatory hypertrophy in persons with chronic pressure or volume overload can bring the systolic wall tension (pressure) to normal or above normal, but the diastolic wall tension may remain abnormal when there is volume overload.[14] Hypertrophy, especially concentric hypertrophy, reduces the compliance of the ventricle, so that elastic recoil and relaxation may be impaired. In eccentric hypertrophy, there is myocyte elongation that leads to a spherical shape of the heart.[14, 17] Figure 25-3 shows the changes in left ventricular configuration depending on the basic mechanism producing the hypertrophy. In a standard chest radiograph, these changes may be noted and become more pronounced with progression of heart failure.

Hypertrophy increases the myocardial requirement for oxygen. This is supplied by the coronary arteries, and energy is produced by an increasing number of mitochondria, which proliferate early in the process of developing hypertrophy.[17] As long as the oxygen supply

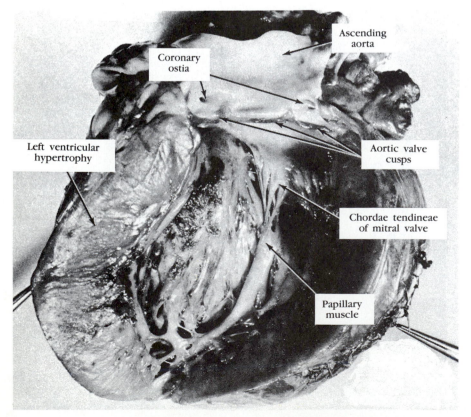

FIGURE 25-2 *Marked thickening of the left ventricular myocardium showing a normal aorta and medial leaflet of the mitral valve. (Reprinted from J. Kernick, B. Bullock, and J. Matthews. Cardiovascular nursing. New York: G.P. Putnam, 1971.)*

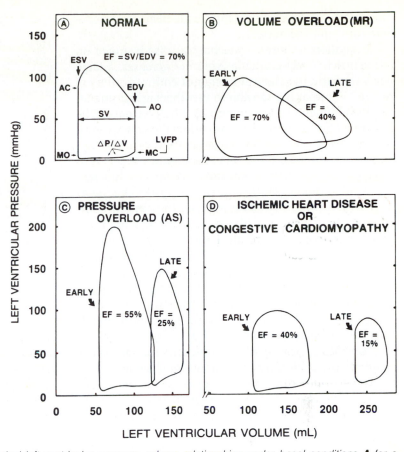

FIGURE 25-3 *Typical left ventricular pressure–volume relationships under basal conditions* **A** *for a normal person and* **B** *for patients with compensated (early) and decompensated (late) congestive heart failure (CHF) due to left ventricular volume overload (mitral regurgitation),* **C** *pressure overload (aortic stenosis [AS]), and* **D** *ischemic heart disease after myocardial infarction or idiopathic congestive cardiomyopathy. The loops progress counterclockwise as they trace the phases of the cardiac cycle. In panel A, normal ventricular systolic ejection occurs from aortic opening (AO) to aortic closure (AC), whereas diastolic filling begins at mitral opening (MO) and terminates just before mitral closure (MC). The stroke volume (SV) for compensated CHF is normal (70 mL), and for decompensated CHF, it is reduced (40 mL), but the forward SV is similar to that in the other CHF examples (70 and 40 mL). The remaining SV is ejected into the left atrium. Left ventricular filling pressure (LVFP) occurs at mitral valve closure and in the examples shown is 18 mm Hg for compensated and 35 mm Hg for decompensated CHF. The upper limit of normal is 12 mm Hg. If heart rate (HR) is normal for compensated CHF (75 beats/ minute) and comparably elevated for each example of decompensated CHF (95 beats/minute), then cardiac output (HR × forward SV) is normal in compensated and equivalently depressed in decompensated CHF. However, there are marked differences between the six CHF examples with respect to the ejection (EF), the percentage of end-diastolic volume ejected during systole, and the chamber volumes at end-systole (ESV) and end-diastole (EDV). This is due to the particular pattern of cardiac compensatory mechanism (hypertrophy and dilatation) activated by each of the examples of CHF depicted in panels B, C, and D. Diastolic stiffness can be estimated from the ratio of changes in pressure to the change in volume (P/V) at different points during diastole. (Source: W.N. Kelley, Textbook of Internal Medicine [2nd ed.] Philadelphia: J.B. Lippincott, 1992).*

from the coronary arteries and the mitochondrial production of adenosine triphosphate keep up with the enlarging muscle, the ventricle will pump efficiently. When an imbalance between oxygen supply and demand occurs, ischemia and cardiac dysfunction result.

Dilatation of the Heart

Dilatation refers to enlargement of cardiac chambers. It often occurs because of increased volume of blood that enters the heart. The ventricles are always dilated in acute CHF. Dilatation often coincides with hypertrophy, especially if the stressful event causing the failure is chronic, such as chronic systemic hypertension.

Radiographic enlargement of the cardiac shadow characterizes heart failure. In the normal heart, increased input to the ventricle results in increased ventricular force of contraction, but no permanent enlargement occurs. As the cardiac reserve fails, the ventricle is unable to pump out all of its contents and thus enlarges.

The cardiac reserve is the ability of the heart to increase its output under stress.

Dilatation imposes a mechanical disadvantage on the ventricles. As ventricular volume increases, a large portion of the mechanical energy of contraction is expended in imparting tension to the fibers and a smaller portion for fiber recoil or shortening. This concept can be illustrated by comparison of the contractile power of two left ventricles. If one ventricle had twice the diameter of another, it would take four times the contractile power to produce the same systolic pressure in the larger ventricle.[14]

A heart that is greatly dilated also works at a metabolic disadvantage, because its need for oxygen is increased. More blood to the myocardium is required, which may not be supplied by the coronary arteries.

Dilatation is characteristic of cardiomyopathy, in which separation of the trabeculae carneae may occur together with fibrosis of the myocardium. Usually, the greater the dilatation, the more ineffective the cardiac contraction. Ineffective left ventricular contraction is called *hypokinesis of the left ventricle.*

In persons with valvular insufficiency, septal defects, or other abnormal communications, the diastolic inflow to one or both ventricles is permanently augmented. In such conditions, dilatation of cardiac chambers occurs to maintain normal or near-normal circulation even if a defect is quite large.

Summary of Compensatory Mechanisms

The compensatory mechanisms described above may preserve the life of the individual, but they usually aggravate the underlying condition.

Sympathetic regulation tends to preserve circulation to the brain and heart but increases the cardiac workload by increasing the afterload, which may depress the effectiveness of cardiac contraction. Activation of the RAA system also increases afterload because of the peripheral vasoconstriction produced. The aldosterone effect increases blood volume and thus increases preload. Increased oxygen consumption needs may not be provided by improved cardiac output. The Frank–Starling effect increases the energy requirements of the myocardium. Hypertrophy increases the oxygen need of each myocardial muscle cell, which is problematic if the blood flow is reduced from coronary artery disease.

The *cardiac reserve* is accomplished by increasing the stroke volume and heart rate. The normal heart can increase its output four to five times that of normal under conditions of stress. As heart failure ensues, the reserve falls, so that the individual may first have symptoms of heart failure when experiencing significant stress. Later in the course of the disease, symptoms develop when only minor stress is encountered. Heart failure manifestations at rest indicate that there is no cardiac reserve for any stressful situation at all.

CLASSIFICATION OF HEART FAILURE

Heart failure has been classified as left-sided and right-sided on the basis of clinical manifestations. It has further been divided into forward and backward effects to explain its low-output and venous congestion components. In some cases, the forward or low-output syndrome dominates, whereas in others, the congestive phenomenon is the major manifestation. In reality, both features are present in heart failure, just as both left- and right-sided effects necessarily must be present. Biventricular failure refers to failure of both ventricles. Usually, right heart failure (RHF) follows left heart failure (LHF). This discussion divides LHF and RHF into separate entities. However, the reader must keep in mind that the heart and lungs are interconnected; what affects one side of the heart eventually affects the other (Fig. 25-4).

LEFT HEART FAILURE

Left heart failure occurs when the output of the left ventricle is less than the total volume of blood received from the right side of the heart through the pulmonary circulation. As a result, the pulmonary circuit becomes congested with blood that cannot be moved forward, and the systemic blood pressure falls.

Causes

The most common cause of predominantly left ventricular failure is MI. Other causes include systemic hypertension, aortic stenosis or insufficiency, and cardiomyopathy. Mitral stenosis and mitral insufficiency also cause the symptoms of LHF. Flowchart 25-1 illustrates the different causes of left-sided congestive failure and how they produce the condition.

Pathophysiology

Because the left ventricle cannot pump out all of its blood, blood dams back to the left atrium into the four pulmonary veins and the pulmonary capillary bed. As the volume of blood in the lungs increases, the pulmonary vessels enlarge. The pressure of blood in the pulmonary capillary bed increases. When it reaches a certain critical point (approximately 25–28 mm Hg), fluid passes across the pulmonary capillary membrane into the interstitial spaces around the alveoli and finally into the alveoli (Flowchart 25-2). Actual alveolar pulmonary edema occurs when the rate of fluid transudation exceeds the ability of the plentiful lymphatic drainage to remove it from the interstitial spaces.[14] Acute pulmonary edema results as the alveoli fill with fluid; this impairs gas exchange, which can be life-threatening. Higher pulmonary capillary bed pressures may cause microhemorrhages in the sacs or rust-colored sputum due to the

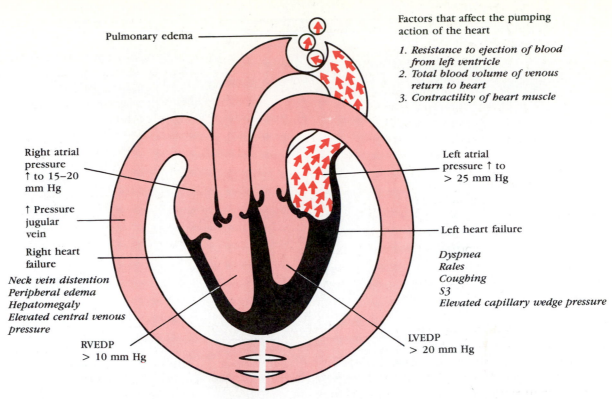

Pulmonary edema

Factors that affect the pumping action of the heart

1. Resistance to ejection of blood from left ventricle
2. Total blood volume of venous return to heart
3. Contractility of heart muscle

Right atrial pressure ↑ to 15–20 mm Hg

↑ Pressure jugular vein

Right heart failure

Neck vein distention
Peripheral edema
Hepatomegaly
Elevated central venous pressure

RVEDP > 10 mm Hg

Left atrial pressure ↑ to > 25 mm Hg

Left heart failure

Dyspnea
Rales
Coughing
S3
Elevated capillary wedge pressure

LVEDP > 20 mm Hg

FIGURE 25-4 *Biventricular failure usually results when left ventricular failure occurs, with elevated pulmonary pressures and subsequent elevation of the right-sided pressures leading to right-sided failure. (Adapted from Dossey, B., Guzzetta, C., Kenner, C., Critical Care Nursing: Body, Mind, Spirit [3rd ed.] Philadelphia: J.B. Lippincott, 1992)*

presence of hemosiderin-laden alveolar macrophages.[4] The presence of large amounts of these hemosiderin-laden macrophages (heart failure cells) is often indicative of long-standing cases of pulmonary congestion, as with mitral stenosis.[4]

These phenomena just described are the congestive phenomena of LHF that result from the volume overload of the left ventricle. They are also called the *backward effects of LHF*.

The left ventricle also cannot pump its normal stroke volume out to the aorta. Thus, the systemic blood pressure decreases. This decrease is sensed by the baroreceptors that cause a reflex stimulation of the SNS. The result of SNS stimulation is increased heart rate and peripheral vasoconstriction. The RAA system is stimulated, leading to further vasoconstriction, together with sodium and water retention (see Flowchart 25-2).

The phenomena described above result from the inherent compensatory mechanisms of the body to preserve blood volume and pressure, even at the expense of organs and tissues. The vasoconstriction helps to centralize blood volume while the aldosterone mechanism increases blood volume through sodium retention. These are the main manifestations of the *forward effects of LHF*.

Chronic LHF often occurs in mitral valve disease, and it may occur progressively in cardiomyopathy and

post-MI. In the last two conditions, pulmonary congestion may be evidenced, but acute pulmonary edema does not occur unless additional stress increases the cardiac demand. Individuals with mitral stenosis, for example, have been shown to have pulmonic pressures greater than 30 mm Hg without symptoms of acute pulmonary edema. This is mainly due to increased lymphatic absorption of interstitial pulmonary fluid, as previously described. In conditions of sudden onset, however, this level would cause acute pulmonary congestion.

Signs and Symptoms

In the early stages of LHF, *dyspnea* is exhibited when the cardiac reserve is exceeded. As fluid begins to accumulate in the pulmonary capillary bed, the formation of interstitial edema causes a defect in oxygenation.[12] The oxygen saturation of blood decreases, causing the chemoreceptors to stimulate the respiratory center. The respiratory rate increases at first during exercise and later even at rest. Shortness of breath on exertion (dyspnea on exertion) is a common and relatively early symptom. The person may complain of breathlessness when walking or after eating a heavy meal.

Because of decreased cardiac output and decreased oxygen saturation of the blood, hypoxia of the body

Flowchart 25-1   Left-Sided Congestive Heart Failure

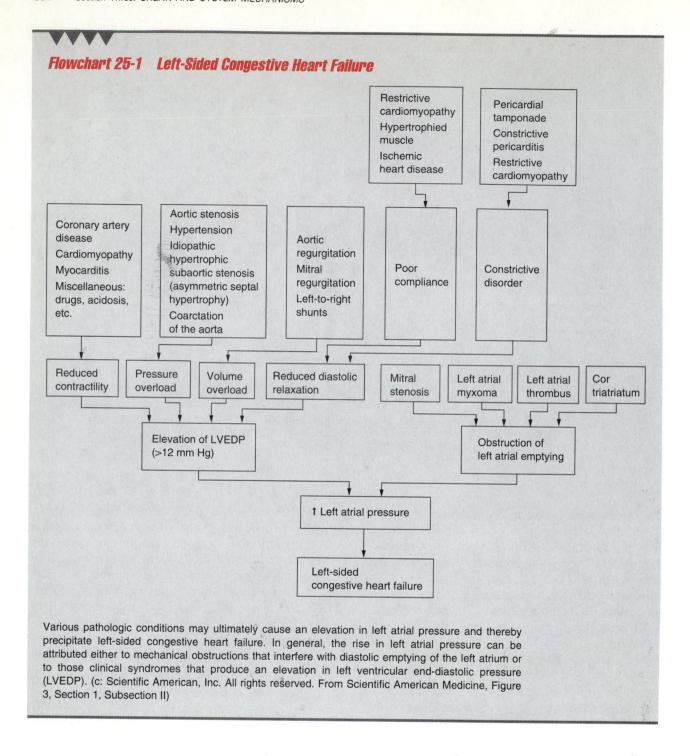

Various pathologic conditions may ultimately cause an elevation in left atrial pressure and thereby precipitate left-sided congestive heart failure. In general, the rise in left atrial pressure can be attributed either to mechanical obstructions that interfere with diastolic emptying of the left atrium or to those clinical syndromes that produce an elevation in left ventricular end-diastolic pressure (LVEDP). (c: Scientific American, Inc. All rights reserved. From Scientific American Medicine, Figure 3, Section 1, Subsection II)

tissues occurs, which results in easy fatigue, weakness, and dizziness. Dizziness is the result of hypoxia to the brain. As failure and hypoxia worsen, disorientation, confusion, and ultimately unconsciousness can occur. Loss of potassium induced by increased levels of aldosterone also causes muscle weakness. Aldosterone conserves sodium at the expense of potassium and is often called potassium-wasting hormone.

Inability to breathe in a supine position is called *orthopnea.* In chronic LHF, interstitial and alveolar pulmonary edema may be present all of the time; the up-

right position is assumed so that fluid gravitates to the bases of the lungs, making breathing easier.

Auscultation of the heart reveals an S_3 gallop and a paradoxical split of the second sound on expiration. A *pulsus alternans,* characterized by alternating weaker and stronger pulsations in the peripheral arteries, often occurs and indicates a poorly functioning ventricle.

Paroxysmal nocturnal dyspnea refers to the onset of acute episodes of dyspnea at night. The cause of this condition is unknown, but it is thought to result from improved cardiac performance at night during recum-

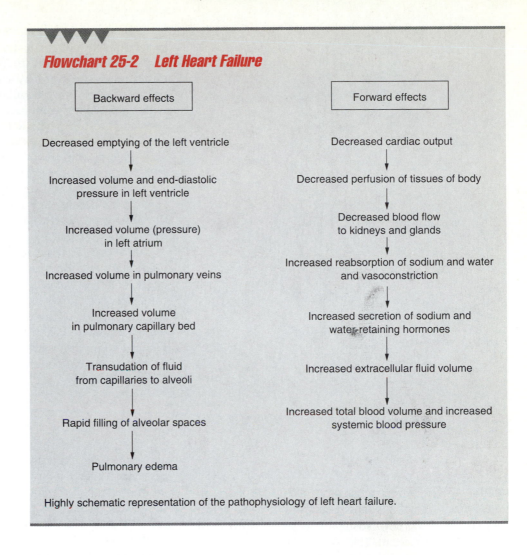

Flowchart 25-2   Left Heart Failure

Backward effects	Forward effects

Backward effects

Decreased emptying of the left ventricle

↓

Increased volume and end-diastolic pressure in left ventricle

↓

Increased volume (pressure) in left atrium

↓

Increased volume in pulmonary veins

↓

Increased volume in pulmonary capillary bed

↓

Transudation of fluid from capillaries to alveoli

↓

Rapid filling of alveolar spaces

↓

Pulmonary edema

Forward effects

Decreased cardiac output

↓

Decreased perfusion of tissues of body

↓

Decreased blood flow to kidneys and glands

↓

Increased reabsorption of sodium and water and vasoconstriction

↓

Increased secretion of sodium and water-retaining hormones

↓

Increased extracellular fluid volume

↓

Increased total blood volume and increased systemic blood pressure

Highly schematic representation of the pathophysiology of left heart failure.

bence. This causes increased reabsorption of fluid that has accumulated in the lower half of the body into the systemic veins, where it is returned to the heart. The increased fluid returns to and overloads the left ventricle, causing acute pulmonary congestion until the individual assumes the orthopneic position. Acute breathlessness and a feeling of smothering are described (Fig. 25-5).[12] This particular breathing difficulty is considered to be a specific symptom of LHF.[6]

Cardiac asthma is a term that has been used to describe wheezing due to bronchospasm induced by heart failure. The bronchioles may react to the increased fluid in the alveoli, constrict, and produce the characteristic wheezing.[3]

Pulmonary edema is an acute, life-threatening condition that most frequently results from LHF but may also result from abnormal permeability of the alveolo-capillary membrane. Signs and symptoms of acute pulmonary edema include dyspnea of sudden onset, basal rales, gasping respirations, extreme anxiety, rapid weak pulse, increased venous pressure, and decreased urinary output. The skin is cool and moist to the touch, ashen-gray, or cyanotic. A cough accompanied by expectoration of frothy white, pink-tinged, or bloody sputum may be present. Most attacks gradually subside in 1 to 3 hours, usually with treatment, but they may progress rapidly to shock and death.[3]

RIGHT HEART FAILURE

Right heart failure occurs when the output of the right ventricle is less than the input from the systemic venous circuit. As a result, the systemic venous circuit is congested, and output to the lungs decreases.

Causes

The major cause of RHF is LHF; the right ventricle fails because of the excessive pulmonary pressures generated by failure of the left heart. Other causes include chronic obstructive lung disease, pulmonary embolus, right ventricular infarction, and congenital heart defects, especially those that involve pulmonary overloading and pulmonary hypertension. Flowchart 25-3 illustrates the pathways that can lead to RHF. Right heart failure that results from lung disease is called *cor pulmonale.*

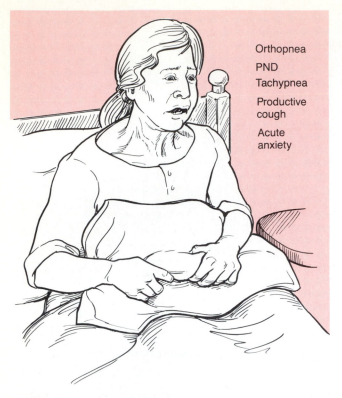

Orthopnea

PND

Tachypnea

Productive cough

Acute anxiety

FIGURE 25-5 *Pulmonary signs and symptoms of left heart failure.*

Pathophysiology

In RHF, the right ventricle cannot pump all of its contents forward, so blood dams back from the right ventricle to the right atrium, causing increased pressure in the systemic venous circuit. The increased volume and pressure are transmitted to distensible organs, such as the liver and spleen. Increased pressure in the peritoneal vessels leads to transudation of fluid into the peritoneal cavity. Increased pressure at the capillary line causes fluid to move into the interstitial space, and systemic peripheral edema results (Flowchart 25-4). The cardinal signs of RHF are jugular venous distension, hepatomegaly, splenomegaly, and peripheral, dependent edema. These are considered the *backward* or *congestive* effects of RHF.

The right ventricle also cannot maintain its output to the lungs. This results in decreased pulmonary circulation and decreased return to the left side of the heart. These *forward effects of RHF* cause all of the forward effects of LHF (see Flowchart 25-2).

Signs and Symptoms

The signs and symptoms of RHF reflect both forward and backward effects. Dependent, pitting edema is characteristic and may be noted in the sternum or sacrum of a bedridden person as well as in the feet and legs of a person in the sitting position.

Enlargement of the spleen and liver can cause pressure on surrounding organs, respiratory impingement, and organ dysfunction. Inadequate deactivation of aldosterone by the liver may lead to additional fluid retention. Jaundice and coagulation problems may result with severe, long-standing, decompensated RHF. Ascites also occurs when RHF is severe and may cause restriction of respiratory excursion and abdominal pressure. Pleural effusions also may appear due to the increased capillary pressure.

Jugular venous distension occurs and can be measured at the bedside. It is measured in centimeters when the head is elevated to a 30-degree, 45-degree, or 90-degree angle (Fig. 25-6).

With pure RHF (that not precipitated by LHF), the pulmonary symptoms are minimal to absent, whereas engorgement of the venous and portal systems is significant.[4] The peripheral edema may be massive and gradually affect most of the tissues of the body, a condition termed *anasarca*. When RHF is caused by lung disease, the underlying lung problem will present its symptoms as well as the cardiac dysfunction.

BIVENTRICULAR CONGESTIVE HEART FAILURE

As stated previously, CHF usually affects both the left and right sides. Because the right and left sides of the heart are connected by a vascular circuit, there is no way for one side to pump more blood than the other for any significant period of time without affecting the other side.[14] The clinical picture almost always shows components of both LHF and RHF. The manifestations may be more low output or congestive, but they affect almost all of the organs and tissues of the body. Table 25-2 summarizes the clinical abnormalities of CHF.

DIAGNOSIS OF CONGESTIVE HEART FAILURE

Radiologic Changes

Radiologic evidence of pulmonary congestion usually precedes the development of audible rales in LHF. Cardiac enlargement is noted by an increased size of the left ventricular shadow. The left ventricle extends past the midclavicular line, and fluid effusion may be present throughout the lung fields (Fig. 25-7). In RHF, the right ventricular shadow can be seen extending out from the right sternal border. Pulmonary markings may be decreased due to decreased pulmonary circulation (Fig. 25-8).

Hemodynamic Monitoring

The balloon-tipped flow-directed catheter (Swan-Ganz) is an effective monitoring system for assessing pulmo-

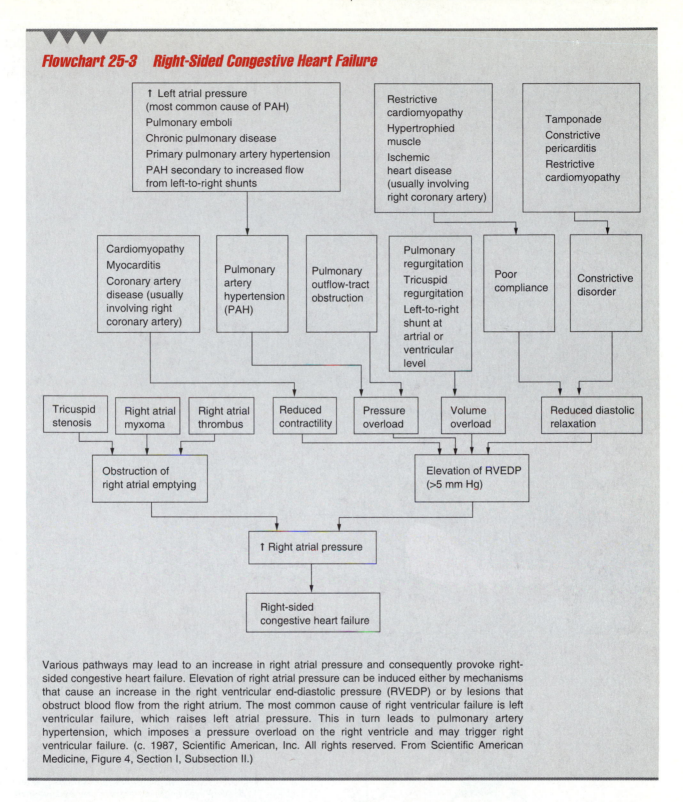

Flowchart 25-3   Right-Sided Congestive Heart Failure

Various pathways may lead to an increase in right atrial pressure and consequently provoke right-sided congestive heart failure. Elevation of right atrial pressure can be induced either by mechanisms that cause an increase in the right ventricular end-diastolic pressure (RVEDP) or by lesions that obstruct blood flow from the right atrium. The most common cause of right ventricular failure is left ventricular failure, which raises left atrial pressure. This in turn leads to pulmonary artery hypertension, which imposes a pressure overload on the right ventricle and may trigger right ventricular failure. (c. 1987, Scientific American, Inc. All rights reserved. From Scientific American Medicine, Figure 4, Section I, Subsection II.)

nary and systemic circulations. The Swan-Ganz catheter is threaded into the pulmonary artery, where it finally halts in a vessel slightly smaller than the inflated balloon tip, blocking the flow of blood from the right ventricle.[16] A pressure reading at this time reflects the diastolic pressures of the left ventricle if there is no concomitant mitral valve disease. This pulmonary artery wedge pressure reflects its pressures because of the continuous circuit to the left heart. Thus, pressure measurements reflect the left ventricular end-diastolic pressure (Fig. 25-9).

The end-diastolic volume, normally 70 mL per m² of body surface, is elevated in the failing heart. Because an increase in end-diastolic volume is often associated with an increase in end-diastolic pressure, the end-diastolic

Flowchart 25-4   Right Heart Failure

Backward effects	Forward effects
Decreased emptying of the right ventricle	Decreased volume from the right ventricle to the lungs
↓	↓
Increased volume and end-diastolic pressure in the right ventricle	Decreased return to left atrium and subsequent decreased cardiac output
↓	↓
Increased volume (pressure) in right atrium	All the forward effects of left heart failure
↓	↓
Increased volume and pressure in the great veins	Expansion of blood volume and vasoconstriction
↓	
Increased volume in the systemic venous circulation	
↓	
Increased volume in distensible organs (hepatomegaly, splenomegaly)	
↓	
Increased pressure at capillary line	

Highly schematic illustration of the pathophysiology of right heart failure.

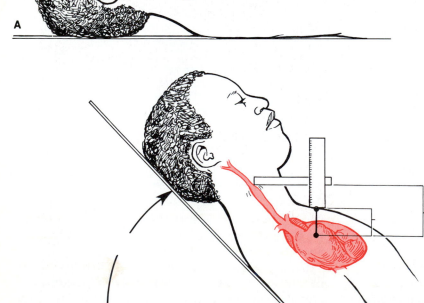

FIGURE 25-6 *Measuring jugular venous pressure.* ***A.*** *Neck veins are normally distended when the person is supine.* ***B.*** *Place the person at a 45-degree angle, so that the sternal angle is approximately 5 cm above the right atrium. Place a ruler on the sternal angle and measure the distance in centimeters from the sternal angle to the horizontal level of the highest visible pulse of the distended neck vein. The value obtained by this measurement plus 5 cm (distance from sternal angle to right atrium) provides an approximate measure of central venous pressure.*

TABLE 25-2 *Clinical Abnormalities in Congestive Heart Failure*

Abnormality	Organ/Tissue	Symptoms and Signs
Low output (reduced regional blood flows)	Kidneys	Salt and water retention; azotemia; hyponatremia; impaired drug excretion
	Skeletal muscle	Fatigue; tiredness; decreased aerobic capacity; lactic acidemia; tachypnea from somatic afferent nerve stimulation
	Skin	Cold, pale, cyanotic, sweaty extremities; impaired heat loss
	Brain	Sleep reversal; Cheyne-Stokes respiration; reduced central ventilatory drive; confusion; stupor (late)
	Gut	Early satiety; postprandial discomfort
	Liver	Centrilobular necrosis (rare)
Congestion (increased pulmonary and systemic venous pressures)	Lungs	Shortness of breath (dyspnea) on exertion, when recumbent (orthopnea), awakening the patient from sleep (paroxysmal nocturnal dyspnea); pulmonary edema; tachypnea; rales, pleural effusions; redistribution of blood flow from base to apex of lungs; ventilation-perfusion mismatch; hypoxemia
	Jugular veins	Distension; prominent V waves
	Skin	Dependent pitting edema
	Liver	Enlargement; tenderness; ascites; reduced drug metabolism; splenomegaly (late)
	Kidney	Proteinuria; hypoalbuminemia
	Gut	Ascites; poor absorption; anorexia; protein and lymphocyte loss; constant fullness
	Skeletal muscle	Fatigue

Source: W. N. Kelley, Textbook of Internal Medicine (2nd ed.). Philadelphia: J.B. Lippincott, 1992.

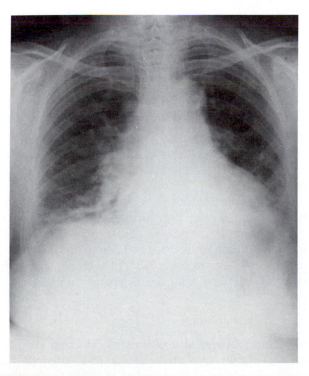

FIGURE 25-7 *Radiologic changes in left heart failure. Note left ventricular enlargement and fluid effusion in lung fields.*

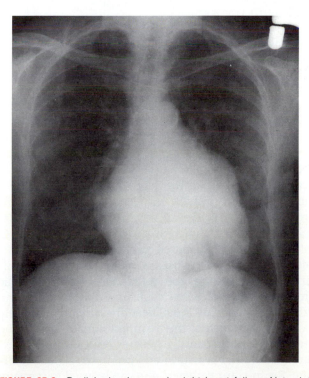

FIGURE 25-8 *Radiologic changes in right heart failure. Note right ventricular shadow extending from the right sternal border.*

A. Catheter advanced to right atrium, balloon is inflated. Pressure is low, usually 2–5 mm Hg.

B. Catheter is floated to right ventricle with the balloon inflated. Wave-forms indicate a systolic pressure of 25–30 mm Hg and a diastolic pressure of 0–5 mm Hg.

C. As the catheter moves into the pulmonary artery, the systolic pressure remains the same but the diastolic pressure elevates to 10–15 mm Hg.

D. The balloon is deflated and the catheter is moved until it can be wedged in a smaller vessel. When the balloon is inflated, the pressure recorded is that pressure in front of the catheter. It is an approximate measure of the left ventricular end diastolic pressure.

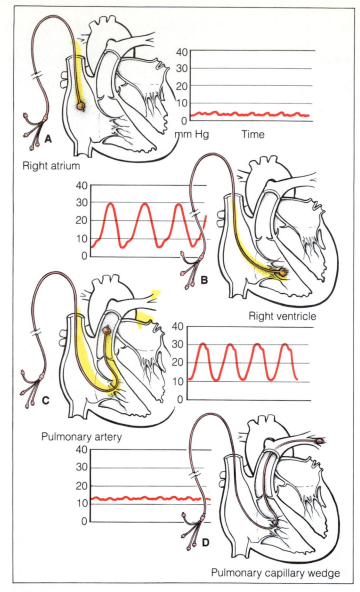

FIGURE 25-9 Insertion of a flow-directed cardiac catheter.

pressure can be used as an indicator of ventricular function. The end-diastolic pressure of the left ventricle is usually 12 mm Hg or less and in the right ventricle 5 mm Hg or less. A high left ventricular end-diastolic pressure can be the result of increased left ventricular volume or reduced left ventricular compliance or both. In the absence of increased pulmonary vascular resistance and mitral valve disease, mean pulmonary capillary wedge pressure and pulmonary artery diastolic pressure reflect left ventricular end-diastolic pressure. When the balloon tip is deflated, the catheter tip usually locates in a branch of the main pulmonary artery. The Swan-Ganz catheter also measures central venous pressure (right atrial pressure) and pulmonary artery pressure. Swan-Ganz catheters also can be used to measure cardiac output by the thermodilution method, in which

a computer analyzes a temperature differential between two points on the catheter. The normal cardiac output is approximately 4 to 8 liters per minute. The level of decreased cardiac output in persons with CHF helps to determine the necessary treatment. Levels of 2.2 to 3.0 liters per minute or below may indicate cardiogenic shock, depending on the size and age of the individual.

Table 25-3 lists normal values of hemodynamic data that can be derived from hemodynamic monitoring.

Arterial Blood Gases

The normal arterial and venous blood gases are presented in Table 25-4. Hypoxemia (decreased partial pressure of oxygen or Po2) is often the only change that is noted with CHF. Oxygen saturation often remains

TABLE 25-3   Normal Values of Hemodynamic Data

Hemodynamic Data	Normal Values
Right atrial pressure (RAP) or central venous pressure (CVP)	1–5 mm Hg
Pulmonary artery pressure (PAP)	17–32 mm Hg systolic
	4–13 mm Hg diastolic
	9–19 mm Hg mean
Left ventricular end-diastolic (LVEDP) pressure or pulmonary capillary wedge pressure (PCWP)	5–12 mm Hg
Cardiac output (CO)	
Heart rate × stroke volume	4–8 L/min
Cardiac index (CI)	
CO ÷ body surface area (square meters)	2.8–4.2 L/min/m²
Arterial blood pressure	100–140 systolic
	60–80 diastolic
Mean arterial pressure	
Diastolic + ⅓ pulse pressure	70–100
Systemic vascular resistance (SVR) or peripheral vascular resistance (PVR)	1100–1400 dyne/sec/HRU

normal until decompensation is severe. The partial pressure of carbon dioxide (P_{CO_2}) may be low due to hyperventilation. In end-stage CHF, the P_{CO_2} may be elevated. Table 25-4 also shows the comparison of the values between arterial and venous blood. Note that the venous pH is normally somewhat more acidic than arterial blood, the oxygen saturation is 20% to 25% less, and the carbon dioxide level is higher. Arterial blood gases are discussed in detail in Chapter 28.

TABLE 25-4   Arterial and Venous Blood Gas Studies (Normal Values in Healthy Adults)

	Arterial Blood	Mixed Venous Blood
pH	7.40* (7.35–7.45)	7.36* (7.30–7.41)
P_{O_2}	80–100 mm Hg	35–40 mm Hg
O_2Sa	95%	70–75%
P_{CO_2}	35–45 mm Hg	41–51 mm Hg
HCO_3	22–26 mEq/L	22–26 mEq/L
Base excess	−2 to +2	−2 to +2

*Indicates the mean.

Other Laboratory Tests

Serum sodium levels are often low in CHF, even though body sodium levels are almost always elevated. This lab picture results from the retention of sodium and water and is called *dilutional hyponatremia. Serum potassium* may be decreased due to the aldosterone effect and the administration of potassium-depleting diuretics. Electrolyte imbalances are discussed in Chapter 10. Other laboratory values may be altered depending on the underlying cause of the CHF.

▼ Cardiogenic Shock

CAUSES OF CARDIOGENIC SHOCK

Heart failure may lead to cardiogenic shock with a low-output component, the congestive phenomena, or both. The most common cause of cardiogenic shock is MI; however, cardiomyopathy, dysrhythmias, cardiac tamponade, pulmonary embolism, or any factor that can depress myocardial function may precipitate this syndrome.

Cardiogenic shock always carries a grave prognosis. If it develops after MI, mortality is approximately 60% to 80%, which correlates well with the amount of ventricular mass lost.[1] A 40% or greater loss of left ventricular mass due to infarctions, both new and old, is highly correlated with cardiogenic shock. It carries a mortality rate of greater than 75%.[8]

PATHOPHYSIOLOGY OF CARDIOGENIC SHOCK

Cardiogenic shock results from decreased ability of the left or right ventricle to maintain adequate cardiac output. This results in decreased systolic blood pressure, with reduced peripheral perfusion manifested by cold, clammy skin, diaphoresis, tachycardia, mental confusion, and decreased urinary output. The cold, clammy skin and tachycardia result from sympathetic stimulation. The effects of SNS stimulation increase the taxation on an already overtaxed heart but enhance cerebral and coronary blood flow. SNS stimulation markedly decreases renal perfusion and increases the risk for acute renal failure (see Chapter 13).

w/out O₂ Anaerobic metabolism begins in peripheral cells as vital oxygen deprivation occurs. The effect of this energy production is to keep cells viable, but the production of lactic acid as a byproduct leads to metabolic acidosis (see p. 220). Acidosis depresses cardiac function. Further depression of cardiac function may result from a *myocardial depressant factor* released from the pancreas in shock situations.[4]

Cardiogenic shock is often described in stages. If the compensatory mechanisms can restore arterial pressure and urinary output, it is termed *compensated shock*. If the underlying cause of the shock is not corrected, the response of the body to poor tissue perfusion results in continuation of the shock state, which is called *progressive shock*. When arteriolar tone is finally destroyed and peripheral pooling occurs, death is inevitable. This condition is called *irreversible* or *decompensated shock*. Pooling is enhanced by loss of arteriolar tone before loss of venular tone, which encourages fluid movement into the interstitial spaces. Anaerobic energy production and lactic acidosis eventually cause cellular failure and death.

DIAGNOSIS OF CARDIOGENIC SHOCK

Diagnosis of cardiogenic shock is often one of exclusion. Sometimes hypovolemic or even septic shock must be ruled out. The symptoms and signs presented by the affected individual are analyzed. Physical examination reveals gallop rhythms, sometimes venous engorgement, and the effects of acute hypotension. The ECG often shows cardiac dysrhythmias and evidence of MI. The chest x-ray usually shows a dilated or enlarged heart, which may be accompanied by the pulmonary infiltrates of acute pulmonary edema. The Swan-Ganz catheter reveals elevated pulmonary wedge pressures and decreased cardiac output.[1] Chapter 13 gives a detailed explanation of the pathophysiology of the different types of shock along with signs and symptoms and diagnostic tests.

▼ Diseases Affecting Myocardial Contractility

DEFINITIONS

The term *cardiomyopathy* refers to a group of myocardial diseases that primarily affect the pumping ability of the heart that is not caused by disease or dysfunction of other cardiac structures (eg, valves, coronary artery disease).[10] Box 25-2 lists the World Health Organization classification of cardiomyopathy. *Myocarditis* is the word used for myocardial disease associated with inflammation of the myocardium.

CARDIOMYOPATHY

Primary or *idiopathic myocardial disease* refers to conditions affecting the ventricular muscle that have no known origin. *Secondary* cardiomyopathy designates conditions in which the causative factors are known. The cardiomyopathies have been classified as congestive, restrictive, and hypertrophic (Fig. 25-10).[10]

Congestive or Dilated Cardiomyopathy

Congestive or dilated cardiomyopathy, also called *idiopathic dilated cardiomyopathy*, is usually of unknown etiology but has been described in association with beriberi, thyrotoxicosis, alcoholism, childbirth or the postpartum period, diabetes mellitus, drug toxicity (especially from daunorubicin), cobalt therapy, and certain neuromuscular disorders. The incidence of this type of

---

BOX 25-2 ▼ World Health Organization Classification of Cardiomyopathy

I. Cardiomyopathy of unknown cause
   Dilated cardiomyopathy
   Hypertrophic cardiomyopathy
   Restrictive cardiomyopathy
   Unclassified cardiomyopathy
II. Specific heart muscle disease
   Infective
   Metabolic
   General systems diseases
   Heredofamilial
   Sensitivity and toxic reactions

From a report of the WHO/ISFC task force. This is a listing of major categories only; specific disorders are not listed.

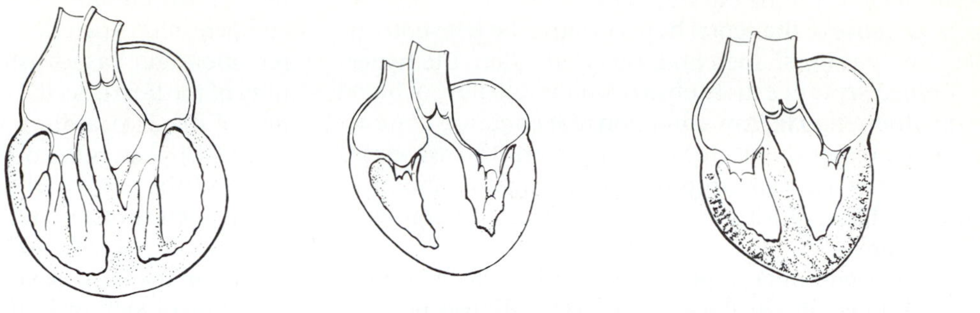

	Dilated (congestive)	Hypertrophic	Restrictive
Morphologic	Biventricular dilatation	Marked hypertrophy of left ventricle, occasionally also of right ventricle, and usually but not always, disproportionate hypertrophy of septum	Reduced ventricular compliance; usually caused by infiltration of myocardium (e.g., by amyloid, hemosiderin, or glycogen deposits)
Hemodynamic			
Cardiac output	↓ ↓	Normal	Normal to ↓
Stroke volume	↓ ↓	Normal or ↑	Normal or ↓
Ventricular filling pressure	↑ ↑	Normal or ↑	↑ ↑
Chamber size	↑ ↑	Normal or ↓	Normal or ↑
Ejection fraction	↓ ↓	↑ ↑	Normal to ↓
Other findings	May have associated functional mitral or tricuspid regurgitation.	Obstruction may develop between interventricular septum and septal leaflet of mitral valve. Mitral regurgitation may be present.	Characteristic ventricular pressure tracings resemble those recorded in constrictive pericarditis, with early diastolic dip-and-plateau configuration.

FIGURE 25-10 *Morphologic and hemodynamic characteristics of the cardiomyopathies. (Source: c. 1987, Scientific American Inc. All rights reserved from Scientific American Medicine, Table I, Section I, Subsection XIV).*

cardiomyopathy is estimated to be 3 to 10 cases per 100,000, with 20,000 new cases diagnosed every year in the United States.[5] The striking effect of this type of cardiomyopathy is immense cardiomegaly. The enlargement is a combination of dilatation and hypertrophy of the heart. This dilatation leads to a hypokinetic myocardium, with the usual onset of biventricular CHF.[5] Symptoms include exertional dyspnea, fatigue, paroxysmal nocturnal dyspnea, and pulmonary edema with symptoms of RHF late in the course of the disease. Atrial and ventricular gallops may be noted on auscultation. Peripheral edema and hepatomegaly are signs of RHF.

Restrictive Cardiomyopathy

Restrictive cardiomyopathy describes the clinical picture of constrictive pericarditis, the underlying cause of which is actually myocardial.[15] The etiology is generally unknown but has been described in association with such diverse conditions as amyloidosis, hemosiderosis, and glycogen storage disease. In the systemic myocardial disorders, the myocardial muscle becomes infiltrated with abnormal substances that apparently cause dys-

function of the ventricle. In the idiopathic form there is extensive fibrosis, but no pathologic substrate can be identified.[15]

Congestive and restrictive cardiomyopathies are mostly differentiated on the basis of the presence or absence of cardiomegaly. Symptoms of biventricular failure are common. Ventricular filling is impeded and the end-diastolic pressure of the ventricles usually becomes exceedingly high. The prognosis for survival is poor and death often results from CHF.

Hypertrophic Cardiomyopathy

Hypertrophic cardiomyopathy usually refers to an asymmetric increase in ventricular muscle mass. It has also been termed *idiopathic hypertrophic subaortic stenosis* and *hypertrophic obstructive cardiomyopathy*.[2]

The etiology of this condition is unknown. Familial occurrence is noted with no predominance for either sex. Certain studies support a genetic abnormality of protein synthesis.[2] The pathologic features include greater hypertrophy of the ventricular septum than of the ventricular chambers. Small or normal ventricular chamber size and disorganization of septal muscle cells, especially of the myofibrils, may occur.

Because of the septal hypertrophy, the left ventricular cavity is misshapen and, on contraction, the hypertrophied septum causes obstruction to the flow of blood from the ventricle. Any condition that enhances contractility increases the degree of obstruction. The associated left ventricular hypertrophy causes impairment of ventricular filling during diastole and reduced ventricular compliance.[1]

The signs and symptoms are due to 1) left ventricular outflow obstruction; 2) diastolic dysfunction; 3) myocardial ischemia; and 4) dysrhythmias.[9] These dysfunctions cause symptoms of LHF, including exertional dyspnea, angina, periods of syncope, and orthopnea. Obstruction of ventricular outflow is more severe under stress, and when beta-blocking drugs are given, the obstruction may be reduced or abolished.[9] The diastolic dysfunction results from abnormalities in relaxation and filling, which cause a prolongation in the rapid filling phase of diastole. Myocardial ischemia is indicated by the electrocardiographic changes of decreased blood flow. Various forms of rhythm alterations may result and are related to myocardial ischemia and/or conduction system effects. Right-sided effects occur later in the course of the disease. The prognosis is variable due to the complexity of the disease expression, and sudden cardiac death is common in persons with this condition.[9]

MYOCARDITIS

Inflammation of the myocardium may result from an infectious process; chemical agents, such as chemotherapeutic drugs; and hypersensitivity responses. Viruses, especially the Coxsackie viruses, bacteria, protozoa, metazoa, and fungal infections, have been implicated in its causation. Myocarditis is often a self-limiting condition that is manifested by tachycardia, symptoms of heart failure, and gallop rhythm on auscultation. Flulike symptoms occur in approximately 60% of persons diagnosed with myocarditis, and they usually occur before the onset of the cardiac symptoms.[12] Many types of myocarditis resolve with bed rest, fluid restriction, and limited drug therapy. In a small percentage of affected persons, the disease is progressive and leads to all of the manifestations of dilated congestive myocardiopathy.

▼ Chapter Summary

▼ Congestive heart failure is a clinical syndrome characterized by abnormal retention of sodium and water resulting from decreased cardiac output. Circulatory overload may be seen systemically in the tissues with edema or in the lungs with pulmonary congestion or edema. The causes are varied, with the syndrome being secondary to intrinsic or extrinsic causes.

▼ Onset of CHF may be insidious or acute. In all cases, there is an attempt by the body to compensate. This compensation includes sympathetic stimulation, fluid retention and vasoconstriction, and increased contractility of the heart. As the condition progresses, hypertrophy of the myocardium may increase contractility, but this also increases the need for myocardial oxygen. Dilatation of the cardiac chambers is always a component and is seen on chest x-ray.

▼ CHF is divided into left-sided and right-sided heart failure on the basis of symptoms. In most cases, there is symptomatology of both LHF and RHF. Symptoms of LHF are mainly of pulmonary congestion, which may progress to pulmonary edema. The main symptom of RHF is systemic congestion manifested by peripheral edema.

▼ CHF is diagnosed through clinical manifestations, chest x-ray, arterial blood gases, and especially through the use of the flow-directed pulmonary artery catheter.

▼ Untreated CHF may progress to cardiogenic shock. The cardiac output is insufficient to maintain adequate tissue perfusion. It is often fatal if not appropriately treated.

▼ Cardiomyopathy is a term used for a group of myocardial diseases that affect the pumping ability of the heart. Many of these conditions are of unknown origin, but they may be associated with an inflammatory process, especially virally induced.

▼ References

1. Alpert, J.S., and Becker, R.C. The pathophysiology of cardiogenic shock. In R.C. Schlant and R.W. Alexander (eds.), *Hurst's The Heart* (8th ed.). New York: McGraw-Hill, 1994.
2. Bristow, M.R., and O'Connell, J.B. Myocardial diseases. In W.N. Kelley (ed.), *Textbook of Internal Medicine* (2nd ed.). Philadelphia: J.B. Lippincott, 1992.
3. Cheitlin, M.D., Sokolow, M., and McIlroy, M.B. *Clinical Cardiology* (6th ed.). Norwalk, Conn.: Appleton-Lange, 1994.
4. Cotran, R.S., Kumar, V., and Robbins, S.L. *Robbins' Pathologic Basis of Disease* (4th ed.). Philadelphia: W.B. Saunders, 1989.
5. Gilbert, E.M., and Bristow, M.R. Idiopathic dilated cardiomyopathy. In R.C. Schlant and R.W. Alexander (eds.), *Hurst's The Heart* (8th ed.). New York: McGraw-Hill, 1994.
6. Guyton, A.C. *Textbook of Medical Physiology* (8th ed.). Philadelphia: W.B. Saunders, 1990.
7. Hurst, J.W., and Morris, D.C. The history: Symptoms and past events related to cardiovascular disease. In R.C. Schlant and R.W. Alexander (eds.), *Hurst's The Heart* (8th ed.). New York: McGraw-Hill. 1994.
8. Leier, C.V. Approach to the patient with hypotension and shock. In W.N. Kelley (ed.), *Textbook of Internal Medicine* (2nd ed.). Philadelphia: J.B. Lippincott, 1992.
9. Maron, B.J., and Roberts, W.C. Hypertrophic cardio-

myopathy. In R.C. Schlant and R.W. Alexander (eds.), *Hurst's The Heart* (8th ed). New York: McGraw-Hill, 1994.

10. Mason, J.W. Classification of cardiomyopathy. In R.C. Schlant and R.W. Alexander (eds.), *Hurst's The Heart* (8th ed). New York: McGraw-Hill, 1994.

11. McCall, D. Congestive heart failure. In J.H. Stein (ed.), *Internal Medicine* (4th ed). St. Louis: C.V. Mosby, 1994.

12. O'Connell, J.B., and Renlund, D.G. Myocarditis and specific myocardial diseases. In R.C. Schlant and R.W. Alexander (eds.), *Hurst's The Heart* (8th ed). New York: McGraw-Hill, 1994.

13. Rowell, L.B. *Human Cardiovascular Control.* New York: Oxford Press, 1993.

14. Schlant, R.C., and Sonnenblick, E.H. Pathophysiology of heart failure. In R.C. Schlant and R.W. Alexander (eds.), *Hurst's The Heart* (8th ed.). New York: McGraw-Hill, 1994.

15. Shabetai, R. Restrictive cardiomyopathy. In R.C. Schlant and R.W. Alexander (eds.), *Hurst's The Heart* (8th ed.). New York: McGraw-Hill, 1994.

16. Wiedemann, H.P. Intensive care monitoring and mechanical ventilation. In J.H. Stein (ed.), *Internal Medicine* (4th ed.). St. Louis: C.V. Mosby, 1994.

17. Zelis, R., and Sinoway, L.I. Pathophysiology of heart failure. In W.N. Kelley (ed.), *Textbook of Internal Medicine.* Philadelphia: J.B. Lippincott, 1989.

Chapter 26

Hypertension

Barbara L. Bullock

▼ **CHAPTER OUTLINE**

▼ **LEARNING OBJECTIVES**

1 Define **hypertension** as it relates to different age groups.
2 Compare the definitions of borderline, mild to moderate, labile, benign, and malignant hypertension.
3 List and describe briefly the factors that are related to the cause of hypertension.
4 Describe briefly the significance of altered levels of serum lipoproteins.
5 Explain how blood pressure levels are normally maintained in the arterial system.
6 Describe the abnormal renin theory in the production of essential hypertension.
7 Compare the pathophysiology of essential and secondary hypertension.
8 List the typical symptoms of hypertension.
9 Explain the major clinical complications of hypertensive disease.
10 List the diagnostic tests used in hypertensive disease.

Barbara L. Bullock: PATHOPHYSIOLOGY: ADAPTATIONS AND ALTERATIONS IN FUNCTION, 4th ed.
© 1996 J.B. Lippincott-Raven Publishers

Hypertension is the most common disease in the United States, afflicting two of every five American adults.[12] It is a direct risk factor for and contributor to heart and vascular disease, especially myocardial infarction, congestive heart failure, and cerebrovascular accident. The etiology of the disorder is poorly understood, treatment is lifelong, and the condition is generally asymptomatic until complications develop. The frequency of sudden death is markedly increased among hypertensive persons.

▼ Definitions

Hypertension is defined as abnormal elevation of the systolic arterial blood pressure (BP). Levels that are considered to be hypertensive vary with age (Table 26-1). Blood pressure levels fluctuate within certain limits depending on body position, age, and stress. Blood pressure varies widely during the course of the day, with a surge in readings early in the morning after arising from sleep. This may, in part, account for the early morning increase in sudden death, heart attacks, and strokes.[9, 11] Variations are noted with activity, such as running, when the systolic pressure elevates and diastolic pressure may fall. Borderline hypertension in adults is considered to be consistent readings (three or more) between 140/90 and 160/95, with readings above 160/95 being definitely hypertensive. Hypertension is also frequently classified as mild, moderate, or severe on the basis of the diastolic pressure. Mild hypertension has a diastolic pressure in the range of 90 to 95; moderate, 95 to 100; and severe, 110 or greater. The diagnosis is made by high readings (>140/90) on three separate occasions after 20 minutes or more of rest.[1] Sustained hypertension occurs when the BP remains elevated over hours or days.[8] Persons who have occasional BP elevation should be considered to have borderline hypertension rather than la-

TABLE 26-1 Hypertension As It Relates to Different Age Groups

Age Group	Normal	Hypertensive
Infants	80/40	90/60
Children 7–11 y	100/60	120/80
Teenagers 12–17 y	115/70	130/80
Adults 20–45 y	120–125/75–80	135/90
45–65 y	135–140/85	140/90–160/95
Over 65 y	150/85	160/90 (borderline)

TABLE 26-2 Causes of Hypertension

Types of Hypertension	Causes
Essential, idiopathic, or primary	Related to obesity, hypercholesterolemia, atherosclerosis, high-sodium diet, diabetes, stress, type A personality, familial history, smoking, and lack of exercise

Secondary	Renovascular
	  Parenchymal disease, such as acute and chronic glomerulonephritis
	  Narrowing, stenosis of renal artery—due to atherosclerosis or congenital fibroplasia
	Cushing's disease or syndrome
	Oral contraceptives
	  May be due to increased secretion of glucocorticoids as result of adrenal disease or pituitary dysfunction
	Primary aldosteronism
	  Increased aldosterone secretion, often a result of adrenal tumor
	Renin-secreting tumors
	Pheochromocytoma
	  Tumor of adrenal medulla causing increased secretion of adrenal catecholamines
	Coarctation of the aorta
	  Congenital constriction of aorta usually at the level of the ductus arteriosus with increased blood pressure above the constriction and decreased pressure below the constriction

bile hypertension and be advised to make lifestyle modifications and keep a close check on the readings.[9]

The most common feature of hypertension is a mixed elevation of systolic and diastolic BPs. Occasionally, the diastolic pressure is elevated without a significant increase in systolic pressure. This indicates an increase in systemic vascular resistance (SVR) and is most common in young persons. Increase in systolic pressure without diastolic elevation may occur in elderly persons or in persons with hyperdynamic circulation (eg, hyperthyroidism) or aortic insufficiency. This type of hypertension is called *isolated systolic hypertension*.

Other definitive terms include *essential* (idiopathic) *hypertension*, which has no specific etiologic basis, and *secondary hypertension*, which is due to a known cause (Table 26-2). Benign and malignant hypertension refer to the course of the disease, and either may result from essential or secondary hypertension. Benign hypertension is a misnomer because it causes permanent damage, even though it has a gradual onset and begins with BP levels only slightly above normal. It is chronic with secondary effects that are not clinically evident for a long time.[2] Malignant hypertension is rapidly progressive, uncontrollable BP elevation that causes rapid onset of end organ complications, including renal failure, cerebrovascular accident, retinal hemorrhages, congestive heart failure, and encephalopathy.

▼ Etiology of Hypertension

AGE

There is a positive relationship between age and the frequency of hypertension with the prevalence increasing as the individual ages. More than 60% of the American population over age 65 years is hypertensive.[13] Hypertension in those below age 35 years markedly increases the frequency of heart disease or coronary artery disease (CAD) and premature death.

SEX

Overall, men have a higher frequency of hypertension than women. However, at middle age and beyond, the prevalence begins to change, and disease in women exceeds that in men at the older ages (over age 65 years). The risk of complications in women is less than that of men at any age.

RACE

Blacks have at least twice the frequency of hypertension as whites.[9, 13] The consequences of the disease are usually more severe in blacks, both men and women. The prevalence and severity of hypertension as well as the death rate from hypertension is greater than that in whites. This may be due to decreased access to adequate treatment but it also may relate to genetic differences, psychosocial or nutritional factors.[1]

HEREDITY

Genetic influences play a role in the development of hypertension. Prevalence of the disease is clustered in families. For example, if both parents have essential hypertension, prevalence in offspring is one out of two. One hypertensive parent produces a one in three frequency while normotensive parents produce a one in 20 frequency in their children.[1]

LIFESTYLE

The relationship between hypertension and factors such as education, income, diet, and aspects of lifestyle has been studied with inconclusive results. Low income, low educational levels, and stressful lives or occupations seem to be related to greater frequency of hypertension. Family history of the disease has always been considered a risk factor. However, this relationship may be related more to lifestyle than to a straight genetic link, especially with respect to essential hypertension. Obesity is considered to be a major risk factor. When weight reduction is achieved, BP often returns to the normal range. Cigarette smoking is implicated as a high risk factor for both hypertension and CAD. Dietary intake of saturated fats is thought to be a major factor in the development of high serum cholesterol levels. Hypercholesteremia and hyperglycemia are both major factors in the development of atherosclerosis, which is closely associated with hypertension. The lipoproteins responsible for hyperlipidemia and hypercholesteremia are thought to foster the development of atherosclerosis through increasing the deposition of lipid on the intimal surfaces (see pp. 525–528).[1]

DIABETES MELLITUS

The relationship between diabetes mellitus and hypertension is obscure but the statistics support a definite link between hypertension and CAD. The main cause of death in diabetes mellitus is cardiovascular disease, especially with early onset and poor control of the diabetic condition. Diabetes mellitus is the third leading cause of mortality in the United States and leading cause of chronic renal failure and blindness.[5]

SECONDARY HYPERTENSION

As described earlier, hypertension can develop secondary to known diseases (see Table 26-2). When the causative factor is treated, the BP may return to normal. Of secondary forms of hypertension, renal parenchymal and renovascular disease are the most common causative factors.[9] Oral contraceptives have been linked to mild hypertension related to an increase in renin substrate and increased levels of angiotensin II and aldosterone.[9] Endocrine hyperfunction related to cortical and medullary hypersecretion accounts for less than 0.5% of all hypertension.[9]

▼ Pathophysiology of Hypertension

BLOOD PRESSURE DETERMINANTS

To understand the pathophysiology of hypertension, one must review normal arterial pressure determinants. Blood pressure is normally maintained within rather narrow limits. During sleep, however, it may fall to 60/40 mm Hg or less; during exercise, marked increases may be noted that often correspond to changes in heart rate and cardiac output (CO).

Total peripheral resistance (TPR) or SVR is an important factor in the regulation of arterial BP. It is the sum of all resistances offered by the vascular beds of the body. These vary with different organs, but the systemic peripheral resistance has the greatest effect on the mean arterial BP. Very small changes in arteriolar diameter, also called the precapillary sphincter diameter, cause significant effects on both systemic arterial pressure and blood flow. Mean arterial pressure (MAP) can be calculated by using the following formula[7]: CO × TPR = MAP.

A more simple way to calculate MAP is to add the diastolic pressure and one-third of the pulse pressure (which is the difference between systolic and diastolic pressures). For example, if the BP is 160/100, then 100 + 1/3(60) = 20 + 100 = 120 (MAP). The normal MAP is from 70 to 100 mm Hg.[4]

Arterial pressure is maintained by 1) the CO, which is the main determining factor for systolic BP and is determined by the volume pumped from the heart; 2) blood volume, which is the amount of blood in the vascular tree that can be pumped; and 3) peripheral resistance, which is mainly determined by the caliber of the arterioles.[7] When the arterioles are more constricted, it takes more pressure to pump blood through them and, conversely, less pressure when they are dilated.

Aortic impedance is another factor that affects systolic and diastolic pressure. It is regulated by the aortic valve and the elasticity of the aortic wall. Each time the heart pumps, it meets some resistance from the aortic valve and the distension of the aortic wall. If the wall is stiff or thickened, it will offer more resistance to CO.[3]

Other factors have an influence on arterial pressure through affecting CO and systemic resistance. The sympathetic nervous system causes increased SVR and increased cardiac contractility which, in turn, increase the BP. The sympathetic nervous system also influences the renin-angiotensin-aldosterone system, which causes arteriolar constriction through the release of angiotensin II and increased blood volume through the liberation of aldosterone (see below).

COMPENSATORY MECHANISMS FOR INCREASED AFTERLOAD

In hypertension, there is usually an elevation of the afterload (resistance) against which the ventricle must empty. A higher afterload requires the ventricle to develop more pressure to empty its contents. Consistent increase in workload requires thicker heart muscle, so the ventricular muscle hypertrophies.[3] This hypertrophy is often concentric, with enlargement occurring from the epicardium to the endocardium (see Figure 25-2). The chamber size does not increase, thus the heart does not appear enlarged on radiographs, but the increased muscle mass may increase the weight of the heart significantly. Hypertrophy can be demonstrated electrocardiographically by increased amplitude of the R waves of the precordial leads. The increased muscle mass in-

creases the myocardial need for oxygen and usually reduces the compliance of the ventricle. Together with a muscle mass needing more oxygen to sustain its increased workload is an acceleration of coronary atherosclerosis from the hypertensive process. This then reduces myocardial blood flow and increases the risk of cardiac ischemia and infarction.[3]

ESSENTIAL HYPERTENSION

There is no real agreement as to the etiology of essential hypertension; 90% of all hypertension has no definite identifiable cause. It is known that arterioles offer abnormally increased resistance to blood flow. This increases SVR, causes a decreased capillary flow, and results in increased resistance against which the heart must pump. Numerous theories have been offered to explain hypertension, including 1) changes in the arteriolar bed itself, causing chronically increased resistance; 2) abnormally increased tone of the sympathetic nervous system from the vasomotor centers causing increased systemic vascular resistance (SVR); 3) increased blood volume resulting from renal or hormonal dysfunction; and 4) a genetic increase in arteriolar thickening causing the abnormal SVR. It is more likely of multifactorial etiology.[1, 9, 13]

One theory that has been studied extensively is the abnormal renin theory. It has been demonstrated that when blood flow to the kidneys is decreased, the juxtaglomerular cells release renin (a proteolytic enzyme), which reacts with angiotensinogen (a plasma protein formed by the liver) to form angiotensin I, which is then converted to angiotensin II in the lungs. Angiotensin I elaborated in an intermediate step of the process exhibits no physiologic activity, but angiotensin II is a potent vasoconstrictor. The target for angiotensin II effect is the arterioles. Circulating angiotensin II also stimulates aldosterone secretion, which, in turn, increases blood volume by conserving sodium and water (Flowchart 26-1). Renin synthesis is increased by sodium deprivation and decreased by sodium overloading. Angiotensin II, the end product of the cascade, besides its vasoconstrictive and aldosterone effects, increases the activity of the sympathetic nervous system and inhibits sodium excretion.[3]

Increased serum renin levels are not present in every form of hypertension, but they correlate well with some types, especially the accelerated or malignant form.[1, 8] Renin levels are ascertained from peripheral or renal venous blood. The renin studies can help determine if a renal artery lesion is the cause of the hypertension. The renal vein blood allows more accurate sampling, and the ratio of renin activity in blood samples drawn from each renal vein is determined. A renal vein renin ratio of 1.5 or greater on the stenotic side is abnormal and generally indicates a significant renal artery stenosis, a secondary form of hypertension.[8] High-renin essential hypertension is often associated with high plasma norepineph-

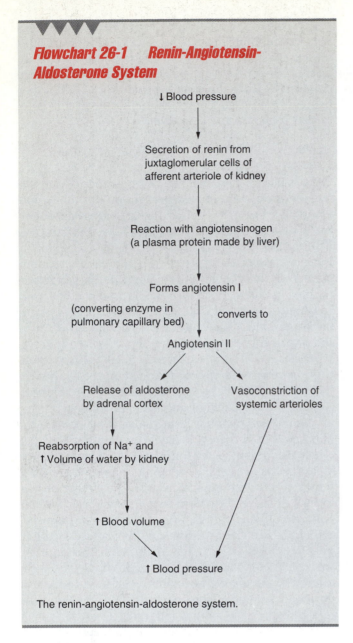

Flowchart 26-1   Renin-Angiotensin-Aldosterone System

↓ Blood pressure

Secretion of renin from
juxtaglomerular cells of
afferent arteriole of kidney

Reaction with angiotensinogen
(a plasma protein made by liver)

Forms angiotensin I

(converting enzyme in
pulmonary capillary bed)   converts to

Angiotensin II

Release of aldosterone   Vasoconstriction of
by adrenal cortex   systemic arterioles

Reabsorption of Na+ and
↑ Volume of water by kidney

↑ Blood volume

↑ Blood pressure

The renin-angiotensin-aldosterone system.

Renovascular Hypertension

Renovascular hypertension has been studied extensively. It results from atherosclerotic or fibrous dysplastic stenosis of one or both renal arteries.[8] The resultant decrease in renal perfusion causes activation of the renin-angiotensin-aldosterone system. The degree of hypertension is closely related to the amount of renal ischemia produced by the obstruction. Serum renin levels are usually elevated, but the amount of aldosterone secreted in relation to the amount of angiotensin II present is inappropriately increased for no known reason.[3] The result of this type of hypertension is a marked increase in SVR and CO with very high levels of systemic BP. Drug therapy with beta blockers, angiotensin-converting enzyme (ACE) inhibitors, and calcium channel blockers can control the severe BP disturbances caused by the stenosis, but the functional impairment of the involved kidney continues. Most centers use one of several surgical options to improve renal blood flow to the affected side. The usage of the percutaneous transluminal angioplasty in the renal artery has provided a less invasive method of enlarging the renal artery through a balloon procedure, much the same as that used in coronary vessels.[13]

Renal Parenchymal Disease

Renal parenchymal disease, such as glomerulonephritis and renal failure, often causes a renin-dependent or sodium-dependent type of hypertension. The pathophysiology varies depending on the extent of renal insufficiency and type of renal disease. Hypervolemia with normal SVR may appear, or normal or diminished circulation with a very increased SVR or both increased volume and SVR may result.[10]

Cushing's Disease

Cushing's disease is a disease of the adrenal cortex that causes an increase in blood volume and pressure. Excess adrenocorticotropic hormone with bilateral adrenal hyperplasia accounts for most secondary hypertension due to Cushing's disease (see pp. 701–702).

Primary Aldosteronism

Primary aldosteronism is caused by aldosterone excess from an adenoma of the adrenal gland and accounts for less than 1% of persons with hypertension.[13] High BP that results from increased production of aldosterone is a classic example of volume-related hypertension. The major criterion for the diagnosis of this condition is excess aldosterone in the presence of low plasma renin activity. Plasma renin is not a good screening test because approximately 30% of persons with essential hy-

rine levels. High-renin hypertension is more common in whites than blacks, and the condition may respond to beta-blocker medication as the initial therapy. Blacks usually have a lower plasma renin level and are more responsive to diuretic therapy than are whites. In conditions of accelerated malignant hypertension or hypertensive encephalopathy, there is usually an elevated plasma renin activity, which may respond to a converting enzyme inhibitor such as captopril.[6, 13]

SECONDARY HYPERTENSION

Secondary hypertension develops from a specific underlying cause (see Table 26-2). Approximately 5% to 10% of cases of hypertension are due to secondary causes.

pertension have subnormal plasma renin activity.[8] Although hyperaldosteronism promotes salt and water retention, the ultimate mechanism that sustains the hypertension is unknown.

Pheochromocytoma

Pheochromocytoma is a secreting tumor of chromaffin cells, usually of the adrenal medulla. This tumor causes hypertension as a result of increased secretion of epinephrine and norepinephrine. Epinephrine mainly increases cardiac contractility and rate, while norepinephrine mainly increases the SVR. The hypertension produced by a pheochromocytoma is usually severe and runs a very malignant course.[13] Surgery offers a potential cure but should be undertaken only when BP is completely controlled.

Coarctation of the Aorta

Coarctation of the aorta is a congenital constriction of the aorta, often at the level of the ductus arteriosus. This produces a syndrome of markedly elevated pressures in the upper extremities and a decrease in perfusion of the lower extremities (see pp. 493–494). Sometimes the plasma renin activity is increased, but this finding is inconsistent and the SVR may not be elevated.[3]

Estrogen-Induced Hypertension

In the normotensive female, the administration of estrogen in the form of birth-control pills or for postmenopausal symptoms may cause a slight increase in the systemic BP. If this drug is given to the borderline hypertensive female or one who has overt hypertension, there may be a significant elevation in the BP. The administration of low-dose combinations of estrogen–progesterone has decreased the incidence of estrogen-induced hypertension. In rare situations, there is precipitation of accelerated forms of hypertension and the sequelae of that is elevated BP.[13]

CLINICAL MANIFESTATIONS OF HYPERTENSION

Hypertension is often categorized as mild or moderate; severe, accelerated, or malignant; labile; or isolated systolic hypertension. Mild or moderate hypertension is often asymptomatic or vague symptoms may be described. It is frequently discovered on a screening BP check. When mild or moderate hypertension is sustained, target organ damage is likely (see below). The presence of family history; arterial bruits, especially carotid, renal, and femoral; and cardiac signs or symptoms

provides a basis for further studies. If a cause cannot be delineated, treatment measures are begun to prevent target organ dysfunction. Severe, accelerated, or malignant hypertension often is seen in the emergency setting where the BP is extremely high and the diastolic pressure is usually over 125 mm Hg.[8] Very rapid renal, cardiac, and cerebral damage may occur if the BP is not controlled quickly. Assessment of the status of end-organ function and rapid treatment can be lifesaving.[13] Labile hypertension is a common result of stress or other disease conditions. It is characterized by wide fluctuations in BP. Assessment should be much like that for mild or moderate hypertension, especially to make sure that there is no evidence of target organ damage. Isolated systolic hypertension may be associated with many disease conditions and is common in the elderly individual. It carries the same risks for cardiovascular damage as does mild or moderate hypertension.[8]

When symptoms do occur, hypertension is usually far advanced. The classic symptoms of headache, epistaxis, dizziness, and tinnitus thought to be associated with high BP are no more common in hypertensive than in normotensive individuals. Unsteadiness, waking headache, blurred vision, depression, and nocturia have been shown to be increased in persons with untreated hypertension.[8]

Changes in the retina (retinopathy) provide some objective clues to the clinical course of the disease. The Keith-Wagener-Barker funduscopic classification indicates a I rating for minimal arteriolar narrowing; II for more significant narrowing and arteriovenous nicking; III for flame-shaped hemorrhages and cotton wool exudates; and IV for the above changes with papilledema. Retinopathy has been shown in studies to be associated with 5-year survival rates of 85% for Group I, 50% for Group II, 13% for Group III, and 0% for Group IV.[8] Papilledema is always associated with malignant hypertension.[8]

The pathologic sequelae of hypertension, regardless of the cause, involve the target organs of the brain, eyes, kidneys, and heart. Untreated hypertension damages the small arterioles, which, in turn, causes *target organ dysfunction*. The organs are most acutely affected by vascular damage from the small arterioles. Hypertensive effects on the target organs are the result of prolonged elevation of the systemic BP. These are summarized in Table 26-3.

The BP remains consistently above the normal level for the age of the person. Many affected persons complain of angina pectoris, especially on exertion or during stressful situations. Headache is occasionally described, especially an occipital type that may be present on waking and may be associated with nausea, vomiting, and mental confusion. Renal dysfunction may be the first sign with nocturia or hematuria. Symptoms of left ventricular failure are common, especially dyspnea on exertion.

TABLE 26-3 *Hypertensive Effects on Target Organs*

Organ	Effect	Manifested By
Heart	Myocardial infarction	ECG changes; enzyme elevations
	Congestive failure	Decreased cardiac output; S3 or summation gallop auscultated; cardiomegaly on radiograph
	Myocardial hypertrophy	Increased voltage R wave in V_3-V_6; increased frequency of angina; left ventricular strain, manifested by ST and T wave changes
	Dysrhythmias	Usually ventricular dysrhythmias or conduction defects
Eyes	Blurred or impaired vision	Nicking arteries and veins; hemorrhages and exudates on visual examination
	Encephalopathy	Papilledema
Brain	Cerebrovascular accident	Severe occipital headache, paralysis, speech difficulties, coma
	Encephalopathy	Rapid development of confusion, agitation, convulsions, death
Kidneys	Renal insufficiency	Nocturia, proteinuria, elevated blood urea nitrogen level, creatinine
	Renal failure	Fluid overload, accumulation of metabolites, metabolic acidosis

ECG: electrocardiogram.

Accelerated (malignant) hypertension is a state in which end-organ damage from the disease occurs within a short time. It is manifested by a rapid increase in diastolic pressure (130 mm Hg or greater). This is a true emergency, causing symptoms of hypertensive encephalopathy: nausea, vomiting, restlessness, blurred vision, and headache. Renal damage is inevitable. Left ventricular failure, seizures, or coma may develop. Death often ensues without immediate, appropriate treatment.

The end result of hypertensive disease may include several major complications. These are end effects of target organ damage and include 1) hypertensive cerebrovascular disease manifested by stroke; 2) hypertensive encephalopathy; 3) myocardial infarction; and 4) renal failure.

Stroke

Vascular lesions may cause either a hemorrhagic or ischemic stroke. The increasing pressures may cause dilatation of the small, sometimes nonelastic, and aged vessels. This, in turn, causes breaks in the vessel and hemorrhage into the brain parenchyma. The dilatations of the smaller intracerebral arteries are called *Charcot-Bouchard microaneurysms*. These microaneurysms may rupture and cause signs of intracerebral hemorrhage. In the process of aneurysm formation, the vessels undergo some repair, which eventually leads to thickening and tortuosity of the endothelium.[2]

Ischemic infarcts often occur from associated atherosclerosis of the extracranial vessels (carotids and vertebrals). The thickened endothelium of the small vessels decreases or obstructs the blood flow to an area. Stroke, or cerebrovascular accident, is described in detail in Chapter 50.

Hypertensive Encephalopathy

This ominous manifestation results from leakage of water and electrolytes from the brain capillaries into the tissues of the brain. This leakage produces cerebral edema and is often associated with papilledema (optic disk swelling). Encephalopathy is most commonly seen in malignant hypertension or when a hypertensive state assumes a malignant, uncontrolled pattern. The condition may be heralded by severe headache, confusion, or lethargy followed by agitation, convulsions, coma, and frequently death.[8]

Myocardial Infarction

Myocardial infarction may result from atherosclerosis of the coronary arteries or from the same type of hyaline sclerosis previously described in relation to arterioles of the brain. It is believed that hypertension accelerates atherosclerosis because it causes injury to the endothelium, which increases lipid accumulation and atheroma formation.[1] The associated left ventricular hypertrophy increases the risk for developing a myocardial infarction. All of these factors lead to a much increased incidence of congestive heart failure.[8,13]

Renal Failure

Renal failure from primary hypertension frequently results from progressive damage to the arcuate arteries and the afferent arterioles. Progressive hyaline sclerosis leads to ischemic death of nephrons and to fibrosis, which leads to contracted kidneys. With significant loss of nephrons, renal failure ensues. This process is markedly accelerated with fibroid necrosis of the larger arteries when it is associated with malignant hypertension.[10]

▼ Diagnosis of Hypertension

Unlike many other diseases, hypertension is usually asymptomatic, and the disease may not be recognized for years unless the person seeks medical attention for another health problem or has a routine BP reading. Correct and accurate measurement of BP is the key element in making the diagnosis. Blood pressure should be measured after at least 5 to 20 minutes of rest in a quiet, familiar environment. Several positions are usually recommended to attain the most accurate readings: right and left arms with the person sitting, right arm with the person supine, and right leg with the person prone. As noted earlier, arterial BP is determined by CO and resistance to blood flow. The higher pressure is the systolic pressure and the lower pressure is the diastolic. An error factor of a few millimeters for both systolic and diastolic pressures is accepted because they are indirect measures.

Examination for vascular insufficiency, including peripheral pulses, is essential. Evidence of cardiac involvement may be revealed by gallop rhythms on auscultation or displacement of the point of maximal impulse, indicating cardiomegaly. Changes in the vascular bed of the eyes may be noted on ophthalmic examination.

A complete health history should be taken, including family history, age at onset of hypertension, presence of risk factors, diet, symptoms of atherosclerotic disease, and symptoms relating to hypertension. Tests, including an electrocardiogram, intravenous pyelogram, blood urea level, and creatinine level, provide supportive objective data. An electroencephalogram may also be indicated. All of the tests are to determine presence and extent of target organ damage.

The prognosis for uncontrolled hypertension is dismal. Statistics of premature death correlate with levels of BP elevation. The risk of cerebrovascular accident, for example, is five times higher for hypertensive than for normotensive individuals. Better case findings and proper treatment have improved the outlook for victims of systemic hypertension.

▼ Chapter Summary

▼ Hypertension is the general designation for an elevated BP that remains above designated levels for the person's age and activity.

▼ Systemic hypertension is extremely common, and the cause, in most cases, is unknown. When the cause is unknown, the hypertension is termed essential or idiopathic hypertension. If the BP elevation is secondary to a specific etiologic agent, it is termed secondary hypertension. Essential hypertension is closely associated with increased age, male gender, black race, heredity, diabetes mellitus, and destructive lifestyles (smoking, obesity, high dietary intake of saturated fats).

▼ In all cases of hypertension, there is increased afterload, which means that the heart consistently must pump against increased resistance. This forces the heart to compensate by hypertrophy of cardiac muscle to meet the increased demand. In some cases, renin has been isolated as the initiator of the process. Renin-associated hypertension usually presents as very high pressures and causes early onset of complications.

▼ Clinical manifestations of hypertension are rare until it is far advanced. Then the classic symptoms of headache, epistaxis, dizziness, and tinnitus may or may not occur. Unsteadiness, waking headache, blurred vision, depression, and nocturia are more common in untreated hypertension. Retinopathy frequently occurs, especially in uncontrolled hypertension.

▼ Complications of hypertension include cerebrovascular accident (ischemic or hemorrhagic), hypertensive encephalopathy, myocardial infarction, and renal failure. Diagnosis is essential for treatment and can prevent many complications. The disease is asymptomatic, in most cases, so BP screening is critical in identifying an at-risk population.

▼ References

1. Cheitlin, M.D., Sokolow, M., and McIlroy, M.B. *Clinical Cardiology* (6th ed.). Norwalk, Conn.: Appleton-Lange, 1994.
2. Cotran, R.S., Kumar, V., and Robbins, S.L. *Robbins' Pathologic Basis of Disease* (4th ed.). Philadelphia: W.B. Saunders, 1989.
3. Frohlich, E.D. Pathophysiology of systemic arterial hypertension. In R.C. Schlant and R.W. Alexander, *Hurst's The Heart* (8th ed.). New York: McGraw-Hill, 1994.
4. Ganong, W.F. *Review of Medical Physiology* (16th ed.). Los Altos, Calif.: Appleton & Lange, 1994.
5. Garber, A.J. Diabetes mellitus. In J. Stein, *Internal Medicine* (4th ed.). St. Louis: C.V. Mosby. 1994.
6. Gifford, R. W. Treatment of patients with systemic arterial hypertension. In R.C. Schlant and R.W. Alexander, *Hurst's The Heart* (8th ed.). New York: McGraw-Hill, 1994.
7. Guyton, A.C. *Textbook of Medical Physiology* (8th ed.). Philadelphia: W.B. Saunders. 1991.
8. Hall, W.D., Wollam, G., and Tuttle, E. Diagnostic evaluation of the patient with hypertension. In R.C. Schlant and R.W. Alexander (eds.), *Hurst's The Heart* (8th ed.). New York: McGraw-Hill, 1994.
9. Kaplan, N.M. Arterial hypertension. In J. Stein, *Internal Medicine* (4th ed.) St. Louis: C.V. Mosby. 1994.
10. Kelleher, S.P., and Schrier, R.W. The kidney in hypertension. In R.W. Schrier (ed.), *Renal and Electrolyte Disorders* (3rd ed.). Boston: Little, Brown, 1986.
11. Rubin, E. and Farber, J.L. *Pathology* (2nd ed.). Philadelphia: Lippincott. 1994.
12. Tortora, G. and Grabowski, S.R. *Principles of Anatomy and Physiology* (7th ed.). New York: Harper-Collins. 1993.
13. Weinberger, M.H. Systemic hypertension. In W.N. Kelley (ed.), *Textbook of Internal Medicine* (2nd ed.). Philadelphia: J.B. Lippincott, 1992.

TABLE 27-2   *Mechanisms of Atherogenic Risk Factors*

Risk Factor	Cellular Mechanism
Hypertension	Increased systemic vascular resistance (SVR), endothelial damage, increased platelet adherence, increased permeability of endothelial lining. Renin-angiotensin system may induce cellular changes.
Cigarette smoking	Endothelial damage from carbon monoxide. Platelet aggregation. Smoking-induced increased SVR leads to endothelial damage.
Elevated serum cholesterol level, especially with low HDL cholesterol levels	Increased LDL cholesterol damages endothelium and causes accumulation on endothelial lining and proliferation of smooth muscle cells.

HDL: high-density lipoprotein; LDL: low-density lipoprotein.

THE RELATIONSHIP OF LIPID METABOLISM TO ATHEROSCLEROSIS. The lipids of the body are mostly in the form of lipoprotein particles, and these have been divided into classes according to their density. The major classes of particles are chylomicrons, very low-density lipoproteins, intermediate-density lipoproteins, low-density lipoproteins (LDLs), and high-density lipoproteins (HDLs). These particles have a lipid core with associated proteins, called apolipoproteins.[12] Table 27-3 details the functions and normal values of each of these particles. Each class of lipoprotein particles contains different amounts of cholesterol, and this relates to its atherogenic propensity. Two metabolic pathways for lipoprotein synthesis and release have been identified. These are the exogenous and endogenous cholesterol transport pathways, which work together in the formation of cholesterol. Figure 27-1 illustrates the function and relationship of these pathways with the end result of increasing or decreasing the serum cholesterol. As can be seen from the figure, the liver hepatocyte is essential in the formation of LDL and this lipoprotein is the major factor in the transport of cholesterol in the plasma.[13] The

TABLE 27-3   *Function and Normal Values of Lipoprotein Particles*

Lipoprotein	Value	Function
Total cholesterol	<200 mg/dL	Serum lipoprotein, metabolized by the liver. Necessary for the production of steroid hormones, cellular membranes, and bile acids.
Chylomicrons		Source is exogenous dietary. Dominant core is triglyceride, not thought to play a part in atherogenesis.
Very low density lipoprotein (VLDL)		Endogenous, synthesized by the liver. Core is triglyceride, may play a part in high density lipoprotein (HDL) structure when catabolized.
Intermediate-density lipoprotein (IDL)		Catabolized by liver through interaction with low density lipoprotein (LDL) receptors on hepatocyte membranes. Triglyceride removed from lipoprotein until LDL particles are formed.
Low density lipoprotein (LDL)	<160 mg/dL	LDL supplies cholesterol to cells for cell membrane and steroid hormone synthesis. Many cell membranes have receptors for LDL. High-fat diet may suppress LDL receptor activity so that particles circulating in plasma are not removed. Exposure of LDL to endothelial cells causes peroxidation and increased negative charge. This may cause chemotaxis for blood monocytes and accumulation of cholesterol esters in macrophages and smooth muscle cells, leading to atherosclerotic plaque.
High density lipoprotein (HDL)	>35 mg/dL	In two forms. Larger HDL carries more cholesterol and returns it to liver for excretion in the bile. Larger form can be converted back to smaller form, which increases its atherogenic potential. Normally, HDL is thought to be preventive in atherosclerosis development.

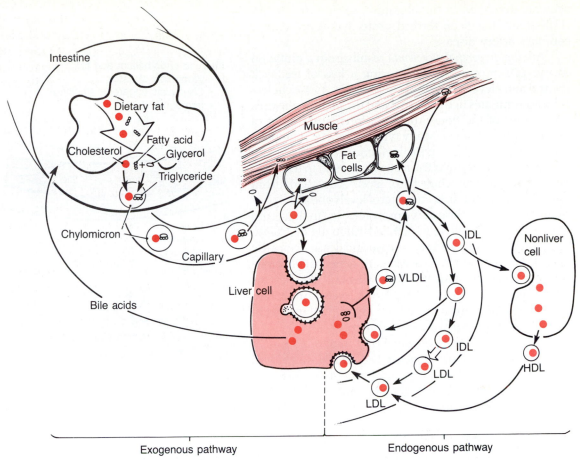

FIGURE 27-1 *Exogenous and endogenous cholesterol transport pathways. In the exogenous pathway, dietary fat is absorbed as cholesterol and fatty acids from the intestinal mucosa. Triglycerides are formed from fatty acid and glycerol linkages. Both triglycerides and cholesterol are packaged into chylomicrons that are absorbed into the circulation. In the capillaries the bonds holding the fatty acids in triglycerides are split by lipoprotein lipase. Fatty acids are removed, leaving cholesterol-rich lipoprotein. These are taken up by liver cells and either secreted into the intestine (as bile acids) or packaged as very low density lipoproteins (VLDL) which are secreted into the circulation. This first step in the endogenous cycle is followed by the removal of triglyceride from the VLDL leaving the intermediate density lipoprotein (IDL) in the circulation. Some IDL is taken up by the liver or non-liver tissues to form low-density lipoproteins (LDL). Most of the LDL in circulation binds to hepatocytes or other cells and are removed from the circulation. High density lipoproteins (HDL) take up cholesterol from cells. This cholesterol is esterified by a specific enzyme causing the esters to be transferred to LDL and taken up by cells.*

intermediate-density lipoproteins are the major source of plasma LDL. Approximately 70% of plasma LDL is cleared by the liver by binding it to surface receptors. LDL can also be transported through other receptor pathways in most cells of the body, and this causes the entire lipoprotein to move to the inside of the cell to be used for cellular structural purposes.[7] The cell controls its own internal cholesterol concentration by decreasing absorption of LDL when the concentration becomes too great within the cell.[7] The LDL that remains in the blood has the highest concentration of cholesterol of all of the lipoproteins. Some of this is degraded by scavenger cells of the mononuclear phagocyte system, which may make cholesterol available to contribute to the pathology of

atherosclerosis.[2] The cells of the mononuclear phagocyte system are mainly macrophages, and macrophage-derived foam cells are a main part of atherosclerotic lesions. It has been shown that each of the cell types of atherosclerotic lesions is able to oxidize LDL, which may significantly affect the formation of the atherosclerotic plaque.[12] HDL functions to carry cholesterol to the liver so that it can be removed from the body. This cholesterol is principally free cholesterol, which is rapidly degraded in the liver.[13] Persons who have defects in this degradation process are seen to have dyslipoproteinemias, increased intracellular cholesterol esters, and premature atherosclerosis. An inverse relationship between coronary artery disease and HDL cholesterol levels has been repeatedly described in the literature, so that this "good cholesterol" has been termed protective in preventing coronary artery disease.[13]

Familial hypercholesterolemia results from a mutation in the LDL receptor gene, causing a loss of feedback control and elevated levels of cholesterol.[2] As the cholesterol accumulates in the plasma and throughout the cells and tissues of the body, there is a premature onset of atherosclerotic lesions. Many types of genetic mutations have been described, but the incidence is about 1 in 500 persons and the result is from birth a twofold to threefold elevation in plasma cholesterol level.[2] The relationship between the circulating cholesterol levels and the development of atherosclerosis is closely released to the serum LDL levels: levels between 600 and 1,000 mg/dL lead to early-onset coronary artery disease and death before the age of 20 years in persons who are genetically homozygous for familial hypercholesterolemia.[13] The heterozygous persons with LDL cholesterol levels from 250 to 500 mg/dL suffer from premature myocardial infarction usually at about age 40 to 45 in men.[13]

Other defects in lipoprotein and in apolipoprotein synthesis may lead to changes in LDL or LDL-like serum concentrations and in early-onset atherosclerosis. It is important to identify the genetic source of the atherogenic lesion, because some types respond to cholesterol-lowering drugs whereas others may be improved by nicotinic acid therapy.[13]

Pathology

The possible precursor of the lesion of atherosclerosis is the fatty streak that often develops within the first decade of life.[2] This streak is composed of lipid droplets, called *foam cells*, that are deposited on the intima of arteries. Early fatty streaks have been shown to consist of macrophages, and as the lesions expand there appear to be smooth-muscle cells that migrate into the intima.[3, 12] When the actual atherosclerotic lesion forms, it is referred to as an atheroma or an atheromatous plaque. It is composed of fatty and fibrofatty material that is white to yellow. It protrudes into the artery and may compromise the vascular supply to the involved tissue.[12] As shown in Figure 27-2, plaques have essentially three components: 1) cells of smooth muscle, macrophages, and other leukocytes; 2) connective tissue with collagen, elastic fibers, and proteoglycans; and 3) lipid deposits both intracellularly and extracellularly.[2] The center of the plaque becomes necrotic and contains cellular debris, lipid-laden foam cells, calcium, cholesterol crystals, and a mass of lipid material. The smooth-muscle cells form on the surface and make a fibrous cap.[2]

Atherosclerotic lesions differ in different areas of the body and in different persons. Coronary artery lesions, for example, are very fibrous, and in long-standing lesions, the fibrosis may convert the atheroma to a fibrous

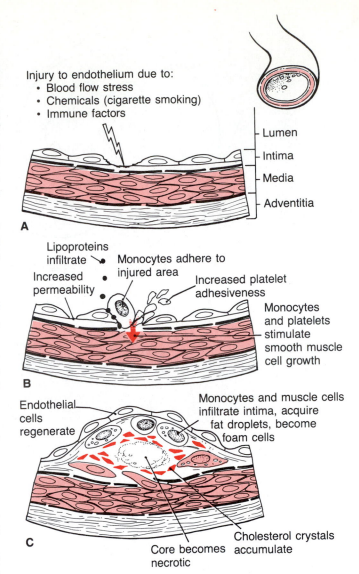

FIGURE 27-2 *The process of atherogenesis and formation of an atheroma. **A.** Endothelial injury initiates process. **B.** Platelets and monocytes adhere and stimulate growth of smooth muscle. **C.** Regeneration and migration of smooth muscle cells add to formation of the atheroma. Lipid deposits are both intracellular and extracellular. The center of the atheroma becomes necrotic.*

scar.[2] Plaques are labeled as complicated when they have become significantly calcified, ulcerated or thrombosed or when they undergo a hemorrhage or cause a weakened medial wall (Fig. 27-3).[2] The calcium can account for a stiff, brittle artery that does not accommodate well the dynamic flow of blood through it. Ulceration on the surface may dislodge the debris within the plaque and cause embolization to a smaller artery. Thrombosis is very common and occurs with initiation of the intrinsic clotting cascade, gradual accumulation of blood cells, and, finally, obstruction of the lumen of the vessel. Thrombi are also frequently incorporated into the plaque; the thrombosis gradually grows until the lumen is occluded and the blood supply stopped. Hemorrhage

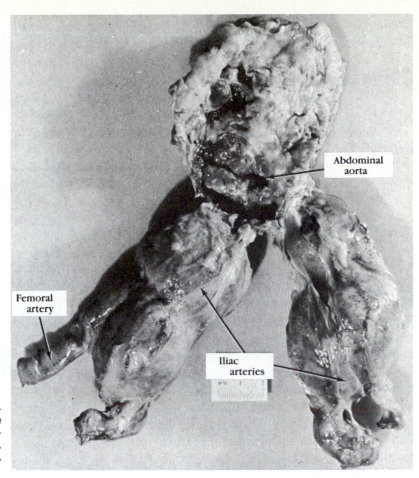

FIGURE 27-3 *Opened abdominal aorta showing diffuse atherosclerotic plaques with ulceration. There are aneurysms of both common iliac arteries. (Reprinted from J. Kernicki, B. Bullock, and J. Matthews, Cardiovascular Nursing. New York: G.P. Putnam, 1971.)*

into the plaque results from disruption of thin-walled capillaries that provide blood to the plaque.[2] The hematoma may occlude the lumen or be localized in the plaque. Medial atrophy accounts for the association of atherosclerosis and aneurysm formation. It may be caused by disruption of medial blood supply or the calcium infiltration of the endothelium and, to some extent, the medial layer.[2]

Because atherosclerosis can be induced in most animals by feeding them a diet high in cholesterol, and because the disease process rarely occurs in humans unless the cholesterol level is greater than 160 mg per dL, hyperlipidemia can be considered as a major causative factor. The lipid in the atheroma is derived from serum lipoproteins, as discussed earlier.

Even though any vessel in the body may be affected by atherosclerosis, the aorta and coronary, carotid, and iliac arteries are involved with the greatest frequency. The abdominal aorta is involved more frequently than the thoracic, and the lesions tend to locate at ostia and bifurcations.[2] A wide range of clinical effects may result from the ischemia and infarction of specific areas. Table 27-4 summarizes some of the common clinical and pathologic effects.

Embolization from a thrombosed atheroma causes

TABLE 27-4 *Clinical and Pathologic Effects of Atherosclerosis in Different Anatomic Sites*

Site	Clinical and Pathologic Effects
Abdominal/terminal aorta	Ischemic effects in lower extremities; gangrene of toes, feet; effects of fusiform abdominal aneurysm; embolism of atherosclerotic debris to smaller arteries
Aortoiliac and femoral arteries	Intermittent claudication; gangrene of toes, feet; aneurysm formation in iliac arteries
Coronary arteries	Angina pectoris; conduction disturbances; myocardial infarction
Carotid and vertebral arteries	Transient ischemic attacks; cerebrovascular accident (CVA) or stroke
Renal artery	Hypertension; renal ischemia (hematuria, proteinuria)
Mesenteric arteries	Intestinal ischemia (ileus, bowel perforation with peritonitis)

the characteristic signs of arterial occlusion: 1) diminished or absent pulses; 2) skin pallor, cyanosis, or both; 3) pain; and 4) muscle weakness. A large embolus may arise from a thrombosed atheroma in the descending aorta and may travel to the terminal aorta. If the embolus occludes the iliac arteries and terminal aorta, it is known as a *saddle embolus*. Its source is usually the heart, either from a myocardial infarction involving the endocardial surface or from mitral valve disease.

ATHEROSCLEROTIC OCCLUSIVE DISEASE OF THE LOWER EXTREMITY

Pathogenesis

Gradual occlusion of an atherosclerotic terminal aorta or of other large vessels can cause symptoms and signs of ischemia to the part supplied. If the terminal aorta is affected, clinical manifestations include intermittent claudication, loss of peripheral hair, shiny skin, and impotence. Atherosclerotic occlusive disease other than coronary artery disease most commonly affects the terminal portion of the aorta and the large and medium arteries, especially those of the lower extremities. It predominantly occurs in men between ages 50 and 70 years. The prevalence and severity of this disorder are increased if the person suffers from concomitant diabetes mellitus.

When a large artery is obstructed, the pressure in the smaller arteries distal to the obstruction decreases and blood flow declines. As the main arterial trunk progressively becomes narrowed, collateral circulation develops to maintain blood flow. This may provide circulation to the limb for an extended time (Fig. 27-4). Limb-threatening arterial insufficiency may result as the lesion progresses, leading to gangrene if the cellular deprivation of oxygen is critical enough to cause cell death.[16]

Pain

Various types of pain are described that are related to the degree of impairment of circulatory supply. Intermittent claudication is an aching, persistent, cramplike, squeezing pain that occurs after a certain amount of exercise of the affected extremity.[4] It is relieved by rest without change of position and occurs in almost all persons at some stage of the disease. It is frequently the first symptom noticed and often begins in the arch of the foot or calf of the leg.

Rest pain is usually localized in the digits. It is described as a severe ache or a gnawing pain, often occurring at night and persisting for hours at a time. Rest pain is caused by severe ischemia of tissues and sensory nerve terminals. It may herald the onset of gangrene.[8] It is aggravated by elevation of the extremity and often relieved by dependency.

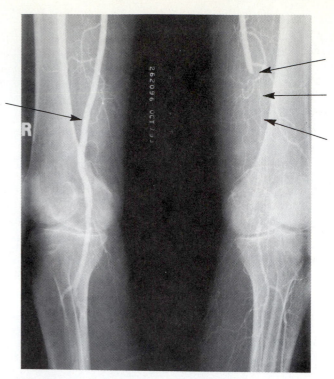

FIGURE 27-4 *Arteriogram showing arterial obstruction and collateral circulation. Arrow on left shows normal right femoral artery circulation; arrows on right show complete blockage of left femoral artery and profuse collateral circulation.*

Pain of ischemic neuropathy usually occurs late in the course of progressive disease with severe ischemia. This severe pain is often associated with various types of paresthesia. It may be described as a lightening, shock-like sensation that usually occurs in both the foot and leg and follows the distribution of the peripheral sensory nerves. The pain of ulceration and gangrene is usually localized to the areas adjacent to ulcers or gangrenous tissue. It is severe, persistent, and frequently worse at night. The pain is described as an aching sensation and sometimes may be associated with sharp, severe stabs of pain.

Coldness or Cold Sensitivity

Coldness or sensitivity to cold is a frequent symptom of occlusive disease. Complaints of coldness in the digits of the feet with exposure to a cold environment may be associated with color changes such as blanching or cyanosis. The temperature of the feet is colder to the touch than the body, and this may vary with the level of activity and complaints of ischemic leg pain.

Impaired Arterial Pulsations

Pulsation in the posterior tibial and dorsalis pedis arteries is impaired or absent in most lower-extremity occlusions. Impairment of pulsations in the popliteal and femoral arteries is less frequent. Pulsations may improve on rest, which indicates that some of the altered blood flow may be due to spasm of the artery.

Color Changes

Affected extremities may be of a normal color; however, in advanced disease, cyanosis or an abnormal red color called *rubor* may be seen, particularly when the extremity is placed in a dependent position. Postural color changes are often asymmetric, and affected extremities or digits become abnormally blanched after being elevated for a few minutes. When the extremity is placed in a dependent position, a delay of 5 to 60 seconds may be required for color to return to the skin. The part first becomes abnormally red and then gradually the rubor lessens. The rubor is caused by maximal dilatation of the arterioles and capillaries of the part.[9]

Ulceration and Gangrene

Ulcerative lesions may occur spontaneously on an ischemic extremity, or they may result from trauma, such as pressure on the toenails from shoes. In the absence of diabetes mellitus, gangrene is rare unless there is some traumatic event.[10] Bruises, nicks, or cuts in the skin; freezing; burning; or application of strong, irritating medicines or chemicals may cause the initial injury that will not heal. It is usually confined to one extremity at a time. The lesion may be manifested by small spots on a digit or it may involve a whole extremity.

Ulcers may develop on the tips of digits, between the toes, or at the base of the flexor surface of the toes. The area around the ulcer is painful and may be swollen or exhibit redness at the margin. Secondary infections are common and lead to abscess formation, cellulitis, and spread of infection. Gangrene and ulceration related to diabetes are discussed on pages 738–739.

Edema

Edema of the feet and legs may occur when there is severe obstruction. It is most evident when the legs are in a dependent position. The edema is not as dominant as that seen with venous occlusions (see pp. 537–538). Associated ischemic skin lesions, capillary atony, deep venous thrombosis, and lymphangitis contribute to the edema.

Sexual Dysfunction

Occlusive disease of the terminal aorta can decrease the blood supply to the vascular tree supplying penile circulation. The problem of inability to attain or maintain an erection is reported, especially in cases of total occlusion of the terminal aorta.[10]

Other Changes

As a result of moderate to severe chronic ischemia, small scars, depressions, or pitting may form on the tips of the pedal digits. Nail growth is slow and nails may become thickened and deformed. They also may be paper-thin. The digits or an entire foot may appear shrunken and the muscles atrophy. Therefore, the calf or thigh may get smaller.

Superficial Thrombophlebitis

At some stage of the disease, superficial nonvaricose veins are involved in a type of thrombophlebitis. This occurs in approximately 40% of persons with atherosclerotic occlusive disease. The smaller veins are usually involved with lesions or are red, raised, indurated, tender, cordlike veins that measure approximately 0.5 to 3.0 cm long. The lesions usually cause permanent occlusion of the veins, but the redness and symptoms of thrombophlebitis subside, usually in 1 to 3 weeks after onset.[8]

ATHEROSCLEROTIC OCCLUSIVE DISEASE OF THE UPPER EXTREMITY

Just as atherosclerosis is the major cause of lower extremity occlusion, it also is the main cause of brachiocephalic, carotid, and subclavian artery occlusion.

CASE STUDY 27-1

Mr. Joe Brown is a 60-year-old Caucasian male who sought medical attention due to increasing problems with intermittent claudication and loss of color in the left leg. He was found to have absent pulses in the left foot even with Doppler studies. A femoral arteriogram showed complete occlusion of the femoral artery several inches above the left knee. Extensive collateral circulation could be seen and the dorsalis pedis artery was weakly outlined. Except for a history of tobacco smoking, no other risk factors were identified. No other atherosclerotic lesions were noted. A femoral popliteal bypass was recommended to restore circulation to the left foot.

1. *Describe the process of atherosclerotic occlusion of a vessel.*
2. *What is the basis for the development of collateral circulation?*
3. *Why did Mr. Brown have the symptoms described?*
4. *What is the relationship between smoking and atherosclerotic arterial disease?*
5. *Describe the principle of Doppler studies and how a femoral arteriogram is done.*
6. *How would the surgical procedure recommended restore arterial circulation?*

See Appendix G for discussion.

Lesions tend to be located at the bifurcations of the arch vessels and the common carotid arteries.[10] The proximal left subclavian artery is the most frequently affected, excluding the common carotid artery occlusions, which are described in Chapter 50. Upper extremity ischemia is very uncommon due, in part, to the *subclavian steal.* This phenomenon refers to cerebral ischemia that results from a flow off of blood from the circle of Willis back through the affected side vertebral artery to the ischemic arm. The steal is invariably produced by exercising the arm and diversion of cerebral flow retrograde to the arm.[10] The syndrome usually presents with the typical picture of transient ischemic attacks or other central nervous system dysfunction. Diagnostic studies, especially using Doppler techniques, will demonstrate obstruction to blood flow.

AORTIC AND ARTERIAL ANEURYSMS

An aneurysm is a localized dilation of the wall of an artery. It develops at a site of weakness of the medial layer of the artery. Aneurysms may be classified as abdominal or thoracic according to their location on the aorta. Pathologically, they may be described as fusiform, dissecting hematomas, or saccular on the basis of their appearance. Some aneurysms are found on the peripheral arteries, especially those in the cerebral circulation or at sites of surgical incisions (false aneurysms). Most aneurysms are atherosclerotic, but they may result from congenital defects, infections such as syphilis, and trauma.

Fusiform aneurysms produce circumferential dilatation of the vessel. The wall balloons out on all sides (Fig. 27-5). As the process is occurring, the aneurysmal sac fills with necrotic debris and thrombus. Calcium infiltrates the area. The sac dilates because of a weakened medial layer. The dangers of this type of aneurysm include rupture, embolization to a peripheral artery, pressure on surrounding structures, and obstruction of blood flow to organs supplied by the tributary arteries.

Abdominal Aortic Aneurysms

Almost all abdominal aortic aneurysms are fusiform and atherosclerotic, and most arise at a level below the branchings of the renal arteries. They often extend to and include the iliac arteries (see Figure 27-5).[9] These aneurysms are three to four times more common in men than in women and are often found in persons in the seventh or eighth decade of life.[10, 17] Clinical manifestations are usually nonexistent. Occasionally, the person discovers a pulsatile abdominal mass. More frequently, the aneurysm is discovered when a physical examination is performed for some other reason, such as vague abdominal symptoms or poor peripheral circulation. Pain of recent onset may herald an expanding aneurysm with impending rupture.[10]

Rupture may cause the initial symptoms, with bleeding frequently occurring into the retroperitoneal space. In such instances, exsanguination is generally prevented due to the location of the hemorrhage. The initial symptoms of this type of hemorrhage include abdominal pain and symptoms of hemorrhagic shock. Pressure from a large or enlarging abdominal aortic aneurysm on surrounding abdominal organs, together with lack of blood supply to the intestines, can precipitate ileus or intestinal obstruction.

Physical examination reveals a pulsatile abdominal mass. This is almost a diagnostic finding. Due to intra-aneurysmal clot, the size of the aneurysm may not be appreciated on angiographic studies.[9] A radiograph of the abdomen often confirms the presence of the aneurysm due to a rim of calcification that is seen in the wall of the vessel.

Thoracic Aneurysms

Thoracic aortic aneurysms may be caused by atherosclerosis, necrosis of the medial layer, and syphilis. Atherosclerotic aneurysms are usually fusiform and may be located in the ascending, arch, or descending segments of the aorta. Those that result from medial necrosis are usually dissecting in nature, whereas syphilitic aneurysms are often saccular (see below).

Most thoracic aneurysms are asymptomatic and are detected incidentally on chest radiograph.[10] The most common clinical manifestation of thoracic aneurysms is deep, aching back pain. This may be associated with erosion of the ribs or may be an indication that the aneurysm is expanding and that rupture may be imminent.[10] Compression of respiratory structures and of the

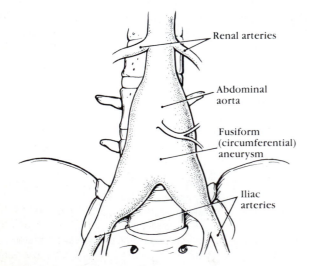

FIGURE 27-5 *Fusiform aneurysm of the aorta.*

Renal arteries

Abdominal aorta

Fusiform (circumferential) aneurysm

Iliac arteries

recurrent laryngeal nerve may cause dyspnea, hoarseness, and coughing. Rupture as the initial manifestation is usually fatal.

Dissecting Aneurysms

Dissecting aneurysms are also called *dissecting hematomas*. An intimal tear and degeneration of the medial layer allow blood to separate the intimal layer from the adventitial layer (Fig. 27-6). Weakening of the medial layer appears to be essential in the production of dissection.[5] Aortic dissection most frequently occurs in the ascending aorta.[2, 10] Eighty percent of persons with this problem also have systemic hypertension. It also may be associated with the hereditary disorder called *Marfan syndrome*, which is characterized by degeneration of the elastic fibers of the aortic media, usually beginning at the aortic root and spreading segmentally throughout the aorta. Physical examination reveals long arms and legs, thin hands and feet, lax ligaments, and deformities of the thoracic cage.[2]

The clinical manifestations of dissection often present a striking change in appearance. External rupture may lead to exsanguination, but more often, the process involves dissection from the initial point away from the heart. As it dissects through the aortic segment, it often causes obstruction to vessels branching off the aorta. If it occurs across the arch of the aorta, color changes and cerebral ischemia may be noted suddenly. Aortic regurgitation may result if the dissection occurs through the aortic valve. The affected person usually complains of the sudden onset of severe, tearing chest pain that radiates to the back, abdomen, and hips.[4, 10] Mortality of

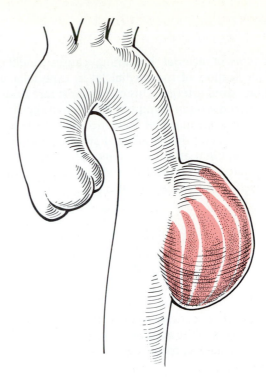

FIGURE 27-7 *Saccular aneurysm of the descending aorta.*

dissecting hematomas is very high. In the initial 24 hours after dissection, it is 35% and continues to be high in the first and second weeks. Two of the main factors that determine mortality are the place of origin of dissection and whether the process is self-limiting.[2]

Saccular Aneurysms

Saccular aneurysms are more frequently associated with syphilis or congenital malformations rather than atherosclerosis. They are characterized by an outpouching on one side of an artery (Fig. 27-7). Common congenital saccular aneurysms are described as *berry aneurysms* when they occur on the arteries of the circle of Willis. The danger of the intracerebral aneurysms is intracranial rupture and bleeding, which often is fatal (see Chapter 52).

Saccular syphilitic aneurysms most frequently arise on the ascending and descending thoracic aorta. These can compress the mediastinal structures, cause pressure on the surrounding skeletal structures, thrombose, or rupture. Syphilitic or luetic aneurysms are rarely reported in the United States because of improved treatment and measures to control syphilis.[1]

One of the most common aneurysms is the *false aneurysm* that may form at a surgical site for arterial repair. These have been reported after revascularization surgeries, such as aorto-iliac bypass of the lower extremities and repair of arteries damaged by trauma. This aneurysm may erode into a surrounding structure and rupture, causing grave effects.[4]

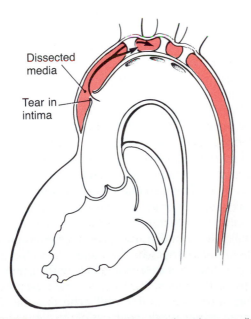

Dissected media

Tear in intima

FIGURE 27-6 *Consequences of dissection from the ascending aorta across the arch of the aorta.*

MÖNCKEBERG'S SCLEROSIS (MEDIAL CALCIFIC SCLEROSIS)

This type of arterial hardening causes ringlike, focal calcification of the medial layer, especially in the medium-sized arteries. This condition is rare under age 50 years and is often asymptomatic even in aged individuals.[2] It is seen in equal incidence in both sexes. The vessels most commonly affected are the femoral, tibial, radial, and ulnar arteries. In some cases, atherosclerosis is associated with the calcification process, but the process itself is not atherosclerotic.

ARTERIOLOSCLEROSIS

Arteriolosclerosis, as its name implies, involves degeneration of the intima and media of small arteries and arterioles. When this affects the kidney, hypertension results, but hypertension often is the initiator of the condition. It also may occur in the peripheral arteries and arterioles of the aged and is often considered to be a part of the aging process.

ARTERIOSPASTIC DISORDERS

Raynaud's phenomenon is the clinical syndrome of episodic constriction of the small arteries or arterioles of the extremities, resulting in intermittent pallor and cyanosis of the skin of the extremities. After an episode of constriction, hyperemia may produce rubor. Raynaud's phenomenon may occur in association with several conditions and diseases. Thus, it is a vasospastic disorder that produces temporary changes in skin color and is often secondary to some underlying disorder.[14] A large group of seemingly unrelated conditions may share this as one of their features (Table 27-5). The link with connective tissue disease, especially scleroderma, is notable in that Raynaud's phenomenon may precede the skin changes by months or years.[14] This type of Raynaud's phenomenon is termed secondary Raynaud's phenomenon, and when the symptoms are present the evaluation for the presence of an underlying condition is critical in its diagnosis.

Raynaud's phenomenon (primary Raynaud's phenomenon or Raynaud's disease) occurs predominantly in women, and heredity may play a role in its development. Onset of symptoms usually begins between ages 20 and 40 years. Because investigators rarely are able to examine sections of the blood vessels in cases of early Raynaud's disease, little is known of the pathologic changes in the initial stages. In advanced stages, the intima of the digital arteries is thickened.

The typical clinical picture of primary Raynaud's phenomenon is color changes on exposure to cold. At first, only the tips of the fingers are involved, but later, the more proximal parts also exhibit color changes. All of the fingers of both hands usually undergo color changes that include pallor, cyanosis, and rubor. The sequential change from pallor to cyanosis and finally to rubor is characteristic.[15]

Pallor is caused by spasm of the arterioles and possibly the venules. During this time, blood flow into the capillaries is decreased or absent, causing the affected part to appear dead white. Cyanosis results from capillary dilatation, which occurs later in the course of the disease. Blood flow becomes sluggish with extraction of more oxygen. Rubor indicates excessive hyperemia due to reactive vasodilatation. Exposure to emotional or thermal (cold) stimuli initiate vasoconstriction with subsequent color changes in the digits. Pain characterizes advanced disease, often associated with ulceration on the tips of the digits. Paresthesia, such as numbness, tingling, throbbing, and a dull ache may be present. During an actual attack, coldness of the digits is evident, sensory acuity is decreased, and the involved digits may swell. Table 27-6 compares the clinical features of pri-

---

TABLE 27-5 *Mechanistic Classification of Raynaud's Phenomenon*

Vasospastic
    Primary (idiopathic) Raynaud's phenomenon
    Drug-induced
        β-Adrenergic blockers
        Ergot
        Methysergide
    Pheochromocytoma
    Variant angina
    Migraine
Structural
Vibration syndrome
    Arteriosclerosis
    Thromboangiitis obliterans
    Cold injury (frostbite, pernio, immersion foot)
    Neurovascular compression (thoracic outlet syndrome, carpal tunnel syndrome, crutch pressure)
    Chemotherapy (bleomycin, vinblastine)
    Polyvinyl chloride disease
    Connective tissue disease
        Systemic sclerosis
        Systemic lupus erythematosus
        Overlap syndrome
        Polymyositis/dermatomyositis
        Rheumatoid arthritis
Hemorrheologic
    Cryoglobulinemia
    Cryofibrinogenemia
    Cold agglutinin disease
    Paraproteinemia (plasma cell dyscrasia)
    Polycythemia (essential thrombocythemia, polycythemia vera)

Source: W. N. Kelley, *Textbook of Internal Medicine*, 2nd ed. Philadelphia: J.B. Lippincott, 1992.

TABLE 27-6 *Clinical Features Helpful in Distinguishing Primary Raynaud's Phenomenon From Raynaud's Phenomenon of Early Connective Tissue Disease*

Feature	Primary Raynaud's Phenomenon	Raynaud's Phenomenon Secondary to Connective Tissue Disease
Sex	Overwhelmingly female	Male or female
Age of onset	Menarche	Mid-20s and later
Extent of involvement	Usually all digits	Frequently a single digit to start
Frequency of attacks*	Usually >10/d	Usually 0–5/d
Symptoms	Mild to moderate	Moderate to severe
Symptoms also precipitated by emotional stress	Yes	Rarely
Evidence of ischemic injury (eg, ulcers or loss of finger pulp)	No	Yes
Finger edema	Rare	Common
Periungual erythema	Rare	Common
Evidence of other vasomotor syndromes (eg, migraine or livedo reticularis)	Yes	No

*Frequency of attacks is somewhat variable and depends on climate.
Source: W. N. Kelley, *Textbook of Internal Medicine.* Philadelphia: J.B. Lippincott, 1992.

mary Raynaud's phenomenon with that picture associated with connective tissue disease.

THROMBOANGIITIS OR BUERGER'S DISEASE

Buerger's disease affects the small and medium-sized arteries and medium-sized, mostly superficial, veins of the extremities. It is mainly seen in young men between ages 20 and 35 years, but the frequency is increasing in women. It is almost invariably a disease that affects persons who use tobacco. It frequently results in arterial occlusion, causing ischemia and gangrene to the extremities. The nonatherosclerotic lesion consists of microabscesses that have a central focus of polymorphonuclear leukocytes usually surrounded by mononuclear cells.[2] Histopathologic evidence indicates that Buerger's disease has some of the characteristics of a collagen or autoimmune disease.[8]

Clinical manifestations include frequent coexisting migratory phlebitis, early tenderness over the involved vessels, upper extremity involvement, absence of heart disease, marked early venospasm, and generally a low serum cholesterol concentration.

Pathologically, the disease has the following outstanding characteristics:

1. Thromboangiitis is primarily a disease of the blood vessels of the extremities. It involves the lower extremities more severely than the upper extremities.

2. The disease almost always develops in medium-sized or small arteries. Arteries commonly involved are the posterior tibial, anterior tibial, radial, ulnar, plantar, palmar, and digital. Larger arteries, such as the femoral and brachial, are affected late and only when the disease is severe. Small and medium-sized veins are affected less commonly and large veins, rarely.

3. The lesions are focal or segmental and not diffuse.

4. The lesions appear to be of different ages but, in general, the disease throughout a single affected segment seems to be of essentially the same age.

5. The disease produces occlusions of the vessels, followed by development of collateral and anastomotic vessels.[2, 8, 9]

The gross characteristics of the vessels affected by thromboangiitis obliterans vary depending on the age of the lesions at the time they are examined. The vessels appear contracted at the site of destruction. The occluded segments are indurated but not brittle. The arteries are more frequently obliterated than their accompanying veins. In the diseased vessel, the occlusion may extend for variable lengths and then stop abruptly. Occlusions may occur at two different levels in the same vessel, and between these sites the vessel may be completely patent.

The most striking physiologic change is the impairment of arterial blood flow. Blood flow through peripheral arteries in the extremities is reduced, particularly in more distal portions. Another factor that contributes to ischemia is arteriolar spasm. The degree of spasm varies among individuals and perhaps with the stage of disease. The degree of arterial insufficiency in the affected extremities depends on two factors: 1) the amount of arterial occlusive disease and 2) the tone of the arterioles, which may vary from normal to moderate or severe spasm.

Venous obstruction, the result of thrombophlebitis, may be an associated factor in the circulatory disturbance in thromboangiitis obliterans. The obstruction is often minor because the venous circulation has a great capacity to develop collateral circulation. In some cases, venous obstruction contributes to malnutrition of capillaries and a tendency to develop edema in the affected extremity if it remains in a dependent position for a long time.

Dependent rubor is caused by the presence of numerous dilated capillaries in skin that contain blood of high oxygen content.[9] Rubor is seen in thromboangiitis that is associated with chronic and moderately severe arterial insufficiency. One explanation, supported by studies of the oxygen content of venous blood, is that capillaries suffer from malnutrition and become atonic, and their capacity to interchange oxygen and other metabolic products is impaired.

▼ Pathologic Processes of Veins

The veins have walls that contract or relax, an intact endothelium to prevent clotting, and valves that promote blood flow to the heart. Normally, the valves of the larger veins and communicating veins prevent retrograde flow of blood in the superficial and deep veins, which promotes the forward flow of blood.[6] The system provides a venous pump, which makes it possible for the person to be in an upright position. When a person is standing, the pressure of blood in the feet rises to about 90 mm Hg. When standing is continued, as much as 15% to 20% of the blood volume can be sequestered and effectively lost from the circulation.[6] Walking causes the muscles to contract and squeeze blood into the veins and propel it toward the heart. When the muscles relax the venous valves prevent the backflow of blood to the periphery.[6] The structure of the veins, discussed on page 429, provides the basis for normal return of blood to the heart.

OBSTRUCTIVE DISEASE OF VEINS

Obstructive lesions of the veins may be permanent or temporary, partial or complete. Obstruction to some portion of the main trunk causes the distal large veins to become dilated, causing incompetent valves. The small veins and venules may be damaged permanently as a result of pressure, stretching, hypoxemia, and malnutrition. Permanent impairment in interchange of fluid may result from disruption of small vessels. Damaged venous capillaries may function normally when the person is in a recumbent position but show inadequacy in a standing position. This inadequacy is due to increased hydrostatic pressure and sometimes to associated incompetent valves.

Venous Thrombosis

Lesions in veins may produce localized thrombi in small veins or extensive thrombi in the larger veins. Classically, it is associated with Virchow's triad: 1) venous stasis; 2) changes in the wall of the vein; and 3) a hypercoagulable state.[6] Venous thrombosis may develop as a result of an inflammatory or traumatic lesion of the endothelium of the vein wall. In most cases, however, there is no evidence of either. An inflammatory reaction may develop in the wall of the vein as a reaction to primary thrombosis, so that phlebitis may ensue several hours after the thrombus is formed.

The lesions of the endothelium, relative stasis of venous blood flow, and hypercoagulability of blood are three identified factors that precipitate venous thrombosis. One or a combination of these factors may produce a thrombus. A thrombus develops as a result of slowed flow in the venous bloodstream and is associated with platelet aggregation. After several days and after development of a secondary reaction in the wall of the thrombosed vein, a sudden proximal extension may protrude from the end of the original organizing thrombus. Emboli may develop at this time from the proximal extension, or the new clot may stick and become organized. Emboli may be small or large and tend to lodge in the vessels of the pulmonary circulation (see pp. 604–606).[2]

A thrombus organizes from its outer margins centrally. In some veins, the entire thrombus becomes organized, with complete and permanent occlusion of the lumen. In a large thrombus, involution usually occurs by a process of partial fibrosis and partial lysis, which is probably due to the action of naturally occurring fibrinolysins in the blood. In most cases, the center disappears and a varying portion of the periphery may organize on a fibrous ring. In other instances, bands of fibrous tissue extend across the old lumen of the vein and divide it into many small lumina. The result is usually some restoration of function of the vein, but the lumen is partially obstructed by the remaining fibrous tissue and decrease of its circular diameter.[16]

The degree of inflammatory reaction in the different layers of the veins varies. In some persons, the thrombus causes minimal reaction, whereas in others an intense reaction extends throughout all layers. Inflammatory cells, leukocytes, lymphocytes, and fibroblasts accumulate and cause congestion of capillaries in and around the venous wall. Venous thrombosis causes obstruction to venous blood flow and relates to the size and location of the involved vein. If it occurs in superficial veins and in short segments, collateral circulation will compensate.

This may also be true in obstruction of the saphenous vein of the leg or a larger vein of the arm (eg, median basilic or cephalic) because of the numerous anastomoses that occur. Collateral channels may become evident even after obstruction of the superior or inferior vena cava.[8]

When thrombosis occurs in the iliofemoral or axillary veins, the collateral circulation compensates only partially, and venous pressure increases in the veins distal to the thrombosis. This increased pressure results in distension of all veins and even venules of the limb. The increased pressure in the venules and capillaries causes intense congestion of these areas. Pressure changes inhibit normal reabsorption of fluid and electrolytes from the tissues in the venous end of the capillaries. Edema of the affected limb then develops.

THROMBOPHLEBITIS AND PHLEBOTHROMBOSIS

Thrombophlebitis refers to an inflamed vein as a result of a thrombus. Phlebothrombosis is probably the same entity but does not exhibit a marked inflammatory component. Deep venous thrombosis refers to either thrombophlebitis or phlebothrombosis in the deep venous system of the legs.[13] Thrombosis in a vein ultimately causes inflammatory changes.[2]

Idiopathic thrombophlebitis is a recurrent condition that produces segmental lesions in the small and medium-sized veins. The thrombus may be recanalized and the lumen restored, but more frequently the vein becomes completely obliterated. *Suppurative thrombophlebitis* differs in that it usually results from bacterial invasion. The wall of the vein becomes markedly inflamed and leukocytes infiltrate the area. Bacteria within the thrombus and portions of the endothelium ultimately lead to abscesses. The abscesses may rupture into the bloodstream. *Chemical thrombophlebitis* may result from venous irritation from drugs (eg, antibiotics or potassium) or other chemicals that gain access to the venous circulation. The thrombus becomes adherent and completely organized, resulting in a vein that is contracted, fibrotic, and cordlike.

The symptoms and signs of thrombophlebitis develop acutely and usually persist for 1 to 3 weeks. In small or medium-sized veins, acute thrombophlebitis rarely produces systemic reactions. With involvement of the larger vessels, temperature may rise to as high as 102°F (39°C). Thrombosis of superficial veins often involves redness, pain, tenderness, and localized edema.

Thrombosis of the deep veins of the legs may produce calf pain and tenderness in the calf muscles. Enlargement of the calf and a positive Homans' sign may result. Homans' sign refers to pain in the calf muscle when the foot is dorsiflexed. Thrombosis of the iliofemoral vein usually produces a typical, acute, clinical picture. Moderate to severe pain in the thigh and groin with diffuse pain throughout the limb is described. Superficial veins may be prominent and distended in an enlarged limb. The skin of the leg and thigh may be slightly cyanotic. Thrombosis may be accompanied by impaired or absent pulses from associated arterial spasm. Fever and tachycardia may also be associated. Pitting edema is characteristic with onset a few days after the obstruction ensues. As the edema becomes chronic, it may be associated with skin changes and brawny edema (thick, hardened skin with nonpitting edema).

Thrombosis of the axillary and subclavian veins produces a clinical picture similar to that of iliofemoral thrombosis. The axillary vein becomes tender, prominent, and enlarged with pitting edema in the forearm and hand. Superficial veins of the entire arm are prominent, and those of the pectoral region on the affected side may be distended.

Diagnosis of venous thrombosis involves tests, such as venous Doppler studies, that identify venous patency through Doppler ultrasound, which detects the movement of red blood cells through the vein. The Doppler studies are usually used in the deep venous system of the ankle, calf, thigh, and groin.[11]

VENOUS INSUFFICIENCY AND STASIS

Chronic venous insufficiency results from stasis of venous blood flow, especially of the iliofemoral veins. Old iliofemoral thrombophlebitis leaves behind a thickened, inelastic vein wall, damaged venous valves, and a partially or sometimes completely obstructed lumen. In the lower extremity, the three groups of veins—deep, communicating, and superficial—normally have thin, elastic walls and segmentally spaced valves of the bicuspid type. As described earlier, venous flow against gravity in the lower limbs is possible by action of the calf muscle and the competent valves. Muscular compression of the elastic veins forces blood upward, and the valves prevent retrograde flow. This mechanism fails in chronic venous insufficiency, usually because of incompetent valves. The result is venous hypertension in the affected system.

Ambulatory venous pressure becomes high, and this upsets the normal equilibrium of capillary fluid exchange, causing congestion and edema. Stasis also results from the high ambulatory pressures, as manifested by changes in the skin and subcutaneous tissues around the distal one-third of the leg and around the ankle. Changes that may occur include edema, hyperpigmentation, dermatitis, induration, stasis cellulitis, and, ultimately, venostasis ulcers (Fig. 27-8). The amount of edema varies according to length of dependency of the affected limb. There is characteristically a light brown pigmentation in white skin and a darker pigmentation in black skin. The edema is brawny and

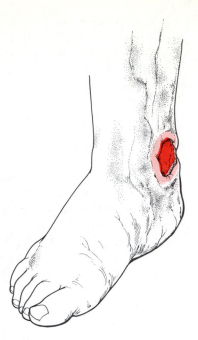

FIGURE 27-8 *Stasis dermatitis with a stasis ulcer from long-term venous stasis.*

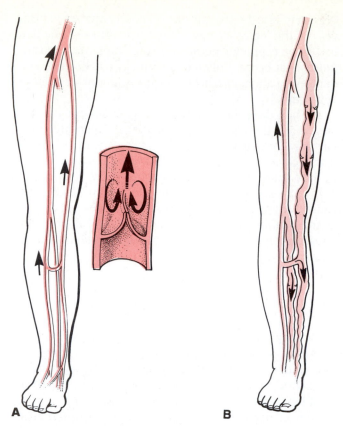

FIGURE 27-9 *Varicose veins.* **A.** *Normal vein with competent valves.* **B.** *Incompetent valves with tortuous, dilated segments. Promotes stasis of blood in lower extremities.*

often feels hard to the touch. Pain may be present. A dull ache in the affected leg may develop after the person has been standing for variable periods. Pain is usually described as being more severe when standing still rather than when walking. The pain usually disappears within 5 to 30 minutes after assumption of a recumbent position with the leg elevated. Nocturnal muscular cramps may be reported.

VARICOSE VEINS

Varicose veins are dilated, elongated, and tortuous superficial veins of the lower extremities.[13] They are produced by incompetent valves and increased intraluminal pressure (Fig. 27-9). Varicose veins vary from a small group of dilated veins to a distension of the whole venous system of the leg.[13] Varicosities probably develop because of an inherent weakness in the structure of the vein. Superficial veins dilate when normal resistance against intraluminal pressure is lacking. Primary varicose veins may develop from hereditary predisposition, pregnancy, standing for a long time, and marked obesity. Prolonged periods of standing favor development of varicosities because of the high gravitational pressure within the veins. Obesity tends to place external pressure on the veins, especially the iliofemoral veins. An estimated 10% to 20% of the general population have varicose veins, with women affected four times more often than men.[2]

Deep thrombophlebitis often gives rise to secondary varicosities. Loss of valve sufficiency produces unusual strain on the superficial veins. A common finding is the presence of localized dilations just distal to the venous valves. Valve incompetency is due primarily to extreme dilatation in the affected veins, which causes separation of the valve cusps. In primary varicose veins, the incompetency tends to progress downward in the saphenous main channel and in its tributaries. In secondary varicose veins, which arise because of deep vein insufficiency, the incompetency tends to progress upward from incompetent perforating veins in the lower one-third of the leg.[9]

Varicose veins can lead to chronic venous insufficiency. In the early stages, localized pain and heat may be noticed after prolonged standing. Persistent edema may develop, together with trophic skin changes and stasis ulcers. The stasis ulcers heal slowly and often become infected.

Diagnosis of venous insufficiency can be made by assessment of physical findings and, occasionally, phlebography. *Phlebography* involves injecting radiopaque material into the venous system and taking radiographs of the injected area. It is performed to localize deep-vein thrombosis or to evaluate varicosities.

▼ Pathologic Processes of the Lymphatic System

The lymphatic system serves the essential function of draining excess fluids and proteins from the interstitial space. It provides the only means for returning plasma proteins that have leaked into this space to the general circulation. Whenever tissue fluid levels increase, lymphatic drainage also increases.

In this way, lymphatic flow is an essential method for control of tissue fluid volume. Venous obstruction and congestive heart failure have been identified as factors that can alter capillary pressure and produce edema. When fluids continually escape into the interstitial spaces, edema may not be noted because of this increased lymphatic drainage, which is a compensation by the lymphatic system.

Obstruction of the lymph vessels interferes with this control mechanism and may precipitate or contribute to edema. Numerous factors may cause lymphedema, and these are categorized as inflammatory or noninflammatory. *Lymphangitis* refers to inflammation of the lymph vessels, usually by bacterial organisms. *Lymphadenitis* refers to inflammation of the lymph nodes. *Lymphedema* specifies edema resulting from lymphatic obstruction.[5] Primary or idiopathic lymphedema is rare. Milroy's disease, a congenital lymphedema noticeable at birth, is usually caused by faulty development of lymphatic channels. *Lymphedema praecox* affects females predominantly between ages 9 and 25 years. It is characterized by swelling of one or both feet that becomes progressive and unremitting. The lymphatic channels are dilated due to incompetent lymph valves.

Secondary lymphedema is much more common than the primary form. Obstruction of the lymph channels may result from malignant metastatic infiltration of the lymph nodes and channels. Inflammation or infection of the channels may result in fibrosis and obstruction. A common cause of lymphedema is the surgical removal or irradiation of lymph nodes to prevent the spread of a malignancy.

Lymphedema is essentially the result of stasis. Chronic stasis often leads to *brawny edema*, which describes the appearance of the skin subjected to continual stretch. The skin becomes thick, hardened, infiltrated with plasma proteins, and often "orange peel" in appearance. This edema is different from cardiac edema in that it does not pit on digital pressure.

Inflammatory lymphedema usually occurs after an acute infection of the lymphatic system. Lymphangitis is characterized by painful red streaks following the lymph vessels, which may eventually involve the lymph nodes as well. The agent that most commonly causes lymphangitis is betahemolytic streptococcus, but any virulent pathogen may initiate it. Systemic effects include a marked temperature elevation, malaise, and chills. Localized edema occurs and may become progressive if attacks are recurrent. *Chronic lymphangitis* may follow, causing fibrosis of the affected area, further edema, skin changes, and sometimes ulcerations.

Diagnosis of lymphedema is done primarily to differentiate it from edema of venous origin. Lymphangiography involves injecting radiopaque dye into the affected lymph vessel and monitoring its passage radiologically. This procedure may localize the source of the obstruction.

▼ Diagnostic Procedures for Vascular Lesions

PHYSICAL EXAMINATION

Diagnosis of vascular system problems is usually based on the signs and symptoms of arterial occlusion or of venous insufficiency. Palpation of the peripheral pulses is important in estimating blood flow in the peripheral arterial circuit. Systolic bruits over the abdominal area and femoral artery are common and, in association with other signs, may indicate peripheral arterial disease. Bruits refer to sounds produced in the blood vessels, usually only audible if some factor is obstructing blood flow. Tenderness to palpation or tenderness with the inflation of a blood pressure cuff over the calf or thigh (Löwenberg's cuff sign) gives high suspicion for deep-vein thrombosis. Pain on dorsiflexion of the foot with stretching of the gastrocnemius muscle (Homans' sign) also may be present.[8] Ankle edema, especially unilateral, may be seen. Many procedures may be performed to diagnose vascular lesions.

DOPPLER ULTRASOUND

This procedure involves the use of a Doppler recorder to hear flow over the larger veins. Flow is normally increased by distal compression of the vein and decreased by Valsalva's maneuver and varies with respiration. Lack of flow sound may indicate venous thrombosis. Arterial lesions also may be evaluated by Doppler studies. The proximal and distal pressures of the suspected lesion are auscultated to determine the pressure gradient. The Doppler flowmeter is used at the ankle to compare arterial pressure there with brachial systolic pressure.

ANGIOGRAPHY

Angiography involves the use of a contrast material of high opacity to outline the great vessels, particularly the aorta and its branches. The contrast material may be injected into an artery, vein, or chamber of the heart.

In persons with symptoms of obstruction involving the superior vena cava, angiography shows the site and extent of obstruction and may give other important data about it. Angiography also may be of great value in studying known aneurysms of the thoracic aorta.

Peripheral Arteriography and Aortography

In this procedure, the femoral artery is cannulated and the catheter is placed in the appropriate position. This approach may be used to pass a catheter retrograde up the aorta to the desired position for radiopaque dye injection, or the catheter may be left in the femoral artery to visualize the lower arterial circulation (see Figure 27-4). The clinical usefulness of this procedure is in the precise localization of atherosclerotic disease or in thromboangitis obliterans and aneurysms. This method may be used to selectively inject dye into any aortic tributary by moving the catheter to the ostium of the selected artery and injecting dye. The risk of bleeding is less than in other approaches and can be more quickly assessed.

Venography

Venography, also called phlebography, is an x-ray contrast study that identifies thrombi in the venous system. It is accomplished by injecting dye into the venous system, and films are taken of the area to visualize a filling defect. The procedure is performed by catheterizing a superficial vein on the foot and injecting dye. The subsequent films follow the movement of the dye through the venous system up to the inferior vena cava.[11]

▼ Chapter Summary

▼ Peripheral vascular disease is a term used to describe disease of the arteries, veins, or lymphatics. In practice, it is used to describe arterial disease.

▼ The most common cause of arterial disease is atherosclerosis, which results from a disorder of lipid metabolism and the deposition of fibrofatty plaque on the inner lining of the arteries. It is thought that the plaque development is a reaction to the laying down of the fatty material on the intimal surface. The atherosclerotic lesions gradually enlarge, ulcerate, hemorrhage, and become thrombosed. As this happens, circulation to the area supplied by the artery becomes compromised. The induction of atherosclerosis is mainly dietary but may be familial (genetic).

▼ Occlusive disease of the lower extremities is usually in the larger arteries and is seen in persons over the age of 50. It is increased in severity when associated with diabetes mellitus. The clinical manifestations include pain, coldness, color changes, ulceration, and gangrene. De-

pending on the location, there may be associated thrombophlebitis or sexual dysfunction.

▼ Arterial aneurysms are most commonly seen in the aorta, especially the abdominal aorta, and are caused by atherosclerotic weakening of the vessel.

▼ Dissecting hematomas involve weakness of the medial layer of the artery and are often associated with hypertension.

▼ Saccular aneurysms are most commonly caused by congenital weakness of the vessels, especially of those on the circle of Willis in the brain.

▼ Syphilis can cause weakening of a portion of the arterial wall, or the "false" aneurysm may form at the site of a surgical incision.

▼ Arteriospastic disorders are either idiopathic or associated with various connective tissue diseases.

▼ Buerger's disease is a special condition that affects the small and medium-sized arteries and veins, with phlebitis and arterial involvement of lower and upper extremities, including vasospasm and thrombotic occlusion.

▼ Venous diseases include venous thrombosis, thrombophlebitis, and phlebothrombosis. These may be associated with varicose veins and may promote venous insufficiency and stasis.

▼ The lymphatic system may be affected by obstruction, which causes lymphedema, a brawny edema that does not pit on digital pressure. Inflammatory lymphedema is characterized by painful red streaks that follow the lymph vessels and usually is caused by a virulent microorganism.

▼ References

1. Cheitlin, M.D., Sokolow, M., and McIlroy, M.B. *Clinical Cardiology* (6th ed.). Norwalk, Conn: Appleton-Lange. 1993.
2. Cotran, R.S., Kumar, V., and Robbins, S.L. *Robbins' Pathologic Basis of Disease* (5th ed.). Philadelphia: W.B. Saunders, 1994.
3. Fogelman, A.M., Murphy, F.L., and Edwards, P.A. Pathogenesis of atherosclerosis. In W.N. Kelley (ed.), *Textbook of Internal Medicine* (2nd ed.). Philadelphia: J.B. Lippincott, 1992.
4. Glover, J.L. Aneurysms and occlusive diseases of the aorta and peripheral vessels. In W.N. Kelley (ed.), *Textbook of Internal Medicine* (2nd ed.). Philadelphia: J.B. Lippincott, 1992.
5. Glover, J.L. Diseases of the veins. In W.N. Kelley (ed.), *Textbook of Internal Medicine* (2nd ed.). Philadelphia: J.B. Lippincott, 1992.
6. Glover, J.L. Miscellaneous vascular problems. In W.N. Kelley (ed.), *Textbook of Internal Medicine* (2nd ed.). Philadelphia: J.B. Lippincott, 1992.
7. Guyton, A. *Textbook of Medical Physiology* (8th ed.). Philadelphia: W.B. Saunders, 1991.

8. Joyce, J.W. The diagnosis and management of diseases of the peripheral arteries and veins. In R.C. Schlant and R.W. Alexander (eds.), *Hurst's The Heart* (8th ed.). New York: McGraw-Hill, 1994.

9. Juergens, J.L., Fairbairn, J.E. II, and Spittell, J.A. Jr. *Peripheral Vascular Diseases* (5th ed.). Philadelphia: W.B. Saunders, 1986.

10. Lindsay, J., DeBakey, M.E., and Beall, A.C. Diseases of the aorta. In R.C. Schlant and R.W. Alexander, et al. (eds.), *Hurst's The Heart* (8th ed.). New York: McGraw-Hill, 1994.

11. Pagana, K.D., and Pagana, T.J. *Mosby's Diagnostic and Laboratory Test Reference*. St. Louis: C.V. Mosby, 1992.

12. Ross, R. Factors influencing atherogenesis. In R.C. Schlant and R.W. Alexander, et al. (eds.), *Hurst's The Heart* (8th ed.). New York: McGraw-Hill, 1994.

13. Rubin, E. and Farber, J.L. *Pathology* (2nd ed.). Philadelphia: J.B. Lippincott, 1994.

14. Seibold, J.R. Management of Raynaud's phenomenon and scleroderma. In W.N. Kelley (ed.), *Textbook of Internal Medicine* (2nd ed.). Philadelphia: J.B. Lippincott, 1992.

15. Silver, R.M. Raynaud's phenomenon. In J.H. Stein (ed.), *Internal Medicine* (4th ed.). St. Louis: C.V. Mosby, 1994.

16. Spittell, P.C., and Spittell, J.A. Diseases of the peripheral arteries and veins. In J.H. Stein (ed.), *Internal Medicine* (4th ed.). St. Louis: C.V. Mosby, 1994.

17. Zabalgoitia, M., and O'Rourke, R.A. Diseases of the aorta. In J.H. Stein (ed.), *Internal Medicine* (4th ed.). St. Louis: C.V. Mosby, 1994.

▼ *Unit Bibliography*

Baker, J.D. Assessment of peripheral arterial occlusive disease. *Crit. Care Clin. North. Am.* 3:493, 1991.

Barnett, D.B., Pouleur, H. and Francis, G.S. *Congestive Cardiac Failure: Pathophysiology and Treatment*. New York: M. Dekker, 1993.

Cheitlin, M.D., Sokolow, M., and McIlroy, M.B. *Clinical Cardiology* (6th ed.). Norwalk, Conn.: Appleton & Lange, 1994.

Conover, M.B. VT or SVT? *Crit. Care Nurse* 9:2, 1989.

Cotran, R., Kumar, V., and Robbins, S. *Robbin's Pathologic Basis of Disease* (5th ed.). Philadelphia: W.B. Saunders, 1994.

Das, D.K. *Pathophysiology of Reperfusion Injury*. Boca Raton: CRC, 1993.

Evans, C.A., and Burdon, R.H. *Free Radical Damage and Its Control*. New York: Elsevier, 1994.

Fink, B.W. *Congenital Heart Disease: A Deductive Approach to Its Diagnosis* (2nd ed.). Chicago: Year Book, 1985.

Fletcher, G.F. *Cardiovascular Responses to Exercise*. Mt. Kisco, NY: Futural, 1994.

Fray, J.C.S., and Douglas, J.G. *Pathophysiology of Hypertension in Blacks*. New York: American Physiology Society by Oxford University Press, 1993.

Ganong, W.F. *Review of Medical Physiology* (16th ed.). Norwalk, Conn.: Appleton-Lange. 1993.

Govan, A.D.T., Macfarlane, P.S., and Callander, R. *Pathology Illustrated* (3rd ed.). New York: Churchill-Livingstone, 1991.

Gravanis, M.B. *Cardiovascular Disorders: Pathogenesis and Pathophysiology*. St. Louis: Mosby Year Book, 1993.

Gwathmey, J.K., Briggs, G.M., and Allen, P.D. *Heart Failure: Basic Science and Clinical Aspects*. New York: M. Dekker, 1993.

Hosenpud, J.D., and Greenberg, B.H. *Congestive Heart Failure: Pathophysiology, Diagnosis, and Complications, Approach to Management*. New York: Springer Verlag, 1994.

Isselbacher, K.J. (ed.). *Harrison's Principles of Internal Medicine* (13th ed.). New York: McGraw-Hill, 1994.

Juergens, J.L., et al. *Peripheral Vascular Disease* (6th ed.). Philadelphia: W.B. Saunders, 1986.

Katz, A.M. *Physiology of the Heart* (2nd ed.). New York: Raven, 1992.

Killip, T. Arrhythmias in myocardial infarction. *Med. Clin. N. Am.* 60:233, 1976.

Langman, J. *Medical Embryology: Human Development: Normal and Abnormal* (2nd ed.). Baltimore: Williams & Wilkins, 1969.

Little, R. *Physiology of the Heart and Circulation* (3rd ed.). Chicago: Year Book, 1986.

Moslen, M.T., and Smith, C.V. *Free Radical Mechanisms of Tissue Injury*. Boca Raton: CRC Press, 1992.

Opie, L.H. *The Heart: Physiology and Metabolisms* (2nd ed.). New York: Raven Press, 1991.

Rowell, L.B. *Human Cardiovascular Control*. New York: Oxford, 1993.

Rubin, E., and Farber, J.L. *Pathology* (2nd ed.). Philadelphia: J.B. Lippincott, 1994.

Schlag, G., and Redl, H. *Pathophysiology of Shock, Sepsis, and Organ Failure*. New York: Springer Verlag, 1993.

Schlant, R.C., and R.W. Alexander. *Hurst's The Heart* (8th ed.). New York: McGraw-Hill, 1994.

Silverman, M.D., et al. *Electrocardiography: Basic Concepts and Clinical Application*. New York: McGraw-Hill, 1983.

Sodeman, W., and Sodeman, W. *Pathologic Physiology* (2nd ed.). Philadelphia: W.B. Saunders, 1986.

Summers, G. The clinical and hemodynamic presentation of the shock patient. *Crit. Care Nurs. Clin. North Am.* 2:2, 1990.

Tarr, M., and Lamson, F. *Oxygen-Free Radicals in Tissue Damage*. Boston: Birkhauser, 1993.

Visant, M., and Spence, M. *Common Sense Approach to Coronary Care* (4th ed.). St. Louis: C.V. Mosby, 1985.

Weber, P.C., and Leaf, A. *Atherosclerosis: Cellular Interactions, Growth Factors, and Lipids*. New York: Raven Press, 1993.

Wilson, J.E. *Vascular Surgery: Principles and Practice*. New York: McGraw-Hill, 1987.

Yellon, D.M., and Jennings, R.B. *Myocardial Protections: The Pathophysiology of Reperfusion and Reperfusion Injury*. New York: Raven Press, 1992.

Respiration

THIS UNIT is divided into four chapters; each deals with aspects of the pulmonary system. Chapter 28 discusses the normal anatomy and physiology of the pulmonary system. It is a review that provides the basis for the material in Chapters 29, 30, and 31, which cover various aspects of pathophysiology of the pulmonary system.

Diseases of the pulmonary system have been categorized as restrictive, obstructive, and other alterations. There is necessarily some overlap among these categories, but an attempt has been made to classify them according to functional impairments. The chapters contain discussion of pathologic, clinical, and diagnostic aspects of pulmonary disease.

The reader is encouraged to use the learning objectives as study guides and to supplement the material with references listed in the unit bibliography. Several case studies are included to provide application of learning concepts.

Chapter *28*

Normal Respiratory Function

Darlene H. Green

▼ **CHAPTER OUTLINE**

▼ **LEARNING OBJECTIVES**

1 Describe the normal basic pulmonary anatomy.
2 Describe the action of the pulmonary pumping mechanism.
3 Identify the mechanisms of nervous control in the respiratory tract.
4 Compare the concepts of compliance and elastance in the normally functioning pulmonary system.
5 Describe the importance of the anatomic dead space in pulmonary function.
6 Identify the major muscles of respiration and their function.
7 Compare tissue resistance and airway resistance.
8 Relate the concept of work of breathing to oxygen consumption and carbon dioxide production.
9 Describe the major patterns of airway resistance.
10 Describe the anatomy and dynamics of pulmonary perfusion.
11 Compare normal ventilation and perfusion from the apex to the base of the lung.
12 List factors that alter normal ventilation and perfusion.
13 List the normal pressures in the heart and pulmonary vascular system.
14 Relate the oxyhemoglobin dissociation curve to tissue oxygenation.
15 Outline the pattern of normal gas exchange.
16 Describe the function of surfactant in the alveoli.
17 Describe the function of alpha$_1$-antitrypsin in the lungs.
18 List the major protective reflexes of the lungs.
19 Explain the function of the mucociliary transport system in the defense of the lungs.
20 Distinguish between humoral and cell-mediated immunity in the lungs.
21 Describe the role of the macrophages in the lungs.

Barbara L. Bullock: PATHOPHYSIOLOGY: ADAPTATIONS AND ALTERATIONS IN FUNCTION, 4th ed.
© 1996 J.B. Lippincott-Raven Publishers

To delineate clearly the pathophysiology of respiratory diseases, this chapter reviews the anatomy and physiology of the pulmonary system and includes an in-depth discussion of the following essential concepts: compliance, elastance, resistance, ventilation, perfusion, diffusion, and alveolar airway clearance in health. A description of pulmonary function tests is also included. To live is to breathe. Between a newborn's first breath and the last expiration is a lifetime of respiration. Breathing is the only bodily function that occurs automatically and can be controlled voluntarily as well. It is also the only bodily function that immediately interacts with the environment, whatever it may be: a fresh ocean breeze, stale cigarette smoke, noxious automobile exhaust, a damp cellar, or a dusty workplace. Normally, breathing occurs below the level of consciousness, rhythmically and inconspicuously, unless some kind of physical stress interferes, such as breathlessness after running, swimming, or climbing a mountain, or when the lungs are impaired by diseases, such as asthma, emphysema, bronchitis, pneumonia, or fibrosis.

The human body must adapt itself continually to an unfriendly environment. The lungs especially are constantly attacked by irritants, gases, and microorganisms. Consequently, the respiratory apparatus has developed an elaborate defense system to protect itself and the body from these inhalants.

The main function of the lungs is to take oxygen from the air and deliver it across the alveolar–capillary membrane to the hemoglobin. Oxygen is transported on hemoglobin by circulating red blood cells to the tissues. At the tissue line, it diffuses across the cellular membrane to the mitochondria to aid in producing energy to support the metabolic processes of life. As a result of these metabolic processes, carbon dioxide is produced, and is transported back to the lungs and expelled into the environmental air.

▼ *Anatomy of the Pulmonary Tree*

AIRWAYS

Air normally enters the body through the nose or the mouth. Here and in the pharynx it is warmed, moistened, and filtered. Even though air has been filtered in the upper respiratory tract, it is not sterile when it reaches the lower respiratory tract. Much debris remains, as evidenced by autopsies of the lungs of cigarette smokers or those exposed to heavy air pollution.

The air passes through the larynx and into the respiratory tree, which is a series of successively smaller, branching tubes (Fig. 28-1). Immediately below the larynx is the trachea, which divides at a point called the carina into the right and left main stem bronchi. The right main stem bronchus is shorter and wider than the left, coming off the trachea in a nearly straight line (see Figure 28-1). This explains why aspirated objects and fluids lodge more frequently in the right lung than

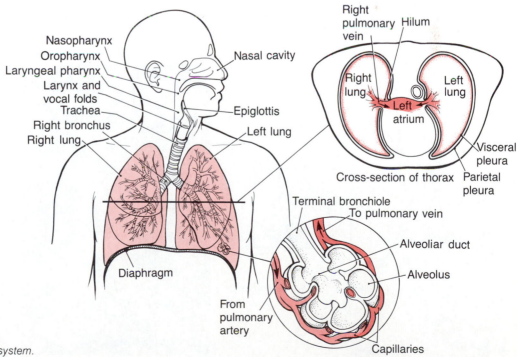

FIGURE 28-1 *The respiratory system.*

in the left. It also makes suctioning of the left main stem bronchus difficult.

The right and left main stem bronchi divide into the lobar bronchi, which divide into the segmental bronchi. The segmental bronchi then divide into the terminal bronchioles. The diameter of each of these successive segments is smaller than the last, but the number of airways in the smaller segments is greater than in the larger ones, providing a broader surface area. This anatomic division, called the *generations of bronchi*, ends at approximately the 16th generation from the trachea. The lower airway divisions are termed bronchi from the main stem (largest) down to the smallest division that contains cartilage. Thereafter, they become bronchioles. The terminal bronchioles branch into the respiratory bronchioles, which open into alveolar ducts and are completely surrounded by alveoli, where gas exchange takes place.

ANATOMY OF THE LUNGS

The lungs lie in the thoracic cavity, separated from each other by the mediastinum. The lungs are cone-shaped with the narrow ends, or *apices*, directed upward and the wide *bases* at the lower portion. Each lung is composed of lobes: three on the right and two on the left. The lobes are divided into smaller compartments called *lobules*. The lobules are further divided into smaller segments and terminate finally in the alveolar sacs.

Surrounding the lungs is the pleural membrane, which provides a covering over the lungs and lines the thoracic wall. The layer overlying the lung parenchyma is called the *visceral pleura* and the outer layer is the *parietal pleura*. Between these layers is a thin film of serous fluid that allows the visceral layer to move on the

parietal layer without friction during normal ventilation. Fluid between these two slick surfaces causes movement like two pieces of wet glass, friction free, but the presence of negative pressure causes the surfaces to adhere tightly to each other. The pleurae glide easily over each other but cannot easily be pulled apart. Between the layers is a potential space called the *intrapleural* or *pleural* space.

PARENCHYMA OF THE LUNGS

The alveolar ducts, the final generation, are totally lined with alveoli (Fig. 28-2). Respiratory exchange of gas (diffusion) takes place only in the alveoli. Therefore, these structures are designated collectively as the respiratory zone of the lungs. Because of their tiny size and large numbers, the alveoli have a volume of about 2,500 mL in the adult. They have a diffusing area (surface area) about the size of a tennis court (approximately 70 m^2). Each terminal bronchiole supplies its own unit which consists of several respiratory bronchioles, each with alveoli arising from its walls. These alveoli do not have separate connections with the terminal bronchiole but are of various shapes and are interconnected, resembling a long corridor with adjacent rooms (the alveoli) on each side.

The individual alveolus is one layer of cells thick and is built on a structure of elastin and muscle fibers. Each alveolus communicates with the pulmonary capillary bed to move gases by diffusion across the *alveolocapillary interspace* (Fig. 28-3). Interconnecting the alveoli are tiny openings called the *pores of Kohn* (Fig. 28-4), which allow air to circulate among the alveoli so that within a second after inspiration all alveoli in an acinus have the same gas concentration. In young children, the pores of

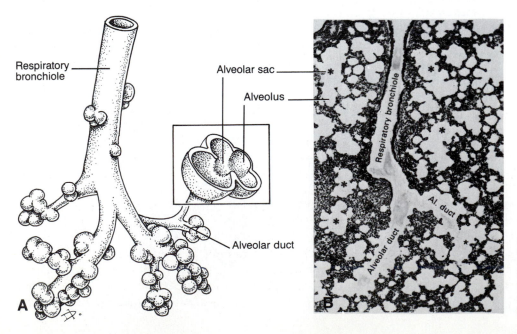

Respiratory bronchiole

Alveolar sac

Alveolus

Alveolar duct

Respiratory bronchiole

Al. duct

Alveolar duct

A

B

FIGURE 28-2 A. *Schematic diagram and* **B.** *low-power view of a respiratory bronchiole leading into alveolar ducts (child's lung). Asterisks in* **B** *indicate alveolar sacs. (Source: D.H. Cormack, Essential Histology. Philadelphia: J.B. Lippincott, 1993)*

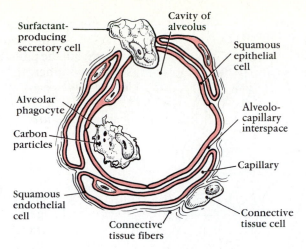

FIGURE 28-3 *Representation of a single alveolus with surrounding capillaries and other cells. Note alveolocapillary interspace.*

Kohn are few in number and poorly developed, but with age these structures increase in number and size.

The pores of Kohn are helpful in the event of obstruction of a small airway. In a process called *collateral ventilation*, if an airway smaller than a lobar bronchiole is obstructed, the alveoli that the airway normally supplies can continue to be ventilated by the pores of Kohn.[3] Collateral ventilation appears to be more effective in adults than in young children.

▼ *Pulmonary Circulation*

The lung has two blood supplies: the *bronchial* and *pulmonary circulations*. The first consists of the bronchial arteries, which arise in the thoracic aorta and upper intercostal arteries. As a part of the systemic blood supply, these arteries nourish the trachea and bronchi to the level of the respiratory bronchioles. After forming capil-

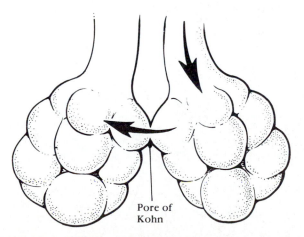

FIGURE 28-4 *Schematic demonstration of collateral communication between the alveoli through pore of Kohn.*

lary plexuses, some of the bronchial circulation returns through a pulmonary vein to the left atrium, while some empties into the bronchial vein that terminates in the azygos vein which, in turn, empties into the superior vena cava.

The bronchial circulation supplies the lung's supporting tissues, its nerves, and the outer layers of the pulmonary arteries and veins. Normally, it supplies neither the alveolar walls and ducts nor the respiratory bronchioles. In the event of interruption of the pulmonary circulation, the bronchial circulation can support the metabolic needs of these tissues, but the tissues lose the ability to participate in gas exchange.

The second blood supply to the lungs is the pulmonary circulation. From the pulmonary artery, the lungs normally receive the entire output of the right ventricle, approximately 70 mL of blood. Imagine this volume spread over the surface area of the lung (70 m²), and one can see how rapidly diffusion of gases with blood can take place. This blood circulates through the pulmonary capillary bed and then returns to the left heart by way of the pulmonary veins (Fig. 28-5).

▼ *Major Muscles of Ventilation*

The major muscle of ventilation, which enlarges the chest cavity, is the *diaphragm*. Innervated by the phrenic nerves, this flat, dome-shaped muscle lowers approximately 1 cm in quiet respiration. In forced inspiration, it may descend as much as 10 cm. This diaphragmatic movement temporarily compresses the abdominal contents. Consequently, the movement of the diaphragm can be impeded by abnormalities in the abdominal cavity, such as ascites and hepatomegaly. If abdominal pain is present, diaphragmatic action is reduced because of the *splinting effect*, a voluntary limitation of ventilatory movements.

The thoracic cavity is further enlarged by an upward and outward motion of the lower ribs accomplished by the *external intercostal muscles*. The upper ribs also move outward. The ribs are attached to the vertebrae in such a way that they rotate on an axis as they are moved by these muscles.

Whereas inspiration normally is an active effort, expiration is a passive one in which the muscles relax and allow the lungs and chest wall structures to return to resting size. The pressure in the thorax gradually rises and air moves out of the lungs.

The *internal intercostal muscles* are used in forced expiration to stiffen the intercostal spaces during straining. The *muscles of the abdominal wall* are also powerful aids to forced expiration. Normally, they are used only to generate the explosive pressure that is necessary for coughing. They also contract at the end of forced inspiration in synchrony with glottic closure to limit and stop

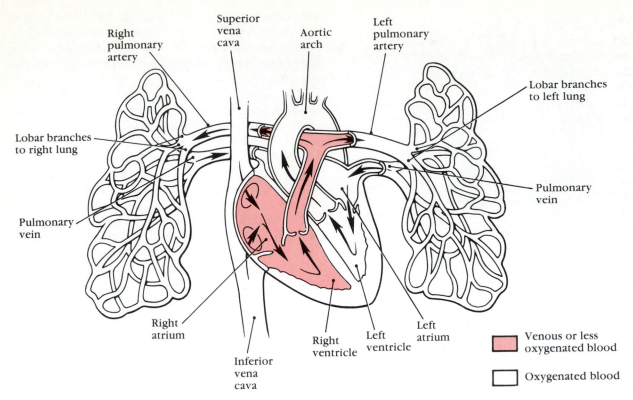

FIGURE 28-5   *Circulation from the right heart to the lungs to the left heart.*

the inspiration abruptly. The *accessory muscles*, scalene and sternomastoid, are used during labored breathing to raise the first two ribs and sternum and increase the size of the thoracic cavity.

▼ Nervous Control of Respiration

NERVE SUPPLY

The major nerve supply to the diaphragm is through the two *phrenic nerves*. Each half of the diaphragm is innervated by one of these nerves, which originate mainly from the fourth cervical nerve of the respective side. The 11th cranial nerve, the accessory, innervates most of the larynx and pharynx.

Bronchial smooth muscle is innervated by both *parasympathetic (vagus) and sympathetic nerve supply.* Increased vagal influence causes bronchoconstriction, whereas increased sympathetic stimulation causes bronchodilation. Any factor that decreases the caliber of the airway (bronchoconstriction) increases resistance and work of breathing, whereas increased caliber of the airway (bronchodilation) has the opposite effect.

The vagus nerve also transmits the appropriate signal to limit inspiration when an overstretch signal is received from the lungs. This reflex, called the *Hering-Breuer reflex*, serves as a protective mechanism to limit lung inflation.

RESPIRATORY CENTERS

The nervous system adjusts alveolar ventilation to the demands of the body. This occurs through the *respiratory centers* that are located in the medulla oblongata and the pons (Fig. 28-6). Normally, these areas of the brain regulate ventilatory rate and depth through the chemical signals of carbon dioxide and hydrogen ion levels.

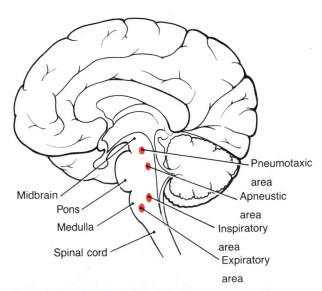

FIGURE 28-6   *Location of respiratory centers.*

CENTRAL CHEMORECEPTORS

Respiratory neurons located in the medulla oblongata are the major chemosensitive areas (chemoreceptors). Figure 28-6 shows separate areas responsible for inspiration and expiration. The major stimulus for the *inspiratory area* is the carbon dioxide concentration of the blood. This area also transmits input from the peripheral chemoreceptors. The regular rhythm of the ventilatory effort is generated in the inspiratory area. The effort continues below the conscious level, although the conscious control of breathing always overrides the unconscious.

The *expiratory area* is located in a separate part of the medulla but is usually not active unless there is some respiratory distress. When pulmonary ventilation becomes excessive, the expiratory muscles are activated to aid the expiratory effort. How the interaction occurs between the inspiratory and expiratory areas is not known.[5]

The *pneumotaxic center* is located in the pons and participates continually in the inspiratory effort by directly limiting the tidal volume of air inspired. Activation of this center increases rate of respiration, whereas decreased stimulation decreases the respiratory rate. Another center in the pons, the *apneustic center*, functions in some brain pathology to cause excessive inflation of the lungs with occasional expiratory efforts.

PERIPHERAL CHEMORECEPTORS

Decreased oxygen tension levels in arterial blood are sensed by the peripheral chemoreceptors of the carotid bodies and aortic arch (Fig. 28-7). The hypoxic stimulus, described as 30 mm Hg oxygen tension less than that which is normal for the person, is transmitted to the respiratory center. It results primarily in stimulation of inspiratory neurons and effects an increased respiratory rate through the phrenic nerve. The peripheral chemoreceptors are also sensitive to changes in carbon dioxide and hydrogen, but the direct effect of the central respiratory center overrides the sensitivity from the peripheral receptors.

▼ *Compliance and Elastance*

To understand pulmonary pathology, it is important to understand the concepts of *compliance* and *elastance*, also called *elasticity*. Generally, it can be said that the respiratory system behaves like a pump with a flow-resistive mechanism. The pumping part of the mechanism can be thought of as two separate components: the lungs and the chest wall with its associated structures.

Compliance is a measurement of distensibility or how easily a tissue is stretched; the fewer elastic forces to be overcome to stretch a substance, the more compliant it is. Compliance is measured and recorded by the amount

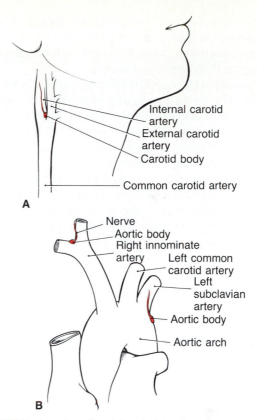

FIGURE 28-7 *Location of peripheral chemoreceptors.*

of volume change that results from pressure applied. Compare the blowing up of an old balloon with that of a new one.

Less pressure is needed to make a large volume change in the old balloon, whereas more pressure is required to make a smaller volume change in the new one. Compliance is, thus, important because the more compliant a tissue is, the less pressure is required to stretch it. Using delta (Δ) as a symbol for change, compliance is expressed as follows:

$$C = \frac{\Delta V \text{ (volume in liters)}}{\Delta P \text{ (pressure in centimeters of water)}}$$

Using the balloon analogy, one can discover which balloon is more compliant if arbitrary numbers are assigned as follows:

Old Balloon
Small pressure needed: 1
Large volume change: 10
$$C = \frac{10}{1}$$
C = 10
New Balloon
Large pressure needed: 10
Small volume change: 3
$$C = \frac{3}{10}$$
C = 0.30

From these figures, one finds that the old balloon is much more compliant or more easily stretched than the new one. Therefore, it has fewer elastic forces to oppose the stretch than the new balloon.

Elastance is the opposite of compliance. Compliance refers to the forces promoting expansion of the lung, whereas elastic forces are those promoting the return to the normal resting position or original shape. Compliance and elastance are closely related in pulmonary dynamics. The lungs inherently tend to be elastic, so without normal aids to expansion, they will tend to collapse. Compliance refers to the amount of force necessary to produce the volume change or stretch. The amount depends on the elastic forces at work. A highly compliant rubber band, for example, has few elastic forces, whereas a less compliant (thicker) rubber band has more.[3] The thick rubber band takes more work to stretch it and returns much more readily to its original shape than the thin one. Therefore, the thick rubber band is less compliant and more elastant than the thin one. The following formula is used to calculate elastance:

$$\frac{E}{\text{(elastance)}} = \frac{\Delta P \text{ (pressure)}}{\Delta V \text{ (volume)}}$$

The chest wall also has the properties of elastance and compliance, but they differ from those of the lungs. To illustrate this difference, one can imagine that the lungs and chest wall could be separated but remain as living and moving structures retaining all of their properties. Each of the two structures could be separated from the pull of the other and could seek its own resting size at an equilibrium between elastance and compliance. In the case of the chest wall freed from the lungs, it would seek a much larger resting size than when it was attached to the lungs. Without the inward pull of the lungs, the chest wall would be abnormally large.

Conversely, the lungs separated from the chest wall would tend to relax to a much smaller size than when they rested against the chest wall. They have more elastic recoil than might be expected from the amount of elastin and fiber they contain, due to a meshlike network, the structure of which itself increases elastic recoil. This arrangement is termed *nylon stocking elasticity*.

Taking the properties of the lungs and chest wall together, it can be seen that elastance of the lungs prevents overdistension of the thorax, whereas chest wall compliance prevents collapse of the lungs. Contraction of the diaphragm, discussed earlier, lowers that muscle and increases the size of the thoracic cage. All of this creates a negative intrapleural pressure, causing air to move from the atmosphere to the lungs. Relaxation of the diaphragm, a passive process, causes the muscle to move to its resting position, intrapleural pressure to increase, and air to move from the lungs to the atmosphere. These properties account for the finding that expiration is normally a passive process, whereas inspiration is an active process.

Many diseases alter the compliance and elastance of either the lungs or chest wall, but disease may not affect *both* properties of either structure. In general, bronchopulmonary diseases affect lung compliance, whereas chest wall obesity and diseases of the thoracic skeleton or respiratory nerves affect chest wall compliance. Alveolar edema and atelectasis reduce compliance by reducing the number of inflated alveoli.

Compliance of the lung is increased by emphysema and is somewhat increased in the aged person. Usually, dynamic measurements of compliance are used rather than estimates of elastance, and changes are referred to as *decreased* or *increased* compliance. In the case of pulmonary fibrosis, where there is increased fibrous tissue and stiffening of the lung tissues, compliance is reduced. More pressure than usual is needed to stretch this lung and chest wall system. The total compliance of this lung and chest wall system is then less than normal.

If a person is being mechanically ventilated, measurements of compliance provide useful objective assessment data. *Dynamic lung compliance* calculated in this way is not entirely accurate because the true calculation requires static conditions. It is accurate enough to be a useful tool for assessing gross changes in total compliance, however. The following method is used to calculate dynamic compliance:

$$\frac{\text{Effective dynamic}}{\text{compliance}} = \frac{\text{expired tidal volume (mL)}}{\text{inspiratory pressure (cm } H_2O)}$$

The measurement of compliance may be even more useful if related to lung volume. Compliance per lung volume is called *specific compliance*. Decreased specific compliance means that the lung tissue has become more rigid, and, in severe cases, the pressures needed to expand the lungs adequately over time are more than the person can produce or maintain. This results in hypoventilation. Many disorders, including obstructions, pulmonary edema, and pneumonia, may decrease both compliance and lung volume. Specific compliance is also related to lung size and is reduced by 50% in pneumonectomy.

▼ *The Mechanics of Breathing*

As stated previously, a particular pressure is necessary to cause a change in the volume of the lungs. Volume can be changed by either a high pressure from outside the body forcing air in or a negative pressure from inside the body causing air to move into the lungs. Normally, humans breathe by using negative pressure.

PHASES OF VENTILATION

The phases of ventilation involve the movement of the diaphragm and the other respiratory muscles (Fig. 28-8). As the diaphragm descends, it enlarges the intrapleural space, which causes a negative intrapulmonary pressure. The air then flows into the lungs to equalize the pressure. The subatmospheric or negative pressure, which is necessary for air to flow into the lungs, is achieved by enlarging the lung and chest cavity. When the chest and lungs enlarge, the pressure inside the thorax is lower than it was before the enlargement. At the end of active effort, the diaphragm relaxes and moves upward, which increases intrapulmonary pressure to above atmospheric level. The air moves passively out of the lungs. The elastic recoil of the lung tissue moves the lungs to their resting or unstretched state.

Thus, inspiration is an active process initiated by the contraction of the diaphragm and the outward pull by the intercostals. Air moves from greater to less pressure. Expiration is a passive process that occurs when the respiratory muscles relax and the intrapulmonic pressure increases above the atmospheric level. Even when the system is relaxed, the lungs are continually pulling in and attempting to return to their smaller relaxed size. This process creates a negative intrapleural pressure and explains one of the reasons why air is pulled into the chest when the chest wall is punctured.[8]

CHANGES IN AIRWAY SIZE

The size of the airways is also affected by the process of ventilation. The airways are attached to and supported by the lung parenchyma. Because the lungs expand to fill a larger space on inspiration, all of these structures, including the airways and alveolar ducts, are pulled to a larger size. The size of the airways and alveolar ducts is reduced as lung volume decreases during expiration. During quiet ventilation, some of the smaller airways close during expiration. Because of the effects of gravity, airway closure is more pronounced in the supine position.

AIRWAY RESISTANCE

During respiration, the volume of the thorax and consequently of the airways is changing. Airways offer resistance to airflow, the amount of which directly affects the amount of pressure needed to move air in and out of the lungs.

Pressure–flow relationships may be quite complex even in simple straight tubes. Because the respiratory tree is a series of branching tubes of varying sizes, the relationships become more complex.

The amount of pressure lost because of friction depends on the flow pattern of the air. The two major airflow patterns are laminar and turbulent (Fig. 28-9). In laminar (or streamline) flow, the gas in the airways is like very thin cylinders moving inside each other. The cylinder on the outside moves slowly, and each inner cylinder of air moves progressively faster. Gas density has no influence on the velocity of this type of flow. Basically, the gas flows along a straight line with little friction to the molecules. When airway caliber changes, however, the laminar pattern is altered. Additional pressure may be required to reaccelerate the gas and to reestablish a laminar flow pattern. Laminar flow occurs more readily in the small peripheral airways, which are generally straight and smooth.

When flow rates are high or when airways are partially obstructed or collapsed, airflow becomes turbu-

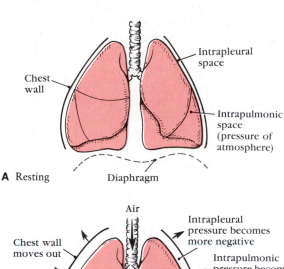

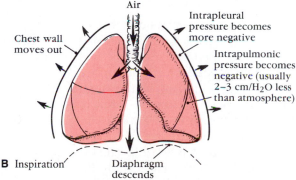

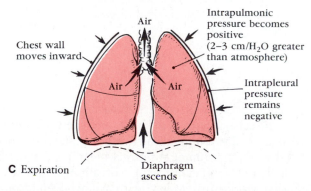

FIGURE 28-8 *Phases of ventilation.* **A.** *No air movement (resting).* **B.** *Air moves from the environment to the intrapulmonic space (inspiration).* **C.** *Air moves from the intrapulmonic space to the environment (expiration).*

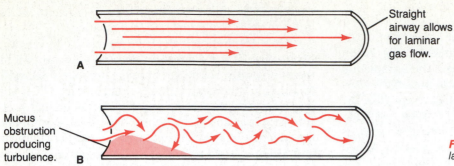

Straight airway allows for laminar gas flow.

Mucus obstruction producing turbulence.

FIGURE 28-9 **A.** *Schematic representation of laminar gas flow and* **B.** *turbulent gas flow.*

lent. In normal lungs, turbulent flow occurs in the large central airways because of molecular collision and resistance at the sides of the tubes. In turbulent flow, gas density becomes important. The pressure difference for a given flow is reduced by lowering gas density. Much of the airflow in the lungs is probably transitional between turbulent and laminar.[11] The work required for maintaining turbulent airflow is greater than that required to maintain laminar flow.[7]

Change in airway width greatly alters resistance. When airways widen, resistance is greatly diminished and air flows through easily. When airways narrow, resistance is increased and air moves through them with much more difficulty. It takes more pressure to move air through a narrow airway than a wide one. In the area of the lung where flow is laminar, if airway radius is reduced by one-half, resistance is increased by 16 times.[11] This finding has great importance for persons whose airways are narrowed by bronchospasm or pressure from tumors or infectious processes, because increased airway resistance increases the work of breathing.

Because airways normally widen on inspiration and narrow on expiration, resistance is generally greater on expiration than on inspiration. This normal change in resistance helps to explain why air becomes trapped on expiration in asthma or other chronic obstructive lung diseases.

Although there are many extremely small peripheral airways, they are so tiny that they make little difference in the resistance factors that can be measured. It is postulated that the initial changes of chronic lung disease occur in these small airways where they cannot be measured.[15] These airways make up areas called silent zones, where diseases can be present without detection.

In normal respiration in the upright position, the bases of the lungs tend to ventilate better than the apices. This has been demonstrated by having a person inhale radioactive xenon gas and monitoring its diffusion with a radiation camera. During the inspiratory phase, the bases undergo a larger change in volume and have a smaller resting volume than the apices. In the supine position, this difference disappears and the ventilations become the same. In abnormalities such as pulmonary

edema, the apices tend to ventilate better and the smaller airways in the bases often close.[15]

Airway resistance can be altered by many factors. A sigh or deep inspiration usually reduces resistance, whereas forced expiration even in the healthy person increases it. Airway compression is the usual cause of increased resistance during forced expiration; this factor is markedly enhanced in persons with diseased or weakened airway walls.[11] The presence of mucus or inflammation of the airway as well as endotracheal intubation will increase resistance to airflow.

Measurements of resistance are the *forced expiratory volume in one second* (FEV_1) and *forced vital capacity* (FVC) (see pp. 565–567).

TISSUE RESISTANCE

In addition to airway resistance, there is some resistance in the lung and chest wall tissues called *tissue resistance*. Although the frictional resistance of tissue movement cannot be measured directly, it can be calculated. In the healthy young adult man, tissue resistance is about 20% of total pulmonary resistance. Tissue resistance is rarely increased to the point of being limiting by itself. It is increased in pulmonary sarcoidosis, pulmonary fibrosis, diffuse carcinomatosis, asthma, and kyphoscoliosis. Tissue resistance may be particularly high where movement of the thoracic cage is severely limited, as in neurologic disease, musculoskeletal disease, or deformity of the chest structures.

▼ The Work of Breathing

The act of breathing requires muscular work to overcome the elastic forces of the lungs and chest wall. Work is also needed to overcome airway and tissue resistance. Initial work is minimal at normal breathing frequency but increases significantly at high breathing frequencies. Resistive work is minimized with a slow, deep respiratory pattern and increases with respiratory frequency. The opposite is true of elastic work. Two-thirds of the work of breathing is against elastic forces, prompting the lungs to return to the resting position. Slow deep breathing greatly increases the work necessary to overcome elastic forces. When the work forces are summarized, respiratory work is the least at a frequency of 14 breaths per minute.

The work of breathing, as described earlier, is proportional to the pressure change times the volume change. Volume change is the amount of air moved in and out with each breath, called *tidal volume*. The pressure change is that pressure needed to overcome the *elastic* and *resistive* forces. During quiet breathing, 65% of the work done overcomes elastic forces and 35% overcomes frictional resistance.[7] The elastic forces are mainly the elastic recoil of the chest wall and lungs themselves. Resistive forces are mainly those of airway and tissue resistance.

Respiratory pathology usually alters breathing patterns. The pattern finally adopted by the person will be the one that requires the least work, although it always requires more work than the normal pattern. For example, if flow resistance increases, the breathing may be slow and deep. If compliance is reduced, a rapid, shallow pattern of breathing may be adopted.

The work of breathing, as in other body work, consumes oxygen. Normally, at rest, respiration accounts for less than 5% of the total metabolic rate. This increases moderately with normal ventilatory changes, but with significant respiratory pathology, the work of breathing may increase many times.[15] In advanced disease states, the oxygen cost of ventilation can be 25% to 30% of the total metabolic rate. In this situation, the ventilatory effort may cost the person more oxygen than it delivers and may produce more carbon dioxide than can be eliminated. This progressive process, without appropriate intervention, continues until respiratory failure ensues.

▼ *Substances Important in Alveolar Expansion*

SURFACTANT

Surfactant is a mixture of phospholipids composed of phosphatidylcholine (lecithin) and phosphatidylglycol. It is synthesized in the type II or granular pneumocytes lining the alveolus and is secreted to form a film across the alveolar surface. Surfactant provides surface stability and prevents collapse of the alveolar structures, despite their extreme smallness.[4]

Surface tension is the force required to tear liquid apart at the surface where fluid interfaces with air. In the lungs, instead of water surrounded by air, there are millions of air bubbles (alveoli), each with an air–liquid interface. Surface tension can be illustrated by blowing soap bubbles. The pressure required to blow the bubble causes it to distend, but when the pressure is released, the surface tension causes the bubble to collapse.

A deficiency of surfactant results in an increase in the surface tension in the alveolus during expiration that leads to collapse or atelectasis of the alveoli. Amounts of surfactant in the lungs vary according to the diameter of the alveoli. As the alveoli inflate, the surfactant spreads out over the surface of the alveolar membrane. As the alveoli empty, the surfactant layer becomes thicker in relation to the decreased space. Smaller alveoli have a thicker layer, whereas larger alveoli have a thinner layer. This promotes expansion and stability of the alveoli.[5]

To be effective, the surfactant layer must be replenished continually. The half-life of pulmonary lecithin is 14 hours, which suggests that active synthesis must continually take place in the type II cells of the alveoli. Normal ventilation seems to be the most important factor in the replenishment of surfactant, which probably is due to the need for oxygen in the production of this substance. Hypoventilation may lead to atelectasis due to diminished renewal of surfactant. A sigh or a deep breath normally provides renewal of surfactant. In hypoventilation, a decreased supply of oxygen with decreased synthesis of surfactant leads to decreased surface tension in the alveoli. The result is widespread collapse of the alveoli.

Surfactant also acts as a waterproof material and may prevent the transudation of fluid across the alveolar capillary membrane during the respiratory cycle. Fluid exudation from capillary to alveolus has been shown to result from a decrease in the surfactant levels. Therefore, surfactant helps keep the alveoli dry. The absence of surfactant leads to a tendency to pull fluid into the alveoli, causing severe pulmonary edema.

Without surfactant, the surface tension of the alveoli would be fixed. Greater pressure would be necessary to keep an alveolus open because its volume and radius would decrease on expiration. Atelectasis would regularly occur at low lung volumes due to collapse of small alveoli. Large inspiratory pressures would be required to reopen the alveoli. The point of collapse is referred to as the *critical closing pressure*; the pressure necessary to open a collapsed alveolus must be enough to overcome surface tension. Without surfactant, each breath would require as much work as the first breath at birth.

Disorders that involve destruction, inactivation, or insufficient production of surfactant cause marked changes in pressure–volume relationships, even without changes in lung or chest wall tissues. Possibly, the best known instance of surfactant deficiency is in the *infant respiratory distress syndrome*, also called *hyaline membrane disease*, although the presence of the membrane seems to be secondary to the pathology rather than the cause of the disease. The condition is closely associated with prematurity and appears to be caused by immaturity of the

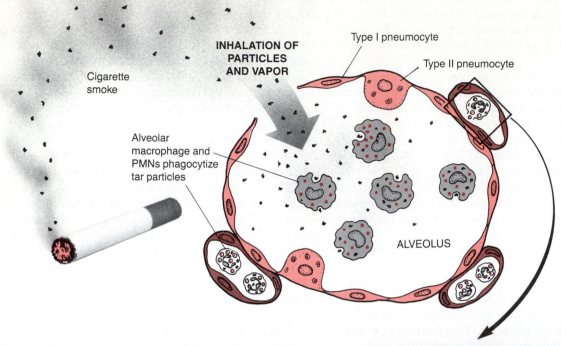

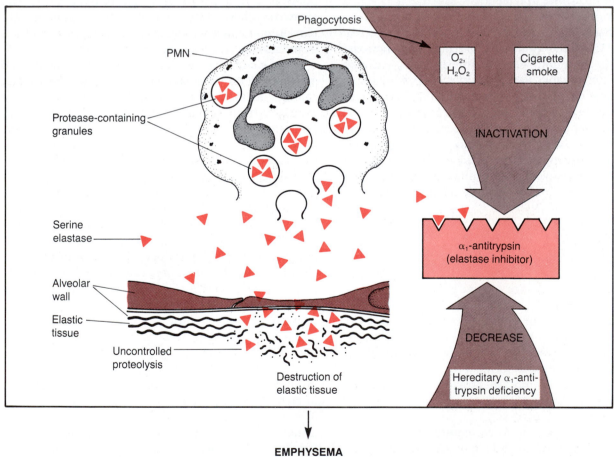

FIGURE 28-10 *The proteolysis-antiproteolysis theory of the pathogenesis of emphysema. Some product in tobacco smoke induces an inflammatory reaction. The serine elastase in polymorphonuclear leukocytes, which is a particularly potent elastolytic agent, injures the elastic tissue of the lung. Normally, this enzyme activity is inhibited by α_1-antitrypsin, but tobacco smoke directly or through the generation of free radicals inactivates α_1-antitrypsin (proteinase inhibitor). (Source: E. Rubin and J.L. Farber Pathology [2nd ed.]. Philadelphia: J.B. Lippincott, 1994).*

type II cells and deficiency of surfactant synthesis. Further discussion of a similar problem, adult respiratory distress syndrome, appears on pages 587–589.

ALPHA₁-ANTITRYPSIN

In the search for the cause of emphysema, clinicians noted that some families had a high frequency of the disease and that the onset was at an early age. The correlation between the absence of alpha₁-antitrypsin (a glycoprotein synthesized by the liver) and familial early-onset emphysema was first studied in 1962, when the level of alpha₁-antitrypsin was found to be genetically controlled.[2] The *homozygous* state is linked with early onset of panlobular emphysema. The *heterozygous* or intermediate state may have greater susceptibility to emphysema, particularly in the presence of repeated inflammatory reactions.

Produced by the liver, the primary function of alpha₁-antitrypsin is to inhibit proteolytic enzymes, including elastase, collagenase, trypsin, and chymotrypsin. Deficiency of the enzyme decreases the protective action and tips the balance in favor of the proteolytic enzymes and leads to tissue destruction.[10] A widely accepted hypothesis (protease–antiprotease mechanism) for the tissue destruction states that leukocytes and macrophages release proteases, mainly elastases, in the inflammatory response (Fig. 28-10). That these proteases are capable of producing emphysema has been well established in animal research.[1,6] Proteases are neutralized by alpha₁-antitrypsin. Without this inhibitor, these enzymes attack and destroy the alveolar membrane. The protease–antiprotease hypothesis is supported in studies of cigarette smoking. Smokers have increased numbers of neutrophils in the alveoli, and the condensates of smoke stimulate the release of their elastases into the alveoli. Decreased antielastase activity in these persons results from inhibition of alpha₁-antitrypsin activity by oxidants in cigarette smoke and other factors, resulting in disease despite normal levels of alpha₁-antitrypsin. Research related to the role of protease–antiprotease imbalance in the development of emphysema in the alpha₁-antitrypsin sufficient person (the most common form of emphysema) is hampered by the fact that the process occurs over 30 to 40 years.[16]

▼ Defenses of the Airways and Lungs

MUCOCILIARY TRANSPORT, OR THE MUCOCILIARY ESCALATOR SYSTEM

The mucociliary escalator system, or *mucous blanket*, provides the major defense of the respiratory tract against disease. The components of this system include the goblet cells, which secrete mucus; the ciliated epithelial cells; and mucus itself.

The *ciliated epithelial cells* of the respiratory tract clear the airways by moving fluid forward (Fig. 28-11). These cells line the entire respiratory tract with the exception of the anterior one-third of the nose, part of the pharynx, and the alveoli. The surface of each ciliated cell contains about 200 cilia. The cilia move in a continuous wave to carry mucus and debris up the airway to the larynx.

From an upright position, the cilia sweep forward about 30 to 35 degrees and then bend to make their recovery (see Figure 28-11B). The movement has been likened to strokes of the oars of a boat. Each cilium makes a forceful, fast effector stroke forward, followed by a less forceful, slower stroke backward to get in position again. There is precise timing and coordination of the strokes of a row of cilia; together they move as a wave. Beating in sequential waves as high as 1,000 cycles per minute, cilia move mucus up the airway. Because the beat is rapid, the mucous layer does not have time to recoil between beats.

A mucous blanket, made up primarily of the secretions of goblet cells that line the airways and mucus-secreting glands located in the larger ciliated bronchi, moves forward on the cilia. Cells in the alveoli may also contribute secretions to the mucous blanket. The rate of secretion of these cells is difficult to estimate because of resorption and expectoration of mucus. The mucous blanket consists of two layers: the *sol layer*, which surrounds the cilia, and the *gel* (surface) *layer*. The less

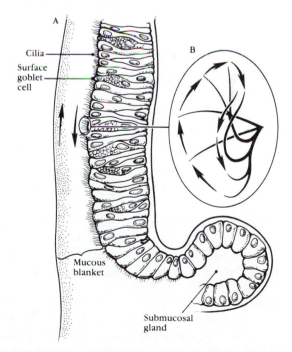

FIGURE 28-11 **A.** *The mucociliary escalator.* **B.** *Conceptual scheme of ciliary movement, which allows forward motion to move the viscous gel layer and backward motion to occur entirely within the more fluid sol layer.*

viscous sol layer provides a medium in which the cilia can move. With power strokes, the tips of the cilia strike the bottom of the gel layer and propel it toward the mouth to either be swallowed or expectorated.[7] Smoking a cigarette paralyzes the cilia for approximately 30 minutes. Chronic smoking leads to loss of cilia.

The mucous layers retain a constant depth, and the rate of transport of mucus increases rapidly as the mucus moves toward the trachea. Some mucus is resorbed in the large airways to maintain a constant depth with little removed by evaporation, because inspired air is virtually 100% saturated with moisture by the time it reaches the pharynx. Mucociliary transport is known to be altered by depressed ciliary activity, changes in the property of mucus, and injury to the respiratory epithelium cells.

Mucus is produced primarily by the goblet or mucus-secreting cells that lie along the tracheobronchial tree. In the healthy person, these cells produce an estimated 100 mL of mucus per day, continually humidifying and protecting the respiratory passages. Disease such as chronic bronchitis can increase mucus production to 200 mL or more per day. The mucous covering of the epithelium in the respiratory passages is normally uninterrupted. Adhesive properties of mucus allow particles that bind particulates to adhere so that they can move out of the respiratory tract. Respiratory tract mucus has been likened to well-engineered paint, which flows easily when brushed rapidly. But when the brushing ceases, it sticks to the wall to which it was applied.[7] Mucus is normally composed of water, electrolytes, and several types of mucopolysaccharides, which account for its viscosity.

ALVEOLAR CLEARANCE

Mucociliary transport, lymphatic drainage, blood flow, and phagocytosis all contribute to creating a sterile environment within the alveoli. Macrophage activity is the principal *alveolar* defense against particulates. These alveolar macrophages regularly scavenge the surface of the epithelium, digesting foreign material (represented schematically in Fig. 28-12).

Surface tension may play a part in removing particulates from the lungs. Particulates move from an area of low surface tension to an area of higher surface tension. Therefore, particulates may move from the environment of alveolar surfactant to the higher surface tension of the respiratory bronchioles and up the mucus escalator to the pharynx.[7]

Some particulates are removed to perivascular, peribronchial, and hilar lymph nodes. The lymphatics probably transport the particulates engulfed in macrophages. It is unclear to what extent blood flow is responsible for alveolar clearance.

Some particulates remain in the lungs for protracted periods, whereas others stay for an intermediate period

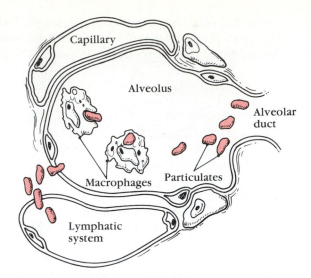

FIGURE 28-12 *Alveolar clearance effected by macrophage ingestion of particulate matter, particles traveling in the alveolar duct, lymphatic clearance of particulate matter, blood flow clearance, and carriage of particulates within the macrophages.*

and are cleared. This seems to depend on a number of factors, such as deposition site, nature of the particulate, and host resistance. A small number of particulates remain in the lungs indefinitely. Those such as asbestos, silica, and carbon may stimulate fibroblast proliferation; over time this can create severe restrictive pulmonary disease.

DEPOSITION OF PARTICULATES IN THE AIRWAYS

Under normal conditions, an individual inspires 10,000 to 12,000 liters of air daily. Each liter of urban air may have several million particles suspended in it, most of which are deposited along the respiratory tract and are cleansed by the defenses of the lung. Particles smaller than 0.5 μm in diameter usually remain suspended in inhaled air and are expelled from the lungs during expiration.

The first site of deposition of particulates in the airway is the nose (Fig. 28-13). Particulates larger than 10 μm in diameter are filtered out in the nares or trapped in the nasal mucosa. It is the inertia of large particles that determines deposition at these sites. Their large mass and high linear velocity force them to rain out in the nasal mucosa. Together with being filtered, the warming and moistening of air in the nose allows the defense mechanisms of the lower respiratory tract to function more effectively.

As the inhaled air flows over the tonsils and adenoids, particulates are deposited by impaction. These structures are ideally located in the airway to entrap debris that passes over them. In addition to mechanical defense, the tonsils and adenoids may function in the

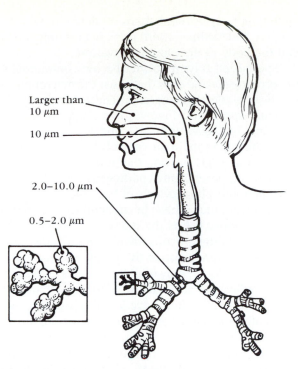

FIGURE 28-13 *Deposition of particulates in the airways depends on their size.*

Larger than 10 µm

10 µm

2.0–10.0 µm

0.5–2.0 µm

immunologic reaction. Farther along the respiratory tract, linear velocity of air decreases as the surface area increases, which allows particulates in the range of 2 to 10 µm to be deposited on the mucociliary blanket by sedimentation.

Particulates smaller than 2 µm reach the alveoli by gravitational forces and, to a lesser extent, by brownian movement, which describes the random movement of molecules due to thermal energy. The particulates are removed primarily by mucociliary transport and phagocytosis. Smaller particles may present more of a threat to the lungs than larger ones, because they penetrate more deeply and remain longer in the tissue.

Together with size, the aerodynamic properties of particulates and deposition sites must be considered. For example, asbestos particles up to 300 µm have been shown to reach the lung periphery where, because of their aerodynamic properties rather than their size, they behave like particles of about 1 µm.[11] This explains why asbestos often severely damages the distal portions of the lung.

REFLEXES OF THE AIRWAYS

The respiratory tract is equipped with reflexes that rid it of debris and protect it from inhaled foreign substances. As is true of other mechanisms, hypoactivity or hyperactivity of these reflexes create conditions that are detrimental to the host.

The *sneeze reflex* is one of the defenses against irritant materials. Particulates or irritants stimulate sensory receptors of the trigeminal nerves, resulting in the sneeze response. The sneeze is characterized by a deep inspiration, followed by a violent expiratory blast through the nose.

The *cough reflex* is important in clearing the trachea and large bronchi of foreign matter. Irritants cause different impulses to be carried by the vagus nerve to the medulla. Conscious control can also initiate the cough mechanism. The cough reflex initiates a deep inspiration. The glottis then closes, the diaphragm relaxes, and the muscles contract against the closed glottis. Maximum intrathoracic and interairway pressures are produced that cause the trachea to narrow. When the glottis opens, the large pressure differential between the airways and the atmosphere, coupled with tracheal narrowing, creates airflow through the trachea at velocities as high as 100 miles an hour.[5] This is very effective in propelling secretions toward the mouth. While the cough is more effective in clearing the major airways, it also may help clear the peripheral airways through a milking action created by the high intrathoracic pressures. This may deliver secretions from the peripheral airways to the main bronchi for expulsion by coughing.

Together with other mechanisms, reflex *bronchoconstriction* protects the upper and lower airways from mechanical and chemical irritants. Both cough and reflex bronchoconstriction are initiated in the subepithelium of the airways by receptors sensitive to irritants. For example, when the receptors are exposed to dust, the reflex narrowing of the airways, along with cough, increases the linear velocity of airflow and assists in the removal of dust from the airways. Reflex bronchoconstriction also protects the alveoli from harmful fumes and prevents gases from entering the pulmonary circulation.

Removal of gases from the inspired air depends on their solubility in water. Highly soluble gases, such as sulfur dioxide and acetone, are removed in the upper respiratory tract. Less soluble gases, such as nitrous oxide and ozone, reach the peripheral lungs. This accounts for the observation that sulfur dioxide inhalation results in bronchitis, whereas nitrous oxide inhalation may lead to pulmonary edema. The protection offered by reflex bronchoconstriction is dose-related and time-related, which means that if exposure to the toxic fumes is brief or of low concentration, reflex bronchoconstriction may protect the lungs.

▼ Defenses Against Infection

DEFENSE AGAINST MICROBIAL AGENTS

Invasion of the lungs by microbial agents presents special problems in defense. Microorganisms have the ability to replicate themselves, and, conceivably, one organism could multiply and completely permeate lung tissue. The defenders against infectious agents must act quickly to kill the organisms before they have sufficient opportunity to multiply, which can be in minutes to hours.

Under normal circumstances, the alveolar macrophage system is the primary bactericidal mechanism for clearing infectious agents from the lungs.[6] The *alveolar macrophages* ingest bacteria at such a rapid rate that most are destroyed in situ. The rate of bacterial killing in the lungs exceeds the rate at which the bacteria are transported out of the lungs. This has been demonstrated by radioactive tracer-labeled bacteria. In 24 hours, 30% to 40% of the radioactivity is cleared, but nearly all bacteria are killed. This is known as *net bacterial lung clearance*. Three factors contribute to this process: 1) physical transport of bacteria out of the lung; 2) in situ bacterial killing; and 3) bacterial multiplication.[12]

The rate of bactericidal activity by the macrophages is influenced by different bacterial strains. For example, *Staphylococcus aureus* is removed at a faster rate than *Proteus mirabilis*. Some organisms are readily inactivated by phagocytosis, whereas others appear resistant to this process. *Klebsiella pneumonia* and *Pseudomonas aeruginosa* are slowly killed in the lungs, resulting in a net increase, rather than a net clearance, of these organisms.[12] Conditions in the metabolic environment, such as hypoxia, acidosis, and high levels of cortisol, slow net bacterial lung clearance. Ethyl alcohol and tobacco smoke have been shown to depress clearance, but all organisms are not depressed equally. For example, alcohol completely suppresses the killing of *P. mirabilis* but not of *S. aureus* or *S. albus*. This selective action on the alveolar macrophages has important clinical ramifications. In chronic obstructive lung disease, mixed flora are constantly present in the respiratory tract, but one predominant organism will be responsible for lung infection when it occurs.

Acute viral infections predispose the host to bacterial infections in the lungs. Viruses appear to interfere with alveolar macrophages and suppress their bactericidal ability. The greatest susceptibility appears between the 6th and 10th day after the acute viral infection, during which time superimposed bacterial pneumonias frequently develop.

The dynamics of different responses to bacteria, fluctuations in host resistance, and environmental changes may permit an organism to multiply at any given time.[9] All of these factors influence the fate of the microorganism, that is, whether it remains in a localized area, is disseminated throughout the body, or is killed and thus eliminated from the body.

IMMUNOLOGIC DEFENSE

Closely associated with the macrophage system is the *immunologic defense of the lungs*. The cells involved in the specific immune response are described in Chapter 14. These include the T lymphocytes (thymic-dependent) and B lymphocytes (bone marrow–derived), which in a complex, interacting pattern provide immunity and defend the body against foreign invasion.

Specialized B lymphocytes become immunoglobulin-secreting plasma cells that assist the macrophages in inactivating infectious material. This action is called the *humoral response* and involves five classes of immunoglobulins: IgG, IgM, IgA, IgD, and IgE. The first three classes are important in the control of infectious diseases. Both IgM and IgG provide the primary and secondary antibody responses against pathogens by facilitating opsonization and phagocytosis of bacteria.

Two types of IgA have been identified: *secretory* and *serum*. Secretory IgA is the major immunoglobulin on the surfaces of the mucous membranes. On the respiratory mucosa, IgA protects the lungs against viral and bacterial invasion. It may inhibit the ability of the organisms to adhere to the mucosal surfaces. Persons with chronic bronchitis often have low levels of IgA, which apparently contributes to a high frequency of recurrent pulmonary infections.

The T lymphocytes provide for cell-mediated immunity. They play a major role in attracting macrophages to the site of an infection. Tuberculosis is an excellent prototype for understanding this response. Inhaled tuberculosis bacilli travel from the lungs to the lymph nodes, where the macrophages engulf, process, and concentrate the antigens of the bacilli. A few T lymphocytes bearing receptors for tuberculin antigens react with the bacillus and undergo multiplication. These T cells circulate back to the lungs and release chemical mediators that induce macrophages and other leukocytes to kill the bacteria (see pages 575–576).

The presence of *Pneumocystis carinii* pneumonia is found only in the immunocompromised host, especially in acquired immunodeficiency syndrome (AIDS), which targets the T helper cell. *P. carinii* has emerged as the leading opportunistic pathogen in persons with AIDS who have depressed T cell function.[14]

Humoral and cell-mediated immunity function together to protect the lungs from infection. Both are essential for a fully competent immunologic defense.

INTERFERON

Interferon is a protein that inhibits viral replication. It appears to be produced and regulated within the cells. Cells react to viruses by producing interferon, which causes unaffected surrounding cells to synthesize another protein that protects the cells by preventing viral replication. All cells seem to produce interferon when exposed to a virus, but viruses differ in their ability to act as interferon inducers. It is thought that lymphocytes assist the host to counteract viruses, and these lymphocytes can produce interferon. Because of this, it has been suggested that interferon may be the mediator of the cellular immune response with certain viruses.[9]

Interferon may also be important in protecting the organism against bacteria and tumors. It has been used experimentally in the treatment of cancer and viral infections in immunosuppressed persons.

▼ *Normal Gas Exchange*

Oxygen makes up about 21% of the atmospheric air, and most of the remaining 79% is composed of nitrogen. Carbon dioxide makes up only a minute percentage (approximately 0.02%) of atmospheric air, and the remainder consists of minuscule amounts of other trace gases, such as argon, neon, and helium, are present.

OXYGEN TRANSPORT TO THE TISSUES

The oxygen tension, or partial pressure of oxygen at sea level, is equal to the barometric pressure of 760 mm Hg multiplied by the fraction of oxygen in dry air (20.93%), which equals 159 mm Hg. As the inspired air is warmed and humidifed in the upper airways, however, it is diluted by water vapor, and this causes the oxygen tension to fall to 149.3 mm Hg. The inspired air is then further diluted by carbon dioxide in the lower airways and alveoli. Factors that lower inspired oxygen concentration or that raise alveolar carbon dioxide levels also lower alveolar oxygen levels and hence lower arterial blood oxygen tension, which may reduce the delivery of oxygen to the tissues. Table 28-1 displays the blood gas pattern seen when normal arterial blood is analyzed.

Oxygen is delivered by a linked chain of transfers from the atmosphere to the alveoli to the blood and then to the tissues and cells of the body. It diffuses from areas of higher partial pressure to areas of lower pressure. It is transported initially from the air of the atmosphere to the larger airways by movements of the diaphragm and chest wall that cyclically lower the intrathoracic pressure. This results in air moving in and out of the lungs (*ventilation*) and then being delivered by the smaller peripheral airways to the alveoli (*distribution*). Air then crosses the alveolar–capillary membrane (*diffusion*) and is carried in the plasma, bound chemically to hemoglobin. During *perfusion*, blood is delivered through the pulmonary capillary system past the alveoli for the purpose of gas exchange. At the capillary level, it diffuses into the tissue fluid surrounding the cells and then to the cells themselves, where it is metabolized.

Oxygen is essential for cellular metabolism, and the cells have no capability to store it. Without constant delivery of oxygen, tissue hypoxia and anaerobic metabolism result. *Tissue hypoxia* is defined as inadequate critical oxygen tension to meet the needs of the cell. *Critical oxygen tension* is that cellular oxygen tension which causes mitochondrial dysfunction.[13]

Tissue hypoxia is not synonymous with *arterial hypoxemia*, which refers to decreased oxygen tension in the arterial blood. Tissue hypoxia and arterial hypoxemia may exist simultaneously or independently of each other. Arterial hypoxemia can be measured via arterial blood gas analysis. Tissue hypoxia cannot be directly measured but is assessed on the basis of clinical signs and symptoms.

The relationship between arterial and tissue oxygenation is explained in large part by the relationship between hemoglobin and oxygen. Oxygen and carbon dioxide diffuse across a membrane along a gradient from higher pressure to lower pressure. Most of the oxygen is transported to the body cells in chemical combination with hemoglobin. *Hemoglobin* is a complex spheric molecule that is made up of four heme groups, each of which is enfolded in a chain of amino acids. Each heme group can combine with an oxygen molecule, which gives hemoglobin the capability of carrying four oxygen molecules per hemoglobin molecule. Hemoglobin combined with oxygen is called *oxyhemoglobin*, whereas oxygen-free hemoglobin is called *reduced* hemoglobin (see p. 376).

In the adult, normal hemoglobin levels range from 12 to 16 g/dL of blood. It has been found that 1 g of hemoglobin fully saturated can carry 1.34 mL of oxygen. Each milliliter of blood with an oxygen tension of 100 mm Hg can carry about 0.03 mL of dissolved oxygen. This means that 100 mL of blood with a hemoglobin of 15 g and 100% saturation has an oxygen content of about 20.4 mL of oxygen, which is expressed as *volumes percent*. A very small percentage of oxygen is carried dissolved in the plasma, but hemoglobin is by far the most important method of oxygen transport in the blood.

OXYHEMOGLOBIN DISSOCIATION CURVE

The relationship between oxygen and hemoglobin is nonlinear. The affinity of hemoglobin for oxygen has been plotted on an oxyhemoglobin dissociation curve, an S-shaped curve (Fig. 28-14). It is derived by plotting

TABLE 28-1 *Arterial Blood Gas Values*

Substance	Values
Oxygen	
Tension (P_{O_2})	75–100 mm Hg breathing room air
Saturation (Sa_{O_2})	96–100% of capacity
Carbon dioxide	
Tension (P_{CO_2})	35–45 mm Hg
pH	7.35–7.45
Bicarbonate (HCO_3^-)	22–26 mEq/L
Carbonic acid (H_2CO_3)	1.05–1.35 mEq/L (always 3% of P_{CO_2})
Base excess/deficit	+2/−2

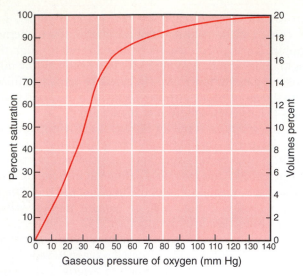

FIGURE 28-14 *The oxyhemoglobin dissociation curve.*

oxyhemoglobin saturation (the percentage of hemoglobin that has combined with oxygen) against the oxygen tension (mm Hg) to which it is exposed. Because oxyhemoglobin dissociation is readily reversible, the curve reflects the ease with which hemoglobin gives up oxygen as well as the ease with which it takes up oxygen. This is important because, to a large extent, oxygen delivery to the tissues depends on the ease with which hemoglobin gives up its oxygen once it reaches the tissues.

Study of the oxyhemoglobin dissociation curve reveals that it is initially very steep and then flattens. The upper portion of the curve is flat, showing that when the oxygen tension (Po_2) is 70 mm Hg or above, hemoglobin becomes nearly fully saturated. When the available oxygen begins to fall below 60 mm Hg, the degree of saturation also falls rapidly. Note in Figure 28-14 that when the Po_2 falls to 40 mm Hg, the saturation of hemoglobin is about 70% or approximately the level of venous blood. At 20 mm Hg Po_2, the saturation is about 30%, which will not sustain life.

Many factors alter the affinity of hemoglobin for oxygen. An increase in hemoglobin affinity for oxygen makes the curve shift to the left, and oxygen is given up less readily to the tissues. Alkalemia, hypothermia, and hypocarbia are among factors that can cause a leftward shift. Conversely, acidemia, hypercarbia, and hyperthermia reduce the affinity of hemoglobin for oxygen and cause, by inference, increased oxygen availability to the tissues, noted on the curve as a shift to the right. This is a desirable situation permitting the oxygen demands of a person with increased metabolism to be more easily met. Figure 28-15 shows the effects of pH, Pco_2, and body temperature on the affinity of hemoglobin for oxygen.

The factors that affect tissue oxygenation are sum-marized in Box 28-1. Oxygen content of arterial blood is determined by a combination of alveolar oxygenation, hemoglobin level and quality, and hemoglobin affinity for oxygen. Oxygen delivery to the tissues depends on the status of the cardiovascular system and regional perfusion. At the tissue level, oxygenation depends on vascularity, diffusion characteristics, and intracellular mechanisms.

CARBON DIOXIDE TRANSPORT

Carbon dioxide is the product of metabolic combustion and travels the pathway opposite to oxygen, along pressure gradients from tissues to blood to alveoli to airways and then out to the atmosphere. Total amounts of oxygen consumed and carbon dioxide produced are *not* determined by the quantity of ventilation but by the actual *metabolic demands* of the cells. The body at rest requires about 250 mL of oxygen per minute and produces about 200 mL of carbon dioxide per minute as a result of its continuing metabolic cellular requirements. Heavy exercise may increase the production of carbon dioxide up to 20 times this volume.

The normal match between ventilation and perfusion serves the ultimate purpose of supplying oxygen and eliminating carbon dioxide from the cells and eventually from the body. Alveolar ventilation is about 4 liters of air per minute. Cardiac output (and resulting tissue perfusion) is about 5 liters of blood per minute.

Because carbon dioxide diffuses about 20 times more readily than oxygen, tissue carbon dioxide diffuses rapidly into the venous end of the capillaries with a gradient of less than 1 mm Hg. Venous blood entering the lungs with a Pco_2 of 46 mm Hg readily transfers carbon dioxide into the alveoli (Fig. 28-16).

With normal alveolar ventilation, alveolar carbon dioxide ($Paco_2$) of 40 mm Hg is in equilibrium with the resulting arterial carbon dioxide ($Paco_2$) of 40 mm Hg. The levels of both alveolar and arterial carbon dioxide are directly and inversely proportional to the volume of alveolar ventilation ($\dot{V}A$). Thus, in alveolar hypoventilation, halving the alveolar ventilation from 4 to 2 liters per minute doubles the $Paco_2$ from 40 to 80 mm Hg. In hyperventilation, doubling the alveolar ventilation from 4 to 8 liters a minute halves the $Paco_2$ to 20 mm Hg.[4, 5]

Blood carries carbon dioxide in three different forms: 1) 5% or less is transported to the lungs in the *plasma* as *dissolved carbon dioxide*; 2) nearly 70% diffuses into the red blood cells (RBCs) and is carried in the form of *bicarbonate*; and 3) approximately 25% is carried in the RBCs bound to the hemoglobin.[8]

Figure 28-17 illustrates the reaction of carbon dioxide as it is carried dissolved in the RBCs. It is important to note that this is a reversible reaction that occurs rapidly at the tissue level, where carbon dioxide is picked up and in the lungs where it is released. Most carbon dioxide

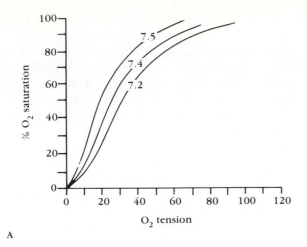

A

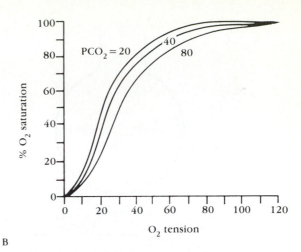

B

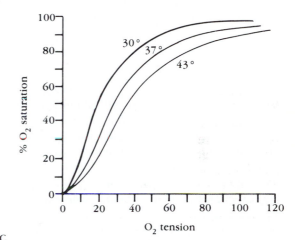

C

FIGURE 28-15 *Effects of **A** pH, **B** PCO_2, and **C** temperature on the oxyhemoglobin dissociation curve.*

diffuses into the RBCs, where it is catalyzed in a reaction with carbonic anhydrase and water to form carbonic acid. This carbonic acid immediately dissociates into hydrogen ions (H^+) and bicarbonate ions (HCO_3^-) that can diffuse back into the plasma or may stay in combination with a positive ion in the RBCs. The excess hydrogen ion formed in this reaction usually binds with the hemoglobin molecule to form hydrogen hemoglobin. If significant amounts of (HCO_3^-) diffuse into the plasma, a negative ion is drawn into the RBCs to equalize the

---

BOX 28-1 ▼ Factors That Affect Tissue Oxygenation

Oxygen tension arterial blood
Hemoglobin content
Hemoglobin saturation
Blood flow to tissues
Diffusion of oxygen to tissues
Diffusion of carbon dioxide
Arterial pH
Body temperature

---

electrochemical gradient. This ion is usually chloride, and the mechanism of its movement is called the *chloride shift*.[5] This process can provide bicarbonate to the plasma when the pH is decreased. Normally, in the lungs a reverse process occurs very rapidly. Hydrogen is released from hemoglobin and recombines with bicarbonate to form carbonic acid, which dissociates into carbon dioxide and water. Carbon dioxide diffuses out of the RBCs into the alveoli and is blown off in the exhaled air.

Carbon dioxide may react directly with hemoglobin and be carried in a loose chemical bond on the hemoglobin molecule. This is referred to as *carbaminohemoglobin* and accounts for about 25% of the carriage of carbon dioxide to the lungs. In the pulmonary capillary bed, carbon dioxide is simply released to the alveoli and blown off in exhaled air.

VENTILATION–PERFUSION RELATIONSHIPS

Arterial oxygenation is affected not only by ventilation but also by the *blood supply to the lungs*. Abnormalities in pulmonary blood flow (perfusion) or in relationships between ventilation and perfusion ($\dot{V}A/\dot{Q}$ ratio) alter

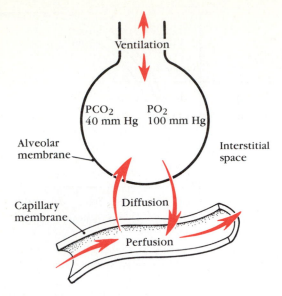

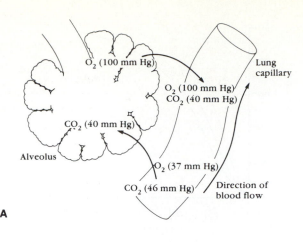

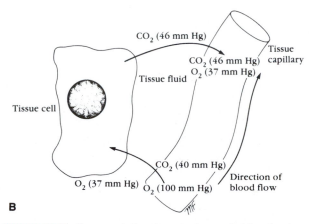

FIGURE 28-16 *Movement of gases across the alveolocapillary membrane due to ventilation, diffusion, and perfusion.*

arterial oxygen tension and, subsequently, oxygenation of body tissues.

Oxygen and carbon dioxide are exchanged as blood circulates through the pulmonary capillary bed. The capillaries are arranged such that each is adjacent to an alveolus. The capillaries are very small, approximating the size of an RBC. The capillary wall and alveolar wall are each only one cell thick, so the diffusing membrane is very thin. Gases, therefore, diffuse across the membrane with little difficulty (Fig. 28-18).

Each RBC stays in the pulmonary capillary bed

FIGURE 28-18 *Representation of gas exchange **A** at the alveolus and **B** at the tissue level. (Source: R.S. Snell, Clinical Histology for Medical Students. Boston: Little, Brown, 1984)*

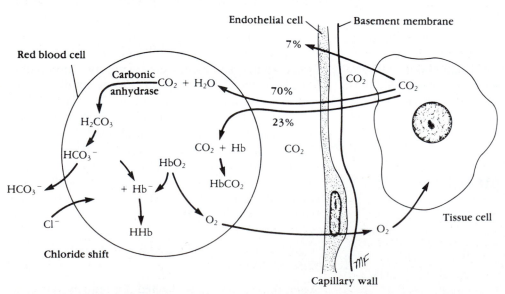

FIGURE 28-17 *Methods of carbon dioxide transport in the red blood cell. Seventy percent of CO_2 is combined with H_2O) to form carbonic acid and bicarbonate, 23% is carried in combination with Hb, and 7% is carried in the plasma. (Source: R.S. Snell, Clinical Histology for Medical Students. Boston: Little, Brown, 1984).*

TABLE 28-2 *Differences Between Pulmonary and Systemic Circulations*

Factor	Pulmonary	Systemic
Pressures	Low (pulmonary artery mean 14 mm Hg)	High (aortic mean 100 mm Hg)
Pressure changes	Symmetric and of low magnitude within lungs	Asymmetric and of great magnitude depending on system supplied (eg, renal arteriole pressure much higher than hepatic circulation)
Pressure determined by	Arteriolar/alveolar gradient and/or or arteriolar/venular gradient	Arteriolar/venular gradient
Vascular resistance	One tenth of that of systemic circulation; can decrease resistance as pulmonary pressure rises	Resistance 10 times that of pulmonary circulation; less ability to lower resistance when pressure rises
Capillary support	Capillaries surrounded by gas-filled alveoli; collapse or distend depending on pressure in and around	Capillaries surrounded by tissue; less tendency to collapse or distend
Directing blood flow	System rarely directs blood between regions	Regulates and distributes blood to specific areas throughout body

about 1 second and exchanges gases with two or three alveoli during this time. Approximately 70 mL of blood is normally exchanging gases at a given moment in the pulmonary capillary bed of an adult, in contrast to the large volume of air that is moved by the alveoli with each breath. This is an important, if temporary, safeguard against lack of oxygen. Storing oxygen, even for a few moments, guards against the extra oxygen needs encountered during breath holding.[15]

In addition to moving blood to the blood–gas barrier for gas exchange, the pulmonary circulation also provides a reservoir for blood, filters small thrombi from the blood, and traps white blood cells.

Generally, the pulmonary circulation is a low-pressure system with pressures much lower than the systemic circulation. The normal mean pulmonary artery pressure is 14 mm Hg. Because the mean left atrial pressure of the heart is about 5 mm Hg, the driving pressure across the pulmonary bed is only about 9 mm Hg.

Pressure in the pulmonary artery or in the pulmonary capillary bed may be increased by pathology, but an increase in one does not necessarily mean a corresponding increase in the other. The pulmonary and systemic circulations are compared in Table 28-2. Table 28-3 lists the normal pressures within the heart and the pulmonary circulation.

Both acidemia and hypoxemia can stimulate constriction of the pulmonary arteries and, thus, increase resistance in the pulmonary capillary bed. Either of these conditions causes vasoconstriction alone; together they provide a synergistic effect. Once this vasoconstriction occurs and persists for some time, it may cause an adverse effect on the right ventricle because of increased work needed to pump blood into the constricted pulmonary vasculature. Over time, this may lead to right ventricular hypertrophy and subsequent right ventricular failure (known as cor pulmonale).

Approximately 10% to 20% of the total blood volume is present in the pulmonary vascular bed at any given time. The bed is capable of accepting several times this amount, which allows it to accommodate variations in cardiac output or blood volume. The distensibility of the bed is accomplished both by dilating pulmonary vessels and by opening closed or unused vessels. Distension of the pulmonary vascular bed reduces pulmonary

TABLE 28-3 *Approximate Normal Pressures in the Heart and Pulmonary Circuit*

Location	Pressure (mm Hg)		
	Systolic	Diastolic	Mean
Superior vena cava			6–10
Inferior vena cava			6–10
Right atrium			2–5
Right ventricle	25	0–5	
Pulmonary artery	25	10	
Pulmonary capillary bed			8–12
Left atrium			5–10
Left ventricle	120	0–10	
Aorta	120	80	
Systemic arteriole			30

vascular resistance until its capacity is reached. Then, as increases in blood flow cannot be accommodated, pulmonary vascular resistance increases.

Perfusion changes more rapidly from the top to the bottom of the upright lungs than does ventilation. Therefore, the ventilation–perfusion ratio decreases down the lungs (Fig. 28-19). If the individual is in the upright position, pulmonary blood flow increases linearly from top to bottom due to gravitational forces. At the apex, the pulmonary arterial pressure is just sufficient to raise minimal amounts of blood to the top of the lungs and perfuse the apices. Capillary pressure is very low. If blood volume is reduced for some reason, such as systemic loss or pulmonary capillary destruction, apical perfusion may decrease or cease altogether.[15]

Blood flow to the lungs changes with exercise and position. With exercise, all areas of the lung receive increased blood flow. When a person lies down, flow from apices to bases becomes uniform.

The concept of regional differences in ventilation has important ramifications for the person with asymmetric lung pathology. An example might be the person whose left lung appears to be radiographically *whited out* by a process such as pneumonia. To maximize ventilation, perfusion, and gas exchange, the person should not be positioned on the left side. Instead, the person should be turned onto his or her right side or back to capitalize on the abilities of the unaffected lung. Arterial blood gas values can be significantly affected with this type of positioning.

As previously mentioned, the perfusion gradient down the lung exceeds the ventilation gradient. To state a $\dot{V}A/\dot{Q}$ ratio, ventilation and perfusion must be expressed in the same units. For example, blood flow of 4 liters/minute and ventilation of 5 liters/minute in the average adult male results in a $\dot{V}A/\dot{Q}$ ratio of about 0.8:1.0, or 0.8. In the healthy person, the deviation from a ratio of 1 is largely due to anatomic dead space. Nor-

mally, a portion of the air inspired does not come in contact with the alveoli and does not participate in gas exchange. This *anatomic dead space* usually remains relatively constant, but *alveolar dead space* (where alveolar gas does not participate in blood–gas exchange) may be significantly altered in pathologic states. The $\dot{V}A/\dot{Q}$ ratio is altered in conditions in which alveolar *dead space ventilation* and thus physiologic dead space ventilation are increased. A higher than normal amount of inspired gas is wasted, resulting in a lower-than-normal amount of inspired gas exchanged with the blood. To compensate for this wasted ventilation and to maintain normal PaO_2 and $PaCO_2$, total ventilation must increase. This moves more inspired gas per minute to improve exchange with blood. If the body is incapable of increasing ventilation and blood flow enough to maintain adequate gas exchange, carbon dioxide retention and hypoxemia may result. In any case, the work of breathing is increased. If the body is incapable of altering ventilation and blood flow to meet this need, altered blood gases, decreased cellular oxygenation, and clinical symptoms occur.[8]

The opposite of dead space ventilation is *shunting*. All cardiopulmonary and pulmonary disease leads to problems with dead space ventilation or shunting or both. Shunting refers to an area that is perfused but not ventilated (Fig. 28-20). A small amount of shunting (less than 2.5% of cardiac output) is normal; it occurs because not all blood is exchanged at the alveolocapillary line. This accounts for the fact that normal oxygen saturation of hemoglobin in arterial blood gases is 96% to 100%. Pathologic amounts of shunting may be caused by such problems of nonventilation as atelectasis and pneumonia (see Chapter 29).

In shunting, the $\dot{V}A/\dot{Q}$ is decreased. Blood returning from the affected areas of the lung mixes with blood returning from the oxygenated areas. This lowers the total level of oxygen in the arterial blood, resulting in a lowered PaO_2.

If shunting is not severe, the body can compensate for the amount of carbon dioxide that is not excreted by the shunted areas. Hyperventilation of the unaffected areas can blow off enough carbon dioxide to compensate. Oxygen exchange cannot be compensated for so readily, because carbon dioxide is much more diffusible than oxygen. If compensation occurs, it leads to a blood gas pattern of normal $PaCO_2$ with hypoxemia. If the body is unable to compensate adequately for the carbon dioxide exchange, blood gases show acidemia, hypoxemia, and hypercapnia. A compromised pulmonary or cardiovascular system could lead to loss of ability to compensate for the demands of shunting or other abnormalities.

Both shunt and dead space defects are often referred to as $\dot{V}A/\dot{Q}$ mismatching. All other factors being equal, the lung with a $\dot{V}A/\dot{Q}$ mismatch is unable to exchange as much oxygen and carbon dioxide as the lung with a normal $\dot{V}A/\dot{Q}$ ratio.

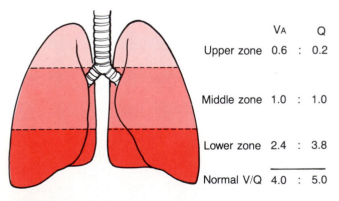

	VA		Q
Upper zone	0.6	:	0.2
Middle zone	1.0	:	1.0
Lower zone	2.4	:	3.8
Normal V/Q	4.0	:	5.0

FIGURE 28-19 *The lungs can be divided into three zones. Ventilation-perfusion ($\dot{V}/\dot{Q}$) differs according to the position assumed. In the upright position, the upper segments are hypoperfused, and in the lower segments they are hypoventilated. The relationship between ventilation and perfusion varies in the zones.*

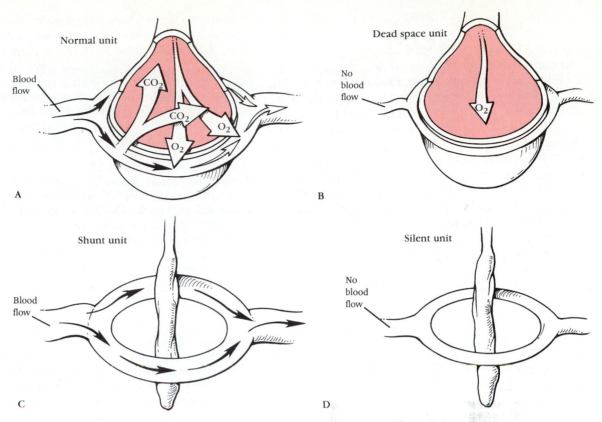

FIGURE 28-20 *A. Schematic representation of normal alveolar-capillary unit, of B ventilation without perfusion, C of perfusion without ventilation, and D of neither perfusion nor ventilation.*

▼ Respiratory Regulation of Acid–Base Equilibrium

As is described in Chapter 11, the major blood buffers are hemoglobin, the plasma proteins, and the carbonic acid––bicarbonate system. Any increase in carbon dioxide concentration in the blood causes a shift in its pH toward the acidic side; any decrease causes it to shift toward the alkaline side. Therefore, the amount of carbon dioxide present in the blood affects the pH significantly. Carbon dioxide, usually in the form of carbonic acid (H_2CO_3), is closely regulated by the physiologic buffer system of the lungs.

If the metabolic rate increases, the rate of carbon dioxide formation increases. Conversely, if the rate of metabolism decreases, the formation of carbon dioxide also decreases. Alveolar ventilation changes according to nervous control of respiration through the *chemoreceptors* in the medulla. These chemoreceptors are extremely sensitive to minute changes in the carbon dioxide level and stimulate an increase or decrease in the respiratory rate. If the blood pH declines to 7.0, alveolar ventilation may increase up to five times above the resting value. An increase in pH to above 7.5 may decrease alveolar ventilation to one-half the normal value. Thus, the respiratory rate and depth of respiration physiologically can retain or blow off excess carbon dioxide according to the pH of blood (Fig. 28-21).

The two major alterations in acid–base balance related to pulmonary function are *respiratory acidosis* and *alkalosis*. Respiratory acidosis is due to some factor that compromises ventilation. Thus, hypoventilation leads to retained carbon dioxide and causes an excess of carbonic acid in the blood. The excess carbon dioxide or hydrogen ion is a powerful stimulus for the central chemoreceptor in the medulla oblongata, which initiates a response increasing respiratory rate and depth, which is designed to blow off the rising amount of CO_2 in the blood.

Respiratory alkalosis results from hyperventilation, which blows off carbon dioxide, leading to decreased carbonic acid and a shift of the pH to alkaline.

▼ Pulmonary Function Testing

Pulmonary function tests (PFTs) measure many variables, including lung volume. They are important tools in the diagnosis and evaluation of pulmonary status. Spirometric tests are limited to disclosing abnormalities only when they are relatively diffuse. Therefore, results of these studies may be normal in early disease states or in localized, rather than diffuse, conditions. When results of a pulmonary function test are abnormal, other

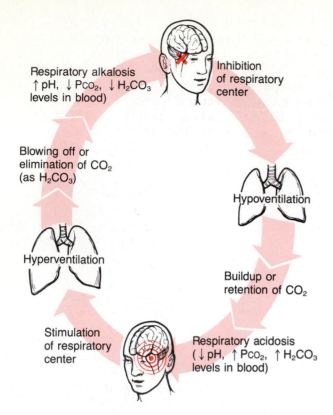

FIGURE 28-21 *Changes in pH, Pco₂, and Hco₃ according to respiratory rate and depth. Note the continuum of respiratory center.*

clinical data must be collected before an accurate diagnosis can be made.[15] The effectiveness of spirometry also is totally dependent on the ability and cooperation of the persons being tested. Pulmonary function study results are evaluated in relation to predicted normal results. Tables of norms based on age, sex, and size are used to predict normal values for each person. The tables are not totally reliable because of individual differences among persons.

Pulmonary function tests provide a yardstick in establishing the amount of disability in the course of pulmonary disease. They are used in many settings to diagnose and manage patients with pulmonary or cardiac disability and in epidemiologic surveys for industrial hazards or community disease risks.

Lung contents can be divided into four capacities or compartments, each of which is made up of two or more volumes. Figure 28-22 illustrates average values for the various tests. The *lung volumes* usually are measured as follows:

1. *Tidal volume* (*VT*) is the volume of gas moved in and out of the lungs with each breath. The normal V_T ($\pm$ 500 mL) is only a small percentage of the amount of air that the lungs are capable of moving.
2. *Expiratory reserve volume* (*ERV*) is the additional amount of gas or air that can be forcefully exhaled after a normal expiration is complete ($\pm$ 1,200 mL).
3. *Residual volume* (*RV*) is the amount of air remaining in the lungs after a forced expiration ($\pm$ 1,200 mL).

4. *Inspiratory reserve volume* (*IRV*) is the maximum volume of air that can be inhaled after a normal resting inspiration ($\pm$ 3,100 mL).

The *lung capacities* are as follows:

1. *Total lung capacity* (*TLC*) is the maximum volume of gas that the lungs can hold. All of this gas is not available for exchange, because it includes dead space gas. The TLC equals the IRV plus the V_T plus the ERV plus the RV (TLC = IRV + V_T + ERV + RV). Given the figures above, the TLC equals approximately 6,000 mL of air.
2. *Functional residual capacity* (*FRC*) refers to the volume of gas remaining in the lungs at the end of a spontaneous expiration and includes the ERV and the RV (FRC = ERV + RV). The FRC decreases in such conditions as obesity that affect the chest wall mass. With an increased FRC, it would take more change in the ventilatory rate or more time to reduce a given high carbon dioxide level than with a normal FRC. The FRC equals approximately 2,400 mL of air.
3. *Vital capacity* (*VC*) can be measured either as expiratory or inspiratory. *Expiratory VC* is the maximum volume of gas that can be exhaled after the deepest possible inspiration. Usually, expiratory VC equals *inspiratory VC*, which is the maximum amount of gas that can be inhaled after the fullest possible expiration. *Total vital capacity*, therefore, equals IRV plus V_T plus ERV (VC = IRV + V_T + ERV). It equals about 5,000 mL in males. In severe obstructive pulmonary disease, the inspiratory VC may be much greater than the expiratory. The VC increases with height, usually is greater in men, and is roughly proportional to lean body weight in young adults. It decreases slightly in the supine position due to the splinting of posterior rib movement and reduced diaphragmatic action. On quiet breathing, the lungs are roughly one-third inflated in the supine position and one-half inflated in the upright position.
4. *Inspiratory capacity* (*IC*) is the maximum volume of air that can be inhaled from a resting position. It equals the V_T plus the IRV (IC = V_T + IRV). A reference value for IC is approximately 3,600 mL of air.

The RV, TLC, VC, and FRC are not anatomically fixed but depend on elastic characteristics and muscle forces. All

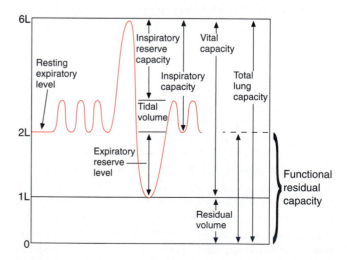

FIGURE 28-22. *Pulmonary function tests showing normal lung volumes.*

lung volumes and capacities change with aging due to the associated decrease of elastic recoil in the elderly person's lungs. The resting position (at the end of quiet expiration) shifts in the direction of inspiration. Therefore, with age, the RV and FRC increase slightly and the VC decreases. This decrease is partially due to stiffening of the thoracic cage and decreased chest mobility.

Besides lung volumes, the forced vital capacity (FVC) can yield much information in persons with chronic obstructive disease. The amount of air that can be forced out of the lungs on expiration is measured first at 1 second and then at the time it takes to complete the expiratory effort. The 1-second measurement is called the forced expiratory volume in 1 second (FEV_1). The shape of the curve is important in indicating abnormalities. Generally, in obstructive disease, expiration takes much longer than normal and is less complete because of premature airway closure and subsequent air trapping. In restrictive disease, the shape of the curve may be normal but compressed due to the smaller chest volume without changes in the actual airflow. The volume obtained by the FEV_1 is placed over the FVC to get a ratio or percentage. Normally, the FEV_1/FVC is 80%, which means that 80% of the total volume can be expired in the first second. Generally, in restrictive lung disease, both FVC and FEV_1 are reduced. In contrast, obstructive disease tends to reduce the FEV_1 much more than the FVC. Mixed restrictive and obstructive patterns are common, and the FEV_1 may also be affected by changes in airway resistance, elastic recoil, and lung compliance.

Alveolar ventilation, or the amount of gas actually reaching the exchange area, refers to the V_T minus the dead space. This is calculated as follows: $\dot{V}_A = (V_T - V_D) \cdot f$, where V_A is alveolar ventilation in 1 minute; the dot indicates that it is a timed measurement; and f equals respiratory frequency. Dead space (V_D) is usually estimated from standard tables, but it can be approximated to equal an adult's ideal weight in pounds.

Minute ventilation is the total amount of air entering or leaving the body per minute. It is calculated by multiplying the V_T by the respiratory rate. It includes the anatomic dead space. The formula for this calculation is as follows: $\dot{V}_E = V_T \times R$.

▼ Chapter Summary

▼ The structures that make up the pulmonary tree provide a passageway for air from the environment to the alveoli, where gas exchange takes place. In the process of entering, air is filtered and humidified. At the alveoli, exchange of gases from the circulation to the alveoli occurs, with the movement of gas always following diffusion from higher to lower concentration of the gas. Oxygen moves from the alveolus to the capillary, whereas carbon dioxide moves in the opposite direction.

▼ Air movement depends on an intact ventilatory system and normal compliance and elastance of the pulmonary structures. The alveoli depend on surfactant to maintain distension.

▼ The pulmonary system has a large defensive system that prevents infection and foreign material from entering the body. Gas exchange depends on normal oxygen transport across the alveolar–capillary interface and the exchange in the tissues. The oxyhemoglobin dissociation curve can be used to predict tissue oxygenation. Ventilation–perfusion relationships vary within the lung zones but normally are maintained at about 0.8.

▼ Diagnostic tests that are used for pulmonary function include the arterial blood gases and testing for the various lung volumes. These are helpful in diagnosing pulmonary pathologies.

▼ References

1. Cotran, R.S., Kumar, V., and Robbins, S.L. *Robbins' Pathologic Basis of Disease* (5th ed.). Philadelphia: W.B. Saunders, 1994.
2. Eriksson, S. Alpha1-antitrypsin deficiency: Lessons learned from the bedside to the gene and back again. *Chest* 90:181, 1989.
3. Farzan, S. *A Concise Handbook of Respiratory Diseases* (3rd ed.). Reston, Va.: Reston, 1992.
4. Ganong, W.F. *Review of Medical Physiology* (16th ed.). Los Altos, Calif.: Lange, 1993.
5. Guyton, A.C. *Textbook of Medical Physiology* (8th ed.). Philadelphia: W.B. Saunders, 1991.
6. Kuhn, C., and Askin, F.B. Lung and mediastinum. In J.M. Kissane (ed.), *Anderson's Pathology* (9th ed.). St. Louis: C.V. Mosby, 1990.
7. Martin, D., and Youtesy, J. *Respiratory Anatomy and Physiology*. St. Louis: C.V. Mosby, 1988.
8. Nunn, J.F. *Applied Respiratory Physiology* (4th ed.). London: Butterworths, 1993.
9. Roitt, I.M., Brostoff, J. and Male, D. *Immunology* (3rd ed.). St. Louis: C.V. Mosby, 1993.
10. Scoggin, C. Hereditary lung diseases. In W.N. Kelley (ed.), *Textbook of Internal Medicine* (2nd ed.). Philadelphia: J.B. Lippincott, 1992.
11. Seaton, A., Seaton, D., and Leitch, A. *Crofton and Douglas's Respiratory Diseases* (4th ed.). Oxford: Blackwell Scientific, 1989.
12. Toews, G. Pulmonary clearance of infectious agents. In J.E. Pennington (ed.), *Respiratory Infections: Diagnosis and Management* (2nd ed.). New York: Raven Press, 1989.
13. Walter, J.B. *An Introduction to the Principles of Disease* (2nd ed.). Philadelphia: W.B. Saunders, 1982.
14. Walzer, P. Pneumocystis carinii infections. In W.N. Kelley (ed.), *Textbook of Internal Medicine* (2nd ed.). Philadelphia: J.B. Lippincott, 1992.
15. West, J. *Respiratory Physiology: The Essentials* (4th ed.). Baltimore: Williams & Wilkins, 1990.
16. Wewers, M. Pathogenesis of emphysema: Assessment of basic science concepts through clinical investigation. *Chest* 90:190, 1989.

Chapter 29

Restrictive Alterations in Pulmonary Function

Darlene H. Green

▼ **CHAPTER OUTLINE**

▼ **LEARNING OBJECTIVES**

1 Describe compression and absorption atelectasis.
2 Discuss the role of surfactant in the development of atelectasis.
3 Discuss ventilation–perfusion abnormalities in atelectasis.
4 List the organisms and the areas that they affect in upper respiratory tract infections.
5 Discuss the pathophysiology of pneumococcal pneumonia.
6 List the causes of tuberculosis and the role of individual susceptibility in acquiring the disease.
7 Describe the pathophysiology of primary and reinfection tuberculosis.
8 List two causes of aspiration pneumonia and describe the danger of each.
9 Describe in detail the pathophysiology of alveolar and interstitial pulmonary edema.
10 Discuss how restrictive pulmonary disease can occur in a person having a simple rib fracture.
11 Describe the hemodynamics of flail chest abnormality.
12 List and describe disease-induced pleural effusion.
13 Outline the clinical manifestations of pleural effusion.
14 Describe tension pneumothorax.
15 Review central nervous system control of respiration.
16 Indicate how a head injury may affect respiration.
17 Describe the pulmonary problems that may occur with Guillain-Barré syndrome.
18 Describe the onset of respiratory failure in Duchenne muscular dystrophy.
19 Outline the ways in which silicosis and asbestosis can cause a restrictive process.
20 Indicate how particulate matter is cleared in coal worker's pneumoconiosis.
21 Relate the development of pulmonary fibrosis to emphysematous changes in the pneumoconioses.
22 Indicate two chest deformities that may cause restrictive pulmonary disease.
23 Explain why restrictive pulmonary disease can occur in obese individuals, especially those afflicted by the Pickwickian syndrome.
24 Define the role of surfactant in the development of idiopathic respiratory distress syndrome of newborns.
25 Describe in detail the pathophysiology of adult respiratory distress syndrome.

Restrictive pulmonary disease is an abnormal condition that causes a decrease in total lung capacity and vital capacity. It involves difficulty in the inspiratory phase of respiration. In this chapter, several conditions are considered, some of which do not precisely fit the above definition but may lead to significant restriction. Table 29-1 classifies the conditions and their pathogenesis.

▼ *Atelectasis*

Atelectasis is a common, acute, restrictive disease that involves the collapse of previously expanded lung tissue or incomplete expansion at birth. It is usually described as a shrunken, airless state of the alveoli.

The two major alterations that occur with atelectasis are compression of lung tissue from a source outside the alveoli and absorption of gas from the alveoli. *Compression atelectasis* may be produced by such conditions as pneumothorax, pleural effusion, and tumors within the thorax (Fig. 29-1A). *Absorption atelectasis* occurs when secretions, pus, or mucosal edema in the bronchi and bronchioles obstruct these airways and prevent the movement of air into the alveoli (see Figure 29-1B). The air trapped in the alveoli is absorbed and the alveolar sacs collapse. Stasis of secretions in the larger airways, the most common cause of obstruction, provides an excellent medium for bacterial growth and stasis pneumonia. Breathing 100% oxygen will result in more rapid collapse of alveoli, because pure oxygen is more readily absorbed than the normal mixture of gases.

Atelectasis is a common postoperative complication due to retained secretions. After surgery, the patient's protective cough response decreases due to medications and pain. An ineffective cough reflex, which diminishes the tidal volume, and decreased sigh mechanism lead to inadequate alveolar expansion. Increased viscosity of sputum results, with a tendency for secretions to gravitate to the dependent areas.

Adults are susceptible to atelectasis, particularly in the right middle lobe, which is most vulnerable because of the angle of convergence of its bronchus with the right main bronchus. The right middle lobe also seems to have increased susceptibility to bacterial pneumonia, which tends to flourish in copious pooled secretions.

The natural tendency of the lungs is to collapse, because elastic forces are constantly trying to force the lung tissue inward. These forces are opposed by the negative intrapleural forces and chest wall expansion. When airflow into the alveoli is obstructed, alveolar sacs collapse and produce little or no surfactant. Surfactant, due to its short half-life, must be constantly replenished, and this requires normal ventilation. To offset the tendency to collapse, collateral communication often occurs through the pores of Kohn. The amount of commu-nication partly depends on the overall degree of inflation of the lungs (Fig. 29-2). Eventually, airways to adjacent alveoli will also be obstructed, and this collateral communication becomes ineffective.

Initially, perfusion to the collapsed airways is not affected, so blood shunts by the ineffective alveoli and is not oxygenated. This results in a *perfusion-without-ventilation* shunt or a direct right-to-left shunt across the lungs (Fig. 29-3). Depending on the amount of atelectasis present, the ventilation/perfusion ratio will be altered (less than 0.8) and if atelectasis is significant, hypoxemia will also be significant (see p. 564).

One can readily see that the process of atelectasis may occur in many situations, including the obstructive conditions in which a portion of lung tissue is hyperinflated and adjacent sections are collapsed. Clinical manifestations depend on the amount of atelectasis. Rales in the bases and/or diminished breath sounds are common in postoperative atelectasis. A mild case may produce no symptoms, but as it progresses or becomes more widespread, dyspnea, tachycardia, cough, fever, and disturbances in chest wall expansion may occur. Blood gas analysis shows hypoxemia when significant atelectasis is present. Hypercapnia and decreased pH may herald a progression toward respiratory failure (see pp. 610–611).

▼ *Infectious Disease of the Respiratory Tract*

Infectious processes can involve either the upper or lower respiratory tract or both. They may be caused by viruses, bacteria, rickettsiae, fungi, or protozoa and be mild, self-limited, or debilitating.

UPPER RESPIRATORY TRACT INFECTION

The upper respiratory tract warms, humidifies, and filters the air. In this process, it is exposed to a wide variety of pathogens that may lodge and grow in various areas depending on the susceptibility of the host. Pathogens may lodge in the nose, pharynx (particularly the tonsils), larynx, or trachea and may proliferate if the defenses of the host are depressed. The spread of the infection depends on the resistance mounted by the host and on the virulence of the organism. Figure 29-4 shows the defensive anatomy and physiology of the upper respiratory tract, including the mucociliary blanket, which normally provides a very efficient cleansing mechanism for expelling foreign material.

An example of an upper respiratory tract infection is a sore throat (nasopharyngitis), which, if caused by the bacteria beta-hemolytic streptococci, leads to suppuration in the nasopharynx and tonsils that may spread to

TABLE 29-1 Restrictive Diseases

Category	Examples	Pathogenesis	Assessment of Findings
Respiratory center depression	Narcotic and barbiturate dependence	Direct depression of respiratory center	Respiratory rate: <12/min; associated signs of hypoventilation
	Central nervous system lesions, head trauma	Injury to or impingement on respiratory centers	Hyper- or hypoventilation; cerebral edema and its signs
Neuromuscular	Guillain-Barré syndrome	Acute toxic polyneuritis; intercostal paralysis leads to diaphragmatic breathing; vagal and SNS paralysis lead to reduced ability of bronchioles to constrict, dilate, react to irritants	Reduced negative inspiratory pressure, V_T, V_C, compliance, breath sounds; hypoxemia, hypercapnia
	Duchenne muscular dystrophy	Genetic; thoracoscoliosis; paralysis of intercostals, abdominal muscles, diaphragm, accessory muscles	Pulmonary symptoms appear late; reduced IC, ERV, V_C, V_T, FRC, compliance P_{O_2}; elevated P_{CO_2}; abnormal respiratory patterns
Restriction of thoracic excursion			
Thoracic deformity	Kyphoscoliosis, pectus excavatum	Deformity of chest compresses lung tissue and limits thoracic excursion	Reduced breath sounds in affected areas, probably with rales; reduced compliance, TLC, V_C, ERV; signs of hypoventilation, hypoxemia, increased work of breathing
Traumatic chest wall instability	Flail chest	Fracture of a group of ribs leads to unstable chest wall; reduced intrathoracic pressure on inspiration pulls area in and causes pressure on parenchyma; this increases work of breathing and hypoventilation	Obvious flail, unequal chest excursion, bruising, skin injuries, localized pain on inspiration, dyspnea, reduced breath sounds with rales and rhonchi; reduced compliance, ERV, TLC, V_C, P_{O_2}
Obesity	Obesity hypoventilation syndrome (Pickwickian syndrome)	Excess abdominal adipose tissue impinges on thoracic space and diaphragmatic excursion; reduced respiratory drive; increased weight of chest restricts thoracic excursion	Somnolence, twitching, periodic respirations, polycythemia, right ventricular hypertrophy/failure; reduced compliance, ERV, TLC, V_C, P_{O_2}; elevated P_{CO_2}; distant breath sounds
Pleural disorders	Pleural effusion	Accumulation of fluid in pleural space secondary to altered hydrostatic or oncotic forces	Unequal chest expansion; dullness and reduced breath sounds in affected area; may be constant chest discomfort; dyspnea if amount of fluid large; if over 250 mL, shows on radiographs; if large, bulging of intercostal space
	Pneumothorax	Accumulation of air in pleural space with proportional lung collapse	Hyperresonance; reduced breath sounds; tracheal deviation away from pneumothorax; tachycardia; unequal chest expansion; breath sounds reduced or absent; shows on radiographs

(continued)

TABLE 29-1 (continued)

Category	Examples	Pathogenesis	Assessment of Findings
Disorders of lung parenchyma	Pulmonary fibrosis	Many possible causes: occupational sarcoid, etc.	Reduced compliance, hypoxemia, hypercapnia, and their consequences
	Tuberculosis	Bacterial invasion leads to scarring, reduced compliance, and reduced lung function	Visible on films; positive skin test, sputum; malaise, weight loss, fatigue, evening fever with night sweats, cough, hemoptysis
	Atelectasis	Obstruction of bronchioles, shrunken airless alveoli; reduced compliance; right-to-left shunting	Dyspnea, tachycardia, cough, fever, decreased chest wall expansion, hypoxemia, radiologic evidence
	Adult respiratory distress syndrome (ARDS)	Widespread atelectasis; loss of surfactant; interstitial edema, formation of hyaline membrane	Dyspnea, tachypnea, grunting, labored respirations, hypoxemia, occasional hypercapnia, cyanosis; radiographs show bilateral patchy infiltrates
	Pulmonary edema	Increased pulmonary capillary pressure leads to interstitial and alveolar edema	Hypoxemia, tachypnea; signs of congestive heart failure, radiologic butterfly infiltrates, rales
	Aspiration pneumonia	Chemical irritant from aspirant leads to bronchoconstriction, necrosis, and fibrosis of airways	Hypoxemia, signs of ARDS, wheezing, tachypnea, tachycardia
	Pneumoconiosis	Inhalation of pollutants, results in scarring, fibrosis, and secondary emphysema	Slow developing pulmonary signs of dyspnea, hypoxemia, hypercapnia, cor pulmonale
	Bacterial pneumonia	Virulent bacteria, especially pneumococcal; inflammatory exudate with congestion and edema; poor ventilation in consolidated areas	Rapidly developing fever, chest pain, cough, blood-streaked or rusty-colored sputum; responds well to antibiotic treatment
	Viral pneumonia	Rapid onset of inflammation of alveoli and terminal and respiratory bronchioles; secondary bacterial infection common	Respiratory distress with or without fever; much more severe in children with fever, dehydration, and respiratory failure, especially under 2 y of age

SNS: Sympathetic nervous system

the sinuses. Susceptible individuals may later develop a reaction to the organism that is manifested as rheumatic fever (see pp. 484–486).

Viruses also cause pathology of the upper respiratory tract. Influenza, for example, is characterized by an acute inflammation of the nasopharynx, trachea, and bronchioles and leads to edema, congestion, and necrosis of these structures. The common cold is characterized by an acute inflammation of the nasopharynx, pharynx, larynx, and trachea, resulting in swelling of the mucous membranes and mucopurulent serous exudate. The purulence is due to secondary bacterial infection.

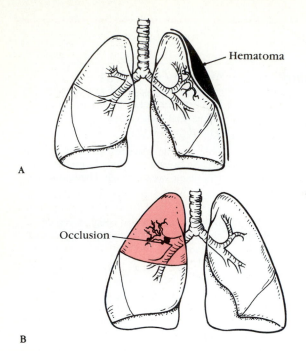

FIGURE 29-1 **A.** *Compression of lung tissue by hematoma.* **B.** *Right upper lobe atelectasis caused by bronchial occlusion.*

LOWER RESPIRATORY TRACT INFECTION

Infectious processes of the lower respiratory tract can be caused by any of the pathogens that affect the upper respiratory tract. These lead to a variety of pathologic and clinical features depending on host resistance and virulence of the organism.

Bacterial Pneumonia

Bacterial pneumonia is a common infection that is life-threatening for much of the population, especially the aged, chronically ill, and immunosuppressed. This threat has been drastically reduced by antimicrobial preparations, which have decreased the death rate, shortened the course of the disease, and prevented many serious complications, such as empyema. However, pneumonia is the most common cause of death among the infectious diseases.[1] Pneumonias can be classified as either *hospital-acquired* or *community-acquired*. Pneumonia is considered to be hospital-acquired (nosocomial) if the onset occurs 48 hours or more after the person's admission to the hospital. Community-acquired pneumonia is typically treated on an outpatient basis.

For bacteria to invade the lung successfully, there must be an alteration in net bacterial lung clearance. This alteration may occur as a result of decreased bactericidal ability of the alveolar macrophages, the extreme virulence of the bacteria, or increased susceptibility of the

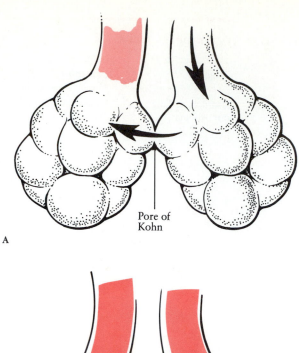

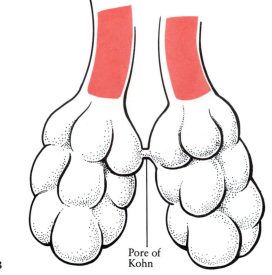

FIGURE 29-2 **A.** *Demonstration of collateral circulation between the alveoli through the pores of Kohn.* **B.** *Atelectasis occurring with obstruction to both bronchioles.*

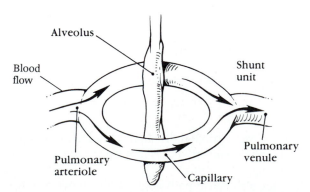

FIGURE 29-3 *Schematic demonstration of a right-to-left shunt across the pulmonary bed.*

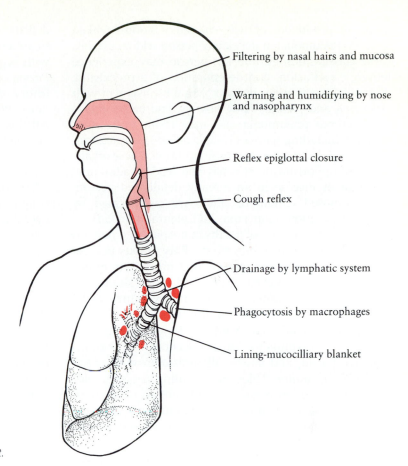

Filtering by nasal hairs and mucosa

Warming and humidifying by nose and nasopharynx

Reflex epiglottal closure

Cough reflex

Drainage by lymphatic system

Phagocytosis by macrophages

Lining-mucocilliary blanket

FIGURE 29-4 *Defense of the respiratory tract.*

host to infection. Normally, the bactericidal activity of macrophages is extremely important in supplementing the mucociliary escalator system in removing pathogens. Pneumococcal pneumonia (*Streptococcus pneumoniae*), once considered synonymous with bacterial pneumonia, is still the most common bacterial pneumonia. It is responsible for 40% to 80% or more of community-acquired pneumonias.[1] It follows an orderly sequence in the lung; its severity depends greatly on host resistance, medical intervention, or both. Although infection may develop in healthy persons, underlying factors such as malnutrition, alcoholism, and aging increase risk. Pathophysiologically, an initial, acute, inflammatory response occurs that brings excess water and plasma proteins to the dependent areas of the lower lobes. Red blood cells, fibrin, and polymorphonuclear leukocytes infiltrate the alveoli. The bacteria are contained within segments of pulmonary lobes by this cellular recruitment, causing leukocytes and fibrin to consolidate within the involved area.

The inflammatory exudate progresses through stages including *hyperemia* and *red* and *gray hepatization*, and finally terminates in resolution. Hyperemia, also called the stage of congestion, is characterized by engorgement of the alveolar spaces with fluid and hemorrhagic exudate. The outpouring of edema fluid provides a rich medium for proliferation and rapid spread of the organism through the lobe.[5] In the stage of red hepatization, the exudate coagulates, resulting in a red appearance of affected lung tissue, which demonstrates the consistency of liver tissue.

The stage of gray hepatization occurs when the number of red blood cells in the exudate decreases and they are replaced by increased numbers of neutrophils, which infiltrate the alveoli, causing the tissue to become solid and grayish.[5,11] During resolution, polymorphonuclear leukocytes are replaced by macrophages that are highly phagocytic and destroy the organisms. The exudate liquefies and is coughed up or absorbed.

The filling of alveoli with exudate (consolidation) causes them to become airless. Sustained perfusion with poor ventilation occurs in the consolidated area, but this rarely is severe enough to cause a true hypoxemia. The infection resolves as exudate is lysed and reabsorbed by the neutrophils and macrophages. The lymphatics carry exudate away from the site of infection, resulting in restoration of both structure and function of the lung. In some cases, resolution does not occur and the exudate is converted to fibrous tissue, rendering the affected alveoli functionless.[11]

The clinical manifestations of pneumococcal pneumonia include fever, tachypnea, cough, pleuritic chest pain, and production of rusty-colored or blood-streaked sputum. Pneumonia in the elderly person seldom exhibits these classic findings, and the person may experience lethargy, confusion, and deterioration of a preexisting disease.[1] Complications include pleural involvement with empyema and pleuritis, lung abscess, and bacteremia.[11]

Bacterial pneumonia also may result from other bacteria, including species of *Staphylococcus*, *Streptococcus*, *Klebsiella*, *Pseudomonas*, and *Escherichia coli*. These organisms are opportunistic at times and lead to additional infection or disease in an already debilitated person. Such imposed conditions often are complicated by abscess formation, empyema, and pleural effusion.

An estimated 15% of deaths in hospitalized persons are due to nosocomial pneumonia. Fifty to sixty percent of all hospital-acquired pneumonias are due to gram-negative bacilli. Tracheal intubation, both short-term for surgery and long-term for respiratory failure, is the single most consistent factor in the development of nosocomial pneumonia. Antibiotic treatments, predisposing the individual to "super infections" with gram-negative bacilli, and gastric alkalinization with either antacid or histamine-2 blockers, resulting in gastric colonization with gram-negative bacilli, are also important risk factors of severe nosocomial pneumonia. Surgery, obesity, concurrent disease, and advanced age also increase the risk.[12]

Legionella Pneumonia (Legionnaires' Disease)

During a 1976 American Legion convention in Philadelphia, 221 persons developed a strange type of pneumonia resulting in the death of 34 people.[2] By January 1977, the bacterium that caused the outbreak had been identified. *Legionella pneumophila* is a fussy organism that refuses to grow unless its precise requirements are met but proliferates when conditions are right (warm, aquatic environments).[2] Initially, it was thought to be a new bacterium, but previously unclassified organisms were subsequently recognized to belong to the same family. Legionella pneumonia often occurs in minor sporadic epidemics probably arising by spread from contaminated water, such as that from the air conditioning cooling tower of a public building. The disorder is not spread from person to person. Although the disease may be subclinical, symptoms that appear after a 2- to 10-day incubation include flulike complaints, a dry nonproductive cough, and headache that may be severe. An elevated temperature is common and may be associated with a relative bradycardia. Diagnosis is often difficult in a nonepidemic setting.[2]

Pneumocystis carinii Pneumonia

Although *Pneumocystis carinii* causes pneumonia in individuals with a wide variety of underlying immune deficits, with rare clusters of cases occurring in cancer treatment centers, the high susceptibility of patients with acquired immunodeficiency syndrome (AIDS) to *Pneumocystis carinii* pneumonia (PCP) has changed it from a medical curiosity to a disease of central importance. PCP accounts for 85% of pulmonary infections in AIDS patients and is the most common cause of death among these patients. Five to 30 percent of first episodes of PCP are fatal, and the mortality rate for those requiring mechanical ventilation is from 50% to 100%.[18] In AIDS, the manifestations include dyspnea, fever, and cough, which, in the initial episode, progress gradually over 2 to 4 weeks. Pathologically, there is intraalveolar inflammation that results in a decreased diffusion capacity leading to the development of hypoxemia.[8]

Histoplasmosis

Histoplasmosis is caused by the fungus *Histoplasma capsulatum*, which is common in the Mississippi and Ohio River valleys of the United States because it is found primarily in the soils of the river valleys of temperate zones. The growth of the organism is enhanced when it is mixed with bird droppings. It is more common in rural areas where chicken coops and other farm buildings are found, but it also may be found in urban and suburban areas that have been contaminated by bird droppings. Outbreaks of histoplasmosis may also be associated with excavation of infected soil during construction of roads or buildings. Bats may be infected with the organism, and inhalation of infected bat droppings by cave explorers may result in "cave fever," or histoplasmosis.

A minor disturbance of dry contaminated soil may scatter spores into the air, resulting in direct inhalation of the fungus. In the immunocompetent person, the spores are engulfed by macrophages, and within 7 to 14 days, specific lymphocyte-mediated cellular immunity develops. This results in rapid limitation of infection with no symptoms and no intervention required. However, any condition that alters cellular immunity, such as corticosteroid therapy, lymphomas, AIDS, or organ transplants, will promote widespread dissemination of the organisms with a pathologic course quite different from the typical benign course of the acute or primary disorder. The primary form of the illness cannot be passed from person to person.

Progressive disseminated histoplasmosis has a grave prognosis, often ending in death within weeks. This relatively rare disease is found in the immunocompromised individual and may also be seen in very young children and the elderly. The clinical picture is variable, but it is a febrile, wasting illness with hepatosplenomegaly. Progressive disseminated histoplasmosis was accepted as an AIDS-defining illness in 1987, and in some areas of the country it is the second most common form of opportunistic infection, second only to PCP.[14] The third form of the illness, chronic pulmonary histoplasmosis, is evidenced by a chronic cough producing purulent sputum, occasional hemoptysis, and persistent fever. It occurs most often in middle-aged male smokers with emphysema, with the fungus colonizing in the abnormal pulmonary spaces.

Mycoplasmal Pneumonia

Mycoplasmal organisms are smaller than bacteria but are not classified as viruses. *Mycoplasma pneumoniae* is a common cause of upper respiratory tract infections, with pneumonia occurring in less than 10% of infected subjects.[16] It normally affects younger persons with a fibrinous pleurisy and interstitial pneumonia. The disease tends to be self-limited and is rare after age 45 years.[11] However, adulthood does not prevent the disease and it should be considered even in the elderly who have contact with children.

Viral Pneumonia

Viral pneumonias are frequently mild and self-limited in adults but may be rapidly proliferative and fatal in children. The pediatric diseases include bronchiolitis and pneumonia. Epidemics of this viral infection occur in winter and often affect children under 2 years of age.[11] In adults, viral pneumonias may affect the alveolar epithelial cells or the bronchioles. The course may be very rapid, causing an acute clinical picture of respiratory distress with or without fever. A major concern with viral infection is that the terminal and respiratory bronchioles may become damaged and then become susceptible to secondary bacterial invasion that spreads to the surrounding alveoli. The common types of viruses are the influenza, adenovirus, chickenpox virus, and respiratory syncytial virus.

Tuberculosis

Tuberculosis (TB) has afflicted the human race since the dawn of civilization. Known as the White Plague, TB reached epidemic levels during the 19th century. By 1882, Robert Koch had isolated the tubercle bacilli, dispelling the prevailing theory that TB was hereditary. Improved living conditions and the advent of chemotherapy effective against the organism resulted in a sharp decline in the incidence of the disease, with an annual decrease in the number of new cases. This decline continued until 1985 when, despite a slight increase, it was believed that with new diagnostic and treatment technologies, TB could be essentially eliminated in the United States by the year 2000. However, the rate continued to rise, and by 1990 reports of TB outbreaks with strains of bacteria resistant to many of the antituberculous drugs began to emerge. With the realization that current drugs may no longer be effective came the dread that TB would once again become the public health threat it was at the beginning of the century when, without antimicrobial therapy, 50% of those with active TB died of the infection and TB was the leading cause of death in the United States.[6]

Concurrent with identification of drug-resistant TB, human immunodeficiency virus (HIV) co-infection became recognized as a contributing factor to the increased number of TB cases. Tuberculosis, known to be highly associated with the poor housing, undernutrition, poor hygiene, and lack of access to health care as a consequence of poverty, has an increased incidence among the indigent, the homeless, and those in overcrowded housing and in sites where persons infected with HIV and those immigrating from countries of high prevalence of drug-resistant TB organisms may also be located.[17] Typically, these groups include persons who are noncompliant with therapy and unaccessible by the public health system. A lack of appropriate therapy leads to continued transmission of the disease with increased numbers of persons with infection and active disease as well as the development of drug-resistant bacteria leading to drug-resistant disease. Before 1990, outbreaks of drug-resistant TB were rare; between 1990 and 1993, eight hospitals documented nosocomial spread of multiple drug-resistant TB, leading to revision of the Centers for Disease Control guidelines of prevention of TB transmission in health care facilities.[3]

The first encounter that an individual has with tubercle bacilli, the primary infection, sets the stage for possible future development of active (clinical) TB. *Mycobacterium tuberculosis*, an aerobic, rod-shaped, acid-fast bacterium, is transmitted by means of aerosolized droplet nuclei when a person harboring the organism speaks, coughs, laughs, or sneezes. Because of their small size, the organisms are deposited in the lung periphery, usually in the lower part of the upper lobe or the upper part of the lower lobe (Fig. 29-5). The establishment of infec-

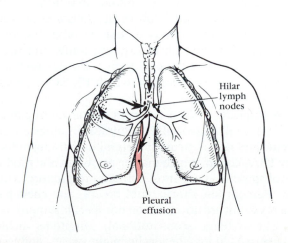

FIGURE 29-5 *Tuberculosis organisms are usually deposited in the lung periphery, either in the lower part of the upper lobe or the upper part of the lower lobe. Arrows indicate putrance, deposition, spread to hilar lymph nodes, and pleural effusion.*

tion depends both on the virulence of the bacteria and the microbicidal ability of the alveolar macrophages that ingest it. In primary infection in the immunocompetent individual, the mycobacteria become surrounded by polymorphonuclear leukocytes, and inflammation results. After a few days, macrophages replace the polymorphonuclear leukocytes. Some mycobacterial organisms are carried off by the lymphatics to the hilar lymph nodes. The combination of the initial lesion and lymph node involvement is called the *Ghon complex*, but this rarely results in spread to other body organs.

Macrophages called *epithelioid cells* engulf the mycobacteria. These cells join together to form giant cells that ring the foreign cell. Within the giant cell, caseous necrosis develops, probably a result of acquired hypersensitivity to the organism. Caseous necrosis has a characteristic granular, cheesy appearance. The area surrounding the central core of necrosis is ringed with sensitized T lymphocytes. Fibrosis and calcification develop as the lesion ages, resulting finally in a *granuloma*, which is called a *tubercle*. Collagenous scar tissue encapsulates the tubercle, effectively separating the organisms from the body. The organisms may or may not be killed in the process, but sensitized T lymphocytes develop to enhance the bactericidal ability of the macrophages. This results in cell-mediated immunity that usually lasts through life and can be demonstrated by administering purified protein derivative of the bacilli. A positive inflammatory wheal response indicates the presence of memory T cells for the mycobacteria.

Typically, the defense mechanisms of the body control the infection and the person is unaware of the initial exposure (primary infection); however, a small proportion, usually children, develop progressive primary disease. The lifetime risk of developing active TB after exposure is 5% to 10% in the healthy person in contrast to the 50% or greater rate in the HIV-positive individual.[4] It is generally agreed that active TB results from reactivation of dormant infection under certain circumstances that include diabetes, cancer, chronic alcoholism, pregnancy, malnourished state, corticosteroids or other immunosuppressive therapy, silicosis, gastrectomy, and stress. Because active TB is the only form of the disease that is contagious, it is the means by which TB can perpetuate itself.

A suspicion of TB is the most important step in the diagnosis and control of TB. Physical findings are not specific and not particularly helpful in defining pulmonary TB. A cough, which may be persistent and productive of sputum, is the most common respiratory symptom. Hemoptysis, shortness of breath, and chest pain may occur but are not common nor specific symptoms of TB. The systemic (constitutional) symptoms include malaise, weight loss, headache, night sweats, and fever. The person may simply complain of not feeling well, and may have no symptoms but seek intervention because of

abnormal results of a chest x-ray, often performed for an unrelated reason. Before the beginning of the epidemic of HIV, only 15% of reported TB cases showed extrapulmonary symptoms. In the population of HIV-infected persons with TB, about one-third have both pulmonary and nonpulmonary involvement.[10] Listed in order of descending frequency, nonpulmonary sites include lymph nodes, pleura, genitourinary tract, bone, meninges, and intraabdominal organs. The epidemic of HIV has altered the frequency and description of disseminated or miliary TB, which is a result of the systemic proliferation of the organism affecting multiple organs due to inadequate host defenses.[10]

When TB is suspected, an acid-fast bacterium smear on sputum should be done quickly, because smear-positive individuals can spread the disease. Advanced culture technology has increased the accuracy and speed of definitive diagnosis through positive sputum cultures. With the use of radiometric culture methods identification of a positive culture can be completed in a two-week time frame. Tests that identify specific *M. tuberculosis* DNA should be available and soon will be especially useful in identifying extrapulmonary TB.[16]

CASE STUDY 29-1

Mr. Josiah Fine is a 28-year-old black male who was admitted to the intensive care unit in respiratory distress. He has a known history of HIV which has not been treated and the patient has had no apparent symptoms since diagnosis 3 years ago. The respiratory distress was of insidious onset, with night sweats and a dry, hacking cough for the past week. The x-ray pattern appears to be compatible with *Pneumocystis carinii*. Mr. Fine was tested for tuberculosis and after two weeks was diagnosed with active TB.

1. *What is the relationship between TB and HIV infection?*
2. *How is TB spread? What measures can be used to prevent the spread of this disease?*
3. *Describe the pathophysiology of pulmonary tuberculosis.*
4. *How would the signs and symptoms differ in this man from other individuals with TB?*
5. *Describe the treatment protocol for TB. What might interfere with the progress of treatment in this case?*

See Appendix G for discussion.

▼ *Aspiration Pneumonia*

Aspiration usually refers to the inhalation of gastric contents, food, water, or blood into the tracheobronchial system. Aspiration pneumonia results when the material is propelled into the alveolar system and most frequently occurs after vomiting or near-drowning.

Aspiration of gastric contents is relatively common and

is especially associated with impaired consciousness, which includes such conditions as cardiac arrest, seizure, alcoholic intoxication, stroke, and general anesthesia. The gastric contents are very acidic, having a pH of less than 3. Aspiration of this material results in chemical irritation and destruction of the mucosa of the tracheobronchial tree. In the lungs, areas of hemorrhage and edema occur, especially in dependent portions.

The severity of the response depends on the person's physiologic status and the quantity and acidity of the aspirant. Nosocomial cases of aspiration are more likely to contain gram-negative bacteria, particularly if the person is intubated or has received histamine-2 blockers or antacids. Persons receiving nasogastric tube feeding are at particular risk of aspiration.

After aspiration, respiratory distress usually begins abruptly with evidence of bronchospasm, dyspnea, tachycardia, and cyanosis. Severe hypoxemia frequently occurs and may precipitate adult respiratory distress syndrome (ARDS).

Aspirated foodstuffs may be diagnosed by their content or appearance. Lipid-laden macrophages, for example, indicate that fats have been aspirated and have caused an acute or chronic pneumonia. Foods may cause mechanical obstruction of the airway or chemical irritation of the mucosal lining, especially if they are mixed with acid gastric secretions.

In *drowning* or *near-drowning*, aspiration of water usually causes intense laryngospasm, which does not adequately protect the alveoli from fluid. The result of near-drowning is severe hypoxemia and acidosis. Seawater aspiration may lead to secondary pulmonary edema because of the high sodium content of the water.[7] The close relationship between near-drowning and ARDS may, in part, be due to washing out of surfactant from the alveolar linings.

▼ *Pulmonary Edema*

The pulmonary vascular system has a great capacity to accommodate amounts of blood up to three times its normal volume, but at a critical pressure point, fluid moves across the alveolocapillary line and pulmonary edema occurs. Pulmonary edema is simply an accumulation of fluid in the tissues (interstitium and alveoli of the lungs).

Understanding the mechanism by which pulmonary edema occurs is enhanced by the understanding of *Starling's equation*. Hydrostatic and osmotic pressures are the major forces that affect movement of water across the capillary membrane. The normal hydrostatic pressure in the pulmonary capillaries is approximately 7 to 10 mm Hg. The plasma oncotic pressure is approximately 25 mm Hg. Therefore, the alveoli tend to stay dry, because the pressures oppose fluid movement into the interstitium and alveoli.

Pulmonary edema fluid is distributed positionally. Normally, when a person is in the upright position, the hydrostatic pressures are higher in the lung bases than at the apices. Acute pulmonary edema may show bizarre patterns of distribution because of variations in the transmission of pleural pressures in different areas of the lungs. However, in chronic pulmonary edema, the fluid tends to accumulate at the lung bases.

Hydrostatic pressure in the pulmonary bed must increase to a level of approximately 25 to 30 mm Hg for pulmonary edema to occur when capillary permeability is normal and the alveolar system is intact. Lymphatic drainage of a few milliliters per hour is usually sufficient to drain any excess protein and fluid that does not move back into the capillary. Lymphatics are probably sparse in the alveolar regions and more plentiful in the peribronchial and perivascular spaces, but these can increase lymph-carrying capacity 6-fold to 10-fold, so that a sustained increase in hydrostatic pressure can be compensated for by increased lymphatic drainage.[15]

The most common cause of pulmonary edema is left ventricular failure. This is discussed in more detail on pages 502–505. Left ventricular failure may be due to such pathology as acute myocardial infarction, hypertension, or mitral valve disease. Pulmonary edema may also result from acute inflammation, poisoning with certain gases (especially chlorine and nitrogen peroxide), pulmonary aspiration of gastric juice, excessive volume overload, some types of cerebral damage, and smoke inhalation (Table 29-2). The mechanisms for producing edema differ, but all result in increased interstitial or alveolar fluid (Fig. 29-6).

In the case of pulmonary edema from acute inflammation, the result is alveolar damage, which leads to increased permeability and fluid exudation into the alveoli. In cerebral damage, the reaction of the body is to increase sympathetic nervous system stimulation, resulting in diversion of blood to the lungs, which increases the hydrostatic pressure and causes edema. Fluid overloading is rare with a normal heart but occurs when the fluid volume exceeds the heart's ability to pump it all. Smoke inhalation may be injurious due to chemical pneumonitis from the fumes, gases, and particulate matter.[15] Intraalveolar hemorrhage; congested, edematous alveoli; and interstitial edema may all result from this type of injury.

Pulmonary edema due to heart failure occurs when the left side of the heart is no longer able to accept all of the output sent to it from the right side of the heart. As a result, a small amount of blood is dammed back into the pulmonary circulation with each beat of the heart. Gradually, the amount of accumulated blood exceeds the distensible capacity of the pulmonary vasculature. The excess blood in the pulmonary tree increases pulmonary

TABLE 29-2 *Causes of Pulmonary Edema*

Cause	Condition
Left ventricular failure (increased pulmonary capillary pressure)	Myocardial infarction, mitral valve disease, cardiomyopathy, mitral stenosis, dysrhythmias
Alveolar damage and increased capillary permeability	Acute inflammation, sepsis, inhalation of poisonous gases, smoke fumes and particulates, aspiration of toxic fluids
Drug-induced injury	Oxygen radicals produced by chemotherapeutic agents; alveolocapillary cytotoxicity due to heroin, oxygen toxicity; allergic reactions causing increased alveolocapillary permeability by antibiotics, inhalants, and iodinated radiocontrast media, for example; hydrochlorothiazide and tocolytic induced, mechanism unknown
High altitude	Mechanism unknown, diffuse pulmonary edema
Post head injury	Autonomic nervous system stimulation, volume diverted to heart and lungs
Fluid overloading	Massive transfusions, intravenous fluids, electrolyte (especially sodium) imbalance
Lymphatic obstruction/insufficiency	Diffused carcinomatous infiltration lymphatic channels, silicosis, lymphangitis
Decreased colloid osmotic pressure	Hypoalbuminemia from liver, kidney, wasting diseases

capillary hydrostatic pressure. This pressure increase is most severe in the dependent areas of the lungs, accounting for increased fluid buildup in the bases.

Pulmonary blood pressure is also raised by reflex vasoconstriction of the pulmonary vessels that occurs in response to hypoxemia, which may result from the decreased cardiac output. As pressure in the pulmonary circulation increases, fluid is forced into the pulmonary interstitial spaces. This phenomenon is known as *transudation*.

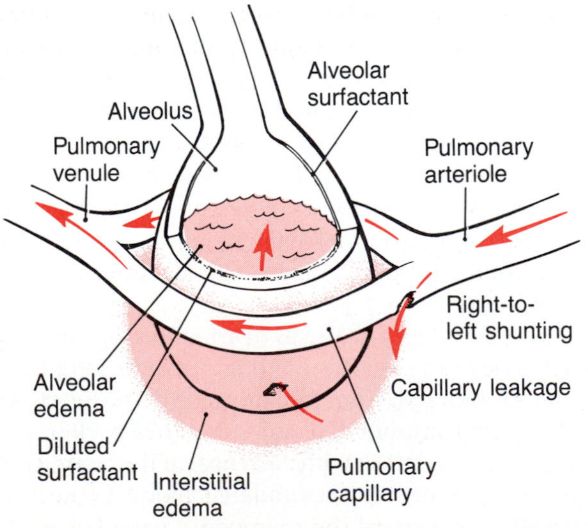

Pulmonary edema actually occurs in two stages (Fig. 29-7). The first stage is *interstitial edema*, in which fluid accumulates in the peribronchial and perivascular spaces. The lymphatics attempt to decrease this fluid by widening their lumina and increasing the rate of flow. Some widening of the alveolar walls may also occur at this stage. Interstitial pulmonary edema widens the distance between the alveoli and pulmonary capillaries but has little effect on gaseous exchange in the early stages.

The second stage occurs when interstitial hydrostatic pressure is so high that it pushes fluid into the alveoli, resulting in *alveolar edema*. The alveoli fill one at a time, diluting surfactant with the incoming fluid. This reduces the surface tension in the alveoli and predisposes them to collapse. Some alveoli may be compressed by surrounding edematous alveoli, whereas others are not aerated because the airways that supply them are filled with fluid. When no oxygen is present in the alveoli, right-to-left shunting occurs. Sometimes the shunt may be as large as 50%, resulting in severe hypoxemia and, later, hypercapnia. This ventilation–perfusion abnormality is called a *shunt unit* (see Figure 29-6).

The symptoms of pulmonary edema are directly attributable to its pathophysiology. The onset of symptoms may be sudden or gradual. If pulmonary edema is mild and develops slowly, the major symptoms are wheezing, paroxysmal nocturnal dyspnea, and dry

FIGURE 29-6 *Schematic representation of interstitial alveolar edema, right-to-left shunting, alveolar edema, and surfactant interference.*

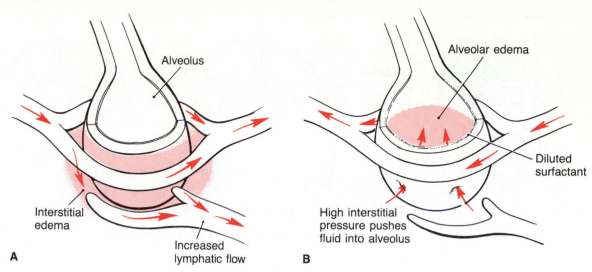

FIGURE 29-7 *Illustration of stages of pulmonary edema.* **A.** *Interstitial pulmonary edema and increased lymphatic flow.* **B.** *Alveolar pulmonary edema.*

cough. When it is fully developed, there is dyspnea, orthopnea, wheezing, and productive cough. The person expectorates profuse amounts of sputum that initially may be white and frothy but becomes pink-tinged or bright red. The pink-tinged fluid results from microvascular leaking of red blood cells. Bloody, frothy sputum comes from pulmonary capillaries that have ruptured under high pressure if the underlying cause is heart failure. Hemoptysis (bloody sputum) also may occur with severe alveolocapillary damage due to substances such as toxins and smoke.

The elastic work of breathing is greatly increased, because the accumulated interstitial fluid causes lung stiffening and loss of compliance. This, together with hypoxemia, leads to a pattern of rapid, shallow breathing. The lungs fill with fluid, which causes moist bubbling, rales, and wheezing. Abnormal heart sounds are common due to heart failure. Chest roentgenograms show cardiomegaly and the fluid accumulation appears as confluent patchy opacifications that are concentrated centrally in the lungs, having the appearance of a butterfly or bat's wing.[15] Arterial blood gases reflect the degree of hypoxemia, hypercapnia, or both.

▼ *Traumatic Injuries of the Chest Wall*

Traumatic injuries of the chest wall are common results of automobile accidents or other injuries. The injuries may be simple, such as a rib fracture, or as serious as flail chest abnormality.

The most common chest wall injury is *simple rib fracture*. Because it causes inspiratory pain, there is voluntary splinting, which results in restricted tidal volume and an increased respiratory rate. The victim voluntarily inhibits the urge to cough. The young, previously healthy person usually tolerates a fractured rib well, but a person with underlying pulmonary disease or an elderly person may develop impaired clearance of secretions, atelectasis, pneumonia, or even respiratory failure. The condition is further aggravated if the chest is strapped and narcotic analgesics are used. Chest strapping limits the ability to take a deep breath and, thus, enhances the risk for atelectasis and pneumonia. Compliance and all measurements of lung volume are reduced. The respiratory drive and the cough reflex may be depressed by administration of narcotic analgesics.

If several adjacent ribs in an area are fractured, the stability of that area of chest wall may be lost (Fig. 29-8). As a result, on inspiration the intrathoracic pressure is lowered and that area of the chest wall is sucked in. The underlying lung tissue does not expand, and gas exchange becomes impaired. Compliance is reduced. When the victim exhales, the affected area of the chest is elevated somewhat because of the increased intrathoracic pressure, creating a paradoxic movement during the ventilatory cycle.

This injury increases the work of breathing and impairs ventilatory efficiency. The more the person works to maintain adequate ventilation, the more paradoxic the respiratory motion. In severe cases, a pendulum movement of the mediastinum may occur with each breath, putting pressure on the otherwise unaffected lung. The paradoxic motion may increase central venous pressure while decreasing venous return to the heart, resulting in decreased blood pressure. Normal breathing is impaired and coughing is impossible, resulting in hypoventilation, hypoxemia, and even respiratory failure. Clinical manifestations of *flail chest* abnormality include

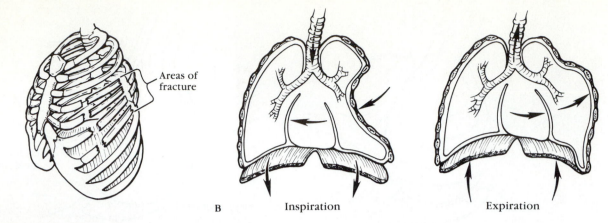

FIGURE 29-8 *A. Chest wall injury that can produce flail chest abnormality.* **B.** *Physiology of flail chest abnormality resulting in paradoxical breathing.*

the obvious signs of chest wall trauma; "flail" movement with unequal chest excursion; severe dyspnea; pain, especially on inspiration; rales; and reduced breath sounds. Chest radiographs show evidence of fractured ribs, and blood gases indicate the degree of hypoxemia.

▼ *Pleural Effusion*

Pleural fluid is normally produced in quantities just sufficient to lubricate the surfaces of the visceral and parietal pleura to provide a smooth sliding surface. This small amount of fluid is continually replenished and reabsorbed, maintaining a constant amount in the pleural space.

Pleural fluid accumulation or effusion may result from disease or trauma. Conditions that may lead to fluid accumulation include neoplasms, infections, thromboemboli, and cardiovascular and immunologic defects. Thoracic trauma may cause bleeding into the pleural space.

Pleural effusions are frequently categorized as transudates and exudates. Generally, inflammatory diseases and those of tissue destruction produce exudates with a specific gravity of above 1.017 and a high concentration of protein and lactic dehydrogenase. Transudates, which are produced by such diseases as congestive heart failure, show lower values for these components, with protein below 3.5 g/dL and lactic dehydrogenase below 200 U.[5]

The accumulation of pleural transudates is sometimes referred to as *hydrothorax*. If the effusion contains purulent material, it is called *empyema*. If empyema ultimately leads to fibrous fusing of the lung and chest wall, it is called *fibrothorax*. If the pleural fluid contains blood, it is called *hemothorax*.

Fluid in the intrapleural space occupies space and displaces lung tissue by reducing the amount of lung expansion possible by direct pressure on the tissue, resulting in compression atelectasis (Fig. 29-9). It may cause a mediastinal shift, which puts pressure on the opposite lung as well. Compliance decreases, altering ventilation and perfusion on the affected side. When fluid is removed from the pleural space, lung tissue reexpands, allowing ventilation and perfusion to return to normal. This removal is often performed through a *thoracentesis* (Fig. 29-10). Clinical manifestations depend on the rate of effusion. A hemothorax from a ruptured thoracic aneurysm, for example, causes rapid accumulation of blood as well as dramatic signs and symptoms of blood loss and a mediastinal shift. In a slower process, 2,000 mL of fluid in the pleural space may accumulate before dyspnea is noted. Common symptoms relate to the amount of pulmonary embarrassment and include dyspnea, blood gas abnormalities, cyanosis, and jugular vein distension.

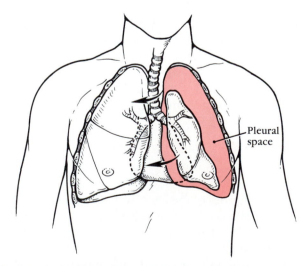

FIGURE 29-9 *Pleural effusion. Fluid has collected in the pleural space and has displaced lung tissue. Also note the shift of fluid into the mediastinum and torsion of the bronchus.*

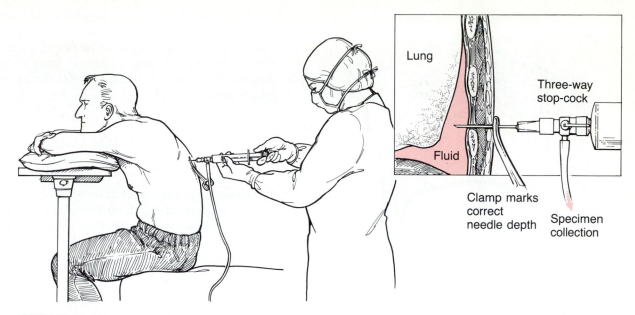

FIGURE 29-10 *Thoracentesis. A method for obtaining a sample of fluid in pleural effusion. It may be used for diagnosing a pleural effusion or for improving ventilation when larger amounts are removed.*

▼ *Pneumothorax*

Pneumothorax occurs when air enters the pleural space. Once this takes place, lung tissue is displaced in much the same way as if fluid had entered the space.

Air may enter the pleural space from an opening in the chest wall or from the lungs themselves (Fig. 29-11). Some of the causes of pneumothorax from the lungs are puncture by a fractured rib, spontaneous rupture of a superficial bleb, and rupture of a bleb during vigorous mechanical ventilation. Tracheobronchial rupture due to trauma may also cause pneumothorax. Surgical pneumothorax occurs as a part of every thoracotomy. *Spontaneous pneumothorax* may occur secondary to disease, such as emphysema, when a bleb on the surface of the lung ruptures and releases air into the pleural spaces (Fig. 29-12A). Primary spontaneous pneumothorax may occur in healthy young adults with no preexisting lung disease.

Pressure in the potential intrapleural space is nor-

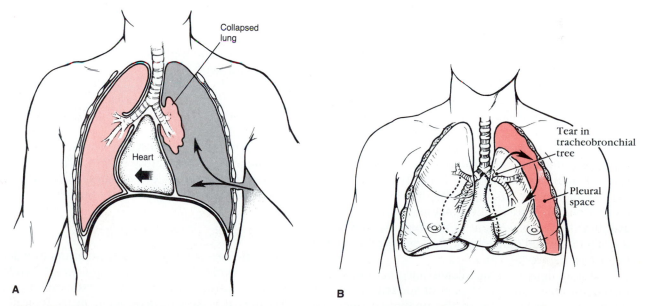

FIGURE 29-11 **A.** *Air has entered the pleural space through an opening in the chest wall.* **B.** *A tear in the tracheobronchial tree has caused air to move into the pleural space. The lung collapses, and the mediastinum shifts to the unaffected side.*

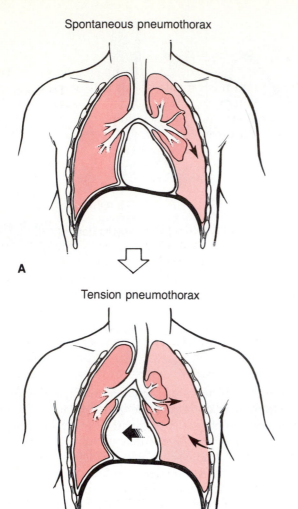

Spontaneous pneumothorax

A

Tension pneumothorax

B

FIGURE 29-12 **A.** *Spontaneous pneumothorax.* **B.** *Tension pneumothorax.*

mally lower or more negative than intraalveolar pressure. Therefore, if there is a break in either the integrity of the lung through the visceral pleura or the chest wall through the parietal pleura, air rushes to the area of lowest pressure, the pleural space. This continues as long as the air leak is present. Sometimes air leaks into the pleural space on inspiration, but the tissue seals itself on expiration, and outward leakage does not occur. This results in *tension pneumothorax*, which is a life-threatening condition of air buildup in the space, with displacement of and pressure on the structures within the mediastinum. This displacement to the opposite side affects the other lung and may impede the venous return to the heart (see Figure 29-12B).

Clinical signs of a significant pneumothorax may include dyspnea and chest pain of sudden onset. The trachea may deviate toward the unaffected side, and vesicular or bronchial breath sounds on the affected side may be reduced. Arterial blood gases may reveal acute

hypoxemia at the outset. The degree of all of the clinical signs depends on the extent of the pneumothorax. Symptoms of tension pneumothorax include increasing respiratory distress and cyanosis, bulging sternum, distended neck veins, elevated central venous pressure, and hypotension.

▼ Central Nervous System Depression

The respiratory center is made up of groups of nerve cells that are scattered through the reticular formation in the medulla oblongata. This center is responsible for respiratory rhythm. Although this structure is the major respiratory control, the pons coordinates breathing. The respiratory neural structure in the pons is called the *pneumotaxic center*. Stimulation of this center increases respiratory frequency, whereas depression slows respiration. The apneustic center also modifies the respiratory pattern. Cranial or cerebral trauma or central nervous system lesions, such as malignancies, brain abscesses, and other conditions, may result in injury to or impingement on the mediators of respiration and result in alterations of respiratory patterns.

If head injury affects the pneumotaxic center in the medulla, it may alter the rate, rhythm, and depth of respiration. Apnea may also occur. If central nervous system depression results because of trauma or disease, it frequently leads to decreased ventilatory drive, decreased responsiveness to ventilatory stimuli, and absence of the sigh mechanism. The result is a restrictive pathology that decreases total lung capacity.

Increasing intracranial pressure may lead to pressure on the respiratory center and change in breathing patterns, but more common is hypoxemia in obtunded persons due to the acute restrictive disease. The airway reflexes are depressed, increasing the risk of obstruction and aspiration.

▼ Neuromuscular Diseases

Many types of neuromuscular diseases may cause impairment of the respiratory system. The most common are summarized in Table 29-3. These can lead to an acute or chronic restrictive pulmonary process.

GUILLAIN-BARRÉ SYNDROME

Guillain-Barré syndrome (acute inflammatory demyelinating polyradiculoneuropathy, or Landry's syndrome), which is named after the two persons who originally described it, is an acute toxic polyneuritis. Typically, in its early stages, it is mistaken for a flu syndrome. As it progresses, it is accompanied by varying degrees of mus-

TABLE 29-3 *Neuromuscular Diseases Exhibiting Respiratory Insufficiency*

Disease	Example

Spinal cord disease	Trauma
	    Quadriplegia
	    Paraplegia
	Poliomyelitis

Motor nerve disease	Acute inflammatory demyelinating
	    polyradiculoneuropathy,
	    Guillain-Barré syndrome, or
	    Landry's ascending paralysis
	Tick-bite paralysis
	Porphyria

Myoneural junction disease	Myasthenia gravis Myasthenic syndrome
Muscle-wasting disease	Muscular dystrophy Congenital myotonia
Infectious disease	Tetanus

cular weakness and paralysis. This condition appears in some cases to result from an individual hypersensitivity response to a particular type of virus (see pp. 278–281). It has been described as occurring after a wide variety of conditions, such as upper respiratory tract infection or mononucleosis, or it may have no antecedent event.[5] The respiratory muscles typically become involved, and death, if it occurs, is most frequently due to respiratory complications.

The pulmonary problems in Guillain-Barré syndrome are threefold. First, paralysis of the internal and external intercostal muscles reduces functional breathing ability. Breathing then becomes entirely diaphragmatic, leading to reduced tidal volume, hypoxemia, and hypercapnia. Second, there is paralysis of the preganglionic fibers of the vagus nerve and of the postganglionic fibers of the sympathetic nervous system. Vagal paralysis causes loss of the normal protective mechanisms that respond to such stimuli as bronchial irritation and foreign bodies. The reflex bronchoconstriction is also lost. Paralysis of the sympathetic postganglionic fibers causes loss of bronchodilation. Third, the gag reflex is diminished or absent.

Pathologically, segmental loss of myelin sheath in the peripheral nerves may occur. Other body areas are also affected by paralysis but this is not life-threatening. Even though the syndrome may last for a few weeks, recovery may be complete if respirations are adequately supported during the acute stage.

Clinical manifestations include the rapid onset of symmetric weakness beginning in the legs and moving upward. The muscles are flaccid, and sensory changes may or may not be present. This effect on muscles of the pharynx and larynx may lead to impaired swallowing and gag reflexes. Cough reflex is depressed, and superimposed respiratory infection frequently occurs. Functional return is variable and usually progresses in a reverse pattern, with respiratory improvement occurring first, followed by functional improvement beginning in the upper extremities and finally in the lower extremities. Various types of residual impairment have been described.

DUCHENNE'S MUSCULAR DYSTROPHY

The most common, rapidly progressive type of muscular dystrophy is Duchenne's muscular dystrophy. Two types of the disease are described according to its progression: one form progresses rapidly and the other more slowly. Both forms of Duchenne's muscular dystrophy are hereditary, being X-linked recessive. Women are the carriers and their sons tend to manifest the disorder.

Muscular weakness results, leading to difficulty walking in the early years of life. Thoracoscoliosis and respiratory muscle weakness then progress rapidly. The muscles seem to weaken in this order: intercostals, abdominals, diaphragm, and accessory muscles of respiration. Despite respiratory impairment, studies show that alveolar hypoventilation occurs only as an acute or terminal event. As the severity of respiratory involvement increases, many patients are left with the use of only the accessory muscles of respiration. As a result, they may display unusual breathing patterns, such as frog breathing, gulping air, head bobbing, and pursed-lip breathing. The final acute respiratory failure is often triggered by an acute respiratory infection.[7]

▼ Respiratory Diseases Caused by Exposure to Organic and Inorganic Dusts

Many organic and inorganic dusts have been identified as being injurious to the lungs. The group of diseases caused by these dusts are collectively called the *pneumoconioses*.

SILICOSIS

Silicosis is the oldest and most widespread of the industrial diseases. It results from inhalation of silicon dioxide (silica), the most abundant compound in the earth's crust. Workers with high silica exposure include stone masons, potters, sand blasters, and foundry workers.

The main characteristic of silicosis is fibrosis, which is manifested initially as hard nodules of about 1 mm in diameter in lung parenchyma that increase in size and coalesce as the disease progresses. It usually takes 20 years or more of exposure for silicosis to progress to interstitial fibrosis and respiratory insufficiency.[11]

Silicosis causes defects in the immune response, both humoral and cellular. The reason for the defects is unknown. It is believed that the silica particles cause lysis of the macrophages that ingest them.[11] Immune response may then be responsible for the development of the fibrotic lesion. Among the industrial inhalants, silica is particularly dangerous because of its effect on macrophages, allowing the fibrotic lesions to proceed unchecked. This causes a very severe restrictive pulmonary disease. Persons with silicosis have an increased susceptibility to TB.

COAL WORKERS' PNEUMOCONIOSIS (BLACK LUNG DISEASE)

Most of the coal dust (carbon and silica) inhaled by miners is removed by the alveolar macrophages, with the remainder accumulating in the macrophages. Over time, the dust-laden macrophages gather at the perivascular structures, and local fibrosis ensues. Early in the disease, the process is manifested as a restrictive process with progressive fibrosis. As the disease progresses, the respiratory bronchioles dilate as a result of traction created by the contracting fibrous tissue. Centrilobular emphysema ensues from the dilatation and destruction of the respiratory bronchioles. The walls of the bronchioles break down, forming single spaces. If exposure to coal dust continues, centrilobular emphysema may occur throughout the lungs. Panlobular or primary emphysema characterized by destruction of the alveoli rather than the more central respiratory bronchioles is not observed in relationship to dust inhalation. A small percentage of those afflicted with simple pneumoconiosis due to silica or coal dust develop a more complicated form of the disease characterized by massive pulmonary fibrosis and chronic restrictive pulmonary disease. Although it is generally accepted that simple pneumoconiosis is related to the quantity and composition of dust retained in the lungs, the etiology of complicated pneumoconiosis is not as clear. It has been suggested that the process involves an immunologic mechanism and that it results in the development of massive fibrotic lesions. In the past, the recovery of the TB bacillus from the lungs of miners with complicated pneumoconiosis led researchers to conclude that the bacillus was the mediator of the immunologic defense. This theory, however, has not been substantiated, and the pathogenesis of the condition remains obscure.

BYSSINOSIS (BROWN LUNG DISEASE)

Bronchoconstriction also occurs due to hypersensitivity to inorganic and organic dusts. An example is byssinosis, which results from long-term exposure to cotton dust.

Cotton dust extracts have been shown to cause bronchoconstriction; it is now believed that exposure leads to a discharge of naturally produced histamine, leading to bronchospasm. When histamine stores are depleted, reactivity to cotton dust decreases, which explains the dynamics of byssinosis.

The described syndrome involves complaints of chest tightness, low-grade fever, and dyspnea by textile workers. The symptoms are more pronounced on Monday after a weekend away from the factory and the syndrome has become known as *Monday fever*. Later in the week, the symptoms gradually disappear. Researchers have demonstrated that the textile workers in the study group exhibited decreased ventilatory capacity and increased airway resistance during the Monday workday.

Eventually, the worker may complain of chest tightness on subsequent days of the week until symptoms may be accompanied by permanent incapacity. Further study in the areas of epidemiology and the mechanisms of bronchial inflammation is necessary before the mechanism of byssinosis can be fully understood.[15]

ASBESTOSIS

Occupational exposure to asbestos has occurred in the mining, manufacturing, and application occupations. The main use of asbestos is in cement products for construction, but it is also used in insulation and fireproofing. The most important health-related effects from asbestos exposure are pulmonary fibrosis and tumors.

The minerals known as asbestos vary considerably in length and diameter. Chrystotile is a type of serpentine fiber with a curly configuration able to shear into many small fibrils. It accounts for 95% of the asbestos in the world. All other forms of asbestos are amphiboles, straight fibers that do not shear. Crocidolite, an amphibole, can penetrate deep into the lung and is implicated in the development of mesothelioma, a cancer of the pleura with a grim prognosis.[9]

Particles of asbestos may be cleared by the mucociliary escalator system or, if deposited deep within the lung parenchyma, may be partially or completely engulfed by alveolar macrophages.[9] Some of the fibers may be removed through lymphatic circulation.

Diffuse pulmonary fibrosis resulting from asbestos exposure is termed *asbestosis* (white lung). The fibrosis initially affects the alveolar walls and gradually involves the interstitium. Prominent symptoms include exertional dyspnea, severe nonproductive cough, clubbing of the fingers, and, ultimately, symptoms of respiratory failure.[9] Rales and restriction of lung inflation are common clinical findings. Pleural changes may be associated and include hyaline plaques that undergo calcification. Recurrent exudative pleural effusions may also be present.

Although it is uncertain whether asbestos acting alone can cause lung cancer in nonsmokers, asbestos and smoking appear to combine in a multiplicative fashion to produce lung cancer.[9]

▼ Pulmonary Fibrosis

Pulmonary fibrosis is a chronic restrictive condition that involves diffuse fibrosis of the lung tissue and results in severe loss of compliance with lung stiffness. As indicated above, fibrosis is frequently due to occupational exposure to substances, such as coal dust. In cases where the cause is unknown, the disease may be referred to as the *Hamman-Rich syndrome* or, preferably, *idiopathic pulmonary fibrosis*.

Sarcoidosis is another disease that includes among its features a severe, diffuse, pulmonary fibrosis. It produces bilateral hilar lymphadenopathy or lung pathology that is visible on chest x-ray in 90% of cases.[5] This disease has a characteristic granulomatous tissue response that must be distinguished from TB or fungal infections. It presents a number of immunologic abnormalities and macrophage changes. Systemic effects are common, with the lungs being the most severely affected, followed by eye and skin lesions.[5] Severely decreased compliance and diffusing capacity may lead to hypoxemia and cor pulmonale. The clinical course may exhibit periods of progression and periods of remission that may be initiated by steroid therapy.[5] The cause of sarcoidosis is unknown, and the prognosis depends on the amount of pulmonary infiltrate with or without lymphadenopathy.

▼ Thoracic Deformity

Many chest deformities are not severe enough to compromise pulmonary status. Severe deformities do compress lung tissue in one or more areas of the chest, however, and may limit thoracic excursion. Severe *kyphoscoliosis*, in which the body is essentially twisted over to one side, is one example. Another is *pectus excavatum*, or funnel chest, in which the lower end of the sternum is caved in because of attachment to the spine by thick fibrous bands. *Pectus carinatum* (pigeon breast) causes abnormal prominence of the sternum, and the rib structure may limit respiratory movement. Many other deformities also restrict pulmonary status.

In general, severe thoracic deformities compress portions of lung tissue and limit chest expansion, leading to areas of small lung volume and atelectasis. Compliance, total lung capacity, and other volume measurements are reduced. The pulmonary vascular bed in the affected areas is also reduced, resulting in increased work of breathing, alveolar hypoventilation, and the consequences of hypoxemia.

Because of the wide variety of deformities and their effects on pulmonary status, the pulmonary function of each affected person must be assessed carefully. Gener-ally, the effect of pectus excavatum is not severe, whereas the effect of kyphoscoliosis varies from mild to very severe.

▼ Sleep-Related Breathing Disorders

The normal effects of sleep on breathing vary according to the stages of sleep (see pp. 185–188). During rapid eye movement sleep, an increased rate and even paradoxical breathing frequently occurs. During nonrapid eye movement, the rate of breathing may decrease and the rhythm may become irregular.[7]

SLEEP APNEA SYNDROME

Sleep apnea is classified as *central*, when airflow ceases due to absence of ventilatory efforts, *obstructive*, when there are chest and abdominal movements with no airflow, or *mixed*, when there is initial loss of ventilatory effort followed by ventilatory efforts without airflow.[7] The pathophysiologic effects depend on the duration and frequency of the apneic episodes. Flowchart 29-1 illustrates the pathogenesis of the syndrome.

OBESITY HYPOVENTILATION SYNDROME

Obesity hypoventilation syndrome is recognized as a part of the spectrum of sleep-related breathing disorders. Severe obesity may result in restricted ventilation, especially in the supine position. Obesity hypoventilation syndrome (once referred to as *Pickwickian syndrome*) is related to morbid obesity and presents a picture of hypoventilation, somnolence, severe hypoxemia, polycythemia, and cor pulmonale.[7] The term comes from Charles Dickens' description of Joe, a fat boy notorious for falling asleep in *Posthumous Papers of the Pickwick Club*.

Severe obesity causes pulmonary restriction by two means. First, the extreme excess of adipose tissue in the abdomen tends to force the thoracic contents up into the chest and, thus, restricts diaphragmatic excursion. Second, the weight of the chest wall greatly increases the amount of work required to move the chest for inspiration. This is especially true for a woman with pendulous breasts. Severe obesity results in reduced compliance, expiratory reserve volume, total lung capacity, and vital capacity, with all of these reductions due to a great increase in the work of breathing and great susceptibility to respiratory infections. Arterial blood gas studies reveal hypercapnia and hypoxemia.

Obesity alone does not provide an adequate explanation of the disorder, because some massively obese persons have the syndrome and some do not. Obstructive sleep apnea occurs in persons who are not obese as well as in those who are, and although weight loss

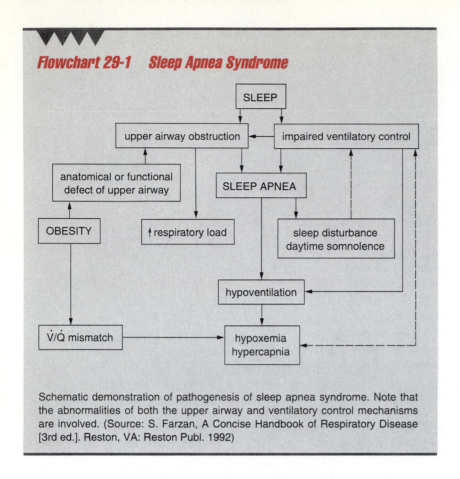

Flowchart 29-1   Sleep Apnea Syndrome

Schematic demonstration of pathogenesis of sleep apnea syndrome. Note that the abnormalities of both the upper airway and ventilatory control mechanisms are involved. (Source: S. Farzan, A Concise Handbook of Respiratory Disease [3rd ed.]. Reston, VA: Reston Publ. 1992)

typically relieves this condition, sometimes it does not. Severely affected persons have depression of the ventilatory drive and may experience apneic episodes due to upper airway obstruction during sleep. Somnolence is characteristic and may be related to sleep deprivation that occurs as a result of frequent awakenings after the airway-obstructive episodes.

Therapy for sleep apnea depends on whether there is upper airway obstruction for which tracheostomy may be used. A second, newer surgical approach is a procedure which involves removal of the uvula, part of the soft palate, and pharyngeal tissue. Whether it will prove to be effective in treating the disease remains to be seen. Nasal continuous positive airway pressure is a less invasive way to maintain upper airway patency with promising results.[20]

▼ Idiopathic Respiratory Distress Syndrome of the Newborn

Idiopathic respiratory distress syndrome (IRDS) of the newborn is the most clearly understood abnormality that involves surfactant deficiency. The surfactant layer develops late in fetal life, at about the 28th to 32nd week. Infants born before the 28th week are at a greater risk for developing acute respiratory distress. This is still a major

cause of death in premature infants. The severity of the respiratory distress and the mortality are related to gestational age at birth.

The pathology of IRDS includes inadequate pulmonary expansion and diffuse atelectasis, which is of a primary type because the lungs have never been expanded. Pulmonary vascular resistance increases because of high pulmonary arterial pressures, presumably due to increased pulmonary arteriolar resistance. The resulting increased pressure creates a higher than normal pressure on the right side of the heart. This high pressure perpetuates fetal circulation by keeping the foramen ovale and the ductus arteriosus patent. Idiopathic respiratory distress syndrome, or hyaline membrane disease, is characterized by large right-to-left shunting that accentuates hypoxemia and hypercapnia in later stages and is increased by hypoxemia, which leads to increased right heart pressures. Ischemic injury in the lung fields causes fluid to leak into interstitial and alveolar spaces and the hyaline membrane to form. Vascular engorgement occurs, the lymphatics dilate, and cellular debris lines the alveoli, with evidence of degenerating epithelial and endothelial cells in the alveolocapillary membrane. The hyaline membranes are apparently composed of plasma, fibrin, necrotic epithelial cells, and amniotic fluid and contribute to the respiratory distress.[11] Atelectasis is extensive, with widespread infiltration of the pulmonary tissue (Flowchart 29-2).[7]

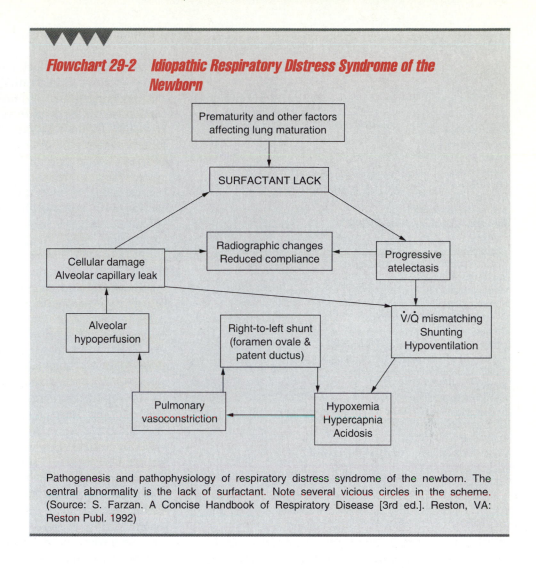

Flowchart 29-2 Idiopathic Respiratory Distress Syndrome of the Newborn

Pathogenesis and pathophysiology of respiratory distress syndrome of the newborn. The central abnormality is the lack of surfactant. Note several vicious circles in the scheme. (Source: S. Farzan. A Concise Handbook of Respiratory Disease [3rd ed.]. Reston, VA: Reston Publ. 1992)

Clinical manifestations include dyspnea from the first moments of life and rapid, shallow respirations. The lower ribs retract on inspiration and an expiratory grunt usually is heard.

Hypoxemia is characteristic, and an elevated P_{CO_2} level with respiratory or metabolic acidosis may complicate the picture.

Treatment measures are improving the prognosis in this condition. Continuous positive airway pressure is used with good results to improve oxygenation, and replacement of surfactant appears to be beneficial. However, the condition still carries a high mortality rate.

▼ Adult Respiratory Distress Syndrome

Adult respiratory distress syndrome (ARDS) is a condition characterized by severe hypoxemia and progressive loss of lung compliance. It causes severe restrictive disease. It has been known by a number of other names, including shock lung, traumatic wet lung, capillary leak syndrome, postperfusion lung, congestive atelectasis, and posttraumatic pulmonary insufficiency. This syndrome is never a primary disease, but rather, occurs secondary to some other insult to the body. General etiologic factors have been identified and classified as to the mechanism of causation (Table 29-4). The following categories are described: 1) reduced perfusion; 2) increased capillary permeability; 3) direct tissue and capillary insults; and 4) others, with obscure mechanisms. Regardless of the etiology, the response of the lung to injury occurs predictably, consisting of three phases:

1. Exudative phase (24–96 hours): Alveolar capillary and epithelial injury with increased permeability and edema.
2. Early proliferative phase (3–10 days): Proliferation of type II alveolar cells; hyaline membrane organizes and alveolar septum thickens.
3. Late proliferative phase (7–10 days): Fibrosis of hyaline membranes and alveolar septum, respiratory ducts, and bronchioles.[19]

In the injury phase, the effects of ARDS are similar despite the initiating underlying condition (Flowchart 29-3). The insult leads to capillary congestion and con-

TABLE 29-4 *Underlying Causes That Can Precipitate Adult Respiratory Distress Syndrome (ARDS)*

Reduced Perfusion
Cardiogenic shock
Trauma
Major burns
Fat embolus
Hemorrhage
Severe hypovolemia
Increased Capillary Permeability
Sepsis
Pneumonia
Noxious fume or smoke inhalation
Reactions to drugs
Venoms or toxins
Immune complex diseases
Overtransfusion of crystalloids
Uremia
Direct Tissue and Capillary Insults
Aspiration of gastrointestinal contents
Rapid decompression
Near-drowning
Oxygen toxicity
Hypoxemia
Fluid overload
Starvation
Other Mechanisms, Not Well Understood
High-altitude reactions
Sudden changes in intrathoracic pressure
Central nervous system injuries
Narcotic overdose
Cardiopulmonary bypass

sequent alteration of capillary permeability. Endothelial cell damage occurs, as does malfunction of the type II pneumocytes. The activity of these cells decreases, which results in decreased production of surfactant. Fluid leaks into the pulmonary interstitium and eventually into the alveoli. This causes stiffening of the lungs (loss of compliance) and dilution of surfactant. The altered compliance and diluted surfactant work together to lead to widespread atelectasis, which causes hypoxemia. In addition, there may be pulmonary interstitial edema and hemorrhage, the formation of alveolar exudate or hyaline membrane, and a predisposition to secondary pulmonary infection. Widespread atelectasis leads to an increased right-to-left shunt across the pulmonary capillary bed, causing critical hypoxemia. In the early proliferative phase, the major manifestations are much like an acute pneumonia, with major problems relating to oxygen saturation and poor pulmonary compliance. Pulmonary infections may result from life-support measures, such as oral intubation, and must be diagnosed and treated. In the fibrotic phase, the goal of treatment is to prevent permanent damage. Most sur-

vivors of ARDS have resolution of the fibrosing condition.[19]

A special pulmonary pathophysiologic process has been described in individuals exposed to high levels of oxygen for more than 36 hours. Continuous breathing of high concentrations of oxygen leads to *oxygen toxicity*, with diffuse parenchymal damage resulting in interference with the production of surfactant and formation of hemorrhagic exudate, with fibrin in the alveoli, alveolar ducts, and respiratory bronchioles. The earliest change is thickening of interstitial spaces with fluid containing fibrin, polymorphonuclear leukocytes, and macrophages. Two special processes explain the resulting dysfunction. First, breathing pure oxygen results in absorption of the gas from the alveoli. Nitrogen, normally present in atmospheric gas, is not present under these circumstances and, therefore, does not exert its function of keeping the alveoli expanded. The result is alveolar collapse. Second, oxygen has a toxic effect on the surfactant-producing cells, so that this vital substance is not produced in adequate quantities. Without adequate surfactant, the alveoli collapse and fluid exudes from the capillaries to the alveolar sacs.

The results of ARDS are progressive hypoxemia and reduced lung compliance, despite the administration of high levels of oxygen. Any person whose oxygen tension decreases while receiving high concentrations of oxygen should be considered a prime candidate for ARDS.

Those at a high risk for ARDS should be observed for onset of the condition throughout the first 96 hours after insult. No previous history of lung disease may be obtained, but persons with previous lung pathology are somewhat more susceptible to development of ARDS. Observable symptoms include extreme dyspnea, tachypnea and grunting, and labored respirations that occur late in the phenomenon. Therefore, the arterial blood gases of persons who develop the disease indicate decreasing P_{O_2} despite oxygen therapy. Venous oxygenation falls early in the course of the disease and may be seen to drop below 60% (normal 70%). If the arterial P_{O_2} is not correctable to above 50 when a person is receiving 100% oxygen, there should be a high index of suspicion for this condition. Usually, clinical deterioration is rapid and progressive. Hemoptysis and cyanosis may or may not occur. The hypoxemia and increased work of breathing may initially lead to metabolic acidosis. As respiratory muscles tire, respiratory acidosis occurs. Chest films show progressive, patchy, bilateral infiltrates.

It has been proposed that the event which initiates ARDS affects multiple organs simultaneously, but because alveolar flooding is immediately life-threatening as opposed to other organ edema, respiratory symptoms are seen first. If there is failure to reverse the initial event or if secondary infections occur the extrapulmonary signs of multiple organ failure may be seen.[13] The prognosis for affected individuals, formerly reported as a

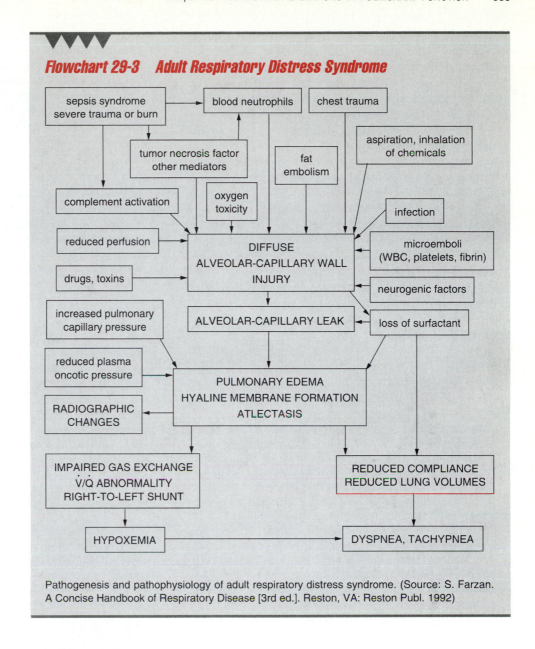

Flowchart 29-3　Adult Respiratory Distress Syndrome

Pathogenesis and pathophysiology of adult respiratory distress syndrome. (Source: S. Farzan. A Concise Handbook of Respiratory Disease [3rd ed.]. Reston, VA: Reston Publ. 1992)

mortality rate of 70% to 90%, has improved to about 40% to 50%, and depends on extrapulmonary involvement. Treatment primarily includes intermittent mandatory ventilation with positive end-expiratory pressure and management of underlying etiology, if possible. Other therapies being studied include surfactant replacement, inhaled nitric oxide, and extracorporeal membrane oxygenation.[13, 19] If the underlying cause is treatable or self-limiting and treatment is initiated at an early stage, a higher survival rate can be expected.[15]

▼ *Chapter Summary*

▼　Respiratory disorders have been divided into those that cause restriction of lung volumes and those that cause obstruction to airflow within the lungs.

▼　The most common cause of restrictive pulmonary disease is atelectasis, which is a shrunken, airless state of the alveoli. It may be found in conjunction with infections of the pulmonary system or as a response to inadequate inflation (eg, postsurgical) or hypoxemia (ARDS).

▼　A variety of conditions can cause restrictive pulmonary alterations, including upper and lower respiratory tract infections, aspiration pneumonia, and pulmonary edema.

▼　Of current, special concern is the emergence of TB as a major health threat. It is seen in alarming numbers in the immunocompromised populations and often is drug-resistant. The opportunistic infections of PCP and histoplasmosis are also a great threat to the immunocompromised populations.

▼　Traumatic injuries can cause thoracic wall damage or damage to intrapleural structures, which can result in pneumothorax or hemothorax. Neuromuscular diseases can decrease the ability of the respiratory muscles to perform adequately. Environmental or work-related exposure to organic and inorganic dusts can produce a restrictive process that also may be associated with some of the obstructive conditions.

▼ Sleep apnea syndrome and obesity hypoventilation syndrome are problems increasingly seen in the sick, obese population. These syndromes can produce severe respiratory failure unless they are properly recognized and treated.

▼ The IRDS of the newborn and the ARDS of the adult result from surfactant deficiency. IRDS occurs when the cells have not matured sufficiently to produce surfactant. ARDS occurs secondarily to a condition that suppresses surfactant production.

▼ ARDS is increasingly being described as a part of multiple organ dysfunction and often is the terminal event that was initiated by another mechanism (eg, trauma, liver failure).

▼ References

1. American Thoracic Society. Guidelines for the initial management of adults with community-acquired pneumonia: Diagnosis, assessment of severity, and initial antimicrobial therapy, *Am. Rev. Respir. Dis.* 148:1418–1426. 1993.

2. Bernstein, M.S., and Locksley, R.M. *Legionella* infections. In K.J. Isselbacher (ed.)., *Harrison's Principles of Internal Medicine* (13th ed.). New York: McGraw-Hill, 1994.

3. Bloch, A. Cauthen, G., Onorato, I, Dansbury, K., Kelly, G., Driver, C., and Snider, D. Nationwide survey of drug-resistant tuberculosis in the United States. *JAMA* 271(9): 665–671, 1994.

4. Bloom, B.R., and Murray, C.J.R. Tuberculosis: Commentary on a reemergent killer. *Science* 257:1055–1064, 1992.

5. Cotran, R.S., Kumar, V., and Robbins, S.L. *Robbins' Pathologic Basis of Disease* (5th ed.). Philadelphia: W.B. Saunders, 1994.

6. Daniel, T.M., Bates, J.H., and Downes, K.A. History of tuberculosis. In B.R. Bloom (ed.), *Tuberculosis: Pathogenesis, Protection, and Control*. Washington: ASM Press (American Society for Microbiology), 1994.

7. Farzan, S.A. *A Concise Handbook of Respiratory Diseases* (3rd ed.). Reston, Va.: Reston, 1992.

8. Fishman, J.A. *Pneumocystic carinii* pneumonia. In A.P. Fishman (ed.), *Update: Pulmonary Diseases and Disorders*. New York: McGraw-Hill, 1992.

9. Gee, J.B.L. Occupational lung disease. In D.H. Simmons and D.F. Tierney (eds.), *Current Pulmonology, Volume 13*. St. Louis: Mosby Year Book, 1992.

10. Hopewell, P.C. Overview of clinical tuberculosis. In B.R. Bloom (ed.), *Tuberculosis: Pathogenesis, Protection, and Control*. Washington, D.C.: ASM Press, 1994.

11. Kuhn, C., and Askin, F.B. Lung and mediastinum. In J.M. Kissane (ed.), *Anderson's Pathology* (9th ed.). St. Louis: C.V. Mosby, 1990.

12. Pennington, J. Hospital-acquired pneumonias. In J.E. Pennington (ed.), *Respiratory Infections: Diagnosis and Management* (2nd ed.). New York: Raven Press, 1989.

13. Rinaldo, J. The adult respiratory distress syndrome. In D.F. Tierney (ed.), *Current Pulmonology Volume 15*. St. Louis: C.V. Mosby, 1994.

14. Sarosi, G.A., and Davies, S.F., Fungal diseases. In D.H. Simmins and D.F. Tierney (eds.), *Current Pulmonology Volume 13*. St. Louis: Mosby Year Book, 1992.

15. Seaton, A., Seaton, D., and Leitch, A. *Crofton and Douglas's Respiratory Diseases* (4th ed.). Oxford: Blackwell, 1989.

16. Schluger, N.W., and Rom, W.N. Current approaches to the diagnosis of active pulmonary tuberculosis. *Am. J. Respir. Crit. Care Med* 149:264–267, 1994.

17. Smith, P.G., and Moss, A.R. Epidemiology of tuberculosis. In B.R. Bloom (ed.), *Tuberculosis: Pathogenesis, Protection, and Control*. Washington, D.C.: ASM Press, 1994.

18. Staikowsy, F. Lafon, B., Guidet, B., Dennis, M., Mayaud, C., and Offenstadt, G. Mechanical ventilation for *Pneumocystic carinii* pneumonia in patients with the acquired immunodeficiency syndrome: Is the prognosis really improved? *Chest* 104:756–762, 1993.

19. Taylor, R.W., and Norwood, S.H. The adult respiratory distress syndrome. In J.M. Civetta, T.W. Taylor, and R.R. Kirby (eds.), *Critical Care* (2nd ed.). Philadelphia: J.B. Lippincott Co., 1992.

20. White, D.P. Sleep apnea syndrome. In W.N. Kelley (ed.). *Textbook of Internal Medicine* (2nd ed.). Philadelphia: J.B. Lippincott Co., 1992.

Chapter 30

Obstructive Alterations in Pulmonary Function

Darlene H. Green

▼ CHAPTER OUTLINE

▼ LEARNING OBJECTIVES

1. Define **obstructive pulmonary disease**.
2. Differentiate between acute and chronic bronchitis.
3. Describe the pathophysiology of an acute asthmatic attack.
4. Describe the symptoms that result from bronchoconstriction.
5. Discuss pulsus paradoxus.
6. Compare the conditions that are classified as chronic obstructive pulmonary disease.
7. Explain the pathology of bronchiectasis.
8. Describe the signs and symptoms of bronchiectasis.
9. Discuss the basis for the development of cystic fibrosis.
10. List the criteria used in diagnosing cystic fibrosis.
11. List at least two risk factors in the development of chronic bronchitis.
12. Describe the pathophysiology of chronic bronchitis.
13. Differentiate chronic bronchitis from emphysema on the basis of pathologic and clinical features.
14. Relate similarities of chronic bronchitis and emphysema.
15. Describe the interrelationships of all the obstructive pulmonary diseases.
16. Describe the pathology of the different types of emphysema.
17. Discuss the pathophysiologic course of emphysema.
18. Define **hypoxia, hypoxemia**, and **hypercapnia**.
19. Explain why polycythemia occurs with chronic obstructive pulmonary disease.
20. Differentiate between compensated and uncompensated respiratory acidosis.

Barbara L. Bullock: PATHOPHYSIOLOGY: ADAPTATIONS AND ALTERATIONS IN FUNCTION, 4th ed.
© 1996 J.B. Lippincott-Raven Publishers

In general, obstructive pulmonary conditions obstruct airflow within the lungs, leading to less resistance to inspiration and more resistance to expiration. This results in prolongation of the expiratory phase of respiration. Many conditions can obstruct airflow; the more prominent ones are detailed in this chapter.

▼ Acute Obstructive Airway Disease

The classification of an acute obstructive airway disease is dependent on the episodic nature of the condition. The two major entities in this classification are *acute bronchitis* and *asthma*. In both, the obstruction is intermittent and reversible.

ACUTE BRONCHITIS

Acute bronchitis is a common condition caused by infection and inhalants that results in inflammation of the mucosal lining of the tracheobronchial tree. The most common infectious causes of acute bronchitis include influenza viruses, adenoviruses, rhinoviruses, and the organism *Mycoplasma pneumoniae*. Increased mucus secretion, bronchial swelling, and dysfunction of the cilia lead to increased resistance to expiratory airflow, usually resulting in some air trapping on expiration.

Bronchitis causes cough and production of large amounts of usually purulent mucus with associated wheezing if there is significant air obstruction. Coughing that produces purulent material may indicate a superimposed bacterial infection if the underlying etiology was viral. Once the stimulus for bronchitis is treated or removed, bronchial swelling decreases and the airways return to normal.

ASTHMA

Asthma is an episodic, acute airway obstruction that results from stimuli that would not elicit such a response in healthy persons. It has been defined as a disorder characterized by recurrent paroxysms of wheezing and dyspnea that are not attributable to underlying cardiac disease or other disease. This means that the person with asthma has a tendency toward bronchospasm as a response to a variety of stimuli. An estimated 5% of the population of the industrialized world is affected by asthma.[4] The common characteristics of all asthmatic reactions are hyperresponsiveness and an inflammatory response in the airways. The current view is that asthma is basically an inflammatory disease with airway hyperresponsiveness as a secondary feature.[2, 11] Between acute attacks, the lungs are usually normal or relatively normal.

Although asthma is characterized by wheezing, not all wheezing is related to asthma. Unilateral localized wheezing may be caused by aspiration of foreign bodies or by a tumor. Other causes include pulmonary emboli, infections, left ventricular failure, cystic fibrosis, immunologic deficiency, and viral respiratory illnesses. Wheezing is always a significant sign that should be investigated.

Pathophysiologic Mechanisms

Although there may be significant overlap between the two groups, the causes of asthma may be divided into two major categories: extrinsic and intrinsic.

Extrinsic (allergic) asthma commonly affects the child or young teenager who frequently relates a personal or family history of allergy, hives, rashes, and eczema. Results of skin tests are usually positive for specific allergens, indicating the probability that extrinsic asthma is allergic.

Childhood asthma attacks are usually self-limited and frequently are precipitated by exposure to specific antigens. A major allergen is the mite found in house dust. Seasonal asthma suggests pollen allergies. It is common for the person who "outgrows" asthma in childhood to develop other allergic manifestations in adulthood. Usually, the asthmatic attacks decrease in severity and frequency as the person matures. However, the more severe the childhood asthma, the less likely it is to remit in adulthood.

The pathophysiology of asthma attacks is related to the release of chemical mediators in an IgE-mast cell interaction (see pp. 349–350). This results in constriction of the bronchial smooth muscle, increased bronchial secretion from the goblet cells, and mucosal swelling, all of which lead to significant narrowing of the air passages.[5] It is basically an IgE-associated immune reaction in which the allergen evokes immediate production of histamine and other chemicals by the target organ, which is the lung. The acute respiratory obstruction, resistance to airflow, and turbulence of airflow are due to the following three responses: 1) bronchospasm, which involves rhythmic squeezing of the airways by the muscle bands surrounding them; 2) production of abnormally large amounts of thick mucus; and 3) the inflammatory response, including increased capillary permeability and mucosal edema (Fig. 30-1).

Allergy alone as a basis for the attacks is rare, and many mechanisms may be involved. Exercise, infection, and emotional upset are factors that often amplify the symptoms. Whatever the mechanisms, once bronchospasm is induced by one agent, the airway response to superimposed stimuli is greatly enhanced. For example, if a person with a subclinical response to pollen becomes emotionally upset, the airway response to the emotions may be greatly magnified because of the pollen sensitivity already established. Without a tendency toward

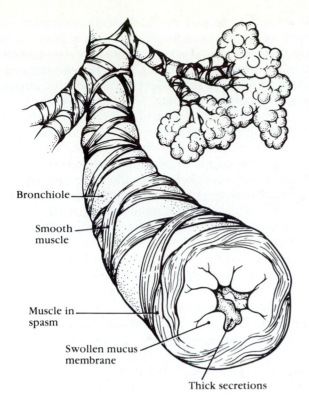

Bronchiole

Smooth muscle

Muscle in spasm

Swollen mucus membrane

Thick secretions

FIGURE 30-1 *Bronchial asthma. The bronchiole is obstructed on expiration, particularly by muscle spasm, edema of the mucosa, and thick secretions.*

bronchospasm, emotions, pollen, or other substances will not produce asthma.

Intrinsic (idiosyncratic) asthma usually affects adults, including those who did not have asthma or allergy before middle adulthood. There is a negative family or personal history for allergy, eczema, hives, and rashes.

In either type, respiratory infection may be a major precipitator of a severe asthma attack. Bacterial and viral infections may precipitate the attack, but viruses seem to be more important in this respect.

Clinical Manifestations

Asthma is considered to be a clinical syndrome characterized by cough, wheezing, and breathlessness and chest tightness initiated by allergens, infection or other stimuli. The stimuli can include drugs (particularly aspirin and beta-adrenergic blockers), exercise (especially in dry, cold climates), emotional stress, gastroesophageal reflux with microaspiration, active and passive cigarette smoke, occupational exposure to chemicals, and air pollution.[6]

The signs and symptoms of an asthmatic attack are closely related to the status of the airways. The only certainties about the manifestations of asthma are its variability and unpredictability. Bronchospasm leads to

both obstruction of the airways and air trapping. Air trapping is probably due to the acute increase in expiratory flow resistance, which means that the inspired air simply cannot be exhaled in the time available before metabolic demands trigger another inspiration. As a result, a portion of each breath is retained. The hyperinflated alveoli exert lateral traction on the bronchiolar walls so that inspiratory airway diameter is further increased. This may aid slightly in gas exchange, but it requires more inspiratory energy to overcome the tension of the already stretched elastic tissue.

The pressure of the trapped air tends to flatten the diaphragm's ability to function as the major organ of respiration and may oppose expansion of the lower chest. The costal fibers that are attached to the lower ribs are pulled into a horizontal, rather than upright, position. They can no longer move up and out, so the lower chest cannot expand normally. With the flat, fixed diaphragm, the accessory muscles are called on to enlarge the chest with each inspiration. This increases energy cost and also causes increased inflation of the apices rather than the bases. Figure 30-2 shows characteristic pulmonary function studies before, during, and after an acute asthmatic attack.

Wheezing, a common sign, can be likened to pulling on the opening of a balloon full of air to make it squeak. The smaller the opening past which the air is rushing, the more squeaking occurs. In the chest, wheezing results from air squeezing past the greatly narrowed airways. Narrowing is caused by bronchospasm plus mu-

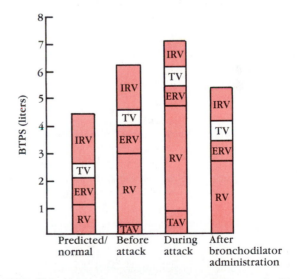

FIGURE 30-2 *Pulmonary function before, during, and after an asthma attack. The normal values are indicated as predicted values: inspiratory reserve volume (IRV), tidal volume (TV), and expiratory reserve volume (ERV). Before the attack, there is a small volume of trapped air (TAV) with a larger than usual residual volume (RV). During the attack, the residual volume increases dramatically. After bronchodilator therapy, the trapped air volume and residual volume decrease markedly.*

cosal edema and obstructive secretions. Because the airways are normally smaller on expiration, expiratory wheezing occurs first. As the attack progresses, wheezing is both inspiratory and expiratory. Wheezes are *adventitious lung sounds,* which are musical, louder than the underlying sounds, and continuous. They are often described as *expiratory* or *inspiratory* to indicate the phase of respiration in which they are loudest.

Pulsus paradoxus, or paradoxic pulse, is an objective measure of bronchospasm in a severe attack. The amplitude of the arterial pulse normally decreases with inspiration and is produced by the pooling of blood in the pulmonary vessels. Due to respiratory distress in the asthmatic attack, the amount of pooling apparently increases.

The paradoxic pulse is an exaggeration of the normal amplitude change of the arterial pulse with a fall of arterial blood pressure more than 10 mm Hg on inspiration. It is measured by pumping up the blood pressure cuff to above the systolic pressure and lowering the pressure very slowly while the person breathes quickly. If a paradoxic pulse is present, Korotkoff's sounds become audible first during expiration and then during all phases of respiration.[5] The point at which all beats are equally loud is recorded as the bottom of the paradoxic pulse. Paradoxic pulse is recorded as follows: 140 − 120/60.

The point at which beats can be heard on expiration is 140. The point at which all beats are equally loud is 120, and the diastolic pressure is 60. Therefore, the pulsus paradoxus is 20. The normal difference is less than 8 mm Hg. Although assessment of pulsus paradoxus can help to evaluate the severity of airway obstruction, the time and effort required to obtain an accurate measurement may not be clinically warranted. A simple measurement of the peak expiratory flow rate is often more practical.[5] Peak expiratory flow rate, a measure of the expiratory flow rate, is decreased during an asthma attack and can reflect the severity of airway obstruction and air trapping.

Fatigue is a major problem in an acute asthma attack. The increased work of breathing leads to increased oxygen consumption until a point is reached at which the individual begins to tire and is no longer able to hyperventilate enough to meet the increased oxygen demand. The degree of hypoventilation that results can be accurately assessed by monitoring arterial carbon dioxide levels, which may indicate the onset of respiratory failure.

A large amount of yellow or green sputum is produced by the bronchial mucosa in an asthma attack. It tends to be thick and obstructive due to its volume and the associated bronchoconstriction and dehydration. Inflammation is responsible for mucosal edema, which may be due to infection, a common precipitator of the attack.

Once the attack has subsided and underlying precipitators have cleared, the lungs usually return to normal. There is, however, a significant relationship between asthma and the development of chronic obstructive lung disease (COLD) or chronic obstructive pulmonary disease (COPD) later in life. Table 30-1 summarizes the symptoms of asthma and the underlying pathophysiology.

The term *status asthmaticus* has been used to describe a severe episode of asthma that is not relieved by usually effective treatment. It implies that inflammatory changes have occurred that are not easily reversed. Although infection may be the more common precipitating factor

TABLE 30-1 *Clinical Manifestations of Asthma and Underlying Pathophysiology*

Symptoms	Pathophysiology
Dyspnea; orthopnea; coughing; wheezing; chest tightness; elevated paradoxic pulse; reduced breath sounds; hyperresonance, hypoxia	Bronchospasm; air trapping; diaphragmatic flattening
Tachycardia; labored breathing; air hunger; intercostal retractions	Increased work of breathing; fatigue; increased oxygen consumption
Thick, sticky sputum; poor skin turgor; other signs of dehydration	Increased sputum production; dehydration; fever associated with infection
Thick green or yellow sputum	Infection
Bronchospasm, eosinophilia, if allergy present	Inflammation
Apprehension/panic	Anxiety

in intrinsic asthma, status asthmaticus may be provoked by any of the usual factors, and for most affected persons, it begins as any other asthma attack and only reveals its true nature as it becomes refractory to therapy.[8] Typically, breathlessness builds until the affected person cannot do anything other than breathe. Anxiety, extreme orthopnea, loud wheezing, sweating, tachycardia, and obvious increased work of breathing develop. Tachycardia, paradoxic pulse, and altered blood gases are indicators of severity and prognosis. Objective measures of airflow limitations, such as peak expiratory flow rate, are important to gauge response to therapy. Onset of respiratory failure may be signaled by cyanosis, decreased wheezing with progressive hypoventilation, and decreased levels of consciousness. Status asthmaticus is a life-threatening medical emergency that requires hospitalization. The recent increase in the asthma death rate has been alarming. Table 30-2 summarizes the risk factors for mortality in asthma.[8]

TABLE 30-2 *Risk Factors for Mortality in Asthma*

Demographic factors
    Adolescent or young adult
    Non-Caucasian
Historic factors
    Prior life-threatening attacks (prior intubation for asthma)
    Hospitalizations or emergency room visits (three or more) within the past year
    Emergency room visits or hospitalizations in past month
    Use of three or more asthma drugs
    Marked decrease in PEFR
    Corticosteroid use (past/present)
    History of syncope/hypoxic seizures
    Coexisting severe lung disease
Psychosocial factors
    Poor compliance with medications; inability to use devices
    Denial
    Alcoholism
    Continued smoking
    Depression or other major psychiatric illness
    Procrastination in seeking medical care
Physician-related factors
    Failure to diagnose or appreciate severity of attack
    Underuse of corticosteroids
    Failure to adequately follow up and monitor using objective measures
    Inappropriate use of sedatives or other drugs
    Failure to identify high-risk patient
    Failure to educate patient

PEFR: peak expiratory flow rate.
From Hill, N. S. and Weiss, E. B. Status Asthmaticus. In E. B. Weiss and M. Stein. *Bronchial Asthma: Mechanisms and Therapeutics* (3rd ed.). Boston: Little, Brown 1993.

▼ Chronic Obstructive Pulmonary Disease

Chronic obstructive pulmonary disease (COPD) is the fourth leading cause of death in the United States; mortality has more than tripled in the last 30 years.[3] The age-adjusted death rate for COPD has been increasing, whereas rates for the leading causes of death have decreased. Mortality from COPD is inversely related to education and income. In the near future, COPD is expected to decrease in men and increase in women due to the history of increased smoking by women begun in the 1950s.[7] Additionally, disability due to COPD is enormous, causing an estimated 250 million hours lost from work annually.[9]

Chronic obstructive lung diseases are similar to asthma in that expiratory airflow is obstructed and exacerbations and remissions are common. The acute and chronic obstructive diseases differ in that the lung tissues do not return to normal between exacerbations in chronic conditions. Instead, pulmonary damage is a slowly progressive process.

The abbreviations *COPD* and *COLD* refer to a group of conditions associated with chronic obstruction to airflow within the lungs. Usually they refer to emphysema or chronic bronchitis, but they may include inflammation of the small bronchi, bronchiectasis, and cystic fibrosis. Asthma, considered in this chapter to be an acute obstructive condition, is also often grouped with the chronic conditions. Of these diseases, the obstruction of chronic bronchitis, bronchiectasis, and cystic fibrosis chiefly results from secretions, whereas that in emphysema is anatomic. Pneumoconiosis is often classified with chronic obstructive diseases, but because its underlying pathogenesis differs, it is discussed on page 584.

BRONCHIECTASIS

Bronchiectasis is a chronic disease of the bronchi and bronchioles, characterized by irreversible dilatation of the bronchial tree and associated with chronic infection and inflammation of these passageways. Once a common disease in the United States, postinfectious bronchiectasis has become rare since the introduction of antibiotics. Most persons with bronchiectasis have an underlying systemic disease, such as cystic fibrosis, primary ciliary dyskinesia, or immunodeficiency, in which airway infection is superimposed. It is generally agreed that bronchiectasis is associated with a defect in the bronchial walls, which may be congenital or acquired. Because some degree of infection generally always exists, bronchiectasis can best be described as a combined congenital and acquired process characterized by inflammation that results in the replacement of bronchial mucosa by fibrous scar tissue.[10] This process leads to destruction of the bronchi and permanent dilatation of the bronchi and bronchioles, which allows the areas affected to be targets for a chronic, smoldering infection (Fig. 30-3).

The lower lobes are the most vulnerable and usually are filled with a yellow−green infected material that may spread to the pleural cavity. It may or may not be associated with an acute inflammatory exudate with bronchial ulceration or abscess.[4]

The most common symptom is a chronic cough that is productive of purulent sputum, especially with severe disease and an acute infection. Typically, the purulent sputum is also bloody and foul-smelling. Dyspnea, fever, weakness, and weight loss may also be present. This disease, which can affect all ages and both sexes, had a dismal prognosis in the preantibiotic era. Currently, the progression of the disease is variable, directly related to the severity of the disease and how effectively it is managed.[5]

CYSTIC FIBROSIS (MUCOVISCIDOSIS)

Cystic fibrosis is a hereditary disorder in which large quantities of viscous material are secreted. It affects the sweat glands, bronchi, pancreas, and mucus-secreting glands of the small intestine (see pp. 755−759). Although a genetic disorder is present at birth, the disease in some affected persons is not detected until adolescence or early adulthood due to unusual, subtle, or absent symptoms.

The pathologic features include a high concentration of sodium and chloride in the sweat and abnormal mucus secretion and elimination. Secretion of tenacious mucus throughout the airways produces airway obstruction that leads to various combinations of atelectasis, pneumonia, bronchitis, emphysema, and other respiratory conditions. Secondary bacterial infection is common.

Associated pancreatic insufficiency causes abnormal stools, malnutrition, and abdominal distension. Intestinal obstruction is common in the neonate.

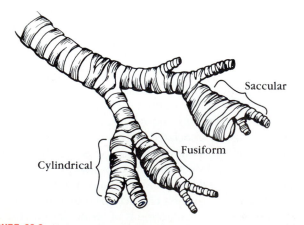

FIGURE 30-3 *Various types of bronchiectasis; the morphology varies.*

The clinical manifestations are variable, with some persons having mainly gastrointestinal symptoms and others developing severe pulmonary problems. All of the manifestations relate to inability to handle excessive secretions. Pulmonary signs and symptoms are common and include chronic cough, persistent lung infections, and cor pulmonale.

To diagnose the disease, at least three of the following four criteria are essential:[4] 1) increased sodium and chloride in the sweat; 2) deficient pancreatic enzymes in the gastrointestinal secretions; 3) chronic pulmonary infections, especially with opportunistic organisms such as *Pseudomonas aeruginosa* and *Staphylococcus aureus;* and 4) family history of the problem. The prognosis is variable, with survival past age 20 years increasing. Gastrointestinal and pulmonary problems are encountered throughout life.

CHRONIC BRONCHITIS

Continued bronchial inflammation and progressive increase in productive cough and dyspnea not attributable to specific causes are classic features of *chronic bronchitis.* The term has usually been applied to persons who have a productive cough on most days for at least 3 consecutive months in 2 successive years. Usually, the inflammation and cough are responses of the bronchial mucosa to chronic irritation from cigarette smoking, atmospheric pollution, or infections.[9]

Pathophysiologically, thickening and rigidity of the bronchial mucosa result from vasodilatation, congestion, and edema. The mucosal areas may be infiltrated with lymphocytes, macrophages, and polymorphonuclear leukocytes. Excessive secretion plus narrowing of the passageways causes obstruction first to maximal expiration and later to maximal inspiratory airflow. Bacteria, especially *Haemophilus influenzae* and *Streptococcus pneumoniae*, are often cultured from the airways.[9]

This bronchitis is closely related to emphysema but is usually defined as an abnormality that involves excessive secretion of mucus and bronchial inflammation, whereas emphysema involves degeneration of the alveolar parenchyma. Bronchitis may lead to the following: 1) increased airway resistance with or without emphysematous changes; 2) right heart failure (cor pulmonale); and 3) dysplasia of the respiratory epithelial cells, which may undergo malignant change.[4]

The clinical manifestations include cyanosis, copious production of sputum, mild degrees of hyperinflation, marked hypercapnia, and severe hypoxemia. Heart failure with manifestations of right-sided failure occurs as the disease progresses. These manifestations include jugular venous distension, cardiac enlargement, liver engorgement, and peripheral edema. Bronchitic persons have often been called ''blue bloaters'' because of the presence of marked cyanosis and edema. The clinical picture varies depending on the amount of associated emphysema. Table 30-3 compares the clinical and physiologic features of the two conditions. Bronchitis and emphysema rarely occur in isolation from each other. Some mixture of clinical signs and symptoms is usually present.

PULMONARY EMPHYSEMA

Emphysema is the most common chronic pulmonary disease and is frequently classified with chronic bronchitis because of the simultaneous occurrence of the two conditions. In anatomic terms, emphysema involves the portion of lungs distal to a terminal bronchiole (*acinus*) where gas exchange takes place. Emphysema results in permanent, abnormal enlargement of the acinus with associated destructive changes.[4] It may be classified as *vesicular* when it involves the spaces distal to the terminal bronchioles and *interlobular* or *interstitial* when it affects the tissue between the air spaces.[9] The common

term *pulmonary emphysema* usually designates the vesicular type.

Pathophysiology

Emphysema seems to be due to many separate injuries that occur over a long time. Prevalence and severity are greatest in elderly persons. The elastin and fiber network of the alveoli and airways is broken down. The alveoli enlarge, and many of their walls are destroyed. Alveolar destruction leads to the formation of larger than normal air spaces (pools), which greatly reduce the alveolar diffusing surface. Once the process begins, it progresses slowly and inconsistently. Alveolar destruction also undermines the support structure for the airways, making them more vulnerable to expiratory collapse. There may be associated airway inflammation and consequent increase in mucus production, although many persons with emphysema produce little or no sputum.

The exact mechanism of injury is yet to be deter-

TABLE 30-3 *Features That Distinguish and Show Similarity Between Bronchial and Emphasematous Types of Chronic Obstructive Lung Disease*

Clinical Manifestations	Bronchitis	Emphysema
History	Tobacco smoking usual; frequent "colds," "flu," chest infections. Dyspnea, progressive. Cough invariable.	Tobacco smoking usual, insidious onset of dyspnea, which becomes incapacitating; cough, dry, nonproductive related to smoking.
Chest exam	Rales and rhonchi, wheezing. Increased A-P diameter, especially in late stages	Breath sounds quiet. Heart sounds distant. Marked increase in A-P diameter, dorsal kyphosis. Expiratory phase prolonged. Increased resonance.
Sputum	Copious, purulent common	Scant and thick
Weight loss	Not early symptom	Often early, marked weight loss
Chest x-ray	Evidence of old inflammation	Depression and flattening of diaphragm. Decreased vascular markings. Bullous lesions.
Heart/respiratory failure	Right heart failure common with edema, cyanosis. "Blue bloater" appearance. Respiratory failure common in late stages.	Heart failure late sign. Respiratory failure common. "Pink puffer" appearance.
Arterial blood gases	Decreased Po^2. Intermittently increased Pco^2, especially in late stage	Decreased Po^2, in late stage, chronic increase in Pco^2
Pulmonary function tests	Increased residual volume. Prolonged FEV_1.	Increased residual volume. Prolonged FEV_1.

A-P: anterior-posterior
 * Weight loss for emphysema

mined. Ischemia may cause alveolar breakdown, although specific vascular lesions have not been found. Repeated injuries from smoking, infection, and air pollution often lead to emphysema, but the exact mechanism of injury has not been identified. Most, but not all, of those affected are cigarette smokers.

Specific types of emphysema have been shown to be related to a deficiency in the enzyme alpha$_1$-antitrypsin, which inhibits the proteases of elastase and collagenase. These proteases are normally major contributors to tissue destruction during the inflammatory process. Without the inhibition of alpha$_1$-antitrypsin, the destruction or digestion of pulmonary tissue occurs more at the bases than at the apices of the lungs. This circumstance leads to the onset of severe obstructive lung disease early in adult life, often before age 40 years. The onset of hypoxia and cor pulmonale in these persons heralds a poor prognosis.

The types of emphysema have been classified according to the area of lung affected; that is, classification is anatomic and may describe lobules or acini (Tables 30-4 and 30-5). Many types of emphysema can only be classified with certainty by autopsy report. Pulmonary interstitial emphysema is an associated condition that involves overdistension of the alveoli and dissection of air into the perivascular spaces. The dissection may continue into the mediastinum, causing *pneumomediastinum*, or into the pleural cavity, causing *pneumothorax*. Figure 30-4 illustrates the appearance of alveoli in the main types of emphysema.

Emphysema has a major effect on compliance and elasticity. The major abnormality is loss of *elastic recoil*.[9] Because alveolar walls are destroyed, fibrous and muscle tissues are lost, making the lungs more distensible. Even in severe disease, inspiratory airway resistance tends to be normal. Air trapping occurs because of loss of elastic recoil, which increases airway size on inspiration and causes collapse of the small airways on expiration. Thus, a minor obstruction on inspiration is a serious obstruc-

TABLE 30-4 *Classification of Emphysema*

Classification	Description
Diffuse or generalized	Lobules or acini through affected lung
Focal	Associated with focal dust deposition (eg, coal dust)
Irregular	Associated with shrinkage of fibrotic scars, usually from old disease
Obstructive	Accompanied by demonstrable bronchial obstruction
Bulla	Emphysematous space of more than 1 cm in an inflated lung; may occur in any type of emphysema

TABLE 30-5 *Lobular and Acinar Terminology of Emphysema*

Lobules	Acini
Panlobular: all lung affected; diffuse throughout lung	Panacinar: whole acinus affected; diffuse throughout lung
Centrilobular: spaces around central bronchioles affected; usually affects apices	Centriacinar: area around alveolar ducts affected; usually affects apices
Periseptal: occurs at periphery of lobule; less common than above types	Periacinar: occurs at periphery of acinus; less common than above types
Irregular: scarring throughout the acinus irregularly	

tion on expiration. If expiration is forced, a sharp rise in pressure on the airways leads to compression of the bronchi and bronchioles. The resultant distension eventually leads to disruption in the alveolar walls and surrounding musculoelastic tissue around the small airways. Figure 30-5 illustrates the difference between normal alveoli and distended alveoli of emphysema. The loss of gas-exchanging surface with associated vascular changes results in decreased diffusion capacities.[9]

Clinical Manifestations

The clinical manifestations of emphysema are usually absent in the early stages and very insidious in onset. They may overlap with those of bronchitis. The person with emphysema has often been called the "pink puffer" on the basis of the pink appearance of the skin resulting from hyperventilation and adequate tissue oxygenation in the early stages. Dyspnea ("puffer") is characteristic. In the early stages, it occurs with exertion and later progresses to dyspnea at rest. Severe hyperinflation of the lungs due to the alveolar destruction and overdistention may lead to an increased anteroposterior chest diameter, resulting in the typical barrel chest. Dorsal kyphosis, prominent anterior chest, and elevated ribs all contribute to this appearance (Figure 30-6). The accessory muscles are used to raise the thorax on inspiration, and the abdominal muscles are developed to force air out actively. As a result, the expiratory cycle is prolonged. Pulmonary function tests show a prolonged FEV_1 with decreased vital capacity, despite an increase in total lung capacity. Respiratory sounds are frequently very quiet unless a superimposed infection accounts for expiratory wheezes and rales.

Chronic bronchitis and emphysema coexist in most persons with COPD. Figure 30-7 shows how the clinical manifestations of chronic bronchitis and emphysema

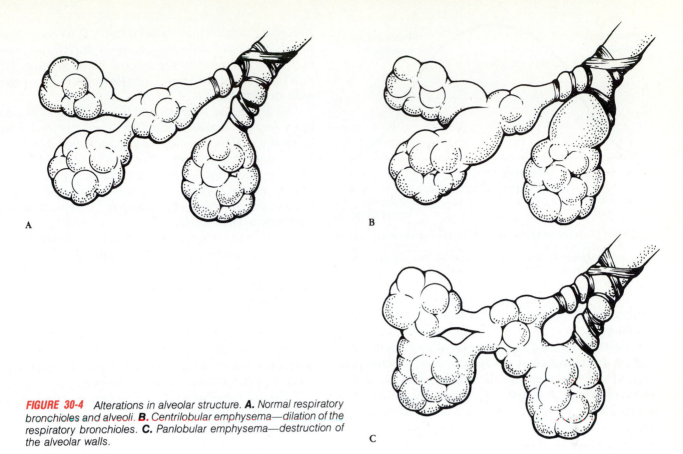

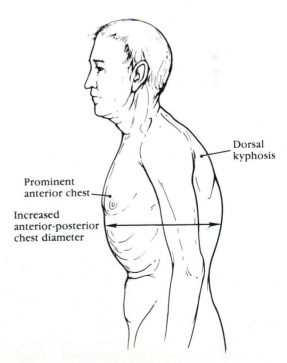

FIGURE 30-4 *Alterations in alveolar structure.* **A.** *Normal respiratory bronchioles and alveoli.* **B.** *Centrilobular emphysema—dilation of the respiratory bronchioles.* **C.** *Panlobular emphysema—destruction of the alveolar walls.*

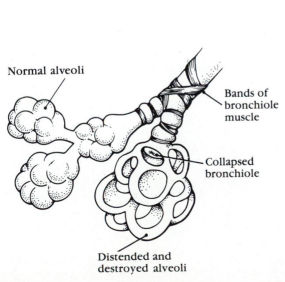

Normal alveoli

Bands of bronchiole muscle

Collapsed bronchiole

Distended and destroyed alveoli

FIGURE 30-5 *Distended and destroyed alveoli versus normal alveoli.*

Dorsal kyphosis

Prominent anterior chest

Increased anterior-posterior chest diameter

FIGURE 30-6 *Barrel chest of emphysema.*

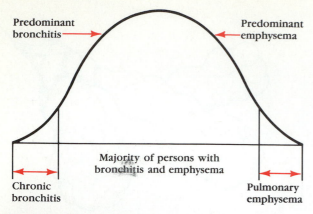

FIGURE 30-7 *The overlap of clinical manifestation of chronic bronchitis and emphysema in chronic obstructive pulmonary disease. (Source: D. Mahler, P. Barlow, and R. Mathay, Chronic obstructive diseases. Clin Geriatric Med 2:2, May, 1986.)*

overlap. Most persons exhibit manifestations of both conditions.

Hypoxia is a very common result of emphysema. It is defined as inadequate delivery of oxygen to satisfy the metabolic requirements of the organs and cells of the body. Direct measurement of oxygen in the tissue is impossible, so hypoxia is usually diagnosed by its end-organ effects. Hypoxia of the brain, for example, causes clinical signs, such as mental changes, stupor, and coma.

Hypoxemia is defined as reduced levels of oxygen in the blood. Blood gas levels are measured directly, and normal oxygen tension in the arterial blood is 80 to 100 mm Hg. A value of 55 to 60 mm Hg or lower for oxygen indicates hypoxemia.[1]

As a response to prolonged hypoxia, the individual may develop cyanosis, clubbing, and polycythemia. Clinically, evident cyanosis is a late and unreliable sign of hypoxemia. It does not occur unless reduced hemoglobin is more than 5 g/100 mL of capillary blood. In the anemic person, cyanosis may not occur at all. In the polycythemic person, cyanosis may be present despite adequate oxygen levels.

The human brain, which accounts for about 20% of total oxygen consumption while comprising only about 2% of body weight, is very sensitive to hypoxia. Therefore, cerebral symptoms may be induced by hypoxemia. A small degree results in restlessness, change in personality, and impaired judgment. Moderately severe hypoxemia causes impaired motor function and confusion. Severe hypoxemia, at levels between 20 and 30 mm Hg, often causes delirium and coma. If persistent and severe, it can cause permanent cortical damage.

Chronic hypoxemia causes a release of renal erythropoietic factor, which reacts with a plasma protein to form erythropoietin. This substance stimulates increased production of red blood cells, and blood volume increase

TABLE 30-6 *Physiologic Effects of Hypoxemia*

Pao_2 (mm Hg)	Function	Abnormality	Sign or Symptom
<60	Heart rate	↑	Tachycardia
	Respiratory rate	↑	Tachypnea
	Na^+ and H_2O excretion	↑	Edema
<55	Cardiac output	↑	Bounding pulses
	Dysrhythmias	↑	Tachyarrhythmias
			Bradyarrhythmias
	Mentation	↓	Somnolence
			Confusion
			Pinpoint pupils
	RBC mass	↑	Plethora
			Erythrocythemia
			Thromboemboli
	PA pressure	↑	Jugular venous distention
			Edema
			RV S_4
			Hepatomegaly
			Abnormal ECG*
<30	Cardiac output	↓	Cyanosis
			Pulse pressure
			Shock
	Metabolism	↓	Lactic acidosis

ECG: electrocardiogram; RBC: red blood cell; PA: pulmonary artery; RV: right ventricular.
*ECG findings of cor pulmonale (RAE, RVE, rightward shift in ventricular or atrial vectors).
Source: W. N. Kelley (ed.). *Textbook of Internal Medicine* (2nd ed.). Philadelphia: J.B. Lippincott, 1992.

TABLE 30-7 *Comparative Values for Compensated and Uncompensated Respiratory Acidosis*

Arterial Blood Gas Components	Normal Values	Compensated Respiratory Acidosis (An Example)	Uncompensated Respiratory Acidosis (An Example)
pH	7.35–7.45	7.35	7.22
P_{CO_2}	35–45 mm Hg	54 mm Hg	74 mm Hg
P_{O_2}	80–100 mm Hg	62 mm Hg	40 mm Hg
O_2 saturation	95–100%	83%	69%
HCO_3	22–26 mEq/L	32 mEq/L	28 mEq/L
H_2CO_3	1.05–1.35 mEq/L	1.8 mEq/L	2.9 mEq/L

(see pp. 377–379). The resulting *polycythemia* characteristically develops and leads to increased blood viscosity, which further impedes oxygenation of the tissues. The oxygen-hemoglobin dissociation curve shifts to the right with hypoxemia, allowing for increased release of oxygen to the tissues. Table 30-6 summarizes the general effects of hypoxemia.

Hypercapnia (retention of carbon dioxide) is also common with COPD when the disease becomes severe, usually when FEV_1 is less than 1 liter.[12] It results from hypoventilation, mostly due to an uneven match-up of ventilation and perfusion in the lungs. At normal ventilatory rates, inadequate carbon dioxide is excreted and carbon dioxide is retained. Increasing P_{CO_2} levels lead to increased ventilation due to the central chemoreceptor in the medulla. When pulmonary disease is severe, ventilation changes do not usually return P_{CO_2} levels to normal, that is, the work of breathing becomes too great to sustain the high ventilatory rate.

Hypercapnia becomes chronic and depresses the receptiveness of the medullary chemoreceptor. The person may lose most of the stimuli for breathing from the central chemoreceptor and depend on the peripheral chemoreceptors on the aortic arch and carotid sinuses to stimulate a ventilatory drive. The peripheral chemoreceptors are stimulated by hypoxemia of less than 60 mm Hg oxygen tension.

The normal pH change that would accompany the retention of carbon dioxide is counteracted by renal retention of bicarbonate, leading to a normal or near-normal pH (see p. 217). This adaptation is protective and assists the body function, even though the P_{CO_2} remains excessively high. The adjusted pH reflects *compensated respiratory acidosis.* Table 30-7 shows examples of compensated and uncompensated respiratory acidosis.

Any of the chronic lung diseases may lead to respiratory failure, which is discussed further in Chapter 31.

▼ *Chapter Summary*

▼ Acute obstructive airway disease is usually caused by infectious agents and is characterized by increased mucus secretion, bronchial swelling, cilia dysfunction, and resistance to expiratory airflow with air trapping.

▼ Asthma is an acute, inflammatory, episodic airway obstruction that is precipitated by an exaggerated response to a variety of stimuli. It is characterized by wheezing, which may be initiated by an environmental agent along with other factors, such as exercise, infection, and emotional upset. Between acute episodes, the airways are normal with no pathologic changes. Clinical manifestations of an asthmatic attack relate to the amount of airway constriction involved and may be minor or life-threatening. Asthma may progress to chronic lung disease.

▼ Chronic obstructive pulmonary disease is a general term for conditions associated with chronic obstruction to airflow within the lungs. These conditions include chronic bronchitis, bronchiectasis, cystic fibrosis, and emphysema. There is considerable overlap in pathology and clinical manifestations between bronchitis and emphysema. Causative conditions include tobacco smoking, atmospheric pollution, and infections.

▼ Lack of alpha₁-antitrypsin, as discussed in Chapter 28, causes early development of emphysema. Emphysema causes permanent, abnormal destruction of the acinus of the lungs with an insidious onset and chronic retention of carbon dioxide and hypoxemia.

▼ Clinical manifestations of bronchitis include chronic, productive cough with hypoxemia and right-sided heart failure as the disease progresses. Bronchiectasis is a chronic disease associated with chronic infection of the terminal bronchioles causing cough and large amounts of purulent sputum.

▼ Cystic fibrosis is a multisystem disease whose pulmonary symptoms relate to production of excessive secretions and chronic infections. It is sometimes classified with the restrictive pulmonary disorders.

▼ *References*

1. Albert, R.K. Approach to the patient with cyanosis and/or hypoxemia. In W.N. Kelley (ed.), *Textbook of Internal Medicine* (2nd ed.). Philadelphia: J.B. Lippincott, 1992.
2. Barnes, P.J. Inflammation. In E.B. Weiss and M.Stein (eds.), *Bronchial Asthma: Mechanisms and Therapeutics* (3rd ed.). Boston: Little, Brown, 1993.
3. Centers for Disease Control, Mortality patterns—United States, 1991. *MMWR* 42(46), 1993.
4. Cotran, R.S., Kumar, V., and Robbins, S.L. *Robbins' Pathologic Basis of Disease* (5th ed.). Philadelphia: W.B. Saunders, 1994.
5. Farzan, S.A. *A Concise Handbook of Respiratory Diseases* (3rd ed.). Reston, Va.: Reston, 1992.
6. Freitag, A., and Newhouse, M.T. Management of asthma in the 1990s. In D.F. Tierney (ed.), *Current Pulmonology, Volume 15*. St. Louis: Mosby-Year Book, 1994.
7. Higgins, M., and Thom, T. Incidence, prevalence, and mortality: Intra- and intercountry differences. In M. Hensley and N. Saunders (eds.), *Clinical Epidemiology of Chronic Obstructive Pulmonary Disease*. New York: Marcel Dekker, 1989.
8. Hill, N.S., and Weiss, E.B. Status asthmaticus. In E.B. Weiss and M. Stein (eds.), *Bronchial Asthma: Mechanisms and Therapeutics* (3rd ed.). Boston: Little, Brown, 1993.
9. Kuhn, C., and Askin, F.B. Lung and mediastinum. In J.M. Kissane (ed.), *Anderson's Pathology* (9th ed.). St. Louis: C.V. Mosby, 1990.
10. Luce, J.M. Bronchiectasis. In J.F. Murray and J.A. Nadel (eds.), *Textbook of Respiratory Medicine* (2nd ed.). Philadelphia: W.B. Saunders Co., 1994.
11. McFadden, E.R. Asthma. In K.J. Isselbacher et al. (eds.), *Harrison's Principles of Internal Medicine* (13th ed.). New York: McGraw-Hill, 1994.
12. Seaton, A., Seaton, D., and Leitch, A. *Crofton and Douglas's Respiratory Diseases* (4th ed.). Oxford: Blackwell, 1989.

Chapter 31

Other Alterations Affecting the Pulmonary System

Darlene H. Green

▼ LEARNING OBJECTIVES

1   Describe the ventilation-perfusion abnormality that occurs with pulmonary embolus.
2   Discuss the underlying risk factors for the development of pulmonary embolus.
3   Describe the clinical manifestations that may occur in the process of pulmonary embolization.
4   Explain briefly how resolution of emboli occurs.
5   Describe the development of pulmonary hypertension.
6   Define **rhinitis, pharyngitis, sinusitis, and laryngitis**.
7   Explain briefly the dangers of laryngeal edema.
8   Classify and briefly describe cancer of the larynx.
9   Discuss some factors that predispose to the onset of malignancy in the lung.
10 Describe the pathology, major clinical manifestations, and prognosis of four major types of intrapulmonary malignancy.
11 List the most common sites of metastasis of lung cancer.
12 Differentiate between respiratory insufficiency and respiratory failure.
13 Explain how adaptation can occur in chronic respiratory insufficiency.
14 Describe the clinical manifestations of respiratory failure.
15 Discuss the prognoses in acute and chronic respiratory failure.

Barbara L. Bullock: PATHOPHYSIOLOGY: ADAPTATIONS AND ALTERATIONS IN FUNCTION, 4th ed.
© 1996 J.B. Lippincott-Raven Publishers

Several of the pulmonary disease processes do not easily lend themselves to strict classification as restrictive or obstructive. This chapter discusses some of these conditions, including pulmonary embolus, tumors of the lung, and respiratory insufficiency and failure. Respiratory failure may result from many intrapulmonary and extrapulmonary diseases. It is frequently the cause of death in chronic pulmonary disease.

As discussed in Chapter 28, the normal ratio of alveolar ventilation (4 L/min) to volume of blood flow in the pulmonary capillaries (V/Q) is about 0.8 because cardiac output averages about 5 L/min. A decrease of alveolar ventilation in relation to perfusion occurs in any part of the lung in which airways are obstructed by secretions (bronchitis), expiratory dynamic collapse (emphysema), or muscular spasm (asthma), or in which alveoli are collapsed (atelectasis) or are filled with fluid (pulmonary edema). These conditions cause increased venous blood flow past nonventilated alveoli. The oxygen-poor mixture is added to the arterial blood, and the result is hypoxemia. As stated previously, hypoxemia resulting from underventilated alveoli is, in essence, a form of right-to-left shunting of venous blood past the alveoli (see pp. 561–564).

Another type of ventilation–perfusion abnormality is the reduction of perfusion in relation to ventilation. This occurs most commonly when pulmonary emboli obliterate arteriolar blood supply but may occur if cardiac output is reduced because of congestive heart failure. In these examples, ventilated but nonperfused alveoli increase the physiologic dead space because a significant number of alveoli receive inspired air but do not participate in the exchange of oxygen or carbon dioxide.

In conditions in which hypoxemia is the result of a ventilation-perfusion abnormality, the pressure of carbon dioxide (Pco_2) often is normal or low, because compensatory hyperventilation is able to lower the more easily diffusible Pco_2. Thus, the clinical pattern of ventilation-perfusion inequality is often one of hypoxemia with hyperventilation, lowered Pco_2, and even respiratory alkalosis. This picture is directly related to the degree of the ventilation-perfusion defect and eventually may result in hypoxemia, hypercapnia, and respiratory acidosis.

▼ Pulmonary Embolus

A pulmonary embolus is defined as an occlusion of one or more pulmonary vessels by matter that has traveled from a source outside the lung. Any foreign material freely traveling in the systemic venous system must finally terminate in the pulmonary vascular bed. For example, if a clot in a small vein dislodges, it travels through progressively larger vessels until it reaches the right ventricle, from which it is pumped by the pulmonary artery to the lungs. The usual cause of pulmonary embolus is a thrombus from the deep veins of the legs or pelvis that dislodges and travels with the flow of blood to the lungs. It may also be caused by a fat embolus, amniotic fluid embolus, or air embolus, by particulate matter injected intravenously, or, rarely, by gas, parasites, or foreign objects.

Pulmonary embolus is probably the third most common acute cause of death in the United States, but the diagnosis is often missed.[3] Many persons may have thrombi in the venous system that actually embolize but are diagnosed as a pulmonary infection or pleurisy, or are not diagnosed at all. Pulmonary emboli rarely strike the young and healthy but occur in a high-risk group that includes bedridden persons, the obese, the elderly, and those with a history of prior emboli or thrombosis. Persons who suffer from congestive heart failure, who undergo abdominal or pelvic surgery, or who have sustained trauma to the legs are also at high risk. The risk factors are cumulative: the more factors present, the greater the risk of developing pulmonary emboli. Although pulmonary embolism is often an unexpected cause of death in hospitalized patients, as many as 95% of these patients have identifiable risk factors.[8]

SEQUENCE OF EVENTS IN PULMONARY EMBOLIZATION

The right lung is more frequently involved in the embolic process than the left, and the degree of obstruction is related to the size of the embolus. The physiologic consequences of pulmonary embolus are greater than can be explained by the degree of occlusion alone. A large embolus may cause infarction of the lung parenchyma, but this is not directly related to the size of the embolus because the bronchial arteries continue to nourish the lung tissue.[5]

Most pulmonary emboli are the result of thrombi that dislodge from the deep veins of the legs and pelvis. Phlebothrombosis is the most common type of deep vein thrombosis and frequently occurs in immobilized or obese persons and in those who have sustained surgical or accidental trauma. For a thrombus of this nature to form, an abnormality must be present, because clotting rarely occurs if blood flow and vascular integrity are normal. Three conditions, known as Virchow's triad, favor clot formation: 1) venostasis, 2) endothelial disruption of the vessel lining, and 3) hypercoagulability.

Local concentration of coagulation factors, together with an injury to the venous wall, may provide a place for clots to form. As the flow of blood slows or stops over the injured area, the clot begins to form and extends or propagates itself up the vein (Fig. 31-1). It may then retract and pull away from the vessel wall and become a free-floating embolus. Vagal stimulation or minor physi-

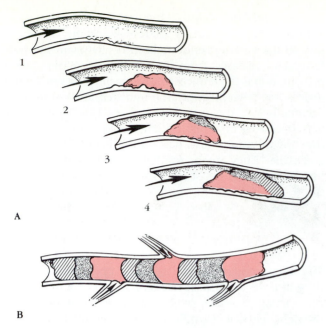

FIGURE 31-1 *A. Sequence of clot formation on area of intimal damage. B. Propagation of clot up the length of the vein wall may lead to pulmonary embolus.*

cal exertion may immediately precede embolization. Small fragments of the clot may break off and produce several areas of embolization on the lungs. Multiple embolization of the pulmonary capillary bed is more common than occlusion of the main pulmonary artery or its branches.

After the blood clot lodges in the pulmonary capillary bed, it impedes blood flow beyond the point of the obstruction. Perfusion in the pulmonary capillary bed stops. If large areas are affected, infarction of lung tissue may occur; infarcts of various sizes occur in 5% to 10% of patients with pulmonary embolism. The newly formed infarct becomes hemorrhagic but later is filled with scar tissue.[3]

A wide variety of pathophysiologic responses to a pulmonary embolus occur, depending on the size of the embolus and the ability of the host to compensate. Small obstructions to the blood supply usually create no hemodynamic changes and are called *silent pulmonary emboli.* Larger obstructions cause increased resistance to pulmonary blood flow, which can lead to *cor pulmonale* (right ventricular heart failure resulting from lung disease). Studies show that more than 50% of the pulmonary vasculature must be obstructed to cause significant increase in pressure in the pulmonary artery.[9] However, in individuals with preexisting lung disease, increased pulmonary artery pressure leading to cor pulmonale may occur with much less of the vasculature obstructed. Vasoconstriction in the smaller pulmonary arterial vessels is apparently common and may be caused by the liberation of vasoactive substances, such as serotonin.

Vasoconstriction enhances the risk for pulmonary ischemia and infarction.

The increase in pulmonary artery pressure leads to an increased workload for the right side of the heart as it pumps blood into the pulmonary circulation. The result is tachycardia, which progresses to signs of right ventricular failure, including jugular venous distention, hepatomegaly, and peripheral edema. A large saddle embolus obstructing the main pulmonary artery at its bifurcation to the right and left branches leads to acute cor pulmonale, severe shock, and, often, sudden death.[5]

The process of embolization may be continuous, with small emboli being released from a thrombotic focus over months or years. Often undiagnosed, this process can lead to pulmonary embarrassment.

The lungs are capable of clearing emboli more rapidly than any other organ. The pulmonary endothelium is rich in both plasmin activator and heparin.[9] Resolution of the pulmonary embolus occurs by absorption and fibrosis. Activation of the intrinsic fibrinolytic system may restore the pulmonary circulation within a few hours or days.[7] This process begins as early as a few hours after a small embolic episode. Fibrous replacement converts infarcted lung tissue to scar tissue. Clots are partly or totally dissolved by the fibrinolytic system. Residual material, resistant to fibrinolytic attack, may organize and become small, scarred areas.

CLINICAL MANIFESTATIONS

The signs and symptoms of pulmonary embolus vary greatly and depend on both the amount of lung tissue affected and the state of health of the heart and lungs before to the event (Box 31-1).

The embolus may be clinically silent with no manifestations at all. The most frequent symptom is the sudden onset of mild, moderate, or severe dyspnea that may be transient. Tachypnea that persists is highly suggestive of pulmonary embolus. Fever and cough, sometimes with associated hemoptysis, often occur. Pain may be absent, mild, or severe, and may be manifested as pleural pain or as deep, crushing, substernal pain mimicking that of myocardial infarction. The pain often occurs with pulmonary infarction and may be oppressive and substernal. Anxiety, apprehension, and restlessness are common responses to hypoxemia. Palpitations and weakness associated with profuse perspiration, nausea, and vomiting often are present. If embolization is massive, cardiovascular collapse may result, leading to sudden shock, seizures, or cardiopulmonary arrest.

Clinical signs of pulmonary embolus may include splinting of the involved side, cyanosis, distended neck veins, tachycardia with an increased pulmonic sound, or an S_3 or S_4 gallop. Rales, wheezing, and decreased breath sounds in the affected areas are frequent findings.

Definitive diagnosis is often difficult. The chest ra-

BOX 31-1 ▼ Signs and Symptoms of Pulmonary Embolus

Initial manifestations
  May be clinically absent
  Dyspnea of sudden onset
  Cough
  Fever
  Pain—pleuritic or deep and crushing
  Hemoptysis
  Tachypnea
  Anxiety, apprehension, restlessness
  Palpitations
  Weakness
  Diaphoresis
  Nausea and vomiting
  Shock
Physical examination findings
  Splinting of involved side
  Cyanosis
  Distended neck veins
  Area of dullness over involved side
  Tachycardia
  S_3 or S_4 gallop
  Atrial fibrillation, right bundle branch block
  Right axis deviation on 12-lead
  Rales
  Localized decreased breath sounds
  Localized wheezing
  Chest film may be normal or show patchy areas of infiltration
Lung scan and pulmonary arteriogram definitive
Arterial blood gases frequently show hypoxemia and hypercapnia

---

diograph often appears normal, and any abnormalities may be general, such as elevated diaphragm, atelectasis, or pleural effusion. The serum enzyme lactic dehydrogenase (LDH) level is often elevated. Arterial blood gases may show hypoxemia, hypocapnia, and respiratory alkalosis as a result of the marked tachypnea. Hypoxemia correlates well with the extent of the area occluded.

The radioisotope lung scan shows perfusion defects in areas of the lung and supports the diagnosis. A pulmonary arteriogram is occasionally performed to provide visualization of the vessels of the pulmonary tree.

FAT EMBOLIZATION

Fractures of the long bones are the major source of emboli composed of fat particles. Fat embolism can be demonstrated in approximately 90% of cases of severe skeletal injury but only about 1% exhibit signs and symptoms.[3] The origin of the embolus appears to be the bone marrow, and the particles enter the bloodstream through the ruptured veins 12 to 24 hours after fracture. Fat also may be mobilized from the injured site and may form large globules in the plasma.[7] Alveolar edema often

occurs, exhibiting a clinical picture much like that seen with the adult respiratory distress syndrome. Toxic injury to the vascular endothelium results from the free fatty acids released from the fat globules.[3] The classic presentation is the clinical triad of dyspnea, mental confusion, and petechiae; arterial hypoxemia is commonly present before dyspnea occurs. Petechiae, present in 50% of cases of fat embolization, characteristically occur over the anterior chest, base of the neck, conjunctiva, and axilla.[4] They are the result of a rapid onset of thrombocytopenia, the cause of which is not clearly understood.

▼ Pulmonary Hypertension

Pulmonary hypertension can result from heart disease, lung disease, or both. It refers to an increase in pulmonary artery pressure, which increases the workload of the right ventricle. Significant pulmonary vascular obliteration must be present for pulmonary artery pressure to be elevated because there is normally a large reserve in the pulmonary capillary bed.

As a rule, pulmonary hypertension involves progressive disease, either of the pulmonary vessels or of the lung parenchyma. The medial layer of the pulmonary arteries usually hypertrophies, and the system loses its ability to adapt to stress factors, such as increased blood flow or hypoxia. Hypoxic vasoconstriction is both a cause and a result of pulmonary hypertension.[7]

As the process becomes persistent, end-diastolic pressure in the right ventricle becomes elevated. The right ventricle hypertrophies and further increases its systolic pressure. In the early stages, symptoms of right ventricular failure or cor pulmonale occur only during periods of increased stress. As it progresses, cor pulmonale is present all of the time, manifested by jugular venous distention, hepatomegaly, and peripheral edema (see pp. 505–506).

The pulmonary artery pressure, which is normally approximately 25/10 mm Hg, is elevated to above 40/15 mm Hg and may be much higher as the disease progresses. At a certain critical point, the right ventricle cannot compensate for the increased pressure, and intractable cardiac failure occurs.

Death from chronic respiratory disease may result from heart failure or respiratory failure. Nearly all persons with these diseases exhibit some symptoms of chronic cor pulmonale.

Causative conditions besides chronic obstructive lung diseases include congenital cardiac left-to-right shunts that overload the pulmonary vascular system, valvular conditions such as mitral stenosis, any condition in which hypoxia is sustained, pulmonary emboli, and long-standing left-sided heart failure can cause this condition. The mechanism for the development of pulmonary hypertension may be volume and pressure overload or sustained vasoconstriction.

▼ Upper Respiratory Tract Alterations

Alterations in the upper respiratory tract are very common and usually self-limiting conditions; they include rhinitis, pharyngitis, sinusitis, and laryngitis. Cancer of the larynx is a more serious disease that affects the upper respiratory tract.

Rhinitis refers to inflammation of the nasal cavities that results in a persistent nasal discharge caused by secretory hyperactivity of the submucosal glands of the nasal cavities. The cause of rhinitis is commonly viral, bacterial, or allergic. The viral form is recognized as the common cold. Allergies or exposures to irritants injure the normal cilia of the nasal mucosa. Bacterial growth often occurs after an initial viral attack.

Pharyngitis is usually caused by viral or bacterial invasion of the pharynx that produces a sore throat. The appearance of the throat varies depending on the causative agent. Tonsils are often affected; they become reddened and swollen and exude a suppurative discharge. Most pharyngitis is relatively innocuous, but untreated streptococcal infections can have systemic effects in some persons. These effects may be manifested as scarlet fever, rheumatic fever, rheumatic heart disease, or glomerulonephritis. Other organisms, such as the *Corynebacterium diphtheriae* and *Haemophilus influenzae*, can also cause grave effects.

Sinusitis is an inflammation of the sinus cavities that often spreads from a rhinitis infection to the sinuses. The most common organisms causing this condition are group A *Streptococcus pyogenes*, *Staphylococcus aureus*, and *H. influenzae*. The infection usually causes localized pain in the frontal, maxillary, ethmoid, or sphenoid sinuses (Fig. 31-2). A purulent exudate indicates bacterial infection that, when severe, is associated with the constitutional symptoms of fever, chills, pain in the sinuses, and nasal obstruction. Chronic disease may be indicated by a postnasal discharge and tenderness over the sinus cavity.

Laryngitis often occurs in persons who overuse the voice in singing or other vocal activities. It may also be caused by any organism that affects the upper respiratory tract. It involves both vocal cords and is manifested by cough and hoarseness with loss of the voice. Laryngitis can also be chronic, precipitated by overuse of tobacco, straining of the voice, or inhalation of toxic gases. Rarely, this condition causes *laryngeal edema* and obstruction to airflow. Complete obstruction causes asphyxia; incomplete obstruction causes laryngeal stridor and acute respiratory distress.

CARCINOMA OF THE LARYNX

Polyps of the vocal cords are not usually premalignant, but the *laryngeal papilloma* is a true neoplasm that has the potential of undergoing malignant transformation. Most affected persons are or have been heavy tobacco smokers.

Most cancers of the larynx arise on the vocal cords and are clinically manifested by hoarseness. This malignancy is closely associated with chronic laryngitis and

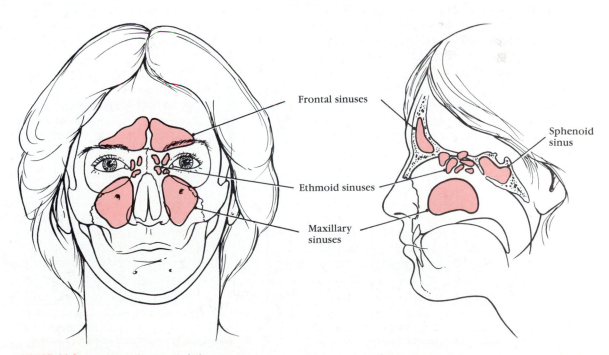

Frontal sinuses

Sphenoid sinus

Ethmoid sinuses

Maxillary sinuses

FIGURE 31-2 *Location of paranasal sinuses.*

smoking. Its frequency is greatest in men after the fourth decade.

Clinical manifestations of cancers of the larynx include pain, a palpable lump, dysphagia, and, occasionally, respiratory distress. The tumor, being a relatively slow-growing malignancy of the squamous epithelium, is curable in the early stages.

▼ Lung Tumors

Tumors of the lung may be benign or malignant. The majority are malignant and have an unremitting, progressive course leading ultimately to death. The only benign tumor that is discussed in this section is the hamartoma, which is often difficult to differentiate from a malignancy. The malignant tumors are described according to histologic classification and pathogenesis.

BENIGN TUMORS

The *hamartoma* is not a true neoplasm but a congenital anomaly that in the bronchi or lung tissue frequently leads to tumorlike lesions containing connective tissue, cartilage, and bronchial epithelium.[7] The lesions are encapsulated, firm, and grayish-white with a rough, nodu-

lar surface. They appear on chest films on the periphery of the lung, in the subpleural area, and endobronchially, making them difficult to distinguish from malignant tumors. These uncommon lung tumors rarely cause any clinical symptoms but must be differentiated from malignancies.

MALIGNANT TUMORS

Factors Predisposing to Malignancy

Cigarette smoking, air pollution, and industrial chemicals seem to account for the increasing frequency of bronchogenic carcinoma. Statistical evidence supports the relation between cigarette smoking and certain types of lung cancer. The death rate from lung cancer is twice as high in urban areas as in rural areas, implicating air pollution as an etiologic factor. Figure 31-3 shows the phenomenal increase in lung cancer deaths since 1930.[1] Lung cancer mortality increased almost fourfold between 1950 and 1990. For men, the death rate from lung cancer increased from 21.6 per 100,000 to 75.6; for women, it increased from 4.8 to 31.8 per 100,000 persons.[2] Lung cancer has now overtaken breast cancer as the leading cause of cancer death in women. Although the incidence of breast cancer is greater, the mortality rate for lung cancer surpassed that of breast cancer

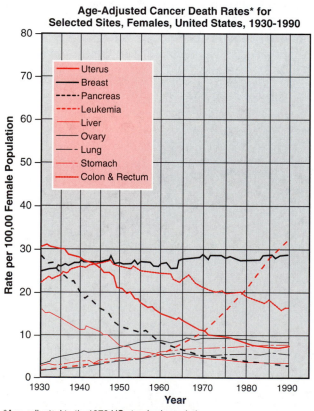

A *Age-adjusted to the 1970 US standard population.

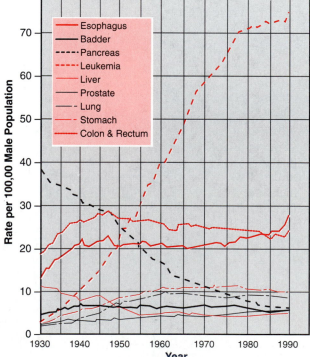

B *Age-adjusted to the 1970 US standard population.

FIGURE 31-3 *Cancer death rates for (**A**) females and (**B**) males.*

among white women in 1986 and among black women in 1990.[2]

Lung cancer *alone* is responsible for the increased cancer mortality rate from 1950 to 1990. Excluding lung cancer, cancer mortality has actually been falling by 14%. The increase in lung cancer reflects the patterns of cigarette smoking in this country. The lung cancer death rate for men is expected to begin to decline before the year 2000; for women, it will continue to rise into the next century.[2] Reducing cigarette smoking is clearly the single most important means of reducing lung cancer in the United States. Although other factors are associated with lung cancer, each of the other agents is potentiated by cigarette smoking.

Certain occupations apparently predispose persons to lung cancer. Asbestos workers have about a 10 times greater risk of developing the disease than the general population. More startling, an asbestos worker who smokes has a 90 times greater risk of developing lung cancer than the general population. Other industrial agents that increase risk are uranium, chromate, arsenic, and iron.

Studies suggest a correlation between chronic bronchitis and bronchogenic carcinoma, and the differences in mortality from lung cancer reported among various countries is related to their varying frequency of chronic bronchitis.[3] The excess mucus secretion characteristic of chronic bronchitis may interfere with the bronchial epithelial cells, making them likely to undergo malignant change. Also, the bronchial mucosa, which is chronically inflamed, exhibits depressed ciliary activity, and airway cleansing is decreased.[7]

Gross Appearance of Pulmonary Malignancy

The appearance of pulmonary carcinoma, although variable, falls into one of three types: 1) the *hilar, infiltrating form*, which causes a large tumor mass that presses on the bronchi; 2) the *peripheral* or *nodular form*, which may appear as a single tumor or as multiple nodular masses through the lung; or 3) the *diffuse type*, which looks very much like pneumonia and may be difficult to see on gross examination.[7] Squamous cell and small cell carcinomas tend to be centrally located and of the hilar, infiltrating type; adenocarcinoma and large cell carcinoma are more commonly peripheral.

Microscopic Appearance of Pulmonary Malignancy

The four major types of pulmonary neoplasms account for about 95% of lung cancers. The relative frequency of each type varies considerably at different research centers, owing to different classification guidelines and the difficulty of analyzing small amounts of biopsy material obtained from fiberoptic bronchoscopy. Some sources classify cancers as simply small cell or non–small cell because the behavior and treatment of the two types is so different.

The *squamous cell carcinoma* is the most common morphologic type of bronchogenic carcinoma. It causes 35% to 60% of lung malignancies. The cell type may be well differentiated, but, more frequently, it is undifferentiated and quite pleomorphic in appearance. It tends to have large, well-outlined areas of tumor growth arising from the bronchi.[3] These invade surrounding tissue in the early stages of the disease but later metastasize readily to the lymph nodes, brain, bone, adrenal glands, and liver. This tumor type has a very high correlation with heavy cigarette smoking, occurring almost exclusively in smokers. The 2-year prognosis is poor, with a survival rate of less than 50%. Unfortunately, it has the best prognosis of the four major types of pulmonary malignancy.

Adenocarcinoma of the lungs, accounting for about 30% of lung tumors, is increasing in relative and absolute frequency, especially among women, in whom this tumor represents 40% of the total.[3] The rare nonsmoker who develops lung cancer usually develops this type. Although the tumor is comparably slow-growing, its tendency for early invasion of lymphatics and blood vessels produces its low survival rate. The overall 2-year prognosis is poor, with a survival rate of only about 20%.

Large cell, undifferentiated, or giant cell carcinoma is distinct from the previous two tumors in that the cells involved are large and very anaplastic. The cells do not secrete hormones and also do not tend to grow at the same rate as the small cell type. The tumor is most often located in the peripheral areas of the lungs. These tumors account for about 15% of lung cancers. The overall prognosis remains very poor with a survival rate of only about 12% after 2 years.

The *small cell (oat cell) carcinoma* consists of small, dark cells located between the cells of the mucosal surfaces. They are characterized by rapid growth and early metastasis through the lymphatic system and blood. This disease is rare in the peripheral areas and frequently exhibits large, obstructive growths in the main bronchi.[7] Small cell carcinomas often secrete substances like those normally found in other areas of the body, including adrenocorticotropic hormone and antidiuretic hormone. The result of adrenocorticotropic hormone secretion is Cushing syndrome, which causes obesity, osteoporosis, hypokalemia, alkalosis, and other problems. Secretion of antidiuretic hormone leads to retention of water, hyponatremia, renal sodium loss, anorexia, nausea, and lethargy. The prognosis in this malignancy is the worst of the four lung cancer types, with a survival rate of only 3% to 5% after 2 years. The median survival rate after diagnosis is 2 to 4 months. Small cell carcinomas account for about 25% of lung cancers; they occur almost exclusively in cigarette smokers.

The propensity for metastasis is very common with lung cancer, although the rate may vary. More than one-half of afflicted persons (perhaps as many as 75%) have metastasis at the time of diagnosis.[7] The spread commonly occurs to the pleura, mediastinum, lymph nodes, liver, bone, brain, and adrenal glands.

The clinical manifestations of carcinoma of the lung are difficult to classify. Most individuals are asymptomatic for a long time or develop signs of metastasis. The most common symptoms of the primary tumor are cough and expectoration of bloody sputum. Because most persons with lung cancer are heavy smokers, they tend to dismiss the symptoms as routine. Hemoptysis may be severe. Lymph node enlargement may cause encroachment on the superior vena cava, obstruction, and dramatic signs and symptoms. Chest pain, dyspnea, and hoarseness may be present. Often the first symptoms are those caused by distant spread of the malignancy; these may include obstruction of the superior vena cava, recurrent nerve paralysis, bone lesions, or neurologic symptoms. Radiologic evidence on a routine chest film is often the first sign. However, by the time a lung tumor is radiologically evident, it has usually invaded surrounding structures. Sputum cytology and bronchoscopy help to confirm the diagnosis.

▼ Respiratory Failure

RESPIRATORY INSUFFICIENCY

Respiratory insufficiency is said to occur when the lungs are not able to exchange adequate amounts of carbon dioxide and oxygen to carry out the normal activities of daily living. In chronic respiratory insufficiency, the body gradually adapts to the pulmonary dysfunction. This process of adaptation includes hyperventilation, use of accessory muscles to breathe, circulatory changes to adjust the oxygen delivery to vital organs, and renal compensation to maintain the blood pH.[5] In *acute respiratory insufficiency*, hypoxemia and hypercapnia become severe and the compensatory mechanisms instituted by the body do not adjust the oxygen and carbon dioxide levels sufficiently to supply the body's needs. Without immediate treatment, inadequate tissue oxygen and severe respiratory acidosis ensue.

RESPIRATORY FAILURE

Respiratory failure is the inability of the lungs to meet the basic demands for tissue oxygenation at rest. Respiratory failure can occur as a result of a wide variety of intrapulmonary or nonpulmonary disorders (Table 31-1). Table 31-2 indicates that certain precipitating factors may cause the exacerbation of preexisting respiratory insufficiency.

The definitive diagnosis of respiratory failure depends on the arterial blood gases. A Po_2 of less than 50 mm Hg and a Pco_2 of more than 50 mm Hg often are accepted as determining values.[5] These are related also to the age, past history, and overall condition of the person. Acute deterioration of blood gases in a person with chronic lung disease indicates failing compensation and respiratory failure.[5] The disorder may exist with hypoxemia as the predominant problem or with a combination of hypoxemia and hypercapnia.

As respiratory failure ensues, the Pco_2 begins to rise, which leads to significant respiratory acidosis, indicating the inability of the lungs to eliminate the excess carbon dioxide. It may develop rapidly or slowly depending on

TABLE 31-1   *Some Common Conditions That May Cause Ventilatory Failure With Hypercapnia*

Conditions That Decrease Neuromuscular Function	Conditions That Increase Ventilatory Load
DEPRESSED RESPIRATORY DRIVE	**INCREASED AIRWAY RESISTANCE**
Sedative drugs	Upper airway obstruction
Hypothyroidism	Increased bronchial secretions and edema
Brain stem lesion	Bronchospasm
	Dynamic airway obstruction
ALTERED NEUROMUSCULAR TRANSMISSION	
Poliomyelitis	**DECREASED LUNG COMPLIANCE**
Myasthenia gravis	Increased lung water
Guillain-Barré syndrome	Infection
Amyotrophic lateral sclerosis	Atelectasis
Cord or phrenic nerve injury	Interstitial fibrosis
Pancuronium bromide	Acute lung injury
Aminoglycosides	Infarction
Anticholinesterase insecticides	Intrinsic positive end-expiratory pressure
MUSCLE WEAKNESS	**DECREASED CHEST WALL COMPLIANCE**
Myopathies	Chest wall trauma
Muscular dystrophy	Pleural effusion
Malnutrition	Pneumothorax
Shock, hypoxemia	Kyphoscoliosis
Hypokalemia	Ascites
Hypocalcemia	Peritoneal dialysis
Hypophosphatemia	Upper abdominal surgery
Hypomagnesemia	Ileus
	Obesity

(Kelley, W. N. *Textbook of Internal Medicine* [2nd ed.]. Philadelphia: J.B. Lippincott, 1992.)

TABLE 31-2 *Precipitating Factors That May Result in the Development of Respiratory Failure*

Factor	Example
Pulmonary infection, especially in presence of chronic obstructive pulmonary disease	Bacterial pneumonia Viral pneumonia Fungal pneumonia
Trauma	Automobile accident Gunshot/knife wound Burns
Infection	Sepsis Wound infection
Cardiovascular event	Myocardial infarction Aortic aneurysm Pulmonary embolism
Allergic reaction	Transfusion reaction Drug allergy Bee sting or other venom
Pulmonary aspiration	Vomitus Near drowning
Surgical procedure	Abdominal or thoracic surgery
Drug reaction	Overdose barbiturates or narcotics Anesthetic reaction
Mechanical factor	Pneumothorax Pleural effusion Abdominal distention
Iatrogenic factor	Endotracheal intubation/failure of clearance of tracheobronchial secretions
Neuromuscular disorders	Guillain Barré syndrome Multiple sclerosis Muscular dystrophy

renal compensation. The normal chemoreceptors for carbon dioxide may become inoperative, and the hypoxic stimulus may be the only stimulus for the respiratory effort. Oxygen should be administered with caution to these persons.

The clinical manifestations are dependent on the underlying cause but especially involve the resulting oxygen-carbon dioxide imbalance.[5] Dyspnea may not occur if there is depression of the respiratory center, so the respiratory rate may be either very rapid or slow. Hypoxemia leads to inadequate tissue perfusion with varying degrees of cyanosis, depending on the amount of right-to-left shunting. This is seen especially when the respiratory failure results from severe atelectasis or the adult respiratory distress syndrome (see pp. 587–589). Hypercapnia refers to P_{CO_2} levels above 45 mm Hg. It indicates inadequate alveolar ventilation and the inability to release carbon dioxide. The symptoms, which are often associated with hypoxemia, include increased pulse and blood pressure, dizziness, headache, mental clouding and central nervous system depression, muscle twitching, and tremor.

Carbon dioxide narcosis, which occurs as levels of carbon dioxide progressively increase to levels of 70 mm Hg or higher, leads to dilation of cerebral blood vessels, increased blood flow to the brain, increased intracranial pressure, and constriction of the pulmonary vessels.[5] This severe hypercapnia causes symptoms of confusion, convulsions, coma, and even death.

The prognosis of acute respiratory failure depends on the underlying causative mechanisms and whether or not lung function can improve. It may be the initial manifestation of the multisystem organ failure dysfunction syndrome. Respiratory failure is often the cause of death in pulmonary and nonpulmonary conditions.

▼ *Chapter Summary*

▼ Included among the other alterations of the pulmonary system are very important conditions that can lead to respiratory failure. Restrictive, obstructive, and other conditions can lead to this difficult problem.

▼ Pulmonary embolism usually is a result of deep venous thrombosis in the lower extremities and is caused by any number of factors that produce venostasis and thus, thrombosis. The resulting embolus can only go with the flow of blood to the filter provided in the lungs. The lungs then react to the lodged embolus with the clinical manifestations depending on the size and location of the lodged embolus.

▼ Fat embolization is a special form that occurs with fracture of the long bones in which the fatty marrow embolizes to the lungs.

▼ Pulmonary hypertension also is secondary to other conditions such as chronic obstructive lung disease, congenital heart disease or pulmonary fibrosis.

▼ The upper respiratory tract alterations include sinusitis, rhinitis, and others including carcinoma of the larynx, which usually arises on the vocal cords.

▼ Most lung tumors are malignant and most are related to cigarette smoking. This malignancy is still increasing in incidence in the U.S., especially in women. The most common form is the squamous cell type that arises in the bronchi, but the adenocarcinoma, the giant-cell, and the oat-cell types also are increasing in incidence. The prognosis for all of the lung cancers is dismal despite treatment measures.

▼ Many systemic diseases cause respiratory failure as their terminal event. Respiratory insufficiency usually is progressive to respiratory failure without treatment. Respiratory failure causes an oxygen–carbon dioxide imbalance which often results in respiratory acidosis. It is often the initial part of the multisystem organ failure dysfunction syndrome.

▼ *References*

1. Boring, C., Squires, T., Tong, T., and Montgomery, S. Cancer statistics, 1994. *CA Cancer J. Clin.* 44:7–9, 1994.
2. Centers for Disease Control. Current trends: Mortality trends for selected smoking-related cancers and breast cancer—United States, 1950–1990. *MMWR* 42, 1993, p. 44.
3. Cotran, R.S., Kumar, V., and Robbins, S.L. *Robbins' Pathologic Basis of Disease* (5th ed.). Philadelphia: W.B. Saunders, 1994.
4. Deppe, S., Barrette, R., and Thompson, D. Other embolic syndromes. In Civetta, J., Taylor, R., and Kirby, R., *Critical Care* (2nd ed.). Philadelphia: J.B. Lippincott, 1992.
5. Farzan, S.A. *A Concise Handbook of Respiratory Diseases* (2nd ed.). Reston, Va.: Reston, 1985.
6. Fedullo, P. Pulmonary embolism. In Tierney, D.F. (ed.), *Current Pulmonology, Vol. 1*. St. Louis: Mosby, 1993.
7. Kuhn, C., and Askin, F.B. Lung and mediastinum. In Kissane, J.M. (ed.), *Anderson's Pathology* (9th ed.). St. Louis: Mosby, 1990.
8. Mehra, M., and Bode, F. Pulmonary embolism. In Civetta, J., Taylor, R., and Kirby, R. (eds.), *Critical Care* (2nd ed.). Philadelphia: J.B. Lippincott, 1992.
9. Nunn, J.F. *Applied Respiratory Physiology* (4th ed.). London: Butterworth, 1993.

▼ *Unit Bibliography*

Albelda, S.M. The alveolar-capillary barrier in the adult respiratory distress syndrome. In Fishman, A.P. (ed.), *Update: Pulmonary Diseases and Disorders*. New York: McGraw-Hill, 1992.

Albert, R.K. Approach to the patient with cyanosis and/or hypoxemia. In Kelley, W.N. (ed.), *Textbook of Internal Medicine* (2nd ed.). Philadelphia: J.B. Lippincott, 1992.

Augustine, A., Harris, R., and Wynder, E. Compensation as a risk factor for lung cancer in smokers who switch from nonfilter to filter cigarettes. *Am. J. Public Health* 79:188, 1989.

Barnes, P. A new approach to the treatment of asthma. *N. Engl. J. Med.* 321:1517, 1989.

Baum, G., and Wolinsky, E. *Textbook of Pulmonary Diseases* (5th ed.). Boston: Little, Brown, 1994.

Bloom, B.R. (ed.). *Tuberculosis: Pathogenesis, Protection, and Control*. Washington: ASM Press, 1994.

Boutotte, J.T.B.: The second time around. *Nursing 93* 23:42–49, 1993.

Braun, S.R. *Concise Textbook of Respiratory Physiology*. New York: Elsevier, 1989.

Brock, E.T., and Shucard, D.W. Sleep apnea. *Am. Fam. Physician* 49:385–394, 1994.

Brown, L.H. Pulmonary oxygen toxicity. *Focus Crit. Care* 17:68, 1990.

Bruderman, I. Bronchogenic carcinoma. In Baum, G., and Wolinsky, E. (eds.), *Textbook of Pulmonary Diseases* (4th ed.). Boston: Little, Brown, 1989.

Burton, G.G., Hodgkin, J.E., and Ward, J.J. *Respiratory Care: A Guide to Clinical Practice* (3rd ed.). Philadelphia: J.B. Lippincott, 1991.

Caruthers, D.D. Infectious pneumonia in the elderly. *Am. J. Nurs.* 90:56, 1990.

Civetta, J., Taylor, R., and Kirby, R. (eds.). *Critical Care* (2nd ed.) Philadelphia: J.B. Lippincott, 1992.

Connor, P., Berg, P., Flaherty, N., et al. Two stages of care for pleural effusion. *RN* 52:30, 1989.

Cotran, R.S., Kumar, V., and Robbins, S.L. *Robbins' Pathologic Basis of Disease* (5th ed.). Philadelphia: W.B. Saunders, 1994.

Crystal, R.G., et al. The alpha1-antitrypsin gene and its mutations. *Chest* 95:196, 1989.

Dunlap, N.E., and Briles, D.E. Immunology of tuberculosis. *Med. Clin. North Am.* 77:1235–1251, 1993.

Eriksson, S. Alpha1-antitrypsin deficiency: Lessons learned from the bedside to the gene and back again. *Chest* 90:181, 1989.

Farzan, S.A. *A Concise Handbook of Respiratory Diseases* (3rd ed.). Reston, Va.: Reston, 1992.

Fishman, A.P. *Update: Pulmonary Diseases and Disorders*. New York: McGraw-Hill, 1992.

Flenley, D. *Respiratory Medicine* (2nd ed.). London: Bailliere Tindall, 1990.

Ganong, W.F. *Review of Medical Physiology* (16th ed.). Los Altos, Calif.: Lange, 1994.

Golden, et al. A randomized comparison of once-monthly or twice-monthly pentamidine prophylaxis. *Chest* 104:743–750. 1993.

Guyton, A.C. *Textbook of Medical Physiology* (8th ed.). Philadelphia: W.B. Saunders, 1991.

Hensley, M., and Saunders, N. *Clinical Epidemiology of Chronic Obstructive Pulmonary Disease*. New York: Dekker, 1989.

Holgate, S.T., et al. *The Role of Inflammatory Processes in Airway Hyperresponsiveness*. Oxford: Blackwell, 1989.

Hudgel, D.W., and Cherniack, N.S. Sleep and breathing. In Fishman, A.P. (ed.), *Update: Pulmonary Diseases and Disorders*. New York: McGraw-Hill, 1992.

Ioli, J.G. Giving surfactant to premature infants. *Am J Nurs* 90:59, 1990.

Isselbacher, K.J., et al. (eds.). *Harroson's Principles of Internal Medicine* (13th ed.). New York: McGraw-Hill, 1994.

Janson-Bjerklie, S. Status asthmaticus. *Am. J. Nurs.* 90:52, 1990.

Kelley, W.N. *Textbook of Internal Medicine*. (2nd ed.). Philadelphia: J.B. Lippincott, 1992.

Kissane, J.M. *Anderson's Pathology* (9th ed.). St. Louis: Mosby, 1990.

Madsen, L.A. Tuberculosis today. *RN* 53:44, 1990.

Martin, R.A. AIDS with disseminated histoplasmosis. *J. Fam. Pract.* 29:628, 1989.

Martin, R.J. *Cardiorespiratory Disorders During Sleep* (2nd ed.). Mt. Kisco, N.Y.: Futura, 1990.

Mines, A.H. *Respiratory Physiology* (3rd ed.). New York: Raven Press, 1993.

Mossman, B., and Gee, J. Asbestos-related diseases. *N. Engl. J. Med.* 320:1721, 1989.

Murray, J.F., and Nadel, J.A. (eds.). *Textbook of Respiratory Medicine* (2nd ed.). Philadelphia: W.B. Saunders, 1994.

Nunn, J. *Applied Respiratory Physiology* (4th ed.). London: Butterworth, 1993.

Pachon, J., Prados, D., Capote, F., et al. Severe community-acquired pneumonia: Etiology, prognosis, and treatment. *Am. Rev. Respir. Dis.* 142:369, 1990.

Pennington, J. *Respiratory Infections: Diagnosis and Management* (2nd ed.). New York: Raven Press, 1989.

Riechman, L.B., and Hershfield, E.S. (eds.). *Tuberculosis: A Comprehensive International Approach*. New York: Dekker, 1993.

Rinaldo, J. Adult respiratory distress syndrome. In Rippe, J.M., Irwin, R.S., Alpert, J.S., and Fink, M.P. (eds.), *Intensive Care Medicine* (2nd ed.). Boston: Little, Brown, 1991.

Roitt, I. *Essential Immunology* (7th ed.). Oxford: Blackwell, 1991.

Roitt, I., Brostoff, J., and Male, D. *Immunology* (3rd ed.). St. Louis: Mosby, 1993.

Sarosi, G., and Davies, S. *Fungal Diseases of the Lung* (2nd ed.). New York: Raven Press, 1993.

Schluger, N.W., and Rom, W.N. Current approaches to the diagnosis of active pulmonary tuberculosis. *Am. J. Respir. Crit. Care Med.* 149: 264–267, 1994.

Seaton, A., Seaton, D., and Leitch, A. *Crofton and Douglas's Respiratory Diseases* (4th ed.). Oxford: Blackwell, 1989.

Selwyn, P.A. Tuberculosis and AIDS: Epidemiologic, clinical and social dimensions. *J. Law Med. Ethics* 21:279–288, 1993.

Shapiro, B.A., et al. *Clinical Application of Blood Gases* (4th ed.). Chicago: Year Book Medical Publishers, 1989.

Shapiro, B.A., et al. *Clinical Application of Respiratory Care* (4th ed.). Chicago: Year Book Medical Publishers, 1991.

Shovein, J.T., Land, L.P., Richter, G., and Leedom, C.L. Near-drowning. *Am. J. Nurs.* 89:680, 1989.

Snapper, J. Inflammation and airway function: The asthma syndrome. *Am. Rev. Respir. Dis.* 141:531, 1990.

Stratton, M.B. Ventilation-perfusion scintigraphy in diagnosis of pulmonary thromboembolism. *Focus Crit. Care* 17:287, 1990.

Sturm, J.A. *ARDS: An Aspect of Multisystem Organ Failure.* New York: Springer-Verlag, 1991.

Thurlbeck, W.M. *Pathology of the Lung.* New York: Thieme, 1988.

Virella, G. *Introduction to Medical Immunology* (3rd ed.). New York: Dekker, 1993.

Walter, J.B. *Pathology of Human Disease.* Philadelphia: Lea & Febiger, 1989.

Warner, K. Smoking and health: A 25-year perspective. *Am. J. Public Health* 79:141, 1989.

Weinberger, S., Schwartzstein, R., and Weiss, J. Hypercapnia. *N. Engl. J. Med.* 321:1223, 1989.

Weiss, E.B., and Stein, M. (eds.). *Bronchial Asthma: Mechanisms and Therapeutics* (3rd ed.). Boston: Little, Brown, 1993.

West, J.B. *Pulmonary Pathophysiology: The Essentials* (4th ed.). Baltimore: Williams & Wilkins, 1992.

West, J.B. *Respiratory Physiology: The Essentials* (4th ed.). Baltimore: Williams & Wilkins, 1990.

Urinary Excretion

THE URINARY system maintains the appropriate concentration of electrolytes and water in the blood and eliminates many waste products. Chapter 32 explains normal renal function and provides a basis for the subsequent chapters that discuss different forms of renal pathology. Chapter 33 details the immunologic, infectious, and toxic alterations that can affect renal function. Chapter 34 describes the common causes of micturition dysfunction and genitourinary obstruction with emphasis on the formation of different types of calculi. Benign prostatic hyperplasia and renal and bladder tumors are included. Chapter 35 describes renal failure, its causes, and its clinical course.

The reader is encouraged to use the learning objectives to provide a systematic method for study. The extensive bibliography provides a current and historical perspective on general and specific aspects of renal function and dysfunction.

Chapter 32

Normal Renal and Urinary Excretory Function

Barbara L. Bullock

▼ CHAPTER OUTLINE

▼ LEARNING OBJECTIVES

1 Explain the internal structure of the kidneys, including the lobes, lobules, cortex, medulla, and renal pelvis.
2 Relate the main layers of the glomerular membrane, including the epithelial, glomerular basement membrane, and endothelial layers, to the formation of ultrafiltrate.
3 Describe the juxtaglomerular apparatus.
4 Discuss the function of the various parts of the nephron.
5 Describe the blood supply to the kidneys.
6 Describe in detail the mechanisms responsible for urine formation, including glomerular filtration, tubular reabsorption, and secretion.
7 Define **filtration, filtrate, tubular reabsorption, transport maximum**, and **secretion**.
8 Describe the pressures responsible for filtration.
9 Calculate the net filtration pressure and relate it to the glomerular filtration rate.
10 Describe active transport of glucose ions and protein from the proximal convoluted tubules.
11 Describe hypotonic and hypertonic urine formation and explain the countercurrent mechanism in the loop of Henle.
12 Discuss antidiuretic hormone and its relation to water regulation in the distal convoluted tubules and collecting tubules.
13 Explain the secretion of hydrogen ions and its relation to acid-base balance.
14 Discuss the functions of the kidney in erythrocyte production, vitamin D_3 activation, and gluconeogenesis.
15 Explain renal regulation of the renin-angiotensin-aldosterone system.
16 Explain the physical characteristics of urine.
17 Describe the structure and purpose of the ureters.
18 Explain the micturition reflex.

Barbara L. Bullock: PATHOPHYSIOLOGY: ADAPTATIONS AND ALTERATIONS IN FUNCTION, 4th ed.
© 1996 J.B. Lippincott-Raven Publishers

The renal system must function normally in order to sustain life. Human kidneys convert more than 1,700 L of blood per day to about 1 L of variably concentrated urine.[5] This system removes waste products from the blood and maintains critical levels of water and electrolytes in the blood. Urine, produced by the kidneys, is transported to the ureters, which empty into the bladder. Urine is excreted from the body through the urethra.

▼ Anatomy of the Kidneys

MACROSCOPIC ANATOMY

The kidneys are bean-shaped, reddish-brown organs that are located retroperitoneally on either side of the vertebral column, extending from the 12th thoracic vertebra to the third lumbar vertebra. Each kidney weighs about 150 g and is about 10 cm long, 5 cm wide, and approximately 2.5 cm thick.[9] The right kidney is slightly lower than the left because the liver is located above it (Fig. 32-1). Surrounding the kidneys is a layer of adipose tissue, or perirenal fat, that helps protect and support them. A fibrous layer of connective tissue called *renal fascia* encapsulates and anchors the kidneys in place in the abdomen.

Located externally at the concave portion of the kidney is a notch called the hilum. Structures at the hilum of each kidney are the renal artery and vein, lymphatics, nerves, and renal pelvis. The renal pelvis is the funnel-shaped extension of the upper ureter that provides a passageway for urine to the bladder (Fig. 32-2).

Internally, the kidneys are composed of the cortex and the medulla. The cortex, the outer portion, lies under the renal fascia. Substantial portions of the inner medullary layer are separated by cortical substances that are called renal columns or columns of Bertin.[3] Also, originating in the cortex and extending into the medulla are the uriniferous tubules, which are made up of the parenchymal (functioning) units of the kidneys, the nephrons. The medulla, the inner portion of the kidney, contains an estimated 8 to 18 *renal pyramids*, so-called because they are triangular. They are striated because of the collecting ducts, nephrons, and blood vessels of which they are composed. The apex of each pyramid is called the papilla. Below the papillae is a large cavity called the renal pelvis, which is interrupted by cuplike extensions called the minor and major calices. These structures are lined with transitional epithelium. The minor calices (approximately 10 in number) have openings that collect urine from the collecting ducts of the

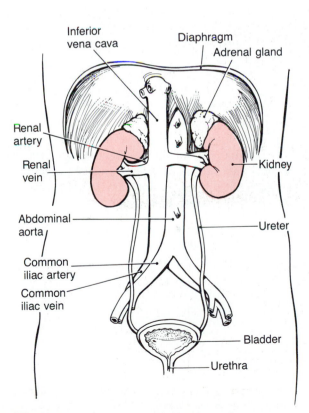

FIGURE 32-1 *Urinary system, with blood vessels.*

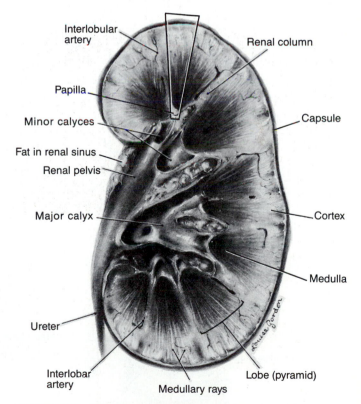

FIGURE 32-2 *Cut surface of the kidney, showing the renal pelvis. (Cormack, D. Essential Histology. Philadelphia: J.B. Lippincott, 1993.)*

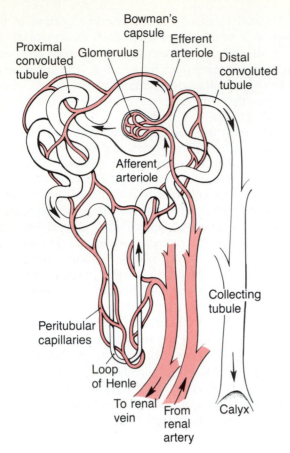

FIGURE 32-3 *Structure of the nephron and glomerulus.*

MICROSCOPIC ANATOMY: THE NEPHRON

It is estimated that a pair of kidneys contains 2.5 million nephrons. The nephron is a unique and complex structure. It is composed of Bowman's capsule, the proximal convoluted tubule (PCT), the loop of Henle, and the distal convoluted tubule (DCT). Many distal tubules empty into one collecting tubule or duct (Fig. 32-3).

Bowman's capsule is a cuplike structure that surrounds a capillary network called the glomerulus; the two together are called the renal corpuscle. The renal corpuscle has been likened to a fist (glomerulus) pushed into a balloon (Bowman's capsule).[12] There is an inherent space between the two structures where ultrafiltrate is received from the blood through the membrane of the glomerulus (Fig. 32-4).

The membrane of the glomerular capillaries is composed of three main layers: the epithelial layer, glomerular basement membrane, and the endothelial layer. The main function of the glomerular membrane is to form glomerular filtrate, a solution like plasma but without plasma proteins (see pp. 621–623). Formation of glomerular filtrate is the initial step in urine formation.

Nephrons are classified as either cortical or juxtamedullary (Fig. 32-5). The glomeruli of the cortical nephrons are in the outer two-thirds of the cortex. The tubules of the cortical nephrons penetrate into the outer region of the medulla.[11] The remaining one-third of the cortical area consists of glomeruli of the juxtamedullary nephrons, which contain a long loop of Henle that extends deep into the medulla. Lining the inner layer of Bowman's capsule, adjacent to the glomerulus, is a thin layer of epithelial cells called podocytes. These podocytes have projections called pedicles (foot processes) that cover the glomerular basement membrane. Between the pedicles are narrow regions called slit pores (filtration slits), through which proteins with a molecular weight of less than 50,000 can pass (Fig. 32-6).[6] Because plasma proteins have a slightly higher molecular weight, they normally cannot cross the glomerular membrane. Because of the location, numbers, and arrangement of slit pores, there is a large surface area that

pyramids and empty urine into the major calices (approximately three in number) and then into the renal pelvis, from which it is excreted to the ureters (see Figure 32-2).

The human kidney has up to 18 lobes, each of which is made up of cortical tissue and a conical medullary pyramid. Each pyramid of the kidney corresponds to a single lobe.[4] The lobes are well-defined structures and are made up of a number of lobules. The lobules are the parts of the kidney containing the nephrons that drain into common collecting tubules.

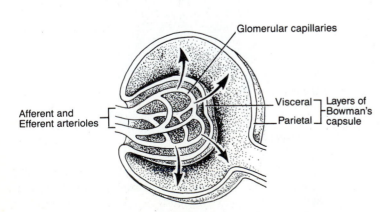

FIGURE 32-4 *Simplified organization of a renal corpuscle. (Cormack, D. Essential Histology. Philadelphia: J.B. Lippincott, 1993.)*

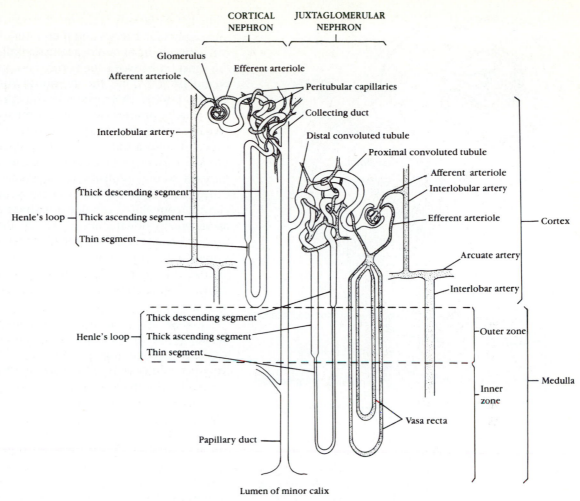

FIGURE 32-5 *Structure of cortical and medullary nephrons. Blood supply to the nephron, the vasa recta is shown schematically; this capillary structure normally surrounds Henle's loop. (Borysenko, M., et al. Functional Histology [2nd ed.] Boston: Little, Brown, 1984.)*

allows for rapid filtration of fluid. Diseases that affect the foot processes allow plasma proteins and sometimes cells to pass into the glomerular filtrate.[10]

Adjacent to the layer of epithelial cells is the glomerular basement membrane, which consists of a continuous meshwork of fibrillae that contain mucopolysaccharides. This meshwork prevents large proteins and molecules from passing into Bowman's capsule, a function that prevents protein loss in the urine.

The inner layer of the glomerular capillary is composed of endothelial cells. This layer consists of thousands of pores (fenestrations) that line the glomerulus and aid in membrane permeability (see Figure 32-6). The glomerular filtrate passes through three layers before it arrives in Bowman's capsule, but each layer is several hundred times more permeable than the usual capillary membrane.[6,11]

After the glomerular filtrate passes through the glomerulus into Bowman's capsule, it enters the PCT, which is located in the cortex and is approximately 14

mm long. Cuboidal epithelial cells line the PCT. On the luminal surface of these cells is a brush border of microvilli that increases the surface area available for secretion and absorption of fluids and solutes. Also located in the PCT cells are mitochondria. More than 65% to 80% of the glomerular filtrate is reabsorbed in the PCT, and the remaining 20% to 35% proceeds to the loop of Henle.

The two major portions of the loop of Henle are the descending and ascending limbs (see Figure 32-3). The thickened descending limb begins in the cortex. As it dips into the medulla, it becomes thinner and varies in length from 4.5 to 10.0 mm.[2] The descending limb loops and makes a tight hairpin turn upward, where it becomes thin and is called the thin portion of the ascending limb. The main function of both limbs of the loop of Henle is to concentrate urine. After urine passes through the limbs, it proceeds to the DCT, which is located in the renal cortex.

The DCT is lined with cuboidal cells containing mitochondria and fewer microvilli than are present in the PCT. As the cuboidal cells change to columnar cells,

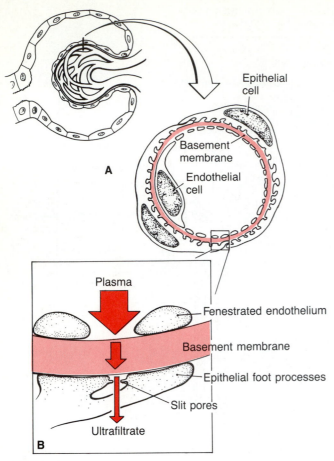

Epithelial cell

Basement membrane

Endothelial cell

A

Plasma

Fenestrated endothelium

Basement membrane

Epithelial foot processes

Slit pores

Ultrafiltrate

B

FIGURE 32-6 *A. Schematic illustration of the three layers of the glomerular capillary.* ***B.*** *The dense layer of the glomerular basement membrane (GBM) prevents passage of large molecules into the ultrafiltrate.*

the area becomes very dense, thus forming the macula densa. The macula densa lies in close contact with the vascular component of the juxtaglomerular apparatus (Fig. 32-7). Located within the apparatus are juxtaglomerular cells that produce the enzyme renin, which transforms angiotensinogen to angiotensin I (see pp. 519–520). The macula densa cells also contribute to the control of the glomerular filtration rate.[12]

The main function of the DCT is to transport electrolytes and water. Two or more DCTs join together to form the collecting duct, which conducts the formed urine. The collecting ducts are lined with cuboidal cells that terminate in the renal medulla. Urine is transported from the collecting duct to a papillary collecting duct, which opens into the minor calix. Urine is then excreted from the minor to the major calix and into the renal pelvis, ureters, bladder, and urethra.

BLOOD SUPPLY TO THE KIDNEYS

In a resting state, it is estimated that the kidneys receive 20% to 25% of cardiac output, which is more than 1,000 mL per minute. From the aorta, blood enters the hilum of the kidney by way of the renal artery, which branches into segmental arteries and then interlobar arteries that run between the pyramids of the medulla (Fig. 32-8). At the junction between the cortex and medulla (corticomedullary junction), the interlobar arteries convert to arcuate arteries that penetrate the cortex and branch into smaller arteries called interlobular arteries, which give rise to the afferent arterioles. The afferent arterioles subdivide into a tuft of capillaries called a glomerulus. Blood leaves the glomerulus by the efferent arteriole and forms a second network of capillaries; this network, called the peritubular capillary network, mainly encircles the convoluted tubules (proximal and distal). The arrangement of capillaries between these arterioles is unique because it allows a higher pressure to be maintained in the glomerulus. Also, the efferent arterioles are smaller in diameter than the afferent arterioles, again causing higher glomerular pressure because of increased vascular resistance.

The deeper-lying (juxtamedullary) glomeruli also break up into the peritubular network but have a set of capillaries penetrating the medulla. These thin-walled vessels are in close proximity to the thin ascending and descending loops of Henle and are referred to as the vasa recta (see Figure 32-5). The vasa recta aid in concentrating urine.

The interlobular veins are formed from the peritubular capillary network and empty into the arcuate veins and then the interlobar veins, which converge to form the renal vein. Blood from the renal vein leaves the kidneys and drains into the inferior vena cava.

INNERVATION OF THE KIDNEYS

Nerve fibers reach the kidneys through the renal plexus, which extends along the renal artery. The kidneys are innervated mostly by the sympathetic division of the autonomic nervous system, but smaller numbers of parasympathetic fibers are also present. The nerve supply generally follows the distribution of the arterial vessels in the renal parenchyma. The nerve supply comes mostly from the celiac plexus and the mesenteric, upper splanchnic, and thoracic nerves.[11] The sympathetic nerves, when stimulated, constrict the afferent arteriole and cause an increase in blood pressure. The parasympathetic system has important effects on the ureters and urinary bladder but no noted effects on the kidneys themselves.[12]

▼ Physiology of the Kidneys

The kidneys maintain a constant plasma concentration of substances by removing some from the blood and adding some back to it (Box 32-1).[12] These functions are essential to maintain life, even though the kidneys do not regulate all inorganic or organic substances. The

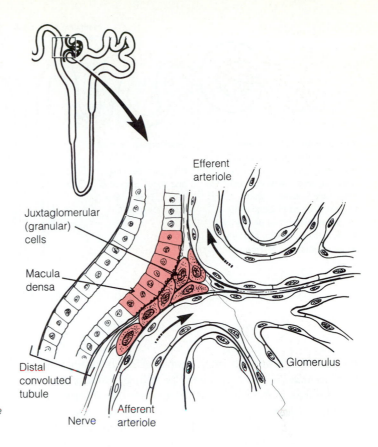

FIGURE 32-7 *The relation of the juxtaglomerular apparatus, the distal convoluted tubule, and the glomerulus.*

kidneys have a large reserve in renal function owing to the large number of nephrons. The critical functions of blood pressure regulation, erythropoietin production, secretion of 1,25-dihydroxyvitamin D_3, and gluconeogenesis are discussed later in this chapter.

The kidneys use three major mechanisms to main-tain a balance that alters the composition of urine and thereby keeps the composition of plasma within strict limits. These mechanisms are glomerular filtration, tubular reabsorption, and tubular secretion. Figure 32-9 provides a reference for the major functions of each portion of the nephron.

GLOMERULAR FILTRATION

Filtration, the initial step in urine formation, is the result of pressures that force fluids and solutes through a membrane. The filtration process occurs between the layers of

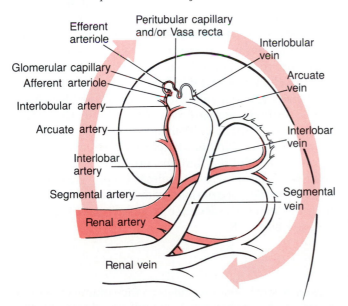

FIGURE 32-8 *Pathway of blood flow from its entrance in renal artery to exit through renal vein. (Adapted from R. Memmler, B. Cohen, and D. Wood. The Human Body in Health and Disease [7th ed]. Philadelphia: J.B. Lippincott, 1992.)*

BOX 32-1 ▼ Functions of the Kidneys

Regulation of water and electrolyte balance
Removal of metabolic waste products from the blood and their excretion in the urine
Removal of foreign chemicals from the blood and their excretion in the urine
Regulation of arterial blood pressure by altering both sodium excretion and the secretion of renin and possibly other vasoactive substances
Secretion of erythropoietin
Secretion of 1,25-dihydroxyvitamin D_3
Gluconeogenesis

Vander, A. J. *Renal Physiology*. New York: McGraw-Hill, 1991.

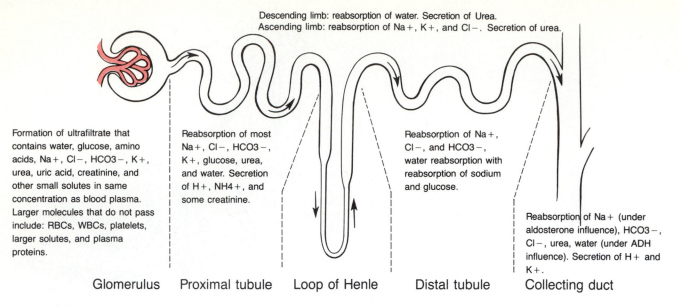

Descending limb: reabsorption of water. Secretion of Urea.
Ascending limb: reabsorption of Na+, K+, and Cl−. Secretion of urea.

Formation of ultrafiltrate that contains water, glucose, amino acids, Na+, Cl−, HCO3−, K+, urea, uric acid, creatinine, and other small solutes in same concentration as blood plasma. Larger molecules that do not pass include: RBCs, WBCs, platelets, larger solutes, and plasma proteins.

Reabsorption of most Na+, Cl−, HCO3−, K+, glucose, urea, and water. Secretion of H+, NH4+, and some creatinine.

Reabsorption of Na+, Cl−, and HCO3−, water reabsorption with reabsorption of sodium and glucose.

Reabsorption of Na+ (under aldosterone influence), HCO3−, Cl−, urea, water (under ADH influence). Secretion of H+ and K+.

Glomerulus   Proximal tubule   Loop of Henle   Distal tubule   Collecting duct

FIGURE 32-9 *Functions in each portion of the nephron.*

the glomerulus and Bowman's capsule. The resulting fluid is *glomerular filtrate*, a relatively protein-free solution.

Approximately 125 mL of glomerular filtrate per minute (180 L per 24 hours) is produced. Normally, urine output equals 1 to 2 L/d, which means that the tubules and peritubular capillaries are responsible for reabsorbing approximately 179 L, an amount greater than 99% of the filtrate received. The quantity of glomerular filtrate produced each minute is called the *glomerular filtration rate* (GFR).

The quantity of filtrate and the filtration process are dependent on several factors. Various pressures contribute to the outward flow of filtrate into Bowman's capsule and retention of fluid within the glomerulus. The *hydrostatic pressure* is a simple outward force created by the systemic blood pressure. This pressure is normally about 75 mm Hg which is equivalent to the mean arterial pressure (MAP). The *colloid osmotic pressure* or *oncotic pressure* is the inward force, exerted by plasma proteins, that holds fluid within the glomerulus (see Figure 32-9).

The pressure that is chiefly responsible for filtration is the *glomerular blood hydrostatic pressure* (GBHP). This refers to the MAP described above. This pressure forces filtrate out of the glomerulus into Bowman's capsule and normally is approximately 60 to 80 mm Hg. If the hydrostatic pressure decreases to 42 mm Hg, filtration usually does not take place.[11] Working in opposition to the hydrostatic pressure is the *capsular hydrostatic pressure* in Bowman's capsule, which is normally about 18 mm Hg. This pressure is exerted by the walls of Bowman's capsule and the fluid in the renal tubule. Increased capsular pressure causes the GFR to decrease.[6] The other pressure that works in opposition to the glomerular pressure is the *blood colloidal osmotic pressure*, which is normally about 30 mm Hg. Because blood contains more protein

than filtrate does, the colloidal property constantly exerts an inward force.

The net result of all these pressures—glomerular, capsular, and colloidal osmotic—is the *net filtration pressure*. The net filtration pressure is equal to the forces inducing filtration minus the forces opposing filtration:

$$NFP = GBHP - (CHP + BCOP)$$

where NFP is the net filtration pressure, GBHP is the glomerular capillary hydrostatic or hydraulic pressure, CHP is the hydrostatic or hydraulic pressure in Bowman's capsule, and BCOP is the oncotic or colloid osmotic pressure in glomerular-capillary plasma.[11] For example, if the GBHP is 60 mm Hg, the CHP is 15, and the BCOP is 27, NFP = 60 − (15 + 27), or 18 mm Hg.

The net filtration pressure in the kidney is considerably higher than in other systemic capillaries. Many factors can change the GFR by changing the net filtration pressure. Increased hydrostatic pressure or decreased colloid osmotic pressure can increase the GFR (Fig. 32-10). Sympathetic nervous system stimulation results in vasoconstriction of the afferent and efferent arterioles, which affects the net filtration pressure. Because constriction of the afferent arterioles is usually greater than that of the efferent arterioles with sympathetic stimulation, the result is a decrease in glomerular hydrostatic pressure and GFR.

Renal Clearance

The term renal clearance refers to the volume of plasma from which a substance is completely cleared by the kidneys per unit time.[12] Measurement of the clearance of substances is extremely useful in the evaluation of renal function. It has been used successfully to evaluate the

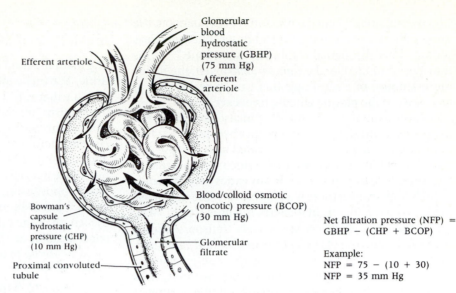

Efferent arteriole

Glomerular
blood
hydrostatic
pressure (GBHP)
(75 mm Hg)

Afferent
arteriole

Bowman's
capsule
hydrostatic
pressure (CHP)
(10 mm Hg)

Blood/colloid osmotic
(oncotic) pressure (BCOP)
(30 mm Hg)

Glomerular
filtrate

Proximal convoluted
tubule

Net filtration pressure (NFP) =
GBHP − (CHP + BCOP)

Example:
NFP = 75 − (10 + 30)
NFP = 35 mm Hg

FIGURE 32-10 *Schematic representation of the relation between hydrostatic pressure and colloid osmotic pressure. The end result is the net filtration pressure, which forms the ultrafiltrate.*

GFR. A polysaccharide called *inulin* is freely filtered at the glomerulus and not reabsorbed in any way in the tubules. It can, therefore, be used to determine the GFR. It must be administered intravenously at a constant rate for several hours to produce a constant level in the blood plasma. The GFR can then be calculated by the following formula:

$$GFR = (U_{In} \times V) \div P_{In}$$

where U_{In} is the concentration of inulin measured in the urine, V is the volume of urine produced over a specified time, and P_{In} is the plasma inulin concentration. To use an example cited in Vander[12], if the U_{In} is 360 mg/L, 0.2 L of urine is produced in 2 hours, and P_{In} is maintained at 4 mg/L during that period:

$$GFR = (360 \times 0.2) \div 4 = 18 \text{ L in 2 hours,}$$
$$\text{or 150 mL/min}$$

In clinical practice, estimating the GFR from inulin is inconvenient, so an endogenous substance, creatinine, is used to estimate it. Creatinine is almost totally excreted. Using it to calculate GFR usually overestimates the true value, but the value is very close to actual GFR. It can be calculated by collecting a 24-hour urine sample and a blood sample.[7] The formula then becomes:

$$\text{Estimated GFR} = U_{cr} \times V \times P_{cr}$$

U_{cr} is the amount of creatinine excreted in the urine in 24 hours, and P_{cr} is the measured level of serum creatinine; both of these terms are expressed in mg/dL. V is the volume of urine excreted during the 24-hour period, expressed in mL/min (total volume divided by 1440 minutes). For example, if 1,800 mL of urine is excreted in 24 hours, V = 1,800 mL/24 hr = 1.25 mL/min. If the concentration of creatinine is 104 mg/dL in the urine and 1.0 mg/dL in the blood;

$$GFR = 104 \times 1.25 \times 1.0 = 130 \text{ mL/min}$$

TUBULAR REABSORPTION

As described in the previous section, of the 180 L of glomerular filtrate produced each day, approximately 179 L is reabsorbed in the tubules. The kidneys are able to change the composition of urine by excreting different concentrations of substances.[6] This is achieved by reabsorption and secretion. For example, if a person ingests a large volume of water, the resulting urine is very dilute; on the other hand, if a person is in a dehydrated state, the urine output is markedly decreased and the urine becomes very concentrated. *Tubular reabsorption*, the second step of urine formation, requires movement of solutes between the filtrate and the blood in the surrounding vasa recta and peritubular capillaries.

Reabsorption in the Proximal Convoluted Tubules

In the *proximal convoluted tubules*, tubular reabsorption is accomplished by active and passive transport of ions. Some ions passively follow the active transport of other ions.[6] Approximately 70% of glomerular filtrate is reabsorbed in the PCT.

ACTIVE TRANSPORT. Active transport is the movement of molecules against a concentration gradient, and it requires an expenditure of energy. Active transport causes movement of substances from PCT to plasma. The PCTs are able to carry on active transport because of their epithelial cells that contain mitochondria. These cells also have a brush border that increases the surface area for reabsorption and secretion. Some of the substances that are moved actively or permissibly with active transport include glucose, many electrolytes, amino acids, proteins, and vitamins.[11]

Glucose is actively transported from the tubules into the plasma, and normally none appears in the urine.

Glucose apparently binds with, and is dependent on, the same sodium carrier in the brush border that transports sodium ions through the tubular membrane.[6, 11] This transport is limited by the *transport maximum*, the maximum amount of a substance that can be reabsorbed at any time.[2] If the plasma glucose level exceeds the *threshold* of approximately 175 mg/dL, glucose appears in the urine (glycosuria). Glycosuria occurs because the transport mechanism has become saturated with glucose and must leave it in the tubules, from which it is excreted in the urine. The transport maximum varies between individuals, especially if there is a chronic increase in glucose load, as often happens in diabetes mellitus (see p. 741).

Sodium and *potassium* are actively transported from the tubules into the plasma of the peritubular capillaries by way of the basal channels of the epithelial cells. Because sodium and potassium are positive ions, they set up an electronegative cytoplasm in the epithelial cells. This allows negative ions, such as chloride and phosphate, to follow the positive ions.[6]

Proteins are reabsorbed in the PCT through the energy-dependent process of endocytosis.[12] The proteins attach to the membrane of the brush border of the PCT, are ingested by the tubular cells, and are broken down into amino acids, which are transported into the plasma. If permeability of the glomerular membrane increases, large protein molecules can leak into the filtrate, causing proteinuria.

PASSIVE TRANSPORT. Passive transport, including osmosis and diffusion, involves the movement of substances across a membrane without the expenditure of energy. It is accomplished by the establishment of an electrical gradient of positive ions, mainly sodium, which allows negative ions and water to diffuse across the tubular membrane.

Water is removed from the tubules as the result of the *isosmotic process*, which maintains equal osmotic pressures of fluid inside the tubules and in the plasma. When the solutes are actively reabsorbed into the plasma, the concentration of solute in the tubules decreases and the concentration in the peritubular capillaries increases, causing water to move into the peritubular capillary. Approximately 70% of water is reabsorbed by passive transport in the PCT. The role of the kidneys in controlling osmolality of the plasma through the transport of water is critical in maintaining fluid balance. The excretion of excess water or conservation of water maintains the plasma osmolarity at a fixed specific gravity of 1.010. This regulation is greatly influenced by antidiuretic hormone in the distal convoluted and collecting tubules (see p. 526).

Chloride and *bicarbonate* apparently diffuse across the tubular membrane into the peritubular capillaries. In the PCT, their diffusion occurs because of an electrochemical gradient created by positive ions.

Concentration of Urine in the Loop of Henle

The main function of the loop of Henle is to concentrate urine. For this concentration to occur, the countercurrent mechanism is used. The two components of this mechanism are the countercurrent multiplier and the countercurrent exchanger. The concept of the countercurrent multiplier system was proposed by Drs. Kuhn and Ruffel in 1942. The hypothesis states that a small difference in osmotic concentration between fluids flowing in opposite directions in two parallel tubes connected in a hairpin fashion can be multiplied many times along the length of the tubes.[1] The nephrons involved in renal concentration are the juxtamedullary nephrons whose loops of Henle extend into the medulla of the kidney, about 20% to 30% of the total number of nephrons. Their loops of Henle are surrounded by vessels of the vasa recta, which can reabsorb substances into the blood.[11] The loops of Henle and the juxtamedullary capillary system (vasa recta) work together to concentrate urine.

COUNTERCURRENT MULTIPLIER. In the PCT, tubular fluid is neither concentrated nor diluted because reabsorption is caused by water permeability of the tubular epithelium.[1] As fluid progresses down the descending limb of the loop of Henle, it is still isotonic to plasma. The excretion of excess solutes (concentration of urine) requires a hyperosmolality of the medullary interstitial fluid. This hyperosmolality is greater in the long segments of the loop of Henle and may increase to as much as 1,200 mOsm/L at the turn of the loop. Sodium and chloride are transported from the thin segment (descending and loop portions) into the medullary interstitium. Current research indicates that this movement occurs when the interstitial concentration of urea is high, causing water to move into the interstitial area. Approximately half of the medullary osmolarity is determined by urea.[12] The sodium and chloride concentrations become increased in the thin segment, and these ions probably diffuse passively out of this area and into the interstitium. Urea is poorly absorbed by the vasa recta and becomes trapped in the medullary interstitium. It is partly reabsorbed by ascending limbs of the loop of Henle.

As sodium, chloride, potassium, and water move up the ascending limb (thick portion), sodium, chloride, and potassium are transported out of the tubule into the interstitium. Thus, the distal tubule receives hypotonic fluid.[11, 12] Water is not removed because the ascending limb is almost impermeable to it. Because this process continuously concentrates the filtrate with sodium chloride and urea in the section of the loop of Henle that is located in the medulla, it is called the *countercurrent multiplier*. As fluid moves up the ascending loop, sodium is transported out and the filtrate becomes more dilute. As the filtrate passes to the distal and collecting tubules, water is reabsorbed under the influence of antidiuretic hormone, resulting in the final regulation of the specific gravity of the urine. Figure 32-11 summarizes the process for countercurrent multiplication.

Urea is also exchanged by this mechanism, and excess is excreted in the urine. Urea is produced through degradation of amino acids, and the amount formed usually depends on the protein intake in the diet and the ability of the liver to convert ammonia to urea. Normally, the body produces 25 to 30 g of urea each day but maintains only 8 to 20 mg/dL in the plasma. Approximately half of the urea that is filtered remains in the interstitial fluid of the medulla. The ascending thin limb of the loop of Henle is permeable to urea, but the DCT and collecting ducts are not. Therefore, urea remaining in the tubules at this point is excreted.

COUNTERCURRENT EXCHANGER.　As discussed above, the vasa recta are important in carrying out the countercurrent mechanism. The vasa recta run parallel to the loops of Henle. Because of the hairpin loops, blood entering the system follows the same gradients as those produced in the loops. The looped vessels do not create the gradient, but they do protect it.[12] Blood enters the descending limbs of the vasa recta with a solute concentration of approximately 300 mOsm/L. At this point, sodium, chloride, and urea diffuse from the interstitial fluid into the blood, thus creating a higher osmolality in the blood, which causes water to move back into the blood. At the tip of the hairpin turn of each vessel in the vasa recta, osmolality can reach 1,200 mOsm/L for a maximum concentration, which is also the concentration in surrounding interstitium.

As blood ascends the vasa recta, water returns to the blood, and sodium, chloride, and urea move back by diffusion into the interstitial fluid. By the time blood leaves the medulla, its osmolality is slightly higher than that of blood that enters the vasa recta.[1] This mechanism provides a precise balance between the countercurrent systems and prevents sodium from accumulating in the interstitium.[12] This entire action by the vasa recta is called the *countercurrent exchange mechanism.*

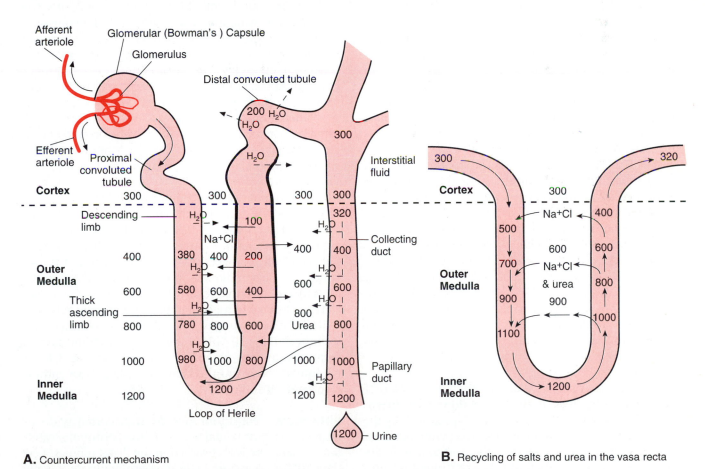

A. Countercurrent mechanism

B. Recycling of salts and urea in the vasa recta

FIGURE 32-11　*Mechanism of urine concentration. The thick ascending limb of the loop of Henle is relatively impermeable to water and urea.* **A.** *Countercurrent mechanism.* **B.** *Recycling of salts and urea in the vasa recta. All concentrations are in milliosmoles per liter (mOsm/L). (Tortora, G., and Grabowski, S. Principles of Anatomy and Physiology [7th ed.]. New York: Harper Collins, 1993.)*

CLINICAL CONSIDERATIONS IN URINE CONCENTRATION. In any form of renal disease, the inability to achieve maximal urinary concentration occurs early.[12] The medullary gradient is almost invariably affected, and conditions such as changes in renal blood flow alter the gradient by carrying away too much or too little water or solute. Osmotic diuresis can wash out the gradient and prevent concentration of the urine.

The concentration of urine is usually reported as specific gravity which, by usual measurement methods, measures urine density, not concentration. Urine osmolarity may be quite different from the specific gravity. For example, if there is protein in the urine, the specific gravity is increased with no significant change in osmolarity.[12]

The osmolarity of urine may be increased as a result of increased concentrations of urea, creatinine, uric acid, potassium, or other substances. Because of the effect of aldosterone, there may be small amounts of sodium in the urine even when the urine appears maximally concentrated.[12]

Reabsorption in the Distal Convoluted Tubules

SODIUM, CHLORIDE, AND POTASSIUM REABSORPTION. The DCT and collecting tubules reabsorb smaller amounts of sodium than do the loops of Henle. The release of aldosterone, stimulated by serum potassium concentration and the renin-angiotensin-aldosterone system, affects sodium reabsorption at the DCT. Both potassium and angiotensin II apparently are necessary for aldosterone biosynthesis[8] (see pp. 698–699).

The final urine product normally contains less than 1% of total filtered sodium and chloride.[12] Sodium is reabsorbed by primary active transport. Chloride reabsorption is both passive (following sodium) and active. Active chloride transport is usually with bicarbonate ion; it may involve reabsorption of chloride in deficiency states with loss of bicarbonate or the reverse.[12]

An increase in serum potassium from increased intake provides a direct stimulus for the release of aldosterone. Aldosterone then causes retention of sodium ion and urinary excretion of potassium. This is an important mechanism in maintaining the serum concentration of potassium.[8]

WATER REABSORPTION. Water is regulated in the DCT and collecting tubules by the production of *antidiuretic hormone* (*vasopressin*). This hormone is produced by the hypothalamus and stored and released by the posterior pituitary gland. It is secreted by the posterior pituitary when the osmoreceptors in the anterior hypothalamus respond to an increase in the osmolarity of the plasma (see pp. 684–685). The hormone directly regulates the permeability of the membranes of the renal epithelial cells. This occurs by binding to receptors in the membranes of the collecting duct.

If amounts of antidiuretic hormone in the blood are increased, water is osmotically moved from the tubules into the capillaries by means of increased permeability of the tubular membrane to water. This results in more concentrated urine and adds water to the plasma. Without antidiuretic hormone, the permeability is decreased, causing water to stay in the tubules, which results in very dilute urine.

TUBULAR SECRETION

Secretion, the final step in urine formation, is the movement of fluid and solute from the blood back into the glomerular filtrate; it usually requires an expenditure of energy to cross the electrochemical gradient. Active and a few passive secretory mechanisms are present at various points in the tubules.

HYDROGEN IONS. Hydrogen ions (H^+) are secreted in the PCT, DCT, and collecting tubules. The number of H^+ ions secreted depends on the pH of the extracellular fluid and the amount of buffer in the glomerular filtrate. The normal pH of urine varies from 4.5 to 8.0 depending on dietary intake and metabolism. If the urine pH decreases to 4.4, secretion becomes inhibited. If the hydrogen ion concentration is high in extracellular fluid (plasma), large quantities of hydrogen are secreted. Low concentrations cause small amounts of H^+ secretion.

When ammonia (NH_3) is passively secreted by the tubules, it can combine with the actively secreted hydrogen, forming ammonium ion (NH_4^+). Ammonium ion is secreted into the filtrate, and sodium (Na^+) is replaced. The exchange of Na^+ and H^+ causes Na^+ to move into the renal capillaries and combine with bicarbonate ion to form sodium bicarbonate. This is one way the renal cells maintain acid-base balance and buffer excess H^+ (see pp. XX). Carbonic anhydrase, a special enzyme in the renal cells, is necessary in this process and causes water and carbon dioxide to combine, resulting in the formation of carbonic acid (H_2CO_3). When H_2CO_3 dissociates, it forms hydrogen and bicarbonate ions (H^+ and HCO_3^-). The hydrogen ions are then exchanged for sodium in the cell. This ammonia-ammonium mechanism is especially important when excess acid loads continually bombard the kidneys, such as with chronic respiratory insufficiency.

POTASSIUM. Potassium ions are transported with sodium from the proximal tubules to the peritubular capillaries, and more is reabsorbed in the distal tubules. Less than 10% of potassium in the glomerular filtrate actually arrives at the distal tubules. Excretion of excess potassium requires active secretion of potassium from the capillaries into the cortical and collecting ducts. This is partly under the control of aldosterone. The reabsorption of sodium leaves a negative electrochemical gradient in the tubules. Electrochemical neutrality must be maintained, so positive potassium takes the place of sodium. Excess potassium is ingested in the normal diet, up to several hundred milliequivalents per day. The secretion method for potassium excretion is essential to maintain the normal serum value of 3.5 to 5.0 mEq/L. Levels of 7.0 mEq/L or higher may precipitate cardiac dysrhythmias and death (see p. 201).

Flowchart 32-1 shows pathways by which excess potassium intake leads to increased excretion. If a person is on a very low potassium diet or is potassium depleted, the cortical collecting duct does not secrete potassium.[12] The medullary collecting duct also reabsorbs some potassium. This is the only mechanism for the conservation of potassium, causing its value to be depleted rather easily in dietary deficiency or when osmotic diuretics are administered.

BLOOD PRESSURE REGULATION BY THE KIDNEYS

The regulation of arterial blood pressure by the kidneys involves the retention and excretion of sodium as well as the *renin-angiotensin-aldosterone system*, which combines the activities of the enzyme renin and the hormone aldosterone. Sodium effects on blood volume and blood pressure are discussed in Chapters 25 and 26.

Located in each kidney are special cells called *juxtaglomerular cells*, which make up the juxtaglomerular apparatus. This apparatus produces *renin*, an enzyme, and secretes it into the blood. The stimulus for this secretion is decreased perfusion pressure in the afferent arteriole. Renin then causes angiotensinogen, a plasma protein, to split and produce *angiotensin I*, a polypeptide that is transformed into *angiotensin II* in the lungs. Angiotensin II causes vasoconstriction throughout the body and stimulates the adrenal cortex to release *aldosterone*. With the release of aldosterone, sodium is transported from the tubules to the blood, passively followed by water. These movements increase blood volume and blood pressure (see Flowchart 32-2). The increased volume of circulating blood causes the renal cells to receive increased amounts of oxygen. Vasoconstriction increases the peripheral resistance and blood pressure.

The release of renin is the primary initiator of the mechanism for blood pressure control. Its release basically depends on four interrelated mechanisms:

1. Intrarenal baroreceptors that respond to stretch and vary renin secretion inversely to the degree of stretch. If blood volume (and thus blood pressure) decreases, more renin is released from the granular juxtaglomerular cells.
2. Sodium or chloride receptors in the macula densa respond to increased concentrations by inhibiting renin release and to decreased concentrations by stimulating release.

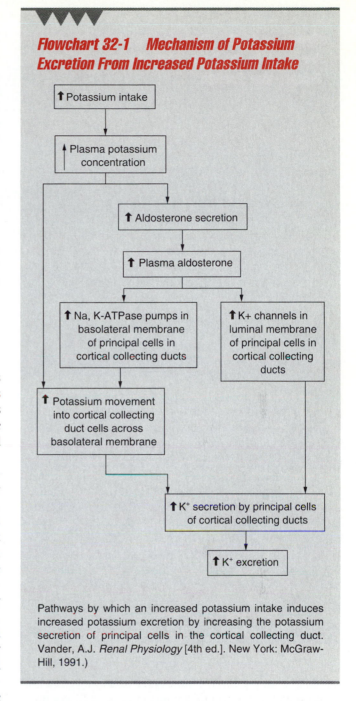

Flowchart 32-1   Mechanism of Potassium Excretion From Increased Potassium Intake

Pathways by which an increased potassium intake induces increased potassium excretion by increasing the potassium secretion of principal cells in the cortical collecting duct. Vander, A.J. *Renal Physiology* [4th ed.]. New York: McGraw-Hill, 1991.)

3. Renal sympathetic nerves, besides causing a decrease in renal blood flow, which leads to baroreceptor and macula densa response, cause direct stimulation of the juxtaglomerular cells and release of renin.
4. Angiotensin II directly inhibits renin secretion, which is a negative feedback process that controls its production.[12] It also constricts efferent arterioles, stimulates the release of aldosterone, increases thirst through the hypothalamus, and stimulates the release of antidiuretic hormone from the posterior pituitary.[11]

The kidney functions as a critical part of blood pressure regulation through chemical mediators and blood

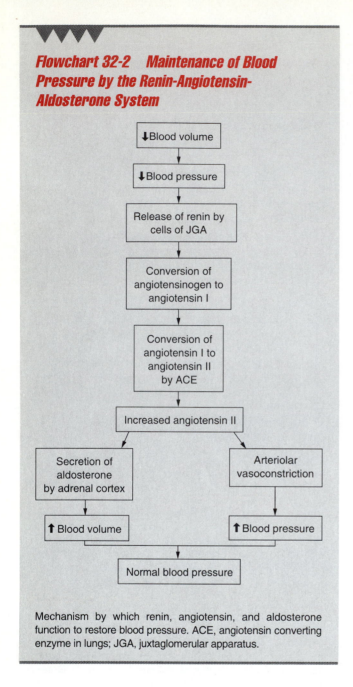

Flowchart 32-2   Maintenance of Blood Pressure by the Renin-Angiotensin-Aldosterone System

Mechanism by which renin, angiotensin, and aldosterone function to restore blood pressure. ACE, angiotensin converting enzyme in lungs; JGA, juxtaglomerular apparatus.

volume manipulation. Alterations to kidney function often have profound effects on the arterial blood pressure; these effects are discussed in the other chapters in this unit.

ERYTHROPOIETIN SECRETION

The hormone erythropoietin has been identified as a major factor in the control of erythrocyte production (see p. 376). The location of cells that secrete this hormone has not been precisely identified, but the stimulus for its secretion is hypoxia to the renal cells.[12] Erythropoietin directly stimulates the bone marrow to cause production of erythrocyte progenitors, which then mature to erythrocytes.[10] Without this hormone, anemia results

and is usually very severe, such as that seen in end-stage renal failure. Chronic hypoxia, such as that seen with COPD, causes increased erythrocyte production and erythrocytosis.

SECRETION OF ACTIVATED VITAMIN D

Cholecalciferol (vitamin D) is either produced by the effects of ultraviolet light on the skin or ingested in certain foods. It must undergo several changes, by means of hydroxylation in the liver and kidneys, before it can stimulate active absorption of calcium by the intestine. The effects of activated vitamin D (1,25-dihydroxychole-calciferol, or vitamin D_3) on calcium balance and bone reabsorption are discussed in detail on pages 851–852.

GLUCONEOGENESIS IN THE KIDNEYS

The kidneys have been shown to be gluconeogenic organs in cases of prolonged fasting.[11] They can synthesize glucose from amino acids and release it into the bloodstream.[12]

PHYSICAL CHARACTERISTICS OF URINE

Box 32-2 summarizes some specific characteristics of urine. Variations relate to diet and fluid intake. The color of urine varies according to how concentrated or dilute it is. It normally ranges from pale yellow to amber, which is the result of the pigment urochrome. It often varies with the specific gravity, being more deeply colored when the specific gravity is increased. The urine may become discolored from certain disease conditions or from foods or medicines. The most common change is dark or bright red urine from bleeding along the upper or lower urinary tract. Dark yellow urine may be associated with increased concentration of conjugated bilirubin in the blood. Drugs such as phenazopyridine and phenytoin can produce a pink, red, or red-brown urine. Severe

BOX 32-2 ▼ Physical Characteristics of Urine

Appearance	Clear, amber yellow
pH	4.6–8.0
Odor	Aromatic to ammonia-like
Specific gravity	1.005–1.030
Ketones	Negative
Protein	50–80 mg/24 hours at rest
	<250 mg/24 hours after strenuous exercise
Glucose	Negative
	<0.5 g/day or <2.78 mmol/day
Red blood cells	<2 per microscopic slide
	0 red blood cell casts
Bacteria	Negative culture and sensitivity
Urobilinogen	0–4 mg/24 hours

Pseudomonas infection, especially of the entire urinary tract, may produce a blue-green or green, often cloudy, urine.

The normal volume of urine is one to two liters per day, with water accounting for about 95% of the total volume.[11] Abnormal constituents or high concentrations of normal constituents may affect the appearance and odor of urine. The specific gravity of urine is normally from 1.001 to 1.035. The lower numbers indicate a dilute urine, whereas the higher specific gravities indicate a high concentration of solutes.

▼ Accessory Urinary Structures and Bladder

When urine is excreted from the kidneys, it is transported from the renal pelvis to the ureters by peristaltic contractions. It is emptied into the bladder, which releases it into the urethra.

URETERS

The ureters vary in length from 25 to 30 cm and are approximately 1.25 cm wide. They enter the bladder at oblique angles. They are composed of three layers of smooth muscle, including an inner layer of longitudinal muscle, a middle layer of circular muscle, and an outer layer that is a fibrous coat. The ureters also are lined with a layer that is composed of mucous membrane. This layer, because of mucus secretion, cannot be permeated by the constituents of urine (Fig. 32-12).

The ureters are innervated by both sympathetic and parasympathetic nerves. Each has an intramural plexus of nerve fibers that extend along its entire length.[6] As urine is formed, it collects in the renal pelvis, and as pressure increases, peristaltic movement forces the urine down the ureter toward the bladder. The peristaltic contractions occur at a rate that ranges from once every 10 seconds to once every 2 to 3 minutes.[6] These cause a spurting action by which urine fills the bladder.

BLADDER

When empty, the bladder is like a deflated balloon. When filled with urine, it rises into the abdomen and becomes pear-shaped. The bladder is located behind the symphysis pubis. It is composed of several layers: mucosa, submucosa, detrusor muscle, and serous layer. The mucosal layer contains *transitional epithelium*, which, in combination with the rugae (multiple folds in the mucosa), allows the bladder to stretch during urinary filling.[4] The submucosa contains connective tissue that

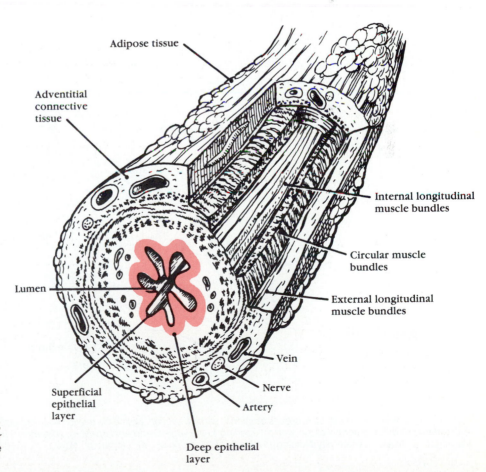

FIGURE 32-12 *Structure of the ureter, including smooth muscle layers, outer connective tissue, and blood nerve supply.*

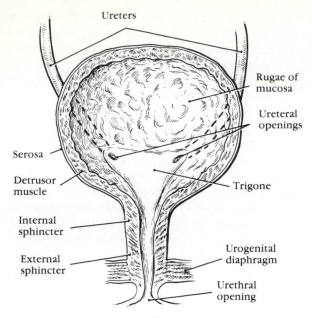

FIGURE 32-13   *Structure of the bladder and its internal and external urethral sphincters.*

connects the mucous and muscular layers. The serous layer coats the superior portion of the bladder and is formed by the peritoneum. The detrusor muscle is composed of longitudinal and circular muscles, allowing for contractility. The contractions of the detrusor muscle of the bladder can increase its pressure as high as 40 to 60 mm Hg. This muscle is, therefore, the one that causes bladder emptying.[6]

An area called the *trigone* is located at the base of the bladder and is formed by the two ureters and the urethra. Between the bladder and the urethra is an *internal urethral sphincter*; below it is an *external urethral sphincter*. These sphincters are formed by circular muscles and, when stimulated, allow urine to pass from the bladder into the urethra (Fig. 32-13).

The principal nerve supply to the bladder is through the sacral plexus, which mainly connects with spinal cord segments S2 to S4.[6] Sensory fibers respond to stretch of the bladder walls. The motor nerve fibers are mainly parasympathetic. Sympathetic fibers connect with the lumbar portion. The pudendal nerves supply the external sphincter.[6]

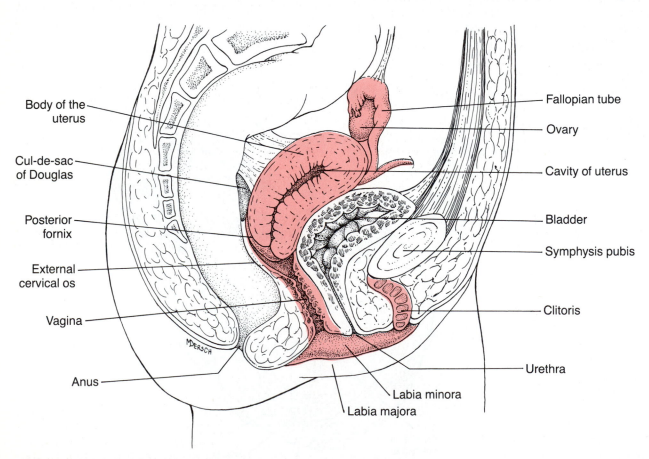

FIGURE 32-14   *Female reproductive organs as seen in sagittal section. Notice the relation of the bladder to the uterus and the proximity of the urethral opening to the vaginal and anal openings. (Reeder, S.J., Martin L.L., Koniak, D. Maternity Nursing [17th ed.]. Philadelphia: J.B. Lippincott, 1992.)*

MICTURITION REFLEX. Micturition (voiding) is the result of a spinal reflex from the sacral portion of the spinal cord. Stretch receptors become stimulated when there is 150 to 300 mL of urine in the bladder. The bladder pressure increases with increased filling, and the parasympathetic nerves become stimulated. This causes the micturition reflex, which results in contraction of the detrusor muscle and relaxation of the internal sphincter. Urination proceeds unless it is stopped by voluntary contraction of the external sphincter, which is under cerebral control. The cerebral centers keep the micturition reflex partly inhibited until micturition is desired. The higher centers can inhibit the reflex by continual tonic contraction of the external sphincter. The centers also can facilitate the reflex by relaxing the external sphincter.[6]

URETHRA

The urethra, located at the apex of the bladder, is the final excretory passageway for urine. The urethral opening to the exterior is the urinary meatus. The female urethra is located posteriorly to the symphysis pubis and anteriorly to the vagina. The urethra is approximately 3.75 cm long and is composed of smooth muscle (Fig. 32-14).

When the male urethra leaves the bladder, it passes through the prostate gland, then between a membranous portion that extends from the prostate gland to the corpus spongiosum of the penis. Finally, the urethra passes through the corpus spongiosum and terminates at the urinary meatus. The male urethra is approximately 20 cm long and transports both urine and semen (Fig. 32-15).

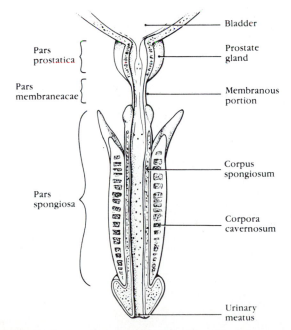

Pars prostatica

Pars membraneacae

Pars spongiosa

Bladder

Prostate gland

Membranous portion

Corpus spongiosum

Corpora cavernosum

Urinary meatus

FIGURE 32-15 *Structure of the male genitourinary anatomy.*

▼ *Chapter Summary*

▼ The macroscopic and microscopic structure of the kidney provide the structure in which the formation of ultrafiltrate and the urine end product can occur. This requires a diffuse network of blood and lymphatic vessels, nerves, nephrons, glomeruli, and collecting areas for the urine. The nephron is composed of Bowman's capsule, the proximal convoluted tubule (PCT), distal convoluted tubule (DCT), and collecting duct in cortical nephrons. In medullary nephrons there is, additionally, a loop of Henle which makes possible the concentration of urine. The blood supply to the kidney is a high pressure, high flow system which terminates in the glomerulus, a system of capillaries through which blood is filtered and ultrafiltrate arrives in Bowman's capsule. The main structure responsible for this filtration is the glomerular basement membrane.

▼ The kidneys function to make urine which is of a markedly different composition than plasma. Through ion exchanges and excretion of substances, the kidneys regulate the electrolyte and water balance of the body. Glomerular filtrate is formed; the rate of its formation is the glomerular filtration rate (GFR). Reabsorption goes on throughout the tubules with approximately 70% being reabsorbed in the PCT. Active transport and endocytosis are other important processes throughout this system. The loop of Henle has as its main function the concentration of urine through the countercurrent multiplier effect in its exchanging with the vasa recta. The DCT and collecting tubules reabsorb sodium depending upon the amount of aldosterone in the blood which increases sodium reabsorption and increases potassium excretion. Water is regulated in the DCT and collecting tubules by the production of antidiuretic hormone (ADH) which causes the reabsorption of water.

▼ The kidneys function in blood pressure regulation through the secretion of renin which leads to the formation of angiotensin II, vasoconstriction and release of aldosterone. Increased renin secretion leads to increased blood pressure through increased systemic vascular resistance and increased blood volume. The kidneys also provide a major mechanism for the control of erythrocyte production. This hormone directly stimulates the bone marrow to cause production of erythrocytes. Another function of the kidney is in the activation of 1,25 dihydroxycalciferol (activated vitamin D) which affects calcium balance and bone reabsorption.

▼ From the kidney, urine flows through the accessory urinary structures to the bladder. Urine can accumulate in the bladder until micturition occurs. The reflex is inhibited by cerebral centers. Relaxation of the internal sphincter allows the passage of urine through the urethra to the exterior.

▼ *References*

1. Berl, T., and Schrier, R.W. Disorders of water metabolism. In Schrier, R.W., *Renal and Electrolyte Disorders* (3rd ed.). Boston: Little, Brown, 1986.
2. Brenner, B.M., and Rector, F.C. *The Kidney* (5th ed.). Philadelphia: Ardmore, 1994.
3. Cormack, D.H. *Essential Histology*. Philadelphia: J.B. Lippincott, 1993.
4. Cormack, D.H. *Ham's Histology* (10th ed.). Philadelphia: J.B. Lippincott, 1991.
5. Cotran, R.S., Kumar, V., and Robbins, S.L. *Robbins' Pathologic Basis of Disease* (5th ed.). Philadelphia: W.B. Saunders, 1994.
6. Guyton, A.C. *Textbook of Medical Physiology* (8th ed.). Philadelphia: W.B. Saunders, 1991.
7. Kee, J.L. *Handbook of Laboratory and Diagnostic Tests* (2nd ed.). Norwalk, Conn.: Appleton & Lange, 1994.
8. Linas, S.L., and Schrier, R.W. Disorders of the renin-angiotensin-aldosterone system. In Schrier, R.W., *Renal and Electrolyte Disorders* (3rd ed.). Boston: Little, Brown, 1986.
9. Memmler, R.L., Cohen, B.J., and Wood, D.L. *The Human Body in Health and Disease* (7th ed.). Philadelphia: J.B. Lippincott, 1992.
10. Spargo, B.H., and Haas, M. The Kidney. In Rubin, E., and Farber, J.L., *Pathology* (2nd ed.). Philadelphia: J.B. Lippincott, 1994.
11. Tortora, G.J., and Grabowski, S.R. *Principles of Anatomy and Physiology* (7th ed.). New York: HarperCollins, 1993.
12. Vander, A.J. *Renal Physiology* (4th ed.). New York: McGraw-Hill, 1991.

Chapter 33

Immunologic, Infectious, Toxic, and Other Alterations in Function

Barbara L. Bullock

▼ **LEARNING OBJECTIVES**

1 List the major organisms that can cause cystitis.
2 Differentiate between hemorrhagic and suppurative cystitis.
3 Explain the normal protections against infection in the male and female urinary systems.
4 Differentiate between acute and chronic pyelonephritis, pathologically and clinically.
5 Describe antiglomerular basement membrane disease using Goodpasture syndrome as a model.
6 Explain the significance of crescents in renal pathology.
7 Describe the cause, pathology, clinical manifestations, and prognosis for poststreptococcal glomerulonephritis.
8 Describe briefly the pathology of rapidly progressive glomerulonephritis.
9 Discuss the pathophysiology of **nephrosis**.
10 Describe the development of edema in nephrotic disease.
11 Describe the relations among idiopathic nephrotic syndromes, minimal change disease, focal glomerulosclerosis, membranous glomerulopathy, and membranoproliferative glomerulonephritis.
12 Describe how aspirin, phenacetin, codeine, and caffeine can cause nephritis.
13 Outline the mechanisms by which hyperuricemia, hypercalcemia, and hypokalemia can cause tubular or parenchymal alterations.
14 Review the immunologic mechanisms that can cause tubulointerstitial alterations.
15 Describe the mechanisms that can result in renal tubular acidosis.
16 Explain briefly polycystic disease of the kidneys.

Barbara L. Bullock: PATHOPHYSIOLOGY: ADAPTATIONS AND ALTERATIONS IN FUNCTION, 4th ed.
© 1996 J.B. Lippincott-Raven Publishers

Many factors affect the genitourinary system and can cause problems ranging from the relatively innocuous to progressive conditions that lead to renal failure. The most common genitourinary disease is infection of the bladder mucosa, which may ascend to the pelvis of the kidney. Conditions of kidney dysfunction are often divided into those that affect the glomeruli, the tubules, the interstitium, and the blood vessels. The early manifestations of disease affecting the specific areas tend to be distinct.[5] Some agents affect more than one structure, and damage to one structure almost always affects the others. These concepts are presented in this chapter and in the following two chapters.

▼ Infections of the Genitourinary Tract

Urinary tract infections (UTIs) are extremely common and account for up to 6 million physician office or clinic visits yearly in the United States.[17] These infections are diagnosed by culture of the causative microorganism. Active infection is usually considered to be present when more than 100,000 bacteria per milliliter of urine appear in a clean-voided specimen. The most common cause of urinary tract infection is *Escherichia coli*, an aerobic organism present in large numbers in the lower intestinal area. Infections also may be caused by other organisms, such as *Klebsiella, Proteus*, and *Staphylococcus* species, especially in the presence of an indwelling catheter. Recurrent infections are more often caused by these organisms. Hospital-acquired infections often result from the presence of an indwelling urethral catheter and are found in persons receiving antimicrobial agents. These persons often develop infections with bacteria which have become resistant to the effects of the antimicrobials.[17]

CYSTITIS

Cystitis, or inflammation of the bladder, is more common in women than in men because of the proximity of the urethral opening and vagina to the anal area. Normally, the urethra contains diphtheroids and *Streptococcus* and *Staphylococcus* organisms. Gram-negative organisms may gain access to the bladder during sexual intercourse, after urethral trauma, or as a result of poor hygiene. Normally, these organisms are rapidly expelled by voiding because urine is acidic and flushes away excess bacteria. In men, prostatic secretions have antibacterial properties.

Risk factors for cystitis include sexual intercourse, pregnancy, neurogenic bladder, kidney disease, obstructive conditions, chemotherapy agents, radiation therapy, and diabetes mellitus. The most dangerous sequel of cystitis is pyelonephritis, which is thought to result from

organisms in the bladder that have ascended to the renal pelvis (see below). Vesicoureteral reflux increases the risk of pyelonephritis from cystitis. This condition involves the retrograde flow of urine from the bladder into the ureters. It often occurs in children who have abnormalities of the bladder or urinary tract that allow urine to reflux from the bladder to the renal pelvis. It also may follow a UTI in an adult.

The pathology of cystitis varies. If bloody urine is present, it is called *hemorrhagic cystitis*; this is a frequent sequel of chemotherapy or radiation therapy over the bladder area. *Suppurative cystitis* occurs when suppurative exudate accumulates on the endothelial lining of the bladder (Fig. 33-1). The exudate is composed of polymorphonuclear leukocytes in early stages, but mononuclear infiltrates appear if the condition progresses to chronic cystitis. Ulcerations may be present in either the acute or chronic phase.

Clinical manifestations include significant bacteriuria in 60% to 70% of cases. Some persons may have symptomatic cystitis with no definitive diagnosis of an organism by culture.[5] Dysuria, frequency, urgency, and suprapubic pain are classic symptoms. Any individual who has an indwelling catheter for more than 96 hours has a high risk for developing cystitis with organisms that become resistant to therapy.[9]

PYELONEPHRITIS

Inflammation of the renal pelvis, called pyelonephritis, is mainly caused by bacterial kidney infection.[15] Because the genitourinary system is continuous from the urethra to the bladder to the kidneys, ascending infection from

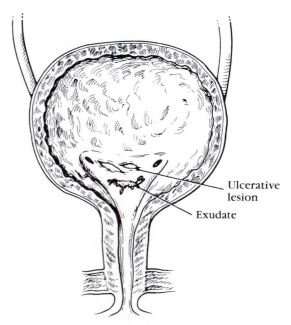

FIGURE 33-1 *Suppurative cystitis with ulceration of the bladder mucosa and suppurative exudate on the lining of the bladder.*

the bladder is the most common cause of pyelonephritis.[17] In addition to ascending infection, pyelonephritis may be caused by septicemia (hematogenous) or by vesicoureteral reflux, or the cause may be unknown. As with cystitis, the infection most commonly is caused by gram-negative bacteria. Two forms of pyelonephritis have been described: acute and chronic.

ACUTE PYELONEPHRITIS. Acute pyelonephritis usually occurs suddenly with onset of fever, chills, nausea, vomiting, diarrhea, and pain at the costovertebral angle. It may follow a symptomatic or asymptomatic bladder infection, or it may result from vesicoureteral reflux. Occasionally, acute pyelonephritis is initiated by a blood-borne, virulent organism, but this route of infection almost always signifies the presence of other kidney injury.

Pathologically, acute pyelonephritis gives rise to abscesses on the cortical surface of the kidney that often surround the glomeruli. Glomerular damage is rare, but the tubules may rupture. The infection also may follow urinary tract obstruction, with suppurative exudate filling the renal pelvis. Healing usually involves replacement of affected areas of the cortical surface by scar tissue.

Clinical manifestations of acute pyelonephritis include the sudden onset of high fever and chills, with marked tenderness on deep pressure of one or both costovertebral areas. Leukocytosis and pyuria with leukocyte cases are common. The urinalysis does not differentiate upper parts of the urinary tract from the lower UTIs. The urine may actually be sterile.[16] In the acute phase, some hematuria may be present but it usually does not persist after the acute manifestations have abated. The symptoms of acute pyelonephritis subside with or without treatment, but urine colonization by nonpathogenic organisms may persist for weeks or months. Uncomplicated acute pyelonephritis usually responds well to treatment, but there is a high incidence of recurrence.[5]

CHRONIC PYELONEPHRITIS. Chronic pyelonephritis is difficult to diagnose except when a history of urinary tract infections, pyuria, and bacteriuria can be elicited. Chronic pyelonephritis may follow obstructive conditions, such as congenital anomalies or renal calculi. It is often the cause of renal insufficiency in vesicoureteral reflux. Chronic pyelonephritis is a common cause of chronic renal failure and is found in 11% to 20% of persons having chronic renal dialysis for end-stage renal disease (see pp. 662–666).[5]

Pathologically, the kidneys have become scarred and irregular, and the calices and renal pelvis are deformed (Fig. 33-2). Gradual atrophy and destruction of the tubules lead to impairment of function that results in chronic renal failure.[15] Chronic pyelonephritis has been reported to follow vascular and hypertensive conditions that affect the glomeruli.

The clinical manifestations of chronic pyelonephritis vary, sometimes manifesting recurrent episodes of acute pyelonephritis or gradual onset of renal insufficiency and failure. Mild proteinuria with lymphocytes and plasma cells is characteristic. Although chronic pyelonephritis has been linked to bacterial infections, not all affected

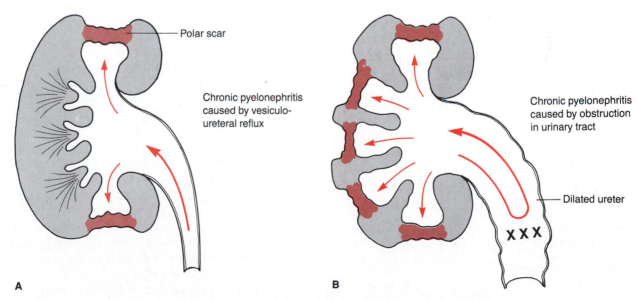

A   B

FIGURE 33-2   *The two major types of chronic pyelonephritis.* **A.** *Vesiculoureteral reflux causes infection of the peripheral compound papillae and scars in the poles of the kidney.* **B.** *Obstruction of the urinary tract leads to high-pressure backflow of urine, which causes infection of all papillae, diffuse scarring of the kidney, and thinning of the cortex. (Rubin, E., and Farber, J.L. Pathology [2nd ed.]. Philadelphia: J.B. Lippincott, 1994.)*

persons relate a history of urinary tract infection. Damage can result from asymptomatic bacterial infection.[5]

▼ Glomerular Disease

Glomerular injury is the most common cause of chronic renal failure, with immunologically induced glomerulonephritis causing 25% to 30% of all cases of end-stage renal failure.[3] Diabetes mellitus and hypertension are the leading diseases that cause renal failure through their effects on the glomerular basement membrane (GBM).[2] Glomerular injury may also result from chemicals, irradiation, hypoxemia, and other agents. Table 33-1 lists the most common forms of glomerular diseases. These forms may be primary or secondary. Primary glomerular disease is often idiopathic or immunologically mediated; secondary forms result from systemic or hereditary diseases.

Glomerular disease may be nephritic or nephrotic, or both. In *nephritic disease*, there is active proliferation of glomerular cells and an extensive inflammatory process. When there is increased permeability of the GBM, proteinuria and possibly nephrosis result. *Nephrosis* refers to the sequelae of albuminuria that is usually greater than

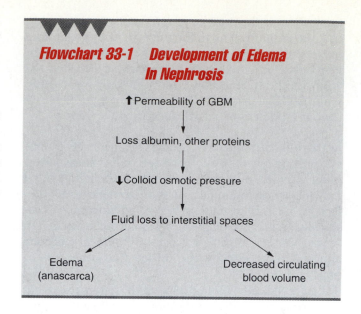

Flowchart 33-1 Development of Edema In Nephrosis

↑Permeability of GBM
↓
Loss albumin, other proteins
↓
↓Colloid osmotic pressure
↓
Fluid loss to interstitial spaces
↓   ↓
Edema   Decreased circulating
(anascarca)   blood volume

3.5 g/day. The result of the urinary loss of large amounts of albumin is hypoalbuminemia. A serum albumin level of less than 3 g/dL results in generalized body edema. Flowchart 33-1 shows the process of the development of edema in nephrosis. Hyperlipidemia results from hepatic lipoprotein synthesis, which is stimulated by the decreased serum protein levels. The excess lipids formed are mostly cholesterol in the early stages; in late stages, triglycerides also become elevated.[5]

TABLE 33-1 Glomerular Diseases

PRIMARY GLOMERULONEPHRITIS
Acute diffuse proliferative glomerulonephritis (GN)
   Poststreptococcal
   Nonpoststreptococcal
Crescentic (rapidly progressive) GN
Membranous GN
Lipoid nephrosis (minimal change disease)
Focal segmental glomerulosclerosis
Membranoproliferative GN
IgA nephropathy
Focal proliferative GN
Chronic GN

SYSTEMIC DISEASES
Systemic lupus erythematosus
Diabetes mellitus
Amyloidosis
Goodpasture's syndrome
Polyarteritis nodosa
Wegener's granulomatosis
Henoch-Schonlein purpura
Bacterial endocarditis

HEREDITARY DISORDERS
Alport's syndrome
Fabry's disease

Cotran, R. S., Kumar, V., and Robbins, S. L. *Robbins' Pathologic Basis of Disease* (5th ed.). Philadelphia: W.B. Saunders, 1994.

IMMUNE-MEDIATED GLOMERULAR DISEASE

Many types of glomerular damage are caused by antigen-antibody complexes precipitated in the glomeruli. Table 33-2 presents a general classification of immune mediated glomerulopathies. Antigen-antibody responses to infectious agents are frequent causes of immune complex disease, but the condition can be associated with many types of autoimmune disease, malignancies, and thyroiditis.

POSTSTREPTOCOCCAL GLOMERULONEPHRITIS. Group A, β-hemolytic streptococci have been shown to possess nephrotoxic surface proteins. Glomerulonephritis develops 1 to 2 weeks after an infection with this streptococcal organism. Nasopharyngeal infection is the usual source, but occasionally it may be a streptococcal skin infection. Development of poststreptococcal glomerulonephritis (PSGN) requires an individual sensitivity to β-hemolytic streptococci, as is evidenced by the fact that no active infection can be demonstrated by blood or urine cultures. Increased antistreptolysin or other streptococcal exoenzyme titers and depressed serum complement levels are common findings.

TABLE 33-2 *General Classification of Immune-Mediated Glomerulopathies*

Clinical Presentation	Most Common Histologic Variants	Most Likely Primary Pathogenetic Mechanism	Major Causative Agents on Entities
NEPHRITIC SYNDROMES			
Acute (postinfectious) glomerulonephritis	Proliferative glomerulonephritis	Trapped immune complexes	Streptococci Other bacteria Viruses Parasites
Rapidly progressive glomerulonephritis	Crescentic glomerulonephritis	Anti-GBM antibodies	Anti-GBM antibodies including Goodpasture syndrome
		Trapped immune complexes	Lupus erythematosus Mixed cryoglobulinemia Subacute bacterial endocarditis Henoch-Schönlein purpura Idiopathic, immuno-fluorescence-positive
		Uncertain	Wegener granulomatosis Polyarteritis Idiopathic, immuno-fluorescence-negative
Slowly progressive glomerulonephritis	Membranoproliferative glomerulonephritis (also presents as nephrotic syndrome)	Uncertain (see text)	Partial lipodystrophy Miscellaneous (see text)
NEPHROTIC SYNDROME	Minimal change nephropathy (minimal change disease, nil disease, lipoid nephrosis)	Uncertain	Allergy Hodgkin disease
	Focal and segmental glomerulosclerosis and hyalinosis ("focal sclerosis"; also presents as slowly progressive glomerulonephritis)	? Trapped immune complexes	Heroin addiction
	Membranous nephropathy	Formation of immune complexes in situ	Hepatitis Gold, penicillamine Non-Hodgkin lymphoma Carcinomas (bronchogenic, GI, kidney, thyroid, etc.) Collagen vascular diseases
PERSISTENT URINARY ABNORMALITIES (HEMATURIA AND PROTEINURIA)	Mesangial proliferative glomerulonephritis (also presents as nephrotic syndrome)	Trapped immune complexes	IgA nephropathy (Berger disease and Henoch-Schönlein purpura) IgM nephropathy

GBM, glomerular basement membrane; GI, gastrointestinal.
Kelley, W. N., ed. *Textbook of Internal Medicine* (2nd ed.). Philadelphia: J.B. Lippincott, 1992.

Pathologically, enlarged hypercellular glomeruli can be demonstrated, with proliferation of cells on the epithelial side of the GBM. Infiltration of the area with polymorphonuclear leukocytes and monocytes is followed by interstitial edema and inflammation. "Humps" can be seen on the epithelial side of the GBM; they probably represent precipitated antigen–antibody complexes.[16] Increased permeability of the GBM results in loss of red blood cells and protein in the urine. A decrease in glomerular filtration rate leads to retention of sodium and water. Hypocomplementemia is frequently associated with and results from large amounts of precipitated complement in the complexes.

The clinical manifestations of PSGN include the

acute onset of edema, oliguria, proteinuria (which is usually mild or moderate but may reach nephrotic levels, 73.5 g/24 hr), anemia, and a characteristic cocoa-colored urine with red blood cell casts. Hypertension is usual and probably results from fluid retention. A markedly elevated antistreptolysin-O titer indicates the presence of circulating antibody to the hemolysin streptolysin O, which is usually elevated 1 week to 1 month after a streptococcal infection. Other streptococcal exoenzymes include deoxyribonuclease, β-hyaluronidase, and nicotinamide adenine dinucleotidase. These titers are often increased and are measured by the streptozyme test, a combination of tests that is used to screen individuals for recent streptococcal infection. The erythrocyte sedimentation rate is usually increased, indicating inflammation.

Acute PSGN occurs most frequently in children, most of whom totally recover within a week and then exhibit immunity to further infection. Occasionally, PSGN converts to either a rapidly or slowly progressive form of glomerulonephritis; with either form, renal failure results. Adults who develop PSGN have a higher frequency of persistent proteinuria, hematuria, and renal failure than children do.[10]

NONSTREPTOCOCCAL GLOMERULONEPHRITIS. In addition to the *Streptococcus* organisms, other bacteria, viruses, and parasites have been implicated as causes of acute glomerulonephritis. These also presumably cause the precipitation of immune complexes and lead to a variety of lesions, including crescentic glomerulonephritis and proliferative glomerulonephritis.[6, 10] As with PSGN, this type of glomerulonephritis occurs after infection and usually responds well to treatment.

RAPIDLY PROGRESSIVE GLOMERULONEPHRITIS

Rapidly progressive glomerulonephritis (RPGN) leads to renal failure over weeks to months. It may occur as a complication of acute or subacute infectious disease, from multisystem disease such as systemic lupus erythematosus, or from Goodpasture syndrome. It also may occur as an idiopathic or primary condition (Box 33-1).

Pathologically, characteristic capillary overgrowths with focal or necrotizing proliferations called *crescents* involve more than 70% of the glomeruli. Gaps or discontinuities of the GBM also may be associated with the crescents. Anti-GBM antibodies or deposits of immunoglobulins may be demonstrated on the glomerulus (Fig. 33-3). Circulating antibodies are not usually detected unless the condition is associated with a specific process for which antibody production can be demonstrated.

The idiopathic form of disease is common and may be identified by enlarged, pale kidneys with cellular proliferation in Bowman's space. Crescents form very

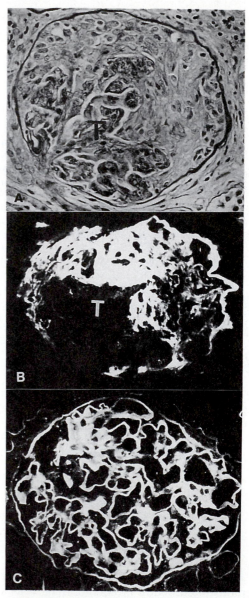

FIGURE 33-3 *Rapidly progressive glomerulonephritis.* ***A.*** *A cellular crescent compresses the adjacent glomErular capillary tuft.* ***B.*** *The crescent is stained with antifibrinogen antiserum, and the compressed capillary tuft (T) is unstained.* ***C.*** *A continuous (linear) pattern Of immunofluorescence staining for IgG is seen along glomerular capillary basement membranes and in Bowman's capsule in a patient with Goodpasture syndrome. (Kelley, W.N. [ed.]. Textbook of Internal Medicine [2nd ed.]. Philadelphia: J.B. Lippincott, 1992.)*

BOX 33-1 ▼ *Causes of Rapidly Progressive Glomerulonephritis*

Acute or subacute infection
  β-hemolytic streptococci
  Bacteria, viruses, parasites
Idiopathic or primary disease
Multisystem or autoimmune disease

rapidly, and they distort and compress the capillary lumina with fibrin deposition throughout.[5] The GBM is disrupted; interstitial edema with infiltration of leukocytes leads to degenerative changes of the tubules. Crescent formation indicates severe glomerular disease. Widespread crescent formation carries a bleak prognosis, with more than 90% of affected persons developing chronic renal failure.[10]

Clinical manifestations include a rapid, progressive diminution in renal function, severe oliguria, or anuria with irreversible renal failure in weeks or months. Hypertension, proteinuria, and hematuria are common.

RAPIDLY PROGRESSIVE GLOMERULONEPHRITIS CAUSED BY HEREDITARY OR MULTISYSTEM DISEASE.

Many systemic conditions are associated with glomerular injury, and this problem is a major clinical complication in some diseases. Most of these conditions are discussed in other chapters of this text, but some of the renal pathology is discussed here.

Lupus nephritis, with subsequent chronic renal failure, is a very common complication of systemic lupus erythematosus (see pp. 359–360). It is probably caused by trapped immune complexes in the GBM that produce destruction and nephrosis. It is associated with a low serum complement level and is diagnosed by kidney biopsy.[19] The pathology in the kidneys can vary from minimal changes to crescent formation and renal failure.[3] Diagnosed nephritic syndrome is usually treated with high-dose steroid therapy, which markedly increases the risk for systemic infection.[3]

Henoch-Schönlein purpura has a pathology that is similar to that of IgA nephropathy (see below). This condition is characterized by purpuric skin lesions that involve the arms, legs, and buttocks. Abdominal manifestations include pain, vomiting, and intestinal bleeding.[5] Joint pain and RPGN with deposition of IgA in the GBM are characteristic. This condition is more commonly seen in children and may respond to treatment with corticosteroids.

Wegener granulomatosis is a systemic vasculitis that involves the respiratory and genitourinary systems. Renal involvement may be mild or may progress to RPGN and renal failure. Antibodies to neutrophil cytoplasmic antigens are very common. Other laboratory findings are nondiagnostic, but characteristic pulmonary findings include nodular infiltrates, which may cavitate.[3]

Diabetic glomerulosclerosis is a major cause of end-stage renal disease in persons with diabetes mellitus. The most common lesions involve the glomeruli and cause the nephrotic syndrome and chronic renal failure. Proteinuria is common in all types of diabetics.[5] The clinical manifestations of diabetic renal disease are discussed on p. 739.

Amyloidosis may produce glomerulonephritis by precipitation of amyloid within the glomeruli. Individuals with this condition often have significant proteinuria and the nephrotic syndrome and then develop chronic renal failure.[5].

Hereditary nephritis refers to a group of hereditary diseases that involve the glomeruli in a pattern of segmental proliferation with an increase in the mesangial matrix. The end result is defective GBM synthesis. The best known of these conditions is Alport syndrome, which includes nerve deafness, eye disorders, and nephritis as its components. The mode of inheritance is heterogenous, either X-linked or autosomal in nature.[5]

GOODPASTURE SYNDROME.

Goodpasture disease is a term used for RPGN caused by anti-GBM antibody. This rare autoimmune disorder affects young men (ages 18 to 35 years) more often than women. It begins abruptly and is often preceded by a flulike illness or exposure to hydrocarbon fumes.[6] It may progress rapidly, causing severe and sometimes fatal hemoptysis, or it may exhibit long remissions. More than 90% of affected individuals exhibit anti-GBM antibodies, usually of the IgG class.[6] Pathologically, the glomeruli may have nearly normal configuration, or they may exhibit crescent formation. Deposits of fibrin, complement fragments, and immunoglobulins may be present within the crescents. Anti-GBM antibodies may be bound to the alveolar basement membrane. These antibodies can cause alveolar damage and intrapulmonary and extrapulmonary hemorrhage that may be massive and life-threatening.

Clinical features include hematuria, red cell casts, proteinuria, and nephrosis. Pulmonary bleeding often recurs in episodes and may be fatal even without evidence of renal disease.[6] Rapidly progressive or insidious renal failure may result.

The prognosis for this condition is improving and depends on the severity of pulmonary and renal involvement. Treatment with steroids and plasma exchange therapy has induced remissions and halting of the disease progression.[6] Renal failure and uremia have been controlled by hemodialysis. Pulmonary hemorrhage usually decreases after bilateral nephrectomy.

IGA NEPHROPATHY (BERGER SYNDROME)

This type of glomerulonephritis is characterized by IgA deposits in the mesangial cells of the glomeruli. These cells are found in the central part of the glomerulus and function as phagocytes. They are able to contract when confronted with various stimuli, and thus, they influence the filtration process.[18] IgG or IgM, or both, may accompany the deposits of IgA. This form of nephropathy is characterized by gross or microscopic hematuria or at least proteinuria.[5] The process of renal dysfunction is caused by entrapment of IgA complexes in the glomeruli, probably as a result of an abnormality of immune regulation.[5] The disease appears to be slowly progressive, and 50% of affected persons develop renal failure over a period of 20 years.[5] Treatments with steroids, cytotoxic agents, and phenytoin (which has been shown to lower serum IgA) have had variable results.[3] The disease may be associated with minimal change disease.

MINIMAL CHANGE DISEASE (LIPOID NEPHROSIS)

Lipoid nephrosis is the most common nephrosis in children between the ages of 2 and 8 years.[4] It results in decreased glomerular filtration rate and loss or binding together of adjacent glomerular foot processes. The epithelial cells of the GBM form pedicles or projections called *foot processes*. Normally, these structures are involved with preventing large protein and fat molecules from escaping into the urine. Loss or binding of these structures allows the leakage of albumin and fat particles into the urine. No antibodies have been demonstrated in this condition, but a relation with respiratory infections or routine immunization has led to the theory that it is a hypersensitivity reaction.[5] Because lipoid nephrosis also responds to steroid therapy and is associated with other atopic diseases, it is thought to involve defects in T-cell-–mediated immunity (see pp. 326–327).[5]

The disease is named for its pathologic features, which show few changes except that the adjacent glomerular foot processes bind together and allow plasma proteins and fats to pass into the urine. The kidneys appear edematous and pale.

The clinical course is variable and usually includes massive proteinuria without hypertension or hematuria. The progression of minimal change disease is characterized by periods of remission and exacerbation with a 10-year survival rate of 90% to 95%, especially for corticosteroid-responsive persons.[10] In a few persons, minimal change disease progresses to focal glomerulosclerosis and then to renal failure.

FOCAL SEGMENTAL GLOMERULOSCLEROSIS

Focal segmental glomerulosclerosis involves sclerosis and hyalinization of some of the juxtamedullary glomeruli. Deposits of IgM and C3 complement fragments are seen on immunofluorescence of the segmental sclerosing lesions. It may be a separate entity from minimal change disease or IgA nephropathy, or it may just be a more severe form.[10] Idiopathic focal segmental glomerulosclerosis accounts for 10% and 20% of cases of nephrotic syndrome in children and adults.[10] Secondary focal segmental glomerulosclerosis may occur as a complication of systemic diseases such as diabetic nephropathy. A progressive decline in glomerular filtration rate with increasing albuminuria and hypoalbuminemia occurs, and renal failure finally results, especially in adults.

Children usually have a better initial response to therapy but still usually progress slowly to renal failure.[10]

MEMBRANOUS NEPHROPATHY

Membranous nephropathy (membranous glomerulonephritis) is most common in middle-aged adults, with a male-to-female occurrence ratio of 2:1.[10] Protein is deposited uniformly in the outer glomerular capillary wall, with the deposits usually containing IgG and complement.[5] Capillary thickening with GBM projections accounts for the loss of protein in urine. The kidneys usually are large, swollen, and pale. If nephrosis with edema and hypoalbuminemia occurs, the disease usually progresses to renal failure. Hematuria and mild hypertension may be present. This disease is usually idiopathic, but it may develop in association with systemic lupus erythematosus, exposure to inorganic (gold or mercury) or organic (penicillamine, captopril) drugs, solid tumors, or some infections. It may progress with increasing renal impairment, or it may show repeated exacerbations and remissions or a spontaneous, complete remission.

MEMBRANOPROLIFERATIVE GLOMERULONEPHRITIS (SLOWLY PROGRESSIVE GLOMERULONEPHRITIS)

In membranoproliferative glomerulonephritis (mesangiocapillary or tubular glomerulonephritis), the GBM thickens and mesangial cells proliferate. The mesangial cells normally help to support the capillary loops in the glomerulus. Membranoproliferative glomerulonephritis apparently does not occur after a streptococcal infection but does account for 5% to 10% of cases of idiopathic nephrosis in children and adults, between the ages of 5 and 30.[5, 10] Abnormalities of the immune system seem to account for circulating immune complexes. In some persons, *hypocomplementemia*, especially of the C3 component, occurs.[6] The pathology of this condition may be seen in association with miscellaneous conditions such as malaria, bacterial endocarditis, chronic hepatitis B, systemic lupus erythematosus, collagen diseases, and certain malignancies.[10]

Clinical manifestations include any of the manifestations of the nephrotic syndrome. The disease assumes several forms but tends to be slowly progressive and unremitting. At least 50% of affected persons develop chronic renal failure within 10 years.[5, 10]

CHRONIC GLOMERULONEPHRITIS

Chronic glomerulonephritis is an insidiously developing, progressive dysfunction that usually terminates in end-stage renal failure after years of increasing renal insufficiency. It may result from any type of glomerular disease and exhibits both nephrotic and nephritic characteristics. Figure 33-4 indicates the variety of primary

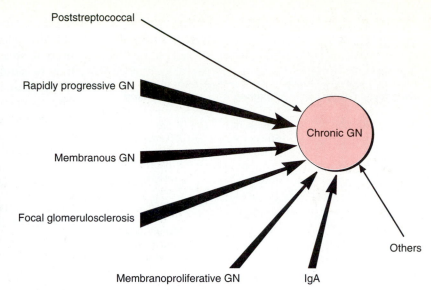

FIGURE 33-4 *Primary glomerular diseases leading to chronic glomerulonephritis (GN). The thickness of the arrows reflects the approximate proportion of patients in each group who progress to chronic GN. Poststreptococcal, 1%–2%); rapidly progressive (crescentic), 90%; membranous, 50%; focal glomerulosclerosis, 50%–80%; membranoproliferative , 50%; IgA nephropathy, 30%–50%. (Cotran, R., Kumar, V., and Robbins, S., Pathologic Basis of Disease [5th ed.]. Philadelphia: W.B. Saunders, 1994.)*

glomerular diseases that may lead to chronic glomerulonephritis.

Pathologically, the glomeruli become scarred and may become totally obliterated. The tubules are atrophic. The glomeruli and renal capsules become infiltrated with lymphocytes and plasma cells. Hyalinization of the glomeruli leads to obliteration of the pathology of the original disease. Vascular sclerosis of arteries and arterioles probably contributes to the arterial hypertension that is almost always associated with this disease.

The progression of the condition is related to the underlying disorder, but it almost always continues relentlessly to uremia. Proteinuria, hypertension, and azotemia are common with later manifestations of uremia (see pp. 667–669).

CASE STUDY 33-1

Ms. Mary Lee, a 49-year-old secretary, was seen by her physician for complaints of fatigue, weight gain, and anorexia. She related a history of glomerulonephritis as a child with no apparent residual problems. Urinalysis showed marked proteinuria. Her blood pressure was 150/105 and serum creatinine was 4.1 mg/dL, with a blood urea nitrogen of 56 mg/dL.

1. *If this condition is related to the glomerulonephritis seen in childhood, why is it manifest so many years later?*
2. *Describe the different types of glomerular diseases that may lead to this condition.*
3. *Describe the pathophysiology of the condition. (Look ahead to chapter 35 to understand the stages of development of this condition).*
4. *What measures can be utilized to delay the ultimate outcome of this condition?*
5. *What are appropriate treatments that may be used during the various stages?*

See Appendix G for discussion.

▼ Tubular and Interstitial Diseases

Histologic and functional abnormalities of the renal tubules and parenchyma can be caused by many factors. If the cause is infectious, the term *pyelonephritis* is usually used to describe the process (see pp. 634–636). Nonbacterial factors such as toxins, metabolic imbalances, and immunologic derangements can cause impairment of renal concentrating ability, metabolic acidosis, and loss of sodium, chloride, potassium, and water. Acute and chronic forms of tubular and interstitial diseases are described here. The acute process may account for as many as 10% to 15% of persons having acute renal failure. Primary chronic interstitial nephritis may be the cause of up to 25% of cases of end-stage renal disease.[14] Table 33-3 indicates causes of acute interstitial nephritis, and Table 33-4 indicates causes of chronic interstitial nephritis.

TOXIC MECHANISMS

The renal tubules and parenchyma sustain damage from nephrotoxic substances because of the large quantities of renal blood flow and the concentration of the substances in the tubules. Toxins that can cause acute tubular damage include heavy metals, organic solvents, radiolabeled contrast agents, cyclosporin A, antibiotics, antifungals, and other pharmaceutic agents. The most common toxic substances are pharmaceutic agents, including phenacetin, aspirin, certain antibiotics, and diuretics.

Chronic analgesia nephritis is a common cause of renal insufficiency in some countries, such as Australia and New Zealand. It occurs most frequently in persons who ingest mixtures of aspirin, caffeine, phenacetin, and codeine. The mechanism may include inhibition of the vasodilatory effect prostaglandins by aspirin, which can lead to renal ischemia.[5, 14] Phenacetin may have a direct toxic effect on the vasa recta, or it may cause papillary

TABLE 33-3 Causes of Acute Interstitial Nephritis

Diagnostic Group	Common	Uncommon
Systemic infection	Diphtheria Streptococci	Leprosy Rickettsia Legionella Syphilis Leptospira Toxoplasma Brucella Mycoplasma Measles virus Epstein-Barr virus

Drug reaction	Antibiotics
	  Methicillin
	  Penicillin
	  Ampicillin
	  Cephalosporins
	  Sulfonamides
	  Rifampin
	  Cyclosporin A
	  Phenindione
	  Nonsteroidals
		Antibiotics
		  Oxacillin
		  Nafcillin
		  Tetracycline
		Diuretics
		  Thiazides
		  Furosemide
		  Triamterene
		  Ethacrynic acid
		  Phenytoin
		  Allopurinol
		  Cimetidine

Idiopathic immune lesion		Anti-TBM disease TINU syndrome Sarcoid

TBM, tubular basement membrane; TINU, acute interstitial nephritis and associated uveitis.

Kelley, W. N., ed. Textbook of Internal Medicine (2nd ed.). Philadelphia: J.B. Lippincott, 1992.

necrosis. The result is fibrosis, necrosis, and calcification of the papillary areas. The papillae of the kidneys have necrotic areas and calcification fragments. Entire papillae may be sloughed off and excreted in the urine. Headache, anemia, gastrointestinal symptoms, and hypertension also can occur. The kidneys first lose the ability to concentrate urine; severe renal insufficiency then leads to azotemia and electrolyte imbalance. If the drugs are discontinued, renal function tends to improve over time.

ALLERGIC INTERSTITIAL NEPHRITIS

Hypersensitivity reactions to antibiotics and furosemide or thiazide diuretics usually begin about 15 days after exposure to the drug.[1] Allergic reactions are not dose-dependent but mostly depend on T-lymphocyte reactions in the interstitial areas. The reactions are characterized by fever, eosinophilia, hematuria, sterile pyuria, proteinuria, and skin rash, but absence of these reactions does not exclude their existence.[1] Cortical tubulointerstitial nephritis occurs secondary to the papillary necrosis.[5] Oliguria and azotemia develop transiently, or acute renal failure may develop. After the drug is discontinued, recovery usually is complete.[16]

Immune mechanisms can cause a reaction to the renal tubular cells. This often occurs in transplant rejections. The immune antibodies that have been implicated in causation of glomerulonephritis may affect the renal tubules.[5]

METABOLIC IMBALANCES

Abnormal body metabolism can lead to the production of metabolites that are toxic to the renal tubules. The imbalances that most frequently cause renal dysfunction

TABLE 33-4 Causes of Chronic Interstitial Nephritis

Common	Uncommon	Rare
Urinary obstruction	Uric acid	Stones
Urinary reflux	Oxalate	Hypercalcemia
Analgesics	Light chain nephropathy and myeloma	Hypokalemia
Heavy metals	Balkan nephropathy	Granulomatous disease
Arteriolar nephrosclerosis	Radiation	Tuberculosis
	Sickle cell anemia	Xanthogranulomas
	Medullary cystic disease	Malacoplakia
	Granulomatous diseases	Sjögren's syndrome
	Wegener granulomatosis	Urinary tract infection
	Sarcoidosis	
	Infiltrative leukemia or lymphoma	
	Transplant rejection	

Kelley, W. N., ed. Textbook of Internal Medicine (2nd ed.). Philadelphia: J.B. Lippincott, 1992.

are hyperuricemia, hypercalcemia, hypokalemia, and hyperoxaluria.

HYPERURICEMIA. The most common cause of hyperuricemia is gout (see pp. 876–877). Gouty nephropathy results from prolonged elevations of the serum uric acid level. Crystalline deposits of uric acid are left in the tubules, especially the distal tubules and collecting ducts. The result is intrarenal obstruction with inflammation and fibrosis of the tubules. Nephropathy is characterized by insidious renal insufficiency with proteinuria and decreased renal concentrating ability. The precipitated urate bodies induce a *tophus*, which is the urate bodies surrounded by mononuclear giant cells. Tophi commonly occur in the ear, the patellar bursae, and around connective tissues. In the kidney, they tend to be deposited in the medulla or pyramids and evoke a typical inflammatory reaction.[5] This may result in tubular destruction and scarring.

Acute uric acid nephropathy has been reported after the administration of cytotoxic drugs in the therapy of certain leukemias and lymphomas.[1] Volume depletion, such as after severe vomiting, can contribute to the process. Uric acid crystals precipitate in the collecting ducts, leading to partial or total tubule obstruction. The obstruction can result in acute renal failure. Uric acid nephrolithiasis occurs in about 15% of persons with uncontrolled gout and chronic hyperuricemia.

HYPERCALCEMIA. Acute hypercalcemia produces a vasopressin defect that results in hypertension, decreased renal blood flow, and volume depletion that can cause acute renal failure.[1] Chronic deposition of calcium on the tubules and in the interstitium can lead to renal insufficiency.[1] Any condition that causes an increase in circulating calcium can result in increased frequency of calcium stones, obstruction, and nephropathy. Intracellular accumulation of calcium can disrupt the cellular processes, causing cell death and consequent obstruction of nephrons by cellular debris.

HYPOKALEMIA. If moderate or severe hypokalemia persists for several weeks, it can lead to a functional decrease in concentrating ability. Chronic hypokalemia may occur with gastrointestinal diseases, adrenal hyperfunction, and long-term diuretic therapy. Function usually returns to normal after potassium levels are restored.

HYPEROXALURIA. Oxalate nephropathy can occur from defective glyoxylic acid metabolism and from ethylene glycol, methoxyflurane, and massive ascorbic acid overdose.[1] Inherited enzyme deficiencies can produce hyperoxaluria with progressive interstitial fibrosis and recurrent renal stones. Systemic poisoning with ethylene glycol (antifreeze) resembles acute alcohol intoxication but can cause chronic tubulointerstitial nephritis.[1] Normal oxalate values are determined from a 24-hour urine collection and are about 8 to 40 mg per 24 hours, or 110-440 μmol per 24 hours.[7]

RENAL TUBULAR ACIDOSIS

The term renal tubular acidosis refers to a group of disorders, either primary renal or systemic, characterized by defective secretion of hydrogen ions with normal glomerular filtration. The metabolic acidosis may occur because of failure to secrete hydrogen ion in the collecting duct or failure to reabsorb bicarbonate in the proximal tubule.[8] Numerous conditions can produce renal tubular acidosis (Table 33-5). Renal tubular acidosis is often described as type I, which is that produced by distal tubule failure, or type II, in which the dysfunction is in the proximal tubule. Type I renal tubular acidosis is caused by impaired distal tubular hydrogen ion secretion and decreased bicarbonate regeneration.[13] The daily accumulation of acid exhausts the serum buffers, and eventually bone calcium is used to buffer the serum. Because of the inability to secrete hydrogen, the urine pH remains high. Type II renal tubule acidosis involves impairment at the proximal tubule with a resultant loss of bicarbonate.[11] A hyperchloremic metabolic acidosis and alkaline urine result. If the distal tubule is not affected, the serum bicarbonate falls to about 14 mEq/L, at which point secretion of hydrogen occurs and the acid–base balance is preserved.[12, 13] Table 33-6 compares the clinical features of the two types of renal tubule acidosis.

TABLE 33-5 *Causes of Renal Tubular Acidosis*

Distal (Type I)	Proximal (Type II)
Hypokalemic or normokalemic	Primary (idiopathic)
Primary (idiopathic)	Cystinosis
Hypercalcemia	Wilson's disease
Nephrocalcinosis	Lead toxicity
Multiple myeloma	Cadmium toxicity
Hepatic cirrhosis	Mercury toxicity
Lupus erythematosus	Amyloidosis
Amphotericin B	Multiple myeloma
Lithium	Nephrotic syndrome
Toluene	Early renal transplant injury
Renal transplant rejection	Medullary cystic disease
Medullary sponge kidney	Outdated tetracycline
Hyperkalemic	
Hypoaldosteronism	
Obstructive nephropathy	
Sickle cell nephropathy	
Lupus erythematosus	

Schrier, R. W. *Renal and Electrolyte Disorders* (3rd ed.). Boston: Little, Brown, 1986.

TABLE 33-6 *Clinical Features of Renal Tubular Acidosis (RTA)*

Proximal RTA (Disordered Reclamation)	Distal RTA (Disordered Regeneration)

Defect in H^+ secretion causing:
  Sodium bicarbonaturia
  Hyperchloremic metabolic acidosis
  High urine pH (>6)
  Contracted extracellular volume
  Hypokalemia
	Defect in H^+ secretion causing:
	  Hyperchloremic metabolic acidosis
	  Cellular (bone) H^+ buffering
	  Hypercalciuria/hyperphosphaturia
	  Nephrolithiasis/calcinosis
	  Natriuresis/contracted extracellular volume
	  Kaliuresis/hypokalemia

Acid–base balance (and low urine pH) at new steady state of metabolic acidosis	Always positive H^+ balance (urine pH >6)
Treatment: Hydrochlorothiazide and KCl	Treatment: K^+, HCO_3

Muther, R. S., Barry, J. M., and Bennett, W. M. *Manual of Nephrology*. Philadelphia: Dekker, 1990.

▼ Congenital Disorders Leading to Renal Dysfunction

Renal malformations are very common at birth but may not cause significant clinical problems until adult life. Congenital renal disease most often results from a developmental defect arising during gestation rather than from a hereditary defect. An exception to this is polycystic disease, which is clearly hereditary.[5] Simple renal cysts are common in the aged individual; they usually remain asymptomatic but may occasionally cause abdominal masses, abdominal or back pain, or infection.[8] Renal malformations may result from failure of renal development (renal agenesis or hypoplasia), displacement of the kidneys (abdominal or pelvic), or renal cysts. Developmental malformations account for about 20% of chronic renal failure in children.

Autosomal dominant polycystic kidney disease accounts for 6% to 12% of renal transplantations or chronic dialysis; it is an autosomal dominant inherited condition. It affects both kidneys, and renal function usually begins to deteriorate after the third decade of life. The kidneys appear to be largely infiltrated with cysts that encroach on the calices and renal pelvis.[5] Clinical manifestations may include recurrent urinary tract infections, hypertension, abdominal or flank pain, hematuria, and proteinuria. It is often asymptomatic for years and is difficult to diagnose. In about 90% of cases, renal failure develops by the age of 70.[8] Persons with polycystic kidney disease also tend to have other congenital anomalies, such as cystic disease of the liver and intracranial berry aneurysms.[5, 8]

Renal cystic disease has been seen to develop in persons receiving chronic hemodialysis. The pathogenesis is unknown. There is also a high correlation of these cysts to the development of renal cell carcinoma along with a potential for hemorrhage from the cysts.[8]

▼ Chapter Summary

▼ Infections of the urinary tract are common and are most commonly caused by *E. coli*. Lower urinary tract infections usually affect the bladder, causing cystitis, which is much more common in females due to the length of the urethra.

▼ Pyelonephritis can result from ascending infection from the bladder and refers to inflammation of the renal pelvis. It may be acute or chronic in nature. Acute pyelonephritis responds well to treatment but may progress to chronic pyelonephritis. The chronic form is difficult to diagnose (because not all affected persons relate a history of urinary tract infection), but is a common cause of chronic renal failure.

▼ Glomerular injury is the most common cause of chronic renal failure and immunologically mediated glomerular disease is the main pathology. Glomerulonephritis may be poststreptococcal, which occurs most frequently in children and recovery is nearly 100%. In adults it may progress to the rapidly or slowly progressive form, culminating in chronic renal failure. There are many causes of RPGN.

▼ Other glomerular diseases include minimal change, focal segmental glomerulosclerosis, membranous nephropathy, and chronic glomerulonephritis. Chronic glomerulonephritis is insidious, progressive, and usually terminates in end-stage renal failure.

▼ Tubular and interstitial diseases affect the renal parenchyma and tubules. This may be the result of nephrotoxicity from multiple causes. When it is severe it can cause acute renal failure. Renal tubular acidosis is a group of disorders caused by defective secretion of hydrogen ions.

▼ Congenital disorders are common but may not manifest themselves until adult life. Most congenital renal disorders are due to a problem during gestation with the exception of the very common hereditary problem of polycystic disease.

▼ *References*

1. Albert, S., and Neilson, E.G. Tubulointerstitial diseases. In Stein, J. (ed.), *Internal Medicine* (4th ed.). St. Louis: Mosby, 1994.

2. Badalamenti, J. Chronic renal failure. In Levine, D.Z., *Care of the Renal Patient* (2nd ed.). Philadelphia: W.B. Saunders, 1991.

3. Cattran, D.C. Acute nephritic syndrome. In Levine, D.Z., *Care of the Renal Patient* (2nd ed.). Philadelphia: W.B. Saunders, 1991.

4. Coggins, C.H. Hematuria, proteinuria, and nephrotic syndrome. In Levine, D.Z., *Care of the Renal Patient* (2nd ed.). Philadelphia: W.B. Saunders, 1991.

5. Cotran, R.S., Kumar, V., and Robbins, S.L. *Robbins' Pathologic Basis of Disease* (5th ed.). Philadelphia: W.B. Saunders, 1994.

6. Couser, W.C. Glomerular diseases. In Stein, J. (ed.), *Internal Medicine* (4th ed.). St. Louis: Mosby, 1994.

7. Fischbach, F. *A Manual of Laboratory and Diagnostic Tests.* (4th ed.). Philadelphia: J.B. Lippincott, 1992.

8. Kaehy, W.D. Renal cysts and cystic diseases. In Kelley, W.N. (ed.), *Textbook of Internal Medicine* (2nd ed.). Philadelphia: J.B. Lippincott, 1992.

9. Kaye, D., Tunkel, A.R., and Fournier, G.R. Urinary tract infections. In Stein, J. (ed.), *Internal Medicine* (4th ed.). St. Louis: Mosby, 1994.

10. Knutson, D.W., and Abt, A.B. Immune-mediated glomerulopathies. In Kelley, W.N. (ed.), *Textbook of Internal Medicine* (2nd ed.). Philadelphia: J.B. Lippincott, 1992.

11. Laski, M.E., and Kurtzman, N.A. Disorders of acid-base balance. In Stein, J. (ed.), *Internal Medicine* (4th ed.). St. Louis: Mosby, 1994.

12. Levine, D.Z., Burns, K.D., and Goldstein, M.B. Acid-base disturbances in azotemic patients. In Levine, D.Z., *Care of the Renal Patient* (2nd ed.). Philadelphia: W.B. Saunders, 1991.

13. Muther, R.S., Barry, J.M., and Bennett, W.M. *Manual of Nephrology.* Philadelphia: B.C. Decker, 1990.

14. Neilson, E.G., and Kelly, C.J. Tubulointerstitial diseases. In Kelley, W.N. (ed.), *Textbook of Internal Medicine* (2nd ed.). Philadelphia: J.B. Lippincott, 1992.

15. Rubin, R.H., Tolkoff-Rubin, N.E., and Cotran, R.S. Urinary tract infection, pyelonephritis, and reflux nephropathy. In Brenner, B.M., and Rector, F.C. (eds.), *The Kidney* (5th ed.). Philadelphia: Ardmore, 1994.

16. Spargo, B.H., and Haas, M. The kidney. In Rubin, E., and Farber, J.L., *Pathology* (2nd ed.). Philadelphia: J.B. Lippincott, 1994.

17. Toye, B., and Ronald, A. Approach to infections of the genitourinary tract including perinephric abscess and prostatitis. In Kelley, W.N. (ed.), *Textbook of Internal Medicine* (2nd ed.). Philadelphia: J.B. Lippincott, 1992.

18. Vander, A.J. *Renal Physiology* (4th ed.). New York: McGraw-Hill, 1991.

19. Wolfish, N.M. Pediatric nephrology. In Levine, D.Z., *Care of the Renal Patient* (2nd ed.). Philadelphia: W.B. Saunders, 1991.

Chapter 34

Disorders of Micturition and Obstruction of the Genitourinary Tract

Barbara L. Bullock

▼ CHAPTER OUTLINE

▼ LEARNING OBJECTIVES

1. Compare obstructive and irritative mechanisms of voiding dysfunction.
2. Review the micturition reflex and relate dysfunction to voiding patterns.
3. Describe the patterns and causes of incontinence.
4. Discuss the pathogenesis of benign prostatic hyperplasia, including hormonal influences (testosterone, estrogen, and dihydrotestosterone).
5. Relate the symptoms and complications of benign prostatic hyperplasia to the pathogenesis of the process.
6. Describe the composition of renal calculi.
7. Explain the factors that cause stone formation.
8. Discuss the factors that contribute to the production of calcium stones.
9. Explain the factors that contribute to the production of uric acid stones.
10. Identify the major causes of cystine and struvite stones.
11. Discuss the pathogenesis of renal cell carcinoma.
12. Identify the staging mechanism for renal cell carcinoma.
13. Describe the histology of Wilms' tumor.
14. Discuss the etiologic factors that contribute to carcinoma of the bladder.
15. Identify the clinical manifestations of bladder cancer.

Barbara L. Bullock: PATHOPHYSIOLOGY: ADAPTATIONS AND ALTERATIONS IN FUNCTION, 4th ed.
© 1996 J.B. Lippincott-Raven Publishers

▼ Disorders of Micturition

Voiding difficulties—including difficulty initiating a stream, painful urination, and incontinence—are among the most common problems that are brought to medical attention. It is thought that a vast number of voiding problems are not diagnosed because of the embarrassing nature of the problem. Some of these problems, such as stress incontinence, are intermittent. They usually occur in response to a sudden increase in bladder pressure without an adequate pressure increase in the sphincter control by the bladder.

The cerebral centers inhibit or facilitate the micturition reflex voluntarily when urination is either suppressed or desired. Emptying of the bladder is at least partly caused by contractions of the detrusor muscle of the bladder (see pp. 630–631). Voiding requires an intact central nervous system, functional sphincter and bladder muscles, and an unobstructed pathway to the external portion of the body. Female voiding occurs at lower intrabladder pressure than for males because of the short, straight female urethra. The neurologic connections to accomplish micturition are complex. Disturbance of any of these connections produces a disorder of micturition.[18]

INTERFERENCE WITH EMPTYING OF THE BLADDER

Difficulty starting and maintaining a urinary stream is a common symptom of benign prostatic hyperplasia (BPH). Urinary symptoms are the presenting complaint of most men with this condition (see p. XX). The difficulty in urination may be associated with uninhibited bladder contractions, which result in dribbling incontinence or difficulty in stopping the urinary stream.[19] Individuals who have had prostatic surgery, prostatitis, or denervation injury also may have this problem.

Acute inflammation of the bladder, or of the vulva and vagina in females, may be associated with urinary retention owing to incomplete bladder emptying.[18] The presence of edema at the urethra increases outflow resistance. Chronic infections can cause urethral scarring and subsequent stenosis. Inflammation or hypersensitivity of the urethra produces a low voiding flow rate and raised voiding pressure, together with symptoms of frequency, nocturia, and urgency.[18] Surgical procedures for stress incontinence may result in difficulty in bladder emptying. Bladder overdistention can be caused by repression of the urge to void or after surgical procedures if a catheter is not used to drain the bladder. The bladder muscle may become overdistended; as a result, it becomes poorly contractile. Incomplete emptying is common after suprasacral spinal cord injury or lesion. If reflex activity is initially lost, then reflex voiding is not coordinated with sphincter function.[19]

INTERFERENCE WITH URINE STORAGE IN THE BLADDER

Frequency and incontinence are common problems that affect both men and women, especially after the age of 50. The problems can be transient or persistent and may be related to conditions such as urinary tract infections or prostatic problems.

Frequency refers to voiding more often than every 2 hours. Persons affected often complain of urgency (intense need to void), dysuria (discomfort or pain on voiding), or incontinence (involuntary voiding). These symptoms are often called irritative symptoms.[19]

Urinary incontinence is a very common health problem in the adult population, especially in the elderly group. Recent data indicate a 10% to 20% incidence of significant urinary incontinence among community-dwelling elderly persons.[16] The problem is more common in women and is associated with cognitive and functional impairment.[16] It can be divided into overlapping categories of stress, urge, overflow, and functional incontinence (Table 34-1).

Stress urinary incontinence refers to the loss of urine on physical effort, such as sneezing, coughing, or running.[20] It occurs most frequently in women, affecting 5% to 15% of this population. The cause is not known, but it results from decreased urethral resistance and is related to multiple childbirth, estrogen deprivation, congenital bladder neck malformation, surgical procedures for prolapse, denervation of sphincter muscles, or multiple bladder infections.[22, 23] In men, stress incontinence most commonly occurs after surgical procedures for BPH or denervation injuries. Loss of urine occurs when the pressure in the bladder exceeds that generated by the urinary sphincter muscle.[22]

Urge or urgency incontinence is often associated with stress incontinence in that leakage of urine occurs because of inability to delay voiding after bladder fullness is perceived.[16] It is associated with sphincter dysfunction but also may be associated with detrusor muscle motor or sensory instability. This type of incontinence may occur temporarily with bladder infections, stones, or tumors, or it may be continuous, such as with central nervous system disorders.[23] Lesions in the frontal lobes, internal capsule, and reticular formation of the pons and cerebellum affect voiding function variably according to the severity of the lesion.[18] Spinal cord lesions above the sacral area usually produce a hyperreflexic detrusor muscle with uncoordinated sphincter activity, making control of urinary output very difficult. Lesions below the sacral root tend to produce an acontractile bladder.[10, 18] Pelvic plexus injuries may result from pelvic surgeries, and the bladder impairment may be incomplete and unpredictable.[16]

Overflow incontinence may be associated with the previous two types or it may be manifested by the loss of small amounts of urine when the bladder is full.[12] It also

TABLE 34-1 *Basic Types and Causes of Persistent Geriatric Urinary Incontinence*

Type	Definition	Common Causes
Stress	Involuntary loss of urine (usually small amounts) simultaneously with increases in intraabdominal pressure (eg, cough, laugh, or exercise)	Weakness and laxity of pelvic floor musculature Bladder outlet or urethral sphincter weakness
Urge	Leakage of urine (usually larger volumes) because of inability to delay voiding after sensation of bladder fullness is perceived	Detrusor motor or sensory instability, isolated or associated with one or more of the following: local genitourinary conditions, such as cystitis, urethritis, tumors, stones, and outflow obstruction; central nervous system disorders, such as stroke, dementia, parkinsonism
Overflow	Leakage of urine (usually small amounts) resulting from mechanical forces on an overdistended bladder or from other effects of urinary retention on bladder and sphincter function	Anatomic obstruction by prostate, stricture, cystocele Acontractile bladder associated with diabetes mellitus or spinal cord injury Neurogenic (detrusor-sphincter) dyssynergy associated with multiple sclerosis and other suprasacral spinal cord lesions
Functional	Urinary leakage associated with inability to toilet because of impairment of cognitive or physical functioning, psychological unwillingness, or environmental barriers	Severe dementia and other neurologic disorders Psychological factors, such as depression, anger, and hostility

Kelley, W. N., ed. *Textbook of Internal Medicine* (2nd ed.). Philadelphia: J.B. Lippincott, 1992.

may occur in association with neurologic disorders, especially the neurogenic bladder of diabetes mellitus.[8] Strictures or BPH may impede the flow of urine, resulting in small amounts of dribbling when the bladder is distended and the muscles contract.

Functional or total incontinence occurs when there is no conscious control of voiding behavior. It occurs with severe central nervous system disorders and occasionally with severe psychologic dysfunction.[12,16] This type of incontinence is diagnosed when the other types have been ruled out, and it is probably the leading cause of incontinence among hospitalized persons.[12] Loss of urine occurs reflexively, much as in infants. Constant dribbling of urine is unusual, but normal bladder filling and distention stimulate bladder contractions with smaller than normal urine volumes. The desire to void, if noted, occurs immediately before uncontrolled bladder emptying. Return to normal voiding patterns can occur after the neurologic or psychologic status improves.

▼ Obstruction of the Genitourinary Tract

Obstructive disorders can cause considerable renal dysfunction, including hemorrhage and renal failure, if they are left untreated. The principal obstructive conditions are prostatic hyperplasia, renal calculi, and renal tumors.

BENIGN PROSTATIC HYPERPLASIA

BPH affects most men older than 50 years of age. In years past, the word *hypertrophy* was used, which was misleading because the increase in the size of the prostate gland is caused by hyperplastic proliferation of glandular and cellular tissue (Fig. 34-1). Normally, the prostate gland weighs 20 g, surrounds the urethra, and consists of four lobes. By age 70 years, the prostate may weigh from 60

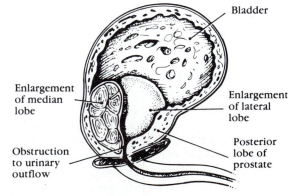

FIGURE 34-1 *Enlargement of median and lateral lobes of the prostate gland. Notice the obstruction to urinary outflow.*

to as much as 200 g.[6] Further discussion of function and diseases of the prostate is found in Chapter 55.

Pathogenesis

The cause of BPH is unknown, but it is believed to result from an imbalance between the male and female sex hormones that occurs with advancing age. Normally, testosterone is the main androgen in the blood, and it forms two metabolites: dihydrotestosterone and 17β-estradiol. Dihydrotestosterone is responsible for mediating many of the actions of testosterone. Estradiol is a steroid that possesses estrogenic properties and acts with androgens for many physiologic activities. It can act independently and causes effects opposite to those of androgens. Testosterone metabolites and estradiol have been shown to act together to produce prostatic hyperplasia in the dog.[3]

Plasma testosterone levels decrease in men older than age 60 years, but BPH can occur, possibly because of increased estradiol levels, which may sensitize the prostate gland to growth promotion from dihydrotestosterone.[11] The plasma levels of estradiol and dihydrotestosterone apparently do not cause BPH, but their effects in the prostate may initiate the process.

In the plasma, testosterone binds to two proteins: globulin and albumin. A small percentage of free hormones is in balance with a protein-bound steroid and is able to enter the cells. Within the cells, testosterone is converted by a 5α-reductase enzyme to dihydrotestosterone. It is then bound to a specific androgen receptor protein, and the hormone-receptor complex changes before entering the nucleus.[2,3] Study of both BPH and carcinoma of the prostate gland has demonstrated these specific receptor complexes in both stromal and glandular components. They are responsive to estradiol and dihydrotestosterone stimulation.[11]

Estrogen levels increase in men with aging. The estrogen binds to specific receptors in the cytoplasm and moves into the nucleus as a hormone-receptor complex. Dihydrotestosterone is apparently the hormonal mediator in BPH, partly because of decreased catabolism of the molecule and partly because of increased intracellular binding of the molecule. Therefore, prostate growth is accelerated because of increased estrogen, which increases the level of the androgen receptor in the gland.[6,11]

Hyperplasia usually occurs in the median and lateral lobes, with the posterior lobe not affected. Seventy-five percent of prostatic carcinomas arise in the posterior lobe.[6] In BPH, the lobes vary in size and are separated from each other by stroma, including connective tissue and smooth muscle fibers. Enlargement of the lateral lobes compresses the urethra, and enlargement of the medial lobe obstructs urine outflow by obstructing the urethral orifice (Fig. 34-2).

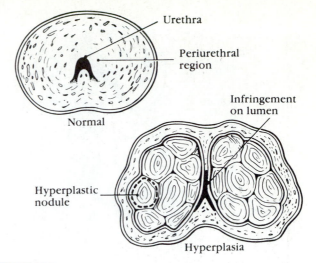

FIGURE 34-2 *Relation to the urethra of normal and of hyperplastic prostate. Notice infringement on the lumen in the latter.*

Hyperplasia, which may be fibromuscular or glandular, results in a proliferation of cells that begins in the periurethral region and causes a smooth and regular appearance of the gland. Located in the adjacent prostatic tissue are areas of ischemia and necrosis encircled by margins of squamous metaplasia. As the periurethral lobes enlarge, the normal tissue and the urethra are compressed.

Clinical Manifestations

If hyperplasia causes significant obstruction, frequency of urination, decrease in force and size of stream, hesitancy, straining to urinate, difficulty in starting and stopping the stream, and inability to empty the bladder are noted. Urinary obstruction complications that may arise from BPH include hydroureter, acute urinary retention of sudden onset, acute renal failure, hematuria, calculi, cystitis, reflux, urinary tract infection, and thickening of the bladder muscles.

RENAL CALCULI

Calculi can form in various areas of the renal system. Crystallization in the renal pelvis or calices is called nephrolithiasis. Urolithiasis refers to stones anywhere in the urinary tract. The stones may be composed of calcium salts, uric acid, oxalate, cystine, xanthine, or struvite.[6]

Symptoms of urolithiasis vary from hematuria or oliguria to renal colic. Hematuria results from the damage done by the stone in the urinary tract. Oliguria may result when the stone obstructs the flow of urine. Renal colic results from spasms as calculi are passed, causing flank pain that radiates to the abdomen and groin.

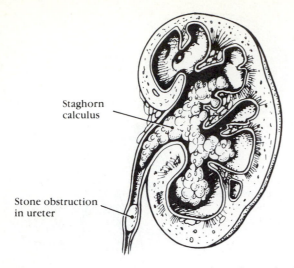

FIGURE 34-3   Staghorn calculus obstructing the entire renal pelvis.

Urinary stones or calculi are common in the United States, with more than 5% of the population developing them at least once.[21] The frequency is higher in men, in persons leading a sedentary lifestyle, and in families with a history of stones. The average age for the occurrence of renal stones is between 20 and 30 years, but they can occur at any age.[6]

Structure and Composition

Calculi vary in shape and size; some are as small as grains of sand, and others entirely fill the renal pelvis (staghorn calculi). They also vary in color, texture, and composition (Figs. 34-3 and 34-4). Stones may be either unilateral or bilateral and may be single or multiple. Stones contain an organic matrix or framework and crystalloids such as calcium, oxalate, phosphate, urate, uric acid, struvite, or cystine. Stones may be associated with infection of the urinary tract, and these stones usually are composed of magnesium ammonium phosphate hexahydrate, struvite, and carbonate apatite (a calcium-containing compound). These stones result from kidney or bladder infection by bacteria that produce urease.[13]

Factors That Cause Stone Formation

Stone formation may result from alteration in urine pH, decrease in inhibitors, or supersaturation of urine. The urine almost always shows an increase in concentration of the stones' constituents. Some constituents act as promoters for stone formation; for example, uric acid promotes calcium oxalate stones.[21] Some individuals have hypercalciuria, hyperoxaluria, or hyperuricosuria without forming clinically apparent stones.[6]

ALTERATIONS IN pH.   The solubility of crystalloids is affected by alterations in pH that cause them to leave the urine and attach to the matrix, resulting in crystallization. Stones that form in an acid urine contain uric acid, cystine, oxalate, or xanthine. In alkaline urine, most stones contain calcium phosphate or struvite. Persistent use of medications containing aluminum hydroxide, calcium carbonate, ascorbic acid, and sodium bicarbonate affect urinary pH and thus increases the risk of stone formation.

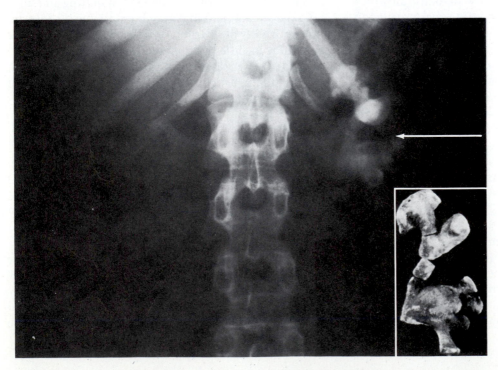

FIGURE 34-4   Radiologic appearance of a large staghorn calculus. Arrow shows location of stone. Insert picture shows actual appearance on removal.

DECREASE IN INHIBITORS. A decrease in inhibitors (magnesium, sodium, pyrophosphate, urea, citrate, amino acids, and trace metals) may cause stone formation. The stone must be stable to grow to a size that is clinically significant. Urine contains inhibitors for calcium oxalate and calcium phosphate but not for uric acid, cystine, or struvite.[4] It was concluded in one study that calculi be caused by from alterations in several urine components that result in abnormal formation or abnormal accumulation of crystals.[4]

SUPERSATURATION OF URINE. The main cause of stone formation is breakdown of the balance between conservation of water and excretion of materials that are poorly soluble. If urine becomes saturated with certain materials, crystals may form, aggregating to create a stone.[5] As the insoluble material accumulates, urine reaches a critical point at which it can no longer keep the material in solution; it is at this point that stone growth occurs. Urine pH affects the formation of stones because some precipitate in acid urine and others require alkaline urine.[13]

Types of Stones

Even though many stones are composed of mixtures of substances, they usually have distinctive characteristics. The majority contain calcium, but uric acid, oxalate, cystine, struvite, and xanthine also may predominate. Table 34-2 categorizes the main types of renal stones.

CALCIUM STONES. Calcium stones are often formed in the presence of hypercalciuria or hypercalcemia (Box 34-1). Hypercalciuria occurs with increased excretion of urinary calcium. Calcium stones are radiopaque, white to gray, and usually small and soft. Normally, the calcium level in urine is approximately 100 to 300 mg per 24 hours (in SI units, 2.5–7.5 mmol/d), depending on the preparatory diet, which affects the reference values.[17] Hypercalcemia occurs when the total serum calcium exceeds 11 mg/dL (3 mmol/L) in adults. Calcium is excreted in the urine in increased amounts, or it may precipitate into the kidney substance (nephrocalcinosis).

Hypercalciurias have been classified according to cause as absorptive, resorptive, and renal. These classifications overlap and may represent a continuum.[5] Despite these limitations, the classifications may clarify the source of the excess calcium and stone formation.

Absorptive hypercalciuria is caused by exaggerated absorption of calcium from the bowel as a result of an increased rate of conversion of vitamin D, which often occurs with hyperparathyroidism. The serum calcium level is usually elevated, with associated hypophosphatemia and parathyroid hormone level increases. Nephrocalcinosis is common and should be a cause for investigation of parathyroid function.[9]

TABLE 34-2 *Types of Renal Stones*

	Percentage of All Stones
CALCIUM STONES (OXALATE, PHOSPHATE)	75
Hypercalcemia and hypercalciuria (5%)	
Hypercalciuria without hypercalcemia (55%)	
Absorptive	
Renal	
Idiopathic	
Hyperuricosuria (20%)	
Hyperoxaluria (5%)	
Enteric	
Primary	
Hypocitraturia	
No known metabolic abnormality	
STRUVITE (Mg^{++}; NH_3; Ca^{++}; PO_4)	10–15
Renal infection	
URIC ACID	6
Associated with hyperuricemia	
Associated with hyperuricosuria	
Idiopathic	
CYSTINE	1–2
OTHERS OR UNKNOWN	± 10

Cotran, R., Kumar, V., and Robbins, S. J. *Robbins' Pathologic Basis of Disease* (5th ed.). Philadelphia: W.B. Saunders, 1994.

Resorptive hypercalciuria results when calcium is removed or reabsorbed from the bone. This can occur in persons who are immobilized, such as after spinal cord injury. Five to ten percent of persons who are immobilized for prolonged periods develop renal calculi.[4] Stones produced by reabsorption abnormality develop over a long time.

A *renal defect* that causes hypercalciuria is usually a tubular defect resulting in a calcium leak. An example of this defect is renal tubular acidosis, in which the distal convoluted tubule and collecting duct are not able to maintain acid urine (see pp. 643–644). Calcium is not as soluble in alkaline urine and may precipitate to form stones. In renal tubular acidosis, stones may also result from low levels of urinary citrate, an inhibitor of calcium.

Several disorders of calcium metabolism result in hypercalcemia, including Paget disease, multiple myeloma, and primary hyperparathyroidism. Nephrocalcinosis and renal calculi are common in these conditions.[6]

Ninety percent of all calcium-containing stones are composed of calcium oxalate.[9] Mild degrees of hyperoxaluria can increase the rate of calcium oxalate stone formation.[9] Oxalates are present in certain green leafy

BOX 34-1 ▼ *Causes of Hypercalcemia*

Primary hyperparathyroidism
Cancer
   Parathyroid hormone-related protein
   Ectopic production of 1,25-dihydroxyvitamin D_3
   Other factors produced ectopically
   Lytic bone metastases
Nonparathyroid endocrine disorders
   Thyrotoxicosis
   Pheochromocytoma
   Adrenal insufficiency
   Vasoactive intestinal polypeptide hormone—producing tumor
Granulomatous diseases (1,25-dihydroxyvitamin D_3 excess)
   Sarcoidosis
   Tuberculosis
   Histoplasmosis
   Coccidioidomycosis
   Leprosy
Medications
   Thiazide diuretics
   Lithium
   Estrogens and antiestrogens
Milk-alkali syndrome
Vitamin A intoxication
Vitamin D intoxication
Familial hypocalciuric hypercalcemia
Immobilization
Parenteral nutrition
Acute and chronic renal insufficiency

Stein, J., ed. *Internal Medicine* (4th ed.). St. Louis: Mosby, 1994.

vegetables, but stones are rarely caused by excess consumption of these foods. Stones can be caused from intestinal diseases, increased amounts of ethylene glycol, hereditary disorders, or renal insufficiency.[5] Hyperoxaluria may occur after intestinal bypass surgery and with Crohn disease. Oxalate, the product of glycine metabolism, is produced from glyoxylate or glycolate.

Calcium stone disease may result from no known cause, and this occurs in about 15% of calcium stone-formers.[9] These patients have normal urinary pH, serum electrolyte, and urine values. Many times these persons have recurrent stone disease, which may be caused by an absence of inhibitors to stone growth.[9]

URIC ACID STONES. Calculi composed of uric acid cause approximately 5% to 10% of all kidney stones in persons living in the United States.[13] These stones are yellow to brown, smooth and soft, and are formed in acid urine. Both supersaturation of urine with uric acid and decreased urinary pH contribute to their formation. The urinary concentration of free uric acid determines the probability of stone formation. Normal total uric acid excretion is about 500 mg per 24 hours. If the urinary pH increases, for example from 5.0 to 6.0, the amount of free acid decreases and crystal formation does not occur.[5, 9]

Persons with uric acid stones excrete less urinary ammonia than normal, and acid urine results.[9]

Uric acid stone formation is much more common in persons with gout than in normal persons. In most cases, this is a result of a low urinary pH and a decreased production of ammonia rather than an increase in uric acid production.[9] Hypovolemia, from dehydration or other causes, contributes to stone formation because of the concentrated uric acid and low urinary pH that result. Diseases such as the leukemias cause cell necrosis, which results in hyperuricosuria because purines convert mostly to uric acids. Massive hyperuricosuria is fairly common after chemotherapy for certain tumors. Idiopathic uric acid stone formation may follow an autosomal dominant inheritance pattern that contributes to stone development at an early age.[9]

Uric acid stones are usually radiolucent and may be of any size, from small, gravel-like particles to staghorn calculi that fill the renal pelvis.[4] Renal function declines rapidly with the larger, space-occupying stones. Their size may be reduced with medical intervention.

CYSTINE STONES. Cystine stones are formed in acid urine and are white or yellow, small and soft. They are characterized by hexagonal crystals that eventually form staghorn calculi. They usually do not occur in adults unless cystine excretion exceeds 300 mg/day. However, affected persons often excrete 600 to 1,800 mg/day.[6] Cystinuria is caused by an inherited renal tubular defect affecting the absorption of the urine amino acids, including cystine, which is the least soluble. Cystine stones are usually radiopaque because of the amount of sulfur contained within the stones.[9]

STRUVITE OR MAGNESIUM AMMONIUM PHOSPHATE STONES. Struvite stones are caused by urinary tract infection, most commonly with bacteria of the *Proteus* species. They may form after bladder catheterization and cystoscopy. Long-term antibiotic therapy may predispose the individual to *Proteus* infection. Other organisms that produce urease include *Klebsiella, Pseudomonas, Serratia, Enterobacter,* and *Staphylococcus*.[13] Struvite stones are more frequent in women and tend to be recurrent.

The causative bacteria contain the enzyme urease, which splits urea into ammonia and causes elevated urinary pH (Flowchart 34-1). The organisms are often called *urea-splitters*. Staghorn calculi fill the renal pelvis and are difficult to treat. Sometimes nephrectomy must be performed to relieve the obstruction.

RENAL TUMORS

Tumors of the renal system can cause damage to the renal parenchyma whether they are benign or malignant. A renal tumor is usually larger when found by palpation than when it is discovered on a routine radiologic examination. Symptoms are usually late in de-

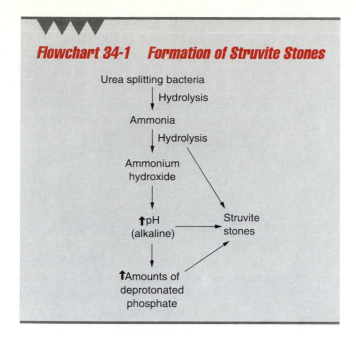

Flowchart 34-1   Formation of Struvite Stones

Urea splitting bacteria

↓ Hydrolysis

Ammonia

↓ Hydrolysis

Ammonium hydroxide

↓

↑pH (alkaline) → Struvite stones

↓

↑Amounts of deprotonated phosphate → Struvite stones

veloping and may include complaints of dull pain in the flank area or hematuria. Renal tumors are classified as benign or malignant and also according to their area of involvement.

Benign Tumors

Cortical adenomas are usually found during postmortem examination of elderly people and are the most prevalent benign tumors of the kidneys. They are usually not larger than 3 cm in diameter and do not produce symptoms unless they enlarge. These adenomas are believed to originate from the tubular epithelium and may be responsible for painless hematuria. They may be difficult to distinguish histologically from small, well-differentiated renal cell carcinomas.[6]

Oncocytomas are large, encapsulated, benign tumors composed of large eosinophilic cells.[6] These tumors may grow to a large size, and biopsy becomes essential to differentiate them from renal cell carcinomas.

Hamartomas or angiomyolipomas are rare, benign neoplasms that are composed of vascular, smooth muscle and mature adipose tissue.[15] They are often seen in adults with tuberous sclerosis, which is characterized by cerebral cortex lesions, epilepsy, and mental retardation, along with many skin abnormalities.[6]

Malignant Tumors

RENAL CELL CARCINOMAS.   Renal carcinomas usually occur in persons between 50 and 70 years of age, are most common in men, and account for 85% to 89% of tumors of the kidney. About 25,000 cases of kidney cancer are diagnosed every year, with about 10,600 deaths.[14] A higher percentage of renal adenocarcinomas

is reported among users of tobacco products. There is increased incidence in families, which has led to a search for a genetic link. Renal carcinomas or cysts often occur in association with von Hippel–Lindau disease, which is a hereditary defect involving angiomas of the retina and cerebellum.[6] Environmental factors related to the development of this malignancy include asbestos exposure and gasoline exposure. There is also an increased risk among persons with end-stage renal disease who develop acquired cystic disease.[14]

Renal carcinomas arise from tubular epithelium and can occur anywhere in the kidney. They vary in size from a few to several centimeters, and their weight may be in kilograms (Fig. 34-5). The tumors may proliferate throughout the kidneys to the ureters, the hilum, the renal vein and the inferior vena cava. Their color varies from white to yellow to gray, and cells may be clear, granular, or sarcomatoid in appearance.[14]

The tumor margins are usually clearly defined and cause pressure on the renal parenchyma. The tumors often spread or bulge into the renal calices and may extend to the ureter. They characteristically invade the venous system and spread by vascular metastases to the lungs, bone, lymph nodes, liver, and brain. Metastases may occur to almost any organ. Morphologically, the cells may be very anaplastic giant cells or clear cells, or they may be more well-differentiated.

Another characteristic of renal cell carcinoma is that the abnormal cells frequently produce hormones or hormonelike substances such as erythropoietin, parathyroid-like hormone, renin, gonadotropins, or glucocorticosteroids.[6] These secretions produce *paraneoplastic syndromes* that may be the first manifestations of disease and may lead to diagnosis of the tumor.

The behavior of the tumors is unpredictable, with

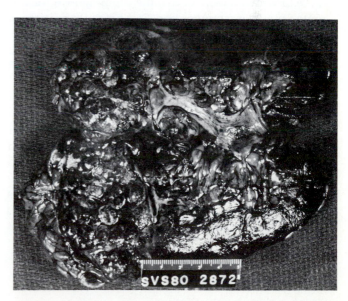

FIGURE 34-5   *Renal carcinoma showing enlargement and infiltration of the kidney parenchyma.*

rapid growth and metastases being followed by years of slow growth. Metastases may resolve after nephrectomy. Symptoms are variable; microscopic or macroscopic hematuria is the most consistent feature. Other symptoms include flank pain, fever, weight loss, and tumor mass that may be palpated. The combination of hematuria, flank pain, and palpable mass is labeled "the classic triad" and represents a poor prognosis.[14] About 30% of persons with renal cell carcinoma have metastasis at the time of diagnosis, with 75% of these being to the lung.[14]

Regardless of type and pattern, there is significant consistency in the staging of renal cell tumors (Table 34-3). Prognosis is based on several factors, including staging, the number of metastases, cell type, and size and weight of the tumor.

WILMS' TUMOR. Wilms' tumor is a malignant tumor that accounts for 6% to 30% of abdominal tumors in children, usually occurring between 2 and 4 years of age.[6] By the time the tumor is discovered, a very large abdominal mass is often palpable. Symptoms that may develop include microscopic hematuria, pain, fever, vomiting, and hypertension resulting from renal ischemia. Pulmonary metastasis is often present at the time of diagnosis.

Wilms' tumors are gray to yellow, are circular, have a fibrous capsule, and frequently have solid, cystic, and hemorrhagic areas. Histologically, they contain proliferating embryonic connective tissue with dense nuclei. The glomeruli are primitive, with a poorly formed Bowman's capsule, and they lack a basement membrane.[1] At first, the tumor is surrounded by a dense capsule and grows by pushing the renal parenchyma out of its path. When the capsule ruptures, metastasis to the lungs, lymphatic system, liver, and brain occurs rapidly.

Numerous factors determine the prognosis for this tumor, but of great importance is the stage at the time of diagnosis. The National Wilms' Tumor Study has adopted the staging system reproduced in Table 34-4. Long-term survival rates have improved to 90% with treatment by chemotherapy, radiotherapy, and surgery.[6]

TUMORS OF THE RENAL PELVIS. Of the malignant tumors of the kidneys, those of the renal pelvis account for 5% to 10%. Their frequency is increased in persons with analgesia-induced nephropathy and among tobacco users, but the precise carcinogen is unknown. Infiltration of the pelvic wall and renal calices is common, as is renal vein involvement. Five-year survival rates are from 5% to 100%, depending on the stage and spread of the tumor.[14]

TUMORS OF THE BLADDER

Bladder cancer is the sixth most common malignancy in the United States, with 50,000 new cases annually and about 9,500 deaths.[7] Most tumors of the bladder are

TABLE 34-3 *TNM Classification for Tumors of the Kidney*

PRIMARY TUMOR (T)

TX	Minimum requirements cannot be met
T0	No evidence of primary tumor
T1	Small tumor, minimal renal and caliceal distortion of deformity; circumscribed neovasculature surrounded by normal parenchyma
T2	Large tumor with deformity or enlargement of kidney or collecting system
T3A	Tumor involving perinephric tissues
T3B	Tumor involving renal vein
T3C	Tumor involving renal vein and infradiaphragmatic vena cava

Note: Under T3 tumor may extend into perinephric tissues, into renal vein, and into vena cava as shown on cavography. In these instances, the T classification may be shown as T3A, B, and C, or some appropriate combination, depending on extension (*e.g.*, T3A–B is tumor in perinephric fat and extending into renal vein).

T4A	Tumor invasion of neighboring structures (eg, muscle, bowel)
T4B	Tumor involving supradiaphragmatic vena cava

NODAL INVOLVEMENT (N)

The regional lymph nodes are the paraaortic and paracaval nodes. The juxtaregional lymph nodes are the pelvic nodes and the mediastinal nodes.

TX	Minimum requirements cannot be met
N0	No evidence of involvement of regional nodes
N1	Single, homolateral regional nodal involvement
N2	Involvement of multiple regional or contralateral or bilateral nodes
N3	Fixed regional nodes (assessable only at surgical exploration)
N4	Involvement of juxtaregional nodes

Note: If lymphography is course of staging, add *1* between *N* and designator number; if histologic proof is provided, + if positive, and − if negative. Thus, *N1*+ indicates multiple positive nodes seen on lymphography and proved at operation by biopsy.

DISTANT METASTASIS (M)

MX	Not assessed
M0	No (known) distant metastasis
M1	Specify

Specify sites according to the following notations: Pulmonary, PUL; osseous, OSS; hepatic, HEP; brain, BRA; lymph nodes, LYM; bone marrow, MAR; pleura, PLE; skin, SKI; eye, EYE; other, OTH.

Note: Add "+" to the abbreviated notation to indicate that the pathology (p) is proved

DeVita, V. T., Hellman, S., and Rosenberg, S.A. *Cancer Principles and Practice of Oncology* (4th ed.). Philadelphia: J.B. Lippincott, 1993.

TABLE 34-4 *Wilms' Tumor Study: Staging of Tumors of the Kidney*

Stage	Description
I	Tumor limited to kidney and completely resected
II	Tumor extending beyond kidney but completely resected
III	Residual nonhematogenous tumor confined to abdomen
IV	Hematogenous metastasis
V	Bilateral renal involvement either initially or subsequently

Forland, M. *Nephrology* (2nd ed.). Garden City, NJ: Medical Examination, 1983.

---

malignant, and an increased number are reported each year. There is a prolonged period of progressively atypical cells that precedes the appearance of these neoplasms. Carcinoma of the bladder usually affects the transitional epithelium and may be classified as transitional cell papilloma, invasive or noninvasive transitional cell carcinoma, or other forms such as squamous cell or adenocarcinoma.[1]

Bladder cancer occurs much more frequently in industrialized countries and is definitely associated with dyes and pigments used in textile, printing, plastic, rubber, and cable industries.[6] The risk is two to four times greater among tobacco users and persons who abuse analgesics.[7] The parasite, *Schistosoma haematobium*, in the bladder probably accounts for the very high frequency of bladder cancer in Egypt. Certain metabolites, such as L-tryptophan, and certain drugs, such as cyclophosphamide, have been linked to an increased risk of cancer.

TABLE 34-5 *Bladder Epithelial Tumors and Frequency Distribution*

BENIGN	
Transitional cell papilloma	2–3%
Inverted papilloma	rare
MALIGNANT	
Transitional cell carcinomas	90%
Grade I	20%
Grade II	} 60%
Grade III	
Carcinoma in situ (in the absence of other cancers)	5–10%
Squamous cell carcinomas	3–7%
Mixed	
Undifferentiated small cell carcinoma	rare
Adenocarcinoma	1%

Cotran, R., Kumar, V., and Robbins, S. *Robbins' Pathologic Basis of Disease* (5th ed.). Philadelphia: W.B. Saunders, 1994.

A general grading and staging system for bladder tumors is indicated in Table 34-5. The papillary lesions are usually grade I, whereas the grade III are usually invasive in nature.

The usual presentation of bladder cancer is gross or microscopic hematuria that causes no pain. Dysuria, urinary frequency, or urgency may accompany the hematuria.[7] Other symptoms are rare until late in the course of the disease. Long-term survival depends on early diagnosis and adequate treatment.

▼ Chapter Summary

▼ Voiding difficulties are among the most common problems seen and the incidence may be much greater than is reported. Some of the voiding problems are intermittent and most are slowly progressive.

▼ The most common problem in elderly males is benign prostatic hyperplasia which is, to a greater or lesser extent, invariable with the aging process.

▼ Frequency and incontinence of significant proportion are seen in 10% to 20% of the elderly population. It is more common in women and may be classified as stress, urge, overflow, or total incontinence.

▼ Obstructive disorders include benign prostatic hyperplasia, renal calculi, renal tumors, and tumors of the bladder. BPH is thought to result from an imbalance between the male testosterone and the female estrogen, but the relationship is not clear.

▼ Renal calculi can form anywhere in the renal system and can be of different compositions. The common stones are composed of calcium, uric acid, struvite, and cystine. Some are formed in alkaline urine, while others may form in acid urine.

▼ Most tumors of the urinary system are malignant. Renal cell carcinomas are most common in men and arise from tubular epithelium anywhere in the kidney. They are unpredictable and may grow rapidly and metastasize early, or they may grow slowly, causing few symptoms. Wilms' tumor is a malignant tumor that occurs almost exclusively in young children and has responded well to treatment.

▼ Bladder cancer is a very common malignancy in the U.S. and is associated with industrialized areas using carcinogenic agents. The cancer usually grows slowly and long-term survival depends on early diagnosis and treatment.

▼ References

1. Anderson, W.A.D., and Scotti, T.M. *Synopsis of Pathology* (12th ed.). St. Louis: Mosby, 1990.
2. Bartsch, G., Mikuz, G., Dietz, D., and Rohr, H.P. Morphometry in the abnormal growth of the prostate. In

Fitzpatrick, J.M., and Krane, R.J. (eds.), *The Prostate*. New York: Churchill-Livingstone, 1989.

3. Chanadian, R. Hormone receptors in the prostate. In Fitzpatrick, J.M., and Krane, R.J., *The Prostate*. New York: Churchill-Livingstone, 1989.

4. Coe, F.L., and Favus, M.J. Disorders of stone formation. In Brenner, B.M., and Rector, C.C. (eds.), *The Kidney* (5th ed.). Philadelphia: Ardmore, 1994.

5. Coe, F.L., and Favus, M.J. Nephrolithiasis. In Wilson, J.D. (ed.), *Principles of Internal Medicine* (12th ed.). New York: McGraw-Hill, 1991.

6. Cotran, R.S., Kumar, V., and Robbins, S.L. *Robbins' Pathologic Basis of Disease* (5th ed.). Philadelphia: W.B. Saunders, 1994.

7. Fair, W.R., Fuks, Z.Y., and Scher, H.I. Cancer of the bladder. In DeVita, V.T., Hellman, S., and Rosenberg, S.A., *Cancer: Principles and Practice of Oncology* (4th ed.). Philadelphia: J.B. Lippincott, 1993.

8. Garber, A.J. Diabetes mellitus. In Stein, J. (ed.), *Internal Medicine* (4th ed.). St. Louis: Mosby, 1994.

9. Garrick, R.E., and Goldfarb, S. Renal lithiasis. In Kelley, W.N. (ed.), *Textbook of Internal Medicine* (2nd ed.). Philadelphia: J.B. Lippincott, 1992.

10. Guyton, A. *Textbook of Medical Physiology* (8th ed.). Philadelphia: W.B. Saunders, 1991.

11. Horton, R. Benign prostatic hypertrophy in the elderly. In Kelley, W.N. (ed.), *Textbook of Internal Medicine* (2nd ed.). Philadelphia: J.B. Lippincott, 1992.

12. Katz, M.S., Gerety, M.B, and Lichtenstein, M.J. Gerontology and geriatric medicine. In Stein, J., *Internal Medicine* (4th ed.). St. Louis: Mosby, 1994.

13. Lemann, J. Nephrolithiasis. In Stein, J., *Internal Medicine* (4th ed.). St. Louis: Mosby, 1994.

14. Linehan, W.M., Shipley, W.U., and Parkinson, D.R. Cancer of the kidney and ureter. In DeVita, V.T., Hellman, S., and Rosenberg, S.A., *Cancer: Principles and Practice of Oncology* (4th ed.). Philadelphia: J.B. Lippincott, 1993.

15. Natale, R. Tumors of the kidney, ureter, and bladder. In Kelley, W.N. (ed.), *Textbook of Internal Medicine* (2nd ed.). Philadelphia: J.B. Lippincott, 1992.

16. Ouslander, J.G. Incontinence in the elderly. In Kelley, W.N. (ed.), *Textbook of Internal Medicine* (2nd ed.). Philadelphia: J.B. Lippincott, 1992.

17. Pagana, K.D., and Pagana, T.J. *Mosby's Diagnostic and Laboratory Test Reference*. St. Louis: Mosby, 1992.

28. Shah, P.J.R. Pathophysiology of voiding disorders. In Drife, J.O., Hilton, P., and Stanton, S.L. (eds.), *Micturition*. New York: Springer-Verlag, 1990.

19. Stafford, S.J. Disorders of micturition. In Schrier, R.W., and Gottschalk, C.W. (eds.), *Diseases of the Kidney* (4th ed.). Boston: Little, Brown, 1988.

20. Stanton, S.L. Stress urinary incontinence. In *1990 Neurobiology of Incontinence*. Wiley, Chichester: Ciba Foundation Symposium, 1990.

21. Sutton, R.A.L. Stone disease. In Levine, D.Z., *Care of the Renal Patient* (2nd ed.). Philadelphia: W.B. Saunders. 1991.

22. Swash, M. The neurogenic hypothesis of stress incontinence. In *1990 Neurobiology of Incontinence*. Wiley, Chichester: Ciba Foundation Symposium, 1990.

23. Warrell, D.W. Pathophysiology of genuine stress incontinence. In Drife, J.O., Hilton, P., and Stanton, S.L. (eds.), *Micturition*. New York: Springer-Verlag, 1990.

Chapter 35

Renal Failure and Uremia

Barbara L. Bullock

▼ **LEARNING OBJECTIVES**

1 Describe prerenal, renal, and postrenal causes of acute renal failure.
2 Discuss the two major causes of acute tubular necrosis.
3 Describe the pathologic features of nephrotoxic and ischemic acute tubular necrosis.
4 Explain the three mechanisms that have been proposed to explain the reduction in glomerular filtration rate in acute renal failure.
5 Discuss arterial vasoconstriction and prostaglandins in relation to oliguria.
6 Differentiate among the three stages of acute renal failure.
7 Discuss the pathogenesis of water imbalance, hyponatremia, hyperkalemia, metabolic acidosis, anemia, and elevated levels of creatinine, phosphate, and urea during the oliguric stage of acute renal failure.
8 Identify the clinical manifestations characteristic of the diuretic phase of acute renal failure.
9 Describe the causes and stages of chronic renal failure.
10 Discuss the intact nephron theory and its relation to chronic renal failure.
11 Explain fluid and electrolyte imbalances in chronic renal failure.
12 Discuss the causes and effects of metabolic acidosis in chronic renal failure.
13 Describe hyperparathyroidism and vitamin D metabolism in relation to bone disease in chronic renal failure.
14 Explain the factors leading to anemia in chronic renal failure.
15 Relate the multisystem effects of the uremic syndrome to the biochemical alterations caused by the process.
16 Discuss gastrointestinal abnormalities in relation to uremia, including ulcerations, oral changes, and bleeding.
17 Describe the cause of renal osteodystrophy in the uremic syndrome.

Renal failure occurs when the kidneys are unable to remove accumulated metabolites from the blood. The process causes alterations in electrolyte, acid-base, and water balances, as well as the accumulation of substances that normally are totally excreted by the body. Renal failure is a process of cessation of renal function. It can occur abruptly, as in acute renal failure (ARF), or over a long period, as in chronic renal failure (CRF). This chapter details the effects of both processes.

▼ Acute Renal Failure

ARF is a clinical syndrome in which the kidneys are unable to excrete the waste products of metabolism, usually because of renal hypoperfusion. The syndrome usually has an abrupt onset. It may lead to *azotemia*, which is the accumulation of nitrogenous waste products in the blood, and to *oliguria*, in which urine output is less than 400 mL per 24 hours. About 40% of ARF is nonoliguric. ARF can result from different causes. These have been divided into the major categories of *prerenal functional*, *intrarenal structural*, and *postrenal obstructive* disease (Box 35-1).

CAUSES

ARF is broadly defined as any condition that causes sudden suppression of kidney function. It is related to a number of factors, including ischemic disorders, nephrotoxic disorders, diseases of the small blood vessels, diseases of the major blood vessels, and acute interstitial nephritis. The most common causes are ischemia and nephrotoxicity.

Prerenal functional disease refers to any condition that diminishes renal perfusion pressure, such as hypovolemia or shock. Acute azotemia is caused by hypotension, hypovolemia, and decreased renal perfusion. This may be acutely reversed by immediate intervention. Hepatorenal syndrome is renal failure that occurs in the patient with hepatic failure. It often occurs in association with a gastrointestinal hemorrhage, dehydration, excessive diuresis, or massive paracentesis.[14] The features of hepatorenal syndrome include no apparent pathologic changes in the kidney, but a functional ARF.[18]

Intrarenal ARF results from acute parenchymal changes that damage the nephrons. Many conditions can cause parenchymal damage, including acute glomerulonephritis, vascular diseases, interstitial nephritis, and acute tubular necrosis (ATN). *Acute intrinsic renal failure*, or *vasomotor nephropathy*, can be induced by renal hypoperfusion and ischemia, nephrotoxins, and other mechanisms. It also is called ATN, which is a syndrome of abrupt and sustained decline of glomerular filtration rate (GFR) (see later sections of this chapter).

The postrenal obstructive category includes any

BOX 35-1 ▼ Causes of Acute Renal Failure

Prerenal Functional
Hypotension
Extrarenal sodium loss
    Gastrointestinal loss (vomiting, diarrhea, nasogastric suction, intestinal fistula, acute bleeding)
    Skin loss (heat exposure, burns, inflammatory diseases)
Renal sodium loss
    Extrinsic (osmotic diuresis, diuretic administration, mineralocorticoid deficiency)
    Intrinsic (salt-wasting nephropathy)
Third-space fluid accumulation
    Generalized edematous disorders (congestive heart failure, cirrhosis, nephrotic syndrome)
    Gastrointestinal (pancreatitis, peritonitis)
    Miscellaneous (crush injury, skeletal fracture)
Hepatorenal syndrome
Drug-induced
    Nonsteroidal antiinflammatory drugs or aspirin
    Angiotensin-converting enzyme inhibitor

Intrarenal Structural
Ischemic acute tubular necrosis
Nephrotoxic acute tubular necrosis
    Antibiotics (aminoglycosides, amphotericin B)
    Heavy metals (cisplatin)
    Radiocontrast agents
    Endogenous toxins (myoglobin, hemoglobin, myeloma light chains)
Vascular processes
    Atheroembolic disease
    Renal artery occlusion
    Vasculitis
Acute glomerulonephritis
Acute tubulointerstitial nephritis

Postrenal Obstructive
Intrarenal
    Acute uric acid nephropathy
    Drugs (methotrexate)
Extrarenal

Kelley, W. N. *Textbook of Internal Medicine* (2nd ed.). Philadelphia: J.B. Lippincott, 1992.

---

condition that obstructs excretion of normally elaborated urine. The most common intrarenal causes of postrenal ARF are uric acid crystal precipitation and methotrexate toxicity.[14] The extrarenal causes of obstructive ARF are much more common and include benign prostatic hyperplasia, renal calculi, and any condition that obstructs urine flow.

PATHOGENESIS

ARF results in a severe reduction in GFR and oliguria or sometimes anuria, associated with a rise in the blood urea nitrogen and creatinine levels.[24] Several mechanisms have been proposed, most of which relate to the intrarenal type of ARF, which has multiple causes. The pathophysiologic abnormalities include hemodynamic alterations, usually from hypotension; tubular obstruction by casts and debris; back-leak of filtrate through damaged tubules; and decreased glomerular capillary permeability.[16] The underlying process results in the renal injury.

The back-leak theory of increased permeability proposes that the lack of urine output is caused by disruption of tubular epithelium rather than GFR. Substances are reabsorbed from the tubular lumen and interstitium into the peritubular circulation. Tubular obstruction by intraluminal casts, debris, or interstitial edema may cause a decrease in GFR because of the increased hydrostatic pressure in Bowman's capsule. Filtration failure theories relate to a decrease in renal blood flow that leads to increased renovascular resistance. Afferent arteriolar vasoconstriction initially may cause a 60% to 80% decrease in renal cortical blood flow.[21] In the initial stage, renal blood flow is definitely decreased. In the established phase, the GFR decreases out of proportion to renal blood flow. Loss of renal autoregulation seems to be the major occurrence; it may be related to disruption of the renin-angiotensin-aldosterone system or other phenomena.

ACUTE TUBULAR NECROSIS

ATN is the term given to ARF caused by destruction of tubular epithelial cells.[24] It is the most common cause of ARF.

Etiology

The two most common causes of ATN are ischemia and exposure to nephrotoxic agents (Box 35-2). Ischemia is the more frequent cause, with its duration determining the extent of damage and the prognosis for return of urinary function. According to one study, ischemia present for 25 minutes or less caused mild and reversible damage.[6] Others showed that 2 hours of ischemia caused severe and irreversible damage.[13] ATN most frequently appears after an episode of shock, usually subsequent to conditions such as sepsis, burns, crushing injuries, and peripheral circulatory collapse.[24] It seldom occurs as a result of massive hemorrhage alone. Another form of ischemic ATN results from hemolysis or skeletal muscle breakdown. Hemoglobin and myoglobin precipitate in the blood and urine. These substances are toxic to the tubules, and are almost always associated with dehydration and oxygen deprivation.[9]

Nephrotoxic agents destroy tubular cells by direct cellular toxic effects, lysis of red blood cells (RBCs), intravascular coagulation, precipitation of oxalate and uric acid crystals, and tissue hypoxia.[5, 24] Factors that affect nephrotoxicity of agents include the hydration status, preexisting renal disease, and the person's age. Dehydra-

---

BOX 35-2 ▼ *Ischemia and Nephrotoxins That Are Implicated in Acute Tubular Necrosis*

Ischemia
Severe congestive heart failure: cardiogenic shock
Hemorrhagic, septic, neurogenic shock
Burns
Dehydration
Hepatic failure with ascites
Complications of pregnancy: toxemia

Nephrotoxins
Antibiotics such as gentamicin
Antibacterials such as sulfonamides
Diuretics such as furosemide
Antineoplastic drugs such as methotrexate
Contrast media, especially those containing iodine
Organic solvents such as carbon tetrachloride
Hemoglobin/myoglobin products
Fungicides such as amphotericin B
Heavy metals such as gold therapy
Anesthetic agents such as methoxyflurane
Antitubercular drugs such as isoniazid
Narcotic analgesics such as heroin
Antigout drugs such as colchicine
Anti–heavy metal poisoning agent such as calcium edetate disodium

---

tion leads to increased susceptibility of renal tissues to nephrotoxic agents. When there is preexisting renal insufficiency, functional renal tissue may be further compromised by the toxic agents. As one ages, the number of nephrons decreases, so that drugs become more concentrated in the tubules. People older than 75 years of age who are exposed to nephrotoxic drugs have a much higher frequency of nephrotoxicity than younger individuals.[10]

Antibiotics, including the aminoglycosides, penicillins, cephalosporins, tetracyclines, amphotericin B, and sulfonamides, are principal causes of renal disruption. Radiographic contrast materials that contain iodine, solvents, heavy metals, and pigments of hemoglobin and myoglobin also can cause ATN.[17]

Pathology

In the *ischemic type of ATN*, patchy necrosis occurs in the tubules (Fig. 35-1A). The main area of necrosis is in the straight portion of the proximal tubules, but lesions also occur in the distal tubules. If severe injury has been sustained, injury to the basement membrane occurs, and this exposes the tubular lumen to the interstitial space. The mitochondria in the epithelium appear swollen when viewed through the electron microscope. The areas that have no lesions have dilated tubules and

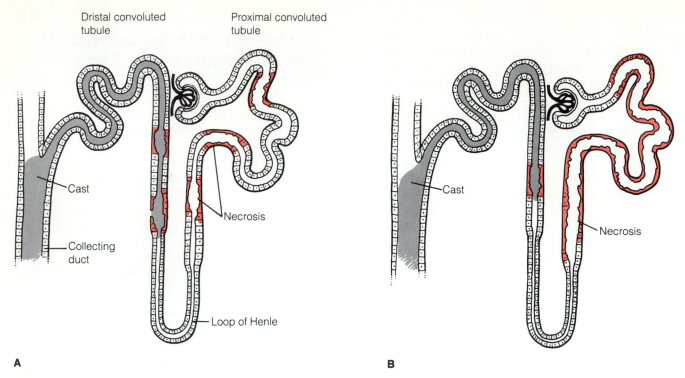

Dristal convoluted tubule   Proximal convoluted tubule

Cast

Necrosis

Collecting duct

Loop of Henle

A

B

Cast

Necrosis

FIGURE 35-1 **A.** *Patchy ischemic necrosis of the proximal tubules.* **B.** *Characteristic nephrotoxic injury of large segments of proximal tubule.*

flattened epithelium. Damage to the brush border of the proximal tubule cells also results.[9]

A characteristic finding of ischemic ATN is blockage of tubule lumina by casts. Other abnormalities include leukocytes in the vasa recta, dilation of Bowman's spaces of the glomeruli, interstitial edema, and inflammatory cells in the interstitium. The glomeruli appear to be normal.[23]

In the *nephrotoxic type of ATN*, a more uniform appearance is characteristic (see Figure 35-1B). Lesions are located in the proximal tubules but may occur in the basement membrane and distal tubules if severe injury has been sustained. Less basement membrane disruption usually occurs with nephrotoxic ATN than with ischemic ATN.[13] Casts, which are debris from cells, obstruct the distal tubules, and necrosis is present in all nephrons. Interstitial edema, leukocytes in the vasa recta, and inflammatory cells in the interstitium are characteristic.

Pathophysiology

Oliguria is a cardinal feature of the early stages of ARF, with either vascular or tubular origin. Approximately 30% to 50% of persons with ARF do not exhibit oliguria, but progressive azotemia occurs because of the impaired renal function. Most of the others are oliguric rather than anuric.[16] The pathophysiology of ATN with the production of oliguria is shown in Flowchart 35-1 and described in the following sections.

Research suggests that *tubular factors* are the primary sources in the pathogenesis of renal insufficiency (Flowchart 35-2).[6] If oliguria is caused by a tubular abnormality, it is believed to be the result of either back-leakage or intratubular obstruction.

Tubular obstruction is believed to be caused by casts, debris, or interstitial edema. Tubular obstruction occurs as a result of tubular ischemia, which causes swelling and necrosis of the cells of the tubules. The necrotic cells are sloughed off, causing obstruction to the tubules and increased pressure in Bowman's capsule. This pressure opposes the glomerular hydrostatic pressure and results in a decreased GFR. Oliguria results, often progressing to anuria. Together with output decline, there is dysfunction in the ability to excrete urea, creatinine, potassium, sodium, and water.

Oliguria also may result from *vascular changes*, especially renal artery vasoconstriction. In early stages of ARF, renal vasoconstriction occurs in the renal cortex, resulting in ischemia and a reduction in GFR, and leading to oliguria. The renin-angiotensin-aldosterone system may contribute to the vasoconstriction and oliguria. Renin is released when plasma volume is low. The secretion of renin causes conversion of angiotensinogen to angiotensin, finally leading to vasoconstriction. The afferent arteriole constricts, which leads to decreased GFR and oliguria (see Flowchart 35-2).

The arterial vasoconstriction also may be enhanced by the loss of the vasodilator effects of some of the prostaglandins.[9] Early in the course of renal vaso-

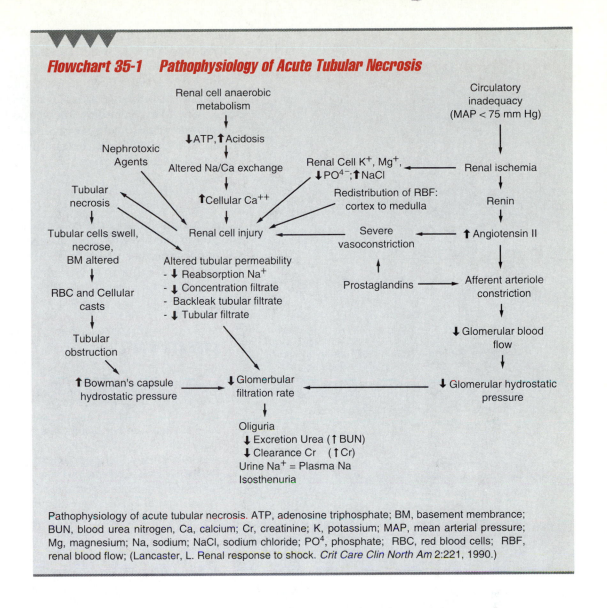

Flowchart 35-1   Pathophysiology of Acute Tubular Necrosis

Pathophysiology of acute tubular necrosis. ATP, adenosine triphosphate; BM, basement membrance; BUN, blood urea nitrogen, Ca, calcium; Cr, creatinine; K, potassium; MAP, mean arterial pressure; Mg, magnesium; Na, sodium; NaCl, sodium chloride; PO^4, phosphate; RBC, red blood cells; RBF, renal blood flow; (Lancaster, L. Renal response to shock. *Crit Care Clin North Am* 2:221, 1990.)

constriction, autoregulation, partly through the effect of prostaglandin release, retains blood flow through the kidneys and prevents tubular necrosis. As the constriction continues, this mechanism may be lost.

STAGES OF ACUTE RENAL FAILURE

The course of ARF can vary tremendously among persons with different physiologic problems. The three stages of ARF are initiation, maintenance, and recovery. The *initiation stage* is the initial or inciting event that causes necrosis of the convoluted tubules. The course of ARF is related to the magnitude of the inciting insult, the period of hypotension, and the length of time the hemodynamics are altered.[9]

The *maintenance stage* is characterized by oliguria and electrolyte imbalances. If urine production ceases (anuria), bilateral renal obstruction may be the cause. The urine specific gravity often remains at about 1.010,

which is the same as plasma. The renal blood flow decreases causing a marked decrease in GFR. As the GFR decreases, the fluid and electrolyte balances become greatly altered. Water excess may initially result from exogenous administration of fluids during the early critical stage, or it may be related to fat catabolism, with associated mild to moderate hyponatremia. As much as 300 mL of water per day may result from protein and fat catabolism.[23] The hyponatremia that occurs is mainly caused by the dilution of extracellular fluid. Hyperkalemia often occurs during the maintenance stage; it is mostly caused by decreased renal excretion but may be related to excessive breakdown of muscle protein. Metabolic acidosis results from inappropriate excretion of hydrogen by the kidneys. After 2 to 3 days of ARF, most persons develop moderate to severe anemia because of suppressed erythropoiesis (probably caused by lack of erythropoietin and uremic toxins). Elevations of creatinine, phosphate, and urea result from breakdown of muscle protein and inability to excrete metabolites.

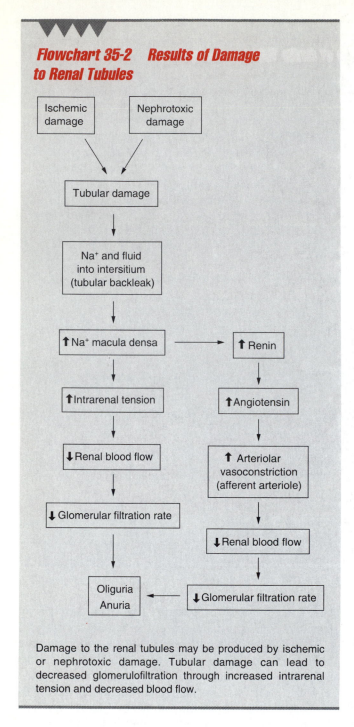

Flowchart 35-2 Results of Damage to Renal Tubules

Damage to the renal tubules may be produced by ischemic or nephrotoxic damage. Tubular damage can lead to decreased glomerulofiltration through increased intrarenal tension and decreased blood flow.

days of diuresis. Dehydration may occur as a result of the inability to conserve water. Laboratory values indicate a progression toward normal levels and increased production of RBCs. Wide fluctuations in fluid and electrolyte balance are common during this stage. Recovery is gradual, with GFR, renal blood flow, and tubular function improvement occurring over a 6- to 12-month period of time. The ability to concentrate urine appropriately is the final stage of recovery.[17]

Prognosis

The prognosis for ARF depends on the underlying cause, the onset and severity of the disease, and medical intervention. Mortality varies from 10% to 75%, with the highest risks being in the traumatized, postoperative, and aged populations.[14]

CASE STUDY 35-1

Ms. Serena Jones is a 20-year-old black female who was brought to the emergency room in a comatose state following the ingestion of a large amount of barbiturate drugs and alcohol in an apparent suicide attempt. At the time of admission her blood pressure was 50/32, pulse weak and thready at 88, apneic and supported by ventilatory assistance. Despite routine therapeutic measures her blood pressure remained low during the first 36 hours after admission. Her renal output decreased from 20 mL/hour to 1–2 mL/hour. Serum creatinine became elevated to 5.2 mg/dL and blood urea nitrogen 76 mg/dL. Serum potassium climbed from 4.8 to 6.5 in this period of time.

1. *As far as renal status is concerned, what is the apparent diagnosis of the problem described?*
2. *Describe, in detail, the pathophysiology of the diagnosis selected.*
3. *Considering the laboratory results, is there any emergent problem seen? If so, what is the danger and what should be done to prevent complications?*
4. *What are the possible ultimate outcomes of the condition described above?*
5. *Select some appropriate treatment options and indicate a rationale for their institution.*

See Appendix G for discussion.

With the increase of urea and other nitrogenous wastes in the blood, *azotemia* progresses.

The *recovery stage* is characterized by gradual increase of urine output. Diuresis may begin as early as 24 hours after the onset of ARF, or it may begin much later. The increased output, as much as 6 L/day, does not indicate total return of renal function. Tubular function remains altered, which is indicated by large amounts of sodium and potassium lost in urine. Serum urea, creatinine, and other accumulated substances act as osmotic diuretics. They also continue to rise during the first

▼ Chronic Renal Failure

CRF is a slowly progressive condition characterized by irreversible reduction in the GFR. Renal impairment is relentlessly progressive and leads to *end-stage renal disease* (Table 35-1). Numerous conditions that cause CRF primarily affect the renal parenchyma (Box 35-3). Regardless of the cause, the result is damage to the

TABLE 35-1 *Stages of Chronic Renal Failure*

Stage	Description
1. Decreased renal reserve	Homeostasis maintained; no symptoms; residual renal reserve 40% of normal
2. Renal insufficiency	Decreased ability to maintain homeostasis; mild azotemia and anemia; may be unable to concentrate urine and conserve H_2O; residual renal function 15%–40% of normal; GFR decreases to 20 mL/min (normal 100–120 mL/min)
3. Renal failure	Azotemia and anemia severe; nocturia, electrolyte and fluid disorders; residual renal function 5%–15% of normal
4. Uremia (end-stage renal disease)	No homeostasis; becomes symptomatic in many systems, residual renal function less than 5% of normal

GFR, glomerular filtration rate.

nephrons and glomeruli. This damage may be diffused throughout both kidneys, or it may be focal. Progressive loss of nephrons leads to greater dysfunction and more difficulty in maintaining an adequate fluid and electrolyte balance. Systemic effects occur in all of the organs of the body. The progression toward *uremia* (urine in the blood) usually is gradual because it is controlled by diet and fluid restrictions for long periods (Flowchart 35-3). After the kidneys can no longer maintain the fluid and electrolyte balance, dialysis therapy becomes necessary.

PATHOPHYSIOLOGY

The intact nephron theory aids in explaining the pathophysiology of CRF. Experiments support an *orderliness* of impaired renal function in the diseased kidney, which means that total nephron units are lost.[19] This finding lends support to the theory that the manifested loss of renal function is the result of a decreased number of correctly functioning nephrons, rather than being reflective of the number of diseased nephrons. A crucial feature of this theory is that the balance between glomeruli and tubules must be maintained. As the nephrons receive more filtrate, they also must be able to reabsorb more to maintain the steady state (Flowchart 35-4).

The progressive nature of nephron loss accounts for the sustaining of kidney function in the early stages due to a compensatory increase in reabsorption and excretion. As the number of nephrons declines to numbers inadequate to sustain the homeostatic balance, physiologic disruptions occur. Renal failure eventually affects all of the body systems through the inability of the kidney to perform its metabolic functions and to clear toxins from the blood. These problems are discussed in the next section.

BOX 35-3 ▼ Causes of Chronic Renal Failure

Glomerulopathies
Primary glomerular diseases
Focal and segmental glomerulosclerosis
Membranous nephropathy
Membranoproliferative glomerulonephritis
IgA nephropathy
Idiopathic crescentic glomerulonephritis
Other
Secondary glomerular diseases
Diabetes mellitus
Amyloidosis
Postinfectious glomerulonephritis
Heroin-abuse nephropathy
Collagen vascular diseases (systemic lupus erythematosus, systemic sclerosis, polyarteritis nodosa, Wegener granulomatosis)
Sickle cell glomerulopathy

Tubulointerstitial Renal Diseases
Nephrotoxic (antibiotics, nonsteroidal antiinflammatory agents, heavy metals, diuretics)
Analgesic nephropathy
Reflux/chronic pyelonephritis
Hypercalcemia nephropathy/nephrocalcinosis
Renal tuberculosis
Myeloma kidney
Lymphoma/leukemia (with infiltration)
Multisystem disorders (sarcoidosis, Sjögren syndrome)

Hereditary Diseases
Polycystic kidney diseases
Alport syndrome
Medullary cystic disease
Fabry disease

Vascular Diseases
Renal artery obstruction
Hypertensive nephrosclerosis
Chronic radiation nephritis

Obstructive Nephropathy
Prostatic diseases
Nephrolithiasis
Retroperitoneal fibrosis/tumor
Congenital
Other

Kelley, W. N. *Textbook of Internal Medicine* (2nd ed.). Philadelphia: J.B. Lippincott, 1992.

PHYSIOLOGIC PROBLEMS CAUSED BY CHRONIC RENAL FAILURE

FLUID IMBALANCE. Early in CRF, when the kidneys lose renal function, they are unable to concentrate urine appropriately, and this results in excess water loss. The solute load per nephron is increased, and normal solute concentration in the blood is maintained until the GRF is reduced to about 25% of normal or less.[19] Osmotic diuresis may result, and the affected person may become dehydrated.

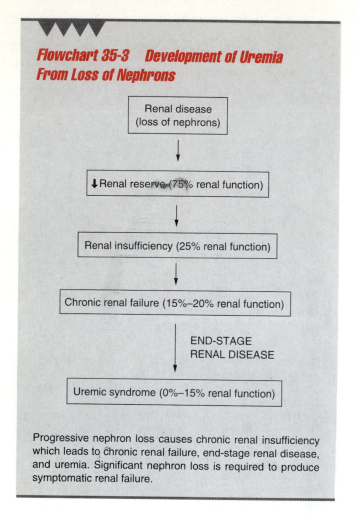

Flowchart 35-3   Development of Uremia From Loss of Nephrons

Renal disease
(loss of nephrons)

↓Renal reserve (75% renal function)

Renal insufficiency (25% renal function)

Chronic renal failure (15%–20% renal function)

END-STAGE
RENAL DISEASE

Uremic syndrome (0%–15% renal function)

Progressive nephron loss causes chronic renal insufficiency which leads to chronic renal failure, end-stage renal disease, and uremia. Significant nephron loss is required to produce symptomatic renal failure.

As greater numbers of nephrons become dysfunctional, an inability to dilute urine results. This results in a condition called *isosthenuria* which refers to urine and plasma having the same osmolality (about 1.010), called a *fixed specific gravity.*

Urine with a fixed specific gravity always denotes severe renal damage. Fluid overload with water and sodium retention may result when the GFR decreases to less than 5 mL/min. Anuria is seen when the GFR falls to this level.[1]

SODIUM IMBALANCE.   Maintenance of sodium balance is a serious problem, in that the nephrons may excrete as little as 20 to 30 mEq of sodium daily or up to 200 mEq/day. The varying amounts of sodium lost may be explained by the intact nephron theory. In other words, the damaged nephrons are unable to exchange sodium, so the intact nephrons receive the excess, causing an excess amount to be excreted in the urine. This increased elimination is accompanied by osmotic diuresis, which causes a reduction in blood volume and GFR and subsequent dehydration. Sodium loss may be enhanced by gastrointestinal disturbances, especially vomiting and diarrhea, that may aggravate the hyponatremia and dehydration.

In severe CRF, sodium balance can be maintained even though flexibility in adjusting to sodium levels is lost. A healthy person can reduce urinary excretion of sodium practically to zero or increase it to above 500 mEq/day when faced with sodium deficit or excess. If the GFR of a person with CRF decreases to less than 25 to 30 mL/min, obligatory sodium excretion of about 25 mEq/day may occur, with maximum excretion of 150 to 200 mEq/day. If water intake is restricted, hypernatremia may result. If water intake is excessive, dilutional hyponatremia may occur, often associated with edema and weight gain.[1, 15]

POTASSIUM IMBALANCE.   Before end stage renal disease, hyperkalemia is seldom a problem if water balance is maintained and metabolic acidosis is controlled. Potassium balance is believed to result from the adaptations made in response to the increased potassium presented to each functioning nephron. The mechanism for maintaining potassium balance is not understood, but it may be related to enhanced aldosterone secretion. As long as urine output is maintained, the potassium level usually is maintained. However, hyperkalemia may result from excessive intake of potassium, certain medications, hypercatabolic illness (infection), or hyponatremia. In acute acidosis, either metabolic or respiratory, the serum potassium level rises. For every 0.1 decrease of pH unit, the serum potassium increases by about 0.6 mEq/L.[25] Elevated serum potassium also is characteristic in uremia or end-stage renal disease.

Hypokalemia also can occur in association with a number of factors, including poor intake, diuretic therapy, hyperaldosteronism, vomiting, and excessive diarrhea.[1, 12] In tubular renal disease, the nephrons may fail to reabsorb potassium, leading to increased potassium excretion. Hypokalemia causes a functional inability of the nephron to concentrate urine. It also increases the renal excretion of ammonium to promote potassium conservation.[12] The result is metabolic alkalosis, a characteristic feature of hypokalemia.

ACID-BASE IMBALANCE.   Metabolic acidosis develops because the kidneys are unable to excrete enough hydrogen ion to keep the pH of the blood in a normal range. Renal tubule dysfunction leads to progressive inability to excrete hydrogen ion. In general, the decreased hydrogen excretion is proportional to the decreased GFR.[1] Acids, which are continually being formed by metabolism in the body, are not filtered as effectively through the glomerular basement membrane; the production of ammonia decreases, and the tubular cell becomes dysfunctional. Failure to form bicarbonate also may contribute to this imbalance. Part of the excess serum hydrogen is buffered by the bone salts. As a result, chronic metabolic acidosis increases the possibility of osteodystrophy (Fig. 35-2).[7]

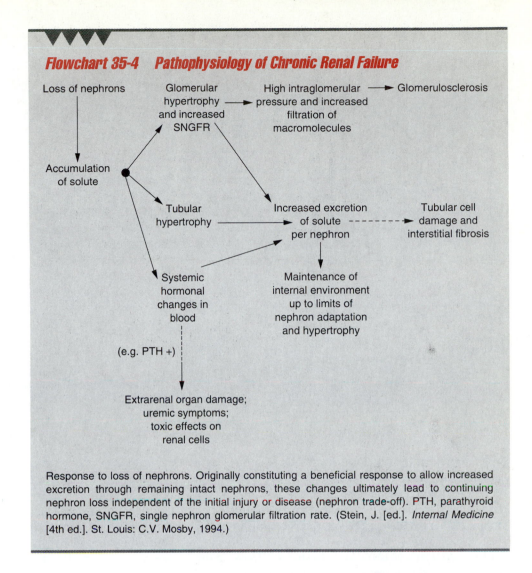

Flowchart 35-4   Pathophysiology of Chronic Renal Failure

Response to loss of nephrons. Originally constituting a beneficial response to allow increased excretion through remaining intact nephrons, these changes ultimately lead to continuing nephron loss independent of the initial injury or disease (nephron trade-off). PTH, parathyroid hormone, SNGFR, single nephron glomerular filtration rate. (Stein, J. [ed.]. *Internal Medicine* [4th ed.]. St. Louis: C.V. Mosby, 1994.)

MAGNESIUM IMBALANCE. The magnesium level is normal in early CRF, but progressive reduction in urinary excretion may cause accumulation. A combination of decreased excretion and high intake of magnesium may result in neuromuscular depression and cardiac or respiratory arrest.[22]

PHOSPHORUS AND CALCIUM IMBALANCE. Calcium and phosphorus levels normally are maintained by the parathyroid hormone, which causes renal reabsorption of calcium by the kidneys, mobilization of calcium from bone, and depression of tubular reabsorption of phosphorus. When the renal function deteriorates to 20% to 25% of normal, hyperphosphatemia and hypocalcemia occur, leading to secondary hyperparathyroidism. This secondary hyperparathyroidism also is associated with altered vitamin D metabolism. If prolonged, it results in renal osteodystrophy (see p. 668).

Activated vitamin D normally is responsible for enhancing calcium absorption in the gastrointestinal tract and increasing reabsorption of calcium from bone.

When CRF is present, hypocalcemia develops because of decreased absorption of calcium.[1] Figure 35-2 summarizes the development of renal osteodystrophy in CRF.

ANEMIA. A decreased hemoglobin in patients with CRF is the result of several factors: 1) short life span of RBCs because of altered plasma; 2) increased loss of RBCs because of gastrointestinal ulceration, dialysis, and blood taken for laboratory analysis; 3) reduced erythropoietin because of decreased renal formation and inhibition from uremia; 4) folate deficiency if the person is undergoing dialysis; 5) iron deficiency; and 6) elevated levels of parathyroid hormone, which stimulates fibrous tissue or osteitis fibrosis, taking up bone marrow space and causing decreased production by the marrow.[2] The normocytic, normochromic anemia, with hematocrit in the range of 15% to 30%, usually is proportionate to the degree of azotemia.[25]

BLEEDING DISORDERS. Bleeding disorders are common in CRF, and are mainly caused by thrombocyto-

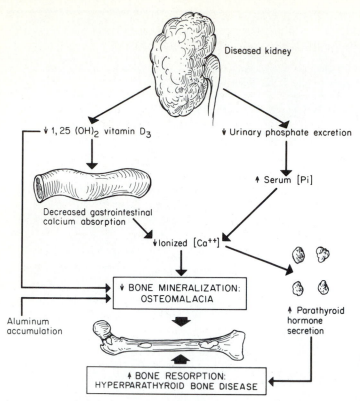

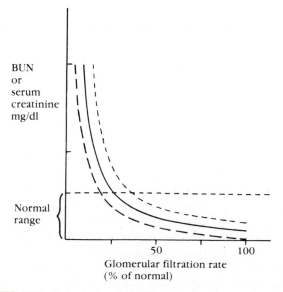

FIGURE 35-2 *Evolution of uremic osteodystrophy showing the roles of 1,25-dihydroxyvitamin D₃, parathyroid hormone, and aluminum accumulation. (Kelly, W.N. [ed.]. Textbook of Internal Medicine [2nd ed.]. Philadelphia: J.B. Lippincott, 1992.)*

penia or platelet dysfunction. As the nitrogenous wastes accumulate, there is increased risk of hemorrhage. Bleeding often is manifest by purpura, which is characterized by hemorrhage into the skin. Factor VIII deficiency also may play a role in the bleeding disorder.[1]

UREA AND CREATININE ALTERATIONS. Urea, a by-product of protein metabolism, accumulates as the uremic stage develops. The blood urea nitrogen (BUN) level is not an adequate indicator of renal disease because it is elevated not only whenever the GFR decreases but with increased protein intake, with shock, dehydration, infection, gout, and renal impairment.[11]

Serum creatinine level is a better indicator of renal dysfunction because urinary excretion of creatinine equals the amount produced in the body. Therefore, the GFR can be estimated by changes in the serum creatinine level (Fig. 35-3). With normal renal function, an increase of serum creatinine from 1 to 2 mg/dL represents a fall of GFR from 120 to 60 mL/min. With severe renal failure, plasma creatinine stabilizes at about 10 mg/dL.

The serum creatinine and BUN levels are referred to as *renal function studies*. If the BUN is elevated and the creatinine is normal, the source is not renal. If both values are elevated it confirms renal dysfunction. Because BUN is formed by the liver as an end product of protein metabolism, it may be low in liver disease and it does not elevate in hepatorenal syndrome, but the creatinine does increase.

CARBOHYDRATE INTOLERANCE. Carbohydrate intolerance can occur in persons with CRF and may be caused by impaired degradation of insulin by diseased kidneys and decreased uptake of hepatic glucose. Hyperglycemia correlates with the extent of renal failure and is probably caused by insulin resistance, because insulin levels are normal or increased.[1]

FIGURE 35-3 *The relation of blood urea nitrogen (BUN) or serum creatinine concentration to glomerular filtration rate. The broken lines indicate that there is a family of curves rather than a single one for all. (Papper, S. Clinical Nephrology [2nd ed.]. Boston: Little, Brown, 1978.)*

▼ *Uremic Syndrome*

As renal failure progresses, it eventually becomes symptomatic, and the prognosis is poor without dialysis. The uremic syndrome represents the fourth stage of CRF, or end-stage renal disease (see Table 35-1). Uremia is defined as symptomatic renal failure associated with metabolic events and complications.[6] The symptoms are described according to the effects they have on all body systems (Fig. 35-4).

NEUROLOGIC ALTERATIONS

Diverse changes in the central and peripheral nervous systems affect nerve conduction time and sleep patterns and cause uremic encephalopathy. The process of uremic encephalopathy exhibits a number of subtle to obvious changes. Some sort of uremic neuropathy occurs in at least 50% of all persons who have end-stage renal disease or are on long-term hemodialysis.[19]

Peripheral neuropathy, an early symptom of uremia, begins in the lower extremities. Affected persons gradually develop a delayed sensory and motor response, burning sensations, and numbness in the feet and legs. Even in the absence of peripheral neuropathy, evidence of autonomic dysfunction (eg, hypotension or impotence) may be present.[3] Peripheral neuropathy may be generalized, or it may occur in isolated areas; usually the manifestations are symmetric and include both motor and sensory effects. Restless leg syndrome or constant leg motion is present in 40% of cases.[1] Complaints of a crawling sensation, prickling, or pruritus are common. A specific uremic neurotoxin has not been identified.[3]

As renal failure progresses, central nervous system effects vary, and include drowsiness, inability to concentrate, poor memory, hallucinations, seizures, and coma. The alterations are believed to be related to the accumulation of uremic toxins, to deficiency of ionized calcium in spinal fluid with retention of potassium and phosphates, to hypertensive crises, and to altered fluid loads.[6]

Dialysis dementia is a progressive and frequently fatal neurologic disease that affects some persons on long-term hemodialysis. The cause of the condition is unclear, but it has been linked with aluminum intoxication and, in the growing child, exposure of developing brain tissue to uremia. Personality changes, dementia, seizures, and death may result. Electroencephalographic changes are common.[3]

CARDIOVASCULAR ALTERATIONS

Cardiovascular disease in the form of stroke, myocardial infarction, congestive heart failure, and cardiac tamponade is the most common cause of death for persons with end-stage renal disease.[4] Hypertension is present in

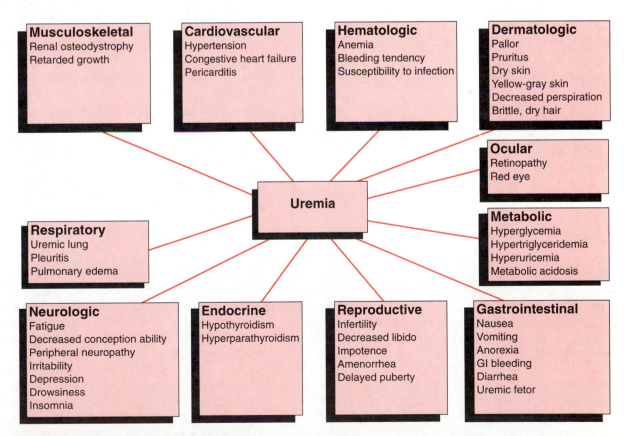

FIGURE 35-4 *Uremia affects all body systems.*

most persons with uremia; it may result from fluid overloading but usually is related to vascular changes (nephrosclerosis) or increased renin secretion.[6] It is caused by increased cardiac output or increased systemic vascular resistance.[4] Fluid overloading is the result of sodium and water imbalance. Vascular changes include accelerated atherosclerosis and narrowing of the arterioles. *Hyperreninemia* often occurs.

Fibrinous pericarditis may develop in end-stage renal disease and may be associated with an excess of pericardial fluid and fibrin formation on the epicardial surface.[1] The fluid can cause cardiac restriction and even tamponade. Fibrinous pericarditis may be asymptomatic, associated with substernal pain, or symptomatic of cardiac tamponade. Cardiomyopathy with patchy degeneration of muscle fibers may occur. Pericarditis may be caused by the uremia, and it is associated with elevated serum urea and creatinine levels. It also may result after dialysis, arising acutely with elevated temperature and pain. Persons who do not comply with routine dialysis therapy tend to have a high frequency of pericarditis.[4, 20]

Congestive heart failure may develop as a result of salt and fluid overloading, together with the characteristic hypertension. Pulmonary edema often results from the heart failure.

RESPIRATORY ALTERATIONS

The *uremic lung* seen on radiologic examination characteristically exhibits "bat wings" and involves perihilar congestion. The term is a misnomer, because the syndrome is not always present with uremia. Uremic pneumonitis is another term that may be used for the vascular congestion seen in the absence of circulatory overload in uremia.[19] An end-stage pattern has been noted that resembles the respiratory distress syndrome and is related to high serum urea levels. Pneumonia also is a major threat in CRF because the uremic environment depresses the immune response.

GASTROINTESTINAL ALTERATIONS

The most common gastrointestinal symptoms are nausea, vomiting, hiccups, and anorexia. Their cause is not well understood, but they are related to the degree of uremia and may improve if hydration is maintained. Ulcers may form in the oral mucosa (*uremic stomatitis*). These probably form from the production of ammonium by bacterial ureases from high levels of salivary urea.[1] Uremic fetor, or urine breath, occurs when the salivary urea is broken down to ammonia, causing an unpleasant metallic taste. The oral mucosa often is dry, and the tongue is yellow–brown. Gastritis, peptic ulcer disease, esophagitis, and colitis are common localizations of gastrointestinal lesions.[9] Gastrointestinal bleeding is a complication that may result from ulcerations and capillary fragility.

MUSCULOSKELETAL ALTERATIONS

The effects of altered levels of calcium and phosphorus are shown in Figure 35-2. The resulting faulty bone metabolism, called *renal osteodystrophy*, is caused by a combination of hyperparathyroidism, calcium and phosphorus alterations, and decreased synthesis of the active form of vitamin D. Several resulting bone lesions include osteomalacia, osteitis fibrosa, soft-tissue calcification, and osteosclerosis.

Hyperparathyroidism is a response to decreased ionized calcium in the serum. The causes of decreased calcium include phosphate retention, altered vitamin D metabolism, altered feedback with calcium and parathyroid hormone, and other factors. Phosphate retention is a consequence of decreased renal function and higher levels of parathyroid hormone. Phosphaturia results at the expense of high parathyroid hormone levels. Phosphate retention also leads to hypocalcemia and increased hormone levels. Calcium feedback is altered, and excessive levels of calcium are required to suppress parathyroid hormone in persons with uremia.[8]

Osteomalacia is the result of poor tissue use of vitamin D, which causes accumulation of osteoid material after calcification has ceased. *Osteitis fibrosa* occurs when fibrous tissue replaces bone tissue. It may result from secondary hyperparathyroidism. Soft-tissue *metastatic calcification* refers to the deposition of calcium and phosphate crystals in the synovial tissues and soft tissues, especially the eyes, joints, muscles, and lungs. *Osteosclerosis*, believed to be similar to soft-tissue calcification, is caused by bone redistribution and remodeling. This lesion causes enhanced bone density, mainly affecting the face, skull, and spine.

Renal osteodystrophy causes an enhanced tendency to spontaneous fractures. Many of the complications of this condition can be prevented by using phosphate-binding agents, administering activated vitamin D, and supplementing dietary calcium.[19]

HEMATOLOGIC ALTERATIONS

The hematologic effects of uremia include a normocytic, normochromic anemia and altered hemostasis. Anemia is usually severe. It results from decreased erythropoietin production by the kidneys.[4] Hemolysis of RBCs is common; it is related to a decreased survival time of erythrocytes in uremic plasma. Uremic plasma interferes with the ability of the erythrocyte membrane to pump sodium out, leading to swelling and hemolysis of RBCs. Dialysis also may cause hemolysis by mechanical destruction or reaction to the dialysate.[6, 19] Coagulation defects, caused by platelet defects, occur in most persons with uremia. Abnormal bleeding results cause a wide range of problems, including epistaxis, purpura, and frank hemorrhage.[2] Depressed immune response leads to a high incidence of infection and inhibition of phagocytosis.[19]

DERMATOLOGIC ALTERATIONS

The most common dermatologic disorders associated with end-stage renal disease include pruritus, dry skin, pruritic papules called Kyrle disease, and skin discoloration or pigmentation. Skin pallor results from anemia, and there also is a characteristic sallow, yellow pigmentation. Retention of pigmented urochromes results in their deposition in the subcutaneous fat. Dryness of the skin, or xerosis, is caused by atrophy of the sweat glands and dehydration. Uremic itching or pruritus is unexplained but possibly is related to excess parathyroid hormone, skin deposits, or peripheral neuropathy.[4] Kyrle disease describes lesions that are pruritic and irregular, with hyperkeratotic plugs on most surfaces except the face, mucous membranes, and palms and soles[4]. Uremic frost may occur in advanced uremia when the urea deposits are excreted in sweat and crystallize. Soft-tissue calcification results from secondary hyperparathyroidism, which leads to chalky plaque deposits under the skin.[20]

OTHER SYSTEM ALTERATIONS

Other organ and system alterations also occur, as noted in Figure 35-4. Uremia does not spare any system, so endocrine, reproductive, ocular, and other effects may be seen.

▼ Chapter Summary

▼ Renal failure occurs when the kidneys are unable to maintain the water and electrolyte balance of the body. The kidneys also are unable to remove metabolites and toxins from the blood. Abrupt decline in renal function is termed acute renal failure and progressive renal failure is termed chronic renal failure.

▼ Acute renal failure causes immediate disruption of the body's metabolism. It may be caused by prerenal, intrarenal, or postrenal alterations. In all cases there is a severe reduction of glomerular filtration which causes oliguria and anuria.

▼ Acute tubular necrosis refers to ARF caused by ischemia or nephrotoxic destruction of the renal tubules. The most common type is ischemic ATN which has a higher incidence of chronic renal failure associated with it. The stages of ARF depend on the success of the treatment and the extent of the damage.

▼ Chronic renal failure is a slowly progressive condition characterized by irreversible reduction of the GFR. The renal impairment is progressive from damage to insufficiency to renal failure to end-stage renal disease and uremia. CRF causes multiple system-wide problems that affect fluid and electrolyte balance, and the nervous, cardiovascular, respiratory, gastrointestinal, musculoskeletal, hematologic, and dermatologic systems. Progression to uremia will cause death unless treatment measures are instituted to prevent the accumulation of toxic metabolites.

▼ References

1. Alfrey, A.C. Chronic renal failure: Manifestations and pathogenesis. In Schrier, R.W. (ed.), *Renal and Electrolyte Disorders* (4th ed.). Boston: Little, Brown, 1992.
2. Anagnostou, A., and Kurtzman, M.A. Hematologic consequences of renal failure. In Brenner, B.M., and Rector, F.C. (eds.), *The Kidney* (5th ed.). Philadelphia: Ardmore, 1994.
3. Arieff, A.I. Neurologic manifestations of uremia. In Brenner, B.M., and Rector, F.C. (eds.), *The Kidney* (5th ed.). Philadelphia: Ardmore, 1994.
4. Badalamenti, J., and DuBose, T.D. Chronic renal failure. In Levine, D.Z., *Care of the Renal Patient* (2nd ed.). Philadelphia: W.B. Saunders, 1991.
5. Bonventre, J.V. Pathophysiologic pathways for renal injury. In Kelley, W.N. (ed.), *Textbook of Internal Medicine* (2nd ed.). Philadelphia: J.B. Lippincott, 1992.
6. Brenner, B.M., and Rector, F.C. (eds.). *The Kidney* (5th ed.). Philadelphia: Ardmore, 1994.
7. Coburn, J.W., and Llach, F. Renal osteodystrophy. In Narins, R.G., *Maxwell and Kleeman's Clinical Disorders of Fluid and Electrolyte Metabolism* (5th ed.). New York: McGraw-Hill, 1994.
8. Coburn, J.W., and Slatopolsky, E. Vitamin D, parathyroid hormone, and renal osteodystrophy. In Brenner, B.M., and Rector, F.C. (eds.), *The Kidney* (5th ed.). Philadelphia: Ardmore, 1994.
9. Cotran, R., Kumar, V., and Robbins, S.L. *Robbins' Pathologic Basis of Disease* (5th ed.). Philadelphia: W.B. Saunders, 1994.
10. Davis, K.M., and Minaker, K.L. Disorders of fluid and osmolality regulation in the elderly. In Kelley, W.N. (ed.), *Textbook of Internal Medicine* (2nd ed.). Philadelphia: J.B. Lippincott, 1992.
11. Fischbach, F. *A Manual of Laboratory and Diagnostic Tests* (4th ed.). Philadelphia: J.B. Lippincott, 1992.
12. Gabow, P.A., and Peterson, L.N. Disorders of potassium metabolism. In Schrier, R.W. (ed.), *Renal and Electrolyte Disorders* (4th ed.). Boston: Little, Brown, 1992.
13. Harris, R.C., Meyer, T.W., and Brenner, B.M. Nephron adaptation to renal injury. In Brenner, B.M., and Rector, F.C. (eds.), *The Kidney* (5th ed.). Philadelphia: Ardmore, 1994.
14. Humes, H.D., and Messana, J.M. Evaluation and treatment of oliguria and acute renal failure. In Kelley, W.N. (ed.), *Textbook of Internal Medicine* (2nd ed.). Philadelphia: J.B. Lippincott, 1992.

15. Innerarity, S.A. Electrolyte emergencies in the critically ill renal patient. *Crit. Care Clin. North Am.* 2:89, 1990.

16. Kumar, S., and Stein, J.H. Acute renal failure. In Stein, J. (ed.), *Internal Medicine* (4th ed.). St. Louis: Mosby, 1994.

17. Lancaster, L. Renal response to shock. *Crit. Care Clin. North Am.* 2:221, 1990.

18. Levy, M. Edematous states and hepatorenal syndrome. In Levine, D.Z., *Care of the Renal Patient* (2nd ed.). Philadelphia: W.B. Saunders, 1991.

19. Luke, R.G., and Strom, T.B. Chronic renal failure. In Stein, J. (ed.), *Internal Medicine* (4th ed.). St. Louis: Mosby, 1994.

20. Mujais, S.K., Sabatini, S., and Kurtzman, N.A. Pathophysiology of uremia. In Brenner, B.M., and Rector, F.C. (eds.), *The Kidney* (5th ed.). Philadelphia: Ardmore, 1994.

21. Oken, D.E., Wolfert, A.J., and Gehr, T.W. The pathophysiology and differential diagnosis of acute renal failure. In Shoemaker, W.C., et al. (eds.), *Textbook of Critical Care* (2nd ed.). Philadelphia: W.B. Saunders, 1989.

22. Quamme, G.A., and Dirks, J.H. Magnesium metabolism. In Narins, R.G., *Maxwell and Kleeman's Clinical Disorders of Fluid and Electrolyte Metabolism* (5th ed.). New York: McGraw-Hill, 1994.

23. Schrier, R.W. *Renal and Electrolyte Disorders* (4th ed.). Boston: Little, Brown, 1992.

24. Spargo, B.H., and Haas, M. The kidney. In Rubin, E., and Farber, J.L., *Pathology* (2nd ed.). Philadelphia: J.B. Lippincott, 1994.

25. Ziyadeh, F.N., and Agus, Z.S. Approach to the patient with chronic renal failure. In Kelley, W.N. (ed.), *Textbook of Internal Medicine* (2nd ed.). Philadelphia: J.B. Lippincott, 1992.

▼ *Unit Bibliography*

Abuelo, J.G. *Renal Pathophysiology*. Baltimore: Williams & Wilkins, 1989.

Anderton, J.L., and Thomson, D. *Nephrology*. New York: Churchill-Livingstone, 1988.

Bach, P.H., and Locks, E.A. *Nephrotoxicity In Vitro and In Vivo*. New York: Plenum, 1989.

Blandy, J.P., and Moors, J. *Urology for Nurses*. Boston: Blackwell, 1989.

Brenner, B.M., and Rector, F.C. (eds.). *The Kidney* (5th ed.). Philadelphia: Ardmore, 1994.

Burgio, K.L., Pearce, K.L., and Lucca, A.J. *Staying Dry: A Practical Guide to Bladder Control*. Baltimore: Johns Hopkins University Press, 1989.

Cattell, W.R. *Clinical Renal Imaging*. New York: Wiley, 1989.

Catto, G.R., and Rower, W.A. *Nephrology in Clinical Practice*. Baltimore: Arnold, 1988.

Cotran, R., Kumar, V., and Robbins, S. *Robbins' Pathologic Basis of Disease* (5th ed.). Philadelphia: W.B. Saunders. 1994.

Davison, A.M. *Nephrology*. London: Heinemann, 1988.

Drife, J.O., Hilton, P., and Stanton, S.L. *Micturition*. New York: Springer-Verlag, 1990.

Fitzpatrick, J.M., and Kram, R.J. *The Prostate*. New York: Churchill-Livingstone, 1989.

Freeman, R.M., and Malvern, J. *The Unstable Bladder*. Boston: Wright, 1989.

Gabriel, R. *Renal Medicine* (3rd ed.). Philadelphia: Bailliere Tindall, 1988.

Jelter, K.F. *Nursing for Continence*. Philadelphia: W.B. Saunders, 1990.

Kelley, W.N. (ed.). *Textbook of Internal Medicine* (2nd ed.). Philadelphia: J.B. Lippincott, 1992.

Krane, R.J., Fitzpatrick, M., and Siroky, J.M. *Clinical Urology*. Philadelphia: J.B. Lippincott, 1994.

Levine, D.Z. *Care of the Renal Patient* (2nd ed.). Philadelphia: W.B. Saunders, 1991.

Mandelstan, D. *Understanding Incontinence: A Guide to the Nature and Management of a Very Common Complaint*. London: Disabled Living Foundation, Chapmans Hall, 1989.

Massry, S.G. *Textbook of Nephrology* (2nd ed.). Baltimore: Williams & Wilkins, 1989.

Muther, R.S., Barry, J.M., and Bennett, W.M. *Manual of Nephrology*. Philadelphia: Dekker, 1990.

Narins, R.G. *Maxwell and Kleeman's Clinical Disorders of Fluid and Electrolyte Metabolism* (5th ed.). New York: McGraw-Hill, 1994.

1990 Neurobiology of Incontinence. Wiley, Chichester: Ciba Foundation Symposium 151, 1990

Rose, B.D. *Pathophysiology of Renal Disease* (2nd ed.). New York: McGraw-Hill, 1987.

Rose, B.D. *Renal Pathophysiology: The Essentials*. Baltimore: Williams & Wilkins, 1994.

Rubin, E., and Farber, J.L. *Pathology* (2nd ed.). Philadelphia: J.B. Lippincott, 1994.

Schrier, R.W. *Manual of Nephrology* (3rd ed.). Boston: Little, Brown, 1990.

Schrier, R.W. *Renal and Electrolyte Disorders* (4th ed.). Boston: Little, Brown, 1992.

Schrier, R.W., and Gottschalk, C.W. *Diseases of the Kidney* (5th ed.). Boston: Little, Brown, 1993.

Selding, D.W. *Clinical Disturbances of Water Metabolism*. New York: Raven Press, 1993.

Stein, J. (ed.). *Internal Medicine* (4th ed.). St. Louis: Mosby, 1994.

Sweny, P., Farrington, K., and Moorhead, J. *The Kidney and Its Disorders*. Boston: Blackwell, 1989.

Tischer, C., and Brenner, B.M. *Renal Pathology with Clinical and Functional Correlations*. (2nd ed.). Philadelphia: J.B. Lippincott, 1994.

Uldall, R. *Renal Nursing* (3rd ed.). Boston: Blackwell, 1988.

Ulrich, B.T. *Nephrology Nursing*. Norwalk, Conn.: Appleton & Lange, 1989.

Vander, A.J. *Renal Physiology* (4th ed.). New York: McGraw-Hill, 1991.

Endocrine Regulation

THE ENDOCRINE system is a complex system that coordinates and maintains the balance of the metabolic activities of the body through secretion of hormones. The secretion of hormones usually is activated by other hormones or neural influences, or both, and follows a closely regulated feedback mechanism. Chapter 36 describes pituitary function and explains how alterations can cause major effects on other body functions. Chapter 37 details the activity of the adrenal gland, its role in the stress response, and major alterations in function. Chapter 38 follows normal thyroid activity, with discussion of hyperthyroidism, hypo-

thyroidism, and thyroid cancer. Parathyroid function also is included in this chapter. Chapter 39 discusses the normal endocrine secretion activities of the pancreas (exocrine activities are discussed in Chapter 42). Diabetes mellitus, pancreatitis, carcinoma of the pancreas, and cystic fibrosis are major pathologies presented in Chapter 39.

The reader is encouraged to use the learning objectives at the beginning of each chapter to organize the study of this unit. Several case studies are included to enhance learning. The unit bibliography is helpful in providing direction for further study.

Chapter 36

Pituitary Regulation and Alterations in Function

Camille Stern

Camille Stern

▼ CHAPTER OUTLINE

▼ LEARNING OBJECTIVES

1 Describe the basic structure and function of hormones.
2 Differentiate the structure and function of the adenohypophysis and the neurohypophysis.
3 List and describe the functions of the hormones of the adenohypophysis.
4 Describe the functions of the two hormones of the neurohypophysis.
5 Draw the feedback method of control between the hypothalamus and pituitary.
6 Briefly outline the vascular supply to the pituitary and hypothalamus.
7 Discuss the function of at least four known hormones released by the hypothalamus.
8 Differentiate clearly between specific pituitary hormones and secretions of the target gland.
9 List and describe the effects of growth hormone.
10 Describe the physiologic effects of antidiuretic hormone.
11 Explain the different factors that cause the release of antidiuretic hormone.
12 Briefly describe the effects of oxytocin on uterine contractility and lactation.
13 Explain the mechanical and hormonal effects of pituitary malfunction.
14 Briefly describe conditions that cause enlargement of the sella turcica and their effects.
15 Explain the multitude of problems that result from deficiency conditions of the anterior pituitary.
16 Describe Sheehan syndrome.
17 Describe the results of hypersecretion of single pituitary hormones.
18 Differentiate between gigantism and acromegaly.
19 Define and explain the clinical syndrome of diabetes insipidus.
20 Clearly explain the syndrome of inappropriate antidiuretic hormone secretion.
21 Describe the pathophysiology produced by pituitary tumors.

Barbara L. Bullock: PATHOPHYSIOLOGY: ADAPTATIONS AND ALTERATIONS IN FUNCTION, 4th ed.
© 1996 J.B. Lippincott-Raven Publishers

The human organism contains complex systems of communication that coordinate and maintain its functions. Through these systems, the body monitors the activities and needs of each of its parts and responds accordingly to maintain normalcy. Through these systems of communication, it is possible for one cell to influence the functions of other adjacent and distant cells. When studying the mechanisms of the endocrine glands, one must relate neural control to the functions of the endocrine glands themselves. Research in the past two decades has determined that the neurologic and endocrine systems and their functions are multiple, complex, and closely interrelated.[9, 10] This interrelation is clearly evident in both normal physiology and disease pathophysiology. Neuroendocrinology investigates the pathway mechanisms of neural control and endocrine secretions.

Endocrine cells primarily secrete hormones into the bloodstream. Hormones may act directly on specific organs, or they may have more generalized effects on different and widespread tissues of the body. Each component of the endocrine system has specific functions, coordinating with other cells to create an environment conducive to survival of the total organism. Figure 36-1 shows the anatomy and location of the endocrine glands.

Many of the endocrine glands have neural inputs that control their flow and secretory activity, and endocrine function, in turn, regulates many functions within the nervous system.[10] The balance of neuroendocrine function is intricate and precise. Neural control of endocrine function is maintained by three mechanisms: input to neurons that secrete hypothalamic hormones, activity of the intermediate lobe of the pituitary, and autonomic innervation of glands (such as the pancreatic islets) that are not directly controlled by trophic hormones.[9]

This chapter describes the characteristics of hormones and clarifies their effects on target cells. The major focus is on the pituitary gland, its anatomic structure and physiologic function, its role within the complex communication system for maintaining a balance, its relation to the overall endocrine system, and pathologic manifestations of functional imbalance.

▼ Hormones

The word hormone stems from the Greek root *ormaino*, which means "to excite, arouse, set in motion." Hormones are chemical substances that exert a physiologic

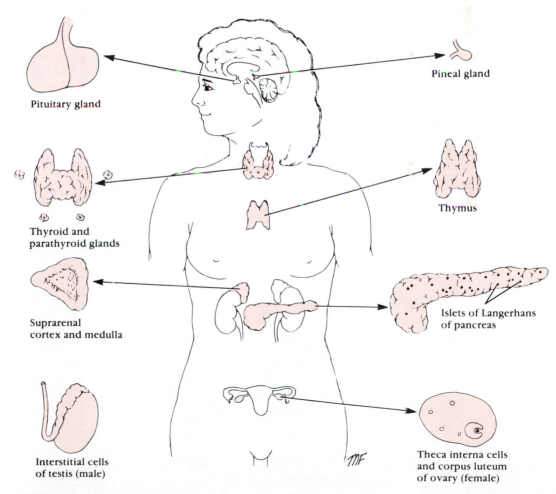

Pituitary gland

Pineal gland

Thyroid and parathyroid glands

Thymus

Suprarenal cortex and medulla

Islets of Langerhans of pancreas

Interstitial cells of testis (male)

Theca interna cells and corpus luteum of ovary (female)

FIGURE 36-1 *Location of the endocrine glands.*

effect on other cells. The capacity to synthesize these substances is not limited to endocrine organs but may be a characteristic of peripheral tissues or even of precursors in the bloodstream.

Secretion of a given hormone usually is activated by hormonal or neural influences on specific target cells by feedback mechanisms. Secreted hormones that act selectively on other specific target cells to regulate and maintain normal function are called *trophic hormones*. Hormones affect function in four broad physiologic areas: reproduction, growth and development, maintenance of the internal environment of the organism, and regulation of available energy.[10] Hormonal action can be either diffuse and complex or limited and tissue-specific.

The actions of hormones in endocrine tissues may occur in one of four modes: endocrine, neural, paracrine, and autocrine. Classically, *endocrine* influence is carried out by hormonal messengers that are secreted into and carried by circulating body fluids. *Neural* communication occurs when chemical messengers transmit cell-to-cell communication across synaptic junctions. *Paracrine* influence is the result of messenger hormones acting locally by diffusion onto contiguous cells. *Autocrine* influence occurs when the messenger hormones are able to modify the secretory activity of the cells that produced them. Figure 36-2 shows the modes of hormone action.

Hormones also are classified according to chemical structure. The basic types are steroids, derivatives of tyrosine (amines), and protein-based hormones. *Steroid hormones* are derived from a basic precursor, cholesterol. Steroids are lipids and can move through the cell membranes of target tissues to exert their action by affecting the cytoplasm or nucleus. Steroids enter the cell, bind with a cytoplasmic receptor, and then enter the nucleus to form messenger ribonucleic acid. This promotes translation at the ribosomes to form new proteins.[11]

The amines, or derivatives of the amino acid tyrosine, enter the cell through specific cell membrane receptors and combine with a nuclear receptor. These hormones, which synthesize proteins, include the thyroid hormones, epinephrine, and norepinephrine.[23]

The proteins, or peptides, are classified according to whether they have long or short chains. The short chains are peptides, and the more complex long chains are proteins. Peptide linkage is a major way by which amino acids are joined to form proteins. The average protein has about 400 amino acids. Most protein hormones bind directly with nuclear deoxyribonucleic acid (DNA).

Table 36-1 lists the major endocrine hormones as to type, target tissue, and action. The actions of hormones are highly selective because of binding of specific receptor sites in target tissue. Some, such as epinephrine and glucagon, act on cell membrane receptors, whereas the lipid-soluble steroids act on intracellular nuclear and cytoplasmic receptors.

▼ *Morphology of the Pituitary Gland*

GROSS ANATOMY

The human adult pituitary is about 1 cm long, 1.0 to 1.5 cm wide, and 0.5 cm thick. It is round or ovoid and weighs about 0.5 g. Because of its position beneath the hypothalamus of the diencephalon, it also is called the *hypophysis*, taken from the Greek roots *ypo*, meaning "under," and *phyo* meaning "to grow." The gland rests in a small depression (hypophyseal fossa) of the sphenoid bone called the *sella turcica*. It is covered by a tough membrane, the diaphragma sellae, through which passes the structure joining the pituitary to the hypothalamus, the hypophyseothalamic stalk. This structure also is called the infundibular stalk. Because disorders of the hypothalamus often are expressed as malfunctions of

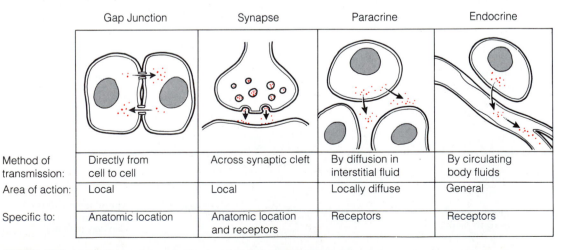

	Gap Junction	Synapse	Paracrine	Endocrine
Method of transmission:	Directly from cell to cell	Across synaptic cleft	By diffusion in interstitial fluid	By circulating body fluids
Area of action:	Local	Local	Locally diffuse	General
Specific to:	Anatomic location	Anatomic location and receptors	Receptors	Receptors

FIGURE 36-2 *Intercellular communication by chemical mediators.*

TABLE 36-1 *General Endocrine Glands and their Hormones*

Gland	Hormone	Target Organ or Tissue	Principal Functions
Pituitary (hypophysis cerebri)			
Adenohypophysis	Growth hormone, somatropic hormone (GH)	General	Accelerates rate of body growth, particularly growth of bone and muscle; exerts anabolic effect; affects metabolism of carbohydrate and lipid; elevates blood glucose
	Thyroid-stimulating hormone (TSH)	Thyroid	Controls synthesis and secretion of thyroid hormones
	Adrenocorticotropic hormone (ACTH)	Adrenal cortex	Controls synthesis and secretion of adrenal cortical steroids
	Follicle-stimulating hormone (FSH)	Ovaries, testes	Stimulates of ovarian follicle in female; stimulates spermatogenesis in male
	Luteinizing hormone (LH); Interstitial cell-stimulating hormone (ICSH)	Ovaries, testes	Stimulates development of corpus luteum after ovulation and progesterone synthesis therein; in male, stimulates development of interstitial tissue of testes and secretion of androgen
	Prolactin (PRL)	Mammary glands	Initiates and promotes milk secretion by mammary glands
	Melanostimulating hormone (MSH)	Melanocytes of skin	Dispersion of melanin in melanocytes
Neurohypophysis	Antidiuretic hormone (vasopressin) (ADH)	Renal tubes Arterioles	Facilitates water absorption by distal and collecting ducts of nephron Produces vasoconstriction, causes a pressor effect
	Oxytocin	Smooth muscle, especially of uterus	Contraction, parturition
Thyroid	Thyroxine (T_4)	General	T_3 and T_4 accelerate the metabolic rate and oxygen consumption of all bodily tissues
	Triiodothyronine (T_3)	General	
	Thyrocalcitonin (CT)	Skeleton	Metabolism of calcium and phosphorus Increase calcium absorption into bone
Parathyroid	Parathyroid hormone (PTH)	Skeleton, kidneys, gastrointestinal tract	Metabolism of calcium and phosphorus; increases serum calcium
Endocrine pancreas	Insulin	General	Regulates carbohydrate metabolism, decreases blood sugar, stimulates protein synthesis, lipogenesis
	Glucagon, pancreatic	Liver	Stimulates hepatic gluconeogenesis, glycogenelysis; raises blood sugar
Adrenal cortex	Glucocorticoids	General	Metabolism of carbohydrate, regulates metabolism, depresses inflammation
	Aldosterone	Renal tubules	Increases serum Na^+, decreases serum K^+
Adrenal medulla	Epinephrine	Heart muscle, smooth muscle, arterioles	Accelerates heart rate; causes arteriolar vasoconstriction of most smooth muscle
		Liver, skeletal muscle	Stimulates glycogenolysis
		Adipose tissue	Stimulates lipolysis
	Norepinephrine	Arterioles	Causes arteriolar vasoconstriction
Testes	Testosterone	Accessory sex organs	Stimulates normal growth, development, and functions; regulates spermatogenesis
		General	Stimulates maturation of secondary sex characteristics

(continued)

TABLE 36-1 *(continued)*

Gland	Hormone	Target Organ or Tissue	Principal Functions
Ovaries	Estrone, estradiol	Accessory sex organs	Stimulates normal growth, development, and cyclic functions, female sex characteristics
		Mammary glands	Development of system of ducts
		General	Stimulates maturation of secondary sex characteristics
	Progesterone (from corpus luteum)	Uterus	Prepares endometrium for implantation of fertilized ovum
		Mammary glands	Development of alveolar system

pituitary secretion, one must appreciate the functional and anatomic relation of the hypothalamus to the pituitary gland.[6]

Anatomically and physiologically, the pituitary is divided into regions that function as distinct and different endocrine organs. The anterior lobe is called the *adenohypophysis*, and it is subdivided into two regions: the pars tuberalis, which is made up of a small mass of tissue running up along the infundibulum and surrounding the stalk, and the pars distalis, which forms the bulk of the anterior lobe. The posterior lobe is called the *neurohypophysis*. It includes three regions: the neural lobe, the infundibular stalk, and the median eminence of the tuber cinereum, which forms the attachment with the hypothalamus (Fig. 36-3A).

The intermediate lobe (pars intermedia) lies between the anterior and posterior lobes and often is considered to be separate and distinct. Because it is poorly developed in the adult human, its function is questionable. The only known secretion of the intermediate lobe is melanocyte-stimulating hormone, which is synthesized from a large prohormone that also is a precursor of corticotropin.[18] These hormones do not seem to be of major importance in skin pigmentation in humans.

The two parts of the pituitary develop from a common germ layer, the ectoderm, but originate from two distinctly different embryologic anatomic sources. The adenohypophysis derives from an upward diverticulum of the ectodermal layer of the roof of the mouth or pharyngeal epithelium known as the Rathke pouch. The neurohypophysis originates as a downward ectodermal diverticulum from the hypothalamic portion of the diencephalon. These two lobes come together to form the hypophysis. Whereas the Rathke pouch loses its connection with the pharyngeal membrane, the neurohypophysis retains neural tract connections with the hypothalamus. These neural fiber connections are crucial in the secretory functions of the neurohypophysis.

The functioning pituitary remains connected to the hypothalamus through the neural tracts of the infundibular stalk and by an elaborate vascular system. These neural and vascular pathways are essential to the function of the pituitary, which is the bridging of the nervous system with the endocrine system.[18]

HISTOLOGY

ADENOHYPOPHYSIS. Traditionally, anterior pituitary cells were classified on the basis of their staining properties. Many of these cells contain secretory granules, but some are sparsely granulated or are considered to be agranular. This classification was replaced after the development of assays to measure the levels of hormones in the blood. Radioimmunoassays are highly successful in measuring the levels of specific hormones. The ideal test is probably the demonstration of hormone action on target tissues.[23]

Table 36-2 summarizes the anterior pituitary cell types with respect to hormones secreted. The interactions are not entirely clear-cut. In several instances, two hormones are secreted by the same type of cell. Secretion of one or more hormones may be stimulated by general or specific factors. These factors are clarified, if not simplified, in the discussions in this chapter.

NEUROHYPOPHYSIS. The neurohypophysis contains neuroglial cells and cells known as *pituicytes*. The pituicytes serve no endocrine function but act as supporting structures for the terminal nerve fibers and tracts of the hypothalamus.[22] The bulk of the posterior lobe consists of the hypothalamicohypophyseal tract (see Figure 36-3B). This tract consists of a bundle of nonmyelinated nerve fibers whose cell bodies are located in the supraoptic nucleus of the hypothalamus near the optic chiasma and in the paraventricular nucleus in the wall of the third ventricle.

Axons from these cell bodies traverse the hypophyseal stalk to terminate in the posterior lobe in proximity with the vessels that make up the capillary plexus. The neurohypophysis stores and releases two hormones,

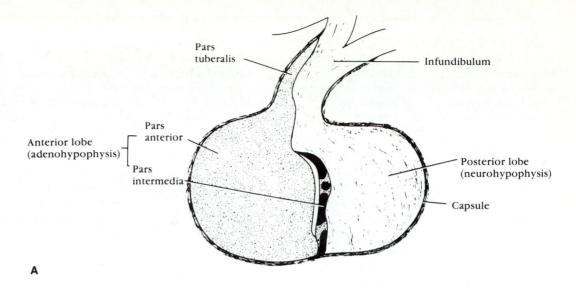

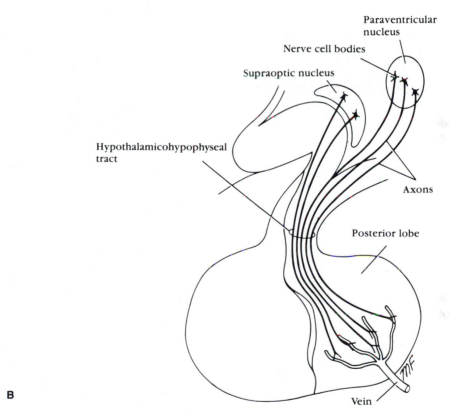

FIGURE 36-3 *A. Divisions of the hypophysis.* **B.** *The hypothalamohypophyseal tract.*

oxytocin and *antidiuretic hormone* (ADH). These hormones are synthesized by the hypothalamus and carried to the posterior pituitary in secretory vesicles through axon terminals.[22]

PARS INTERMEDIA. The intermediate lobe lies between the adenohypophysis and the neurohypophysis. As previously noted, this lobe, which has a major role in pigmentation and coloration in lower animal species,

apparently has little effect on the normal skin pigmentation of humans.[6, 21] The pigmentary changes encountered in several endocrine diseases, such as the abnormal pallor of hypopituitarism and the hypopigmentation of adrenal insufficiency, are attributed to changes in circulating adrenocorticotropic hormone (ACTH). Because ACTH has a common 13-amino acid sequence with melanocyte-stimulating hormone, it has melanocyte-stimulating activity.

TABLE 36-2 *Anterior Pituitary Cell Types*

Hormone	Cell Type	Target Organ	Function
Somatropic hormone, growth hormone (GH)	Somatotrope Acidophil	All tissues	Increases rate of protein synthesis in all cells; decreases rate of carbohydrate use throughout body; increases mobilization of fats and use of fats for energy
Adrenocorticotropic hormone (ACTH)	Corticotrope Basophil, large chromophobe	Adrenal cortex	Regulates secretion of cortisol and corticosteroids; enhances production of adrenal androgen
Prolactin (PRL)	Lactotrope Acidophil	Breasts	Produces lactation; stimulates development of alveolar secretory system
Thyroid-stimulating hormone (TSH)	Thyrotrope Basophil	Thyroid	Increases all known activities of thyroid glandular cells
Gonadotropic hormones: follicle-stimulating hormone (FSH), luteinizing hormone (LH)	Gonadotrope Basophil	Follicles of ovaries, interstitial cells of Leydig in testes, seminiferous tubules of testes	Regulates spermatogenesis; regulates maturation of ovarian follicle and ovulation production of testosterone
Nonsecretory	Other cell types. (Primitive, nonsecretory)	Unknown	Some 15% to 20% of anterior pituitary cells are either nonsecretory or function is unknown

▼ Relation of the Pituitary to the Hypothalamus

Although the pituitary has been called the "master gland," most of its functions are controlled by the hypothalamus. Secretion of pituitary hormones is activated by signals from the hypothalamus through a complex humoral and neural communication system.

HYPOTHALAMIC SECRETION OF RELEASING AND RELEASE-INHIBITING FACTORS

Through feedback and other mechanisms of communication, specialized neurons in the hypothalamus are stimulated to synthesize and secrete substances called releasing and inhibiting hormones. The function of these agents is to regulate the secretion of pituitary hormones; the pituitary hormones, in turn, control the secretion of hormones of the target endocrine glands. Figure 36-4 shows the target organs of the pituitary hormones.

The hypothalamus secretes a corresponding releasing hormone or factor for each anterior pituitary hormone (Table 36-3). In addition, the hypothalamus exerts dual influence, because it also secretes inhibiting hormones for prolactin (PRL) and growth hormone (GH). Dopamine, which exerts the dominant influence, is the inhibiting hormone secreted for PRL. Somatostatin is the inhibiting hormone for GH. An inverse relation exists between the blood levels of hormones of the target organs and the stimulation of synthesis and secretion of the

related pituitary hormones. The mechanism of control occurs through a negative feedback system that involves the hypothalamus, anterior pituitary, and trophic (target) gland (Fig. 36-5). Flowchart 36-1 shows the negative feedback for hormone balance and the specific mechanism for the regulation of ACTH secretion.

If the circulating plasma concentration level of any given target organ hormone is elevated above body need, the hypothalamus senses this imbalance and suppresses the secretion of the corresponding releasing hormone. Accordingly, the anterior pituitary responds by decreasing hormone secretion, thereby decreasing the stimulus to the target gland hormone. Conversely, if the circulating plasma level concentration of a target organ hormone falls below some critical level, the hypothalamus secretes a releasing hormone, triggering hormone secretion from the anterior pituitary gland, which in turn stimulates the target organ hormones. Through this feedback system, hormone balance is carefully regulated and controlled.

Because the neuroendocrine regulation of hormonal balance is extremely sensitive, other influences on the body's internal and external environment may produce changes in circulating hormone levels during periods of stress. Emotion, trauma, and diurnal changes create hormonal and other variations.

HYPOTHALAMIC-PITUITARY NEURAL AND CIRCULATORY STRUCTURES

To clearly understand the influence of the hypothalamus on the pituitary, it is necessary to understand the neural and circulatory structures essential to their interrelation.

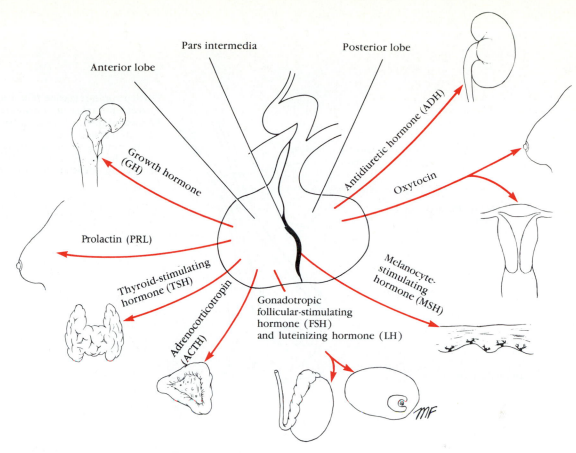

FIGURE 36-4 *Diagram showing the target organs of pituitary hormones.*

As has been stated, each lobe of the pituitary functions as a distinct and different endocrine gland. Therefore, the structural relation of each with the hypothalamus is different. The modes of transmission of signals from the hypothalamus are through neural connections for the neurohypophysis and through a complex vascular portal system for the adenohypophysis.

TABLE 36-3 *Anterior Pituitary Hormones and their Associated Releasing Hormones (Factors)*

Anterior Pituitary Hormone	Hypothalamic Releasing Hormone
Thyroid-stimulating hormone	Thyrotropin-releasing hormone
Luteinizing hormone	Luteinizing hormone–releasing hormone
Follicle-stimulating hormone	Luteinizing hormone–releasing hormone
Adrenocorticotropic hormone	Corticotropin-releasing hormone
Growth hormone	Growth hormone–releasing hormone
Prolactin	Prolactin-releasing hormone (no single hormone identified)

ADENOHYPOPHYSIS. The adenohypophysis secretes or fails to secrete its hormones into the circulation as a result of signals from the hypothalamus that arrive by the hypothalamicohypophyseal portal system. This communication system uses two capillary plexuses organized in series within the structures. Branches of the internal carotid and posterior communicating arteries of the circle of Willis give origin to the superior hypophyseal arteries. These arteries immediately branch to form a network of fenestrated capillaries called the *primary plexus*, located on the ventral side of the hypothalamus (Fig. 36-6). Some capillary loops also penetrate into the median eminence, where they serve the dual functions of supplying nerve cells around the base of the hypothalamus and receiving regulating factors secreted by hypothalamic cells.

The primary plexus drains into the sinusoidal hypophyseal portal vessels that carry blood down the infundibular stalk to the anterior pituitary. After reaching the adenohypophysis, the vessels again form a capillary network called the *secondary plexus*. These vessels maintain the cells of the anterior pituitary and deliver the regulatory factors from the hypothalamus to each cell. Vessels of the secondary plexus drain into the anterior hypophyseal veins. From here, hormones ultimately are transported to their target glands. The system begins and

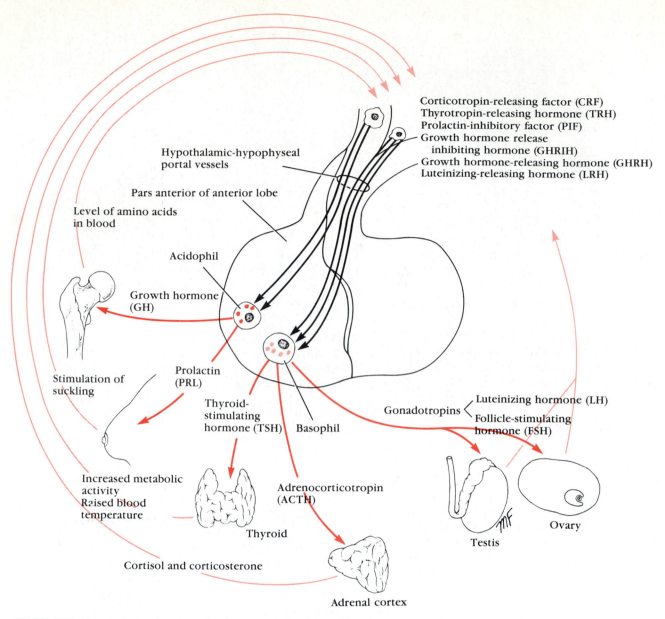

FIGURE 36-5   *The mechanisms involved in controlling the activities of the pars anterior of the anterior lobe of the pituitary gland. Notice the important feedback mechanisms.*

ends in capillaries and is called the *hypothalamicohypophyseal portal system.*[11]

Anterior pituitary function is achieved through neural as well as vascular communication. The anterior pituitary, however, is poorly supplied with neural tracts from the hypothalamus. It has no secretomotor nerve fibers and only sparse vasomotor fibers.

The following is a summation of the probable mechanism through which neural transmissions take place. The unusual vascular system of the pituitary facilitates transmission of signals from the central nervous system (CNS) to the adenohypophysis. Before reaching secretory cells of the gland, arterial blood passes through the primary plexus, which extends into the median emi-

nence. Significant numbers of nerve fibers terminate in the vicinity of these capillaries. These nerve fibers release neurosecretory products that are carried through the capillary sinusoids of the anterior lobe through hypophyseal portal vessels to effect release of anterior pituitary hormones.[11]

Neural signals may arise from external stimuli such as heat or cold or from internal stimuli such as emotion. Other neural stimuli that exert an influence but are as yet poorly understood include sleep-related and diurnal or circadian rhythms.

Another unique feature of the pituitary gland is that the blood–brain barrier is incomplete in the area in which the major plexus of the portal system originates.

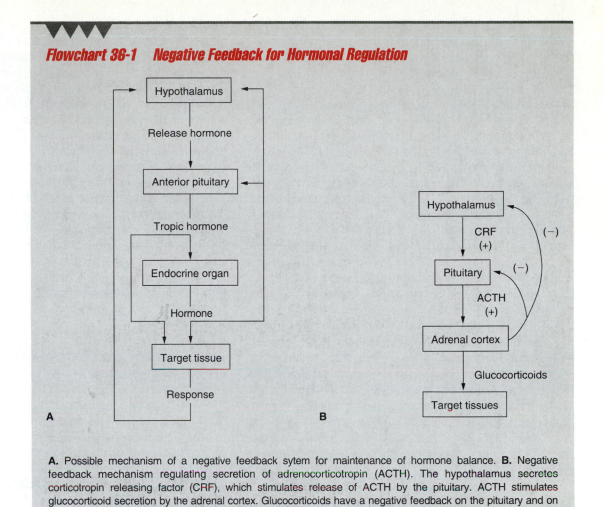

Flowchart 36-1   Negative Feedback for Hormonal Regulation

A. Possible mechanism of a negative feedback sytem for maintenance of hormone balance. **B.** Negative feedback mechanism regulating secretion of adrenocorticotropin (ACTH). The hypothalamus secretes corticotropin releasing factor (CRF), which stimulates release of ACTH by the pituitary. ACTH stimulates glucocorticoid secretion by the adrenal cortex. Glucocorticoids have a negative feedback on the pituitary and on the hypothalamus.

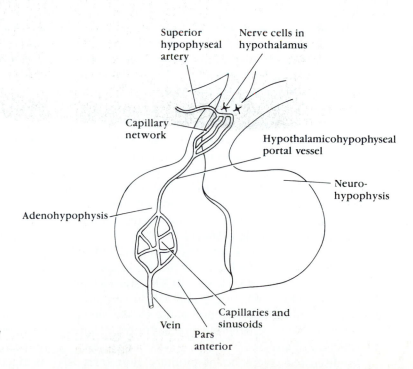

FIGURE 36-6 *The hypothalamicohypophyseal portal system.*

Endothelial fenestrations provide access for hormone molecules to the hypothalamus and pituitary. This allows for the feedback regulation of pituitary function described in the previous section.[6]

NEUROHYPOPHYSIS. The neurohypophysis, unlike the adenohypophysis, contains no cells with secretory granules. Embryologically, the posterior pituitary arises essentially as an invagination from the hypothalamus and retains neural tract connections from this area. Cell bodies located in the supraoptic nucleus of the hypothalamus synthesize ADH. Synthesis of oxytocin, the second hormone secreted by the posterior lobe, takes place in the paraventricular nucleus.[11]

The neurosecretory process occurs in the following sequence. Hormone biosynthesis takes place within the cell bodies of the hypothalamus in the form of hormonally inactive precursors. The active hormone is thought to be cleaved from the precursors during the 1 to 2 hours in which they are transported down the axons of the neuron fibers to the posterior pituitary. The posterior pituitary contains two distinct carriers essential for the transport of ADH and oxytocin.[6] Hormones are stored in the posterior pituitary until release is triggered by the hypothalamus. Because neurosecretory cells retain their capacity to conduct electrical impulses, stimuli from the cell bodies in the hypothalamus are conducted down the axons of the neurosecretory fibers to trigger hormone release.

▼ Functions of the Anterior Pituitary

The adenohypophysis secretes at least six hormones, four of which directly control the functioning of specific target glands—the thyroid, adrenals, and gonads. Hormones that control the functioning of target glands are called *trophic* hormones, from the Greek *trophos*, meaning "to nourish," or *tropos*, meaning "to turn toward." The six peptide hormones secreted by the anterior pituitary are 1) growth hormone (GH), also called somatotropin; 2) adrenocorticotropic hormone (ACTH), also called corticotropin; 3) thyroid-stimulating hormone (TSH), also called thyrotropin; 4) follicle-stimulating hormone (FSH); 5) luteinizing hormone (LH); and 6) prolactin (PRL), also called lactogenic hormone (see Figure 36-5 and Table 36-1).

All anterior pituitary hormones except GH and PRL regulate the functions of other endocrine glands and are, therefore, trophic hormones. GH, ACTH, and PRL are polypeptides, whereas TSH, LH, and FSH are glycoproteins. GH stimulates the secretion of the somatomedins from the liver. These small proteins act as intermediaries in the action of GH itself.

As discussed, secretion of pituitary hormones is regulated by hypothalamic release of "releasing" hormones. These include thyrotropin-releasing hormone, growth hormone–releasing hormone, corticotropin-releasing factor, and luteinizing hormone–releasing hormone, also called gonadotropin-releasing hormone. In addition, two release-inhibiting substances are liberated by the hypothalamus. These are growth hormone release–inhibiting hormone, also called somatostatin, and prolactin-inhibiting factor.

Release factors are liberated by neurosecretion, which is the release of a substance from nerve endings directly into the bloodstream. Liberated release hormones are carried to the sinuses of the anterior pituitary. Within the adenohypophysis, the release hormones act on the gland's cells to control their secretions. The mechanisms that trigger synthesis and release of the hormones include feedback as well as various other stimuli in the internal and external environments.

HORMONES SECRETED

THYROID-STIMULATING HORMONE (TSH). The physiologic role of TSH is to activate synthesis and secretion of the hormones of the thyroid and to maintain the size of the gland and its rate of blood flow (see pp. 712–719). The pathologic problems that result from derangements in TSH secretion are the same as those of hypersecretion or hyposecretion of the thyroid hormones.

ADRENOCORTICOTROPIC HORMONE (ACTH). The physiologic role of ACTH is to regulate synthesis and secretion of adrenal steroids by adrenal cortical tissue. It also maintains the size and blood flow of the adrenal cortex. Excessive secretions of the cortex result in enlargement of the gland, and absence or marked diminution results in atrophy. Pathologic problems that stem from imbalance in ACTH secretion are equivalent to those caused by hypersecretion or hyposecretion of adrenal hormones (see pp. 701–704).

FOLLICLE-STIMULATING HORMONE (FSH). In men, the target organs for FSH are the testes. The hormone directly stimulates the germinal epithelium of the seminiferous tubules to activate and facilitate the rate of spermatogenesis. For optimal effects, it appears to require the concomitant presence of LH. Sometimes, these hormones are used to treat infertility in men or in women.

In women, the target organs for FSH are the ovaries; FSH is essential for the normal cyclic growth of the ovarian follicle. It is responsible for the development and growth of a large number of graafian follicles and for an increased ovarian weight.

The gonadotropins stimulate the synthesis of testosterone in men and of estradiol and progesterone in women. As with other anterior lobe hormones, secretion is triggered from the hypothalamus and is mediated by feedback mechanisms. Therefore, increased circulation levels of androgens and estrogens inhibit FSH secretions (see Unit 15).[7]

LUTEINIZING HORMONE (LH). Target organs for LH in men are the testes, where LH stimulates the growth and secretory activity of the testicular interstitial cells (Leydig cells). This action stimulates the synthesis and secretions of the male androgen testosterone. The female target organs are the ovaries, where LH is essential for ovulation. Action of the hormone readies the ovarian follicle and forms the corpus luteum from the ruptured follicle. As noted previously, the presence of FSH is required to accomplish these functions.[21]

PROLACTIN (PRL). The predominant physiologic roles for PRL are in breast development and lactation. The hormone acts in synergy with estrogen to promote growth and development of the female mammary glands; therefore, it is said to have a dual role in lactation. It acts with estrogen to prepare the mammary glands for lactation, and then it initiates secretion of the nutrients of these glands. PRL secretion increases during pregnancy, reaching a peak with delivery. The secretion is regulated by a release-inhibiting factor. Release also may be initiated by suckling. The initiation and adequacy of secretion show physiologic variations associated with sleep, stress, and other stimuli, as do those of other pituitary hormones.

GROWTH HORMONE (GH). GH is the only hormone secreted by the anterior pituitary that has no specific target organ. All cells of the human body may be considered target cells for this hormone. GH, or somatotropin, is regulated by release hormones from the hypothalamus and by somatomedin, a substance synthesized in the liver. Because growth is a complex phenomenon, many other factors play a role in the rate and mode of growth. Variation of growth also exists between ethnic groups, so height and weight charts from one ethnic group may not be applicable to others.[2] Action of GH is influenced by other hormones, such as thyroid hormone, insulin, the steroids, and androgens. It also is influenced by nutritional status, exercise, stress, diurnal variations, and sleep. Secretion of GH is suppressed by an inhibiting factor (somatostatin). GH varies from the other hormones in that it is species-specific. It has been synthesized from *Escherichia coli* through recombinant DNA technology. This type of GH can be used to treat deficiency.[6] Effects of GH are summarized in the next section.

ACTIONS OF GROWTH HORMONE

EFFECTS ON GROWTH OF BONE AND CARTILAGE. GH exerts an indirect rather than a direct effect on the growth of bone and cartilage. It stimulates growth of these structures by promoting the synthesis of several proteins that are collectively called somatomedin. These proteins are known to be formed in the liver and probably in the muscle and kidneys also. Somatomedin acts directly on the bone and cartilage to promote growth. It is essential to the deposition of chondroid sulfate and collagen.[11] Because the formation of cartilage is accelerated and the epiphyseal plates widen, additional matrix is formed at the ends of long bones. Through this mechanism, linear structure is increased. After the epiphyses close, linear growth is no longer possible. Therefore, excessive GH after adolescence results in thickening of bones and tissues.

INCREASED PROTEIN SYNTHESIS. GH facilitates the transport of amino acids through the cell membrane. This increase in amino acid concentrations in the cells is thought to be partially responsible for increased protein synthesis. It also is believed to exert a direct effect on ribosomes to cause the production of greater numbers of protein molecules.[11] As a result of these mechanisms, GH creates a positive nitrogen and phosphorous balance and is, therefore, an anabolic protein hormone.

EFFECTS ON RIBONUCLEIC ACID METABOLISM. GH stimulates the transcription process in the nucleus, causing increased formation of ribonucleic acid. This, in turn, promotes growth by promoting protein synthesis.

DECREASED CATABOLISM OF PROTEINS. In addition to an increase in protein synthesis, a decrease in the breakdown of cell proteins occurs. The reduction is believed to result from the ability of GH to mobilize free fatty acids from adipose tissue to supply energy. This response acts as a protein-sparer as well as a carbohydrate-sparer.[11]

EFFECTS ON ELECTROLYTE BALANCE. GH increases gastrointestinal absorption of calcium and reduces sodium and potassium excretion.[21]

EFFECTS ON FAT AND GLUCOSE METABOLISM. GH exerts a strong influence on stimulation of fat catabolism in adipose tissue. This action results in the production of large amounts of acetylcoenzyme A, which acts as a ready source of energy and has the effect of reducing the use of glucose for energy (glucose-sparing). In the presence of excessive quantities of GH, several potential problems may develop from this action. The response may result in increased ketone levels in the blood (ketogenic effect) or in increased concentration of liver lipids (fatty liver). The glucose-sparing effect of fat catabolism results in storage of increased amounts of glucose in the cells as glycogen. When cellular capacity becomes saturated, circulating blood levels of glucose are elevated (diabetogenic effect), resulting in increased demand for insulin. If this effect persists long enough, the β cells of the islets of Langerhans are exhausted and diabetes mellitus results.[21] GH is not the only anterior pituitary hormone that increases blood glucose levels, however; ACTH, TSH, and PRL all have this capacity.

OTHER ACTIONS OF GROWTH HORMONE. Two additional facts seem important to the understanding of GH. First, GH fails to cause growth if carbohydrate is lacking. Second, secretion of GH is increased during episodes of hypoglycemia *except* those that occur in adult hypopituitarism.

All of this information indicates that GH has many functions other than those of stimulating and supporting growth in the developing child. Although secretion and the subsequent physiologic effects are most pronounced during the early developing years, secretion and release are essential to many bodily functions throughout life.

CIRCADIAN PATTERNS OF ANTERIOR PITUITARY SECRETIONS

The secretions of the pituitary are cyclic and can be demonstrated on a regular rhythmical basis called a *circadian* or *diurnal rhythm* (see pp. 181–182). Secretion of GH and PRL is greatest in the early hours of sleep; ACTH regulates cortisol secretion, reaching maximum between 2 AM and 4 PM and causing peak levels at about 8 AM; TSH reaches a maximum level between 8 PM and midnight.[11] Loss of diurnal rhythm can be an early diagnostic feature of hypothalamic or pituitary dysfunction. Measurement of hormone levels and supplemental replacement should be governed by the susceptibility of the pituitary at different times.[21]

▼ Functions of the Neurohypophysis

Unlike the adenohypophysis, the neurohypophysis does not function as an endocrine gland. Posterior pituitary hormones are synthesized in the hypothalamus and stored in the posterior lobe to await the signal from the hypothalamus for release. Cell bodies located in the supraoptic nuclei of the hypothalamus are considered to be largely responsible for synthesis of ADH, whereas cell bodies located in the paraventricular nuclei synthesize oxytocin. It is recognized, however, that both supraoptic and paraventricular nuclear cell bodies synthesize some amount of both of the hormones secreted by the neurohypophysis (Fig. 36-7).

Synthesis and secretion of posterior lobe hormones takes place in a two-step process. In the first step, a hormonally inactive precursor is synthesized in the specified cells of the hypothalamus. This precursor is transported by way of secretory granules down the neural fibers of the hypothalamicohypophyseal tract. The actual hormone is believed to be separated from the precursor during the period in which the granules traverse the axons of this tract to reach the posterior lobe. Hormones are then stored in the posterior pituitary until appropriate stimulus for secretion is initiated by the hypothalamus. Because neurosecretory cells and fibers also have the capacity to conduct electrical impulses, action potentials initiated by stimulus to cell bodies of the hypothalamus are conducted down the axons of the neuron fibers to stimulate release of the hormones.[18]

ANTIDIURETIC HORMONE

PHYSIOLOGIC ACTION. The kidneys are the specific target organs of ADH (also called *vasopressin*). In the presence of ADH, the distal tubules and collecting ducts of the nephrons become more permeable to water, causing increased water reabsorption. This results in decreased concentration (osmotic pressure) of the extracellular fluid (plasma). In the absence of ADH, tubules and collecting ducts of the nephrons are almost impermeable, and little or no water is reabsorbed.[11] In addition, ADH has a vasopressor effect if administered in large doses and may cause hypertension. The effect is caused by direct action of ADH on smooth muscles in the vascular wall. It may improve systemic fluid volume by reducing the size of the vascular bed.

REGULATION BY THE HYPOTHALAMUS. Increased osmolarity of plasma and decreased circulating vascular volume are the major physiologic stimuli for initiation of ADH secretion. Both osmoreceptors and volume receptors influence the hypothalamus to initiate the signal for release of ADH.[11]

Osmoreceptors located in the hypothalamus consist of small vesicles surrounded by a semipermeable membrane in which nerve endings are embedded. Increased osmolarity of plasma in the vicinity of the hypothalamus causes water to move out of these osmoreceptors, decreases their volume, and reduces the degree of stretch sensed by neurons. This response presumably stimulates the hypothalamus and initiates the electrical impulse that signals for pituitary release of ADH.

Although the location of *volume receptors* is unknown, they are thought to be outside the CNS, probably predominantly in the thoracic cavity. The circulating vascular volume sensed in the thoracic region, rather than the vascular volume of the total body, apparently is the crucial factor in ADH release. For example, a shift in blood volume caused by pooling of blood in the periphery is accompanied by ADH release, as is change from a supine to a sitting or standing position. Exposure to high temperatures, which shifts blood from deeper to more superficial regions, increases ADH secretion, whereas exposure to cold temperatures, which shifts blood from superficial to deeper regions, reduces its secretions. Positive-pressure respiration, which decreases blood volume in the great veins of the thorax, also results in ADH release.

OTHER FACTORS THAT REGULATE SECRETION AND RELEASE. As previously noted, feedback mechanisms protect blood osmolarity and volume balance through influence on ADH secretion. If all factors are in balance,

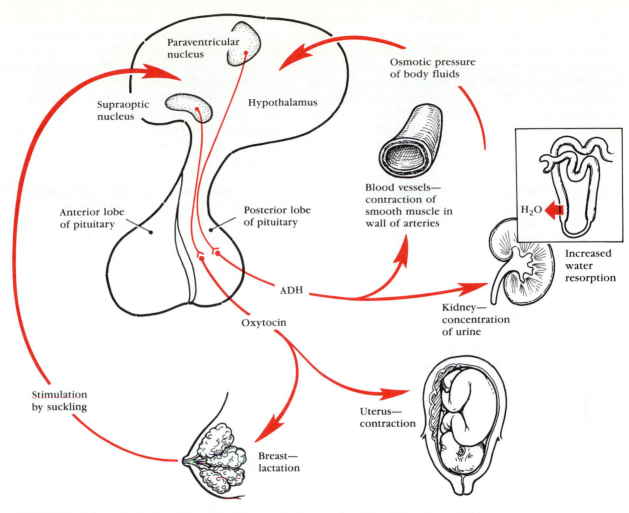

FIGURE 36-7   *Schematic drawing of the mechanisms involved in controlling the activities of the posterior lobe of the pituitary gland. ADH, antidiuretic hormone.*

uniform secretion of ADH maintains the fluid balance. If body fluids are depleted or osmotic pressure rises, appropriate mechanisms are activated and ADH is released. This stimulates the kidneys to reabsorb more water, which restores blood volume or reduces osmotic pressure, and balance is achieved. The state of balance inhibits release of ADH until further need arises.

Other factors that may influence ADH secretion include trauma, pain, anxiety, and drugs such as nicotine, morphine, and tranquilizers. Alcohol inhibits secretion, which partially accounts for the diuresis associated with excess intake of alcohol.

OXYTOCIN

EFFECTS ON THE UTERUS.   Oxytocin stimulates the contraction of smooth muscle in a number of organs in the human body. A major physiologic role of this hormone is to stimulate smooth muscle cells in the pregnant uterus. It is released in large quantities during the expulsive phase of parturition. The mechanism by which oxytocin release is triggered has been described as follows.

When labor begins, the tissues of the uterine cervix and vagina distend and become stretched. This stretch reflex initiates afferent impulses to the hypothalamus and stimulates the synthesis of oxytocin in cell bodies of the paraventricular nucleus. Oxytocin then migrates down the nerve fibers of the hypothalamicohypophyseal stalk to the neurohypophysis. From there, it is released into the circulation and carried by the blood to the uterus, where it acts on smooth muscle cells to reinforce uterine contraction. Because the greatest amounts of oxytocin are present in the blood during the expulsive stage of labor, it appears that the quantity released depends on the forcefulness of uterine contractions and the degree of stretch of cervical and vaginal tissues. It is recognized that oxytocin may be one of the factors that precipitate labor.[18]

EFFECTS ON LACTATION.   A second major role of oxytocin is to eject milk from lactating breasts. Milk formed by cells of the breasts is stored until suckling begins. For about 30 seconds to 1 minute after suckling is initiated, no milk is ejected. This is called the latent period. During this period, suckling stimuli to the nipple initiate signals that are transmitted to neuron cell bodies in the paraventricular and supraoptic nuclei to initiate posterior pituitary release of oxytocin. Circulating blood transports oxytocin to the breasts, where it initiates contraction of myoepithelial cells to force milk out of the alveoli into the ducts and lacteal sinuses opening to the nipple.[11] Because epinephrine inhibits oxytocin secretion, emotion, anxiety, and pain can inhibit oxytocin release and, thus, lactation.

EFFECTS ON FERTILIZATION. In lower animals, distention and stretch of vaginal and cervical tissues during copulation increases the secretion of oxytocin. Uterine contractions experienced during orgasm have been attributed in part to this increased secretion. It also has been postulated that oxytocin facilitates fertilization by causing the uterus to propel semen upward through the fallopian tubes. It is unknown if this process occurs in the human female.[11]

▼ Introduction to Pituitary Pathology

Malfunctions of the pituitary gland result from one or more of the following conditions: 1) invasive or impinging tumors of the pituitary or hypothalamus; 2) vascular infarction within the gland; 3) mechanical damage from trauma or surgery; 4) inflammatory processes; 5) genetic or familial predisposition; 6) developmental and structural anomalies of the gland itself; 7) feedback from prolonged malfunction of one or more of its target glands; 8) autoimmune responses; and 9) conditions of idiopathic origin.[5, 21]

Symptoms of pituitary malfunction may be precipitated by changes in hormonal balance or by purely mechanical forces. For example, tumors of the pituitary cause malfunction because of pressure from their space-occupying properties, destruction of tissue, and contributions to hypersecretion as a result of tumor cell secretory capacity. More advanced or larger lesions may impinge on surrounding tissues, such as the optic chiasma or the area of the third ventricle, producing visual disorders, headaches, or other neurologic changes.[21] Vascular and tumor infarctions, structural and developmental anomalies or inflammatory processes, and autoimmune responses influence functioning by compromising or destroying tissue. Feedback from malfunction of a target gland can result in hyperplasia of the pituitary gland.

Because the pituitary is a crucial link in the production of several hormones, abnormalities of the gland often alter normal hormone secretion. Pressure or tissue destruction may compromise function and result in problems associated with hyposecretion. Conversely, because many tumors of the pituitary secrete hormones, the presence of these lesions may result in symptoms stemming from hypersecretion.

Factors that influence hormone secretions of the pituitary inevitably influence functions of the specific endocrine gland, depending on the hormone. For example, conditions that stimulate hyperfunctioning of the pituitary initiate excessive activation of the target organs, whereas suppression or destruction of pituitary tissue with loss of hormone secretions results in hypofunction of target organs.

For convenience, pituitary pathologies may be divided into disorders of the adenohypophysis and those of the neurohypophysis. These may be subdivided further as disorders of hyperfunctioning or hypofunctioning. Because the anterior and posterior lobes of the pituitary operate as distinct and separate functional units, malfunctions of each have different characteristics.

▼ Pathology of the Anterior Pituitary

Four types of anterior pituitary disorders usually are described: enlargement of the sella turcica with or without evidence of a space-occupying lesion, visual disorders, hypopituitary hormone secretion, and hyperpituitary hormone secretion.[6] Hormone deficiencies resulting in malfunction may be classified as primary, secondary, or tertiary. Primary deficiencies are the result of disease of the target gland; secondary deficiencies result from pituitary lesions or disorders; tertiary deficiencies result from hypothalamic disorders.[6]

DIAGNOSTIC ASSESSMENT OF THE ANTERIOR PITUITARY

Evaluation of persons with pituitary diseases may include physical examination and radiologic, neuroophthalmic, and endocrine diagnostic studies. The types of tests used and the extent of testing depend on the symptoms. Radiologic studies include plain skull films, computed tomography, pneumoencephalography, and arteriography (see pp. 964–967). Neuroophthalmic evaluation is done by formal visual field examination with tangent screening. Endocrine studies include plasma levels and urinary excretion levels of each of the pituitary and target gland hormones. Radioimmunoassay is an important advance in diagnosis of endocrine problems. Antibodies that are specific for certain chemical groups are used; the accuracy of assay results depends on the specificity of the antibody and its ability to bind the hormone.[1] Other assays include protein-binding and radioreceptor assays that use proteins to bind to the hormones.

Chemical assays and free hormone levels are other methods of determining certain hormone concentrations. Free hormone can be assessed directly or by measuring bound hormone and calculating the free level. Plasma or urinary levels indicate marked excess or deficiency. To evaluate the results, the normal circadian pattern, stress reaction, and other factors must be taken into consideration. Urine measurements are much more effective for steroid hormones than for protein-derived hormones because the metabolites of the former are excreted in urine. Dynamic testing assesses the ability of the gland to respond to stimulation. Hormones that stimulate a response may be administered, or suppressive drugs or substances may be given. Many other tests provide indirect information, and include serum glucose, calcium, and potassium.[1]

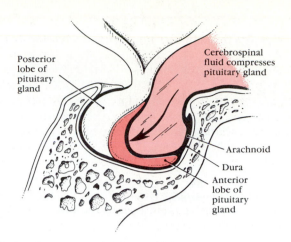

FIGURE 36-8 *Empty sella syndrome.*

ENLARGEMENT OF THE SELLA TURCICA

An increase in the size of the sella turcica often results from erosion of this structure caused by pressure from lesions in the pituitary region. Enlargement may be caused by pituitary adenomas, craniopharyngiomas, meningiomas, epithelial cysts, granulomas, malignant tumors of primary origin, or metastases from carcinomas of the breast. Enlargement may result from nontumorous enlargement of the sella, called *empty-sella syndrome*. Sella enlargement also may result from primary hypothyroidism or hypogonadism, which may be attributed to hyperplasia of the thyrotropes or gonadotropes because it is accompanied by elevated thyrotropin or gonadotropin levels.[6] This condition is seen more commonly in children.

Endocrine evaluation for an enlarged sella turcica should include assessment of thyroid and adrenal hormone levels together with basal gonadotropin levels. Basal PRL levels are important, because more than one-half of pituitary tumors secrete PRL.

EMPTY-SELLA SYNDROME

The empty-sella syndrome is classified as primary or secondary, according to its underlying cause. *Primary, or idiopathic, empty-sella syndrome* results from an abnormally large opening through which the hypophyseal stalk passes. This often is a developmental defect. With increased intracranial pressure, the arachnoid membrane tends to herniate through the opening, creating a sac filled with cerebrospinal fluid. This compresses the pituitary gland against the wall of the sella turcica, creating the appearance of an empty sella (Fig. 36-8). The condition also may occur as a consequence of necrosis of a pituitary adenoma or of Sheehan syndrome, which are discussed on page 689. *Secondary empty-sella syndrome* can develop as a result of spontaneous infarction or of regression of a tumor. The secondary variant of the syndrome results from ablation of the gland by irradiation or surgery.

Radiographically, the sella may appear enlarged or normal in size. The primary disease seldom is manifested as pituitary hypofunction. If hypofunction occurs, it usually is evidenced by depressed GH and gonadotropin secretion.

About 90% of persons with primary empty-sella syndrome are female. Most often, it is asymptomatic.[12] It is diagnosed most often in obese, hypertensive, middle-aged women who have borne many children. The tendency for the pituitary to enlarge during pregnancy and regress afterward may be the basis of pathogenesis. Headache is a common symptom. Visual field defects are rare but do occur in persons who have infarction of a pituitary tumor with subsequent development of empty-sella syndrome or if the optic chiasma prolapses into the sella.

HYPOPITUITARISM

Hypopituitarism may be initiated by extremely low secretion of pituitary hormones or by pituitary or hypothalamic disease.[19] *Panhypopituitarism* refers to the failure of all cell types in the pituitary gland. Surgical hypophysectomy (removal of the pituitary) causes dramatic clinical features of both anterior and posterior hormone deficiency.[7] The most common processes are Sheehan pituitary necrosis, nonsecreting adenoma, and craniopharyngioma. These, along with other causes are indicated in Table 36-4. Evaluation and diagnosis are by physical examination, neuroophthalmic evaluation, and measurement of baseline hormone levels.

Anterior pituitary hormone deficits may occur singly or in various combinations. The speed of onset and extent of hormone deficiency depend on the nature and size of the precipitating cause. Onset may be acute and life-threatening, as in acute adrenocortical insufficiency. More often, however, onset is slow, and it may occur over a period of months or years. Clinical signs and symptoms seldom manifest until at least 75% of the anterior lobe is destroyed.[5]

TABLE 36-4 *Pituitary Lesions Causing Hypopituitarism*

TUMORS
Pituitary adenoma
Craniopharyngioma
Metastatic carcinoma
Primary pituitary carcinoma
Meningioma

PITUITARY INFARCTION
Pituitary apoplexy (pituitary tumor)
Postpartum pituitary necrosis (Sheehan's syndrome)
Diabetes mellitus
Shock
Sickle cell anemia (crisis)
Infections (malaria, epidemic hemorrhagic fever)
Cavernous sinus thrombosis
Vasculitis (temporal arteritis, Takayasu's arteritis)
Trauma (stalk section or sella fracture)

INFILTRATIVE DISEASES
Sarcoidosis
Tuberculosis
Leukemia
Lymphoma
Hemochromatosis
Autoimmune hypophysitis

MISCELLANEOUS
Hypophysectomy
Radiation necrosis
Carotid artery aneurysm
Pituitary abscess
Congenital anomalies (hypoplasia, aplasia)

Kelley, W.W. *Textbook of Internal Medicine* (2nd ed.). Philadelphia: J.B. Lippincott, 1992.

Signs and symptoms of anterior pituitary insufficiency depend on the age of the affected person, the underlying destructive process, and the extent and rapidity of hormone loss.[17] In adults, the clinical features of panhypopituitarism include absence of axillary and pubic hair, genital and breast atrophy, skin pallor, pallor of nipples, fine skin wrinkling (especially of the face), intolerance to cold, premature aging, poor muscle development, amenorrhea in premenopausal women, loss of previously normal libido and potency in men, and several endocrine deficiencies. Shortness of stature may be evident if onset occurs before puberty. If hypothyroidism is marked, overweight is common. Reduced visual acuity, optic atrophy, and hemianopsia may occur if there is suprasellar expansion of a lesion or mass.

Diagnosis is made on the basis of history and physical examination, neuroophthalmic examination, and plasma immunoassay. Treatment consists of hormone replacement to reestablish function. Thyroid replacement hormones, cortisone, or hydrocortisone may be used as indicated. In women, diethylstilbestrol or preparations of conjugated estrogens (Premarin) help to maintain secondary sex characteristics; androgens or testosterone can restore libido and potency in men.

DEFICIENCIES OF SINGLE ANTERIOR PITUITARY HORMONES

PROLACTIN DEFICIENCY. Postpartum failure to lactate is the only symptom of clinical significance in deficient PRL secretion. This condition has classically been associated with Sheehan syndrome, the postpartum pituitary necrosis that results from hemorrhage and shock during delivery (see next page).

GONADOTROPIN DEFICIENCY. As previously stated, hypogonadism is the most common pituitary deficiency among adults. Its occurrence in the premenopausal woman is manifested by amenorrhea, atrophy of the breasts and uterus, and cornification of the vaginal orifice. A man experiences testicular atrophy associated with decreases in libido, potency, beard growth, and muscle tone. If onset of the deficiency occurs before puberty, the manifestations include eunuchoid appearance, lack of development of secondary sex characteristics, and infertility. Men fail to develop facial hair, an adult male voice, and normal genitalia. Women fail to manifest normal breast development and onset of menses. Both sexes may exhibit absence of axillary and pubic hair. The most common tumors responsible for the syndrome are the craniopharyngioma, a congenital tumor in the suprasellar region, and the chromophobe adenoma, which arises in the pituitary chromophobes.[6, 7]

Fröhlich syndrome is a severe gonadotropin deficiency that usually affects prepubertal boys. It includes obesity and hypogonadism associated with diabetes insipidus, retardation, and visual problems, all of which are related to hypothalamic rather than pituitary dysfunction. The obesity is probably the result of hypothalamic-induced overeating.[15]

THYROTROPIN DEFICIENCY. Hypothalamic or pituitary hypothyroidism exhibits some symptoms in common with primary hypothyroidism but usually is less severe. Isolated TSH deficiency is rare, however, and symptoms of other anterior lobe hormone deficiency usually are present concomitantly. This factor differentiates pituitary from primary hypothyroidism. In pituitary hypothyroidism, fine wrinkling of the skin and loss of secondary sex characteristics, which are related to gonadal insufficiency, are distinguishing characteristics. Menstrual history is significant, because menorrhagia is common in primary hypothyroidism, whereas amenorrhea is expected in the pituitary form.[21]

DEFICIENCY OF ADRENOCORTICOTROPIC HORMONE. Deficiency of ACTH is the most serious of the endocrine deficiencies in persons with anterior pituitary disease.[21] Like pituitary hypothyroidism, ACTH deficiency usually is associated with deficiency of other pituitary hormones; this can be a characteristic that differentiates pituitary origin from adrenal origin of disease. Symptoms include poor response to stress, nausea, vomiting, hyperthermia, and collapse. Decreased skin and nipple pigmentation is exhibited, which also differentiates pituitary hypoadrenalism from primary adrenal disease (see pp. 703–704).

DEFICIENCY OF GROWTH HORMONE. GH deficiency affects children in their formative years. It is caused by a suprasellar cyst or craniopharyngioma that impedes thalamic or pituitary function. Genetic transmission of GH deficiency accounts for about 10% of pituitary dwarfism and results from an autosomal recessive trait.[21] It often is associated with evidence of sella turcica destruction seen radiographically. It also can be caused by ischemic necrosis and inflammatory changes.

Deficiency of GH is considered in children whose proportional short stature (below the third percentile) is far below that of their normal counterparts. Other characteristics include delayed sexual development associated with bright rather than dull mentality. Most children with this condition exhibit excess subcutaneous fat, poorly developed muscles, thin hair, and underdeveloped nails. In some cases, an appearance of premature aging is evident, with dry, wrinkled skin.

The characteristics of normal mentality and anatomic symmetry without gross deformity differentiate the person with GH deficiency from one with *cretinism* resulting from thyroid deficiency.[5]

SHEEHAN SYNDROME. Sheehan syndrome, or postpartum pituitary necrosis, was first described as pituitary necrosis occurring after a delivery complicated by hemorrhage and shock. In the course of pregnancy, the pituitary gland enlarges and develops increased circulation. In the event of acute blood loss, which sometimes accompanies labor and delivery, sudden systematic hypotension can precipitate ischemia and destruction of the anterior lobe.[5] The result is hypofunction of the gland. There may be a lag of months or years between the intrapartum incident and full development of symptoms. Characteristic symptoms are common to a variety of pathologic processes that destroy a significant proportion of pituitary function. Therefore, the syndrome may be produced by any destructive lesion of the pituitary.

Symptoms depend on the degree of impairment of pituitary function relative to the extent of tissue destruction. These symptoms initially include evidence of increased intracranial pressure, headache, visual deficits, stiff neck, papilledema, and convulsions, later followed by symptoms of hormone deficiency, including gonadal, thyroidal, and adrenal effects.[6]

HYPERPITUITARISM

Pituitary hypersecretion normally involves overproduction of only a single hormone except in certain hormone-secreting tumors.[21] It often is caused by a decreased feedback signal when there is hypofunction of a target gland. The pituitary responds to the decreased hormone level by increasing production of the stimulating hormone. Pituitary adenomas also may secrete primarily one type of hormone. These almost exclusively involve the somatotropic (GH), lactotropic (PRL), or corticotropic (ACTH) cells.[21]

HYPERPROLACTINEMIA. Women with PRL-secreting adenomas may exhibit galactorrhea, amenorrhea, or depressed libido. Some exhibit evidence of decreased estrogens and hirsutism (excessive hair growth in inappropriate places), which are believed to be the result of depression of ovarian function or stimulation of adrenal androgen function. Men with PRL-secreting adenomas do not exhibit galactorrhea because of lack of development of acini in the male breasts. These lesions in men usually occur only as space-occupying lesions with hypogonadism. The hypogonadism apparently occurs because of a defect in endogenous gonadotropin-releasing hormone.[7] Diagnosis and evaluation are by radiologic studies and studies of basal PRL level.

HYPERSECRETION OF ADRENOCORTICOTROPIC HORMONE. Excess secretion of ACTH by the pituitary gland results in *Cushing disease*. Excess ACTH stimulates excess cortisol, which causes alteration in the distribution of fat and blood glucose along with other disruptions (see p. 701). If the excess cortisol is caused by adrenal overproduction, the condition is called *Cushing syndrome*. Manifestations of Cushing syndrome are detailed on page 702. Cushing disease of pituitary origin is most frequently caused by a basophil ACTH-secreting adenoma of the gland. Excess ACTH causes hyperplasia and hyperfunction of the adrenal cortex.

HYPERSECRETION OF GROWTH HORMONE. Hypersecretion of GH that occurs before puberty results in *gigantism*. This pituitary abnormality has been defined as height exceeding 80 in (203 cm) in adults or exceeding three standard deviations above the mean for age in children. The disorder is the result of oversecretion of GH by a pituitary adenoma in a growing child before closure of the epiphyses. Before epiphyseal closure, growth is linear and symmetric. Hypogonadism often is associated and leads to delayed epiphyseal closure and a more prolonged growth period.[7]

Clinical features of gigantism include symmetric growth of stature to enormous proportions, sometimes reaching 8 to 9 ft (244 to 274 cm) in height. Growth is symmetric because both epiphyseal and oppositional bone growth occur concurrently. Affected people also may develop the distortions that are characteristic of acromegaly. Cardiac hypertrophy often is associated with mild hypertension that eventually may lead to cardiac failure.[7] Thyroid enlargement and adrenocortical hyperplasia occasionally occur. Early in the course of the disease, people with gigantism may be unusually strong, but osteoporosis and muscle weakness are characteristic in later stages.[6, 7]

Acromegaly occurs when GH-secreting tumors of the pituitary develop after puberty and after fusion of the epiphyses. After epiphyseal closure, linear growth of bones is no longer possible. Tissues thicken and growth takes place in the acral areas (hands, feet, nose, and mandible).[6] The clinical signs and symptoms associated with acromegaly result from 1) the local effects produced by tumor growth on other pituitary hormones, producing hypopituitarism; 2) the effects of tumor growth on extrasellar CNS structures; and 3) the effects of hypersecretion of GH.[13, 14]

Somatotropic adenomas are predominantly responsible for acromegaly. Growth of the tumor ultimately may destroy normal cells. As a consequence, hypopituitarism may develop as the disease progresses. Both sexes are affected equally, and the condition most often is detected in the third or fourth decade of life. The disease progresses slowly and insidiously and often goes undetected for years. Affected persons may first notice progressive increase in ring, shoe, hat, and glove sizes. The skull and head increase in size, and the fingers and hands become broad and spadelike. Increased growth of subcutaneous connective tissue of the face leads to coarsening of the features (Fig. 36-9). The face assumes a thick, fleshy appearance. The lips are thickened and enlarged, and have accentuated skin folds. The ears and nose become enlarged because of hypertrophy of the cartilages. There is overgrowth of the supraorbital ridge, and the cheeks become prominent. Overgrowth of the maxilla results in lengthening of the face, and alveolar bone growth results in separations of the teeth. Overgrowth of the mandible results in prognathism (jaw projection).

Hypertrophy of the costal cartilage leads to an increased circumference of the chest. Absorption of bone is rapid, and osteoporosis occurs. Acromegalic arthritis develops from proliferation of joint cartilage and affects the joints of the long bones and the spine. Long bones thicken and become massive. There often is bowing of the legs.

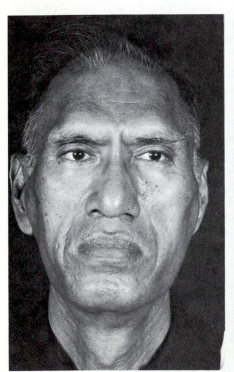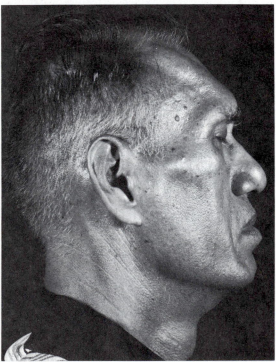

FIGURE 36-9 *A 64-year-old man with acromegaly. Note the prominent, "lantern-like" jaw, the large zygomatic arches and supraorbital ridges, and the sloping "beetle brow." The bony overgrowth often results in a comparative hollowing of the temporal region. The nose and ears are enlarged, and the latter may be calcified. The skin folds are exaggerated, the skin is tough and oily, and there is enlargement of the sebaceous glands and pores. (Becker, K.L. Principles and practice of endocrinology and metabolism [2nd ed.]. Philadelphia: J.B. Lippincott, 1995.)*

The skin becomes thickened, and hirsutism occurs in females. The tongue enlarges and may protrude from the mouth. The lungs, liver, spleen, kidneys, and intestines enlarge twofold to fivefold. Hypertension, coronary artery atherosclerosis, and marked cardiomegaly occur. Congestive heart failure often develops. The gonads enlarge, but their function is subnormal. The adrenals, thyroid, and parathyroid become enlarged.[6]

The typical physical picture is one of a big, burly person with forward carriage of the head, prognathism, kyphosis, bowlegs, prominent forehead, thickened chest, and husky, cavernous voice (Fig. 36-10). Many men develop impotence and women develop amenorrhea. Growth of the adenoma apparently impinges on the normal cells and induces insufficiency of other hormones.

Diagnosis is by assessment of physical characteristics, serial radiographs, and photographs. Laboratory immunoassay of plasma GH levels and response to glucose stimulation during a glucose tolerance test can help in diagnosis. People normally suppress GH after ingestion of 100 g of glucose, but the acromegalic patient may show increased levels.[13]

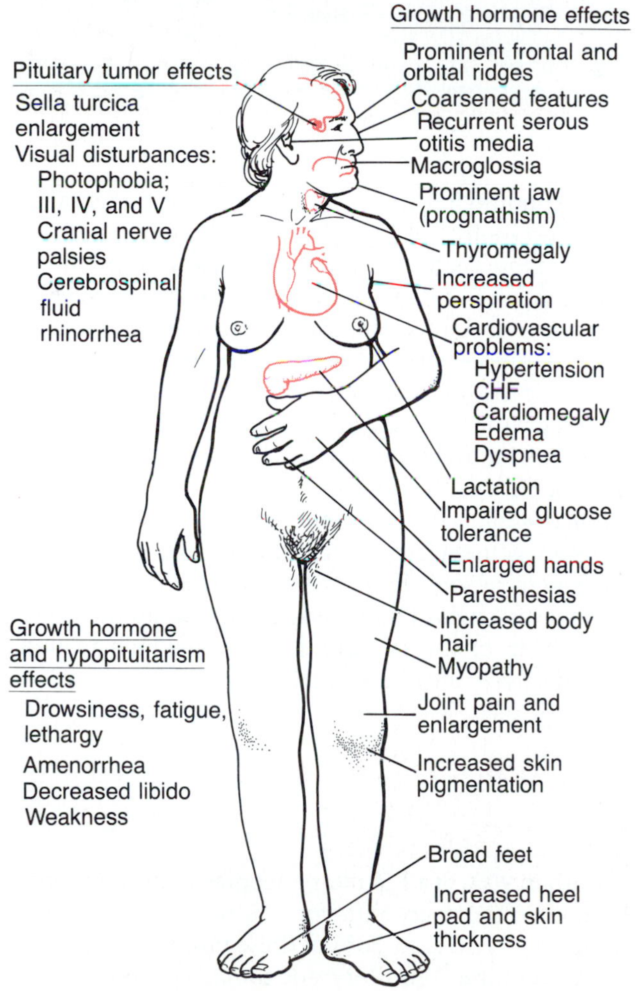

▼ Pathology of the Posterior Pituitary

Pathologic conditions stemming from lesions of the neurohypophysis are rare. Posterior lobe pathology is almost always related to primary disease or other processes outside the gland itself. The posterior lobe releases two hormones, ADH and oxytocin, which are synthesized and secreted by the hypothalamus.

DIABETES INSIPIDUS

A deficiency in ADH release causes the condition known as diabetes insipidus. The underlying causes of ADH deficiency have been categorized as follows: 1) neoplastic or inflammatory processes that impinge on the hypothalamoneurohypophyseal axis, such as adenomas, metastatic carcinoma, abscesses, meningitis, tuberculosis, and sarcoidosis; 2) surgical or irradiation injury to the hypothalamoneurohypophyseal axis, such as hypophysectomy; 3) severe head injuries; and 4) idiopathic influences (Box 36-1). Rarely, the syndrome is familial and is inherited as a mendelian dominant.[5, 20]

Lack of ADH causes a failure of the distal and collecting ducts of the nephrons to reabsorb water. Water is lost through a dilute, low-osmolarity urine despite hyperosmolarity in the serum and extracellular fluid.[8] The resulting clinical features of diabetes insipidus include polyuria, excessive thirst, and polydipsia. Polyuria causes a rise in serum osmolarity that stimulates the thirst center. In persons who are unable to respond with the thirst mechanism, such as those with severe head injuries, hypernatremia and hyperosmolarity rapidly develop.[4] Normal function of the thirst center ensures that polydipsia replaces water lost through polyuria.[20] Symptoms usually are sudden in onset and pronounced, with urine output reaching 10 L or more in a 24-hour period. Urine is pale, and its concentration is very dilute, with a specific gravity less than 1.005. Diagnosis is on the basis of clinical manifestations, dehydration tests, and response to vasopressin administration. Treatment is administration of ADH (vasopressin), usually by nasal spray.

SYNDROME OF INAPPROPRIATE ANTIDIURETIC HORMONE

The syndrome of inappropriate ADH (SIADH) is the persistent release of ADH unrelated to plasma osmolarity or volume deficit. The normal feedback inhibition of the posterior pituitary is hypoactive or inactive, caus-

Growth hormone effects

Prominent frontal and orbital ridges
Coarsened features
Recurrent serous otitis media
Macroglossia
Prominent jaw (prognathism)
Thyromegaly
Increased perspiration
Cardiovascular problems:
  Hypertension
  CHF
  Cardiomegaly
  Edema
  Dyspnea
Lactation
Impaired glucose tolerance
Enlarged hands
Paresthesias
Increased body hair
Myopathy
Joint pain and enlargement
Increased skin pigmentation
Broad feet
Increased heel pad and skin thickness

Pituitary tumor effects

Sella turcica enlargement
Visual disturbances:
  Photophobia;
  III, IV, and V
  Cranial nerve palsies
Cerebrospinal fluid rhinorrhea

Growth hormone and hypopituitarism effects

Drowsiness, fatigue, lethargy
Amenorrhea
Decreased libido
Weakness

FIGURE 36-10 *Appearance of acromegaly. Clinical manifestations relate to growth hormone secretion and effects from tumor encroachment in small pituitary space.*

BOX 36-1 ▼ *Causes of Diabetes Insipidus*

I. Vasopressin deficiency (neurogenic or central diabetes insipidus)
   A. Decreased secretion
      1. Idiopathic
         a. Sporadic (? autoimmune)
         b. Familial (autosomal dominant inheritance)
      2. Traumatic (accidental or surgical)
      3. Malignancy
         a. Primary (craniopharyngioma, germinoma, meningioma, pituitary adenoma with suprasellar extension)
         b. Metastatic (lung, breast, leukemia)
      4. Granuloma (sarcoid, histiocytosis, xanthoma, dissemination)
      5. Infectious (meningitis, encephalitis, syphilis)
      6. Vascular (aneurysm, Sheehan's syndrome, cardiac arrest, vasculitis)
      7. Psychobiologic (anorexia nervosa)
      8. Toxic (carbon monoxide)
      9. Congenital malformations
   B. Increased metabolism
      1. Pregnancy
II. Vasopressin resistance (nephrogenic diabetes insipidus
   A. Idiopathic
      1. Sporadic
      2. Familial (X-linked recessive inheritance)
   B. Post obstructive
   C. Malignancy (retroperitoneal fibrosarcoma)
   D. Granuloma (sarcoid)
   E. Infectious (pyelonephritis)
   F. Vascular (sickle cell disease or trait)
   G. Metabolic (hypokalemia, hypercalciuria)
   H. Toxic (lithium, demeclocycline, methoxyflurane, methicillin)
   I. Malformations (polycystic disease)
   J. Pregnancy
III. Excessive water intake (primary polydipsia)
   A. Psychogenic (schizophrenia, affective disorders)
   B. Dipsogenic
      1. Idiopathic
      2. Traumatic
      3. Granuloma (neurosarcoidosis)
      4. Infectious (meningitis)
      5. Other (multiple sclerosis)

(J. Stein [ed.]. *Internal Medicine, 4th ed.* St. Louis. CV Mosby, 1994.)

BOX 36-2 ▼ *Differential Diagnosis of the Syndrome of Inappropriate Antidiuretic Hormone (SIADH) Secretion*

Neoplasms
    Lung (small cell in 80%), pancreas, duodenum, lymphoma, ureter, prostate, Ewing sarcoma
Pulmonary
    Infection (viral, bacterial, fungal), abscess, asthma, respirator therapy
Central nervous system
    Trauma, neoplasms, infections, vascular, degenerative diseases (including aging), psychoses
Cardiac
    Atrial tachycardias, post–mitral commissurotomy syndrome
Metabolic
    Myxedema, adrenal insufficiency, acute porphyria, anterior pituitary insufficiency, angiotensin II
Stress
Drugs
    Hypoglycemic agents (chlorpropamide, tolbutamide) antineoplastic drugs (cyclophosphamide, vincristine), narcotics (morphine, barbiturates), psychotropics (phenothiazine derivatives)

Stein, J. (ed.). *Internal Medicine* (4th ed.). St. Louis. Mosby, 1994.

Other conditions capable of this ectopic secretion include carcinoma of the pancreas, lymphoma, bronchogenic tuberculosis, Hodgkin disease, and thymoma. Disorders and trauma of the CNS, such as subdural hematoma and infection, may be the basis of malfunction. Conditions such as stress, pain, and hypovolemia may cause the physiologic release of ADH in the absence of a hypertonic plasma.[20] Diagnosis is made on the basis of serum sodium levels and the clinical picture of hypervolemia. It should be suspected in any person with hyponatremia who has hypertonic urine.

Management includes fluid restriction, diuretics, assessment of sodium balance, assessment for evidence of congestive heart failure, and treatment for the underlying cause of the syndrome. No drugs are available that effectively suppress ADH.

▼ Tumors of the Pituitary

ADENOMAS

More than 90% of all pituitary neoplasms are adenomas. Pituitary tumors account for 6% to 18% of all brain tumors. Only 10% to 20% of these pituitary tumors are nonfunctioning.[7] Pituitary adenomas can be classified according to predominant cell type and also according to their secretory qualities. They may interfere with pituitary functions by virtue of their space-occupying properties or by secretions of various hormones. In general,

ing continued release of ADH. The result is excessive reabsorption of water in the renal system and excessive retention of water with expansion of fluid volume. Fluid overload, hyponatremia, and hemodilution result.

The syndrome may occur from a stimulus either inside the hypothalamicohypophyseal system or from an outside source (Box 36-2). It may occur as a result of a tumor of the hypothalamus or hypophysis that impinges on tissues that control secretions. SIADH also may result from a paraneoplastic syndrome in which nonendocrine tumors demonstrate inappropriate secretion of ADH.[3] Oat cell bronchogenic carcinoma is the most common ADH-secreting lesion causing SIADH.

problems stemming from the space-occupying factor are the result of destruction or suppression of surrounding tissue. Those stemming from secretory properties result in hypersecretion or hyperfunction. All lesions can produce CNS symptoms or visual problems because of their space-occupying properties, depending on the size and location of the lesion.

The growth pattern of adenomas is variable and is unrelated to hormone secretion. The tumors often become apparent clinically because of their compressive effect or because of impingement on adjoining structures. Pituitary adenomas are almost always benign but may exhibit aggressive growth so that surgical removal is difficult or impossible.[7]

Pituitary adenomas can cause neurologic or endocrinologic clinical signs and symptoms, including visual or neurologic deficits, headaches, or impaired gonadal function. Because of the anatomic location of the pituitary, a tumor may impinge on the opthalmic nerve, causing neuroophthalmic symptoms.[16] The tumors may be discovered accidentally on review of skull films. Growth disturbances such as acromegaly or gigantism may be the major sign of a GH-secreting adenoma. PRL-secreting adenomas cause gonadal dysfunction, and ACTH-secreting adenomas may produce Cushing disease.

Craniopharyngiomas (*Rathke pouch tumors*) are tumors of congenital origin derived from remnants of the Rathke pouch. These lesions commonly occur in young children and usually are cystic, although some are solid. They normally are well encapsulated and benign, although some become malignant. Many contain sufficient calcification to be visualized on radiography. They may reach considerable size (8–10 cm in diameter). Because of location, they frequently compress the optic nerve, leading to visual impairment.[7, 21]

MALIGNANT TUMORS

Although they are rare, primary malignant lesions do occur in the anterior lobe of the pituitary. They occasionally arise in preexisting benign adenomas or craniopharyngiomas. Characteristically, they are fast-growing and rapidly exhibit clinical manifestations. These tumors are massive and extensively invade nearby structures. Distant metastases are common, especially to the liver. The histologic distinction between rapidly growing adenoma and carcinoma often is difficult.[5] Neoplastic metastasis to the pituitary is rare; it may occur with carcinoma of the breast, lung, or thyroid.

▼ *Chapter Summary*

▼ The endocrine system primarily functions through hormone interaction in the tissues. It is controlled by and controls many functions within the nervous system. There is a constant feedback process which allows for precise regulation of bodily functions. Hormones function through various mechanisms depending upon the target organ or cell. The basic types of hormones are steroids, tyrosine based, and protein-based. The actions of hormones are highly selective due to specific binding of receptors sites in target tissue.

▼ The pituitary gland or hypophysis is composed of two separate functional areas, the adenohypophysis (anterior) and neurohypophysis (posterior). The adenohypophysis secretes growth hormone, adrenocorticotropic hormone, prolactin, thyroid stimulating hormone, follicle-stimulating hormone, and luteinizing hormone. It also contains nonsecretory cells whose function is unknown. Most of the hormones of the adenohypophysis are under the influence of releasing hormones from the hypothalamus. The neurohypophysis contains neuroglials cells that store and secrete hormones made by the hypothalamus.

▼ The growth hormone is secreted under various stimuli and causes growth of bone and cartilage, increased protein metabolism, fat catabolism, elevation of blood glucose. All of these promote growth which is also influenced by nutritional status, exercise, stress, other hormones and other factors. Adrenocorticotropic hormone regulates synthesis and secretion of adrenal steroids by adrenal cortical tissue and it maintains the size and blood flow of the adrenal cortex. Prolactin functions in breast development and lactation. Thyroid stimulation activates synthesis and secretion of the hormones of the thyroid gland. Follicle stimulating hormone activates and stimulates the germinal epithelium of the seminiferous tubules to facilitate the rate of spermatogenesis. Leuteinizing hormone is necessary for the growth and secretory activity of the testicular interstitial cells. These hormones in women are essential for cyclic growth of the ovarian follicle and ovulation.

▼ The neurohypophysis secretes antidiuretic hormone (ADH) which is made in the hypothalamus. This hormone is essential to cause renal water reabsorption and thus keep the osmolarity of the plasma normal. Osmoreceptors regulate the amount of ADH secretion. Oxytocin stimulates the contraction of smooth muscle, especially the uterus. It is also essential to lactation.

▼ Pathology of the anterior pituitary may be described according to space occupying lesions which may cause neurologic defects or visual disorders or hormone secretion. Hypopituitarism may be initiated by low secretion of pituitary hormones or by hypothalamic disease. It may affect all of the pituitary hormones or specific hormone deficit. The signs and symptoms relate to the target organ effect. Hyperpituitarism normally involves overproduction of only a single hormone and may be due to target organ dysfunction or pituitary adenomas.

▼ Pathology of the posterior pituitary is mainly manifest in ADH secretion, either hyper or hypo secretion. The manifestations are directly related to fluid volume retention or deficit.

▼ Pituitary neoplasms are mainly adenomas and are classified according to predominant cell type or secretory qualities.

▼ *References*

1. Baxter, J.D. Principles of endocrinology. In Wyngaarden, J.B., and Smith, L.H. (eds.), *Cecil's Textbook of Medicine* (18th ed.). Philadelphia: W.B. Saunders, 1988.
2. Becker, K.L. *Principles and Practice of Endocrinology and Metabolism*. Philadelphia: J.B. Lippincott, 1991.
3. Bunn, P.A., and Ridgway, E.C. Paraneoplastic syndromes. In DeVita, V.T., Hellman, S., and Rosenberg, S.A. (eds.), *Cancer: Principles and Practice of Oncology* (4th ed.). Philadelphia: J.B. Lippincott, 1993.
4. Buonocore, C.M., and Robinson, A.G. The diagnosis and management of diabetes insipidus during medical emergencies. *Endocrinol Metab Clin North Am* 22:411–423, 1993.
5. Cotran, R.S., Kumar, V., and Robbins, S.L. *Robbins' Pathologic Basis of Disease* (5th ed.). Philadelphia: W.B. Saunders, 1994.
6. Daniels, G.H., and Martin, J.B. Neuroendocrine regulation of the anterior pituitary and hypothalamus. In Wilson, J.D., et al. (eds.), *Harrison's Principles of Internal Medicine* (12th ed.). New York: McGraw-Hill, 1991.
7. Frohman, L.A. The anterior pituitary. In Wyngaarden, J.B., and Smith, L.H. (eds.), *Cecil's Textbook of Medicine* (18th ed.). Philadelphia: W.B. Saunders, 1988.
8. Germon, K. Fluid and electrolyte problems associated with diabetes insipidus and syndrome of inappropriate antidiuretic hormone. *Nurs. Clin. North Am.* 22(4):785–796, 1987.
9. Greenspan, F.S. (ed.). *Basic and Clinical Endocrinology* (3rd ed.). Norwalk, Conn.: Appleton & Lange, 1991.
10. Griffin, J.E., and Ojeda, S.R. Organization of the endocrine system. In Griffin, J.E., and Ojeda, S.R. (eds.), *Textbook of Endocrine Physiology*. New York: Oxford University Press, 1988.
11. Guyton, A. *Textbook of Medical Physiology* (8th ed.). Philadelphia: W.B. Saunders, 1991.
12. Kannan, C.R. *The Pituitary Gland, Vol. 1*. New York: Plenum, 1987.
13. Mendelsohn, G. *Diagnosis and Pathology of Endocrine Diseases*. Philadelphia: J.B. Lippincott, 1988.
14. Molitch, M.E. Acromegaly. In Collu, R., Brown, G.M., and Van Loon, G.R. (eds.), *Clinical Neuroendocrinology*. Boston: Blackwell, 1988.
15. Olefsky, J.M. Obesity. In Wilson, J.D., et al. (eds.), *Harrison's Principles of Internal Medicine* (12th ed.). New York: McGraw-Hill, 1991.
16. Piziak, V.K., and Gilliland, P. F. Pituitary tumors: Look for early signs and symptoms. *Emerg Med* 25: 124–132, 1993.
17. Reasner, C.A. Anterior pituitary disease. *Crit Care Nurs Q* 13:62–66, 1990.
18. Reichlin, S. Neuroendocrinology. In Wilson, J.D., and Foster, D.W. (eds.), *Williams' Textbook of Endocrinology* (8th ed.). Philadelphia: W.B. Saunders, 1992.
19. Slaunwhite, W.R. *Fundamentals of Endocrinology*. New York: Dekker, 1988.
20. Streeten, D.H.P., Moses, A.M., and Miller, M. Disorders of the neurohypophysis. In Wilson, J.D., et al. (eds.), *Harrison's Principles of Internal Medicine* (12th ed.). New York: McGraw-Hill, 1991.
21. Thorner, M.O., Vance, M.L., Horvath, E. and Kovacs, K. The anterior pituitary. In Wilson, J.D., and Foster, D.W. (eds.), *Williams' Textbook of Endocrinology* (8th ed.). Philadelphia: W.B. Saunders, 1992.
22. Tortora, G., and Grabowski, S.R. *Principles of Anatomy and Physiology* (7th ed.). New York: HarperCollins, 1993.
23. Wilson, J.D. Hormones and hormone action. In Wilson, J.D., et al. (eds.), *Harrison's Principles of Internal Medicine* (12th ed.). New York: McGraw-Hill, 1991.

Chapter *37*

Adrenal Mechanisms and Alterations

Camille Stern

▼ **CHAPTER OUTLINE**

▼ **LEARNING OBJECTIVES**

1 Discuss the normal anatomy of the adrenal gland.
2 Describe the mechanisms that regulate adrenocortical hormone secretions.
3 Identify the pattern of synthesis of each of the major hormones of the adrenal cortex.
4 Outline the physiologic effects of mineralocorticoids, glucocorticoids, and androgen hormones.
5 Identify the process that results in Cushing syndrome.
6 Define **Cushing syndrome** and its major clinical manifestations.
7 Differentiate between primary and secondary aldosteronism.
8 Describe the pathologic process and resulting physical changes of the adrenogenital syndromes.
9 Outline the clinical manifestations of primary adrenocortical insufficiency.
10 Compare primary and secondary adrenocortical insufficiency.
11 Discuss the clinical features of adrenal crisis.
12 Describe catecholamine biosynthesis and storage.
13 Explain the cause of pheochromocytoma.
14 Outline the major clinical features of pheochromocytoma.
15 Discuss multiple endocrine neoplasia syndrome and its relation to pheochromocytoma.

The adrenal cortex and adrenal medulla and their associated hormones probably developed as protections from immediate stress or injury and against prolonged food and water deprivation. One of the primary functions of the adrenal glands remains protection of the body against both acute and chronic forms of stress.[9] The adrenal cortex and the adrenal medulla share adjacent sites but have no similar functions.

▼ Anatomy of the Adrenal Glands

The adrenal, or suprarenal, glands are located retroperitoneally at the superior pole of each kidney. Although structurally connected, the adrenal cortex and adrenal medulla are separate organs in both tissue origin and physiologic function. The adrenals are rather flat, with the right gland having a pyramidal appearance and the left a curved, semilunar shape (Fig. 37-1). A thick, fibrous capsule surrounds the glands, and peritoneal fasciae, independent of the kidneys, provide support. The usual weight of each gland in a healthy adult is between 3 and 6 g, and the adrenals tend to be slightly heavier in males.

Arterial blood supply is from the renal, or inferior, phrenic arteries or directly from the abdominal aorta. Inside the glands, the vessels break up into sinusoids and drain medially into the glands. Venous drainage is different for right and left glands. The right adrenal empties venous blood directly into the vena cava, whereas the left empties into the left renal vein. Nervous innervation is both sympathetic and parasympathetic. Nerves enter through the cortex and progress to the medulla.

The golden yellow adrenal cortex surrounds the medulla, which is more medially located. Three distinct layers make up the cortex. The first is the *zona glomerulosa*, composed of a thin layer of irregularly shaped cuboidal cells. Immediately beneath is the second layer, the *zona fasciculata*. Cuboidal cells of this layer run in long strands and are separated by the sinusoidal spaces. The third layer of the cortex, the *zona reticularis*, is composed of groups of cells of irregular shape (Fig. 37-2). Both the zona fasciculata and the zona reticularis are regulated so closely by adrenocorticotropic hormone (ACTH) that deficiency or excess alters their structure and function. During periods of adrenal inactivity, when ACTH is deficient, the cells of the zona fasciculata and reticularis atrophy and become filled with vacuoles; during periods of active function, when ACTH is present in large or excess amounts, hyperplasia and hyperactivity result.[19]

The adrenal medulla lies central to and is surrounded by the adrenal cortex. It is flat and gray and is composed of sheets of irregularly shaped masses of cells with small nuclei. The cells are surrounded by sinusoidal blood vessels.

▼ The Adrenal Cortex

ADRENOCORTICAL HORMONES

The adrenal cortex is responsible for the secretion of three major groups of steroid hormones. The *mineralocorticoids* and *glucocorticoids* are the two most important of these, with the third and less significant being the *androgens*. The major glucocorticoid is *cortisol*, which is secreted mostly by the zona fasciculata. The major mineralocorticoid is *aldosterone*, which is secreted by the zona glomerulosa almost independently of ACTH influence; ACTH is necessary only to maintain the viability of the glomerulosa cells. Androgens are produced by the

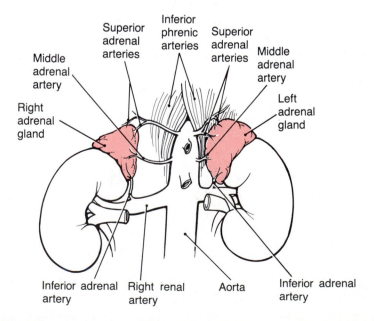

FIGURE 37-1 *Location and appearance of adrenal glands in anterior view.*

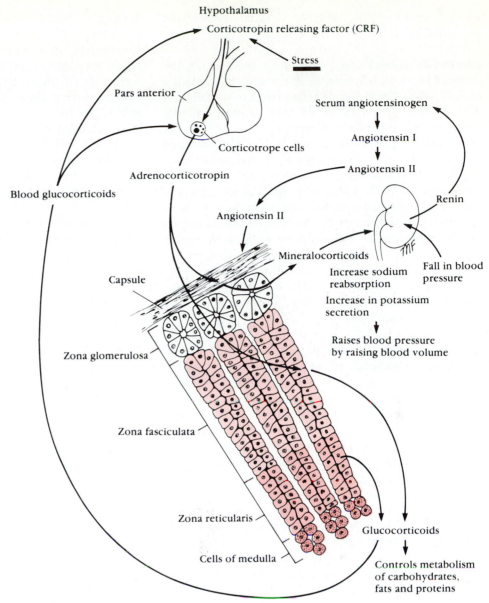

FIGURE 37-2 *Mechanisms involved in the control of mineralocorticoid secretion and glucocorticoid secretion of the adrenal cortex.*

cells of the zona fasciculata and probably also by the zona reticularis.

Regulation of adrenocortical hormone secretion is accomplished mainly through ACTH, which exerts direct control over the glucocorticoids and sex steroids. Aldosterone secretion is primarily controlled by the renin-angiotensin-aldosterone system and by serum potassium and sodium levels (see Figure 37-2).

Adrenocorticotropic Hormone

ACTH is produced by the anterior pituitary gland. Its release is controlled by corticotropin-releasing factor, which is produced by the hypothalamus (see pp. 678–682). The amount of circulating ACTH normally is controlled by three factors: circulating levels of cortisol, individual bio-rhythms, and stress. These factors, together with states of dysfunction, stimulate corticotropin-releasing factor to release ACTH into the bloodstream.

FEEDBACK SYSTEM OF CORTISOL AND ADRENOCORTICOTROPIC HORMONE. Cortisol regulates the activity of the hypothalamic-pituitary-adrenal axis by its feedback effects on both ACTH and corticotropin-releasing factor.[1] When circulating levels of cortisol decrease, ACTH acts directly on the adrenal cortex to stimulate production. Increased secretion of cortisol occurs within a few minutes after ACTH initiates production of the hormone. Low levels of ACTH result in decreased hormone biosynthesis and decreased renal blood flow. Thus, circulating levels of cortisol respond directly to a feedback system with ACTH. Decreased cortisol levels result in stimulation of ACTH, whereas elevated levels cause decreased release of ACTH.

EFFECTS OF BIORHYTHMS.   Individual biorhythms, the *circadian* or *diurnal rhythms*, affect the normal circulating level of ACTH. The pattern is related to sleep periods and may be altered by changes in daily activity.[21] In the hours before and just after waking, the ACTH level reaches the highest peak of the 24-hour day. The level decreases continuously during the remainder of the day. In relation to this pattern, cortisol level rises at about the same time as ACTH and also declines as the day progresses. The plasma cortisol concentration usually is highest on awakening in the morning, falls later during the day, and reaches the lowest level during the first 2 hours of sleep.[21] From this point, cortisol gradually returns to its maximum level before the period of waking (see pp. 181–182). Although the basic pattern of biorhythms is similar for all humans, wide variations can occur in any individual.

EFFECTS OF STRESS.   Any physical or emotional stress increases the secretion of ACTH, which results in increased production and secretion of cortisol. Stresses that may initiate this reaction include illness, hypotension, and exposure to extreme cold. The mechanism behind this effect is thought to be related to the ability of the glucocorticoids to provide the body with the materials needed for energy. These materials include amino acids, protein, fatty acids, glucose, sodium, and water, levels of all of which increase in a stressful situation.[2]

Specific stress responses of the body occur with the stages of the general adaptation syndrome as defined by Selye (see p. 178–182). Corticotropin-releasing hormone and ACTH often are referred to as the "stress hormones," and they are routinely measured as indicators of levels of stress and coping ability.[16] During the initial stages of the alarm phase of the general adaptation syndrome, acute release of epinephrine produces characteristic catecholamine effects. This is followed by changes that resemble adrenocortical insufficiency, such as decreased blood pressure, decreased levels of serum glucose and serum sodium, and increased levels of serum potassium. The period of insufficiency is followed by a period of active adrenocortical function that continues until a stable baseline has been reestablished. Stable levels of hormone production occur during the resistance phase. If the stage of exhaustion is reached, adrenocortical hormone insufficiency may once again be encountered.

Renin-Angiotensin-Aldosterone System

The renin-angiotensin-aldosterone (RAA) system is the major influence over the production of aldosterone by the zona glomerulosa. The enzymelike substance renin is released from the juxtaglomerular apparatus in the nephrons of the kidneys in response to changes in perfusion pressure and solute delivery in the renal distal tubules. Through a complex process of hydrolysis, renin undergoes chemical changes to become angiotensin II, which exerts a strong control over the regulation of aldosterone secretion (see Figure 37-2). The mechanism by which this is accomplished is not completely understood. It is known that the action is rapid and that the production of aldosterone stops when angiotensin II is removed. The renin-angiotensin-aldosterone system does not influence cortisol production or secretion.

EFFECT OF ELECTROLYTES ON ALDOSTERONE SECRETION.   The electrolyte with the most influence on aldosterone secretion is potassium. If serum potassium levels are elevated, aldosterone secretion increases. An increase in potassium of less than 1 mEq/L triples aldosterone secretion.[12] Lowered levels of potassium decrease the rate of aldosterone release.

Sodium functions by similar, but reverse, principles. Decreased sodium levels stimulate aldosterone secretion, and increased sodium concentrations inhibit aldosterone secretion.

Biosynthesis and Transport of Steroid Hormones

Biosynthesis of adrenocortical hormones, or steroids, uses cholesterol as the initial precursor (Flowchart 37-1). Cholesterol is obtained both from blood and from the adrenal cortex. Within the cortex, during normal states of activity, cholesterol is stored in lipid droplets in the cytoplasm of the cells. Although the adrenal cortex is capable of synthesizing cholesterol for steroid production, most is taken from these cholesterol stores that were obtained from cholesterol circulating in the bloodstream. During periods when the cortex is not being stimulated by one of the regulating mechanisms, available cholesterol remains in storage, and the production of steroid hormones is minimal.[12]

Stimulation from any of the adrenal regulators begins the process of steroid biosynthesis. Cholesterol undergoes many chemical and enzymatic conversions in the steroid manufacturing process. In this series of changes, the one step through which all steroids must pass is the conversion of cholesterol to pregnenolone. At this point, the production of the major hormones occurs by different and individual mechanisms.

After steroid biosynthesis, the steroid hormones are released into the bloodstream to be carried to the tissue cells. In the blood they bind to specific proteins known as *transcortins*, or *corticosteroid-binding globulins*, which have an affinity for all major steroids. Binding causes inactivation of the steroid hormones, excretion of the steroids by the kidneys, and prevention of excess tissue uptake. At

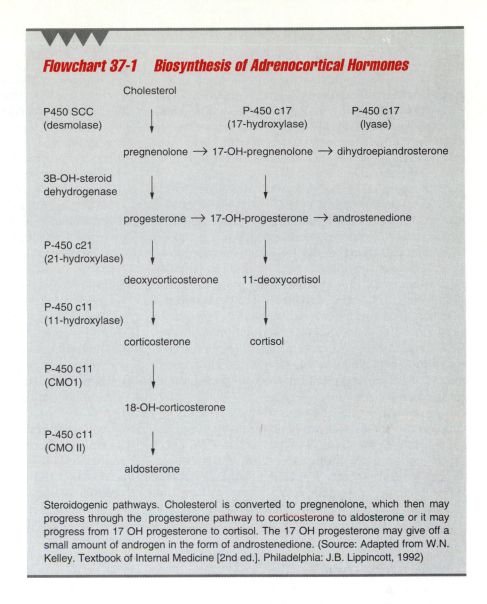

Flowchart 37-1 Biosynthesis of Adrenocortical Hormones

Cholesterol

P450 SCC
(desmolase)

P-450 c17
(17-hydroxylase)

P-450 c17
(lyase)

pregnenolone → 17-OH-pregnenolone → dihydroepiandrosterone

3B-OH-steroid
dehydrogenase

progesterone → 17-OH-progesterone → androstenedione

P-450 c21
(21-hydroxylase)

deoxycorticosterone   11-deoxycortisol

P-450 c11
(11-hydroxylase)

corticosterone   cortisol

P-450 c11
(CMO1)

18-OH-corticosterone

P-450 c11
(CMO II)

aldosterone

Steroidogenic pathways. Cholesterol is converted to pregnenolone, which then may progress through the progesterone pathway to corticosterone to aldosterone or it may progress from 17 OH progesterone to cortisol. The 17 OH progesterone may give off a small amount of androgen in the form of androstenedione. (Source: Adapted from W.N. Kelley. Textbook of Internal Medicine [2nd ed.]. Philadelphia: J.B. Lippincott, 1992)

the target site, the steroids are released to exert their physiologic action.

Physiologic Actions

MINERALOCORTICOIDS. The principal mineralocorticoid that exerts a physiologic action is aldosterone. Almost all mineralocorticoid activity is produced by this steroid, but cortisol contributes slightly. The single most important action of aldosterone is sodium retention. Because of this action and its resultant effect on intracellular and extracellular fluid volume, aldosterone has a profound effect on fluid balance.

Sodium retention results in a simultaneous loss of potassium by excretion in the urine. This exchange of ions takes place in the distal renal tubules. Together with sodium, water is retained. Thus, higher circulating levels of aldosterone cause sodium retention, increased plasma volume, and higher blood pressure; decreased circulat-

ing levels have opposite effects. Any excess or deficit in normal circulating aldosterone can lead to a variety of basic electrolyte disturbances with resultant effects on body functions.

In addition to the tubules, aldosterone acts on other tissues to retain sodium. Salivary and sweat glands are influenced to conserve sodium in extreme heat. Absorption of sodium by the intestinal mucosa prevents excess loss in fecal waste. Aldosterone also conserves sodium by influencing the exchange of intracellular and extracellular water.

GLUCOCORTICOIDS. Glucocorticoids are named for their ability to regulate serum glucose levels by several mechanisms. Their effect is not as pronounced or prolonged as that of the regulating ability of insulin. The primary action in the tissues is *catabolic*, with increased breakdown of proteins and increased excretion of nitrogen. In the liver, *anabolic* actions occur, such as increased amino acid uptake and increased synthesis of ribonucleic acid and protein.

The activities generated by the glucocorticoids are accomplished by the production and secretion of cortisol. Cortisol is important in the control and metabolism of carbohydrates, lipids, and proteins; also, it assists in metabolic reactions to stress. The daily secretion rate varies very little in nonstressful situations.[1] In greater than physiologic amounts, the effect of cortisol in inflammation and allergies is vital.

The action of cortisol on carbohydrate metabolism may be primarily viewed by its two major effects on glucose production and use. The first major effect of cortisol is to increase the amount of glucose released by enhancing the ability of the liver for gluconeogenesis (glucose production). This is accomplished by stimulating adipose tissue to release free fatty acids, the gluconeogenic substrate needed by the liver. The second major action of cortisol is to decrease the use of glucose by the tissues. In muscle, adipose, and lymphatic tissues, uptake and metabolism are reduced. Through these actions—increased gluconeogenesis and the inhibition of glucose use by tissues—serum glucose concentrations are increased.

The release of free fatty acids from tissue stores into the plasma makes lipids available for energy use. This mobilization of fat stores is one aspect of a metabolic alteration that occurs in times of stress or deprivation: the change from the use of glucose to the use of fatty acids for energy.[7] It is not understood how cortisol initiates the mobilization of fatty acids or why fat deposits are removed from one area of the body and deposited in another, as may easily be seen in adrenocortical dysfunction.

The effects of cortisol on protein are twofold. First, it decreases protein stores in all tissues of the body except the liver. This is carried out by preventing the synthesis of protein and by breaking down protein stores in the cells into amino acids. Second, protein synthesis in the liver is stimulated. Amino acids are released into the liver from cell protein catabolism, thereby increasing the amount of amino acids available to the liver for protein synthesis.

The mechanism by which cortisol responds to stress is not understood, yet it is recognized as being almost essential for survival of the human organism. Any extreme physical or emotional stress can initiate the response, including severe trauma, emotional upset, chronic or debilitating disease, infection, or extreme temperatures (Fig. 37-3).

Administration of glucocorticoids—specifically cortisol—in larger than normal amounts decreases the inflammatory response to infection or injury. Each step of the inflammatory process is blocked by steroids. Cortisol reduces the passage of water into and out of the cell. Also, allergic processes are stopped with the administration of cortisol, which alters the inflammatory process that occurs in response to any allergen. The mechanisms by which the components of the inflammatory process are blocked are not understood, but they are thought to be related to the ability of the glucocorticoids to stabilize cell membranes and prevent rupture of the lysosomes.

Cortisol affects the blood cells in a variable manner.

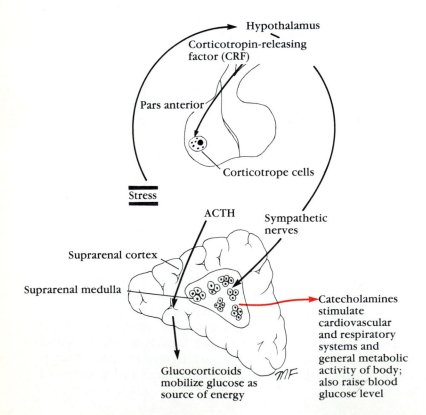

FIGURE 37-3 *The effects of stress on the activities of the adrenal gland. ACTH, adrenocorticotropin.*

The circulating levels of eosinophils and lymphocytes are decreased, and production of red blood cells and platelets is increased. Because of the decreased lymphocyte level, humoral immunity is decreased and infection may occur.[7]

ANDROGENS. The adrenal androgens, or male sex hormones, that are produced in the adrenal cortex have little physiologic significance in the healthy adult. Some of the androgens produced are converted to testosterone, the major male sex hormone, and hypersecretion of the adrenal cortex can cause the appearance of dramatic masculinizing changes as a result of the androgens.

▼ *Adrenocortical Hyperfunction*

CUSHING SYNDROME

CAUSES. The term *Cushing syndrome* refers to the clinical manifestations that result from excess glucose production caused by hypersecretion of cortisol from the adrenal cortex. Although the results are clinically similar, three separate factors may cause Cushing syndrome: adrenal neoplasms, hypersecretion of ACTH by the anterior pituitary (this condition is called *Cushing disease*), and ectopic ACTH syndrome.[21] The therapeutic administration of synthetic glucocorticoids can induce the symptoms of Cushing syndrome.[6]

Adrenal neoplasms that secrete cortisol cause excessive circulating cortisol. As cortisol secretion increases, it is no longer controlled by ACTH. Cortisol secretion by the neoplasm eventually exceeds that of normal adrenocortical cells, at which point the normal cells may cease producing cortisol altogether. Nonmalignant, cortisol-secreting tumors of the adrenal glands seldom secrete excessive androgenic hormones.[11]

Pituitary tumors are the most common cause of Cushing syndrome.[13] In pituitary-dependent Cushing disease, cortisol oversecretion is caused by excessive release of ACTH from the anterior pituitary gland.[2] This causes increased secretion and release of both cortisol and androgenic hormones.

Cushing syndrome may occur from excess production of ACTH by a neoplasm not located in the adrenal gland. This particular form occurs in approximately 2% to 3% of persons afflicted with oat cell carcinoma of the lung.[8] Other malignant neoplasms can secrete ACTH and cause this peculiar paraneoplastic syndrome (see pp. 609–610). In addition to hypersecretion of cortisol, persons with Cushing syndrome exhibit the absence of circadian rhythm changes in the release of ACTH and cortisol.

With increased cortisol secretion there is an increased rate of gluconeogenesis, resulting in elevated serum glucose levels. The islet cells of the pancreas eventually are unable to produce sufficient amounts of insulin, and diabetes mellitus may result.[7] Loss of protein occurs almost everywhere in the body except the liver. In the muscular system, protein loss results in decreased strength and muscle wasting. Humoral immunity is reduced, decreasing the threshold to infection. Skin tissues lose collagen and become very thin, tearing and bruising easily. In the bones, osteoporosis can cause weakness and bone fractures. Hyperpigmentation may be seen, and it is caused by the melanostimulating properties of ACTH.

CLINICAL MANIFESTATIONS. The clinical signs and symptoms vary only slightly with the cause of the disease. Although scattered in the population, Cushing syndrome is more frequently seen in women, especially those of childbearing age.[18] Androgens are responsible for a few of the bodily changes, but most of the abnormalities are direct results of hypercortisolism. The three classic manifestations are truncal obesity, purple striae, and round facial features.

Truncal obesity results from the mobilization of fat in the lower parts of the body to the trunk, causing the abdomen to be greatly protuberant, even as the extremities become thin and wasted. Many persons with Cushing's syndrome cannot rise from a squatting position without assistance. The enlarged abdomen is characteristic, and it may be an extension of thoracic accumulation of fat, the buffalo torso. Fat accumulation around the neck and cervical area is termed the *buffalo hump*. Purple striae appear on the abdomen as a result of the stretching of the abdominal skin when the fat cells are being deposited. They are purple because of the collagen deficit in the skin tissues. Round and full facial features, often called moon facies, also result from the hypercortisolism.

Figures 37-4 and 37-5 show the major clinical manifestations of Cushing syndrome. Excessive androgen secretion results in excess hair growth, often on the face, which is especially prominent in women. Androgen hormones may cause acne and oligomenorrhea. Extreme androgen excess may result in coarsening of the voice, recession of the hairline, and hypertrophy of the clitoris. Psychiatric disturbances may surface, with personality alterations or more severe changes. Polyuria may result from hyperglycemia. Varying degrees of hypertension are exhibited, often with the development of left ventricular hypertrophy.

The mortality rate of Cushing syndrome is 50% or greater unless treatment is initiated. Death usually results from severe infection. If Cushing syndrome occurs in children, growth ceases. If treatment is not begun before the epiphyses of the bones have sealed, short stature is permanent.[21]

Cushing syndrome secondary to pharmacologic therapy with glucocorticoids is extremely common in individuals with systemic connective tissue disease (eg, lupus erythematosus, rheumatoid arthritis) and in persons who have had organ transplantation and are re-

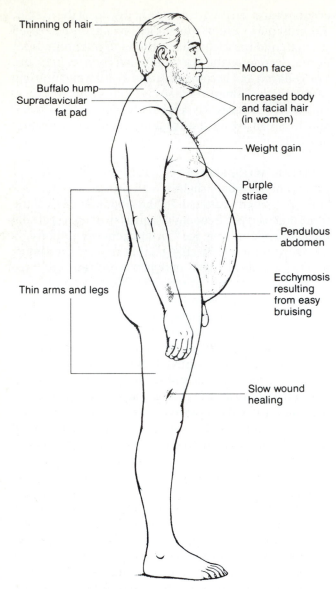

FIGURE 37-4 *The major clinical manifestations of Cushing syndrome. (Smeltzer, S.C. and Bare, B.G. Brunner and Suddarth's Textbook of Medical-Surgical Nursing. [7th ed.]. Philadelphia: J.B. Lippincott, 1992.)*

ceiving the therapy to prevent rejection of the graft. Glucocorticoid therapy also may be used in some cancer therapies or pulmonary conditions. Long-term glucocorticoid therapy reproduces most of the signs and symptoms of Cushing syndrome, with changes in fat distribution, muscle weakness, striae, bruising, poor wound healing, and osteoporosis being common.[6] Hypertension, diabetes mellitus, and opportunistic infections are seen at a greatly increased rate, but androgenic effects are rare.[6]

PRIMARY ALDOSTERONISM

Primary aldosteronism, also known as *Conn syndrome*, is the result of excessive and uncontrolled secretion of the mineralocorticoid aldosterone. The usual cause is an adrenocortical adenoma; rarely, it results from adrenal hyperplasia. Aldosterone conserves sodium and wastes potassium, and the clinical features of this disorder are a direct result of those functions.

The principal features of primary aldosteronism are hypertension, hypernatremia, and hypokalemia. Therefore, this condition may be suspected in any hypertensive patient who concurrently exhibits hypokalemia (less than 3.5 mEq/L). Conservation of sodium leads to retention of water, resulting in increased volume in the extracellular and vascular compartments, which in turn results in arterial hypertension. This condition may resemble hypertension originating from cardiovascular disease.

Loss of potassium may produce a variety of manifestations, depending on the severity of the depletion. The most common result is muscle cramps and weakness. Hypokalemia may progress to tetany and even muscle paralysis. Changes in the pattern of cardiac conduction may develop.

Alterations in renal function are apparent because the kidney is the primary site of sodium conservation. Polydipsia, polyuria, and nocturia occur in response to the sodium-induced increased fluid volume and volume-dependent hypertension.

SECONDARY ALDOSTERONISM

Secondary aldosteronism results from stimulation of aldosterone secretion outside the adrenal cortex, usually by the renin-angiotensin-aldosterone system. Almost any factor that decreases the blood supply to the kidneys results in increased plasma renin levels. The mechanism is somewhat compensatory: increased renin levels lead to increased aldosterone secretion and sodium conservation; water retention results from sodium conservation, leading to increased blood flow to vital organs. Edema occurs only in the presence of preexisting or underlying cardiovascular disease. Secondary aldosteronism leads to a combination of elevated levels of plasma renin and aldosterone.[3]

ADRENOGENITAL SYNDROMES

The adrenogenital syndromes are uncommon conditions caused by adrenocortical overproduction of androgens. The ultimate result is virilization. The age and sex of the affected person determine the nature and severity of the disorder. The causes of adrenogenital syndromes include congenital adrenal hyperplasia, adrenal adenoma, and adrenal carcinomas.[3]

Androgens ultimately are converted to the male hormone testosterone. Testosterone is extremely potent, and only small amounts are required to produce bodily changes. In men, masculinizing effects are masked by the production of testosterone from the testes. It is in children and women that virilization becomes most

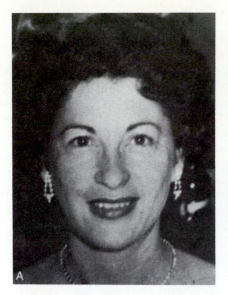 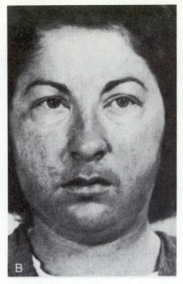 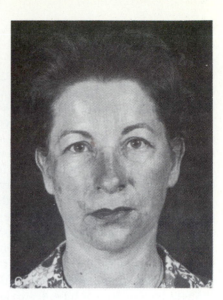

FIGURE 37-5 *Progressive facial changes in a woman with Cushing disease.* **A.** *Before onset of the illness.* **B.** *Preoperative.* **C.** *One year after surgery. (Becker, K.L.* Principles and Practice of Endocrinology and Metabolism [2nd ed.]. *Philadelphia: J.B. Lippincott, 1995.)*

apparent. Young boys begin to develop secondary sex characteristics, regardless of their age at the time of onset. Females respond to androgen stimulation with hirsutism, clitoral hypertrophy, and other masculinizing effects.

CONGENITAL ADRENAL HYPERPLASIA. This is one of the most common adrenogenital syndromes. It is caused by a congenital deficiency in the enzymes that causes adrenocortical biosynthesis and occurs most often in the pediatric age group.[3] There is not an absence of the enzymes but an error in metabolic pathways of steroid production. The appearance of clinical manifestations depends on the point at which synthesis of cortisol, aldosterone, and androgens is blocked. There may be clinical signs and symptoms of either glucocorticoid or mineralocorticoid deficiency or excess. Also, androgen excess and virilization or sexual ambiguity and infantalism may occur. In the most frequently encountered of these conditions, a defect in 21-hydroxylase, excessive androgen production in the female fetus causes the external genitalia to resemble those of a male, but the internal structures—uterus, ovaries, and fallopian tubes—are normal and functional.

▼ *Adrenocortical Hypofunction*

PRIMARY ADRENOCORTICAL INSUFFICIENCY

Also known as *Addison disease*, primary adrenocortical hypofunction results from insufficient secretion of adrenocortical hormones because of insidious and profound destruction in the adrenal glands. It is not a common disorder, and it becomes evident only after 90% of the functioning adrenocortical cells have been destroyed.[3] The two major causes of adrenal destruction that produce this condition are idiopathic atrophy (80%) and tuberculosis (20%). In regions where tuberculosis is poorly controlled, the frequency of Addison disease is high.

Idiopathic atrophy has been attributed to an autoimmune disorder, and many affected people have adrenal autoantibodies. Primary adrenocortical failure, associated with organ-specific immunity, results from progressive destruction of both adrenals by an autoimmune process.[3,6] Further, autoimmune failure may be an isolated problem, or it may appear as part of an autoimmune alteration in several endocrine glands, including the ovaries, parathyroids, thyroid, and β cells of the pancreas.[10] The principal feature of autoimmune adrenal failure is atrophy of the adrenal glands and thickening of the capsule as a result of lymphatic infiltration of the adrenal cortex.

Adrenocortical insufficiency primarily results from deficient cortisol secretion and, in some cases, deficient aldosterone and androgen production.[18] Clinical manifestations depend on the degree of hormonal deficiency; in many persons, the onset is slow and insidious, with the principal features being weight loss, fatigue, and muscle weakness.[20] Changes in the skin are the most dramatic; they occur in about 98% of affected people, and help to diagnose the primary (adrenocortical) insufficiency.[3] Skin color changes result from increased ACTH production, which is uninhibited by steroid response from the adrenal cortex. Areas of hyperpigmentation become visible because the pituitary increases the production of ACTH in an attempt to compensate, and ACTH also has melanostimulating properties. These darkened areas are especially visible in the body areas most exposed to light, pressure areas, hand creases, and buccal mucosa.[17] Areas of vitiligo (pale patches surrounded by excess pigmentation) also are apparent.

Many affected persons experience hypotension as a result of volume depletion. Orthostatic hypotension and tachycardia are present in all persons with acute primary adrenal insufficiency.[14] Sodium loss results in depletion of extracellular volume, which in turn causes decreased cardiac output and decreased blood pressure.[6] Hypoglycemia also can result from the decrease in gluconeogenesis caused by the reduction in cortisol levels. Hyperkalemia results from aldosterone deficiency. Nausea, vomiting, weight loss, and diarrhea are the most common gastrointestinal disturbances. Other body changes include loss of hair, decreased sexual function, and mental disturbances, which range from mild neuroses to deep depressions.[17] Because the symptoms often are vague and the disease onset insidious, the potential for adrenocortical insufficiency should be evaluated in any person who is seriously ill without a specific, identifiable cause.[10] Box 37-1 lists the major clinical manifestations of Addison's disease.

It has been reported with increasing frequency that other physiologic disorders may be associated with primary adrenocortical insufficiency. This association has been called *Schmidt syndrome*, which refers to autoimmune endocrine failure together with polyglandular failure.[21] Disorders that may be associated include gonadal failure, thyroid dysfunction, diabetes mellitus, hypoparathyroidism, and pernicious anemia.

ADRENAL CRISIS

Adrenal crisis (Addisonian crisis, acute adrenal insufficiency) usually occurs because of a sudden decrease or absence of adrenocortical hormones. It is most commonly seen following abrupt withdrawal of long-term corticosteroid therapy.[17] Chronic administration of corticosteroids causes adrenal atrophy, and withdrawal of these drugs suddenly causes a life-threatening alteration (see next section). It may also affect people with both treated and undiagnosed Addison disease if they are exposed to major stresses such as trauma, infection, surgery, or severe illness. Affected people may develop severe dehydration from nausea and vomiting. Weakness, confusion, and hypovolemic shock also are associated.[21] Without immediate intervention, death rapidly ensues. For the person with underlying adrenal insufficiency, the cause of the crisis is not understood, but it may be related to hemorrhage, infection, or infarction in the gland itself.[15]

Waterhouse-Friderichsen syndrome is acute, bilateral, fulminant hemorrhagic infarction of the adrenal cortex. It mainly follows septicemia and shock caused by meningococcal or pseudomonal organisms.[17] The syndrome produces progressive hypotension and is closely associated with disseminated intravascular coagulation. The process may respond to early treatment with antibiotics and the use of steroids. Without early treatment, death follows within hours to a few days.[3]

SECONDARY ADRENOCORTICAL INSUFFICIENCY

Secondary adrenocortical insufficiency results from decreased cortisol secretion because of atrophy of the adrenal cortex. The disorder is a result of decreased ACTH secretion caused by pituitary or hypothalamic disease or by therapeutic pharmacologic doses of glucocorticoids. Mineralocorticoid secretion usually is not affected. Clinically, the features may resemble those of primary insufficiency, except for the absence of hyperpigmentation. The most common cause of secondary adrenocortical insufficiency is acute withdrawal of exogenous steroid therapy. If a person is receiving steroid therapy, slow tapering off is required to allow the adrenal glands to return to active production of their own corticosteroids.

▼ The Adrenal Medulla

CATECHOLAMINES

The most important human catecholamines are epinephrine, norepinephrine, and dopamine, which are synthesized in the brain, sympathetic nerve endings, and chromaffin tissues. The adrenal medulla produces and secretes the catecholamines epinephrine (adrenaline) and norepinephrine (noradrenaline) from the chromaffin cells of the medulla. In relation to these two catecholamines, the adrenal medulla functions as part of the autonomic nervous system. These cells stain readily

---

BOX 37-1 ▼ Clinical Manifestations of Addison's Disease

Weight loss
Fatigue and weakness
Hyperpigmentation of skin, especially that which is light exposed
Vitiligo
Orthostatic hypotension due to hypovolemia
Anorexia
Nausea and vomiting
Diarrhea
Hyponatremia
Hypoglycemia
Hyperkalemia
Cardiac dysrhythmias related to K^+ retention

with chromium salts and secrete adrenaline. Adrenal medullary secretion is about 80% epinephrine and 20% norepinephrine.[7]

Epinephrine exerts its greatest effect on the heart, increasing both rate and contractility. It is a potent mediator of the metabolic rate. Norepinephrine, on the other hand, is secreted by both the adrenal medulla and the sympathetic nerve terminals. It exerts its greatest influence on the arterioles, causing vasoconstriction that leads to increased blood pressure. Stimulation of the sympathetic nervous system causes both direct sympathetic effects and release of the adrenal medullary hormones.

CATECHOLAMINE BIOSYNTHESIS AND STORAGE. The precursor for catecholamine biosynthesis is tyrosine. Through hydroxylation, decarboxylation, and methylation, tyrosine yields norepinephrine and, ultimately, epinephrine (Fig. 37-6). The sequence of the process is as follows: tyrosine → dihydroxyphenylalanine (dopa) → dopamine → norepinephrine → epinephrine.[21] The tyrosine hydroxylase reaction is probably the factor that controls the rate of catecholamine production. Catecholamine is stored by subcellular particles, called granules, which are present in most adrenomedullary cells in the chromaffin granules.

CATECHOLAMINE SECRETION. Catecholamines may be released with acetylcholine stimulation of calcium passage into the chromaffin granules and subsequent liberation into the extracellular fluid. As the adrenal medulla produces the major portion of circulating epinephrine, a small amount is released into the bloodstream almost continuously. Norepinephrine is primarily produced by the sympathetic ganglion cells. Release of large amounts of catecholamines occurs after stimulation of the sympathetic nervous system. Other substances and conditions that may stimulate the release of epinephrine and norepinephrine include serotonin, bradykinin, exercise, hypovolemia, glucagon, and hypoglycemia.[17] Catecholamines participate in metabolic processes together with insulin and glucagon.[21] The action of the catecholamines is opposite that of insulin and similar to that of glucagon, so that it is the interaction that is important.

Extremely stressful situations cause a massive release of epinephrine and norepinephrine, which results in the fight-or-flight reaction. This enables the body to react effectively to any severe hazard or threat to survival. Physiologic response to this massive release of epinephrine includes increased blood pressure and heart rate, pupil dilatation, decreased peristalsis, and circulatory constriction in all major organ systems except the muscular and cardiovascular systems. The response to norepinephrine stimulation is similar, but with the major action being increased arterial blood pressure, a result of vigorous vasoconstriction. These responses are apparently normal catecholamine actions that are accelerated to meet the unusual and immediate cellular demands.

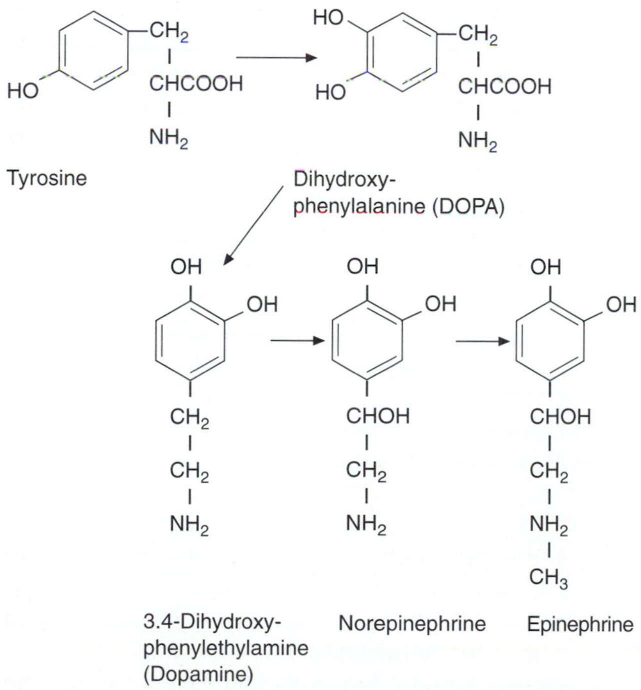

ALTERED FUNCTION OF THE ADRENAL MEDULLA

The only significant disorders of altered function of the adrenal medulla are neoplasms. The gland itself is not considered necessary for life because the body has other sources of catecholamines. The presence of a neoplasm called a *pheochromocytoma* in the adrenal medulla produces apparent states of hyperfunction of the adrenomedullary catecholamines.

PHEOCHROMOCYTOMA. Pheochromocytomas are rare tumors of the adrenal medulla whose primary clinical manifestation is hypertension. Pheochromocytomas originate in the chromaffin cells of the medulla. During fetal life, the chromaffin cells are widespread in the developing body, and their function is associated with the sympathetic ganglia. After birth, most of these cells disappear. Those that remain cluster in the adrenal medulla. Although more than 95% of all functioning chromaffin tumors are located in the adrenal medulla, others have been found in extraadrenal sites, including areas near the kidney and heart and within the cranial vault.[5]

FIGURE 37-6 *Steps in the synthesis of norepinephrine and epinephrine from tyrosine. (From I. Danishefsky, Biochemistry for Medical Science. Boston: Little, Brown, 1980.)*

Pheochromocytomas occur in either sex, usually between ages 25 and 50 years. Children seldom are affected. It is not uncommon for this disorder to affect more than one member of the same family. The tumors usually are benign and bilateral, but a small percentage are malignant with metastasis. Most tumors are well encapsulated and extremely vascular; sometimes, the tumor is palpable. Because of their high vascularity, rupture can cause massive hemorrhage that can be fatal.[17]

Pheochromocytomas produce and secrete excessive quantities of epinephrine and norepinephrine into the bloodstream, resulting in clinical manifestations of catecholamine excess. Therefore, the affected person remains in an accelerated state of response similar to the fight-or-flight reaction. Symptoms may occur spontaneously or may be induced with increased physical or emotional activity or stress.

The primary finding is systemic arterial hypertension. Elevated blood pressure may be sustained or intermittent, mild or malignant, depending on the rate and amount of catecholamine secreted. These persons also may exhibit clinical signs and symptoms of headache, pallor, palpitations, and sweating because of the direct effects of the elevated blood pressure and increased epinephrine and norepinephrine.[4] Most pheochromocytomas secrete a greater amount of norepinephrine, which is then responsible for the hypertension.[23] Together with this, the smaller amounts of epinephrine produced are responsible for the myocardial side effects. Sustained elevation of catecholamine secretion can lead to cardiomegaly, left ventricular failure, cardiomyopathy, and, ultimately, death from heart failure. Some persons with pheochromocytoma may develop chest pain, angina, or even an acute myocardial infarction in the absence of coronary artery disease.[22] Cardiac dysrhythmias also may be observed. Other metabolic effects include excessive perspiration, palpitations, headaches, hyperventilation, and flushing. Increased frequency of neurofibromatosis, a familial disorder, has been associated with pheochromocytoma.

MULTIPLE ENDOCRINE NEOPLASIA. Pheochromocytomas also may be associated with a disorder known as multiple endocrine neoplasia syndrome (see pp. XX). This complicated group of disorders is termed multiple because of the multicentricity and bilateral growth of the tumors as well as the involvement of several glands.[17] One of the important aspects concerning the association of symptoms is that 85% of persons with either familial or sporadic pheochromocytomas who also have medullary thyroid carcinomas are normotensive, whereas more than 60% of persons with familial or sporadic pheochromocytomas not associated with medullary carcinoma have chronic hypertension.[21]

▼ Chapter Summary

▼ The adrenal cortex secretes glucocorticoids and mineralocorticoids that are essential for life. These hormones are steroid hormones and are synthesized from cholesterol.

▼ The glucocorticoids regulate serum glucose levels through a primarily catabolic process. They function in the stress response to stabilize the cell membrane and block the inflammatory process. This mechanism may be life-saving in the acute situation. The secretion of the glucocorticoids is under the direct influence of ACTH from the pituitary.

▼ The mineralocorticoids, mainly aldosterone, function to retain sodium and thus, water. The secretion of aldosterone is under the direct influence of serum sodium or potassium levels or the RAA system.

▼ Hyperfunction of the adrenal gland is called Cushing syndrome. The clinical picture may result from pituitary stimulation, adrenal neoplasms, or ectopic ACTH syndrome. By far the most common cause of the clinical picture of Cushing's syndrome is long-term administration of corticosteroids for other diseases.

▼ Aldosteronism results from uncontrolled secretion of aldosterone, which causes hypertension, hypernatremia, and hypokalemia.

▼ Hypofunction of the adrenal gland is also known as Addison's disease. It is most frequently due to autoimmune destruction, but may also result from tuberculosis. The clinical picture is opposite that of Cushing syndrome, with hypotension, hyperkalemia, and lack of glucocorticoid response to stress.

▼ Adrenal crisis results with a sudden loss of adrenocortical hormones which most commonly is seen when a person who has been taking corticosteroids suddenly stops taking the drugs. The adrenal gland, having been suppressed by the exogenous drugs, cannot provide the corticosteroids necessary for life.

▼ The adrenal medulla produces the catecholamines epinephrine and norepinephrine. These hormones are under the direct influence of the sympathetic nervous system and are released in stress to achieve the "fight or flight" response. Neoplasms of the adrenal medulla will produce a pheochromocytoma which places the body in a chronic state of catecholamine excess, and hypertension is a major manifestation.

▼ References

1. Becker, K.L. *Principles and Practice of Endocrinology and Metabolism.* Philadelphia: J.B. Lippincott, 1991.
2. Carrieri, V.K., Lindsey, A.M., and West, C.M. *Pathophysiological Phenomena in Nursing: Human Responses to Illness* (2nd ed.). Philadelphia: W.B. Saunders, 1993.

3. Cotran, R.S., Kumar, V., and Robbins, S.L. *Robbins' Pathologic Basis of Disease* (5th ed.). Philadelphia: W.B. Saunders, 1994.

4. DeQuattro, V., Myers, M., and Campese, V.M. Pheochromocytoma: Diagnosis and therapy. In DeGroot, L.J. (ed.), *Endocrinology* (2nd ed.). Philadelphia: W.B. Saunders, 1989.

5. Goldfien, A. Adrenal medulla. In Greenspan, F.S. (ed.), *Basic and Clinical Endocrinology* (3rd ed.). Norwalk, Conn.: Appleton & Lange, 1991.

6. Grekin, R.I. Adrenocortical disorders. In Kelley, W.N. (ed.), *Textbook of Internal Medicine* (2nd ed.). Philadelphia: J.B. Lippincott, 1992.

7. Guyton, A. *Textbook of Medical Physiology* (8th ed.). Philadelphia: W.B. Saunders, 1991.

8. Ihde, D.C., Pass, H.I., and Glatstein, E.J. Small cell lung cancer. In DeVita, V.T., Hellman, S., and Rosenberg, S.A., *Cancer: Principles and Practice of Oncology* (4th ed.). Philadelphia: J.B. Lippincott, 1993.

9. Kaplan, N.M. The adrenal glands. In Griffin, J.E., and Ojeda, S.R. (eds.), *Textbook of Endocrine Physiology*. New York: Oxford University Press, 1988.

10. Kendall, J., and Loriaux, D.L. Disorders of the adrenal cortex. In Stein, J. (ed.), *Internal Medicine* (4th ed.). St. Louis: Mosby, 1994.

11. Norton, J.A., Levin, B., and Jensen, R.T. Cancer of the endocrine system. In DeVita, V.T., Hellman, S., and Rosenberg, S.A., *Cancer: Principles and Practice of Oncology* (4th ed.). Philadelphia: J.B. Lippincott, 1993.

12. Parker, K.I. Steroid hormone biosynthesis. In Kelley, W.N. (ed.), *Textbook of Internal Medicine* (2nd ed.). Philadelphia: J.B. Lippincott, 1992.

13. Piziak, V.K., and Gilliland, P.F. Pituitary tumors: Look for early signs and symptoms. *Emerg Med Clin North Am* 25:124–132, 1993.

14. Reasner, C.A. Adrenal disorders. *Crit Care Nurs Q* 13: 67–73, 1990.

15. Reichlin, S.D. Neuroendocrinology. In Wilson, J.D., and Foster, D.W. (eds.), *Williams' Textbook of Endocrinology* (8th ed.). Philadelphia: W.B. Saunders, 1992.

16. Reus, V.I., and Collu, R. Endocrine effects of stress. In Collu, R., Brown, G.M., and Van Loon, G.R. (eds.), *Clinical Neuroendrocrinology*. Boston: Blackwell, 1988.

17. Rubin, E., and Farber, J.L. *Pathology* (2nd ed.). Philadelphia: J.B. Lippincott, 1994.

18. Tuck, M.L., and Stern, N. Adrenal disease. In Hershman, J.M. (ed.), *Endocrine Pathophysiology: A Patient-Oriented Approach*. Philadelphia: Lea & Febiger, 1988.

19. Tyrell, J.B., Aron, D.C., and Forsham, P.H. Glucocorticoids and adrenal androgens. In Greenspan, F.S. (ed.), *Basic and Clinical Endocrinology* (3rd ed.). Norwalk, Conn.: Appleton & Lange, 1991.

20. Werbel, S.S., and Ober, K.P. Acute adrenal insufficiency. *Endocrinol Metab Clin North Am* 22:303–328, 1993.

21. Wilson, J.D., and Foster, D.W. (eds.). *Williams' Textbook of Endocrinology* (8th ed.). Philadelphia: W.B. Saunders, 1992.

22. Winer, N. Pheochromocytoma. *Crit Care Nurs Q* 13:14–22, 1990.

23. Yucha, C., and Blakeman, N. Pheochromocytoma: The great mimic. *Cancer Nurs* 14:136–140, 1991.

Chapter *38*

Thyroid and Parathyroid Functions and Alterations

Camille Stern

▼ **CHAPTER OUTLINE**

▼ **LEARNING OBJECTIVES**

1   Describe the normal anatomy of the thyroid gland.
2   Explain the process by which the thyroid hormones are formed.
3   Identify the function of the iodide pump.
4   Describe the mechanisms for releasing and transporting the thyroid hormones.
5   Describe the function of calcitonin.
6   Describe the effects of the thyroid hormones on metabolic processes, carbohydrate metabolism, and vitamin metabolism.
7   Identify the clinical manifestations of hyperthyroidism.
8   Relate the signs and symptoms of Graves' disease to underlying pathophysiology.
9   Differentiate between toxic multinodular goiter and toxic adenoma.
10 Identify the clinical manifestations of hypothyroidism.
11 Describe the physical changes and underlying causes of adult hypothyroidism.
12 Compare thyrotoxic crisis and myxedema coma.
13 Describe the causes and symptoms of each of the thyroid carcinomas.
14 Describe the normal anatomy and function of the parathyroid glands.
15 Describe hypoparathyroidism.
16 Compare the effects of primary, secondary, and tertiary hyperparathyroidism.

Barbara L. Bullock: PATHOPHYSIOLOGY: ADAPTATIONS AND ALTERATIONS IN FUNCTION, 4th ed.
© 1996 J.B. Lippincott-Raven Publishers

The thyroid gland is primarily responsible for controlling the rate of metabolic processes in the body. The parathyroid glands control calcium levels and bone reabsorption. These two glands are related by proximity and, as recently discovered, by function. In this chapter, normal structure and physiology are explored and the major disorders of these glands are examined.

▼ Anatomy of the Thyroid Gland

The primary function of the thyroid gland, the second largest endocrine gland in the human body, is to regulate and control the rate of metabolism. The thyroid is located in the anterior neck, between the larynx and the trachea (Fig. 38-1). In the normal thyroid, two lobes lie slightly lateral to the trachea, one on either side, and are connected by a thin band of tissue known as an isthmus. The isthmus lies just below the cricoid cartilage of the trachea. Characteristically, the superior portion of each lobe is somewhat pointed, whereas the inferior portion is rounded and blunt.

The thyroid is reddish and beefy in appearance and has a rubbery texture on palpation. In the average adult, the gland weighs 20 to 30 g. It is enclosed in two layers of connective tissue, with the outer layer being

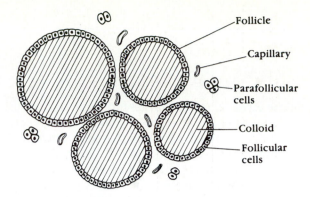

FIGURE 38-2 *Follicles of thyroid gland showing colloid filling each sac.*

continuous with the cervical fascia of the neck and the inner layer of connective tissue closely adhering to the gland itself.

Thyroid tissue originally develops from the oral epithelium. In an adult, the foramen cecum, a depression on the dorsum of the tongue, points to the location from which thyroid tissue evolved. Rarely, the duct that connects the thyroid and the foramen cecum, known as the *thyroglossal duct*, may remain.

Blood supply to the thyroid arises from two main pairs of arteries. Branching from the external carotid arteries, the superior thyroid arteries enter and supply the upper portions of the lobes. The inferior thyroid arteries, arising from the subclavian arteries, supply the lower portion of the lobes. An estimated 4 to 6 L of blood per hour circulate through the thyroid.

Nervous system control is accomplished primarily by the second through fifth thoracic spinal nerves and by the superior and middle ganglia of the thoracolumbar nervous system. Cervical ganglia provide the thyroid with adrenergic stimulation, and the vagus nerve provides cholinergic stimulation.

The body of the thyroid is composed of a mass of tiny follicles that are all about equal in size (Fig. 38-2). These follicles, or sacs, are each, in effect, separately functioning glands the size of a pinhead. The iodine-accumulating capacity of each follicle is directly proportional to its individual surface area.[21] Although the sacs do not have outside openings, rich vascular, lymph, and nervous networks surround them, exchanging iodine for hormones. The follicles have a single-layer epithelial lining, and an amorphous secretory fluid (colloid) fills each sac. The primary component of thyroid colloid is a large protein molecule called *thyroglobulin*, from which the thyroid hormones are released.

Another distinct cell type in the thyroid gland is the *parafollicular* cell. These cells have an ovoid and irregular shape and are scattered among the other, more numerous thyroid cells.

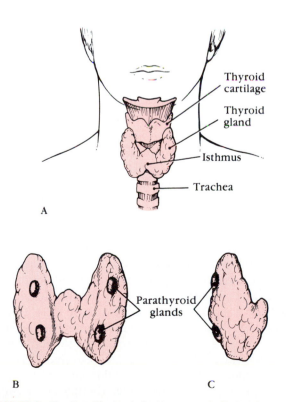

FIGURE 38-1 *The thyroid gland.* **A.** *Anterior view.* **B.** *Posterior view showing parathyroid gland.* **C.** *Lateral view.*

▼ *Physiology of the Thyroid Gland*

THYROID IODIDE PUMP

Iodide is essential to the normal functioning of the thyroid gland. After iodide enters the body through eating or drinking, it is absorbed into the bloodstream from the gastrointestinal tract within about an hour. Circulating in the blood, iodide is competed for by the thyroid and the kidneys. About two-thirds of the iodide circulating in the bloodstream is excreted in the urine, and the remaining one-third is selectively removed from the blood by the thyroid.

Removal of iodide from the circulation is accomplished by means of an iodide pump or trap. Thyroid-stimulating hormone (TSH) enhances and is most influential in the iodide transport, although other factors also affect the mechanism.[21] The iodide pump normally is able to concentrate iodide to about 25 times the concentration in the blood, but at those times when the thyroid gland becomes maximally active, the concentration can increase to as high as 350 times blood concentration.[8] After iodide is taken into the thyroid cell, it is oxidized to iodine.[18]

To prevent a basic iodine deficiency, sufficient intake of iodine is necessary. Ingested quantities of iodine vary, depending on the natural content in the soil and water in any given environment and on the intake of iodine-enriched salt and foods. Iodinized table salt contains 1 part sodium iodide to 100,000 parts of sodium chloride.

STRUCTURE AND STORAGE OF THYROID HORMONES

The thyroid iodide trap is an active, energy-requiring mechanism. At the beginning of this process, iodine is removed from the circulation in the form of sodium or potassium iodide. It then passes through the follicular cells and into the colloid. The thyroglobulin molecules in the colloid contain an active amino acid, tyrosine, which combines with the iodine in the process of forming the thyroid hormones.

Two separate combinations of these molecules form the two main thyroid hormones, triiodothyronine (T_3) and thyroxine (T_4). Nearly 10 times more T_4 than T_3 is secreted from the thyroid gland, but as it circulates, some of the T_4 deiodinates, making two to three times as much available to the tissues. T_3 is three to five times more active than T_4, but the duration of T_4 is three to five times longer. The T_3 hormone causes increased synthesis of total ribonucleic acid in some tissues and increases in specific messenger ribonucleic acid synthesis in others.[20] The overall effect of both hormones is similar, and their functions appear to be identical.

The thyroid hormones are stored in the follicular colloid as part of the thyroglobulin molecule. The thyroid gland is unique in its ability to store hormones in the thyroglobulin molecule. Colloid in the normal thyroid is composed primarily of thyroglobulin molecules. In effect, this is a storage mechanism, which functions if synthesis of the thyroid hormones should cease.

RELEASE AND TRANSPORT OF THYROID HORMONES

The thyroid hormones are regulated through a complex interaction. The hypothalamus, pituitary, and thyroid glands are part of the interaction, which is further controlled by higher centers in the brain. The major regulator of thyroid hormone secretion is TSH, or thyrotropin, which is a glycoprotein hormone secreted by the anterior pituitary gland. It is thought to be responsive to slight changes in thyroid hormone levels. The release of TSH is mediated by the thyroid-releasing hormone (TRH) from the hypothalamus. This hormone stimulates the synthesis and release of TSH. Thyroid hormones inhibit these functions, thereby exerting influence on the feedback regulation of TSH secretion. The relation of TRH, TSH, and the thyroid hormones exists as a feedback system (Flowchart 38-1). Whenever T_3 and T_4 levels become too low in the circulating bloodstream, TRH triggers the release of TSH to increase the secretion of T_3 and T_4. It accomplishes this by increasing all of the known activities of the thyroid gland cells.[8] As the blood levels of T_3 and T_4 begin to rise, the anterior pituitary decreases secretion of TSH, thereby decreasing the rate of thyroid hormone production. TSH stimulates an increase in the size and number of the follicular cells, thereby increasing their ability to absorb iodide.[18] It also increases the breakdown of thyroglobulin, releasing T_4 and T_3 from the thyroid gland. Through these mechanisms, adequate levels of hormones are maintained in the bloodstream at all times. When the hormones are needed, an enzymatic reaction splits the thyroglobulin molecule and frees the hormones for entry into the bloodstream.

In the blood, T_4 and T_3 immediately combine with circulating plasma proteins. The affinity of circulating hormones and proteins is so great that the hormones are released to the tissue cells slowly. As the hormones enter the cells, both T_4 and T_3 bind with intracellular proteins, where they are again stored. They are then inside tissue cells and are available to nourish those cells. The hormones have a direct effect on the mitochondria of the cells, resulting in an increased total number and an increased concentration of oxidative enzymes.[18] Through these actions, the hormones directly influence cell metabolism and metabolic rate. The thyroid hormones are used within several days to several weeks.

Measurement of T_3, T_4, and TSH are used to diag-

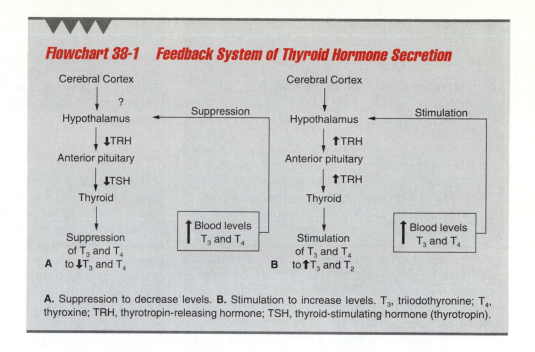

Flowchart 38-1   Feedback System of Thyroid Hormone Secretion

A. Suppression to decrease levels. **B.** Stimulation to increase levels. T_3, triiodothyronine; T_4, thyroxine; TRH, thyrotropin-releasing hormone; TSH, thyroid-stimulating hormone (thyrotropin).

nose hypo- or hyperthyroidism. TSH levels are normally 2–10 μU/mL or 2–10 mU/L (SI units) and reflect pituitary function. T_3 is measured with T_4 which assesses that bound to albumin as well as free T_4. Normal levels by different methods are about 5–10 μg/dL.

▼ Formation and Function of Calcitonin

In the 1960s, another thyroid hormone, calcitonin, was discovered. Its formation and mechanisms of action are so different that it must be considered separately from T_4 and T_3. Calcitonin is a large polypeptide that contains 32 amino acids. It is synthesized in the parafollicular, or C, cells of the interstitial tissue between the follicular cells of the thyroid.[8]

Calcitonin has a direct effect on bone tissue by counteracting hypercalcemia. Increased serum calcium levels stimulate the release of this hormone from the thyroid gland. After it is released, it inhibits bone reabsorption, thus inhibiting the rate of release of calcium from bone tissue to plasma. This process causes a reduction in blood calcium levels. The action of calcitonin is essentially the reverse of the action of the parathyroid hormone (PTH) from the parathyroid glands (see pp. 720–722). Whereas the action of PTH is long-acting and continually maintains constant levels of circulating calcium, calcitonin only begins to act when there is excess calcium in the blood. It does not block PTH or prevent its release. Calcitonin merely exerts an opposite action on both bone and kidneys. Bone reabsorption by osteoclasts is inhibited, and, in

response to calcitonin, the loop of Henle allows calcium to be filtered out and excreted in urine.

▼ Physiologic Effects of the Thyroid Hormones

EFFECTS ON METABOLIC PROCESSES. Because the thyroid hormones are carried to all body tissues, their effects are widespread and varied. They exert influence over all major body systems, as well as the most intricate of cell functions. Their major influence is to increase basal metabolic rate (BMR), which is the rate of heat production and energy expenditure in the body. A test to measure BMR is actually a measurement of oxygen consumption. Several nonthyroid factors can affect the usefulness of this test. The BMR rises during periods of increased hormone production and secretion, thus increasing energy expenditure and heat production. When this occurs, calorigenesis (the use of food for energy) also is increased. Calorigenesis increases the consumption of oxygen by the body.

EFFECTS ON PROTEIN METABOLISM. The thyroid hormones increase protein synthesis and therefore are essential for normal growth and development in children and young adults. They also stimulate the synthesis of many enzymes and hormones.[20] After stores of fat and carbohydrate have been depleted, proteins may be used for energy. This protein depletion results in a negative nitrogen balance. It is not clear whether this is a direct result of the thyroid hormone or caused by a negative caloric balance.[21] Releasing proteins also releases amino acids, making them available for energy, and increases the rate of gluconeogenesis.

EFFECTS ON CARBOHYDRATE METABOLISM. Thyroid hormones affect virtually every function of carbohydrate metabolism. They are responsible for an increased rate of gluconeogenesis, rapid cellular uptake of glucose, increased intestinal absorption of glucose and galactose, and an increased rate of glucose uptake by adipose tissue. Especially in carbohydrate metabolism, thyroid hormones are interactive with or dependent on other hormones. Insulin secretion is increased, which also enhances carbohydrate metabolism.

EFFECTS ON LIPID METABOLISM. Thyroid hormones essentially stimulate all aspects of lipid or fatty metabolism. The major result of their influence is depletion of fat storage, especially of lipids. This leads to increased plasma concentration levels of free fatty acids. Serum cholesterol, however, is lowered by the action of thyroid hormones, probably because of increased intestinal excretion and conversion of cholesterol into bile acids.

EFFECTS ON VITAMIN METABOLISM. Because thyroid hormones increase the rate of metabolic processes, they increase the physiologic need for vitamins. Many vitamins contain enzymes or coenzymes. Increased secretion of thyroid hormones causes depletion of vitamins because of the liberation of enzymes, unless the intake of vitamins by ingestion is increased.

▼ Altered Thyroid Function

GOITER

The presence of a goiter, or enlarged thyroid gland, is not necessarily indicative of thyroid dysfunction, but it may demonstrate insufficient iodine intake.[19] Goiters may appear in states of hypofunction as well as hyperfunction. The gland enlarges in an attempt to produce sufficient amounts of thyroid hormones. Various types of disorders can alter the size and state of the thyroid (Fig. 38-3). In the absence of identifiable clinical manifestations, an enlarged thyroid gland is referred to as a *nontoxic goiter*.

HYPERTHYROIDISM

Hyperthyroidism, also known as *thyrotoxicosis*, is characterized by increased T_3 and T_4 production, often 5 to 15 times the normal rates. As a result, excess amounts of thyroid hormones are circulated to the tissues. Hyperthyroidism may be related entirely to disease of the thyroid, or it may originate from outside the thyroid. Exogenous hyperthyroidism is most commonly caused by self-medication with thyroid hormone drugs.[19] In years past, these drugs were prescribed for weight loss through increased BMR, and they still are taken for weight loss, even though the side effects can be severe. Hyperthyroidism may be permanent or temporary, mild or severe.

The severity of the disease is affected by the person's age, duration of hyperthyroid function, and presence of other disease processes in any other organ systems. It is much more common in women than in men, with an estimated incidence of 2 to 3 per 1,000 women.[19] Because increased amounts of thyroid hormones reach the cells, all metabolic activities are accelerated. The BMR rises, energy expenditure is increased, and heat production rises.

CLINICAL MANIFESTATIONS. The clinical manifestations of hyperthyroidism are varied, and they may arise in any major organ system (Fig. 38-4). One of the primary features is development of a palpable goiter or growth of a preexisting goiter. The skin becomes flushed, warm, and moist. Hair tends to be fine and breaks easily;

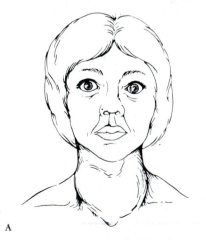
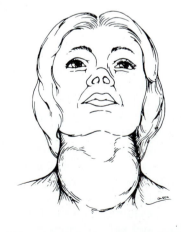
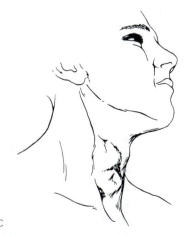

A   B   C

FIGURE 38-3 *Thyroid abnormalities.* **A.** *Diffuse toxic goiter (Graves disease) with exophthalmos.* **B.** *Diffuse nontoxic goiter.* **C.** *Nodular goiter. (Judge, R.D., Zuidema, G.D., and Fitzgerald, F.T. [eds.]. Clinical Diagnosis [4th ed.]. Boston: Little, Brown, 1982.)*

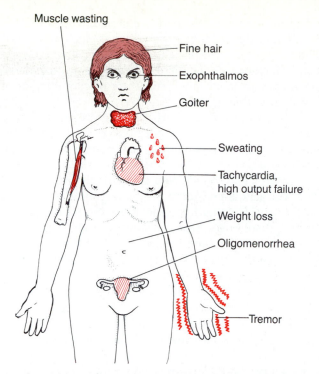

Muscle wasting

Fine hair

Exophthalmos

Goiter

Sweating

Tachycardia,
high output failure

Weight loss

Oligomenorrhea

Tremor

FIGURE 38-4 *The major clinical manifestations of hyperthyroidism. (Rubin, E., and Farber, J.L. Pathology [2nd ed.]. Philadelphia: J.B. Lippincott, 1994.)*

in some instances, hair is lost. Nails of the fingers and toes break easily and often separate from the beds.

Hyperthyroidism is often associated with endocrine ophthalmopathology, resulting in a characteristic stare. This is caused by upper eyelid retraction and frequently occurs with thyrotoxicosis. Movements of the eyelids are

jerky and irregular. Most people with hyperthyroidism develop some *exophthalmos*, or protrusion of the eyeballs, which may cause difficulty in closing the eyelids. Exophthalmos is commonly caused by massive swelling, interstitial inflammatory edema, and local muscle infiltration (Fig. 38-5).[1] Degenerative changes in the muscles that control the eye may result over time.[5]

Cardiovascular changes are pronounced because of the increased metabolic demands on the heart. Pronounced tachycardia always is present, even during sleep. Systolic blood pressure often rises.[6] Palpitations occur because of the increased force of cardiac contractions. Atrial or supraventricular dysrhythmias are not uncommon. Most people who have no underlying or preexisting cardiac failure can maintain the increased rate of cardiovascular function required. Hyperthyroidism eventually may precipitate congestive heart failure, however.

Changes in nervous system function are indicated by increasing restlessness and nervousness, decreased attention span, and the need to be almost constantly in motion, even though fatigue occurs rapidly. Afflicted people also become emotionally labile, having bursts of temper and rapid mood changes.

In the gastrointestinal system, increased appetite is apparent, but there usually is associated weight loss. Increased food intake may be insufficient to meet the increased metabolic demands, and there also may be complaints of nausea, vomiting, or diarrhea. The affected person usually is thin, even emaciated.

Other systemic changes may become apparent. Dyspnea occurs during periods of increased physical activity. Mild polyuria, heat intolerance, excessive per-

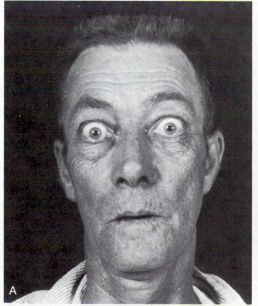
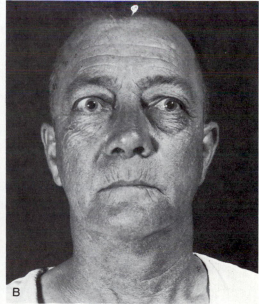

FIGURE 38-5 *Patient with Graves disease treated with antithyroid drug. **A.** Appearance before therapy. **B.** Four months after commencement of therapy. Notice the markedly decreased stare. Eventually, radioactive iodine treatment was required for permanent cure. (Source: Becker, K.L. Principles and Practice of Endocrinology and Metabolism [2nd ed]. Philadelphia: J.B. Lippincott, 1995.)*

spiration, and increased susceptibility to infection may be manifested. Table 38-1 summarizes the effects of thyrotoxicosis.

THYROID STORM. Thyrotoxic crisis, or thyroid storm, is an uncommon but life-threatening complication of hyperthyroidism. It may occur in people with untreated hyperthyroidism or after surgery in those who are inadequately prepared for surgical thyroidectomy. At one time, thyroid storm was a common complication of thy-

roidectomy in the postoperative period. Now it usually arises after the onset of extreme stress, such as a major illness, injury, or, especially, infection. Other medical causes include trauma, diabetic ketoacidosis, toxemia of pregnancy or labor, and premature discontinuation of antithyroid therapy.[11]

The symptoms of thyroid storm are caused by a sudden increase in thyroid hormone levels in the bloodstream, which results in a marked increase in all of the clinical manifestations of hyperthyroidism. Other clinical features may result from sympathetic overactivity.[6] The hallmark is considered to be uncontrolled fever of 100° to 106°F. Other hypermetabolic symptoms include profuse diaphoresis, shock, vomiting, and dehydration. Central nervous system symptoms also may be exacerbated, including hyperkinesis, anxiety, and confusion.[11] The physiologic effects of the hypermetabolic processes are so devastating to the body tissues that those in crisis must receive immediate intervention or death rapidly ensues. Treatment includes aggressive antithyroid drug therapy and measures to reduce the high fever.

GRAVES' DISEASE. The most common and well-known form of hyperthyroidism is Graves' disease. Also known as exophthalmic goiter, diffuse toxic goiter, Basedow disease, and primary hyperthyroidism, it is the most common form of thyrotoxicosis in persons younger than 50 years of age.[3] It is not simply a disease of the thyroid but a multisystem syndrome that may include major manifestations of hyperthyroidism, diffuse thyroid enlargement, infiltrative ophthalmopathy, infiltrative dermopathy, and generalized lymphoid hyperplasia. These features may occur individually or in any combination. Graves' disease may occur at any age but primarily strikes those between 30 and 50 years of age. Women have the disease more frequently than men, and more than one member of the same family often is affected.

It is now accepted that there is an autoimmune component to this disease. The T lymphocytes become sensitized to antigens within the thyroid gland and stimulate the B lymphocytes to synthesize antibodies to these antigens.[7] In the 1950s, a substance was discovered in the serum of many people with Graves' disease. It was an immunoglobulin G1, later called *long-acting thyroid stimulator*. This antibody is also referred to as thyroid-stimulating immunoglobulin.[7] It has all of the functions of TSH, but the effects last longer and are not subject to the control of rising levels of thyroid hormones in the blood. This antibody is detected in almost every person with untreated Graves' disease. Although the reason is unknown, autoimmune thyroiditis is more common in women.[3] More recently, a thyroid-stimulating autoantibody has been found to be the functional analogue to TSH, binding so strongly to TSH receptor sites that it can prevent the binding of TSH.[11] Because the autoantibody is not under feedback control, thyroid hy-

---

TABLE 38-1 *Effects of Thyrotoxicosis*

System	Effects
General	Nervousness, insomnia, fatigue, tremulousness, heat intolerance, weight loss
Skin	Warm and moist, hyperhidrosis, alopecia, hyperpigmentation, onycholysis, acropachy, pretibial myxedema, preradial myxedema, urticaria, pruritus, vitiligo
Eyes	Exophthalmos, conjunctivitis, chemosis, ophthalmoplegia, optic nerve involvement
Cardiovascular	Tachycardia, shortness of breath, palpitations, atrial fibrillation, heart block, high output congestive heart failure, angina pectoris, increased pulse pressure, Means–Lerman "scratch" murmur
Gastrointestinal	Tremor of tongue, hyperphagia, increased thirst, diarrhea or hyperdefecation, elevated liver function tests, hepatomegaly
Metabolic	Elevated serum calcium, decreased serum magnesium, increased osseous alkaline phosphatase, hypercalciuria
Neuromuscular	Fine tremor of hands, weakness of proximal muscles, myopathy, muscle atrophy, creatinuria, periodic paralysis
Osseous	Osteoporosis
Neurologic	Fever, delirium, stupor, coma, syncope, choreoathetosis
Reproductive/sexual	Irregular menses, gynecomastia, decreased fertility
Hematopoietic	Anemia (usually normochromic, normocytic), lymphocytosis, lymphadenopathy, enlarged thymus, splenomegaly
Mental	Restlessness, irritability, anxiety, inability to concentrate, lability, depression, psychiatric reactions
Influence on vitamins	Decreased serum vitamin A, prealbumin, and retinol-binding protein; increased requirement for pyridoxine and thiamine; decreased serum vitamin D_2

Becker, K. L. *Principles and Practice of Endocrinology and Metabolism.* Philadelphia: J.B. Lippincott, 1990.

persecretion results. The exact mechanism is not clearly understood.

Heredity and genetic factors also are accepted contributors to the development of Graves' disease. This form of hyperthyroidism frequently occurs in more than one family member and may affect several generations of the same family. Both genetic and autoimmune components are of major influence. It also has been suggested that severe emotional stress may be a factor, because the disease frequently arises after severe emotional or physical trauma.

The outstanding clinical features of Graves' disease are diffuse and palpable goiter, unilateral or bilateral exophthalmos, pretibial myxedema, and signs of hypermetabolism or thyrotoxicosis.[23] Mild to moderate skeletal or muscular myopathies are fairly common.[1] The onset of symptoms usually is gradual. Complaints of nervousness, irritability, fatigue, heat intolerance, and weight loss are common. These symptoms are a result of the increased metabolic rate. The thyroid gland is enlarged to two to three times the normal size in most cases. It may, however, be massively enlarged, or it may remain near normal size. Enlargement usually is symmetric, and the surface is smooth.

Exophthalmos, the most common ocular change, normally is accompanied by periorbital edema. The person has a characteristic bulging, wide-eyed stare. The eye musculature often is so affected that the cornea and sclera are damaged because of an inability to close the eyes (see Figure 38-5). Affected persons often complain of a ''sandy'' sensation or of retroorbital pressure.[3] In most cases, exophthalmos gradually disappears with treatment of the hyperthyroidism. Infiltrative ophthalmopathy is a more serious and extensive involvement and may cause permanent changes in eye function. It also may cause especially difficult problems in treatment.

Infiltrative dermopathy, commonly called *pretibial myxedema*, is a rare but dramatic manifestation that affects the pretibial area of one or both legs, causing a barklike appearance of the skin. The appearance may range from mild, without clinical symptoms, to severe and limiting.[1] Localized edema and swelling of the skin and subcutaneous tissues occur. Hyaluronic acid accumulates in the interstitial spaces and, combining with water, forms edema that is boggy and nonpitting. Persons having pretibial myxedema have a profound immunologic disruption, and it is thought that these dermatologic changes are a direct result of that immunologic reaction.[11]

TOXIC MULTINODULAR GOITER. In some people with a long-standing history of nontoxic goiter, hyperthyroidism may appear insidiously. This disorder is known as toxic multinodular goiter, or *Plummer disease*. Women older than 50 years of age are most frequently affected.

The mechanism that causes nontoxic goiter to become toxic is not known.

The clinical manifestations are mild in comparison to Graves' disease. Thyrotoxicosis signs are less prominent, and serum thyroxine levels are only marginally elevated. Cardiovascular symptoms are the most pronounced. Atrial fibrillation, tachycardia, and congestive heart failure may develop. Also apparent are muscle weakening and fatigue. It often is difficult to diagnose toxic multinodular goiter because of its slow onset. The signs and symptoms may be attributed to lethargy and aging.

TOXIC ADENOMA. Toxic adenoma is a less common form of hyperthyroidism. It usually results from the development of a follicular adenoma. These adenomas are subdivided according to the size of the follicles into macrofollicular, microfollicular, and embryonal varieties.[21] They may occur in pairs or triplets. The function of the adenoma may be more or less than that of normal thyroid gland tissue, but it secretes thyroid hormone without the stimulation of TSH. As the adenoma grows, it begins to take over the function of normal thyroid tissue. Without intervention, complete atrophy and suppression of the remainder of the thyroid gland eventually occurs.[21] The adenoma must reach the size of 2 to 3 cm before it is capable of producing a state of hyperthyroidism. The lesion may undergo necrosis and hemorrhage of its center. If this occurs, symptoms of thyrotoxicosis recede, and the remainder of the thyroid gland tissue resumes normal functioning. Most persons affected with toxic adenoma are between 30 and 40 years of age, and they usually have a history of a lump in the neck that has been growing slowly for many years. Clinical features are not pronounced; cardiovascular symptoms are probably the most prominent.

HYPOTHYROIDISM

Hypothyroidism is the result of a deficiency of thyroid hormone, which leads to a decreased rate of body metabolism and a general slowing down of body processes. Any of the following factors may contribute to the onset of hypothyroidism: hypothalamic dysfunction, TRH or TSH deficiency, pituitary disorders, specific idiopathies, thyroid deficiencies, and thyroid destruction.[11] The degree of dysfunction is related to the relative amount of hormone deficiency in the tissues. Hypothyroidism is fairly common, and it is recognized as an underdiagnosed health problem, particularly in elderly persons.

CLINICAL MANIFESTATIONS. Changes in the skin occur with hypothyroidism when hyaluronic acid binds with water. The combination produces the characteristic baggy, full, edematous skin. Edema is most apparent in the face, hands, and feet. The skin is pale, cool, and dry.

CASE STUDY 38-1

Ms. Karen Randolph is a 48-year-old business executive in a large national firm. She is married and has three children, ages 16, 14, and 11. Ms. Randolph reports that she has been under a great deal of stress in her work setting for approximately the last year.

Ms. Randolph reports the onset 4 to 5 months ago of symptoms which have continued to intensify. Although her weight is usually stable at 130 lb, she has experienced a gradual and persistent weight loss despite increasing food intake. She also complains of being "hot all the time." Although her usual energy level is high, she now feels extreme fatigue and has difficulty accomplishing routine daily tasks at home and at work. Her husband and children state that she has been extremely irritable.

She states that she has always been healthy and has had no significant illnesses in the past. Her family medical history is unremarkable with the exception of her mother and two maternal aunts, who had thyroidectomies.

A physical examination reveals that her height is 5 ft 7 in (170 cm) and her current weight is 112 lb (50.4 kg). Her vital signs are as follows: blood pressure 185/92, heart rate 92/min, respirations 22/min, and temperature 99.4°F orally. Her hair is fine and brittle, with a lack of luster or shine. Although her facial features and expressions are symmetrical, she very clearly has bilateral exophthalmos. A large, diffuse goiter is found on palpation of the thyroid gland. Electrocardiography shows sinus tachycardia. Other systems are negative. On examination, Ms. Randolph appears very anxious and is constantly fidgeting with the jewelry on her hands.

1. *Ms. Randolph was diagnosed with Graves' disease. Discuss the pathophysiology.*
2. *Graves' disease is considered to have an autoimmune component. What does this mean?*
3. *What, if anything, is the significance of Ms. Randolph's family history?*
4. *Why is exophthalmos characteristic of Graves' disease?*
5. *What is the basis for the noted irritability and fidgeting?*
6. *What findings would be apparent with pretibial myxedema?*
7. *Which hormones trigger the changes that occur with Graves' disease?*
8. *Explain the basis for the weight loss and the hot feelings.*

See Appendix G for discussion.

Wounds or breaks in the skin heal slowly. Often, cold intolerance results from decreased energy expenditure and calorie consumption.[1]

Cardiovascular symptoms may closely resemble those of congestive heart failure. Cardiac output is decreased, as are heart rate and circulating blood volume. Peripheral vascular resistance is increased, ultimately resulting in decreased flow of blood to the tissues. The term *myxedema heart* refers to the clinical picture of an enlarged heart with electrocardiographic and serum enzyme changes.

The gastrointestinal tract, together with other body functions, slows down under the influence of a hypothyroid state. Most persons have a decreased appetite and, contrary to popular belief, only a slight increase in weight. Decreased peristalsis leads to an accumulation of gas and complaints of constipation.

Hypothyroid effect on the nervous system also decreases function. Thinking and movement begin to slow down. Mental dullness often is apparent. Personality changes may occur, resulting in severe depression or extreme agitation and anxiety. Movements are slow and disorganized, causing the appearance of clumsiness.

Other body system changes also result from hypothyroidism. Muscle pains are common, and strength decreases. Reduced renal blood flow and glomerular filtration contribute to the cardiovascular changes. Anemia and changes in clotting factors occur. In both sexes, hypothyroidism decreases sexual drive.

Exactly the opposite of hyperthyroidism, hypothyroidism causes decreased thyroid function and reduced energy metabolism, resulting in a lower BMR. Protein synthesis and degradation are reduced, resulting in retarded growth of bone and muscle tissue. Glucose absorption from the stomach and intestines is delayed, resulting in delayed insulin time. As with protein, the synthesis and degradation of lipids are decreased. The net result is a decreased rate of energy metabolism.

CRETINISM. Thyroid hormone deficiency during embryonic and neonatal life results in a state known as cretinism in infants and young children. This deficiency is not readily apparent at birth, and it may take several weeks to several months before hypothyroidism is discovered. The infant becomes sluggish and falls behind the normal rate of growth and development. Mental retardation and delayed growth patterns are characteristic.

Cretins are dwarflike. Their arms and legs are short in relation to the trunk (Fig. 38-6). The face of a cretin is broad and puffy, and the teeth usually are malformed; the skin is coarse and dry with sparse hair. The abdomen is protuberant, which often results in umbilical hernias. Early recognition and treatment reverse the effects of hypothyroidism in an infant, preventing the onset and development of cretinism.

ENDEMIC GOITER. In some areas of the world, an iodine deficiency exists in the environment to the degree that goiters may be common among the people dwelling in that region. The term *endemic goiter* refers to an enlargement of the thyroid gland to twice normal size or

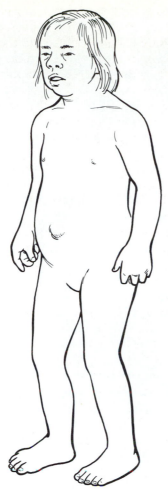

FIGURE 38-6 *Cretinism caused by hypothyroidism.*

larger in at least 10% of the population of an area (Fig. 38-7).[10] The Great Lakes region of the United States and mountainous areas of other countries, such as the Swiss Alps, are noted for iodine deficiency of their soil and water. Because of the lack of iodine, the thyroid cannot synthesize T_4 and T_3, and the result is decreased serum levels of thyroid hormones. Secretion of TSH is increased, and the thyroid gland becomes hyperplastic, leading to the formation of a goiter, which represents the attempt by the gland to produce thyroid hormones.

ADULT HYPOTHYROIDISM. Severe hypothyroidism in the adult often is called *myxedema*. Its onset is slow and may not be recognized for many years. Primary adult hypothyroidism results from the loss or destruction of thyroid gland tissue. This may be caused by an autoimmune or disease process within the thyroid or by removal of the gland, or it may occur after treatment for Graves' disease.[5] Secondary hypothyroidism results from pituitary TSH insufficiency, usually because of a lesion in the pituitary gland.

Early symptoms of adult hypothyroidism are fatigue and lethargy. Marked sensitivity to cold temperatures occurs, as well as gradual slowing of mental

and physical function. These progress through the course of the disease. The skin, hair, and nails become dry, with the hair and nails becoming brittle and breaking easily. The muscles and joints are stiff and aching, especially in the morning after waking. Slight weight gain often is noted despite decreased appetite. Table 38-2 summarizes the clinical presentation of thyroid hormone deficiency.

As the clinical signs and symptoms continue to develop, the full picture of myxedema may appear (Fig. 38-8). Thickness, especially in the face, hands, and feet, becomes apparent, caused by the same process that results in pretibial myxedema in the person with Graves' disease. The voice becomes hoarse and the tongue thickens. The body temperature is lower than normal, resulting in mild hypothermia. Finally, mental and physical lethargy progress to extremes. If untreated, this process continues for many years.

SICK EUTHYROID SYNDROME. A clinical condition that may occur in acutely or chronically ill people has been called the sick euthyroid syndrome.[11,21] The common finding is depressed T_3 and T_4 levels, deficient enough to be well within the definition of hypothyroidism. Sick euthyroid syndrome is distinct from primary hypothyroidism, however, in that the TSH levels are not elevated. The TSH response to TRH may be slightly elevated but is not above the normal range. Sick euthyroid syndrome is rather common in intensive care units after a variety of illnesses and disorders, such as surgery, myocardial infarction, renal insufficiency, ketoacidosis, cirrhosis, thermal injury, and other critical problems.[11] Therefore, it is important that this problem be differentiated from true thyroid disease as quickly as possible.

MYXEDEMA COMA. Myxedema coma is a medical emergency in persons with hypothyroidism. The comatose state is the most severe expression of profound hypothyroid function.[11] It usually occurs during the winter months and affects mostly elderly myxedematous persons. Any stress, such as extreme cold, trauma, infection, central nervous system depressants, or physical stress, may precipitate this crisis. There are three distinct features necessary for diagnosis: altered mental status, defective thermoregulation, and a precipitating illness or event.[14] Myxedema coma also may occur as the end stage of adult hypothyroidism.[13] Lethargy progresses to coma, with hypotension and hypothermia on examination. Hypothermia is considered the most characteristic symptom. The coma results from a continuous slowing of the vital centers; the respiratory center becomes more depressed, cardiac output continues to drop, and cerebral hypoxia increases as a result. Other changes include hypotension, severe hypothermia, bradycardia, hypoventilation with respiratory acidosis, and carbon dioxide

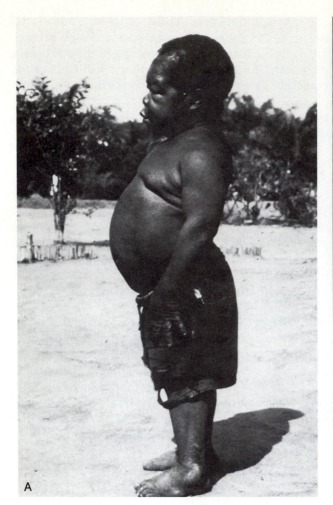
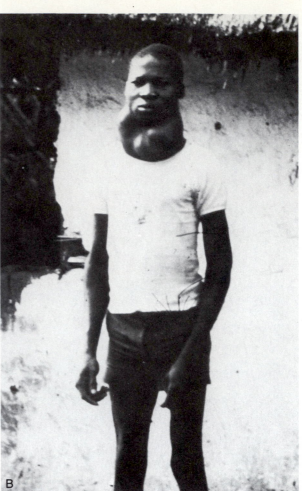

FIGURE 38-7   *A. Endemic cretinism of Zaire. These children, born in areas of severe iodine deficiency have marked mental retardation, short stature, muscle weakness, and motor incoordination. They may or may not have a goiter. Notice the obesity, the protuberant abdomen, and the dry skin of the hands. This condition is caused by prenatal iodine deficiency, probably combined with the maternal ingestion of cassava; the thiocyanate content of this plant crosses the placenta and further injures the developing fetal thyroid gland. Myxedematous endemic cretinism may be prevented by an injection of iodized oil to the pregnant mother.* **B.** *Other members of the community are clinically euthyroid but, as in this youth, some of them have very large, multinodular goiters. (Becker, K.L.* Principles and Practice of Endocrinology and Metabolism. *Philadelphia: J.B. Lippincott, 1990.)*

narcosis, together with various fluid and electrolyte disorders.[11] Without intervention, the mortality is as high as 50%. Although myxedema coma is rare now, its frequency may increase in the future because of the increasing use of radioiodine for the treatment of Graves' disease. Reaction to radioiodine can result in permanent hypothyroidism.[7]

CHRONIC AUTOIMMUNE THYROIDITIS.   The chronic autoimmune form of thyroiditis, also known as *Hashimoto disease*, primarily occurs in women 30 to 50 years of age, but it can occur at any age and is thought to be a major cause of hypothyroidism.[21] It is the most common of the inflammatory thyroid diseases.[16] The two most characteristic findings are a large, palpable goiter and high levels of circulating autoantibodies.

The goiter results from defects of hormone biosynthesis in the thyroid. Because of the failure to produce adequate hormone levels, the pituitary produces TSH abundantly. The result is a goiter without clinical evidence of thyrotoxicosis. Chronic autoimmune thyroiditis may lead to hyperthyroidism but usually results in thyroid hypofunction. The thyroid gland enlarges very gradually. The goiter becomes firm and rubbery and usually is minimally tender, although extreme pain can occur. Left untreated, the gland continues to enlarge for years. There often is a family history of chronic autoimmune thyroiditis or a history of family members with Graves' disease, nontoxic goiter, or primary hypothyroidism. Also, families may show an increased frequency for other autoimmune disorders, such as rheumatoid arthritis and pernicious anemia.

TABLE 38-2 *Clinical Presentation of Thyroid Hormone Deficiency*

	Symptoms	Signs
General	Cold intolerance Fatigue Mild weight gain	Hypothermia
Nervous system	Lethargy Memory defects Poor attention span Personality change	Somnolence Slow speech Myxedema wit Psychopathology: myxedema madness Diminished hearing and taste Cerebellar ataxia
Neuromuscular	Weakness Muscle cramps Joint pain	Delayed relaxation of deep tendon reflexes Carpal tunnel syndrome
Gastrointestinal	Nausea Constipation	Large tongue Ascites
Cardiorespiratory	Decreased exercise tolerance	Hoarse voice Bradycardia Mild hypertension Pericardial effusion Pleural effusion
Reproductive	Decreased libido Decreased fertility Menstrual disorders	
Skin and appendages	Dry, rough skin Puffy facies Hair loss Brittle nails	Nonpitting edema of hands, face, and ankles Periorbital swelling Pallor Yellowish skin (carotenemia) Coarse hair Dry axillae

Becker, K. L. *Principles and Practice of Endocrinology and Metabolism.* Philadelphia: J.B. Lippincott, 1990.

NONTOXIC GOITER.   Sometimes the thyroid gland enlarges without evidence of alterations in rate of body metabolism. This is termed a *nontoxic*, or simple, goiter. It commonly occurs at puberty, during adolescence, or during pregnancy. This disorder occurs in 10% of all North American women.[5] Several causes may be responsible for the goiter, such as iodine deficiency or genetic enzymatic defects. They result in a decreased rate of production of thyroid hormones, which in turn results in increased secretion of TSH from the pituitary. Hyperplasia of thyroid tissue occurs in compensation, and, in mild cases, there usually is no clinical evidence of alteration in function. If thyroid hypertrophy is severe, there may be signs of hyperthyroidism. Usually, the only clinical evidence is the enlarged, palpable thyroid.

MALIGNANT THYROID TUMORS

Carcinoma of the thyroid gland is not common and accounts for only a small percentage of the total number of diagnoses of cancer. No existing evidence supports a familial tendency or predisposition to thyroid carcinoma other than the parafollicular type; some identified predisposing factors are female gender, goiter, and a positive family history for multiple endocrine neoplasia.[11] It has been shown that radiation therapy in childhood dramatically increases the risk of at least two forms of thyroid carcinoma.

PAPILLARY CARCINOMA.   Papillary carcinoma originates in the papillary cells of the thyroid and is the most common type of thyroid cancer, accounting for about 70% to 80% of all thyroid cancers.[19] It is most common in children and young adults and especially affects women. Radiation exposure in childhood contributes to the causation of this cancer. It is a slow-growing cancer and may remain in the gland for many years. The first indication may be a palpable node in the thyroid or enlarged lymph nodes in the neck region. Metastasis can occur through the lymphatics to other areas of the thyroid or, in some cases, to the lungs.

FOLLICULAR CARCINOMA.   Follicular carcinoma, as the name implies, originates in the follicular cells; it

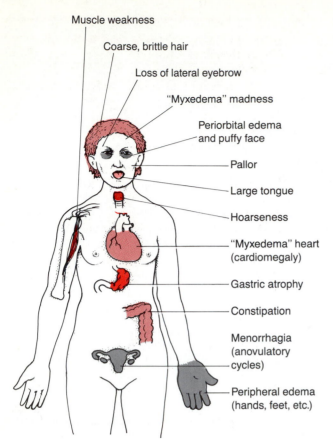

Muscle weakness
Coarse, brittle hair
Loss of lateral eyebrow
"Myxedema" madness
Periorbital edema and puffy face
Pallor
Large tongue
Hoarseness
"Myxedema" heart (cardiomegaly)
Gastric atrophy
Constipation
Menorrhagia (anovulatory cycles)
Peripheral edema (hands, feet, etc.)

FIGURE 38-8 *The dominant clinical manifestations of hypothyroidism. (Rubin E., and Farber, J.L. Pathology [2nd ed.]. Philadelphia: J.B. Lippincott, 1994.)*

accounts for 10% to 20% of thyroid carcinomas.[19] It affects an older population, usually those older than age 40 years; it occurs in women two to three times more often than in men.[5] Childhood exposure to radiation increases the risk of this cancer. The initial feature is an asymptomatic thyroid nodule that exhibits slow patterns of growth. This tumor is more invasive than the papillary carcinoma and may spread through the area blood vessels. Common sites of metastasis are the lungs and bones.

ANAPLASTIC CARCINOMA. Anaplastic carcinoma is a highly malignant form; it accounts for about 10% of thyroid cancers. The tumors usually arise in the seventh to eighth decade of life.[5] It is slightly more common in women than in men. Metastasis occurs rapidly, first to the surrounding areas and then to all parts of the body. The person initially may complain of a mass in the region of the thyroid. As the cancer involves structures adjacent to the thyroid, hoarseness, stridor, and difficulty in swallowing may occur. Tracheal deviation and tumor ulceration may develop.[15] Life expectancy after diagnosis usually is only a few months.

PARAFOLLICULAR CARCINOMA. Parafollicular, or medullary, carcinoma is unique among the thyroid cancers.

Only a small number of cases are of this type. It affects women more than men and is most common in those older than age 50 years. Parafollicular carcinoma also metastasizes quickly, often to distant sites of the body, such as the lungs, bones, and liver. Its distinctive feature is its ability to secrete calcitonin because of its origin in the parafollicular cells.[5, 19] This carcinoma frequently has familial tendencies and may be associated with multiple endocrine neoplasia.

▼ *The Parathyroid Glands*

ANATOMY

The parathyroid glands, four in number, lie posterior and adjacent to the thyroid gland. There is one parathyroid gland in each superior and inferior lateral area of the thyroid. Each gland is small, about the size of a pea, and their combined total weight is about 120 mg. The glands are reddish brown or yellowish brown, and each is enclosed in a small fibrous capsule (see Figure 38-1).

There are two cell types in the parathyroid gland—the *oxyphil cell* and the *chief cell*, or principal cell. Oxyphil cells are slightly larger but are not actually engaged in the secretion of hormones and do not have a known function.[5] Chief cells are responsible for producing and secreting PTH (Fig. 38-9).

FUNCTION

The parathyroid glands regulate the serum levels of calcium in the body and control the rate of bone metabolism. Vitamin D and calcitonin also affect calcium metabolism. Normal total serum calcium is 9–10.5 mg/dL or 2.25–2.75 mmol/L (SI units). Total calcium levels refer to that which is free (ionized) and that albumin bound. The parathyroid glands secrete *PTH (parathor-*

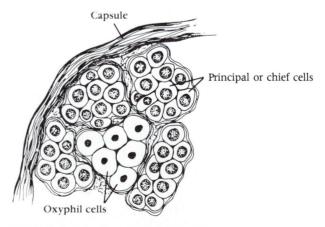

Capsule
Principal or chief cells
Oxyphil cells

FIGURE 38-9 *Parathyroid glands. The cells are arranged in cords by loose connective tissue. The principal cells are predominant in number. Oxyphil cells are recognized by their smaller, more condensed nuclei and larger relative cytoplasmic volume. (Borysenko, M., et al. Functional Histology [2nd ed.]. Boston: Little, Brown, 1984.)*

mone). Secretion of this hormone is not under the control of the pituitary gland but is directly regulated by a negative feedback system of the circulating blood levels of calcium. The major function of PTH is the maintenance of a normal level of extracellular fluid calcium.[1] As calcium levels fall, more PTH is secreted; as calcium levels rise, hormone secretion is reduced. Almost any factor that reduces serum calcium levels stimulates the release of PTH (Fig. 38-10A).[5]

Vitamin D is obtained through dietary ingestion of foods with a high content of the vitamin and through synthesis in the skin. Foods that contain vitamin D include milk products and fish-liver oils. Many vitamin D-enriched foods also are available. Vitamin D synthesized in the skin, known as calciferol, is activated on direct exposure to sunlight. Vitamin D is essential for calcium absorption from the intestinal tract into the

bloodstream. It also increases retention of calcium and phosphorus and controls the mineralization of bone matrix. It is therefore important in controlling and maintaining circulating levels of calcium.[8]

Calcitonin, or thyrocalcitonin, which is produced and secreted by neuroendocrine cells throughout the body and in the parafollicular cells of the thyroid gland, opposes the action of PTH and lowers blood calcium levels.[1] Serum calcium levels are decreased when calcium circulating in the blood is transferred back to the bones (see Figure 38-10B). Although the physiologic role of calcitonin is not clear and is almost certainly minor, calcitonin secretion is stimulated by a rise in serum calcium.[6] To maintain calcium levels, PTH acts on bones, kidneys, and intestines to induce reabsorption of calcium. Some of PTH's most important effects are 1) to increase plasma calcium concentration and decrease

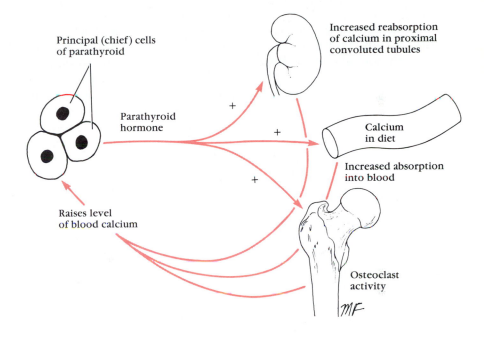

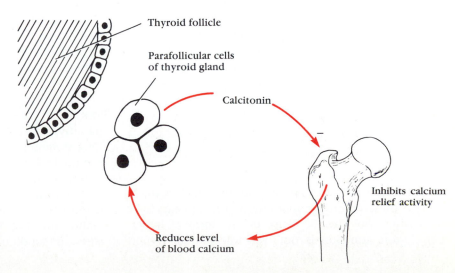

FIGURE 38-10 *A. Regulation and action of the parathyroid hormone. B. Regulation and action of calcitonin secretion by the parafollicular cells of the thyroid gland.*

plasma phosphate concentration; 2) to increase urinary excretion of phosphate but decrease urinary excretion of calcium; 3) to increase the rate of skeletal remodeling and the net rate of bone reabsorption; 4) to increase the number of osteoblasts and osteoclasts on bone surfaces; 5) to cause an initial increase in calcium entry into the cells of its target tissues; 6) to alter the acid-base balance of the body; and 7) to increase gastrointestinal absorption of calcium.[21]

EFFECT ON BONE REABSORPTION. Because the greatest storage of calcium in the body is in bone, it is here that PTH has its greatest effect, increasing the rate of metabolic breakdown of bone tissue. This action primarily is exerted on osteoclasts, which are large cells with several nuclei that participate in the reabsorption of bone.[8] After the release of PTH, osteoclasts reabsorb an area of mineralized bone to release calcium. PTH also stimulates the formation of new osteoclasts and delays the conversion of osteoclasts into osteoblasts, which are the principal cells of bone formation. The overall strength of bone is not substantially altered by this process in a healthy person with normally functioning parathyroid glands.

EFFECT ON REABSORPTION IN THE KIDNEYS. The action of PTH on the kidneys involves increased reabsorption of calcium ions and decreased reabsorption of phosphate ions. These actions occur at different sites in the kidneys and by different mechanisms. Decreased reabsorption of phosphate is caused by the direct effect of PTH on tubular absorption, and the increase in calcium reabsorption is caused by a direct effect on the distal convoluted tubule. In early research, the effect of PTH on the tubular absorption of phosphate was considered to be the primary and most important role. Currently, it is recognized that this action is secondary to the hormone's role in bone reabsorption of calcium.

EFFECT OF PARATHYROID HORMONE ON INTESTINAL REABSORPTION. PTH also influences the reabsorption of calcium from the small intestine. It is necessary for activated vitamin D to be present for this process to occur. Reabsorption of calcium from the intestine also increases absorption of calcium phosphate, thus decreasing the amount of phosphate elimination.

▼ Altered Function of the Parathyroid Gland

HYPERPARATHYROIDISM

The incidence of hyperparathyroidism, which is much more common than hypoparathyroidism, appears to be increasing. The specific cause of any form of hyperparathyroid function is not well understood. Hyper-

secretion of PTH results in elevated serum calcium levels and excessive secretion of phosphorus by the kidneys. In most cases, a single benign adenoma is the cause. A history of long-standing hypocalcemia may contribute to a predisposition for hyperparathyroidism. Three forms of hyperfunction of the parathyroid glands usually are recognized: primary, secondary, and tertiary.

PRIMARY HYPERPARATHYROIDISM. Primary hyperparathyroidism is characterized by hypercalcemia that results from failure of the normal feedback mechanism to decrease secretion of PTH. The three most common causes are parathyroid adenomas (80% of all cases), hyperplasia of all four parathyroid glands, or some form of parathyroid carcinoma.[1,2] As the serum calcium concentrations rise, parathyroid secretion is no longer reduced, and calcium levels continue to increase.

The clinical manifestations are variable and nonspecific. Some people experience mild symptoms, and others have severe symptoms. The most common manifestation is the presence of renal calculi in the genitourinary system, which probably result from precipitation of calcium and phosphate in the kidneys.[5] Other variable symptoms include renal symptoms, skeletal changes, and hypercalcemia. In addition to the formation of renal stones, hematuria may be noted. Gastrointestinal complaints include anorexia, nausea, vomiting, and constipation, as well as generalized abdominal pain.[2] Changes within the skeletal system are diverse. Sometimes new bone is laid as quickly as calcium is reabsorbed, and the patient has only mild complaints of vague skeletal pains. At other times, various bone diseases such as osteoporosis or osteomalacia may result.

SECONDARY HYPERPARATHYROIDISM. In secondary hyperparathyroidism, levels of circulating PTH are high, perhaps initiated by a variety of causes that result in a low serum calcium concentration. Although renal disease is the most common cause of secondary hyperparathyroidism, other causes include low-calcium diet, pregnancy or lactation, rickets, and osteomalacia. In the Western world, the usual cause is renal failure. Low calcium levels cause the parathyroid glands to become hyperplastic to compensate. After compensation attempts, calcium may remain low or may attain normal levels.

TERTIARY HYPERPARATHYROIDISM. Tertiary hyperparathyroidism results from previously developed, long-standing secondary hyperparathyroidism, which eventually leads to elevated serum calcium levels.[12] Autonomous secretion of PTH continues without regard for serum calcium levels. In most instances, adenomas have developed in the already hyperplastic parathyroid glands after the onset of secondary hyperparathyroidism. This condition is accompanied by abnormally high calcium levels. Tertiary hyperparathyroidism often is described in persons with renal failure who develop hypercalcemia.

Renal osteodystrophy, which may occur with tertiary hyperparathyroidism, arises in persons with chronic renal failure who develop hyperphosphatemia.[9] Parathyroid hyperfunction then occurs and increases serum calcium concentrations (see pp. 665–666). Metastatic calcifications may occur in the soft tissues, such as the eyes, lungs, and joints.[5]

HYPOPARATHYROIDISM

Hypoparathyroidism results when insufficient amounts of PTH are secreted or when the hormone fails to act at the tissue level. Without circulating PTH, calcium is not resorbed from bone, kidneys, or intestines. The result is a decreased serum concentration of calcium. This in turn causes increased neuromuscular excitability and the symptoms of tetany. All of the clinical manifestations result from decreased levels of serum calcium concentration. Affected persons whose serum calcium levels have slowly dropped to abnormal levels are less likely to develop symptoms than are those who experience acute hypocalcemia.[17]

CLINICAL MANIFESTATIONS. In 70% of cases of hypoparathyroidism, tetany becomes the major clinical manifestation.[21] It begins with numbness and tingling of the extremities and progresses to stiffness, cramps, and spasms. Carpal spasms are common and are the most prominent symptoms. If serum calcium levels continue to fall, the neuromuscular manifestations become more severe and pronounced. Laryngeal muscles are susceptible to spasms, and death by asphyxiation can result if intervention is not immediate. At the very least, wheezing caused by bronchospasm occurs. Hypocalcemia seldom presents as an acute crisis, except in the postoperative when the glands have been in advertently removed during thyroidectomy.[4]

After hypoparathyroidism has existed for several months to several years, other physical changes may become apparent. Nails become brittle and may atrophy, and horizontal ridges are apparent on their surfaces. Alopecia occurs in patches on the head, and there may be almost complete loss of eyebrows. The skin becomes coarse and dry with patches of brownish pigment. Papilledema often is present and may occur with increased intracranial pressure. Electrocardiography in hypocalcemia may show a lengthening of the QT interval. Serum calcium levels fall and remain subnormal. Sometimes, personality changes and psychiatric symptoms occur, such as emotional lability, extreme irritability and anxiety, depression, and delirium. Convulsions and grand mal seizures may occur.

Three clinical signs are used to diagnose tetany and hypoparathyroidism. The first test is for a positive Chvostek sign. A quick tap or light blow over the parotid gland near the ear produces twitching of the facial muscles, especially the upper lip, nose, and eye (Fig. 38-11). A Trousseau sign is elicited by occluding blood supply to the arm for 3 minutes; the result is positive if carpopedal spasms occur (Fig. 38-12). The Erb sign is considered positive if a 6-mV current produces a motor response. A specific positive response to any of these clinical signs usually is considered diagnostic.

IDIOPATHIC HYPOPARATHYROIDISM. Idiopathic hypoparathyroidism is relatively uncommon. The course of dysfunction is variable. It may be congenital or acquired, mild or severe, transient or lifelong. The congenital form is related to defective or absent parathyroid glands. Children are most commonly diagnosed, with females being affected twice as often as males. An autoimmune state also may be involved in idiopathic hypoparathyroidism. The symptoms, including tetany, usually are severe.

POSTOPERATIVE HYPOPARATHYROIDISM. More common than the idiopathic form is hypoparathyroidism related to damage or removal of the parathyroid glands during thyroid surgery. Removal of the thyroid gland without detachment of the parathyroids is the most frequent cause. Any surgery that involves manipulation of the structures of the throat, such as radical neck dissection, can result in clinical features of hypoparathyroidism. With damage or partial removal, the remaining parathyroid tissue usually is able to compensate. Therefore, the loss of PTH is transient. Complete

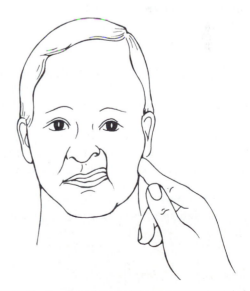

FIGURE 38-11 *Tapping of the facial nerve approximately 2 cm anterior to the earlobe elicits the Chvostek sign (unilateral twitching of the facial muscles) in some patients with hypocalcemia or hypomagnesemia. (Metheny, N.M. Fluid and Electrolyte Balance [2nd ed.]. Philadelphia: J.B. Lippincott, 1992.)*

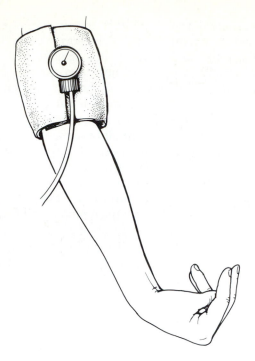

FIGURE 38-12 *Carpopedal spasm (Trousseau's sign) elicited when blood supply is occluded to the arm for 3 minutes. It is a characteristic sign of hypocalcemia.*

removal of the glands results in total loss of parathyroid function, and severe hypocalcemia rapidly follows.

PSEUDOHYPOPARATHYROIDISM. Pseudohypoparathyroidism, also known as *Albright's hereditary osteodystrophy*, is a form of hypoactive functioning that is familial in origin. It is widely believed to be transmitted by an X-linked dominant gene. Hypocalcemia and hypophosphatemia are characteristic of this disorder. The parathyroid glands are normal in size or slightly enlarged, and there is no deficit in circulating levels of PTH, but there is some abnormality in the PTH receptor interaction, causing failure of a response to PTH.[5] Women are affected twice as frequently as men. Persons with this condition have developmental skeletal abnormalities and usually exhibit a mild to moderate degree of mental retardation. They are short and stocky, often less than 5 ft (152 cm) tall, and usually exhibit obesity. The face is very round because of structural abnormalities in the development of the facial and cranial bones. The metacarpal bones are short and stubby. There normally is some degree of widespread subcutaneous soft-tissue ossification and calcification.

▼ *Chapter Summary*

▼   The thyroid gland is important to regulate and control the rate of metabolism. The hormones thyroxine (T_4) and triiodothyronine (T_3) are the main hormones se-

creted to increase metabolism. They are under the direct influence of TSH from the anterior pituitary which is under the influence of TRF from the hypothalamus.

▼   There is a closely regulated feedback process for the maintenance of adequate thyroid hormone in the blood. Formation of the hormones depends on adequate iodine which is supplied in the diet.

▼   The thyroid gland also secretes calcitonin which is secreted directly in relation to serum calcium levels. Increased calcium causes calcitonin secretion which moves the calcium from the serum into the bones.

▼   Hyperthyroidism, or thyrotoxicosis, is a condition which is characterized by increased T_3 and T_4 production. The resulting clinical picture is one of hypermetabolism. A goiter may or may not be present and other manifestations depend on the amount of hypersecretion that occurs.

▼   Graves' disease is the most common form of severe hyperthyroidism and is characterized by goiter, exophthalmos, pretibial myxedema, and hypermetablism.

▼   Hypothyroidism is the result of thyroid hormone deficiency and all of the clinical manifestations result from the slowing of the metabolic processes. Severe hypothyroidism in the adult is called myxedema and in the infant and child, cretinism. Goiter may be present due to TSH stimulation of the thyroid that is unable to produce hormones due to lack of iodine.

▼   Malignancy of the thyroid gland is not common and the prognosis depends on the form of the malignancy and how early it was detected.

▼   Parathyroid hormone is essential in regulating calcium metabolism. It is secreted when the calcium level is decreased and causes the reabsorption of calcium from bones, gut, and kidneys.

▼   Hyperparathyroidism results in hypercalcemia and is most commonly caused by a parathyroid adenoma or by renal disease. Hypoparathyroidism causes hypocalcemia and may be idiopathic or surgically induced. It causes dangerous tetany and laryngeal spasm.

▼ *References*

1. Becker, K.L. *Principles and Practice of Endocrinology and Metabolism.* Philadelphia: J.B. Lippincott, 1991.
2. Bilezikian, J.P. Primary hyperparathyroidism. In Stein, J. (ed.), *Internal Medicine* (4th ed.). St. Louis: Mosby, 1994.
3. Braverman, L.E., and Utiger, R.D. *The Thyroid: A Fundamental and Clinical Text.* Philadelphia: J.B. Lippincott, 1991.
4. Bybee, D.E. Saving lives in parathyroid crises. *Emerg Med* 19:62, 1987.
5. Cotran, R., Kumar, V., and Robbins, S.L. *Robbins' Pathologic Basis of Disease* (5th ed.). Philadelphia: W.B. Saunders, 1994.
6. Gavin, L.A. Thyroid crises. *Med Clin North Am* 75:179–193, 1991.

7. Greenspan, F.S., and Rapoport, B. Thyroid gland. In Greenspan, F.S. (ed.), *Basic and Clinical Endocrinology* (3rd ed.). Norwalk, Conn.: Appleton & Lange, 1991.

8. Guyton, A.C. *Textbook of Medical Physiology* (8th ed.). Philadelphia: W.B. Saunders, 1991.

9. Hahn, T.J. Calcium, phosphate, magnesium, and bone: Physiology and disorders. In Hershman, J.M. (ed.), *Endocrine Pathophysiology: A Patient-Oriented Approach* (3rd ed.). Philadelphia: Lea & Febiger, 1988.

10. Hershman, J.M. Thyroid disease. In Hershman, J.M. (ed.), *Endocrine Pathophysiology: A Patient-Oriented Approach* (3rd ed.). Philadelphia: Lea & Febiger, 1988.

11. Levey, G.S., and Klein, I. Disorders of the thyroid. In Stein, J. (ed.), *Internal Medicine* (4th ed.). St. Louis: Mosby, 1994.

12. Lloyd, R.V. Parathyroid glands. In Lloyd, R.V. (ed.), *Endocrine Pathology*. New York: Springer-Verlag, 1990.

13. McMillan, J.Y. Preventing myxedema coma in the hypothyroid patient. *Dimens Crit Care Nurs* 7:136, 1988.

14. Nicoloff, J.T., and LoPresti, J.S. Myxedema coma: A form of decompensated hypothyroidism. *Endocrinol Metab Clin North Am* 22:279–290, 1993.

15. Rubin, E., and Farber, J.L. *Pathology* (2nd ed.). Philadelphia: J.B. Lippincott, 1994.

16. Singer, P.A. Thyroiditis: Acute, subacute, and chronic. *Med Clin North Am* 75:61–77, 1991.

17. Tohme, J.F. Hypocalcemic emergencies. *Endocrinol Metab Clin North Am* 22:363–375, 1993.

18. Tortora, G., and Grabowski, S. *Principles of Anatomy and Physiology* (7th ed.). New York: HarperCollins, 1993.

19. Utiger, R. Disorders of the thyroid gland. In Kelley, W.N. (ed.), *Textbook of Internal Medicine* (2nd ed.). Philadelphia: J.B. Lippincott, 1992.

20. Utiger, R. Thyroid hormone production, transport, and action. In Kelley, W.N. (ed.), *Textbook of Internal Medicine* (2nd ed.). Philadelphia: J.B. Lippincott, 1992.

21. Wilson, J.D., and Foster, D.W. (eds.). *Williams' Textbook of Endocrinology* (8th ed.). Philadelphia: W.B. Saunders, 1992.

Chapter 39

Normal and Altered Functions of the Pancreas

Doris Heaman

▼ **LEARNING OBJECTIVES**

1 Describe the macroscopic and microscopic anatomy of the pancreas.
2 Explain the physiologic regulation of insulin secretion.
3 Describe the metabolic effects of insulin.
4 Explain the actions of glucagon and somatostatin and their effects on metabolism.
5 Discuss the frequency and cause of diabetes mellitus.
6 Explain the differences in genetic characteristics between insulin-dependent diabetes mellitus and non–insulin-dependent diabetes mellitus.
7 Explain the pathophysiology of diabetes mellitus and its complications.
8 Relate the clinical manifestations of diabetes to the pathophysiologic changes.
9 Distinguish between ketoacidosis; hyperglycemic, hyperosmolar, nonketotic coma; and lactic acidosis.
10 Outline the physiologic responses to hypoglycemia.
11 Identify tests used in the diagnosis and evaluation of diabetes mellitus.
12 Explain the pathophysiology of pancreatic islet cell diseases: hyperinsulinism, Zollinger–Ellison syndrome (gastrinoma), and multiple endocrine neoplasia (Werner syndrome).
13 Discuss the frequency and cause of acute pancreatitis.
14 Describe the chemical and pathologic changes characteristic of pancreatitis.
15 Relate the clinical manifestations of acute pancreatitis to the histologic alterations.
16 Discuss the complications of acute pancreatitis, and relate laboratory findings of acute pancreatitis.
17 Discuss the frequency, cause, types, and clinical course of carcinoma of the pancreas.
18 Discuss the frequency and genetics of cystic fibrosis.
19 Describe the pathophysiologic changes that occur in various body systems in cystic fibrosis.
20 Relate the clinical manifestations of cystic fibrosis to the pathophysiologic changes.
21 Discuss laboratory and diagnostic findings related to cystic fibrosis.

Barbara L. Bullock: PATHOPHYSIOLOGY: ADAPTATIONS AND ALTERATIONS IN FUNCTION, 4th ed.
© 1996 Lippincott-Raven Publishers

This chapter describes the anatomy, physiology, pathology, and alterations in function of the pancreas. The pancreas consists of both exocrine and endocrine portions. It is important in the digestion and metabolism of food, and much of its anatomic structure serves gastrointestinal function. The most common disorders of the exocrine pancreas are cystic fibrosis, pancreatitis, and tumors. Special cells in the islets of Langerhans influence metabolism through the secretion of insulin and glucagon. Diabetes mellitus is the most common disorder associated with pancreatic islet dysfunction of the endocrine portion, and it is a leading cause of disability and death in the United States.

▼ Anatomy and Physiology

The pancreas is an elongated retroperitoneal gland that lies in the upper portion of the posterior abdominal wall. It resembles a fish, with its head and neck lying in the C-shaped curve of the duodenum, its body extending horizontally behind the stomach, and its tail touching the spleen (Fig. 39-1). The head is at the level of the second lumbar vertebra, makes up about 30% of the gland, and lies within the concavity of the duodenum. The neck, the narrowed portion between the head and the body, joins to the body, which accounts for the largest portion of the gland. The tail tapers off from the body. The pancreas is firm and has a characteristic lobular appearance with a light yellow and slightly pink coloration.

In the adult, the total length of the pancreas is 12 to 20 cm, with a width of 3 to 5 cm and a maximal thickness of 2 to 3 cm. Its weight is between 60 and 140 g. The pancreas is composed of the acini (grapelike formations), which secrete digestive juices into the duodenum, and the islets of Langerhans, which secrete insulin and glucagon into the blood.

The exocrine portion of the pancreas forms the largest mass (about 80%) of the gland. Major enzymes secreted include trypsin, chymotrypsin, peptidases, amylases, lipases, phospholipases, and elastase. Trypsin is critical in enzyme activity because it activates other enzymes. Exocrine secretion varies from 1.5 to 3.0 L daily, depending on demands of intestinal volume and contents.

The acini form a network of larger ducts that eventually drain into the major secretory ducts of Wirsung and Santorini. The duct of Wirsung extends from the surface of the tail of the pancreas to the duodenum at the ampulla of Vater, usually alongside the common bile duct. It empties into the duodenum at the same place as the common bile duct, the duodenal papilla. In most cases, the sphincter of Oddi surrounds both ducts. In one-third of cases, the duct of Wirsung and the common bile duct form a common channel before terminating at the ampulla of Vater. The accessory duct of Santorini exits from the main duct near the neck of the pancreas and enters the duodenum about 2 cm above the main duct.

The endocrine portion of the pancreas, the islets of Langerhans, is embedded between exocrine units like small islands. The islets contain three major types of cells: the *alpha* (α), *beta* (β), and *delta* (δ) cells (Fig. 39-2). These types compose 20%, 70%, and 6% to 12% of islet cell population, respectively. All of these cells empty their secretions into the bloodstream. The α cells secrete

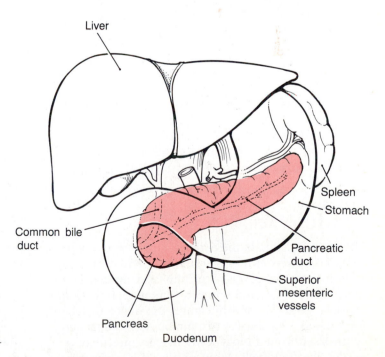

FIGURE 39-1 *Relation of pancreas to other abdominal organs.*

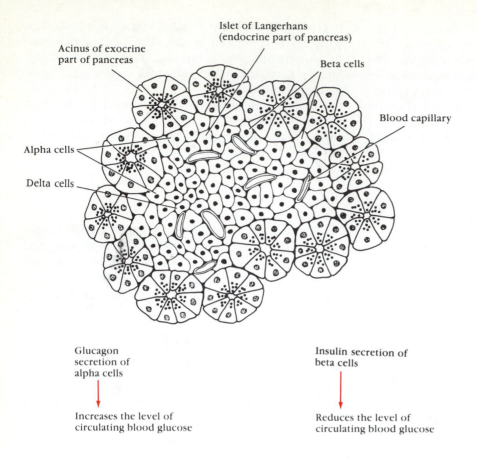

Islet of Langerhans
(endocrine part of pancreas)

Acinus of exocrine
part of pancreas

Beta cells

Blood capillary

Alpha cells

Delta cells

Glucagon
secretion of
alpha cells

Insulin secretion of
beta cells

Increases the level of
circulating blood glucose

Reduces the level of
circulating blood glucose

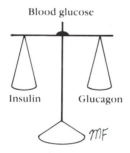

Blood glucose

Insulin   Glucagon

FIGURE 39-2 *Regulation of the secretion of insulin and glucagon from the cells of the islets of Langerhans.*

glucagon, the β cells secrete *insulin,* and the δ cells contain secretory granules that secrete gastrin or *somatostatin.* Although there are as many as 2 million islets, each 20 to 300 μm in diameter, the endocrine portion makes up only about 1% of the weight of the pancreas.

PHYSIOLOGIC REGULATION OF INSULIN SECRETION

The main function of the endocrine portion of the pancreas is to secrete *insulin,* a hormone essential for normal carbohydrate metabolism. Insulin also influences the metabolism of fats and proteins. Therefore, it is a prime anabolic hormone and integrates the major metabolic fuels. Insulin consists of two amino acid chains and is synthesized from a biologically inactive precursor, *proinsulin,* by the β cells. Proinsulin itself is derived from an even larger polypeptide, *preproinsulin.*[30] The average adult pancreas secretes an estimated 35 to 50 units of insulin daily.

Carbohydrates (primarily glucose), fats, and proteins influence insulin output during meals. Insulin is the only known hormone that reduces the circulating glucose levels. Although numerous physiologic factors can alter insulin secretion, output is regulated mainly by blood glucose level through a negative feedback mechanism (Fig. 39-3). If the glucose concentration in the blood that is perfusing the pancreas exceeds about 100 mg/dL, an immediate β-cell response extrudes the granule's contents from the β cell. If blood glucose levels fall, the rate of insulin secretion also decreases. The release of insulin is biphasic. Glucose prompts both an immediate and a sustained release as more insulin is synthesized. The feedback mechanism is rapid-acting, and insulin

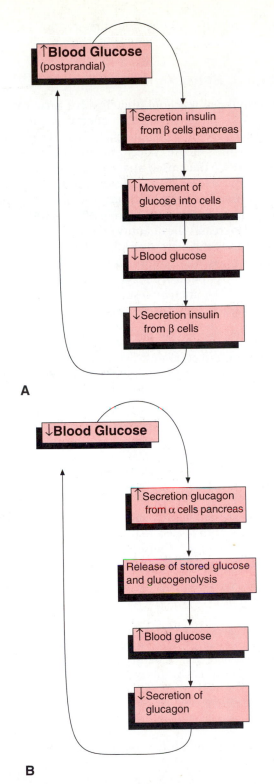

A

B

FIGURE 39-3 *Negative feedback system of* **A** *Insulin, and* **B** *Glucagon.*

ginine, lysine, and phenylalanine. Insulin in turn promotes transport of the amino acids into the tissue cells. Fats, although weak stimulators of insulin release, promote sufficient amounts to prevent ketoacidosis. Oral ingestion of fat triggers release of gastrointestinal hormones that augment insulin secretion.

Although insulin secretion is mostly considered in terms of response to nutrients, measurable amounts are secreted at a low basal rate between meals and during prolonged fasting. The gastrointestinal hormones secretin, cholecystokinin, gastrin, and gastric-inhibiting peptide, which are released by the gastrointestinal tract after a meal, stimulate pancreatic insulin release. These hormones, released during digestion, cause an anticipatory increase in blood insulin in preparation for the glucose and amino acids absorbed from the meal.

Other hormones that either directly increase the secretion of insulin or potentiate glucose stimulation of insulin are glucagon, cortisol, growth hormone, progesterone, and estrogen. Prolonged increased amounts of these hormones can lead to exhaustion of the β cells and diabetes. The hormone glucagon, which is synthesized in the pancreatic α cells, affects hepatic glucose production. High pharmacologic doses of corticosteroids also may induce diabetes, especially in susceptible individuals.

The autonomic nervous system plays a major role in modulation of insulin secretion between meals, during times when there is no intake, and in response to stressors. Norepinephrine and acetylcholine, transmitters of the autonomic nervous system, and the adrenomedullary hormone epinephrine influence secretion by the α, β, and δ cells of the islets of Langerhans. The α-adrenergic activities of the sympathomimetic amines (epinephrine and norepinephrine) inhibit insulin secretion. Although catecholamine stimulation of β-adrenergic sites increases insulin secretion, the α-adrenergic action of epinephrine predominates.

Other factors, primarily pharmacologic, stimulate insulin secretion, including sulfonylurea drugs and theophylline. In contrast, β-receptor blocking agents and diazoxide inhibit secretion. Table 39-1 lists factors that increase or decrease insulin secretion.

EFFECT OF INSULIN ON FACILITATED DIFFUSION

Insulin is an influential hormone that affects the biochemical function of every organ in the body. Its most important action is to accelerate the transport of glucose across most cell membranes in the body. In the absence of insulin, the rate of transport of glucose into body cells is about 25% of the normal rate; if excess insulin is secreted, the rate may increase to five times normal. Figure 39-4 shows the transport of glucose through the cell membrane by means of a carrier-mediated mechanism called *facilitated diffusion*, or carrier transport. Insu-

levels reach 10 to 20 times the basal rate with blood glucose levels of 300 to 400 mg/dL. The cessation of secretion is equally rapid, occurring within minutes after restoration of blood glucose to fasting level.[17]

Amino acids also can stimulate insulin secretion in varying degrees. The most potent stimulants are ar-

TABLE 39-1 *Factors That Affect Insulin Secretion*

Increased Secretion	Decreased Secretion
↑ Serum glucose	Norepinephrine
↑ Glucagon	Epinephrine
Cortisol—adrenocorticotropic hormone	Somatostatin
Growth hormone	Fasting and starvation
Gastrointestinal hormones— especially secretin	Sympathetic nervous stimulation
Parasympathetic nervous stimulation	Pharmacologic agents: Diazoxide
Pharmacologic agents:	β-Receptor blocking agents
β Stimulators	
Theophylline	
Sulfa drugs	
α-Receptor blocking agents	

lin influences this transport of glucose into the cell by combining with a receptor protein in the cell membrane. It is the activated receptor that results in glucose transport within seconds or minutes. After the glucose concentration inside the cell is equal to that on the outside, additional glucose is not transferred into the cell. Insulin is especially effective in facilitating transport of glucose in skeletal and adipose tissue, the liver, and the heart. Adipose and skeletal tissues alone make up 65% of body weight.

Insulin does not enhance glucose transport into the brain, erythrocytes, leukocytes, intestinal mucosa, or epithelium of the kidneys. The brain continues to function normally even if insulin deficiency causes hyperglycemia. In erythrocytes and leukocytes, the level of free glucose is close to that in plasma. These cells do not

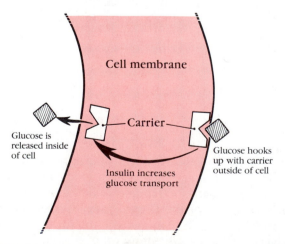

FIGURE 39-4 *Insulin increases glucose transport by facilitated diffusion, a passive process.*

suffer from insulin deficiency, but they cannot survive glucose deficiency.

METABOLIC EFFECTS OF INSULIN

Insulin stimulates reactions that involve fats, carbohydrates, and proteins. Insulin affects *carbohydrate metabolism* by increasing the rate of glucose metabolism, decreasing blood glucose concentration, and increasing glycogen stores in the muscle and liver. Insulin affects *fat metabolism* by increasing the rate of glucose transport into fat cells, forming lipids from fatty acids, and promoting storage in adipose tissue. Insulin affects *protein metabolism* and increases the quantity of protein by increasing translation of the messenger ribonucleic acid (RNA) code in the ribosomes to form more protein, and by enhancing transcription of deoxyribonucleic acid (DNA) to form more RNA, thereby resulting in additional protein synthesis. Insulin's diverse effects are integrated so that it is the prime synthesis and storage hormone in metabolism. Its actions are focused on three metabolically important target tissues: liver, adipose tissue, and muscle. The effects on these tissues are summarized in Table 39-2 and in the following discussion.

Liver

The liver is an important blood-glucose buffer system. It is the major site for synthesis of glycogen, lipids, and proteins, and is the major endogenous source of glucose. Insulin is secreted by the pancreas into the portal system and enters the systemic circulation through the liver. The role of the liver with respect to insulin and carbohydrate homeostasis is unique because of the following aspects:

1. Insulin promotes glycogen storage by inhibiting the action of an enzyme, phosphorylase, which is responsible for breakdown of liver glycogen and release of glucose into circulation.
2. Insulin increases glycogen synthesis by stimulating the actions of enzymes necessary for formation of glycogen.
3. Insulin is not necessary for transport of glucose into the liver because the liver cells are freely permeable to glucose. The uptake is increased by glucokinase, an enzyme that is responsible for "trapping" glucose inside liver cells so that the intracellular concentration is roughly equal to the plasma concentration.
4. In the basal state, glucose is continuously released from the liver. The ability of the liver to release free glucose derives from its capability for glycogenolysis (breaking down stored glycogen) and gluconeogenesis (forming new glucose) and from its possession of an enzyme that promotes further breakdown of glycogen into glucose. This process is critical during prolonged fasting, when glucose is oxidized minimally in most tissues and is used almost exclusively by the brain.
5. In the basal state, between meals, when blood glucose level falls and the pancreas secretes less insulin, glycogen synthesis and storage are halted.

TABLE 39-2 *Target Sites and Metabolic Actions of Insulin*

Substance	Liver	Adipose Cell	Muscle
Carbohydrate	Glycogen synthesis Gluconeogenesis Glycogenolysis	Glucose transport Glycerol synthesis	Glucose transport Glycolysis Glycogen synthesis
Fat	Lipogenesis	Triglycerides Fatty acid synthesis Promotes storage	
Protein	Proteolysis for gluco- neogenesis		Amino acid uptake Protein synthesis Protein anabolism

6. Absorbed hexoses have direct access to the liver through the portal vein before circulating to peripheral tissues.

Because of these characteristics, the liver is important in buffering blood glucose. If there is an excess of insulin or glucose, the hepatic cells take up large quantities of glucose, which are deposited as glycogen as well as being converted to fat. About 60% of glucose ingested in a meal is stored in this manner.[17] If there is an absence of insulin or the blood glucose concentration falls too low, the hepatic cells release quantities of glucose into the blood by glycogenolysis and gluconeogenesis. In this manner, insulin enables the organism to maintain a stable blood glucose balance.

Adipose Tissue

Maintenance of energy balance is a major role of adipose tissue. It is the only tissue that can store a variable amount of "fuel" in the form of fat. The oxidation of 1 g of fat yields 9 calories. Unlike that of the liver cell, the membrane of the fat cell (adipocyte) is capable of excluding glucose. Adipose tissue does not release glucose but can release free fatty acids and certain amino acids. Insulin greatly enhances the transport of glucose into fat cells and promotes fat storage in adipose tissue. The metabolism of glucose within fat cells occurs in several steps:

1. Glucose is rapidly phosphorylated within the fat cell.
2. Glucose is further metabolized to 2-carbon fragments (acetylcoenzyme A), which are converted to fatty acids.
3. A larger portion is degraded by glycolysis into α-glycerophosphate. The latter readily combines with free fatty acids to form triglycerides, the primary storage form of fat within the adipose cell.

Insulin promotes fat storage by inhibiting the action of the enzyme lipase within the fat cell, which results in inhibition of both lipolysis and release of fatty acids into the circulation, and by promoting glucose transport into the cell. Through its action on glucose metabolism, insulin provides the precursors necessary for combining and storing fatty acids as triglycerides. Fatty acids and all of the lipid components of plasma greatly increase in the absence of insulin. High lipid concentrations in the plasma, especially cholesterol, increase the risk of developing atherosclerosis.

Muscle

As in adipose tissue, insulin increases transport of glucose across the membrane into muscle cells through facilitated diffusion. Within the cell, the glucose is metabolized completely to carbon dioxide or, if oxygen is limited, to lactic acid. After the glucose molecule that enters the cell is phosphorylated, it is used for energy or stored as glycogen. Unlike the liver, muscle cannot release glucose from stored glycogen into the body fluids because it lacks the necessary enzyme, glucose phosphatase, to convert glycogen into glucose. Little glucose is stored in the form of triglyceride.

Quantitatively, muscle cell consumption of glucose is small during a resting state. Muscle tissue uses mostly fatty acids for energy because the normal resting muscle membrane is almost impermeable to glucose except in the presence of insulin. During exercise, glucose use greatly increases. This usage of glucose requires smaller amounts of insulin because exercising muscle fibers are more permeable to glucose in the absence of insulin. The contraction process itself increases permeability of fibers. Muscles also use large amounts of glucose in the first few hours after a meal. Food intake increases the blood glucose level, which stimulates the secretion of large amounts of insulin and the transport of glucose into muscle cells.[17]

Summary of Effects of Insulin

In summary, insulin is primarily a storage hormone. Its diverse metabolic actions on various target tissues demonstrate the integrated and synergistic effect it has on the metabolism of fats, carbohydrates, and proteins. Each molecule of glucose that enters a cell is immediately phosphorylated. Adipose tissue and muscle take up glucose only under the influence of insulin, phosphorylate it, and either store it in the form of glycogen or convert it to triglycerides (fatty acids). At the same time, the presence of free fatty acids impedes glucose oxidation and decreases the release of amino acids from muscle for hepatic gluconeogenesis. Glucose uptake by muscle is also stimulated, providing fuel to replace fatty acids whose release from adipose tissue is inhibited by insulin. Fat accumulation also is increased by release of fatty acids at the adipose cell from lipoproteins that arrive by way of the circulation from the liver and gastrointestinal tract. The antilipolytic action of insulin on the adipose cell increases fat storage; this inhibits gluconeogenesis in the liver by depriving the liver of fatty acids and cofactors used in gluconeogenesis.

PHYSIOLOGY OF GLUCAGON

Glucagon, a hormone secreted by the α cells of the islets of Langerhans, is important in the regulation of carbohydrate metabolism. The action of glucagon is opposite to that of insulin, and its secretion results in an increase in blood glucose concentration. The major effects of glucagon are stimulation of *glycogenolysis* and *gluconeogenesis* (see Figure 39-3). Glucagon is a powerful hormone that can increase blood glucose about 20% within minutes.[17] It also promotes proteolysis and ketogenesis.

Glucagon secretion is regulated by blood glucose concentration. Changes in blood glucose levels have the opposite effect on glucagon secretion that they do on insulin secretion. A decrease in the level of blood glucose increases glucagon secretion. In almost every instance, glucagon has a metabolic effect directly opposite that of insulin: insulin promotes storage of glycogen in liver and muscle, glucagon inhibits it; insulin inhibits glycogenolysis, glucagon promotes it; insulin inhibits lipolysis, glucagon stimulates it. Thus, a negative feedback system with opposing actions of insulin and glucagon maintains the blood glucose levels (see Figure 39-3).

Glucagon secretion is increased by exercise, starvation, insulin lack, and amino acid ingestion. It is important in the maintenance of glucose levels during fasting, exercise, and stressful situations to help to protect the body against hypoglycemia.

SOMATOSTATIN

Somatostatin, a hormone excreted by the δ cells of the pancreas, is essential in the metabolism of fats, carbohydrates, and proteins. It acts as a neural agent by inhibiting secretions of insulin and glucagon and other nonislet hormones. Although not a neurotransmitter, its actions are opposite to those of acetylcholine. The release of somatostatin is stimulated by epinephrine. Somatostatin also is widely present in the central nervous system, primarily the hypothalamus. Smaller amounts have been noted in the cells of the thyroid and gastrointestinal tract. The precise function of somatostatin in metabolic processes is not clearly defined, but it is postulated that it acts in concert with insulin and glucagon to control the flow of nutrients into and out of circulation.[40]

REGULATION OF BLOOD GLUCOSE

In the healthy person, the blood glucose ranges between 60 and 100 mg/dL in the fasting state. This concentration rises to 120 to 140 mg/dL after a meal. The feedback system returns the concentration to normal within about 2 hours after the last absorption of carbohydrates. The blood glucose level is vital in maintaining nutritional balance in the brain, retinae, and germinal epithelium of the gonads because glucose is the only nutrient that can be used to supply adequate energy. More than one-half of all glucose formed by gluconeogenesis during the interdigesting period is used by the brain.[17]

The liver acts as a reservoir and buffering system for glucose. The liver stores sufficient glycogen to maintain a normal blood sugar for 12 to 24 hours. If blood glucose levels are high, almost two-thirds of the glucose is stored; if the blood glucose concentration falls below normal, the stored glucose is released to maintain the blood level. If the blood glucose level is high (eg, after meals), insulin secretion is increased to return the concentration to normal.

The glucagon feedback system assists in maintaining the range of glucose concentration by stimulating glycogenolysis and gluconeogenesis. Under normal circumstances, the insulin feedback mechanism is the most important, but in starvation states or excessive use of glucose during stress and exercise, the glucagon system becomes important.

Stimulation of the sympathetic nervous system causes a rise in blood glucose level. The release of the catecholamines epinephrine and norepinephrine stimulates glycogenolysis in the liver, resulting in rapid release of glucose into the circulation.

Growth hormone and cortisol increase blood glucose levels less rapidly than the insulin-glucagon system. Both hormones decrease use of glucose in peripheral cells. Cortisol also stimulates gluconeogenesis, thereby resulting in an increased blood glucose level. Growth hormone and glucocorticoids are secreted during periods of hypoglycemia, and the decrease the rate of glucose use by most cells of the body. These hormones are less powerful in regulating blood glucose than insulin and glucagon, and they require hours rather than minutes to effect a change in the serum glucose.

▼ *Diabetes Mellitus*

Diabetes is a metabolic disorder characterized by a relative or absolute lack of the hormone insulin, or by insulin resistance, or both, which results in impaired use of carbohydrates and altered metabolism of fats and protein. The word *diabetes*, from a Greek term meaning "a siphon," suggests excessive urine formation; the word *mellitus*, from the Greek word for "honey," suggests sweetness.

HISTORY

Writings about diabetes go back more than 3,000 years, to the Ebers papyrus, in which afflicted people were described as passing frequent and large amounts of urine. Ayur Veda described the sweetness of the urine and noted that ants were attracted to it. He wrote of weakness, emaciation, polyuria, and carbuncles in affected people. Aretaeus, a first-century Greek physician, is credited with naming the disorder. He described the disease as a "melting down of the flesh and limbs into urine." Lipemia of diabetic blood was noted by Helmunt sometime between 1573 and 1664 A.D. The first diagnostic sign of the disease was established by Thomas Willis in the seventeenth century, when he tasted the urine of his patients and noted its sweetness. A French physician, Michel Chevreul, discovered that the sweetness was caused by sugar.

In 1869, Langerhans, while a medical student, described the group of cells in the pancreas that produce insulin. Elliot Joslin was prescribing dietary restrictions long before the discovery of insulin. In 1921, Banting and Best were able to purify islet cell tissues from dogs, and they obtained a decrease in blood sugar levels when the tissue was injected into diabetic animals. Within 6 months, insulin was administered to humans, and the "rapid melting" and "speedy death" described by Aretaeus were alleviated.

CLASSIFICATION

In 1979, the National Diabetes Data Group and National Institutes of Health, endorsed by the World Health Organization and the American Diabetes Association, outlined a classification of diabetes (Box 39-1).[29] Most cases consist of one of two variants: *type I, insulin-dependent diabetes mellitus* (*IDDM*) and *type II, non–insulin-dependent diabetes mellitus* (*NIDDM*) (Table 39-3).

Type I diabetes, previously called juvenile-onset diabetes, has an onset before age 30 in people who are not obese. Only 10% of these persons have a positive family history of a diabetic parent or sibling, although there may be a family history of the disease. Plasma insulin levels are low, and they respond little or not at all to insulin stimulators such as glucose and oral hypoglycemics. These persons are ketosis-prone and require exogenous insulin. The pancreas contains little or no endogenous insulin, and the overall β cell mass is reduced. Ability to synthesize insulin is evident at birth, but the level falls with time. About one-third of these patients experience a "honeymoon" period, a remission characterized by temporary restoration of insulin secretion, which is reflected in release of C peptide (a measure of residual β-cell secretory capacity). This period is followed by a relapse within weeks or months.

Type II diabetes, previously called adult-onset diabetes, usually occurs after age 30, and about 70% to 80%

BOX 39-1 ▼ *Classification of Diabetes Mellitus and Other Types of Glucose Intolerance*

1. Insulin-dependent (IDDM) type I
2. Non–insulin-dependent (NIDDM), type II
   Nonobese NIDDM
   Obese NIDDM
   Maturity-onset diabetes of the young (MODY)
3. Secondary: Other types, including diabetes mellitus associated with certain conditions and syndromes that may be (a) pancreatic disease, (b) hormonal, (c) drug- or chemical-induced, (d) insulin receptor abnormalities, (e) certain genetic syndromes, or (f) other.
4. Impaired glucose tolerance (IGT). Previously called chemical, latent, or subclinical diabetes.
   Nonobese IGT
   Obese IGT
5. Gestational diabetes mellitus (GDM)
6. Normal glucose tolerance but risk classes
   Previous abnormality of glucose tolerance
   Potential abnormality of glucose tolerance

TABLE 39-3 *Comparison of Insulin-Dependent (IDDM, Type I) and Non–Insulin-Dependent (NIDDM, Type II) Diabetes Mellitus*

Variables	IDDM (Type I)	NIDDM (Type II)
Incidence	~10%	~90%
Age at onset	Usually before 20 years	Usually after 30 years
Heredity	Inherited susceptibility	Stronger familial tendency than type I
HLA association	Chromosome 6 HLA-DR3, HLA-DR4 linked	No HLA association
Onset	Abrupt	Insidious
Seasonal distribution	Increased onset during fall and winter	No known association
Body weight	Normal or underweight	Usually obese (~80%)
Control	Wide fluctuations of blood sugar in relation to growth, diet, insulin, and exercise	Stable, usually easily controlled
Exogenous insulin	Needed by all	May be needed during stress or initial management
Oral hypoglycemics	Not useful	May be useful in 30%–40% of cases
Beta cells of pancreas	Destruction or inability of cells to secrete insulin	Secrete inadequate or varying amounts of insulin
Ketoacidosis	Common	Uncommon
Insulin reactions	Common	Uncommon

HLA, human leukocyte antigen.

of affected people are obese. This type accounts for about 80% of total cases of diabetes. In contrast to IDDM, patients with NIDDM have a positive history of diabetes in the immediate family. At birth, these people synthesize insulin, but the level falls as they age and β-cell function deteriorates. Insulin resistance also may occur, together with relative insulin deficiency. Persons with NIDDM are not ketosis-prone. *Maturity-onset diabetes in young people* (*MODY*) is a rare form of type II diabetes. In these persons, diabetes is mild, ketosis-resistant, and non–insulin-dependent and occurs before age 25. It affects children as young as 10 years, and there is an autosomal dominant inheritance pattern.

Patients with type I or type II disease comprise the majority of diabetic cases. Diabetes also can occur in association with other conditions and syndromes, such as pancreatic disease, Cushing syndrome, insulin-receptor abnormalities, genetic syndromes, and hormone- or drug-induced disorders. Gestational diabetes occurs only during pregnancy. Pregnancy may be a diabetogenic condition. Women demonstrate varying degrees of glucose intolerance related to metabolic effects of hormones secreted during pregnancy. Clinical manifestations may be evident in people who have a predisposition for diabetes. "Impaired glucose tolerance" is a clinical class that includes those whose glucose tolerance tests are abnormal. They are asymptomatic but are recognized as being at higher risk for diabetes than the general population.

Diabetes and other states of glucose intolerance have been recognized in association with a large number of genetic disorders. Table 39-4 summarizes the more common disorders.

INCIDENCE AND CAUSE

Diabetes is a common disorder of the endocrine system, with an estimated 8 million affected persons in the United States alone. Of these, approximately 600,000 have the insulin-dependent type.[20] Diabetes ranks as the third leading cause of death in the United States. The incidence is higher among African Americans than among Caucasians. Diabetes is more common in women than in men, especially among persons age 60 years or older.

In recent decades, the incidence has increased. Some of the probable causative factors are changes in lifestyle and obesity, which are predisposing to diabetes; increased life expectancy and an older population, who have a higher incidence of the disease; and decreased

TABLE 39-4 *Genetic Disorders or Syndromes Related to Diabetes Mellitus or Glucose Intolerance*

Disorder or Syndrome	Inheritance Pattern
Cystic fibrosis	Autosomal recessive
Glucose-6-phosphate dehydrogenase (G6PD) deficiency	Autosomal recessive
Type 1 glycogen storage disease	Autosomal recessive
Hemochromatosis	Autosomal recessive
Hereditary relapsing pancreatitis	Autosomal dominant
Familial hypertriglyceridemia	Autosomal dominant
Muscular dystrophy	X-linked recessive (autosomal dominant, autosomal recessive)
Pheochromocytoma	Autosomal dominant
Prader-Willi syndrome	Chromosomal
Retinitis pigmentosa, neuropathy, ataxia, and diabetes	Autosomal dominant
Autosomal recessive	Autosomal recessive
Turner syndrome	Chromosomal
Klinefelter syndrome	Chromosomal
Down syndrome (trisomy 21)	Chromosomal

mortality rates in the affected childbearing population, who have children with a hereditary predisposition to the disease.

INSULIN-DEPENDENT DIABETES

This form of diabetes, formerly known as juvenile-onset or ketosis-prone diabetes, usually develps in childhood with a peak incidence at puberty. Current research inplicates β-cell destruction and absence or severe lack of insulin as the cause of IDDM. Genetic predisposition to β-cell destruction, infection, autoimmunity, and environmental factors have been postulated as causative mechanisms.[40] Flowchart 39-1 shows the pathogenesis of IDDM.

Multifactorial genetic, metabolic, microbiologic, and immunologic etiologies have been cited for the variants of the diease. Abnormalities may occur in the β *cell* (inadequate insulin secretion, abnormal insulin), in the *plasma* (abnormal binding, destruction), and in the *target cell* (cell membrane or intracellular abnormalities).[8, 41]

GENETIC PREDISPOSITION. Susceptibility is polygenetic in nature and is indicated by the association of IDDM with human leukocyte antigen (HLA) alleles. The

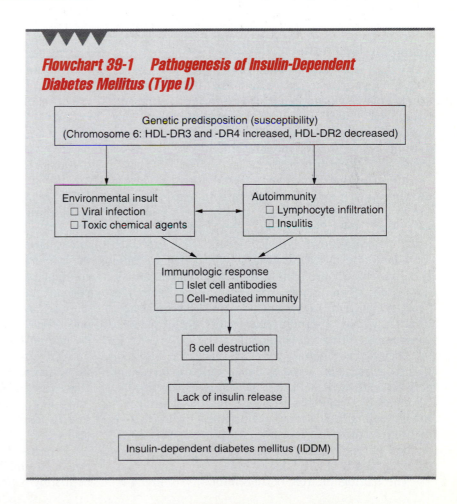

Flowchart 39-1 Pathogenesis of Insulin-Dependent Diabetes Mellitus (Type I)

disorder is not passed on in true Mendelian fashion. Several genes that code for alleles of leukocyte antigens and complement components have been located on the histocompatibility region of chromosome 6. Certain antigens, HLA-DR3 and -DR4, are found with increased frequency in individuals with IDDM, compared with controls (95% versus 50%, respectively). Other HLA alleles (eg, DR2), which may provide a resistance to the disorder, are noted less frequently.

The concordance rate (both twins affected) among identical twins is only about 50%.[23] Twins who are HLA-identical are at greater risk for IDDM than HLA-non-identical siblings. Also, individuals with more than one of the alleles associated with IDDM (eg, DR3 and DR4) are at higher risk for the disorder.[32] Because the precise mode of inheritance for IDDM is unknown, the inheritance connection is still being investigated.[7] Environmental factors also are thought to contribute to the disorder, and more than one gene may be involved.

ENVIRONMENTAL FACTORS. Environmental factors operating in a genetically susceptible person play a significant role in this type of diabetes. Agents such as viruses, dietary factors, and β-cell toxins, which lead to acute insulitis and damage to β cells, have also been implicated in the destructive immune process of IDDM.[7]

Many types of infections have been reported to precede the onset of diabetes mellitus. These include mumps, rubella, varicella, measles, influenza, coxsackievirus, cytomegalovirus, viral pneumonias, and, occasionally, bacterial pneumonias. In addition, the number of cases diagnosed increases during autumn and winter, when viral infections are most frequent. This temporal association of onset of IDDM with an infection may be related to genetic susceptibility of β cells to viruses and other toxic agents.

The exact role of viruses is not established, but investigations have implicated either virus-induced injury of the β cell and autoimmunity against the islet cell or breakdown of β cell mass caused by prior autoimmune reactions of unknown origin.[32] Specific HLA types are more common in IDDM, especially in children. These children tend to have high levels of islet cell antibodies, lymphocytes, monocytes, and eosinophils. With the peak incidence of IDDM between 5 and 15 years of age, it is likely that environmental factors are of greatest consequence during childhood.[24, 38]

Diet during infancy may influence the onset of IDDM in later life. Some evidence supports a relation between IDDM diabetes and exposure to cow's milk, exhibited by antibodies to bovine serum albumin.[7, 14] Breast feeding could protect against infection destructive to β cells by providing immune factors. Also, early introduction of foreign antigens such as cow's milk protein and solid foods may be diabetogenic.[21, 41]

The pathogenic role of autoimmunity is strengthened by findings of islet cell antibodies and sensitized T cells and by the association of other immune disorders (eg, Graves' disease, Addison disease, pernicious anemia) with IDDM. The person with NIDDM lacks this antigenic tendency.[13] Autoimmune diabetes is associated largely with individuals who carry HLA-DR3 and -DR4 antigens. Antibodies from the autoimmune process are considered to be indicators rather than causes of pancreatic destruction. Autoimmune diabetes progresses slowly and becomes clinically evident only after more than 90% of β cells have been destroyed. The β cells are greatly affected by free radicals, and the precise role of antioxidants in preventing damage from free radicals is being researched. Antioxidants have been shown to decrease β-cell destruction in animal studies.[40]

In summary, the pathogenesis of IDDM is most often related to a combination of environmental, genetic (HLA-linked), and immunologic factors probably triggered by viruses.

NON–INSULIN-DEPENDENT DIABETES MELLITUS

NIDDM is the most common type of diabetes and accounts for approximately 80% of all cases. Although the incidence is low in certain populations living in tribal societies unaffected by urban technology, members of those same populations living in an urban setting experience an increased incidence.[15] Lifestyles that accompany urbanization frequently result in obesity, which increases insulin resistance in tissues and predisposes to the onset of the disease. Maturity-onset diabetes of the young (MODY), an uncommon form of NIDDM with onset at a young age (<25 years), is caused by mutations in the glucokinase gene transmitted in an autosomal dominant inheritance pattern.[12, 40] Persons with NIDDM are not insulin-dependent and are ketosis-resistant. NIDDM is not thought to be associated with HLA antigens, with the exception of some subtypes.[32]

PATHOGENESIS. The pathogenesis of NIDDM, in which the lack of insulin is not severe, has been explained as a consequence of various causative factors. Genetic predisposition and environmental factors such as nutrition and exercise have been implicated in β-cell dysfunction. The pathogenesis lacks specificity, but two alterations in endocrine function have been identified: inadequate insulin secretion and insulin resistance, which is a defect in the response of peripheral tissues to insulin. NIDDM is characterized by these two metabolic defects.[4, 9, 23] Obesity has a profound diabetogenic influence and contributes to insulinemia and tissue insensitivity to insulin (Flowchart 39-2).

Patterns in insulin secretion are the first changes noted. In unaffected persons, insulin is secreted in an oscillating pattern. With inadequate function of β cells,

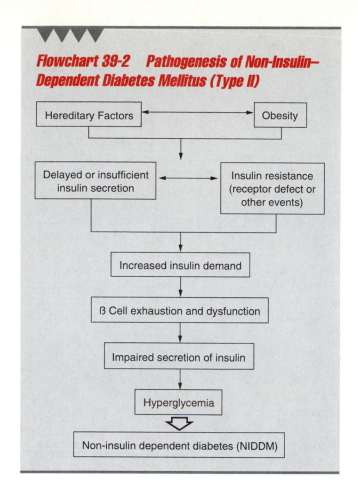

Flowchart 39-2 Pathogenesis of Non-Insulin–Dependent Diabetes Mellitus (Type II)

human insulin-receptor gene is believed to have a role in insulin resistance, and glucose intolerance is believed to contribute to the disorder.[36,38] Family histories, twin studies, and studies of histocompatibility of antigens confirm a strong genetic component.[32]

The genetic influence is greater in NIDDM than in IDDM, as evidenced by an almost 100% concordance rate in identical twins with NIDDM, compared with less than 50% for IDDM. The environmental factor of urban lifestyle must also be considered as part of the interaction.[32,40] Inheritance is multifactorial, with persons having mutations in more than one gene. The specific inheritance pattern is not known. Occurrence risks for siblings or offspring of persons with NIDDM are 5% to 10% for having the disorder and 15% to 25% for having an abnormal glucose tolerance.[32]

The inheritance pattern in MODY is autosomal dominant. A gene on chromosome 7 and a genetic region of chromosome 20 are implicated.[32] Heterogeneity may also be present because of variable insulin responses in MODY. There is no association between HLA antigens and NIDDM.

AGE. Except for persons with IDDM, increasing age is related to a decline in glucose tolerance and an increase in insulin resistance, along with an increased prevalence of diabetes. The frequency rises sharply after 40 years of age, probably reflecting a general change in glucose tolerance. The blood glucose is low in childhood and rises progressively; after 70 years of age, about 15% of the population show a mild abnormal glucose tolerance. The separation between diabetes and nondiabetes may present a problem if tolerance is not adjusted for age. This increasing frequency has been explained as a decrease in body function that occurs in all body cells with senescence.

BODY WEIGHT. About 80% of persons with NIDDM are obese, and the frequency of diabetes in obese people is greater than in the general population. The interrelation occurs because obesity is associated with insulin insensitivity in target tissues (ie, muscle, liver, and adipose cells). It is well known that blood levels of insulin are higher in an obese person and take longer to return to the fasting state. Obesity acts as a diabetogenic factor because the accompanying insulin resistance increases the need for insulin. In practice, because obese persons are resistant to the effects of insulin, the obese diabetic patient responds poorly to treatment with insulin. Weight loss increases glucose tolerance.

GENDER. Diabetes is more frequent in women than in men. Between 40 and 60 years of age, women diabetics outnumber men by almost 2 to 1. In Japan, Malaysia, and India, diabetes is 50% to 100% more common in men. In the West Indies, the sex distribution is equal, but

however, these patterns do not occur. This is demonstrated after oral glucose intake when the rise in plasma insulin is delayed and the peak insulin level is reached after the glucose peak. It is believed that there is an abnormality of glucose receptors on the β cells as well as inadequacy of insulin.[23] Most persons with NIDDM are hyperinsulinemic early in the course of the disorder, but plasma levels usually decline later in the course of the disease.[39]

Insulin resistance is a pathological condition in which the biological response to insulin is decreased. Persons with NIDDM have a diminished response to both exogenous and endogenous insulin.[26] Resistance of cells to insulin effects is a major factor. At the cellular level, there is a decrease in insulin receptors as well as impaired postreceptor influences in transmembrane diffusion of glucose.

Most persons with NIDDM are both insulin-deficient and insulin-resistant. Both factors contribute to the hyperglycemia of NIDDM.

HEREDITY. For centuries, it has been noted that diabetes "runs in families" because about 40% of people who develop the disease have a positive family history. A genetic component is accepted in the etiology. The black women with diabetes outnumber black men with diabetes. The reason for increased occurrence in women may be related to the late effects of high parity, which may not be manifested until after 45 years of age.

DIET. Certain factors implicate diet as a possible causative factor in the onset of diabetes. The frequency is great in wealthier communities in the United States. The effects of high-carbohydrate and high-fat diets have been studied extensively. Modification of dietary intake of carbohydrates minimizes hyperglycemia in this population, and limitation of saturated fat intake delays the onset of atherosclerosis. Results of the Diabetes Control and Complications Trial resoundingly emphasize the benefits of tight control of blood glucose in preventing complications of IDDM. These findings apply to NIDDM as well. Therefore, diet is a major variable in the pathophysiology.[1, 29, 34]

STRESS. Any form of stress with the neuroendocrine response increases gluconeogenesis and glycogenolysis. Infection, life changes, and various environmental factors can be stressors that induce or worsen a diabetic state.

GESTATIONAL DIABETES. Gestational diabetes is a state of carbohydrate intolerance that occurs during pregnancy. Affected women may develop overt diabetes later in life. Pregnancy causes changes in metabolism because of hormonal changes. In the first half of pregnancy, there is hypertrophy of the pancreas, with an increase in the number of β cells, increased glyconeogenesis, and decreased gluconeogenesis. Therefore, the action of insulin is enhanced.[27] During the second half of pregnancy, there are increased levels of human chorionic somatomammotropin hormone, which causes peripheral resistance to insulin. In addition, circulating cortisol and other metabolic changes lead to the breakdown of complex carbohydrates to simple sugars. These simple sugars cross the placenta and may produce fetal hyperinsulinemia because maternal insulin does not cross the placenta.[27] Vaginal and urinary infections are more common during pregnancy. Pregnancy-induced hypertension is seen more frequently among diabetics, and diabetic ketoacidosis occurs at a lower blood glucose level during pregnancy.

PATHOPHYSIOLOGY OF COMPLICATIONS OF DIABETES

Few diseases have as many widespread and systemic lesions as diabetes. Essentially all tissues and organs are altered by the hyperglycemia of diabetes. Changes in the pancreas, blood vessels, peripheral nerves, kidneys, and eyes account for the major complications of this disease.[29]

Pancreas

Changes in the pancreas are more frequently associated with IDDM than with NIDDM. Metabolic alterations are greater in IDDM because of the greater deficiency of insulin. In classic IDDM, the number of islet cells is reduced, degranulation of β cells and fibrosis of the islets occur, and there is lymphocytic infiltration. In NIDDM, the number of islet cells usually is normal, and the degree of β-cell granulation is somewhat reduced or may be normal.

HYALIN. A frequent pancreatic lesion is hyalinization of the islets. Hyalin, an eosinophilic, glassy, translucent material, may infiltrate small areas or the entire islet. It may have the fibrillar structure characteristic of amyloid.[7] Progressive accumulation of the deposits reduces β-cell mass. Hyalinization occurs in IDDM but is more common in NIDDM, and it correlates with the duration of disease. It may also occur in nondiabetics.

FIBROSIS. Thickening of the capsule and islets by fibrous connective tissue is a common change, and the islet cells may be replaced by collagen tissue. These changes are related to the duration of diabetes. Fibrosis also occurs in nondiabetics who have pronounced atherosclerotic changes and in people with other types of pancreatic lesions.

DEGRANULATION OF β CELLS. A reduction in β cells is a consistent finding in IDDM. The amount of β-cell granulation correlates with the amount of insulin stored. In NIDDM, the number of islets is usually normal, and β-cell granulation is reduced or absent.

LEUKOCYTIC INFILTRATIONS. Eosinophils and lymphocytes infiltrate the islets in an inflammatory type of reaction that is referred to as insulitis. The inflammatory infiltrates are considered a type of immunologic reaction.

Vascular System

Vascular lesions are a hallmark of diabetes. Vessels of all sizes are affected. The atherosclerotic lesions in the diabetic are like those in nondiabetics but are usually more severe. The sclerosis and capillary basement membrane thickening are related to hyperglycemia.[7] It is believed that glycosylation of phospholipids, coagulation factors, and hypertension contribute to the development of arteriolar lesions.

The lipid deposits, called atheromas or plaque, which are laid down on the intimal surfaces consist of cholesterol, triglycerides, and phospholipids. Lipids circulating in plasma as large molecules combine with proteins and are called lipoproteins. Low-density lipoprotein carries about 75% of circulating cholesterol, whereas high-density lipoprotein carries about 15% to 20% (see pp. 526–528). Electron microscopic studies have revealed microangiopathy (thickening of the walls of the arterioles, capillaries, and venules) in the kidney, retinae, and neural and epidermal vascular beds.

The atherosclerosis is the major factor in the high frequency of myocardial infarction, cerebrovascular accidents, and gangrene of the extremities in diabetes. Coronary atherosclerosis is up to five times more prevalent than in the general population, and myocardial infarction is the most common cause of death.[23] Atherosclerosis is most prevalent in obese and hypertensive individuals. Atherosclerosis develops within a few years of the onset of the disease. People who have had diabetes for a few years, whatever the age of onset, usually have significant atherosclerosis.[7]

The principal clinical manifestations of peripheral arterial disease are ischemic lesions of the feet and the lower extremities. In addition, neurotrophic changes cause loss of sensation, which may decrease attention to small injuries that become infected. A small break may lead to cellulitis, lymphangitis, infection, and necrosis of tissue.

Kidneys

Approximately 30% to 40% of persons with IDDM develop renal failure; a smaller proportion of persons with NIDDM are affected.[33] The predominant renal changes are glomerular lesions, renal vascular atherosclerosis, phelonephritis, and renal tubular alterations from glycogen and fatty changes.

DIABETIC GLOMERULOSCLEROSIS. Diabetic glomerulosclerosis may appear in a nodular form or as Kimmelstiel-Wilson disease, which results from a focal thickening of the basement membrane surrounded by peripheral capillary loops.[7] There also may be a diffuse glomerulosclerosis; this is the most common form, and it is characterized by an overall thickening of the glomerular basement membrane. Because the diabetic capillaries permit leakage of plasma proteins, proteinuria is characteristic.

OTHER LESIONS. Other common renal lesions affect the vascular supply, renal pelvis, and medulla. Lesions that consist of masses containing lipid material and debris deposited throughout the glomerulus ultimately cause alterations of the glomerular tuft and progressive renal insufficiency.[33] Atherosclerosis and arteriolosclerosis of the renal artery or arterioles are common and may be related to hypertension. Pyelonephritis usually is a bacterial ascending infection of the kidneys, and it occurs most frequently in diabetics. *Necrotizing renal papillitis*, or renal medullary necrosis, involves unilateral or bilateral necrosis of the renal pyramids, which may result in sloughing of necrotic papillae in urine.

Pathology of the Eye

RETINOPATHY. Diabetic retinopathy, the inclusive term for several retinal changes related to diabetes, is a leading cause of blindness in the United States. Whether visual handicap occurs depends on whether the maculae are involved. This condition is rare before the growth-spurt years and develops slowly, corresponding to the duration of the disease. Retinopathy follows alterations in blood flow through the retinae and has various manifestations: thickening of retinal capillaries, microangiopathies, and microaneurysms, which are discrete saccular dilatations or outpouchings of vessels (Fig. 39-5). The microaneurysms are asymptomatic; they are seen as discrete, dark red, circular spots near retinal vessels, and they are diagnostic of diabetes mellitus.

Hemorrhages usually are present in the macular area between the superior and inferior temporal vessels, and they resemble red blotches. If located in the area of

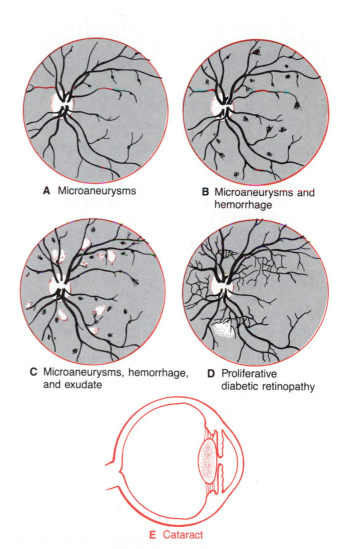

A Microaneurysms

B Microaneurysms and hemorrhage

C Microaneurysms, hemorrhage, and exudate

D Proliferative diabetic retinopathy

E Cataract

FIGURE 39-5 *Eye changes of diabetes: **A**, Microaneurysms; **B**, Microaneurysms and hemorrhage; **C**, Microaneurysms, hemorrhage and exudate; **D**, proliferative diabetic retinopathy; **E**, Cataract.*

the fovea, they can destroy central vision. Exudates occur as a result of abnormal porosity of the retinal vessels and seepage of fluid into the retinae. Soft exudates, called cotton-wool spots, are large, fluffy, and gray-white and may resolve in several weeks. The more common hard exudates are yellow, with discrete sharp edges that may coalesce; they take longer to develop, and they produce retinal degeneration. Venous changes include enlarged, irregular veins, sometimes resembling strings of sausages.

LESIONS OF THE VITREOUS. Lesions of the vitreous are a serious complication that includes neovascularization (formation of new vessels) and fibrous tissue in the fundus. In time, atrophy of new vessels and contraction of fibrous tissue affect central and peripheral vision. Changes between fibrovascular tissue and the vitreous may lead to hemorrhage and retinal detachment.

CATARACTS. Accumulation of sorbital (polyhydroxy alcohol formed from glucose) in the lens causes cataracts. Opacities of the lens are common in diabetics. They usually are of gradual onset and are similar to senile cataracts (see Figure 39-5). Transitory lens changes caused by dehydration also occur in diabetics.

Nervous System

Neurons are vulnerable to the ketoacidosis of uncontrolled diabetes and the hypoglycemia of insulin reactions. Neuropathy may involve the peripheral nerves, brain, spinal cord, cranial nerves, or autonomic nervous system. Peripheral and autonomic nerve dysfunction frequently contribute to complications of diabetes. The relation between metabolic aspects of disease and diabetic neuropathy remains unknown. Failure of affected people to improve with management of hyperglycemia supports the proposed relation between peripheral neuropathy and a process independent of glucose and insulin metabolism. A correlation has been found between duration of disease and diabetic control.[11] Accumulation of sorbitol is probably responsible for injury to the Schwann cell and pericytes of retinal capillaries.[7]

Polyneuropathy, characterized by myelin degeneration and eventual irreversible injury to axons, is caused by an accumulation of abnormal metabolites and by depletion of substances necessary for nerve cell conduction. The associated sensory loss and motor weakness usually occur first and most severely in the feet.

Mononeuropathy is probably related to ischemia and infarction of the vessels that supply the nerves. Manifestations of nervous system involvement include pain, paresthesias, decreased proprioceptive sensations, motor impairment, and muscle weakness and atrophy.

Alterations in the autonomic nervous system may lead to nocturia and atony of the bladder, postural hypotension, and delayed gastric emptying. Disturbances in neural innervation of the pelvic organs lead to sexual impotence in men and orgasmic difficulties in women.

Because of peripheral arterial ischemic disease and neurotrophic changes, there is loss of sensation in the feet, and they are therefore more susceptible to infection. A pathologic condition may not be noticed and may progress rapidly.

A *Charcot joint*, or neuropathic joint disease, develops because of the trauma and stress of joint motion. Relaxation of supporting structures of the joint leads to cartilage degeneration, disorganization, and collapse of bones. Neuropathic joint disease usually involves the feet.

Skin Changes

The skin of the diabetic is structurally different from that of the nondiabetic. Dryness is caused by dehydration and occurs in poorly controlled diabetes. Poor skin turgor may be related to protein wasting and dehydration. Impaired granulocyte function and decreased circulation lead to skin changes and also may contribute to infection.

NECROBIOSIS LIPOIDICA EPIDERMIS. Most common on the shins, this lesion usually develops after diabetes has been present for years. It begins as a papule that progresses to a soft, yellow, ulcerated plaque. Histologically, the lesion consists of collagen surrounded by an inflammatory infiltrate composed of lipid-laden macrophages.[22]

DIABETIC DERMOPATHY. Dermopathy, or shin spots, is seen microscopically as atrophy of the epidermis and fibrosis of the dermis. These hemorrhagic-like areas are brown, scaly, round patches, and look as though the person has been struck time and time again in the shins. There is no associated pain or ulceration.[22]

INFECTIONS. Bacterial infections are more frequent in diabetics than in nondiabetics.[35] Infections that arise from acne may expand and progress into cellulitis. Furuncles and carbuncles are of serious concern. Dermatophytosis (athlete's foot) is common, and although relatively harmless in the nondiabetic, it may lead to serious infection and loss of a foot in the diabetic. Monilial infections occur in the diabetic, often in the genitalia and groin and under the breasts. The high moisture, the glucose content of the skin, and chafing support the growth of *Candida albicans*, especially in an obese person. Severity of infections may be worsened by reduction of circulation and nerve degeneration.

LIPODYSTROPHY. Lipodystrophy is characterized by general or partial loss of body fat and may be caused by insulin injections. Scar and lipoma-like accumulations beneath the skin form large bumps (lipohypertrophy) with repeated injection of insulin. These sites tend to become fibrous and insensitive, and insulin is absorbed poorly from these areas.

XANTHOMAS. Firm, yellowish-pink nodules develop under the epidermis of knees and elbows and on the periorbital areas and buttocks as a result of the hyperlipemia of diabetes. The lesions may be as large as 5 mm, and the papule is surrounded by an inflammatory-type halo. Although these nodules are not limited to persons with diabetes, they signify high serum triglyceride levels and disappear with return of triglycerides to normal.

Hepatic Fatty Changes

In long-standing diabetes, fatty changes develop, and the size of the liver increases. Infiltration of fat causes it to appear yellowish, and glycogen vacuoles may be present in nuclei of the cells. These liver changes are related to elevated serum lipid levels.

Muscle Changes

Degenerative changes occur in striated muscle in persons who have long-standing, poorly controlled diabetes. The pathology is probably related to microangiopathy and neuronal degeneration. Diabetic amyotrophy, a syndrome of muscle weakness, pain, and atrophy, occurs in the elderly, especially in men. The disorder usually is limited to the psoas and quadriceps muscles.

CLINICAL MANIFESTATIONS AND COMPLICATIONS

Most diabetics have polydipsia, polyuria, polyphagia, weight loss, and weakness. Many also have infections. A hyperglycemic person is at risk for infection because neutrophil functions are handicapped by high glucose levels. Infection is a leading cause of morbidity and mortality. Prominent pathogens are *Staphylococcus aureus* and *Candida albicans*. *Candida* secretes a protein that diminishes phagocytosis by the host.[18]

The predominant pathophysiology of diabetes is related to impaired use of glucose by cells; to increased mobilization, abnormal metabolism, and abnormal deposition of fats; and to depletion of protein in body tissues. These manifestations occur because of insulin deprivation, which results in *hyperglycemia* (blood glucose as high as 200–1,000 mg/dL) owing to the impaired uptake of glucose, especially into muscle and adipose tissue, and increased gluconeogenesis and glycogenolysis by the liver. These factors, together with increased dietary intake of carbohydrate, result in an increased blood sugar level.

With hyperglycemia, osmotic pressure of the plasma increases, fluid shifts to the intravascular compartment, and cells become dehydrated. After the blood glucose

level reaches about 160 to 180 mg/mL, the renal tubules cannot reabsorb all of the glucose filtered by the glomeruli, and glycosuria occurs. If the blood glucose level reaches 300 to 400 mg/mL, a common occurrence in untreated diabetes, a person may lose as much as 100 g of glucose into the urine each day. The renal excretion of glucose requires accompanying water and produces excessive urination, or *polyuria*. Excessive urination also increases loss of water, potassium, sodium, and chloride, resulting in extracellular fluid depletion and compensatory intracellular dehydration. As sodium and potassium are lost, electrolyte imbalance, weakness, fatigue, and malaise occur. Loss of water causes an increase in serum osmolality, which stimulates the thirst center in the hypothalamus and the body's response of *polydipsia*. With the loss of large quantities of glucose and semistarvation of the cells, there is a compensatory increase in hunger, *polyphagia*. As the level of insulin, an anabolic hormone, decreases, protein and fat catabolism increase, resulting in the release of ketones, nitrogen, and potassium into the circulation. Weight loss is common, especially in IDDM. Figure 39-6 shows a typical example of a young, thin man with clinical features of IDDM. Figure 39-7 shows a typical example of an elderly, obese woman with the clinical features of NIDDM.

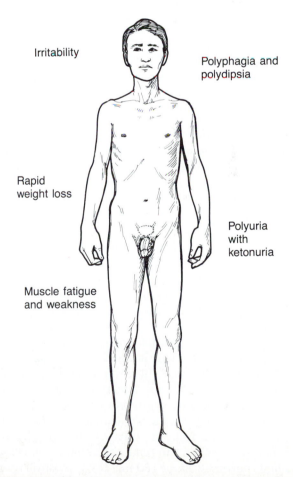

Irritability

Polyphagia and polydipsia

Rapid weight loss

Polyuria with ketonuria

Muscle fatigue and weakness

FIGURE 39-6 *Clinical features of insulin-dependent diabetes (type I).*

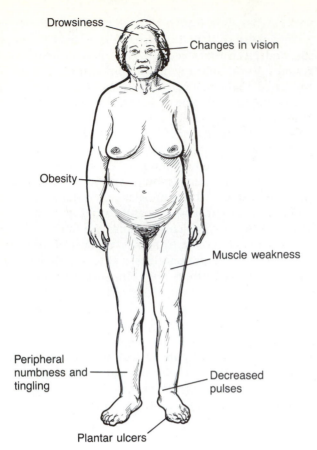

Drowsiness

Changes in vision

Obesity

Muscle weakness

Peripheral numbness and tingling

Decreased pulses

Plantar ulcers

FIGURE 39-7 Clinical features of non-insulin–dependent diabetes (type II).

Diabetic Ketoacidosis

The metabolic result of lack of insulin and severe dehydration is ketoacidosis. With the stress response, there is increased secretion of counterregulatory hormones, including corticosteroids, catecholamines, and glucagon, which further increase glucose production. The signs and symptoms are pronounced manifestations of uncontrolled diabetes. Polyuria, polydipsia, polyphagia, weakness, and anorexia, in addition to nausea, vomiting, and abdominal pain, occur in increasing severity. Ketonemia, gastric dilatation, and decreased peristalsis from potassium loss contribute to nausea and vomiting. The gastrointestinal symptoms and tender abdomen may mimic a surgical emergency. Ketonuria increases electrolyte loss.

The most important pathogenic element in ketoacidosis is marked decrease in insulin production, which leads to hyperglycemia, glycosuria, and progressive metabolic acidosis. Without insulin, glucose cannot enter the cells, and a form of intracellular starvation occurs. Glucose accumulates in the blood, increasing osmolality and pulling water from the cells into the intravascular compartment. When the renal threshold for glucose is reached (normally about 180 mg/dL), glycosuria results

and this induces an osmotic diuresis with polyuria and a profound loss of electrolytes and water.[7] The body enters a catabolic state, and there is a shift from carbohydrate to protein and fat metabolism. Fats are broken down (lipolysis) for energy faster than they can be metabolized. The ketone acids (acetoacetic and β-hydroxybutyric acids) are strong and dissociate to yield hydrogen ions, consequently causing a drop in pH. As the plasma pH decreases, the respiratory center is stimulated to prevent further decline in pH, and breathing becomes deep and rapid (Kussmaul respiration). The acetone formed during ketosis is volatile and is blown off during expiration, giving the breath a sweet or fruity odor. When acidosis depresses their action, ketones are not well metabolized, so that acidosis and catabolism are enhanced. Hypovolemia and increased blood viscosity also may cause systemic thrombi or emboli, a myocardial infarction, or a cerebrovascular accident.

Protein catabolism results in the breakdown of amino acids and electrolytes from muscle tissue. The liver, the primary site for glucose synthesis, converts amino acids to glucose, perpetuating the hyperglycemic and acidotic states. The metabolic derangement also is increased by the presence of glucoregulatory hormones (cortisol, catecholamines, glucagon, and growth hormone) during diabetic ketoacidosis. The antagonistic activity exhibited by these hormones promotes gluconeogenesis and worsens the hyperglycemia.

After the lungs are no longer able to maintain pH by blowing off carbon dioxide, plasma carbonic acid levels rise and acidosis progresses. Further decrease in pH, accompanied by hyperosmolality, dehydration, hypotension, and tissue breakdown, contributes to depression of cerebral function and eventually leads to coma and death (Flowchart 39-3). Persons with NIDDM seldom develop ketoacidosis.

Hyperglycemic, Hyperosmolar, Nonketotic Coma

Hyperglycemic, hyperosmolar, nonketotic coma (HHNK) has been recognized with increasing frequency. This variation in hyperglycemic diabetic coma is characterized by extreme hyperglycemia (800–2,000 mg/dL) and hyperosmolality (>350 mOsm/kg), mild or undetectable ketonuria, and absence of acidosis. The syndrome occurs almost exclusively in older people and in persons with mild diabetes that does not require insulin.

The mechanism of HHNK is best understood by considering the principles of osmolality. Without insulin to lower blood glucose, the blood becomes more concentrated because glucose is a large molecule that does not easily pass cell walls and draws large amounts of water. The profound hyperglycemia is largely responsible for the increased plasma osmolality that causes an osmotic diuresis. The intracellular fluid is drawn out to help

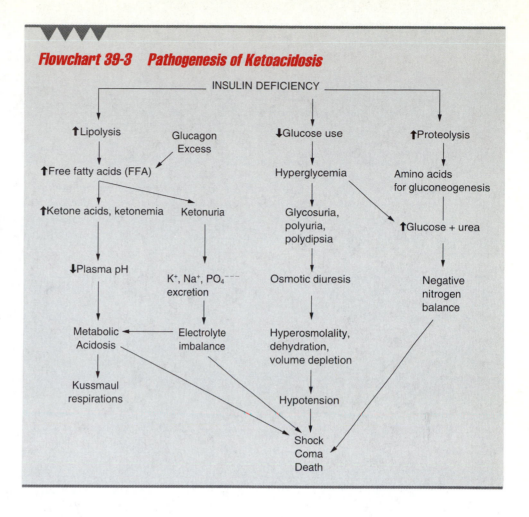

Flowchart 39-3   Pathogenesis of Ketoacidosis

equalize the increasing osmotic pressure of blood hypertonic with sugar. Water in the intracellular fluid moves from cells into the bloodstream, leaving cells dehydrated and shrunken. Dehydration stimulates secretion of the glucoregulatory hormones glucagon, cortisol, and epinephrine. If hypokalemia also occurs, it further decreases insulin secretion. These two events cause severe hyperglycemia. Fluid intake initially balances the fluid lost to glycosuria. Later, intake is insufficient and dehydration ensues. The person gradually becomes more obtunded and cannot respond to thirst. Without treatment with insulin and fluids, the process becomes self-perpetuating. Hyperosmolality leads to hemoconcentration and is conducive to thrombus formation. Fluid losses lead to hypovolemia and shock. If these are not corrected, death may result (Flowchart 39-4).

Similarities exist between HHNK and ketotic coma. In both, a shortage of insulin and a defect in use of glucose result in hyperglycemia, osmotic diuresis, and dehydration. Elevation of urea nitrogen levels usually occurs in both, although the causes may be different. Metabolic acidosis occurs in both, but it is less severe in the hyperosmolar disorder. The major difference is that large quantities of ketone bodies are produced in ketotic

coma but not in HHNK. No insulin is secreted in ketotic coma, but some residual ability to secrete insulin remains in HHNK. The small quantities of circulating insulin probably prevent the mobilization of fat from tissues and the release of ketone bodies. The cortisol and growth hormone levels are not as elevated in HHNK as in DKA which may explain the decreased number of ketone bodies formed.

The clinical manifestations of HHNK are polyphagia, polydipsia, polyuria, glycosuria, dehydration, abdominal discomfort, hyperpyrexia, hyperventilation, electrolyte imbalance, central nervous system dysfunction, postural hypotension, and shock. Impaired mental status is related to dehydration or electrolyte imbalance. The skin has decreased turgor, mucous membranes are dry, and the eyes are sunken and soft. Some degree of renal impairment occurs in many affected persons.

The onset of HHNK may be triggered by an acute illness or surgery as well as by stressful events, for example pancreatic disease, myocardial infarction, hemodialysis, renal dialysis, severe burns, and hyperalimentation. A number of drugs (eg, corticosteroids, diuretics, diphenylhydantoin, immunosuppressive agents) also may induce or contribute to the syndrome.

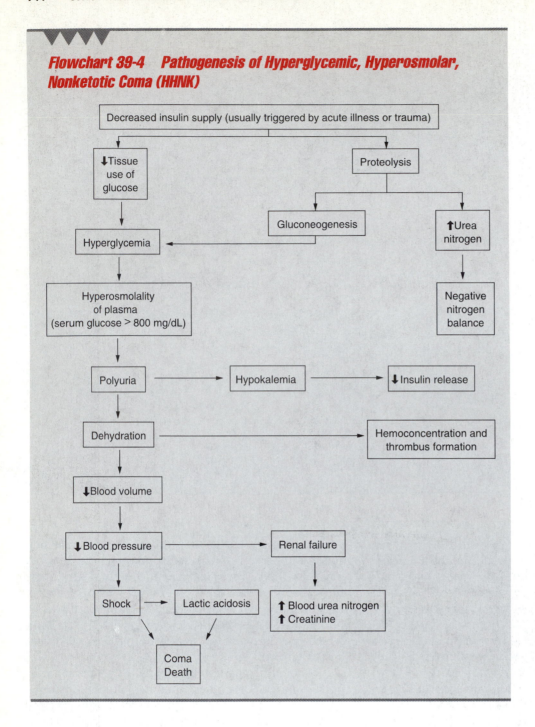

Flowchart 39-4   Pathogenesis of Hyperglycemic, Hyperosmolar, Nonketotic Coma (HHNK)

The laboratory results are similar to those of keto-acidosis, except that the serum glucose levels usually are higher (often >1,000 mg/dL) and serum osmolalities also are more elevated (>350 mOsm/kg H_2O). Bicarbonate concentrations and pH often are normal but may decrease as the syndrome progresses. Severe hypokalemia is common. There usually is no ketoacidosis in classic cases, but lactic acidosis may result from hypovolemic shock. Plasma acetone is absent or slightly elevated; creatinine and blood urea nitrogen levels become elevated with renal impairment. Compared with keto-acidosis, there is less elevation of the plasma free fatty acids, growth hormone, and cortisol. The prognosis in HHNK is not as good as in diabetic ketoacidosis, and death often is attributed to the underlying or associated disease that precipitated the coma.

Lactic Acidosis

If anaerobic glycolysis in the body produces more lactic acid than can be used or converted to glucose, lactic acidosis occurs. It frequently occurs with sustained hypoxia or hypotension (eg, shock, septicemia, hemorrhage, renal insufficiency, starvation). Lactic acidosis may develop in diabetics as a spontaneous syndrome or in association with diabetic ketoacidosis or HHNK when marked hypoperfusion occurs. Lactic acidosis should be suspected in any stuporous or comatose person whose blood gases show metabolic acidosis. Diagnosis is confirmed by a plasma lactate level in excess of 7 mmol/L, with a low plasma bicarbonate level, absence of ketosis, and an anion gap produced by the excess lactate (see pp. 224–226).

Insulin Reactions

Hypoglycemia is a rather frequent metabolic complication of diabetes, although it is largely a consequence of insulin therapy. Most diabetics who take insulin experience a hypoglycemic reaction at some time. Reactions can result from an overdose of insulin, inadequate food intake, increased amounts of exercise, or nutritional and fluid imbalances caused by nausea and vomiting.

The symptoms of hypoglycemia reflect glucose deprivation to the brain. The following physiologic responses occur: epinephrine release (sweating, shakiness, nervousness, headache, palpitations, and increased blood pressure, heart rate, and respirations); parasympathetic nervous system response (hunger, nausea, eructation); and cerebral function decline (bizarre behavior, dulled sensorium, lethargy, convulsions, coma). Clinical signs and symptoms may not correlate with blood glucose level, and they may occur when the glucose level drops rapidly from a very high to a still-elevated level.

The adrenergic response results in increased liver glycogenolysis to raise blood glucose concentration and stimulation of the reticular activating system to a state of wakefulness and alertness. If the liver glycogen supply is exhausted and glucose is not replaced, convulsions and permanent brain damage result.

Hypoglycemia also can occur independently of insulin. The following conditions can cause low blood glucose levels: severe *liver disease*, which impairs glycogen uptake and release; *adrenocortical insufficiency*, in which the glucocorticoids (cortisol and cortisone) are unavailable to stimulate gluconeogenesis; and *islet cell tumors*, which overproduce insulin. Some medications, such as salicylates, oral antidiabetic agents, propranolol, monoamine oxidase inhibitors, and certain sulfonamides, contribute to hypoglycemia. Alcohol (ethanol) has long been recognized as an agent that can induce hypoglycemia. It also potentiates the effects of insulin and oral antidiabetic agents. Table 39-5 offers a comparison between hypoglycemia and different types of comas seen in diabetes.

Somogyi Effect

Somogyi described a syndrome of nighttime hypoglycemia follwed by rebound hyperglycemia in the morning. It occurs most often in persons who receive

TABLE 39-5 *Comparison of Hypoglycemia, Diabetic Ketoacidosis, Lactic Acidosis, and Hyperglycemic, Hyperosmolar, Nonketotic Coma*

Variables	Hypoglycemia	DKA	Lactic Acidosis	HHNK
Physical response	Trembly, weak; difficulty talking	Nausea, vomiting; polyuria; polyphagia; polydipsia; headache	Similar to DKA (varied, depending on factors contributing to development)	Similar to DKA
Mental status	Anxious, confused; behavioral changes	Irritable; comatose	Acute changes in state of consciousness; stuporous; comatose	Similar to DKA; stuporous; focal motor seizures
Blood pressure	Normal	Low	Low	Low
Skin	Cold, moist, pale	Hot, flushed, dry	Pallid, dry	Very dry
Mucous membranes	Normal	Very dry	Dry	Extremely dry
Respiration	Normal	Hyperventilation	Hyperventilation	Normal
Blood sugar	40 mg or less	300–800+ mg	80–200 mg	800–2000 mg
Serum ketones	0	4+	0–2+	0–2+
Blood CO_2	24–30	5–16 or less	5–16	18–24
Plasma lactic acid	Normal	Normal	High	Normal
Plasma pH	7.4–7.5	7.0–7.3	6.8–7.2	7.4

DKA, diabetic ketoacidosis; HHNK, hyperglycemic, hyperosmolar, nonketotic coma.

large amounts of insulin. The syndrome may be caused by increased sensitivity to insulin. It occurs more frequently in children and in persons with type I diabetes.

Some persons have wide variations in blood sugar level that occur when insulin dosage is increased to control elevated levels. The exogenous insulin produces hypoglycemia. These people often have nocturnal hypoglycemia, followed by hormone-mediated hyperglycemia in the morning. Epinephrine, glucagon, adrenal corticosteroids, and growth hormone are secreted as part of the body's response to the excessive action of insulin. Epinephrine and glucagon spur glycogenolysis in the liver, corticosteroids stimulate gluconeogenesis in the liver, and hyperglycemia occurs. The blood sugar usually is elevated, but periods of severe hypoglycemia may be experienced. If this *rebound hypo-hyperglycemia* is suspected, the insulin dose may be slowly reduced, divided into smaller doses, or administered at different times.

CLINICAL COURSE

The course of diabetes may be insidious or abrupt. The ketosis-prone insulin-dependent type that usually affects younger people sometimes undergoes transient remission after onset, called a honeymoon period, which may last a few weeks to a few months; then glucose intolerance becomes unstable or brittle. The person is sensitive to changes in exogenous insulin, dietary deviations, growth spurts, unusual physical activity, infection, and stress and is vulnerable to hypoglycemia and ketoacidosis.

Maturity-onset, nonketosis-prone diabetes may have few, if any, symptoms, and it follows an insidious course. The person with nonketosis-prone NIDDM usually does not experience the acute metabolic syndrome but suffers from the other complications previously described.

DIAGNOSTIC EVALUATION

Numerous laboratory tests are performed to diagnose and follow the course of diabetes mellitus.

FASTING BLOOD SUGAR.   Normal test values rule out significant diabetic problems but do not completely exclude diabetes, because only about 30% to 40% of cases can be diagnosed by measurement of fasting blood sugar. The fasting blood sugar should be measured in the early morning, at least 8 hours after a meal. Normal values are 65 to 100 mg/dL using a method specific for glucose, or 80 to 120 mg/dL using a method that measures all blood sugars and reducing substances. A fasting blood sugar above 120 mg/dL should be further investigated with a glucose tolerance test.

TWO-HOUR POSTPRANDIAL BLOOD SUGAR.   This test is a measurement of the amount of glucose in the person's blood 2 hours after a meal. Values may range from 200 to 2,000 mg/dL, depending on duration and severity of the diabetes. Glucose levels seldom are elevated 2 hours after carbohydrate intake in nondiabetics.

GLUCOSE TOLERANCE TEST.   The glucose tolerance test is based on the principle that a nondiabetic person can absorb a test amount of glucose from circulation at a faster rate than a diabetic. As demonstrated in Figure 39-8, when a nondiabetic fasting person ingests 1 g glucose per kilogram of body weight, the blood glucose rises to peak levels of 150 to 160 mg/dL and falls to normal within 2 to 3 hours. The urine usually remains free of glucose. In the diabetic, the blood sugar peak levels are much higher, and the return to fasting levels is delayed 5 to 6 hours because of a lack of insulin response to the glucose.

GLYCOSYLATED HEMOGLOBIN.   Measures of glycosylated hemoglobin (glycohemoglobin) provide an accurate long-term indicator of an individual's average blood glucose and reflect the metabolic control of the diabetic condition. It is elevated in persons with hyperglycemia.

Glycosylated hemoglobin is formed slowly and irreversibly through the 120-day life span of the red blood cell. The process occurs through a nonenzymatic reaction that results in the attachment of glucose to amino groups of the hemoglobin molecule as red blood cells circulate in the bloodstream. Glycosylated hemoglobin consists of components A_{1a}, A_{1b}, and A_{1c}, which make up about 4% to 8% of the total hemoglobin. Many laboratories measure the sum of the three glycohemoglobins when reporting results. Others report values for hemoglobin A_{1c}.[20, 31] The higher the blood glucose level, the more hemoglobin A_{1c} is present in the red cell. In nondiabetic adults, the normal level is 2.2 to 4.8%; in children, it is 1.8 to 4.0. Good diabetic control should maintain a level of 2.5 to 6.0. A value above 8.0 reflects poor control.[31]

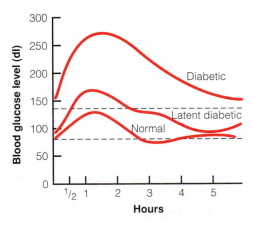

FIGURE 39-8   *Glucose tolerance curves.*

PLASMA INSULIN ASSAY.   This test measures insulin by radioimmunoassay. The insulin assay, when compared with the oral glucose tolerance test, reflects characteristic curves in diagnosing conditions. Insulin-dependent diabetics have low fasting insulin levels as well as flat glucose tolerance test curves because of lack of insulin.[31]

URINE GLUCOSE.   In normal kidneys, the glucose filtered through the glomeruli from the blood is reabsorbed in the proximal tubules. The renal tubules have a maximum absorptive capacity (renal threshold) of about 160 to 180 mg/dL of blood. At blood levels greater than this, sugar is spilled into the urine and can be detected by screening methods. Glucose may appear in the urine at normal blood levels in people without diabetes if the ability of the renal tubules to absorb glucose is impaired. Many diabetics, especially those with a history of atherosclerosis, may have a higher renal threshold, which prevents the appearance of glucose in urine until the blood level is quite high.

URINE KETONES.   Ketonuria refers to the loss of ketone bodies, such as acetone, β-hydroxybutyric acid, and acetoacetic acid, in the urine. This reflects the abnormal oxidation of fats and may occur in persons with diabetes, glycogen storage disease, starvation, or high-fat diets. Ketones occasionally are present with fever or other conditions that increase metabolic requirements. Accumulation of acidic ketones in the blood leads to metabolic acidosis and an acetone smell to the breath.

VOLUME OF URINE IN A 24-HOUR PERIOD.   A nondiabetic person secretes an average of 1,200 to 1,800 mL of urine in 24 hours, whereas the uncontrolled diabetic excretes 2,000 mL or more in 24 hours.

▼ Hypoglycemia

Hypoglycemia is a common condition that is diagnosed in the symptomatic person with a blood sugar level of less than 50 mg/dL. The symptoms presented are those caused by the counter-regulatory hormones which include glucagon, cortisol, growth hormone, and catecholamines.[38] These symptoms include tachycardia, shakiness, weakness, and diaphoresis which are especially noted when the glucose levels fall rapidly. The causes of hypoglycemia are presented in Table 39-6. They are from multiple sources so diagnosis requires a specific history and usually a positive glucose tolerance test, especially with reactive hypoglycemia. Treatment of the cause of hypoglycemia may include better insulin control in the diabetic individual or to localize and resect neoplasms. Dietary treatment of idiopathic hypoglycemia includes a low carbohydrate diet with frequent, small meals. When systemic conditions are treated there is often an improvement in the hypoglycemia.[38]

▼ Pancreatic Islet Cell Disorders

HYPERINSULINISM

A major pathophysiologic characteristic associated with hyperplasia or tumors (insulinomas) of the β cells is unregulated insulin secretion and hypoglycemia. Glucose transporter proteins are believed to be responsible for the continued release during hypoglycemia in these persons.[3] Three chracteristics, known as the *Whipple triad*, describe the classic presentation: fasting hypoglycemia, symptoms of hypoglycemia, and immediate relief after intravenous glucose administration.[28]

When hyperplasia or tumors (insulinomas) of the β cells occur, enough insulin may be secreted to induce

TABLE 39-6 *Differential Diagnosis of Hypoglycemia in Adults*

Reactive Hypoglycemia

Idiopathic (functional)
Alimentary (post-gastric surgery or functional)
Early diabetes mellitus (adult-onset)
Hereditary fructose intolerance (rare mild forms)

Fasting Hypoglycemia

Endogenous Causes
Insulinoma
Islet cell hyperplasia
Extrapancreatic neoplasms
Adrenocortical insufficiency
Growth hormone deficiency
Glucagon deficiency (?)
Hepatic failure
Renal failure
Autoimmune (antiinsulin or antireceptor antibodies)
Exogenous Causes
Insulin reactions
Surreptitious insulin injections
Oral hypoglycemic agents
Ethanol
Other medications (eg, β-blockers, pentamidine)

Artifactual Hypoglycemia

Leukocytosis (secondary to glycolysis in improperly stored blood samples)
Hyperlipidemia (mild, secondary to glucose exclusion from nonaqueous phase)

(W.N. Kelley (ed.). *Textbook of Internal Medicine* [2nd ed.]. Philadelphia: J.B. Lippincott, 1992.)

hypoglycemia. Most islet cell tumors are benign, but a small percentage are metastasizing malignant tumors. Most persons with insulinomas are women, and the median age at diagnosis is 50 years. An exception is multiple endocrine neoplasia syndrome, in which the median age at diagnosis is between 20 and 30 years.[37]

The insulin-producing adenomas, or insulinomas, vary from minute lesions to large masses. They occur singly or scattered throughout the pancreas; they usually appear as encapsulated, firm nodules that are distributed throughout the pancreas and compress the surrounding tissue. Histologically, they do not differ from the normal islet cell.[7]

Hyperinsulinism also may be caused by hyperplasia of the pancreatic islets, an alteration that occurs in infants born of diabetic mothers. The infant responds to the elevated blood sugar levels of the mother by producing increased numbers of cells and an increase in size of the cells. After delivery, the increased secretion causes serious episodes of hypoglycemia.

Postprandial hypoglycemia may occur in persons who have undergone surgical procedures such as gastrectomy, gastrojejunostomy, and vagotomy. Rapid emptying of gastric contents may lower glucose levels far more rapidly than insulin levels and produce hyperinsulinism and hypoglycemia.[37]

ZOLLINGER–ELLISON SYNDROME (GASTRINOMA)

A syndrome described by Zollinger and Ellison is a clinical condition of peptic ulceration associated with a non–β-cell islet tumor (see pp. 785–787). It is characterized by gastric secretion of large amounts of hydrochloric acid and pepsin. The stimulus for the hypersecretion is attributed to gastrin; hence, the tumor also is known as a gastrinoma. Most of the tumors occur in the pancreas, but they may be located in the duodenum. These tumors are the most common hormone-secreting tumors of the pancreas. They are characterized by hypergastrinemia in the presence of excessive gastric acid secretion. Almost all persons with Zollinger–Ellison syndrome have ulcer disease.[26]

Approximately half of gastrinomas are malignant and metastasize to regional lymph nodes. There may be metastasis to bones, mediastinum, and skin. Morbidity and mortality usually are attributed to the effects of the secretion of gastrin from the tumor and its metastases, and to complications of ulcer disease such as bleeding and perforation. The tremendous gastric hypersecretion leads to intractable ulcers. The sites of the ulcers are similar to those of peptic ulcers; symptoms are similar but more progressive and less responsive to treatment. The high acidity of the small intestine causes inactivation of pancreatic lipase; this precipitates bile salts and causes fluid and electrolyte imbalance. Large volumes of acid gastric juices promote diarrhea. As a result, many affected persons develop malabsorption syndromes. Alteration in the intestinal mucosa from acidity affects absorption of nutrients.

Gastrinomas may occur in association with multiple endocrine neoplasia, type I (MEN I) syndrome. Because hyperparathyroidism is a component of MEN I, gastrinoma patients should be screened for MEN I (see next section).[26]

WERNER SYNDROME

Werner syndrome is familial and has an autosomal dominant pattern of transmission with incomplete penetrance. Clinical features resemble early senescence, and it is referred to as adult progeria. Multiple adenomas are present in the parathyroid glands, pituitary, and pancreas. The disorder often is associated with peptic ulcer and gastric hypersecretion (Zollinger–Ellison syndrome). Both Zollinger–Ellison and Werner syndromes have been found in some families, implying that the syndromes are variants of the same mutant gene. Some of the tumors are malignant, and the term *multiple endocrine neoplasia* (*MEN*) has replaced the previously used term, *multiple endocrine adenomatosis*. The major syndromes that are caused by multiple endocrine hyperfunction are the MEN syndromes. Several of the conditions are familial with an autosomal dominant pattern. There are three types of MEN syndromes:

1. MEN, type I (Werner syndrome) includes tumors or hyperplasia of the parathyroids, thyroid, pancreatic islet cells, pituitary, and adrenal cortex. The clinical manifestations vary, depending on the systems involved. More than one-half of those affected have adenomas in two or more endocrine glands, and three or more glands are involved in one-fifth of these persons. The fundamental defect has been postulated to be an excess of a circulating growth factor.[6]
2. MEN, type IIA (Sipple syndrome) includes pheochromocytoma, medullary thyroid carcinoma, and parathyroid hyperplasia.
3. MEN, type IIB includes medullary thyroid carcinoma and pheochromocytoma but may be accompanied by distinct dysmorphic features such as neuromas of the lips, buccal mucosa, tongue, and gastrointestinal tract.

Clinical manifestations of MEN include intractable peptic ulcers, hyperparathyroidism, hyperinsulinism, Cushing syndrome, and hypertension related to pheochromocytoma.[7]

▼ *Pancreatitis*

ACUTE PANCREATITIS

Pancreatitis, or inflammation of the pancreas, is characterized by hemorrhage, necrosis, and suppuration of pancreatic parenchyma. Pathologic changes occur in varying degrees of severity and are caused by activation of proteolytic enzymes within the pancreas rather than in the intestine.

Frequency and Cause

This condition has an overall prevalence in the United States of 0.5%.[16] Acute pancreatitis occurs most frequently in middle life and more often in women than in men. Two major causes, *alcoholism* and biliary tract disease, especially *cholelithiasis* (gallstones), are responsible for the largest number of cases, but in many instances the cause is obscure. Factors in the origin of pancreatitis are listed in Box 39-2. In men, pancreatitis often is associated with high consumption of alcohol, but the condition develops only after years of alcohol abuse. Gallstones have been demonstrated in the feces of 40% to 60% of patients with acute pancreatitis.[7] Pancreatitis also may occur as a result of surgical trauma, particularly

---

BOX 39-2 ▼ *Factors in the Origin of Pancreatitis*

Alcoholism
Biliary tract disease
Postoperative (abdominal, nonabdominal)
Postendoscopic retrograde cholangiopancreatography (ERCP)
Trauma (abdominal injury; intraoperative)
Metabolic (hyperlipidemia, uremia, renal failure, after renal transplantation, hypercalcemia, pregnancy, cystic fibrosis, kwashiorkor)
Vascular (shock, lupus erythematosus, thrombocytopenic purpura, polyarteritis, atheromatous embolism)
Drugs
   Association
      Immunosuppressive—corticosteroids, L-asparaginase, azathioprine
      Diuretics—thiazides, furosemide, ethacrynic acid
      Estrogens, oral contraceptives
      Antibodies—tetracyclines, sulfonamides
   Possible association
      Acetaminophen
      Isoniazid, rifampin
      Propoxyphene
      Valproic acid, procainamide
      Anticoagulants
Infections (mumps, viral hepatitis, coxsackievirus, echovirus, *Ascaris*, *Mycoplasma*)
Mechanical (duct obstruction, duodenal obstruction)
Penetrating duodenal ulcer
Hereditary pancreatitis
Idiopathic

that involving the pancreas and adjoining organs. Other possible causes are certain metabolic conditions (hyperparathyroidism, pregnancy, uremia, kidney transplantation), certain drugs (opiates, thiazides, steroids, oral contraceptives, sulfonamides), vascular disease, infection, and nutritional and hereditary factors.

Pathology

The chemical and pathologic changes characteristic of pancreatitis reflect the destructive effects of pancreatic enzymes. The precise mechansim that triggers the activation of enzymes and autodigestion is unknown. The major histologic alterations in pancreatitis are *necrosis of fat and cells, proteolytic destruction of pancreatic parenchyma (proteolysis), edema, hemorrhage*, and *inflammation*.

The exocrine pancreas secretes more than 20 enzymes. The proteolytic enzymes are secreted in a proenzyme or inactive form that prevents autodigestion of the pancreas. Trypsin plays a major role because it activates the major proteolytic enzymes involved in autodigestion (Flowchart 39-5). Trypsin normally is secreted from the pancreas in the form of trypsinogen and is activated in

the duodenum (see pp. 772–774). The major initiating pathology is premature activation of trypsinogen in the pancreas. Significant amounts of trypsin, chymotrypsin, and elastase have been detected in the diseased pancreas.

Elastase exists in high concentrations in granules of acini cells, and it is present in pancreatic secretions as an inactive precursor. After activation by trypsin, it causes elastic fibers of blood vessels and ducts to dissolve. Hemorrhage caused by breakdown of elastic fibers of the vessels may be minor or extreme, varying from red blood cells and fibrin clots to large masses of blood over large areas. Prekallikrein is converted to kallikrein by trypsin. Kallikrein leads to the release of bradykinin and kallidin (a plasma kinin), which further increase vasodilatation and vascular permeability. Phospholipase A acts on phospholipids, with a resultant release of compounds that have strong cytotoxic effects and damage cell membranes and the ductal system, leading to necrosis.

A leukocytic reaction appears around the areas of hemorrhage and necrosis. Secondary bacterial invasion may produce a suppurative necrosis or abscess. Milder lesions may be absorbed, or they may calcify cr become

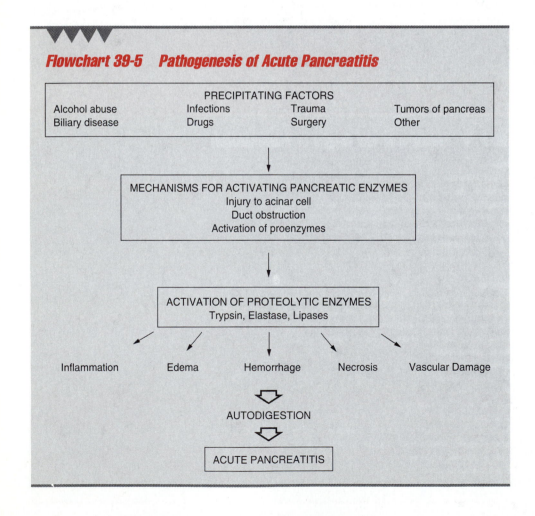

Flowchart 39-5   Pathogenesis of Acute Pancreatitis

PRECIPITATING FACTORS

| Alcohol abuse | Infections | Trauma | Tumors of pancreas |
| Biliary disease | Drugs | Surgery | Other |

↓

MECHANISMS FOR ACTIVATING PANCREATIC ENZYMES
Injury to acinar cell
Duct obstruction
Activation of proenzymes

↓

ACTIVATION OF PROTEOLYTIC ENZYMES
Trypsin, Elastase, Lipases

Inflammation   Edema   Hemorrhage   Necrosis   Vascular Damage

⇩

AUTODIGESTION

⇩

ACUTE PANCREATITIS

fibrotic if they are more severe. If fluid is walled off by fibrous tissue during the inflammatory process, a pancreatic cyst known as a pseudocyst is formed.

Alcohol-induced changes are major factors in the pathogenesis of pancreatitis. Alcohol is a stimulator of pancreatic secretions and also causes duodenal edema of the ampulla of Vater, obstructing flow of secretions. Long-term alcohol ingestion increases the protein concentration of secretions, which leads to formation of protein plugs in the ducts and subsequent obstruction by the precipitates, resulting in degeneration and fibrosis of acini cells. Alcohol may decrease the tone of the sphincter of Oddi and cause duodenal reflux. Another factor that predisposes alcoholics to pancreatitis may be the elevated serum triglyceride levels that occur after a meal.[16] Most alcoholic pancreatitis is an acute exacerbation of chronic pancreatitis.[7]

Hyperlipidemia is known to be associated with pancreatitis. Experimental studies indicate that lipolysis of triglycerides by pancreatic lipase in the pancreas leads to high concentration of free fatty acids in tissues. Animal studies indicate that these free fatty acids can initiate pancreatic injury.[7]

Hypercalcemia is thought to be a factor in activating trypsinogen and in the subsequent development of acute pancreatitis. An association of pancreatitis with parathyroid adenomas and carcinomas has been noted.

Acinar cell injury caused by viruses, endotoxins, toxic chemicals, ischemia, or trauma may precipitate activation and release of pancreatic enzymes. This theory is postulated for pancreatitis not caused by alcoholism or biliary disease.[7]

Clinical Manifestations

There are no precise clinical features that differentiate pancreatitis from other disorders. *Abdominal pain* and tenderness are present in almost all cases of acute pancreatitis and frequently occur in chronic pancreatitis. The pain usually has no prodromal symptoms and often occurs after a large meal or an episode of heavy alcoholic consumption. It usually is severe and may reach full intensity in a matter of minutes or gradually over several hours. Pain is frequently localized in the epigastrium, becoming more severe to the right or left of the epigastrium or generalized throughout the upper abdomen. Pancreatic pain usually is steady, boring, and penetrating. Unlike the pain of biliary colic, it radiates straight through to the back in about one-half of affected people. Affected persons are restless, anxious, and may seek relief by flexing the spine, by bending forward and flexing the knees against the chest, or by lying on one side with knees flexed. Characteristically, the pain of acute pancreatitis lasts for hours and days rather than a few minutes or a few hours.

The pain of pancreatitis is related to ductal swelling, extravasation of plasma and red blood cells, and release of digested proteins and lipids into surrounding tissue. The pancreatic capsule is stretched by the edema, exudate, red cells, and digestive products. These substances seep out of the gland into the mesentery, causing a peritonitis that stimulates the sensory nerves and causes intense pain in back and flanks when the gland is damaged extensively. During an acute attack, the pain is generalized over the abdomen because of peritoneal irritation and release of kinins. Large doses of narcotics are avoided because they may induce spasm of the sphincter of Oddi, which aggravates the pancreatitis and increases pain. As pain increases with the spread of intraperitoneal and retroperitoneal inflammation, local or diffuse paralytic ileus may occur. Peripheral vascular collapse and shock may develop rapidly. The stretching of the gland also may cause nausea and vomiting. Vomiting and abdominal distention also are related to intestinal hypomotility and chemical peritonitis.

Other nonspecific findings include low-grade fever, hypotension, tachycardia, and shock. Mild jaundice is sometimes present and becomes severe if the common bile duct becomes obstructed.[10] Bowel sounds usually are diminished. A pancreatic pseudocyst may be palpable in the upper abdomen. In severe necrotizing pancreatitis, discoloration of the flanks (Grey Turner sign) or around the umbilicus (Cullen sign) may be noted. A history of a prior attack of pancreatitis may be valuable in diagnosing the condition.

The extensive injury to tissue, necrosis, and inflammation produce fever in about two-thirds of cases of acute pancreatitis. Fever is caused by absorption of pyrogens into the circulation, but persistent high fever or temperature spikes imply pancreatic abscess or other septic complications.[16]

Complications

CARDIOVASCULAR COMPLICATIONS. With massive exudation of plasma into the retroperitoneal space and in cases of hemorrhage, there is a drop in blood pressure and a rise in pulse. Release of bradykinin results in marked peripheral vasodilatation, which further reduces blood pressure. Accumulation of fluid in the small bowel, a third-space shift, causes additional loss of fluid and leads to systemic hypotension and shock. The decrease in intravascular volume together with hypotension diminishes urine output, and acute tubular necrosis of the kidneys may result. Myocardial and cerebral ischemia also may occur.

COAGULATION DEFECTS. Although not a frequent feature of the disease, hypercoagulability of blood may occur as a result of elevations in levels of platelets, factor VIII, fibrinogen, and, possibly, factor V.

ILEUS.   The large and small bowel may dilate in a general response to inflammation of the peritoneum. The gut may contain air and fluid, contributing to hypovolemia.

PULMONARY-PLEURAL COMPLICATIONS.   Acute pancreatitis frequently is accompanied by a pleural effusion. The fluid may be hemorrhagic. This pleural effusion apparently is caused by the retroperitoneal transudation of fluid, with markedly elevated secretion of amylase into the pleural cavity from the inflamed, swollen pancreas.

GASTROINTESTINAL BLEEDING.   This may occur in association with a pseudocyst or abscess, mucosal bleeding of the duodenum caused by adjacent inflammation from the pancreas, or esophageal or gastric varices related to splenic or portal vein thrombosis. Gastritis and esophagitis in alcoholics may be a source of hemorrhage in pancreatitis.

HYPOCALCEMIA.   Sharp falls in serum calcium levels may occur in acute pancreatitis and levels below 7 mg/dL are a poor prognostic sign.[10] These are related to extensive lipolysis of tissues, which releases free fatty acids that combine with calcium to form soaps in the retroperitoneal area. The parathyroids do not rapidly compensate for the abrupt lowering of calcium by the mechanism of soap formation. Neuromuscular irritability and tetany result from severe hypocalcemia.

ACIDOSIS.   Lactic acidosis may result from the central hypovolemia or from the ketosis that occasionally occurs when there is extensive destruction of the gland.

HYPERLIPIDEMIA.   High levels of serum lipids often are noted during attacks of pancreatitis, especially in persons with alcoholic pancreatitis and in those with pre-existing elevated triglyceride levels. The plasma may have a creamy appearance.

PSEUDOCYSTS.   Inflammatory pseudocysts are a frequent complication during recovery from an episode of severe acute pancreatitis. The cysts are non–epithelium-lined cavities that contain plasma, blood, pancreatic products, and inflammatory exudate. They are solitary and measure 5 to 10 cm in diameter. They occur as a result of destruction of tissue and obstruction in the ductal system. Pancreatic juice may collect in them and leak into the peritoneal cavity. If large, pseudocysts may impinge on neighboring structures such as the portal vein, causing *acute portal hypertension*, and on the bile duct, causing *jaundice*. Sometimes, the cysts rupture and cause generalized peritonitis.

PANCREATIC ABSCESS.   One of the most serious complications of acute pancreatitis is a pancreatic abscess, a collection of purulent and necrotic tissue. It occurs if an episode of pancreatitis is severe enough to cause parenchymal necrosis and if the pancreatic and surrounding tissues become secondarily infected. There usually are several foci of infection rather than a discrete abscess that can be easily drained. Pancreatic abscesses occur most frequently in association with alcohol abuse. Fistulization into an adjacent structure with massive bleeding may occur.

JAUNDICE.   Mild jaundice is common in acute pancreatitis. The swelling of the head of the pancreas impinges on the common bile duct that passes through it. If the bile duct is compressed by pseudocysts or stones, jaundice may be more severe.

Diagnostic Evaluation

The major findings of acute pancreatitis are increases in the activities of *serum amylase* and *serum lipase*. Serum amylase values usually exceed 200 Somogyi units; normal levels are 60 to 180 Somogyi units/dL. The amylase-creatinine clearance ratio is usually increased. There does not appear to be a correlation between elevation of amylase and severity of disease.

Serum lipase activity, most specific for acute pancreatitis, parallels that of serum amylase, and abnormal levels persist for a longer time. Normal serum lipase values depend on the laboratory procedure used, but they usually are below 1.5 U/mL. The increased activity occurs shortly after onset of disease, almost always within the first 24 hours, and may remain high for weeks. *Leukocytosis*, with increased polymorphonuclear leukocytes and a shift to the left, is frequent. The leukocyte counts range from 10,000 to 20,000 but occasionally rise to 50,000 mm^3. The *hematocrit* may be elevated from loss of serum into the peritoneal spaces with resultant hemoconcentration.

Hyperglycemia is related to various factors such as increased glucagon, decreased insulin, and increased glucocorticoid and catecholamine levels. *Hyperlipemia* often occurs, and it may predate the onset of overt pancreatitis. Levels of *serum calcium* and *serum magnesium* decrease, especially in persons having fat necrosis. Blood calcium levels may fall and remain down for 7 to 10 days. Hypocalcemia is an indicator of severe pancreatitis.[10]

Ultrasonic examination of the pancreas in severe pancreatitis may help to confirm a clinical impression, assess degree of resolution of inflammation, and reveal dilatation of the common bile duct secondary to obstruction and presence of gallstones. *Computed tomography scans* may be obtained if unexplained abdominal pain suggests either pancreatitis or pancreatic carcinoma. Scans also may be used in prolonged pancreatitis or recurrent pancreatitis to rule out a pseudocyst or interductal calculi. *Roentgenograms* may be obtained to rule out a perforation and exclude other diagnoses.

CHRONIC PANCREATITIS

Manifestations of chronic pancreatitis are similar to those of acute pancreatitis except for their chronicity and recurrence. This disorder occurs in the same type of person who is prone to developing acute pancreatitis. The person usually is an alcohol abuser and less frequently has biliary disease. Nonalcoholic tropical pancreatitis and hereditary or familial pancreatitis are forms of chronic pancreatitis that are relatively rare. If bouts recur, a pancreatic insufficiency may result, even though the pancreas has considerable functional reserve.

In chronic pancreatitis, histologic changes persist even after the causative agent has been removed. In the United States, the most common cause of chronic pancreatitis is alcohol abuse. The pathologic changes are characterized by the deposition of protein plugs in the small ducts of the pancreas. An inflammatory process is set up, and fibrous tissue is deposited. Eventually there is intraductal calcification and marked parenchymal destruction, with only a few islet cells and some acinar tissue remaining. Exocrine pancreatic insufficiency is manifested by steatorrhea (excess fat in the stools), azotorrhea (excess nitrogenous material in the feces), and weight loss. Microscopically, the stool exhibits fat globules and striated meat fibers that indicate impaired digestion of fats and proteins. Endocrine pancreatic insufficiency may lead to diabetes mellitus. Abdominal pain is a serious problem in chronic pancreatitis and may be responsible for severe weight loss, malnutrition, and general debility. During early stages of the disease, the person may be asymptomatic between attacks.

The predominant complications of chronic pancreatitis that are associated with abdominal pain are pancreatic pseudocyst, stricture and obstruction of the common bile duct or pancreatic duct, and, occasionally, carcinoma of the pancreas. Fat malabsorption, pleural effusions, ascites, and diabetes mellitus are other complications that may be seen (Fig. 39-9).

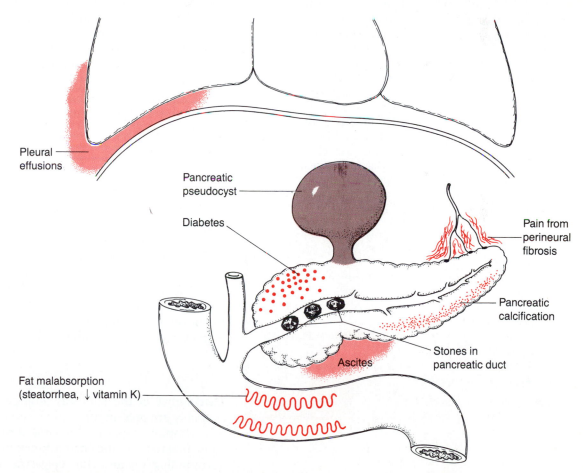

FIGURE 39-9 *Complications of chronic pancreatitis. (Rubin, E., and Farber, J.L. Pathology [2nd ed.]. Philadelphia: J.B. Lippincott, 1994.)*

CASE STUDY 39-2

Mr. S., 55 years of age, comes to the emergency room (E.R.) of a large urban hospital. This is Mr. S.'s third admission to the E.R. within 3 years. He is complaining of severe epigastric pain radiating to his back. There is guarding of the abdomen. Nausea and vomiting are associated with the pain. He is disoriented when responding to the triage nurse.

Physical examination revealed poor skin turgor; other signs of dehydration were evident. Slight jaundice, fever, tachycardia, orthopnea, midline tenderness and guarding were present.

Mr. S. denies taking any medications. He states he drinks socially but does not get intoxicated.

History— Employed as a painter. Lives alone. Visits sister frequently. His wife died 3 years ago from ovarian cancer. His only son lives over 500 miles away. Mr. S. had an oral cholecystectography 6 months PTA. Results were normal.

Dignostic Evaluation:

Routine laboratory values	Within normal limits (WNL), except for WBC, which was 16,000/mm³ (normal = 5,000–10,000/mm³
Serum glucose	150 mg/dl (normal 80–115 mg/dl)
Serum amylase test	640 IU (normal = 56–190 IU/L)
Urine amylase test	1240 IU/hr (normal = 3–35 IU/hr)
Serum lipase test	240 units/L (normal = 0–110 units/L)
Ultrasound of pancreas	Head of pancreas enlarged and edematous
CT of abdomen	Pancreas enlarged
ERCP	Normal pancreatic duct

Radiograph revealed pleural effusion.

1. What are risk factors for the development of pancreatitis?
2. What is the pathophysiologic basis for Mr. S.'s clinical manifestations of pancreatitis?
3. What triggers the autodigestive process which characterizes pancreatitis?
4. What is the major enzyme involved in activating the pathologic process?
5. What is pancreatic pseudocyst? Differentiate between a pseudocyst and a pancreatic abscess.
6. Which of Mr. S.'s laboratory values would indicate a diagnosis of pancreatitis?

See Appendix G for discussion.

▼ Carcinoma of the Pancreas

Carcinoma of the pancreas occurs mainly in the exocrine portion of the gland in the ductal epithelium; the most common site is the head of the pancreas. Cancer of the pancreas is the fifth most common cause of death from cancer in the United States. Pancreatic cancers have a poor prognosis, causing about 5% of all neoplastic deaths in the United States.[2] The incidence is increasing; about 25,000 new patients are identified annually, and more than 24,000 of these will die within 5 years.[2,23] A significant increase in frequency has been attributed to smoking, consumption of alcoholic beverages, history of pancreatitis, and consumption of fat. There is a higher incidence in African Americans and in males. Chemists and people exposed to industrial agents also are at higher risk for pancreatic cancer. Most tumors occur in people older than age 60 years; they seldom occur before age 40.

Clinical symptoms of cancer of the pancreas depend on its site of origin and manifestations of metastasis. Tumors of the head of the pancreas tend to obstruct the bile duct and duodenum and lead to early symptoms of obstructive jaundice. Carcinoma of the body and tail are less easily recognized clinically and become apparent only if adjacent structures are involved or after metastatic dissemination produces symptoms. Most carcinomas of the pancreas grow in well-differentiated glandular patterns and are *adenocarcinomas*. About 10% assume an *adenosquamous* pattern or an uncommon pattern of extreme anaplasia with *giant cell* formation. About 0.5% arise in cysts and are called *cystadenocarcinoma*. An *acinar cell carcinoma* occasionally occurs in children.[5,7]

CARCINOMA OF THE BODY AND TAIL OF THE PANCREAS

These tumors usually are large and invade the entire tail and body of the pancreas; they may even be palpable in a thin person. They spread more extensively than tumors of the head, crowd the vertebral column, spread into the retroperitoneal spaces, and may even invade the spleen, adrenals, colon, or stomach. Metastases spread by way of the splenic vein, which lies on the margins of the organ, to surrounding nodes and the liver. The liver may be enlarged two to three times its normal size.[7]

CLINICAL MANIFESTATIONS

Carcinomas of the pancreas progress insidiously and probably are present for months and perhaps years before symptoms appear. The clinical manifestations are those that relate to the encroachment of the pancreas on surrounding organs. Dull epigastric abdominal pain, which may radiate to the back; weight loss with anorexia, generalized malaise, and weakness; and jaundice are among the few characteristic signs or symptoms that point to a diagnosis of pancreatic cancer. Anorexia occasionally is accompanied by a curious aversion to meats and a metallic taste in the mouth.[5] Large tumors that arise from the head of the pancreas often encase the common bile duct. Jaundice is common and often is accompanied by pruritus and weight loss.

Nausea, vomiting, weakness, fatigue, diarrhea, and dyspepsia also are fairly common. Vomiting may indicate gastric or duodenal encroachment or peritoneal metastasis. Hematemesis and melena indicate invasion of the tumor into duodenal or gastric organs that are vascular. About one-fourth of persons with pancreatic cancer have a palpable abdominal mass. They often complain of both constipation and diarrhea, and emotional disturbances may be noted. Thrombophlebitis and diabetes mellitus are other clinical features. An abdominal bruit may be auscultated in the periumbilical area and left upper quadrant because of compression of the splenic artery by a tumor.

Spontaneously appearing phlebothrombosis, also called migratory thrombophlebitis, is noted in carcinoma of the pancreas. This is called the Trousseau sign; it was so named by Trousseau when he developed migratory thrombophlebitis during the course of his own fatal disease. Thromboses appear and disappear in other forms of cancer, but the two highest correlations are in pancreatic and pulmonary neoplasms. The thromboses are attributed to confinement to bed and surgical treatment. Thromboplastic factors have been identified in the serum that lead to a hypercoagulable state because of thromboplastic properties of the necrotic products of the tumor.[7]

DIAGNOSTIC EVALUATION

Laboratory procedures are important in providing clues to the presence of these cancers in their early stages. About 80% to 90% have elevated levels of carcinoembryonic antigen. Measurement of this antigen may be helpful in following the course of pancreatic cancer, with titers of greater than 20 mg/mL usually being associated with metastases. As with obstructive jaundice, serum bilirubin levels increase, stools become clay-colored, and urine urobilinogen levels fall. Alkaline phosphatase levels are elevated.[5] Ultrasonography can help localize tumors and differentiate them from cysts. A computed tomographic scan and magnetic resonance imaging of the pancreas are helpful in confirming presence of tumor. Percutaneous needle biopsy is useful in diagnosis after tumors are localized.

▼ Cystic Fibrosis

Cystic fibrosis (CF), formerly referred to as mucoviscidosis or fibrocystic disease of the pancreas, is a multisystem disorder of infants, adolescents, and young adults. CF has been clearly recognized as a disease entity only since the late 1930s. Historical notes tell of the midwife licking the forehead of the newborn to identify any salty taste. CF is characterized by alterations in the secretory process of the exocrine (mucus-producing) glands that result in pulmonary disease, pancreatic insufficiency, and elevated sweat electrolytes.

INCIDENCE

CF is a common inherited condition and the most fatal genetic disease in Caucasians of European origin. The incidence is about 1 in 2,000 in white populations, with a carrier rate of 1 in 25. Black and oriental races are seldom affected. There is no difference in sex distribution.

GENETIC CHARACTERISTICS

CF is transmitted by the autosomal recessive mode of inheritance. If both parents are carriers of the gene, there is a 25% chance with each pregnancy that the child will have CF, a 50% chance that the child will carry the gene but not have the disease, and a 25% chance that the child will neither have CF nor carry the gene. Chromosome number and structure are normal. Clinical manifestations are evident only in homozygotes; carriers of the gene (heterozygotes) show no symptoms of the disease. More children with CF are surviving to adulthood, marrying, and reproducing; therefore, genetic risks are important considerations.

CF results from mutations of a gene located on chromosome 7q31. The deletion of an amino acid accounts for most mutations and results in a protein (CF gene product) called the cystic fibrosis transmembrane conductance regulator (CFTR). The gene *F503* is expressed only in exocrine organs. The CFTR molecules are normally found on the endoplasmic reticulum of cells lining ducts of exocrine organs, especially the lungs, pancreas, intestine, and sweat ducts of the skin. They function as regulators of ion and water channels through which electrolytes can pass. The CF gene is found in 75% of non-Jewish and 30% of Jewish CF carriers who are of northern European descent.[32]

PATHOGENESIS

CF is a disorder of secretory epithelia of the lungs, sweat glands, pancreas, intestine, liver, reproductive tract, and other organs. CFTR molecules are normally found on the endoplasmic reticulum of cells lining the ducts of exocrine organs. With sympathetic stimulation of the CFTR-containing exocrine cells, there is secretion of mucus, electrolytes, and water into the duct opening. It is the combination of water and electrolytes that assists in hydration of exocrine secretions, and mucus enables them to move along the ducts and be released. In persons with CF gene mutations, there is inadequate synthesis of CFTR. Therefore, pores are lacking for release of electrolytes at cell surfaces. This alteration affects chloride transport and is manifested by an increase in sodium chloride in sweat.[19,25] On stimulation, these ducts produce thick, viscous secretions that plug the ducts of the exocrine organs.

CF is characterized by 1) pancreatic enzyme deficiency leading to malabsorption of fat-soluble vitamins A, D, E, and K; 2) large volumes of thick, viscous bronchial mucus resulting in chronic pulmonary disease; and 3) elevated sodium and chloride concentrations in sweat. Anatomic changes of CF result from obstruction of exocrine ducts by thick, heavy, dehydrated mucus. Flowchart 39-6 shows the multisystem effects of CF.

Gastrointestinal Tract

The extent of changes is related to whether secretions are carried to the gastrointestinal tract from cells with nar-row necks, such as the goblet cells; from wide-mouthed ducts, such as glands in the duodenum; or from narrow ducts, such as those in the pancreas, liver, and salivary glands. The thick, tenacious secretions tend to cause more problems in long, narrow ducts, with resultant changes in tissues and alterations of function. The greatest alterations in structure and function occur in the pancreas.

STRUCTURAL CHANGES IN THE PANCREAS. Abnormalities in the pancreas occur in most affected people. These changes are evident microscopically and macroscopically as early as the neonatal period. The changes are variable and depend on the age at onset and the severity of disease. They may consist of accumulation of mucus or, as the disease progresses, blockage of the collecting ducts, damage to acinar tissue, fibrosis and duct dilatation, and degeneration of the parenchyma. The ducts may be replaced by fat and fibrous tissue and converted into cysts. These changes in appearance are

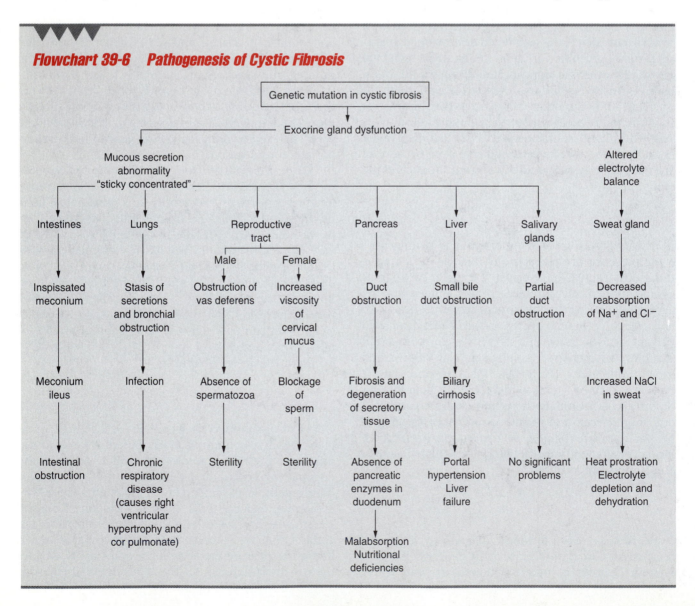

Flowchart 39-6   Pathogenesis of Cystic Fibrosis

the bases for the designation fibrocystic disease of the pancreas.

Pathologic changes begin during fetal life and frequently are severe enough by birth to prevent exocrine secretions from reaching the duodenum. The development of diabetes mellitus in some older people is suggestive of impairment of the blood supply by progressive fibrosis.

Functional changes occur as a result of structural alterations. There is a lack of enzymes (trypsin, amylase, lipase) in the duodenum. As a result, proteins are not completely digested and nitrogen is excreted in the stools; starch is not completely broken down and appears as granules; and fats are largely undigested and are excreted in the stools in excessive amounts. The stools are large and oily, and have a pungent odor, caused in part by breakdown products of protein produced by bacteria in the intestine.

LIVER. Blockage of the bile duct by mucus and mononuclear periportal cell infiltration leads to cirrhosis and portal hypertension. Esophageal varices and splenomegaly may result.

INTESTINE. Absence of pancreatic enzymes and altered gastrointestinal mucous secretions produce thick, tenacious plugs of viscid mucus that obstruct the lumen of the small intestine, causing meconium ileus.

SALIVARY GLANDS. The salivary glands frequently undergo histologic changes such as dilatation of ducts and glandular atrophy and fibrosis.

OTHER GLANDS. Pathologic changes also occur in other glands. Plugging occurs in the bile ducts, leading to fibrosis and liver dysfunction. CF is an important cause of hepatic cirrhosis and portal hypertension in adolescents and young adults.

Respiratory System

Pulmonary changes occur in almost all affected persons and usually are the primary determinants of the ultimate outcome of the disease. Both upper and lower respiratory tracts are involved because of the presence of mucus-secreting glands and cells. The lungs are structurally normal at birth, but problems begin in the small bronchioles, where the thick, tenacious mucus collects and provides a medium for bacterial growth. The most common organisms are *Staphylococcus aureus*, *Haemophilus influenzae*, and *Pseudomonas aeruginosa*. The mucoid form of the last is especially troublesome.

Infection alters the integrity of the bronchial epithelium and invades the peribronchial tissues. Bronchiectasis develops in the terminal bronchioles. Trapping of air produces an overinflated, barrel-shaped chest. Mucopurulent exudates also are present in the upper respiratory tract. Nasal polyps occur with increased frequency and often are associated with sinus infections. Pulmonary hypertension results from thickened arterioles, which, together with the obstructive bronchial disease, leads to right ventricular hypertrophy and cor pulmonale.

Reproductive System

Abnormalities include atresia or obstruction of the vas deferens and epididymis in the male. Spermatogenesis is decreased or absent. In the female, mucus-producing glands of the cervix also may produce viscid mucus that blocks the entry of sperm. The frequency of cervical polyps is increased.

Sweat Glands

Although there is a high electrolyte content of the sweat and an alteration in reabsorption of sodium chloride in the sweat ducts, no structural abnormalities are noted in the ducts.

CLINICAL MANIFESTATIONS

Clinical manifestations differ among children depending on disease progression and age of the child. Because CF affects several organ systems in varying degrees, sometimes it is difficult to recognize. Most persons are diagnosed in early childhood because of symptoms related to the respiratory and gastrointestinal systems. An early manifestation of CF is meconium ileus in the newborn, which blocks the small intestine with thick, tenacious, puttylike meconium. The degree varies from a delay in passing meconium (meconium plug syndrome) to an obvious intestinal obstruction, usually in the area of the ileocecal valve, which may be accompanied by atresia, volvulus, or perforation and peritonitis. Prolapse of the rectum related to chronic constipation is a common complication in children with untreated CF.

As the child grows older, the impaired pancreatic function results in malabsorption of fats and the fat-soluble vitamins. The child has a good appetite but appears malnourished. Bleeding disorders may occur as a result of vitamin K deficiency from malabsorption.

In the classic case, the child is examined after several months of life because of respiratory symptoms, failure to thrive, and foul-smelling, bulky, greasy stools. Any one or all of these characteristics may be noted. In some cases, symptoms are not apparent until several years have passed. Many infants have a dry, repetitive cough that occurs in an attempt to remove the sticky secretion. Vomiting may follow a bout of coughing. Classic progression of chest infection occurs, with increased coughing and sputum, development of barrel chest, finger-clubbing, dyspnea, and cyanosis. Sputum is thick, sticky, and difficult to expectorate. In the early stages, it is yellow, particularly if caused by *S. aureus*. With the mucoid strain, *P. aeruginosa*, sputum is greenish and slimy. Poor gas exchange leads to hypoxemia and pulmonary complications and may progress to cor pulmonale.

Uncommonly, CF may be diagnosed during adolescence or adulthood. Diagnosis is difficult, because the sweat test is less reliable in the older than the younger affected population. Persons affected with CF who have not had severe chest infection may have abdominal problems, diabetes, or liver disease.

DIAGNOSTIC EVALUATION

Molecular genetic testing for CF has revolutionized diagnosis and genetic counseling. Of the approximately 200 mutations, the six that can be identified through gene testing account for 85% to 90% of carriers. Therefore, relatives can now determine whether they carry the mutant gene present in the affected person.[32] Direct and indirect testing are available to diagnose CF and to determine carrier status. Direct testing is done by linkage analysis, which uses the strong association of the primary CF mutation with a specific haplotype (linked genes inherited as a unit). This method is useful for intrauterine diagnosis if a DNA sample from the affected child is unavailable.[32]

Prenatal diagnosis is possible through chorionic villus sampling or amniocentesis. It is important to know which mutation is present in the family in order to diagnose accurately. Otherwise, only 70% of affected fetuses can be identified. If the index case (affected child) is unavailable, information can be obtained from testing of intestinal enzymes such as intestinal alkaline phosphatase in the amniotic fluid.

Neonatal screening can be done by examination of a drop of dried neonatal blood for elevated levels of serum immunoreactive trypsinogen. However, there are significant numbers of false-positive and false-negative results. DNA mutation analysis can be done on dried blood.[32]

Criteria for diagnosis of CF include increased electrolyte concentration of sweat, absence of pancreatic enzymes, impaired fat absorption, chronic pulmonary involvement, and family history of the disorder. Most children have both pulmonary and pancreatic involvement, but one may exist without the other.

The *pilocarpine iontophoresis sweat test* is the simplest and most reliable method to confirm the diagnosis. Up to age 20, a level of more than 60 mEq of sweat chloride per liter is diagnostic of CF. Values between 50 and 60 mEq/L are highly suggestive. The sweat test is repeated if results are questionable or if they are negative and clinical manifestations are strongly suggestive of CF. Reliable sweat tests are difficult to obtain in the first 3 to 4 weeks of life because the sweat glands are not yet well developed functionally.

Chest radiographs reveal changes in the respiratory system. Chest films reveal slightly increased diameter of upper chest, with overaerated lungs, widespread consol-

idation, and fibrotic changes. There may be areas of lobar or segmental collapse. Pulmonary function tests assist in evaluating the therapeutics and monitoring progress of the disease.

Changes in radiologic patterns of the small intestine are noted in CF as in other malabsorptive diseases.

CASE STUDY 39-3

Kara, a blue-eyed, blond-haired female, age 14 months, is admitted to the pediatric unit with paroxysmal coughing and a respiratory infection. Kara is the second child of a 32-year-old father and a 30-year-old mother. Kara has a history of recurrent respiratory infections. She is pale and thin, especially her extremities. Her abdomen is distended and her mother reports that her stools are large, frothy in appearance, and foul smelling. She is in the 5th percentile for weight and the 10th percentile for height.

Family history- both parents and older sister, age 4, are well. A maternal uncle died in his late twenties from pneumonia and heart failure secondary to cystic fibrosis.

Physical examination—Wheezing, rhonchi, tachypnea with a prolonged expiratory phase.

Diagnostic Evaluation: chest radiograph revealed patchy atelectasis, hyperinflation, and air trapping.

Sweat electrolytes (iontophoresis)

Sodium	90 mEq/L (normal <70 mEq/L)
Chloride	70 mEq/L (normal < 50 mEq/L)
Secretin-pan creozymin Test (duodenal aspirate)	Absence of trypsin
Fecal fat test 72-hr	Fat retention coefficient 80% (normal > 95%)

Oximetry readings were 88%—92% in oxygen tent Antibiotics and chest physiotherapy are ordered. Parents are instructed in pancreatic enzyme therapy. A high-protein diet with moderate fat and multiple vitamin supplements is ordered. Genetic testing and counseling are recommended.

1. *What in Kara's history and clinical manifestations would explain why she has cystic fibrosis?*
2. *What is the genetic inheritance pattern? Could prenatal testing identify the disease prenatally? How?*
3. *Which two body systems are primarily affected and how?*
4. *What in the pathogenesis of cystic fibrosis leads to right ventricular hypertrophy development?*
5. *What pathophysiological changes account for the appearance of Kara's stools?*
6. *Why would a sweat electrolyte test be ordered?*
7. *Why would a pancreatic enzyme test be ordered?*
8. *Why would a fat test be ordered?*
9. *How would genetic counseling benefit the family?*

See Appendix G for discussion.

Fibrosis abnormalities also are evident in barium studies of the duodenum.

Pancreatic deficiency is noted on examination of duodenal contents for pancreatic enzyme (trypsin and chymotrypsin) activity. Trypsin is absent in about 80% of affected people. Chemical examination of feces reveals marked steatorrhea. Normal stools should not contain more than 4 g of fat per day. Stools of children with CF often contain 15 to 30 g/d.

▼ Chapter Summary

▼ The endocrine secretion of the pancreas governs much of the glucose metabolism of the body. It is regulated through the hormones insulin and glucagon, which are secreted by the beta and alpha cells of the islets of Langerhans.

▼ Diabetes mellitus is a disease of absolute or relative lack of insulin secretion. It is categorized as insulin-dependent diabetes mellitus (IIDM, or Type I) and non-insulin-dependent diabetes mellitus (NIDDM, or Type II). The etiology of the disorder varies according to the type and the onset of complications may be earlier in the Type I form. Either disorder is prone to system-wide complications that involve the pancreas, vascular system, eye, nervous system, skin, liver, and muscles. Diabetic ketoacidosis and HHNK are manifestations of major glucose metabolism problems and may be life threatening.

▼ Other disorders of the pancreatic islet cell include hyperinsulinism, Zollinger–Ellison syndrome, and Werner's syndrome. These have various forms which include blood glucose regulation problems and hypersecretion of gastric acid along with other problems.

▼ Pancreatitis is a relatively common problem that is increasing in incidence. It is often related to alcohol ingestion and the clinical manifestations may be chronic or very acute, causing gastrointestinal bleeding, ileus, and many other problems.

▼ Carcinoma of the pancreas also is increasing in incidence and has a poor prognosis. Clinical manifestations may be obscure or may be similar to those of pancreatitis.

▼ Cystic fibrosis is a multisystem disorder that is genetically induced. It affects the gastrointestinal tract, respiratory system, reproductive system, and sweat glands. The lifespan of children with the disease is improving, but death usually occurs before the age of 30.

▼ References

1. American Diabetes Association. Diabetes control and complications. *Diabetes Forecast*, September 1993, pp. 41–62.
2. Black, J.M., and Matassarin-Jacobs, E. *Luckman and Sorensen's Medical-Surgical Nursing: A Psycholophysiologic Approach*. Philadelphia: W.B. Saunders, 1993.
3. Boden, G., Mauer, E., and Mozzoli, M. Glucose transporter proteins in human insulinoma. *Ann. Intern. Med.* 121:109–112, 1994.
4. Bogardus, C. Insulin resistance in the pathogenesis of NIDDM in Pima Indians. *Diabetes Care* 16:228–231, 1993.
5. Cello, J.P. Carcinoma of the pancreas. In Wyngaarden, J.B., and Smith, L.H. (eds.), *Cecil's Textbook of Medicine* (18th ed.). Philadelphia: W.B. Saunders, 1988.
6. Ch'ng, J.L. Multiple endocrine neoplasia. In Kelley, W.N. (ed.), *Textbook of Internal Medicine* (2nd ed.). Philadelphia: J.B. Lippincott, 1992.
7. Cotran, R.S., Kumar, V., and Robbins, S.L. *Robbins' Pathologic Basis of Disease* (4th ed.). Philadelphia: W.B. Saunders, 1989.
8. Craighead, J.E. Diabetes. In Rubin, E., and Farber, J.L, *Pathology* (2nd ed.). Philadelphia: J.B. Lippincott, 1994.
9. DeFronzo, R.A. Pathogenesis of type 2 (non-insulin-dependent) diabetes mellitus: A balanced overview. *Diabetologia* 35:389–397, 1993.
10. Dimagno, E.P. Pancreatitis. In Kelley, W.N. (ed.), *Textbook of Internal Medicine* (2nd ed.). Philadelphia: J.B. Lippincott, 1992.
11. Eisenbarth, G.S. Type I diabetes. In Kelley, W.N. (ed.), *Textbook of Internal Medicine* (2nd ed.). Philadelphia: J.B. Lippincott, 1992.
12. Foster, D.W. Diabetes mellitus. In Wilson, J.D., et al. (eds.). *Harrison's Principles of Internal Medicine* (12th ed.). New York: McGraw-Hill, 1991.
13. Froguel, P., et al. Familial hyperglycemia due to mutations in glucokinase: Definition of a new subtype of non-insulin-dependent (type 2) diabetes mellitus. *N. Engl. J. Med.* 328:697–702, 1993.
14. Gerstein, H.C. Cow's milk exposure and type 1 diabetes mellitus: A critical review of the clinical literature. *Diabetes Care* 17:13–18, 1994.
15. Go, V.L. Pancreatic secretion. In Stein, J. (ed.), *Internal Medicine* (4th ed.). St. Louis: C.V. Mosby, 1994.
16. Greenberger, N.J., and Toskes, P.P. Disorders of the pancreas. In Wilson, J.D., et al. (eds.), *Harrison's Principles of Internal Medicine* (12th ed.). New York: McGraw-Hill, 1991.
17. Guyton, A.C. *Textbook of Medical Physiology* (8th ed.). Philadelphia: W.B. Saunders, 1991.
18. Hostetter, M.K. Handicaps to host defense: Effects of hyperglycemia on C3 and *Candida albicans*. *Diabetes* 39:271, 1990.
19. Jetten, A.M., Yankaskas, J.R., Stutts, M.J., et al. Persistence of abnormal chloride conductance regulation in transformed cystic fibrosis epithelia. *Science* 244:1472, 1989.
20. Karam, J.H. Diabetes mellitus and hypoglycemia. In Tierney, L.M. Jr., McPhee, S.J., and Papadakis, M.A. (eds.), *Current Medical Diagnosis and Treatment* (33rd ed.). Norwalk, Conn.: Appleton & Lange, 1994.
21. Kostraba, J.N., et al. Early exposure to cow's milk and solid foods in infancy, genetic-predisposition and risk of IDDM. *Diabetes* 42:288–295, 1993.
22. Kozak, G.P., and Krall, L.P. Disorders of the skin. In Marble, A., et al. (eds.), *Joslin's Diabetes Mellitus* (12th ed.). Philadelphia: Lea & Febiger, 1985.
23. Kumar, V., Cotran, R.S., and Robbins, S.L. *Basic Pathology* Philadelphia: W.B. Saunders, 1992.

24. Leslie, R.D., and Elliot, R.B. Early environmental events as a cause of IDDM: Evidence and implications. *Diabetes* 43:843–850, 1994.

25. Levitan, I.B. The basic defect in cystic fibrosis. *Science* 244:1423, 1989.

26. Martin, B.C., et al. Role of glucose and insulin resistance in the development of type 2 diabetes mellitus: Results of a 25 year follow-up study. *Lancet* 340:925–929, 1992.

27. May, M., and Mahlmeister, L. *Maternal and Neonatal Nursing: Family Centered Care* (3rd ed.). Philadelphia: J.B. Lippincott, 1994.

28. Mayer, R.J. Pancreatic cancers. In Wilson, J.D., et al. (eds.), *Harrison's Principles of Internal Medicine* (12th ed.). New York: McGraw-Hill, 1991.

29. National Diabetes Control and Complications Trial Research Group. The effect of intensive treatment of diabetes on the development and progression of long-term complications in insulin-dependent diabetes mellitus. *N. Engl. J. Med.* 329:977–986, 1993.

30. Olefski, J.M. Diabetes mellitus. In Wyngaarden, J., and Smith, L.H. (eds.), *Cecil's Textbook of Medicine* (18th ed.). Philadelphia: W.B. Saunders, 1988.

31. Pagana, K.D., and Pagana, T.J. *Diagnostic Testing and Nursing Implications*. St. Louis: Mosby, 1992.

32. Robinson, A., and Linden, M. *Clinical Genetics Handbook*. Boston: Blackwell, 1993.

33. Rubin, E., and Farber, J.L. *Pathology* (2nd ed.). Philadelphia: J.B. Lippincott, 1994.

34. Santiago, J.V. Lessons from the Diabetes Control and Complications Trial. *Diabetes* 42:1549–1554, 1993.

35. Sauer, G.C. *Manual of Skin Diseases* (6th ed.). Philadelphia: J.B. Lippincott, 1991.

36. Seino, S., Seino, M., and Bell, G.I. Human insulin-receptor gene. *Diabetes* 39:243, 1990.

37. Service, F.J. Hypoglycemic disorders. In Wyngaarden, J., and Smith, L.H. (eds.), *Cecil's Textbook of Medicine* (18th ed.). Philadelphia: W.B. Saunders, 1988.

38. Smith, R.J. Approach to the patient with hypoglycemia. In Kelley, WN. *Textbook of Internal Medicine* (2nd ed.). Philadelphia: J.B. Lippincott, 1992.

39. Tajima, N., Matsushima, M., and LaPorte, R.E. Population studies. In Lesslie, R.D.G. (ed.), *Causes of Diabetes*. New York: Wiley, 1993.

40. Taylor, S.I., Accili, D., and Imai, Y. Insulin resistance or insulin deficiency: Which is the primary cause of NIDDM? *Diabetes* 43:735–740, 1994.

41. Unger, R.H., and Foster, D.W. Diabetes mellitus. In Wilson, J.D., and Foster, D.W. (eds.), *Williams' Textbook of Endocrinology* (8th ed.). Philadelphia: W.B. Saunders, 1992.

42. Virtanen, S.M., et al. Early introduction of dairy products associated with increased risk of IDDM in Finnish children. *Diabetes* 42:1786–1790, 1993.

▼ *Unit Bibliography*

Anmuth, C.J., et al. Chronic syndrome of inappropriate secretion of antidiuretic hormone in a periatric patient after traumatic brain injury. *Arch. Phys. Med. Rehabil.* 74:1219–1221, 1993.

Bardin, C.W. *Current Therapy in Endocrinology and Metabolism* (5th ed.). St. Louis: Mosby, 1994.

Becker, K.L. *Principles and Practice of Endocrinology and Metabolism.* Philadelphia: J.B. Lippincott, 1991.

Braverman, L.E., and Utiger, R.D. *The Thyroid: A Fundamental and Clinical Text* (6th ed.). Philadelphia: J.B. Lippincott, 1991.

Brownlee, M. Glycation and diabetic complications. *Diabetes* 43:836–841, 1994.

Chambers, J.K. Metabolic bone disorders: Imbalances of calcium and phosphorus. *Nurs. Clin. North Am.* 22:861, 1987.

Chernow, B., Wiley, S., and Zaloga, G. Critical care endocrinology. In Shoemaker, W., et al. (eds.), *Textbook of Critical Care* (2nd ed.). Philadelphia: W.B. Saunders, 1989.

Chipps, E. Transsphenoidal surgery for pituitary tumors. *Crit Care Nurs* 12:30–39, 1992.

Cotran, R.S., Kumar, V., and Robbins, S.L. *Robbins' Pathologic Basis of Disease* (5th ed.). Philadelphia: W.B. Saunders, 1994.

Dubrey, S.W., et al. Risk factors for cardiovascular disease in IDDM: A study of identical twins. *Diabetes* 43:831–834, 1994.

Epstein, C.D. Fluid volume deficit for the adrenal crisis patient. *Dimens. Crit. Care Nur.* 10:210–217, 1991.

Featherston, W.E., and Ram, C.V.S. Secondary causes of hypertension: Health and cost benefits of making these diagnoses. *Consultant* 27:109, 1987.

Feek, C., and Edwards, C. *Endocrine and Metabolic Disease.* New York: Springer-Verlag, 1988.

Few, B.J. Corticosteroids and respiratory distress syndrome. *Matern. Child Nurs. J.* 13:17, 1988.

Findling, J.W., and Mazzaferri, E.L. Cushing syndrome: An etiologic workup. *Hosp. Pract.* 27:107–118, 1992.

Fitzgerald, P.A. *Handbook of Clinical Endocrinology* (2nd ed.). Norwalk, Conn.: Appleton & Lange, 1992.

Frank, R.N. The aldose reductase controversy. *Diabetes* 43:169–172, 1994.

Greenspan, F.S. *Basic and Clinical Endocrinology* (3rd ed.). Norwalk, Conn: Appleton & Lange, 1994.

Gusek, A. Ten commonly asked questions about diabetes. *Am. J. Nurs.* 94:19–20, 1994.

Goodman, H.M. *Basic Medical Endocrinology* (2nd ed.). New York: Raven, 1994.

Guyton, A.C. *Textbook of Medical Physiology* (8th ed.). Philadelphia: W.B. Saunders, 1990.

Hadley, Mac E. *Endocrinology* (3rd ed.). Englewood Cliffs, N.Y.: Prentice-Hall, 1992.

Harper, J. Use of steroids in cerebral edema: Therapeutic implications. *Heart Lung* 17:70, 1988.

Haupt, H.A. Anabolic steroids and growth hormone. *Am. J. Sports Med.* 21:468–474, 1993.

Hoekelman, R.A. Juvenile diabetes: Prevention, control, and cure. *Pediatr Ann* 23:278–280, 1994.

Holmes, E.W. Endocrinology, metabolism, and genetics. In Kelley, W.N. (ed.), *Textbook of Internal Medicine* (2nd ed.). Philadelphia: J.B. Lippincott, 1992.

Hung, W. *Clinical Pediatric Endocrinology.* St. Louis: Mosby-Year Book, 1992.

Isley, W.I. Serum sodium concentration abnormalities. *Crit. Care Nurs. Q.* 13:23–33, 1990.

Jeffcoat, W. *Lecture Notes in Endocrinology.* Boston: Blackwell, 1993.

Johnstone, M.T., and Creager, M.A. Impaired endothelium-dependent vasodilation in patients with insulin-dependent diabetes mellitus. *Circulation* 88:2510–2516, 1992.

Kaplan, S.A. *Clinical Pediatric Endocrinology* (2nd ed.). Philadelphia: W.B. Saunders, 1994.

Karry, M.S., Blozzard, P.M., and Migeon, C.I. *Wilkins The Diagnosis and Treatment of Endocrine Disorders in Childhood and Adolescence* (4th ed.). Springfield: Charles C. Thomas, 1994.

Kern, W., et al. Evidence for effects of insulin on sensory processing in humans. *Diabetes* 43:351–354, 1994.

Kovaks, L., and Robertson, G.L. Syndrome of inappropriate antidiuresis. *Endocrinol. Metab. Clin. North Am.* 21:859–875, 1992.

Leslie, R.D., and Elliot, R.B. Early environmental events as a cause of IDDM: Evidence and implications. *Diabetes* 48:843–850, 1994.

Newgard, C.B. Cellular engineering and gene therapy srategies for insulin replacement in diabetes. *Diabetes* 43:341–350, 1994.

Rhodes, C.J., and Alarcon, C.A. What B cell defect could lead to hyperproinsulinemia in NIDDM? *Diabetes* 43:511–517, 1994.

Rosenbloom, A.L., and Scatz, D.A. Diabetic ketoacidosis in childhood. *Pediatr. Ann.* 23:284–288, 1994.

Rubin, E., and Farber, J.L. *Pathology* (2nd ed.). Philadlephia: J.B. Lippincott, 1994.

Sarsany, S.L. Thyroid storm. *RN* 51:46, 1988.

Schatz, D.A. Hypoglycemia in childhood diabetes. *Pediatr. Ann.* 23:289–291, 1994.

Service, F.J. Hypoglycemic disorders. In Wyngaarden, J., and Smith, L.H. (eds.), *Cecil's Textbook of Medicine* (18th ed.). Philadelphia: W.B. Saunders, 1988.

Sizonenko, R.C. *Pediatric Endocrinology* (2nd ed.). Baltimore: Williams & Wilkins, 1993.

Thorens, B., and Waeber, G. Glucagon-like peptide-1 and the control of insulin secretion in the normal state and in NIDDM. *Diabetes* 42:1219–1224, 1993.

Tucker, S.M., Canobbio, M.M., Paquette, E.V., and Wells, M.F. Hyperthyroidism: Thyroid crisis. *J. Emerg. Nurs.* 15:352, 1989.

Waskin, J., et al. Risk factors for hypoglycemia associated with pentamidine therapy for pneumocystis pneumonia. *JAMA* 260:345–347, 1988.

Wilson, J.D., et al. (eds.). *Harrison's Textbook of Internal Medicine* (12th ed.). New York: McGraw-Hill, 1991.

Wilson, J.D., and Foster, D.W. (eds.). *Williams' Textbook of Endocrinology* (8th ed.). Philadelphia: W.B. Saunders, 1992.

Wyngaarden, J.B., and Smith, L.H. (eds.). *Cecil's Textbook of Medicine* (19th ed.). Philadelphia: W.B. Saunders, 1992.

Chapter 40

Normal Function of the Gastrointestinal System

Barbara L. Bullock

▼ CHAPTER OUTLINE

Appetite, Hunger, and Satiety
Anatomy of the Gastrointestinal Tract
Oral or Buccal Cavity
Pharynx
Esophagus
Stomach

Small Intestine
Large Intestine
Physiology of the Digestive System
Oral Secretions and Movement of Food to the
   Stomach
Gastric Motility and Secretion

Emesis
Secretion and Absorption in the Small Intestine
Secretion, Absorption, and Excretion in the Large
   Intestine
Chapter Summary

▼ LEARNING OBJECTIVES

1 *Differentiate appetite, hunger, and satiety.*
2 *Describe the function of salivary ptyalin.*
3 *Briefly define* **functional syncytium** *as applied to the gastrointestinal system.*
4 *Locate and describe the functional significance of the sphincters in the gastrointestinal tract.*
5 *Locate and clearly describe the function of the gastric glands.*
6 *Explain the important characteristics of chyme as it moves into the small intestine.*
7 *Describe the appearance and function of the intestinal microvilli.*
8 *Locate the blood supply, nerve supply, and lymphatic drainage of the gastrointestinal system.*
9 *Relate the importance of oral secretions to digestion.*
10 *Describe the process of swallowing.*
11 *Clearly delineate the purposes of all of the gastric secretions in digestion.*
12 *Describe the relation of nervous and hormonal mechanisms in digestion.*
13 *Briefly outline the cephalic, gastric, and intestinal phases of gastric secretions.*
14 *Define and list examples of* **secretagogues**.
15 *Explain the mechanisms that cause emesis.*
16 *Describe how the intestines inhibit gastric secretions.*
17 *Describe specifically where nutrients are absorbed in the small intestine.*
18 *Relate the mechanisms necessary for the absorption of carbohydrates, proteins, and fats.*
19 *Briefly list the form and mechanism for the absorption of nutrients, vitamins, and minerals.*
20 *Briefly explain the role of the large intestine in regulating water balance.*

Barbara L. Bullock: PATHOPHYSIOLOGY: ADAPTATIONS AND ALTERATIONS IN FUNCTION, 4th ed.
© 1996 Lippincott-Raven Publishers

Normal functioning of the human body depends on an intact digestive system. In the broadest sense, the gastrointestinal tract is a tubular structure called the *alimentary canal*, which extends from the pharynx to the anus. Throughout this tubular structure, ingested food is processed, digested, and absorbed. The nutrients absorbed may be further processed by accessory organs, used for energy, or stored to be used later for energy. For digestion to occur, the vital functions of motility, secretion, and absorption must proceed in a regulated manner. Finally, by participating in the excretion of waste products, the gastrointestinal system helps to rid the body of unusable and, in some cases, toxic materials.

▼ Appetite, Hunger, and Satiety

Appetite refers to a desire for specific types of food. Learned patterns of behavior alter the appetite, creating a desire for food beyond the needs of the body. Hunger refers to the desire for food that results from the manifest need for energy. Satisfaction of hunger is called satiety.

The hunger center is in the *hypothalamus*, as is the *satiety center*, but the two are in separate locations.[7] The feeling of hunger frequently is generated by rhythmic contractions of the stomach, which may cause a painful sensation called hunger pangs. Stimulation from the hunger center is related to the nutritional status of the body. Especially important in this process is the concentration of glucose in the blood. A decreased concentration of blood glucose intensifies the hunger response. Serum fat levels and amino acids tend to promote satiety. Distention of the gastrointestinal tract suppresses the hunger center through inhibitory signals, probably from sensory signals by the vagal nerves.

The appetite center is more subtly controlled by the cortical areas and is stimulated by sight, touch, and smell. Even thoughts of food can stimulate the appetite center. Alterations of appetite for specific foods are conditioned by culture, environment, and socioeconomic circumstances.

▼ Anatomy of the Gastrointestinal Tract

The activities of the gastrointestinal tract are accomplished through a continuous structure that begins with the oral cavity and terminates with the anal sphincter (Fig. 40-1). The activities are carried out through the processes of ingestion, movement or passage of food, digestion, absorption, and removal or defecation.[15]

ORAL OR BUCCAL CAVITY

The lips, tongue, cheeks, teeth, taste buds, and salivary glands are associated with the oral cavity and contribute to the preparation of food for eventual absorption. This preparation includes reducing food particles to manageable size, stimulating salivary glands to increase saliva secretion, and moving food to the appropriate position for swallowing. Table 40-1 summarizes the oral structures and their participation in preparing food for digestion.

The submandibular, parotid, and sublingual salivary glands lie outside the oral cavity and pour their secretions into the mouth through ducts (Fig. 40-2). The glands continuously secrete *saliva*, which contains large amounts of water and small amounts of sodium, potassium, chloride, bicarbonate, phosphates, urea, and a few other solutes. Saliva also contains *ptyalin* (salivary amylase), an enzyme that digests starches, and *lysozyme*, a bacteriolytic enzyme that helps to protect the teeth from decay and to decrease the number of bacteria in the mouth. The average amounts of salivary secretion range from 1,000 to 1,500 mL/day. Stimulation for this secretion is relayed to the medulla by the parasympathetic fibers of the facial, trigeminal, glossopharyngeal, and vagus nerves. Efferent parasympathetic stimulation leads to increased secretion of saliva. Stimulation of the sympathetic system causes localized vasoconstriction and a decrease in salivary secretion.

PHARYNX

The pharynx actively moves food into the esophagus, while closing and sealing off the nasopharynx, during the process of swallowing. As the bolus of food moves toward the esophagus, respiration is inhibited and the *epiglottis* moves downward to protect the trachea (see later section). After the swallowing reflex is initiated by voluntary movement of food to the back of the mouth, swallowing continues as a reflex activity (see pp. 770–771).

ESOPHAGUS

The esophagus provides a passageway for food from the pharynx to the stomach. An *upper esophageal sphincter* prevents food or fluid movement into the posterior pharynx and trachea. It is a muscular, pliable tube that is easily affected by intrathoracic or intraabdominal pressures or volumes. The esophagus is lined with a mucosal layer composed of squamous epithelium.[4] Glands along its length secrete mucus to lubricate the bolus of food passing through.

The construction of the smooth muscle of the esophagus and other structures in the alimentary canal has been described as a *functional syncytium* because the smooth muscle fibers lie close to one another. This con-

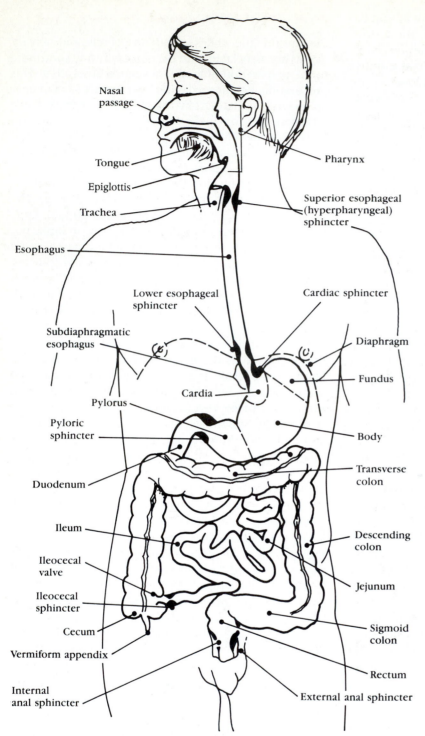

Nasal passage

Tongue

Epiglottis

Trachea

Esophagus

Lower esophageal sphincter

Subdiaphragmatic esophagus

Pylorus

Pyloric sphincter

Duodenum

Ileum

Ileocecal valve

Ileocecal sphincter

Cecum

Vermiform appendix

Internal anal sphincter

Pharynx

Superior esophageal (hyperpharyngeal) sphincter

Cardiac sphincter

Diaphragm

Fundus

Cardia

Body

Transverse colon

Descending colon

Jejunum

Sigmoid colon

Rectum

External anal sphincter

FIGURE 40-1 *The digestive system.*

struction allows for waves of muscular contraction called *peristalsis*.[7]

About 5 cm above the esophageal entry to the stomach is a narrowed area called the *gastroesophageal, cardiac,* or *lower esophageal sphincter* (see Figure 40-1). A sphincter is an opening that has an extra amount of muscle surrounding it. The gastroesophageal sphincter cannot be identified on anatomic dissection, but it acts as a sphincter. It normally remains constricted but relaxes when a peristaltic wave is conducted through it, allow-

ing food to pass to the stomach. The gastroesophageal sphincter seems to prevent acid reflux into the esophagus. Table 40-2 defines the functions of the various sphincters along the passageway.

STOMACH

The stomach is a pear-shaped, hollow, distensible organ whose parts consist of the cardia, fundus, body, antrum, and pylorus. Figure 40-3 shows the positions of the

TABLE 40-1 Participation of the Oral Structures in Digestion

Structure	Process
Teeth	Reduce food to sizes appropriate for swallowing; break down dense particles
Tongue	Places food in proper position for swallowing; mixes secretions to moisten food
Salivary glands	Moisten and lubricate foods in the mouth; add ptyalin enzyme for digestion of starches
Muscles of mastication, or chewing	Provide movement for the grinding of food to smaller particles; provide more surface area for the digestive enzymes to act

TABLE 40-2 Sphincter Function

Sphincter	Function
Upper esophageal	Prevents expulsion of food into posterior pharynx
Lower esophageal	Transports food bolus from esophagus to stomach and prevents gastric reflux into upper esophagus
Pyloric	Coordinates organized emptying of stomach and prevents reflux of duodenal contents
Ileocecal	Prevents retrograde expulsion of intestinal contents
Anal	Inhibits expulsion of colonic contents unless voluntary relaxation is established

greater and lesser curvatures of the stomach. The upper portion of the stomach is continuous with the esophagus and lies close to the diaphragm; the lower portion is continuous with the duodenum through the lower pyloric sphincter.

The interior lining of the stomach lies in mucosal folds called *rugae*. Within the mucosal folds are glands that secrete gastric juices (Fig. 40-4). Gastric juice is composed of secretions from four major cell types: *chief cells, parietal cells, mucus-producing cells,* and *gastrin-producing cells (G cells).* The chief cells secrete the pro-enzyme *pepsinogen,* which, when activated, digests proteins. The parietal cells secrete *hydrochloric acid,* which has a pH of about 0.8. It is thought that these cells also secrete the intrinsic factor, a glycoprotein that binds with vitamin B_{12} and makes it available for absorption in the small intestine.[7] Mucous cells located in the gastric surface epithelium constantly secrete a thin mucus film. Mucous neck cells, located in the middle and upper portions of gastric glands, have as their major function

regeneration of mucus-secreting cells. When stimulated, gastrin-producing or G cells release gastrin into the bloodstream.[4]

About 1,500 to 3,000 mL of gastric juice is secreted daily and mixes with the food entering the stomach. The combination of food and gastric juice makes a semiliquid mass called *chyme,* which is propelled into the small intestine through the pyloric sphincter (Fig. 40-5).

The nervous supply to the stomach is through the intrinsic and the autonomic nervous systems. The intrinsic system begins in the esophagus and continues all the way to the anus. The layers involved in this system include the *myenteric* and the *submucosal plexuses.* These control the tone of the bowel, rhythmic contractions, and the velocity of excitation of the gut. The autonomic nervous system increases excitation through the parasympathetic branches, especially in the esophagus, stomach, large intestine, and anal region. The main function of the sympathetic portion of the autonomic nervous system is to inhibit activity of the gastrointestinal system.

The arterial blood supply to the stomach comes mainly from the celiac artery. Venous blood is drained through the gastric veins, which connect to and terminate

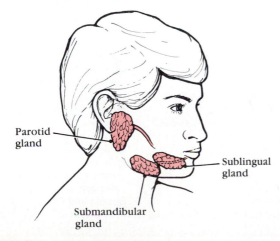

FIGURE 40-2 Salivary glands.

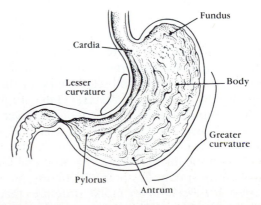

FIGURE 40-3 Segments of the stomach. Notice the greater and lesser curvatures.

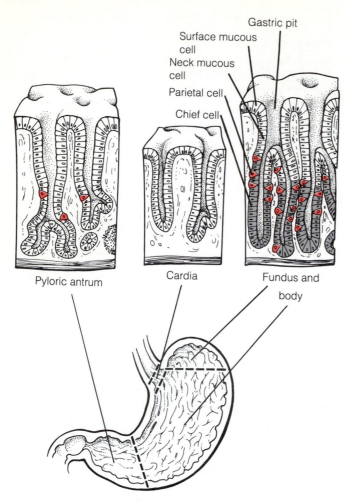

FIGURE 40-4 *Four anatomic and three histologic regions of the stomach. The depths of the gastric pits and the glandular composition are different in the various areas of the stomach. (Adapted from Fenoglio-Preiser, C.M. et al. Gastrointestinal Pathology: An Atlas and Text. New York: Raven, 1989.)*

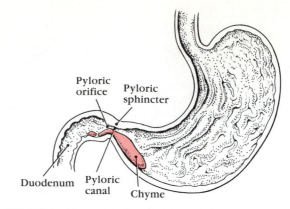

FIGURE 40-5 *Movement of chyme through the pyloric sphincter.*

tive cells and mucus-producing goblet cells. The absorptive cells are columnar and have a brush border on the luminal side. These cells have a marked power for regeneration; they differentiate from intestinal epithelial cells into absorptive cells. An intestinal epithelial cell lives about 5 days, after which it is shed into the intestinal secretions.[16]

Blood circulation to the small intestine occurs through the gastroduodenal, superior pancreaticoduodenal, and celiac arteries. Venous drainage is through the superior mesenteric vein, which empties into the portal vein and travels to the liver. The entire small intestine is richly supplied with lymphatic vessels. The intestinal cells form large quantities of secretions that have a neutral pH. These secretions contain enzymes and hormones that function to break down nutrients.

The liver, gallbladder, and pancreas, which are considered in greater detail in Chapter 42, are essential

in the portal vein. The stomach has profuse lymphatic drainage through lymphatic vessels and nodes.

SMALL INTESTINE

The small intestine extends from the pylorus to the ileocecal valve. It is about 12 feet (3.6 m) long in the living human. In the cadaver, it is longer because the muscles of the intestinal wall are relaxed.[4] The small intestine is divided into sections: *duodenum, jejunum,* and *ileum* (see Figure 40-1). Absorption and secretion occur throughout the length of the small intestine (Table 40-3).

The intestinal wall is composed of four layers: mucosa, submucosa, muscularis, and serosa (Fig. 40-6). Fingerlike folds of the mucosa, called *villi,* project into the lumen of the interior of the intestines and increase the absorptive surface by about 600 times (Fig. 40-7). The *crypts of Lieberkuhn* are pitlike structures that lie in grooves between the villi and are composed of absorp-

TABLE 40-3 *Principal Sites of Absorption*

Nutrient	Absorptive Site
Carbohydrates	Jejunum
Protein	Jejunum
Fat	Jejunum
Water	Jejunum; also duodenum, ileum, and colon
Fat-soluble vitamins—A, D, E, K	Duodenum
Vitamin B_{12}	Terminal ileum
Other water-soluble vitamins	Duodenum
Iron	Duodenum
Calcium	Duodenum
Sodium	Jejunum by passive diffusion; ileum and colon by active transport
Potassium	Jejunum and ileum
Magnesium	Distal ileum

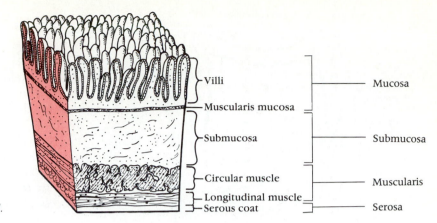

Villi

Muscularis mucosa — Mucosa

Submucosa — Submucosa

Circular muscle — Muscularis

Longitudinal muscle
Serous coat — Serosa

FIGURE 40-6 *Layers of the intestinal wall.*

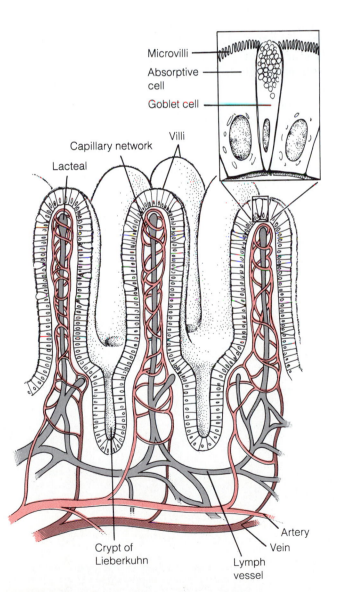

Microvilli

Absorptive cell

Goblet cell

Villi

Capillary network

Lacteal

Crypt of Lieberkuhn

Lymph vessel

Artery

Vein

FIGURE 40-7 *Structure of the intestinal villi.*

organs in the promotion of digestion. Chyme entering the small intestine stimulates a hormone, called cholecystokinin, by distending the small intestine. This hormone, in turn, stimulates the pancreas to release its enzymatic secretions into the duodenum. The stimulation from cholecystokinin causes the gallbladder to contract and push bile into the small intestine.

LARGE INTESTINE

The large intestine begins with the end of the ileum at the ileocecal valve (Fig. 40-8). The area of meeting is called the cecum. A small structure, called the *vermiform appendix*, extends from the cecum; it is a relatively nonfunctional pouch. The colon portion of the large intestine is subdivided into the ascending, transverse, descending, and sigmoid areas. The large intestine itself begins with the cecum, contains the colon, and terminates in the rectum and anal canal.

The number of mucus-secreting goblet cells is increased in the large intestine. The mucous material secreted helps prevent trauma to the bowel, provides material that causes feces to form a mass, and protects the bowel against resident bacteria. Most of the liquid and electrolytes from the semiliquid material of the small intestine are absorbed in the large intestine, especially in the ascending and transverse colon. Feces usually consist of about three-fourths water and one-fourth solid matter, of which about 30% is dead bacteria. The brown color of fecal material is produced by breakdown products of bilirubin.

The rectum is about 20 cm of the final descending portion of the large intestine and terminates in the anal canal. There is an internal anal sphincter 2 to 3 cm from the termination of the rectum and an external sphincter, the *sphincter ani*, which opens to the outside of the body.

The blood supply to the large intestine is profuse and arises from branches of the superior and inferior mesenteric arteries. Venous drainage is mainly through the mesenteric veins, terminating in the portal veins. This

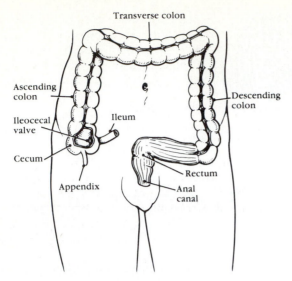

FIGURE 40-8   *Segments of the large intestine.*

system is important in the pathology of portal hypertension because increased portal pressure is reflected in the veins surrounding the esophagus and anal canal. The entire large intestine is supplied with an extensive lymphatic drainage system of vessels and nodes (see Figure 40-9).

▼ *Physiology of the Digestive System*

Digestion takes substances in one form and breaks them down into molecules that are small enough to pass through the intestinal wall to the blood and lymphatic systems. This activity requires chemical secretions and mechanical movements, all working together in a coordinated manner. The molecules may be moved by simple diffusion, active transport, or facilitated diffusion. *Motility, secretion,* and *absorption* work together to make the process of digestion work.

ORAL SECRETIONS AND MOVEMENT OF FOOD TO THE STOMACH

The major digestive secretion of the salivary glands is the enzyme *ptyalin,* which breaks down starches. Not only is this amylase, or carbohydrate digester, active in the mouth, but it continues its function in the stomach. The action continues until the digestive secretions of the stomach begin to alter the chyme. It is estimated that 30% to 40% of starches are broken down by ptyalin.

The liquid saliva contains water and mucus needed to liquefy and lubricate ingested food. The amount of

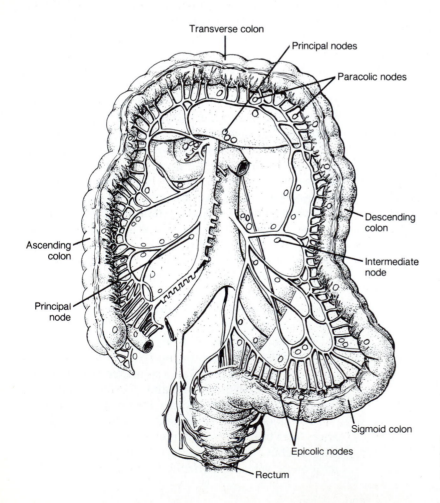

FIGURE 40-9 *Diagram of the blood supply and lymphatic drainage of the large intestine. (Fenoglio-Preiser, C.M., et al. Gastrointestinal Pathology: An Atlas and Text. New York: Raven, 1989.)*

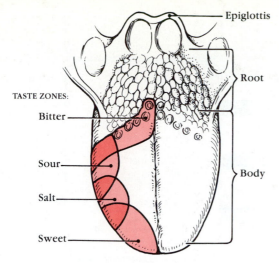

FIGURE 40-10   *The tongue and areas of taste.*

saliva secreted is regulated by the parasympathetic nervous pathways. Irritation of stomach mucosa initiates a reflex increase in salivation.

The movements of the tongue are important to position the *bolus* of ingested food, which has been reduced to smaller sizes by the teeth, into proper alignment for swallowing. The taste buds, scattered over the mucous membrane of the tongue surface, carry sensory input through the seventh and ninth cranial nerves to the brain, where taste is interpreted. Perception of taste is a complex process, with various areas of the tongue being sensitive to different tastes. Figure 40-10 shows the areas of the tongue that respond to sweet, sour, salty, and bitter tastes. The major motor nerve of the tongue is the hypoglossal, which is closely aligned with the vagus nerve. It innervates the extrinsic and intrinsic muscles that move the tongue into various positions.

Swallowing is the key event in the initiation of digestion because it increases esophageal peristaltic motion, decreases pressure in the lower esophagus, and initiates the gastroenteric reflex. This reflex increases small-bowel motility and assists in moving nutrients along the alimentary canal. Swallowing, or deglutition, is initiated

when the tongue moves a bolus of food to the pharynx. The cricopharyngeal sphincter relaxes for 1 second or less, and the *primary peristaltic wave* is initiated. This wave begins in the pharynx and spreads to the esophagus.[7] The respiratory passages are protected by the epiglottis to prevent food from moving into them. The bolus of food then passes through the pharynx to the esophagus in about 1 second (Fig. 40-11). The respiratory passages reopen and breathing resumes.

As food passes into the esophagus, peristalsis and pressure changes move it toward the stomach. Peristalsis, which occurs throughout the gastrointestinal tract, is a series of sequential muscular movements. The primary wave moves down the esophagus, and *secondary peristalsis* continues until all of the food is in the stomach.[7] The coordination (functional syncytium) of the entire system allows for wavelike movements of the smooth muscle. As the food moves toward the lower esophageal or gastroesophageal sphincter, the wave of peristalsis causes the normally constricted area to relax, and the food moves into the stomach. The peristaltic waves are initiated by vagal reflexes from the esophagus to the medulla oblongata and back to the esophagus.[7]

GASTRIC MOTILITY AND SECRETION

The fundus of the stomach increases its volume as it fills with food. This distensibility allows the stomach to maintain a low intragastric pressure. The antrum is responsible for mixing food through contraction waves that push the food (now chyme) toward the pylorus.

GASTRIC MOTILITY AND EMPTYING.   Solids must be broken down to less than a millimeter in size before they can pass through the pyloric sphincter. Gastric motility patterns occur in phases: phase I occurs 1.5 to 2 hours after meals, when gastric contractions decrease to one every 4 to 5 minutes; phase II is a 30-minute span of irregular contractions; this is followed by phase III, which is 5 to 15 minutes of sweeping contractions.[11] Hunger pangs may be experienced during phases II or III. Contractile movements in the full stomach are of

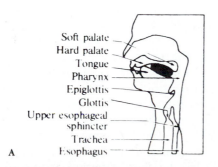
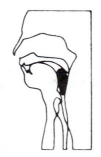
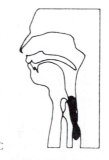
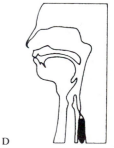

FIGURE 40-11   *Illustration of the structures involved in moving a bolus of food through the pharynx and upper esophagus during swallowing and the initiated peristaltic movements that help to move the bolus down the esophagus.*

three types: peristaltic waves, contractions of the antrum, and contractions of the fundus and body.

Peristaltic activity in the stomach arises from a pacemaker located high on the greater curvature of the stomach. Electrical slow waves are propagated through the longitudinal muscle layer to the pylorus. This cyclical wave of partial depolarization and repolarization, also called the *basic electrical rhythm*, occurs in humans about three times per minute.[5, 11]

GASTRIC SECRETION. The glands of the stomach secrete 1,500 to 3,000 mL of gastric juice per day. Secretory activity follows a regular daily pattern, with the least secretion occurring in the early morning. The amount of gastric secretion also varies with individual dietary habits, other stimuli that provoke secretions, and the strength of the inhibitory mechanisms.

Gastric juice contains mucus, intrinsic factor, hydrochloric acid, pepsinogen, and the electrolytes sodium, potassium, magnesium, chloride, and bicarbonate. Certain other enzymes, such as gastric lipase, urease, lysozyme, and carbonic anhydrase, also are present in the secretions. The cells that make up the gastric glands secrete mucus, pepsinogen, and hydrochloric acid (see Figure 40-4).

The parietal cells in the fundus and body of the stomach secrete *hydrochloric acid* as a highly concentrated liquid with a pH of about 0.8. A suggested mechanism for the formation of hydrochloric acid is shown in Figure 40-12. The theory relating hydrochloric acid secretion to bicarbonate replenishment in the blood is supported by the observation that each hydrogen ion secreted is matched by a bicarbonate ion that is returned to the blood. This means that the amount of bicarbonate entering the blood during the gastric secretory phase is directly proportional to the amount of acid secreted. Carbon dioxide enters the cell or is formed in the cell during metabolism, reacts with water catalyst by using carbonic anhydrase, and forms carbonic acid. This carbonic acid then dissociates to bicarbonate and hydrogen. The hydrogen ion enters the parietal cell canaliculi by active transport, whereas bicarbonate is diffused back into the blood. The chloride ion also is actively transported from blood to the canaliculi.[3, 14] Only during periods of relative gastric inactivity is adequate carbon dioxide produced to make a small amount of hydrochloric acid. During digestion, the parietal cell takes its needed carbon dioxide from the circulating blood. This elevates the venous pH after eating, which has been called the *postprandial alkaline tide*. The urine also becomes more alkaline.[5, 11]

Pepsin is the main proteolytic enzyme of gastric juice. It is secreted by the chief cells of the gastric glands in the form of pepsinogen. It has no digestive activity until it is activated into pepsin, which occurs in the presence of hydrochloric acid and previously activated pepsin. Pep-

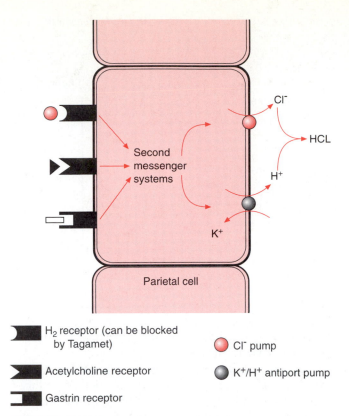

FIGURE 40-12 *Numerous stimuli can initiate the secretion of hydrochloric acid into the lumen of the stomach. These require H_2 receptors, gastrin receptors, and acetylcholine receptors. These receptors can be blocked by pharmacologic agents which results in a decrease of the production of hydrochloric acid.*

sin is most active in a highly acid medium. It functions optimally in a pH of 2.0 and is almost inactive in secretions with a pH greater than 5.0.

Mucus is produced by the columnar cells of the surface epithelium. The surface of the stomach mucosa has a continuous layer of columnar epithelial cells that secrete large amounts of viscous and alkaline mucus to coat the mucosa and create a protective sheet. The epithelial lining of the stomach has remarkable properties of repair and can reproduce itself in 36 to 48 hours. The mucous cells secrete a thin mucus, and the amount of this secretion varies with vagal stimulation and irritation. This additional line of defense lubricates the passage of food, absorbs pepsin, and washes away noxious substances. Failure to secrete mucus in adequate quantities to protect the underlying mucosa increases the susceptibility of the mucosa to the actions of hydrochloric acid and pepsin.[7]

Gastric juices contain small quantities of the enzymes gastric lipase, gastric amylase, gastric urease, gelatinase, carbonic anhydrase, and lysozyme. Gastric lipase acts primarily on butterfat and has little effect on other fats, which require bile for their digestion. Gastric amylase has a minor role in digestion of starch. Gastric urease, formed by the bacteria that contaminate the gastric mucosa, splits urea to produce ammonia. Gelatinase helps to liquefy some of the proteoglycans in meats.[7] Carbonic anhydrase, present in the epithelial cells and in high concentrations in parietal cells, is thought to be produced by the disintegration of desquamated epithelial cells and is essential in the formation of hydrochloric acid. Lysozyme is a carbohydrate-splitting enzyme present in small amounts in the gastric juice. Its cellular origin is not known.

FORMATION OF CHYME. Gastric motility is governed by the peristaltic waves that occur every 15 to 25 seconds and mix ingested food with gastric secretions. The result of this movement and mixing is the thin, highly acidic liquid chyme. Chyme is moved into the small intestine mostly because of the higher pressure gradients in the stomach that exceed the duodenal pressure. The acidity and amount of chyme entering the duodenum help to regulate the duodenal and pancreatic secretions.

NERVOUS AND HORMONAL INFLUENCES. Digestion also is regulated by nervous and hormonal mechanisms. Innervation through the vagus nerve excites stomach excretion directly by stimulating the gastric glands. Distention of the stomach wall activates local reflexes to stimulate gastric secretion. The local reflexes elicit autonomic nervous system activity and cause the release of the hormone gastrin. This hormone is absorbed into the bloodstream and stimulates the gastric secretory glands to cause a marked increase in gastric acid secretion. Gastric secretion is thought to occur in three phases: cephalic, gastric, and intestinal (Fig. 40-13).

The cephalic phase prepares the stomach for food and digestion. It is under nervous control and is initiated by stimuli such as the sight, smell, or thought of food. Impulses from receptors such as the retinae, taste buds,

and olfactory glands travel to the cerebral cortex, and the motor fibers of the vagal nerves of the stomach stimulate the glands of the stomach to secrete juice rich in hydrochloric acid and gastrin.[11]

The *gastric phase* is initiated when food enters the stomach. Gastrin is released by acetylcholine stimulation of the gastrin-producing cells. The process is triggered by distention of the stomach caused by food and by exposure of the mucosa to substances called *secretagogues*. Examples of secretagogues are caffeine and alcohol. Gastrin is absorbed in the blood and stimulates acid and pepsin secretion from parietal and chief cells, which produce about two-thirds of the total gastric secretions.[7,11] Food in the stomach initiates local reflexes in the intramural plexus of the stomach, and vasovagal reflexes induce parasympathetic stimulation to increase the secretion. The rate of secretion in response to gastrin continues for several hours while food remains in the stomach. Both the gastrin and vagal mechanisms are important in gastric secretion. Gastrin also has extragastric action, including the stimulation of insulin and release of calcitonin. It causes muscle contraction of the lower esophageal sphincter, small intestine, colon, and gallbladder. It inhibits smooth muscle contraction of the pyloric, ileocecal, and Oddi sphincters.

The *intestinal phase* of gastric secretion is less active than the cephalic or gastric phases, but once it is initiated, it may last for 8 to 10 hours while food remains in the duodenum. This phase begins with the entrance of acidic chyme into the small intestine, which leads to an increase in gastrin secretion.

The intestines also inhibit gastric secretion when there are partially digested proteins, acid, fat, or hypertonic solutions in the duodenum. Distention, caused by the presence of food, initiates the *enterogastric reflex*, which slows the influence of the vagus nerve. The pur-

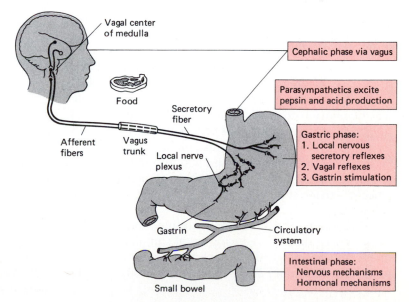

FIGURE 40-13 *The phases of gastric secretion and their regulation. (Guyton, A.C. Textbook of Medical Physiology (8th ed.). Philadelphia: W.B. Saunders, 1991.)*

pose of the enterogastric reflex appears to be to delay stomach emptying until some emptying can occur in the small intestine. Intestinal hormones, especially secretin and cholecystokinin, oppose the stimulatory effects of gastrin and slow the movement of chyme from the stomach to the small intestine.[7] This inhibitory feedback prevents excessive acid secretion and protects the intestinal mucosa from injury.

During the interdigestive phase, while no digestion is occurring in the gastrointestinal tract, the stomach secretes only a few milliliters of gastric juice per hour.[15] Secretions in the stomach normally follow a steady, dynamic course regulated by both nervous and hormonal factors that foster structural and functional integrity in the mucosa. Pathologic conditions, drugs and chemicals, or surgery can disrupt the balance between secretion and inhibition.

The best-known chemical stimulant of gastric secretion is *histamine*, which is released in response to injury by cells such as mast cells, basophils, and blood platelets. Although less potent than gastrin, histamine causes the parietal cells to secrete large amounts of gastric juice. Large amounts of endogenous histamine may be present in the gastric mucosa, and, during active secretion, small amounts are present in gastric juice and urine. Physical or emotional stress increases the release of histamine.

OTHER INFLUENCES ON GASTRIC SECRETION AND MOTILITY. Caffeine and nicotine are secretagogues that increase the amount and acidity of gastric secretion. Alcohol has been found to stimulate only the amount of gastrin secretion. Aspirin, alcohol, and bile salts alter the permeability of the epithelial barrier and allow back-diffusion of hydrochloric acid, which may result in injury to tissue and blood vessels. Aspirin produces changes in the gastric mucosa and decreases the total output of mucus, which reduces its protective effect on the gastric mucosa. Prolonged administration of large quantities of corticotropic and adrenal steroids increases gastric secretion, which favors the development or recurrence of peptic ulcers.[10,14] A number of studies have reported a slight increase in frequency of peptic ulcers in persons treated with adrenocortical steroid drugs.[6] Nonsteroidal antiinflammatory drugs have been implicated in acute gastric injury with erosive and hemorrhagic gastritis; of the drugs studied, aspirin has been shown to cause both acute and chronic injury.[16] Parasympathetic agents such as acetylcholine, reserpine, and pilocarpine also are secretory stimulants. Insulin, through its hypoglycemic effects, excites the vagus nerve and increases gastric gland activity.

Belladonna and its alkaloids, atropine and hyoscine, depress secretions by reducing vagal stimulation. Synthetic anticholinergic drugs such as propantheline bromide (Pro-Banthine) are used to control gastric activity and secretion.

Emotional disruptions have long been recognized as exerting an important influence on the secretory and motor functions of the stomach. Studies seem to indicate that prolonged anxiety, guilt, conflict, hostility, and resentment lead to engorgement of the gastric mucosa and increased secretion. The significant decrease in gastric secretion after complete vagotomy suggests that hypersecretion is caused by excessive stimulation of the vagus nerve.[16]

EMESIS

Emesis is a complex reflex, triggered by the central nervous system, that involves a sequential and coordinated contraction of many muscles. The central nervous system has a diffuse group of neurons located on the dorsal surface of the floor of the fourth ventricle called the *chemoreceptive trigger zone*. This zone is not a discrete anatomic structure, but disruption of neural pathways in this area abolishes the emetic response. The neurons in this zone sense the presence of chemicals such as morphine or other stimuli in the blood and activate the vomiting center in the medulla. The vomiting center also can be directly activated by the stomach during gastrointestinal irritation by way of the sympathetic and vagal afferent neurons.[1] Varied conditions can stimulate the emesis response, and individuals are unique in their propensity for emesis. It may be associated with a pathologic condition, or it may be a response to stress, offensive odors, or other conditions of daily life (Box 40-1).

Activation of the vomiting center causes active contraction of the somatic muscles, with inhibition of gastric tone, opening of the esophageal sphincters, and closing of the glottis. This muscular activation is accomplished

BOX 40-1 ▼ Stimuli for Emesis Response

Drugs
Toxins
Pregnancy
Motion
Alcohol consumption
Radiation therapy
Ketosis
Pain
Psychogenic conditions
Infections
Anesthesia
Acute head injury
Increased intracranial pressure
Brain tumors
Migraine headache
Overdistention of gastrointestinal tract
Obstruction of gastrointestinal tract
Vestibular disease
Fever

through the motor pathways from the fifth, seventh, ninth, tenth, and twelfth cranial nerves. Figure 40-14 summarizes the physiology of the emesis response.

A person experiences the emesis response within its three components of nausea, retching, and expulsion. These components can occur in sequence, but nausea and retching often occur without expulsion. The person commonly experiences the perception of nausea at the onset of this response. Other associated symptoms include pallor, cold sweats, and hypotension caused by sympathetic nervous system stimulation. Nausea and the accompanying sensations often diminish after expulsion of the stomach contents.[1]

SECRETION AND ABSORPTION IN THE SMALL INTESTINE

The major nutrients are mostly absorbed in the small intestine, with the simpler substances usually being absorbed in the first portion of the small bowel. Substances that require greater hydrolysis and simplification are absorbed at later points in the small intestine. Table 40-3 shows the specific absorption sites of major nutrients.

The anatomic structure, previously detailed, provides the mechanism for this to occur. In the small intestine, secretions are received from the pancreas and liver and supplemented by intestinal secretions. Secretions of the small intestine include enzymes, hormones, and mucus. These substances, listed in Tables 40-4 and 40-5, include secretions from the pancreas and liver. The major effects of all of the enzymes and hormones are detailed in the tables. All of the secretions work together to digest carbohydrates, proteins, and fats. Absorption depends on the proper hydrolysis of nutrients by secretions that increase the movement from the intestinal lumen to the bloodstream.

Biliary secretions include bile salts, lipids, water, electrolytes, and bilirubin. Of these, bilirubin is a waste product that gives color to the feces. Bile salts exert a detergent-like effect on fat and emulsify it. The pancreatic secretions contain enzymes and large amounts of bicarbonate and water. Formation of pancreatic and biliary secretions is detailed in Chapter 42.

The chyme that enters the duodenum is highly acidic because it was mixed with large amounts of hydrochloric acid in the stomach. All of the intestinal enzymes

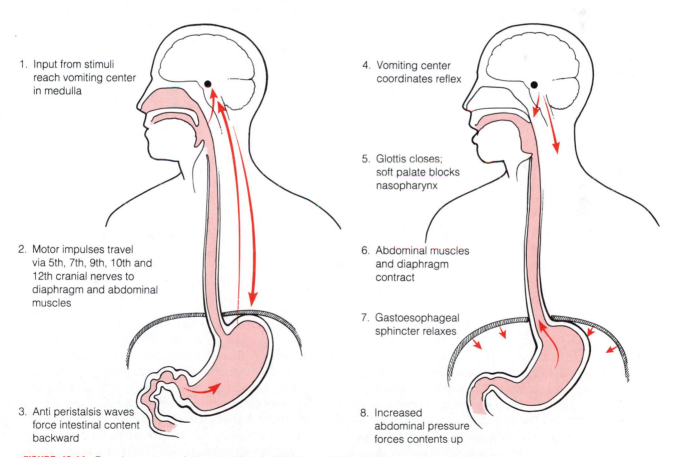

1. Input from stimuli reach vomiting center in medulla

2. Motor impulses travel via 5th, 7th, 9th, 10th and 12th cranial nerves to diaphragm and abdominal muscles

3. Anti peristalsis waves force intestinal content backward

4. Vomiting center coordinates reflex

5. Glottis closes; soft palate blocks nasopharynx

6. Abdominal muscles and diaphragm contract

7. Gastoesophageal sphincter relaxes

8. Increased abdominal pressure forces contents up

FIGURE 40-14 *Emesis response. Antiperistalsis is the first stage. Antiperistaltic waves travel backward from the intestine or stomach. Vomiting itself involves closure of the glottis, lifting of the soft palate to close the nares, and contraction of the diaphragm and abdominal muscles. The result of this is relaxation of the gastroesophageal sphincter, allowing expulsion of gastric contents through the esophagus.*

TABLE 40-4 *Digestive Enzymes*

Enzyme	Source	Substrate	Products	Remarks
Ptyalin	Salivary glands	Starch	Smaller carbohydrates	
Pepsin	Chief cells of stomach mucosa	Protein (nonspecific)	Polypeptides	Activated by hydrochloric acid
Gastric lipase	Stomach mucosa	Triglycerides (lipids)	Glycerides and fatty acids	
Enterokinase	Duodenal mucosa	Trypsinogen	Trypsin	Activates or converts trypsinogen to trypsin; trypsinogen hydrolyzed to expose active site
Trypsin	Pancreas	Protein and polypeptides	Smaller polypeptides	Converts chymotrypsinogen to chymotrypsin
Chymotrypsin	Pancreas	Proteins and polypeptides (different specificity than trypsin)	Smaller polypeptides	
Nuclease	Pancreas	Nucleic acids	Nucleotides (base + sugar + PO$_4$)	
Carboxypeptidase	Pancreas	Polypeptides	Smaller polypeptides	Cleaves carboxy terminal end
Pancreatic lipase	Pancreas	Lipids, especially triglycerides	Glycerides, free fatty acids, glycerol	Very potent
Pancreatic amylase	Pancreas	Starch	2 disaccharide units = maltose	Very potent
Aminopeptidase	Intestinal glands	Polypeptides	Smaller peptides	
Dipeptidase	Intestine	Dipeptides	2 amino acids	
Maltase	Intestine	Maltose	2 glucose	
Lactase	Intestine	Lactose	1 glucose, 1 galactose	
Sucrase	Intestine	Sucrose	1 glucose, 1 fructose	
Nucleotidase	Intestine	Nucleotides	Nucleosides and phosphates (base + sugar)	
Nucelosidase	Intestine	Nucleosides	Base and sugar	
Intestinal lipase	Intestine	Fats	Glycerides, fatty acids, glycerol	

Note: Enzymes act on one another during and after digestion, but it is only after digestion (after their substrates are removed) that they have any marked effect on one another.

work best in an alkaline medium, which requires chyme to be neutralized and alkalinized. The amount of the alkaline pancreatic secretion is closely correlated with the pH of the chyme entering the small intestine.

Chemical and mechanical digestion require that food be changed into the forms that can be moved by absorption through the mucosal lining cells to the blood and lymph vessels. The diffusible forms include monosaccharides, amino acids, fatty acids, glycerol, and glycerides.[7] Figure 40-15 shows schematically where materials are absorbed in the entire gastrointestinal system. Almost all of the nutrients are absorbed in the small intestine, and 90% of all absorption occurs there.

CARBOHYDRATE ABSORPTION. Carbohydrates are ingested primarily as disaccharides, starches, and polysaccharides. Polysaccharides are hydrolyzed into their component disaccharides by the actions of ptyalin and the gastric, intestinal, and pancreatic amylases. Intact disaccharides can be passively absorbed by the small intestine, but relatively few are absorbed in this manner. Most are first split into monosaccharides by enzymes located in the intestinal microvilli. These monosaccharides are then actively absorbed into the blood capillaries of the villi. Absorption occurs against a concentration gradient and apparently requires active transport, although the method by which this occurs is obscure. It is known that

TABLE 40-5 *Hormones of Digestion*

Hormone	Source	Agents That Stimulate Production	Action
Gastrin	Gastric mucosa (primarily pylorus)	Distention of stomach and some protein derivatives	Stimulates production of hydrochloric acid
Enterogastrone	Mucosa of small intestine and duodenum	Fats, sugars, or acids in intestine	Inhibits gastric secretion and mobility
Secretin	Duodenal mucosa	Polypeptides, acids, etc., in intestine (duodenum)	Stimulates pancreas to produce a watery, enzyme-poor juice, with high HCO_3^- content
Cholecystokinin	Duodenal mucosa	Fats in duodenum	Stimulates pancreas to produce enzyme-rich juice and stimulates gallbladder to contract and release bile

sodium increases cellular permeability to glucose, so that glucose transport is related to sodium transport. Some monosaccharides are transported by facilitated diffusion through the intestinal wall (Fig. 40-16).

PROTEIN ABSORPTION. Protein absorption mostly occurs in the duodenum and jejunum. As a result of gastric pepsin and pancreatic enzymes, 70% of protein ingested in the diet is presented to the intestinal absorptive membrane in the form of small peptides, and 30% is in the form of amino acids. The amino acids are immediately absorbed, but only a small amount of peptide is absorbed intact. Most of the peptides are reduced by peptidases in the microvilli to amino acids, and absorption rapidly follows. The sodium transport mechanism also probably provides for amino acid transport (see Figure 40-16). Many amino acids apparently need pyridoxine, a component of vitamin B_6, to aid in transport.

FAT ABSORPTION. Dietary fat consists mainly of long-chain triglycerides, which are hydrolyzed intraluminally into fatty acids and monoglycerides. Hydrolysis occurs in the jejunum through the action of lipase. The most important lipase is secreted from the pancreas. Bile salts and fatty acids aggregate to form *micelles*, which are water-soluble structures. A major function of bile salts is to make fat globules fragmentable by agitating them in the small bowel.[7, 12] These fragments attach themselves to the surface of the epithelial cells. The fatty acids leave the micelles and enter the cell by diffusion, while the bile salts are released to return to chyme to aid in the absorption of more fats. When the fats in the duodenum and upper jejunum have been removed, bile salts are reabsorbed and eventually returned to the liver.

Lipids are resynthesized into triglycerides in the endoplasmic reticulum of intestinal epithelial cells. Molecules of triglycerides then organize into minute fat droplets, which contain small amounts of phospholipid and cholesterol and a protein-coated surface. These droplets, called *chylomicrons*, then pass out of the base of the epithelial cells and enter either the bloodstream or the lymphatic system. About 80% to 90% of all fatty acids enter the bloodstream in the form of chylomicrons (see Figure 40-16). Small amounts of fats are not digested and are excreted in the feces.

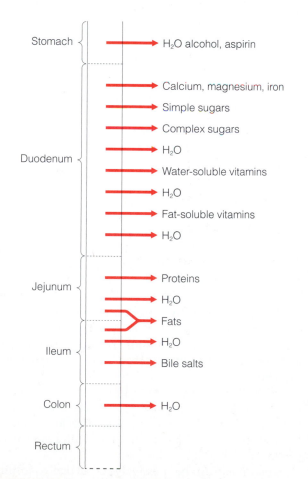

FIGURE 40-15 *Schematic representation of absorption of nutrients in the digestive tract.*

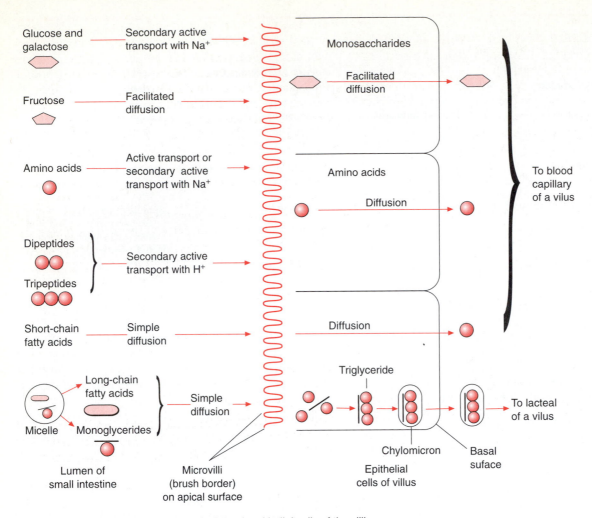

Mechanisms for movement of nutrients through epithelial cells of the villi

FIGURE 40-16 *Absorption of digested nutrients in the small intestine. For simplicity, all digested foods are shown in the lumen of the small intestine, even though some nutrients are digested by brush border enzymes. (Source: G. Tortora and S. Grabowski,* Principles of Anatomy and Physiology, *[7th ed.]. New York: Harper Collins, 1993.)*

WATER ABSORPTION. About 8 L of water per day are absorbed from the small intestine into the portal blood entirely by diffusion.[7] The greatest amount of this absorption occurs in the jejunum. Water crosses the intestinal cell membrane by passing through the pores of this membrane. The rate of absorption is great and probably is enhanced by glucose and oxygen. Therefore, active transport may increase water absorption through shifting of other ions.

ELECTROLYTE ABSORPTION. Electrolytes, must cross the intestinal cell membrane by passing through its pores or by using a membrane carrier. Like water, electrolytes are primarily absorbed into the portal blood rather than into the lymphatic system, and the absorption rate is greater in the proximal than in the distal portion of the small bowel. Monovalent electrolytes, such as sodium, chloride, potassium, nitrate, and bicar-

bonate, are more easily absorbed than polyvalent electrolytes, such as calcium, magnesium, and sulfate.

Most of the *sodium* is absorbed in the jejunum, with less being absorbed in the ileum and the colon. The mechanism for this is active transport of sodium from the epithelial cells into the intercellular spaces. This requires a carrier and energy. Increased sodium concentration in the intercellular spaces creates an osmotic gradient for water, which follows the sodium passively. Both sodium and water are finally absorbed into the capillaries of the villi.[7]

Chloride passively moves through the membranes of the duodenum and jejunum. It is actively transported in the large bowel, where it is exchanged in close relation to bicarbonate ions, which are used to neutralize any acid products in the large intestine.

Potassium can be passively or actively absorbed through the intestinal mucosa.[5,7] Most absorption occurs in the jejunum and ileum through a system not clearly identified.

Calcium is absorbed by active transport throughout the small intestine, but most actively in the duodenum. The solubility of calcium salts is increased in duodenal acid, rather than in the more alkaline medium lower in the intestines. The rate of calcium absorption is altered by the level of parathyroid hormone in the blood (see pp. 720–723). Vitamin D is important in stimulating the rate of intestinal absorption; it is activated by a specific process in the kidneys and then increases calcium absorption.

Magnesium absorption and regulation are tied to both calcium and potassium balance; however, the specific stimuli for magnesium absorption are not well delineated.[2] The distal small bowel is the primary site for magnesium absorption. Because this area often is affected by bowel resection and inflammatory bowel disease, persons with these problems must have supplemental dietary intake. Alcoholism also disrupts magnesium absorption from the intestine, and kidney excretion is accelerated.[9]

Most *iron* is absorbed in its ferrous form in the duodenum. An acid medium facilitates iron absorption. Iron uptake is an active process that is facilitated by *ascorbic acid*, which reduces the ferric to the ferrous form. The rate of absorption is extremely slow, but the rate increases with iron deficiency and decreases with excessive dietary intake of iron.

The *vitamins* are primarily absorbed in the proximal intestine, except for vitamin B_{12}, which is absorbed in the ileum. Most vitamins are passively absorbed. Some are stored in the body, and some have to be replenished on a regular basis. Vitamin B_{12} forms a complex with the intrinsic factor, which, in the ileum, is bound to a specific, unknown receptor in the mucosa and, finally, is absorbed into the blood.

SECRETION, ABSORPTION, AND EXCRETION IN THE LARGE INTESTINE

The function of the large intestine (colon) is mainly to absorb water, but it also is vital in the synthesis of vitamin K and some B-complex vitamins and in the formation and excretion of feces.[13] Electrical activity within the colon is more irregular than in the small intestine. Structurally, the colon has no smooth muscle gap junctions and does not function as a syncytium. Contraction and motility in the colon depend on the individual integration of groups of smooth muscles by neural mechanisms. Proximal colon motility is antiperistaltic to augment water removal from the feces.[8]

The movements of the large intestine are part of the peristaltic activity initiated by the ingestion of food. The final movement of the large intestine is *mass peristalsis*, which drives digested waste material into the rectum.

This usually occurs three to four times a day. The glands of the lining of the large intestine secrete mucus, which lubricates the material and protects the lining of the bowel. Active bacteria in the bowel ferment any remaining carbohydrates, releasing hydrogen, carbon dioxide, and methane gas, and break proteins down into amino acids. This activity gives fecal material its odor.

Water (1,800–3,000 mL) is absorbed daily in the large intestine, along with a few electrolytes. This absorption regulates the consistency of the feces and provides for final water balance in the gastrointestinal system.

Defecation is the process of emptying the rectum, and it is initiated by distention of rectal walls. The external sphincter is under voluntary control and relaxes when intraabdominal and intrathoracic pressures increase, pushing the fecal material out of the body. Increased rectal and intraabdominal pressures may increase the vagal tone and reflexively decrease the heart rate.

▼ *Chapter Summary*

▼   The hunger center is found in the hypothalamus, as is the satiety center. Appetite is more subtle and is found in the cortical areas of the brain, stimulated by sight, touch, and smell.

▼   The gastrointestinal tract is a continuous structure that begins with the oral cavity and terminates with the anal sphincter. The processes of ingestion, movement of food, digestion, absorption, and excretion are carried out through this system. Throughout the process, enzymes, hormones, and various secretions are used to accomplish the function of the system.

▼   Accessory organs that are essential in the process of digestion include the liver, gallbladder, and pancreas and these are considered in Chapter 42.

▼   The major digestive enzymes are ptyalin, pepsin, enterokinase, trypsin, chymotrypsin, pancreatic lipase, pancreatic amylase, lactase, sucrase, and intestinal lipase. Associated hormones are gastrin, enterogastrone, secretin, and cholecystokinin. These function to stimulate secretion of hydrochloric acid, bicarbonate, or to enhance absorption of certain nutrients.

▼   Most of the nutrients are absorbed in the small intestine. The large intestine absorbs water and synthesizes vitamin K and some B-complex vitamins. It also regulates the excretion of waste products.

▼   The nervous system participates in the gastric phases which are the cephalic, gastric, and intestinal. The cephalic phase prepares the stomach for food and digestion, the gastric causes increased secretions, and the intestinal phase slows movement so that absorption can occur.

▼ *References*

1. Carpenter, D.O. Emesis. In Schultz. S.G., *Handbook of Physiology: The Gastrointestinal System, Vol. 1, Part 1.* Bethesda, Md.: American Physiological Society, 1989.
2. Culpepper, R.M. and Schoolwerth, A.C. Approach to the patient with altered magnesium concentration. In Kelley, W.N. *Textbook of Internal Medicine* (2nd ed.). Philadelphia: J.B. Lippincott, 1992.
3. Dharmsathaphorn, K. Transport of water and electrolytes in the gastrointestinal tract. In Narins, R.G., *Maxwell and Kleeman's Clinical Disorders of Fluid and Electrolyte Balance* (5th ed.). New York: McGraw-Hill, 1994.
4. Fenoglio-Preiser, C.M., Lantz, P.E., Listrom, M.B., et al. *Gastrointestinal Pathology: An Atlas and Text.* New York: Raven, 1989.
5. Ganong, W.F. *Review of Medical Physiology* (16th ed.). Norwalk, Conn.: Appleton & Lange, 1994.
6. Greenberger, N.J. *Gastrointestinal Disorders: A Pathophysiologic Approach* (3rd ed.). Chicago: Year Book Medical Publishers, 1986.
7. Guyton, A.C. *Textbook of Medical Physiology* (8th ed.). Philadelphia: W.B. Saunders, 1991.
8. Livingston, E.H., and Passaro, E.P. Postoperative ileus. *Dig Dis Sci* 35:121, 1990.
9. Metheny, N. *Fluid and Electrolyte Balance* (2nd ed.). Philadelphia: J.B. Lippincott, 1992.
10. Morson, B.C., Dawson, I.M., Day, D.W., et al. *Morson and Dawson's Gastrointestinal Pathology.* Oxford: Blackwell, 1990.
11. Nord, H.A., and Sodeman, W.A. The stomach. In Sodeman, W.A., and Sodeman, T.M., *Sodeman's Pathologic Physiology* (7th ed.). Philadelphia: W.B. Saunders, 1985.
12. Shearman, D.J., and Finlayson, N.D. *Diseases of the Gastrointestinal Tract and Liver.* Edinburgh: Churchill Livingstone, 1989.
13. Sodeman, W.A., and Watson, D.W. The large intestine. In Sodeman, W.A., and Sodeman, T.M., *Sodeman's Pathologic Physiology* (7th ed.). Philadelphia: W.B. Saunders, 1985.
14. Spiro, H.M. *Clinical Gastroenterology* (3rd ed.). New York: Macmillan, 1986.
15. Tortora, G.J., and Grabowski, S.R. *Principles of Anatomy and Physiology* (7th ed.). New York: HarperCollins, 1993.
16. Yardley, J.H. Gastritis. In Goldman, H., Appelman, H.D., and Kaufman, N., *Gastrointestinal Pathology.* Baltimore: Williams & Wilkins, 1988.

Chapter 41

Alterations in Gastrointestinal Function

Barbara L. Bullock

▼ **LEARNING OBJECTIVES**

1 List the major sources of inflammation of the gums.
2 Describe the anatomic and functional changes that occur with achalasia.
3 Outline the mechanism for mucosal damage that occurs with esophagitis.
4 Describe pathophysiologically a rolling hiatal hernia and a sliding hiatal hernia.
5 Differentiate between acute and chronic gastritis.
6 Differentiate the types of peptic ulcerations according to underlying etiology, symptomatology, and relationship to malignancy.
7 Briefly describe the pathology of gastric carcinoma.
8 Describe the pathophysiologic changes that result in malabsorption.
9 Discuss nausea, vomiting, and diarrhea in terms of etiology and physiologic effects.
10 Differentiate regional enteritis and ulcerative colitis on the basis of etiology, pathology, symptomatology, and course of the disease.
11 Explain how adynamic or paralytic ileus may lead to ischemia and infarction of the bowel.
12 Distinguish between paralytic ileus and bowel obstruction.
13 Describe the appearance and complications of the various types of hernias.
14 Describe Hirschsprung's disease.
15 Explain why diverticula are common in elderly persons.
16 List some common conditions that can cause hemorrhoids.
17 Discuss the relationship of the American diet and carcinoma of the colon.
18 Differentiate the pathology and symptomatology of carcinoma arising in different areas of the colon.

Barbara L. Bullock: PATHOPHYSIOLOGY: ADAPTATIONS AND ALTERATIONS IN FUNCTION, 4th ed.
© 1996 Lippincott-Raven Publishers

▼ Diseases of the Oral Cavity

ALTERATIONS IN THE GUMS AND TEETH

The gums, or *gingiva*, are subject to localized inflammatory diseases, and they may react to other systemic diseases or drug therapy. *Gingivitis*, an inflammation of the borders surrounding the teeth, may result in pain, bleeding, and destruction of gingival tissue. When this inflammation spreads to the underlying tissues, bones, or roots of the teeth, it is called *periodontitis*. This destructive disease may result in purulent drainage, loss of teeth, spread and infection of the surrounding lymph nodes, and even sepsis.

Overgrowth of the gingiva occurs in persons having long-term treatment with phenytoin (Dilantin). Hormonal and metabolic conditions may cause an increased inflammatory response, with enlarged gingiva noted especially at puberty, during pregnancy, and with conditions such as leukemia and thrombocytopenia.

CHANGES IN THE ORAL MUCOSA

Changes in the oral mucosa often reflect systemic changes in the body. Various conditions may cause these mucosal changes, and the manifestations vary. For example, in scarlet fever the tongue becomes bright red (strawberry tongue), whereas in a *Candida albicans* infection (thrush), localized white lesions of the oral mucosa occur.

Tumors of the oral mucosa are uncommon and are much like skin tumors, except that many of the oral growths are benign rather than malignant lesions.[3] The salivary glands may also develop benign or malignant tumorous growths.

▼ Esophageal Alterations

ACHALASIA

Achalasia is an uncommon disorder of esophageal motility characterized by the inability of the cardiac sphincter of the stomach to relax (Fig. 41-1A). Degeneration of the myenteric ganglion cells in the esophagus and alteration in vagal tone are the precipitating causes. As a result, motility problems occur and food is retained within the area. Hypertrophy and dilatation of the lower esophagus become marked.[19]

This condition becomes chronic and slowly progressive, causing dysphagia, vomiting, nausea, and weight loss. Pain occurs in about one third of the cases.[20] Lung changes, regurgitation, and infections due to unusual organisms (eg, mycobacteria) are probably related to repeated episodes of nocturnal aspiration. The degree of swallowing difficulty in the early stages is increased by stress and anxiety. Increasing dysphagia results, and finally even liquids become difficult to swallow.

Diagnostic tests usually include a barium swallow, which reflects a normally functioning pharynx and cricoesophageal sphincter. However, after a few centimeters, peristaltic action stops or decreases to ineffectual motions. The distended, nonemptying lower esophagus is easily identified as a pouch that narrows into the esophagogastric junction (see Figure 41-1B). Although the lower esophageal sphincter does not open in response to swallowing, it may open slightly as food moves into the area to allow some contents to pass through. Frequent follow-up examinations are required, because affected persons have a statistical increase in frequency of esophageal carcinoma. Surgical intervention may be required to decrease the amount of obstruction.

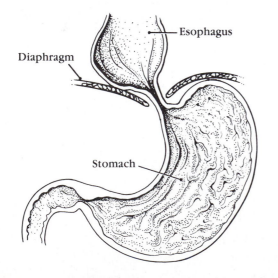

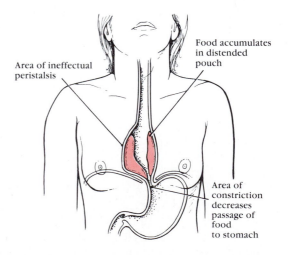

A

B

FIGURE 41-1 *A. Location and appearance of achalatic esophagus. B. Nonemptying or poorly emptying lower esophagus resulting from achalasia.*

ESOPHAGEAL DIVERTICULUM

An *esophageal diverticulum* is an outpouching of the esophagus at any level that can result in trapped food, dysphagia, and regurgitation. It may be caused by a congenital weakness of the esophageal wall, by high pressure developing proximal to an esophageal spasm, or by a hyperactive upper esophageal sphincter.[13] In the pharyngeal portion of the esophagus, it is called *Zenker's pouch* or *diverticulum*. Symptoms are usually insidious, with dysphagia and regurgitation being common. Other diverticula may develop after esophageal or tracheal infection or they may be associated with esophageal motility abnormalities.[2]

ESOPHAGEAL SPASM

Diffuse esophageal spasm is characterized by functional rather than pathologic obstruction of the esophagus characterized by intermittent dysphagia and sometimes spasmotic pain.[2] Spasm is commonly seen with gastroesophageal reflux as a reaction to the acid from stomach contents passing into the lower esophagus.

GASTROESOPHAGEAL REFLUX AND ESOPHAGITIS

Gastroesophageal reflux is the movement of gastric contents into the esophagus. Normally, pressure on the lower esophageal sphincter prevents backflow, or secondary peristalsis moves gastric contents from the esophageal mucosa before damage occurs. An incompetent lower esophageal sphincter is believed to be the primary cause of reflux esophagitis. Other causes include prolonged gastric intubation, ingestion of corrosive chemicals, uremia, infections, mucosal alterations, and systemic diseases, such as systemic lupus erythematosus.[3] Frequent regurgitation through the gastroesophageal junction causes substernal pain. The reflux may be accentuated by postural changes, such as assumption of a supine position. Pulmonary aspiration is a common complication when the condition is severe.[11]

Esophagitis, inflammation of the esophageal mucosa, most often results from gastroesophageal reflux due to prolonged vomiting or an incompetent lower esophageal sphincter. Mucosal damage is related to the contact time between the esophageal mucosa and gastric contents, as well as the acidity and quantity of gastric secretions. Gastric hydrochloric acid alters the pH of the esophagus and permits mucosal protein to be denatured. The pepsin in the gastric secretion has proteolytic properties that are enhanced when the pH is around 2.0. The combination of pepsin and hydrochloric acid increases the capability for damage. Often, an increase in bile salts is associated with gastroesophageal reflux and enhances the effect of the hydrogen ion on the mucosa. This reflux has been shown to cause an inflammation that penetrates to the muscularis layer, resulting in motor dysfunction and decreased esophageal clearance. The results are increased esophageal contact time, more muscle damage, and increased amounts of reflux.[13, 20]

The most common symptoms of esophageal inflammation include heartburn, retrosternal discomfort, and the regurgitation of sour, bitter material. These symptoms are frequently precipitated by ingestion of large amounts of fatty or spicy foods or alcohol. Symptoms correlate with the amount and acidity of reflux. Dysphagia for both solids and liquids increases when severe obstruction occurs. Permanent strictures may develop that make food passage difficult. Irritation of the mucosa may cause bleeding and eventually produce an iron-deficiency anemia. Nocturnal reflux of material into the pharynx may lead to aspiration into the lungs. Reflux may occur in the upright or supine positions or both.[13]

Diagnosis is difficult but may be based on clinical, radiographic, and endoscopic findings. The most effective tests are measurement of pH in the esophagus and biopsy to demonstrate inflammatory changes.[20] Barium swallow may show a poorly distensible, shortened, strictured, and/or ulcerated esophagus.[21] The gastroesophageal scintiscan is a radioisotope study used to document reflux and to provide an assessment of the amount of reflux experienced.[2]

HIATAL HERNIA

A *hiatal hernia* is a condition in which part of the stomach protrudes through the opening of the diaphragm (Fig. 41-2). This condition may be continuous or occur sporadically. The continuous type is called a *rolling para-*

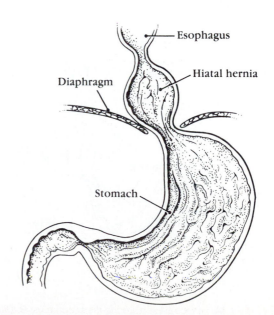

FIGURE 41-2 *Location and appearance of hiatal hernia.*

esophageal hernia and occurs in fewer than 10% of persons with this condition. Part or all of the stomach and even the intestines may herniate, causing dyspnea, severe pain, and often gastric ulceration.[20] The sporadic type, or *sliding hernia*, accounts for 80% to 90% of hiatal hernias and occurs with changes in position or with increased peristalsis. The stomach is forced through the opening of the diaphragm when the person lies down and moves back to its normal position when the person stands upright. This type of hernia may be associated with a congenitally short esophagus or may be secondary to postgastritis scarring.

Many persons with a hiatal hernia exhibit no symptoms. Symptoms such as heartburn, gastric regurgitation, dysphagia, and indigestion are accentuated when the person assumes the supine position postprandially or after overeating, physical exertion, or sudden changes of posture.

Radiographs or endoscopy will reveal a hernia. Surgery is usually recommended with the continuous type of hernia, and it involves affixing the stomach to the abdominal wall by suture (gastropexy).[20]

ESOPHAGEAL VARICES

This condition is closely related to portal hypertension and involves protrusion of the esophageal veins into the esophageal lumen (Fig. 41-3). The distended, thin-walled veins become subject to rupture, a catastrophic event that may occur spontaneously or after a sudden increase in intraabdominal pressure, such as occurs with vomiting (see pp. 820–822).[12]

Rupture of these vessels creates a very large amount of bleeding into the gastrointestinal system and usually leads to large-volume hematemesis. A first bleeding event results in 40% mortality; subsequent episodes are equally catastrophic.[3]

CARCINOMA OF THE ESOPHAGUS

Approximately 5% to 10% of malignancies of the gastrointestinal tract arise in the esophagus, with a marked variability in incidence depending on country of origin. Turkey and eastern China, for example, have rates of 20% to 25%.[20] These malignancies usually remain asymptomatic until they become surgically unresectable. This type of malignancy usually occurs after age 50 years and occurs more often in men. A strong correlation between heavy alcohol intake, cigarette smoking, and esophageal carcinoma has been recorded.[14]

Squamous cell carcinoma is the most common morphologic form. The malignancy may grow around the esophagus at the level of the diaphragm, impinging on the lumen or the tube, or it may cause a bulky, ulcerating tumor mass. Most tumors are located in the middle and lower one third of the esophagus. Adenocarcinomas of the esophagus, the second most common form, most frequently are found in the lower third of the esophagus and may arise from the gastric fundus.[19]

This disease is usually asymptomatic for long periods, with the earliest complaint being a mild dysphagia that becomes progressively worse. Postprandial regurgitation may motivate the person to seek medical assistance. Weight loss is a common complaint; hematemesis and guaiac-positive stools are relatively uncommon. Invasion of surrounding structures may result in back pain, and pressure on respiratory structures may cause varying degrees of respiratory distress.

Definitive diagnosis is made through esophagoscopy with biopsy of the tumor mass. Other diagnostic

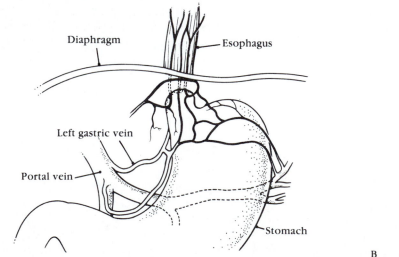

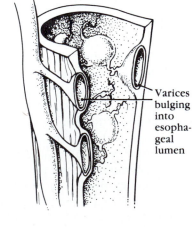

FIGURE 41-3 *A. Venous plexus around the esophagus. B. Dilated venous channels from portal hypertension. These varices bulge into the lumen of the esophagus and rupture easily.*

measures, such as barium swallow, chest film, and blood tests, provide additional information. Prognosis for this malignancy is very poor, with only about 3% surviving for 5 years.[3, 20]

▼ Alterations in the Stomach and Duodenum

GASTRITIS

Gastritis is a general term for an inflammation of the gastric mucosa. It may occur with excessive or completely absent gastric acid secretion. The classification into *acute* and *chronic gastritis* describes the onset and course of the disease. Chronic gastritis may be associated with gastric mucosal atrophy, achlorhydria, and peptic ulceration.

Acute gastritis causes transient inflammation of the gastric mucosa, mucosal hemorrhages, and erosion into the mucosal lining. It is frequently associated with alcohol or aspirin ingestion, smoking, and severely stressful conditions, such as trauma, burns, central nervous system damage, chemotherapy, and radiation therapy.[5] Hydrochloric acid is present in gastritis, but its secretion is not necessarily excessive.[25] Erosion of the gastric mucosa can result in a massive gastric hemorrhage. Therefore, acute gastritis may be associated only with temporary discomfort, or it may have a very serious outcome.

GASTRIC EROSIONS

Gastric erosions, or *stress ulcers*, occur after a major insult to the body. Causes include hypovolemic or septic shock, peritonitis, serious brain injury, drug ingestion (usually aspirin, corticosteroids, or nonsteroidal anti-inflammatory drugs), or major burn injury.[20] Gastric ulcerations after brain damage are called *Cushing's ulcers*; those after burn injury are called *Curling's ulcers*. Ulceration can usually be attributed to ischemia of the stomach mucosa.

When gastric erosions occur, they are multiple and superficial and are present in large areas of the gastric mucosa. Superficial erosions and discrete ulcers form, especially in the fundus. An *erosion* is a superficial mucosa defect of the stomach that does not penetrate the muscularis layer, a feature that helps to distinguish these ulcers from acute peptic ulceration. Such injury permits damage by continual activation of pepsinogen. Gastric acid secretion is sometimes increased, and the erosions often localize in the acid-secreting portion of the stomach. Two mechanisms for production of stress ulcers have been proposed: 1) mucosal ischemia, which relates to lack of blood supply to the gastric mucosa during the poststress period and results from a sympathetic vasoconstrictive action; and 2) enhanced back-diffusion of hydrogen ions due to increased sensitivity of the disrupted gastric mucosa to hydrochloric acid and pepsin. The surface mucosal cells are disrupted, and stimulation of the myenteric plexus leads to hypersecretion of gastric acid and pepsinogen.[17] Histamine is also released from damaged cells, and its effects increase the damage (Flowchart 41-1).

Lipid mediators play a role in either amplifying or delaying ulcerative repair that has been triggered by another factor.[23] In ischemic injury, platelet-activating factor or prostaglandins may promote gastric ulceration (Flowchart 41-2). The role of cortisone and aspirin in causing ulceration may be through lipid mediators.[23]

The major clinical manifestation of gastric erosions or ulceration is massive, painless, gastric bleeding with an onset 2 to 15 days after the original insult.[20] This bleeding, from multiple sites in the gastric mucosa, is very difficult to control. Because of the danger of bleeding after acute stress, such as major trauma, preventive measures are routinely used to decrease hydrogen ion secretion and to neutralize gastric acid.

PEPTIC ULCER DISEASE

Peptic ulcers (peptic ulcer disease) are ulcerative conditions of the gastrointestinal tract that result from *acid–pepsin imbalance*. They are thought to develop when the aggressive proteolytic activities of the gastric secretions are greater than their normal protective abilities. An increase in acid and pepsin from any cause may produce ulcerations if the protective mechanisms are inadequate. Major factors that alter the mucosal barrier include the failure to regenerate the mucous epithelium at a sufficient rate, a decrease in quantity and quality of mucus, and poor local mucosal blood flow. Possibly, vascular occlusion of small nutrient vessels in the mucosa or submucosa causes localized necrosis and subsequent ulcer formation. Peptic activity alone is not responsible for ulcerations; individual susceptibility is necessary.

The most common site for peptic ulcers is the pyloric region of the duodenum, but lesions also occur in the greater curvature of the stomach (Fig. 41-4). Duodenal ulcers constitute 80% of all peptic ulcers. Ulcerative conditions affect approximately 10% to 15% of the general population. Table 41-1 presents some differential features of peptic ulcer disease.

Gastric Ulcers

The primary problem with gastric ulcers appears to be decreased resistance of the gastric mucosa to ingested substances. The level of hydrochloric acid secretion is usually normal or reduced. True *achlorhydria* (lack of hydrochloric acid secretion) is rare with these ulcers and usually indicates a gastric carcinoma. Because gastric ulcers often occur in conjunction with gastric atrophy, the secretions may contain mostly water and small

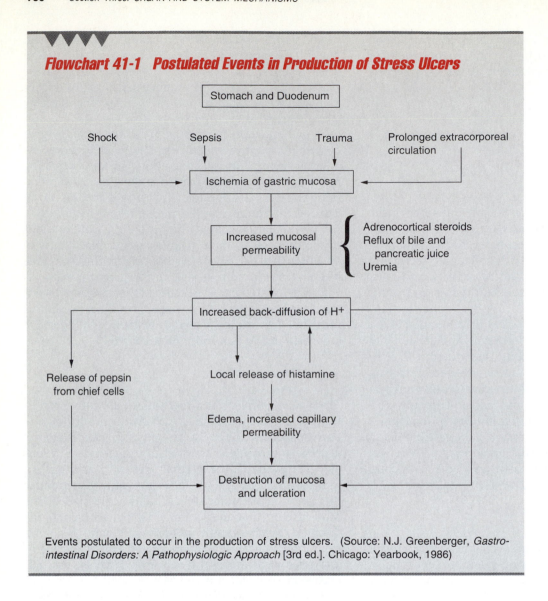

Flowchart 41-1   Postulated Events in Production of Stress Ulcers

Events postulated to occur in the production of stress ulcers. (Source: N.J. Greenberger, *Gastrointestinal Disorders: A Pathophysiologic Approach* [3rd ed.]. Chicago: Yearbook, 1986)

amounts of mucus. The intrinsic factor may not be secreted, causing decreased absorption of vitamin B_{12} and pernicious anemia (see pp. 384–385). As described below, there appears to be an association with the organism *Helicobacter pylori*.

Pathologically, gastric ulcers are often associated with atrophy of the gastric glands. Gastritis always surrounds the ulcerated area. The classic ulcer has a sharply punched-out appearance with a smooth, clean base. The mucosa surrounding it is often edematous. Bleeding may occur if the ulceration erodes through a vessel. Malignant gastric ulcers exhibit a shaggy, necrotic base, as opposed to the smooth base of nonmalignant ulcers. Gastric ulcers transform into malignant tumors often enough to call them premalignant and to encourage frequent follow-up.

Gastric ulcers can be diagnosed by barium swallow (upper gastrointestinal series) and direct endoscopy. Biopsy and routine cytologic studies can be performed with endoscopy. Gastric analysis may reveal a normal or lower-than-normal output of hydrochloric acid, but the large overlap of values among different persons makes this an obsolete test for gastric ulcers except in diagnosing Zollinger–Ellison syndrome.[20] Benign ulcers frequently localize on the greater curvature of the stomach and are usually smaller than malignant lesions. If there is associated achlorhydria, the ulcers are almost always malignant.

The most common symptom with gastric ulcer disease is epigastric pain. The pain may or may not be relieved by eating or it may be precipitated when food is ingested. Gastric ulcers that localize in the pyloric area often relay symptoms of duodenal ulcers. Nausea, vomiting, and weight loss are common. Hemorrhage occurs in approximately 25% of persons with gastric ulcers and is often profound. Perforation of the ulcer through the stomach wall into the peritoneal cavity is less frequent than with duodenal ulcers. Healing and recurrence are

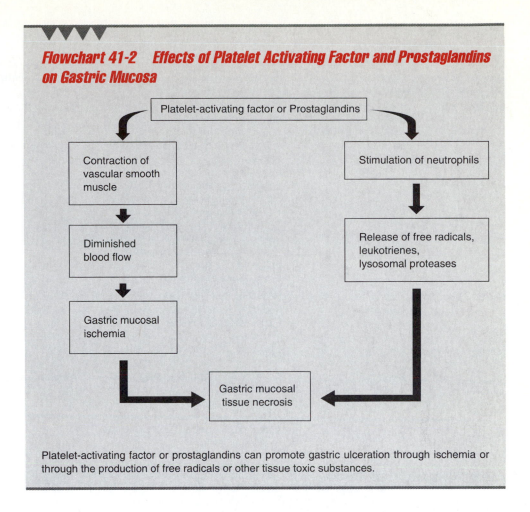

Platelet-activating factor or prostaglandins can promote gastric ulceration through ischemia or through the production of free radicals or other tissue toxic substances.

common, with lack of healing or failure to decrease in size suggesting gastric malignancy. Healing or shrinkage of the ulcer by 50% should occur within 3 months after initiating therapy.[11, 20]

Zollinger-Ellison Syndrome

This disease is usually the result of a gastrin-secreting tumor of the pancreas (see pp. 748–749). It also can be

caused by a primary gastrinoma of the stomach or intestines. Serum gastrin levels are markedly elevated, and large amounts of hydrochloric acid are produced. The tumors of Zollinger-Ellison syndrome are malignant and may produce ulceration in any portion of the stomach or duodenum. The ulcerations carry a high risk of hemorrhage and rupture.[20]

Duodenal Ulcers

Numerous causes and predisposing factors in combination upset the balance between the protective mechanism and the acid–pepsin proteolytic action in the duodenal wall. Duodenal ulcers occur in the presence of acid, but hyperacidity is not always a significant component. Persons with excess acid secretion may also have excess secretion of gastrin or gastrinlike substances from the duodenal wall as well as from the parietal cells. Evidence that the disease has a strong family history and occurs among the type O blood group supports a theory of genetic weakness.[3] Elevated serum pepsinogen level is under study as a significant indicator of predisposition to duodenal ulcer. The genetic trait for hypersecretion of pepsinogen is autosomal dominant and may be a marker for predisposition to duodenal ulcers.[3]

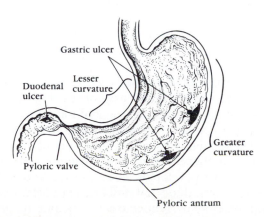

FIGURE 41-4 | *Common locations of gastric and duodenal ulcers.*

TABLE 41-1 *Differential Features of Peptic Ulcer Disease*

Type of Lesion	Frequency	Pathophysiology	Clinical Features	Course
Duodenal ulcer	Men:women, 3:1* Peak frequency 5th–6th decades Prevalence 10%–12%	Normal to increased parietal cell mass Normal to increased gastric acid secretion Normal to mildly elevated circulating gastrin levels Excessive gastrin response to meals; excessive parietal cell sensitivity Genetic factors—familial tendency, frequent blood group O, nonsecretor Positive associations—chronic obstructive lung disease, hepatic cirrhosis, pancreatic insufficiency, hyperparathyroidism Located in duodenal bulb, pyloric channel, postbulbar area	Pain: rhythmicity, periodicity, chronicity Pain-food-relief-pain pattern	Remissions and exacerbations for 10–25 years after onset. "Once an ulcer, always an ulcer." Seasonal trend (spring and fall).
Gastric ulcer	Men:women, 3–4:1 Peak frequency 6th–7th decades	Normal to decreased parietal cell mass Normal to decreased gastric acid secretion (not achlorhydria)	Pain-food-relief-pain pattern, or food-pain pattern	Remissions and exacerbations less than in duodenal ulcer; high recurrence rate. No seasonal trend.
	Duodenal ulcer: gastric ulcer was 4:1; is now 3:2	Normal to elevated circulating gastrin level Presence of gastritis Abnormal gastric mucosal barrier Abnormal pyloric function, bile reflux Ulcerogenic drugs	Weight loss, anorexia	
Gastric erosions or stress ulcer	No sex difference Related to severe stress, sepsis, burns, trauma, head injuries	Head injuries—marked gastric acid hypersecretion Others—gastric mucosal ischemia, acid back-diffusion, acute gastritis	Bleeding frequent in recognized cases; may be severe, persistent (actual frequency unknown)	Half of those who bleed require surgery.

(Reproduced with permission from N.J. Greenberger, *Gastrointestinal Disorders: A Pathophysiologic Approach* [4th ed.]. Copyright © 1991 by Yearbook Medical Publishers, Inc., Chicago.)

* Ratio has recently changed from 3:1 to 1:1.

The emotional factors that increase gastric secretions and influence the pathogenesis of duodenal ulcerations often precipitate the onset or recurrence of symptoms. Studies have been conducted to identify an "ulcer personality," but the findings are inconclusive.[22] Numerous instances have been reported where the disease has been reactivated when the affected person suffers undue stress, anxiety, or fatigue.[3] Endocrine factors, such as estrogen and the adrenal steroids, also may contribute to the formation of ulcerations.

Evidence that *Helicobacter pylori* bacteria is a causative agent is increasing, because virtually all persons with active duodenal ulcer have *H. pylori*. About 80% of persons with gastric ulcers have the organism, and the incidence of recurrence declines when the organism is eradicated. This intriguing theory fails to answer why many persons with the organism do not develop peptic ulcer disease.[18] Figure 41-5 summarizes the gastric and duodenal factors implicated in the pathogenesis of duodenal peptic ulcers. It is thought that several of these factors must be working together in the production of an ulceration.

Duodenal ulcers are usually deep, with a sharp line of demarcation from uninvolved tissue. Most of these ulcerations occur in the first portion of the duodenum, close to the pylorus. Disruption of the integrity of the mucosal wall caused by the acid–pepsin imbalance penetrates the entire thickness of the mucosal membrane, including the muscularis mucosa. Healing requires the formation of granulation tissue and scar. Secretory cellular functions are lost in the area of scarring. A typical duodenal ulcer is round or oval and indurated, with a funnel-shaped lesion that extends into the muscularis layer. It is frequently located within 3 cm of the pyloric junction on either the anterior or posterior wall. Acute ulcerations may develop on chronic ulcers, and perforations through the duodenal wall in active ulcers result in spilling of gastric or duodenal contents into the peritoneum and peritonitis. Erosion of an artery or a vein at the base of the lesion may cause a hemorrhage. The amount

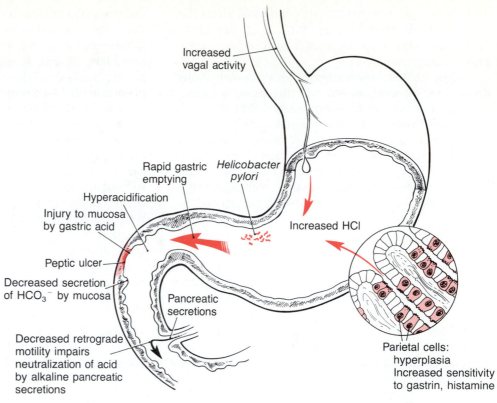

Increased vagal activity

Rapid gastric emptying

Helicobacter pylori

Hyperacidification

Injury to mucosa by gastric acid

Increased HCl

Peptic ulcer

Decreased secretion of HCO_3^- by mucosa

Pancreatic secretions

Decreased retrograde motility impairs neutralization of acid by alkaline pancreatic secretions

Parietal cells: hyperplasia Increased sensitivity to gastrin, histamine

FIGURE 41-5 *Pathogenesis of peptic ulcers.*

of bleeding depends on the vessel involved, and the effects are related to the rapidity and amount of blood loss. Scar formation may cause deformity, shortening, and stiffening of the duodenum, which may interfere with normal emptying of the stomach. Actual obstruction may result from stenosis, spasm, edema, and inflammation.

Clinical manifestations of duodenal ulcerations include a documented pattern of remissions and exacerbations over varying periods of time. An attack is frequently triggered by stress, and exacerbations have been observed to occur most frequently in the fall and spring. A pain-food-relief pattern is characteristic of duodenal ulcer. Pain usually develops 90 minutes to 3 hours after eating, often waking the person at night. This pain is immediately relieved by food or antacids. Pain on awakening in the early morning is rare and is thought to be due to decreased gastric secretions.[11] The pain is usually described as steady, boring, burning, aching, or hunger-like and is localized in the midepigastrium, the right epigastric area, and sometimes in the back. The pain mechanism in duodenal ulcers is thought to be related to irritation of exposed sensory nerve endings by hydrochloric acid. It may result from increased motility or spasm of the muscles at the ulcer site. In rare cases, no pain is described, and the ulcer is discovered when complications arise.

Other gastrointestinal symptoms include heartburn and regurgitation of sour juice into the back of the mouth. Anorexia is not a usual complaint because the individual seeks relief of pain through eating. A duodenal ulcer may rupture because of erosion through the duodenal wall, and this leads to contamination of the peritoneal cavity. As in gastric ulcer disease, hemorrhage may lead to profound blood loss and hypovolemic shock; a slowly bleeding ulcer may be detected by guaiac-positive stools. Localized tenderness around the epigastric area is the only common finding on physical examination.

Diagnosis of duodenal ulcer requires a reliable and accurate history of the characteristic pain. Radiologic and fluoroscopic examinations with barium swallow demonstrate ulcer craters and niches as well as outlet deformities. Gastric endoscopy, direct visualization of the gastric mucosa through a lighted scope, is useful in revealing lesions too small or superficial to be seen on radiographs. Tissue for histologic studies may also be taken during the procedure. Gastric juice analysis may be helpful for persons who do not have typical duodenal ulcer disease to determine the cycle of hydrochloric acid and pepsin secretion. Basal acid output and maximal histamine stimulation analysis may be performed. Basal acid output measures the acidity of gastric secretions without known or intentional stimulation. Achlorhydria after histamine stimulation demonstrates loss of secretory function and almost never occurs with duodenal ulcerations. A 12-hour nocturnal test provides information regarding secretion during a prolonged basal state. Nocturnal levels of hydrochloric acid and pepsin are frequently higher in persons with duodenal ulcers than in those with gastric ulcers. With Zollinger-Ellison syndrome, very high levels of gastric acid secretion may be measured.

All of the therapeutic approaches for duodenal ulcer disease are directed toward relieving pain, promoting healing, and preventing complications. The histamine antagonist drugs that reduce gastric acidity promote healing in a significant number of cases, evidence that supports excess gastric acid as a cause.[6] Helping the person recognize lifestyle and personal factors that precipitate symptoms may enhance compliance with therapy and thus help prevent disease recurrence.

Complications of Peptic Ulcer Disease

Hemorrhage occurs in 15% to 20% of cases of peptic ulcer disease. It may be manifested by melena (occult blood in the stools), hematemesis and/or hemorrhagic shock. Ulcers located posteriorly are more likely to bleed than those in other locations, and the bleeding is often arterial and massive.[6] Other complications include perforation of the wall, which is most common with duodenal ulcer disease and causes abdominal pain and peritonitis. Penetration of the ulcer into surrounding structures is relatively uncommon but may affect the pancreas, liver, and abdominal wall. Symptoms of penetration are those of damage to the affected area.

The inlet and outlet of the stomach may become obstructed; this is most common in the pyloric area. Obstruction may cause severe pain, vomiting, weight loss, and anorexia. The ulcer may be intractable, with frequent recurrence or lack of response to therapy. Other complications, especially obstruction and penetration, may lead to intractable ulcers. When ulcers continue despite therapy, Zollinger–Ellison syndrome must be ruled out.

GASTRIC CARCINOMA

Of all malignancies of the stomach, 90% to 95% are classified as carcinomas. The frequency of gastric carcinoma has been declining steadily in the United States since the 1930s. It is postulated that this is due to a decrease in the consumption of smoked foods. The incidence remains high in such countries as Iceland, Finland, and Japan.[4] Gastric cancer generally occurs between the ages of 60 and 65 years. Survival rates are poor, with less than 5% to 15% surviving for 5 years after diagnosis. Early diagnosis has improved the mortality figures, so that if the lesion is confined to the mucosa and submucosa, 5-year survival improves to 60% to 90%.[20]

Environmental factors evidently play a large part in the origin of gastric cancer, although the significance of each factor is unknown. These factors include diet, socioeconomic class, occupation, and urban residence.[3] Diet has been implicated in gastric carcinoma, especially

with regard to the nitrates that are used as food preservatives. These convert to nitrites in the body, which convert to nitrosamine, a well-known carcinogen.[22] Genetic or hereditary linkage is supported by an increased risk among families and the preponderance of occurrence in persons with blood type A. Gastric carcinoma also is associated with atrophic gastritis or polyps of the stomach.

Pathologically, these carcinomas may arise anywhere on the mucosal surface. They begin as *in situ* (localized) lesions that progress to lesions called *early gastric carcinoma*, which are limited to the mucosa and submucosa. Early spread to regional lymph nodes may occur. As the lesions progress, they may infiltrate the wall or protrude as bulky masses into the outlet of the stomach.[20] Ulceration may occur, with a shaggy, necrotic-appearing base. Carcinomatous masses may be polypoid or ulcerating in appearance (Fig. 41-6). Early metastasis or spread may be to lymph nodes in the region. An infiltrating, diffuse form of carcinoma, the *leather-bottle stomach*, causes thickening of the entire stomach. Distant metastasis is common and is found most often in the liver, lungs, ovaries, and peritoneum. These metastases are often established at the time of diagnosis.

The clinical manifestations are often vague and nonspecific, including early satiety, loss of appetite, weight loss, abdominal pain, vomiting, and change in bowel habits. Anemia and guaiac-positive stools may be discovered. Bleeding may result from vascular erosion as the tumor ulcerates. Pain in gastric carcinoma may mimic ulcer pain or be related to partial outlet obstruction. Massive hemorrhage may cause hemorrhagic shock.

The only definitive diagnostic test for gastric carcinoma is gastric biopsy, usually obtained through gastric endoscopy. Other studies may be helpful, such as barium swallow, blood work, and additional tests to demonstrate a mass in the gastric area.

▼ Alterations in the Small Intestine

Most nutrient absorption occurs in the small intestine. Any alteration of the integrity of the small bowel can result in malabsorption or maldigestion or both, whether the source is motor or mucosal. The common conditions of vomiting, diarrhea, and enteritis can also result in fluid, electrolyte, and nutritional imbalances.

Malabsorption refers to inadequate absorption of ingested nutrients and water. *Maldigestion* is the inability to absorb foodstuffs because they have been broken down inadequately. Box 41-1 outlines some of the major causes of malabsorption. Many disorders can cause malabsorption through differing mechanisms, and the categories of these disorders are not entirely separate. The more common conditions are discussed below. Table

EARLY GASTRIC CANCER

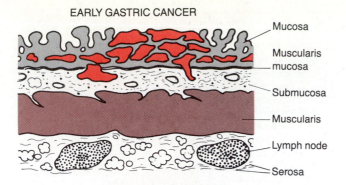

- Mucosa
- Muscularis mucosa
- Submucosa
- Muscularis
- Lymph node
- Serosa

POLYPOID CARCINOMA

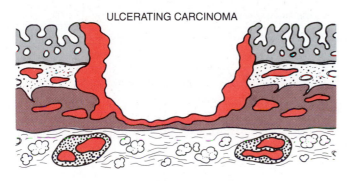

Lymph node metastasis

ULCERATING CARCINOMA

INFILTRATING CARCINOMA (LINITIS PLASTICA)

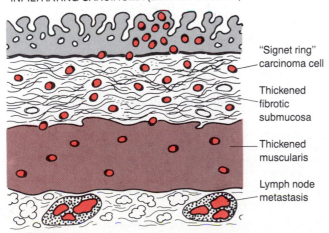

- "Signet ring" carcinoma cell
- Thickened fibrotic submucosa
- Thickened muscularis
- Lymph node metastasis

FIGURE 41-6 *The major types of gastric cancer. (Source: Rubin, E. and Farber, J.L. Pathology [2nd ed.] Philadelphia: J.B. Lippincott, 1994)*

41-2 summarizes the laboratory tests most commonly used to detect malabsorption.

VOMITING AND DIARRHEA

Because 3 to 6 liters of gastrointestinal secretions fill the gastrointestinal lumen every day, excessive vomiting or diarrhea can lead to volume depletion and electrolyte abnormalities.[14] Triggers of gastrointestinal losses include bacteria, viruses, drug reactions, toxins, and excessive use of laxatives and enemas.

Vomiting is usually preceded by nausea. Many clinical states have nausea and vomiting as common manifestations, but the precise mechanisms that trigger the vomiting reflex are poorly understood (see pp. 774–775). The main categories associated with nausea and vomiting are 1) acute abdominal emergencies, such as intestinal obstruction of appendicitis; 2) chronic indigestion, such as ulcer disease or food intolerance; 3) acute systemic infections of viral, bacterial, or parasitic nature; 4) central nervous system disorders associated with increased intracranial pressure or inner ear disorders; 5) acute myocardial infarction or congestive heart failure; 6) endocrine disorders, such as diabetic ketoacidosis; 7) side effects of drugs and chemicals; and 8) psychogenic vomiting due to stress of psychic disturbances.[7]

Vomiting and diarrhea often are components of an acute disease condition, such as viral or bacterial infection. Vomiting may be the primary symptom, or vomiting and diarrhea may be seen. The process may be accompanied by elevated body temperature, achy joints, and shaking chills. The condition may be self-limiting, or it may require fluid, electrolyte, and antibiotic therapy. At high risk are elderly persons and young children, because they have less fluid in reserve and can suffer rapid depletion of fluid and electrolyte balance.

Diarrhea can be classified as *osmotic, secretory*, or of *mixed origin* (Box 41-2). Osmotic diarrhea occurs when there is a poorly absorbable solute in the alimentary tract. It contains large quantities of water and potassium. Copious osmotic diarrhea can lead to rapid fluid and potassium depletion. Secretory diarrhea results when the normal secretory processes are stimulated and electrolytes and water are not absorbed. Depletion of electrolytes, including sodium, bicarbonate, and potassium, occurs along with the water loss. Diarrhea of mixed origin may be due to rapid intestinal transit, and the underlying cause may be difficult to identify.[8]

ENTERITIS

Enteritis, or *gastroenteritis*, is an inflammatory process of the stomach or small intestine caused by viruses, bacteria, or allergic reactions. It may be caused by the ingestion of contaminated food, especially food contaminated by staphylococci, which produce a toxin that reacts with the small intestine mucosa. Dysentery caused by bacteria affects the colon. The pathologic process has varying

BOX 41-1 ▼ *Causes of Malabsorption*

Incomplete Digestion of Nutrients
   Primary—deficient production of pancreatic enzymes
      Chronic relapsing pancreatitis
      Cancer of the pancreas
      Cystic fibrosis
      Extensive pancreatic resection
   Secondary—defective use of pancreatic enzymes
      Post-Billroth II
      Zollinger–Ellison syndrome

   Deficiency of Conjugated Bile Salts
      Severe liver disease
      Extrahepatic biliary tract obstruction

   Abnormal Loss of Nutrients or Bile Salts
      Ileal resection
      Ileectomy
      Ileal bypass
      Severe disease of the terminal ileum

   Abnormal Bacterial Overgrowth in the Small Bowel
      Surgically created blind loops
      Fistulas—enteroenteric, enterocolic, gastrojejunocolic
      Chronic intestinal obstruction due to adhesions or strictures
      Small bowel diverticula
      Motor abnormalities except scleroderma

   Drug-induced Precipitation or Sequestration
      Neomycin
      Calcium carbonate
      Cholestyramine

   Inadequate Mechanical Mixing of Chyme with Digestive Enzymes
      Post-Billroth II
      Post-total gastrectomy

Abnormalities of the Absorptive Surface
   Biochemical or genetic
      Disaccharidase deficiency
      Abetalipoproteinemia
      Primary vitamin B_{12} malabsorption
      Cystinuria
      Hartnup disease
      Celiac sprue
   Inflammatory or infective disorders
      Tropical sprue
      Regional enteritis
      Eosinophilic enteritis
      Infectious enteritis

Lack of Absorptive Surface
   Intestinal resection
   Gastroileostomy

Lymphatic Obstruction
   Whipple's disease
   Intestinal lymphangiectasia
   Lymphoma

Cardiovascular Disorders
   Mesenteric vascular insufficiency
   Congestive heart failure
   Constrictive pericarditis

Endocrine and Metabolic Disorders
   Diabetes mellitus

Hypoparathyroidism

Adrenal insufficiency

Hyperthyroidism

Carcinoid syndrome

(Summarized from Greenberger, N.J. and Isselbacher, K.J. Disorders of absorption. In J.D. Wilson et al., *Harrison's Principles of Internal Medicine* [12th ed.]. New York: McGraw-Hill, 1991.)

TABLE 41-2 *Laboratory Tests Specific to the Detection of Malabsorption*

Test	Normal Finding	Meaning of Abnormal Findings
Fecal fat balance: quantitative determination of stool fat	5 g (or fewer) of fatty acids extracted from stool in 24 hours	More than 6 g/24 hours—clinically significant steatorrhea
D-xylose tolerance test	4 g (or more) D-xylose excreted by kidneys in 5 hours; or 25 mg (or more) D-xylose/dL of blood in 1–2 hours	Decreased values in diseases of intestinal mucosa and in intestinal stasis; values normal in pancreatic insufficiency
Schilling test	Greater than 7% of radioactive vitamin B_{12} excreted in urine/24 hours	Decreased value can indicate lack of intrinsic factor, or malabsorption of ileum
With administration of intrinsic factor		Pernicious anemia abnormal 1st stage, normal 2nd stage. Malabsorption will have abnormal 1st and 2nd stage.

BOX 41-2 ▼ *Classification and Causes of Diarrhea*

Osmotic Diarrhea

Surgical

Gastric: rapid gastric emptying; pyloroplasty; gastroenterostomy; antrectomy

Intestinal: resection or bypass of jejunum and proximal ileum

Disease with histopathologic lesions

Mucosal: celiac (nontropical) sprue, collagenous sprue; tropical sprue; dermatitis herpetiformis and other cutaneous diseases; nutritional (protein calorie malnutrition or *kwashiorkor*; marasmus)

Submucosal (obstructive): Whipple's disease; lymphoma; intestinal lymphangiectasia; amyloidosis

Inflammatory: granulomatous enterocolitis; ulcerative colitis

Infectious or parasitic disease: postgastroenteritis; *Giardia lamblia*; coccidia; *Endolimax nana*; *Strongyloides stercoralis*; *Capillaria philippinensis*

Biochemical mucosal disease

Membrane digestive defects: lactase deficiency (alactasia, congenital lactose intolerance with lactosuria, prematurity, diarrhea of breastfed newborns, adult primary lactase deficiency); sucrase-isomaltase deficiency; sucrase deficiency; enterokinase deficiency

Membrane transport defects: glucose-galactose malabsorption; congenital chloridorrhea

Immune deficiency states

Specific immunoglobulin deficiency: IgA deficiency with normal villi; IgA deficiency with celiac sprue type flat mucosa; IgA deficiency with ataxia-telangiectasia; IgA and IgM deficiency with nodular lymphoid hyperplasia

General immunoglobulin deficiency (acquired): decreased IgA, IgM, IgG

Immunoglobulin metabolism abnormality: IgA heavy-chain disease

Drug-induced

Osmotic cathartics: sorbitol, lactulose; sodium sulfate purge; antacids

Other: colchicine; neomycin; para-aminosalicylic acid; phenformin; lincomycin; tetracycline

Secretory Diarrhea

Exogenous: enteric infections

Toxigenic diarrhea: *Vibriocholerae*; *Escherichia coli* strains; *Shigella dysenteriae I*; *Staphylococcus aureus* strains; *Clostridium perfringens*; *Pseudomonas aeruginosa*

Invasive diarrhea: shigella strains; salmonella strains; *Escherichia coli* strains; *Entamoeba histolytica*

Endogenous

Secretagogues and inhibitors of absorption

Deconjugated and dehydroxylated bile salts

Acting on small intestine and colon: bacterial overgrowth; surgical (vagotomy-pyloroplasty; intestinal blind loop); anatomic defects (small bowel diverticula; stricture; fistula; blind loop); inflammatory bowel disease; hypomotility (diabetic autonomic neuropathy; scleroderma; submucosal disease)

Acting on colon: surgical (ileal resection; ileal bypass); inflammatory bowel disease involving distal ileum

Hydroxy fatty acids, steatorrhea

Surgical: post-gastric surgery

Pancreatic insufficiency

Small intestinal mucosal disease

Methionine malabsorption (metabolized to hydroxybutyrate)

Neoplasms: villous adenoma; ganglioneuroma; medullary carcinoma of the thyroid; pancreatic islet cell tumors (Zollinger–Ellison syndrome, watery diarrhea hypokalemia achlorhydria syndrome)

Defective electrolyte transport: colectomy

Diarrhea of Mixed Origin

Hypermotility

Exogenous: cholinergic drugs

Endogenous: hypocalcemia; hyperthyroidism; hypoadrenalism; hypopituitarism; carcinoid syndrome

(N.J. Greenberger. *Gastrointestinal Disorders: A Pathophysiologic Approach* [3rd ed.]. Chicago: Yearbook, 1986.)

---

manifestations that result in abdominal cramping, diarrhea, and vomiting.

A fluid and electrolyte imbalance often results from enteritis. Parasites may localize in the gastrointestinal tract or invade the circulation. Eosinophilic enteritis is uncommon but may result from an allergy. It is manifested by the accumulation of eosinophils in the gut wall.[24] In general, enteritis causes inflammatory changes in the intestinal mucosa that return to normal when the precipitator is removed.

MALABSORPTION

Causes of Malabsorption

Malabsorption can occur in the luminal or the intestinal phase of transport through the small intestine. Virtually all nutrients are absorbed in the small intestine, thus malabsorption syndromes are those affecting this area. The luminal phase consists of those processes that alter nutrients so that they can be absorbed. Examples include changes by pancreatic enzymes and secretion and the changes promoted by biliary secretions. The intestinal phase includes those processes involved in transport of nutrients through the intestinal wall.[19] Malabsorption may involve a single specific nutrient, such as vitamin B_{12}, or it may involve several or all major nutrient classes. Generalized malabsorption leads to weight loss, malnutrition, and the cachectic state.[19]

Celiac Enteropathy (Nontropical Sprue)

Celiac enteropathy has many names and is thought to be related to gluten intolerance. It occurs more often in women than in men, and the onset of symptoms usually occurs in young adulthood.

Histopathologic changes in the absorptive surface in response to exposure to the protein gluten or its break-down products, found mostly in wheat, are responsible for the manifestations of a general malabsorption syndrome. The mechanism underlying this reaction is unknown, but the data support a hypersensitivity reaction to gluten and its derivative, gliadin.[3]

Gluten proteins have been shown to have antigenic properties, and circulating antibodies to dietary gluten have been demonstrated in persons with active celiac enteropathy. The lamina propria of affected mucosa contains mononuclear leukocytes and plasma cells. In some cases, serum levels of IgA are elevated and levels of IgM are depressed. Antibodies cannot be demonstrated in all cases, however, and there is a poor correlation between antibody levels and disease severity.[3] Corticosteroid therapy has been shown to improve intestinal absorption and histologic appearance.

Regardless of cause, the pathologic changes are characteristic. The villi are flattened or absent, and the epithelium is disorganized and consists of cuboidal rather than the normal columnar cells. The brush border is thickened, and the lamina propria is infiltrated with inflammatory cells. Cytoplasmic changes include membrane disruption and rounded mitochondria. All of these changes result in malabsorption, with impaired uptake and transport of nutrients.[2, 19]

Clinical features may include frequent, foul-smelling, steatorrheic stools (ie, the stools have a fatty or greasy appearance). Loss of body weight and malabsorption of fat-soluble vitamins are common. Severe muscle-wasting and hypoproteinemia may occur. The condition is most commonly diagnosed first in children who fail to thrive.

Treatment measures support the theory of gluten hypersensitivity, because a dramatic or delayed remission of symptoms occurs when barley, wheat, rye, and oats are removed from the diet. Restoration of the normal mucosal epithelium occurs, and malabsorption decreases.

Tropical Sprue

Tropical sprue differs in etiology from celiac enteropathy but is usually characterized by identical mucosal changes in the small intestine. It probably results from nutritional and bacterial alterations and occurs with the greatest frequency in certain tropical areas. It may be caused by *Escherichia coli* bacteria. Symptoms may not arise for months or years after exposure.[3] Because the mucosal lesions result in malabsorption, the clinical picture closely resembles that of celiac enteropathy. Treatment with folic acid is restorative in some cases, and antibiotics may be helpful.

REGIONAL ENTERITIS: CROHN DISEASE

Crohn disease is an idiopathic, chronic, inflammatory bowel disease that may affect any segment of the gastrointestinal tract, although it most commonly affects the terminal ileum or colon.[3] The frequency of this chronic inflammatory disease is equal in men and women, is higher in members of the Jewish race, and exhibits a familial predisposition. Onset is most common between the ages of 15 and 20, with a secondary peak between 55 and 60 years. It is much more common in the United States, Britain, and Scandinavia than in Japan, Russia, and South America.[3] Crohn disease and ulcerative colitis have many etiologic similarities and commonly are grouped as *inflammatory bowel disease*. The origins may be infectious, immunologic, psychosomatic, dietary, hormonal, or unknown. Viruses and specific bacteria, such as *Pseudomonas* and atypical mycobacteria, are possible causative factors. The immunologic features of the diseases may be a primary or secondary response to a viral organism.[3] Ulcerative colitis is described in more detail on page 799.

Gross inspection of the affected bowel discloses shallow, longitudinal mucosal ulcers; long or short areas of stricture; and a cobblestone appearance of the mucosa (Fig. 41-7). The cobblestone appearance results from interconnecting fissures that cut deeply into the intestinal wall and create islands of mucosa elevated by the existing transmural (full-wall thickness) inflammation and its accompanying edema. The bowel wall becomes congested, thickened, and rigid, with adhesions involving the peri-intestinal fat.[14] Areas of involvement are localized and interrupted by areas of normal gut. Several segments of bowel are affected and often are separated by normal bowel. These segments are called *skip lesions* and produce chronic partial intestinal obstruction.[19] Fistulas to other parts of the gastrointestinal tract or other adjacent structures may be present.

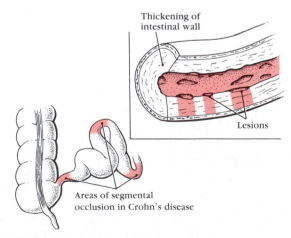

FIGURE 41-7 *Crohn disease showing segmental areas of occlusion and transmural involvement of intestinal wall.*

Microscopically, all layers of the intestinal wall, particularly the submucosa, are edematous and infiltrated with aggregations of lymphocytes and macrophages.[3] Characteristic noncaseating granulomas, which have large mononuclear phagocytes and multinucleated giant cells, form in the bowel wall and often are present in the regional lymph nodes. Dilated lymphatic channels and lymphoid deposits occur at all levels of bowel involvement. The inflammatory changes cause functional disruption of the mucosa, producing malabsorption, especially of bile salts and vitamin B_{12}, which are normally absorbed in the jejunum and ileum. Fluid imbalances occur when large segments of ileum are affected. The strictures and fistulas that occur with this disease predispose the intestine to bacterial overgrowth and abscess formation. Bowel obstruction and peritonitis may result from the strictures and abscesses (Fig. 41-8).

The clinical manifestations of Crohn disease vary. Diarrhea is a dominant symptom and is often accompanied by fever and right lower quadrant or abdominal pain. The apparent linkage with stress and personality factors has been studied extensively, with depression and dependency being seen as typical personality traits. The symptoms usually begin with insidious onset of malaise and diarrhea. As the disease progresses, weight loss, occult blood in the feces, and nausea and vomiting occur. When involvement is diffuse, major features may

be malabsorption and malnutrition. Intestinal obstruction and fistulas develop in 10% to 15% of cases, and peritonitis may result from rupture of the fistulous connection. A significant correlation of this disease with several autoimmune diseases and with adenocarcinoma of the small bowel exists. Chronic debilitation may finally require bowel resection.

Diagnosis of regional enteritis is based on the clinical history, physical examination (which may reveal a right lower quadrant mass), and radiographic results showing a characteristic narrowing, which is called the string sign.

▼ Alterations in the Large Intestine

ADYNAMIC OR PARALYTIC ILEUS

The word *ileus* has come to refer to a functional obstruction of the bowel. It may occur in the small or large intestine and is often classified as physiologic or paralytic. Lack of propulsive peristalsis makes the bowel unable to move contents downward, which leads to absence of bowel sounds and bowel distention.

Peristalsis becomes diminished or absent due in part to a triggering of the sympathetic inhibitory reflex by a noxious stimulus, such as anesthesia, any peritoneal injury, interruption of nerve supply, abdominal injury or surgical manipulation, intestinal ischemia, electrolyte (especially potassium) disturbances, or retroperitoneal pathology.[16] A true ileus can be described as *adynamic*, having absent propulsive motor activity.[19]

The result of ileus is distention of the bowel with gas and fluid. The process is similar to actual bowel obstruction. Colonic bacteria may contribute to the abdominal distention and cause marked alterations of fluid and electrolyte balance. Loss of potassium leads to further intestinal atony. Vomiting and hypotension can cause alteration in the acid–base balance. As fluid shifts to the intestinal area, central blood volume decreases and distention increases.[16] If there is associated mesenteric ischemia, necrosis and rupture of the bowel may occur, causing peritonitis. Clinical findings include abdominal distention, decreased or absent bowel sounds, and signs of dehydration and shock. Symptoms are those of a rapidly progressive colonic obstruction with perforation of the bowel if the individual is not treated by colonoscopic deflation (through an intestinal drainage tube) or surgery.[17]

INTESTINAL ISCHEMIA AND INFARCTION

Intestinal ischemia occurs when tissue demand for oxygen exceeds the supply and toxic metabolites accumulate. Ischemia is particularly prevalent in highly vascular systems, such as the mesentery, which supplies the in-

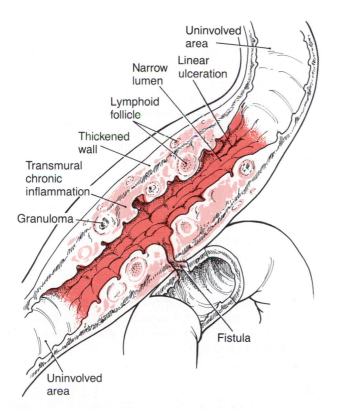

FIGURE 41-8 *Crohn disease. A schematic representation of the major features of Crohn disease in the small intestine.*

Uninvolved area

Linear ulceration

Narrow lumen

Lymphoid follicle

Thickened wall

Transmural chronic inflammation

Granuloma

Fistula

Uninvolved area

testines. Intestinal ischemia can result from any condition that interferes with blood supply to the mesentery (Fig. 41-9). *Occlusive intestinal infarction* usually results from occlusion of the superior mesenteric artery by an embolus or a thrombus. It can also result from inferior mesenteric artery or venous thrombosis. *Nonocclusive intestinal infarction* may result from severe shock, in which blood is shunted away from the mesentery to other vital organs. *Chronic intestinal ischemia* may be produced by atherosclerosis of the superior mesenteric artery, which can produce abdominal angina, especially after eating. Ischemia may lead to patchy areas of infarction. If ischemia or infarction is prolonged, the following events occur in the intestine: 1) the epithelial cells in the intestinal villi detach from the basement membrane; 2) subepithelial blebs of tissue protrude in the villi and, after an hour of continuous oxygen deprivation, the villi have no viable epithelial surface; 3) absorption and processing of nutrients is impaired; 4) the mucosal layer becomes necrotic and is shed into the stool as bloody diarrhea; 5) perforation of the intestine is promoted, leading to peritonitis; and 6) because the mucosal barrier is lost, intestinal bacteria can enter the bloodstream and cause bacteremia.

Symptoms of intestinal ischemia and infarction vary with the area affected and length of time of deprivation. Atherosclerotic ischemia may create an angina-like, cramping, abdominal pain that worsens after meals and then dissipates. Vasospasm and emboli produce an acute, severe abdominal pain with associated vomiting or diarrhea or both. Abdominal distention and tenderness are usually present. Bowel sounds may initially be loud and high-pitched (*borborygmi*) from an increase in rate and force of peristalsis. Hypotension may occur due to displacement of intravascular volume into the intestinal lumen. Prompt diagnosis can prevent shock, peritonitis, or sepsis. Surgery and antibiotics can help salvage the area of intestinal damage.[10]

INTESTINAL OBSTRUCTION

Intestinal obstruction is blockage of the lumen of the bowel by an actual mechanical obstruction. Figure 41-10 illustrates some of the causes, which include volvulus, adhesions, intussusception, hernias, infarction, and neoplasms.

After blockage occurs, gas and air are the primary bowel distenders, and distention occurs proximal to the area of blockage. As the process continues, gastric, biliary, and pancreatic secretions pool. Water, electrolytes, and serum proteins also begin to accumulate in the area. Pooling and bowel distention decrease the circulating blood volume due to a *third-space shift* that moves water into the area proximal to the obstruction and thus decreases plasma volume. Bowel wall edema also interferes with the blood supply to the bowel tissue and depresses normal sodium transport in the mucosa (Fig. 41-11).

Strangulation of a bowel segment may cause necrosis, perforation, and loss of fluid and blood into the inactive bowel. Impairment of blood supply leads at first to increased peristalsis and bacterial invasion of the tissue and finally causes necrosis and peritonitis when intestinal contents are released into the peritoneal cavity. Stasis of the intestinal contents provides an area for increased growth of organisms, with toxins being released into the tissues, further disrupting the intestinal cellular dynamics. Loss of fluids and electrolytes is a major problem and results in decreased systemic circulating fluid volume due to the shift from the vascular to the intestinal lumen. Sepsis and septic shock may result from the release of intestinal gram-negative organisms into the vascular system.

Clinical manifestations include the acute onset of severe, cramping pain that correlates roughly to the area or level of obstruction. Pain may decrease in severity as the distention of the bowel and abdomen increases, which is probably due to impaired motility in the edematous intestine. Increases in the rate and force of peristalsis cause borborygmi in the early period, but these may progress to a silent bowel as the condition persists. Vomiting is almost always present and may be bilious or feculent (having the appearance of feces), depending on the level of the obstruction. Diarrhea may occur if obstruction is not complete.

Hypovolemic shock is the result of a shift of fluid greater than 10% of body weight. Septicemic shock may also result from contamination of the peritoneum when the bowel ruptures. Sepsis and hypovolemic shock produce a life-threatening clinical picture that must be treated aggressively.

Tenderness, rigidity, and fever usually indicate peritonitis. Leukocytosis and elevation of serum amylase level are also common. Distention of the bowel may be noted radiologically, but is not conclusive evidence of the cause or exact level of obstruction.

HERNIAS

A *hernia* is a defect in the abdominal wall. It may occur in the scrotal or inguinal area or in the abdominal wall or diaphragm (Fig. 41-12). Incisional hernias occur in an

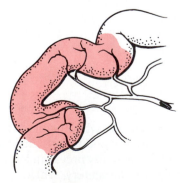

FIGURE 41-9 *Mesenteric occlusion causing intestinal ischemia.*

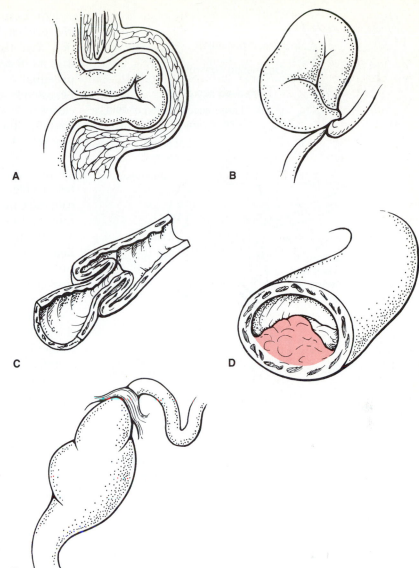

FIGURE 41-10 *Major causes of actual intestinal obstruction.* **A.** *Hernia.* **B.** *Volvulus.* **C.** *Intussusception.* **D.** *Neoplasm.* **E.** *Adhesions.*

area weakened by surgical incision. Whatever the cause, the defect allows abdominal structures (eg, peritoneum, fat, bowel, or bladder) to fill the area, producing a sac filled with the material. Abdominal contents usually move into the defect when abdominal pressure increases. If the bulging of the sac is intermittent, the hernia is called *reducible*. *Incarcerated hernias* contain abdominal contents all the time, and *strangulated hernias* cause necrosis of the abdominal contents due to lack of blood supply. Necrosis of the bowel then leads to all the clinical manifestations of intestinal obstruction.

HIRSCHSPRUNG'S DISEASE

Hirschsprung's disease, also called *congenital megacolon*, is usually manifested in early infancy and is caused by congenital absence of parasympathetic ganglion cells in the submucosal and intramuscular plexuses of one or more segments of the colon. The entire colon and even parts of the small intestine are occasionally involved. When the colon is involved, the bowel becomes greatly dilated, with no peristaltic action in the aganglionic area.

Hirschsprung's disease is a congenital disorder with much higher frequency in boys than in girls. It is associated with other congenital conditions, such as *Down syndrome*. When manifested in early infancy, abdominal distention, constipation, and vomiting occur. Occasionally, this condition is diagnosed in young adults who describe a lifelong problem with constipation.

Megacolon, or enlargement of the colon, may also be produced by any process that inhibits bowel evacuation. Among such processes are psychogenic megacolon, which results from ignoring the urge to defecate, some neurologic disorders, fecal impaction, or chronic depression. The clinical manifestations depend on the degree of aganglionosis or bowel distention. The person is often poorly nourished and anemic and rarely produces fecal material.

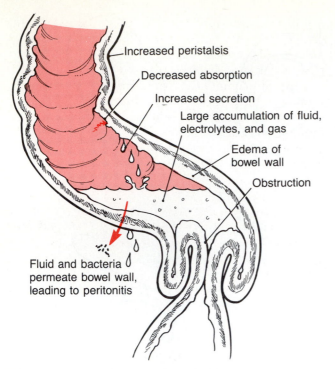

FIGURE 41-11 *Pathophysiology of intestinal obstruction causing peritonitis.*

DIVERTICULAR DISEASE

Diverticula are multiple saclike protrusions of the mucosa along the gastrointestinal tract. Although the terms are loosely used, a *true diverticulum* has all layers of the bowel in its walls, whereas a *false diverticulum* occurs in a weak area of the muscularis of the bowel.

An example of true diverticular disease is *Meckel's diverticulum*, which occurs in 1% to 2% of the population. Two thirds of affected persons are younger than 2 years of age. The diverticular sac, located 1 to 3 feet proximal to the ileocecal junction, is formed by the persistence of a mesenteric structure that normally closes in fetal life. It may be lined with ileal mucosa or contain other types of gastrointestinal mucosal cells. Meckel's diverticulum is usually asymptomatic, but it may cause symptoms that mimic acute appendicitis, Crohn disease, or pelvic inflammatory disease. Gastrointestinal bleeding and intestinal obstruction may complicate the condition.[6,19] False colonic diverticula are common and usually occur in the sigmoid colon.

Because of their frequency in elderly persons, diverticula are thought to be related to the blood supply or nutrition of the bowel in the elderly.[3] Lack of dietary fiber or roughage and decreased fecal bulk also have been correlated with this process.[19]

Diverticulosis refers to the presence of diverticula in the colon that are rarely symptomatic. *Diverticulitis* is inflammation in or around a diverticular sac that results in retention of undigested food and bacteria in the sac. This forms a hard mass called a *fecalith*.[15] Colonic obstruction, fistulas, and abscesses can result. Rupture of the infected material into the peritoneal cavity may lead to peritonitis.

The clinical manifestations of symptomatic diverticular disease vary. Eighty percent of affected persons have no symptoms. Constipation is reported frequently. Fibrosis in the area may develop and cause obstruction by adhesions. The complaint of lower left-sided abdominal pain may be associated with the signs of peritonitis,

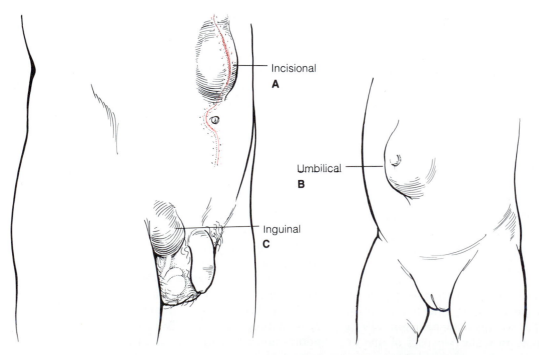

FIGURE 41-12 *Types of hernias.* **A.** *Incisional hernia.* **B.** *Inguinal hernia.* **C.** *Umbilical hernia.*

including guarding, fever, abdominal rigidity, and rebound tenderness. Radiographs and sigmoidoscopy may not indicate the extent of the problem. Surgery may be performed if the process causes obstruction or perforation.

HEMORRHOIDS

Hemorrhoids are dilatations of the venous plexus that surround the rectal and anal areas. These dilatations are very common and develop in susceptible persons due to persistently increased pressure in the hemorrhoidal venous plexus. Hemorrhoids are often related to other types of abnormalities, especially varicose veins. Predisposition may result from constipation or pregnancy. Bleeding hemorrhoids may be a dangerous outcome of portal hypertension (see pp. 820–822).

The dilated venous sacs protrude into the anal and rectal canals, where they become exposed; thromboses, ulcerations, and bleeding then develop. Hemorrhoids may be painful and irritating. Bright red bleeding during defecation or with increased intraabdominal pressure is common. Blood loss is usually insignificant, but chronic anemia may result. Bleeding in association with portal hypertension may be profound and even life-threatening.[12]

ULCERATIVE COLITIS

Ulcerative colitis is primarily an inflammatory disease of the mucous membrane of the colon. The disease may be confined to the rectum, or it may affect segments of the colon or even the entire colon. The bowel fills with a bloody, mucoid secretion that produces a characteristic cramping pain, rectal urgency, and diarrhea.

Pathologically, ulcerative colitis usually begins in the rectal area and extends along the colon. Microscopic inflammatory ulcerated areas may be adjacent to healing areas, but the process is continuous, without the skip lesions characteristic of Crohn disease.[3] In the *acute phase*, the colon mucosa is hyperemic and edematous, and the usual secretions are absent. Small mucosal hemorrhages are evident, and abscesses form into small ulcerations. The mucosa tends to slough off and is lost in the feces. The ulcerations are confined to the mucosa and submucosa, and coalescence of the ulcers can denude large areas of the involved colon.[3] As the disease enters the *chronic phase*, the ulcerations become fibrotic, and thickening of the bowel wall results. Obstruction of the bowel rarely occurs from the fibrous thickening.[9]

Complications of ulcerative colitis include intestinal obstruction, dehydration, and major fluid and electrolyte imbalances. Malabsorption is common, and loss of blood in the stools may cause chronic iron-deficiency anemia. There is a significant relationship between ulcerative colitis and cancer of the colon. Ten percent to 15% of persons who have ulcerative colitis for more than 10 years will develop colon carcinoma.

The etiology of ulcerative colitis is unknown, but a genetic basis has been suggested, because the disease occurs with increased frequency in some families. Its peak occurrence is between ages 15 and 35, and it is much more common in whites than in other races.[9] Agents such as viruses and microorganisms are implicated, and the disease may be associated with autoimmunity. The plasma serum in some persons with the disease has been shown to have an antibody to the colonic epithelial cells. Remissions and exacerbations are common and often can be directly related to major psychological stresses.[9] About 70% of affected persons have complete remissions between attacks, some of which may last for long periods. Approximately 20% have continuous symptoms without remission.[19] Many of the etiologic factors of Crohn disease are also common in ulcerative colitis.

Clinical manifestations vary. The classic symptoms include cramping abdominal pain, bloody diarrhea, fever, and weight loss. Laboratory findings include anemia, leukocytosis, hypoalbuminemia, electrolyte imbalance, and increased serum alkaline phosphatase levels. Despite their evident pathologic differences, ulcerative colitis and regional enteritis may be confused clinically. Table 41-3 shows the major differences between them.

Diagnosis of ulcerative colitis is made on the basis of the clinical features, results of barium enema, and sigmoidoscopic appearance of the mucosa. Biopsy and cultures are essential to exclude carcinoma and bacterial diarrhea.

TABLE 41-3 *Major Differences Between Ulcerative Colitis and Crohn Disease*

Lesion	Crohn Disease	Ulcerative Colitis
MACROSCOPIC		
Thickened bowel wall	Typical	Uncommon
Luminal narrowing	Typical	Uncommon
"Skip" lesions	Common	Absent
Right colon predominance	Typical	Absent
Fissures and fistulas	Common	Absent
Circumscribed ulcers	Common	Absent
Confluent linear ulcers	Common	Absent
Pseudopolyps	Absent	Common
MICROSCOPIC		
Transmural inflammation	Typical	Uncommon
Submucosal fibrosis	Typical	Absent
Fissures	Typical	Rare
Granulomas	Common	Absent
Crypt abscesses	Uncommon	Typical

(Rubin, E. and Farber., J.L. *Pathology* [2nd ed.]. Philadelphia: J.B. Lippincott, 1994.)

POLYPS

A *polyp* in the large intestine is a benign growth that protrudes into the lumen. Polyps are divided into two major categories, *adenomatous* and *hyperplastic*.

Adenomatous polyps are true neoplasms. The growths begin in the mucosa deep within the crypts of the colonic mucosal glands.[22] The polypoidal cells continue to divide and become hyperplastic growths. When reproductive control is lost throughout the mucosal crypt, a neoplasm results. Polyps are very common in the general population. They rarely exceed 5 mm in diameter. These growths may be discovered by routine sigmoidoscopy or barium enema. They may bleed, causing bright red feces. The major clinical significance of hyperplastic polyps is that they have the potential to become neoplastic or adenomatous. Adenomatous polyps may be benign or malignant, and it is difficult to determine the difference unless they have obviously invaded the surrounding mucosa. Smaller growths are called *tubular* or *glandular polyps*, and larger growths are called *villous adenomas*. Twenty-five percent to 50% of villous adenomas harbor carcinomas. These adenomas may be very large, up to 15 cm across.[19] Some researchers view the development as a sequence of events from controlled hyperplasia through a series of stages that terminate in carcinoma.[3] Polyps are usually surgically excised because they have such a close relationship with carcinoma of the colon.

COLORECTAL CARCINOMA

Colorectal carcinoma is second only to lung cancer in causes of death from cancer in the United States. When colon and rectal cancer are detected and treated in early localized stages, there is a 5-year survival rate of 80% to 90%.[1] Factors that predispose a person to colorectal cancer are heredity, fat intake, inflammatory bowel disease, homosexuality, and polyposis of the colon.[8] It is common in both men and women; it occurs at all ages, but the frequency is greatest during the fifth, sixth, and seventh decades. Prevalence is highest in northwest Europe and North America and lowest in South America, Africa, and Asia.

Investigations into causes of colorectal carcinoma have led to the study of animal fat in the diet, anaerobic bacteria of the large bowel, and fiber content of the diet.[7] Each of these factors may partially explain the disease's geographic distribution. The fiber aspect is interesting in that increased bulk in the diet decreases the transit time and also the time of contact between food and bowel. In

---

TABLE 41-4 *Recommendations for Lowering the Risk of Colon and Rectal Cancer*

Action	Mechanisms
1. Regular exercise	Increased intestinal motility
2. Lower total fat intake (20%–25% of calories)	Lower total bile acid and fatty acid flux with promoting and cytotoxic actions
3. Increase proportion of monounsaturated fats (olive oil, special rapeseed oils)	Lower total bile acid flux
4. Increase intake of fish and fish oils	Protective effect of omega-3 fatty acids (prostaglandin synthetases and metabolism)
5. Have optimal intake of bran cereals, whole grain bread, unrefined rice	Avoids constipation, nonneoplastic intestinal diseases antecedent to neoplasia. Optimal amount gives daily stool of about 200 g
6. Have optimal intake of yellow-green and *Brassica* vegetables (cauliflower, brussels sprouts, broccoli)	Specific mechanisms not clear; provides micronutrients and bulk, replacing harmful, more energy-dense foods
7. Have optimal intake of calcium-rich foods (some vegetables, but especially lowfat or nonfat yogurt or milk)	Controls intestinal cell duplication rates
8. Avoid excessive intake of alcoholic beverages	Lower cell turnover rates in rectum
9. Lower intake of highly fried or broiled, browned foods	Possible lower intake of intestine-specific carcinogens

(Frentzel-Beyme, R.R. *Colorectal Cancer.* Berlin: Springer–Verlag, 1989.)

the average American diet, the transit time may be as much as 4 to 5 days compared with 30 to 35 hours in black Africans. Because the American diet is much lower in fiber than the black African diet, colonic cancer is much more prevalent in America.[3] Based on the above observations, Table 41-4 lists nine recommendations for lowering the risk of colorectal cancer. These recommendations focus on ways to reduce production of carcinogens specific to the colon.

About 60% to 70% of these carcinomas arise in the rectum, rectosigmoid area, or sigmoid colon.[3] The type of growth depends on the area of origin. Left-sided carcinoma tends to grow around the bowel, encircling it and leading to early obstruction. On the right side, the tumors tend to be bulky, polypoid, fungating masses. The vast majority of these cancers are adenocarcinomas. Either type may penetrate the bowel and cause abscess, peritonitis, invasion of surrounding organs, or bleeding. These tumors tend to grow slowly, and they remain asymptomatic for long periods of time. Ninety-five percent of carcinomas of the colon are adenocarcinomas that secrete mucin, a substance that aids in extending the

malignancy.[3] Metastasis may occur to the liver, lungs, bones, or lymphatic system.

Clinical manifestations depend on the location of the tumor. The person may have melena, diarrhea, and constipation; these are the most frequent manifestations of left-sided lesions. Right-sided tumors often cause weakness, malaise, and weight loss. Pain is rare with either type and, if present, may result from contractions of the bowel related to partial obstruction of the colon or nerve involvement. The tumor mass is often palpated on physical examination. Obstruction of the bowel may be the first sign of the disease. Metastasis is quite predictable, with invasion of the lymphatic channels, peritoneum, and venous channels producing the spread. The common sites of distant metastasis are the lungs, bones, and brain.[19] At the time of diagnosis, some extension of the tumor often has occurred, but because this malignancy grows slowly, it is considered to be highly curable with early diagnosis and surgical treatment.

Diagnosis requires the standard techniques of proctoscopy, barium enema, radionucleotide scanning, and determination of levels of tumor antigens. Colon cancers

---

TABLE 41-5   *1987 AJCC/UICC Staging Classification of Colorectal Cancer*

PRIMARY TUMOR (T)

TX	Primary tumor cannot be assessed
T0	No evidence of tumor in resected specimen (prior polypectomy or fulguration)
Tis	Carcinoma in situ
T1	Invades submucosa
T2	Invades muscularis propria
T3–T4	Depends on whether serosa is present

Serosa present:

	T3	Invades through muscularis propria into Subserosa
		Serosa (but not through)
		Pericolic fat within the leaves of the mesentery
	T4	Invades through serosa into free peritoneal cavity or through serosa into a contiguous organ

No serosa (distal two thirds rectum, posterior left or right colon):

	T3	Invades through muscularis propria
	T4	Invades other organs (vagina, prostate, ureter, kidney)

REGIONAL LYMPH NODES (N)

NX	Nodes cannot be assessed (*e.g.*, local excision only)
N0	No regional node metastases
N1	1–3 positive nodes
N2	4 or more positive nodes
N3	Central nodes positive

DISTANT METASTASES (M)

MX	Presence of distant metastases cannot be assessed
M0	No distant metastases
M1	Distant metastases present

DUKES STAGING SYSTEM CORRELATED WITH TNM

Dukes' A =	T1N0M0
	T2N0M0
Dukes' B =	T3N0M0
	T4N0M0
Dukes' C =	T(any)N1M0, T(any)N2M0
Dukes' C2 =	T(any)N3M0
Dukes' D =	T(any)N(any)M1

MODIFIED ASTLER-COLLER (MAC) SYSTEM CORRELATED WITH TNM

MAC A =	T1N0M0
MAC B1 =	T2N0M0
MAC B2 =	T3N0M0, T4N0M0
MAC B3 =	T4N0M0
MAC C1 =	T2N1M0, T2N2M0
MAC C2 =	T3N1M0, T3N2M0
	T4N1M0, T4N2M0
MAC C3 =	T4N1M0, T4N2M0

Note: In all pathologic staging systems, particularly those applied to rectal cancer, the abbreviations (m) and (g) may be used: (m) denotes microscopic transmural penetration; (g) or (m + g) denotes transmural penetration visible on gross inspection and confirmed microscopically.

(Modified from American Joint Committee on Cancer. *Manual for staging of cancer* (3rd ed.). Philadelphia: JB Lippincott, 1988; and from Union Internationale Contre le Cancer. *TNM Classification of Malignant Tumors* (4th ed.). Geneva: UICC, 1987)

(Source: DeVita, V.T., Hellman, S., Rosenberg, S.A. *Cancer: Principles and Practice of Oncology* [4th ed.]. Philadelphia: J.B. Lippincott, 1993.)

produce a wide variety of tumor antigens, carcinoembryonic antigen (CEA) being the most well known. The test for CEA is positive in nearly all cases with widespread metastases. The usefulness of the CEA test is being evaluated, because normal levels do not rule out malignancy; however, it can gauge the effectiveness of therapy. Unfortunately, elevated levels are consistently positive only in advanced cancers, and this makes the test's usefulness in screening for colon cancer almost ineffective. "Normal" levels of CEA are less than 2.5 ng/mL, but they may be elevated in nonmalignant inflammatory disease, especially of the gastrointestinal tract.

Prognosis with colorectal carcinoma depends on the extent of bowel involvement, the presence or absence of spread, differentiation of the lesion, and the location of the lesion within the colon. A popular staging system is that of modified Astler and Coller, which uses the following criteria:

Stage A: Tumor confined to the mucosa
Stage B1: Tumor invading the muscularis propria but not penetrating to the serosa
Stage B2: Tumor invading the serosa without lymph node metastases
Stage C1: B1 tumors with metastases to regional lymph nodes
Stage C2: B2 tumors with metastases to regional lymph nodes
Stage D: Distant metastases[19]

Table 41-5 shows the American Joint Committee on Cancer and the Union Internationale Contre le Cancer staging classification of colorectal cancer.

CASE STUDY 41-1

Mr James Fry is a 68-year-old caucasian male who is undergoing evaluation for melena, diarrhea, and constipation. A questionable mass was palpated in the left lower quadrant by the examining physician. Proctoscopy revealed a polypoid lesion which was biopsied and pathology reported carcinoma of the colon. Barium enema showed significant obstruction in the descending portion of the colon. CEA levels were tested and were shown to be 860 ng/mL.

1. *From the symptoms and diagnostic tests, what type of colon cancer does Mr. Frye have?*
2. *What is the significance of the CEA levels?*
3. *When these cancers metastasize, what is the common route for the spread?*
4. *According to the Astler and Coller staging system, what could be the stage for Mr. Fry?*
5. *What are the risk factors for developing cancer of the colon? List at least six recommendations for lowering the risk of developing this type of cancer.*

See Appendix G for discussion.

▼ Chapter Summary

▼   Diseases of the gastrointestinal system include alterations from the oral cavity, esophagus, stomach, and small and large intestines. Some of these are the most common maladies of humankind.

▼   Esophageal alterations include those of motility, spasm, reflux, carcinoma, and structural problems. Reflux of gastric contents causes esophagitis and is common with spasm and hiatal hernia. Esophageal varices are dangerous outpouchings of the esophageal veins into the esophageal lumen and are seen with portal hypertension.

▼   Stomach problems can be temporary gastritis or ulcerative conditions, such as peptic ulcer disease, which may be gastric or duodenal in location. These conditions have characteristic pain patterns and complications. Gastric carcinomas are declining in incidence and have a poor prognosis.

▼   Small intestine disorders may include vomiting or diarrhea, volume depletion, and electrolyte disorders. Malabsorption is a common component and causes nutritional deficits, because virtually all of the nutrients are absorbed in the small intestine.

▼   Crohn disease is a chronic, inflammatory disease that may affect the small intestine. It causes severe diarrhea, weight loss, loss of blood in the feces, and malabsorption, leading finally to chronic debilitation.

▼   Large intestine dysfunction can be functional or pathologic. Functional obstruction of the bowel is due to lack of propulsive peristalsis and is called paralytic ileus. It may be due to intestinal ischemia, nerve supply alteration, or other conditions. Ileus may lead to ischemia and infarction of the bowel, or this may be produced by occlusion of the blood supply to an area of the bowel. Intestinal obstruction refers to mechanical blockage of the lumen of the bowel.

▼   Hernias often affect the large intestine and result when a defect in the abdominal wall allows abdominal structures to fill a sac produced by the defect.

▼   Other common problems of the large intestine are diverticuli, hemorrhoids, polyps, and ulcerative colitis. Ulcerative colitis is often compared to Crohn disease, but the pathology of the conditions is quite different, even though the etiologic factors may be similar.

▼   Colorectal carcinoma is a very common carcinoma and usually occurs after age 50. Many factors increase the risk, but the prognosis is good if the tumor is diagnosed in the early stages.

▼ References

1. *Cancer Facts and Figures, 1990.* New York: American Cancer Society, 1989.
2. Castell, D.O. Diseases of the esophagus. In W.N. Kelley, et

al (eds.), *Textbook of Internal Medicine* (2nd ed.). Philadelphia: J.B. Lippincott, 1992.

3. Cotran, R.S., Kumar, V., and Robbins, S.L. *Robbins' Pathologic Basis of Disease* (5th ed.). Philadelphia: W.B. Saunders, 1994.

4. DeVita, V.T., et al. *Cancer: Principles and Practice of Oncology* (4th ed.). Philadelphia: J.B. Lippincott, 1993.

5. Eastwood, G.L. Gastritis and other gastric diseases. In J.H. Stein (ed.), *Internal Medicine* (4th ed.). St. Louis: C.V. Mosby, 1994.

6. Fenoglio-Preiser, C.M., Lantz, P.E., Listrom, M.B., Davis, M., and Rilke, F.O. *Gastrointestinal Pathology: An Atlas and Text*. New York: Raven Press, 1989.

7. Friedman, L.S., and Isselbacher, K.J. Anorexia, nausea and vomiting. In J.D. Wilson, et al. (eds.), *Harrison's Principles of Internal Medicine* (12th ed.). New York: McGraw-Hill, 1991.

8. Frentzel-Beyme, R.R. Acquired conditions of increased risk of colorectal cancer. In H.K. Seitz, U.A. Simanowski, and N.A. Wright (eds.), *Colorectal Cancer: From Pathogenesis to Prevention*. Berlin: Springer-Verlag, 1989.

9. Glickman, R.M. Inflammatory bowel disease. In J.D. Wilson, et al. (eds.), *Harrison's Principles of Internal Medicine* (12th ed.). New York: McGraw-Hill, 1991.

10. Gottlieb, J.E., Menashe, P.I., and Cruz, E. Gastrointestinal complications in critically ill patients. *Am. J. Gastroenterology* 81:4, 1986.

11. Greenberger, N.J. *Gastrointestinal Disorders: A Pathophysiologic Approach* (3rd ed.). Chicago: Yearbook, 1986.

12. Grozmann, I. Portal hypertension. In I.M. Arias, W.B. Jacoby, A. Popper, D. Schachter, and D.A. Shafritz (eds.), *The Liver: Biology and Pathobiology* (2nd ed.). New York: Raven Press, 1988.

13. Hamilton, S.R. Diseases of the esophagus. In H. Goldman, H.D. Appelman, and W. Kaufman, (eds.), *Gastrointestinal Pathology*. Baltimore: Williams & Wilkins, 1988.

14. Kissane, J.M. *Anderson's Pathology* (9th ed.). St. Louis: C.V. Mosby, 1991.

15. LaMont, J.T., and Isselbacher, K.J. Disease of the small and large intestine. In J.D. Wilson, et al. (eds.), *Harrison's Principles of Internal Medicine* (12th ed.). New York: McGraw-Hill, 1991.

16. Livingston, E.H., and Passaro, E.P. Postoperative ileus. *Digestive Diseases and Sciences* 35(1):121, 1990.

17. Morson, B.C., Dawson, I.M., Day, D.W., Jass, J.R., Price, A.B., and Williams, G.T. *Morson and Dawson's Gastrointestinal Pathology*. Oxford: Blackwell, 1990.

18. Peterson, W.L., and Richardson, C.T. Peptic ulcer disease. In J.H. Stein (ed.), *Internal Medicine* (4th ed.). St. Louis: C.V. Mosby, 1994.

19. Rubin, E., and Farber, J.L. *Pathology* (2nd ed.). Philadelphia: J.B. Lippincott, 1994.

20. Shearman, D.J., and Finlayson, N.D. *Diseases of the Gastrointestinal Tract and Liver*. Edinburgh: Churchill-Livingstone, 1989.

21. Schultze-Delrieu, K.S. and Summers, R.W. Esophageal diseases. In J.H. Stein (ed.), *Internal Medicine* (4th ed.). St. Louis: C.V. Mosby, 1994.

22. Spiro, H.M. *Clinical Gastroenterology* (3rd ed.). New York: Macmillan, 1985.

23. Wallace, J.L. Lipid mediators of inflammation in gastric ulcer. *Am. J. Physiol.* 11:G1, 1990.

24. Watson, D.W., and Sodeman, W.A. The small intestine. In W.A. Sodeman and T.M. Sodeman (eds.), *Sodeman's Pathologic Physiology* (7th ed.). Philadelphia: W.B. Saunders, 1985.

25. Yardley, J.H. Gastritis. In H. Goldman, H.D. Appelman, and N. Kaufman (eds.), *Gastrointestinal Pathology*. Baltimore: Williams & Wilkins, 1988.

normal, glycogenolysis is stimulated, which promotes the release of glucose into the blood to raise the blood glucose level. *Glycogenolysis* is the breakdown of glycogen into glucose.

The liver maintains normal blood glucose levels. After a high-carbohydrate meal, an increased amount of carbohydrate is delivered to the liver, where it is stored and released when the blood glucose level begins to drop. The pancreatic hormone *glucagon* is very important in initiating the release of glucose by the liver.

In the process called *gluconeogenesis*, the liver synthesizes glucose from noncarbohydrate substances, especially proteins. Glucose needs that cannot be met from glycogen stores or exogenous sources must be met through this process. Gluconeogenesis is critically important for cells that cannot use fat for metabolism—the blood cells and the cells of the kidney medulla. The cells of the central nervous system use glucose preferentially but can adapt to fatty acid oxidation in the form of ketones in 2 to 4 days. During fasting, such as between meals and during sleep, the carbon skeleton of amino acids is converted to glucose for energy.

PHAGOCYTOSIS

The sinusoids of the liver are lined with Kupffer cells, which pick up and destroy foreign material circulating through the liver. The portal vein, which circulates the venous blood from the intestine to the liver, carries a higher concentration of toxins and bacteria than other venous blood because, these substances are absorbed when nutrients are absorbed from the intestine. The Kupffer cells, which probably originate in the bone marrow, are highly phagocytic and can remove 99% of bacteria in portal venous blood.[9]

If the level of bacteria or foreign material in the sinusoids increases, the Kupffer cells become active, proliferate, and destroy the foreign material. This activity is crucial to preventing the spread of pathogens to the systemic circulation.

BIOTRANSFORMATION OF FOREIGN SUBSTANCES

Destruction, biotransformation, and inactivation of foreign substances are carried out in the hepatocytes, and substances are changed to acceptable forms for excretion. Many of the endocrine secretions are inactivated in the liver, and many pharmacologic agents are biotransformed here. Some substances are conjugated in the same way as bilirubin, with glucuronic acid, whereas others may be inactivated by proteolysis, deamination, or oxidation. *Proteolysis* refers to the breakdown of proteins into simpler substances. Deamination is the removal of amino acids and may involve transamination or transfer of this group to another acceptor substance. Oxidative deamination causes the release of the amino radical.[5, 14]

The oxidative and conjugative reactions promote the biodegradation or excretion of foreign substances. It has been found that many drugs affect the reactions of other drugs or hormones. These interactions, whether they involve speeding up or slowing down the reactions, occur in hepatocytes. An example of this is the metabolism of warfarin (Coumadin), the effects of which can be potentiated by aspirin. Phenobarbital increases the activity of drug-metabolizing enzymes and hastens the inactivation of warfarin and other agents. Many endogenous hormones, especially corticosterone and aldosterone, are inactivated and conjugated for excretion by the liver. Estrogens impair the secretory activity of the hepatocytes and may alter the results of liver function tests.

Acute alcohol intoxication inhibits drug metabolism by the liver. The chronic alcoholic, however, metabolizes drugs quickly and has an increased tolerance to them, unless there is associated liver failure, which appears to cause decreased drug tolerance. Many drug interactions with alcohol vary according to whether the person is acutely intoxicated or sober. Acute intoxication often significantly potentiates the activity of central nervous system depressants, antihypertensives, antidiabetics, anticoagulants, and anti-inflammatory agents.[11]

Substances that are directly toxic to liver cells are called *hepatotoxins*. One drug that is a known hepatotoxin in excessive dosages is acetaminophen (Tylenol), which causes centrilobular necrosis due to the exhaustion of the glutathione to which it is normally conjugated. If a glutathione precursor is given in response to an overdose of acetaminophen, the liver will be protected from permanent injury. If no treatment is given, however, the rate of liver failure after overdose is very high and often fatal.

Most liver damage resulting from foreign substances is due to hypersensitivity reactions by hepatic cells after exposure to drugs. Some drugs cause jaundice; a notable example is chlorpromazine, which causes cholestasis within the liver. Several other drugs, such as isoniazid and halothane, can cause parenchymal necrosis and hepatitis.[11]

BILE SYNTHESIS

Bile is formed by the liver and stored and concentrated by the gallbladder. The liver secretes 250 to 1,500 mL of bile per day.[1] The hepatocytes make bile, which is a liquid material normally composed of bilirubin, plasma electrolytes, water, bile salts, bicarbonate, cholesterol, fatty acids, and lecithin.

Bilirubin

Bilirubin is a waste product that is excreted from the body only in the form of conjugated bilirubin. Most bilirubin is released in the breakdown of red blood cells. The red blood cell gives off hemoglobin, which further breaks down into its component parts, heme and globin. The globin portion is a protein that probably returns to the intracellular amino acid pool. The heme portion is broken down further into bilirubin and iron. The iron is either stored in the form of ferritin or used to produce new hemoglobin. Except for the iron in the hemoglobin, most iron in the body is stored by the liver in the form of ferritin. When iron is released from the heme of the red blood cell, it combines with apoferritin, a protein synthesized by the liver, and becomes ferritin, or storage iron.[6]

Bilirubin undergoes several reactions and ends up being bound to albumin, on which it travels to the liver. It is called unconjugated, fat-soluble, or indirect bilirubin because it cannot be excreted in bile or through the kidneys. In the liver, it is converted on the smooth endoplasmic reticulum to a water-soluble form when it combines with *glucuronic acid* through the intervention of the enzyme *glucuronyl transferase*.[9] In this water-soluble or conjugated form, it can be secreted into bile and excreted by the intestine or, in special circumstances, by the kidneys. In the intestine, the intestinal bacteria change the excreted bilirubin to *urobilinogen*. Some of this material is reabsorbed and reexcreted by the liver. Most of the bilirubin is converted to *stercobilinogen*, which is oxidized to *stercobilin* before being excreted in the feces.[6] Stercobilin and other bile pigments impart the brown color to the feces. Flowchart 42-1 outlines the process of hemoglobin breakdown and the resulting fate of bilirubin.

In summary, bilirubin must be converted to a conjugated, water-soluble form to cross the cell membrane of the hepatocytes and be excreted in bile. In bile duct obstruction, conjugated bilirubin can cross the membrane of the glomeruli and be excreted by the kidneys. Excess bilirubin in the blood leads to the condition called *jaundice* (see pp. 817–818).

Bile Salts

The bile salts function as detergents and break fat particles into smaller sizes. They aid in making fat more soluble by forming special complexes called *micelles*, which are soluble in the intestinal mucosa (see p. XX). Bile salts are formed by the liver with cholesterol precursors; large amounts can be formed and secreted during periods of increased need. The bile salts are also essential for the absorption of the fat-soluble vitamins A, D, E, and K.

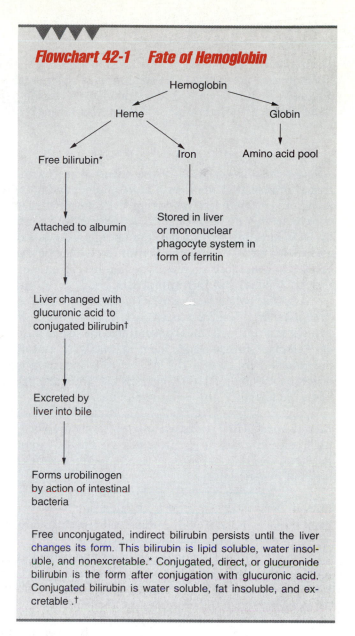

Flowchart 42-1   Fate of Hemoglobin

Free unconjugated, indirect bilirubin persists until the liver changes its form. This bilirubin is lipid soluble, water insoluble, and nonexcretable.* Conjugated, direct, or glucuronide bilirubin is the form after conjugation with glucuronic acid. Conjugated bilirubin is water soluble, fat insoluble, and excretable .†

Other Components of Bile

The electrolytes in bile are partially reabsorbed through the gallbladder mucosa because of the concentrating process that occurs in that organ. Substances that are not absorbed become highly concentrated in the gallbladder bile. For example, liver bile contains about 0.04 g/dL of bilirubin, whereas gallbladder bile contains about 0.3 g/dL. Much of the water in bile is absorbed through the gallbladder mucosa. Reabsorption of water, electrolytes, and free cholesterol in the secreted bile occurs in the small intestine. Cholesterol is excreted through the formation of bile salts and directly in the bile. Imbalance can cause excessive cholesterol in bile and may predispose a person to gallstone formation (see pp. 830–831).

▼ *Major Liver Function Tests*

The major liver function tests provide an index of hepatic function and are helpful in establishing a differential diagnosis in intrahepatic and extrahepatic pathology. The tests discussed below are summarized in Table 42-1.

Serum Enzymes

Alkaline phosphatase (ALP) of the serum is an enzyme that is produced in the liver, kidneys, bone, and other areas and is excreted in bile. Serum levels are elevated in conditions that increase calcium deposits in bone, such as viral hepatitis, obstructive jaundice, malignancies, and many other conditions. Serum levels may be decreased in conditions such as hypoparathyroidism, pernicious anemia, and hypothyroidism.

    Aspartate aminotransferase (AST), formerly called *serum glutamic oxaloacetic transaminase (SGOT)*, is an enzyme that is produced and concentrated in skeletal muscle, cardiac muscle, and liver. It catalyzes certain deamination processes. The AST level is increased in acute myocardial infarction, liver disease, muscular diseases, pancreatitis, and other conditions.

    Alanine aminotransferase (ALT), formerly called *serum glutamic pyruvic transaminase (SGPT)*, is present in high concentrations in the liver and, to a lesser extent, the heart and skeletal muscle. Levels increase with all types of hepatic injury.

    Lactic dehydrogenase (LDH) is present in large quantities in liver tissue. Its level is elevated significantly in liver damage and also with cardiac and muscular damage. The level is increased with certain malignancies and such conditions as pulmonary embolus and pernicious anemia. The LDH isoenzymes are isolated into concentrations of isoenzymes 1 through 5; specific isoenzymes are concentrated in different organs. Increased levels of isoenzyme LDH-5 is the most specific to liver disease, especially hepatitis.

    Gamma-glutamyl transferase (GGT), or gamma-glutamyl transpeptidase (GGTP or GTP), is present throughout the hepatobiliary system and is a sensitive indicator of biliary tract disease. Its levels remain elevated as long as there is hepatocellular damage. GGT levels also elevate with heavy alcohol ingestion and may remain elevated for several days to weeks after alcohol intake ceases.[10]

Bilirubin

Bilirubin is measured as a total value and in its conjugated and unconjugated fractions. These evaluations measure the ability of the liver to conjugate and excrete bilirubin in the intestine. A high level of unconjugated bilirubin with a normal or high level of conjugated bilirubin usually indicates significant intrahepatic cellular damage, but this may also occur with hemolytic jaundice.[12] An increase in conjugated bilirubin and a normal or slight increase in unconjugated bilirubin level, especially in the presence of dark urine and light stools, are almost conclusive evidence of biliary obstruction.

Plasma Proteins

Albumin, the most abundant plasma protein, maintains the plasma colloid osmotic pressure, synthesizes specific amino acids, and binds certain molecules for transport from one area to another. Albumin levels are evaluated by a process called *electrophoresis*. Decreased serum albumin, or hypoalbuminemia, results from severe hepatocellular dysfunction. Hypoalbuminemia results in alteration of colloid osmotic pressure, leading to systemic edema.

    Fibrinogen levels are important in determining the potential for normal blood coagulation. Depletion of this protein occurs in *disseminated intravascular coagulation*, with precipitation of fibrin in the small vessels and rapid depletion of the clotting factors (see p. 411). Deficiency also is noted in conditions that can cause fibrinolysis, such as hemorrhage, burns, poisoning, and cirrhosis.

    The *globulins* are important in the production of antibodies (see pp. 318–320). They also act with albumin to maintain intravascular colloid osmotic pressure. Alterations of globulin levels occur with immunosuppression and with chronic inflammations. Elevation or suppression of globulin levels is not a specific sign of liver disease.

    Another protein that is measured in liver function screening is *prothrombin*. The prothrombin time (PT) reflects the presence of prothrombin, fibrinogen, and other factors. A prolonged PT indicates a deficiency of prothrombin and other clotting factors or impaired uptake of vitamin K. This test measures the factors of the extrinsic system and the common pathway of extrinsic and intrinsic systems (see p. 415). The *partial thromboplastin time (PTT)* measures factors involved in the intrinsic clotting pathway and the common pathway and is a good screening test for bleeding disorders. The other clotting factors can be measured separately, and their levels may be altered in liver dysfunction.

Urine Urobilinogen

Small amounts of bilirubin are usually excreted in the urine in the form of urobilinogen. Conjugated bilirubin may be present in urine when an excessive amount is not being cleared from the plasma. This finding is common in obstructive biliary tract disease and severe cirrhosis of the liver (see p. 824).

Bromsulphalein (BSP) Excretion

This test measures the ability of the liver to remove a dye from the circulation. Liver injury is probable when more

TABLE 42-1 *Major Liver Function Tests*

Test	Normal Level	Abnormalities
Alkaline phosphatase (ALP)	2–5 BU/mL 35–85 ImU/mL	I Biliary obstruction I Early drug toxicity I Cholestatic hepatitis I Extrahepatic inflammatory condition
Aspartate aminotransferase (AST) (formerly called SGOT)	5–40 IU/mL 8–20 U/L (SI units)	I Acute myocardial infarction I Liver damage and most liver disease I Muscle, pancreas, brain, lung, bowel damage D Some severe liver disease D Diabetic ketoacidosis
Alanine aminotransferase (ALT) (formerly called SGPT)	5–35 IU/mL	I Markedly in liver necrosis and acute hepatitis I Slightly in myocardial infarction I Pulmonary, renal, pancreatic injury I Slightly in cirrhosis and chronic liver disease
Lactic dehydrogenase (LDH)	115–225 IU/mL 0.4–1.7 mmol/L (SI units)	I Cardiac injury I Hepatitis, especially LDH isoenzyme 5 I Malignant tumors I Muscle, pulmonary, and renal disease
Bilirubin		I Hepatocellular necrosis or damage
Total	0.1–1.0 mg/dL (5.1–17 mmol/L)	I Cholestasis due to obstruction
Direct	0.1–0.3 mg/dL (1.7–5.1 mmol/L)	I Hemolytic anemia
Indirect	0.2–0.8 mg/dL (3.4–12 mmol/L)	I Liver failure
Serum Ammonia	80–110 µg/dL (47–65 mmol/L)	I Liver failure
Plasma proteins		D Severe liver disease
Total	6–8 g/dL	D Pyelonephritis and nephrosis
Albumin	3.5–4.5 g/dL	D Malnutrition and protein lack
Globulin	2.3–3.4 g/dL	D Chronic inflammation
Fibrinogen	0.2–0.4 g/dL	D Disseminated intravascular coagulation D Congenital afibrinogenemia D With depletion of other coagulation factors D With major alteration of hemodynamics in body (eg, circulatory shock)
Prothrombin time	11–12.5 second (control) 85–100% of control	I (Prolonged) severe liver disease, especially cirrhosis I Fibrinogen deficiency I Warfarin therapy I Biliary destruction
Partial thromboplastin time Activated PTT	60–70 seconds 30–40 seconds	I (Prolonged) in bleeding disorders, especially of the intrinsic pathway I Heparin therapy I Cirrhosis and severe liver disease
Urine bilirubin	Absent/24 hours	I Biliary obstruction I Cirrhosis I Hepatitis
Urine urobilinogen	0–4 mg/24 hours 0.09–4.23 mmol/24 hours	D Biliary obstruction I Hemolysis Normal or cirrhosis
Liver scans Colloidal	Uptake of colloid by Kupffer's cells	Demonstrates large defects; false negative result with small defects

(continued)

TABLE 42-1 *(continued)*

Test	Normal Level	Abnormalities
Rose bengal	Uptake of dye by hepatocytes	Area of reduced intake, "hole" in neoplastic or inflammatory cells
Gallium	Little uptake of dye by normal cells	Uptake by neoplastic and inflammatory cells
Liver biopsy	Normal hepatocytes	Specific pathology of any material sampled; diagnostic of cirrhosis, malignancy, hepatitis, and so forth
Computed tomography	Normal integrity on image of intraabdominal organs	Fluid collections in liver differentiated from tumors; gallbladder or duct enlargement seen

I: test results are increased in these conditions; D: test results are decreased in these conditions.

than 10% of injected dye remains in circulation after 45 minutes.

Liver Scanning (Scintiscans)

Scans are performed to determine the position, shape, size, and structure of the liver. They involve injecting radiopharmaceutical isotopes, which are taken up by hepatocytes, Kupffer cells, or neoplasms. Several scanning procedures are used, with some isotopes concentrating in neoplasms or in areas of inflammation and others concentrating in the hepatocytes. Areas of abscess or tumor produce a void in the scan.

When reading the liver scan, one looks for areas of increased or no uptake, depending on the isotope used. Agents that are excreted in the bile can be followed for bile duct obstruction, whereas those having an affinity for mononuclear phagocytes are concentrated in the spleen. Changes in the liver scan can also assist in following the course of cirrhosis. Persons with early hepatomegaly have even distribution of the radiopharmaceutical agent. As the disease progresses, the left lobe of the liver enlarges, the right lobe becomes smaller, and the spleen takes up increased amounts of the isotope. As liver failure progresses, the liver may exhibit a spotty appearance due to the fibrosis dividing the lobules.

Liver Biopsy

Liver biopsy is performed to make a precise diagnosis of liver disease. It can be beneficial in the diagnosis of hepatitis, cirrhosis, and, sometimes, primary neoplasms. It may be performed as an open biopsy during a surgical procedure or as a needle biopsy using a percutaneous intercostal approach. In the latter, the material aspirated from the needle is examined histologically for abnormalities. Accurate placement of the needle is imperative for precise diagnosis. Care must be taken to prevent laceration of the liver and consequent hemorrhage.

Computed Tomography

The computed tomography (CT) scan is a popular procedure because it provides a radiologic image of the abdominal organs without the need to inject dyes or isotopes. In the initial evaluation of liver disease, CT scans help to differentiate fluid-filled from tumor-filled lesions. The appearance of the surrounding organs and ducts can also be assessed. It is a sensitive scan for determining metastases of primary malignancies but less so for fluid-filled bile ducts.[10]

▼ The Gallbladder

The *gallbladder* is a saclike organ attached to the inferior portion of the liver. It receives bile from the liver that has been diverted from the common bile duct (Fig 42-3). The liver secretes about 700 mL of bile, which flows continuously through the bile duct to the intestine. This flow, called *choleresis*, is increased after meals.[2] The gallbladder's maximum volume is 40 to 70 mL, but its bile is 5 to 10 times more concentrated than that of the liver. Approximately 90% of the water content of gallbladder bile is continually absorbed by the mucosa. Its electrolyte composition includes an increased concentration of potassium and calcium and a decreased amount of chloride and bicarbonate as compared with liver bile.[5, 9] The gallbladder is composed of folds and rugae and can enlarge to accommodate incoming bile.

The gallbladder empties its bile into the common bile duct when a stimulus is received. The major stimulus for this is *cholecystokinin*, a hormone secreted by the duodenal mucosa when fat-containing foods arrive in that area. The cholecystokinin causes bile to move into

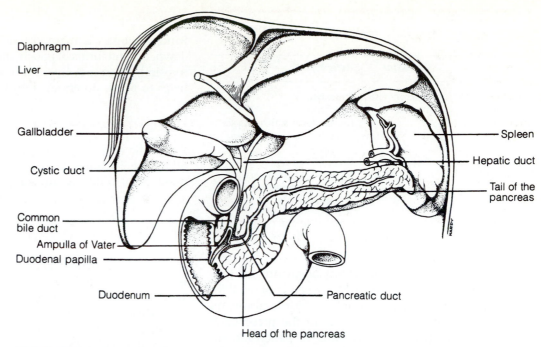

FIGURE 42-3 *The liver and biliary system, including the gallbladder, bile ducts, and pancreas. (Source: Chaffee, E.E. and Lytle, I.M.* Basic Physiology and Anatomy *(4th ed.). Philadelphia: J.B. Lippincott)*

the intestine by causing contractions of the gallbladder and relaxation of the sphincter of Oddi.[2] The gallbladder is also stimulated by the autonomic nervous system. The parasympathetic division is the major mediator for contraction of the gallbladder, whereas stimulation of the sympathetic division causes relaxation of the organ.

Alterations in function of the gallbladder are discussed on page 830. Gallstones and inflammation of the gallbladder are common causes of abdominal pain.

▼ *Exocrine Pancreatic Function*

The *pancreas* is a large organ that lies behind the stomach and extends between the spleen and the duodenum. It is composed of a head, a body, and a tail, which contain the acinar cells and the cells of the islets of Langerhans (see Fig. 42-3). The exocrine acinar cells secrete digestive juices, whereas the endocrine islet cells secrete hormones that are essential in glucose metabolism. The exocrine functions, or those related to digestion, involve the secretion of pancreatic juice into a system of ducts that empty into the pancreatic duct and, in turn, the ampulla of Vater. Pathologic alterations in the pancreas are discussed in Chapter 39.

EXOCRINE PANCREATIC SECRETION

The cells of the pancreas that secrete pancreatic juice are *acinar cells*. The secretion is composed of an alkaline component and enzymes necessary for digesting pro-

teins, fats, and carbohydrates. The alkaline component contains sufficient bicarbonate ion to give the pancreatic juice a pH of about 8. The pancreas normally secretes about 1,500 mL of fluid daily.[5] The enzymes are made by the acinar cells and stored until stimulated for release. The enzymes contained in the secretion are 1) *amylase*, which hydrolyzes carbohydrates to disaccharides; 2) *pancreatic lipase*, which hydrolyzes fats to yield glycerol and fatty acids; and 3) the *preproteolytic enzymes*, mainly trypsinogen and chymotrypsinogen, which, when activated, hydrolyze proteins to amino acids. Table 42-2 summarizes the enzymes and proenzymes of pancreatic secretions.

NERVOUS AND HORMONAL REGULATION OF PANCREATIC SECRETIONS

Nervous stimulation of the pancreas is mainly through the vagus nerve, which transmits impulses to the pancreas during the cephalic and gastric phases of digestion. This results in the secretion of enzymes by the acinar cells. The nervous influences also affect the secretion of the endocrine islet cells.

The hormonal mechanisms are mainly mediated through *secretin* and *cholecystokinin*. When chyme containing fat or amino acids comes into contact with the mucosal cells of the duodenum, the hormone is released, causing the pancreas to secrete large amounts of fluids with large amounts of bicarbonate and few or no enzymes. This alkaline secretion neutralizes the highly acidic gastric juice emptied into the duodenum

TABLE 42-2 *Enzymes of Pancreatic Secretion*

Enzyme	Activator	Action
Trypsin	Enterokinase	Proteolytic
Chymotrypsin	Trypsin	Proteolytic
Amylase		Breaks down starches to di-saccharides and trisac-charides
Carboxypeptidase	Trypsin	Breaks down amino acids
Lipase		Breaks down triglycerides to fatty acids and mono-glycerides

from the stomach, stops the activity of gastrin, and provides an alkalinity of about pH 7, which is optimal for pancreatic enzyme activity. Cholecystokinin also is released from the intestinal mucosa in the presence of food, and it increases the secretion of pancreatic enzymes from the acinar cells. Distention of the intestinal wall by food is the apparent stimulus for the release of cholecystokinin.

Pancreatic polypeptide is gastrointestinal hormone found in the *endocrine cells* of the pancreas. It is released after meals due to vagal and cholecystokinin stimulation. Pancreatic polypeptide is thought to be involved in the regulation of exocrine pancreatic secretion, and gallbladder emptying.[7,9]

PROTEIN DIGESTION

Trypsinogen is converted to the active enzyme trypsin in an alkaline medium through the action of *enterokinase*, which is released by the intestinal mucosa when it comes into contact with chyme. Trypsin then activates other trypsinogen molecules and triggers the conversion of chymotrypsinogen into chymotrypsin. These proteolytic enzymes can split proteins into amino acids for absorption in the intestine.

The two most important protective mechanisms to prevent digestion of the pancreas by the enzymes it secretes are 1) synthesis of enzymes in an inactive form and 2) the presence of a *trypsin inhibitor*, which is secreted by the same cells that secrete the pancreatic enzymes. This trypsin inhibitor is stored in the cytoplasm of the cells surrounding the enzyme granules and prevents the activation of trypsin, thus preventing activation of the other proteolytic enzymes. When the pancreas becomes damaged or when a duct is blocked, pancreatic secretions accumulate. It is hypothesized that the trypsin inhibitor is overwhelmed and the pancreatic enzymes become activated to cause acute pancreatitis.[7]

FAT DIGESTION

Pancreatic lipase is an important ingredient for fat breakdown. Several forms of pancreatic lipase are activated by trypsin.[13] Pancreatic lipase works with the bile salts and helps to break down fats into fatty acids and glycerol.

CARBOHYDRATE DIGESTION

Pancreatic amylase hydrolyzes starches, glycogen, and other carbohydrates into disaccharides. It does not break down plant cellulose into simpler substances.

▼ Chapter Summary

▼ The liver functions in most of the essential processes of life. It is a large organ composed of hepatocytes that synthesize and metabolize protein, carbohydrates, and fats. They also biotransform substances as they pass through the organ and produce and excrete bile, which is essential in digestion. Many hormones are inactivated by the liver, and bilirubin is conjugated so that it can be excreted in the bile.

▼ Within the capillary structure of the liver are a large number of phagocytes, called Kupffer's cells, which destroy foreign material and can remove 99% of bacteria in the portal venous blood. Vitamins, minerals, glucose, and other materials are stored in the liver parenchyma.

▼ The major liver function tests provide an index of hepatic function and help to establish a diagnosis of pathologic conditions. These include studies of liver enzymes, bilirubin, plasma proteins, liver scans, biopsy, and computed tomography.

▼ The gallbladder is an accessory organ that concentrates and secretes bile that is made by the liver. The major stimulus for gallbladder secretion is cholecystokinin, but parasympathetic stimulation from the autonomic nervous system also causes contraction of the organ.

▼ The pancreas is a large organ with endocrine and exocrine functions. The acinar cells of the pancreas secrete digestive juices with enzymes necessary for digesting proteins, fats, and carbohydrates. Large amounts of bicarbonate are secreted in the juices, which gives the pancreatic juice a pH of about 8. Pancreatic secretions are released through stimulus from the parasympathetic nervous system and through the hormones secretin and cholecystokinin.

▼ References

1. Arias, I.M., Jakoby, W.B., Popper, H., Schachter, D., and Shafritz, D.A. *The Liver: Biology and Pathobiology* (2nd ed.). New York: Raven Press, 1988.

2. Bolt, R.J. Pathophysiology of gallbladder disease. In W.A. Sodeman and T.M. Sodeman, *Sodeman's Pathologic Physiology* (7th ed.). Philadelphia: W.B. Saunders, 1985.
3. Cormack, D.H. *Essential Histology*. Philadelphia: J.B. Lippincott, 1993.
4. Fenogliio-Preiser, C.M., Lantz, P.E., Listrom, M.B., Davis, M., and Rilke, F.O. *Gastrointestinal Pathology: An Atlas and Text*. New York: Raven Press, 1989.
5. Ganong, W.F. *Review of Medical Physiology* (16th ed.). Los Altos, CA: Lange, 1994.
6. Greenberger, N.J., and Wenship, D.H. *Gastrointestinal Disorders: A Pathologic Approach* (3rd ed.). Chicago: Yearbook, 1986.
7. Greenberger, N.J., and Wenship, D.H. Approach to the patient with pancreatic disease. In J. Willson, et al. (eds), *Harrison's Principles of Internal Medicine* (12th ed.). New York: McGraw-Hill, 1991.
8. Grundy, S.M. Disorders of lipids and lipoproteins. In J. Stein, et al. (eds), *Internal Medicine* (4th ed.) St. Louis: C.V. Mosby, 1994.
9. Guyton, A.C. *Textbook of Medical Physiology* (8th ed.). Philadelphia: W.B. Saunders, 1991.
10. Podolsky, D.K., and Isselbacher, K.J. Diagnostic tests in liver disease. In J.D. Wilson, et al. (eds) *Harrison's Textbook of Internal Medicine* (12th ed.) New York: McGraw-Hill, 1991.
11. Reynolds, T. B. and Kanel, G.C. Alcoholic liver disease. In J. Stein, et al (eds). *Internal Medicine* (4th ed.). St. Louis: C.V. Mosby, 1994.
12. Saul, S.H. Liver. In V.A. LiVolsi, et al., *Pathology* (2nd ed.). Media, PA: Harwal, 1989.
13. Snodgrass, P.J. Pathophysiology of the pancreas. In W.A. Sodeman and T.M. Sodeman, *Sodeman's Pathologic Physiology* (7th ed.). Philadelphia: W.B. Saunders, 1985.
14. Tortora, G.J., and Grabowski, S.R. *Principles of Anatomy and Physiology* (7th ed.) New York: Harper Collins, 1993.

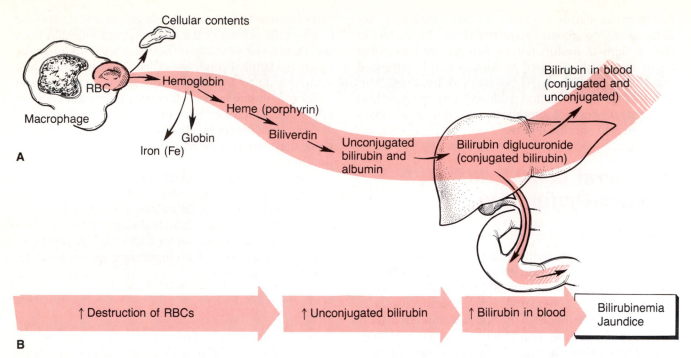

FIGURE 43-1 **A.** *Normal process of conjugation of bilirubin by the liver, which promotes excretion through the bile.* **B.** *With increased destruction of red blood cells, large amounts of unconjugated bilirubin are released and the liver is unable to conjugate all that comes to it. Increased bilirubin in the blood results, which leads to bilirubinemia and jaundice.*

usually results from a hypersensitivity reaction to the drug.

Thalassemias are a group of congenital diseases in which defective synthesis of hemoglobin leads to an increased propensity for hemolysis. Hemolytic anemias are discussed on pp. 381–384.

Obstructive Jaundice

Two major types of obstructive jaundice have been described: 1) *intrahepatic block,* or failure of the hepatocytes to function; and 2) *posthepatic block,* which commonly results from cholestasis as a result of cholecystitis or cholelithiasis (Fig. 43-2). *Cholestasis* is defined as biliary pigment that accumulates in the bile canaliculi and hepatocytes; when they become saturated, accumulation of these pigments in the blood occurs.

Intrahepatic obstruction frequently occurs after hepatitis and hepatocellular failure from cirrhotic fibrosis or hepatic scarring. Some pharmaceutical agents, such as oral contraceptives and chlorpropamide (Diabinese), have been shown to cause intracellular damage and blockage in certain persons.

Extrahepatic obstructive conditions in adults include gallstones, malignancies of an intrahepatic or extrahepatic source, and surgical obstruction of the ampulla of Vater. Obstruction in infancy most commonly results from congenital atresia of the biliary tree.[14] The obstruction limits the excretion of bilirubin in the bile, and an excess of conjugated bilirubin accumulates.[4]

The physiologic effects of obstruction depend on the ability of the liver to conjugate and excrete bilirubin. When the source of jaundice is hepatocellular failure, increased serum levels of unconjugated bilirubin often result due to failure of hepatocytes to produce conjugated bilirubin. Extrahepatic obstruction causes increased levels of conjugated bilirubin with excretion of bilirubin in the urine. As the liver becomes engorged with bilirubin, the activity of the hepatocytes diminishes, and the serum unconjugated and conjugated bilirubin levels increase.

Determining whether jaundice is caused by conjugated or unconjugated bilirubin is important in establishing the source and sometimes the severity of the causative condition. Deposition of pigments in the skin leads to the yellowish or greenish discoloration, which may be most noticeable in the sclera of the eyes. For neonates, increased bilirubin levels may lead to kernicterus and neurologic impairment. In adults, the degree of jaundice often correlates with the severity of liver dysfunction. Assessment of the degree of jaundice is difficult in dark-skinned individuals, but intense yellowish discoloration can be seen in the sclera.

ASCITES

Ascites is the accumulation of fluid in the peritoneal cavity. Box 43-1 list common causes of ascites. It usually results from increasing portal pressure or decreasing plasma protein levels or both. Sodium retention as a

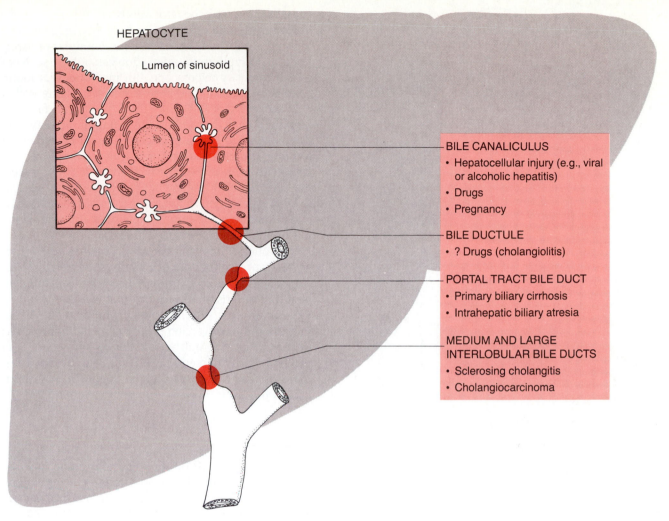

HEPATOCYTE

Lumen of sinusoid

BILE CANALICULUS
• Hepatocellular injury (e.g., viral or alcoholic hepatitis)
• Drugs
• Pregnancy

BILE DUCTULE
• ? Drugs (cholangiolitis)

PORTAL TRACT BILE DUCT
• Primary biliary cirrhosis
• Intrahepatic biliary atresia

MEDIUM AND LARGE INTERLOBULAR BILE DUCTS
• Sclerosing cholangitis
• Cholangiocarcinoma

FIGURE 43-2 *Sites of intrahepatic cholestasis. (Source: Rubin, E. and Farber, J.L. Pathology [2nd ed.]. Philadelphia: J.B. Lippincott, 1994)*

result of aldosterone retention and excessive lymphatic flow may add to the amount of ascitic fluid. Figure 43-3 illustrates the factors that can contribute to the development of ascites.

Portal hypertension, or increased pressure in the portal venous system, can occur because of an intrahepatic block to blood flow through the liver. The resul-

tant increase in capillary pressure leads to disruption of the normal osmotic force at the capillary line, pushing fluid into the peritoneal cavity.

Decreased plasma proteins, especially albumin, are the result of liver dysfunction. This leads to a reduction in the plasma colloid osmotic pressure, which decreases the inward forces or reabsorption pressures. This promotes fluid passage into the peritoneal space.

Ascitic fluid, or transudate, contains large quantities of albumin, the loss of which results in further hypoalbuminemia. Complicating this process is a decrease or depletion of central blood volume as the amount of ascitic fluid increases. As a compensatory mechanism, the body increases the secretion of aldosterone from the adrenal cortex, which leads to retention of sodium and water. The retention indirectly provides more available fluid and increased ascites.

Antidiuretic hormone, which is synthesized by the hypothalamus and released by the posterior pituitary, also is secreted in greater quantities when the central

BOX 43-1 ▼ *Causes of Ascites*

Cirrhosis of the liver
Peritoneal inflammation
Gastrointestinal carcinomas
Ovarian carcinomas
Pancreatitis
Congestive heart failure
Hepatic venous obstruction
Nephrosis and peritoneal dialysis
Myxedema

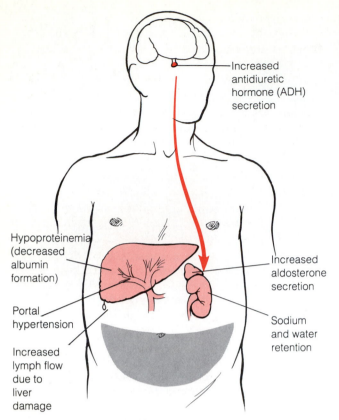

Increased
antidiuretic
hormone (ADH)
secretion

Hypoproteinemia
(decreased
albumin
formation)

Portal
hypertension

Increased
lymph flow
due to
liver
damage

Increased
aldosterone
secretion

Sodium
and water
retention

FIGURE 43-3   *Factors contributing to the development of ascites.*

blood volume is depleted. Increases in renal tubular water reabsorption and blood volume result.

Elevated intrasinusoidal pressure within the liver associated with cirrhosis probably leads to an increase in the lymphatic flow. Lymph fluid may ooze from the hepatic surface and cause increases in the amount of ascitic fluid and in its protein concentration.[4]

Ascites is a self-defeating condition in which the compensatory efforts of the body end up making the condition worse. Without intervention, the course degenerates progressively, leading to greater ascites. Ascites causes abdominal swelling that is noted as increased girth. The extra intraabdominal fluid may cause pressure on the diaphragm and respiratory difficulties. Bacterial peritonitis due mainly to *Escherichia coli* is common, especially when the ascites is associated with alcoholic cirrhosis. Ascitic fluid may be removed by peritoneal tapping, but it frequently reaccumulates rapidly. Generalized edema, or *anasarca*, results mostly from a decrease in the plasma colloid osmotic pressure generated from the decreased albumin levels, which encourages fluid exudation into all of the interstitial compartments.

FATTY LIVER

Fatty liver refers to the infiltration of hepatocytes by fat or lipid material. This infiltration by itself usually does not significantly disrupt the physiologic processes of the

cells, but over time the fatty cells become surrounded by fibrous tissue that separates the liver lobules. The pathologic appearance may be either micronodular or macronodular. Micronodular infiltration can only be seen with a high-intensity microscope, but macronodular lobules have fat infiltration and fibrosis that are grossly visible.[4]

Several factors influence the deposition of fat. A diet high in fat may overwhelm the metabolic activity of the liver, leading to increased triglyceride stores. A diet with too little protein, or starvation, leads to mobilization of fatty acids from adipose tissue. Fatty acids then travel to the liver and infiltrate the hepatocyte. Alcoholism leads to fat accumulation in the parenchymal cells of the liver and distention of the cytoplasm with fat. In certain areas, the infiltrated cells undergo fibrosis.

Alcohol is thought to be a direct hepatotoxin. Large amounts of alcohol have been demonstrated to increase accumulation of lipids within the cells, resulting in a liver that weighs up to 5 kg (normal weight is about 1.5 kg) and appears soft and greasy when cut.[4, 13] Alcohol may affect the conversion of fatty acids to lipoproteins in the liver, but the mechanism for its induction is not precisely known. In addition, alcoholism usually results in nutritional inadequacy, which promotes fatty infiltration of the liver.

CLOTTING DISTURBANCES

Because the liver produces many of the major clotting factors, liver dysfunction of 60% or more leads to depletion of these factors and a tendency to bleed. A decrease in the uptake of vitamin K into hepatocytes leads to defective synthesis of factors II (prothrombin), VII (proconvertin), IX (Christmas factor), and X (Stuart-Prower factor).[14] Vitamin K deficiency may result from fat malabsorption when bile amounts are inadequate. The major clotting dysfunction results from depressed production of prothrombin, and other clotting factors may also be depressed.

Deficiency in clotting factors is one of the earliest signs of liver failure. The platelet count may be inadequate as a result of hypersplenism, which is a frequent companion of liver failure. Hypersplenism results from congestion caused by the portal hypertension.[4] In liver failure, an increased risk of hemorrhage is always present when it is associated with esophageal varices, and the bleeding is very difficult to control with the attendant clotting disturbances.

PORTAL HYPERTENSION
AND ESOPHAGEAL VARICES

Obstruction of blood flow through the liver results in increased pressure in the portal venous system. The term *portal hypertension* refers to high pressures in the portal vein and its tributaries. The main cause of this condition is cirrhosis of the liver, but the various causative conditions have been divided into the following categories:

▼ **Posthepatic**, which results from increased pressure in the inferior vena cava and venous return to the heart. It may be produced by severe right-sided heart failure, constrictive pericarditis, or hepatic veno-occlusive disease.
▼ **Intrahepatic**, which results from blockage to blood flow within the liver. The main cause is cirrhosis of the liver, but other conditions, such as fatty change, biliary tuberculosis, and idiopathic portal hypertension, may be at fault.
▼ **Prehepatic**, which results from blockage of blood flow to the liver, as may be seen in portal vein thrombosis, splenomegaly, or arteriovenous fistula.[4]

Meeting resistance in the portal vein, blood seeks collateral channels around the high pressure areas or through the obstructed liver. In the portal system, the vessels most susceptible to the high pressure are the esophageal and the hemorrhoidal veins (Fig. 43-4). The esophageal veins protrude into the lumen of the esophagus and become thin-walled varices that look like bulging bags on the inner surface of the esophagus.

Esophageal varices can become irritated by gastric acidity or by spasmotic vomiting. Alcohol and other irritants can cause chemical breakdown of the walls of the varices. Any of these situations can result in rupture and massive upper gastrointestinal hemorrhage. The two main factors that encourage hemorrhage are depressed formation of clotting factors and high portal pressures. Continued vomiting after the first bleeding event usually results in additional bleeding. Rupture of esophageal varices may result in exsanguination and death if not treated immediately. Rectal hemorrhoids also may rupture and bleed under pressure, causing a massive amount of bright red bleeding from the rectum. Anything that can cause increased motility of the lower

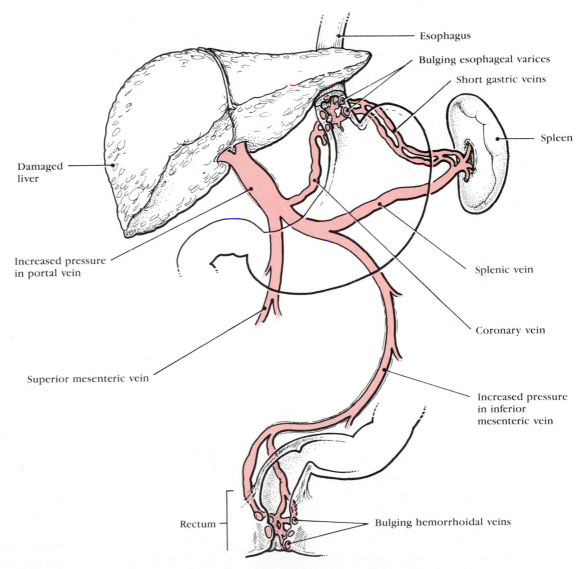

FIGURE 43-4   *Appearance of esophageal varices and dilated hemorrhoidal veins resulting from portal hypertension.*

gastrointestinal tract can increase the risk of hemorrhage from this area.

Collateral channels develop because of the high portal pressure and provide a route for direct shunting of blood from the portal veins to the inferior vena cava, thus bypassing the liver. The shunted blood contains large amounts of ammonia that may precipitate onset of hepatic encephalopathy. The blood-borne bacteria absorbed from the small intestine and normally processed and biotransformed in the liver are also shunted directly into the systemic circulation. Toxic substances may bypass the liver without being metabolized and may accumulate in the body with deleterious effects on the nervous system.

Bleeding from esophageal varices, duodenal ulcers, or other sources may precipitate jaundice and production of ammonia due to the processing and absorption of products of the red blood cell in the intestine. These developments may lead to increased risk of encephalopathy, which, with the bleeding event, is often life-threatening (see below).

HEPATORENAL SYNDROME

In liver failure, the development of associated renal failure indicates a very poor prognosis. The hepatorenal syndrome seems to leave the kidneys almost normal morphologically but functionally impaired. It is diagnosed in persons developing acute renal failure in the presence of significant hepatic disease; frequently it is precipitated by clinical deterioration, such as a gastrointestinal bleeding episode or the onset of hepatic coma.[4] The term *hepatorenal syndrome* should not be used for conditions that produce damage to both the liver and kidneys.[15]

Hepatorenal syndrome begins suddenly, with decreased urinary output and elevated serum urea nitrogen and creatinine levels. It is accompanied by elevated blood ammonia level and increasing jaundice, probably due to the failure of bilirubin to be excreted in the urine. At autopsy, no permanent morphologic change can be demonstrated in the kidneys. The syndrome seems to be an evolutionary process of functional impairment of the kidneys resulting from liver failure. The kidney dysfunction markedly improves with restoration of liver function.[4]

LIVER FAILURE

Liver failure refers to a constellation of clinical manifestations that result from many types of liver disease. The liver has a large reserve, and approximately 80% of its parenchyma can be destroyed before clinical signs of liver failure are evident. Cirrhosis and chronic active hepatitis are the most common causes of liver failure.[6]

Chemicals and drugs, such as carbon tetrachloride and halothane, can cause massive liver necrosis. Reye's syndrome, fatty liver of alcoholism, and antibiotics, such as tetracycline, can cause functional insufficiency.[4] The characteristic physiologic changes of liver failure include the following: 1) jaundice, with increased conjugated and unconjugated bilirubin levels; 2) coagulopathy due to malabsorption of vitamin K and reduced synthesis of clotting factors II, V, VII, IX, and X; 3) changes in neurologic status with hepatic encephalopathy and coma; 4) hypogonadism and gynecomastia due to imbalance of androgen–estrogen levels; 5) palmar erythema with vasodilation in the palms of the hands and feet due to hyperestrogenism; 6) spider angiomas of the skin, probably related to clotting disturbances or hyperestrogenism or both; (7) fetor hepaticus, a peculiar musty odor of the breath often associated with high serum ammonia levels; and 8) ascites and edema related to portal hypertension and hypoalbuminemia.[4] The characteristic wasting of liver disease is manifested by muscular atrophy, weight loss, and loss of plasma proteins and clotting factors. Recovery from liver failure depends on the amount of damage sustained by the liver and the degree to which the liver can regenerate when it is not confronted by multiple toxins, such as alcohol.

Fulminant hepatic failure refers to acute, rapidly developing liver dysfunction. The term is usually reserved for the development of encephalopathy in a person who has experienced no previous liver disease but who develops jaundice and encephalopathy within 4 weeks after the initiating event. This event may include infections, drugs and toxins, ischemia, hypoxia, metabolic disorders, and other conditions, such as autoimmune conditions.[17] A subacute process has been described, especially when the condition is drug or toxin induced, in which the manifestations of liver failure develop 8 to 20 weeks postexposure. Massive liver necrosis and destruction of lobules and even lobes of the liver result. The overall mortality rate is between 75% and 95%, with encephalopathy being the main cause of death.[15]

HEPATIC ENCEPHALOPATHY AND COMA

Hepatic encephalopathy refers to an alteration in the neurologic status in persons with significant liver disease. Its onset may be gradual, but more frequently it is precipitated by a major hemodynamic insult in the marginally compensated individual suffering from cirrhosis of the liver. Conditions that may precipitate encephalopathy include bleeding from esophageal varices; ingestion of narcotics, barbiturates, or anesthetics; excessive protein intake; electrolyte imbalance; and hemodynamic alterations, such as hypovolemia or shock. Anything that can increase the metabolic demands placed on the borderline liver can precipitate liver failure with resultant encephalopathy and coma.

Hepatic encephalopathy occurs because the liver is no longer able to remove neuroactive metabolites from the blood. These metabolites inhibit normal neural functioning by acting as false neurotransmitters.[14] Onset is related to the inability of the liver to metabolize nitrogenous products absorbed from the intestine. These nitrogenous products may include dietary protein or proteins released in gastrointestinal bleeding episodes. Serum ammonia levels are often elevated in encephalopathy, and other substances probably produce the clinical syndrome as well.[8]

Hepatic encephalopathy has been described in terms of phases that vary in length (from days or weeks to months) and may progress insidiously from one level to the next. The earliest phase of encephalopathy is characterized by behavioral changes. Subtle impairment of intellectual abilities is also noted. In the next phase, the person experiences confusion, delusion, and eventual diminished consciousness. As the condition progresses, a phase having the distinct neurologic patterns of hyperreflexia and asterixis occurs. *Asterixis* is a peculiar "flapping tremor" that can be elicited by dorsiflexion of the hands. Violent, abusive behavior, accompanied by changes on the electroencephalogram (EEG), is frequent. Characteristic EEG changes of symmetrical, high-voltage, slow-wave patterns occur one to three times per second and are imposed on a relatively normal reading.

Progression of encephalopathy to coma results in absence of the flapping tremor and depression or decline of the waveforms on the EEG. A positive Babinski's sign and hyperactive reflexes occur with the onset of the comatose phase. Persons exhibiting recurrent or progressive forms of this condition have been found to have distinctive changes in the brain tissue, with proliferation of the astrocytes and patchy cortical necrosis. When these changes occur, areas of permanent damage result.[4] In rapidly occurring liver failure, cerebral edema may be seen, which can cause uncal or cerebellar herniation.[14]

DRUG-RELATED LIVER DAMAGE

Drug reactions are responsible for a number of toxic effects on the human body. Hepatotoxicity can result from formation of toxic metabolites as the liver is biotransforming the drug or from a drug metabolite converting an intracellular protein into an immunogenic molecule. The damage sustained depends on dosage and individual hypersensitivity. Table 43-1 indicates some mechanisms that cause drug-induced hepatotoxicity. Some drugs affect a significant number of persons, and the damage occurs relatively quickly. Many drugs cause problems due only to hypersensitivity reactions, and these problems may not be manifested for weeks to months after initiating therapy. The pathology depends on the amount and location of injury.[4, 17]

TABLE 43-1 *Mechanisms of Drug-Induced Hepatotoxicity*

	Direct	Indirect
Mechanism of liver injury	Protoplasmic poison	Interference with hepatic secretory or excretory processes without parenchymal damage Hepatic necrosis produced by competition or binding with essential metabolites; inhibition of specific enzyme functions
Time interval between exposure and liver damage	Brief	Latent period (1–4 wk) to sensitization
Toxicity	Dose dependent	Independent of dose
Reproducible in experimental animals	Common	Infrequent
Frequency	High	Low
Hepatic lesions	Distinct liver cell necrosis	Variable; hepatitis-like; cholestasis; mixed
Rash, fever, eosinophilia, arthralgia	Unusual	High frequency
Examples	Lomustine (CCNU) phosphorus	Chlorpromazine, chlorpropamide, chlorothiazide

(Adapted from Greenberger, N.J.. *Gastrointestinal Disorders: A Pathophysiologic Approach* [3rd ed.]. Chicago: Yearbook Medical Publishers, 1986.)

REYE'S SYNDROME

Reye's syndrome is an acute illness that occurs most frequently in children between the ages of 6 months and 15 years.[4] The onset of symptoms begins about 3 to 5 days after a viral illness, such as varicella. In nearly every case, the viral fever has been treated with aspirin, which has led to the theory that there is a synergism between aspirin and viral infection.[14] The initial symptoms are vomiting, lethargy progressing to coma, with increased aminotransferases, and ammonia.[4] Pathologically, there is massive infiltration of the liver parenchyma with fat (steatosis). Liver and brain mitochondria are swollen, and cerebral edema occurs in all cases.[4, 14] The amount of cerebral edema corresponds to the severity of the neurologic dysfunction. Fatality rates vary from 10% to 40%, depending on early diagnosis and accurate reporting (see p. 1074).[4] The incidence of Reye's syndrome is declining with education of adults to not treat febrile illness in children with aspirin.

BOX 43-2 ▼ Causes of Cirrhosis

Alcoholic liver disease
Chronic active hepatitis
Primary biliary cirrhosis
Extrahepatic biliary obstruction
Hemochromatosis
Wilson's disease
Cystic fibrosis
α_1-Antitrypsin deficiency
Glycogen storage disease, types III and IV
Galactosemia
Hereditary fructose intolerance
Tyrosinemia
Hereditary storage diseases: Gaucher's, Niemann-Pick, Wolman, mucopolysaccharidoses
Zellweger syndrome
Indian childhood cirrhosis

(Rubin, E. and Farber, J.L. *Pathology* [2nd ed.]. Philadelphia: J.B. Lippincott, 1994.)

▼ Cirrhosis of the Liver

Cirrhosis is a general term for a condition that destroys the normal architecture of the liver lobules. It has the following important structural features: 1) destruction of liver parenchyma; 2) separation of the lobules by fibrous tissue; 3) formation of structurally abnormal nodules; and 4) abnormal vascular architecture.[4, 14] Cirrhosis is classified either according to its causative agent or according to the morphologic changes that result. The morphologic classification includes the *micronodular* type, which exhibits nodules less than 3 mm in diameter, and the *macronodular* type, which exhibits grossly visible, coarse, irregular nodules encircled by bands of connective tissue.[14] The morphologic features of cirrhosis often depend on how long the condition has been present and how extensive the liver damage is. The major causes of cirrhosis are listed in Box 43-2 and indicate a variety of causative conditions that may progress to the ultimate outcome of liver failure. The following discussion includes *biliary* and *alcoholic* causes; *hepatitis* is addressed on pages 827–830. Metabolic disorders, such as iron overload, glycogen storage disease, and Wilson's disease, can cause cirrhosis through deposition of abnormal substances into the hepatocyte, which disrupts its function.

BILIARY CIRRHOSIS

Biliary cirrhosis may be due to an intrahepatic block that obstructs the excretion of bile or may occur secondary to obstruction of the bile ducts. The ultimate outcome differs with each type, and causes vary. Intrahepatic biliary stasis is considered to result from two major mechanisms.

Primary intrahepatic stasis is caused by autoimmune destruction of interlobular bile ducts. This type occurs most often in women older than age 40 years, suggesting an endocrine contribution. Specific and nonspecific immunologic abnormalities have been implicated based on the demonstration of antibodies and impaired T lymphocyte function.[4]

Secondary biliary cirrhosis results from obstruction of the hepatic or common bile duct and produces stasis of bile in the liver. The liver becomes swollen and bile stained. This excess bile may lead to progressive fibrosis, parenchymal cell destruction, and regenerative nodules. The nodules apparently result from a reaction of the interlobular bile ducts to the increased amounts of bile within them. Injury, inflammation, and scarring result from stasis of bile in the lobular compartments.[4, 14] Intrahepatic and extrahepatic biliary cirrhosis show evidence of fibrosis that surrounds hepatocytes and separates the lobules. Scarring and injury are found close to the interlobular bile ducts.

The clinical course is usually more severe in the primary versus the secondary type, because surgical intervention usually relieves the biliary stasis in the latter. Jaundice may be severe with either type and is associated with bilirubinemia and clay-colored stools. Results of liver function tests are abnormal, with alkaline phosphatase and cholesterol levels often becoming markedly elevated. Serum triglycerides and low-density cholesterol levels are often elevated with this condition. Levels of conjugated and unconjugated bilirubin may rise. With increasing liver damage, the signs of hepatocellular failure may appear.

ALCOHOLIC (LAËNNEC'S) CIRRHOSIS

Laënnec's cirrhosis, also called *alcoholic liver disease*, has been shown to be caused by chronic alcoholism, often following a pattern of fatty liver, alcoholic hepatitis, and, finally, alcoholic cirrhosis.[4] At least 10% of persons who are chronic alcoholics have clinical or morphologic evidence of cirrhosis. Significant frequency of the disease is noted in highly civilized countries, among all economic classes, and in all races.

Alcohol has been shown to be a hepatotoxin. It induces metabolic changes within the liver that lead to fat infiltration of the hepatocytes and scarring between the lobules. Alcoholic liver disease usually follows long-term ingestion of more than 80 g/day of ethanol. This amount is found in eight 12-oz beers, 1 liter of wine, or a half-pint of 80-proof whiskey. In susceptible persons, as little as 40 g/day for males and 20 g/day for females can produce alcoholic liver disease.[5] A close association between poor diet and long-term alcohol abuse is often found.

The phases of alcoholic liver disease are usually described as progressing from *alcoholic steatosis* to *alcoholic hepatitis* to *alcoholic cirrhosis*. The steatosis is the fatty liver, which is caused by increased liver synthesis of triglycerides and fatty acids, decreased fatty acid oxidation, and decreased formation and release of lipoproteins.[4] Large fat vesicles appear within the cytoplasm of liver cells and may obscure the appearance of hepatitis.[13] The alcoholic steatosis may be asymptomatic or may be associated with malaise, anorexia, nausea, liver tenderness and enlargement, jaundice, or even sudden death.[4, 13]

When alcoholic hepatitis ensues, acute liver cell necrosis results. Inflammatory cell infiltrates and inclusions called *Mallory's bodies*, or alcoholic hyalin, may lead to pericellular and perivenular (around the cells and veins) fibrosis.[4] The liver becomes enlarged, and hepatocytes degenerate and become infiltrated by leukocytes and lymphocytes. Mallory's bodies produce sclerosing hyaline necrosis.[4, 8] The early disease has an inflammatory character that decreases as the cirrhotic process progresses to the destruction of heptatocytes. Infiltrating fibroblasts and collagen formation lead to early scar formation. Acute exacerbations of alcoholic hepatitis cause inflammation and further damage to the liver parenchyma. The clinical picture of acute alcoholic hepatitis includes general debility (asthenia), jaundice, fever, abdominal pain, ascites, and loss of muscle mass.

As alcoholic cirrhosis ensues, the liver capsule becomes firm, and regenerative nodules form, resulting in a hobnail appearance. As the pathology progresses, the liver shrinks in size and becomes finely nodular in appearance. The nodules are surrounded by evenly spaced, grayish connective tissue.[4, 13] The liver pathology is usually associated with enlargement of the spleen.

The physiologic results of Laënnec's cirrhosis depend on the amount of inflammation, degeneration, infiltration of cells by fat, and scarring. Liver cell degeneration may lead to portal hypertension and ascites. Jaundice and esophageal varices often occur later in the disease. All of the complications associated with liver dysfunction may occur, depending on the degree of parenchymal damage.[5] Some of the more common complications are clotting disorders, hypoproteinemia, biliary obstruction, and gastrointestinal bleeding.

Clinically, cirrhosis of this type is an insidious condition causing abnormal liver function test results, fluid retention, ascites, esophageal varices, and many other manifestations (Fig. 43-5). With abstinence from alcohol, results of liver function tests may return to near normal, but excessive ingestion of alcohol or continued poor diet may lead to decompensation. Alcoholic hepatitis recurs, leading to bouts of decompensation and finally to liver failure. Fifty percent of persons with significant cirrhosis of the liver die of the disease within 5 years. Disease progression can be markedly altered by abstinence from alcohol.[13] Death may be due to hepatic encephalopathy, liver failure, infection, gastrointestinal bleeding, or hepatocellular carcinoma, which appears in 3% to 6% of cases.[4]

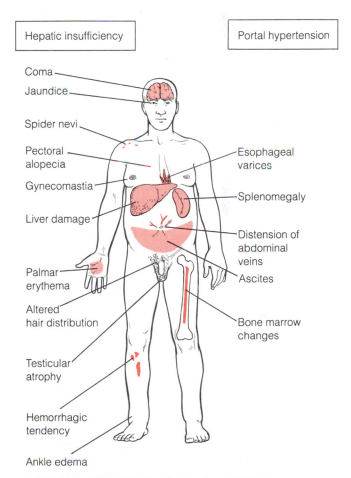

| Hepatic insufficiency | Portal hypertension |

Coma
Jaundice
Spider nevi
Pectoral alopecia
Gynecomastia
Liver damage
Palmar erythema
Altered hair distribution
Testicular atrophy
Hemorrhagic tendency
Ankle edema

Esophageal varices
Splenomegaly
Distension of abdominal veins
Ascites
Bone marrow changes

FIGURE 43-5 *Clinical effects of cirrhosis of the liver.*

▼ Tumors of the Liver

Tumors of the liver that cause functional impairment and hepatomegaly are almost always malignant. The rare benign tumors or tumorlike lesions are described as angiomas, adenomas, or nodular hyperplasias.

BENIGN HEPATIC TUMORS

Most hepatocellular tumors are *adenomas* that occur in women and are related to oral contraceptive use. They cause a well-circumscribed, encapsulated mass that may have a diameter of 5 to 15 cm.[3] These tumors may be discovered as a result of complaints of abdominal pain or bleeding into the peritoneal cavity and do not recur after excision.[14]

Focal nodular hyperplasia, thought to be a hamartomatous malformation, also occurs primarily in women of childbearing age and probably is not related to taking oral contraceptives for a long period of time.[3] Bile duct hamartomas and adenomas are small masses in the ductal structures. Sometimes the gross appearance of multiple hamartomatous malformations may simulate metastatic carcinoma or other conditions, but they do not usually cause symptoms.[4, 14]

Hemangiomas of the liver are very common reddish purple lesions measuring about 2 to 4 cm. These rarely are symptomatic but occur in up to 7% of routine autopsies.[14]

PRIMARY MALIGNANCIES

Primary carcinoma of the liver is relatively rare and may arise within the hepatocytes or the biliary canaliculi, or it may be of mixed type. Hepatocellular carcinoma accounts for 80% to 90% of primary malignancies of the liver.[4]

A study of the epidemiology of primary liver tumors shows that they may be related to diet and other types of liver disease, especially hepatitis. In the United States, the prevalence of primary liver carcinoma is less than 3%, whereas in some parts of Africa this malignancy may represent 50% of all cancers in men and 20% in women. Some of the influences that may contribute to its occurrence are 1) carcinogenic agents in food; 2) cirrhosis of the liver; 3) viral infections of the liver; and 4) parasitic liver infections.[4] Viruses, especially the hepatitis B virus (HBV), can account for the difference in frequency of liver cancers in the United States and Africa. In Africa, markers for HBV are almost invariably present.[14] Hepatitis C antibodies are found in two-thirds to three-fourths of persons with primary hepatocellular carcinoma, making this viral infection an important risk factor for this malignancy.[14]

Pathologically, the growth may be limited to one area, occur in numerous nodules, or occur as infiltrates on the surface of the liver.[3, 10] The tumors may secrete different substances, especially bile products. Paraneoplastic manifestations such as polycythemia, hypoglycemia, and hypercalcemia are very common and result from hormone production by the tumor.[14] Usually the growth rate is very rapid, and the tumor metastasizes early. It often terminates in gastrointestinal hemorrhaging, liver failure, and death.

Physiologically, these tumors interfere with the normal function of the hepatocytes, but they often create no difficulty until they are far advanced. Biliary obstruction with jaundice, portal hypertension with ascites, and different sorts of metabolic disturbances related to the functional impairment of hepatocytes result. Alterations from the paraneoplastic characteristics of the tumor may cause physiologic disturbances, such as hypoalbuminemia, hypoglycemia, and bleeding problems.

Clinically, the affected person exhibits signs of debilitation, weight loss, and cachexia. Typical complaints are of abdominal pain and bloating. Early manifestations may resemble cirrhosis. Jaundice, ascites, and other signs of liver failure are often related to progression of the condition and frequently are seen in the terminal state. Tumors of the liver are rarely considered to be resectable. Precise diagnosis is made by biopsy, but liver and computed tomography scans are helpful.[11] Ultrasound examination is used to detect small, space-occupying lesions.[10] Arteriography is then used to detect small hepatocellular carcinomas or intrahepatic metastases. Liver function tests reflect the degree of disruption of normal function. Alpha-fetoprotein can be used as a screening measure, because its levels are often elevated above 4,000 ng/mL from a normal level of less than 10 ng/mL. This test can also show elevated levels in other neoplastic conditions.

METASTATIC CARCINOMA

The liver is commonly the site of metastases of malignancies arising in other areas of the body, especially those of the pulmonary tract, breast, and gastrointestinal tract. Other types of malignancies metastasize less readily to the liver.

Physiologically, the liver is vulnerable to metastatic carcinoma because of the large volume of blood it receives each minute, the high nutrient level of its blood, and the large reserve of lymphatic drainage. Metastases usually involve large areas of the liver causing disruption to its function. Results of liver function tests are frequently abnormal, especially alkaline phosphatase, and serum enzymes. The level of carcinoembryonic antigen in the serum, which is elevated in many malignancies, is also elevated with many liver malignancies and metastases. Serum levels correlate to some extent with tumor size and degree of metastasis, and levels decrease markedly after successful treatment.

The clinical course depends on the rapidity of growth of the metastatic lesion and the site of the primary malignancy. The nutritional status of the affected person declines rapidly, with marked cachexia, muscle wasting, and hepatomegaly. Obstruction of bile flow may lead to jaundice, and all of the other dysfunctions of liver disease may be present, depending on the amount of liver involvement.

The prognosis for persons with liver metastasis is poor due to the lack of response to treatment and the impossibility of resecting the tumor surgically. Five-year survival has been reported to be less than 5%.

▼ *Viral Hepatitis*

Hepatitis refers to inflammation and injury of the liver. It is a reaction of the liver to a variety of conditions, specifically viruses, drugs, and alcohol. Some of the changes from drugs and alcohol have been previously discussed. *Viral hepatitis* is the term used for infection of the liver by viruses. Identification of the causative viruses is ongoing, but the agents of A, B, C, E, and D viruses account for about 95% of cases of acute viral hepatitis.[9] The viruses E and D are known as non-A, non-B hepatitis.[16] Table 43-2 provides a comparative chart of the characteristics

---

TABLE 43-2 *Characteristics of Viral Hepatitis*

Characteristic	Hepatitis A	Hepatitis B	Delta Virus	Hepatitis C	Hepatitis E
Causative agent	27-nm RNA virus	42-nm DNA virus with surface and core components	36-nm RNA defective virus with HB_sAg coat	RNA virus	32-nm RNA virus
Transmission	Fecal–oral	Parenteral	Parenteral	Parenteral; sporadic also (fecal–oral?)	Fecal–oral; contaminated water supply
Incubation	15–50 days	45–180 days	28–180 days	About 60–180 days	14–56 days
Period of infectivity	Late incubation to early clinical phase	When HB_sAg positive	When anti-HDV seropositive	Unknown	Unknown
Fulminant hepatitis	Rare	Uncommon	Common	Uncommon	Common in third trimester; otherwise uncommon
Chronic hepatitis or carrier state	No	Common (5–10%)	Common	Common	No
Prophylaxis	Hygiene; ISG	Hygiene, HBIG; HBV vaccine	Hygiene; HBV vaccine	Screening blood; hygiene	Hygiene; safe water supply

HB_sAg, hepatitis B surface antigen; HDV, hepatitis delta virus; ISG, immune serum globulin; HBV, hepatitis B virus; HBIG, hepatitis B immunoglobulin.
(Shulman, S.T., Phair, J.P., Sommers, H.M. *The Biological and Clinical Basis of Infectious Diseases* [4th ed.]. Philadelphia: W.B. Saunders, 1992.)

of viral hepatitis. Viral hepatitis is difficult to identify in the elderly because it presents with nonspecific symptoms, such as fatigue, malaise, and diarrhea. Hepatic failure secondary to viral hepatitis is also more common in the elderly and is more difficult to treat.[6]

HEPATITIS A: INFECTIOUS HEPATITIS

Hepatitis A (HAV) infection results most frequently from fecal–oral contamination with the HAV, a single-stranded RNA virus. In rare cases, it is transmitted through blood contamination. It frequently occurs in crowded, unsanitary living conditions, has no sex predilection, and is often epidemic in children or young adults. It has been called the "dormitory disease," because epidemics may break out and infect large numbers of students living close together.[7] This infection may also be transmitted by contaminated, inadequately cooked shellfish. Contaminated water has also been implicated as carrying the organism.

After exposure, an incubation period of 2 to 6 weeks occurs before clinical signs are evident. In children the disease, is usually *anicteric* (without jaundice), and diarrhea, nausea, and malaise are the predominant symptoms. These symptoms usually subside after 3 to 7 days. In adults, the disease is more severe, usually with the onset of jaundice following a flulike syndrome. The clinical course is usually described in three phases: *prodromal*, *icteric*, and *recovery*. The prodromal phase is the period of time when the person first becomes symptomatic with anorexia, nausea, vomiting, and flulike symptoms. It usually precedes jaundice by 1 to 2 weeks. Chronic infection or a fulminant course leading to liver failure is rare.[2] The course is rather predictable. The incubation period is about 3 to 4 weeks, and fecal shedding of infective virions precedes the onset of jaundice by 1 to 2 weeks.[2] As jaundice begins, serum IgM levels begin to rise, followed by an elevation in IgG levels that may last for decades. The liver enzymes alanine aminotransferase (ALT) and aspartate aminotransferase (AST) also rise, indicating hepatocellular necrosis. The jaundice remains present and the transaminases typically remain elevated up to 8 weeks after exposure.[2] The jaundiced or *icteric* phase is usually caused by conjugated hyperbilirubinemia (bilirubin >2.5 mg/dL), causing the urine to become dark, whereas the stools may become lighter due to cholestasis.[4] The icteric phase clears slowly, and usually complete recovery of the liver parenchyma results. Lifetime immunity probably results from hepatitis-A infection.[9]

Hepatitis A does not produce a chronic carrier state or a condition of chronic hepatitis.[9] In such areas as Costa Rica, where the disease is endemic, 90% of the population have anti-HAV antibodies by their teenage years.[4]

HEPATITIS B: SERUM HEPATITIS

Hepatitis B (HBV) results most frequently from blood transfusion or needle virus contamination, but it also may be transmitted placentally and venereally. The fecal–oral route is relatively unimportant.[16] The HBV is a DNA virus that is present in all body fluids of an infected person.[16] It is estimated that there are more than 200 million carriers of HBV worldwide.[2] Populations at high risk for HBV are those exposed to needle contamination, including persons receiving many blood transfusions, personnel and persons in renal dialysis units, and intravenous drug users. Also at high risk are the sexual partners of affected persons, male homosexuals, children with Down syndrome, and persons taking immunosuppressive medications. Families or other close contacts of any of these persons may also be at higher risk. Hepatitis B vaccinations are available and are recommended for most health care workers.

Hepatitis B has a longer incubation period than HAV, averaging 6 weeks, but clinical manifestations can occur up to 6 months after exposure. The HBV organism can be identified by the presence of the surface antigen, the hepatitis B surface antigen (HBsAg), previously called the *Australian antigen*. The HBsAg can be measured in the blood and persists through most of the infection. Its presence can be measured to establish the diagnosis of HBV infection.[9] The intact virion is known as the Dane particle. The particle core is synthesized within the nucleus of the hepatocyte and is composed of HBV core, DNA, and antigen.[4] The first viral antigen to appear is the HBsAg. Another antigen, HBeAg, becomes detectable at about 6 weeks but is rapidly cleared from the serum.[2] If it persists beyond 11 weeks, it indicates a high risk of chronic hepatitis. The core of the virus contains the core antigen, HBcAg, which is not found in the blood, but anti-HBc-IgM antibody is positive in the serum during acute infection and also in a "window period" when the HBsAg is negative.[9] When HBsAg clears from the serum, it indicates clearance of the virus.[2]

Pathologically, HAV and HBV look much alike. Hepatocellular injury and necrosis are usually surrounded by inflammatory cells, mainly lymphocytes and macrophages. The regeneration of hepatocytes begins very early in the disease, and multinucleate hepatocytes, increased mitotic figures, and hepatocyte thickening indicate regeneration.[4] The necrotic pattern may be spotty, confluent (groups of hepatocytes), or massive when most of the liver is affected. The hepatocyte necrosis is probably related to T cell cytotoxicity against the HBV, which would explain why individuals with impairment of T cell function are more likely to have relatively mild necrosis, incomplete elimination of HBV, and often a chronic HBV infection.[16] In general, there is evidence of 1) liver cell injury and scarring, 2) regeneration of liver cells, and 3) proliferation of inflammatory cells, including Kupffer cells.

The clinical syndrome of HBV is unpredictable and can include any of the following syndromes: 1) carrier states, either healthy carrier without evidence of disease or with chronic hepatitis; 2) acute, icteric, or nonicteric hepatitis; 3) chronic persistent or chronic active hepatitis; or 4) fulminant hepatitis with massive or submassive hepatic necrosis. Flowchart 43-1 indicates possible outcomes of infection with HBV.[14] The HBV also has been implicated in 60% to 90% of cases of hepatocellular carcinoma when it has reached a chronic carrier state.[9, 14]

Carriers

"Healthy" carriers can transmit the disease even though they have no evidence of infection themselves. The serum in these individuals is chronically positive for HBsAg and often other antigens, such as anti-HBc. Chronic carrier states are as high as 20% in some Asian populations.[16] Persons who are immune deficient for any number of reasons are more likely to be carriers than are other persons. Children who receive the virus during childbirth are usually carriers.[4]

Acute Hepatitis

The incubation time for HBV varies from 30 to 180 days after exposure. During the preicteric phase, rash, fever, and joint pain occur. The icteric phase may be present in only 50% of cases.[2, 7] Other liver symptoms, such as prolonged prothrombin time and hepatic tenderness, may be present. HBV is often not diagnosed due to lack of specific symptoms. Complete recovery and lifelong immunity is the rule for these persons.[14]

Chronic Hepatitis

Chronic persistent hepatitis is a smoldering infection that may not disrupt liver function severely. Nonspecific symptoms of anorexia and malaise may be noted with variable degrees of jaundice and hepatosplenomegaly.[14] Chronic active hepatitis progresses very rapidly to progressive liver damage, leading to cirrhosis, hepatic failure, and death.[4] Approximately 5% of HBV infections become chronic, and two-thirds of these infections are chronic active hepatitis.[4, 16]

Fulminant Hepatitis

This form of HBV infection progresses very rapidly from onset to fulminant liver failure and death in 2 to 3 weeks. It can result from other causative agents, but viral hepatitis accounts for 50% to 65% of all cases.[4]

HEPATITIS DELTA

The hepatitis delta virus (HDV) is produced by a defective RNA virus distinct from all others. Its onset is abrupt,

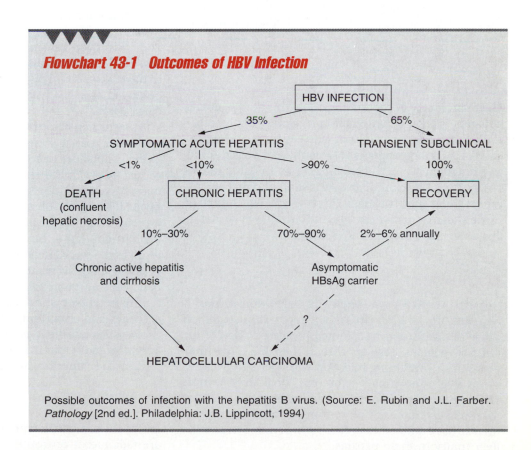

Possible outcomes of infection with the hepatitis B virus. (Source: E. Rubin and J.L. Farber. *Pathology* [2nd ed.]. Philadelphia: J.B. Lippincott, 1994)

with symptoms similar to HBV. The delta agent causes infection only in persons with active infection with HBV.[16] It is associated with more severe infection and a higher rate of fulminant hepatitis than HBV alone. The replication of the HDV is limited to when the HBsAg is found in the sera and the organisms are cleared together.[14] The organism is thought to have a direct cytopathic effect on hepatocytes.[2] It is transmitted by blood, serous body fluids, contaminated needles, and blood transfusions. A chronic state may persist with the combination of HBV and HDV.

The diagnosis is often overlooked or called an exacerbation of chronic HBV. Delta hepatitis is a common and serious cause of fulminant hepatitis, with 25% to 50% of fulminant HBV thought to relate to the delta agent.[9]

NON-A, NON-B HEPATITIS

The term non-A, non-B hepatitis has been used for viral hepatitis not due to HAV, HBV, Epstein-Barr virus, or cytomegalovirus.[16] Most of the non-A, non-B hepatitis cases are probably hepatitis C infection which is described below. At least two modes of transmission are identified for non-A, non-B hepatitis, which suggests that two viral agents exist. These have been labeled hepatitis E, which is transmitted by the fecal–oral route mainly being found in developing countries, and hepatitis C, which is mainly transmitted posttransfusion.[16] An estimated 90% of posttransfusion hepatitis is non-A, non-B hepatitis.

Hepatitis E

The main source of contamination for this non-A, non-B hepatitis is fecal contamination of water supply, especially in developing countries, such as India and southeast Asia. Its target population seems to be young adults and pregnant women. The disease has a fatality rate of 1% to 2%.[16] The clinical disease is similar to that of HAV except the course is usually more severe. No chronic or carrier state seems to exist, and the virus has been identified as a single-stranded RNA virus.[14]

Hepatitis C

Hepatitis C (HCV) was originally called non-A, non-B hepatitis. It is an RNA virus that is apparently a common cause of transfusion-transmitted hepatitis.[16] Half of the infected persons develop chronic hepatitis. This may persist as a continuing infection with elevated liver enzyme levels and minor symptoms, or it may become active and lead to cirrhosis, fulminant hepatitis, or hepatocellular carcinoma. Many chronic alcoholics with liver disease have antibodies to HCV, which may increase the liver injury in these persons.[14]

▼ Gallbladder Disease

CHOLECYSTITIS AND CHOLELITHIASIS

The most common disorders of the gallbladder are *cholecystitis* (inflammation) and *cholelithiasis* (gallstones). Inflammation of the gallbladder is the second most frequent cause of abdominal pain that requires abdominal surgery, the first being appendicitis. Dietary factors, including high fat intake, have long been associated with cholecystitis.

Cholelithiasis refers to biliary tract stones, most of which form in the gallbladder itself. Their major constituents are *cholesterol* and *pigment*, and they often contain mixtures of components of bile. Stones composed primarily of cholesterol account for 80% of gallstones in the United States. Gallstones occur in an estimated 20 million Americans per year, with considerable differences based on race and socioeconomics. Ten percent to 15% of adults in the United States have cholelithiasis, and 50% of these persons are asymptomatic. There is a dramatic increase in frequency among native Americans and Swedes. Some predisposing factors include middle age, female sex, obesity, and possibly multiparity. Pregnancy, oral contraceptives, and estrogen therapy may be contributors.

Clinical Manifestations

The clinical manifestations of gallstones arise when the stones migrate to and obstruct the common bile duct. The obstruction causes pain and blocks bile excretion. Visceral pain is precipitated by biliary contractions and is termed *biliary colic*. This pain is not colicky, but is usually perceived as a steady, severe aching or pressure in the epigastrium.[1]

Obstruction of the bile duct is followed by acute cholecystitis that may be due to increased pressure and ischemia in the gallbladder or to chemical irritation of the organ caused by prolonged exposure to concentrated bile. Primary bacterial infection may cause cholecystitis, but in up to 80% of cases, obstructive stones in the bile duct are present. Therefore, it is thought that bacterial contamination may either be secondary to the stasis or may result from severe infection, such as septicemia. Pancreatic reflux may occur and cause irritation by contact of pancreatic enzymes with the mucosa of the bile duct.[1]

Acute cholecystitis may cause complications with abscesses and/or perforation of the gallbladder. Chronic cholecystitis usually is associated with stones in the biliary ducts and is manifested by intolerance to fatty food, nausea and vomiting, and pain after eating.

Diagnosis

Due to the composition of the stones, about 85% of them are radiolucent on routine x-ray, whereas about 15%

can be visualized by abdominal x-rays, because they are calcified and radioopaque.[1] Abdominal ultrasonography will show stones as small as 3 mm in most affected persons. If the clinical picture remains suspicious after negative ultrasound results, an oral cholecystogram can be performed, which will show nonvisualization of the gallbladder. The white blood cell count may be elevated to 10,000 to 15,000. Bilirubin level is often increased, causing scleral and systemic jaundice. The pain of cholecystitis may mimic myocardial infarction, peptic ulcer, or intestinal obstruction, among other conditions.

▼ Chapter Summary

▼ Liver dysfunction occurs when more than 80% of the parenchyma of the liver has been destroyed. Its manifestations depend on the cause of the dysfunction but include jaundice, ascites, fatty liver, clotting disturbances, portal hypertension and esophageal varices, hepatorenal syndrome, and liver failure with or without hepatic encephalopathy and coma. The basis for all of the signs and symptoms have to do with the interruption of the functions performed by the liver. The liver may also be damaged by hepatotoxins.

▼ Cirrhosis of the liver is a general term for a condition that destroys the normal structure of the liver. It may be caused by intrahepatic block due to biliary obstruction or, more commonly, by alcohol toxicity.

▼ Tumors of the liver are sometimes benign but more frequently malignant, with a very poor prognosis. The course of the disease is very rapid, and response to treatment is minimal.

▼ Viral hepatitis is an inflammation of the liver due to certain specific viruses. The currently identified viruses are HAV; HBV; hepatitis D; non-A, non-B hepatitis, which has at least two forms, hepatitis E, and HCV. Each virus has specific characteristics and epidemiology. Some of the viruses lead to liver failure, some to a chronic carrier state, and some to complete cure.

▼ The most common gallbladder diseases are cholelithiasis and cholecystitis, which are closely related to a high-fat diet and stones composed mostly of cholesterol.

▼ References

1. Apstein, M.D. and Carey, M.C. Biliary tract stones and associated diseases. In J.H. Stein, *Internal Medicine* (4th ed.). St. Louis: C.V. Mosby, 1994.
2. Bain, V.G., Alexander, G.J., and Eddleston, A.L. Immunopathogenesis of viral hepatitis. In S.R. Targan and F. Shanahan, *Immunology and Immunopathology of the Liver and Gastrointestinal Tract*. New York: Igaku-Shoin, 1990.
3. Chopra, S. Hepatic tumors. In J.H. Stein, *Internal Medicine* (4th ed.) St. Louis: C.V. Mosby, 1994.
4. Cotran, R.S., Kumar, V., and Robbins, S.L. *Robbins' Patho-*
logic Basis of Disease (5th ed.). Philadelphia: W.B. Saunders, 1994.
5. Crabb, D.W., and Lumeng, L. Alcoholic liver disease. In W.N. Kelley, *Textbook of Internal Medicine* (2nd ed.). Philadelphia: J.B. Lippincott, 1992.
6. Dam, J.V., and Zeldis, J.B. Hepatic diseases in the elderly. *Gastroenterology Clin. of No. Am.* 19(2): 193, 1990.
7. Dienstag, J.L., Wands, J.R., and Isselbacher, K.J. Acute hepatitis. In J.D. Wilson, et al(eds), *Harrison's Textbook of Internal Medicine* (12th ed), New York: McGraw-Hill, 1991.
8. Greenberger, N.J., and Winship, D.H. *Gastrointestinal Disorders: A Pathophysiologic Approach* (3rd ed.). Chicago: Yearbook, 1986.
9. LaBreque, D.R. Acute and chronic hepatitis. In J.H. Stein. *Internal Medicine* (4th ed.) St. Louis: C.V. Mosby. 1994.
10. Lotze, M.T., Flickinger, J.C. and Carr, B.I. Hepatobiliary neoplasms. V.T. DeVita, S. Hellman, and S.A. Rosenberg. *Cancer: Principles and Practice of Oncology* (4th ed.). Philadelphia: J.B. Lippincott, 1993.
11. Ohtomo, K., and Itai, Y. Early diagnosis of hepatocellular carcinoma. In J.T. Ferrucci and D.G. Mathieu, *Advances in Hepatobiliary Radiology*. St. Louis: C.V. Mosby, 1990.
12. Ostrow, J.D., Jaundice and disorders of bilirubin metabolism. In J.H. Stein. *Internal Medicine* (4th ed), St. Louis: C.V. Mosby. 1994.
13. Reynolds, T.B. and Kanel, G.C. Alcoholic liver disease. In J.H. Stein. *Internal Medicine* (4th ed.) St. Louis: C.V. Mosby. 1994.
14. Rubin, E. and Farber, J.L. *Pathology* (2nd ed.), Philadelphia: J.B. Lippincott, 1994.
15. Schenker, S. and Hoyumpa, A.M. Principal complications of liver failure. In J.H.Stein, *Internal Medicine* (4th ed.), St. Louis: C.V. Mosby, 1994.
16. Shulman, S.T., Phair, J.P., and Sommers, H.M. *The Biologic and Clinical Basis of Infectious Diseases* (4th ed.) Philadelphia: W.B. Saunders. 1992.
17. Zimmerman, H.J. Drug- and toxin-induced liver disease. In J.H.Stein *Internal Medicine* (4th ed.), St. Louis: C.V. Mosby. 1994.

▼ Unit Bibliography

Ahlgren, J. and Macdonald, J. (eds).*Gastrointestinal Oncology*. Philadelphia: J.B. Lippincott, 1992.

Arias, I.M., Jakoby, W.B., Popper, H., Schachter, D., and Shafritz, D.A. *The Liver: Biology and Pathobiology* (2nd ed.). New York: Raven Press, 1988.

Cotran, R.S., Kumar, V., and Robbins, S. *Robbins' Pathologic Basis of Disease* (5th ed.). Philadelphia: W.B. Saunders, 1994.

Dam, J.V., and Zeldis, J.B. Hepatic diseases in the elderly. *Gastroenterology Clin. of No. Am.* 19(2):1990.

DeVita, V.T., Hellman, S., and Rosenberg, S.A. *Cancer: Principles and Practice of Oncology* (4th ed.) Philadelphia: J.B. Lippincott, 1993.

Dornschke, W., and Konturek, S.J. *The Stomach: Physiology, Pathophysiology, and Treatment*. New York: Springer-Verlag, 1993.

Fenoglio-Preiser, C.M., Lantz, P.E., Listrom, M.B., Davis, M., and Rilke, F.O. *Gastrointestinal Pathology: An Atlas and Text*. New York: Raven Press, 1989.

Ferrucci, J.T., and Mathieu, D.G. *Advances in Hepatobiliary Radiology*. St. Louis: C.V. Mosby, 1990.

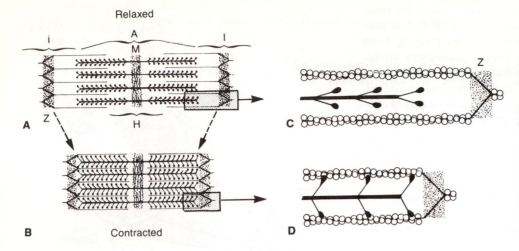

FIGURE 44-2 The components of a sarcomere that may be discerned as striations. The area indicated in **A** is shown in more detail in **C**, and the area indicated in **B** is shown in **D**. In **C**, the cross-bridges on the thick filaments are not interacting with the actin in the thin filaments. In **D**, the interaction of the cross-bridges with the actin is resulting in contraction. (Source: Cormack, D.H. Essential Histology, Philadelphia: J.B. Lippincott, 1993)

produced through a supply of adenosine triphosphate (ATP), which is mostly formed by the extraction of energy from nutrients and oxygen.

The sarcoplasmic reticulum (SR) is similar to the endoplasmic reticulum of other cells. Its major function appears to be to transport calcium into the sarcomere unit to initiate muscle contraction. The SR is composed of tubules running longitudinally and parallel to the myofibrils. The tubules terminate in closed sacs at the end of each sarcomere (terminal cisternae). The SR is highly developed in skeletal muscle but is less well developed in cardiac muscle cells. In smooth muscle, SR is poorly developed with narrow tubules of reticulum beneath which are many vesicles called *caveolae*.[3, 15] The transverse-tubule (T tubule) system is closely associated with the SR. It is composed of tubules that extend across the sarcoplasm but open to and communicate with the exterior of the muscle cell (Fig. 44-3).

NEUROMUSCULAR OR MYONEURAL JUNCTION

Each skeletal muscle fiber is normally innervated by a motor nerve. The nerve fiber branches at its end to form a motor end plate, or myoneural junction, that indents the surface of the muscle fiber membrane (Fig. 44-4). The neuromuscular junction is a type of synapse, a junction of excitable cells that allows a signal to be transmitted from one cell to the next. The junction of the axon terminal with the muscle fiber includes the following structures: 1) the synaptic gutter, the indentation of the fiber membrane where the axon terminal comes in close contact with the fiber; and 2) the synaptic cleft, the small space between the axon and the muscle. Within the axon terminal are synaptic vesicles that contain acetylcholine, the excitatory chemical transmitter. Cholinesterase is present on the surface of the folds of the synaptic gutter and destroys acetylcholine immediately after the response is initiated.

▼ Physiology of Striated Muscle

GENERATION OF AN ACTION POTENTIAL

For a skeletal muscle to contract, a stimulus from the nervous system must be present. When this stimulus arrives from the nerve axon to the myoneural junction, acetylcholine is released into the synaptic gutter space. This neurotransmitter causes the muscle cell membrane to become very permeable to positive ions in the cleft. The channels allow for the movement of sodium, potassium, and calcium.[7] Sodium is the main ion that rushes into the muscle fiber, causing a rise in membrane potential or generation of end-plate potential. The action potential thus generated passes down the sarcolemma, depolarizing the T tubule system and causing the release of calcium ions from the SR. Calcium ions, thus released, strongly bind with troponin-tropomyosin, and the sliding of actin on myosin occurs. This initiates the contractile phase.

SLIDING FILAMENT THEORY

The basis of muscular contraction is the movement or sliding of actin on myosin, which results in shortening of the entire sarcomere unit. Actin and myosin have been shown to have a strong affinity for each other that is inhibited by the proteins troponin and tropomyosin. The structure of myosin facilitates cross-linkages with actin, completing the system needed to perform the muscular contraction (see Figure 44-2).

Pure actin filaments bind strongly with myosin when in the presence of magnesium ions and ATP, which exist in abundance in the myofibrils. When troponin and tropomyosin are added to the thin filaments, binding between actin and myosin is inhibited. When the muscle is at rest, troponin and tropomyosin cover the actin filaments so that they cannot bind with myosin.

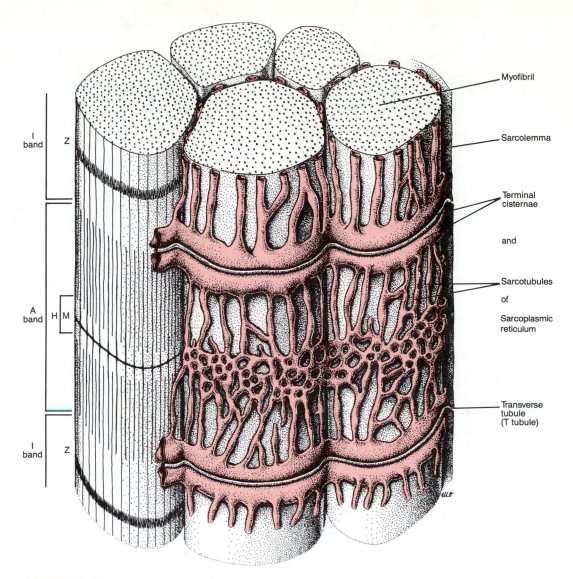

FIGURE 44-3 *Part of a mammalian skeletal muscle fiber, illustrating the sarcoplasmic reticulum surrounding its myofibrils. In mammalian skeletal muscle, two transverse (T) tubules supply a sarcomere. Each T tubule is situated at the junction between an A and an I band, where it is associated with two terminal cisternae of sarcoplasmic reticulum. Terminal cisternae connect with sarcotubules located around the A band, and these anastomose to form a network in the central region of the A band. The triple structure seen in cross-section where terminal cisternae from adjacent sarcomeres flank a transverse tubule is called a triad. (Source: Cormack, D.H.* Essential Histology. *Philadelphia: J.B. Lippincott, 1993).*

Initiation of the contractile process requires that troponin and tropomyosin be inhibited. Calcium ions, released from the SR, bind to sites on troponin molecules. This binding causes the troponin molecule to change shape, which pulls on the tropomyosin strands, moving them to the side and uncovering the cross-bridge binding sites on the actin molecules.[15] Adenosine triphosphate interacts at the site, splits, and activates myosin. Myosin binds to actin, creating a cross-bridge that moves the thin (actin) filaments toward the center. The cross-bridge is broken by the binding on a new ATP molecule. Splitting of this molecule causes the binding to reform at a different place on the actin molecule. This power stroke pulls the actin on the myosin in a step-by-step process described as a ratchetlike movement by Huxley in 1954.[8] The ATP is essential to provide energy through splitting for the cross-bridge movement and to break the myosin–actin connection, which allows the cross-bridge on myosin to return to its original position.

THE "WALK-ALONG" MECHANISM

The mechanism by which the cross-bridges on myosin interact with actin is not completely understood. The cross-bridges attach to and disengage from active sites on the actin filament in a "walk-along" fashion (Fig.

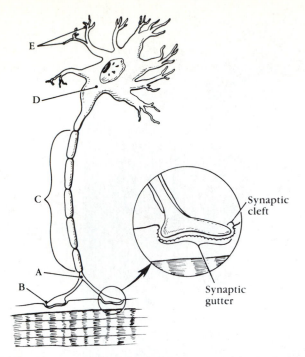

FIGURE 44-4 *Myoneural or neuromuscular junction. **A.** Terminal branching of nerve fibers for the end plate. **B.** Junction of axon terminal and muscle cell membrane. **C.** Axon. **D.** Nerve cell. **E.** Dendrites.*

44-5).[7] The attachment causes dragging of the actin filament (sliding of actin on myosin). After this power stroke, the sites are disengaged and attach to the next active site, pulling the actin filament step by step toward the center of the myosin filament. The cross-bridges theoretically operate independently of each other, so that if more cross-bridges are in contact with the actin filament, the force of the contraction is greater.

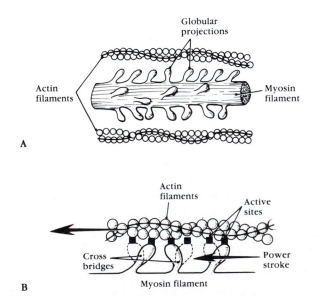

FIGURE 44-5 *"Walk-along" mechanism for muscle contraction. **A.** The relationship between the myosin filament with its globular projections and the actin filaments. **B.** The hinges of the myosin filament attach to successive active sites on the actin filaments.*

RETURN TO MUSCLE RELAXATION

Calcium must be returned to the tubules of the SR so that troponin and tropomyosin can resume their inhibitory function. This is accomplished by an active calcium pump in the walls of the SR. This pump also can concentrate calcium within the tubules, creating a low level of calcium in the myofibrils. As calcium is removed from the troponin, the troponin returns to its original configuration, which then allows tropomyosin strands to recover the actin-binding sites.[15] Without a communication between actin and myosin, the sarcomere unit extends, and the muscle relaxes.

Significant amounts of ATP are required to operate the calcium pump. In addition, the sodium pump is required to restore sodium–potassium balance and water balance within the cell (see pp. 19–20).

Flowchart 44-1 summarizes the processes of muscle contraction and relaxation.

Flowchart 44-1 Summary of Muscle Contraction and Relaxation

Stimulus from nerve axon to myoneural junction

Acetylcholine release in synaptic gutter

Increased permeability of muscle cell membrane to sodium

Rise in membrane potential (action potential generation)

Transmission of action potential through T tubules

Release of calcium from sarcoplasmic reticulum

Binding of calcium with troponin–tropomyosin

Sliding of actin on myosin with shortening of sarcomere unit

Contraction of the muscle fiber

Calcium pump moves calcium back to sarcoplasmic reticulum

Unbinding of troponin–tropomyosin

Inhibition of actin and myosin

Lengthening of sarcomere unit

Relaxation of muscle fiber

Summary of the processes of muscle contraction and relaxation.

ENERGY REQUIREMENTS OF MUSCLE CONTRACTION

Four physiologic reactions are available to provide energy for muscle contraction: 1) use of the limited supply of ATP stores within the cell; 2) conversion of high-energy stores from phosphocreatine (creatine phosphate); 3) generation of ATP through anaerobic glycolysis; and 4) oxidative metabolism of acetyl coenzyme (CoA).

Stored Adenosine Triphosphate

Adenosine triphosphate is a high-energy compound that is supplied mostly through an oxidative process. The ATP existing in the resting muscle cell is rapidly depleted during muscular contraction. Continued demand for energy is met by donation of phosphate from phosphocreatine stores and by anaerobic production of ATP. As exercise is sustained, the increased blood flow to muscle allows for the aerobic production of more ATP.

Phosphocreatine (Creatine Phosphate)

Muscle has a small store of creatine phosphate that can rapidly donate its phosphate to produce ATP and energy. This process occurs very rapidly, but the stores of creatine phosphate are rapidly depleted. Resynthesis in the resting muscle occurs with food metabolism.

Anaerobic Metabolism

Anaerobic metabolism provides ATP when the cellular supply of oxygen is insufficient to produce enough ATP to meet the energy requirements of the cell. In the muscular system, it is often used when the skeletal muscles are taxed, as in athletic exertion. Without the adequate oxygen supply, pyruvate does not enter the citric acid cycle to yield carbon dioxide and water, but rather is reduced to lactic acid (see p. 8). The net ATP formed is much less than with oxygen, but it allows the muscle cells to continue their activity for a short period of time.

Aerobic Production of ATP

As exercise is sustained, blood flow to the area is increased and a new steady state of muscle metabolism is achieved through the initiation of aerobic production of needed ATP.

Once the intense level of activity has stopped, the body consumes excess amounts of oxygen, as evidenced by the labored breathing of runners after a long-distance race. The intake of oxygen oxidizes the excess lactic acid and also aids in the metabolism that replenishes supplies of ATP and creatine phosphate. The amount of excess oxygen required to recover from the intense activity is directly related to the energy demands of the body. The amount of oxygen needed is called the *oxygen debt.*

At rest, the skeletal muscle uses mostly fatty acids for energy production. During exercise, the uptake of glucose and fat increases. An estimated 90% of carbon dioxide is produced through the metabolism of fat.[7]

CIRCULATORY ADJUSTMENTS TO EXERCISE

Exercise performance depends on the ability of the circulatory system to compensate for increased needs. Blood flow to the muscles is increased by opening capillary beds not open at rest. The stimuli for this phenomenon are probably tissue hypoxia and release of local vasodilator agents. Exercise increases cardiac output and heart rate, whereas vasodilation decreases systemic vascular resistance.

Dynamic exercise (isotonic) results in increases in systolic blood pressure, heart rate and stroke volume, and normal or decreased diastolic pressure. This type of exercise includes jogging, running, walking, and playing tennis. Sympathetic nervous system stimulation produces vasoconstriction in other vascular beds, such as the kidneys and gastrointestinal tract. Increased metabolic activity increases the body temperature so that heat loss is initiated. The two main methods of heat loss are through cutaneous vasodilation with radiation from the skin and sweating with evaporation.[9]

In static (isometric) exercise, muscle contractions create tensions but do not move a load. *Isometric exercise* results in elevation of systolic and diastolic blood pressures, increased systemic vascular resistance, and a modest increase in cardiac output and heart rate. *Static exercise* principally increases cardiac afterload stress by increasing systemic vascular resistance, whereas dynamic exercise increases the preload stress by increasing venous return and cardiac output.[12]

Muscles vary according to the work required of them. The speed of contraction is matched with the function of the corresponding muscle. Eye muscles, for example, provide fine, precise movement and react swiftly, whereas large muscles, such as those necessary to maintain posture, react slowly. The larger, slower muscles have smaller fibers and more capillaries and mitochondria than do faster-moving muscles. They are often called *red muscles* because they contain large quantities of myoglobin, an iron-containing protein similar to hemoglobin in red blood cells.[7] Muscle fibers have been classified into three basic types: 1) slow, or type I, which contain large amounts of myoglobin and provide for muscular endurance activities; 2) fast-oxidative-glycolytic, or type IIa; and 3) fast-glycolytic, or type IIb.[14] Types IIa and IIb use slightly different energy sources and are adapted for rapid and powerful muscle contractions, as in sprinting and jumping.[7,9]

Muscle tone is the term applied to the tautness of healthy muscle tissue at rest. This tone is maintained by spinal cord impulses which decreases as neuron excitability decreases or is lost. When tone is lost, the muscle is said to be *flaccid*. Increased excitability of the lower motor unit reflex arc may cause *spasticity* or *rigidity* (see p. 1026).

Exercise training over a period of weeks to months increases the number and size of mitochondria in the muscle cells; the level of mitochondrial enzyme activity; the capacity of muscle to oxidize fat, carbohydrate, and ketones; myoglobin levels; and the capacity to generate ATP.[7] The net effect is to increase the capability of muscles to extract oxygen and to increase aerobic capability at any given workload. The results on the cardiovascular system are decreases in heart rate, blood pressure, and systemic vascular resistance and increased stroke volume at any submaximal workload.[7]

▼ Anatomy of Smooth Muscle

The anatomy of smooth muscle differs somewhat from that of striated muscle, but the greatest difference between the two is functional. The smooth-muscle cell is long and spindle-shaped and has a single nucleus near the center of the cell. A sarcolemma surrounds the fiber, beneath which are many vesicles, or caveolae. These may function like SR storing calcium. Smooth-muscle fibers lack the characteristic striations of skeletal fibers and vary markedly in length. The lack of striations probably is due to a poorly developed SR and T tubule system. Two distinct groups of smooth muscle have been identified: visceral and multiunit (Fig. 44-6). The three different filaments described for smooth muscle are the thin (actin), thick (myosin), and intermediate (dense bodies) filaments, which run continuously through the fiber.[7]

VISCERAL (UNITARY) SMOOTH MUSCLE

Visceral smooth muscle is present in the walls of the hollow visceral organs, such as the uterus, gut, and bile ducts. The cells are closely aligned and form large sheets of tissue. Because of the close proximity of cells, an action potential spreads cell to cell along the muscle until the entire muscle mass is stimulated. These muscles respond to innervation from the autonomic nervous system to increase or decrease the rate of activity, but it is a slow response to this stimulation. When one portion of visceral muscle tissue is stimulated, the action potential is conducted throughout by direct electrical conduction.[7, 15]

MULTIUNIT SMOOTH MUSCLE

Multiunit smooth muscle is present in the ciliary muscles of the eye and in the piloerector muscles of the skin that can cause a gooseflesh appearance. This type of smooth muscle is composed of independent muscle fibers that are individually innervated. They contract more rapidly than the visceral smooth muscle.

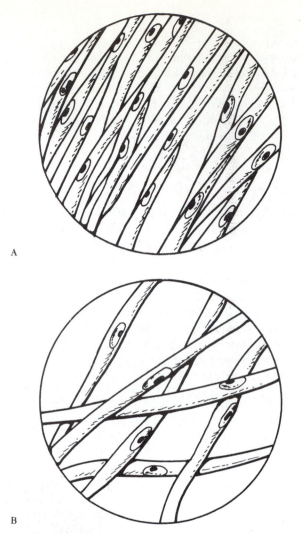

FIGURE 44-6 ***A.*** *Visceral smooth muscle as present in the walls of hollow visceral organs. Note close arrangements of fibers.* ***B.*** *Multiunit cells as present in ciliary muscles of the eyes, for example. Note loose arrangement of fibers.*

▼ Physiology of Smooth Muscle

Four properties distinguish smooth-muscle contractions from other types: 1) the contractile process is relatively slow, with contractions lasting for long periods of time; 2) energy expended during the long contractions is far less than that of striated muscle; 3) in certain circumstances, such as childbirth, the strength of contractions can be very forceful; and 4) slow relaxation follows the slow contraction.

In visceral smooth muscle, electrical excitation proceeds from one muscle fiber to the next due to tight junctions that allow the impulse to pass from muscle cell to muscle cell; this is a *syncytial effect*.

ACTION POTENTIALS IN SMOOTH MUSCLE

Spike Potential

Action potentials develop differently in visceral smooth-muscle tissue. The spike potential, similar to that of striated muscle, can be elicited by 1) electrical stimulation; 2) hormone action; 3) nerve fibers; and 4) spontaneous generation in the muscle fiber itself.[7] A typical spike action potential can be recorded much like that in skeletal muscle.

Slow-Wave Potential

The second type of action potential is the slow-wave potential. Some smooth muscle is self-excitatory, needing no apparent external stimulation. This is evidenced by rhythmic peristaltic waves. The slow waves apparently contribute to the action potential, a type of pacemaker wave.

Action potentials also may involve plateaus, long periods of depolarization, prolonged contraction, and slow repolarization. Prolonged contractions occur in the ureters, the vascular system, and the uterus.[7] Waves of contraction, called *peristalsis*, occur along the gastrointestinal tract. These are inhibited by stimulation of the sympathetic nervous system and augmented by stimulation of the parasympathetic nervous system.

SMOOTH-MUSCLE TONE

Smooth-muscle tone describes the ability of fibers to maintain the long-term contraction that occurs in the peristaltic type of contraction. The smooth muscles of the arterioles exhibit continuous variable degrees of contraction that respond to changing autonomic nervous stimulation. These may also be responsive to local tissue factors or circulating hormones.

NEUROMUSCULAR JUNCTIONS OF SMOOTH MUSCLE

Two types of neuromuscular junctions are present in the innervation of smooth muscle: 1) the *contact type*, in which the nerve fibers come into direct contact with the muscle cells, and 2) the *diffuse type*, which occurs when nerve fibers never come into direct contact with the smooth-muscle fibers. The contraction may be initiated by nerve impulses (through transmitter substances), chemical agents, changes in the muscle itself, and even local stretch or distention.

Smooth muscle has one nerve supply for inhibition and another for excitation. The transmitters for this, acetylcholine and epinephrine, are secreted by the autonomic nervous system. The response to the chemical transmitters varies, but generally, if acetylcholine excites an organ, norepinephrine acts as an inhibitor and vice versa.

▼ Anatomy of Cardiac Muscle

Before advances in microscopic technology, cardiac muscle cells were thought to form a morphologic *syncytium*. *Syn* refers to being together; *cyte* means cell. Light microscopy reveals cardiac tissue to have cross-striations with unique dark bands encircling the fibers at random sites. Seemingly, the cells are incomplete and branch into one another, forming a continuous mass of protoplasm. Electron microscopy, however, reveals that cardiac muscle cells are netlike in appearance, with fibers running together, spreading apart, and again running together in no apparent pattern. The dark bands that can be seen with the light microscope are abutting bands of tissue encircling the cardiac fibers (Fig. 44-7). They are called *intercalated disks* and are located at the sites of the Z bands. The disks represent areas where membranes of adjacent cells approach each other. Functionally, these disks allow a wave of depolarization to pass unhindered from one cell to the next. Although each cardiac fiber branches and anastomoses with other fibers, a plasma membrane actually encases each fiber. Each cell has a single, centrally located nucleus. An abundance of elongated mitochondria are present close to the myofibrils in cardiac tissue. As in skeletal cells, myofibrils and the contractile proteins (actin and myosin) are present.

Structural differences between skeletal and cardiac tissue are apparent. An SR is present in cardiac muscle,

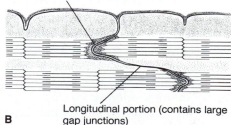

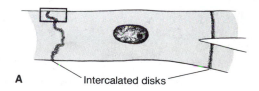

FIGURE 44-7 ***A.*** *Diagram of a cardiac muscle cell with intercalated disks at either end.* ***B.*** *Boxed-in area* ***A*** *as seen in the electron microscope showing the cell junctions in the two different portions of an intercalated disk. The longitudinal portions possess large gap junctions, and the transverse portions possess small gap junctions. (Source: Cormack, D.H. Essential Histology. Philadelphia: J.B. Lippincott, 1993)*

but it is very rudimentary in comparison to that of skeletal muscle. The T tubules are five times larger in cardiac tissue than in skeletal tissue and are lined with mucopolysaccharide filaments. These filaments seem to trap calcium ions that are used by the sarcoplasm once an action potential has been initiated. Because *terminal cisternae* of skeletal tissue are missing in cardiac tissue, scientists believe that the T tubules act as reservoirs for calcium in cardiac muscle, as the terminal cisternae do in skeletal tissue.

Myocardial muscle fibers are structured in such a way that the atria and ventricles, when normal and intact, react individually as syncytial units. The specialized conductive units—the sinoatrial node, atrioventricular node, bundle of His, and Purkinje's fibers—work in concert to cause cardiac contraction. The physiology of cardiac contraction is described in detail in Chapter 22.

▼ Alterations in Muscles of the Body

COMMON PROBLEMS IN MUSCLES

Muscular problems are very common and may result from overuse, especially after an extended layoff from exercise. A temporary soreness is often described, which may result from lactic acid accumulation, small tears in the muscle tissue, muscle spasms, and overstretching of the muscle.[9] The soreness is often delayed in onset and usually goes away with rest and moderate usage. Other muscle problems, described below, include cramps, strain, and injury.

Weakness

Weakness usually is described by the affected person and relates to loss of strength in one or more muscle groups.[16] It may be subjective in nature but is objective when the muscular power is actually decreased on tests of muscular function. This problem is a component of many disorders and is characteristic in chronic illnesses, especially diabetes mellitus. It may reflect primary muscle disease or the underlying disease. Any condition of decreased cardiac output and chronic infectious disease may lead to generalized weakness. Weakness in one limb may be an indicator of multiple sclerosis (see pp. 1090–1091). Muscular atrophy in association may indicate innervation problems or lack of use.

Cramps

Cramps, or spasms, are frequent occurrences in the skeletal muscles. They may be idiopathic or associated with motor system disease, metabolic disease (eg, uremia), tetanus, and electrolyte depletion, especially of sodium, potassium, and calcium. Muscle cramps are often reported at night or during rest and may be due to lowered blood glucose levels at night. Dehydration also may cause cramping, especially if associated with sodium depletion. Cramps are involuntary spasms of specific muscle groups in which the muscles become taut and painful. They may occur in the calf, thigh, hip, or any other major muscle group. Visible fasciculations may also occur before and after cramps.[12]

Strain

Various degrees of muscle damage may be diagnosed as strain, which usually results from overuse. Strains usually occur at the most susceptible part of the muscle–tendon unit and may be very painful or associated with tendinitis. Strains may cause an inflammation of the affected muscle, causing it to swell and become erythematous and hot to the touch.

Injury

Direct trauma may cause a hematoma (bleeding into the muscle tissue) in a muscle, which is identified by localized tenderness, swelling, and pain on movement. Large hematomas can cause damage to the muscle. Muscle tears may result from inadequate warm-up before participating in rigorous sports. Mild tears will heal with rest and splinting, but severe cases may require surgical repair.[13] The most common locations for these tears are in the quadriceps of sprinters, in the hamstrings and biceps of weight lifters, and in the gastrocnemius in tennis players.[13]

Twitches, Fasciculations, and Fibrillations

These reactions are the result of spontaneous discharge of motor units and single muscle fibers. Twitches occurring at rest may be idiopathic or associated with hyperkalemia, motor neuron disease, and peripheral neuropathies.

Fasciculations are involuntary contractions of a single motor unit. They may occur in healthy persons and cause visible dimpling or twitching of the skin. Fasciculations may occur rhythmically, starting and stopping for no apparent reason. Those during contraction of a muscle indicate excessive irritation and may occur years after poliomyelitis or a degenerative nervous system disease. The molecular pathogenesis is not fully understood but apparently involves hypersensitivity of the neuronal membrane to acetylcholine. Continuous fasciculations, called *myokymia*, of unknown etiology may involve all of the voluntary muscles. Fasciculation is often confused with fibrillation, which results from the contraction of single muscle fibers. Fibrillation is not visible and is noted on electromyography.[15] It occurs when the motor unit of the axon is destroyed. The fibers contract rhythmically, often up to 10 times per second. As denervation continues, the muscle fibers atrophy and fibrillation stops.[7]

Tetany

Tetany, a spasmodic condition, most frequently results from hypocalcemia and hypomagnesemia. It is probably due to unstable depolarization of the distal segments of the motor nerves. Hyperventilation may precipitate tetany by lowering serum carbon dioxide level, which reduces the level of ionized calcium.

Myoclonus

Myoclonus is a sudden, unexpected contraction of a single muscle or group of muscles that involves the limbs more than the trunk. This disorder has many causes, from idiopathic benign (sleep) jerks to central nervous system disease.[7]

Tics

Tics differ from myoclonus in that they are sudden, behavior-related, repetitive movements that may be a form of learned behavior or occur as a part of Gilles de la Tourette's syndrome. In the latter, tics may be accompanied by involuntary vocalizations.

HYPERTROPHY

Hypertrophy, the enlargement of individual muscle fibers, is an adaptive condition of the cells that results from an increased demand for work. The cardiac and skeletal muscle cells apparently cannot regenerate to adapt to a need for increased function. Adaptation to increasing loads occurs through enlarging individual fibers, not through the addition of new muscle fibers.[3] Nutrients, such as ATP, creatine phosphate, and glycogen, increase in concentration within the cell when there is need for increased work.

Most hypertrophy is considered to be adaptive in that it results when resistance is continually applied to the muscle walls. A weight lifter or athlete increases the workload through specific muscles that increase size and strength up to a physiologic limit.

Cardiac hypertrophy is a common adaptation for arterial hypertension, aortic valvular stenosis, and co-arctation of the aorta. Hypertrophy increases the force of the cardiac contraction, which can maintain cardiac output for long periods of time. Initially, this is considered to be an adaptive mechanism, but it may become maladaptive if the nutritional needs of the hypertrophied ventricle outstrip the blood supply from the coronary arteries.

ATROPHY

Atrophy refers to the decrease in muscle mass due to diminution in size of the myofibrils. Atrophic muscles can result from such diverse factors as aging, immobilization, chronic ischemia, malnutrition, and denervation.[4] Muscle atrophy can occur very rapidly, with significant wasting occurring in 4 to 6 days when the muscle is immobilized in a shortened position.[12] *Disuse atrophy* describes wasting of muscle tissue due to lack of muscle stress: an example is atrophic changes occurring after a bone fracture and treatment with casting. In one study, after a mean casting period of 131 days, leg volume was reduced by 12% in the casted leg.[12]

Ischemia causes an inadequate blood supply, so that the oxygen and nutrients required for cellular maintenance are diminished. Eventually, ischemic changes may result in infarction of the tissue.

Denervation causes atrophic muscular changes that become irreversible. Loss of normal neural stimulation and reduction of muscle tone seem to be the major factors in these changes, rather than lack of weight bearing. If a muscle cell is reinnervated within 3 to 4 months, full function can be restored. After this time, some of the muscle fibers become permanently atrophied, and after 2 years muscle function is rarely restored (see pp. 1044–1049).

Atrophy of muscle tissue may also occur in malnutrition or in wasting diseases, such as cancer and cirrhosis of the liver. The muscle does not receive adequate nutrition and, consequently, protein wasting occurs.

Widespread muscular atrophy is a consequence of aging and relates to reduction of muscle fiber size and number. Muscle strength decreases an average of 25% after age 60, and the amount of work the muscle can perform decreases even more.[11]

▼ Pathologic Processes Affecting the Skeletal Muscles

Myopathies is the general term given to diseases intrinsic to muscles. The category includes inherited muscular dystrophies, inherited and acquired metabolic myopathies, and inflammatory myopathies. Below is a brief review of the more common myopathies and rhabdomyosarcoma.

MUSCULAR DYSTROPHIES

The muscular dystrophies are genetically determined, progressive diseases of specific muscle groups. They are characterized by progressive weakness of the voluntary muscles.[14] The syndromes are classified mainly by the distribution of involved muscles. Classification may also be based on pattern of inheritance, age of onset, and speed of progression.[4] Several members of the same family may be affected, with males predominating and females carrying the genetic abnormality. Muscle fiber atrophy, necrosis, regeneration, and fibrosis are components of variable frequency depending on the type of muscular dystrophy exhibited.

Duchenne Muscular Dystrophy

This genetic recessive disorder occurs almost exclusively in males. Recent advances in molecular biology have identified the defective gene on the short arm of the X chromosome.[4, 10] The affected gene fails to direct the production of *dystrophin*, a protein normally found adjacent to the sarcolemmal membranes in myocytes and thought to affect muscle fiber contraction.[4] Muscle fibers that do not have dystrophin may lack the normal interaction between the sarcolemma and the extracellular matrix.[14]

Pathologic changes include degeneration of muscle fibers, progressive fibrosis, and an attempt at regeneration by the muscle fibers.[14] As the disease progresses, there is almost complete loss of skeletal muscle fibers, which become replaced by fat and connective tissue.[4, 14]

Duchenne dystrophy is characterized by early development of motor difficulties, inability to walk, symmetric weakness of the arms, and enlargement of the muscles of the calves. Intellectual impairment is common. The disease characteristically begins with lower extremity weakness that progresses upward and finally affects the head and chest muscles. The characteristic pseudohypertrophy of calf muscles is due to infiltration of the fibers with fatty deposits. The muscle becomes significantly weakened. Weakness of the back muscles results in lordosis. Respiratory or cardiac failure often causes death.

Prognosis for this disease is very poor, with death usually occurring before the age of 20. Before that time, increasing disabilities require much medical assistance.

Adult Forms of Muscular Dystrophy

Adult forms of muscular dystrophy, such as Becker's, limb-girdle, and facioscapulohumeral, have a later onset and differ somewhat in the pattern of muscle involvement, heredity, and rate of progression. Becker's muscular dystrophy is less common and less severe than Duchenne muscular dystrophy. Becker's muscular dystrophy shows identifiable dystrophin, which reflects mutations that allow synthesis of some dystrophin.[4] The limb-girdle and facioscapulohumeral forms of the disease have an onset at about 10 to 30 years with weakness of different muscle groups and variable rate of progression. Other forms of muscular dystrophy have been described but are rare.

Laboratory and Diagnostic Tests

Most persons with any form of muscular dystrophy have elevated levels of enzymes normally present in the muscles. These include creatine phosphokinase, lactic dehydrogenase, glutamic transaminase, and glucose phosphate isomerase. All of these findings indicate abnormal muscle plasma membranes.[4] Lymphocyte abnormalities also have been described. Electromyography reveals weak electrical currents present in the muscle cell. Muscle biopsy results are abnormal due to the presence of fatty tissue deposits in the cell.

MYASTHENIA GRAVIS

Myasthenia gravis is a disease related to the inability of the neuromuscular junctions to transmit nerve impulses to the muscle cells effectively (see pp. 1087–1089). There is a defect in the production or release of acetylcholine. This disease is probably autoimmune in causation and is mostly seen in females, with onset of muscle weakness especially of the ocular muscles and muscles of the head and neck.[6]

INFLAMMATORY MYOPATHIES

Polymyositis and *dermatomyositis* are rare inflammatory myopathies of autoimmune or viral origin.[2, 5] Clinically, the onset is usually in adulthood, with proximal limb and neck weakness associated with muscle pain. Muscle necrosis is patchy, and inflammation becomes chronic. In dermatomyositis, cutaneous manifestations of papules, erythematous patches over the joints, and erythema of the face and neck are associated with muscle weakness.[5] Progression of the weakness in polymyositis and dermatomyositis often affects the heart and pulmonary systems. Laboratory findings include elevation of the transaminase levels and myoglobinemia for persons who have lost considerable muscle mass.[2, 5]

Fibrositis-fibromyalgia syndrome is a common condition of musculoskeletal pain without evidence of arthritis.[1] It occurs predominantly in women of childbearing age with the following major complaints: musculoskeletal pain, stiffness, and easy fatigability. The stiffness tends to improve with movement, and a sleep disturbance is often described. Muscle biopsies are inconclusive, but decreased ATP and creatine phosphate levels in areas of described tenderness have been noted. The most commonly related feature is a disturbance of stage 4 (non–rapid eye movement) sleep.[1] Continuing research may clarify this common condition.

INHERITED METABOLIC AND CONGENITAL MYOPATHIES

These diverse myopathies affect muscle tone and produce weakness, often in infants. In the inherited McArdle syndrome, for example, the problem is in the glycolytic pathways for the production of energy. The mitochondrial myopathies exhibit varying pathologies of the mitochondria and a wide range of effects. The congenital myopathies often present as a "floppy infant" who has other associated developmental diseases.[4] Some examples of inherited metabolic myopathies include glycogen storage disease, periodic paralyses, lipid metabolism abnormalities, and mitochondrial myopathies.[6]

ACQUIRED METABOLIC AND TOXIC MYOPATHIES

Acquired metabolic myopathies are often secondary to disorders of the endocrine system. Many endocrine dysfunctions can cause weakness and fatigability, although they usually respond to appropriate endocrine management.[10] Nutritional and vitamin deficiency may lead to myopathy, especially protein deficiency and lack of vitamins D and E.

Toxic myopathies are related to certain drugs and chemicals. Focal, localized myopathies are related to the injection of narcotic analgesics, especially pentazocine and meperidine.[10] Penicillamine, cimetidine, procainamide, and other drugs have been shown to produce weakness, myositis, and even muscle fiber necrosis. In most cases, the mechanism of toxicity to the muscles is poorly understood.[10] Corticosteroid therapy causes steroid-induced muscle weakness, and differentiating it from the initial condition being treated can be difficult.

Excessive alcohol usage can produce a severe rhabdomyolysis (breakdown of striated muscle), which can affect the skeletal and heart muscles.[4] Renal failure may result when there is significant elevation of the myoglobin in the urine.

Polymyositis is an autoimmune disorder in which there is destruction of muscle fibers due to sensitized lymphocytes. It usually begins in women in middle life. Deterioration may be rapid or slow, and remissions are common. Pathologically, muscle fiber damage is seen with chronic inflammatory infiltrate and necrosis and atrophy.[6]

RHABDOMYOSARCOMA

Rhabdomyosarcoma is an uncommon malignant tumor of striated muscle. It occurs most commonly in children and adolescents and may affect the striated muscles of the extremities, head, or neck. This type of sarcoma is very invasive, with extremely anaplastic cells.[4] Five-year survival is 30% to 40%; treatment includes resection, radiation therapy, and chemotherapy.

▼ Chapter Summary

▼ The muscular system is composed of striated skeletal and cardiac as well as nonstriated smooth muscle. The muscles are composed of muscle fibers, which are composed of myofibrils, the contractile units of the muscle. Muscles are metabolically active and depend on a continuous supply of oxygen and multiple mitochondria to produce ATP.

▼ The contraction of a skeletal muscle begins with the release of acetylcholine into the myoneural junction, causing a rise in the membrane potential and release of calcium from the SR. Calcium initiates the actin–myosin shortening, which results in contraction of the muscle. Active pumping of the calcium back into the SR causes the relaxation of the fiber.

▼ Smooth muscle contracts much like striated except in the development of the action potential, causing a slow wave potential in some areas.

▼ Cardiac muscle contracts in much the same manner as striated except that there is a passing of the impulse from muscle fiber to muscle fiber, so that the entire unit contracts as a unit.

▼ Alterations in the muscle include common problems, such as weakness, cramps, strain, and injury. Hypertrophy and atrophy are adaptive mechanisms of the muscle that result from use or disuse in many cases.

▼ The most common inherited pathologic conditions of skeletal muscle are the muscular dystrophies. Other myopathies include inflammatory, metabolic, and toxic myopathies. Rhabdomyosarcoma is a malignant tumor of the striated muscle, which is uncommon.

▼ References

1. Bennett, R.M. The fibrositis-fibromyalgia syndrome. In H.R. Schumacher (ed.), *Primer on the Rheumatic Diseases* (9th ed.). Atlanta: Arthritis Foundation, 1988.
2. Bradley, W.G. Dermatomyositis and polymyositis. In E. Braunwald, et al. (eds.), *Harrison's Principles of Internal Medicine* (12th ed.). New York: McGraw-Hill, 1991.
3. Cormack, D.H. *Essential Histology.* Philadelphia: J.B. Lippincott, 1993.
4. Cotran, R.S., Kumar, V., and Robbins, S.L. *Pathologic Basis of Disease* (5th ed.). Philadelphia: W.B. Saunders, 1994.
5. Cronin, M.E., Miller, F.W., and Plotz, P.H. Polymyositis and dermatomyositis. In H.R. Schumacher (ed.), *Primer on the Rheumatic Diseases* (9th ed.). Atlanta: Arthritis Foundation, 1988.
6. Govan, A.D.T., Macfarlane, P.S., and Callander, R. *Pathology Illustrated* (3rd ed.). New York: Churchill Livingstone. 1991.

7. Guyton, A.C. *Textbook of Medical Physiology* (8th ed.). Philadelphia: W.B. Saunders, 1991.

8. Huxley, H.E. The double array of filaments in cross-striated muscle. *J. Biophys. Biochem Cytol.* 3:631, 1957.

9. McArdle, W.D., Katch, F.I. and Katch, V.L. *Exercise Physiology* (2nd ed.). Philadelphia: Lea and Febiger. 1986.

10. Mendell, J.R., and Griggs, R.C. Muscular dystrophy and other chronic myopathies. In E. Braunwald, et al. (eds.), *Harrison's Principles of Internal Medicine* (12th ed.). New York: McGraw-Hill, 1991.

11. Peppard, R.F., Snow, B.I., and Calne, D. Central and peripheral nervous system alterations in the elderly. In W.N. Kelley (ed.), *Textbook of Internal Medicine* (2nd ed.). Philadelphia: J.B. Lippincott. 1992.

12. Pollock, M.L., Wilmore, J.H., and Fox, S.M. *Exercise in Health and Disease*. Philadelphia: W.B. Saunders, 1984.

13. Pullman, S., and Mooar, P. Sports and occupational injuries. In H.R. Schumacher (ed.), *Primer on the Rheumatic Diseases* (9th ed.). Atlanta: Arthritis Foundation, 1988.

14. Rubin, E., and Farber, J.L. *Pathology* (2nd ed.). Philadelphia: J.B. Lippincott, 1994.

15. Tortora, G., and Grabowski, S. *Principles of Anatomy and Physiology* (7th ed.). New York: Harper Collins, 1993.

16. Vesely, D.L. Weakness. In J. Stein (ed.), *Internal Medicine* (4th ed.). St. Louis: C.V. Mosby, 1994.

Chapter 45

Normal and Altered Structure and Function of the Skeletal System

Barbara L. Bullock

▼ LEARNING OBJECTIVES

1 Differentiate between intramembranous and endochondral ossification in bone formation.
2 Describe the blood supply to a bone, including the nutrient and periosteal arteries.
3 Describe the factors that affect epiphyseal growth.
4 Explain the calcium–parathyroid feedback mechanism.
5 Describe the relationships among bone formation, sex hormones, and age.
6 Discuss the effects of weight bearing on bone structure.
7 Differentiate among the three classifications of joints.
8 Describe the structures of tendons, ligaments, and bursae.
9 Compare the different types of fractures.
10 Describe the process of fracture healing and alterations that can occur.
11 Discuss the symptoms of anterior compartmental syndrome.
12 Describe the clinical syndrome of osteogenesis imperfecta.
13 Describe fibrous dysplasia and Paget's disease of bone.
14 Identify the usual pathogenesis of rickets or osteomalacia.
15 Describe the pathology of avascular necrosis of the head of the femur.
16 Describe the course of osteomyelitis from beginning infection to the chronic stage.
17 Describe the physical changes of scoliosis.
18 Describe the pathogenesis and pathology of rheumatoid arthritis.
19 Describe the metabolic disorder responsible for gout.
20 Describe basic differences between benign and malignant bone tumors.
21 Compare and contrast the sarcomas of cartilaginous origin with those of osteogenic origin.
22 Discuss the skeletal involvement and symptoms of multiple myeloma.

Barbara L. Bullock: PATHOPHYSIOLOGY: ADAPTATIONS AND ALTERATIONS IN FUNCTION, 4th ed.
© 1996 Lippincott-Raven Publishers

▼ *Normal Structure and Function of Bone*

The framework of the human body is the skeletal system. This system of more than 206 bones protects internal organs, provides for support and movement through its muscle attachments, serves as a storehouse for mineral supply, and produces blood cells. A living, dynamic tissue, bone contains blood, nerves, and lymph supplies and provides for the constant movement of calcium, phosphorus, and other minerals into and out of the bloodstream.

Bone is a collagenous protein that is partially composed of complex calcium salts. The organic matrix of bone, called the *osteoid*, is made up primarily of collagen (protein), some polysaccharides, and lipids. The salts, which consist of calcium carbonate and calcium phosphate, form a substance that is a hard crystalline salt. The matrix supplies tensile strength (resistance to being pulled apart), whereas the mineral deposits provide compressive strength (resistance to being crumbled). This combination gives bone the tensile strength of white oak and a compressive strength greater than granite.

BONE FORMATION

Cellular Components

Bone tissue is constantly being formed and reformed. This modeling is facilitated by three types of cells. *Osteoblasts* are formed from osteogenic cells present in the endosteum, periosteum, and epiphyseal plates of long bones. These are bone-forming cells that synthesize the collagenous matrix osteoid in the process of ossification. Osteoid is a protein substance that becomes calcified to produce hard bone. Osteoblasts also help control the calcification of bone. Alkaline phosphatase, which is thought to aid in the mineralization process, is produced by osteoblasts.[11] Osteoblasts synthesize the organic components of bone matrix.[7] When the matrix surrounding the osteoblasts becomes calcified, the cells are called *osteocytes*. *Osteoclasts* are cells of monocyte–macrophage origin whose primary function is the reabsorption of bone. These cells produce acids that make the bone salts soluble and then digest the organic matrix.[7]

Intramembranous Ossification

Bone formation begins in early fetal life. The fetal skeleton is composed mostly of hyaline cartilage that undergoes ossification. The swapping of the cartilaginous material with bone, begun in utero, continues until after puberty. There are two main types of bone formation: intramembranous and endochondral. The more simple and direct type is intramembranous ossification, which occurs in the flat bones of the face and skull. In the cartilaginous fetal structure, osteoblasts secrete organic material that calcifies; from this center of ossification, small bone spicules build up an interlacing network on which more bone is developed. Eventually, the osteoblasts are trapped in small spaces called *lacunae* and become osteocytes. The spongy bone developed is then covered by layers of compact bone.

Endochondral Ossification

The process by which the long bones of the body are formed is called endochondral ossification (Fig. 45-1). The "baby skeleton," which is cartilage, is transformed into bone by ossification, which begins in the center of the shaft (diaphysis) and in each end (epiphysis) of the bone. This formation spreads and with it the destruction of cartilage, until only two thin strips are left at either end of the bone (the epiphyseal plate). These strips remain until bone growth and maturation are completed. Spongy bone is formed in most of the short, flat, irregularly shaped bones and in long bone epiphyses. Marrow is formed in the spaces and the marrow cavity develops in the center of the bone. The osteoblasts on the outside form layers of hard, compact bone. The perichondrium, which is the layer surrounding the early cartilage, becomes the periosteum, and as more layers of compact bone are laid circumferentially, osteoclasts make the marrow, or medullary cavity, larger to support the larger bone. The process has been described in zones as illustrated in Figure 45-1. These are 1) the zone of resting cartilage, which functions to anchor the epiphyseal plate to the bone structure and provide blood supply to much of the calcifying cartilage; 2) the zone of proliferating cartilage, which divides and supplies chondrocytes that are lost at the epiphyseal plate; 3) the zone of maturing cartilage, in which chrondrocytes are filled with glycogen and lipid substances and secrete alkaline phosphatase, which facilitates the calcification of extracellular matrix; and 4) the zone of calcifying cartilage, in which area insoluble calcium salts become deposited and capillaries grow to provide adequate blood supply.[7]

BONE STRUCTURE

Microscopic Structure

Bone has three structural forms: cortical or compact (hard surface area), cancellous or spongy, and medullary (inner core). Whenever bone matrix is laid down rapidly and haphazardly, as occurs after fractures and in fetal growth, the resultant immature form is termed *woven bone*. The microscopic structure of compact bone consists of numerous, parallel, longitudinal canals (haversian canals), which contain blood vessels, lymphatics, and nerves (Fig. 45-2). Around each canal are several layers, or rings, of bone called *lamellae*. Connecting the haver-

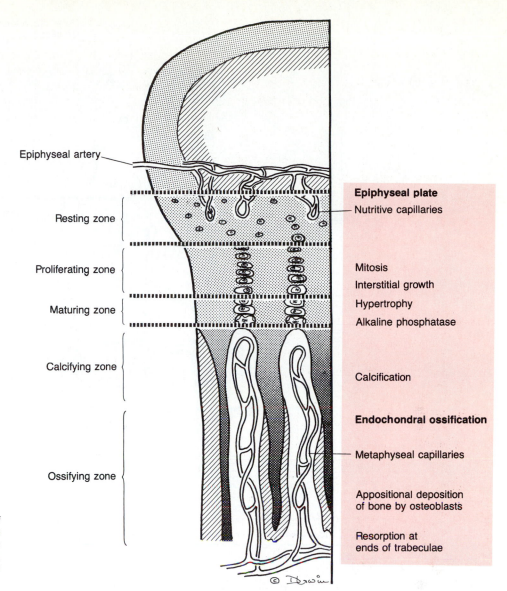

Epiphyseal artery

Epiphyseal plate
Nutritive capillaries

Resting zone

Proliferating zone
— Mitosis
— Interstitial growth

Maturing zone
— Hypertrophy
— Alkaline phosphatase

Calcifying zone
— Calcification

Endochondral ossification

— Metaphyseal capillaries

Ossifying zone
Appositional deposition
of bone by osteoblasts

Resorption at
ends of trabeculae

FIGURE 45-1 *The various parts of an epiphyseal plate, showing the chief processes that occur in this region. (Source: Cormack, D.H. Essential Histology. Philadelphia: J.B. Lippincott, 1993)*

sian canals with the lamellae are the minute canals (canaliculi) that carry oxygen and nutrients to the bone cells. Each canal with its contents and surrounding lamellae makes up a haversian system or *osteon*. Directly under the periosteum and surrounding the medullary canal, several thicknesses of lamellae are laid down, surrounding the entire shaft with hard thickness. The haversian systems run parallel to each other and longitudinally, from metaphysis to metaphysis, and are connected transversely by tubes called *Volkmann's canals*. Blood vessels from the periosteum enter the bone and pass through these canals to enter and leave the haversian system.

Cancellous and Medullary Bone

Cancellous bone is present in short, flat, and irregular bones and in the ends of long bones. It is a collection of

trabeculae, or beams of bone, which gives it a spongy appearance and adds strength due to the many interlacing parts (Fig. 45-3). The spaces in between these trabeculae are filled with bone marrow. The red marrow actively participates in the formation of red blood cells and is present in the adult in the cancellous bone of the ribs, sternum, vertebrae, and pelvis. Red marrow is present in many bones in infants and is gradually converted to yellow marrow composed of fat cells. Most long bones of the adult contain yellow marrow rather than red. Medullary bone is simply a continuation of cancellous bone and is the central area filled with marrow, blood, and lymph vessels.

Nerve and Blood Supply

Because bone is a living tissue, nutrients must be supplied and waste material removed. Total bone blood flow

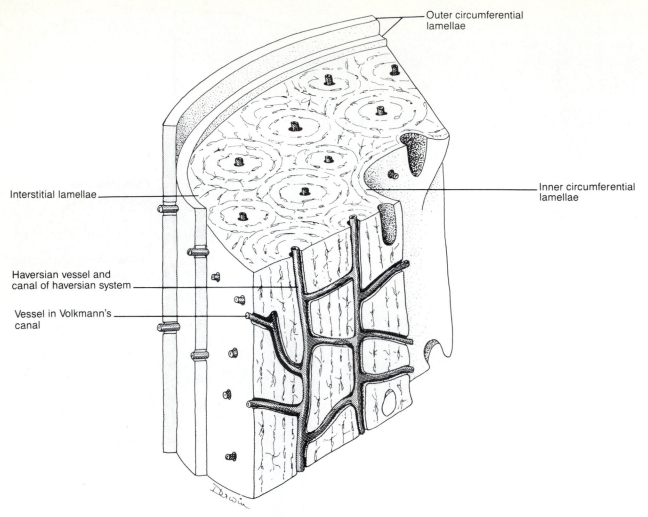

Outer circumferential lamellae

Inner circumferential lamellae

Interstitial lamellae

Haversian vessel and canal of haversian system

Vessel in Volkmann's canal

FIGURE 45-2 *Compact bone organization in the cortex of a long bone (osteon number minimized for clarity). (Source: D.H. Cormack,* Essential Histology. *Philadelphia: J.B. Lippincott, 1993)*

has been estimated to be from 200 to 400 mL per minute. Small bones usually have a single artery and vein entering them, and large bones have several. The chief artery, which enters near the middle of the shaft of long bones, is called the *principal nutrient artery*. After piercing the shaft and reaching the medullary canal, it branches into ascending and descending branches and ends in sinusoidal capillaries. The artery and its branches supply the marrow and cortex as well as the haversian systems.

Nerve supply to bone is sparse and present mainly in the outer layer, the periosteum. It consists of both afferent (sensory) and sympathetic fibers, with the autonomic fibers accompanying and controlling the dilatation of bone blood vessels.

TYPES OF BONES

Bones are most commonly classified as long, short, flat, and irregular. Table 45-1 defines common anatomic terms.

Long Bones

Long bones are the bones of the extremities and are elongated. Each one consists of the following: two epiphyses, or ends, which are knobby areas containing cancellous bone; the diaphysis, which composes the shaft or long portion; and the metaphysis, which contains the epiphyseal plate and newly formed bone. In the adult, the metaphysis and epiphysis are continuous.

The outer and inner surfaces of bone are covered with specialized connective tissue. The dense, white, fibrous membrane wrapping the outside is called the *periosteum* and is composed of two layers. The outer, or fibrous, layer has relatively few cells and is made up of fibrous tissue. The inner layer of the periosteum is very vascular and has an osteogenic function. Lining the marrow and haversian cavities as well as the spaces of spongy bone is a membrane called the *endosteum*. Besides supplying a site of attachment for tendons and ligaments, the periosteum is richly supplied with nerves and blood vessels that are important in nourishing the

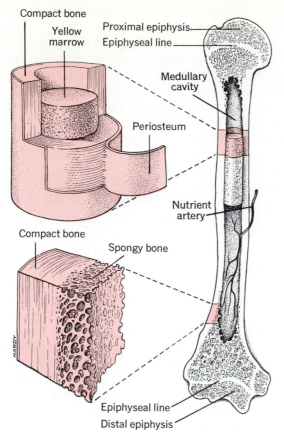

FIGURE 45-3 *A long bone shown in longitudinal section. (Source: Chaffee, E.E., and Lytle, I.M. Basic Physiology and Anatomy* (4th ed.). *Philadelphia: J.B. Lippincott.*

TABLE 45-1 Anatomic Terms in Common Use for Bones

Term	Definition
Process	General term for any bony prominence
Spine or spinous process	Sharp prominence
Tubercle	Rounded prominence on a bone
Tuberosity	Protuberance on a bone
Trochanter	Large process (eg, below the neck of the femur)
Crest	Ridge or linear prominence (eg, iliac crest)
Condyle	Rounded protruding mass that carries an articular surface (eg, knuckle)
Head	The top, beginning, or most prominent part (eg, enlargement beyond the constricted part, as in the femoral head)
Sinus	Cavity within a bone
Foramen	Hole or opening in a bone
Axial skeleton	The 80 bones composing the skull, vertebral column, sternum, and ribs
Appendicular skeleton	The 126 lower bones composing the upper and lower extremities
Proximal	Near the origin of the limb
Distal	Away from the origin of the limb
Medial	Nearer to the midline of the body
Lateral	Farther from the midline of the body

bone. Long bones form most of the appendicular skeleton, such as the femur, humerus, and phalanges (see Figure 45-3).

Short Bones

Short bones, such as those in the wrist, are cube-shaped and consist of cancellous bone enclosed in a thin case of compact bone. These often are combined with other short bones.

Flat Bones

The bones of the skull, ribs, scapulae, and sternum are examples of flat bones. Their function is largely protective. They consist of two plates of hard compact bone covering a thin layer of cancellous bone. These bones, especially those of the ribs and sternum, are important sites for blood formation.

Irregular Bones

Bones that are irregular in shape are similar in composition to the short bones. The vertebrae and the ossicles of the ears are examples of irregular bones.

BONE GROWTH AND FACTORS AFFECTING BONE GROWTH

Location of Bone Growth

The epiphyses of a long bone are separated from the shaft by the epiphyseal plate, which is responsible for the longitudinal growth of bone. On the distal side of this plate, osteoblasts are constantly secreting the bone matrix, which immediately becomes ossified, increasing the length of the bone. Simultaneously, on the proximal side of the epiphyseal plate, new cartilage is being formed. During puberty, ossification exceeds cartilage formation. Gradually, the cartilaginous epiphyseal plate becomes completely ossified, and linear bone growth ceases. Epiphyseal closure occurs about 3 years earlier in women than it does in men, in whom bone length ceases to increase at about the age of 20.[11]

As bones grow longitudinally, they also increase in circumference. Osteoblasts on the inner surface of the periosteum deposit layers of new bone, while osteoclasts in the area next to the medullary cavity make the canal larger to fit the larger bone. Bone activity does not stop when a person reaches puberty. Throughout life, bone continues to form and reabsorb in a process called *remodeling*. In the young adult, approximately one sixth of total skeletal calcium is turned over every year, but when a person reaches the fourth or fifth decade of life, reabsorption begins to outpace formation. Thus, after age 40, approximately 0.5% to 1.0% of the total skeletal mass is lost yearly. Remodeling is influenced by such factors as calcium and phosphorus metabolism, hormones, weight bearing, diet, and environmental influences.

Calcium, Phosphorus, and Parathyroid Hormone

The exact mechanism that causes calcium to deposit and new bone to form remains a mystery. Certain nutritional, endocrine, and environmental states must exist for the process to occur in an orderly fashion.

For new bone to form, adequate amounts of calcium and phosphorus must be present in the plasma and interstitial fluid, which bathes the osteoblasts. These critical amounts are thought to be maintained in part by a partial membrane formed by osteoblasts. This membrane acts as a barrier between bone fluid and the extracellular fluid of the body. The osteoblasts connect with other osteocytes deep in the bone, where calcium can move into and out of the cell. Calcium salts precipitate on the surface of collagen fibers at periodic intervals. These calcium salts become hydroxyapatite crystals, which provide the crystalline structure of bone mineralization.

With a normal diet, a person takes in approximately 1,000 mg of calcium daily, of which 300 mg is absorbed by the intestines into the bloodstream. From there it goes to the extracellular fluid, and some of it is returned to the intestinal tract through bile. A large amount of the daily calcium intake is excreted in the feces and, to a lesser extent, in urine.[15] Despite this large amount of calcium movement into and out of the body, the serum calcium level remains constant at about 10 mg/dL. The serum pH and albumin levels affect the amount of calcium in the blood, with about half of it being bound to serum albumin. This calcium can be released when the serum pH decreases to levels below 7.3.[23] The constancy of extracellular fluid calcium is dependent on vitamin D, parathyroid hormone, and calcitonin (described below).

Phosphorus is a major component of bone and also is involved in many metabolic processes. Serum levels of phosphorus vary according to intake, blood pH, and other factors. Serum samples are accurate only if drawn in the fasting state.[15] Phosphorus is efficiently absorbed by the intestines, and its excretion is regulated by the proximal tubules of the kidney nephrons. If the renal capacity for excreting phosphorus is impaired, hyperphosphatemia results and there is an associated decrease in serum calcium levels (see p. 665).[21]

In the diet, calcium and phosphate are supplied mainly by milk and meats. Phosphate is absorbed with calcium. When calcium is absorbed in abundance, so is

phosphate. Excess phosphate is excreted along with excess calcium in the feces and urine.

When the serum calcium ion concentration is high, production of parathyroid hormone (PTH) is severely curtailed. This results in a lowered serum calcium level. Conversely, when serum calcium levels are lowered, PTH secretion increases, which expands vitamin D activity and absorption of calcium in the intestinal tract. Parathyroid hormone promotes the formation of osteoclasts and retards the production of osteoblasts. The net result is increased reabsorption of bone, which causes the short-term effect of elevating serum calcium levels. Parathyroid hormone increases renal tubular reabsorption of calcium and decreases the reabsorption of phosphate ions.

Vitamin D

Vitamin D is a steroid hormone that is taken in the diet and is formed in the skin by the action of the ultraviolet rays of the sun. Vitamin D is designated as vitamins D_2 and D_3 according to their structural side chains, but they are metabolized identically and have equivalent biologic potencies.[15] For dietary vitamin D to be absorbed, bile must be present. Through a series of events in the liver and kidneys, vitamins D_2 and D_3 are converted to 1,25-dihydroxycholecalciferol (1,25$[OH]_2D_3$), which is the active form of the vitamin. Other metabolites are formed in the complex conversions that take place, but only 1,25(OH)D is thought to have major physiologic action.[15] It affects serum calcium principally by controlling the absorption of calcium by the gut. The feedback mechanism involves increased PTH, increased production of 1,25$(OH)_2D_3$, and increased calcium absorption from the ileum. Vitamin D also increases calcium reabsorption in the kidney nephrons.[13] Renal failure depresses the reabsorption of calcium by the kidneys as well as curtailing the production of 1,25$(OH)_2D_3$. In renal failure, vitamin D is virtually ineffective because of a decrease in the intestinal absorption of calcium.

Parathyroid hormone production increases when serum calcium levels drop, which increases 1,25$(OH)_2D_3$ formation by the kidneys and leads to increased calcium absorption from the gut and from the bone. Lack of either calcium or active vitamin D over a period of time can alter bone formation and cause loss of bone mass.

Calcitonin

Calcitonin is a hormone that is produced and secreted by parafollicular cells of the thyroid gland. The major stimulus for release of calcitonin is hypercalcemia, but its role in normal bone and kidney physiology is unclear.[20] The immediate effect of calcitonin is to reduce bone reabsorption by decreasing osteoclast activity and increasing osteoblast activity. A more prolonged effect is to reduce the quantity of osteoclasts formed from the mesenchymal stem cells. Calcitonin does not significantly alter serum calcium levels in the adult; its effect is more significant in children, who have a more rapid rate of bone remodeling. Calcitonin has been administered in Paget's disease to reduce the rapid rate of bone turnover. Increased calcitonin secretion is triggered by an increase in plasma calcium levels. The resulting decrease in serum calcium levels provides a second feedback mechanism for the control of blood calcium.

Sex Hormones

Estrogen has an osteoblast-stimulating action. At puberty, girls have a rapid growth spurt before the epiphyseal plates close, which is attributed to estrogen. When growth plates close, girls stop growing, and this occurs a few years before their male counterparts on the average. Throughout the premenopausal period, estrogen promotes bone formation by increasing intestinal absorption of calcium and phosphorus and increasing calcitonin production. In the postmenopausal woman, osteoporosis can be caused by the lack of estrogen (see p. 1134–1136).

Testosterone in boys and men increases bone length and thickness and at the same time enhances epiphyseal closure. A decline in testosterone level in the elderly man also can lead to osteoporosis.

Growth Hormone

The anterior lobe of the pituitary gland secretes the growth hormone, somatotropin, which causes a linear increase in long bones by increasing cartilage formation, widening the epiphyseal plates, and increasing the amount of matrix laid down in the ends of the long bones (see pp. 683–684). An excess of growth hormone in the growing person can cause gigantism. In the adult, whose epiphyseal plates are closed, the characteristic bone and soft tissue deformities of acromegaly result. Pituitary insufficiency can result in dwarfism in the child.

Weight Bearing

It has long been observed that muscles atrophy and bones demineralize when a limb is immobilized. Weightlessness experienced by astronauts was noted to cause loss of bone calcium and bone weakness.[8] Physical compression stimulates osteoblastic deposition, probably by generating an electrical potential. This potential at the compression site stimulates osteoblastic activity and increases bone formation. Electrical signals can also stimulate epiphyseal growth. Local skeletal mass increases in the bones most used in physical exertion, such as playing tennis, weight lifting, and dancing.[5]

BOX 45-1 ▼ Factors That Affect Bone Formation

Facilitate Bone Formation
Calcium
Phosphorus
Estrogen
Testosterone
Calcitonin
Vitamins D, A, and C
Growth hormone
Exercise
Insulin

Retard Bone Formation
Estrogen/androgen deficiency
Vitamin deficiency
Starvation
Diabetes
Steroids
Inactivity/immobility
Heparin
Excess parathyroid level

Other Factors

Glucocorticoids cause an increase in protein breakdown in all tissues of the body. Because bone matrix is a protein product, an increase in steroids, as in Cushing's disease, can decrease matrix formation and weaken the bones, causing osteoporosis. Steroids also have the specific effect of depressing osteoblastic activity.[13]

As was described earlier, two-thirds of the volume of bone is made up of osteoid organic material. Because all living tissues contain protein, anything that causes a decrease in protein in the body, such as starvation, retards bone formation and enhances bone loss. Lack of vitamins A and C also decreases the ground substance in bone and leads to decreased bone formation. Persons undergoing long-term heparin therapy develop osteoporosis, because heparin apparently speeds up the breakdown of collagen.[16] Insulin increases the ability of the collagen matrix to produce osteoblasts. A summary of factors facilitating and retarding bone growth is given in Box 45-1.

▼ Normal Structure and Function of Joints

TYPES OF JOINTS

Although individual bones are hard and inflexible, the human body can make graceful, flowing movements. Any motion, whether writing a letter or playing football, is brought about by the simultaneous movement of several *articulations*, or joints. Almost all of the bones of the body are joined to each other in one way or another. Some permit a range of motion and some allow none at all. Joints are classified in several ways, but the most common grouping is according to the degree of movement they permit, as follows: *synarthroses*, immovable; *amphiarthroses*, somewhat movable; and *diarthroses*, freely movable (Fig. 45-4). Joints may also be classified according to the material that connects them, for example, cartilaginous, fibrous, and synovial.

Synarthroses provide little movement, have a rigid surface, and include the bones of the skull. The sutures of the cranial bones are joined together by fibrous tissue and interlocking projections and indentations. These joints are not completed at birth, and an infant has six gaps, or *fontanelles*, between bones. *Synchondrosis*, another type of immovable joint, is cartilage joining two bony surfaces. An example of synchondrosis is the "joint" between the epiphysis and diaphysis of long bones that disappears after puberty. A third type of synarthrosis is a *gomphosis*, which resembles a peg in a hole, an example of which is a tooth in the jaw.

Amphiarthroses are joints that permit very limited motion. A *symphysis* is a joint in which the bones are connected by disks of fibrocartilage. Examples are the symphysis pubis and the intervertebral disks. One can see the benefits of such flexibility of the pelvis in child-

birth and in the backbone with any movement. A *syndesmosis* is a slightly movable joint in which the bones are connected by ligaments, permitting some bending and twisting, an example of which is the articulation between the tibia and fibula.

Diarthroses are often called *synovial* joints. They are freely movable and require lubrication to reduce the friction and abrasion that occur when one surface moves on another. The articulating surfaces of the bone are covered by a white, slick hyaline cartilage, and the entire joint is surrounded by an articular capsule that is filled with viscous synovial fluid. The inner layer of this capsule is a slippery, smooth membrane, whereas the outer layer is a tough, fibrous membrane. This inner, or *synovial*, membrane is rich in capillaries and cells, and is composed of secreting and phagocytic cells. The secretory cells produce synovial fluid, which contains water and protein. The phagocytic cells remove foreign material which may have deposited into the area. The glucose level of the fluid is similar to that of serum. The chief function of this fluid is to lubricate and supply nutrients to the cartilage. The excess protein it contains is returned to the blood by way of the lymphatic system that drains the area. Synovial joints are supplied with sensory nerves that cause pain when there is an accumulation of inflammatory cells in the synovial tissues.

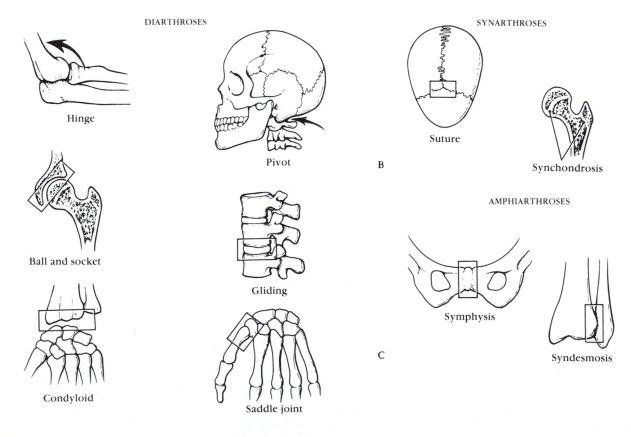

FIGURE 45-4 *Types of joints based on degree of movement.*

CLASSIFICATION OF SYNOVIAL JOINTS

The synovial joints permit a variety of motion and are classified according to the shape of the articulation and the motion it facilitates. Table 45-2 summarizes joint movements and alteration effects. Ball-and-socket joints, such as hip and shoulder joints, allow the greatest degree of motion and are formed by a bone fitting into a cup-shaped cavity of another bone. Condyloid joints are oval-shaped articular surfaces that fit into an elliptical cavity with abduction and adduction limitations. Hinge joints permit movement in one plane only, examples of which are the knee, elbow, and finger joints (Fig. 45-5). Pivot joints allow for rotation and supination and pronation, examples of which are the atlas and axis joints of the head and the juncture between the head of the radius and the radial notch of the ulna. Saddle joints have an articular surface of one bone that is concave in one direction and convex in another; the other bone is just the opposite, so that the two sides fit together smoothly.

TABLE 45-2 *Movements of Joints*

Joint	Type of Movement	Normal Movements	Effects of Alterations
Vertebral	Diarthrotic (may be classified as synarthrotic, cartilaginous, amphiarthrotic)	Bending, stretching, twisting of entire column; slight movement between vertebrae	Pain when moving or lifting; stiffness; low back pain
Clavicular	Diarthrotic	Elevating, protracting, retracting	Pain; inability to move shoulder forward or backward; inability to lift shoulder
Shoulder	Diarthrotic (ball-and-socket)	Flexion, extension, abduction; rotation; circumduction of upper arm	Pain; stiffness; immobility; heat; inability to lift objects; cannot bring arm in toward body; range of activity curtailed
Elbow	Diarthrotic (hinge-and-pivot)	Flexion, extension; supination of lower arm and hand; pronation of lower arm and hand	Immobility; pain; stiffness; heat; activities of daily living greatly diminished; swelling
Wrist	Diarthrotic	Flexion, extension; abduction of hand; adduction of hand	Pain; stiffness; swelling; common complaints of inability to do common activities of daily living such as cooking, opening lids, various grooming activities; may complain of dropping things
Hand	Diarthrotic	Flexion, extension, abduction, adduction, circumduction of thumb; thumb and finger apposition; flexion, extension, limited abduction and adduction of fingers; flexion, extension of fingers	Pain; swelling; stiffness; drops objects; deteriorating writing; ability to perform activities of daily living greatly diminished (buttoning clothes, tying knots or bows, combing hair)
Hip	Diarthrotic (ball-and-socket)	Flexion; extension; abduction; adduction; rotation; circumduction	Pain; stiffness; immobility; heat; limping; loss of range of motion; inability to put on garments that require lifting the legs; cannot climb stairs
Knee	Diarthrotic (hinge)	Flexion; extension; slight tibial rotation	Pain; stiffness; swelling; immobility; limping, falling; redness, swelling; heat
Ankle	Diarthrotic (hinge)	Dorsiflexion; plantar flexion	Pain; stiffness; immobility; limping; unusual discomfort with shoes; foot drop
Foot	Diarthrotic	Flexion; extension; gliding; inversion; slight abduction, adduction	Pain; stiffness; immobility; avoidance of standing and walking; shoes ill-fitting

(Source: Reprinted by permission of J. Moore.)

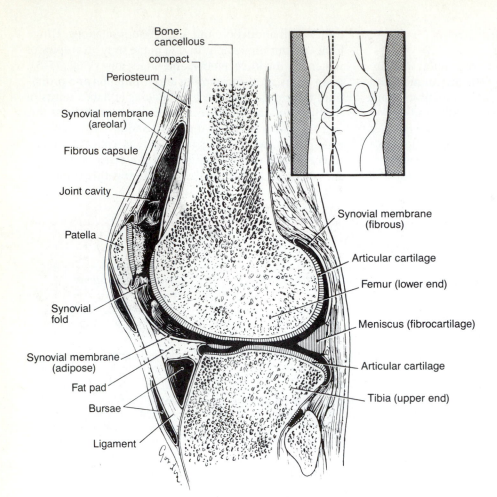

Bone:
cancellous
compact
Periosteum
Synovial membrane
(areolar)
Fibrous capsule
Joint cavity
Patella
Synovial
fold
Synovial membrane
(adipose)
Fat pad
Bursae
Ligament

Synovial membrane
(fibrous)
Articular cartilage
Femur (lower end)
Meniscus (fibrocartilage)
Articular cartilage
Tibia (upper end)

FIGURE 45-5 *Diagram of a knee joint cut in the sagittal plane indicated in the inset. (Source: D.H. Cormack,* Essential Histology. *Philadelphia: J.B. Lippincott, 1993)*

An example of this is the carpometacarpal joint at the base of the thumb. Gliding joints have surfaces that are flat or only slightly curved, thus permitting sliding movement in all directions. Examples of this type of joint are the carpal bones of the wrist and the intervertebral joints.

Movements of joints may be classified as 1) gliding, producing some bone displacement; 2) angular, in which the angle between bones is changed; and 3) rotating, a twisting of a body part.

SYNOVIAL CAVITIES

The joint capsule consists of an outer fibrous layer called the *fibrous capsule* and an inner layer called the *synovial membrane* (see Fig. 45-5). Ligaments may be incorporated into the capsule or separated from it by *bursae*, which are small, flat cavities filled with *synovial fluid*. Synovial fluid is like interstitial fluid except that it contains large quantities of mucopolysaccharides, which accounts for its viscosity and lubricative qualities.[7] The chief function of bursae is to reduce friction between moving parts.

LIGAMENTS AND TENDONS

Ligaments and tendons constitute the connective tissue that hold the body together. There are two types of ligaments, those that connect viscera to each other and those that connect one bone to another.[7] Tendons always connect voluntary muscle to another structure.

Ligaments are composed of distinct bands of connective tissue. Yellow ligaments are elastic (vertebral column) and allow for stretching. White ligaments, such as those in the knee, do not stretch; they provide stability.

Tendons are actual extensions of muscles and attach muscle to bones or to other tissues. The thick, collagenous tissue has fibers that run in one direction so it can withstand a great deal of pull. These parallel bundles give tendons a glistening, shiny, white appearance. When they are part of broad and flat muscles, they have the same general appearance; similarly, when they are part of a long, slender muscle, they are cordlike. The long, hard, cordlike tendons running into the hands and feet are termed *leaders*. Tendons that cross bones or other tendons are lubricated by a slippery solution similar to synovial fluid that contains hyaluronic acid.[7] Tendons receive sensory fibers from muscle nerves, nearby deep

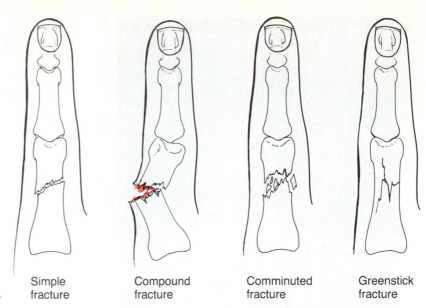

| Simple
fracture | Compound
fracture | Comminuted
fracture | Greenstick
fracture |

FIGURE 45-6   *Types of fractures.*

nerves, and overlying superficial nerves. Blood supply to tendons is scarce, thus injured tendons heal slowly.

▼ Fractures and Associated Soft-Tissue Injuries

Fractures are most commonly defined as breaks in continuity of bone. They are ruptures of living tissue and normally are the result of trauma, but they may be caused by repeated stress and fatigue (stress fracture) or an underlying disease (pathologic fracture). They may have associated extensive soft tissue damage with hemorrhage into muscles and joints, dislocation and rupture of tendons, nerve damage, and disruption of blood supply. Fractures occur when a force (energy) is imposed on a bone that is greater than it can absorb. Fractures are described in terms of types and directions of fracture lines (Fig. 45-6).

CLASSIFICATION OF FRACTURES

Simple fractures do not disrupt the skin overlying the bone. *Compound fractures* break or tear the overlying skin.

Fractures are either *complete*, in which there is complete interruption in the continuity of bone, or *incomplete*, with some part of the bone intact (Figs. 45-7 and 45-8). If a bone is broken in such a manner as to produce three or more fragments, it is called *comminuted* (Fig. 45-9). An *impacted fracture* is one in which one fragment of bone is imbedded in the substance of the other. A fracture characterized by crushed bone is called a *compression* fracture and usually involves the spinal column (Fig. 45-10). A *depressed fracture*, frequently seen in skull fractures, occurs when the bone is driven inward. Re-

peated mechanical stress and strain can result in a *stress fracture* (Fig. 45-11). *Pathologic fractures* occur in diseased bone with little external force or with trivial trauma. Severe twisting or straining may cause a tendon or ligament to pull its bony attachment completely off the main part of the bone, producing an *avulsion* fracture. Fracture

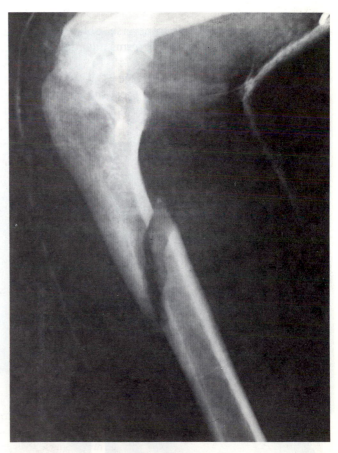

FIGURE 45-7   *Complete fracture of the humerus.*

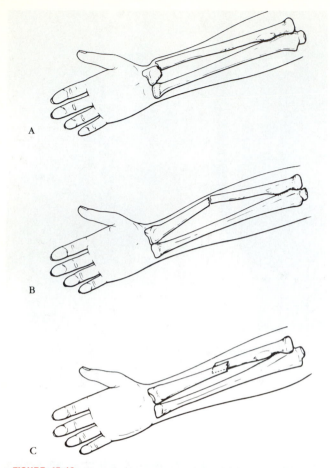

FIGURE 45-13 *Descriptive terms indicating types of fractures.* **A.** *Displacement.* **B.** *Angulation.* **C.** *Overriding.*

within a week are dispersed throughout the soft tissue callus. This temporary bony union is called a provisional or primary union or *procallus*.[1] The procallus creates a balloon or collar over the fracture site and extends well past it. As healing continues, a *bridging external callus* is formed. New bone spicules proliferate as mineral salts are laid down. The late medullary callus appears to be

---

TABLE 45-3 *Mechanical Forces and Related Fractures of Long Bones*

Force	Resulting Fracture
Twisting	Spiral
Angulation	Transverse
Angulation with axial compression	Transverse with separate triangular piece (butterfly)
Twisting, angulation, and compression	Short oblique
Direct blow	Transverse
Crushing blow	Comminuted

---

responsible for the slow growth of new bone across a fracture gap. As the gap in fractured bone is bridged and fracture fragments become united, mature bone begins to replace the callus.[1] The excess callus already laid down is reabsorbed by the osteoclasts. The fracture site becomes firm in about 3 to 4 months, and radiographs show united bone (Fig. 45-14).

The remodeling process is controlled by the weight bearing and muscle stresses put on the bone. Through the processes of formation and reabsorption, bone returns to an architecturally sound state. *Wolff's law* describes a feedback system in which local instability stimulates bone formation and lack of stress stimulates bone reabsorption.[1] If aligned correctly, a simple bone fracture resumes an almost normal appearance within 1 year (Fig. 45-15).

Conditions That Modify Healing

Because fracture healing is a continuous, sequential process, any interruption may modify the final result. This may be due to inadequate immobilization, poor blood supply, distraction of fragments, interposition of soft tissue, or infection.

When the bone is completely transected, *immobilization* is required to hold the fracture fragments rigidly in place. Any movement of the fragments could rupture the fracture hematoma. This reverses and thus prolongs the healing process, because bleeding into the fracture site recurs. Immobilization is the first line of defense in ensuring a solid union.

A poor *blood supply* to the traumatized area can impair the healing process. All tissues of the body need nutrition provided through the bloodstream to maintain life. For the surrounding soft tissue and bones to heal, the blood supply must be adequate to provide the needed nutrition.

Position or *apposition* also can affect healing. *Distraction* describes a situation in which the fracture fragments are pulled apart from each other, so that there is no bony contact. This may be caused by skeletal traction applied to align fragments or by muscle pull on individual fractures. If great enough, distraction may cause excessive tension on the capillaries and decrease the vital blood supply. An increased fracture gap must be bridged with granulation tissue, which increases healing time. When the healing time is increased, the chance of nonunion also increases. Distraction also is associated with the complication of separation of the fracture fragments by soft tissue that seals off the surface of one or both bones. This is known as *interposition of soft tissue*. If one or both of the fragments become covered with soft tissue, the hematoma is unable to form, and growth of granulation tissue is inhibited. This leads to a poor osseous union.

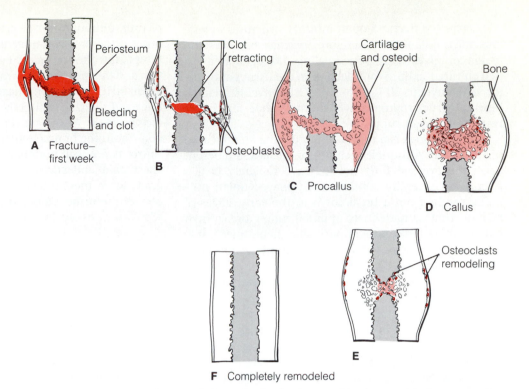

FIGURE 45-14 Healing of a fracture. **A.** Immediately after fracture, blood seeps into the area and a hematoma forms. **B.** After 1 week, osteoblasts begin to form as clot retracts. **C.** After about 3 weeks, a procallus begins to form and stabilizes the fracture. **D.** From 6 to 12 weeks, a callus forms with bone cells. **E.** In 3 to 4 months, osteoclasts begin to remodel the fracture site. **F.** With normal apposition, the bone will be completely remodeled in 12 months.

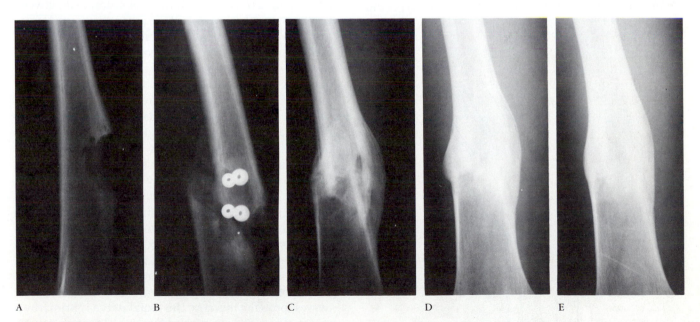

FIGURE 45-15 The sequence of bone healing and remodeling is demonstrated in a 13-year-old bone with a chondromyxoid that was removed surgically. **A.** Initial appearance. **B.** Repaired pathologic fracture 1 month later. **C.** A procallus forms. **D.** Osteogenesis. **E.** Bone remodeling.

Compound fractures open internal structures to various microorganisms; therefore, *infection* becomes the major complication of bone healing. The open area is a rich culture medium for infection in the tissues and also for osteomyelitis (Fig. 45-16). Osteomyelitis retards healing by destroying newly forming bone and interrupting its blood supply (see below).

Delayed union is a term used to denote an increased healing time. Although each person heals at a different pace, the average time needed to completely heal a fracture is generally consistent. A delayed union normally results from a breakdown in the early stages of healing, that is, inadequate immobilization, breakdown in hematoma formation, or poor alignment. Infection at the fracture site delays union, usually until the infectious process is stopped.

Nonunion occurs when the fragments fail to unite, usually because of infection and movement. Infection causes continuous bleeding and breakdown of osteoid matrix. Movement at the fracture site causes repeated bleeding episodes and decalcification at the fragment ends; it may cause the fracture gap to increase to such an extent that the ends no longer touch, leading to a permanent nonunion. *Malunion* is union of the fragments in a position that modifies function.

Pulmonary fat emboli can be identified at autopsy in almost all persons dying soon after receiving fractures of the long bones or pelvis (see p. 606). These may or may not have contributed to the death of the individual.[8] The so-called *fat embolism syndrome* probably has multiple mechanisms of causation. These include chemical injury to the pulmonary vasculature and release of fat deposits from the stores in the fractured long bones. The clinical picture, although not clearly understood, involves the onset of adult respiratory distress syndrome 24 to 72 hours after the traumatic event. Activation of coagulation and the resultant disseminated intravascular coagulation (DIC) often complicate the picture, and it is not known if the DIC is directly related to the fat embolism (see pp. 418–419). The cerebral edema and microembolic fat in the brain circulation are common, but, their source is not well understood.[8] The person experiences chest pain and sudden respiratory difficulty. A low-grade fever, mental confusion, petechiae, and fat globules in the urine support the diagnosis.

COMPARTMENTAL SYNDROMES

Sometimes a fracture causes an injury to adjacent structures. The fragments may rupture and compress nerves that may also be damaged by dislocation or direct trauma. Injuries of the axillary, radial, and peroneal nerves are described as *compartmental syndromes*.

The axillary nerve may be damaged by fractures or dislocations around the shoulder or by penetrating wounds and direct blows. The axillary nerve is composed of C-5 and C-6 fibers and is a branch of the posterior cord of the brachial plexus. It emerges at the level of the humerus head and winds around the neck of the humerus. It supplies the deltoid and teres minor muscles. The deltoid muscle is used as an abductor for the shoulder; therefore, inability to abduct the shoulder indicates damage to the axillary nerve.

The radial nerve is commonly injured in spiral fractures of the humerus. It may be completely severed, impaled on a fractured fragment, or entrapped between the fragments. Lacerations of the arm and proximal forearm and gunshot wounds are also common causes of radial nerve injury. Temporary nerve damage may also result from direct pressure from using crutches or hanging an arm on the back of a chair. The radial nerve is composed of the fibers from some of the cervical spinal nerves (C-5, C-6, C-7, and C-8) and, sometimes, the thoracic spinal nerve, T-1. It is primarily a motor nerve that innervates the biceps, supinates the forearm, and extends the wrist, fingers, and thumb. Therefore, injury usually results in inability to extend the elbow or supinate the forearm. A typical wrist drop occurs that includes inability to extend the fingers. Complete return of function can be expected in most persons with temporary nerve damage. In others, function may not return for as long as 1 year. When function does not return, surgery is usually indicated. However, the radial nerve has a greater ability to regenerate than all other large nerves, probably because the radial nerve is primarily a motor nerve that is involved mainly in gross muscle movements.

Peroneal nerves are classified as common, superficial, and deep. The common peroneal nerve emerges

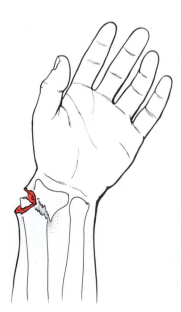

FIGURE 45-16 *Compound fracture of radius with surrounding soft tissue damage.*

from the popliteal fossa and encircles the fibula neck. Damage may be the result of a direct blow, for example, a baseball bat hitting the fibula head with or without the presence of fractures. The result is a footdrop deformity in which the foot returns to normal in a few hours if the nerve is not ruptured.

Compartmental syndromes are uncommon complications of fractures and affect primarily the forearm and tibia. They are generally referred to as *Volkmann's ischemia* or *anterior tibial compartmental syndromes*. Volkmann's ischemia (volar compartmental syndrome) usually is related to the common supracondylar fracture of the humerus in children. Fracture of the tibia is common in anterior compartmental syndrome. Compartmental syndromes may result from a cast that is placed too tight, from intercompartmental bleeding, or from swelling of burns and snake or spider bites.

The compartments of the leg and forearm are composed of bones, muscles, nerves, and other associated structures encapsulated by the fascia and the skin, thus making a closed space (Fig. 45-17). When injury occurs, the pressure builds within the compartment due to bleeding and soft tissue reaction. When the swelling reaches a point at which the fascia permits no further outward enlargement, the increasing pressure is directed inward and compresses blood vessels and other components of the compartment. When tissue pressure increases to equal the diastolic pressure, the microcirculation ceases, although the peripheral pulse is unchanged. Within 30 minutes, damage to nerves begins, and if swelling is allowed to persist for 12 hours, irreversible functional loss occurs. Muscles require an abundant blood supply, and when the microcirculation is severely compromised they become ischemic, with

onset of necrosis in 2 to 4 hours, becoming irreversible in 12 hours.

Anterior compartmental syndrome is heralded by pain in the anterior aspect of the tibia, paresthesia over the distribution of the deep peroneal nerve, and pain on passive dorsiflexion of the toes. The area appears swollen, and blisters may develop on the skin. If the syndrome is allowed to proceed unchecked, paralysis, anesthesia, contractures, footdrop, and gangrene may develop, which in turn may lead to loss of the limb.

Volkmann's ischemia produces a disturbing contracture if untreated. Pain is the predominant symptom; it is referred to the palmar area and is exacerbated on passive extension of the fingers. Some degree of sensory loss in the fingers occurs in the early stages. Contractures (clawlike deformities of the hand), wristdrop, and paralysis result.

OTHER ASSOCIATED SOFT TISSUE TRAUMAS

Tendons may also be damaged by fractures. When ligaments and tendons are involved in fractures, avulsion fractures may result. Damage to the extensor tendon of the distal phalanx can serve as an example. When a fracture occurs, it avulses (pulls apart) a small piece of bone to which the tendon is attached, leading to the inability to extend the distal phalanx. If left untreated, a mallet deformity may result. A dysfunction of the bony attachment may occur in tendon damage that is left untreated. *Visceral damage*, or damage to internal organs, may also occur from fractures. Examples include fracture of the pelvis, in which the bladder is ruptured, and rib fractures causing perforation of the lung.

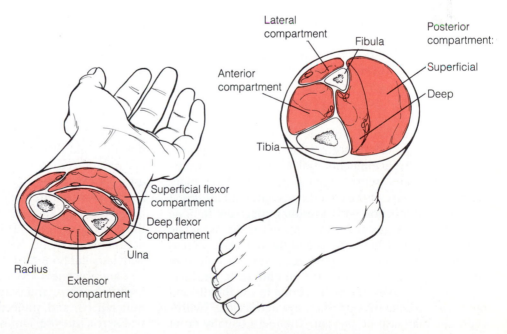

FIGURE 45-17 *Compartments of the forearm and lower leg.*

Superficial flexor compartment

Deep flexor compartment

Radius

Extensor compartment

Ulna

Lateral compartment

Anterior compartment

Fibula

Posterior compartment:

Superficial

Deep

Tibia

▼ Alterations in Connective Tissue Development

OSTEOGENESIS IMPERFECTA

Osteogenesis imperfecta is a group of hereditary disorders in which defective connective tissue formation leads to extremely fragile bones. The disorders have various severity of bone, eye, ear, dental, and cardiovascular involvement. Different types are described, some of autosomal dominant inheritance and some of autosomal recessive inheritance.[24] The bones of the skull and face may be poorly ossified, with numerous fractures occurring in the long bones. The skeletal aspect of this condition is a hereditary form of osteoporosis. Some types have few fractures but exhibit any combination of blue sclerae, deafness, short stature, joint dislocation, and opalescent teeth.[24] In severe cases, death of the infant during childbirth may occur due to trauma to the brain, which is relatively unprotected by the soft, membranous skull.

MARFAN SYNDROME

Marfan syndrome is an autosomal dominant inheritance disorder characterized by abnormal body proportions, including long arms; long digits; thoracic deformity, such as pectus excavatum; curvature of the thoracic spine; and hyperextensibility of the joints.[17] Associated connective tissue defects result in dilatation and dissection of the aorta along with aortic insufficiency (see pp. 483–484).

OSTEOPETROSIS (MARBLE BONES, OR ALBERS-SCHÖNBERG DISEASE)

Osteopetrosis is a familial disease characterized by overgrowth and sclerosing of bone. Although the bones are heavy and thick, they tend to break rather than bend, and fractures often occur. When this disease is due to a recessive trait, it is called *malignant osteopetrosis* and can cause death in utero or in early life. The autosomal dominant trait causes less severe problems that may not be diagnosed until adulthood.[9]

Pathologic changes include an increase in cortical bone to nearly twice its normal density, with the growth almost exclusively endochondral. Crowding of the marrow cavity, often with complete marrow obliteration, results. The cause of the condition is a hereditary defect in osteoclast function with a resultant decrease in bone reabsorption.[9] Signs and symptoms of the disease relate to the skeletal malformations and the defects in hematopoiesis. Optic nerve impingement due to failure of modeling of the skull can result in blindness. Deafness can occur due to overgrowth of bone in the middle and inner ear. Cranial nerve palsies, nystagmus, and hydrocephalus may also be present. The teeth usually erupt late and develop cavities early; osteomyelitis of the jaw often develops. Anemia can be profound due to the small marrow spaces, and the enlarged liver and spleen are sources of extramedullary hematopoiesis. As in osteogenesis imperfecta, treatment is palliative, but children who reach adulthood can look forward to a relatively normal life span.

▼ Idiopathic Alterations in Bone

PAGET'S DISEASE

As early as 1877, Sir James Paget described a disease of chronic bone inflammation that caused softening and bowing of the long bones. Paget's disease existed in ancient times, as shown by the study of bones in archaeologic collections. Evidence of the disease has been found in the skulls of native American Indians and even Neanderthals.

The disease is rare in persons younger than 40 years of age, and men and women are equally affected. The frequency of the disease has ranged statistically from 3% to 4% of the population.[9] The figures include subclinical cases in which the disease was discovered microscopically on autopsy. The possible causes are many, but no exact etiology has been defined. Paget himself thought it was due to a chronic infection, and he called the disease *osteitis deformans*. Viral causation has been investigated, with antigens identical to the respiratory syncytial virus and the measles virus identified.[8, 9] The disease occurs late in life, which allows time for a long period of latency. Other etiologic possibilities include hormonal dysfunction, autoimmune states, vascular disorders, and neoplastic disease.

Pathologically, Paget's disease is characterized by reabsorption of bone followed by rapid overgrowth, a phenomenon that can occur in different stages in the same person and even in the same bone. The histologic features are usually described in phases. The initial, osteolytic, or destructive phase is marked by extensive reabsorption of existing bone, with the presence of numerous multinucleated osteoclasts.[9] The mixed or active phase occurs when the osteoclasts destroy the ordered lamellar bone, and osteoblasts respond to the destruction by rapid disposition of vascular connective tissue and remodeled lamellar bone. During this phase, the area appears to be highly vascular, with cement lines forming at sites where the lamellae are erratically joined, giving a mosaic appearance that may completely replace the preexisting bone.[8] The osteoblastic or sclerotic phase occurs when bone formation outstrips reabsorption, with lamellar bone as the predominant ingredient. Bone size and thickness are increased primarily in the head, femurs, humeri, and scapulae. This bone is soft, poorly mineralized, and subject to fractures. In persons with widespread disease, almost every bone may be affected.[16]

The clinical features progress slowly, and bone deformities can be considered part of the normal aging process. The condition is usually polyostotic (affecting more than one bone). The long bones of the legs become bowed and the pelvis misshapen. The thorax shortens, causing a loss of height. The bones of the skull are often affected, leading to symptoms of vertigo, headache, and progressive deafness due to compression of the eighth nerve. In the early stages of disease, pain in the affected bones may be experienced. Increased vascularity of the rebuilding bone together with cutaneous vasodilatation can produce warmth over affected bone, requiring an increase in cardiac output. Laboratory studies characteristically show elevation in levels of alkaline phosphatase that generally correlate with the extent of the process.[16] Roentgenographic appearance of the bone shows radiolucency with areas of density (lytic areas and areas of increased calcification).

No cure exists for Paget's disease, but newer therapies use calcitonin and diphosphates to inhibit osteoclastic activity. Etidronate disodium, given orally, decreases bone reabsorption, and improvement may last for 6 months or more after discontinuation of therapy. Mithramycin, a drug used in cancer therapy, may also be effective for patients with severe disease.[16] This suggests that the etiology is a virus-induced neoplastic process.

VON RECKLINGHAUSEN'S DISEASE

Osteitis fibrosa cystica, or von Recklinghausen's disease of the bone, is characterized by progressive resorption and destruction of bone brought about by long-standing hyperparathyroidism. Parathyroid hormone (PTH) excretion causes calcium and phosphorus to be removed from bone. Hyperplasia or neoplasia of the parathyroid glands may cause a hypersecretion of this hormone and thus demineralization of bone. Secondary hyperparathyroidism, as in chronic renal insufficiency, leads to decreased conversion of vitamin D to its active form in the kidneys and decreased absorption of calcium in the intestine. The low serum calcium level stimulates PTH secretion (see pp. 720–722).

In the early stages of both primary and secondary hyperparathyroidism, changes in bone resemble osteomalacia or osteoporosis. With advanced disease, there is osteoclastic reabsorption of bone, which is replaced by fibrous tissue in the marrow spaces. The cancellous and cortical bones undergo thinning with resultant deformities. In focal areas of bone reabsorption, large fibrous scars develop, yielding minute to very large cysts, called *brown tumors*. These nonmalignant granulomas receive their brownish color from degeneration and hemorrhage into the site. Because of earlier diagnosis and treatment, only 10% to 15% of persons with primary hyperparathyroidism experience significant skeletal changes.[8] Secondary hyperparathyroidism due to renal failure causes

only a part of the syndrome of *renal osteodystrophy*, which also includes osteomalacia and osteosclerosis.

OSTEONECROSIS

Osteonecrosis in the Adult

Osteonecrosis is synonymous with avascular necrosis, aseptic necrosis, and ischemic necrosis of bone.[27] It has been identified as one of the most common causes of hip pain and incapacity. Table 45-4 lists some associated diseases.

Necrosis of femoral and humeral heads is secondary to various systemic diseases that affect blood supply to the bone. Pathologically, the lesions occur primarily in subcortical areas of long bones that have a narrower capillary circulation than other bones. The initial cause appears to be ischemia, which can be produced by obstruction or compression of the microcirculation.[8] A his-

TABLE 45-4 *Diseases Associated with Osteonecrosis*

Associated Disease	Number of Patients
Systemic lupus erythematosus	82
Rheumatoid arthritis	26
Renal transplant	14
Hemoglobinopathy	12
Trauma	11
Alcoholism	10
Solid tumors	5
Hodgkin's disease	3
Leukemia	2
Gout	9
Asthma	8
Polyarthritis—unknown etiology	7
Polymyositis/dermatomyositis	4
Undifferentiated connective tissue disease	3
Inflammatory bowel disease	4
Giant cell arteritis/polymyalgia rheumatica	3
Arteritis—unspecified	2
Sarcoidosis	2
Cushing's syndrome	2
Systemic sclerosis	1
Raynaud's disease	1
Idiopathic thrombocytopenia	1
Caisson's disease	1
Gaucher's disease	1
Juvenile rheumatoid arthritis	1
Ankylosing spondylitis	1
Sjögrens syndrome	1
Nonassociated diseases	61
Ischemic necrosis of bone only	91
	368

(Adapted from Kelly, W.N., Harris, C.P., & Sledge, G. *Textbook of Rheumatology.* Philadelphia: W.B. Saunders, 1985.)

tory of alcoholism has been reported in 10% to 39% of cases. *Traumatic osteonecrosis* usually occurs with impaired blood supply to femoral or humeral heads. *Nontraumatic osteonecrosis* occurs most frequently in persons receiving glucocorticoids, especially persons with systemic lupus erythematosus and renal transplants.[27] The most common symptom is pain on active motion. Pain at rest and at night is also very common. Limitation of motion also occurs as the disease progresses. Radiographic abnormalities may develop from several months to 5 years after pain is described.[1, 27]

Legg-Calvé-Perthes Disease

Osteochondrosis refers to a set of conditions affecting the epiphyseal region of bone in children during the growth period. The pathology is brought about by avascular necrosis in the area that causes the bone of the epiphysis to soften and die (Fig. 45-18). Various names have been ascribed to avascular necrosis occurring in specific areas, but *Legg-Calvé-Perthes disease* is the most familiar.

The onset of the condition appears to be growth-related. Until age 3 or 4, the predominant blood supply to the femoral head comes across the growth plate from the metaphysis of the femur, with other supply from the lateral epiphyseal vessels. At about 4 years of age, the growth plate begins to block the metaphyseal blood supply, and full development of the ligament artery supply to the femoral head is reached when a child is 7 or 8 years old. This leaves a period of time when the blood supply to the femoral head is dependent on the lateral epiphyseal vessels.

Precipitating causes of avascular necrosis include trauma, infections, or inflammation. In the 2- to 4-year course of the disease, three stages occur:

1. Avascular necrosis causes the bone of the femoral head to soften and die, but the cartilage surrounding it, nourished by synovial fluid, remains viable.

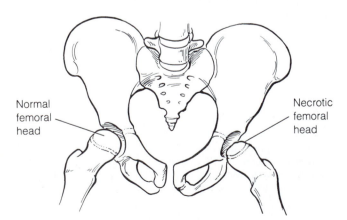

Normal femoral head

Necrotic femoral head

FIGURE 45-18 *Legg-Calvé-Perthes disease. Flattened femoral head is the result of necrosis. Left femoral head is normal.*

2. Blood vessels from adjacent viable tissue grow in through the neck of the femur and begin the slow process of removing dead bone a little at a time, a process called *creeping substitution*.
3. Areas of reabsorbed bone are filled with new bone, and ossification occurs.

All three of these stages—necrosis, removal of dead bone, and reossification—may occur simultaneously within the same bone. Children may complain of aching pain and limited motion early in the disease, but later processes remain painless.

Osgood-Schlatter Disease

Osgood-Schlatter disease usually occurs in boys from 10 to 15 years of age and is characterized by a painful, tender, enlarged tibial tubercle. It is caused by a pull of the patellar tendon on the tibial tubercle epiphysis, caused by sudden or continuous strain during growth. The condition may not be a true osteochondrosis but may be due to injury.[1] Serial films show changes due to aseptic necrosis that results from avascular changes. As in Legg-Calvé-Perthes disease, pain disappears shortly after onset, but the tibial tubercle may remain enlarged for years.

▼ Metabolic and Nutritional Bone Alterations

OSTEOPOROSIS

Osteoporosis is osteopenia due to reduction in both bone matrix and mineralization. *Osteopenia* is a reduction of bone mass greater than that expected for a given age, race, and sex.[14] It results in brittle bones that fracture quite easily. Because bone remodeling, with reabsorption balanced by formation, normally occurs throughout life, anything that either increases reabsorption or decreases formation causes loss of bone mass. The rate of reabsorption follows the surface-volume mass of bones. Therefore, because the trabeculae are composed of sheets of bone and have more surface volume than cortical bone, they are lost more rapidly. This loss leads to increased frequency of fractures in the weight-bearing bones, where trabecular bone predominates. The vertebral bodies, radial head, and femoral neck are examples of this type of bone. Likewise, reabsorption is accelerated on the endosteal surfaces of trabecular bone while formation is occurring at the periosteal surfaces, thus leading to wider bones with a thinner, more porous cortex. The ratio of bone mineral to matrix formation is constant, but there is simply a reduction in both. This contrasts with osteomalacia, in which the matrix is normal but the mineralization is deficient.

Osteoporosis may be caused by genetic, nutritional, mobility, drug-related, hormonal, and age factors. Deficiencies in protein; vitamins C, D, and A; and calcium can lead to reduced matrix and mineralization.[1, 14] Individuals with a family history of fractures due to osteoporosis have a greater risk of developing this condition. Estrogen and testosterone stimulate osteoblastic activity, so that the frequency of osteoporosis increases with menopause. Theories suggest that estrogen may antagonize PTH, which has a bone-reabsorption effect. Estrogen may also affect the absorption and excretion of calcium and phosphorus by direct action on the gastrointestinal tract, possibly through enhancing the metabolism of vitamin D.[8] Women with artificially induced menopause seem to develop the disease faster than those with normal, more slowly declining hormonal levels. Androgen deficiency in men also can lead to later-onset osteoporosis. Endocrine changes, such as diabetes mellitus and thyrotoxicosis, in which protein synthesis is decreased and catabolism is increased, respectively, also cause osteoporosis. Cushing's disease, with its protein catabolic loss, has the same bone results as prolonged steroid therapy. Prolonged therapy with heparin and certain cancer drugs may lead to osteoporosis. Smoking and excess alcohol ingestion increase the incidence of this condition. Irradiation, from radiographs or other exposure to radioactive materials, may affect bone by damage to the osteoblasts. Immobility of a limb and prolonged bed rest can also cause bone loss.

Osteoporosis is estimated to affect one in four women older than age 60. Bone loss begins in women at about age 45 and in men between ages 50 and 60.[14] Complications of the disorder, especially hip fractures, make it the 12th leading cause of death in the United States. Death usually results from respiratory complications secondary to immobility. The decline of estrogen after menopause combines with low bone mass to make certain groups of women more prone to the disease. White women tend to have less bone mass than black women, and thin women have less than obese women. Smokers seem to have less bone mass and tend to undergo menopause earlier than nonsmokers. In general, osteoporosis is most frequent in thin, small-built, fair-complected, freckled blond women with a sedentary lifestyle.[8]

Hip fractures account for more morbidity than all of the other osteoporotic fractures combined. More than 200,000 women suffer hip fractures in the United States each year.[1] In men, hip fractures are often related to long-term immobility, such as after a stroke or head injury. Fractures of the distal forearm are common but rarely cause death. Vertebral fractures, either complete or compression, can occur with a minimal amount of trauma and may cause few symptoms. These vertebrae never regain their normal shape and account for the loss of height and the "dowager's hump" seen in older women and men. Investigations of the appropriate prevention and treatment of osteoporosis have brought about much study and controversy. Studies suggest that various combinations of estrogen, calcium, vitamin D, and sodium fluoride seem to retard bone loss. These treatments are most effective when begun in perimenopausal or early postmenopausal woman.[14] Estrogen appears to stop postmenopausal bone loss for as long as it is taken, although it has side effects. Calcium intake of 1.5 g/day is recommended either in the diet or as a supplement. For persons with vertebral fractures, sodium fluoride induces the formation of new bone and decreases the frequency of other fractures. Vitamin D supplements may retard osteomalacia in the elderly who have deficient diets and minimal sunlight exposure. Studies suggest that regular exercise retards bone loss.[1]

RICKETS/OSTEOMALACIA

Rickets is a disease in the infant or growing child that usually is caused by a lack of vitamin D. Osteomalacia, or adult rickets, results from a calcium or phosphorus deficiency or both. In the United States, vitamin D deficiency alone is rare in adults. The mineral deficiency can result either from a decrease in calcium absorption or an increase in phosphorus loss by the kidneys. In chronic renal failure, the kidneys are unable to activate vitamin D and excrete phosphate. The accompanying hyperparathyroidism increases bone reabsorption of calcium. In elderly persons, low dietary intake of calcium and vitamin D combined with intestinal malabsorption can decrease bone mineralization.

The primary pathology consists of deficient mineralization of bone with a relative increase in uncalcified osteoid. The normal time required for osteoid calcification is 12 to 15 days, but in osteomalacia, the time interval lengthens to several months.[8] The lack of mineralization makes the bones soft, and they bow and break easily. Because bone formation in the growing child is most accelerated at the ends of the long bones, the epiphyseal tissue in rickets is soft, with the normally sharp, narrow line of ossification replaced by a wide, irregular zone of soft, gray tissue. Bowed legs and deformities of the costochondral junction (rachitic rosary) and thorax (pigeon breast), together with defective tooth enamel, are evidence of rickets. In the adult, osteomalacia is displayed by mineral changes and pain in the lumbar vertebrae, pelvic girdle, and long bones of the lower limbs.[25] Fractures occur with only minor trauma. The mineralization defect eventually leads to decreased bone matrix, and a hybrid state of osteomalacia–osteoporosis evolves.[8] Deformities can also occur in adults when the muscles and tendons change the shape of the softened bone.

Vitamin C (ascorbic acid) is necessary for the production of the collagen of fibrous tissue and of bone matrix. A deficiency of vitamin C leads to scurvy, which is characterized by hemorrhages, anemia, and bone and teeth changes. Hemorrhages can occur in any organ and can vary from tiny petechiae to large hematomas. Bone disturbances are evidenced by a defective osteoid and a relative increase in reabsorption over formation. This leads to a decreased density of bone. Bleeding, spongy gums, and loose teeth are common. Scurvy in infants usually does not appear until after 6 months of age, and it takes from 3 months to 1 year of severe vitamin C deficiency to produce scurvy in an adult.

▼ Infectious Diseases of Bone

OSTEOMYELITIS

Osteomyelitis occurs when the bone and bone marrow are invaded by pyogenic organisms, almost always bacteria.[25] Infection of bone can come about in three ways: 1) through the bloodstream (hematogenous); 2) by extension of a contiguous infection; or 3) by direct surgical or traumatic introduction.[1, 25]

In 60% to 70% of cases, the organism that causes osteomyelitis is hemolytic *Staphylococcus*, although streptococci, coliform bacteria, pneumococci, gonococci, or any bacterial or fungal agent may be involved. Immunosuppressed or debilitated persons are at greater risk and may develop infections due to *Salmonella, Pseudomonas, Haemophilus influenzae*, and group B streptococci.[18] The infecting organism enters the bone through the nutrient or metaphyseal vessels and moves into the medullary canal. Vascularity increases, causing edema. Polymorphonuclear leukocytes accumulate in the area. In a few days, thrombosis of local vessels occurs, and ischemia results. Portions of bone tissue die. Pus in this confined space is under pressure and is pushed out through Volkmann's canals to the surface of the bone (Fig. 45-19). It then spreads subperiosteally and can enter the bone at another level or burst out into the surrounding tissue. In infants, before the epiphyseal cartilage seals off the metaphysis, spread can go directly to the joint and cause a suppurative arthritis. In older persons, if joint involvement does occur, it does so through subperiosteal spread. The dead bone is separated from viable tissue, and granulation tissue forms beneath the area of dead bone and infection. The necrotic bone, isolated from viable tissue, is termed *sequestrum*. New bone forms from the elevated periosteum. This bone, called the *involucrum*, envelops the granulation tissue and sequestrum. Small sinuses permit the pus to escape.[25]

In chronic osteomyelitis, the granulation tissue becomes scar tissue and forms an impenetrable area around the infection. The localized area of suppuration is called *Brodie's abscess*.[25] A new area of bone develops to isolate the area further. The process is characterized by chronically draining sinuses with organisms that are resistant to antibiotic therapy.

Hematogenous osteomyelitis often follows urinary tract infection, bacterial endocarditis, respiratory infection, or a large soft tissue infection, such as a decubitus ulcer. Immunosuppressed persons or those with a chronic disease are at high risk for bacteremias and osteomyelitis. Posttraumatic or spreading osteomyelitis is characterized by erythema, local pain, and draining sinuses. Infection of a joint prosthesis may be seen within a few days after surgery. Loosening of fixative appliances for fractures or prostheses in joint replacement is a typical finding, and results of radionuclide scans are nearly always positive.

The person with acute osteomyelitis appears acutely ill, with fever, chills, and variable degrees of leukocytosis. If the osteomyelitis is in a limb, it becomes very painful. The pain is often described as a constant throbbing. Redness and swelling usually occur over the site, and sensitivity to the touch is characteristic. Radiologic evidence is noted after about 10 days and reflects bone destruction. Blood cultures may or may not be positive for the causative organism; massive antibiotic therapy usually arrests the disease. With vertebral osteomyelitis, blood cultures are usually negative and needle biopsy of infected bone is necessary.[18]

TUBERCULOSIS

Tuberculosis is a systemic disease caused by the tubercular bacillus, which spreads through the body through lymphatic or hematogenous routes (see pp. 575–576). Skeletal involvement is rare but may be seen to increase in the future due to drug resistant strains of tuberculosis. It is usually caused by seeding of the bacilli in the marrow cavity. The infection causes destruction of bone tissue and caseous necrosis that may enter the joint cavities or occur under the skin as an abscess with draining sinuses. Tubercular skeletal lesions usually do not wall themselves off, so invasion of joints and intervertebral disks may cause many deformities. Tuberculosis of the spine, called *Pott's disease*, most frequently occurs in children and can lead to kyphosis, scoliosis, or the hunchback deformity.

The onset of skeletal tuberculosis, in contrast to acute pyogenic osteomyelitis, is insidious, beginning with vague descriptions of pain. Complications of tuberculosis of the spine include paraplegia and meningitis. Tuberculosis of the hip and knee joint occurs most often in children.

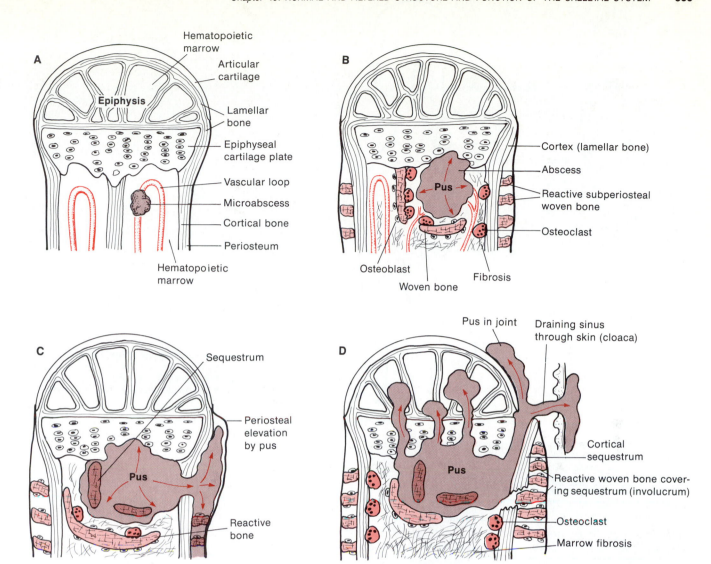

FIGURE 45-19 *Pathogenesis of hematogenous osteomyelitis.* **A.** *The epiphysis, metaphysis, and epiphyseal plate are normal. A small septic microabscess is forming at the capillary loop.* **B.** *The expansion of the septic focus stimulates reabsorption of adjacent bony trabeculae. Woven bone begins to surround this focus. The abscess expands into the cartilage and stimulates reactive bone formation by the periosteum.* **C.** *The abscess, which continues to expand through the cortex into the subperiosteal tissue, shears off the perforating arteries that supply the cortex with blood, thereby leading to necrosis of the cortex.* **D.** *The extension of this process into the joint space, the epiphysis, and the skin produces a draining sinus. The necrotic bone is called a sequestrum. The viable bone surrounding a sequestrum is termed the involucrum. (Source: Rubin, E. and Farber, J.L.* Pathology. *(2nd ed.). Philadelphia: J.B. Lippincott, 1994)*

SYPHILIS

Congenital or acquired syphilis of the bone is rare in the United States. In congenital syphilis, the spirochetes are delivered through the fetal bloodstream to the bones, where they inhibit osteogenesis. The epiphyseal plate is severely damaged and may actually be separated from the metaphysis. Bone syphilis is marked by endarteritis and periarteritis, and reactive bone forms from viable surrounding periosteum. Granulation tissue between the periosteum and cortical bone is laid down. In the tibia, a resulting "saber-shin" deformity gives a curved appearance to the anterior portion of the bone.[25]

Acquired syphilis may also cause osteochondritis or periosteitis; frank syphilitic lesions may appear within the medullary canal. The skull and vertebrae as well as the long bones can be affected in acquired syphilis.

▼ Alterations in Skeletal Structure

ABNORMAL SPINAL CURVATURES

The normal spinal curvature is assessed in routine medical examinations (Fig. 45-20). Changes in its contour give significant clues for underlying musculoskeletal disorders.

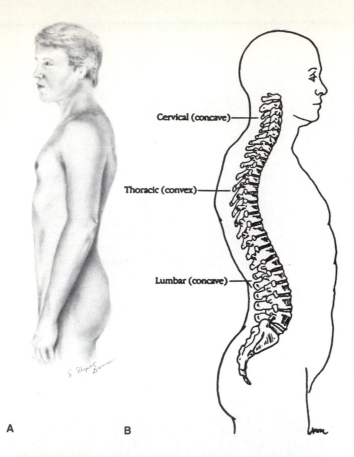

Cervical (concave)

Thoracic (convex)

Lumbar (concave)

A

B

FIGURE 45-20 **A.** Normal curvature of the spine, showing normal posture. **B.** Cervical area is slightly concave, thoracic curve is convex, and lumbar curve concave. (Source: Bates, B. A Guide to Physical Examination and History Taking [6th ed.] Philadelphia: J.B. Lippincott, 1995)

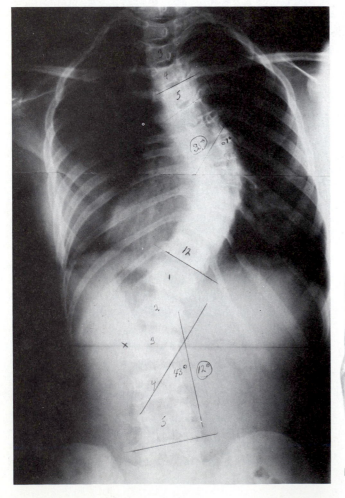

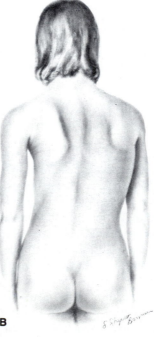

B

FIGURE 45-21 **A.** Scoliosis of the spine with a thoracic primary curve and compensatory curve in the lumbar spine. Vertebral bodies are marked at the approximate beginning and end of each curve and are used to measure the degree of curvature. **B.** Scoliosis may be structural or functional. Structural scoliosis is typically associated with rotation of the vertebrae on each other, and the rib cage is accordingly deformed. (Source: (B). Bates, B. A Guide to Physical Examination and History Taking [6th ed.] Philadelphia: J.B. Lippincott, 1995)

Scoliosis

Scoliosis is a lateral curvature of the spine that can result from another disease, such as polio or cerebral palsy. Most commonly, it is an idiopathic disorder. It is estimated that more than 1 million Americans have some degree of scoliosis, and girls are affected eight times more often than boys. Scoliosis occurs most frequently in the early adolescent years.

The curvatures are classified according to location and consist of a primary, fixed curve with compensatory curves above and below (Fig. 45-21). The deformity occurs slowly and is accelerated by the preadolescent growth spurt. The shoulder blade protrudes, the level of the iliac crests becomes unequal, and the curvature appears to be exaggerated when the person bends over (Fig. 45-22).[2] In general, the younger the age when the curvature is noticed and the higher up in the thorax it occurs, the poorer the prognosis. Severe scoliosis can affect the heart and lungs by restrictive action. It may be markedly improved by surgical procedures.

List

List is a lateral tilt of the spine from the T-1 level (Fig. 45-23). It may result from a herniated disk or a painful spasm of the muscles along the spine.[2]

Gibbous

The angular deformity noted with a collapsed vertebra is a gibbous (Fig. 45-24). Multiple causes include metastatic malignancy of the spine and tuberculosis.[2]

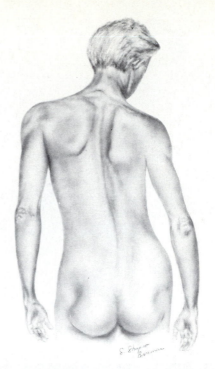

FIGURE 45-23 *List is a lateral tilt of the spine. When a plumb line dropped from the spinous process of T-1 falls to one side of the gluteal cleft, a list is present. Causes include a herniated disk and painful spasms of the paravertebral muscles. Scoliosis is inherent in a list but has not been fully compensated for by a spinal deviation in the opposite direction. (Source: Bates, B. A Guide to Physical Examination [6th ed.] Philadelphia: J.B. Lippincott, 1995)*

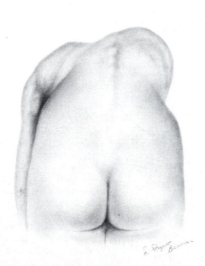

FIGURE 45-22 *The rotary deformity of scoliosis produces a hump or "razorback" deformity. This deviation is best demonstrated by asking the client to bend at the waist. (Source: Bates, B. A Guide to Physical Examination and History Taking [6th ed.] Philadelphia: J.B. Lippincott, 1995)*

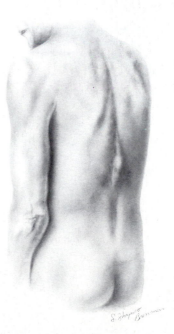

FIGURE 45-24 *Gibbous is an angular deformity of a collapsed vertebra. Causes include metastatic cancer and tuberculosis of the spine. (Source: Bates, B. A Guide to Physical Examination [6th ed.] Philadelphia: J.B. Lippincott, 1995)*

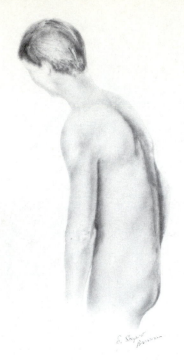

FIGURE 45-25 Flattening of the lumbar curve, muscle spasm in the lumbar area, and decreased spinal mobility suggest the possibility of a herniated lumbar disk or, especially in men, ankylosing spondylitis. (Source: Bates, B. A Guide to Physical Examination [6th ed.] Philadelphia: J.B. Lippincott, 1995)

Flattening of the Lumbar Curve

This contour change suggests a herniated lumbar disk or ankylosing spondylitis.[2] The normal curve in the lumbar area becomes straight (Fig. 45-25).

Lordosis

Lordosis is an accentuation of the normal lumbar curve (Fig. 45-26). It often results from obesity or pregnancy as a compensation for the protuberant abdomen.[2]

Kyphosis

Kyphosis may be the first indication of osteoporosis in the elderly person. It appears as a rounded thoracic convexity, especially in elderly women (Fig. 45-27).[2] It may be accompanied by pain in the vertebral area and radiologic signs of osteoporosis.

CLUBFOOT (TALIPES)

Clubfoot deformities, the most frequent of the orthopedic congenital deformities of the lower extremities, occur with greatest frequency in boys. Two-thirds of the cases are unilateral. Clubfoot may be caused by genetic

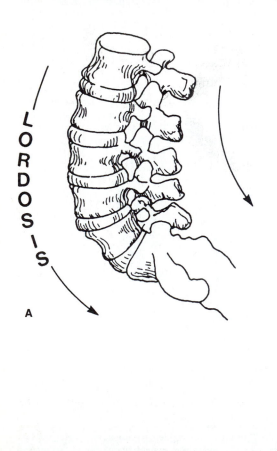

A

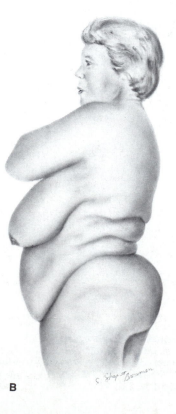

B

FIGURE 45-26 **A.** The normal orientation of the lumbar spine is that of mild lordosis. Exaggerated lordosis may predispose the patient to mechanical back pain. **B.** Lordosis develops to compensate for the protuberant abdomen of pregnancy or marked obesity. It may also compensate for kyphosis and flexion deformities of the hips. A deep midline furrow may be seen between the lumbar paravertebral muscles. (Source: Reilly, A. B. Practical Strategies in Outpatient Medicine [2nd ed.]. Philadelphia: W.B. Saunders, 1991; Bates, B. B. A Guide to Physical Examination and History Taking [6th ed.] Philadelphia: J.B. Lippincott, 1995)

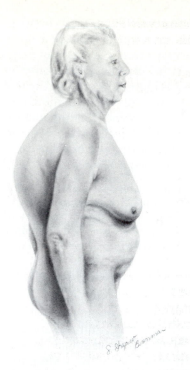

FIGURE 45-27 *Kyphosis, a rounded thoracic convexity, is common in aging, especially in women. (Source: Bates, B.* A Guide to Physical Examination *[6th ed.] Philadelphia: J.B. Lippincott, 1995)*

and environmental factors. Generally, the talus points downward and the foot is adducted. The clinical varieties are *easy* and *resistant*, with the easy cases responding to strapping and stretching alone and the resistant cases requiring surgical intervention.

CONGENITAL DISLOCATION OF THE HIP

Congenital dislocation of the hip is probably caused by a combination of genetic and environmental factors. Genetic factors are linked to both joint laxity and acetabular dysplasia. In addition, just before delivery of a full-term infant, the pregnant woman secretes a ligament-relaxing hormone that crosses the placental barrier and enhances joint laxity. This accounts for the relative rarity of hip dislocation in premature infants. Other environmental factors include intrauterine malposition, breech presentation during delivery, and, in some cultures, swaddling of neonates.

Pathologically, the acetabulum is defective and the femoral head is completely out of the joint, located posterior and superior to the acetabulum. Most frequently, this is a unilateral occurrence. Asymmetric groin skin creases are seen on examination, and the affected leg is shorter than the other. The leg cannot abduct completely. When it is extended and flexed at the hip, a click called *Ortolani's click* may be felt or heard. Because the femoral head must be in correct alignment with the acetabulum for the bones and joint to grow and develop

normally, early detection is necessary. Reduction after age 6 years is almost impossible, and secondary bone changes occur that cause the child to walk with a typical lurching gait. The earlier the child is treated, the more likely that complete hip function will be restored.

▼ Alterations in Joints and Tendons

As discussed earlier, joints allow the body to be mobile. The synovial joints are most affected by alterations. Studies have shown that this type of articular cartilage, which is lubricated and nourished by synovial fluid, has many microscopic spaces filled with fluid, causing it to be elastic and to bounce back despite daily subjection to compression.

ARTHRITIS

The most frequent joint diseases are the arthritides, which affect 1 of every 20 to 30 Americans and constitute a financial and health problem of considerable magnitude. Arthritis simply means inflammation of a joint, and it occurs in many forms. Degenerative joint disease or trauma often is related to an increased incidence of osteoarthritis. Metabolic disturbances may cause gouty arthritis or may be associated with such conditions as psoriasis or bursitis. Suppurative arthritis implies an infection of the joint with pyogenic organisms; tuberculous arthritis is inflammation secondary to tuberculosis. Autoimmune conditions produce many types of arthritis, the most crippling of which is rheumatoid arthritis, which has many forms.

RHEUMATOID ARTHRITIS

Rheumatoid arthritis is an inflammatory disease that has been studied extensively in attempts to uncover an etiologic agent. It occurs throughout the world and affects 1% to 2% of most populations.[28] The incidence is three times greater in women than in men.[25] In recent years, theories have supported an infectious cause or an autoimmune response. Many bacteria and viruses suspected of causing rheumatoid arthritis have been studied, with the inability to demonstrate organisms in the joints of affected persons. There is a high incidence of circulating antibody to Epstein–Barr virus. This antibody is called rheumatoid arthritis–associated nuclear antigen and is similar to the nuclear antigen encoded by Epstein–Barr virus, the Epstein–Barr nuclear antigen.[25] Despite this, the preponderance of evidence supports an autoimmune causation with both cellular and humoral immune factors. Genetic factors also indicate that there is an increased frequency of the disease in close relatives.[25]

Antibodies known as *rheumatoid factor* have been demonstrated in the sera of almost all persons with rheumatoid arthritis. Synovial lymphocytes produce IgG, which is targeted as foreign, and production of IgG and IgM anti-immunoglobulins results. These anti-immunoglobulins are actually the rheumatoid factor. By binding with IgG, the antigenic target, the resulting complex activates the complement system in the joint. The rheumatoid factor titer is in direct relationship to the severity of the disease, although the actual stimulus for the formation of rheumatoid factor is unknown.

The numerous T lymphocytes in the joint may become sensitized to the joint collagens, causing an immunologic response that is enhanced by the release of lymphokines and the presence of prostaglandins.[8, 28] Increased physical or emotional stress has always been recognized as a precipitator of acute exacerbations, but the mechanisms for the stress interaction are unknown.

Joint destruction is the primary pathology of rheumatoid arthritis and may affect any synovial membrane in the body. Joint inflammation with effusion is accompanied by capsular and periarticular soft tissue inflammation, causing swelling, redness, and painful motion of the joint. Proliferative synovitis persists, and the synovium becomes a thickened, hyperemic, densely cellular membrane called a *pannus*, which invades and erodes surrounding cartilage and bone.[28] Joint motion causes bleeding within the cavity. Clots of fibrin and newly formed granulation tissue fill the joint space. Pannus destroys the articular cartilage and underlying bone, resulting in loss of motion. The muscles that pull across the joint give rise to flexion and extension and subluxation deformities. Subcutaneous rheumatoid nodules, which are areas of necrosis surrounded by lymphocytes and plasma cells, are present in about one-fourth of persons affected.

The fluid aspirated from the joint is thin and cloudy and has an elevated white cell level. The lysosomal enzymes released from these neutrophils may be a factor in cartilage destruction. As the acute inflammatory process subsides, granulation tissue becomes scar tissue and eventually bone, causing a true ankylosis (a fixed, stiff joint). Local degenerative muscle is gradually replaced by fibrous tissue, and the involved bones show osteoporosis. Rheumatoid arthritis mostly affects the joints but can affect any system. Small and large arteries anywhere in the system can develop acute necrotizing vasculitis with thrombosis. The vasculitis can cause the vascular insufficiency of Raynaud's phenomenon or obliterative vasculitis from intimal proliferation. The manifestations of cardiac disease include conduction disturbances, pericardial adhesions, myocarditis, and valvular impingement.[3] In the lungs, the person may exhibit pleuritis or interstitial pneumonitis. The eyes may show uveitis, keratoconjunctivitis, or chronic inflammation. Neuropathies, skeletal muscle inflammations, and spleen and liver enlargement may result.

The disease most often occurs between ages 20 and 50 years. The onset can be vague or acute. Fatigue, fever, and malaise may precede actual joint pain, or high fever and aching joints may herald the onset of the disease. Joint stiffness is more noticeable in the morning or after rest. The erythrocyte sedimentation rate is elevated. Classification by the American Rheumatism Association uses four or more of the following symptoms, signs, and laboratory findings for a person whose disease has been continuous for at least 6 weeks:

▼ Morning stiffness in and around the joint for at least 1 hour
▼ At least three joint areas with soft tissue swelling or fluid
▼ At least one joint area swollen in a wrist or joints of the hand
▼ Subcutaneous nodules over bony prominences
▼ Demonstration of abnormal amounts of serum rheumatoid factor
▼ Radiologic changes typical of rheumatoid arthritis on wrist radiographs[28]

Exacerbations are common and often cause increasing damage with greater stiffness and deformities. Any joint may be affected, and spinal cervical involvement may be seen. Hand and wrist deformities with swelling and a zigzag appearance are common (Fig. 45-28).[3]

A variant of rheumatoid arthritis is juvenile rheumatoid arthritis. The onset of juvenile rheumatoid arthritis in persons age 16 years or younger is usually abrupt, with chills and high fever, or it may appear insidiously with typical stiffness of one or more joints. The joint pathology is similar to the adult form, and subcutaneous lesions may also be present. Fortunately, more than one-half of these young persons have a complete remission. Permanent deformities are more com-

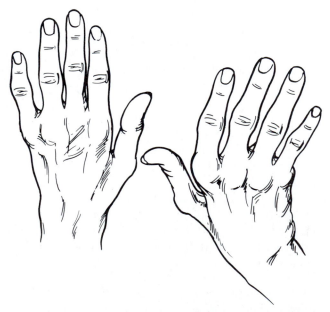

FIGURE 45-28 *Ulnar deviation and subluxation of the metacarpophalangeal joints have occurred in the right hand. These joints also appear swollen. Muscle atrophy has developed in the dorsal musculature of both hands.*

mon in those with acute febrile onset, multiple joint involvement, and a positive rheumatoid factor.[28]

ANKYLOSING SPONDYLITIS

Ankylosing spondylitis is an arthritic condition that is classified as one of a group of seronegative spondylarthrides. Box 45-2 lists the conditions that are placed in this classification. Ankylosing spondylitis is characterized by sacroiliac joint involvement, peripheral inflammatory arthropathy, and the absence of the rheumatoid factor.[6] Destruction of cartilage and bone results in fibrous and bony ankylosing of the spine, giving the patient the typical stiff, or "poker," spine (see Figure 45-25). Mobility of the spine is usually decreased symmetrically but improves somewhat with exercise. Discomfort is insidious in onset and is often described as morning stiffness.[6] If peripheral joints are affected early in the disease, joint replacement procedures may become necessary. The disease is only slightly more prevalent in men than in women, and the symptoms in men are more severe. The peak age range is from 20 to 40 years.[8] An elevated erythrocyte sedimentation rate is characteristic, but evidence of immune complex formation is found less frequently than in rheumatoid disease.[6]

OSTEOARTHRITIS

The term *osteoarthritis* is misleading because inflammation is not a usual component of this condition. The term *degenerative joint disease* more clearly describes the disease, which is the most common rheumatic disease.[22] The frequency usually is age-related, with most persons affected after age 50 years old. Primary osteoarthritis is a disease of unknown etiology, whereas secondary osteoarthritis has a known underlying cause, such as trauma, osteonecrosis, or infection.[25] Joints have a limited way in which to respond to the compressive forces in day-to-day living. In osteoarthritis, it has been found that the matrix in the articular cartilage is depleted, thus "unmasking" the basic collagen structure. Normally, the matrix spreads compression stress hydrostatically, but with its depletion the collagen fibers may rupture, causing flaking, fissuring, and eroding of the articular cartilage. These alterations are characteristic of the disorder.

BOX 45-2 ▼ Seronegative Spondylarthropathies

Ankylosing spondylitis
Reiter's syndrome
Psoriatic arthropathy
Intestinal arthropathy
Juvenile ankylosing spondylitis
Reactive arthropathy

BOX 45-3 ▼ Clinical Features of Primary Osteoarthritis

Age
Usually elderly

Joint Distribution
Monoarthritis or oligoarthritis

Most Frequent Sites
Distal and proximal interphalangeal joints of fingers, first carpometacarpal joint, first metatarsophalangeal joint, hips, knees, cervical spine, lumbar spine

Joints Usually Spared
Metacarpophalangeal joints, wrists, elbows, glenohumeral joints, ankles

Characteristics of Joint Discomfort
Aggravated by use and relieved by rest (but pain also at rest with severe disease); gelling sensation; morning stiffness absent or less than 30 minutes in duration

Joint Examination
Local tenderness, bony or soft tissue swelling, crepitus, effusion

Systemic Manifestations
Absent

Characteristics of Synovial Fluid
Normal viscosity, normal mucin test, mild leukocytosis (<2000 white blood cells/µL), predominantly mononuclear cells

(Kelley, W.N. (ed.). *Textbook of Internal Medicine* [2nd ed.]. Philadelphia: J.B. Lippincott, 1992.)

Laboratory studies rarely show increased erythrocyte sedimentation rate or synovial fluid inflammatory changes. Radiograph results may appear normal or show only narrowing joint space or cyst formation. Osteoporosis is not a direct component of the disease, but because of age considerations it may also be seen. The bone immediately under the affected area shows proliferation of fibroblasts and new bone formation. Periosteal bone growth also increases at the joint margins and at the site of ligament or tendon attachments, developing into bone spurs or ridges called *osteophytes*. The synovial capsule decreases in size, and movement is limited.

Degenerative joint disease generally affects joints that are under much pressure, especially the spine, fingers, knees, hips, and shoulders. Early in the course of the disease, pain, stiffness, and difficulty moving the joint (gelling) occur after joint use and are relieved by rest. Later, pain occurs with motion or rest.[22] Spurs may be formed on the distal interphalangeal joints of the fingers and are termed *Heberden's nodes*. Flexor and lateral deviations of the fingers are common, especially in the elderly (see pp. 168–170). Persons under occupational stress or who are obese or have faulty posture are at greatest risk for the disease. Box 45-3 lists the clinical features of primary osteoarthritis. Trauma, such as sports injuries to a joint at an early age, can render the person more susceptible to osteoarthritis with advancing years. Studies have shown a *wear-and-tear* process, with increased frequency in joints under stress.[4]

HYPERURICEMIA AND GOUT

Gout is a general term for a group of diseases with one or more of the following manifestations: 1) increased serum urate concentration; 2) recurrent attacks of acute arthritis with urate crystals in synovial fluid; 3) aggregated deposits of urate in joints, leading to crippling and deformity; 4) renal disease; and 5) uric acid nephrolithiasis.[10] The prevalence of gout in the United States has been estimated at 275 per 100,000, with the risk increasing with age and serum urate concentrations.[26]

Gout is caused by monosodium urate crystals in the joints, which cause acute arthritis. These crystals precipitate in the joints when body fluids are supersaturated with uric acid. Gout is generally classified as primary or secondary. Primary gout is a genetic disorder in which the exact defect of uric acid metabolism is unknown in the vast majority of cases. Ninety percent of all gout is primary, with men most frequently affected.[25] Secondary gout occurs whenever some superimposed condition either increases the production of uric acid or decreases its excretion.[10] Diseases characterized by rapid breakdown of cells (eg, leukemia), hemolytic anemia, cytolytic agents, and drugs that decrease excretion of urates (eg, thiazides and mercurial diuretics) have all been implicated in secondary gout. Box 45-4 summarizes the mechanisms for hyperuricemia and gout.

In the body, uric acid is made by the enzymatic breakdown of tissue and dietary purines. Gout, a hyperuricemic syndrome, can result from overproduction of uric acid, retention of uric acid due to renal malfunction, or both.[8] Normal purine metabolism is complicated, involving numerous enzymes and two pathways. Although the exact error of metabolism is unknown in most cases, the result is an abnormally large amount of uric acid in the blood. At an excessive point, uric acid crystals precipitate into the joint fluids, kidneys, heart, earlobes, and toes. The mass of urate crystals surrounded by inflammation with lymphocytes, plasma cells, and macrophages is called a *tophus*. Tophi may clump together and form large plaquelike encrustations that invade the articular surface and underlying bone, causing deformities.

Gout is described in four clinical phases: asymptomatic hyperuricemia, acute gouty arthritis, intercritical gout, and chronic tophaceous gout.[25, 26] In asymptomatic hyperuricemia, the serum urate level is elevated even though there are no symptoms. In acute gouty arthritis, there is a sudden onset of severe pain in the great toe or occasionally the heel, ankle, or instep. The affected joint becomes hot, red, and tender. The pain

---

BOX 45-4 ▼ Mechanisms for Hyperuricemia and Gout: Decreased Excretion of Urate

Primary Hyperuricemia
Decreased tubular secretion

Secondary Hyperuricemia
Reduced renal functional mass: chronic renal disease
Increased tubular reabsorption: conditions associated with contraction of extracellular fluid volume
  Dehydration
  Diabetes insipidus
  Diuretics
Decreased tubular secretion
  Conditions associated with increased levels of β-hydroxybutyrate and acetoacetate
  Starvation
  Diabetic ketoacidosis
Conditions associated with hyperlacticacidemia
  Acute ethanol ingestion
  Toxemia of pregnancy
Mechanisms not established
  Lead nephropathy
  Polycystic kidneys
  Associated with drug administration
    Cyclosporine
    Pyrazinamide
    Salicylates (in low dosages)
    Ethambutol
    Diuretics
    Nicotinic acid

(Kelley, W.N. (ed.). *Textbook of Internal Medicine* [2nd ed.]. Philadelphia: J.B. Lippincott, 1992.)

---

becomes intense and intolerable. It may be associated with chills and fever and resolve spontaneously or with treatment. The intervals between attacks are called *intercritical gout*. Crystal deposition persists during this phase. In the fourth phase, tophi occur in many locations, even in the aorta and heart valves. Deforming arthritis is common and can involve any joint.[26] The monosodium urate crystals are deposited in the synovial fluids, and these can rapidly lyse neutrophils, which release lysosomal enzymes and crystals. This makes the inflammatory process continuous.

The association of gout attacks with overeating and alcoholism is well supported. About one-half of gouty persons are more than 15% above their ideal weight, and 75% exhibit hypertriglyceridemia.[26] Ethanol increases urate production through increasing blood lactate, which blocks the renal excretion of uric acid.[10, 26] Therefore, the affected person may describe an excessive consumption of rich foods or alcohol before an attack.

As stated before, acute gouty arthritis is heralded by the sudden onset of acute pain, usually in one joint in the lower extremity. Half of the attacks occur in the metatarsophalangeal joint of the great toe. Persons often relate unusual stress preceding an attack, which could include overeating, overindulgence in alcohol, emotional stress, or physical exertion.[8] A person may be asymptomatic for months or even years between attacks. Over many years, disabling, chronic, gouty arthritis may develop. Atherosclerosis becomes a problem in almost half of persons with gout, and death occurs most frequently from myocardial infarction or renal failure.[26] Treatment consists of a variety of drugs that inhibit uric acid production.

BURSITIS

Bursae are classically described as enclosed sacs containing a small amount of fluid that lubricates and cushions joints (see Figure 45-5). Inflammation of a bursa is common and may be caused by unusual use of a part by trauma, infection, or rheumatoid arthritis. The inflammation results in an excess production of fluid in the sac, which becomes distended and presses on sensory nerve endings, causing pain. Commonly affected bursae are 1) the prepatellar bursa, caused by kneeling (housemaid's knee or nun's knee); 2) the olecranon bursa, subject to the repeated trauma of leaning on one's elbows (bartender's elbow); 3) the bursa located on the plantar aspect of the heel, which is subjected to repeated pressure (postman's heel); and 4) the bursa of the metatarsophalangeal joint of the great toe (bunion).

BAKER'S CYST

Baker's cyst is a firm, cystic mass along the medial border of the popliteal space. It occurs mostly in children and is believed to be caused by fluid distention of the bursal sac associated with local muscles. Some cysts communicate directly with the joint cavity. Swelling is usually the only symptom, and surgical excision, although possible, is often unnecessary.

TUMORS OF JOINTS

Tumors of joints are uncommon, but they may occur on the tendon sheath, the bursae, and around the joints. They are classified as sarcomas of the synovial lining. Primitive mesenchymal cells, rather than synovial membrane cells, form the primary tumor. A gray-white mass invades along muscle and fascial planes, and although the tumor is slow growing, it can metastasize to the lungs, bones, and brain.

TENOSYNOVITIS

Tenosynovitis is an inflammation of the tendon sheath and the enclosed tendon. It primarily affects the wrists, shoulders, and ankles. This condition is thought to be use related, and occupational stresses, such as typing and heavy labor, may precipitate it. Synovial fluid and fibrin constituents within the tendon sheath may cause adhesions. These inflammations cause extreme pain on movement and may exhibit heat and redness or inflammation. Bacterial invasion of pyrogens and tuberculosis also have been implicated as causes of tenosynovitis.

FIBROMATOSIS

Palmar fibromatosis denotes chronic hyperplasia of the fascia in the palm of the hand, leading to fibrosis and a deformity called *Dupuytren's contracture*. The fingers, most often the ring and little fingers, contract into a fixed, flexed position. Usually bilateral, this condition occurs most often in middle-aged men. Heredity is believed to be a major factor in causation.

Plantar fibromatosis is similar to palmar fibromatosis, but it usually does not cause contractures. Nodular masses of fibrocytes arise from the plantar fascia, usually on the medial side of the foot. Trauma is thought to be the cause.

CASE STUDY 45-1

Mr. Ted Smith, a 58-year-old caucasian male, was seen in the outpatient clinic on Monday morning for the sudden onset of acute pain, redness, and swelling of the joint of the right great toe. Mr. Smith is 5'5" tall and weighs 234 pounds. He relates a diet high in fat and drinks approximately 12 beers per night with greater consumption on the weekends. Serum uric acid was 12 mg/dL, serum triglycerides measured 323 mg/dL, and serum cholesterol was 267 mg/dL.

1. *From the clinical situation above, what is the probable diagnosis?*
2. *Describe the pathophysiology of the disorder.*
3. *What are the potential complications of this disease?*
4. *What are the risk factors for developing this condition?*
5. *Discuss modifications in lifestyle that could decrease Mr. Smith's risk of recurrence of symptoms.*

See Appendix G for discussion.

▼ Bone Tumors

Tumors in the skeletal system can be either primary or secondary. Primary lesions can be benign or malignant. Of these, benign tumors are much more common and usually are self-limiting. Malignant tumors of the bone, although rare, are devastating and often fatal. Diagnosis is based on a careful history, tumor location, and radiographic appearance.

Benign bone tumors are usually slow growing, noninvasive, and well localized. Adolescents or young adults are usually affected most frequently, and the tumor growth stops when the skeletal system reaches maturity. Because of their noninvasive characteristics, benign tumors cause little or no pain and are often discovered secondarily to another complaint or a pathologic fracture. Malignant neoplasms grow rapidly, spread and invade Surrounding areas, and cause pain. Classic signs are constant or intermittent pain, usually worse at night; an unexplained swelling over a bone; and a feeling of warmth of the skin over the bone, with prominent veins. Adolescents and young adults are most commonly affected. These tumors metastasize to other parts of the body and are usually fatal without early diagnosis and treatment.

Secondary tumors of the skeletal system are usually metastatic from primary sites in the breasts, lungs, kidneys, or other body systems. As the primary lesion grows and invades surrounding tissue, clumps of cancerous tissues are carried by the blood and lymphatic system to the bone, where they continue to grow and cause destruction.

The growth of tumors in the bone often causes increased radiodensities due to increased osteoblastic activity within the tumor. This can be seen on radiographs, which are helpful in diagnosis. Some tumors cause the bone to appear translucent, indicating increased osteoclast activity.

CLASSIFICATION OF TUMORS

Primary bone neoplasm may be classified according to the skeletal tissue from which it arises: osseous, cartilage, or marrow. Tumors in each of these categories may be benign or malignant. Other bone tumors, such as giant-cell tumors, do not have these origins. This section discusses the more common benign and malignant tumors, which are classified as osteoblastic (bone-forming), chondrogenic (tumors of marrow origin), and of unknown origin.

Fibrous Dysplasia

Fibrous dysplasia, which is characterized by replacement of cancellous bone by fibrous tissue, can affect one bone (monostotic), or many bones (polyostotic). Monostotic forms account for about 70% of cases, and these usually affect the ribs, femur, tibia, maxilla, mandible, or humerus.[8] The condition may be asymptomatic, or disfigurement from bony distortion may be seen. In the polyostotic form, the craniofacial bones are affected most frequently, but crippling deformities also may be associated.

The fibrous lesion begins in the medullary canal and spreads to the cortex, with cancellous bone and marrow replaced by yellow-gray, fibrous tissue. The cortex is thin, and bowing deformities and fractures are common. If this disease occurs in the monostotic form, the lesion grows slowly, but eventually deformity occurs unless the mass is surgically removed. If the polyostotic form of the disease is accompanied by extraskeletal signs and endocrine pathology, it is called *Albright's syndrome.*

Albright's syndrome is differentiated by precocious puberty in girls, café au lait pigmentation of the skin over the bone involvement, and predominant unilateral bone deformity, especially of the skull and long bones.[8] When the facial bones are affected, asymmetry of the face with distortions of the nose, jaw, and even severe displacement of an eye may occur. Although fibrous dysplasia has no proven genetic links, multisystem involvement of the polyostotic form does suggest some basic genetic defect. Many endocrine associations have been identified, including hyperthyroidism, Cushing's syndrome, acromegaly, and hyperparathyroidism.[8]

Bone-Forming Tumors

Benign osteoblastic tumors include *osteomas* and *osteoblastomas. Compact osteoma* is a benign tumor composed of dense bone with a well-circumscribed edge. It frequently arises in the cortical surface of the bone of the skull and paranasal sinuses. Symptoms are caused from impingement of the tumor on the brain or sinuses. The tumors cause the face to become distorted.[8]

Osteoid osteoma most commonly affects the femur and tibia but can grow in any bone in the body except the skull. It is usually located in the diaphyses of long bones. It occurs predominantly in boys and young men between the ages of 5 and 25 years. The tumor consists of a well-rounded, central nidus that is sharply demarcated from a surrounding zone of bone. The nidus may range from a few millimeters to a centimeter and consists of osteoid tissue and trabeculae. The tissue is reddish gray and granular. The main symptom is increasingly severe, localized pain in a lower limb.[12]

Benign osteoblastoma is a rare benign tumor that is sometimes confused with osteoid osteoma or even giant-cell tumors. It occurs most frequently in boys and young men, usually in the first three decades of life. Its most common site is the spinal cord. Pain is a cardinal symptom, usually due to the pressure on adjacent structures, such as the spinal cord or nerve roots. It seems to be less severe than that caused by an osteoid osteoma and may be referred to a site distant from the tumor. Other symptoms depend on the location of the tumor and include weakness and paraplegia. There is no characteristic radiographic appearance. In some cases, one may see bone destruction that is more or less demarcated from normal bone. Surgical removal usually relieves compression on the spinal column and nerve root. When the tumor is in a long bone, it may take on the appearance of an osteoid osteoma with a sclerotic border, except that the nidus may be many times longer.

The most prevalent malignant tumor of osteoid origin is the *osteogenic sarcoma* or *osteosarcoma,* in which tumor cells proliferate osteoid or immature bone. Osteosarcoma is the most common and most fatal primary bone tumor, often affecting people between the ages of 10 and 20 years.[25] It occurs more often in young men than in young women, usually during periods of rapid skeletal growth. It usually arises near the end of a long bone, especially around the knee.[12] Irradiation and oncogenic viruses have been explored in its etiology.[25] When this lesion occurs in later years of life, it is usually related to Paget's disease. Radiation treatment for other tumors has also been indicated in the causation of osteogenic sarcoma in later life. To be classified as a true osteogenic sarcoma, an osteoid substance must be produced. The tumor may show a predominance of elements, with osteoid, chondroid, or fibromatoid differentiation. Bizarre pleomorphic cells with abundant mitoses or multinucleate giant cells are characteristic.[12,25]

Osteosarcomas usually occur in long tubular bones, but the skull, maxilla, spinal column, and clavicles as well as other bones are also affected. The femurs, tibia, and ulnae are the most frequent sites (Fig. 45-29). After the age of 25, its frequency in flat and long bones is nearly equal.[8] The tumor usually is a localized swelling with tenderness associated with a large mass. Pain may or may not be present. Sometimes the tumor is found on incidental radiographic examination of an injury. It tends to recur within 1 to 2 years.

The survival rate of persons with osteosarcoma was dismal when resection or amputation alone was used. Five-year survival of about 60% has been achieved using a combination of aggressive chemotherapy and surgery.[19]

Tumors of Cartilaginous Origin

Benign chondrogenic tumors include osteochondroma and chondroblastoma. Many of these tumors are asymptomatic and are discovered accidentally because of an injury to the area. *Osteochondromas* form a long mass

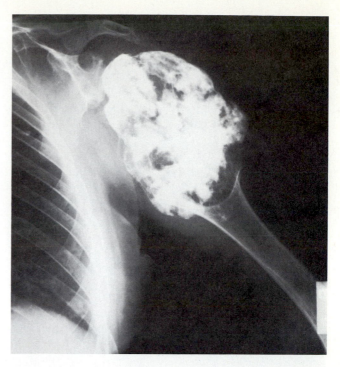

FIGURE 45-30 *Osteochondroma of the proximal right humerus is unusually large. Shows cartilaginous and osteoid matrix being laid down.*

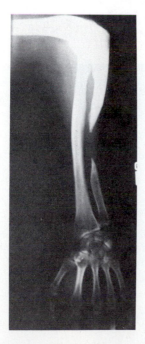

FIGURE 45-29 *Osteogenic sarcoma. Note the complete destruction of the ulna.*

produced by progressive endochondral ossification of a growing cartilaginous cap. The tumor is basically osseous and protrudes from the cortex of the bone with or without a stalk. The caps are usually cauliflower-shaped and occur mainly in persons between the first and second decades of life (Fig. 45-30). The growth of the tumor parallels that of the adolescent, and once the epiphyses have closed, it normally stops. Multiple osteochondromas may occur when more than one bone is affected, with each growth having the same characteristics as the single osteochondroma.

Osteochondromas rarely undergo malignant change to osteosarcomas. This transformation may occur if there are multiple tumors or occasionally after surgical removal of an osteochondroma. The most common site for the tumorous mass is the metaphyseal region of long bones, specifically the femur and tibia, but it can affect any bone that develops by endochondral ossification.

Endochondroma is the term used to describe a tumor when it involves only the medulla and is encapsulated by an intact cortex. It commonly affects the small bones of the hands and feet but may affect the ribs, sternum, spine, and long bones of persons between 20 and 30 years of age. The tumor usually affects the phalanges of the hand, producing a central area of rarefaction (decreasing density and weight). Normally discovered during treatment of a fracture after a trivial injury, the tumor appears radiographically as a well-defined, translucent area with the cortex intact and areas of calcification.

Benign *chondroblastomas* closely resemble giant-cell tumors and affect mainly persons younger than age 20

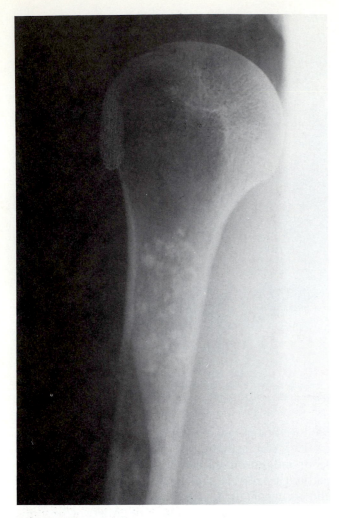

FIGURE 45-31 *Chondrosarcoma of the humerus. Mixed lytic and sclerotic areas give patchy appearance to bone.*

years or before epiphyseal closure, whereas giant-cell tumors are in persons younger than age 20 years. Histologically, chondroblastomas differ from giant-cell tumors in that they contain foci of calcification, trabeculae of osteoid tissue, and well-developed bone as well as more or less well-defined areas of cartilaginous matrix, features that are not usually present in giant-cell tumors. Chondroblastomas are virtually always benign, localized lesions that do not recur and do not invade.

Localized pain may be experienced and is often referred to the adjacent joint region. Wasting of muscle mass due to disuse caused by pain and limping may occur.

Radiographically, an area of central bone destruction is clearly demarcated by surrounding normal bone. There may be margins of increased bone density with mottled areas of calcification within the lesion. The tumor almost always involves the epiphyses and frequently the adjacent metaphyses, which are also seen on the films.[8]

Chondrosarcoma is a malignant bone tumor of cartilaginous origin. It can arise from benign chondrogenic origins, as described earlier, or may develop spontaneously. The tumor occurs more frequently in men than in women.

It is primarily a condition of adulthood and old age and rarely metastasizes until it has grown to a large size.[19]

Chondrosarcomas usually originate in the trunk and the upper ends of the femur and humerus, and points of attachment of muscle to bone at the knee, pelvis, shoulder, and hip are prevalent. Any bone of the body can be affected.

Physical symptoms may include pain, swelling, and a palpable mass due to the active invasive growth of the tumor. Tumors located in the trunk and long bones may be evidenced only by pain, which makes radiographic findings important. These findings usually include mottled areas of calcification and areas of osseous destruction (Fig. 45-31). Even when treated with wide resection, recurrence has been encountered even after 10 years. Metastases may occur many years after initial diagnosis and treatment.[19]

Tumors of Undetermined Origin

Ewing's sarcoma, although rare, is one of the most lethal bone tumors. Approximately 90% of people affected are younger than age 30; the greatest number of tumors occur in the second decade of life. They affect men over women by a 2-to-1 margin.[25] The long tubular bones are most commonly involved, with the innominate bones—the pelvis, ischium, ribs, scapula, and sternum—following in that order, and then virtually any other bone in the body.

Ewing's sarcoma, like many other invasive tumors, results in pain, a tender mass, and venous distension. Some persons may have anemia, temperature elevation, and sometimes leukocytosis.[25] This tumor generally originates in the medullary canal, growing outward and creating a lytic area on radiographs. Ewing's sarcoma is composed of nondistinctive, small, round cells that are

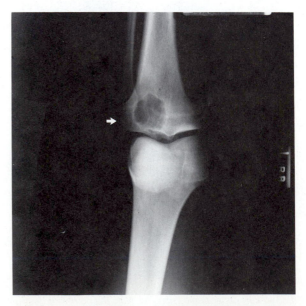

FIGURE 45-32 *Giant-cell tumor of the tibia (arrow).*

not easily identified.[8] Some spicules of bone may be seen, but this is reactive bone and not part of the neoplasm. Elevation of the periosteum is typical, followed by periosteal bone formation, which creates what is known as an onion-skin appearance, seen radiologically.[8]

Giant-cell tumors are poorly understood, apparently malignant, distinct neoplasms. Cases of seemingly benign giant-cell tumors have been reported to undergo malignant transformation. For this reason, a histomorphic grading system has been developed, with Grade I benign, Grade II borderline, and Grade III frankly malignant.[19] Unfortunately, this system is not always accurate, because one part of the tumor may appear benign while another part may appear malignant.

Giant-cell tumors generally affect persons between ages 20 and 55 years. Peak occurrence is in the third decade of life. It affects women somewhat more frequently than men.[19] Most giant-cell tumors arise in the epiphyses of long bones, with more than one-half of the lesions close to the knee in the distal femur and proximal tibia; other sites include the sacrum, vertebrae, humerus, and radius.[19]

Giant-cell tumors usually begin forming within cancellous bone. As they grow and invade, the cortex may be thinned or even broken, but new reactive bone generally preserves the cortex. The expansion of the tumor in the epiphyses classically forms a clublike deformity. Radiographs reveal a somewhat translucent area at the ends of the long bones, with a thin cortex (Fig. 45-32).

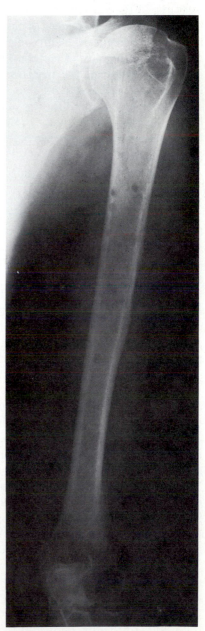

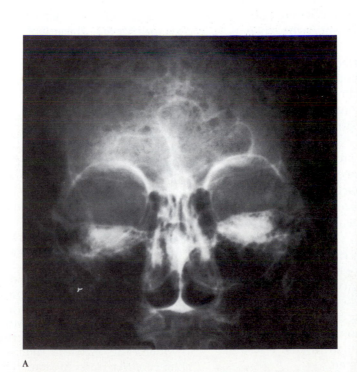

A

FIGURE 45-33 *Multiple myeloma of the* **A** *skull and* **B** *humerus. Note the numerous lytic defects and characteristic diffuse osteoporosis.*

B

HEMATOGENIC TUMORS

Multiple myeloma is the most common neoplasm of the bone. It is composed of plasma cells showing variable degrees of differentiation. The skeletal effects of this condition are discussed in this section (see also pp. 404–405).

Multiple myeloma affects women and men equally, rarely occurs before the age of 50, and has its peak frequency in the fifth and sixth decades. It has a predilection for the vertebral column, but ribs, skull, pelvis, and virtually any bone in the body may be affected. Multiple myeloma appears radiographically as multifocal destructive bone lesions throughout the skeletal system, producing what appear to be rounded, punched-out areas (Fig. 45-33).[8] These areas may measure up to 5 cm, with no surrounding zone of sclerosis. Pathologic fractures of the vertebrae are common.

The person has a history of pain that is often referred to the spinal column. Neurologic symptoms occur because of compression of vertebral bodies or nerve roots due to extension of the neoplasm. Weakness, weight loss, hemorrhagic disorders, and renal involvement are also associated with multiple myeloma. Hypercalcemia, hyperuricemia, and presence of Bence Jones proteins in the urine are frequently noted.[25]

▼ Chapter Summary

▼ Besides being the framework of the human body, the skeletal system is a metabolically active organ that provides for the constant movement of calcium, phosphorus, and other minerals into and out of the bloodstream.

▼ Constant remodeling occurs in bone, causing it to form and reabsorb until the age of about 40, when loss is greater than gain. Many factors influence the growth process. There are many types of bones and joints that provide for the ability to move or protect the internal structures of the body.

▼ Fractures of the bone are usually produced by trauma, and healing requires a sequential process during which a callus is formed to stabilize the fracture. Remodeling occurs with the assistance of the osteoclasts. Many factors can interfere with bone healing, especially loss of apposition and infection.

▼ Connective tissue and bone may exhibit disorders of development, metabolic and nutritional deficits, and defects of unknown origin. Especially common is Paget's disease of bone and osteoporosis. Alterations in skeletal structure may lead to respiratory or cardiac restriction.

▼ Osteomyelitis is the most common infectious disease of bone and usually follows a traumatic injury. It also may result from hematogenous spread.

▼ Arthritis and gout are common maladies that affect the joints and cause pain and disability. Rheumatoid arthritis is thought to be an autoimmune inflammatory condition, whereas gout is caused by hyperuricemia. Osteoarthritis is a disease of aging and may be due to normal wear and tear on the joints of the body.

▼ Malignant tumors of the bones are classified as sarcomas and may be bone forming or cartilaginous in origin. These tumors are found more frequently in young persons and are rapidly growing with a poor prognosis if they are not treated properly. Tumors of blood cell origin arise in the bone marrow. Multiple myeloma is a tumor of B cell origin that causes lytic lesions of the bone.

▼ References

1. An, H.S. *Synopsis of Orthopaedics*. New York: Thieme Medical, 1992.
2. Bates, B. *A Guide to Physical Examination* (5th ed.). Philadelphia: J.B. Lippincott, 1991.
3. Bennett, J.C. Clinical features of rheumatoid arthritis. In H.R. Schumacher (ed.), *Primer on the Rheumatic Diseases* (9th ed.). Atlanta: Arthritis Foundation, 1988.
4. Brandt, K.D. Primary disorders of articular cartilage. In W.N. Kelley (ed.), *Textbook of Internal Medicine* (2nd ed.). Philadelphia: J.B. Lippincott, 1992.
5. Brehm, B.A. *Essays on Wellness*. New York: Harper Collins Publishers, 1993.
6. Calin, A. Ankylosing spondylitis and the spondylarthropathies. In H.R. Schumacher (ed.), *Primer on the Rheumatic Diseases* (9th ed.). Atlanta: Arthritis Foundation, 1988.
7. Cormack, D.H. *Essential Histology*. Philadelphia: J.B. Lippincott, 1993.
8. Cotran, R.S., Kumar, V., and Robbins, S.L. *Pathologic Basis of Disease* (5th ed.). Philadelphia: W.B. Saunders, 1994.
9. Drezner, M.K., McGuire, J.L., and Marks, S.C. Metabolic bone disease. In W.N. Kelley (ed.), *Textbook of Internal Medicine* (2nd ed.). Philadelphia: J.B. Lippincott, 1992.
10. Fox, I.H. Crystal-induced synovitis. In W.N. Kelley (ed.), *Textbook of Internal Medicine* (2nd ed.). Philadelphia: J.B. Lippincott. 1992.
11. Ganong, W. *Review of Medical Physiology* (16th ed.). Norwalk, Conn.: Appleton and Lange, 1994.
12. Govan, A.D.T., Macfarlane, P.S., and Callander, R. *Pathology Illustrated* (3rd ed.). New York: Churchill Livingstone. 1991.
13. Guyton, A.C. *Textbook of Medical Physiology* (8th ed.). Philadelphia: W.B. Saunders, 1991.
14. Hahn, B.H. Metabolic bone disease. In H.R. Schumacher (ed.), *Primer on the Rheumatic Diseases* (9th ed.). Atlanta: Arthritis Foundation, 1988.
15. Holick, M.F., Krane, S.M., and Potts, J.T. Calcium, phosphorus and bone metabolism: Calcium-regulating hormones. In J. Wilson et al., *Harrison's Principles of Internal Medicine* (12th ed.). New York: McGraw-Hill, 1991.
16. Krane, S.M., and Holick, M.F. Metabolic bone disease. In J. Wilson et al., *Harrison's Principles of Internal Medicine* (12th ed.). New York: McGraw-Hill, 1991.
17. Lindsay, J, Debakey, M.E., and Beall, A.C. Diagnosis and treatment of diseases of the aorta. In R.C. Schlant, and

R.W. Alexander. *Hurst's The Heart* (8th ed.). New York: McGraw-Hill, 1994.

18. Mader, J.T. Osteomyelitis. In J.Stein (ed.). *Internal Medicine* (4th ed.). St. Louis: C.V. Mosby, 1994.

19. Malawer, M.M., Link, M.P. and Donaldson, S.S. Sarcomas of bone. In V.T. DeVita, S. Hellman, and S.A. Rosenberg. *Cancer: Principles and Practice of Oncology* (4th ed.). Philadelphia: J.B. Lippincott, 1993.

20. Marx, S.J., and Bourdeau, J.E. Calcium metabolism. In R.G. Narins (ed.). *Maxwell and Kleeman's Clinical Disorders of Fluid and Electrolyte Metabolism* (5th ed.). New York: McGraw-Hill, 1994.

21. Metheny, R.M. *Fluid and Electrolyte Balance* (2nd ed.). Philadelphia: J.B. Lippincott, 1992.

22. Moskowitz, R.W., and Goldberg, V.M. Osteoarthritis. In H.R. Schumacher (ed.), *Primer on the Rheumatic Diseases* (9th ed.). Atlanta: Arthritis Foundation, 1988.

23. Narins, R.G., et al. The metabolic acidoses. In Narins, R.C. (ed.), *Clinical Disorders of Fluid and Electrolyte Metabolism* (5th ed.). New York: McGraw-Hill, 1994.

24. Pyeritz, R.E. Heritable disorders of connective tissue. In H.R. Schumacher (ed.), *Primer on the Rheumatic Diseases* (9th ed.). Atlanta: Arthritis Foundation, 1988.

25. Rubin, E., and Farber, J.L. *Pathology* (2nd ed.). Philadelphia: J.B. Lippincott, 1994.

26. Tate, G., and Schumacher, H.R. Clinical features of gout. In H.R. Schumacher (ed.), *Primer on the Rheumatic Diseases* (9th ed.). Atlanta: Arthritis Foundation, 1988.

27. Zizic, T.M. Osteonecrosis. In H.R. Schumacher (ed.), *Primer on the Rheumatic Diseases* (9th ed.). Atlanta: Arthritis Foundation, 1988.

28. Zvaifler, N.J. Rheumatoid arthritis. In J. Stein (ed.), *Internal Medicine* (4th ed.). St. Louis: Mosby, 1994.

▼ *Unit Bibliography*

An, H.S. *Synopsis of Orthopaedics*. New York: Thieme Medical, 1992.

Apley, A.G. *Apley's system of Orthopaedics and Fractures* (7th ed.). Boston: Butterworth-Heineman, 1993.

Barrett, D. *Essential Basic Sciences for Orthopaedics*. Boston: Butterworth-Heineman, 1994.

Beltran, J. *MRI: Musculoskeletal system*. Philadelphia: J.B. Lippincott, 1990.

Cotran, R., Kumar, V., and Robbins, S.L. *Robbins' Pathologic Basis of Disease* (5th ed.). Philadelphia: W.B. Saunders, 1994.

Cyriax, J.H. *Cyriax's Illustrated Manual of Orthopaedic Medicine* (2nd ed.). Boston: Butterworth-Heineman, 1993.

Dandy, D. *Essential Orthopaedics and Trauma* (2nd ed.). Edinburgh: Churchill Livingstone, 1993.

DeVita, V.T., Hellman, S., and Rosenberg, S.A. *Cancer: Principles and Practice of Oncology* (4th ed.). Philadelphia: J.B. Lippincott, 1993.

Emery, A.E.H. *Duchenne Muscular Dystrophy* (2nd ed.). Oxford: Oxford University Press, 1993.

Gardner, D.L. *Pathological Basis of Connective Tissue Diseases*. Philadelphia: Lea and Febiger, 1992.

Goldie, B.S. *Orthopaedic Diagnosis and Management: A Guide to the Care of Orthopaedic Patients*. Boston: Blackwell Scientific, 1992

Govan, A.D.T., Macfarland, P.S., and Callander, R. *Pathology Illustrated* (3rd ed.). New York: Churchill Livingstone, 1991.

Gould, J.A., and Davies, C.J. *Orthopaedic and Sports Physical Therapy*. St. Louis: C.V. Mosby, 1985.

Gustilo, R.B., Kyle, R.F., and Templeman, D.C. *Fractures and Dislocations*. St. Louis: C.V. Mosby, 1993.

Guyton, A. *Textbook of Medical Physiology* (8th ed.). Philadelphia: W.B. Saunders, 1991.

Hertling, D. *Management of Common Musculoskeletal Disorders* (2nd ed.). Philadelphia: J.B. Lippincott, 1990.

Hoppenfeld, S. and Zeide, M.S. *Orthopaedic Dictionary*. Philadelphia: J.B. Lippincott, 1994.

Howell, E., Widra, L., and Hill, M.G. *Comprehensive Trauma Nursing*. Glenview, Ill.: Scott Foresman, 1988.

Kelley, W.N. *Textbook of Internal Medicine* (2nd ed.). Philadelphia: J.B. Lippincott, 1992.

Kelley, W.N. *Textbook of Rheumatology*. Philadelphia: W.B. Saunders, 1985.

Lewis, C.B., and Knortz, K.A. *Orthopedic Assessment and Treatment of the Geriatric Patient*. St. Louis: C.V. Mosby. 1993.

Magee, D.J. *Orthopedic Physical Assessment*. (2nd ed.). Philadelphia: W.B. Saunders, 1992.

Mourad, L.A. *The Nursing Process in the Care of Adults with Orthopaedic Conditions* (3rd ed.). Albany, NY: Delmar Publications, 1993.

Mourad, L.A. *Orthopedic Disorders*. St. Louis: C.V. Mosby, 1991.

Narins, N.G. (ed.). *Maxwell and Kleeman's Clinical Disorders of Fluid and Electrolyte Metabolism* (5th ed.). New York: McGraw-Hill, 1994.

Newman, R.J. *Orthogeriatrics: Comprehensive Orthopaedic Care for the Elderly Patient*. Boston: Butterworth-Heineman, 1992.

Paton, D.F. *Fractures and Orthopaedics* (2nd ed.). New York: Churchill Livingstone, 1992.

Pollock, M.I., Wilmore, J.H., and Fox, S.M. *Exercise in Health and Disease*. Philadelphia: W.B. Saunders, 1984.

Richardson, J.K., and Iglarsh, Z.A. *Clinical Orthopaedic Physical Therapy*. Philadelphia: W.B. Saunders, 1994.

Rubin, E., and Farber, J.L. *Pathology* (2nd ed.). Philadelphia: J.B. Lippincott, 1994.

Schumacher, H.R. *Primer on the Rheumatic Diseases* (9th ed.). Atlanta: Arthritis Foundation, 1988.

Tortora, G., and Grabowski, S. *Principles of Anatomy and Physiology* (7th ed.). New York: Harper Collins, 1993.

Turek, S.L. *Orthopaedics, Principles, and Their Application* (5th ed.). Philadelphia: J.B. Lippincott, 1994.

Wilson, J.D., et al (eds.). *Harrison's Principles of Internal Medicine* (12th ed.). New York: McGraw-Hill, 1991.

Woessner, J.F., and Howell, D.S. *Joint Cartilage Degradation: Basis and Clinical Aspects*. New York: M. Dekker, 1993.

Protective Coverings of the Body

THE SKIN is the largest and one of the most metabolically active organs of the body, but its function is often underestimated. The skin is part of the integumentary system, which also includes hair, nails, glands, and nerve endings. The integumentary system is a dynamic system that regulates body temperature and fluid balance and prevents microbial invasion. Through these functions, this system serves as a protective covering of the body.

Chapter 46 discusses the protective and complex metabolic activities of skin. Chapter 47 describes common inflammatory processes, tumors, and traumatic alterations in skin integrity.

The reader is encouraged to use the learning objectives as guides to facilitate the study of this important system. The bibliography at the end of the unit provides sources for further study of these topics.

Normal Structure and Function of the Skin

Barbara L. Bullock

▼ CHAPTER OUTLINE

▼ LEARNING OBJECTIVES

1 Describe the characteristics of the layers of the epidermis.
2 Describe the life cycle of the epidermal cell.
3 Discuss the chemical properties of the epidermis.
4 Outline the process for the production of melanin.
5 Discuss the function of the dermis.
6 Relate the structure and function of the subcutaneous tissues to the outer layers of the skin.
7 Describe the process of sweat production and its function in regulating heat.
8 Compare the structure and function of sweat and sebaceous glands.
9 Discuss the growth and development of hair.
10 Describe the purposes for blood supply to the skin.
11 Explain the role of the different nerve receptors in the sensory function of skin.
12 Explain the role of the skin in vitamin D production.

Barbara L. Bullock: PATHOPHYSIOLOGY: ADAPTATIONS AND ALTERATIONS IN FUNCTION, 4th ed.
© 1996 Lippincott-Raven Publishers

The skin is the largest organ of the body, with a surface area of 1.8 m² and comprising 4.5 to 5 kg (10 to 11 lb) of weight in the average adult.[5,12] This surface area increases seven times from birth to maturity. The skin's consistency ranges from the thick (4.0 cm), tough, yet pliable covering of the body to the thin (0.5 cm), delicate, mucous membranes of the mouth, nose, and eyelids. The skin is both pliable and durable, and allows for mobility and protection. At the same time it is one of the most sensitive organs of the body, capable of transmitting a variety of sensations, such as fine touch, pain, temperature, and pressure.[12] The skin functions as a barrier against pathogenic organisms and a protectant against trauma from environmental forces. It is waterproof but can regulate body temperature through sweating. It protects the body from excessive ultraviolet light through production of the pigment melanin. The skin also gives an indication of the general health of a person through color, texture, and alterations in continuity.[4]

▼ Anatomy and Physiology

The skin is composed of three major layers; from the surface inward, these layers are the epidermis, dermis, and subcutaneous tissues (Fig. 46-1). These layers have the following functions: 1) to protect against the external environment; 2) to maintain and regenerate layers; 3) to participate in defending the body against foreign substances; 4) to preserve the internal fluid environment; 5) to participate in excreting wastes; 6) to assist in regulating body temperature; 7) to produce vitamin D; and 8) to affect psychosocial aspects of daily living. The functions of the three layers of the skin are summarized in Table 46-1. Minor factors affecting the skin cause such

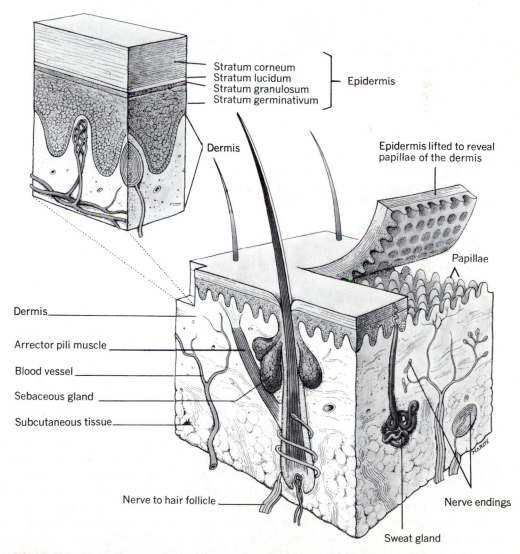

FIGURE 46-1 *Three-dimensional view of the skin. (Source: Chaffee, E. E. and Lytle, I. M. Basic Anatomy and Physiology [4th ed.]. Philadelphia: J.B. Lippincott.)*

TABLE 46-1   *Functions of the Skin*

Function	Epidermis	Dermis	Subcutaneous Tissue
Protection	Keratin provides protection from injury by corrosive materials. Inhibits proliferation of microorganisms because of dry external surface. Mechanical strength through intracellular bonds.	Provides fibroblasts for wound healing. Provides mechanical strength through collagen fibers, elastic fibers, ground substance. Lymphatic and vascular tissues respond to inflammation, injury, and infection.	Absorbs mechanical shock.
Water balance	Low permeability to water and electrolytes prevents systemic dehydration and electrolyte loss		
Temperature regulation	Eccrine sweat glands allow dissipation of heat through evaporation of sweat secreted onto skin surface.	Cutaneous vasculature, through dilation or constriction, promotes or inhibits heat conduction from skin surface.	
Sensory organ	Transmits a variety of sensations through neuroreceptor system.	Encloses extensive network of free and encapsulated nerve endings for relaying sensations to the brain.	Contains large pressure receptors.
Vitamin synthesis	7-Dehydrocholesterol present in large concentrations; photoconversion to vitamin D takes place.		
Psychosocial	Body image alterations result with many epidermal diseases, such as generalized psoriasis.	Body image alterations occur with many dermal diseases, such as scleroderma.	

(Rosen, T. Lanning, M. and Hill, M. *Nurse's Atlas of Dermatology.* Boston: Little, Brown, 1983.)

conditions as wrinkles, hair loss, and rashes. The skin can also reflect major diseases through its color or through malignant neoplasms, for example.[10]

EPIDERMIS

The epidermis consists of stratified squamous epithelium that maintains its constant thickness through coordination of desquamation (loss or shedding) and growth.[5] The shedding property allows for cleansing of the surface while maintaining an intact layer for a protection and permeability barrier.

Layers of the Epidermis

The main layers, or *strata*, of the epidermis, from the dermis to the surface, are the stratum germinativum, stratum spinosum, stratum granulosum, stratum lucidum (present only on the palms and soles), and stratum corneum. These layers are more simply termed the basal, spinous, granular, and keratin layers (Fig. 46-2).

The basal layer is one cell thick and lies in contact with the dermis. Within the basal layer are basal cells, which are cuboidal or columnar, have oval nuclei, and are united to each other by desmosomes, or bridges. These cells are attached to a basement membrane by

tonofibrils, or half-desmosomes. The epidermis is also attached to the dermis by interlocking, irregularly shaped processes of basal cells with corresponding dermal processes that extend different depths into the dermis (dermoepidermal junction). Processes are present in varying numbers throughout the skin. For example, eyelids have few processes, whereas nipples have a complex system of ridges, and fingertips have parallel ridges that form cavernous valleys and tunnels.[3] The highly individualized patterns of fingerprints are the result of these valleys. In the normal epidermis, mitosis of new basal cells is limited to the basal layer. During regeneration, mitosis continues upward into the squamous layer.

Throughout the basal layer are dispersed melanocytes, which form melanin and are responsible for pigmentation of the skin. These cells are wedged between the basal cells. When stained, melanocytes have clear cytoplasm and small, dark nuclei.[2]

The spinous layer contains cells with a polygonal shape. Bridges hold the cells together. As these cells move toward the surface they begin to flatten. Within the cells, fibril or keratin precursors make a three-dimensional framework throughout the cytoplasm.[5]

The granular layer is from two to four cells thick and lies directly above the stratum spinosum. The cells become diamond-shaped and are filled with kerato-

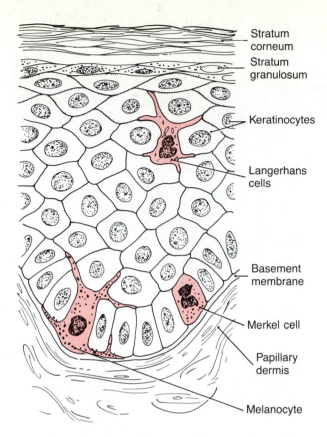

Stratum corneum

Stratum granulosum

Keratinocytes

Langerhans cells

Basement membrane

Merkel cell

Papillary dermis

Melanocyte

FIGURE 46-2 *Normal epidermis is multilayered which prevents fluid loss and protects from environmental insult. Melanocytes provide for skin color and protect against radiation. Langerhans cells provide some immunologic protection. Merkel cells provide sensory function.*

hyalin (hematoxylin) granules.[4] The stratum lucidum is not present in all skin sections but is found in the thick epidermis, such as in the palms of the hands and soles of the feet. The cells in this layer are dead and are little more than cell membranes containing prekeratin filaments and protein.[4] This layer provides for toughness and friction.

The keratin layer varies in thickness from 0.02 mm on the forearm to 0.5 mm or more on the soles of the feet (see Figure 46-2). The cells of this layer are flat and without nuclei. Keratin is a tough, fibrous protein that resists chemical change. This layer shields the body from environmental damage and maintains the internal milieu. The skin has the lowest water permeability of any biologic membrane. This low permeability retards water loss and prevents most toxic agents from entering the body, although some substances are readily absorbed. The horny keratin cells are shed continuously, making way for new cells.

Life Cycle of Epidermal Cells

The life cycle of epidermal cells involves three phases: *mitosis, keratinization,* and *exfoliation.* The major epider-

mal cells are keratinocytes. Epidermal cells are continuously formed in the basal or germinative layer at a rate commensurate with the constant loss. New cells move from the basal layer to the stratum corneum in a random fashion that is influenced by the rate of keratinization and by the time that each cell left the basal layer. Transit time from basal layer to surface is anywhere from 12 to 25 days.[12]

Mitosis is affected by two major factors: the diurnal cycle and hormones. Mitosis seems to occur at a greater rate during periods when the body is at rest or asleep. Hormonal influences include androgens, which cause the growth of hair in the typical masculine locations: over the pubis, on the face, on the chest, and on other locations of the body. Androgens aid in the formation of hair follicles and sebaceous glands. Estrogen hormones aid in the formation of the vaginal epithelium and provide for skin softness. Mitosis may be inhibited by adrenaline, levels of which are increased during times of wakefulness.

The second phase in the epidermal cell life cycle is keratinization. As the epidermal cell from the basal layer moves toward the surface, it loses its ability to undergo mitosis. Instead, it begins to synthesize fibrillar and amorphous proteins, keratin, and membrane-coating granules. The cell finally loses its nucleus and cellular organelles, becomes part of the keratin layer, and is shed. The fibrillar proteins make up the fibrils in the epidermal cell and give the layer strength and chemical inertness. As the cell moves toward the surface, more and more fibrils form, until they make up 50% of the protein in these cells. Amorphous proteins that make up the other 50% are embedded in a matrix and have no definite structure. As the epidermal cell moves closer to the surface, keratohyalin granules form. These granules are present in cells immediately below the horny layer. When a cell reaches the horny layer, its membrane thickens. The nucleus and organelles disintegrate and are eliminated from the cell.

At the end of keratinization, cornified cells are cemented together in varying thicknesses. Those at the surface are shed, resulting in exfoliation, which is the last phase in the life of an epidermal cell.

Keratinocytes provide an environment for other cell types, including nonkeratinocytes such as melanocytes, Langerhans cells, Merkel cells, and, possibly, lymphocytes.[6]

Nonkeratinocytes

Langerhans cells are dendritic nonkeratinocytes that function as a part of the immune system. These cells promote the delayed hypersensitivity reactions seen in the skin.[9, 11] They are present in the basal and suprabasal layers of the epidermis and occasionally in the dermis.[6] *Merkel cells* are present in the deep layers of the epidermis of the hands and feet. They are thought to be mechan-oreceptors.[4] *Lymphocytes,* especially T lymphocytes, have been reported to be part of normal epidermis. Other cells of the immune defense system are present in the dermis and subcutaneous tissues.

Skin Pigmentation

Skin color is determined by *melanocytes,* which originate in the basal layer of the epidermis and in hair follicles. The main function of melanocytes is to synthesize pigment granules, or melanosomes. The main component of melanosomes is melanin, which provides the pigment for skin color. The melanocytes appear in the basal layer of the epidermis as clear cells before they begin to produce melanin.[11]

Melanocytes produce and disperse melanin to keratinocytes (keratinizing basal cells) and hair cells.[1] Melanin is a biochrome of high molecular weight and is produced by oxidation of the amino acid tyrosine with tyrosinase. It forms with a protein matrix in the melanosome to make a melanoprotein. As more melanoprotein is formed, the melanosome grows to become a melanin granule and eventually loses the activity of the enzyme tyrosinase. Formed melanin is transferred to keratinocytes by active phagocytosis of the distal end of the dendritic processes of the melanocyte.[3] The amount of melanin in these melanocyte dendrites determines skin color. In light-skinned persons, melanin is present primarily in the basal layer of the epidermis. In dark- or black-skinned persons, it is present throughout the epidermis, including the outermost horny layer. Melanogenesis increases after exposure to ultraviolet light or x-rays. After exposure, the melanocytes in the basal layer increase activity, become larger, develop longer dendrites, and produce more melanin. They may multiply after exposure to ultraviolet light.[2] Melanin acts as a protective screen to protect the deep layers of the epidermis and the dermis from too much solar ultraviolet radiation.[2]

Skin pigmentation is controlled by genes and hormones. Genes regulate the number and shape of melanocytes in the epidermis and hair follicles. Hormonal influences have been demonstrated through the study of hyperpigmentation, as noted in hyperpituitarism and Addison's disease. Estrogen, progesterone, and melanocyte-stimulating hormone contribute to increased pigmentation in various areas of the body during pregnancy. Apparently, melanocyte-stimulating hormone does not play a major role in pigmentation in humans.[6] Excess amounts of melanocyte-stimulating hormone, however, produce a bronze discoloration of the skin. The exact hormonal mechanism for increasing pigmentation is not known.[8] Figure 46-3 summarizes the process of melanin pigmentation of the skin after exposure to ultraviolet light.

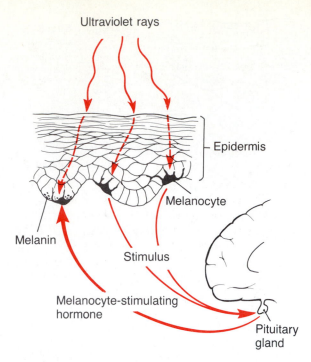

FIGURE 46-3 *Melanin pigmentation of the skin occurs when melanocytes are stimulated by ultraviolet light, causing release of melanostimulating hormone by the pituitary gland which stimulates the cells to produce and disperse melanin in basal layers of the epidermis.*

Chemical Properties of the Epidermis

The epidermis contains carbohydrates and various enzymes that influence skin cell activity. In normal skin, small amounts of glycogen are present, scattered in various areas of the body, such as the scrotum and scalp, and in cells surrounding pilosebaceous and sweat gland openings. After the skin has been traumatized, the amount of glycogen in the epidermis increases.

The epidermis also contains glucose, which diffuses easily into the cells, the amount depending on the serum glucose levels. Eighty percent to 90% of the energy in epidermal cells is derived from adenosine triphosphate, which is generated through respiration and glycolysis. Intense glycolytic activity in the presence of oxygen is a specific feature of the epidermis that is especially important during wound healing and skin regeneration. Enzymes in the epidermis that influence all activity include alkaline phosphatase, acid phosphatase, and esterases. Alkaline phosphatase is not present in normal epidermal cells but is present in a damaged epidermis and disappears after healing. Acid phosphatase is a component of the normal epidermis.[6]

DERMIS

The dermis, or *corium,* lies between the epidermis and subcutaneous tissues (see Figure 46-1). It consists of a matrix of loose connective tissue, a fibrous protein embedded in an amorphous ground substance. The dermis is traversed by blood vessels, nerves, and lymphatics and is penetrated by epidermal appendages. The mass of the dermis accounts for 15% to 20% of total body weight.[6]

Layers of the Dermis

The two main layers of the dermis are 1) the finely textured papillary dermis and 2) the deeper, thicker, coarsely textured reticular layer. The papillary layer lies directly beneath the epidermis. It is composed of thin fibers of collagen, reticular fibers, branching elastic fibers, fibroblasts, abundant ground substance, and capillaries. When the epidermis is removed, the upper surface of the papillary layer forms a negative image of the underside of the epidermis.

The reticular layer lies beneath the papillary layer and extends to the subcutaneous tissue. This layer is composed mainly of thick collagen bundles enmeshed in a network of coarse elastic fibers. It is responsible for the strength and toughness of the skin. There are fewer reticular fibers, blood vessels, fibroblasts, and ground substance in this layer than in the papillary layer.[2, 9] Sensory nerve endings, hair follicles, sweat and sebaceous glands, and some smooth muscle are present in the reticular layer. The combined layers of the dermis vary in thickness. They are thinnest over the eyelids and thickest over the back.[6]

Components of the Dermis

The two layers of the dermis are composed of varying amounts of collagen, elastic and reticular fibers, and ground substance. Collagen fibers lie at the lower portion of the dermis and constitute most of this layer. The molecules form fibers that unite into bundles. These bundles are slightly extensible and wavy, allowing for a certain amount of stretching of the skin.

The elastic fibers are abundant in human skin, entwining with collagen in the reticular layer of the dermis and extending into the papillary dermis. These fibers help secure the epidermis to the dermis and anchor blood vessels. They can be deformed by a small force and then easily recover their original dimensions.[7] Reticular fibers are young, finely formed fibers of collagen. They are present within and under the epidermal basement membrane and also help to secure the epidermis to the dermis.

Ground substance is present in small amounts in normal skin. It is the structureless portion of connective tissue lying outside of cells, fibers, vessels, and nerves that holds all these components together. Ground substance consists of water, electrolytes, glucose, plasma proteins, neutral and acid mucopolysaccharides, and mucoproteins.[6]

Cellular Components of the Dermis

The three major cells that are present in the dermis are fibroblasts, macrophages, and mast cells. *Fibroblasts* are the most abundant of these cells; they secrete procollagen, proelastin, microfibrillar proteins, elastin, and components of ground substance.[1, 6] *Macrophages* probably develop from the blood monocytes and can be fixed or ameboid cells that help rid the dermis of foreign substances and cell residue. Macrophages participate in the immune response and are vital to wound healing, inflammation, tissue reabsorption, and recycling of tissue components (see Chapter 15). *Mast cells* are present in perivascular connective tissue, and their microscopic appearance shows the cytoplasm to be filled with large metachromatic granules. Under certain physical and chemical conditions, these cells degranulate. Such conditions include exposure to cold, heat, x-rays, ultraviolet light, toxins, certain peptides, and protamine sulfate. When degranulation occurs, the substances of heparin and histamine are released. Heparin prevents blood clotting and, in small amounts, accelerates lipid transportation. Histamine increases capillary permeability, contracts smooth muscle, increases chemotaxis, produces an itching sensation, and increases gastric secretion.[7]

Functions of the Dermis

The dermis provides the main protection of the body from external injury. Its flexibility allows joint movement and localized stretching, but resists tearing, shearing, and local pressure. When skin is at rest, the protective collagen network is slack. When exposed to tension, the skin "gives" until the slack is taken up. Skin kept taut for long periods of time becomes fatigued, and stretching results. This is exhibited by the stretch marks or *striae gravidarum* (a pinkish white or gray line seen where skin has been stretched by pregnancy, obesity, or tumor), which are irreversible. The skin also becomes thinner when compressed under force and wells up around the source of compression. Pressure damage may occur from long duration of pressure and distribution of force. Most damage is a result of long duration of pressure, but severe point pressure can injure underlying and cutaneous tissues.

The dermis also provides the necessary base on which the epidermis receives nutrients and grows. It serves as a barrier to infection by way of hyaluronic acid in the ground substance, which prevents bacterial penetration.[7] Hyaluronic acid also binds water and helps maintain dermal turgor. The skin may also store water and electrolytes. Dermal concentrations of cations are slightly higher than those in blood, so that cations stored in the dermis may be tapped to maintain normal levels in blood.

SUBCUTANEOUS TISSUES

The third major layer of skin is the subcutaneous tissue. It is loose-textured, white, and fibrous (see Figure 46-1). Fat and slender elastic fibers are intermingled. Subcutaneous papillae jut into the dermis. These papillae are larger and more dispersed than dermal papillae. It is through subcutaneous papillae that blood vessels and nerves enter the upper layers of skin.

The subcutaneous tissue layer contains blood and lymph vessels, roots of hair follicles, secretory portions of sweat glands, cutaneous and sensory nerve endings, and fat. Subcutaneous fat varies in amount throughout the body and is absent in the eyelids, penis, scrotum, nipples, and areolae. The unequal fat distribution between males and females is partially a result of hormonal influence. Strands or sheets of white, fibrous, connective tissue support the fat tissue.

The subcutaneous tissue contains voluntary and involuntary muscles. Voluntary muscle is present on the scalp, face, and neck. Involuntary smooth muscle is present in the dartos muscle of the scrotum and in the muscle tissue of the areolae and nipples. Subcutaneous tissue is a heat insulator, shock absorber, and calorie-reserve depot.

EPIDERMAL APPENDAGES

The sweat glands, sebaceous glands, and hair compose the epidermal appendages. These extend through layers of the skin (see Figure 46-1). The nails are the protective coverings of the ends of the fingers and toes and are specialized epithelial cells.

Sweat Glands

There are two types of sweat glands: eccrine and apocrine. The *eccrine* sweat glands are present all over the body and are most numerous in thick skin. They open to the surface epidermis and descend through the dermis to just above the subcutaneous layer of the skin. These glands are especially prominent on the soles of the feet, palms of the hand, and axillae.

Eccrine glands are simple, coiled, tubular glands that may be divided into four segments. The lowermost, or secretory, portion has two layers of cells. Of these, myoepithelial cells make up the outer layer and contract to facilitate sweat release. The inner layer is composed of clear large cells and dark small cells, which contain glycogen and polysaccharides, respectively.[6] The secretory layer is one cell thick. In ascending order, the remaining portion of the eccrine unit includes the coiled dermal duct and a straight dermal duct, which opens on the surface of the epidermis through the spiraled intraepidermal duct or pore (see Figure 46-1). The coiled and straight dermal ducts are two cells thick and are composed of cuboidal basophilic epithelium. The duct narrows as it ascends to the surface and widens again as it becomes the intraepidermal spiral duct. The cells lining the spiraling duct are keratinized but have no melanin.

Eccrine glands produce sweat to aid in regulating body temperature. Control of sweating is located in the hypothalamus, which responds to changes in body temperature.[8] Sweat is formed in the secretory coil of the eccrine unit. The solution here is isotonic or slightly hypertonic and contains lactate with small amounts of bicarbonate. In the dermal duct, sodium, chloride, and water are reabsorbed. As sweat exits onto the epidermis, it is hypotonic. As the rate of sweating increases, sodium and chloride concentrations in the sweat also increase, whereas potassium, lactate, and urea concentrations decrease. Not all eccrine glands function all of the time, but they respond promptly to heat stress. The amount of sweat produced depends on the amount of heat to which the person is exposed. Two to 3 liters of sweat per hour may be produced in an adult exposed to extreme heat conditions. Eccrine sweat is a colorless and odorless hypotonic solution that is 99% water and 1% solutes, such as sodium chloride, potassium, urea, protein, lipids, amino acids, calcium, phosphorus, and iron. The specific gravity is 1.005, and the pH ranges from 4.5 to 7.0.[7]

The skin plays passive and active roles in controlling body temperature. Passively, skin is a barrier to the external environment. Actively, the eccrine units, together with the cutaneous blood vessel network, participate in regulatory heat exchange. The sweat glands cool the surface of the skin with the liquid sweat, which evaporates, causing further cooling. The cutaneous vessels dilate or constrict to dissipate or conserve body heat. The control seat for this process is in the hypothalamus, the neural thermostat.

The hypothalamus is stimulated by changes in surface and blood temperatures. An increase in body temperature of 0.5°C. causes the hypothalamus to send a message by way of cholinergic fibers of the sympathetic nervous system to the sweat glands, which pour sweat onto the body surface, causing cooling when it evaporates.[8]

Heat is the primary stimulus to eccrine sweat production, but other physiologic stimuli can stimulate sweating. Gustatory sweating occurs on the face and scalp after eating spicy foods. Emotional stress causes sweating on palms, soles, axillae, and forehead that may extend to the whole body. Pain, nausea, or vomiting also may cause localized or generalized sweating.

Apocrine sweat glands are present in the axillae, around the nipples, in the anogenital region, in the external ear canals (ceruminous glands), in the eyelids (Moll's glands), and in the breasts (mammary glands). These glands make a secretion with an unknown function in humans. In animals, the secretion attracts animals of the opposite sex. The glands remain small until puberty, when they begin secreting.[4] Apocrine gland ducts empty into the pilosebaceous follicle above the entrance of sebaceous gland ducts (see Figure 46-1). The coiled secretory gland is located in the lower dermis or subcutaneous tissues. The straight duct empties into the hair follicle. The apocrine coil has a larger diameter than the eccrine coil. The inner secretory layer of the coil is one cell thick. Surrounding the secretory cells are myoepithelial cells, basement membrane, and elastic and reticular fibers. The straight ductal portion of the gland has two cell layers with no myoepithelium and merges with the epithelium of the hair follicle. Apocrine sweat has a milky color and contains protein and carbohydrates. In the duct, the sweat is sterile and odorless. Only after reaching the surface, where it contacts bacteria, does it assume an odor. The two steps involved in the production of sweat from the apocrine glands are secretion and excretion. Sweat is secreted continuously and fills the duct before being excreted. When the duct is full, peristaltic waves produced by the myoepithelium propel the secretion outward. Excretion may be stimulated by emotional stress or hormones, such as epinephrine.

Sebaceous Glands

Sebaceous glands arise as epithelial buds from the outer root sheath of the hair follicle. The glands are present throughout the body, except in the palms of the hands and soles and dorsa of the feet. Because these glands develop as buds from the root sheath, they are almost always associated with hair follicles, but are found in some hairless skin, such as that of the nipples, prepuce, labia, and glans penis.[4] The size of sebaceous glands is inversely proportional to the diameter of hair in the follicles. They are largest where hair is sparse or absent, such as on the forehead, nose, chest, and back.

Several lobules compose the glands. The lobules are surrounded by a thin, vascular, fibrous tissue capsule in the dermis. The cells next to the capsule provide the germinative layer and correspond to the germinative cells of the basal layer of epidermis (Fig. 46-4). The germ cells change, taking up and filling with lipid, become bloated and disintegrate, and discharge their contents of lipid and cell debris into the sebaceous duct as sebum. Other components of sebum include phospholipids, esterified cholesterol, triglycerides, and waxes. Sebum is then evacuated to the follicle and to the surface. Sebum produces oily skin; it lubricates the hair and skin and prevents drying. Sebaceous glands are holocrine glands, because they have no lumen and form secretions from decomposition of cells.[4]

Hair

Human beings are covered with hair in all areas except the palms, soles, dorsum of digits, lips, glans penis, labia,

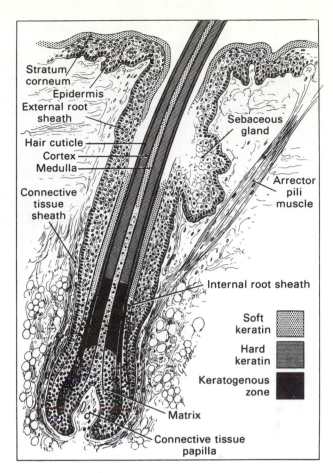

FIGURE 46-4 *Parts of a hair follicle and location of sebaceous gland. (Source: Cormack, D.H.* Essential Histology. *Philadelphia: J.B. Lippincott, 1993)*

and nipples. Hair is needed to screen the nasal passages and protect the scalp and eyes from sun and sweat.

There are several types of hair. Primary hair, or *lanugo*, is present on the human fetus and infant. These same fine hairs may be noted on the adult as *vellus* hairs. An example is the bald man who has fine vellus hair on his scalp. In the adult, coarse pigmented hair is most developed on the scalp, the beard and chest areas in men, and pubic and axillary areas.

Hair varies morphologically and biologically on different parts of the body. It also varies in structure, length, rate of growth, and response to stimuli. For example, sex hormones govern hair growth in the pubic and axillary regions as part of the secondary sex characteristics. Sex hormones do not govern other hair growth. Morphologically, hair is divided into three types: straight, wavy, and woolly, depending on the angle of the hair follicles. Straight hair is found in native Americans, Chinese, and the Mongol races and is coarse.[3] Wavy hair is found in many ethnic groups, whereas woolly hair is found typically in black races.[2, 6]

Hair originates in the hair follicle, and the two may

be considered one structure. The hair bulb lies at the lower end of the follicle and encloses an ovoid, vascular papilla of connective tissue. The matrix cells of the bulb surround the papilla as it juts upward into the bulb (see Figure 46-4). At an outlet at the distal end of the bulb, the papilla emerges and is continuous with the connective tissue sheath that surrounds the follicle. The hair bulb is covered with concentric layers of tissue and enclosed by a thin outer root sheath. A basement membrane of reticular fibers and neutral mucopolysaccharides lies against the external root sheath. A fibrous sheath lies next to the basement membrane and is composed of collagen and fibroblasts. Melanocytes are present in the bulb and in the outer root sheath. The color of hair depends on the amount and distribution of melanin within it. The pigments of the melanin are black, brown, and yellow. The brown and black melanins are called *eumelanin*, and the yellow is called *pheomelanin*. The amounts produced are genetically controlled. It is thought that hair becomes gray when the melanocytes of the bulbs of the hair follicles fail to make tyrosinase.[12]

The mitotic activity of the matrix cells is very great, with hair matrix being replaced every 12 to 24 hours. The hair and inner root sheath are joined, so that they grow at the same rate. When the hair and inner sheath reach the external root sheath, the inner sheath disintegrates and the outer sheath begins to cornify. As the hair reaches the surface opening of the follicle, it is called a *hair shaft* and is a dead cornified structure extending out from the follicle.

The growth of hair occurs in cycles: *anagen*, growing; *catagen*, involuting; and *telogen*, resting. Anagen begins when a papilla joins with cells that enclose it. The papilla juts into the hair bulb, and new matrix cells in the bulb begin to form a hair and push toward the surface. As it pushes to the surface, the old hair in the follicle is loosened, pushed out, and lost. In catagen, the inferior portion disappears, the outer root sheath cornifies around the bulbous end of the hair shaft, melanin synthesis ceases, and the bulb turns white. A cord of epithelial cells replaces the inferior portion and connects the papilla to the bulb. In telogen, the epithelial cord shrinks away from the papilla and disconnects; the epithelial cells of the cord are undifferentiated and wait to join a new papilla and begin anagen. Each hair follicle operates independently; therefore, each hair may be in a different phase of the cycle from its neighbor.[9] The life cycle of hair through the three stages varies in different parts of the body. Scalp hair, which is in anagen from 3 to 10 years, in catagen for 3 weeks, and in telogen for 3 months, has the longest growth period of any hair on the body. The longer the growing period, the longer the hair. Scalp hair grows about 0.4 to 0.5 mm daily and is influenced by factors such as nutrition, light, hormones, and temperature.[2] The phases of the hair cycle may be influenced by illness, which may place growing-phase hairs into resting-phase hairs that can be more easily lost or shed.[1]

Attached to the hair follicle is the arrectores pilorum, a smooth muscle attached to the connective tissue hair sheath and inserted in the dermal papilla. Contraction of this muscle erects hair, squeezes out sebum, and creates gooseflesh during the spasm.

Nails

The nails are composed of specialized layers of epithelial cells and are protective coverings at the ends of the fingers and toes (Fig. 46-5). The rectangular nail plates on the dorsal surfaces of the ends of fingers and toes are composed of closely welded cells of cornified epithelium. They are semitransparent and allow the pink of the vascular nail bed to show. Each nail plate is surrounded by a fold of skin called the *nail bed*. The nail plate rests on top of the nail bed, where fibers attach the nail to the periosteum of the distal phalanx of each digit. The nail bed is abundant with blood vessels and sensory nerve endings. The distal edge of the nail is freely movable. The proximal edge is attached firmly at the base of the nail. The *lunula* is a white, half-moon-shaped area at the base of the nail and is the most actively growing portion of the nail. The epithelium in this area of the nail is thick, and the cells here become keratinized with harder keratin than that present in the hair or the epidermis. From the lunula the nail grows longitudinally over dermal ridges of the nail bed at a rate of about 0.5 mm per week.[4] The soft cuticle that forms over the proximal nail plate is called the *eponychium*.

BLOOD SUPPLY

Blood supply to the skin varies in different parts of the body, depending on such factors as the type of skin perfused, thickness of the skin's layers, and types and numbers of skin appendages. Common to skin throughout the body are a deep subdermal arterial plexus and a superficial subpapillary plexus. Endothelial cells line all parts of the vasculature. In the small capillaries, one endothelial cell surrounds the lumen. Collagen or reticular fibers ensheath the capillaries. Arterioles have an intima, a smooth muscle layer, and an adventitia of

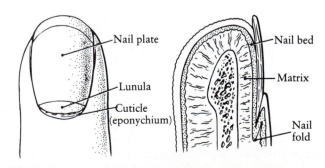

FIGURE 46-5 *Structure of the nail in cross-section of a finger.*

collagen and elastic fibers. Venules consist of epithelium and collagen. In larger veins, smooth muscle and elastic fibers are present. The number of blood vessels is greater than necessary to meet the biologic needs of the skin tissues. The vessels have two functions: 1) to provide oxygen and nutrients to skin cells, together with removing wastes; and 2) to aid in thermal regulation.

The vessels are arranged in a three-dimensional network consisting of the two plexuses (deep and superficial) and the vessels that connect them (Fig. 46-6). The deep plexus is joined to larger vessels in the subcutaneous layer and lies in the lower portion of the dermis. The superficial plexus lies beneath the papillary dermis. A network of capillaries reaches up into the dermal papilla to nourish the upper layers of skin.

A second route of blood flow is through arteriovenous shunts located in the upper part of the reticular dermis. These shunts are important in regulating heat. They are present throughout the skin but are particularly prevalent in the pads and nail beds of fingers and toes, soles and palms, ears, and center of the face. The shunts enable blood to bypass the capillaries and increase blood flow. The plexuses and arteriovenous shunts are controlled by the sympathetic nervous system and constrict and dilate in response to various chemical agents, such as epinephrine and histamine. Under normal thermal conditions, the blood flow to the skin is about 250 mL/minute/m^2 of body surface. This can decrease to 50 mL/minute in severe cold or increase to 2 to 3 L/minute in extreme heat.[8] Vasodilation causes the skin to become hot and red, whereas vasoconstriction causes it to become cold, often with a pale or bluish hue.[8]

NERVOUS CONTROL

The skin is a major sensory organ. Dermal nerve endings receive stimuli from touch, pressure, temperature, pain, and itch. Nerve endings are most numerous on palms, soles, fingers, and mucocutaneous areas of the lips, glans penis, and clitoris.

Temperature, pain, pressure, and itch are perceived by nerves ending in the dermal papilla and surrounding hair follicles (Fig. 46-7). Free nerve endings in the epidermis are both myelinated and unmyelinated and respond to temperature, pain, and pressure.[2] *Merkel endings* are present in the deep layers of the epidermis. The cells have fingerlike cytoplasmic projections between the keratinocytes, and they attach to myelinated afferent fibers. They are thought to function as mechanoreceptors.[2] *Meissner's corpuscles* receive touch stimuli. They lie in the papillary derma on the palms and soles and consist of myelinated and unmyelinated nerve fibers. *Pacinian corpuscles* sense pressure and are located on the soles, palms, nipples, and genital and perianal regions. These encapsulated end organs of myelinated and unmyelinated fibers swiftly send messages to the central nervous system. Mucocutaneous end organs (*Krause's end bulbs*) are present in regions such as the lips, tongue, gums, eyelids, genitalia, and perianal area. These organs probably perceive general sensory stimuli and are present in the subpapillary dermis.

The mucocutaneous end organs, Meissner and Pacinian corpuscles, are specialized sensory nerve end organs in areas of modified hairless skin. The remainder of skin over the body is supplied with sensory and auto-

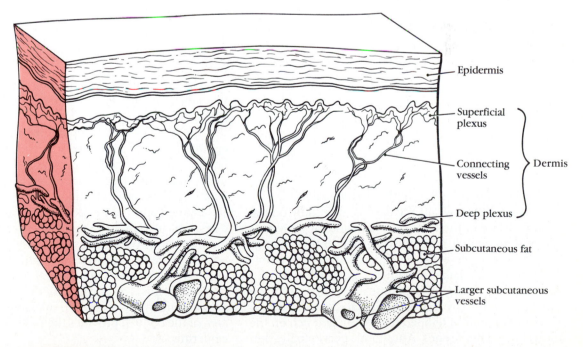

FIGURE 46-6 *Blood vessels of the subcutaneous tissue.*

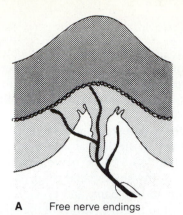

A   Free nerve endings

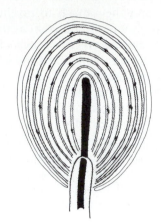

B   Pacinian corpuscle

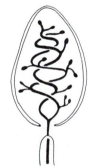

C   Meissner's corpuscle

FIGURE 46-7 *Cutaneous sensory receptors. (Source: Cormack, D.H.* Essential Histology. *Philadelphia: J.B. Lippincott, 1993).*

nomic nerve fibers located in the dermis. *Ruffini corpuscles* are found throughout the dermis, especially on the plantar surface of the feet. They are thought to be mechanoreceptors that respond to tension in the collagen fibers.[2] Sensory nerves are myelinated up to their terminal branches, are large in diameter, and extend toward the epidermis or hair follicle. These nerves arise from the spinal cord, return by way of the dorsal root ganglia, and receive sensations of temperature, pain, and itch on the unmyelinated nerve ends. Autonomic nerves to the skin

are motor nerves, and they do not always have a myelin sheath. Branches of nerves from the sympathetic nervous system innervate blood vessels, arrectores pilorum muscles, and eccrine and apocrine glands.

VITAMIN D SYNTHESIS IN THE SKIN

Vitamin D is an essential fat-soluble vitamin that, when activated, aids in the absorption of calcium and phosphate in the intestine. The activated form of vitamin D (1,25-dihydroxycholecalciferol) is commonly referred to as vitamin D hormone. It improves mineralization of bone by increasing plasma calcium and phosphate concentrations to support forming bone.[8]

Vitamin D hormone is not a single compound but is a family of compounds, the two most important of which are vitamin D_2 and D_3. Vitamin D_3, or *cholecalciferol*, is produced in the skin when it is exposed to ultraviolet irradiation. The skin cells contain 7-dehydrocholesterol in the epidermis. Ultraviolet light penetrates the epidermis and causes 7-dehydrocholesterol to undergo photolysis to form previtamin D, which within a few hours isomerizes to form vitamin D_3. Vitamin D_3 is then transported in the blood bound to serum protein. It is converted in two steps, first by the liver and then the kidneys, to vitamin D hormone and may then be stored in the liver and in body fat.[8] Vitamin D_2, or ergocalciferol, is the therapeutic form of vitamin D and, like vitamin D_3, is transported to the liver and kidneys, where it is converted to vitamin D hormone.[6]

▼ Chapter Summary

▼   The skin is the largest organ in the body and is active in protecting the body against environmental assault and in regulation of body temperature. It actively regenerates its multiple layers through a continuous replacement process.

▼   The layers of the skin are the epidermis, the dermis, the subcutaneous tissues, and the epidermal appendages.

▼   The epidermis is composed of stratified squamous epithelium of various layers in different areas of the body, thickest on the palms and soles and thinnest over the eyelids. The layers are maintained through mitosis, keratinization, and exfoliation.

▼   Pigmentation of the skin is determined by melanocytes, which originate in the basal layer of the epidermis, the number of which are genetically determined. They are stimulated to disperse melanin through the basal layers by ultraviolet radiation.

▼   The dermis is responsible for the strength and toughness of skin and also varies in thickness according to the area of the body. It provides the base for nutrition of the epidermis.

▼ The subcutaneous tissue is the main area for blood and lymph vessels, roots of hair follicles, and secretory portions of glands. This area provides for heat insulation, shock absorption, and calorie reserves.

▼ The epidermal appendages include the sweat glands, sebaceous glands, hair, and nails. The sweat glands are mainly for thermoregulatory control, whereas the sebaceous glands provide lubrication for the hair and skin. Hair allows for heat conservation and improves the appearance of the body. The nails are protective coverings at the ends of fingers and toes.

▼ The blood supply to the dermis is profuse and is critically important in regulating body temperature through vasodilatation and vasoconstriction. Nerves in the skin sense pressure and pain and help to regulate the blood vessel tone.

▼ Activated vitamin D is synthesized in the skin and is produced when it is exposed to the sun.

▼ *References*

1. Bauer, E., Tobas, M., and Goslen, J. Skin: Cells, matrix and function. In W. Kelley (ed.), *Textbook of Internal Medicine* (2nd ed.). Philadelphia: J.B. Lippincott, 1992.

2. Bickers, D.R. Photosensitivity and other reactions to light. In J. Wilson, et al. (eds.), *Harrison's Principles of Internal Medicine* (12th ed.). New York: McGraw-Hill, 1991.

3. Cormack, D.H. *Essential Histology*. Philadelphia: J.B. Lippincott, 1993.

4. Cormack, D. *Ham's Histology* (9th ed.). Philadelphia: J.B. Lippincott, 1987.

5. Farmer, E.R. *Pathology of the Skin*. Norwalk, Conn.: Appleton-Lange, 1990.

6. Fitzpatrick, T.B., et al. *Dermatology in General Medicine* (4th ed.). New York: McGraw-Hill, 1993.

7. Fitzpatrick, T.B., and Soter, N.A. Pathophysiology of skin. In N.A. Soter and H.R. Baden (eds.), *Pathophysiology of Dermatologic Diseases* (2nd ed.) New York: McGraw-Hill, 1991.

8. Guyton, A. *Textbook of Medical Physiology* (8th ed.). Philadelphia: W.B. Saunders, 1991

9. Harrist, T.J., and Clark, W.H. The Skin. In E. Rubin and J.L. Farber (eds.), *Pathology* (2nd ed.). Philadelphia: J.B. Lippincott, 1994.

10. Murphy, G.F., and Mihm, M.C. The Skin. In R.Cotran, V. Kumar, and S. Robbins (eds.), *Robbin's Pathologic Basis of Disease* (5th ed.). Philadelphia: W.B. Saunders, 1994.

11. Sauer, G.C. *Manual of Skin Diseases* (6th ed.). Philadelphia: J.B. Lippincott, 1991.

12. Tortora, G., and Grabowski, S. *Principles of Anatomy and Physiology* (7th ed.). New York: Harper Collins, 1993.

Chapter 47

Alterations in Skin Integrity

Barbara L. Bullock

▼ **LEARNING OBJECTIVES**

1 Identify the two types of skin sensitivity responses.
2 Explain the pathophysiologic process that results in acne.
3 Describe the three types of dermatitis/eczema disease.
4 Discuss the complications of atopic dermatitis.
5 State the cause and precipitating factors of herpes simplex.
6 Describe the features and course of varicella virus disease.
7 Discuss the mechanism of activation of herpes zoster, its target population, and persons at greatest risk of infection.
8 Discuss the cause and treatment of warts (verrucae).
9 Describe the features of rubeola and rubella.
10 Review the common characteristics of impetigo.
11 Compare two examples of scaling disorders of the skin and their treatments.
12 State and discuss briefly the types of benign skin tumors.
13 Differentiate the three major types of malignant skin tumors.
14 Compare and contrast the differences between partial- and full-thickness burns.
15 Describe the changes that occur in the skin as a result of thermal therapy.
16 Discuss the systemic changes that occur as a result of burn injury.
17 Explain the causes, types of injuries, and effects of electrical and chemical burns.
18 Discuss the crucial factors in the formation of decubitus ulcers.
19 Describe the grading of decubitus ulcers.
20 Discuss the skin changes resulting from abrasions, incisions, puncture wounds, and lacerations.

Barbara L. Bullock: PATHOPHYSIOLOGY: ADAPTATIONS AND ALTERATIONS IN FUNCTION, 4th ed.
© 1996 Lippincott-Raven Publishers

Skin diseases have characteristic features called primary lesions. These lesions can be obscured by secondary lesions that result from treatment, scratching, or infection.[22]

Important aspects for determining the pathophysiology of skin disease include the following: 1) characteristics of the lesion; 2) distribution of many lesions; 3) length of time present and recurrence; 4) medications taken, both systemic and topical; 5) family history of disease; and 6) environmental or personal exposure to hazardous material. Table 47-1 lists the basic nomenclature used to describe lesions. Figure 47-1 shows the appearance of various lesions. Description of a lesion may require a combination of these terms.

The usual response of the skin to injury is to generate the inflammatory response. Sources of injury to the skin include bacteria, viruses, temperature extremes, and chemical or mechanical irritants. Inflammation alters the surrounding blood vessels and adjacent tissues and causes redness or erythema. An irritant causes injury to the site, which results in a vascular reaction with fluid exudation and edema. Pressure from the edema or chemical irritation from the release of various mediator substances causes pain due to irritation of the nerve fibers in that area.

Angioedema is a reaction that involves edema not only of the superficial skin but of the subcutaneous tissues. Angioedema can be described as giant wheals, often involving the mucous membranes. It can cause many physical symptoms, including severe respiratory distress, especially when it affects the larynx.

Urticaria is a vascular reaction, commonly called *hives*, that is manifested by transient erythema or whitish swellings (wheals) of the skin or mucous membranes.[1] Skin changes or lesions result from increased vascular permeability and local release of histamine and vasoactive mediators.[28] These changes may result in localized edema, which may begin to resolve within several hours. The lesions are usually erythematous, well-circumscribed wheals. A reddened halo or flare often surrounds the raised part of the lesion.[28] Urticaric lesions often cause pruritus and a stinging sensation. *Acute urticaria* can be defined as a cutaneous vascular reaction that evolves over a short period, from days to several weeks, and usually has a detectable cause. It resolves completely. Urticaria lasting longer than 6 weeks is classified as *chronic urticaria*. It may persist for years; it also may go away and then recur. The underlying cause is usually unknown.

The etiologies of urticaria are numerous and can include such components as foods, inhalants, drugs, injectants (eg, blood, vaccines), chemicals, mechanical and environmental irritants, and psychogenic factors. Cutaneous drug reactions occur in 1% to 3% of all hospitalized medical patients.[29] They usually occur within the first 6 days of drug treatment and have varying clinical features (Table 47-2). Treatment involves removing the causative agent. Antihistamines are often used. Alleviating irritation factors, instituting elimination diets, and preventing and treating dry skin may be of benefit.

TABLE 47-1 *Description of Skin Lesions*

Lesion	Description
Blister	Fluid-filled vesicle or bulla
Bulla	Blister larger than 0.5 cm
Comedo	Plugged and dilated pore, called blackhead or whitehead
Crust	Dried exudate over a damaged epithelium, may be associated with vesicle, bullae, or pustules
Cyst	Semisolid or fluid-filled mass, encapsulated in deeper layers of skin
Desquamation	Shedding or loss of debris on skin surface
Erosion	Loss of epidermis, may be associated with vesicles, bullae, or pustules
Excoriation	Epidermal erosion usually caused by scratching
Fissure	Crack in the epidermis usually extending into the dermis
Macule	Flat area of skin with discoloration, less than 5 mm in diameter
Nodule	Solid, elevated lesion or mass, 5 mm to 5 cm in diameter
Papule	Solid, elevated lesion less than 5 mm in diameter
Plaque	Raised, flattened lesion greater than 5 mm in diameter
Pustule	Papule containing purulent exudate
Scale	Skin debris on the surface of the epidermis
Tumor	Solid mass, larger than 5 cm in diameter, usually extends to dermis
Ulceration	Loss of epidermis, extending into dermis or deeper
Urticarial	Raised wheallike lesion
Vesicle	Small fluid-filled lesion, less than 5 mm in diameter
Wheal	Transient, irregular pink elevation with surrounding edema

▼ Common Inflammatory Alterations of the Skin

DRY SKIN

Dry skin in itself is a noninflammatory condition, but it can become reddened when it persists unrelieved. It is extremely common and consists of roughened, flaky skin with or without pruritus.

Primary Lesions

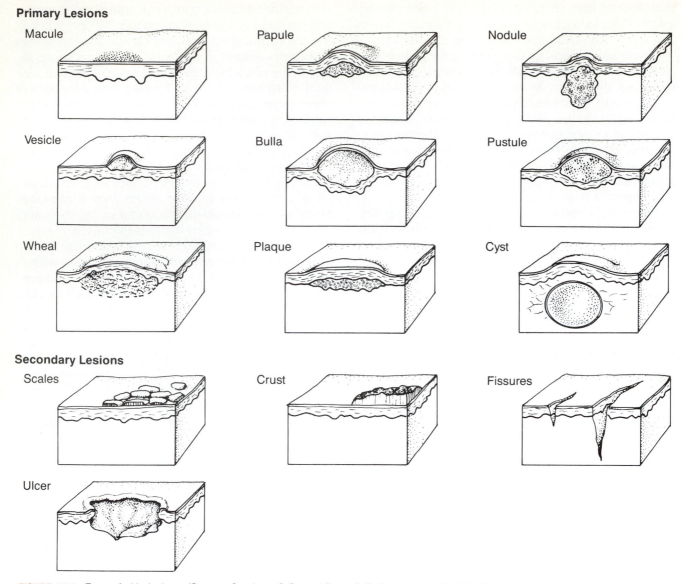

Macule   Papule   Nodule

Vesicle   Bulla   Pustule

Wheal   Plaque   Cyst

Secondary Lesions

Scales   Crust   Fissures

Ulcer

FIGURE 47-1 *Type of skin lesions. (Source: Smeltzer, S.C. and Bare, B.G.* Brunner and Suddarth's Textbook of Medical-Surgical Nursing *[7th ed.]. Philadelphia: J.B. Lippincott, 1992.)*

The defect, which occurs commonly in the aging process, involves loss of water, electrolytes, and skin lipids. It occurs often in dry and cold climates, and environmental conditions aggravate the condition if it previously existed.

Dehydration after sweating dries out the surface keratin, and itching and inflammatory changes can be superimposed.[16] Treatment of dry skin involves rehydration with a moisturizer and water, together with barrier creams used consistently.

ACNE

Acne vulgaris is a common, chronic inflammatory disease of the sebaceous glands and hair follicles of the skin, also known as the *pilosebaceous ducts* (Fig. 47-2). It results from two factors: 1) accumulation of sebum, the fatty secretion liberated by the breakdown of sebaceous cells; and 2) irritation of the area around the hair follicle, leading to a perifolliculitis.

The exact etiology of acne is unknown, but it may be due to either increased activity of the sebaceous glands or inability of the material secreted to escape through a narrow opening. The resulting inflammation is precipitated by the combination of sebum, bacteria, and subsequent release of fatty acids. The release of fatty acids is caused by the hydrolytic action of the lipases, which are furnished by the bacteria on the sebum itself. The inflammatory reaction and resulting edema probably cause the sebaceous follicle to perforate its wall and develop perifolliculitis. The development of acne depends on several factors, including heredity, use of oil-based cosmetics or skin treatments, ingestion of drugs (eg, steroids, androgens), and the presence of bacteria.

TABLE 47-2 *Cutaneous Drug Reactions*

Type of Eruption	Clinical Features	Drugs Potentially Causing the Reaction
Morbilliform	Diffuse, confluent, macular, papular, erythematous Often occur in first week	Penicillins Sulfonamides Phenytoin (with adenopathy, leukocytosis, and liver function abnormalities in hypersensitivity syndrome) Barbiturates Ampicillin (up to 90% of patients with infectious mononucleosis)
Urticaria	Pruritic, erythematous, annular	Penicillins Aspirin Nonsteroidal antiinflammatory agents Radiocontrast media Tartrazine
Erythema multiforme	Multiple urticarial plaques and annular target lesions (±central bullae) Distributed symmetrically with predilection for palms and soles Mucosal erosions common	Sulfonamides (±trimethoprim) Penicillins Barbiturates Phenytoin Carbamazepine
Toxic epidermal necrolysis	Localized or diffuse erythematous or violaceous macules with central (often large) erosions Target lesions sometimes present Mucosal erosions usual	Phenylbutazone Sulfonamides Barbiturates Allopurinol Phenytoin
Fixed drug reaction	Single (or at most a few) lesions, violaceous, annular with dusky center and hyperpigmentation; occasionally vesicular Recur at same location with rechallenge	Phenolphthalein Sulfonamides Tetracyclines Phenylbutazone Barbiturates
Lichenoid	Polygonal papules with overlying fine silvery scale Identical to true lichen planus	Gold Antimalarials Quinidine Thiazides
Vasculitis	Palpable purpura Extremities more than trunk	Penicillins Thiazides Allopurinol Phenytoin
Erythema nodosum	Tender, erythematous nodules Usually anterior tibial surface	Oral contraceptives
Vegetative	Nodular, crusted, purulent, often fungating lesions	Halogens (iodides, bromides)
Acneiform	Superficial papules, pustules	Corticosteroids Phenytoin Halogens
Pityriasis rosea	Oval, slightly scaly papules on trunk and proximal extremities	Gold
Pemphigus foliaceus	Erythematous, scaly, crusted, erosive lesions Upper trunk, face	Penicillamine

(Kelley, W.N. *Textbook of Internal Medicine* (2nd ed). Philadelphia: J.B. Lippincott, 1992.)

Sebaceous glands are hormonally controlled, and the androgenic hormones may increase the development and secretion of sebaceous glands. The lesions are located in the areas of predominant pilosebaceous glands— face, chest, back, neck, and upper arms.

The early, noninflammatory lesions are of two types, white (closed) and black comedones. The white comedo occurs in a closed excretory duct that has a very small, possibly microscopic, opening that prevents drainage. This lesion may lead to an inflammatory process and give rise to a papule or pustule. The black comedo (blackhead) is a widely dilated follicle filled with oxidized

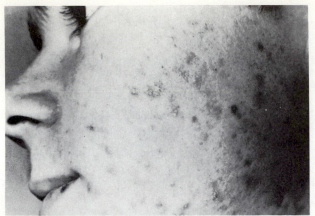

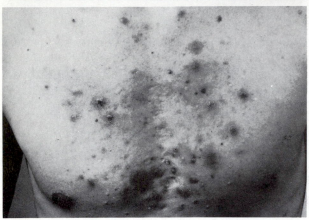

FIGURE 47-2 *Acne of the face and chest. (Source: Sauer, G.C. Manual of Skin Diseases [6th ed.]. Philadelphia: J.B. Lippincott, 1991.)*

melanin that plugs an excretory duct of the skin.[22] Both types of lesions obstruct the emptying of sebum to the surface and may develop into small papules, pustules, nodules, or cysts. Most pustules and cysts eventually open, drain, and heal. If severe, these lesions may result in scarring. The prevalence of acne is increased during adolescence and early adulthood, but it is usually self-limited. The central theme of medical treatment involves reducing the inflammation of the pilosebaceous glands by fostering their free drainage, avoiding rupture, and limiting bacterial growth.

ACUTE ECZEMATOUS DERMATITIS

Dermatitis and eczema are words that are used interchangeably. They constitute the superficial inflammatory diseases of the skin. There are five major classifications (Table 47-3). Morphologically, the changes of acute and chronic dermatitis are specific and recognizable.

Contact Dermatitis

Contact dermatitis includes inflammations that are the result of contact with external agents, either chemical allergens or mechanical irritants. The lesion begins in the area of contact (Fig. 47-3). The irritant removes some of the protective mechanisms of the skin, such as lipids and other hydrophilic material, and causes varying degrees of dryness. When contact is with strong compounds or is prolonged, lesions may evolve. If exposure is continued,

TABLE 47-3 *Classification of Eczematous Dermatitis*

Type	Cause or Pathogenesis	Histology*	Clinical Features
Contact dermatitis	Topically applied chemicals Pathogenesis: delayed hypersensitivity	Spongiotic dermatitis	Marked itching or burning or both; requires antecedent exposure
Atopic dermatitis	Unknown, may be heritable	Spongiotic dermatitis	Erythematous plaques in flexural areas; family history of eczema, hay fever, or asthma
Drug-related eczematous dermatitis	Systematically administered antigens or haptens (eg, penicillin)	Spongiotic dermatitis; eosinophils often present in infiltrate; deeper infiltrate	Eruption occurs with administration of drug; remits when drug is discontinued
Photoeczematous eruption	Ultraviolet light	Spongiotic dermatitis; deeper infiltrate	Occurs on sun-exposed skin; phototesting may help in diagnosis
Primary irritant dermatitis	Repeated trauma (rubbing)	Spongiotic dermatitis in early stages; epidermal hyperplasia in late stages	Localized to site of trauma

* All types, with time, may develop chronic changes.
(Cotran, R., Kumar, V., and Robbins, S. *Robbins' Pathologic Basis of Disease* [5th ed.]. Philadelphia: W.B. Saunders, 1994.)

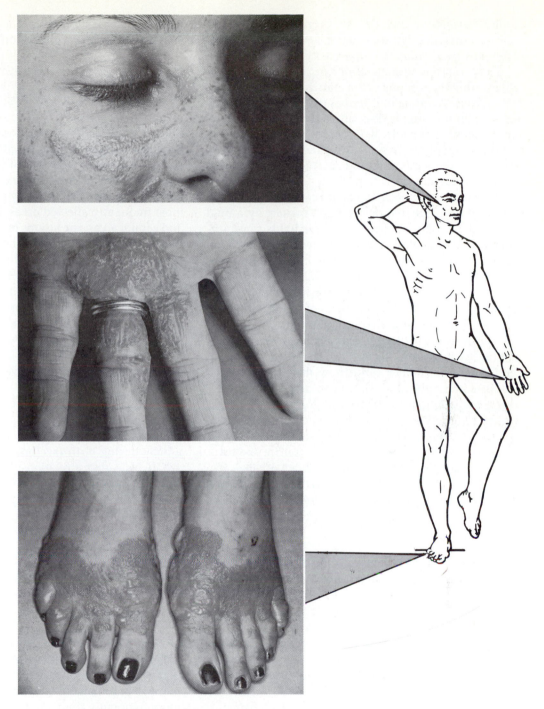

From shoe material

FIGURE 47-3 *Contact dermatitis. (Source: Sauer, G.C.* Manual of Skin Diseases *[6th ed.]. Philadelphia: J.B. Lippincott, 1991.)*

acute dermatitis can progress to the chronic form. In most circumstances, complete tissue repair is possible if the irritant is removed and permanent changes in the skin have not taken place.[15]

Contact dermatitis is a delayed-hypersensitivity dermatitis. It results from exposure of a previously sensitized person to contact allergens. Some of the causes include poison ivy antigens, many industrial chemicals, some drugs, and some metals. The clinical features include marked itching, burning with red blistering, or vesicles at the area of contact. Histologically, there is papillary dermal edema and mast cell degranulation. The pattern is called spongiotic dermatitis.[18]

Removal of the sensitizer is necessary for treatment. The causative agent can be identified by a history, patch testing, or a use test. Unless the condition is severe, medical treatment includes soaks and corticosteroid creams. When dermatitis becomes severe and frequent, systemic steroids may be required.

Drug-related eczematous dermatitis follows a specific hypersensitivity response to a particular drug (see p. 357). It causes a spongiotic dermatitis that usually disappears when the drug is discontinued.[18] In *photoeczematous* reactions, ultraviolet light causes a dermatitis reaction on sun-exposed areas.[18] Some individuals are very sensitive to the sun's rays and react with a significant dermatitis reaction.

Primary irritant contact dermatitis causes a nonallergic skin reaction. Repeated or extended contact by a mild irritant causes skin damage. Strong irritants cause immediate damage on initial contact. Mechanical irritation is due to inflammation from mechanical factors, such as large-size particles of certain materials that cause pruritus. One example is wool, resulting in dermatitis that is due to the mechanical scratchiness of the irritant itself, not the mediation of a chemical substance.

The frequency of chemically caused contact dermatitis has increased. A basic substance such as water can indirectly be a chemical irritant through prolonged exposure and removal of the skin's protective barriers. Soaps and detergents increase the drying and facilitate the irritating action of water. Other chemicals and medications may cause an irritant dermatitis. Various biologic irritants, including human excrement, saliva, and tears, result in dermatitis after prolonged contact. Biologic irritants can also cause a predisposition to the development of yeast and bacterial infections, compounding the problem.

Atopic Dermatitis

Atopic dermatitis is a highly specific disease that results from a genetically determined lowered threshold to pruritus and is characterized by intense itching. The affected areas include the flexural regions, such as the antecubital fossa and wrists.[30] It may appear as a small papule, but evidence points to scratching as the major factor producing the lesion. In acute atopic dermatitis, intense scratching leads to erythema, weeping, scaling, and lichenification. The histology is that of a nonspecific dermatitis. The list of exacerbating factors includes sudden changes in weather, psychological stress, contact with wool or furs, and primary irritant chemicals.

Many complications can develop with atopic dermatitis, including an increase in the severity of viral infections. It is frequently associated with allergic rhinitis or asthma.[30] Affected persons should not be vaccinated against smallpox, as disseminated vaccinia can develop and cause a generalized infection of the skin. These persons are also prone to bacterial and fungal infections, ocular complications, and allergic contact dermatitis. Treatment involves palliation by reducing or controlling precipitating events and providing symptomatic relief of pruritus. Atopic dermatitis tends to decrease in severity as the person approaches adulthood.

▼ Viral Infections of the Skin

HERPES SIMPLEX

Herpes simplex, also known as a fever blister or cold sore, is caused by type 1 herpes simplex virus. Initially, it is an acute condition with groups of vesicles on an erythematous base, which later become purulent and crusting. Distribution may occur to any area of the body, but the most frequently affected areas are the lips and perioral and genital areas; the lesions may be painful and pruritic (Fig. 47-4). They resolve usually within 2 weeks. It is believed that first exposure to infection occurs by the fifth year of life, but is not often observed. Nevertheless, the person has developed antibodies to the virus. A small percentage of children have primary gingivostomatitis or vulvovaginitis as a result. Recurrence throughout life may result from either reactivation of the virus or reinoculation and may be precipitated by stress-producing factors, such as fever, excessive sun exposure, the common cold, illness, and injury.

Herpes progenitalis has become a common infection of the genital area and is caused by the type 2 herpesvirus. It is usually sexually transmitted but can infect a baby during birth (see pp. 1166–1167). Researchers are investigating a relationship of this virus to cervical cancer.

Because no cure has been discovered, treatment of herpes simplex is basically symptomatic relief. Acyclovir (Zovirax) has been shown to be effective in shortening the duration of episodes; it possibly decreases the number of recurrences. The long-term effects are being studied. Prevention can only be aimed at avoiding the identified precipitating factors.

VARICELLA

Otherwise known as *chickenpox*, varicella is caused by the herpes zoster virus. An airborne, highly contagious virus in the prodromal and vesicular stages, it affects children more frequently than adults. The varicella has an incubation period of 10 to 20 days. The prodromal stage often begins with moderate fever and malaise. Pink papules 2 to 4 mm in diameter are surrounded by a reddened halo (dewdrop on a rose petal) that later dries and crusts.[25] Lesions usually occur in groups; their distribution on the face, scalp, trunk, and arms is common. Generalized symptoms of headache, moderate fever, anorexia, and malaise may continue after the lesions erupt. Varicella in adults is much more severe than in children. The usual treatment for varicella in children is aimed at keeping the skin lesions dry and relieving pruritus with lotion as necessary.

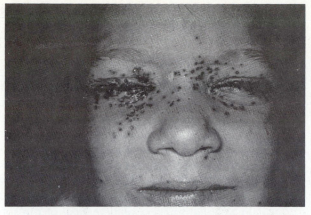

(A) Primary herpes simplex around the eyes in a 5-year-old child

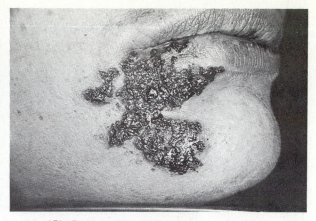

(B) Recurrent herpes simplex on chin with secondary bacterial infection

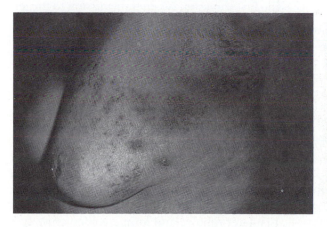

(C) Recurrent herpes simplex on a thumb

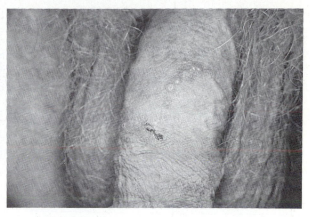

(D) Recurrent herpes simplex on the penis

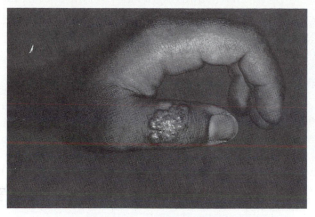

(E) Herpes zoster of left breast area

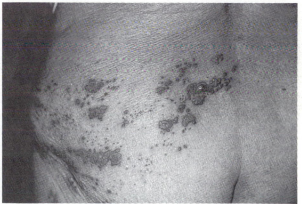

(F) Hemorrhagic zoster of left hip area

FIGURE 47-4 *Herpes simplex and zoster. (Source: Sauer, G.C. Manual of Skin Diseases [6th ed.]. Philadelphia: J.B. Lippincott, 1991.)*

HERPES ZOSTER

Herpes zoster is also produced by a varicella virus and it is often referred to as *shingles*. This acute inflammatory disease occurs when the dormant varicella virus is activated. It occurs most often in the elderly population, but it can occur in any age group. In the older person, pain usually precedes the lesion by 1 to 2 days. The initial features are erythema and discomfort, followed in 1 to 7 days by grouped vesicles along a unilateral dermatome (Fig. 47-5). These vesicles later crust and clear in 2 to 3 weeks. Severe pain can result, and persistence is a feared

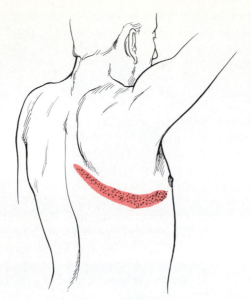

FIGURE 47-5 *Herpes zoster. The inflammatory lesions follow nerve distribution, especially in the thoracic region. Vesicles are apparent for 3 to 5 days, and the crusted lesions remain for about 3 weeks.*

complication. Although uncommon, generalized herpes zoster can result, a condition usually associated with a systemic malignancy of the lymphoma group.[25] A susceptible person may develop chickenpox after exposure to this varicella virus.

WARTS (VERRUCAE)

Verrucae, or warts, are viral infections of the skin by one of 49 different types of human papillomaviruses.[18] These viruses are of the DNA type.[22] There are three main types: verruca vulgaris (common wart), verruca plantaris (plantar wart), and condyloma acuminatum (venereal wart). The etiology of warts is not clearly understood, but they can be transmitted by contact from person to person. They are benign lesions and frequently occur at sites of injury or along a break in the skin.

Verruca vulgaris is a raised, well-circumscribed growth with an irregular gray surface, frequently present on the hands. Although treatment is often unsatisfactory, surgical removal, electrosurgery, and cryosurgery have been used. Many warts resolve without treatment.

Verruca plantaris differs from the common wart by its location and the effect that pressure has on the lesion. The wart tends to grow on the soles of the feet, and pain is frequent due to the irritation of walking. As a result, the wart tends to grow inward.

Condylomata acuminata are lesions established primarily in warm, moist anogenital areas. Also known as venereal warts, they may or may not stem from sexual contact. They are large, pinkish or purplish projections with a rough surface.

RUBEOLA (MEASLES)

Rubeola is a highly contagious infection caused by a myxovirus. The incubation period is approximately 10 to 14 days. Its course usually begins with fever and symptoms of upper respiratory infection that occur 6 to 7 days after inoculation and last 24 hours. The disease then enters the invasion phase, with development of high fever, chills, malaise, headache, photophobia, and dry cough. These symptoms last for 4 to 7 days. Lesions begin as inflammation or petechiae of the soft palate, followed by Koplik's spots, which are blue-white spots surrounded by a bright halo over the buccal mucosa.[16] A macular eruption appears on the face, upper extremities, and trunk.

RUBELLA

Also known as *German measles*, rubella is a common, acute, infectious disease caused by a myxovirus. The incubation period ranges from 12 to 25 days and begins with malaise and mild fever approximately 4 to 5 days before lesions appear. Lesions are small, irregular, pink macules and papules that appear initially on the face, spreading to the entire body. They fade rapidly within 3 days. Adenopathy of the superficial cervical and posterior auricular glands is common.

Rubella is serious in pregnant women, especially in the first trimester, when transmission to the fetus results in fetal anomalies. A titer is available to assess immunity. Vaccination is given to school-aged children and, with caution, to women of child-bearing age with low rubella titers.

▼ Bacterial Infections of the Skin

IMPETIGO

Impetigo is an acute bacterial infection that occurs superficially on the skin as serous and purulent vesicles that later rupture and form a golden crust. It frequently occurs in children, but persons in ill health are also predisposed to it. A common location for lesions is the face, but they may involve the extremities.[22]

Causative organisms include β-hemolytic streptococci and coagulase-positive staphylococci. Impetigo is autoinoculable and can be transmitted among humans. Influencing factors include poor hygiene, tropical climates, and improper sanitation. A serious complication is glomerulonephritis, which may not be prevented by antibiotic treatment.

FOLLICULITIS

Folliculitis is a bacterial infection of the skin that originates within the hair follicle. Staphylococci are the usual causative organisms. Folliculitis appears as a pustule located at the opening of the hair follicle, predominantly on the scalp and extremities. The basic lesion is a reddened macule or papule surrounding the hair follicle. Predisposing factors include poor hygiene and maceration. Immunosuppressed persons or those with diabetes mellitus have a much greater incidence of severe outbreaks of this condition.[22] Folliculitis can extend into the hair bulb and the deeper skin layers if not treated promptly. Systemic antibiotics may be necessary.

FURUNCLES AND CARBUNCLES

Furuncles, also known as *boils*, frequently develop from a preceding staphylococcal folliculitis and are usually located in body areas containing hair follicles. Irritation, maceration, and lack of good hygiene are predisposing factors in their development. The lesions are nodules that are usually tender and red. They frequently remain tense for 2 to 4 days, become fluctuant, and later drain purulent material.[1]

Carbuncles are large staphylococcal abscesses that drain through multiple openings on the skin surface.[22] Some cases of furuncles and almost every case of carbuncles require systemic antibiotic therapy.

▼ Fungal Diseases of the Skin

Fungal diseases of the skin can be classified in three groups: superficial, intermediate, and deep. Some are *opportunistic* and affect a susceptible host, whereas others are truly *pathogenic* and can infect a healthy person.[18] The superficial diseases result in ringworm (tinea capitis), athlete's foot (tinea pedis), "jock itch" (tinea cruris), and tinea versicolor. These fungal diseases are primarily caused by dermatophytes that invade the superficial layers of the epidermis, hair, and nails. They are characterized by areas of scaling and erythema and frequently exhibit vesicles and fissures.[25] Moisture, heat, and maceration are predisposing factors for growth; consequently, lesions appear in areas between toes, the axillae, nails, and groin. Treatment involves local therapy. With certain resistant fungi, griseofulvin, a fungostatic antibiotic, is used.

Intermediate fungal diseases invade both the superficial and deeper tissues. Moniliasis caused by *Candida albicans* is an example. This organism can also produce deep invasion when the host's resistance declines.[18]

Deep fungal infections invade deeper structures of living tissue and include diseases such as sporotrichosis, candidiasis, histoplasmosis, and aspergillosis (see pp. 287–293). A much higher incidence of opportunistic deep fungal infections is being seen after the use of immunosuppressive drugs and invasive procedures.[18]

▼ Scaling Disorders of the Skin

PSORIASIS

Psoriasis is a chronic, genetically determined disease of epidermal proliferation (Fig. 47-6). The increased cell turnover rate and production of immature cells result in the classic features of sharply defined erythematous plaques covered by silvery white, loosely adherent scales.[22]

The precise etiology is not known, but genetic and environmental factors are important in its development. It is viewed as a chronic disease with much diversity in its location, severity, and frequency. Exacerbating factors include local trauma, overexposure to the sun, infection, stress, and physical illness.[22]

Psoriasis affects persons of all ages and is often distributed over the knees, elbows, scalp, and lumbosacral skin. When involved, the nails show pitting and dimpling. Psoriasis may be associated with arthritis. A serious but rare condition known as pustular psoriasis also can occur, causing sterile pustules, high fever, elevated white blood cell count, electrolyte imbalance, and malaise. This condition can be fatal.[3]

Psoriasis usually can be controlled, but remissions are common. Avoiding local skin injury, infection, and stress; maintaining good nutrition; and avoiding excessive weight gain improve the control of this disease.

PITYRIASIS ROSEA

Pityriasis rosea is a common, acute disease of the skin, usually affecting adolescents and young adults. Its course is self-limited and is thought to be infectious, possibly caused by a virus.

CASE STUDY 47-1

Jerry Moore is a 19-year-old caucasian male who has been treated for recurring episodes of psoriasis. He describes a family history of psoriasis on the maternal side. He indicates that exacerbations occur when he is under stress at school or when he has a cold or flu.

1. *What etiologic factors are seen to be important in this disease?*
2. *Describe the pathophysiologic features of the condition.*
3. *What are exacerbating factors?*
4. *Describe some prevention and treatment measures that can improve control of the disease.*

See Appendix G for discussion.

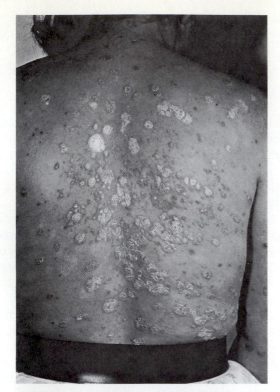

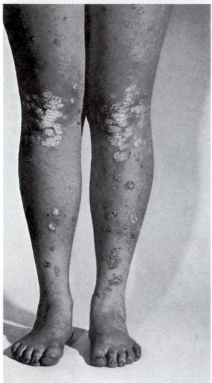

FIGURE 47-6 *Psoriasis in a 17-year-old girl. Moderately extensive psoriasis in classic distribution on back and knees. (Source: Sauer, G.C. Manual of Skin Diseases [6th ed.]. Philadelphia: J.B. Lippincott, 1991.)*

Clinical manifestations often arise after a prodrome of malaise, fatigue, and headache. The first lesion, known as the *herald patch*, is a single, oval, ringlike plaque that is later followed by lesions that are usually flat, erythematous patches covered by fine scales that resemble the primary plaque but are smaller. Lesions are often pruritic. Distribution is commonly on the neck, trunk, and arms.

▼ Skin Tumors

Skin tumors, like all tumors, are of two basic categories, benign and malignant. Benign tumors are slow growing, and growth may stop entirely.[16] Malignant lesions show disorganization and abnormalities. They may grow rapidly and infiltrate surrounding tissues. Metastasis may occur depending on the origin of the tumor.

BENIGN TUMORS

Seborrheic Keratosis

Seborrheic keratosis is the most common tumor in the elderly. A strong predisposing factor is prolonged exposure to the sun. The skin lesion is slightly raised, light brown, and sharply demarcated; pigmentation may deepen and the skin may become thick (Fig. 47-7). The lesion is covered with a greasy crust that is loosely attached.[21] Locations include the trunk, shoulders, face, and scalp. Malignant transformation is uncommon, and most lesions do not require treatment unless they pose cosmetic problems or raise suspicions of malignancy.

Hemangioma

A hemangioma is a benign tumor of newly formed blood vessels. There are many different types. A strawberry hemangioma frequently appears as a dome-shaped, fully red, soft lesion with sharply demarcated edges. It tends to grow slowly and usually regresses completely.

The *nevus flammeus* (ordinary birthmark) is a congenital vascular malformation that is usually unilateral and located on the face and neck. It appears as a light pink to dark purple patch that usually fades and regresses.[18] The *port wine stain* may grow with the child and become unsightly. It is often associated with mental retardation, seizures, hemiplegia, and other problems.[18] *Cavernous hemangiomas* are large, cavernous, vascular channels that may occur in both the skin and subcutaneous tissues. The features of the lesions depend on their extent, varying from round to flat and from bright red to deep purple.

Keratoacanthoma

Keratoacanthoma is a firm, raised nodule with a central crater. It is seen on sun-exposed skin of middle-aged and

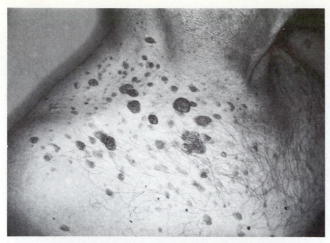

(*A*) Seborrheic keratoses on the neck

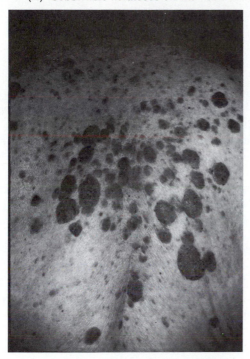

(*B*) Seborrheic keratoses on back

FIGURE 47-7 *Epidermal tumors. (Source: Sauer, G.C. Manual of Skin Diseases [6th ed.]. Philadelphia: J.B. Lippincott, 1991.)*

elderly persons.[21] Because it resembles squamous cell carcinoma, lesions are removed and examined histologically.

Actinic or Solar Keratosis

Actinic keratosis is a premalignant lesion. Lesions are sharply demarcated, rough, and red to brown or gray (Fig. 47-8). At high risk for developing this condition are fair-skinned persons whose skin easily burns with sun exposure.[21] Age of onset is related to the amount of sun exposure. Treatment is necessary, because approx-

imately 20% to 25% of these lesions progress to squamous cell carcinoma.[21] Various methods can be used to destroy them, including curettage, electrodesiccation, cryotherapy, topical chemotherapy, and excisional biopsy.

Leukoplakia, actinic keratosis of the mucous membranes, is a common premalignant lesion, occurring as a whitish patch on the mucosa of the oral cavity.[25] It occurs most often in elderly women.

MALIGNANT DISORDERS

Basal Cell Carcinoma

Basal cell carcinoma is the most common type of skin cancer. Most basal cell carcinomas arise from the epidermis and hair follicles on the head and neck.[14,22] They tend to occur mainly in older persons, and most lesions appear with cumulative, prolonged exposure to the sun.[21] Persons who have had radiation therapy for breast, lung, or other types of internal malignancies have an increased risk. These common tumors are slow growing, and although they rarely metastasize, treatment is necessary, because they may become locally destructive and can erode into vital areas.[18,21] Studies of T-lymphocyte depression in the cutaneous tissues of these individuals support the theory that ultraviolet light impairs host defense mechanisms and allows the tumor to escape immune surveillance.[14,18]

Characteristically, the carcinoma has a smooth surface with a pearly border, often with ulceration of its center (Fig. 47-9). Usually, numerous telangiectasias (localized groups of dilated, small blood vessels) are visible.[18] Treatments include cryotherapy, curettage, electrodesiccation, and topical chemotherapy.

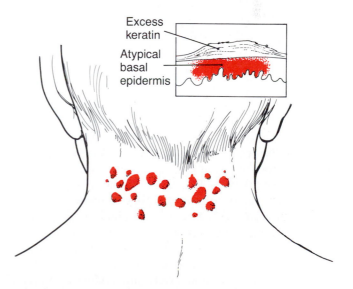

Excess keratin

Atypical basal epidermis

FIGURE 47-8 *Actinic keratoses are commonly seen in the aged individual, often on the back of the neck.*

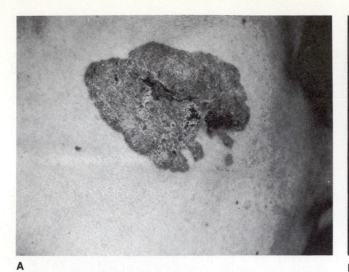

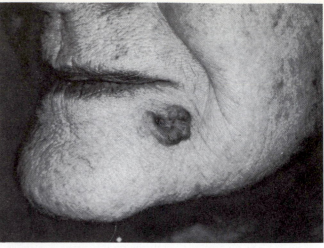

A   B

FIGURE 47-9 **A.** *A large superficial basal cell carcinoma on the back.* **B.** *Basal cell carcinoma on the chin. (Source: Sauer, G.C. Manual of Skin Diseases [6th ed.]. Philadelphia: J.B. Lippincott, 1991.)*

Squamous Cell Carcinoma

Squamous cell carcinoma is a malignant lesion that can affect both the skin and mucous membranes. It most frequently occurs in sun-damaged areas of the body or areas exposed to irradiation or burns. If it remains confined to the epidermis, it is called *Bowen's disease*.[13] The squamous cell carcinoma may also arise in scars, chronic ulcers, fistulas, and sinuses. The burn scar may serve as an initiator, or cocarcinogen, in the production of these malignancies.[14] Immune alterations described include local imbalances of T-cell function that favor tumorigenesis in skin damaged by ultraviolet light.[18]

Characteristically, the carcinoma appears as a rough hyperkeratotic nodule with an indurated base. It may ulcerate and can metastasize. Surgical excision is the treatment of choice. In some instances, curettage and electrodesiccation, irradiation, and chemotherapy can be used.

Malignant Melanoma

Malignant melanoma is a cancer arising from the melanin-producing cells. It is associated with a high risk for invasion and metastasis. Risk of developing some forms of the disease is increased with exposure to the sun. The worldwide frequency of this malignancy is rising more rapidly than any other cancer except lung cancer in women. The at-risk populations are persons with fair complexions and persons with a family history of melanoma.[2] Recognizing the lesion early is important, because prognosis is dependent on such factors as early removal, size, type, and extension. Five-year survival has improved, depending on the clinical type, to 90% to 100% when the tumor is less than 1 mm thick and

is about 50% when the tumor is larger than 3 mm thick.[13] All nevi should be inspected regularly, and self-examination should be taught.

Melanoma occurs most frequently in young and middle-aged adults. The most common location in men is the trunk and in women the legs.[2] The tumors exhibit variable colors and irregular borders and surfaces. Nevi may be brown or black with shades of red, white, or blue. Small satellite lesions 1 to 2 cm from the primary lesion may be seen.[2]

The precursor lesions to melanomas are the congenital nevi and the dysplastic nevi. The congenital nevus rarely becomes malignant if it is small (less than 1.5 cm in diameter). Large congenital nevi (larger than 20 cm in diameter) have a 5% to 20% risk of becoming malignant.[14] Dysplastic nevi are usually larger lesions of various colors with irregular borders and sometimes a central papule.[19] These often appear late in childhood or adolescence but may appear after age 35. When these develop in fair-skinned persons, they will more likely develop into melanoma than will the congenital nevi.

Melanomas are of various types, with the most common being the *superficial spreading melanoma* that usually arises within a nevus (Fig. 47-10). Other types include *nodular*, which is darkly pigmented and may grow from normal skin, and *lentigo maligna melanoma*, which arises on a flat lesion, usually the sun-damaged face of an elderly person.[2, 13] The classification of the tumor is crucial in determining the extent of the surgical dissection for removal. The new staging system adopted by the American Joint Committee on Cancer provides a uniform staging system (Table 47-4).[2]

Melanomas acquire new antigens, some of which are the oncofetal and histocompatibility antigens. The nevi often undergo several morphologic changes before

▼ Traumatic Alterations in the Skin

BURNS

Burns are suffered by approximately 2 million persons annually, of which 130,000 persons require hospitalization and 10,000 die.[4] In a large 5-year study of adult burn patients, the average age was 44 years, 78% were black, and 62% were men. Major causes of burns included flames (44.8%), scalds (28.5%), and chemicals (9.7%). The injuries resulted from direct assault, cooking, smoking, explosion, house fire, contact with hot objects, bathtub accidents, house chores, and various other factors, in that order. Individuals considered to be predisposed to burn injury were the elderly, those living alone, alcohol and drug abusers, and the physically and mentally ill.[4] Burn injuries occur in every age group and both sexes. When they occur, they involve not only the skin tissue but also all of the systems of the body. The depth of thermal injuries depends on the burning agent, temperature, and length of exposure to the heat.[17] The equilibrium point for skin is approximately 44°C (111.2°F.). This temperature can be tolerated for up to 6 hours without burning. The rate of skin destruction doubles with each degree rise, so that at 70°C. (158°F.), fleeting exposure will produce total epidermal necrosis.[17]

Burns are classified as first-, second-, and third-degree. A more precise classification may be made on the basis of partial-thickness, deep dermal, or full-thickness injury (Fig. 47-11). The depth of injury is often difficult to assess in the initial postburn period. To complicate matters further, a partial-thickness injury may convert to a deep dermal or full-thickness injury as a result of wound sepsis and microcirculatory insufficiency with delayed degeneration of deep epithelial appendages. The depth and extent of the burn eventually become more apparent.

Partial-Thickness Burns

Each degree of burn wound depth has various characteristics. Partial-thickness burns include first- and second-degree and deep dermal injuries (Table 47-5). The first-degree burn involves the epidermis. It may be caused by exposure to sunlight, brief exposures to a heat source, splashed hot liquid, high-intensity short-duration explosions, and chemical and electrical injury. A first-degree burn is pink to red, painful, and slightly edematous. The epidermis peels in 3 to 6 days, with itching and redness persisting for a week or more. The wound leaves no scar when healed.[17]

The second-degree, partial-thickness burn may be superficial or deep dermal. It results from intense flash heat, hot liquid, contact with hot objects, chemicals, or electrical injury. The superficial burn involves the epi-

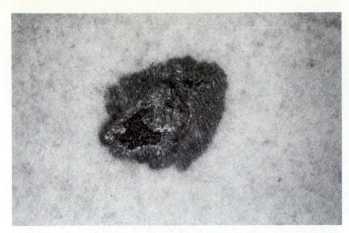

FIGURE 47-10 *Malignant melanoma in a nevus present since birth on the scapular area. (Source: Sauer, G.C. Manual of Skin Diseases [6th ed.]. Philadelphia: J.B. Lippincott, 1991.)*

exhibiting invasive, cancerous properties. Study of the relationship of melanomas to viral carcinogens is intriguing but inconclusive.[10,18] Prognosis depends on the stage of the malignant melanoma at diagnosis, with a 15-year survival of 47% when it is diagnosed in Stage I and decreasing to 2% when it is diagnosed in Stage IV (see Table 47-4). Most melanomas are highly invasive and spread rapidly to the lymphatic system, followed by metastasis to any organ of the body.[2]

TABLE 47-4 *New Staging System for Melanoma Adopted by the American Joint Committee on Cancer*

Stage	Criteria
IA	Localized melanoma ≤0.75 mm or level II* (T1N0M0)
IB	Localized melanoma 0.76–1.5 mm or level III* (T2N0M0)
IIA	Localized melanoma 1.5–4 mm or level IV* (T3N0M0)
IIB	Localized melanoma >4 mm or level V* (T4N0M0)
III	Limited nodal metastases involving only one regional lymph node basin, or fewer than five in-transit metastases without nodal metastases (any T, N1M0)
IV	Advanced regional metastases (any T, N2M0) or any patient with distant metastases (any T, any N, M1 or M2)

* When the thickness and level of invasion criteria do not coincide with a T classification, thickness should take precedence.
(Adapted from American Joint Committee on Cancer. *Manual for Staging of Cancer* [4th ed.]. Beahrs OH, Henson DE, Hutter RVP, and Kennedy BJ, eds. Philadelphia: JB Lippincott, 1992:145.)

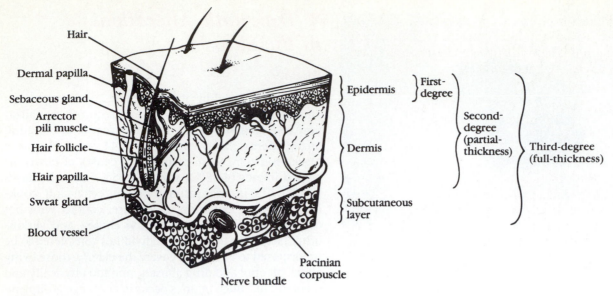

FIGURE 47-11   *Areas affected by partial- and full-thickness burns.*

dermis and dermis. It has a mottled pink to red color. It exhibits blistering and subcutaneous edema and is moist and very sensitive. This burn heals in 10 to 14 days without grafting. If it does not become infected or traumatized, usually no scar forms.

The deep dermal burn varies in color, being mottled with more white than red, a dull white, tan, or cherry red. The red areas blanch and refill. Dark streaks of coagulated capillaries may be seen. The burn extends down to the subcutaneous tissue. If epidermal appendages are intact, the burn has the potential to heal spontaneously without grafting, because viable skin cells are present in the appendages. A deep dermal burn takes several months heal spontaneously. The wound may be blistered and moist or dry; it may or may not be sensitive; and if a hair follicle remains, the hair will not pull

TABLE 47-5 *Classification of Burns*

Type	Tissue	Appearance	Symptoms	Resolution
PARTIAL THICKNESS				
First-degree	Epidermis	Red, pink, slight edema	Pain	Epidermis peels in 3–6 days; itch, redness in a week or so; no scar
Second-degree	Epidermis and upper dermis	Mottled pink to red; blistering edema; moist	Sensitive	Heals in 10–14 days without grafting; no scar if no infection or trauma to wound
• Deep dermal	Epidermis, dermis to subcutaneous tissue	Varies: white, tan, cherry red; red area blanches; dark, coagulated capillary streaks; blister and moist, or dry	May or may not be sensitive; if hair follicles present, hair does not pull out	Has potential to heal spontaneously over several months; may be excised or grafted
FULL THICKNESS				
Third-degree	Epidermis; dermis; subcutaneous layer; no viable epithelial cells remain	White, tan, brown, black, deep cherry red; red areas do not blanch, wet or dry; sunken; eschar; coagulated capillaries	Anesthetic; hair pulls out	Grafting required after debridement
Fourth-degree	Epidermis; dermis; subcutaneous layer; fascia; muscle; bone	Blackened; depressed; bone is dull and dry	Anesthetic; hair pulls out	Grafting required

out. The epithelium produced is extremely thin and may break down easily; the burn may convert to a full-thickness burn if it becomes infected.[5] Many deep dermal burns are excised and grafted.

Full-Thickness Burns

These injuries involve destruction of skin layers down to or including part of the subcutaneous tissue, muscle, or even bone (see Table 47-5).[5] The causes may be the same as for partial-thickness burns. The wound appearance may vary, being white, tan, brown, black, or deep cherry red. The red areas do not blanch. The burn is usually dry and has a sunken, leathery appearance. The leathery covering is called *eschar*. A black network of coagulated capillaries may be seen. The wound itself is anesthetic, and hair pulls out easily. Grafting is required to close the wound. When the full-thickness burn involves the subcutaneous fat layer, fascia, muscle, and bone, it may be classified as a fourth-degree burn.

Tissue damage from this burn depends on the temperature of and duration of exposure to the heat source. The severity of the injury depends on the size of the burned area, its depth and location, the age of the victim, the presence of concomitant illness or injury, and the psychological status of the victim. Further assessment of the burn is aided by knowledge of the circumstances surrounding the injury. Important information includes such aspects as place of injury, exposure to electricity, exposure to fumes, and other factors that may complicate recovery.

Estimation of the percentage of total body surface area that has been burned is crucial to determining fluid and nutritional requirements. The classic rule of nines has been a standard for estimating burn area (Fig. 47-12).[20] This helpful method has some limitations, depending on the age of the burned patient (a child's head represents a greater percentage of body area than an adult's) and the extent of actual third-degree injury.[17]

Localized Changes Due to Burn Injury

When skin is burned, many localized changes occur. Protein in cells is denatured and enzymes are inactivated. The tissue becomes coagulated, desiccated, or carbonized, depending on the temperature of the heat source and the length of exposure to it. Even with mild heat, the normal metabolic activity of a cell is altered. Burns caused by long exposure to low-intensity heat are characterized by major changes in deeper tissues.

The keratin layer is the water vapor barrier in the body. When it is destroyed, large amounts of fluid are lost. In a deep wound, the fluid loss is greater and often continues until the wound finally is closed, usually by grafting.

Burns extending down to and damaging the basal

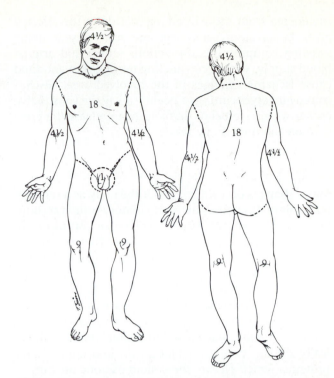

FIGURE 47-12 *The rule of nines. Each arm is 9%; the head, 9%; the torso and abdomen, 18%; the back, 18%; and each leg, 18%. (Source: Dossey, B.M., Guzzetta, C.E., and Kenner, C.V. Critical Care Nursing. [4th ed.]. Philadelphia: J.B. Lippincott, 1992.)*

layer do not regenerate if all parts of this layer are destroyed. Heat extending to the "cement" that binds the epidermis to the dermis causes the epidermis to loosen; lost fluid fills the space and a blister develops. When new epidermis is formed beneath the blister, the blister dries and peels off.

The dermis, composed of collagen fibers, elastin, and mast cells, is damaged when exposed to high degrees of heat. The epidermal appendages, if intact, contain epidermal cells in the external sheaths of the hair follicles. Glands can grow out and form new epithelium. When the burn extends to the subcutaneous tissues, the collagen fibers that normally anchor the dermis to the subcutaneous layer now hold the leathery burn eschar in place. Bacteria that form under the eschar release enzymes that lyse the collagen fibers, making it easier to remove eschar.

The melanocytes in the epidermis do not regenerate well, and in deep burns, the skin color usually does not return. As blood vessels are damaged from the thermal injury, color changes occur in the burn. In sunburn, the vessels in the subpapillary and papillary plexuses dilate, causing reddening. In a severe burn, coagulation of vessels causes the area to lose redness and become whiter, with the vessels themselves coagulating into blackened lines in the wound.

Plasma leaks from damaged blood vessels and provides the fluid for blisters. Lymph vessels, compressed by the edema from the wound, cannot drain the affected area. Escharotomy may become necessary if tissue swelling compromises the venous return and arterial blood supply, so that constricting burned skin and fluid cause ischemic changes in the involved area.[5] Escharotomy involves cutting or peeling away the constrictive eschar with a scalpel or dermatome to release the pressure on the underlying tissue.

Systemic Changes Due to Burn Injury

Many changes occur throughout the body as a result of burn injury. Responses in the circulatory system account for color changes and the edema of burns. Contraction of the skin capillaries causes blanching. The wound appears white if the superficial dermis is coagulated. Later, when arterioles and capillaries dilate, it appears red. The capillaries lose protein-rich fluid through their abnormally permeable walls into the surrounding tissues, creating the most characteristic feature of the burn wound, *edema*. Normally, plasma and interstitial fluid are chemically similar, except for blood cells and large plasma proteins, which elevate the colloid osmotic pressure in the blood. After burn injury, *colloids* (plasma proteins such as albumins and globulins) leak out of the damaged capillaries and into the interstitial spaces. The loss of protein-rich fluid decreases the intracapillary colloid osmotic pressure, causing fluid to shift into the tissues. There is also an accompanying rise in intracapillary pressure as a result of capillary dilatation and increased blood flow of the inflammatory process. The amount of fluid loss into the tissues is correlated with the severity of the burn. The more severe the burn, the more protein is lost. Capillary permeability also increases in tissues around the burn and other areas of the body.[20] The permeability of tissue cells in and around the burn seems to allow abnormal interchange of fluids and electrolytes between cells and interstitial fluid. A limiting factor for extravasation of fluid is increased tissue pressure. Tissue pressure increases as fluid loss increases and reaches a point at which the tissue can hold no more fluid.

The depth of the burn affects the volume and composition of edema fluid. In first-degree burns, protein loss is insignificant and edema slight, because vasodilatation is the only circulatory change. A second-degree burn has more severe capillary damage and more tissue damage. At initial assessment, the surface area of a burn is easily seen, but the depth is not always immediately apparent. Large volumes of fluid can escape beneath the wound before swelling is noted. The third-degree burn involves large injury to skin and the area beneath and around it, which accounts for extensive fluid loss.

Edema can be displaced by pressure, move to dependent areas, and spread beyond the burn. The rate of edema formation depends on temperature of the injuring heat source, duration of exposure, area of the burn, and time since injury. It is difficult to ascertain fluid loss by the amount of visible edema, because such loss occurs deep in the wound beneath it and in the vulnerable third spaces, such as the peritoneal cavity and the lungs.[17] The leathery eschar does not expand with edema pressure, and large amounts of fluid collect beneath it, putting pressure on underlying tissues, causing ischemia as previously described.

Studies show that fluid losses occur rapidly in the period immediately after the burn and decline in about 48 hours.[9] The rate of loss slows when the capillary endothelium returns to its normal state, when the tissue pressure is in balance with capillary hydrostatic pressure, or when capillary stasis occurs. In minor uncomplicated burns, edema is chiefly reabsorbed by the lymphatic system and takes approximately as long as it took the edema to form. Lymphatics also drain larger burns, but this process may take weeks.

The amount of protein lost from plasma varies. Albumin and globulin are lost, with greater amounts of albumin lost than globulin owing to the smaller size of the albumin molecule. Immediately after the burn, the concentration of protein in plasma increases, because there is greater loss of water and electrolytes together with the protein loss. The following compensatory mechanisms exist to counteract fluid loss: interstitial fluid in unburned areas is absorbed by the blood; blood vessels in the spleen and unburned skin constrict, reducing the space that the remaining blood volume must fill; and fluid is absorbed by the gut. Thirst may be intense. In minor burns, these mechanisms suffice. In major large burns, fluids and proteins must be replaced.

Hemoconcentration is a sequel to capillary fluid loss. The fluid portion of the blood is lost to the tissues, allowing the cellular elements to concentrate. The hematocrit level rises; blood flow becomes sluggish, compromising tissue nutrition and oxygenation. Thrombosis sometimes develops in these affected areas.

Water and electrolytes shift back and forth across normal capillary walls. Burn injury alters the shifts by increasing capillary permeability, causing protein loss and altered colloid osmotic pressure. Potassium is released from severely injured cells, causing elevated serum potassium levels and cardiac dysrhythmias. Sodium level may increase in burn tissue, taking water with it. When the victim begins diuresis after approximately 48 hours, potassium and sodium are excreted. Careful monitoring of electrolyte levels is important so that replacement therapy can be initiated.

In some burns, there is a substantial loss of red blood cells, intensifying the effects of plasma loss. This usually occurs in deep burns and seems to be a gradual process. The loss of red blood cells is due in part to hemolysis in the burned area, which results in hemoglobinemia and hemoglobinuria soon after the burn occurs. Free hemoglobin in the plasma indicates a severe burn. For 24 to 48 hours, delayed hemolysis of partially damaged red blood cells occurs. Further decrease in red blood cells results from thrombosis and sludging. Anemia develops as a result of red cell loss as well as with bleeding during debridement and other causes.

Additional fluid is lost as insensible water loss from evaporation from the burn wound surface and through the respiratory system. Respiratory loss also may be enhanced when there is inhalation injury. Signs and symptoms of fluid deficiency include thirst, restlessness, and disorientation. Plain water given to relieve thirst may lead to water intoxication; to avoid this, solutions with balanced electrolytes must be administered. Fluids are usually given intravenously because vomiting and paralytic ileus frequently occur after burn injury.

The fluid loss causes a reduction of circulatory blood volume, which can result in reduced cardiac output and inadequate tissue perfusion. Tissue hypoxia may result, causing a shift to anaerobic cellular metabolism. Acidosis and irreversible burn shock can occur. Blood urea levels may rise if protein catabolism is excessive or if large amounts of nitrogen are released from burned tissue in the presence of oliguria.

The respiratory system is often altered by burn injury, by inhalation injury, and by therapy. Heat exposure and irritants cause swelling and tissue breakdown. Respiratory tissues are irritated by gases from burning materials, such as carbon monoxide. Altered circulation may lead to inadequate pulmonary circulation. Hypoxia may result from the decreased amount of oxygen circulating. Aspiration pneumonia may develop from vomiting episodes. Tracheal or laryngeal obstruction may result from edema in the head and neck region, causing pressure against the trachea and larynx. Also, inflamed linings of trachea and larynx swell and block the airway.[6] Edema under tight eschar in burns of the torso restricts chest movements, which may lead to restrictive respiratory problems. Adult respiratory distress syndrome is an ominous complication of burn injury that frequently results after inhalation injury, shock, or severe hypoxia. Finally, pulmonary emboli are always a danger as a result of changes in the vasculature, sepsis, and immobilization.

Physical findings in the respiratory system include singed nasal hairs and reddened or dark pharynx. Irritation and heat damage to respiratory tissue may lead to respiratory stridor, dyspnea, and copious secretions, often carbonaceous.[6] Deep full-thickness burns of the face also cause burning of pharyngeal tissues. Laryngeal edema, focal erosion, focal laryngitis, and necrosis may be evident. Edema may be exhibited by hoarseness. Respiratory disorders that may occur during the course of therapy include pneumonia, atelectasis, obstruction from mucus plugs, adult respiratory distress syndrome, and septic emboli from infected venosections.

The gastrointestinal tract usually exhibits a decrease

in activity.[5] Secondary pathologies include acute stress (Curling's) ulcers, gastric dilatation, paralytic ileus, and bleeding. Acute gastric and duodenal ulcers in burn victims are morphologically identical to acute stress ulcers in persons without burns. Acute stress ulcers in persons with and without burns are mostly gastric. They occur in 20% to 30% of persons with total body surface burns. Ulcers may occur in the stomach, duodenum, or both. The anatomic location of stress ulcers differs from that of peptic and duodenal ulcers not caused by stress. Stress gastric ulcers are present in the fundic mucosa as opposed to the pyloric mucosa of other gastric ulcers. Stress duodenal ulcers are located in the posterior, rather than the anterior, duodenum. They have several foci when they occur in the stomach and a single focus when they occur in the duodenum.[7] Gastric ulcers are generally smaller than duodenal ulcers. Those measuring 2 to 3 mm are difficult to see during gastroscopy but are deep enough to cause significant bleeding. Many ulcers are hidden in the rugal folds. Stress ulcers exhibit a relative lack of inflammatory response, which may be due to the finding that many occur in the terminal stages of burn illness. Many of these stress ulcers are colonized with gram-negative bacilli. Vascular congestion and submucosal edema are often present. The most commonly held hypothesis for stress ulcers in postburn situations is ischemic hypoxia that may damage the mucosal barrier and allow back diffusion of hydrogen ions.[7] Bleeding and perforation are common complications.

Gastric dilatation and paralytic ileus may appear early after burn injury. These conditions are neurologic in origin, may be secondary to fear or pain, or may occur as a result of hypovolemia or sepsis.[5]

Liver dysfunction often occurs with burn injury. Factors that contribute to liver dysfunction include bacterial infection, lack of proper nutrition, drugs, anesthesia, blood transfusions leading to viral or serum hepatitis, and hepatic hypoxemia. Hepatic hypoxemia seems to result from a decrease in circulating fluid volume. The necrosis that results is usually minimal and focal, of a fatty nature, and reversible.

The kidney changes that occur may be permanent or temporary. Temporary kidney changes are manifested by oliguria, which results from a decreased glomerular filtration rate from the decreased circulating blood volume. Blood urea nitrogen and creatinine levels are elevated, and the level of antidiuretic hormone may be increased (see pp. 658–662). Tubular damage may occur when the kidney is presented with an increased amount of protein breakdown products from the burn. If there is a history of kidney disorder or if the person does not receive adequate treatment, permanent damage may occur. Hematuria may be present as a result of damaged red blood cells. Death may result from acute renal insufficiency despite adequate treatment.

Stress from the burn injury enhances the secretion

of adrenocortical hormones. These hormones, especially cortisone, may help to stabilize the lysosome membranes, decrease inflammation, and prevent an overwhelming response. The long-term effect of adrenocortical stimulation is that these hormones depress the immune response and make the person more vulnerable to infection (see p. 700).

Problems in coagulation may occur after severe burn injury and may result from the burn, from complications secondary to the injury, or from therapy. Abnormalities include decreases in platelet count, altered clot retraction time, and prolonged partial thromboplastin and prothrombin times along with elevated fibrinogen levels. These coagulation defects seem to occur in large burns involving large body surface areas as well as in smaller burns. Consumption or use of clotting factors plays a role in coagulopathies, such as disseminated intravascular coagulation (see pp. 418–419).

Wound infections are a major problem in burns and may lead to sepsis, which is the most common cause of death.[9] The frequency of infection is correlated with the extent and depth of the injury and with the success of treatment measures. Bacteria, both gram-positive and gram-negative, invade the wound surface and eventually reach the viable surrounding tissue. Products liberated by the bacteria can produce septic shock. In a large study of burn wound colonization and treatment, numerous strains of bacteria colonized the wounds within the first 24 hours. If treatment measures were ineffective, penetration into the deeper tissues occurred and sepsis often resulted.[12] The study demonstrated the importance of decreasing the size of open, full-thickness wounds to prevent infection.

Electrical Burn Injuries

Various lesions occur as a result of electrical burns. Six factors determine the extent of these injuries: 1) type of current (direct or alternating); 2) voltage of current; 3) resistance of body tissues; 4) value of current flowing through the tissues; 5) pathway of the current through the body; and 6) duration of the contact with the electrical source.

Direct current does not produce the same contraction of muscle, and low-voltage direct current is not as dangerous as alternating current. High-voltage direct current, however, is often fatal.

Alternating current produces tetanic muscle contraction at low voltages, which prevents the victim from releasing contact with the circuit. These low-voltage currents often result in ventricular fibrillation.[11] Low voltage means less than 500 volts, and high voltage is greater than 500 volts. Low-voltage injuries most often occur in the home and are likely to involve children and infants. The usual source of current is a household plug; a curious child may stick a small object into the outlet. High-

voltage injury commonly occurs in adults working with electric lines or equipment. These injuries have a high mortality, often due to cardiac asystole.

The body tissues offer varying degrees of resistance to electrical current. The resistance of tissues, in order of least to greatest, is as follows: nerves, blood, muscles, skin, tendons, fat, and bone. Skin resistance varies from person to person. The epidermis is nonvascular and offers high resistance when it is dry, but when wet, moisture decreases resistance and enhances the flow of current. The dermis offers low resistance because it is highly vascular.

Thin skin is less resistant than thick skin, making the palms and soles most resistant. Usually, the greater the skin resistance, the greater the local burn, and the less the skin resistance, the more the internal injury. Current in contact with the skin eventually causes blistering. Blisters are moist and conduct current through the skin along the tissues of least resistance—blood vessels and nerves. Vessel walls are damaged and thrombi occur, often at a site far from the site of the electrical injury, making it difficult to evaluate the full extent of damage at the initial evaluation. Progressive tissue necrosis can occur for 12 to 14 days after the injury.[17]

Electric current may flow through the heart, producing ventricular fibrillation and often immediate death. High-voltage current often travels to the respiratory center of the brain, causing respiratory arrest and death.[17] Neurologic complications are the most common results of electrical injury and include varying levels of unconsciousness and spinal cord injuries. In burned extremities, peripheral neuropathies are common.[11]

The value of the alternating current flowing through the body determines the resulting injury. Contact with a circuit produces muscle contraction, which may be severe enough to prevent the victim from releasing himself or herself from the source of current. If cardiac or respiratory arrest does not occur and the victim remains conscious, he or she may report ringing in the ears and deafness for a time or visual disturbances, such as flashes and brilliant luminous spots. The pathway through the body is also important in determining the extent of injury. The longer the contact, the greater the amount of damage.

The injury in electrical burns may be one or more of three types: 1) entry and exit wounds; 2) electrothermal burns (flash or arc burns); and 3) flame burns. The *entry wound* occurs at the contact site. It may be small or large and usually appears as an ischemic, yellow-white, coagulated area, or it may be charred. It is dry and painless, and the edges are well-defined. However, the extent of damage may be far greater than is evident on the surface. Necrosis of subcutaneous tissues and muscle from arterial thrombi may occur, or lack of thrombosis may cause hemorrhaging. Damage may be due to heat from the passage of current or due to the action of the current itself.[31] The *exit wound* appears as a blowout type of injury caused by arcing current between victim and a nearby ground. It is a dry area with depressed edges. This exit wound is usually more severe than the entry wound.[31]

Electrothermal burns are from the heat of the current passing near, but not through, the skin. The depth of the wound depends on the closeness to the electrical source. These are mainly associated with high-voltage current. The electricity arc leaping from the high current has a temperature of 2,500°C. *Flame burns* occur when heat from an electrical current ignites clothing. They may cause more serious injury than the electric injury itself.

The tetanic contractions that lock the victim to the electric source may cause fractures and dislocations of joints. Cataracts often develop months to years after an electrical injury involving the head area. Abdominal injury may occur as a result of electrical trauma to the abdomen. The extent of injury is difficult to determine initially. Abdominal symptoms may not arise until days after the injury. Renal involvement seems to be more prevalent in electrical than in thermal injury. The damage may be caused by the initial electric shock, direct current damage to the kidneys or kidney vessels, abnormal protein breakdown in the damaged tissue, or a combination of all three.[31]

Chemical Burn Injuries

Chemical burns result from exposure to acids or alkaline chemicals (Table 47-6). Most lethal burns result from military conflict and industrial accidents. Domestic and laboratory accidents and criminal assaults usually result in smaller areas of damage.[17] The injury may result from chemical changes as well as from thermal injury to the tissues, depending on the nature of the chemical.

Tissue damage depends on five factors: 1) pH or concentration of the chemical; 2) amount of agent contacting the skin; 3) duration of contact; 4) amount of tissue penetration; and 5) mechanism of action of the chemical.[17] Chemical changes in tissues include denaturation, precipitation, alkalization, edema, separation of the epidermis from the dermis, disorganization of epidermal appendages, and widening and coalescence of collagen bundles.

Chemical agents are often classified by the way in

TABLE 47-6 *Chemical Burns: Pathophysiology and Treatment*

Type	Mechanism	Appearance	Treatment Cleanse	Treatment Neutralize	Treatment Debride
ACID BURNS					
Sulfuric Nitric Hydrochloric Trichloroacetic	Exothermic reaction; cell dehydration; protein precipitation	Gray, yellow; brown, black; soft to leathery eschar	Water	Sodium bicarbonate	Debride
Phenol			Ethyl alcohol	Sodium bicarbonate	Debride
Hydrofluoric			Water	Sodium bicarbonate; magnesium oxide; glycerin paste; calcium gluconate	Debride
ALKALI BURNS					
Potassium hydroxide Sodium hydroxide	Exothermic reaction; cellular dehydration; saponification of fat; protein precipitation	Erythema and blister; soapy, thick eschar; painful	Water	Acetic acid or ammonium chloride	Debride
Lime			Brush off lime powder	Acetic acid or ammonium chloride	Debride
Ammonia	Same as above, plus laryngeal and pulmonary edema	Gray, yellow; brown, black; soft leathery texture	Water	Acetic acid or ammonium chloride	Debride
Phosphorous	Thermal effect; melts at body temperature; runs and ignites at 34°C	Gray, blue, green; flows in dark; depressed, leathery eschar	Water	Copper sulfate	Debride and remove phosphorous particles

(Arndt, K. *Manual of Dermatologic Therapeutics* [4th ed.]. Boston: Little, Brown, 1989.)

which they affect protein. Oxidizing agents are corrosive and cause extensive protein denaturation. Some agents are desiccants and cause cellular dehydration. Others cause anoxic tissue damage.[17] The depth of chemical burns is often difficult to evaluate.

Acid burns most frequently occur in industrial plants as immersion injuries. They are often a result of splattering or spilling of an acid substance. The wound is painful and persists because of the chemical action. Its depth and appearance vary, depending on the amount of acid and length of exposure. Systemic changes are rare, but acid fumes may be inhaled. Treatment is best accomplished by initial dilution of the acid.

Alkali burns result from chemical irritation from a highly alkaline substance. One example is phosphorus burns, which are painful and often occur as a result of warfare. Phosphorus melts at body temperature and penetrates into tissue. When exposed to air, the wound smokes; in the dark, it glows bluish green. Copper sulfate is used to treat these burns by inactivating the phosphorus. The chemical is then removed surgically. Caution must be used in working with copper, as its use may result in copper toxicity with massive hemolysis of red blood cells and acute renal tubular necrosis.

Complications of all types of burn wounds include infection, contractures from scarring, renal failure, ulcers, liver failure, pneumonia, urinary tract infection, and acidosis. The frequency of complications increases with the severity of the burn.

Toxic Epidermal Necrolysis

This is a general term for a group of conditions of varying etiologies, also called Stevens-Johnson syndrome or staphyloccal scalded-skin syndrome, depending on the associated cause. It is very important to determine the causative factor in treating the condition. The condition is characterized by sloughing of the epidermal layer of the skin in response to a triggering agent. The most commonly described etiologic agents are drugs (especially anticonvulsants, sulfonamides, antibiotics, barbiturates, allopurinol, and nonsteroidal anti-inflammatory agents), toxins, graft-versus-host disease, and bacterial and viral infections. The onset of the disease is usually sudden and targets the destruction of the skin and mucous membranes. There is full-thickness destruction of the epidermis and widespread formation of blisters. The skin may peel, and as much as 95% of the epidermis may slough off. Mucous membranes may be edematous, eroded, and bleeding. The mortality of this condition is very high, with death usually being caused by sepsis. Improvement in mortality has resulted from early recognition of the cause of the process and discontinuation of the offending drug with treatment of the cause.

DECUBITUS ULCERS (PRESSURE SORES)

The word *decubitus* derives from the Latin *decumbo*, meaning "lying down."[23] During the late 19th and early 20th centuries, persons with decubitus ulcers generally had wasting diseases, such as tuberculosis, osteomyelitis, and chronic renal failure. Currently, persons at risk have conditions that alter mobility, including individuals with spinal cord injuries, the ill elderly who are incontinent, or persons who are bed- or wheelchairbound. Decubitus ulcers are significant health problems because they increase the length of hospitalization, increase health care costs, and increase the chances of death. Four crucial factors play a role in decubitus formation: 1) pressure; 2) shearing forces; 3) friction; and 4) moisture. Pressure is the most crucial factor, and these ulcers are accurately called *pressure sores*.

Pressure is defined as the exertion of force on a surface by an object in contact with the surface.[26] The force is the weight of the individual applied onto the object on which he or she is lying. Pressure is not evenly distributed over the body when one is lying or sitting. It is greatest over bony prominences, and it is over these areas that decubitus ulcers develop. A balance exists between interstitial pressure and solid tissue pressure to make a total tissue pressure of zero. With an increase in external pressure over an area, the interstitial fluid pressure increases, elevating total tissue pressure. As a result, capillary and arteriolar pressures rise, causing fluid to filter from capillaries. Edema and autolysis of cells follow. As the pressure continues, lymph vessels are occluded, resulting in accumulation of anaerobic metabolic wastes and tissue necrosis.[22] The duration and magnitude of pressure are key factors in the amount of tissue damage. With high pressure, it takes less time for tissue necrosis to occur. Constant pressure of 70 mm Hg for more than 1 hour can produce irreversible tissue damage, depending on the condition of the skin and the person's nutritional status.[26] If pressure is intermittently relieved, tissue change is minimal.

As a pressure sore develops, the first sign is skin erythema from reactive hyperemia. Continuous pressure causes tissue necrosis, and initially an eschar forms that covers and protects the wound. Loss of eschar allows bacterial invasion, and infection results.[26]

The sliding of adjacent tissue layers provides a progressive relative displacement of tissues. These *shearing forces* may be accentuated when the head of the bed is raised and the torso of the person slides down, exerting pressure to the sacrum and deep fascia while the posterior sacral skin is fixed. The shearing force in the deep superficial fascia stretches and angulates blood and lymph vessels, causes thrombosis, and undermines the dermis. The subcutaneous fat layer lacks tensile strength and is vulnerable to the mechanical shearing force. The two surfaces that are in contact move across each other, causing friction. This action removes the outer protective stratum corneum and hastens the onset of ulceration. The friction that occurs when a person is dragged across bed sheets is called *sheet burn*. The sacral ulcer commonly is formed in this way.[23]

Fecal matter, urine, and perspiration irritate and macerate the skin, softening it and making it more vulnerable to pressure sore formation.

Classification and Treatment of Decubitus Ulcers

Decubitus ulcers are graded according to the depth of tissue loss. The usual scale is Grade I to IV, with III and IV putting the affected person at risk for infection and loss of function.[23, 27] Table 47-7 describes these grades, and they are illustrated in Figure 47-13. In Grade I, the sore is reversible. It resembles an abrasion of the epidermis, exposing the underlying dermis. An acute inflammatory response occurs: the wound is irregular in shape; is red, warm, and indurated; and is painful for a normally innervated person. Relief of pressure and local cleansing usually resolve the ulcer in 5 to 10 days.

A Grade II decubitus ulcer is also reversible. As pressure continues, the entire dermis is affected. The wound appears as a shallow full-thickness ulcer with distinct edges, early fibrosis, and skin color changes. The inflammatory response is present. Relief of pressure and local cleansing allow the wound to heal.

In Grade III, the decubitus is extended downward, and the epidermis, dermis, and subcutaneous tissues are involved. This full-thickness skin defect spreads peripherally, because the fascia underlying the subcutaneous layer is resistant to pressure. A small broken area may appear on the surface, with a larger area beneath. The epidermis thickens and rolls over the wound edge toward the ulcer base. The ulcer has a dark-light pigmentation. The skin layers are completely distorted, and the wound begins to drain foul-smelling fluid. Systemic problems begin to occur in a Grade III decubitus ulcer. Fluid and protein are lost, and the person may experience fever, dehydration, anemia, and leukocytosis.

In a Grade IV wound, the fascia underlying the subcutaneous tissue is penetrated and the wound is rapidly undermined. Complications include osteomyelitis of bone, sepsis, joint dislocations, and release of toxins. The condition may be fatal.[27]

A closed decubitus has no external opening but, inside, may act and appear as a Grade III or IV lesion. These ulcers occur after long pressure insults with shear stress. A bursalike cavity forms and is filled with debris from the necrosis of subcutaneous and deeper areas. This type of decubitus ulcer often occurs over ischial tuberosities. Eventually, the overlying skin ruptures.

Another concept that forms the basis of wound care uses a three-color concept for open wounds—red, yellow, and black. *Red* refers to the color of healthy granulation tissue and indicates that normal healing is occur-

TABLE 47-7 *Classification of Decubitus Ulcers*

Grade	Layers of Skin	Wound Appearance	Systemic Changes	Resolution
I	Partial-thickness	Irregular; warm; erythema; painful; edematous	None	Reversible with relief of pressure and local cleansing
II	Partial-thickness Epidermis Dermis	Shallow skin ulcer; edges distinct; fibrosis; skin color changes	None	Reversible with relief of pressure and local cleansing
III	Full-thickness Epidermis Dermis Subcutaneous layer	Thick epidermal ulcer margin; light and dark pigmentation; skin layers distorted; drains foul-smelling fluid	Infection; fat necrosis; loss of fluid and protein; fever; dehydration; anemia; leukocytosis	Relief of pressure; systemic treatment with I.V. fluids; diet; medications; debridement and would graft
IV	Full-thickness Epidermis Dermis Subcutaneous fat Fascia Muscle Bone	Large open area; bone shows through	Osteomyelitis; sepsis; joint dislocation; toxic; can be fatal	Radical surgery to remove necrotic area; general support measures (I.V.; diet; medications)
	Closed subcutaneous tissue and deeper	No external sign until later, when skin ruptures; inside appears as a Grade III or IV wound; bursalike cavity with necrotic debris	Infrequent infection	Wide excision; removal of bursal sac; flap graft with muscle

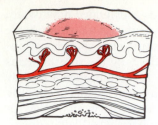

Grade 1

- Resembles an abrasion with epidermal involvement
- Wound red, warm, indurated

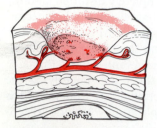

Grade 2

- Entire dermis affected
- Shallow ulcer with red area around margins

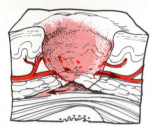

Grade 3

- Epidermis, dermis, and subcutaneous tissue involved
- Spreads along fascial plane
- Wound drains purulent and/or foul smelling fluid
- Systemic infection can occur

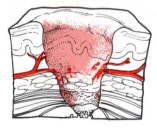

Grade 4

- Invades fascia, bone, muscle, connective tissue
- May cause osteomyelitis, sepsis, and joint dislocation

FIGURE 47-13 *Grading of a decubitus ulcer.*

ring. *Yellow* is the color of suppurative exudate that results from microorganisms in the wound. The presence of this pus interferes with the normal healing process. *Black* is the color of necrotic tissue. The dead tissue also becomes a focus of infection and more tissue loss.[27] The black wound requires debridement, antibiotic therapy, and moist dressings.

OTHER TRAUMAS

Other traumas to the skin include blunt wounds, abrasions (scrapes), incised wounds (as an incision), puncture wounds, and lacerations (cuts). An abrasion is a superficial open wound in which the outer surface layers of skin are scraped off. Nerve endings are exposed and bleeding is minimal. The wound often contains foreign matter that may initiate an inflammatory response. This type of wound normally heals spontaneously. An incision is a clean, straight-edged wound that goes through

all layers of skin; it bleeds freely and heals cleanly when sutured.

Puncture or stab wounds are deeper than they are wide and are caused by such objects as knives, pins, needles, and spikes. Underlying structures may be damaged, with concealed blood loss. A laceration is a cut or tear of tissues and is unlikely to heal without treatment.

In all traumatic skin wounds, tissue viability is crucial and depends on circulation of blood to the area. All open traumatic wounds are contaminated, and host resistance must be supported.[24] The stages of wound healing, discussed on pages 305–308, involve a characteristic inflammatory response initiated by a vasoconstriction that decreases bleeding. This is followed by vasodilatation and increased vascular permeability, leaking plasma proteins into the wound. The final stage involves neutrophilic leukocytes that destroy bacteria.[8] This produces pus and suppuration of surrounding tissues. If the affected tissue can totally regenerate, it replaces the necrotic tissue. Scar formation may become necessary to bridge an area of tissue destruction.

▼ Chapter Summary

▼ Alterations in the integrity of the skin are common problems that may reflect the general health of the individual or skin-specific disorders. Skin conditions may be caused by allergic reactions, infections of all types, or skin tumors. Allergic reactions and other idiopathic conditions include dermatitis and scaling disorders of the skin, such as psoriasis.

▼ Any type of organism can cause manifestations on the skin. These may be vesicles, pustules, nodules, or other lesions. Tumors of the skin are often related to sun exposure. Some are benign and seen as a consequence of aging. Malignant tumors include basal cell and squamous cell carcinoma and malignant melanoma.

▼ Traumatic skin alterations include such common conditions as abrasions, burns, and decubitus ulcers. Burn injury may be partial-thickness or full-thickness, and the systemic response depends on the amount and depth of burn surface. Burns may be caused by heat or flame, electrical injury, or chemical injury.

▼ Decubitus ulcers are common pressure and shear-related skin injuries especially seen among elderly persons and persons with spinal cord injuries. Neglected decubitus ulcers can lead to sepsis and death.

▼ References

1. Arndt, K. *Manual of Dermatologic Therapeutics* (4th ed.). Boston: Little, Brown, 1989.
2. Balch, C.M., Houghton, A.N., and Peters, L.J. Cutaneous melanoma. In V.T. DeVita, S. Hellman, and S.A. Rosen-

berg (ed.), *Cancer: Principles and Practice of Oncology* (4th ed.). Philadelphia: J.B. Lippincott, 1993.

3. Bauer, E.F., Tabas, M., and Goslen, J.B. Psoriasis and other proliferative disorders of epithelium. In W.N. Kelley (ed.), *Textbook of Internal Medicine* (2nd ed.). Philadelphia: J.B. Lippincott, 1992.

4. Brodzka, W., Thornhill, H.L., and Howard, S. Burns: Causes and risk factors. *Arch. Phys. Med. Rehab.* 66(11): 746, 1985.

5. Burgess, M.C. Initial management of a patient with extensive burn injury. *Crit. Care Nurs. Clin. North Am.* (3):2,165, 1991.

6. Cioffi, W.G., and Rue, L.W. Diagnosis and treatment of inhalation injuries. *Crit. Care Nurs. Clin. North Am.* (3):2, 191, 1991.

7. Crawford, J.M. The gastrointestinal tract. In R. Cotran, V. Kumar, and S. Robbins (eds.). *Robbin's Pathologic Basis of Disease* (5th ed.). Philadelphia: W.B. Saunders, 1994.

8. Cuono, C.B. Physiology of wound healing. In F.J. Dagher (ed.), *Cutaneous Wounds*. Mt. Kisco, N.Y.: Futura, 1985.

9. Duncan, D.J., and Driscoll, D.M. Burn wound management. *Crit. Care Nurs. Clin. North Am.* (3):2, 199, 1991.

10. Elder, D.E., and Clark, W.H. Malignant melanoma. In B.H. Thiers and R.L. Dobson (eds.), *Pathogenesis of Skin Disease*. New York: Churchill-Livingstone, 1986.

11. Heimbach, D.M. Electrical injury. In W.N. Kelley (ed.), *Textbook of Internal Medicine* (2nd ed.). Philadelphia: J.B. Lippincott, 1992.

12. Kagan, R.J., et al. Serious wound infections in burned patients. *Surgery* 98(4)10:640, 1985.

13. Katz, S. Approach to the management of skin cancers. In W.N. Kelley (ed.), *Textbook of Internal Medicine* (2nd ed.). Philadelphia: J.B. Lippincott, 1992.

14. Lang, P.C. Nonmelanoma skin cancer. In B.H. Thiers and R.L. Dobson (eds.), *Pathogenesis of Skin Disease*. New York: Churchill-Livingstone, 1986.

15. Lawley, T.J., and Yancey, K.B. Examination of the skin. In J. Wilson et al. (eds.), *Harrison's Principles of Internal Medicine* (12th ed.). New York: McGraw-Hill, 1991.

16. Moschella, S.L., Pillsbury, D.M., and Hurley, H.J. *Dermatology* (3rd ed.). Philadelphia: W.B. Saunders, 1992.

17. Munster, A.M., and Ciccone, T.G. Burns. In F.J. Dagher (ed.), *Cutaneous Wounds*. Mt. Kisco, N.Y.: Futura, 1985.

18. Murphy, G.F., and Mihm, M.C. The skin. In R. Cotran, V. Kumar, and S.L. Robbins (eds.), *Robbins' Pathologic Basis of Disease* (5th ed.). Philadelphia: W.B. Saunders, 1994.

19. Prigel, C. How to spot melanoma. *Nursing 87* 17(6):60, 1987.

20. Rue, L.W., and Cioffi, W.G. Resuscitation of thermally injured patients. *Crit. Care Nurs. Clin. North Am.* (3):2, 181, 1991.

21. Safai, B. Cancers of the skin. In V.T. DeVita, S. Hellmann, and S.A. Rosenberg (eds.). *Cancer: Principles and Practice of Oncology* (4th ed.). Philadelphia: J.B. Lippincott, 1993.

22. Sauer, G.C. *Manual of Skin Diseases* (6th ed.). Philadelphia: J.B. Lippincott, 1991.

23. Sebern, M. Home-team strategies for treating pressure sores. *Nursing 87* 17(4):50, 1987.

24. Shack, R.B., and Manson, P.N. Traumatic wounds. In F.J. Dagher (ed.), *Cutaneous Wounds*. Mt. Kisco, N.Y.: Futura, 1985.

25. Soter, N.A., and Baden, H.P. (eds.). *Pathophysiology of Dermatologic Diseases* (2nd ed.) New York: McGraw-Hill, 1991.

26. Steuber, K., and Spence, R.J. Pressure sores. In F.J. Dagher (ed.), *Cutaneous Wounds*. Mt. Kisco, N.Y.: Futura, 1985.

27. Stotts, N. Seeing red and yellow and black: The three color concept of wound care. *Nursing 90* 20(2):59, 1990.

28. Udey, M., and Goslen, J. Allergic urticaria and erythema multiforme. In W.N. Kelley (ed.), *Textbook of Internal Medicine* (2nd ed.). Philadelphia: J.B. Lippincott, 1992.

29. Udey, M., and Goslen, J. Cutaneous reactions to drugs. In W.N. Kelley (ed.), *Textbook of Internal Medicine* (2nd ed.). Philadelphia: J.B. Lippincott, 1992.

30. Udey, M., Goslen, J., and Tabas, M. Immunologic and allergic cutaneous disorders. In W.N. Kelley (ed.), *Textbook of Internal Medicine* (2nd ed.). Philadelphia: J.B. Lippincott, 1992.

31. Wallace, J. Electrical injuries. In J. Wilson. et al. (eds.), *Harrison's Principles of Internal Medicine* (12th ed.). New York: McGraw-Hill, 1991.

▼ *Unit Bibliography*

Ackerman, A.B. *Differential Diagnosis in Dermatopathology* (2nd ed.). Philadelphia: Lea and Febiger, 1992.

Arndt, K. *Manual of Dermatologic Therapeutics* (4th ed.). Boston: Little, Brown, 1989.

Arnold, H.L., and Odom, R.B. *Andrew's Diseases of the Skin* (8th ed.). Philadelphia: W.B. Saunders, 1990.

Bauer, E., Tabas, M., and Goslen, J. Skin: Cells, matrix and function. In W.N. Kelley (ed.), *Textbook of Internal Medicine* (2nd ed.). Philadelphia: J.B. Lippincott, 1992.

Becker, Y. *Skin Langerhan's (Dendritic) Cells in Virus Infections and AIDS*. Norwell, Mass.: Kluwer, 1991.

Champion, R.H., Burton, J.L., and Ebling, F.J.G. *Textbook of Dermatology*. Boston: Blackwell Scientific, 1992.

Cormack, D. *Ham's Histology* (9th ed.). Philadelphia: J.B. Lippincott, 1987.

Cotran, R.S., Kumar, V., and Robbins, S.L. *Robbins' Pathologic Basis of Disease* (5th ed.). Philadelphia: W.B. Saunders, 1994.

Daghar, F.J. (ed.). *Cutaneous Wounds*. Mt. Kisco, N.Y.: Futura, 1985.

DuVivier, A. *Atlas of Clinical Dermatology* (2nd ed.). New York: Gower, 1993.

Farmer, E.R., and Hood, A.F. *Pathology of the Skin*. Norwalk, Conn.: Appleton-Lange, 1990.

Fitzpatrick, T.B. *Dermatology in General Medicine* (4th ed.). New York: McGraw-Hill, 1993.

Goldsmith, L.A. *Biochemistry and Physiology of the Skin*. New York: Oxford University Press, 1983.

Goldstein, B.G., and Goldstein, A.O. *Practical Dermatology*. St. Louis: Mosby Yearbook, 1992.

Govan, A.D.T., Macfarlane, P.S., and Callander, R. *Pathology Illustrated* (3rd ed.). New York: Churchill Livingstone, 1991.

Guyton, A.C. *Textbook of Medical Physiology* (8th ed.). Philadelphia: W.B. Saunders, 1991.

Habif, T.P. *Clinical Dermatology* (2nd ed.). St. Louis: C.V. Mosby, 1990.

Haponik, E.F., and Munster, A.M. *Respiratory Injury: Smoke Inhalation and Bunrs*. New York: McGraw-Hill, 1990.

Hill, M.I. *Skin Disorders*. St. Louis: C.V. Mosby, 1994.

Lapibere, C.M., and Krieg, T. *Connective Tissue Disease of the Skin*. New York: M. Dekker, 1993.

Lookingbill, D.P., and Marks, J.G. *Principles of Dermatology* (2nd ed.). Philadelphia: W.B. Saunders, 1993.

Martyn, J.A.J. *Acute Management of the Burned Patient.* Philadelphia: W.B. Saunders, 1990.

McLaughlin, E.G. *Critical Care of the Burn Patient.* Rockville, Md.: Aspen Publishing, 1990.

Moschella, S. and Hurley, H. *Dermatology* (3rd ed.). Philadelphia: W.B. Saunders, 1992.

Munster, A.M. *Severe Burns: A Family Guide to Medical and Emotional Recovery.* Baltimore: Johns Hopkins, 1993.

Patterson, J.A. *Skin Disorders: Diagnosis and Treatment.* New York: Igaku-Shoin, 1989.

Patterson, J.W., and Blalock, W.K. *Dermatology: A Concise Textbook.* New York: Medical Exam, 1987.

Richard, R. *Burn Care and Rehabilitation: Principles and Practice.* Philadelphia: F.A. Davis, 1994.

Rosen, K., Lanning, M., and Hill, M. *The Nurse's Atlas of Dermatology.* Boston: Little, Brown, 1983.

Rubin, E., and Farber, J.L. *Pathology* (2nd ed.). Philadelphia: J.B. Lippincott, 1994.

Rylah, L.T.A. *Critical Care of Burned Patient.* New York: Cambridge Univ. Press, 1992.

Sams, W.M., and Lynch, P.J. *Principles and Practice of Dermatology.* Edinburgh: Churchill-Livingstone, 1990.

Sauer, G.C. *Manual of Skin Diseases* (6th ed.). Philadelphia: J.B. Lippincott, 1991.

Soter, N.A., and Baden, H.P. (eds.). *Pathophysiology of Dermatologic Diseases.* New York: McGraw-Hill, 1984.

Stevens, A., Wheater, P., and Lowe, J.S. *Clinical Dermatopathology.* Edinburgh: Churchill-Livingstone, 1989.

Thiers, B.H., and Dobson, R.L. *Pathogenesis of Skin Disease.* Edinburgh: Churchill-Livingstone, 1986.

Tortora, G.J., and Grabowski, S.R. *Principles of Anatomy and Physiology* (7th ed.). New York: Harper Collins. 1993.

Trofino, B. *Nursing Care of Burn Injured Patient.* Philadelphia: F.A. Davis, 1991.

Wardrope, J., and Smith, J.A.R. *The Management of Wounds and Burns.* New York: Oxford University Press, 1992.

Neural Control

THE NERVOUS system is incredibly complex and must be approached from an adequate basic knowledge of neural control. This approach considers the complicated system of connections and interconnections that allow for perception and movement. The advanced nervous system allows for the achievement of complicated thought and reasoning powers. Chapter 48 begins the discussion with the normal structure and function of the nervous system. Chapter 49 adds the normal and altered function of the special senses. Chapter 50 details some alterations that affect higher cortical functions, especially cerebrovascular accident, aphasia, agnosia, and epilepsy. Chapter 51 covers the physiologic phenomena of pain. Chapters 52, 53, and 54 detail traumatic alterations, tumors and infections, and degenerative alterations, respectively. Each chapter presents specific diagnostic tests that may be helpful in delineating these alterations. The most useful approach to the nervous system is to show how alterations in specific areas can disrupt function. Frequently, the location of the alterations rather than their size finally determines the degree of functional difficulty. The reader is again encouraged to use the learning objectives to organize study and to acquire a firm grasp of the material in Chapter 48 before considering the pathophysiology of the nervous system. The unit bibliography provides further resources for learning.

Chapter 48

Normal Structure and Function of the Central and Peripheral Nervous Systems

Reet Henze

▼ CHAPTER OUTLINE

▼ LEARNING OBJECTIVES

1 Describe variations in neuron morphology, and classify neurons according to morphology and function.
2 Explain the events occurring with axon injury and regeneration.
3 Discuss **membrane potential** and action potential.
4 List the major types of nerve fibers and their characteristics.
5 Identify factors that influence conduction velocity in nerve fibers.
6 Identify factors that increase and decrease neuron membrane excitability.
7 Describe the types of **sensory receptors** and the phenomenon of receptor adaptation.
8 Discuss the events occurring at the chemical synapse.
9 Discuss characteristics of neurotransmitters.
10 List the major structures of the central nervous system in hierarchical order from spinal cord to cerebral cortex.
11 Identify the major functions of the central nervous system structures.
12 Trace and identify major information transmitted by the major ascending and descending spinal tracts.
13 List the components of the peripheral nervous system.
14 Differentiate between structure and function of the somatic efferent and the visceral efferent fibers.
15 Contrast the functions of the sympathetic and parasympathetic divisions of the autonomic nervous system.
16 Differentiate between adrenergic and cholinergic effector organs.
17 Describe the function, formation, composition, and flow of cerebrospinal fluid.
18 Discuss the mechanism and function of the blood–brain barrier.
19 List the major arteries supplying blood to the brain.
20 Discuss the factors responsible for a constant cerebral blood supply in the healthy brain.
21 Describe the indications for and procedures performed in the following diagnostic studies in head and spine injuries: radiographs, angiography, digital subtraction angiography, CT scan, MRI, echoencephalography, transcranial Doppler sonography, brain scan, PET, lumbar puncture, myelography, and EEG.

Barbara L. Bullock: PATHOPHYSIOLOGY: ADAPTATIONS AND ALTERATIONS IN FUNCTION, 4th ed.
© 1996 Lippincott-Raven Publishers

Humans interact with the environment through the nervous system, perceiving and responding to the stimuli that continually impinge on them. A complex system of connections and interconnections of nerve cells provides this perception, interim processing, and response. In addition, characteristics that endow humans with the ability to think, feel, reason, and remember evolve from these interacting neuronal networks of the brain.

▼ *The Neuron*

The neuron is the structural and functional unit of nerve tissue, which has the capability to generate and conduct electrochemical impulses (Fig. 48-1). Its cellular and cytoplasmic components and metabolic activities that maintain cell life are similar to those of other cells. The distinctive cellular shapes of neurons and their structural synapses that allow transmission of impulses from one to another are unique to the nerve cells. Unlike other cells, the mature neurons are unable to reproduce themselves. They lack centrosomes and, therefore, are incapable of mitosis. If the cell body dies, the entire neuron dies. Under certain circumstances, however, axons of peripheral nerves regenerate if the cell body is preserved.

Incoming signals to the neuron may be transmitted to dendrites directly, to the cell body, or to the axon by the axon of another neuron (Fig. 48-2). The area of contact between neurons is known as the *synapse*.[5] Dendrites, together with the cell body, contain Nissl bodies, which synthesize cell protein and contain much of the ribonucleic acid of the cytoplasm. Intracellular mitochondria produce adenosine triphosphate for energy. Small vesicles and cisterns known as *Golgi apparatus* are present in the neuron and are thought to be involved in the condensing and storage of secretory substances as well as in the formation of enzymatic substances that digest intracellular materials.

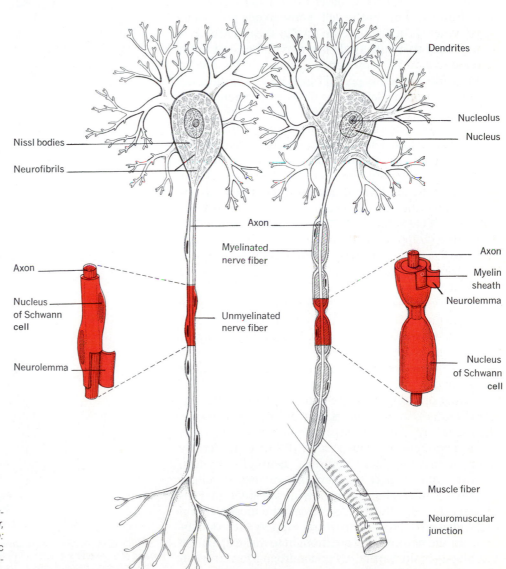

FIGURE 48-1 *Typical efferent neurons:* (Left) *unmyelinated fiber,* (right) *myelinated fiber.* (Source: Chaffee, E.E., and Lyttle, I.M. Basic Physiology and Anatomy, *Philadelphia: J.B. Lippincott.)*

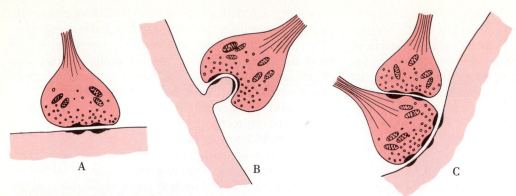

FIGURE 48-2 *Synapses between an axon terminal and* **A.** *a dendritic or cell body,* **B.** *A dendrite spine, and* **C.** *another axon terminal. (Source: Cormack, D.H. Essential Histology. Philadelphia: J.B. Lippincott, 1993.)*

A fibrous axon (nerve fiber) originates from the axon hillock of the cell body (perikaryon) and transmits signals from the cell body to various parts of the nervous system. These long fibers differ from dendrites, which carry transmissions to the cell. Some axons are myelinated, whereas others have no myelin sheath. Myelin is a fatty layer that surrounds the nerve fiber and helps increase conduction of nerve impulses. The myelin sheath is interrupted by periodic gaps known as the *nodes of Ranvier*. Axon collaterals or fibers may emerge from these gaps. Exchange of metabolites occurs between the axon and the extracellular environment at the nodes. The nodes of Ranvier are present in both central and peripheral nervous system neurons. However, they are much easier to identify in the peripheral nervous system. Schwann cells are located along the peripheral axons and produce the myelin sheath of lipoprotein that encases the fiber. Some of these cells produce numerous concentric wrappings around the central core axon and give the axon its characteristic white color (Fig. 48-3). Unmyelinated fibers contain Schwann cells but lack the concentric wrappings. The outermost thin layer of myelin of the myelinated fibers is known as the *neurolemma* of the axon. This neurolemma also enwraps the unmyelinated axon. However, it is lacking in the myelinated fibers within the spinal cord and brain. Myelin provides protective, nutritive, and conductive functions for the axon.

The supporting structure to the neurons of the central nervous system (CNS) is provided by the *neuroglia*. Neuroglia are the counterpart to the Schwann cells in the peripheral nervous system (PNS). Considerably more numerous than neurons, neuroglia protect, nourish, and support the neurons. Astrocytes, oligodendroglia, microglia, and ependyma are different types of glial cells (Fig. 48-4).[12] Astrocytes, the most plentiful of the glial cells, provide structural support and nourishment for the neurons and are thought to make up part of the blood–brain barrier. Oligodendroglia form myelin along axons in the CNS, and microglia have the phagocytic properties of removing cellular debris in the CNS.

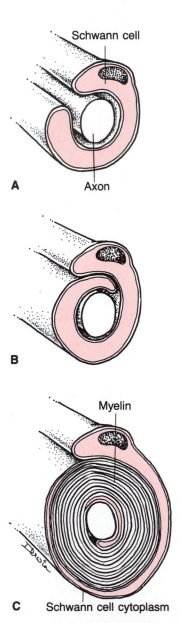

FIGURE 48-3 *Three consecutive stages in the myelination of a segment of an axon by a Schwann cell of the peripheral nervous system. The Schwann cell adheres to its surrounding basement membrane, and its inner margin grows around the axon. (Source: Cormack, D.H. Essential Histology. Philadelphia: J.B. Lippincott, 1993.)*

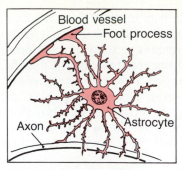

Astrocytes
- Function in metabolism of neurotransmitters
- Star-shaped cells
- Function in formation of blood-brain barrier
- Provide a supporting network in brain and vasculature

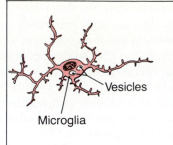

Microglia
- Small glial cells, function in phago-cytosis and clearing injured areas of CNS
- May migrate from one site to another

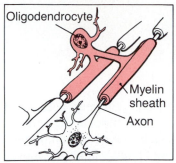

Oligodendrocytes
- Most common glial cell
- Provide support
- Produce myelin sheaths

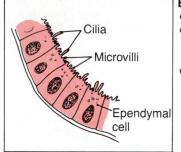

Ependymal cells
- Epithelial cells
- Form continuous epithelial lining for ventricles
- Assist in circulation of cerebrospinal fluid

FIGURE 48-4. *Types of neuroglial cells.*

Ependymal cells line the ventricles of the brain and central canal of the spinal cord, and, in part, provide for the brain–cerebrospinal fluid barrier.

The billions of neurons in the nervous system may be identified according to their morphology and function. Various projections may arise from the body of the cell, leading to their classification as pseudounipolar,

bipolar, or multipolar neurons (Fig. 48-5). The multipolar neuron, most prevalent in the nervous system, consists of one major projection from the cell body, the axon, and generally multiple minor branchings (dendrites). An example of a multipolar neuron is the efferent neuron shown in Figure 48-1.

Neurons can also be classified according to their

A Bipolar

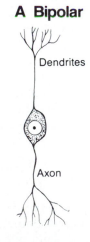

B Pseudounipolar

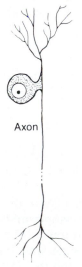

C Multipolar

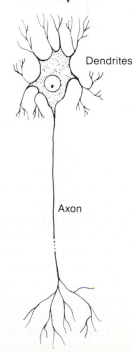

FIGURE 48-5 *The three basic shapes of neurons. (Source: Cormack, D.H. Essential Histology. Philadelphia: J.B. Lippincott, 1993.)*

general function. Sensory (afferent) neurons relay messages about internal and external body environmental changes to the CNS. Motor and secretory (efferent) neurons transmit messages from the CNS to the periphery. Association (internuncial or interneurons) neurons relay messages from one neuron to another within the brain and spinal cord. The relationship of the afferent, association, and efferent neurons and their fibers can be summarized in the following manner:

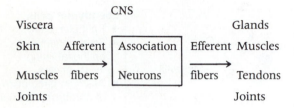

Clusters of neurons within the CNS are called *nuclei* (gray matter). Groups of neurons outside the CNS are known as *ganglia* (see pp. 947–958).

PERIPHERAL AXON DEGENERATION AND REGENERATION

An injured neuron may regenerate as long as its cell body remains relatively unharmed. However, serious damage to the cell body results in death of the entire neuron. A crushed or severed axon of a peripheral nerve fiber triggers certain processes within a few hours of injury. Changes in the axon distal to the injury (wallerian degeneration) are particularly dramatic because that portion has been severed from the metabolic control of the cell body. Initially, the distal portion swells and the terminal neurofilaments hypertrophy. The myelin sheath shrinks and retracts at the nodes of Ranvier, where the remaining nerve fiber becomes exposed. The axon gradually disappears and myelin disintegrates into fragments that are phagocytized.

Changes also occur proximal to the injury in both the axon and the cell body itself (retrograde degeneration). Degenerative changes similar to those in the distal portion of the axon occur at the proximal portion for a few millimeters from the injury. The changes in the cell body (chromatolysis) are in response to repair of damages. The extent of cellular change is related to the location of the injury along the axon. An axon injury near the cell body produces greater changes in the cell than a more distant injury. The cellular cytoplasm swells and the nucleus is eccentrically placed toward the cell wall. Chromatolysis of Nissl bodies, suggestive of increased protein synthesis, takes place, and the number of mitochondria increase. Injured neurofibrils (delicate threads projecting into the axon from the cell body) attempt to grow back into their original placements and begin sprouting from the proximal portion of the injured axon within 14 days after injury. If the fibrils are successful in finding their way into the neurolemma, which generally remains intact, then they grow at a rate of 3 to 4 mm per day. The remaining Schwann cells form a sheet of myelin around the restored neurofibril, and the nodes of Ranvier are reformed as the nerve regenerates. Early surgical repair of severed peripheral nerves facilitates nerve regeneration. Regeneration of injured nerves in the CNS is more difficult due to glial scarring, which frequently inhibits new fibrils from reaching their destinations.

▼ *Neuronal Conduction*

MEMBRANE POTENTIAL

Membrane potentials are generated because of a disparity between cations and anions at the semipermeable and selectively permeable nerve cell membrane. Specific proteins at the cell membrane allow the movement of ions and facilitate the existence of the nerve cell potential and impulse propagation. These proteins include cell membrane pumps and channels. Pumps maintain appropriate ion concentrations in the cell side of the membrane by actively moving ions against concentration gradients (see pp. 19–23). Channel proteins provide selective paths for specific ions to diffuse across the cell membrane.

ACTION POTENTIAL

Unique to nerve, muscle, and gland cells is the change that can occur in a resting cell membrane potential when the cells are stimulated by electrical, chemical, or mechanical means. These stimuli can produce a sudden increase in cell membrane permeability to sodium, which results in a very brief, positive potential within the cell. The sequence of physiochemical events that results in an alteration in the resting potential lasts a few milliseconds and is called the *action potential*. The events of the action potential are described in Chapter 1.

CONDUCTION VELOCITY IN NERVE FIBERS

The velocity of nerve conduction is influenced by the myelinization and diameter of the axon. Myelin acts as an effective insulator and inhibits electrochemical conduction. Therefore, the current passes over the myelin and through the extracellular fluid and enters the nodes of Ranvier at 1-mm to 2-mm intervals, where the membrane is permeable to the ions. This type of current propagation is known as *saltatory conduction*, implying a leaping or hopping phenomenon (Fig. 48-6).

The myelin sheath enhances the velocity of current conduction as capacitance is reduced, which results in

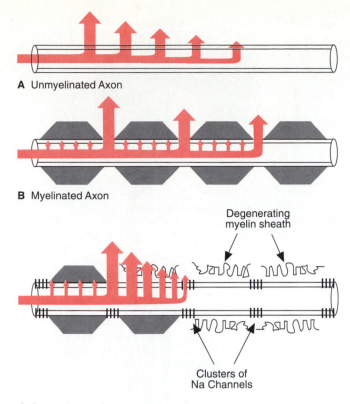

A Unmyelinated Axon

B Myelinated Axon

Degenerating myelin sheath

Clusters of Na Channels

C Demyelinated Axon

*FIGURE 48-6 Excitatory current spreads over a greater distance in a myelinated axon than in an equivalent-diameter unmyelinated axon. **A.** The wave of excitatory-positive current that spreads down an unmyelinated axon head of an advancing action potential leaks out of the axon and dissipates with distance. **B.** The insulating properties of myelin retard this leakage and allow more current to be available at greater distances to depolarize and excite the membrane at the nodes of Ranvier. **C.** Degeneration of the myelin sheath short circuits this insulation and shunts excitatory current to the extracellular space by means of K channels unmasked by the demyelination. Consequently, insufficient charge is available to excite enough nodal sodium (Na) channels to threshold levels, and action potential conduction can fail. (Source: Conn, P.M. Neuroscience in Medicine. Philadelphia: J.B. Lippincott, 1995.)*

reduced numbers of charges propagating the length of the fiber. The heavily myelinated large motor fibers transmit impulses at approximately 100 m per second. In contrast, small unmyelinated fibers may conduct impulses as slow as 0.5 m per second. The wave of action potential leaks out and dissipates with distance (see Figure 48-6).

The diameter of the fiber is an additional important factor contributing to nerve conduction velocity. Velocity is increased in large-diameter nerve fibers due to lower internal resistance and a quicker depolarization time. Table 48-1 presents the relationship of sheathing and diameter to conduction velocities in various types of nerve fibers.

FACTORS INCREASING MEMBRANE EXCITABILITY

Extrinsic and intrinsic conditions affecting the permeability of the sodium ion can profoundly influence cell excitability. Certain drugs can alter the sodium permeability so that facilitory and inhibitory mechanisms of the cell can no longer function normally. Diuretics, for example, can increase sodium loss and alter cell excitability.

Nerve cell membrane excitability is increased with low extracellular calcium levels. Normally, calcium binds with some of the sodium channels and thereby reduces the movement of sodium across the membrane. With less calcium bound to the sodium channels, the movement of sodium becomes less restricted. This increased cell permeability to sodium results in progressively more excitable neuronal tissue. This is manifested clinically by a wide range of signs, including paresthesia, muscular twitching, carpopedal spasms, laryngeal stridor in children, bronchial spasms, tetanic spasms, and convulsions.

TABLE 48-1 *Major Nerve Fiber Classification and Conduction Speed*

Fiber Type	Sheathing	Diameter (μm)	Conduction Speed (m/sec)	Function
A fibers				
Alpha	Myelinated	10–18	60–120	Somatic motor, muscle proprioceptors
Beta	Myelinated	5–10	38–70	Rapid sensory touch, pressure, kinesthesia
Gamma	Myelinated	1–5	15–45	Motor to muscle spindle, rapid sensory (touch, pressure)
Delta	Myelinated	2–5	5–30	Pain, temperature, pressure
B fibers	Thinly myelinated	1–3	3–15	Autonomic preganglionic transmission
C fibers	Unmyelinated	0.5–2	0.5–2	Autonomic postganglionic transmission

FACTORS DECREASING MEMBRANE EXCITABILITY

Increased calcium levels in the extracellular fluid decrease membrane excitability by reducing the membrane permeability that inhibits sodium passage through its channels. Calcium has high protein-binding power as well as positive charges that facilitate repulsion of sodium at the cell membrane. This results in an inhibitory or stabilizing effect on the cell membrane. Clinically, elevated serum calcium levels are reflected by CNS depression. Decreased levels of potassium in the extracellular fluid also decrease membrane excitability by increasing its resting potential. The resting potential is dependent on a constant concentration of potassium. A low extracellular potassium level is reflected clinically by depressed neuromuscular excitation, generalized weakness and fatigability of all muscles, diminished or absent reflexes, and paralytic ileus.

Local anesthetics, such as lidocaine and tetracaine, are other factors that can interfere with the initiation and transmission of the action potential. Depolarization is prevented by decreasing the membrane permeability to sodium, and the negative potential necessary for a propagated discharge does not develop or pass through the anesthetized area. The ease of achieving anesthesia is related to nerve fiber size. Small fibers associated with temperature and superficial pain sensations are most easily anesthetized. Large fibers that transmit sensation of deep pain, touch, and pressure are anesthetized with more difficulty.

▼ Receptors

CHARACTERISTICS OF RECEPTORS

Sensory receptors are specialized nerve cells that respond to specific information from the internal and external environments. The information is then transmitted by spinal or cranial nerves to specific areas of the CNS for interpretation. This is accomplished through conversion of various forms of natural energy from the environment into action potentials in neurons. Common to all receptors is this *transduction* of energy. Mechanical energy is converted by *mechanoreceptors*. Thermal energy is sensed by *thermoreceptors*. Light energy is transmitted by *photoreceptors*, and chemical energy is converted by *chemoreceptors*. Receptors that respond to injury are known as *nociceptors*. *Exteroceptors* give information about the external environment and *interoceptors* and *proprioceptors* are sensitive to internal impulses and changes. *Teleceptors*, such as those found in the eyes and ears, provide information from more distant stimuli.

Receptor cells exhibit a wide range of morphologic and sensitivity differences (Fig. 48-7). Some have free nerve endings with coils, spirals, and branching net-

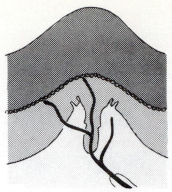

A Free nerve endings

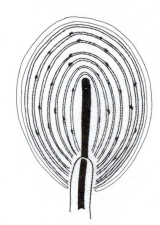

B Pacinian corpuscle

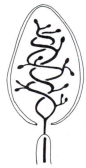

C Meissner's corpuscle

FIGURE 48-7 *Cutaneous sensory receptors. (Source: Cormack, D.H. Essential Histology. Philadelphia: J.B. Lippincott, 1993.)*

works; may be present throughout the body; and detect pain, cold, warmth, and crude touch. Other receptor cells are encased in variously shaped capsules and detect tissue deformation. Each receptor cell has adapted to respond to one specific type or modality of stimulus at a much lower threshold than do other receptors. This response in receptors is referred to as *adequate stimulus*. It remains the same no matter how the receptor is stimulated. Each nerve tract terminates at a specific point in the CNS where the stimulus is interpreted.

When a constant stimulus is applied to a receptor, the frequency of action potentials initiated in the sensory nerve decreases. This phenomenon is known as *adaptation*. Sensory organ adaptation varies widely. The pressure applied to a pacinian corpuscle results in a receptor potential that adapts rapidly. These fast-adapting receptors are called *phasic* receptors. In contrast, the muscle spindles and receptors for pain adapt very slowly. These receptors are known as *tonic* receptors.

RECEPTOR POTENTIAL

The modalities of sensation are converted by specific receptors into electrical energy by action potentials through graded potential changes. The receptor responses are not an all-or-nothing event like the action potentials of neurons. Rather, the magnitude is dependent on the intensity of the stimulus. As the magnitude of the stimulus is increased, the receptor potential increases. Receptor potentials are stationary, producing a local flow of current that spreads electrically to surrounding areas of the cell through a change of ionic conductance of the membrane of the nerve terminal. The ionic permeability change that initiates the receptor potential depends only on the stimulus, not on conductance changes through the function of the membrane potential as brought about in the action potentials. Because the receptor potential is not dependent on the membrane potential, it does not regenerate and remains stationary at the transducer area of the nerve terminal. If the receptor potential is great enough, the axon is depolarized and an action potential is triggered at the first node of Ranvier.

The mechanisms that generate receptor potentials vary with receptors.[6] For example, deformation generates receptor potential in the pacinian corpuscles, and chemicals initiate receptor potentials in the rods and cones of the eyes. Because most receptor terminals are minute and difficult to study, less information is available about their activity than about that of the action potentials.

▼ The Synapse

Information concerning the environment is relayed through a succession of neurons in contact with each other. These areas of contact are known as *synapses*. The terminal portion of the presynaptic axon, the *bouton* or *knob*, may synapse with the cell body, dendrites, axons of other nerve cells, or effector cells of muscles or glands. Impulses at the synapse can be transmitted through chemical or electrical means. Chemical synapses, by far the most common, involve the release of a chemical substance (neurotransmitter) in response to a stimulus. This substance may have an excitatory or inhibitory

effect on the postsynaptic cell membrane. The electrical synapses are fused and are found in invertebrate and lower vertebrates. They propagate uninterrupted impulses. The discussion here is limited to chemical synapses.

The presynaptic fiber conducts impulses toward the synapse and terminates in an enlarged knob called the *synaptic bouton, knob, end-foot,* or *button*. This presynaptic bouton is divided from the postsynaptic membrane by a narrow space of about 2 to 3 nanometers, known as the *synaptic cleft*. The presynaptic bouton contains stored particles of a transmitter substance that is released at the synapse in response to a stimulus. Vesicles open and empty the transmitter substance, which then excites or inhibits the postsynaptic or effector neuron. Mitochondria in the presynaptic bouton provide the adenosine triphosphate for synthesizing the released substance that is continually regenerated. For example, the common transmitter substance acetylcholine is reduced to choline and acetic acid by the action of the enzyme cholinesterase. Choline and acetic acid are reabsorbed by the terminal bouton and, with the enzymatic assistance of choline acetylase, are resynthesized to acetylcholine, which is stored in the presynaptic vesicles until the next adequate stimulus.

Conduction of impulses through synapses is unidirectional, that is, impulses can be transmitted only through terminal boutons of presynaptic membranes to postsynaptic membranes.

EVENTS AT THE CHEMICAL SYNAPSE

As previously noted, the presynaptic terminal bouton contains vesicles with packets of appropriate transmitter substances. A very low level of spontaneous release of this transmitter substance occurs in the resting synapse. This causes spontaneous minidepolarizations at the synapse. When an action potential spreads to the presynaptic bouton, as shown in the neuromuscular junction in Figure 48-8, depolarization of the membrane triggers release of this transmitter substance. It is thought that the trigger release at the terminal bouton requires calcium ions. This theory is supported by observations that low extracellular calcium levels result in diminished amounts of transmitter substance being released. The neurotransmitter substance then attaches to the postsynaptic receptor sites, and the postsynaptic membrane potential is modified. The neurotransmitter substance not taken up by the postsynaptic receptors may be taken up by the presynaptic bouton and stored or inactivated by monoamine oxidase. Some of the unattached neurotransmitter is inactivated at the synaptic cleft or at the postsynaptic membrane by enzymes. In addition, some of the free neurotransmitter is lost through extracellular diffusion.[7]

The presynaptic release of an excitatory transmitter

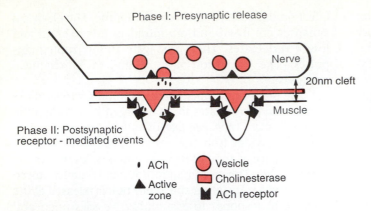

Phase I: Presynaptic release

Nerve

20nm cleft

Muscle

Phase II: Postsynaptic receptor - mediated events

- ACh
- Active zone
- Vesicle
- Cholinesterase
- ACh receptor

FIGURE 48-8 *Overview of cholinergic synaptic transmission at the neuromuscular junction, showing the two major phases of synaptic transmission. Phase I shows presynaptic release of acetylcholine (ACh)-containing vessicles by active zones of the motor nerve terminal. In Phase II, ACh binds to receptors on the postsynaptic or postjunctional muscle membrane. Nerve and muscle are separated by a synaptic 20-nm cleft containing cholinesterase, which hydrolyses ACh. (Source: Conn, P.M. Neuroscience in Medicine. Philadelphia: J.B. Lippincott, 1995.)*

substance can initiate a depolarizing response in the postsynaptic membrane that is referred to as the *excitatory postsynaptic potential* (EPSP).[4,5] The EPSP is graded, nonpropagative, and the result of an increase in the permeability of the postsynaptic membrane to sodium, potassium, chloride, and calcium ions. Sodium ions flow in across the membrane and decrease the negativity of the postsynaptic cell. The threshold voltage change produced in a motoneuron during depolarization in an EPSP is approximately 13 mV, from a resting potential of −70 to −57 mV.

The activity of one terminal bouton is not significant enough to initiate an action potential in the postsynaptic cell. Many active terminals must discharge spontaneously to elicit an action potential. This phenomenon is known as *summation*.[13] Thus, the amplitude of the EPSP depends on the number of activated synapses, and if sufficient numbers are firing, an action potential results.

Threshold is the lowest on the motoneuron at the axon hillock, and the thresholds of the cell body and dendrites are considerably higher. Therefore, action potentials initiated in most neurons originate in the axon hillock.

Some synapses release an inhibitory transmitter, thought to contain gamma-aminobutyric acid at the postsynaptic membrane. This produces limited permeability to potassium and chloride. Potassium effluxes as chloride influxes, and no corresponding inflow of positive sodium ions occurs. This increases the negativity of the already negative postsynaptic cell, and a state of hyperpolarization results. This is called an *inhibitory postsynaptic potential*.[4,5] The permeability change is very brief, because active transport of chloride out of the cell restores resting potential rapidly. Like the EPSP, the inhibitory postsynaptic potential is graded and does not propagate. During the inhibitory postsynaptic potential, the cell is less excitable as the membrane potential is more negative, and increased excitatory activity is needed to reach the threshold level.

In addition to the inhibitory postsynaptic potential, another form of inhibition, called *presynaptic inhibition*, occurs throughout the nervous system. Although concentrated in the peripheral afferent fibers, this type of inhibition occurs at the presynaptic bouton, and no change occurs in the postsynaptic membrane. An inhibitory terminal bouton acts on the presynaptic bouton by releasing a neurotransmitter that partially depolarizes the presynaptic terminal, which greatly reduces the voltage of the action potential and thus reduces the excitability in the membrane. It is thought that presynaptic inhibition provides for a control mechanism of sensory inflow, so less important input is eliminated, and the major signal is relayed more clearly to the CNS.

FACILITATION

Many presynaptic terminals converge on each postsynaptic neuron. A certain number of action potentials must be transmitted simultaneously for a sufficient amount of neurotransmitter to be released to produce an action potential in the postsynaptic membrane. If an insufficient amount of a neurotransmitter is released, the postsynaptic membrane is excitatory, although not to threshold level, and it is said to be facilitated. It is above resting potential but below threshold value and thus very receptive to a stimulus that can activate it with ease.

DIVERGENCE AND CONVERGENCE

Extremely complex networks of neurons exist in the nervous system. Extensive interactions among neurons are mediated through highly organized circuit connections. As axons emerge from the cell body, they divide and subdivide into many collateral branches that synapse with various numbers of other neurons. This presynaptic division is known as *divergence*. For example, the fibers of afferent neurons entering the spinal cord generally divide and subdivide into collateral branches that supply terminal boutons to many other postsynaptic spinal neurons. As a result, no one fiber contributes to an action potential, but rather, many fibers cooperatively produce the innervation. The repetitive subdivision strengthens the afferent information, which is made available to various parts of the CNS through the process of divergence. Similarly, most postsynaptic neurons receive terminal boutons from presynaptic fibers. This postsynaptic anatomic phenomenon is known as *convergence*. Many axons may converge on a single neuron, and the EPSP is dependent on sufficient amplitude of the active boutons converging on it.

NEUROCHEMICAL TRANSMITTER SUBSTANCES

Presynaptic bouton vesicles store specific chemical substances that, when released into the synaptic cleft, either excite or inhibit other cells. Some transmitter substances are present only in the specific parts of the nervous

system, whereas others are widely dispersed. Table 48-2 lists a few of the neurochemical transmitters that have been identified. Since the identification of the first neurotransmitter in 1921, approximately 50 more have been identified.[5] It is thought that many more will be identified in the future. It has been difficult to pinpoint these substances because of the complex structure of the nervous system fibers.

Substances are considered to be neurochemical transmitters if they have the following general characteristics:[14] 1) are released by the presynaptic bouton on stimulation; 2) contain an enzyme in the presynaptic bouton for transmitter synthesis; 3) produce excitation or inhibition in the postsynaptic cell; and 4) have dem-

TABLE 48-2 *Neurotransmitters: Source and Action*

Name	Secretion Source	Action
Acetylcholine First neurotransmitter identified	Neurons in many areas of brain Large pyramidal cells (motor cortex)	Usually excitatory Inhibitory effect on some of the parasympathetic nervous system (eg, heart by vagus)
Chief transmitter of parasympathetic nervous system	Some cells of basal ganglia Motor neurons that innervate skeletal muscles Preganglionic neurons of autonomic nervous system Postganglionic neurons of parasympathetic nervous system Postganglionic neurons of sympathetic nervous system	
Serotonin Controls body heat, hunger, behavior, and sleep	Nuclei originating in the median raphe of brain stem and projecting to many areas (especially the dorsal horns of the spinal cord and hypothalamus)	Inhibitor of pain pathway cord; helps to control mood and sleep
Norepinephrine Chief transmitter of sympathetic nervous system	Many neurons whose cell bodies are located: In brain stem and hypothalamus (controlling overall activity and mood) Most postganglionic neurons of sympathetic nervous system	Usually excitatory, although sometimes inhibitory Some excitatory and some inhibitory
Dopamine Affects control of behavior and fine movement	Neurons on the substantia nigra; many neurons of the substantia nigra send fibers to the basal ganglia that are involved in coordination of skeletal muscle activity	Usually inhibitory
Gamma-aminobutyric acid (GABA)	Nerve terminals of the spinal cord, cerebellum, basal ganglia, and some cortical areas	Excitatory
Glutamate	Presynaptic terminals in many sensory pathways; some cortical areas	Excitatory
Glycine	Synapses in spinal cord	Inhibitory
Enkephalin	Nerve terminals in the spinal cord, brain stem, thalamus, and hypothalamus	Excitatory to systems that inhibit pain; binds to the same receptors in the central nervous system that bind opiate drugs
Endorphin	Pituitary gland and areas of the brain	Binds to opiate receptors in the brain and pituitary gland; excitatory to systems that inhibit pain
Substance P	Pain fiber terminals in the dorsal horns of the spinal cord; also, the basal ganglia and hypothalamus	Excitatory

(Hickey, J.V. *Neurological and Neurosurgical Nursing* [3rd ed.]. Philadelphia: J.B. Lippincott, 1992.)

onstrated a mechanism that diminishes the effects of the transmitter.

Acetylcholine is a well-established neurochemical transmitter, and its activity at the neuromuscular junction is well understood. The terminal bouton of cholinergic nerve fibers contains vesicles, each of which holds about 10,000 molecules of acetylcholine. A vesicle fuses with the presynaptic membrane and results in the release of acetylcholine (see Figure 48-8). This process is known as *exocytosis*. It is thought that the fusion of the vesicle to the presynaptic membrane is brought about by a sudden, transient increase in the concentration of calcium ions in the terminal bouton. The nerve impulse at the terminal bouton opens calcium channels to allow their flow into the bouton to facilitate exocytosis. The exact mechanism of the calcium activity in exocytosis is unknown. When the fused vesicle has discharged its acetylcholine at the presynaptic membrane, it is reclaimed by the bouton and restored with acetylcholine for its future use.[7] The synthesis of acetylcholine occurs in the bouton in the following manner:[14]

$$\text{Acetylcoenzyme A (acetate) + choline} \xrightarrow[\text{ATP}]{\text{choline acetyltransferase}} \text{acetylcholine}$$

The acetylcholine that diffuses across the synaptic cleft binds with an acetylcholine receptor on the postsynaptic membrane. This receptor is a channel protein that, in the presence of acetylcholine, lowers its energy state to an open conformation, allowing passage of sodium and potassium ions. Thus, a postsynaptic potential or voltage change is produced. The chemically gated postsynaptic potentials differ from action potentials of neurons in that their amplitude is smaller and their duration longer, and they are graded in accordance with the amount of transmitter released.

Within 2 or 3 milliseconds of its release into the synaptic cleft, after it has depolarized the postsynaptic membrane, acetylcholine is hydrolyzed by the enzyme acetylcholinesterase:[14]

$$\text{Acetylcholine} \xrightarrow[\text{water}]{\text{acetylcholinesterase}} \text{choline + acetate}$$

Acetylcholinesterase is abundantly present in the membrane of the terminal bouton.

Insights into neurotransmitters and their inhibiting enzymes have been gained through the use of various pharmacologic agents that act on or compete with these substances. For example, the muscle relaxant curare competes with acetylcholine for receptor sites at the postsynaptic membrane. Thus, acetylcholine cannot bring about the membrane permeability for depolarization. Some drugs, such as nicotine, simulate acetylcholine action. Neostigmine and physostigmine inactivate the enzymatic action of acetylcholinesterase. Magnesium affects acetylcholine release. Elevated magnesium levels inhibit acetylcholine release by competing with the calcium ions that are necessary for the process.

Norepinephrine is the transmitter substance at all postganglionic sympathetic fibers, except those innervating sweat glands and skeletal muscle vasculature. This substance is formed through a series of steps catalyzed by enzymes, with the initial active transport of tyrosine from the circulation into the nerve terminals as follows:[6]

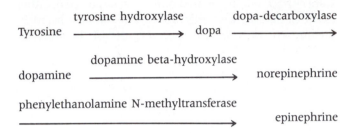

A nerve impulse initiates the release of norepinephrine into the cleft. Norepinephrine activity at the receptor is terminated primarily through its uptake into the terminal bouton and is transported back into the vesicles for reuse. In addition, a small amount of norepinephrine is inactivated by the activity of monoamine oxidase, and an additional small amount escapes the terminal bouton uptake and enters the systemic circulation, where it is metabolized by the liver into vanillylmandelic acid and excreted in the urine. Disease states exhibiting increased production of catecholamines characteristically show increased urinary excretion of vanillylmandelic acid. Minute amounts of released norepinephrine, which escape uptake and metabolic breakdown in the liver, appear unchanged in the urine.

▼ *The Central Nervous System*

PHYLOGENETIC DEVELOPMENT

The human nervous system has a complex major processing system that lends control in a hierarchic manner. The highest level is the cerebral cortex, and the lowest, or most rudimentary, is the spinal reflex arc.

The three distinct regions in the embryonic brain are the *rhombencephalon* or *hindbrain*, the *mesencephalon* or *midbrain*, and the *prosencephalon* or *forebrain* (Fig. 48-9). The most sophisticated activities and complex subdividing occur in the prosencephalon, which includes the cerebral hemispheres, basal ganglia, and olfactory tract. This portion of the brain can be subdivided into the *telencephalon*, or *endbrain*, and the "deep inside" component of the prosencephalon, the *diencephalon*. Optic tracts traverse the prosencephalon and terminate in the optic nerves of the retinae at the inferior surface of the

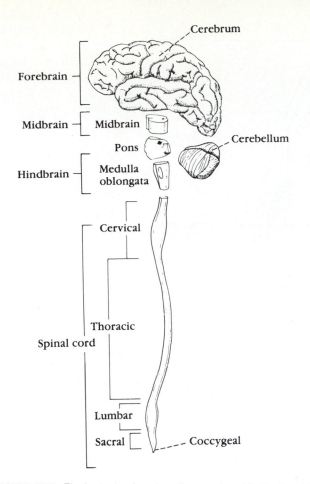

FIGURE 48-9 *The brain develops from three regions: hindbrain, mid-brain, and forebrain. (Source: Snell, R.S.* Clinical Neuroanatomy for Medical Students. *(3rd ed.). Boston: Little, Brown, 1992.)*

forebrain. The diencephalon includes structures such as the thalamus, hypothalamus, subthalamus, and epithalamus. The pituitary complex evolves from the hypothalamus. The mesencephalon connects the forebrain with the hindbrain. Anteriorly, it comprises the cerebral peduncles, and posteriorly, the corpora quadrigemina (also known as superior and inferior colliculi).

Below the mesencephalon is the *rhombencephalon*, which is subdivided into the *metencephalon*, giving rise to the pons and cerebellum encasing the fourth ventricle, and the *myelencephalon* which gives rise to the medulla oblongata. Extending from the rhombencephalon inferiorly is the spinal cord.[9]

PROTECTIVE COVERINGS OF THE BRAIN AND SPINAL CORD

Protection is afforded the brain and spinal cord by bony coverings, the meninges, and the cerebrospinal fluid (CSF). The brain, weighing approximately 3 lb in the adult, is encased within the skull, which is a nonflexible structure composed of several fused bones (Fig. 48-10). Three depressions in the base of the skull are known as the *anterior, middle*, and *posterior fossae*. The frontal lobes are encased in the anterior fossa, the lower portion of the diencephalon and the temporal lobes lie in the middle fossa, and the cerebellum is housed in the posterior fossa.

A major opening, the *foramen magnum*, is at the base of the skull and allows information to be processed between higher and lower centers (Fig. 48-11). At birth,

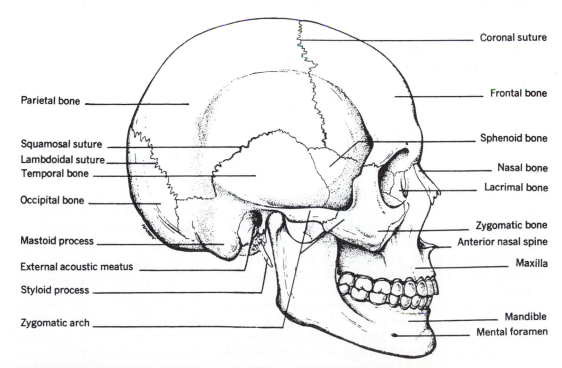

FIGURE 48-10 *Lateral view of the skull. (Source: Hickey, J.* Neurological and Neurosurgical Nursing *[3rd ed.]. Philadelphia: J.B. Lippincott, 1992.)*

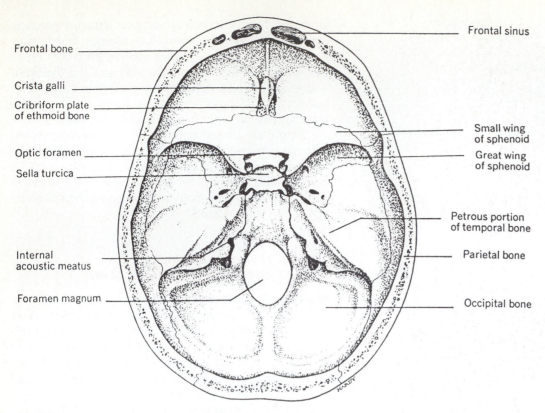

FIGURE 48-11 *View of the base of the skull from above, showing the internal surfaces of some of the cranial bones. (Source: Hickey, J.* Neurological and Neurosurgical Nursing *[3rd ed.] Philadelphia: J.B. Lippincott, 1992.)*

openings within the skull, known as the *fontanelles*, are present. These generally close by 18 months of age.

The spinal cord is encased in the vertebral column, which consists of 24 movable vertebrae—7 cervical, 12 thoracic, and 5 lumbar—and the fused 5 sacral and 4 coccygeal vertebrae. Figure 48-12 shows the relationship of spinal nerves and vertebrae. Intravertebral disks separate each of the vertebrae. The central cartilaginous portion of the intervertebral disk is known as the *nucleus pulposus* and the outer fibrous capsule as the *anulus fibrosus*.

In addition, the brain and spinal cord are protected by three connective tissue membranes called the *meninges*: the *dura mater*, the *arachnoid mater*, and the *pia mater*. The dura mater, a thick, tough, nonelastic fibrous membrane composed of the endosteal and meningeal layers, lies directly below the skull. It serves a protective function for the brain, particularly at times when the integrity of the skull is not intact. The extension of the dura between the cerebral hemispheres is known as the *falx cerebri*. Between the cerebrum and cerebellum it is known as the *tentorium cerebelli*; between the lateral lobes of the cerebellum as the *falx cerebelli* and above the sella turcica as *diaphragma sellae*. A layer of the dura mater, together with the arachnoid and pia mater, extends through the foramen magnum and lines the ver-

tebral column. The *epidural space* is between the inner surface of the skull and the dura mater. The space between the dura and arachnoid is known as the *subdural space*. A network of small blood vessels traverses this space. The delicate arachnoid, consisting of fibrous, weblike tissue, is the middle layer of the meninges wherein the CSF circulates and is reabsorbed. The area below the arachnoid membrane containing the CSF is known as the *subarachnoid* space. The innermost layer, the pia mater, is a delicate, vascular, lacelike membrane directly adherent to the brain and spinal cord. The arachnoid layer projects small extensions called *arachnoid villi* into the dura mater that reabsorb CSF into the blood (Fig. 48-13). Larger blood vessels lie in the subarachnoid space and branch into smaller vessels that pass through the pia mater as they enter the brain tissue.

THE SPINAL CORD PROCESSING SYSTEM

The spinal cord, which is encased in the vertebral canal and protected by the vertebral column, transmits more complex signals from higher centers and responds spontaneously to local sensory information with automatic motor responses called *reflexes*. It is approximately 42 to 45 cm long in the adult and is segmented into cervical,

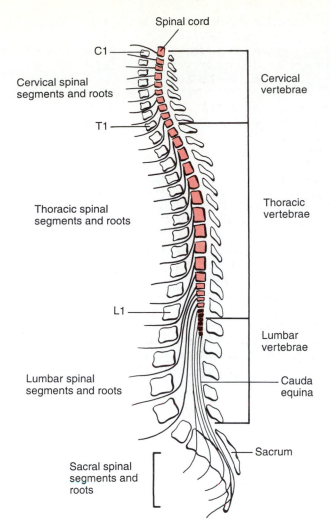

FIGURE 48-12 *The organization of the spinal cord into cervical, thoracic, lumbar, and sacral segments. Notice the exit of the lumbar and sacral roots through intervertebral foramina located caudal to the spinal segment with which the roots are associated. (Source: Conn, P.M. Neuroscience in Medicine. Philadelphia: J.B. Lippincott, 1995.)*

thoracic, lumbar, and sacral sections. Signals are received and transmitted through 31 pairs of spinal nerves, which are named for their corresponding vertebral level. Segments of the spinal cord do not correspond with vertebral levels (see Figure 48-12). The spinal cord is approximately 25 cm shorter than the vertebral canal and ends at the level of the first or second lumbar vertebra in the adult. It emerges from the base of the skull, the *foramen magnum*, and continues to the coccyx, where it ends in a tapered cone called the *conus medullaris*. From the conus extends a thin filamentous connective tissue called the *filum terminale*. Together, the lumbosacral nerve roots project from the conus and are called the *cauda equina*.

The spinal cord enlarges at the lower cervical segments and again at the lower lumbar segments. These enlargements denote the origins of the *brachial* and *lum-*

bar plexuses, respectively. The brachial plexus, extending from C-5 to T-1, innervates the upper extremities, and the lumbar plexus, extending from L-3 to S-2, innervates the lower extremities. The cell bodies are located in the inner, butterfly-shaped, gray portion of the spinal cord, and the ascending and descending projection nerve fibers form the outer white area. The spinal cord is divided into a symmetrical right and left section, with each section containing *anterior, lateral,* and *posterior columns*. These column run the entire length of the cord. Major ascending and descending tracts and their transmissions are presented in Table 48-3. A small opening in the middle of the spinal cord, the *central canal*, is lined by ependymal cells and contains CSF. Afferent spinal nerves enter the cord at the posterior horn (somatic sensory and visceral), and efferent nerves emerge at the anterior horn (motor and autonomic) (Fig. 48-14). The cell bodies of efferent motor fibers are located in the anterior horn, and the cell bodies of the afferent sensory fibers are situated outside the spinal cord in the posterior root ganglion. Contact between the afferent and efferent fibers is made within the spinal cord through interneurons.

Reflex Arc

A fundamental component of the nervous system is the reflex which, in its simplest form, occurs in the spinal cord. A stimulus from the external environment may produce an immediate stereotypical reflex response from the CNS. For a reflex response to occur, the following mechanisms must be functional: an afferent neuron with its receptor, an area for the synapse transmission to occur (one or more central neurons), and an efferent neuron with its effector organ. The impulse passes from receptor to effector and commands a quick organ response. This simple chain of neuronal activity is known as a *reflex arc* and, at its most elemental level, is a *monosynaptic reflex* consisting of only one synapse and two neurons (see Figure 48-14). Most reflexes result from many more synaptic interconnections and are referred to as *polysynaptic reflexes*. The reflex activity encountered at higher levels in the CNS is considerably more complex.

LOW-BRAIN PROCESSING SYSTEM (RHOMBENCEPHALON)

The next level of processing in the CNS takes place in the rhombencephalon. The major components of this region are the medulla oblongata, pons, cerebellum, and fourth ventricle (Fig. 48-15). The processing encountered at this level occurs at the unconscious level and influences such vital activities as respiratory, cardiac, and vasomotor control.

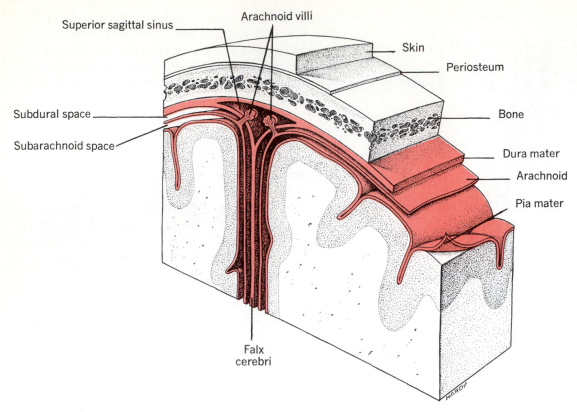

FIGURE 48-13 *The cranial meninges. Arachnoid villi, shown within the superior sagittal sinus, are one site of cerebrospinal fluid absorption into the blood. (Source: Chaffee, E.E. and Lytle, I.M. Basic Physiology and Anatomy [4th ed.]. Philadelphia: J.B. Lippincott.)*

Medulla Oblongata

The medulla extends directly from the cervical spinal cord at the level of the foramen magnum and lies below the pons and fourth ventricle. The medulla is subdivided into three distinct sections: anterior, lateral, and posterior. Fissures and sulci provide landmarks that distinguish these divisions. The anterior portion contains two prominent ridges known as the *pyramids* that contain the *descending pyramidal tract*. These fibers project from the primary motor and somasthetic cortical areas and cross from one side to the other (pyramidal decussation) at the lower medulla before entering the spinal cord. The majority of these fibers decussate and descend as the *lateral corticospinal* tract. The fibers from the motor cortex that remain uncrossed descend into the spinal cord as the *anterior corticospinal* tract.[10] Injury anywhere along the corticospinal tract above the decussation results in motor deficits of the contralateral extremities.

The *olive*, a prominent mass, is located in the lateral section of the medulla. This structure gives rise to the *inferior olivary nuclear complex*, which is important in controlling movement, postural change, locomotion, and equilibrium through an interconnecting network of fibers among the cerebral cortex, spinal cord, and cerebellum. This region contains nuclei for cranial nerves

XVII (hypoglossal), XI (accessory), X (vagus), and IX (glossopharyngeal). Cardiac and vasomotor control evolve from the reticular formation of this region. Respirations are controlled by the medullary center in coordination with the pneumotaxic center in the pons.

The posterior portion of the medulla forms a portion of the floor of the fourth ventricle. The ascending *medial lemniscus* tract arises here from the crossed-over fasciculi cuneatus and *gracilis fibers* (Fig. 48-16). The medial lemniscus is a major ascending brain stem tract that carries discriminative tactile information, pressure sensation, proprioception, and vibration sensation to the sensory thalamic nucleus. Lesions in the medical lemniscus result in contralateral sensory deficits.

Pons

The pons is continuous with the medulla and midbrain, separated by the pontine sulcus from the medulla and the superior pontine sulcus from the midbrain. The pons lies ventral to the cerebellum and is divided into two parts: a *dorsal* portion, the pontine tegmentum, and a *ventral* portion, the pons proper.[1] The dorsal portion is continuous with the medullary reticular formation and, together with the medulla, forms the floor and lateral

TABLE 46-3 *Major Spinal Cord Tracts*

Name	Origin	Termination	Crossed	Function	Dysfunction
ASCENDING TRACTS					
Fasciculus gracilis	Spinal cord at sacral and lumbar level	Medulla→thalamus→cerebral cortex (sensory strip)	Yes	Conscious proprioception, fine touch,* and vibration sense from lower body	Lower body Astereognosis Loss of vibration sense Loss of two-point discrimination Loss of proprioception
Fasciculus cuneatus	Spinal cord at thoracic and cervical levels	Medulla→thalamus→cerebral cortex (sensory strip)	Yes	Conscious proprioception, fine touch,* and vibration sense from upper body	Upper body Astereognosis Loss of vibration sense Loss of two-point discrimination Loss of proprioception
Posterior spinocerebellar	Posterior horn	Cerebellum	No	Conduction of sensory impulses from muscle spindles and tendon organs of the trunk and lower limbs from one side of the body to the same side of cerebellum for the subconscious proprioception necessary for coordinated muscular contractions	Ipsilateral uncoordinated postural movements
Anterior spinocerebellar	Posterior horn	Cerebellum	Some	Conduction of sensory impulses from muscle spindles and tendon organs of the upper and lower limbs from both sides of the body to the cerebellum for the subconscious proprioception necessary for coordinated muscular contractions	Ipsilateral uncoordinated postural movements
Lateral spinothalamic	Posterior horn	Thalamus→cerebral cortex	Yes	Interpretation of pain and temperature	Loss of pain and temperature sensation contralaterally below the level of the lesion
Anterior spinothalamic	Posterior horn	Thalamus→cerebral cortex	Yes	Conduction of sensory impulses for pressure and crude touch† from extremities and trunk	Because one branch of the first neuron immediately synapses with a second, which ascends ipsilaterally for many levels; cord injury rarely results in complete loss of pressure and crude touch sensation

(continued)

TABLE 48-3 *(continued)*

Name	Origin	Termination	Crossed	Function	Dysfunction
DESCENDING TRACTS					
Lateral corticospinal	Motor cortex (area 4)→internal capsule→midbrain→pons→medulla	Anterior horn; all spinal levels in laminae IV through VII and IX	80%–90% cross at the medulla	Controls voluntary muscle activity	Voluntary muscle paresis/paralysis
Anterior corticospinal	Motor cortex (area 4)→internal capsule→midbrain→medulla→anterior funiculus of the cervical and upper thoracic levels	Anterior horn (at each level of cord, axons cross to other side)	Not at medulla; synapse with cells of lamina VIII	Controls voluntary muscle activity	Voluntary muscle paresis/paralysis
Corticobulbar	Areas 4, 6, and 8 of cortex→internal capsule→brain stem	Brain stem; connects with cranial nerves V, VII, IX, X, XI, and XII	Yes	Controls voluntary head movement and facial expression	Because of bilateral innervation, facial expression is usually not affected
Rubrospinal	Midbrain (red nucleus)	Anterior horn	Yes	Facilitates flexor alpha and gamma motor neurons and inhibits extensor motor neurons; also influences muscle tone and posture, particularly of the arms	Altered muscle tone and posture
Reticulospinals Pontine reticulospinal Medullary reticulospinal	Reticular formation (brain stem)	Anterior horn	No	Facilitates extensor motor neurons, particularly of the legs; input to gamma motor neurons	Altered muscle tone and posture
Vestibulospinals	Reticular formation (brain stem)	Anterior horn	No	Conveys autonomic information from higher levels to preganglionic autonomic nervous system neurons to influence sweating, pupillary dilatation, and circulation	Altered muscle tone and sweat gland activity
Lateral vestibulospinal			No	Facilitates extensor alpha motor neurons and inhibits flexors	Altered muscle tone and postural equilibrium
Medial vestibulospinal			No	Inhibits fibers to upper cervical alpha motor neurons; influences extraocular movement and visual reflexes	Altered muscle tone and equilibrium in response to head movement

* Fine touch is the ability to identify various objects (eg, a key) that are placed in the hand while the eyes are closed.
† Crude touch refers to light touch and may be tested with a wisp of cotton placed in the hand while the eyes are closed.
(Hickey, J.V.. *Neurological and Neurosurgical Nursing*. Philadelphia: J.B. Lippincott. 1992.)

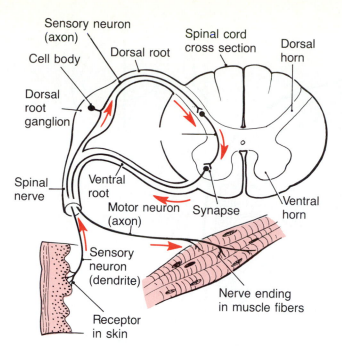

FIGURE 48-14 *Reflex arc showing the pathway of impulses (see text).*

wall of the fourth ventricle. This portion also contains important ascending and descending tracts and nuclei for cranial nerves V (trigeminal), VI (abducens), VII (facial), and VIII (acoustic) (see pp. 947–951). The pons regulates respiration through its pneumotaxic center.

The ventral portion of the pons consists of a large mass of orderly longitudinal and transverse fiber bundles that are interspersed with many pontine nuclei. The longitudinal fiber bundles traversing through this portion of the pons are the corticospinal, corticopontine, and corticobulbar. The ventral portion of the pons is an important relay center between the cerebral cortex and the opposite cerebellar hemisphere in providing smooth, coordinated movements. The transverse fibers arise from the pontine nuclei and cross to the opposite side to form the middle cerebellar peduncle.

Cerebellar Processing

The cerebellum lies in the posterior cranial fossa and is separated from the cerebrum by the tentorium cerebelli (see Figure 48-15). The superior, middle, and inferior cerebellar peduncles connect the cerebellum to the midbrain, pons, and medulla, respectively. The cerebellum exerts ipsilateral control: the right side of the cerebellum controls the right side of the body and the left side of the cerebellum controls the left side of the body. As noted in Figure 48-17, the cerebellar structures are divided into two major lateral hemispheres and an intermediary section, the vermis. Fissures divide the hemispheres into three principal lobes: the *archicerebellum* (flocculonodu-

lar lobe), *paleocerebellum* (anterior lobe), and *neocerebellum* (posterior lobe). The archicerebellum is integrated with the vestibular system and is concerned with muscle tone, equilibrium, and position through its influence on the trunk musculature. The paleocerebellum consists of the cerebellum that lies anterior to the primary fissure, receiving most of the proprioceptive and interoceptive input from the head and body. It helps to maintain equilibrium and coordinate automatic movements as well as to regulate muscle tone. The neocerebellum, phylogenetically the newest, consists of the cerebellum between the primary fissure and the posterior fissure. It coordinates voluntary movements and has extensive connections with the cerebral cortex.

The cerebellum processes and transmits information concerning current body movements, maintains posture, and regulates muscle tone. It does this through information it receives from the motor cortex of the cerebrum by way of the *corticocerebellar* pathway and from various sensory receptors by way of the *anterior* and *posterior spinocerebellar* tracts. Other significant tracts relaying this information to the cerebellum include the *spinoreticular* tract by the reticular area of the brain stem and the *spino-olivary* tract by the inferior olivary nucleus. Fiber-efferent tracts originate in various cerebellar nuclei and transmit information to the cerebral motor cortex, basal ganglia, red nucleus, reticular formation, and vestibular nuclei.[6]

Because the pathways from the cerebral cortex to the cerebellum are indirect descending motor tracts, disruption of cerebellar function does not hinder voluntary movement, although movement no longer is smooth and coordinated. Disruption of cerebellar function can result in ataxia, intention tremor, adiadochokinesia (inability to perform rapid alternating movements), dysmetria (inability to judge distances when reaching out toward an object), hypotonia, tremor, and asthenia.

MIDBRAIN PROCESSING SYSTEM (MESENCEPHALON)

The midbrain extends from the pons and projects briefly between the two cerebral hemispheres, connecting the lower centers with the diencephalon. It, therefore, is a major motor and sensory fiber pathway between the higher and lower centers. The nuclei for the third and fourth cranial nerves originate in this region. The *cerebral aqueduct (aqueduct of Sylvius)*, a small channel between the third and fourth ventricles, lies in the midbrain. The midbrain *tegmentum* is located ventral to the cerebral aqueduct and is continuous with the pontine tegmentum. The reticular formation in this region contains the *substantia nigra* and the *red* nucleus. The substantia nigra is a large pigmented mass containing neurotransmitters, particularly dopamine. It supports motor function through its connections with the thalamus, corpus

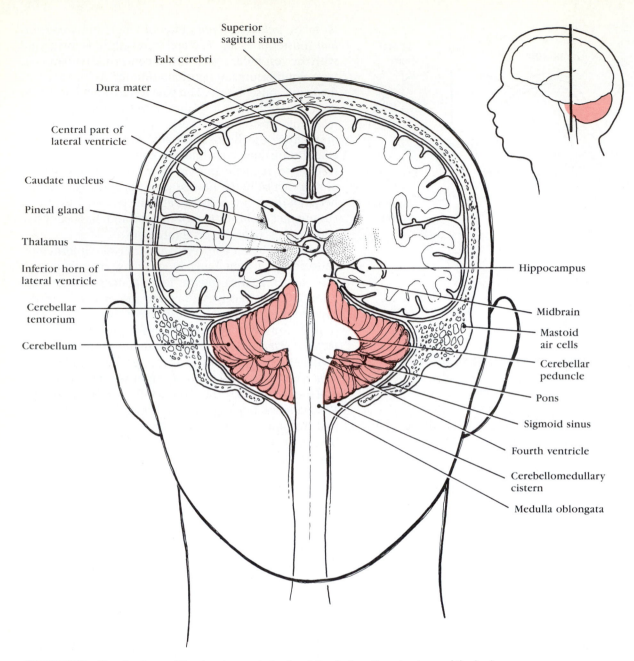

FIGURE 48-15 *The structures of the rhombencephalon in relation to the other structures of the brain, consisting of the medulla oblongata, the pons, and the cerebellum.*

striatum, and superior colliculus.[1] The red nucleus influences head and neck movement as well as motor control by the cerebellum. The *superior colliculus*, a relay center for the optic system, and the *inferior colliculus*, which relays information concerning auditory impulses, are also contained in this area. The superior and inferior colliculi (*corpora quadrigemina*) compose the tectum. The *crus cerebri* are masses on the ventral surface of the midbrain that comprise motor fibers originating in the cerebral cortex as well as corticobulbar fibers projecting to cranial nerve nuclei and reticular formation.[1]

FOREBRAIN PROCESSING SYSTEM (PROSENCEPHALON)

The forebrain consists of the structures of the diencephalon and the telencephalon. The diencephalon arises from the midbrain and is considered to be a part of the forebrain. It lies between the cerebral hemispheres and encases the third ventricle. Included in the diencephalon are the epithalamus, thalamus, hypothalamus, and subthalamus. The telencephalon comprises the basal ganglia and cerebrum.

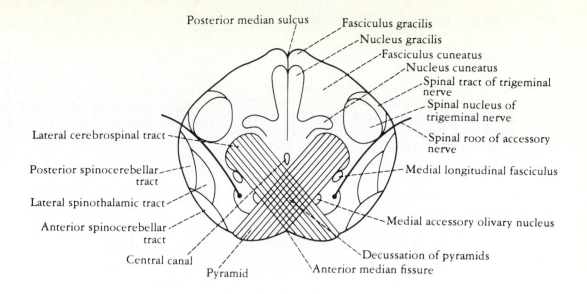

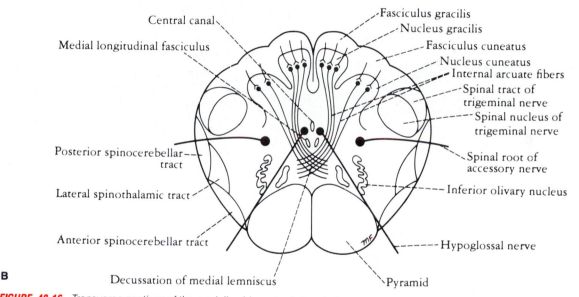

FIGURE 48-16 *Transverse sections of the medulla oblongata.* **A.** *Level of decussation of the pyramids.* **B.** *Level of decussation of the medial lemnisci. (Source: Snell, R.S.* Clinical Neuroanatomy for Medical Students. *Boston: Little, Brown, 1992.)*

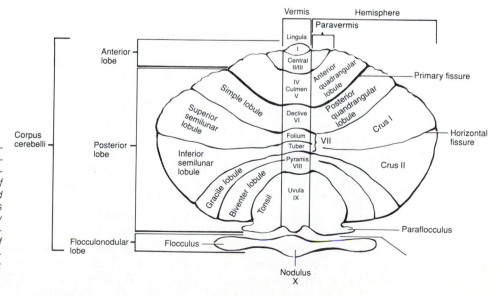

FIGURE 48-17 *Schematic of the flattened cerebellum, showing the fissures, lobes, and lobules of the cerebellum. The terms on the left side of the diagram refer to terminology used for the human cerebellum. The terms on the right side refer to terminology used for animals. The Roman numerals designate the ten lobules of the vermis. (Source: Conn, P.M.* Neuroscience in Medicine. *Philadelphia: J.B. Lippincott, 1995.)*

Thalamic Processing

The thalamus, the largest portion of the diencephalon, is a major center for processing sensations and relaying these to the cerebral cortex. Input from all sensoria, except that for olfaction, is processed here. Numerous afferent nerve tracts from lower levels transmit information to the specific relay nuclei of the thalamus. The thalamus is divided into three sections: *lateral, medial,* and *anterior,* which are separated by the *internal medullary lamina.* Groups of nuclei within the internal medullary lamina are referred to as *intralaminar thalamic nuclei.* Sensory data are relayed through these nuclei.

The reticular activating system continues its upward projection to the thalamic nuclei. From the thalamic nuclei, fibers diffuse to all areas of the cerebral cortex. This system is known as the *diffuse thalamocortical system* (Fig. 48-18). This system, which is also referred to as the nonspecific thalamocortical system, activates the first two layers of neurons of the cortex by partially depolarizing superficial cortical dendrites, resulting in increased facilitation of the cortex.[6] The *paleospinothalamic pathway,* which transmits burning and aching sensations, terminates in the diffuse thalamocortical system. Axons of the optic tract synapse in the lateral geniculate body, which projects from the thalamus. The fibers projecting from the lateral geniculate body pass posteriorly and terminate in the visual cortex.

Hypothalamic Processing

The hypothalamus lies below the thalamus and forms part of the walls and floor of the third ventricle. It consists of a group of nuclei with specific functions and is divided into the anterior and posterior portions. The hypothalamus is connected to the pituitary gland by the pituitary stalk, which provides the route for its neuroendocrine control.

Major processing of internal stimuli evoking the autonomic nervous system is concentrated in the hypothalamus. The functions that maintain the internal milieu processed by the hypothalamus include blood pressure, heart rate, respiratory rate, body temperature, water metabolism, body fluid osmolality, feeding behavior, and neuroendocrine activity. The hypothalamus is a focal structure of the *limbic* system. Figure 48-19 illustrates the structures of the limbic system, which, in concert with the hypothalamus, perform an important role in overall behavior and emotions. Because vital autonomic functions are processed here, destruction of the hypothalamus results in death. The majority of the hypothalamic activity occurs at an unconscious level, but excessive stimulation may evoke a conscious response. An example of this is a person who is chilled and consciously seeks warmth.

Responses to emotions of fear, anger, and excitement reflected by increased pulse rate, increased respiratory rate, increased gastric acidity, and sweating are communicated from the hypothalamus. Prolonged stimulation of the hypothalamus may result in hypertension or ulcers. The *epithalamus* consists of the pineal body, habenular nuclei, stria medularis, and posterior commissure. It is located in the region above the thalamus and contains the roof of the third ventricle. Olfactory impulses are relayed through this region, and visual reflexes are associated with certain fibers in the posterior commissure. The function of the pineal body in the adult is uncertain. It is visible on skull films due to calcified material that accumulates with age, and it can provide useful information in the identification of space-occupying lesions. The *subthalamus* is found between the midbrain tegmentum and dorsal thalamus and serves as an important extrapyramidal motor connecting center.

Basal Ganglia Processing

The basal ganglia (Fig. 48-20), situated deep within the cerebral hemispheres, are responsible for motor control and information processing in the extrapyramidal system. The basal ganglia include the *caudate nucleus, putamen,* and *globus pallidus.* These nuclear masses have complex interconnections with the *subthalamic nucleus, red nucleus,* and *substantia nigra.* The claustrum and amygdaloid body, considered by some authors to be part of the basal ganglia, are not directly involved in motor control. The basal ganglia are intimately related to the thalamus through circular neural pathways that control motor function. They inhibit muscle tone by transmitting inhibitory signals to the bulboreticular facilitory area and excitatory signals to the bulboreticular inhibi-

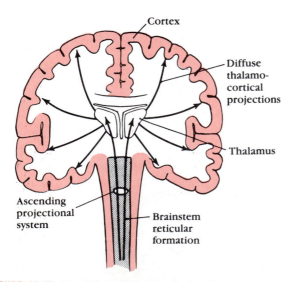

FIGURE 48-18 *The diffuse thalamocortical system.*

Cortex

Diffuse thalamo-cortical projections

Thalamus

Ascending projectional system

Brainstem reticular formation

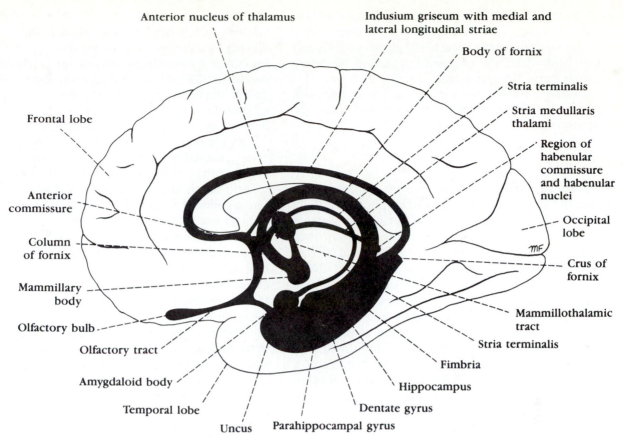

FIGURE 48-19 *Key structures of the limbic system. (Source: Snell, R.S.* Clinical Neuroanatomy for Medical Students *[3rd ed.]. Boston: Little, Brown, 1992.)*

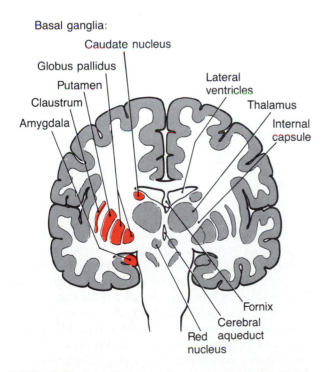

FIGURE 48-20 *Coronal section of brain showing basal ganglia.*

tory area. Lesions in the basal ganglia result in an overactive facilitory area and underactive inhibitory area, resulting in body rigidity. Gross intentional movement that is performed without conscious thought is regulated by the caudate nucleus and putamen (collectively called the *striate body* or *corpus striatum*).

Striate body transmissions are sent to the globus pallidus and relayed to the ventrolateral nucleus of the thalamus and then on to the cerebral cortex. From the cortex, the information travels through the pyramidal and extrapyramidal tracts to the spinal cord. Other impulses travel to the globus pallidus and then on to the substantia nigra and the reticular formation, where the final route transmits down through the reticulospinal tract. The globus pallidus relays impulses through a similar feedback circuit to the ventrolateral nucleus of the thalamus and on to the cerebral cortex and finally to the pyramidal and extrapyramidal tracts to the spinal cord. It also transmits by shorter circuits to the reticular formation and on to the reticulospinal tract of the spinal cord.[6]

The subthalamus nucleus, red nucleus, and substantia nigra are closely related to the globus pallidus and striate body. Their interactions, which control and coordinate motor function, are extremely complex and extensive, and little is known of the exact interconnections.

The neurons transmitting to the globus pallidus and striate body from the substantia nigra are inhibitory through *dopamine* secretion.[3]

Dysfunction or lesions in the region of the basal ganglia are manifested in involuntary tremor, athetosis, and torticollis.

CEREBRAL PROCESSING

Anatomically, the highest and largest portion of the brain, the cerebrum, is thought to be phylogenetically related to the thalamus because of its closely associated structure and function. All areas of the cerebral cortex (surface area of the cerebrum) have afferent and efferent fibers interconnecting with specific areas of the thalamus. As previously noted, this relationship is affirmed through the diffuse thalamocortical system.

The gray cerebral cortex is composed of five basic types of neurons: pyramidal cells, stellate cells, fusiform cells, horizontal cells, and the cells of Martinotti. The pyramidal and stellate cells are the most numerous. Pyramidal cells have pyramid-shaped bodies with axons that extend into the subcortical white matter. The stellate cells have a star-shaped body with short axons and dendrites. The horizontal cells lie entirely on the horizontal plane with axons and dendrites that are parallel to the cortical surface. Polymorph or multiform cells may be modified types of pyramidal cells with a wide variety of shapes and contours. Dendrites often extend into the cortical layers, whereas axons project into the white matter. The cells of Martinotti are multipolar, with short branching dendrites and myelinated axons. They may be modified stellate cells.[1]

The white matter of the cerebral hemispheres is composed of three types of myelinated nerve fibers: projection, transverse, and association. Projection fibers connect the cerebral cortex with lower centers of the brain and spinal cord, transverse fibers connect the two cerebral hemispheres, and association fibers provide interconnections within the same cerebral hemisphere. Convergence of cortical afferent and efferent fibers occurs in the *internal capsule* located adjacent to the thalamus and basal ganglia.

The cerebral surface appears as a series of convolutions (*gyri*) and grooves (*sulci*) that are instrumental in identifying the structural and functional geography of the cortex. Brodmann is credited with mapping specific functional areas on the central cortex (Fig. 48-21).[12] More than 100 of these have been identified. The deeper grooves, called *fissures*, assist in establishing the major cerebral regional divisions: the *frontal, parietal, temporal,* and *occipital* lobes. Similarly, the two cerebral hemispheres are distinguished from each other by the deep *longitudinal fissure* (Fig. 48-22). The cerebral hemispheres, which exhibit *contralateral* body control, are divided by a continuation of the dura mater known as the *falx cerebri*, which projects into the longitudinal cerebral fissure. Directly inferior to the longitudinal cerebral fissure, the fibers of the corpus callosum join the hemispheres. In the great majority of the population, the left hemisphere is dominant in the interpretive functions.

In addition to its anatomic superiority, the cerebral cortex maintains the highest level of information processing in the human. Some functional areas are localized; others are more general and widely dispersed. The significant localized functional areas include the primary motor projection and sensory projection areas. The motor projection area is located on the anterior wall of the central sulcus and adjacent to the precentral gyrus (Fig. 48-23). This area controls voluntary skeletal muscle movements of the contralateral body. The disproportionate representation of body parts on the sensory cortex is illustrated in Figure 48-24. The sensory projection area (somesthetic area) is located on the postcentral gyrus and receives input from the thalamus-projected sensations of the contralateral side of the body.

Other rather well-localized functions processed in the cortex include visual, hearing, olfaction, and somatic interpretations. The mental and intellectual activities in humans are processed and interpreted in widely dispersed association areas of the cortex.

A brief review of the function of the cerebral hemisphere lobes follows (see Figure 48-22). The *frontal* lobe, the largest of the lobes, extends from the central sulcus (fissure of Rolando) forward and from the lateral fissure (fissure of Sylvius) upward. It contains the motor strip (Brodmann's area 4), premotor area (areas 6 and 8), Broca's speech center (areas 44 and 45), and association areas related to higher mental functions and behavior. The *parietal* lobe lies between the central sulcus and the parieto-occipital fissure. The lateral fissure divides the parietal from the temporal lobe. Angular, postcentral, and supramarginal gyri are significant landmarks in the parietal lobe. Primary and secondary somesthetic areas are contained here, as are many sensory association fibers. Interpretations of feeling and hearing are made here (areas 1, 2, and 3). In addition, body image recognition evolves from the parietal lobe.

The *occipital* lobe lies posterior to the parietal lobe and is divided from the cerebellum by the parieto-occipital fissure. Primary visual centers and visual association areas are contained in the occipital lobe (areas 18 and 19). The *temporal lobe* extends downward from the lateral fissure and posteriorly to the parieto-occipital fissure. Auditory receptive centers (areas 41 and 42), auditory association area (area 22, Wernicke's), smell interpretation, and memory storage are contained in the temporal lobe.

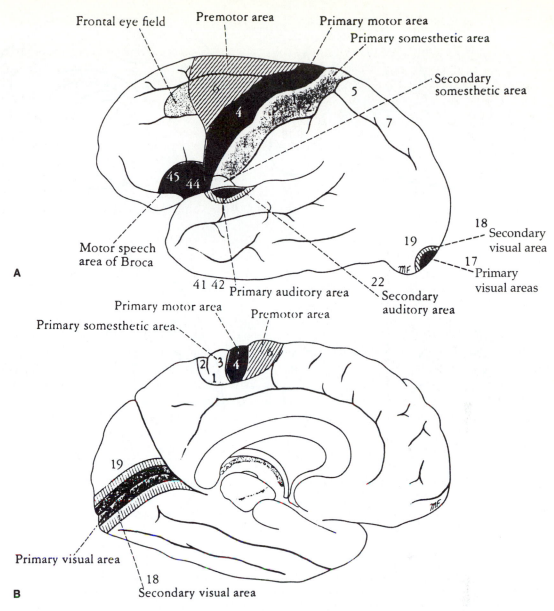

FIGURE 48-21 *Functional localization of the cerebral cortex based on Brodmann's cytoarchitectonic map.* **A.** *Lateral view of the left cerebral hemisphere.* **B.** *Medial view of the left cerebral hemisphere. (Source: Snell, R.S.* Clinical Neuroanatomy for Medical Students. *Boston: Little, Brown, 1992.)*

▼ The Peripheral Nervous System

The peripheral nervous system includes the nerve tissue outside the brain and spinal cord. It is composed of 31 paired spinal nerves and 12 cranial nerves as well as numerous ganglia and plexuses. The cervical spinal nerves are numbered according to the vertebral level below, and the remaining spinal nerves are numbered according to the level of the vertebra at their exit level. Every spinal nerve contains a dorsal (afferent) and ven-

tral (efferent) root. The afferent nerve cells lie within the dorsal root ganglion, and their fibers innervate through spinal nerves and through plexuses of the visceral nervous system. The efferent cell bodies lie within the ventral gray column of the spinal cord and innervate through ventral roots of all spinal nerves to the skeletal muscle and through ventral roots of spinal nerves of the thorax, upper lumbar, and middle sacral region to the viscera.

The cranial nerve nuclei are contained in the brain stem. Some cranial nerves have only sensory components, some only motor components, and some both

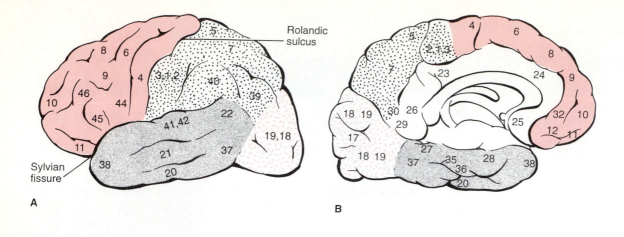

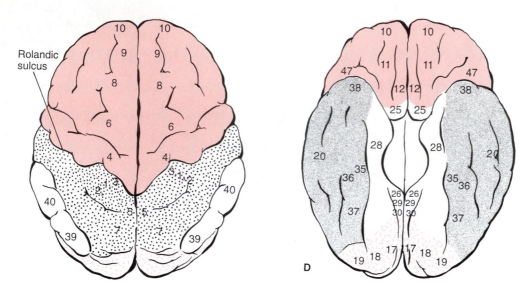

FIGURE 48-22   *Line drawings of **A.** lateral, **B.** mesial, **C.** superior, and **D.** inferior views of the brain, depicting major demarcation points, including the rolandic sulcus and the sylvian fissure. The four main lobes are shown in different shades: red, frontal; dots, parietal; dashes, occipital; shading, temporal. Only the left hemisphere is depicted in the lateral and mesial views, but the mapping would be the same on the right hemisphere. The unmarked zone, including the cingulate gyrus (ie, areas 24 and 23) and areas 25, 26, 27, and 28, corresponds to a region commonly referred to as the limbic lobe. In the superior perspective, the left hemisphere is on the left and the right hemisphere is on the right; the sides are reversed in the inferior perspective. (Source: Conn, P.M. Neuroscience in Medicine. Philadelphia: J.B. Lippincott, 1995.)*

(mixed). Their names and general functions are presented in Table 48-4. Their functions and alterations in function are further described on pp. 1035–1039.

AFFERENT (SENSORY) DIVISION

The afferent (sensory) division of the peripheral nervous system detects, transmits, and processes environmental information from internal and external sources through a variety of specific receptors. The *somatic afferent* fibers carry impulses from the skin, skeletal muscles, joints, and tendons to the CNS. The *visceral afferent* fibers carry impulses from the viscera to the CNS.

The receptors of afferent fibers transmit to the CNS by numerous converging fibers through peripheral nerves. As a result of this convergence of neurons, injury to a nerve fiber does not result in clearly defined sensory deficits. Rather, the area that responds in an altered manner is vaguely defined.

The areas in the skin supplied by specific spinal nerve dorsal roots are called *dermatomes*. Traditionally, these have been arranged to correspond to the spinal cord segments. Thus, a rather loose topographic division of these segments includes the 8 cervical, 12 thoracic, 5 lumbar, and 5 sacral cord regions. Considerable overlapping exists between the dermatomes and, generally,

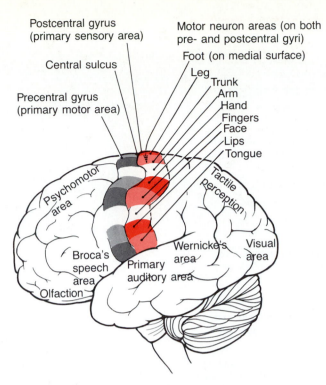

FIGURE 48-23 *Topographic organization of functions of control and interpretation on the precentral and postcentral gyri.*

sensory deficits are identified when more than a single spinal nerve is interrupted. Dermatomes are mapped according to the segmentation of individual dorsal roots (Fig. 48-25).

The first-order afferent fibers carrying sensory data enter the spinal cord by way of the dorsal roots to the dorsal root ganglia and become dispersed according to function. Fibers that transmit pain and temperature are anatomically related, cross over, and ascend through the *lateral spinothalamic tract* to the posterior ventral nucleus of the thalamus. The *ventral spinothalamic tracts* contain many of the fibers from receptors that are sensitive to touch, proprioception, and pressure (Fig. 48-26). From here, these proceed to the somesthetic region of the cerebral postcentral gyrus. Impulses from muscles, tendons, ligaments, and joints (proprioceptive fibers) disperse in a variety of tracts. Some simply cross the cord to the anterior horn (stretch reflex). Others synapse with the posterior gray column and ascend the spinocerebellar tracts to the cerebellum, whereas yet others ascend by way of the posterior white columns, decussate at the medial lemniscus, and continue to the posterior ventral nucleus of the thalamus. The ascent from this region continues to the sensory cortex at the postcentral gyrus. Figure 48-22 identifies the somesthetic projection areas

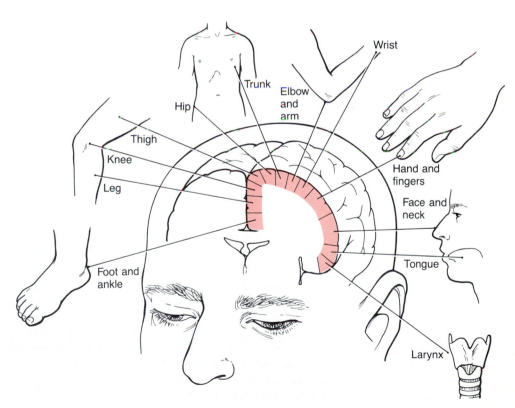

FIGURE 48-24 *Areas of brain that control specific areas of the body. Size indicates relative distribution of control.*

TABLE 48-4   *The Cranial Nerves*

Number	Name and Type of Nerve	General Function
I	Olfactory (sensory)	Sense of smell
II	Optic (sensory)	Vision
III	Oculomotor (motor)	Motor control and sensation for four eye muscles and upper eyelid elevator, pupillary constriction and accommodation
IV	Trochlea (motor)	Movement of major eyeball muscle medially and down
V	Trigeminal (mixed)	Mastication and perception of facial sensations. Blink eye reflex (sensory limb)
VI	Abducens (motor)	Movement of eyeball laterally
VII	Facial (mixed)	Facial expression, salivation, lacrimation, taste sensations from anterior two thirds of tongue. Blink eye reflex (motor limb)
VIII	Acoustic (sensory)	Equilibrium and hearing
IX	Glossopharyngeal (mixed)	Salivation, movement and sensation of pharynx, taste and sensation of posterior tongue, and carotid baroreceptor sensations
X	Vagus (mixed)	Swallowing, phonation, and laryngeal control, and parasympathetic innervation to thoracic and abdominal viscera
XI	Spinal accessory (motor)	Head and shoulder movement
XII	Hypoglossal (motor)	Movement of tongue

on the postcentral gyrus. It is significant that the body areas that contain more sensory receptors are accorded a larger area on the surface of the sensory cortex. For example, the face and fingers, which are rife with receptors, occupy a larger neuronal area in the cortex than does the large body area of the trunk, with its comparatively smaller receptor population.

As noted earlier, an important component of the afferent division is the thalamus, primarily because almost all sensory systems convey impulses to its specific nuclei through either the dorsal column or anterolateral tract. Together with the thalamus, the cortex is concerned with conscious perception of sensory stimuli that occur distantly from it. The thalamus provides perception of touch and pressure, whereas more complex discrimination sensations, such as texture, size, and weight of objects, are interpreted by the cortex.

EFFERENT (MOTOR) DIVISION

Voluntary and involuntary body activities initiated by the efferent division are transmitted in response to the stimuli the CNS has received from the afferent division. These responses may be through the innervation of smooth muscles, cardiac muscle, and glands and arrive by way of the autonomic nervous system. This is referred to as the *visceral efferent system*. The skeletal muscles, tendons, and joints receive innervation from the CNS by the *somatic efferent system*. The somatic responses at the lowest level occur in the spinal cord and are transmitted through the spinal reflex arc from each spinal segment. These responses are automatic and spontaneous.

The efferent fibers emerge from the ventral horn nuclei (motor horn cells) and transmit impulses through the spinal nerves. Both efferent and afferent fibers transmit concurrently in most peripheral nerves. Thus, injury to one of these nerves could result in both sensory and motor deficits.

The efferent fibers receive their impulses from simple spinal reflex circuits or more complicated descending pathways from higher centers. The significant higher centers that are important in relaying efferent responses to the periphery include the precentral gyrus (motor cortex), basal ganglia, brain stem, and cerebellum. The fibers that transmit from these areas do so through two principal tracts: pyramidal and extrapyramidal.

Pyramidal and Extrapyramidal Tracts

The pyramidal tract (Fig. 48-27), both lateral corticospinal and ventral corticospinal, originates in the motor cortex (precentral gyrus) of the cerebrum in large pyra-

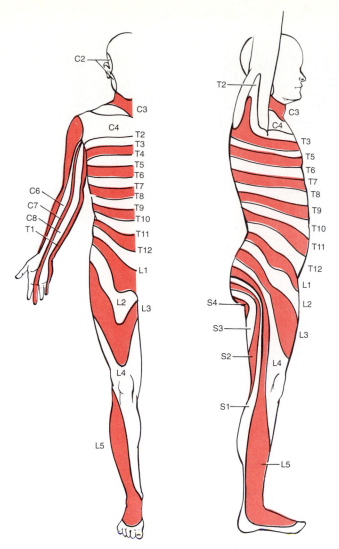

FIGURE 48-25 *A dermatome is the area of skin supplied by axons from a single dorsal root ganglion. (Source: Conn, P.M.* Neuroscience in Medicine. *Philadelphia: J.B. Lippincott, 1995.)*

and joints. The neurons innervating skeletal muscle are known as the *lower motor neurons.*

The remaining efferent fibers that do not traverse the pyramid in the brain stem are part of the extrapyramidal system. Unlike the pyramidal tract, the extrapyramidal tracts do not continue to the cord uninterrupted. The system is more complex, less directed, and highly interconnected and is considered by some authors to be a functional, rather than an anatomic, entity.[1,2] Many of the fibers descend from the cortex directly to specific areas in the basal ganglia and brain stem, whereas others make intermediate synapses. Several extrapyramidal tracts originate in the brain stem and are named for their site of origin. These include the *vestibulospinal tract* from the lateral vestibular nucleus in the medulla, the *rubrospinal tract* from the red nucleus in the midbrain, the *tectospinal tract* from the roof (superior colliculus) of the midbrain, and the *reticulospinal tract* from the reticular formation in the pons and medulla. The majority of the extrapyramidal fibers decussate with the reticulospinal tract. In addition to the named tracts, important fibers of the extrapyramidal system originate in the cerebellum and the vestibular apparatus.

The pyramidal tract processes information regarding voluntary movement dealing with precise and specific activities of muscles, whereas the extrapyramidal tracts provide the "supporting" type of movement that accompanies the more precise movements afforded by the pyramidal tract. For example, the gross movements necessary to engage in the activity of writing are influenced by the extrapyramidal tracts. Included here are such movements as might be necessary for proper body positioning, particularly of the upper arm and shoulder. The more precise movement of holding the pencil effectively is controlled by the corticospinal tract.

▼ The Autonomic Nervous System

The autonomic nervous system, also referred to as the general visceral efferent system, maintains the internal environment in a relatively steady state. Though it is outside the CNS, it is influenced by the CNS and is distinct from the peripheral nervous system. Autonomic fibers project innervations, which are activated involuntarily from the CNS to smooth muscles, cardiac muscle, and glands to regulate activities related to respiration, cardiovascular function, digestion, excretion, body temperature, and sexual function. Centers in the hypothalamus, brain stem, and spinal cord transmit reflex responses to visceral organs to regulate the internal environment. Autonomic fibers differ from somatic efferent fibers in that they consist of a double neuron chain from the CNS to the visceral effectors, whereas the somatic

mid-shaped cells called *Betz cells.* It transmits, uninterrupted, in a descending manner through the basal ganglia and brain stem. The area where it joins other projection fibers, between the basal ganglia and the thalamus, is known as the *internal capsule.* In the brain stem, most of the fibers decussate and project through a structure known as the *pyramid.* The crossed fibers then continue to descend as the *lateral corticospinal tract* and terminate in the ventral horn of the gray matter at a specific spinal cord level. A few fibers continue to descend without decussation by way of the *ventral corticospinal tract* and cross near the level of their termination in the ventral horn. The fibers of the pyramidal tract are contained in the CNS and compose the *upper motor neuron.* The pyramidal fibers synapse with segmental anterior horn cells (motor neurons), which, in turn, synapse with peripheral efferent fibers innervating specific muscles, tendons,

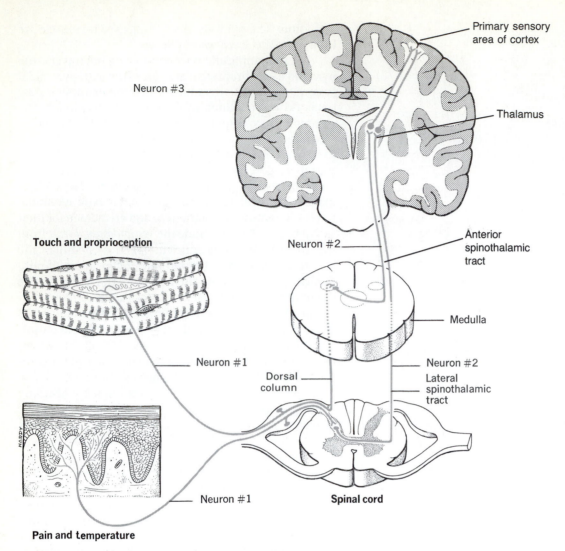

FIGURE 48-26 *Representation of the touch-pressure pathways (Neuron #1) ascending in the dorsal column to the medulla, where they synapse with second-order neurons (Neuron #2) that cross to the opposite side (decussate) and ascend in the anterior or lateral spinothalamic tract to the thalamus. Third-order neurons (Neuron #3) connect the thalamus with the cerebral cortex. (Source: Adapted from Hudak, C.M. and Gallo, B.M. Critical Care Nursing [6th ed.]. Philadelphia: J.B. Lippincott, 1994.)*

efferents transmit through one neuron. Visceral efferent fibers transmit in spinal nerves and in several cranial nerves. Visceral efferent innervation frequently accompanies somatic efferent activity. For example, a jogger receives innervation from the somatic efferent fibers to provide the skeletal muscle responses required in the jogging activity. Simultaneously, the somatic efferent system innervates the cardiac and smooth muscle. The somatic efferent responses can be observed readily, whereas the visceral efferent responses are less obvious.

In addition to the autonomic efferent fibers, certain afferent fibers are sometimes assigned to the autonomic nervous system. These are present in spinal nerves as well as in certain cranial nerves. They innervate receptors in the viscera, thorax, and walls of the blood vessels.

The autonomic nervous system consists of two func-

tionally distinct divisions: *sympathetic* and *parasympathetic* (Fig. 48-28). Many visceral effector organs have a dual nerve supply, one from each division. The sympathetic division assists the body into action during physiologic and psychological stress by supportive activities, such as increasing heart and respiratory rates and mobilizing glucose from glycogen stores to supply the skeletal muscles with additional energy. The parasympathetic division provides a counterbalance for the sympathetic division. Nerve cells of both divisions group outside the CNS in structures known as *autonomic ganglia*. Cell fibers that terminate with a synapse at these ganglia and retain the cell body within the CNS are *preganglionic neurons*. Conversely, nerve cells having cell bodies in the ganglia and axons extending to the organs and glands are known as the *postganglionic neurons*.

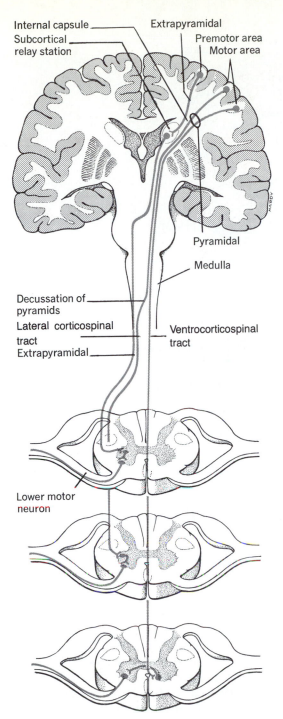

paired ganglia, single ganglia exist surrounding the abdominal aorta and its larger branches, where preganglionic neurons terminate without synapsing in the sympathetic chain. These are known as *collateral (prevertebral) ganglia* and include the celiac and superior and inferior mesenteric ganglia. The terminal ganglia are parasympathetic and are located in proximity to the effector organs.

SYMPATHETIC DIVISION (THORACOLUMBAR)

The cell bodies of the short preganglionic sympathetic neurons arise from the sympathetic motoneurons of the intermediolateral horns of the spinal cord between the first thoracic and second lumbar vertebrae (see Figure 48-29). The fibers of these neurons pass through the intervertebral foramina in conjunction with respective spinal nerves. Shortly, the sympathetic fibers (preganglionic) depart from the spinal nerve and enter a sympathetic chain through the white rami communicans. They may synapse here immediately with a postganglion neuron, pass directly through the sympathetic

FIGURE 48-27 *Descending motor pathways showing the crossed lateral corticospinal tract and the uncrossed ventral corticospinal. (Source: Adapted from Hudak, C.M. and Gallo, B.M. Critical Care Nursing [6th ed.]. Philadelphia: J.B. Lippincott, 1994.)*

The sympathetic system has a chain or trunk of paired ganglia on either side of the spinal cord (*paravertebral ganglia*), extending its full length. These ganglia are connected on each side by nerve trunks and together are referred to as the right and left *sympathetic chains* or *sympathetic trunks* (Fig. 48-29). In addition to these

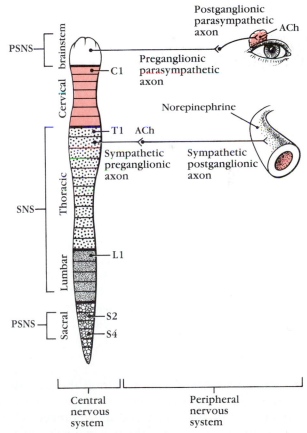

FIGURE 48-28 *Schematic overview of the origins of sympathetic (SNS) and parasympathetic (PSNS) nervous systems with corresponding major transmitter substances at the synapses: acetylcholine (ACh) and norepinephrine (noradrenaline).*

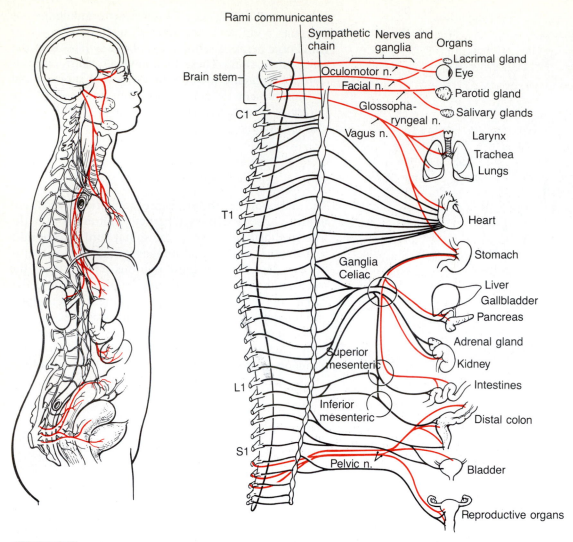

FIGURE 48-29 *Anatomy of the autonomic nervous system. Red indicates the parasympathetic system. (Adapted from: Memmler, R.L. Cohen, B.J. and Wood, D.L.* The Human Body in Health and Disease *[7th ed.]. Philadelphia: J.B. Lippincott, 1992.)*

chain to synapse with a single sympathetic ganglion, or pass up or down the sympathetic chain and synapse at a different level.

Some postganglionic sympathetic fibers, after having synapsed in the sympathetic chain, pass back into the spinal nerve through the gray rami communicans and accompany the spinal nerve to innervate blood vessels, sweat glands, and piloerector muscles in the skin.

PARASYMPATHETIC DIVISION (CRANIOSACRAL)

The autonomic fibers that arise from the cranial and sacral portions of the CNS compose the parasympathetic nervous system (see Figure 48-29). Somatic efferent fibers in the cranial region arise in conjunction with the oculomotor (cranial nerve III), facial (cranial nerve VII), glossopharyngeal (cranial nerve IX), and vagus (cranial nerve X) nerves. The vagus transmits the majority of the

parasympathetic impulses through its wide distribution in the thoracic and abdominal viscera. The remaining cranial nerves innervate organs of the head. The sacral fibers arise from the anterior roots of the second, third, and fourth sacral spinal nerves and innervate pelvic organs and the colon. Most of the preganglionic fibers transmit without interruption to the organs they innervate, where they synapse with the parasympathetic ganglia that are located in the area of the effector organ. In contrast to the sympathetic fibers, the parasympathetic preganglionic fibers are long and the postganglionic fibers are short.

TRANSMITTERS AND RECEPTORS OF THE AUTONOMIC NERVOUS SYSTEM

Chemical mediation is necessary for neuronal transmission between neurons and between neurons and their effector organs. Excitation results from chemical release of transmitter substances between preganglionic and postganglionic neurons and their effectors in the autonomic nervous system. The transmitter substance released at the preganglionic neurons in both the sympathetic and parasympathetic nervous systems is *acetylcholine*. Acetylcholine continues to be the transmitter substance from the parasympathetic postganglionic neurons. Because of the secretion of acetylcholine, these fibers are known as *cholinergic* and their receptors as *cholinoceptive*.

The primary transmitter substance secreted by the postganglionic fibers of the sympathetic nervous system is *norepinephrine*. The fibers are referred to as *adrenergic* and terminate on *adrenoceptive* receptors. These are separated into alpha (α) and beta (β) receptors, based on their sensitivity to certain drugs. They are further subdivided into α_1, α_2, β_1, and β_2. The α_1 receptor activity is associated with vasoconstriction and increased blood pressure, whereas α_2 receptor stimulation is associated with suppression of norepinephrine and relaxation. The β_1 receptor activity is associated with increased heart rate and contractility. The β_2 receptor stimulation results in bronchodilation and vasodilation. Alpha receptors are dispersed widely in various organs but predominate in the precapillary sphincters of smooth muscles of blood vessels. Beta receptors predominate in the heart, coronary arteries, lungs, bronchi, liver, and brain. A few of the fibers of the postganglionic sympathetic nervous system secrete acetylcholine at their terminal fibers, including fibers to sweat glands and postganglionic sympathetic vasodilator fibers to skeletal muscle vasculature.[2] A single postganglionic sympathetic nerve may innervate thousands of receptor sites. This is demonstrated by the diffuse response to the sympathetic nervous system excitation, in contrast to the more localized responses characteristic of parasympathetic activity.

STIMULATION AND INHIBITION ACTION OF THE AUTONOMIC NERVOUS SYSTEM

The actions of the sympathetic and parasympathetic nervous systems on various receptor organs are summarized in Table 48-5.

The dual actions are a cooperative effort to maintain a constant internal environment in response to the everchanging external world. General responses of the sympathetic nervous system are activated under emergency situations to make internal adjustments that facilitate an appropriate response by the body. For example, in response to stressful exercise, the cardiovascular system is stimulated by the sympathetic system to increase cardiac output by increasing heart rate and force, thereby providing additional perfusion to skeletal muscle, brain, and liver while simultaneously reducing the blood supply to the viscera. The parasympathetic system, in contrast, promotes activities that maintain body function from day to day, including digestion and elimination.

The visceral effectors that receive stimulation from both the sympathetic and parasympathetic systems generally receive antagonistic stimulation. An example of this is the effect on bronchial secretions. Sympathetic stimulation decreases bronchial secretions and parasympathetic stimulation increases them. In another example, the sympathetic system dilates the pupils, whereas the parasympathetic system constricts them. The dual system does not function consistently in a cooperative balance, because some organs receive innervation primarily from only one system. Examples include the smooth muscles of the skin, hair, sweat glands, and cutaneous blood vessels, which are primarily innervated from the sympathetic system.

Although most organs and viscera receive innervation from both sympathetic and parasympathetic systems, one of these generally has an inhibitory effect and the other an excitatory effect. There is no consistent rule of thumb for guidance as to which system stimulates and which inhibits.

EFFECTS OF SYMPATHETIC AND PARASYMPATHETIC STIMULATION ON VARIOUS STRUCTURES

Lacrimal Glands

The parasympathetic system vasodilates and stimulates secretion of the lacrimal glands through the postganglionic axons from the sphenopalatine ganglion by the maxillary division of the fifth cranial nerve. The preganglionic axons originate in the superior salivatory nucleus and follow the route of the seventh cranial nerve. The sympathetic system has a vasoconstrictive effect on the lacrimal glands and transmits its impulses through preganglionic neurons, which originate from the intermediolateral cells in the thoracic spinal column and through postganglionic neurons of the superior cervical ganglion. The impulses reach the glands through the maxillary division of the fifth cranial nerve.[11]

Eyes

Pupillary constriction and near-vision accommodation are accomplished through parasympathetic stimulation. The oculomotor nucleus sends preganglionic axons by the oculomotor nerve to the ciliary ganglion. From here the postganglionic axons reach the ciliary muscle and constrictor muscle of the iris by the ciliary nerve. When pupils are reflexively stimulated with light, the pupillary openings decrease and reduce the amount of light reaching the retina.

The sympathetic stimulation dilates the pupils, constricts vessels, and provides far-vision accommodation. The preganglionic axons of fibers accomplishing these

TABLE 48-5 *The Effects of Sympathetic and Parasympathetic Stimulation on Effector Organs*

Organ	Organ Receptor	Sympathetic Stimulation	Parasympathetic Stimulation
EYE			
Radial muscle of iris	α	Contraction (mydriasis)	Contraction (miosis)
Sphincter muscle of iris		Relaxation	Contraction
Ciliary muscle	β	Relaxation	Contraction
HEART			
SA node	β_1	Increases rate	Decreases rate
Atria	β_1	Increases contractility	Decreases contractility
Ventricles	β_1	Increases contractility	
AV node	β_1	Increases conduction	Decreases conduction
Coronary arterioles	β_2	Dilates	
SKIN	α	Constriction	
Mesentery	α	Constriction	
Skeletal muscle	α	Dilates	Dilates
LUNGS			
Bronchial muscle	β_2	Relaxation	Contraction
Bronchial secretions	?	Decreases?	Increases
Sweat glands	α	Localized secretion	Generalized secretion
Pilomotor muscles	α	Contraction	
INTESTINE			
Motility	α, β_2	Decreases	Increases
Sphincters	α	Contraction	Relaxation
LIVER	β_2	Glycogenolysis	
GALLBLADDER AND DUCTS	—	Relaxes	Contracts
PANCREAS			
Acini cells	α	Decreased secretion	Secretion
Islet cells	α, β_2	Inhibits, stimulates	
Salivary glands	α	Thick secretions	Profuse, thin secretions
	β_2	Amylase secretion	
Fat cells	β_1	Lipolysis	
BLADDER			
Detrusor muscle	β	Relaxation	Contractions
Trigone	α	Contraction	Relaxation
			Erection
PENIS	α	Ejaculation	
Basal metabolism	—	Increased	
Adrenal medulla	—	Secretion of epinephrine and norepinephrine	
Mentation	—	Increased	

activities originate in the thoracic spinal segments and ascend by the sympathetic chain to the superior cervical ganglion, where they synapse with the postganglionic neurons. The postganglionic axons travel through divisions of the fifth nerve to the dilator muscles of the irises (levator palpebrae superioris) and radial fibers of the ciliary muscles. Innervation of blood vessels of the retinae, orbits, and conjunctivae is accomplished in the same manner.[13]

Salivary Glands

The superior salivary nucleus projects the preganglionic axons for the submaxillary and sublingual glands, and the inferior salivary nucleus projects preganglionic axons for the parotid gland. The axons from the superior salivary nucleus travel through a branch of the seventh cranial nerve to the submaxillary and sublingual ganglia, and those from the inferior salivary nucleus travel through a branch of the ninth cranial nerve to the otic ganglia. From the submaxillary and sublingual ganglia, axons project to their glands and from the otic ganglia to the parotid gland through the fifth cranial nerve. The parasympathetic system activates these glands to vasodilate and secrete.

The sympathetic system vasoconstricts and promotes secretion of salivary glands. Its preganglionic axons ascend from the upper thoracic spinal cord to the superior cervical ganglia to synapse with the postganglionic neurons. These axons reach the glands along the external carotid and external maxillary arteries.[6]

Heart

The overall effects of the parasympathetic system on the heart are deceleration and coronary artery vasoconstriction. Its stimulation of the heart decreases its effectiveness. However, in the process, it does slow the metabolism and oxygen requirements and thus provides some rest for the cardiac muscle. The parasympathetic preganglionic fibers pass from the dorsal motor nucleus of the vagus and synapse with the postganglionic neurons through the vagal trunk at cardiac plexus ganglia in the atrial walls.

In contrast, the sympathetic system increases the overall activity of the heart, produces both positive chronotropic and inotropic effects, and dilates the coronary arteries. In essence, the sympathetic system makes the heart more effective, although it simultaneously increases workload and metabolic requirements. The upper thoracic spinal cord provides the origin of the preganglionic neurons, which project their axons from the ventral roots and white rami to the sympathetic chain.[10] The postganglionic neurons emerge from higher thoracic and lower cervical ganglia and travel to the cardiac plexus.[14]

Bronchi

The bronchi are constricted by the parasympathetic system. The origin of the parasympathetic neurons and the course of their preganglionic and postganglionic fibers are similar to those of the parasympathetic fibers innervating the heart. The preganglionic fibers synapse with the postganglionic fibers in the pulmonary plexus. The axons of the postganglionic cells terminate in the bronchi and blood vessels.

The sympathetic system dilates the bronchi. The neurons originate in thoracic segments 2 through 6, and their axons enter the pulmonary plexus in a manner similar to that of the parasympathetic system.[6]

Esophagus

The parasympathetic system exerts the main autonomic influence over the function of the esophagus. Stimulation causes smooth muscle of the esophagus to constrict, increasing its overall activity in propelling ingested materials along its course. This stimulation comes from various branches of the vagus nerve.[14]

Abdominal Viscera, Glands, and Vessels

Stimulation of the parasympathetic system promotes peristalsis and increases in secretion by the various gastrointestinal glands. The preganglionic fibers originate from the vagus and synapse with the postganglionic fibers of the various visceral organs in their intrinsic plexus.

In contrast, the sympathetic system inhibits peristalsis and enhances vasoconstriction. The lower thoracic and upper lumbar cord segments provide the origin of the preganglionic neurons. Their axons traverse the splanchnic nerves to synapse with the postganglionic neurons in the prevertebral ganglion plexus. Innervation is provided to the visceral smooth muscle and blood vessels.[11]

Pelvic Viscera

Stimulation of the parasympathetic system assists in urination and defecation by contracting the bladder and lower colon. Penile erection is also facilitated by the parasympathetic system. The neurons that accomplish these functions originate in the sacral cord segments, and their axons transmit to the various organs.

Stimulation of the sympathetic system promotes contraction of the vesicle sphincter, vasoconstriction, and ejaculation. The preganglionic neurons originate in the lower thoracic and upper lumbar segments and travel along the splanchnic nerves similarly to those of the abdominal viscera. The postganglionic fibers travel along the hypogastric nerves of the organs innervated.[11]

Peripheral Vessels and Sweat Glands

The major effect of the autonomic nervous system on the peripheral and deep vessels is stimulation of the sympathetic system. This results in vasoconstriction of cutaneous vessels as well as deep visceral vessels. Sweat glands secrete in response to sympathetic stimulation. The postganglionic fibers to the sweat glands are cholinergic, in contrast with other sympathetic fibers, which are adrenergic.

Adrenal Medulla

In response to sympathetic stimulation, the adrenal medulla secretes epinephrine and norepinephrine, which reach all cells and produce an excitatory effect. This mechanism is part of the diffuse sympathoadrenal system, which is activated in response to stress. In addition to the stimulatory effect on the nervous system, epinephrine and norepinephrine affect metabolism through glycogenolysis in the liver and skeletal muscle and mobilization of fatty acids.

Distinct effects of circulating epinephrine and norepinephrine on heart function include increased force and rate of contraction as well as increased excitability of the myocardium. Norepinephrine produces vasoconstriction in most organs, whereas epinephrine has a dilating effect on the vessels of the liver and skeletal muscle. Other effects observed in response to circulating epinephrine and norepinephrine include increased mental acuity, inhibition of the gastrointestinal tract, and pupillary dilation. Thus, the circulating catecholamines released by the adrenal medulla have functions similar to those of the adrenergic nerve discharges and enhance their action. The effects of the circulating catecholamines linger, because their metabolism or removal from blood takes longer than it does in those released at the adrenergic nerve terminals.[6]

Minimal secretion of epinephrine and norepinephrine occurs at basal conditions, as in sleep. During increased activity and stress or when adrenergic stimulation is increased in such conditions as pain, cold, hypoglycemia, and emotional excitement, secretion is considerably increased. This stimulation is transmitted to the adrenal medulla by the hypothalamic nervous centers as well as by direct sympathetic innervation of the medulla.

Autonomic Reflexes

In response to certain environmental conditions, autonomic reflexes maintain the internal environment appropriate to the demand, that of either action or repair. The actions generally occur at an unconscious level and involve such functions as control of pupillary size, cardiovascular status, and variations in respiratory, gastrointestinal, and genitourinary systems.

▼ The Ventricular System and Cerebrospinal Fluid

FUNCTION OF CEREBROSPINAL FLUID

The CSF that circulates in the subarachnoid space around the brain and spinal cord (Fig. 48-30) provides an important supportive and protective mechanism for the CNS. Together with support from blood vessels, nerve roots, and fine fibrous arachnoid trabeculae, the brain and spinal cord are directly encased within the subarachnoid CSF and receive buoyancy from it that prevents the vessels and nerve roots from stretching in response to movements (Table 48-6). The average weight of the adult brain is approximately 1,450 g in the air, although in the buoyant CSF bath, its weight is reduced to approximately 50 g. This buoyancy allows for relatively effective suspension of the brain and assists in preventing lethal damage under daily traumas.

Pneumoencephalography demonstrates the effects of CSF deficiency on the brain. This diagnostic procedure, rarely performed today, visualizes structural elements of the brain when CSF is removed and replaced by air. Thus, the weight of the brain rests on the vascular, nervous, and meningeal structures and results in a se-

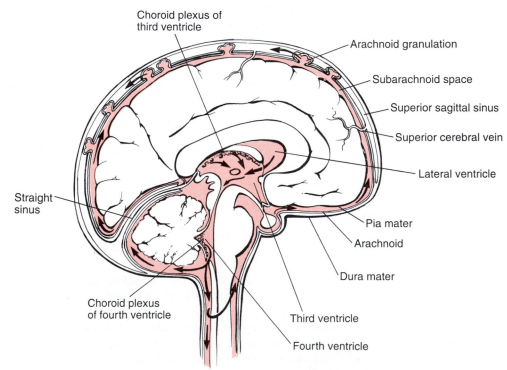

FIGURE 48-30 *Cerebrospinal fluid (CSF) is formed and secreted by the choroid plexuses in the lateral, third, and fourth ventricles. The great vascularity of the plexuses imparts a reddish cast to these tissues. In adult humans, the total weight of the choroid plexus in the four ventricles is 2 to 3 g. Choroidal tissue is not present in the subarachnoid CSF space that surrounds the brain hemispheres and spinal cord. (Source: Conn, P.M. Neuroscience in Medicine. Philadelphia: J.B. Lippincott, 1995.)*

Choroid plexus of third ventricle

Arachnoid granulation

Subarachnoid space

Superior sagittal sinus

Superior cerebral vein

Lateral ventricle

Straight sinus

Pia mater

Arachnoid

Dura mater

Choroid plexus of fourth ventricle

Third ventricle

Fourth ventricle

TABLE 48-6 *Roles of Cerebrospinal Fluid in Serving the Brain*

Cerebrospinal Fluid (CSF) Functions	Examples
Buoyancy effect	Because brain weight is effectively reduced by more than 95%, shearing and tearing forces on neural tissue are greatly minimized.
Intracranial volume adjustment	CSF volume can be adjusted, increasing or decreasing acutely in response to blood volume changes or chronically in response to tissue atrophy or tumor growth.
Micronutrient transport	Nucleosides, pyrimidines, vitamin C, and other nutrients are transported by the choroid plexus to CSF and eventually to brain cells.
Protein and peptide supply	Macromolecules like transthyretin, insulin-like growth factor, and thyroxine are transported by the choroid plexus into CSF for carriage to target cells in brain.
Source of osmolytes for brain volume regulation	In acute hypernatremia there is bulk flow of CSF with osmolytes, from ventricles to surrounding tissue. This promotes water retention by shrunken brain, i.e., to restore volume.
Buffer reservoir	When brain interstitial fluid concentrations of H^+, K^+, and glucose are altered, the ventricular fluid can help to buffer the extracellular fluid changes
Sink or drainage action	Anion metabolites of neurotransmitters, protein products of catabolism or tissue breakdown, and xenobiotic substances are cleared from the central nervous system by active transporters in the choroid plexus or by bulk CSF drainage pathways to venous blood and the lymphatics.
Immune system mediation	Cells adjacent to ventricles have antigen-presenting capabilities. Some CSF protein drains into cervical lymphatics, with the potential for inducing antibody reactions.
Information transfer	Neurotransmitter agents like amino acids and peptides may be transported by CSF over distances to bind to receptors in the parasynaptic mode.
Drug delivery	Some drugs do not readily cross blood–brain barrier but can be transported into the CSF by endogenous proteins in choroid plexus epithelial membranes.

(Conn, P.M.. *Neuroscience in Medicine*. Philadelphia: J.B. Lippincott, 1995.)

vere headache that is greatly intensified by the slightest jarring of the head.

In addition to its mechanical function, CSF provides a medium for passage of substances between blood and the extracellular fluid of the brain. It probably also nourishes brain tissues and removes the metabolites of nerve cell function.

FORMATION AND ABSORPTION OF CEREBROSPINAL FLUID

The CSF is produced, circulated, and reabsorbed continuously. Its principal formation site is in the *choroid plexus* of the lateral ventricle, with most of the remainder being formed in the third and fourth ventricles (Fig. 48-31). Table 48-7 lists the normal composition and pressure of

CSF as well as the significance of common alterations. The choroid plexus is a network of capillary tufts surrounded by cuboidal epithelium. The fluid is produced through filtration, diffusion, and active transport from the blood. A second, lesser source of CSF is from the ependymal cells lining the ventricles and meningeal blood vessels. In the adult human, approximately 500 mL of fluid is produced every 24 hours, and approximately 125 mL is circulating at any given time. Wide fluctuations may occur in the amount produced during any given 24-hour period. Sodium ions are actively transported across the epithelial cells into CSF from blood. This results in a greater osmotic force in the CSF; therefore, to maintain osmotic equilibrium, water passively follows the ions. Thus, water is extracted from the capillaries and is responsible for the secretory function of

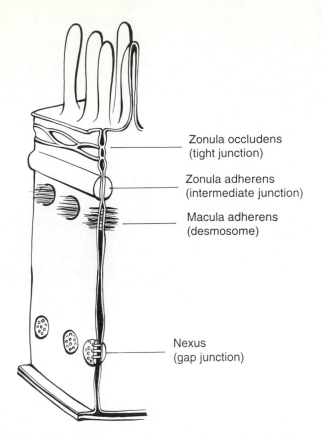

Zonula occludens
(tight junction)

Zonula adherens
(intermediate junction)

Macula adherens
(desmosome)

Nexus
(gap junction)

FIGURE 48-31 *Ultrastructure of the intercellular junctions in the choroid plexus and in ependymal membranes. An integral part of the blood–cerebrospinal fluid (CSF) barrier is the tight junctions or zonulae occludens. These tight junctions are located near the apical (CSF-facing) borders of the choroidal epithelium, where the cells abut each other. The tight junctions are multilayered membranes that completely envelop the cells, offering a physical restriction to the diffusion of most solutes between the plasma and CSF. Gap junctions are between the cells of the ependymal and pia-glial linings. The gap junctions form incomplete belts around the cells, and these intercellular junctions are more "leaky" than their tight junction counterparts in the choroid plexus. Overall, the composition of CSF resembles brain interstitial fluid more than plasma because the gap junctions in the ependyma permit unrestricted diffusion, but the tight junctions in the choroid plexus do not. (Source: Conn, P.M. Neuroscience in Medicine. Philadelphia: J.B. Lippincott, 1995.)*

the choroid plexus. Facilitated diffusion allows transportation of glucose in both directions.

The CSF is reabsorbed into the venous circulation through *arachnoid villi* (see Figure 48-13), granulations that project from the cerebral subarachnoid space into the venous sinuses. The CSF is passively absorbed, because its hydrostatic pressure is greater than that of venous blood in the venous sinuses. Certain particles, such as red blood cells and creatinine, pass unimpeded through the arachnoid villi.

FLOW AND OBSTRUCTION OF FLOW OF CEREBROSPINAL FLUID

The origin of CSF in the choroid plexus of the ventricles and its normal flow to the arachnoid villi (granulations) are illustrated in Figure 48-31. The fluid arrives in the third ventricle from the lateral ventricles through the interventricular foramen, flows on to the fourth ventricle through the cerebral aqueduct, and then goes on to the subarachnoid cisterns through the foramina of Magendie and Luschka. As the fluid flows over the cerebral hemispheres, it passes into the sagittal sinus for rapid reabsorption through the arachnoid villi.

Interference along the pathway of the flow of CSF results in ventricular enlargement and a condition known as *hydrocephalus*. The two types of hydrocephalus are *communicating* and *noncommunicating*. If CSF flows freely between the ventricles and lumbar subarachnoid space, it is communicating hydrocephalus. A problem exists with reabsorption of CSF in this condition. Blockage within the ventricular system that prevents free flow of CSF from one or more ventricles results in noncommunicating hydrocephalus. Ventricular dilation results in both types and leads to increased intracranial pressure (see pp. 1039–1043).

BRAIN BARRIERS

Brain cell function is dependent on a closely controlled environment. Not all circulating substances in the blood pass freely to the brain or CSF. This occurs either because their molecules are too large or the molecules they bind with are too large to cross the CNS membranes. This has been demonstrated with the injection of certain acidic dyes, such as trypan blue, which stain other body tissues but not most brain tissue. The molecules these dyes bind with are too large to enter the brain or CSF. Substances pass into the brain from the blood through capillaries to the extracellular space of the brain or through the choroid plexus into the CSF, from which small amounts are passed into the brain. Barriers exist between the blood and brain, blood and CSF, and brain and CSF.

The materials separating the various cerebral compartments, in essence, are responsible for the entrance and exit of materials to and from the CSF and brain. The choroid plexus and the brain parenchyma (except the hypothalamus) provide the barriers to free movement of substances into the brain. Molecular size, charge, and lipid solubility affect the rate of diffusion across the cerebral membranes and cells. Small molecules and lipid-soluble substances penetrate more rapidly than large molecules and water-soluble polar compounds. Plasma proteins are excluded from the CNS because of their large molecular size. Nonionized substances pass more readily into the brain and CSF than do ionized substances. Substances that penetrate rapidly into the CSF and brain include water, carbon dioxide, and oxygen.

The endothelia of capillary cells of the brain overlap and are fused together by tight junctions, creating a common, thickened basement membrane with adjacent glia and neurons. This dense basement membrane, in conjunction with an additional layer of neuroglial cells

TABLE 48-7 *Normal Characteristics and Common Alterations of Cerebrospinal Fluid*

Component/ Characteristic	Normal Finding	Alteration and Significance
Appearance	Clear, colorless, odorless	Yellowish (xanthochromia)—disintegrating red blood cells from bleed; high protein count
		Cloudiness—infection and increased white blood cells, micro-organisms, and protein
Specific gravity	1.007	
Protein	14–45 mg/dL	Elevated protein—infections, brain tumors, Guillain–Barré syndrome, demyelinating diseases, meningeal hemorrhage
Glucose	40–80 mg/dL (60% of serum glucose)	Changes are related to systemic glucose levels
		Decreases—infections and tumors
		Increases—diabetic ketoacidosis
Leukocytes	0–5/mm³	Increases—infections (meningitis), central nervous system tumors, multiple sclerosis
Chloride	120–130 mEq/L	Decreases—acute tuberculosis
Sodium	140 mEq/L	
Potassium	3.0 mEq/L	
Bicarbonate	23.6 mEq/L	
Pressure	80–180 mm H$_2$O (in side recumbent position)	Low pressure—dehydration, blockage in subarachnoid space
		High pressure—brain tumors, abscesses, hydrocephalus, edema, cerebral hematomas

surrounding the capillaries, restricts diffusion of large molecular substances between the blood and brain (Fig. 48-32). This capillary structure is equated with the blood–brain barrier. The blood–CSF barrier exists as a result of the secretory function of the choroid plexus. This is evidenced by different concentrations of certain substances in the CSF and in plasma, indicating a selective transport by the choroid plexus.

A weaker barrier is afforded by the brain–CSF barrier through the ependymal lining of the ventricular system and its adjacent glial cells. These structures provide some limitation in the transfer of fluids and chemical substances to the interstitial fluids from the CSF.

These barriers protect the brain by inhibiting potentially toxic substances from entering and facilitating entrance to those substances essential for its metabolism. Substances, such as glucose and oxygen, pass to the brain rapidly through the capillary system to maintain a constant environment for the CNS neurons. Certain drugs penetrate the barrier with more ease than others. This is important in the treatment of CNS infections, because certain antibiotics, such as chlortetracyclines and penicillin, have very limited access to the brain. Others, such as erythromycin and sulfadiazine, enter readily. Because proteins are not readily available for binding, drugs generally do not accumulate in the CSF.

Radiotherapy, infections, and tumors interrupt the brain–barrier systems and allow transport of materials that normally are not readily accorded entrance. For this reason, tumor localization with brain scanning is effective. Intravenous radioactive substances are injected and monitored with a scanner. The gamma rays emitted by the substance are recorded on x-ray film and appear as dark areas in the regions of the barrier breakdown.

▼ Brain Blood Supply and Regulation

ARTERIAL AND VENOUS CIRCULATION

The brain receives the blood supply from the internal carotid arteries anteriorly and vertebral arteries posteriorly (Fig. 48-33A). As the internal carotid arteries, which originate from the aorta on the left and common carotid on the right, ascend into the brain, they eventually branch into the anterior and middle cerebral arteries. The vertebral arteries, originating from the subclavian arteries, ascend and become the basilar artery at the pons level. The basilar artery terminates in the right and left posterior cerebral arteries, which supply the posterior regions of the cerebrum. The anterior and posterior cerebral arteries are joined by smaller communicating arteries and form a ring known as the *circle of Willis* (see Figure 48-33B). The blood supply to both cerebral hemispheres is identical. Although anomalies are common, they are usually clinically insignificant. The venous system drains the blood from the cerebrum and cerebellum

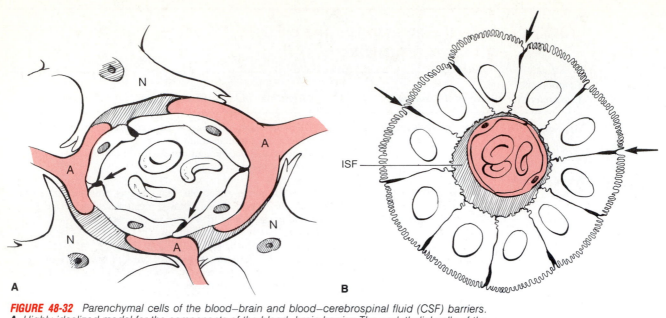

FIGURE 48-32 *Parenchymal cells of the blood–brain and blood–cerebrospinal fluid (CSF) barriers.* ***A.*** *Highly idealized model for the components of the blood–brain barrier. The endothelial cells of the cerebral capillaries lack fenestrations and are tightly joined by zonulae occludens (arrows). Astrocyte foot processes extensively abut the outside surface of the endothelium. The darkened area is the interstitial space surrounding the capillary wall. N: neuron; A: astrocyte foot process.* ***B.*** *Cross-section of a choroidal villus. A ring of choroid epithelial cells surround the interstitial fluid (ISF) and adjacent vascular core. The basolateral surface of the cells has interdigitations, and the outer CSF-facing apical membrane has an extensive microvilli system. Arrows point to the tight junctions between cells at their apical ends. (Source: Conn, P.M.* Neuroscience in Medicine. *Philadelphia: J.B. Lippincott, 1995.)*

through deep veins and dural sinuses that ultimately empty into the internal jugular veins.

AUTOREGULATION AND CEREBRAL BLOOD FLOW

The healthy brain can maintain a fairly constant blood flow, approximately 50 mL/100 g/minute or 20% of the cardiac output, even within widely fluctuating physiologic conditions. Normal cerebral blood flow is provided when the cerebral perfusion pressure (CPP) is maintained between 60 and 130 mm Hg. The CPP commonly ranges around 80 to 90 mm Hg. Cerebral perfusion pressure is determined by subtracting the intracranial pressure (ICP) from the mean systemic arterial pressure (MSAP): CPP = MSAP − ICP.

Autoregulatory mechanisms in the healthy brain maintain the relatively constant blood flow through metabolic and pressure autoregulatory mechanisms. The metabolic autoregulatory mechanism operates in response to increases in carbon dioxide tension and decreases in oxygen tension. Carbon dioxide is the most potent cerebral vessel vasodilator, and its presence in increased amounts results in increased cerebral blood flow. This allows for removal of excess carbon dioxide and restoration of oxygen levels toward normal. Hypercapnia and hypoxia significantly affect vessel diameter

and, thus, intrinsic control of the cerebral blood flow. Likewise, the pH level affects cerebral arteries. Increased hydrogen ion concentrations have a powerful dilating effect on the cerebral vessels.

Pressure autoregulation responds to vessel resistance as a result of changes in intracranial pressure and systemic blood pressure. As a result of this mechanism, a relatively constant blood flow is maintained in the presence of wide fluctuations in systemic arterial blood pressure. Cerebral vessels constrict in response to increased systemic arterial pressure and dilate when the systemic pressure lowers. A mean systemic arterial blood pressure below 60 mm Hg results in decreased cerebral perfusion. Pressure autoregulation is maintained in the healthy brain when ICP is below 30 mm Hg, MSAP is between 60 and 160 mm Hg, and CPP ranges from 50 to 150 mm Hg. Autoregulation ceases when the CPP is less than 40 mm Hg. When the ICP increases significantly and equals the MAP, CPP becomes zero. Marked reduction of cerebral blood flow occurs when intracranial pressure rises rapidly to about 35 mm Hg.

Other factors that affect cerebral blood flow include cerebral outflow, blood viscosity, and cardiac output. Impedance in cerebral outflow may result in increased intracranial pressure and compromise autoregulation. Increases in blood viscosity decrease cerebral blood flow, and decreased blood viscosity increases cerebral blood

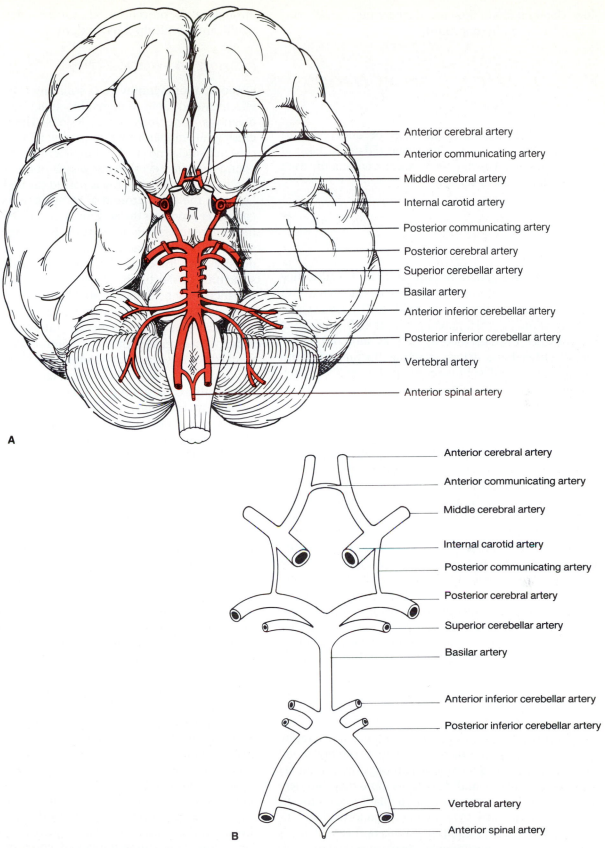

Anterior cerebral artery

Anterior communicating artery

Middle cerebral artery

Internal carotid artery

Posterior communicating artery

Posterior cerebral artery

Superior cerebellar artery

Basilar artery

Anterior inferior cerebellar artery

Posterior inferior cerebellar artery

Vertebral artery

Anterior spinal artery

A

Anterior cerebral artery

Anterior communicating artery

Middle cerebral artery

Internal carotid artery

Posterior communicating artery

Posterior cerebral artery

Superior cerebellar artery

Basilar artery

Anterior inferior cerebellar artery

Posterior inferior cerebellar artery

Vertebral artery

Anterior spinal artery

B

FIGURE 48-33   **A.** *The arterial supply to the brain.* **B.** *The circle of Willis and its connections. (Source: Akesson, E., Loeb, J. and Wilson-Parcevals, L. Thompson's Core Textbook of Anatomy [2nd ed.]. Philadelphia: J.B. Lippincott, 1990.)*

flow. Cerebral blood flow is reduced when cardiac output is decreased by one-third.

▼ Diagnostic Studies of Nervous System Alterations

A variety of diagnostic studies may be undertaken to confirm the diagnosis which is suspected on the basis of the clinical signs. The diagnostic studies commonly used are described in this section.

LATERAL AND POSTEROANTERIOR RADIOGRAPHS OF SKULL AND CERVICAL SPINE

Radiographs are generally done initially because they give certain vital information and can be completed with relative ease. The films can reveal skull fractures and shifting of the calcified pineal gland, thereby indicating the presence of mass lesions, such as subdural hematomas. Other bone defects, such as fractures, fracture compressions, and subluxations of the cervical spine, can be seen on plain films.

CEREBRAL ANGIOGRAPHY

Angiography is particularly useful in diagnosing vascular lesions, such as aneurysms, arteriovenous malformations, vasospasm, vascular tumors, and occlusions of cerebral vessels. It is frequently used in association with computed tomography (CT) studies. Angiography also identifies vessels that have been displaced by hematomas and other mass lesions. This invasive procedure involves injecting a radiopaque dye into an arterial blood vessel to allow visualization of the cerebral circulation. The material that passes through the intracranial and extracranial circulations outlines the arterial, capillary, and venous structures. Usual injection sites of the contrast media are the common carotid, femoral, and brachial arteries. The area of the suspected lesion largely influences the selection of the injection site.

DIGITAL SUBTRACTION ANGIOGRAPHY

Digital subtraction angiography combines radiography and computerized subtraction to evaluate cerebral blood vessels. Because this technique subtracts (by computer) surrounding tissue and structures that may interfere with visualizing vessels, it is particularly useful for diagnosing aneurysms, arteriovenous malformations, tumors, and hematomas. Iodine-based contrast material is injected into an artery or vein to enhance the visualization of the vessels, similar to the method used for standard angiography. Patients must remain motionless throughout the procedure, because movement interferes significantly with the imaging process.

COMPUTED TOMOGRAPHY

Computed tomography (CT) scanning is a very useful, effective, and rapid radiographic modality used for the diagnosis of nervous system lesions. The scans distinguish white matter from gray matter, identify the ventricles and sulci, and, with administration of intravenous contrast media, reveal major vessels of the brain. A narrow moving beam of x-ray is passed through successive layers of the head around a 360-degree axis. A small computer processes the accumulated data by calculating the differences in tissue density in contiguous tissue slices. Pathologic changes can be constructed from the density data in terms of shape, size, and position of structures of the brain. A wide variety of intracranial disorders may be demonstrated by the CT scan, including traumatic intracranial hematomas, neoplasms, cerebral infarctions, hydrocephalus, intracerebral hemorrhage, intracranial shifts, and brain abscesses. Certain spinal disorders, such as fractures, cord tumors, and disk abnormalities, can be effectively diagnosed by scanning. Frequently, CT scanning is used in conjunction with contrast myelography.

As a neurodiagnostic tool, tomography uses low x-ray dosage and has proved to be more efficient in many situations than conventional radiologic and air studies by virtue of its rapidity, noninvasiveness, and high reliability in diagnosis.

MAGNETIC RESONANCE IMAGING

Magnetic resonance imaging (MRI) is a relatively new diagnostic tool that is used to view soft tissue, fluid, and bony structures. It provides views of the successive layers of the brain in any plane within a powerful magnetic field. Protons (hydrogen atoms) of brain tissue and CSF align themselves in the orientation of the magnetic field. A specific radio frequency is introduced into the field that causes protons to resonate and change their alignment. A computer analyzes the absorbed radio frequency energy and projects it as an image on a screen.

The MRI has some distinct advantages over the CT scan. It projects images more clearly in that the gray and white matter are more precisely distinguished, posterior fossa and brain stem tissues are viewed more accurately, and certain lesions involving white matter are more readily identified. Like the CT scan, MRI is noninvasive and poses less hazard to the individual because it does not use radiation. Due to its powerful magnetic field, however, the equipment requires special housing. This procedure may cause implanted chips or rods to be dislodged and is therefore contraindicated for persons who have these.

ECHOENCEPHALOGRAPHY

Echoencephalography (ultrasound) is a safe, noninvasive neurologic diagnostic tool that involves the use of an ultrasound generator and receiver that display echo pulsations on an oscilloscope. Permanent recording is done through an attached camera. Echoes from deep within the skull visualize shifts in midline structures that may reflect intracranial trauma, cerebrovascular alterations, or space-occupying lesions. Lateral shifts of the pineal gland are also determined by echoencephalography as well as by plain radiographs. The echoencephalogram has been useful as an adjunct to more conventional and accurate neurodiagnostic studies, such as the CT scan and angiography. The limitations in echoencephalography lie in the many chances for error in administering and interpreting the test.

TRANSCRANIAL DOPPLER SONOGRAPHY

Transcranial Doppler sonography is a recently developed means for analyzing cranial blood flow that can be used at the bedside. This device allows for the detection of changes in blood vessel size and blood flow velocities. It is particularly useful in detection of cerebral vasospasm. Sound waves are transmitted through thinner areas of the skull or through the orbit of the eye. The speed or velocity of the blood flow is interpreted through the reflected signal.[8] High velocity detection indicates narrowing of the artery (vasospasm). Corresponding low velocity detection may be noted in the collateral arteries. When severe restriction in blood flow occurs, the flow values may actually fall and will correlate well with the amount of vasospasm.

BRAIN SCAN

The brain scan is a neurodiagnostic technique used primarily to detect intracranial tumors, abscesses, and some subdural hematomas. Radionuclide substances are injected intravenously and accumulate in abnormal areas of the brain as a result of breakdown of the blood–brain barrier. The radionuclides emit gamma rays, which are measured by a special scanner. They are not particularly useful in diagnosis of an acute head injury, because the radioactive substance must be injected 1 to 2 hours before scanning. This time span is excessive for persons who require rapid diagnosis and treatment. Positive brain scan findings result when scalp contusions are present. Because many acute head injuries are accompanied by scalp contusions, the scan findings may not present an accurate picture of the underlying brain pathology.

POSITRON EMISSION TOMOGRAPHY

Positron emission tomography (PET) uses radionuclides in assessing physiologic and biochemical processes, such as glucose and oxygen uptake and blood flow in the brain. This diagnostic procedure requires that the patient receive radioactively tagged substances, such as water or glucose, by either inhalation or injection. As the radioactive substance is metabolized, it emits positrons, which then emit gamma rays. This emission is then measured by a gamma scanner. Computer imaging produces a composite picture showing the location of the radioactive material and characteristic patterns of metabolic activity as well as areas of inactivity. Abnormalities in the cerebral vessels, tumors, as well as the physiologic basis for aberrant behavior (eg, dementia) may be detected by PET. The excessive financial and material resources required to house a PET scanner limit its use to large research centers.

LUMBAR PUNCTURE

The lumbar puncture provides information about CSF pressure and provides a means for collecting samples of CSF for laboratory analysis. The patient is positioned in the lateral recumbent position with the neck flexed in the knee–chest position. The region of L4-5 is disinfected and anesthetized. The spinal needle is inserted above the L4 vertebrae in the interspace until it penetrates the dura. A manometer is attached to the needle to measure the opening and closing pressure. CSF samples are collected in tubes for analysis. Table 48-7 lists the normal CSF laboratory findings.

After the completion of the procedure, the patient remains on bed rest for several hours and is encouraged to drink fluids to minimize the headache that is frequently associated with this procedure.

Lumber punctures are contraindicated for persons suspected of having increased ICP, because the release of pressure produced by the lumbar puncture may lead to herniation of the brain structures through the foramen magnum (see pp. 1041–1043).

MYELOGRAPHY

In myelography, radiopaque substance is introduced into the spinal subarachnoid space for the purpose of visualizing the vertebral canal. Before injection of the contrast medium into the subarachnoid space through lumbar puncture, Queckenstedt's test may be done to determine patency of the spinal canal. This is performed by compressing the jugular veins when a lumbar puncture has been made. When the compression is maintained, the CSF pressure is elevated. Unilateral compression results in moderate elevation of CSF pressure, whereas bilateral compression shows an even higher rise. When the compression is terminated, the CSF pressure returns to normal. Failure of the pressure to rise and fall indicates some obstruction within the spinal canal above the lumbar puncture site.

Myelography is performed in the radiology department on a tilt table, so that the person can be manipulated to allow the spinal canal to fill in several positions. With the person in position and lumbar puncture accomplished, approximately 10 mL of CSF is withdrawn and the radiopaque material is injected slowly. Serial films are then taken in various parts of the vertebral canal. On completion of the films, the contrast medium is removed.

Myelography is most commonly used for the diagnosis of intravertebral disk protrusions or bony displacements. Abnormal results indicate incomplete canal filling with contrast medium or total obstruction of its flow. In addition to disk abnormalities, tumors and adhesions encroaching on the spinal canal can be demonstrated.

ELECTROENCEPHALOGRAPHY

The electroencephalogram (EEG) is recorded from the surface of the scalp for the purpose of measuring the electrical potential generated by the brain. The recording is evaluated against previously established norms for location and age. Electrodes are placed on the skull, and variations in potential are recorded between two cortical electrodes (bipolar record) or between a cortical electrode and an indifferent electrode usually placed on the ear (unipolar record). Simultaneous recordings from numerous portions of the cranium are accomplished by systematic electrode placement. The EEG activity reflects the graded potential changes in the cortical neurons. This cortical activity, in turn, is dependent on stimuli reaching it from deeper brain structures, as has been demonstrated by studies that indicate that the cerebral cortex separated from the lower structures lacks the normal EEG patterns. Additional support for deep structure effect on the EEG recording is the finding that both cerebral hemispheres generally demonstrate synchronous activity, suggesting a pacemaker mechanism in the deeper structures of the brain.

The changes observed in the EEG patterns in response to afferent stimulation are referred to as desynchronization of the EEG. This occurs whenever the eyes are opened and alpha rhythm is replaced by a high-frequency, low-amplitude activity that exhibits no dominant pattern. Synchronized alpha activity indicates that many dendrite units are firing simultaneously, resulting in a rhythmic discharge. The frequency and amplitude of the EEG are affected by electrode placement, the activity or behavior and emotional status of the subject, and biochemical and structural status of the cortex. Oscillations vary from 1 to 50 Hz, and scalp voltage amplitude ranges widely according to internal and external environmental conditions.

The EEG evaluations contribute to the diagnostic process of individuals with cranial neurologic problems. Characteristic rhythms are observed with the various epileptic seizures as well as during intervals between the attacks. Focal damage in the cortex, either of internal or external origin, is usually reflected by an irregular and abnormal rhythm, which generally is slow and asymmetric with its corresponding hemispheric position. The EEG is also useful in differentiating psychogenic unresponsiveness (hysteria) from seizure disorders and with tumors, ischemia, metabolic disturbances and sleep disorders as well as the diagnosis of cerebral death.

Types of Brain Waves

Normal EEG results depend on the integrity and normal functioning of the cerebral cortex and certain structures deep in the brain. Four principal wave bands are commonly recorded in the normal individual's brain function: alpha, beta, theta, and delta.

The alpha waves make up alpha rhythm, which ranges at frequencies of 8 to 13 per second but most commonly occurs at frequencies of 9 to 10 per second (Fig. 48-34). Alpha waves are recorded symmetrically in most healthy adults from both the occipital and parietal regions. These are not fully developed until about age 13 years and may exhibit greater amplitude on the right side in younger individuals. Alpha waves are present only in the resting person whose eyes are closed. When eyes are open, the alpha waves disappear and are replaced by an asynchronous rhythm of low voltage. Metabolic aberrations, such as anoxia and hypoglycemia, slow alpha frequency.

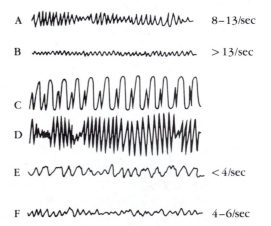

FIGURE 48-34 *Electroencephalogram waves.* **A.** *Alpha waves.* **B.** *Beta waves.* **C.** *Spike and dome waves during petit mal seizures.* **D.** *High-frequency spike waves during grand mal seizure.* **E.** *Delta waves.* **F.** *Theta waves.*

Beta waves are recorded from the frontal lobe of the brain and represent activity of the motor cortex (see Figure 48-34). Their frequency is above 13 cycles per second, and the amplitude is generally low. Beta activity may predominate in some people and is seen to replace alpha waves in those who are tense and anxious. Voluntary movement can block beta wave activity.

Theta waves project a frequency between 4 and 7 cycles per second and an amplitude comparable to that of beta waves (see Figure 48-34). These are recorded primarily in children and in some adults in emotional distress from the parietal and frontotemporal regions of the brain. Visual attention may block theta wave activity.

Delta waves encompass all the electrical rhythms of less than 4 cycles per second (see Figure 48-34). This pattern is observed normally in individuals in deeper stages of sleep and in young children and is the dominant rhythm in infants. Presence of delta waves in the awake adult may signify organic brain pathology.

A significant correlation exists between an individual's level of arousal and the dominant frequency of the EEG. Waves appear at 3 or fewer per second in deep sleep states. As sleep lightens, bursts of 10 to 12 waves per second begin to appear at shorter and shorter intervals until the waking state, when a continuous, more rapid frequency and lower-amplitude rhythm dominate. Thus, a direct correlation can be observed in the person's state of arousal and the cortical electrical activity recorded on the EEG.

Evoked Potentials

Evoked potentials are recorded on the EEG when an external stimulus has been applied to a specific sense organ. These have been useful in demonstrating abnormal sensory organ function. Evoked potentials are commonly used to test the integrity of the visual pathways (pattern-shift visual evoked response), the brain stem (far-field brain stem auditory evoked response), and the somatosensory system (short-latency somatosensory evoked potentials). A computer is used to average and maximize the responses.

The pattern-shift visual evoked response is particularly useful in diagnosing lesions of the optic nerve and its pathways. It is effective in detecting optic neuritis, optic nerve compression, and demyelinization of the optic pathways, such as is associated with multiple sclerosis. Each eye is tested separately as the individual views a pattern of light, while recordings are made on the electroencephalograph.

The far-field brain stem auditory evoked response tests auditory stimuli on the cerebral cortex and is useful for diagnosing peripheral hearing loss and lesions in the auditory tracts and brain stem. A series of clicks is administered to one ear through earphones while an EEG is recorded. This is repeated on the other ear. The ear that is not being tested at the time receives white noise.

The short-latency somatosensory evoked potential diagnoses nerve conduction defects of the somatic sensory system. Peripheral nerves are stimulated by electrodes on overlying skin, and EEG electrodes are placed peripherally and on the scalp. Common stimulation sites are the wrist and ankle. The short-latency somatosensory evoked potential is most useful in diagnoses of lesions in spinal roots, posterior columns, and brain stem involvement, such as may occur with Guillain-Barré syndrome and multiple sclerosis.

▼ Chapter Summary

▼ The functional cell of the nervous system is the neuron. It has sensory and motor functions carrying impulses to and from the cerebral cortex. It also conducts communication throughout the brain and brain stem to integrate reflexes with higher cortical function. The main supporting structure to the neurons are the neuroglia, which protect, nourish and support the neurons.

▼ Impulse transmission throughout the nervous system depends on various types of synapses and chemical neurotransmitters. Numerous receptors respond to internal and external stimulation throughout the body.

▼ The central nervous system is composed of the brain and spinal cord. They are protected by a meningeal layer and cerebrospinal fluid that prevent injury from daily activities and nutrition for the neurons.

▼ The basic neural response is the spinal cord reflex arc, which has an afferent (sensory) neuron and an efferent (motor) neuron. Reflexes at higher levels are much more complex.

▼ The more primitive responses are carried out by brain stem processes, most of which operate below the level of consciousness. In this area are the cranial nerves and thalamic and hypothalamic structures. Basal ganglia, situated deep in the cerebral hemisphere, are important structures for motor control and posture.

▼ The cerebrum is the area of highest thought process and coordinates information processing with both motor and sensory function through the frontal, parietal, temporal, and occipital lobes.

▼ The peripheral nervous system contains afferent and efferent fibers for motor and sensory functions. The pyramidal and extrapyramidal tracts are continuous from brain stem structures to the periphery. Some of the fibers cross over at the level of the medulla, so that motor and sensory responses are on the opposite side of the body.

▼ The autonomic nervous system comprises the sympathetic and parasympathetic nervous systems, which help to regulate the internal environment of the body. These systems affect every organ system of the body, generally with one part increasing while the other decreases the activity of the organs.

▼ Cerebrospinal fluid is of different composition than the blood due to the production in the choroid plexus with reabsorption in the arachnoid villi. It flows in the subarachnoid space throughout the brain and spinal column. The composition of CSF depends on intact brain barriers, which allow some materials to cross while being impermeable to others.

▼ Blood flow to the brain is through the internal carotid arteries and the vertebral arteries, which join in a special way to form the circle of Willis, thus providing a continuous supply to the brain. The venous drainage is through dural sinuses and internal jugular veins.

▼ The diagnostic studies of the nervous system include simple and complex procedures to gain information concerning alterations in cerebral or spinal cord function.

▼ References

1. Carpenter, M., and Sutin, J. *Human Neuroanatomy* (8th ed.). Baltimore: Williams & Wilkins, 1983.
2. Chusid, J. *Correlative Neuroanatomy and Functional Neurology* (19th ed.). Los Altos, Calif.: Lange, 1985.
3. Clark, R. *Essentials of Clinical Neuroanatomy and Neurophysiology* (6th ed.). Philadelphia: F.A. Davis, 1982.
4. Eccles, J. *The Understanding of the Brain.* New York: McGraw-Hill, 1973.
5. Fischbach, G. Mind and brain. *Sci. Am.* 267:50, 1992.
6. Guyton, A.C. *Textbook of Medical Physiology* (8th ed.). Philadelphia: W.B. Saunders, 1991.
7. Iverson, L. The chemistry of the brain. *Sci. Am.* 241:134, 1979.
8. March, K. Transcranial doppler sonography: Noninvasive monitoring of intracranial vasculature. *J. Neurosci. Nurs.* 22:113, 1990.
9. Nauta, W., and Feirtag, M. The organization of the brain. *Sci. Am.* 241:88, 1979.
10. Peele, T. *The Neuroanatomic Basis for Clinical Neurology* (3rd ed.). New York: McGraw-Hill, 1977.
11. Ruch, T., and Patton, H. *Physiology and Biophysics* (20th ed.). Philadelphia: W.B. Saunders, 1973.
12. Snell, R.S. *Clinical Neuroanatomy for Medical Students* (3rd ed.). Boston: Little, Brown, 1992.
13. Stevens, C. The neuron. *Sci. Am.* 241:54, 1979.
14. Willis, W., and Grossman, R. *Medical Neurobiology* (3rd ed.). St. Louis: C.V. Mosby, 1981.

Chapter 49

Adaptations and Alterations in the Special Senses

Reet Henze

▼ **CHAPTER OUTLINE**

▼ **LEARNING OBJECTIVES**

1. Trace the visual pathways from the optic disk to the occipital lobe.
2. Discuss the mechanism of image formation in the eye.
3. Explain the process of accommodation.
4. Discuss factors that influence the pupillary aperture.
5. Identify the functions of rods and cones.
6. Discuss the initiation of receptor potential of the retina.
7. Explain the trichromic theory of color vision.
8. Describe astigmatism, myopia, and hypermetropia.
9. Discuss the pathologic basis of the hemianopsias.
10. Discuss the mechanisms maintaining normal intraocular pressure.
11. Differentiate between chronic simple and acute glaucoma.
12. Discuss the age related changes of vision.
13. Trace sound conduction through the ear and the fiber pathways to the auditory cortex.
14. Differentiate between conduction deafness and sensorineural deafness.
15. Discuss the role of the vestibular system with respect to changes of position and movement.
16. Discuss common clinical findings associated with Meniere's disease.
17. Discuss the age related changes of hearing.
18. Locate the primary sensations of taste on the tongue.
19. Trace taste pathways from innervation of taste buds to cerebral cortex.
20. Discuss pathogenesis of taste disturbance.
21. Identify the receptor cell for the sense of smell.
22. Discuss adaptation of smell receptors.
23. Identify potential causes of anosmia.
24. Discuss the age related changes of taste and smell.

The senses of vision, hearing, taste, and smell provide human beings with the means to perceive the environment and respond in a way that supports adaptation and, at times, even survival. The receptors of the eyes, ears, tongue, and nose are stimulated and messages are transmitted to specific regions of the cerebral cortex for processing. Alterations in the function of these senses, particularly vision and hearing, can result in physiologic, psychological, sociologic, and economic difficulties. Common alterations are described in this chapter; others can be found in specialized texts. Age-related visual changes are delineated in Table 49-1.

TABLE 49-1 *Age-Related Visual Changes*

Structural Change	Functional Change
EYEBALL	
Anterior chamber decreases as lens thickens	Potential for glaucoma increases
Reabsorption of intraocular fluid less efficient	Increase in "floaters"
Decreased water in vitreous humor	
CORNEA	
Becomes flatter, thicker and less smooth	Potential for astigmatism
Arcus senilis	None
EYELIDS	
Loss of elasticity results in eyelid droop	Visual disturbance if significant droop
RETINA	
Decreased rods	Increased lighting required to see objects
LENS	
Increased opacity	Glare from increased light scattering
	Decreased color vision
Loss of elasticity	Decreased accommodation
	Presbyopia
PUPIL	
Pupil size becomes smaller	Decreased amount of light enters retina
	Require more light to see objects
	Visual field decreases
	Dark adaptation less effective
LACRIMAL SECRETIONS	
Secretions diminish	Dull appearance of eye
	Dryness, scratchiness, tightness

Adapted from Ebersole, P., and Hess, P. *Toward Healthy Aging: Human Needs and Nursing Response.* St. Louis: Mosby, 1994.

▼ *Vision*

STRUCTURE AND FUNCTION

The eye is a complex peripheral structure that transmits vision to the visual area of the occipital lobe of the cerebral cortex. It nestles in the orbit, a cone-shaped cavity with fragile walls composed of the frontal, maxillary, zygomatic, sphenoid, ethmoid, lacrimal, and palatine bones. The thinness of the orbital wall makes this area particularly susceptible to fractures. The eyeball occupies the anterior portion of the orbital cavity; its principal structures are identified in Figure 49-1. The area of the orbit not occupied by the eyeball is filled with fascia, fat, nerves, blood vessels, muscle, and the lacrimal gland. Six extrinsic muscles, most of which arise from the apex of the orbit and insert into the scleral lining, allow for the movement and rotation of the eyeball. These are the superior rectus, inferior rectus, medial rectus, lateral rectus, superior oblique, and inferior oblique muscles. Innervation for these muscles arrives from the third, fourth, and sixth cranial nerves.

The three layers of the eyeball are the sclera, choroid, and retina. The outermost supportive and protective layer, the sclera, is composed of dense fibrous tissue and forms a white, opaque membrane around the eyeball except at the cornea, where it becomes transparent. It is through this transparent area that light rays enter the eye to stimulate the rods and cones.

The second (middle) layer of the eyeball is the vascular choroid. Nutrients are exchanged in this heavily pigmented layer. The ciliary muscle, which is important in facilitating light and accommodation reflexes, lies between the sclera and choroid layers. The choroid also contains the iris, the center of which is the pupil. The sphincter and dilator muscles of the iris, together with the ciliary muscle, are known as the intrinsic muscles of the eye. They control the amount of light admitted into the eye. Innervation to these muscles comes from the third cranial nerve and the superior cervical ganglion. The crystalline lens, which is suspended by the suspensory ligament from the inner surface of the ciliary body, bends the rays of light so that they are projected properly on the retina. The anterior chamber is a fluid-filled space anterior to the iris and lens. Along with the posterior chamber, which is located behind the iris and is also fluid-filled, it assists in maintaining constant pressure in the eyeball. Normal intraocular pressure is between 10 and 22 mm Hg, with the most common pressures being 15 or 16 mm Hg. Glaucoma results if drainage of this aqueous humor is insufficient and intraocular pressure rises (Fig. 49-2). Vitreous humor, which is soft and gelatinous, fills the space behind the lens and helps maintain the shape of the eyeball.

The third layer of the eyeball, the retina, consists of two parts. The outer pigmented layer is attached to the

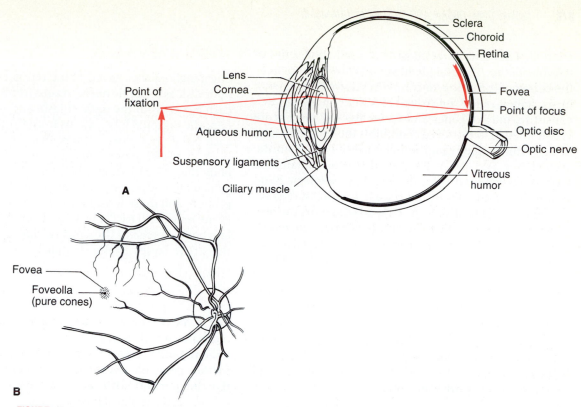

FIGURE 49-1 **A.** Overview of the eye and refraction. The refraction of light rays from the fixation point at the tip of the arrow to the focal point on the retina represents the summed effects of the anterior and posterior surfaces of the cornea and lens. The image of the arrow is projected in an inverted orientation on the retina. **B.** View of the central retina, including the macular region. (Conn, P.M. Neuroscience in Medicine. Philadelphia: J.B. Lippincott, 1995.)

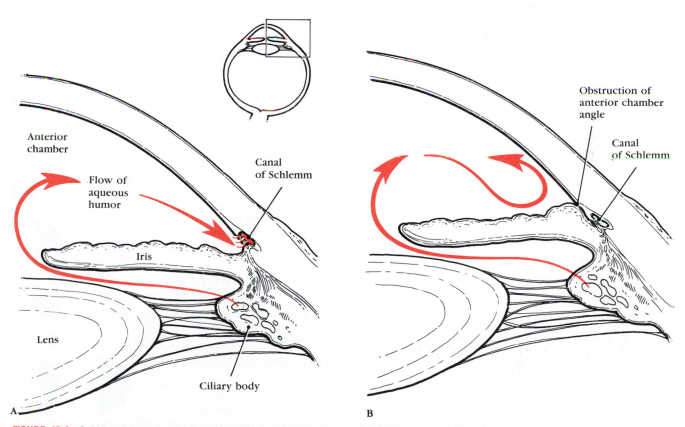

FIGURE 49-2 **A.** Normal flow of aqueous humor. **B.** Obstructed flow in acute (closed or narrow-angle) glaucoma. (Adapted from Lechiger, L., and Moya, F. Introduction to the Practice of Anesthesia [2nd ed.]. New York: Harper & Row, 1978.)

choroid. The inner layer consists of a synaptic series of nervous tissue. The macula lutea, a yellowish spot near the center of the retina, encompasses a small depression in its center called the fovea centralis. This is an area consisting only of cones and projecting the most acute vision. Medial to the fovea centralis is the optic disk. It is at this whitish spot that the optic nerve exits from the eyeball (see Fig. 49-1). Because this area contains no sensory receptors, it is known as the physiologic blind spot of the retina. Increased intraocular pressure is reflected in the optic disk by its cupped shape (ie, the disk appears to be pushed backward). In contrast, increased intracranial pressure produces the opposite effect, an optic disk that is pushed inward, called a *choked disk* or *papilledema*.

The blood supply to the retina enters through the central artery, a branch of the ophthalmic artery. The central artery enters the eyeball with the optic nerve and runs with it to the retina, where it divides in the middle of the disk into superior and inferior branches. The veins in the eyeball are anatomically related to the arteries and empty into the ophthalmic veins.

VISUAL PATHWAYS

The ganglionic cell axons of the retina emerge from the optic disk as the optic nerve. Axons from the nasal half of each eye cross in the optic chiasm and terminate in the opposite occipital lobe. Axons from the temporal half of each eye do not cross but terminate on their respective sides in the superior colliculus and lateral geniculate body (Fig. 49-3).[3] Those fibers terminating in the lateral geniculate body seem to be associated with visual perception, and those terminating in the superior colliculus excite reflex activity.[10] The fibers from the lateral geniculate body emerge as the optic radiation and continue to the striate cortex in the occipital lobe.

IMAGE FORMATION

The refractive surfaces of the cornea and lens initiate the mechanism for image formation. These surfaces and the aqueous and vitreous humors provide varying densities for the light to pass through. This accounts for the refractive phenomenon. If a light ray passes into denser me-

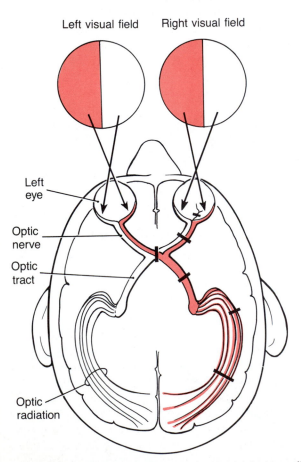

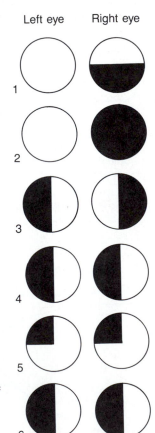

1 **Horizontal defect**
Occlusion of a branch of the central retinal artery may cause a horizontal (altitudinal) defect. Shown is the upper field defect associated with occlusion of the inferior branch of this artery.

2 **Blind right eye** (right optic nerve)
A lesion of the optic nerve, and of course of the eye itself, produces unilateral blindness.

3 **Bitemporal hemianopsia** (optic chiasm)
A lesion at the optic chiasm may involve only the fibers that are crossing over to the opposite side. Since those fibers originate in the nasal half of each retina, visual loss involves the temporal half of each field.

4 **Left homonymous hemianopsia** (right optical tract)
A lesion of the optic tract interrupts fibers originating on the same side of both eyes. Visual loss in the eyes is therefore similar (homonymous) and involves half of each field (hemianopsia).

5 **Homonymous left upper quadrant** (optic radiation, partial)
A partial lesion of the optic radiation may involve only a portion of the nerve fibers, producing, for example, a homonymous quadrantic defect.

6 **Left homonymous hemianopsia** (right optic radiation)
A complete interruption of fibers in the optic radiation produces a visual defect similar to that produced by a lesion of the optic tract.

FIGURE 49-3. *Visual pathways and visual field defects resulting from lesions at various areas along the pathways. (Adapted from: Bates, B.* A Guide to Physical Examination and History Taking *[5th ed.]. Philadelphia: J.B. Lippincott. 1991.)*

dium, it is bent toward the perpendicular and the speed of transmission is slowed. A less dense medium bends the light ray away from the perpendicular and speeds its transmission. The degree of light impediment, or the power of a substance to bend light, is its *refractive index*. The refractive index of air is 1.0; of water, 1.33; of the cornea, 1.38; and of the crystalline lens, 1.40.[8]

Light strikes the cornea at different angles and is bent in different amounts depending on the curvature and refractive indexes of the interposed structures. Refraction of light occurs at the corneal interface, aqueous humor, and crystalline lens, and light is projected on the retina in an inverted and reverted manner that is perceived by the brain as upright.

ACCOMMODATION

Adjustments for distant vision are made by the lens. Normally, parallel light rays from distant objects are focused on the retina. The ciliary muscle contracts to increase the curvature of the lens for viewing of objects closer to the eye. The increased curvature of the lens increases its power, shortens focal length, and focuses near objects on the retina. This is the process of accommodation. The closest point at which a person can clearly focus on an object is called the *near point*. This point recedes with advancing age. For example, the near point for a normal eye of an 8-year-old is approximately 8.6 cm; for a 20-year-old, it is 10.4 cm; and for a 60-year-old, it is approximately 83 cm from the eye. Ocular convergence and pupillary constriction (miosis) are associated with the accommodation reflex. Convergence ensures that images recorded are focused on the macular area at the fovea centralis.[11]

The accommodation reflex is mediated by the third cranial nerve through parasympathetic postganglionic fibers. The stimulus that triggers the accommodation response is perception of an image out of focus. The parasympathetic impulses on the ciliary muscle must, therefore, increase progressively to maintain the image in focus continually. Progressive age reduces the efficiency of accommodation because of the loss of elasticity of the lens. The eye may remain focused almost permanently on a constant distance. This deterioration is known as *presbyopia*. It is readily corrected with proper bifocal lenses for far and near vision.

PUPILLARY APERTURE

The iris controls the amount of light that enters the eye through the action of its two sets of smooth muscles: the sphincter and dilator muscles. Miosis (contraction) is accomplished through the contraction of the sphincter muscle, and mydriasis (dilation) is facilitated through the contraction of the dilator muscle. Innervation for the sphincter muscles comes from the postganglionic para-

sympathetic neurons in the ciliary ganglion. The preganglionic neurons transmit to the ganglion by the third cranial nerve. Innervation for the dilator muscle arrives from the sympathetic postganglionic neurons of the superior cervical ganglion and reaches the eye after following a series of progressively smaller arteries.

The pupillary aperture in the human eye can vary from 1.5 to 8.0 mm in diameter. In normal eyes, the aperture is a reflex response to change in light intensity. Pupils constrict in response to increased light intensities and dilate in response to decreased light intensities (pupillary light reflex). If illumination enters only one eye, both pupils constrict. This simultaneous constriction of the contralateral eye is referred to as the *consensual light reflex*. Photoreceptors of the retina, including rods and cones, are receptors for the light reflex.

Emotional states of alarm produce pupillary dilation. This reaction is initiated by stimulation of the sympathetic fibers and inhibition of the parasympathetic fibers. Darkness inhibits the parasympathetic supply and results in pupil dilation.

Light reflex of the pupil and miosis of accommodation are not identical mechanisms, and they can occur independently of each other. An example of this occurs with the *Argyll Robertson pupil*, which may occur as a complication of syphilis. In this phenomenon, the pupil remains constricted and unresponsive to light but does respond to the accommodation mechanism.[2]

PHYSIOLOGY OF VISION

Rods and cones are receptors of the retina and have distinctly different morphologic compositions and functions (Fig. 49-4). The cones mediate daylight vision, allowing perception of detail and color of objects. The rods mediate night vision, allowing visualization of outlines of objects without revealing color or detail. The rods, however, are very sensitive to movement of objects in the visual field.

The retina is formed by numerous layers of cells, fibers, and ganglia (Fig. 49-5). The nerve cells in the retina include bipolar cells, ganglion cells, horizontal cells, and amacrine cells. The rods and cones, which are adjacent to the pigment epithelium of the choroid, synapse with the bipolar cells, which, in turn, synapse with dendrites of the ganglion cells. Horizontal cells connect receptor cells (rods and cones), and amacrine cells connect ganglion cells to each other and to bipolar cells. The dendrites of the ganglion cells synapse with bipolar cell axons in the inner plexiform layer (see Fig. 49-5), and their axons converge to enter the optic nerve. The fovea centralis is composed of tightly packed cones that connect individually to the optic nerve, whereas in other parts of the retina they share fibers with many other rods and cones. The pigmented layer of the retina is the outermost layer, which decreases light reflection. This

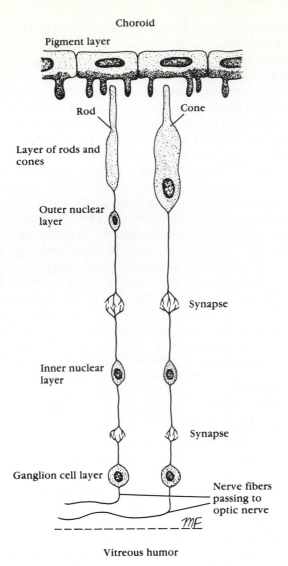

FIGURE 49-4 *Simplified view of rods and cones.*

pigment layer is directly adjacent to the choroid and receives much of its nutritive needs from the choroid vascular supply. Melanin is the black pigment that gives this layer its characteristic dark color.

As light passes through the layers of the retina to reach the light-sensitive portion of the rods and cones deep in the retina, light energy is absorbed by the pigment rhodopsin, or visual purple. Rhodopsin is a light-sensitive protein and aldehyde of vitamin A compound contained in rods that breaks down when light reaches it. This is the initial activity in producing the generator potential. The breakdown of rhodopsin can be visualized by the change in the dark-adapted retina from a dark purple to lack of color on exposure to light. The breakdown of rhodopsin results in the formation of a protein, scotopsin, and a carotene pigment, retinene.[4] In darkness, scotopsin and retinene recombine through a series of intermediary steps and form rhodopsin again, which is stored in the outer segments of the rods and is again photoexcitable.

$$\text{Rhodopsin} \xrightarrow[\text{dark}]{\text{light}} \text{retinene + scotopsin}$$

$$\longrightarrow \quad \text{generator potential}$$

Knowledge about the pigments in the cones is somewhat speculative. Reflection densitometry has demonstrated the presence of pigments in the foveal region of the retina that peak in the blue, green, and red parts of the spectrum. This is accomplished by shining light in the eye and measuring the intensity of energy at different wavelengths in the light reflected from the retina. In this manner, the amount of light absorbed by the visual receptor cells can be determined. Erythrolabe is a pigment identified in the fovea that absorbs light in the red part of the spectrum; chlorolabe is a pigment that ab-

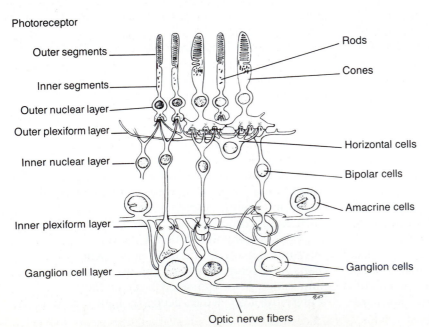

FIGURE 49-5 *Constituent neurons of the neural retina. (Cormack, D.H., Essential Histology. Philadelphia: J.B. Lippincott, 1993.)*

sorbs light in the green part of the spectrum in the fovea. A third cone pigment, iodopsin, a violet-sensitive substance, has been isolated from the retinae of chickens and is also thought to exist in the human eye cones. A pigment receptor for blue substances has also been identified. The cone pigments are similar to rhodopsin in composition, but they vary, allowing absorption of a variety of colors to different extents, and resulting in color-dependent nerve impulses. These impulses are interpreted by the visual cortex as color sensations.

The photochemical decomposition that occurs in response to light striking either cones or rods produces a receptor potential that remains for the duration of the stimulus. The receptor potentials of the retina differ from other receptor potentials in that hyperpolarization is produced rather than depolarization. Each optic nerve fiber connects with many receptors through ganglionic cells. The number of receptor cells on the retina is much greater than the number in the optic nerve. This convergence on ganglionic cells allows summation to occur; therefore, light falling on different parts of the retina together may cause excitation. The more rods and cones that are excited, the more intense the signal. The ganglion cells receive the excitation impulses from the rods and cones through the bipolar cells.

The ganglionic cells produce synaptic depolarization and stimulate all-or-nothing threshold spikes that are propagated along their axons to the lateral geniculate body. Three types of responses are observed in ganglionic cells. One fires only in response to light stimulus on the retina and is known as the "on fiber"; another discharges only in response to light off and is known as the "off fiber." The third, most numerous type responds to both light on and off and is called the "on-off fiber."

The horizontal cells transmit inhibitory impulses laterally from rods and cones to bipolar cells and become most important in detecting visual contrasts and color differentiations. Amacrine cells have a very transient inhibitory effect on the ganglionic cells in response to stimulation from bipolar cells and possibly from rods and cones. Amacrine cell inhibition seems to enhance the contrast experienced in visual images. The neural pathways from the retina to the visual cortex are identified in Figure 49-3.

COLOR VISION

The differentiation of wavelengths of the visible spectrum allows the human eye to detect color in the environment. The precise mechanism that is responsible for color detection has been sought by researchers throughout the past century. Most of the investigation seems to be based on the *trichromatic theory*, which assumes that there are three variations in cones, each containing a different photochemical substance. One type of cone is responsible for red color, another for blue, and the third for green.[4] This theory, also known as the *Young-*

Helmholtz theory, named after its originators more than a century ago, is widely accepted today. Each of these cones gives rise to a distinct impulse that travels to the visual cortex of the occipital lobe. Red, blue, and green are colors that may produce any color in the spectrum by correct proportionate mixture. If all of the cones are stimulated equally, the sensation of white results. In contrast, if no stimulation of the three types of cones occurs, black is experienced. Other colors are perceived as a result of the combined stimulation of the three types of cones to varying degrees.

In summary, color vision evolves from the spectral sensitivity of cones and is most highly developed in the fovea, where cones are concentrated. Each cone is maximally stimulated by a specific color. Color information is transmitted to the brain by common cone pathways of the optic fibers, and the transmission of specific colors is monitored by the stimulation of horizontal cells. Advancing age results in yellowing of the lens, which diminishes the sensitivity of color perception. Blue-green color discrimination seems to be most affected by this progressive change in the aging eye.

COLOR BLINDNESS

Many forms of color blindness exist, but the most common variety is the inability to distinguish between red and green. Color blindness may be hereditary, congenital, or acquired. The most common modality is inheritance through the male sex-linked recessive gene. Congenital color vision defects also tend to be red-green defects with intact yellow-blue vision. A variety of color defects may be acquired.[1] Acquired visual defects may involve partial loss, such as in a quadrant or half of the visual field, or they may involve the entire visual field. If a certain group of color receptors is not present in the retinae, all colors appear the same in the range of missing cones.

Color blindness can be assessed by numerous tests. Those most commonly used are the polychromatic charts and the yarn-matching tests. The former presents a chart, known as the *Ishihara* chart, with numerous look-alike, colored spots in a configuration that a person with normal vision can identify easily. The yarn-matching test involves asking the person to match a skein of yarn with strands from a pile of variously colored yarn.

DARK ADAPTATION

The eyes are said to be *dark adapted* after a period of time in darkness. This decline in visual threshold is at its maximum after approximately 20 minutes in the dark environment. On return to the light environment, the uncomfortable brightness requires the eyes to adapt to light again. This adaptation takes about 5 minutes and is called *light adaptation*. Dark adaptation occurs, in part, as rhodopsin stores are rebuilt in the rods and some similar, yet unknown, process occurs in the cones.[4] Dark adaptation is most effectively maintained by avoiding exposure to light. If visual acuity is necessary in a dark environment, such as for viewing a fluoroscopy screen and radiographs, red goggles may be worn on returning to bright light to avoid having to wait 20 minutes for adaptation. The light wavelengths in the red part of the spectrum allow cone vision to continue while stimulating rods only to a slight degree.

Only the periphery of the retina of the human eye is sensitive to light in the dark-adapted eye; therefore, the sensitivity to darkness is much greater in the rods than the cones. Rods are not exclusively responsible for dark adaptation, however. Because of the presence of both rods and cones, dark adaptation takes place in two stages. First, a small increase in sensitivity occurs, which is accomplished in about 7 minutes and is attributed to dark adaptation of cones. After this, a less rapid but quantitatively greater adaptation occurs in rods.[5]

REFRACTION DEFECTS

Emmetropia (normal refraction) exists when the relaxed eye is capable of clearly focusing distant parallel light rays on the retina (Fig. 49-6). Nearby vision requires

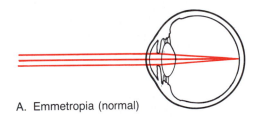

A. Emmetropia (normal)

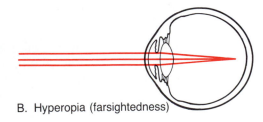

B. Hyperopia (farsightedness)

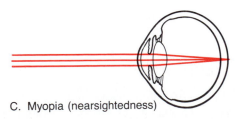

C. Myopia (nearsightedness)

FIGURE 49-6 *A. Emmetropia refers to normal refraction in which the eye can focus on near and distant objects clearly. B. Myopia results from an elongated eyeball and the eye can focus on near objects but not distant objects. C. Hyperopia results from a shortened eyeball that can focus on distant objects but not near objects.*

contraction of the ciliary muscle to bring the object to focus. Defects of vision are present if the light rays converge either in front of or behind the retina, or if the eyeball is abnormally shaped.[4]

Myopia (nearsightedness) occurs when parallel light rays are focused in front of the retina as a result of increased anteroposterior diameter of the eyeball (see Fig. 49-6). Myopic persons cannot focus on a distant object sharply; however, as the individual moves closer to the object, the rays become more focused and the focal point eventually falls on the retina. The excessive refraction of myopia is readily corrected by a *concave* diverging lens, which produces a longer than normal focal point.

Hyperopia (farsightedness) occurs with an abnormally short eyeball; the parallel light rays are focused beyond the retina in the relaxed eye (see Fig. 49-6). Through the mechanism of accommodation, the hyperopic person can focus on distant objects. As objects move closer to the eye, images become blurred and accommodation can no longer compensate. The near point in persons with hyperopia is abnormally distant. This condition is corrected by directing the refraction of light rays through a *convex* lens and shortening the normal focal point.

Astigmatism is a defect of the curvature of the cornea and lens that produces refractive errors in which parallel light rays are imperfectly focused on the retina. Clear focusing requires a spherical cornea and lens on all meridians. In the presence of irregular curvature of these structures, light striking peripheral areas is bent at different angles and is not focused on a single point on the retina. Astigmatism can be corrected with lenses that are cut from a piece of cylindric instead of spheric glass. The axis of the cylinder is placed approximately in relation to the meridian of the eye lens.

VISUAL FIELD DEFECTS

Normally, a person's visual field extends approximately 90 degrees to the temporal side, 60 degrees to the nasal side, and 130 degrees vertically. The *confrontation test* can be used as a crude assessment of visual field acuity. In this test, the examiner is positioned about 2 feet away from the person, who is asked to cover one eye and to fix the gaze of the other eye on the examiner's eye directly opposite. The examiner closes his or her eye so that it roughly superimposes on the person's and then introduces a small object, such as a pencil, from beyond the visual field and asks the patient to indicate when he or she first sees the object. If abnormalities are detected, a standard perimetric test is performed.

Visual field defects occur as a result of lesions in the visual pathway. The specific defect reflects the region of the lesion on the visual pathway (see Fig. 49-3). Blindness in one-half of the visual field is known as *hemianopsia*. Lesions of the decussating fibers of the optic chiasm are commonly a result of pituitary tumors and reflect a *bitemporal hemianopsia*, a mirror-image defect on one side of both visual fields. *Heteronymous* defects are asymmetrical defects in the eyes and usually indicate involvement of the optic chiasm region. Loss of vision in corresponding halves of the visual fields is known as *homonymous hemianopsia* and suggests lesions posterior to the optic chiasm, in the optic tracts that originate on the same side of both eyes. If homonymous hemianopsias can be superimposed on each other accurately, they are said to be *congruous*, and the lesion is probably in the calcarine cortex and subcortical white matter of the occipital lobe.[1] Those homonymous hemianopsias whose boundaries differ are *incongruous* and more likely involve lesions in the parietal or temporal lobe.[1] Defects that affect one quadrant of the visual field are described as *quadrantic hemianopsias*. They involve only a partial area of the optic radiation.

Visual defects may also result from vascular insufficiency. A condition involving recurrent, transient episodes of partial blindness is known as *amaurosis fugax*. It usually is associated with atherosclerotic lesions of the carotid arteries that have dislodged and occluded the arteries that supply the eye. This condition usually involves one eye and reflects ipsilateral carotid artery insufficiency caused by plaque accumulation.

OTHER DISTURBANCES OF VISION

Decreased visual acuity may be associated with various lesions, syndromes, drug therapies, and nutritional deficiencies. Specific types of impairments result from lesions in different locations along the visual pathways.

Scotomas are abnormal blind spots in the visual field which are surrounded by normal vision. They are referred to by their shape and position. These may exist with the person's knowledge (positive scotomas) or without it (negative scotomas). Scotomas may result from vascular disease, toxic effect of certain drugs, nutritional deficiencies, demyelinating diseases, certain hereditary conditions, and glaucoma. *Diplopia*, or double vision, results from an eye muscle imbalance between the eyes, resulting in image reception at different spots on each retina.

Papilledema (choked disk), usually associated with obstruction of venous return from the retina, most commonly occurs with increased intracranial pressure as a result of brain tumor, trauma, hemorrhage, infection, or other causes. In its early stages, minor visual changes, such as fuzziness in vision and engorgement of the retinal vein, may occur, and slight elevation of the optic disk may be seen. As the condition progresses, the entire disk and surrounding tissue become severely elevated and edematous, obscuring the peripheral blood vessels.

Inflammation of the optic nerve, known as *optic neuritis*, is characterized early in its course by a scotoma in the central visual area which is accompanied by intense pain, loss of visual acuity, and photophobia. Optic neuritis may occur in one or both eyes. It is associated most commonly with multiple sclerosis but may also accompany meningitis, polyneuritis, and cerebral tumors.

Optic atrophy results in slow, progressive failure in visual acuity. It is associated with multiple sclerosis, tabes dorsalis, neuritis, glaucoma, increased intracranial pressure, trauma, vascular occlusion, or congenital and hereditary conditions. The optic disk usually appears chalky white with clearly delineated margins. *Degeneration of the retina* may result from drug therapy (particularly the phenothiazine group), infections, or various metabolic or endocrine disorders.

Cerebral tumors, aneurysms, vascular diseases, infections, and degenerative processes can also lead to visual defects, producing a variety of symptoms associated the specific region affected. Defects may result in ocular movement, visual acuity, or interpretation of what is seen. *Amblyopia*, a dimming of vision, may be associated with pituitary tumors, diseases such as diabetes mellitus, renal failure, or exposure to chemical toxins.

Glaucoma

Increased intraocular pressure and loss in the visual field are hallmarks of glaucoma. Several underlying conditions can result in increased intraocular pressure. The most common of these is blockage or stenosis of aqueous outflow channels.[7] Normally, the aqueous humor, which is produced by the ciliary epithelium, flows from the posterior chamber of the eye through the pupil into the anterior chamber. Aqueous humor then leaves the anterior chamber and returns to the venous system by passing through the trabecular mesh of the anterior chamber into the Schlemm canal. A balance between production and absorption of aqueous humor provides for normal intraocular pressure (13–22 mm Hg).

Other potential causes of increased intraocular pressure in glaucoma include increases in systemic vascular pressure, which is reflected in venous engorgement, and decreased drainage through aqueous drainage channels. Increased production of aqueous humor is thought to contribute to glaucoma in a small proportion of cases.[7] The increased intraocular pressure associated with glaucoma may result in atrophy and degeneration of the optic nerve.

Glaucoma is described as *chronic simple* (open-angle) or *acute* (closed-angle or narrow-angle). The angle refers to the area in which the iris meets the cornea in the anterior chamber (see Fig. 49-2). Chronic simple glaucoma is thought to have an hereditary basis and is a common cause of blindness. It may be asymptomatic for years and finally be revealed after the patient experiences peripheral vision loss, difficulty with dark adaptation, blurring of vision, halos around lights, and difficulty focusing on near objects. Although the anterior chamber angle is open in chronic simple glaucoma, an obstruction exists for the flow of aqueous humor through the trabecular mesh. After this type of glaucoma has been diagnosed, the existing visual defects cannot be corrected, but further deterioration can be controlled with miotic drugs.

Acute glaucoma is manifested if an obstruction, either complete or partial, in the flow of aqueous humor is produced by closure of the anterior chamber angle (see Fig. 49-2). This may result from an anteroposterior thickening of the lens or a forward movement of the lens that causes the iris to press against the lens capsule and thereby prevent outflow of aqueous humor. Complete closure of the angle presents a dramatic clinical picture of severe eye pain, blurred or cloudy vision, halos around lights, a hard red eye with cloudy cornea, and nausea and vomiting. Intraocular pressure is elevated. Severe damage can be prevented by laser iridotomy which creates a hole in the iris to prevent attacks of acute-closure glaucoma.

Glaucoma may be primary or secondary to eye conditions associated with infection, tumors, hemorrhage, and trauma. Diagnosis is based on clinical features, tonometry, tonography, and peripheral vision testing.

Cataracts

As noted previously, the normal lens is clear and transparent and acts as a major refractive structure. Certain conditions can cause clouding of the lens and result in loss of vision associated with cataracts. These conditions may result from trauma to the eye, elevated glucose levels in the aqueous humor (diabetes mellitus), irradiation to the lens, viruses, chemicals, infections, and amino acid or vitamin deficiencies. Occasionally, cataracts are congenital, but more commonly they are associated with advancing age (*senile cataracts*). Also, they have been associated with certain disease processes of the skin, skeleton, and nervous system and with chromosomal abnormalities.

Senile cataracts result from the aging process as the lens undergoes changes. New fibers develop continually in the lens, and these slowly increase the lens size. Older lens fibers become dehydrated, compressed, and sclerosed, forming a yellowish-brown pigment that becomes so dense as to result in nuclear sclerosis and decreased transparency. Cataracts produce visual abnormalities as a result of decreased light transmission, abnormal morphology, or biochemical and optical aberrations.[7] Diagnosis of cataracts is confirmed by the clinical features, such as diminished visual acuity associated with blurring, glare, and decreased color perception, as well as by the usual eye tests and ophthalmoscopic examination. They are treated surgically by a lens implant following removal of the cloudy cataract.

Retinal Detachment

The separation of the retina from the choroid is usually spontaneous, although it can occur secondary to trauma. Retinal detachment is common in older persons because aging can cause the vitreous body to shrink, resulting in retinal tearing. As the tear occurs in the retina, choroid vessels transudate and vitreous humor seeps under the retina, stripping it from the choroid. The person with a detached retina experiences "floaters" and lines in the visual field. In addition, flashes of light and blurred black spots appear suddenly in conjunction with defects in vision. If the macula is involved, severe vision loss results. There are often complains of the sensation of a curtain coming over the eye. Usually, there is no pain or redness of the eye.

Diagnosis of retinal detachment is made by clinical symptoms and ophthalmoscopy. A binocular indirect ophthalmoscope and scleral depressor are used to produce a three-dimensional view of the retina and its damage.

Retinitis Pigmentosa

Retinitis pigmentosa is a degenerative inherited disease of the eyes that manifests itself initially by night blindness. The disease may be inherited through an autosomal dominant, autosomal recessive, or X-linked gene.[9] Progression of symptoms can be so slow that it is difficult to detail an accurate course of the disease. Visual field constriction (tunnel vision) is commonly associated with the night blindness. Other symptoms include photophobia and disturbance in color vision. The disease may progress to total blindness, although some individuals retain reading vision in a small central part of the visual field. Changes in the fundus may be identified early in the course of the disease by a disturbance in the pigment epithelium of the retina. Areas of hyperpigmentation and atrophy may be identified by angiography, although the hallmark of retinitis pigmentosa is degeneration of the rods and cones associated with loss of pigmentation.[9] The waxy-appearing optic disk, thinning of retinal arteries, and choriocapillary atrophy are other associated changes.

Diagnosis of retinitis pigmentosa is based on signs and symptoms of the disease, characteristic changes of the fundus, and a family history of the disease.

▼ Hearing

STRUCTURE AND FUNCTION

The ear is a mechanoreceptor; it is sensitive to rapid changes in pressure that are transmitted to its fluid medium. In essence, the ear is a mechanical transducer. Sound at various frequencies is converted into nerve impulses through the cochlear component of the acoustic (eighth cranial) nerve, and these impulses are transmitted into the central nervous system for interpretation. Sound is conducted through air, ossicles, and fluid and is measured in number of vibrations per second, which is recorded as *cycles per second (cps)* or *Hertz (Hz)*. The human ear is able to perceive frequencies to 20,000 Hz. Aging reduces the number of frequencies perceived. The greatest sensitivity of the human ear is in the range of 1,000 to 4,000 Hz.

In addition to the hearing function of the ears, their receptors mediate a sense of position and equilibrium through the vestibular component of the eighth cranial nerve.

SOUND CONDUCTION THROUGH THE EAR

The ear is anatomically segmented into *outer, middle,* and *inner* areas (Fig. 49-7). The outer ear funnels sound waves to the *tympanic membrane* (eardrum). Its canal is an S-shaped, 3-cm tube that is supplied with ceruminous and sebaceous glands as well as hair follicles. The canal has resonance properties because sound waves are reflected from the tympanic membrane; it may enhance or dampen incoming waves. The external canal is lined with squamous epithelium, and cartilage and bone provide support and maintain its patency.

At the terminal end of the external ear, the tympanic membrane separates it from the middle ear. This fibrous tissue vibrates freely with all audible sound frequencies

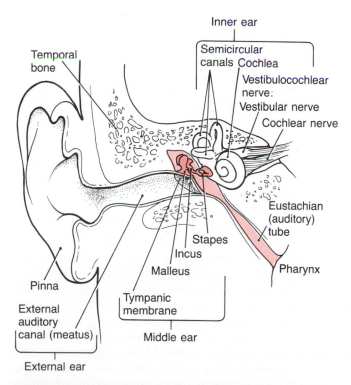

FIGURE 49-7 *Structures of the ear including the external, middle, and inner ear.*

and transmits these to the three auditory ossicles of the middle ear: the *malleus, incus,* and *stapes.* The middle ear with its three ossicles is situated in an air cavity of the temporal bone. It communicates with the nasopharynx by means of the auditory or eustachian tube; the mucous membrane that lines the middle ear extends to line the pharynx and the air cells of the mastoid. The auditory tube, normally closed, also equalizes pressure in the middle ear with atmospheric pressure. Swallowing and yawning open the tube; high atmospheric pressures tend to close the tube. Microorganisms from the oropharynx often travel through the auditory tube to the middle ear, causing infections in this area.

The manubrium of the malleus is attached to the tympanic membrane, and its short process articulates with the incus to produce vibratory movements in the stapes, which is attached to the walls of the oval window (Fig. 49-8). The *tensor tympani* and *stapedius muscles* of the middle ear prevent the bones from transmitting excessive vibrations by pulling on the bones to decrease contact with the tympanic membrane and oval window. The former muscle is innervated by the fifth cranial nerve and the latter by the seventh.

The inner ear is encased in the petrous part of the temporal bone and mediates sound-induced nerve impulses, position orientation, and balance. It is composed of two labyrinths, one within the other. The outer labyrinth is bony and is separated from the inner membranous one by perilymph fluid; it contains the cochlea, the vestibule, and the three semicircular canals (Fig. 49-9). The membranous labyrinth, which lies within the bony labyrinth, contains fluid called *endolymph.* The anterior portion of the membranous labyrinth contains the cochlea, which receives the sound waves from the oval window. The cochlea, a small, shell-shaped structure, is divided into three chambers by the *basilar* and *Reissner membranes.* These chambers are the *scala vestibuli, scala tympani,* and *cochlear duct* (see Figure 49-8). Posteriorly, the cochlea opens into the osseous vestibule, which, in turn, extends to the three semicircular canals (Fig. 49-10).

The *organ of Corti,* located on the basilar membrane within the cochlea, contains the receptor cells of audition. These are hair cells that generate nerve impulses in response to sound vibrations from the oscillations of the oval window. Impulses that stimulate the dendrites of the cochlear division of the acoustic nerve are transmitted to the hearing center in the temporal lobe of the cortex. The various frequencies of sound generate different patterns of vibrations and allow sounds to be differentiated from each other. Subjective interpretation of the frequency of sound waves results in the recognition of *pitch.* The higher frequencies are identified as higher pitch. In addition to frequency, the location of the stimulation of cells on the basilar membrane affects pitch. Low-frequency sounds generate greater activity of the basilar membrane near the apex of the cochlea, and

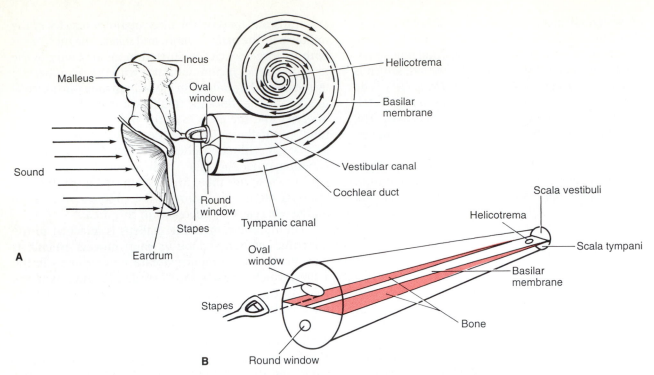

FIGURE 49-8 *The major structural features of the cochlea. **A.** Coupling of the middle ear to the coiled cochlea through the oval and round windows. **B.** The cochlea is shown uncoiled. The basilar membrane is narrow near the round window and wider near the helicotrema, a taper opposite the cross-sectional area of the cochlea. (Conn, P.M. Neuroscience in Medicine. Philadelphia: J.B. Lippincott, 1995.)*

high-frequency sounds activate the basilar membrane near the base of the cochlea. Other frequencies fall between these extremes. This explanation of pitch discrimination is known as the *place theory.*

The amplitude of vibrations affects the perception of loudness at a constant frequency in that greater amplitude produces greater loudness. This does not hold true if two sounds of different frequency are contrasted simultaneously, however, because auditory sensitivity is a function of frequency. Frequency and amplitude are both significant in determining the perception of loudness if there are two or more simultaneous sounds.

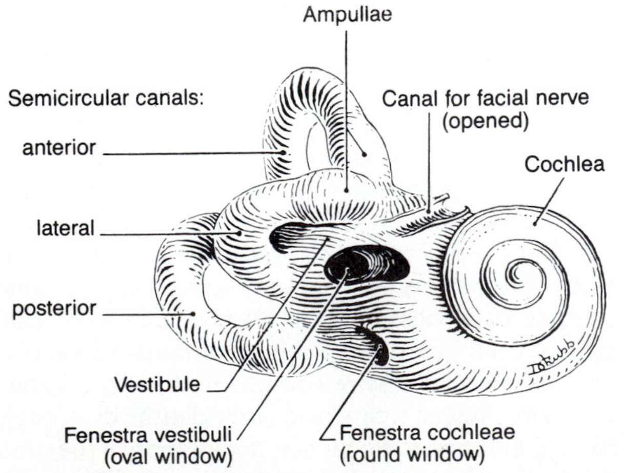

HEARING PATHWAYS

The axons of bipolar neurons from the cochlea enter the pons and divide into the dorsal and ventral cochlear nuclei. Second-order neurons cross here and ascend by the lateral lemniscus to the inferior colliculus. From there, they transmit to the medial geniculate body and on to the auditory cortex in the temporal lobe by the auditory radiations (Fig. 49-11).

The auditory cortex allows a person to recognize tone patterns, analyze characteristics of sound, and localize sound. Low-frequency tones are recognized anteriorly and high-frequency tones posteriorly in the auditory cortex. Neurons throughout the auditory cortex respond to onset, duration, and direction of stimulus.

The auditory association area lies inferior to the primary auditory center and is thought to associate auditory information with other sensations, as well as different sound frequencies with each other. Lesions in this area prevent a person from comprehending the meaning of sounds heard; words can be heard but not understood. The origin (location) of sound is determined by the pattern of the sound's arrival to the two ears. One ear receives information before the other, and the ear that is closer to the sound source receives a louder sound.

FIGURE 49-9 *The bony labyrinth of the inner ear (right ear, lateral view). (Source: Cormack, D.H. Essential Histology. Philadelphia: J.B. Lippincott, 1993.)*

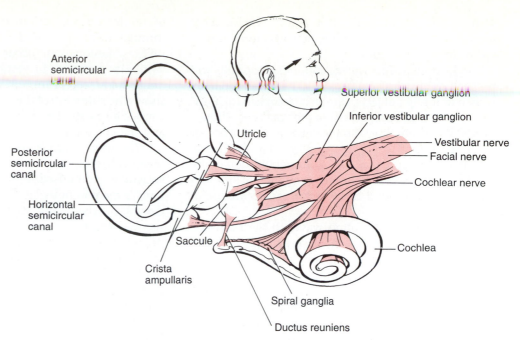

FIGURE 49-10 *Components of the membranous labyrinth include the three semicircular canals (horizontal, anterior, and posterior), the otolith organs (saccule and utricle), and the cochlea. The spiral-shaped cochlea winds around a central bony modiolus. Bipolar neurons in the spiral ganglion innervate the hair cells in the organ of Corti, and their central processes form the cochlear nerve. Peripheral processes of bipolar neurons in the superior and inferior vestibular (Scarpa) ganglia innervate hair cells in the cristae ampullaris of the semicircular canals and the maculae of the saccule and utricle, and their central processes form the vestibular nerve. The arrow indicates the plane of the horizontal semicircular canal. (Conn, P.M. Neuroscience in Medicine. Philadelphia: J.B. Lippincott, 1995.)*

HEARING LOSS

Hearing loss can result from disorders of the central hearing mechanisms or of the peripheral pathways. Peripheral hearing loss involves impairment of sound transmission in the external and middle ear and is referred to as *conduction hearing loss*. Lesions in the neural pathway produce *sensorineural hearing loss*. Problems involving both conductive and sensorineural components result in *mixed hearing loss*; these losses reduce both sensitivity and discrimination of sound in varying degrees. Lesions involving the cochlear nuclei and their

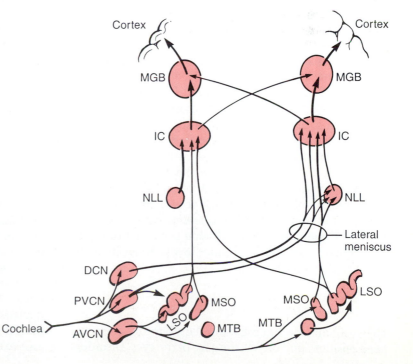

FIGURE 49-11 *The ascending (afferent) neuronal chain from the cochlea to the cortex involves the spiral ganglion cell, cochlear nucleus neuron, superior olivary complex neuron, inferior colliculus neuron, and medial geniculate neuron. Notice the many crossed pathways that allow interactions between the outputs of the two ears. AVCN, anteroventral cochlear nucleus; DCN, dorsal cochlear nucleus; IC, inferior colliculus; LSO, lateral superior olive; MGB, medial geniculate body; MSO, medial superior olive; MTB, medial nucleus of trapezoid body; NLL, nucleus of lateral lemniscus; PVCN, posteroventral cochlear nucleus. (Conn, P.M. Neuroscience in Medicine. Philadelphia: J.B. Lippincott, 1995.)*

connections in the brain result in *central hearing loss*.[13] With this type of hearing loss, the person cannot understand or interpret sounds.

Conduction deafness affects loudness of sounds and can result from obstruction of the external canal by cerumen or foreign objects, tumors, damage to the tympanic membrane, congenital malformations, cholesteatoma, or immobility of the tympanic membrane or ossicles secondary to chronic otitis media. *Otosclerosis* results in conduction deafness by immobilization of the stapes in the oval window. Because conduction loss does not interfere with sound clarity, hearing aids are useful to restore hearing.

The transmission of sound waves in sensorineural hearing loss occurs normally; however, the perception of sound acuity and speech discrimination is impaired. People with sensorineural hearing loss frequently experience a constant, high-pitched ringing in the ears. These people do not perceive the loudness of their own voices and, therefore, tend to speak in louder tones than seems appropriate. Sensorineural hearing loss can be caused by long-term therapy with certain antibiotics in the mycin group, pathology of the hair cells of the cochlea, aging process, infections, persistent exposure to loud noise, or disease processes in the auditory nerve pathway. Sensorineural hearing loss is usually permanent and unresponsive to medical and surgical treatment.

AGE-RELATED HEARING CHANGES

Elderly persons have varying hearing impairments. It is estimated that more than half of the population older than age 65 years has a hearing loss problem. A gradual loss begins in early adulthood and progresses until 80 years and older. The changes in hearing that accompany the aging process are related to structural changes of the outer and middle ear as well as the sensory and neural components of the ears. The ear canal of the outer ear widens, and its skin lining thins and loses elasticity. These changes accompany increased hair growth and dryness of the ear canal and contribute to excessive cerumen collection, the most common correctable hearing loss problem in elderly persons.

Hearing loss changes associated with aging are known as *presbycusis*. *Neural presbycusis* is a sensorineural hearing loss associated with the aging process. It occurs as a result of degeneration of the cochlear nerve fibers and spiral ganglia, which results in diminished speech discrimination. *Sensory presbycusis* occurs as a result of degenerative hair cell changes and atrophy of the organ of Corti, which produce in loss of sensitivity to high frequency tones.

THE VESTIBULAR SYSTEM

The vestibular system maintains equilibrium, preserves head position, and directs the gaze of the eyes. Disorders of coordination may originate from the vestibular system through disruption of the labyrinthine and righting reflexes. Lesions can occur in the labyrinths, in the vestibular nerve, or in vestibular pathways within the brain stem, cerebrum, or cerebellum. Figure 49-12 shows the pathways of the vestibular nerve and its interconnections with the cerebellum, parts of the labyrinths, and the cerebrum.

The *utricle, saccule*, and *semicircular canals* function together to maintain equilibrium (see Fig. 49-10). These structures are housed in a bony labyrinth, which contains a membranous labyrinth composed of the semicircular canals and the two chambers: the utricle and the saccule. Within the utricle and saccule are maculae that provide sensory areas that detect the relation of the head to gravitational pull and other forces. Internal and external hair cells synapse with a network of cochlear nerve endings that terminate in the *cochlear nerve*. Within the semicircular canals, endolymph flows and stimulates the sensory nerve fibers that join up with the vestibular nerve. Fluid flow in the opposite direction inhibits these sensory nerve fibers.

The vestibular portion of the eighth nerve has its peripheral endings on the hair cells of the maculae of the utricle and saccule and on the cristae in the ampullae of the three semicircular canals. The maculae of the utricle and saccule record linear acceleration and static phenomena; the semicircular canals record angular acceleration.[6] Recent evidence implies that the utricle is more related to the semicircular canals' vestibular functions and the saccule has a closer association with hearing.

The ganglion cells of the vestibular division of the eighth nerve are in the internal auditory meatus, and the dendrites end in the specialized epithelium of the hair cells. The axons pass back to the upper medulla, accompanied by the cochlear nerve. On entering the medulla, the fibers pass directly to the cerebellum and to four vestibular nuclei that communicate with the medial longitudinal fasciculus and with the nuclei of the third, fourth, and sixth cranial nerves and the upper cervical and accessory nerves. This connection results in vestibular influence on movement of the neck, eyes, and head.

A close interrelation exists between the vestibular nerves and the cerebellum. This relation accounts for the equilibrium changes that occur with rapid changes in direction. The maculae of the utricle and saccule provide vestibular input to the cerebellum. The influence of the two-way communication results in coordination of the muscles of the neck and the coordination required for posture. Interconnection of vestibular nerves to the reticular system may account for the nausea, vomiting, and sweating that result if the vestibular system is stimulated.

Two vestibulospinal tracts arise from the vestibular nuclei. The lateral tract comes from the lateral vestibular nucleus and extends to the sacral level of the cord. The medial tract comes from the medial vestibular nucleus and extends through the cervical level. Impulses de-

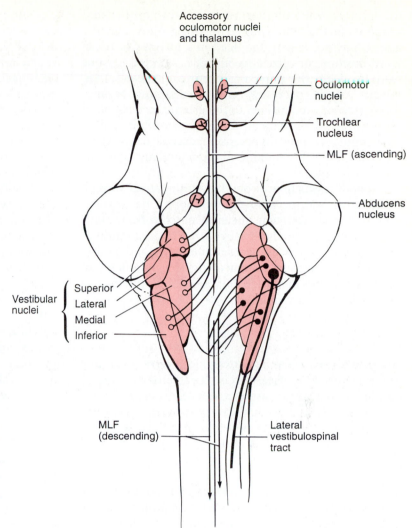

FIGURE 49-12 *The ascending (left) and descending (right) vestibular pathways. Ipsilateral inhibitory and contralateral excitatory ascending projections from the vestibular nuclei course through the medial longitudinal fasciculus (MLF) and target motor neurons in the abducens, trochlear, and oculomotor nuclei. The ascending connections mediate the vestibuloocular reflex. Bilateral descending fibers in the MLF project primarily to motor neurons in the cervical spinal cord that innervate the dorsal neck muscles, forming the basis for the vestibulocollic reflex. The lateral vestibulospinal tract arises from the lateral vestibular nuclei and descends ipsilaterally in the spinal cord, targeting primarily motor neurons that innervate axial extensor muscles that maintain posture. (Conn, P.M. Neuroscience in Medicine. Philadelphia: J.B. Lippincott, 1995.)*

scending in these tracts assist in local myotactic (muscle-stretching) reflexes and reinforce the tonus of the extensor muscles of the trunk and limbs, producing extra force to support the body against gravity and to maintain an upright posture.

Communication between the vestibular nuclei and the cerebral nuclei is not established but may exist because vertigo and dizziness have resulted from cortical stimulation of posterior aspects of the temporal lobe. Disturbances of function of the vestibular system may result in vertigo, nystagmus, and ataxia.

Vertigo

Vertigo is a disturbance of equilibrium that results in sensations of whirling, rotation, weakness, lightheadedness, or faintness. Posture is maintained by the normal interaction of several structures: labyrinths, eyes, muscles, joints, and higher neural centers. Causes of vertigo are multitudinous and include disorders of the labyrinth,

vestibular nerve, vestibular nuclei, cerebellum, brain stem, eyes, and cerebral cortex.

There are several types of vertigo: acute paroxysmal, chronic, and benign positional. Acute paroxysmal vertigo is exemplified by sudden onset of acute sensation of rotatory movement, which is either objective or subjective. If external objects seem to be rotating while the person is stationary, the sensation is said to be that of objective rotatory movement. In subjective rotatory movement, the person feels that he or she is rotating in relation to the external environment. In addition to rotation, sensations of spinning, falling through space, or being pushed are experienced. Movement of objects or of oneself may appear in any plane—horizontal, oblique, or vertical.

Single attacks of vertigo may occur in acute labyrinthitis. Chronic vertigo is experienced as transient sensations of rotation with sudden turning of the head. Another type of attack, which may persist for months, is a constant sense of imbalance. Benign positional vertigo occurs only when the head is in certain postures and ceases when the head is moved out of these positions. An attack may occur with the head in a forward or backward position, or turned to one side. Affected persons learn to avoid the particular posture that causes the attack. Attacks of vertigo can be disabling because the person may be thrown to the ground in reaction to false clues of movement. Nausea, vomiting, pallor, nystagmus, sweating, hypotension, excessive salivation, and difficulty with walking may accompany acute attacks of vertigo.

Rapid destruction of one labyrinth causes vertigo, nystagmus, and, occasionally, temporary nausea and vomiting. The vestibular nuclei seem to work by comparing signals from both labyrinths. If a labyrinth is destroyed, the other side overcompensates for the missing input. Bilateral destruction of the labyrinths does not cause nystagmus or vertigo, but the equilibrium may be disturbed for many months.

Meniere's Disease

Meniere's disease is a classic example of vertigo resulting from labyrinthine disease. It is characterized by recurrent attacks of vertigo associated with disordered autonomic activity and gradual loss of hearing, which frequently begins before the appearance of the first bout of vertigo. Vertigo, which is of the whirling and rotation type, appears abruptly and lasts from minutes to more than an hour. It is usually severe enough to cause the person to lie down. Nausea, vomiting, tinnitus, feeling of fullness in the ears, loss of the sense of proprioception, hypotension, sweating, and nystagmus may accompany the attacks. Considerable variation exists in the frequency and severity of attacks. They may occur for a while and then go into remission for a considerable time.

The mechanism of vertigo is unknown at this time, although it is theorized that the autonomic nervous system control of the labyrinthine circulation is impaired. Caloric testing (irrigation of the ear canal) reveals loss of thermally-induced nystagmus on the involved side, and audiometry shows decreased air and bone conduction. Meniere's disease affects both sexes equally and usually appears in the fifth decade.

Nystagmus

Nystagmus is characterized by rhythmic oscillation of the eyes, and it occurs both in physiologic and pathologic circumstances. Nystagmus can be induced in healthy persons by irrigation of the external auditory canal with hot or cold water or by rotation in a revolving chair. One form of physiologic nystagmus is *opticokinetic nystagmus*, which is induced by having the person look at a repeating pattern passed in a horizontal or vertical direction in front of the eyes.

Pathologically, *vestibular nystagmus* occurs as a response to some disturbance of the synergistic action of the two vestibular organs or their central connections. The nystagmus is always phasic. There is a slow phase in one direction of eye movement and then an opposing quick phase. The direction of nystagmus is based on the direction of the fast component. If the slow phase is to the right and the quick one is to the left, the person is said to exhibit nystagmus to the left. The movement of the eye may be horizontal, vertical, or rotary. The rotary tendency is most prominent if a lesion involves the labyrinth.

Vestibular nystagmus is associated with vertigo and is increased by turning the head or eyes in the direction of the quick phase. This occurs in dysfunction of the semicircular canals or their peripheral neurons. It is limited in duration because central compensation occurs. If it should persist longer than a few weeks, it is usually because of change in the vestibular pathway.[3] Other causes of pathologic nystagmus are abnormal retinal or labyrinthine impulses, lesions of the cervical spinal cord, lesions involving the central paths concerned in ocular posture (particularly those in the midbrain and midbrain tegmentum), weakness of the ocular muscles, drug treatment, and congenital abnormalities of unknown origin.

Labyrinthine Ataxia

Ataxia is often striking in vestibular disease. It is characterized by disturbances of equilibrium in standing and walking and does not affect isolated limb movements. It has many features of cerebellar ataxia, such as the broad-based, staggering gait, the tendency to lean over backward or to one side, and the deviation from direction of gait. It can usually be differentiated from cerebellar ataxia through association with nystagmus and vertigo. Causes of ataxia include degenerative, demyelinating, or inflammatory lesions and lesions in the thalamus and subthalamic region near the main cerebellar and sensory pathways. The most common mixed ataxias are the cerebellar and vestibular forms and the posterior column and cerebellar forms. In multiple sclerosis, symptoms of ataxia are mainly of the cerebellar and vestibular forms.

ASSESSMENT OF HEARING AND BALANCE

A single effective means of assessing hearing ability is to have the patient cover one ear with the hand while the examiner whispers a few words softly near the opposite ear; this procedure is then repeated for the other ear. If the patient is able to perceive the words, the hearing is probably normal. In addition, auditory loss can be determined through the use of equipment, such as the tuning fork and the audiometer. These tools can assist in differentiating sensorineural hearing loss from conductive loss.

A simple test for conductive loss can be demonstrated through the use of a tuning fork. A tuning fork vibrating at 256 Hz is placed on the person's mastoid process until he or she no longer hears it and is then held in the air next to the external auditory canal. This is known as the *Rinne test*. In persons with normal hearing, air conduction is acute and vibrations are heard after bone conduction through the mastoid process has ceased. If vibrations are not heard in the air, the person has conductive hearing loss. If the vibrating tuning fork is heard in the air, the conducting mechanisms through the middle ear are intact and the problem is in the inner ear or its transmissions; the person therefore has sensorineural loss.

The *Weber test* is also effective in identifying hearing loss. A vibrating tuning fork is placed at the vertex of the person's head; normal perception of the sound is equal in both ears. If conductive loss is present, the sound is louder in the affected ear owing to the masking effect of environmental noise. With sensorineural damage, sound is heard better in the normal ear.

Audiometry tests the sensitivity of the ear to pure tones at different frequencies through earphones. The audiometer, which is an electronic oscillator, measures hearing objectively and plots it on a graph that represents the percentage of normal hearing based on the average threshold of normal hearing of a population. Conductive and sensorineural hearing impairments can be differentiated by this means.

The vestibular component of the eighth cranial nerve may be assessed if the person's history reveals vertigo with nausea and vomiting. Vestibular function is evaluated by the *caloric test*. The person is placed supine at a 30-degree elevation. After ascertaining no observable defects of the external auditory canal, the examiner introduces first cold and then warm water alternately into the canal. The ear is irrigated with water at 30°C and 44°C with a minimal pause of 5 minutes between each irrigation. Tonic deviation of the eyes is normally induced to the side being irrigated with cold water; after a short latent period, nystagmus occurs toward the opposite side. Warm-water irrigation produces nystagmus toward the irrigated side. An absent or decreased response indicates impairment of the vestibular system.

▼ *Taste*

STRUCTURE AND FUNCTION

The sense of taste is a specialized function that is concerned with identification of food. The four primary taste sensations are *sweet, sour, bitter,* and *salt*. The other, more complex sensations that human beings perceive are combinations of the primary sensations together with the olfactory sensation. Even though the tip of the tongue perceives all four tastes, specific areas of the tongue are more sensitive to particular sensations (Fig. 49-13).

Taste buds are the organs of taste (Fig. 49-14). These oval structures are most numerous in the fungiform papillae of the tongue and are also present in the palate, pharynx, and epiglottis. Microvilli project from the buds to the surface and come into contact with the substances dissolved in the fluids of the mouth. This contact is thought to be the basis for the generator potentials. Innervation for the taste buds arrives from their base through small myelinated fibers. Each taste bud is innervated by several nerve fibers, and each nerve fiber receives innervation from several taste buds. The life span of a taste bud is approximately 5 to 10 days. As buds degenerate, new buds are formed and innervated. The total number of taste buds diminishes with aging, accounting for the diminished sense of taste in elderly persons.

In addition to taste buds, the sense of smell contributes significantly to taste perception. Odors of substances taken into the mouth pass to the nasopharynx and stimulate olfactory receptors. Consistency and temperature of ingested substances also contribute to the overall taste perception.

Because taste affects what is consumed, it contributes significantly to the nutritional status and internal environment of the body. Nutritional needs are not solely dependent on taste, however. Researchers have shown that people tend to select foods and liquids containing substances in which they are deficient. This conclusion is supported by studies showing that adrenalectomized animals tend to develop a preference for salty substances. Animals that have had the parathyroid gland removed usually show an increased appetite for calcium-containing substances.[4]

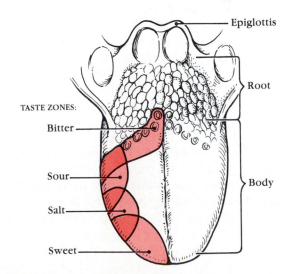

FIGURE 49-13 *The dorsal surface of the tongue showing the areas for perception of sweet, sour, bitter, and salt tastes.*

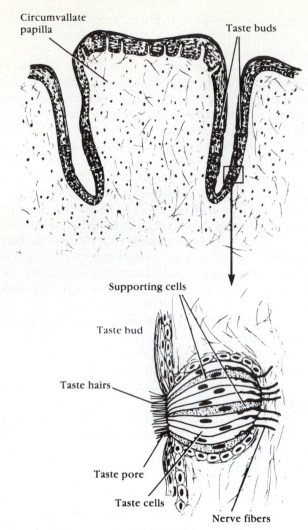

FIGURE 49-14 *Microscopic appearance of a taste bud.*

TASTE PATHWAYS

Innervation from the taste buds to the central nervous system is through the seventh, ninth, and tenth cranial nerves. The taste buds of the anterior two-thirds of the tongue transmit by way of the chorda tympani, a branch of the seventh cranial nerve. The posterior one-third of the tongue, the soft palate, transmits through the ninth cranial nerve, and the remainder of the areas (extreme dorsal portion of tongue, pharynx, and larynx) transmit by means of the 10th cranial nerve. All three of these nerves terminate in the medulla oblongata and form the *tractus solitarius*. From this region, second-order neurons transmit to the thalamus and then on to the postcentral gyrus of the cerebral cortex, where taste sensation shares projection sites with other somatic sensations.

TASTE DISTURBANCES

The sense of taste may be diminished (*hypogeusia*) or absent (*ageusia*) secondary to other underlying problems, such as dryness of the tongue, irradiation of the

head, respiratory infections, and aging. Alterations in taste are associated with heavy smoking and may accompany Bell palsy. Lesions of the thalamus and parietal lobe may result in impairment or loss of taste on the opposite side of the tongue, and parietal lobe seizures may be heralded by an aura of a specific taste. Certain medications can alter the interpretation of taste.

Idiopathic hypogeusia is a syndrome associated with hyposmia, dysosmia (impaired smell), and dysgeusia (perversion of taste), in conjunction with diminished taste acuity. The smell and taste of food are most unpleasant for these people. They often experience weight loss, depression, and anxiety. One identified cause of this syndrome is depression of zinc content in the parotid saliva.[1]

As a result of age-related changes in the taste buds of elderly persons, the threshold necessary to transmit taste rises. The perceptions of sour, salt, and bitter tastes diminish somewhat. For this reason, elderly persons may be observed to use excessive seasoning on their food. Taste perceptions may also be affected by the numerous medications ingested by this group.

TASTE ASSESSMENT

To assess taste, one examines the functioning of the seventh, ninth, and tenth cranial nerves. The discrimination of taste in human beings is relatively crude, and approximately a 30% concentration of a substance is necessary before a taste is detected. Thresholds of response to substances vary, and sensitivity to bitter tastes, in particular, is much higher than to other tastes. This protective mechanism is significant in that many poisonous alkaloids are characteristically bitter.

In assessing taste, substances that are sweet, sour, salty, and bitter are assembled. They are individually swabbed on the appropriate area of the person's tongue, and the patient is asked to identify the taste sensation. To prevent mixing of the substances applied to the tongue, the person is asked to rinse the mouth after each sensation has been identified.

▼ Smell

STRUCTURE AND FUNCTION

In human beings, the sense of smell is closely associated physiologically with the sense of taste. Many foods are perceived partially by both senses, which are chemoreceptors that are stimulated by substances in the nose and mouth. Anatomically, these perceptions differ in that the apparatus perceiving smell is not relayed to the thalamus or to a cortical projection area.

The receptor cells of olfaction are the *bipolar olfactory cells*, which are located in the olfactory mucous membrane. Unlike other nerve cells, the olfactory cells are continuously dying and being replaced by newly generated ones. Peripherally, these cells have dendrites that terminate on the surface of the mucus of the nasal cavity and project a group of cilia. The axons of the olfactory neurons pass through the *cribriform plate* of the ethmoid bone and enter the olfactory bulb. Here they synapse with second-order neurons, the *mitral cells*, and form a plexus of fibers called the *olfactory glomeruli* or *synaptic glomeruli* (Fig. 49-15). Olfactory signals are transmitted from there along the olfactory tract through the axons of the mitral cells and terminate in two principal areas: the prepiriform area and parts of the limbic system.

Olfactory receptors are stimulated by volatile lipids and water-soluble substances that are inhaled into the mucosa of the nasal cavity. Little is known about the excitatory process of the individual receptor cells, although researchers have elicited several potentials in response to different odors. The conduction to the prepyriform cortex and frontal cortex through the thalamus causes the perception of odor and the sensation of smell.[10]

Although the physiologic basis for odor discrimination and differentiation is still unknown, several theories have been proposed. Some physiologists have proposed the existence of primary odors that excite specific cells. An attempt to explain how this excitation takes place is proposed by the proponents of the *stereochemical* theory.

They believe that the odor molecules fit into specifically-shaped receptor sites on the surface of the olfactory microvilli membranes. Other theorists have attempted to explain odor discrimination by the physical properties of the stimulant, such as its molecular vibrations. Electrophysiologic studies have ascertained that different odors stimulate different parts of the olfactory mucosa to varying degrees. On the basis of this, it would appear that olfactory receptors are not specific for a single odor but for a variety of odors to different degrees.[1] The limbic system connections probably account for emotional and memory-related responses to odors.[10]

Adaptation is quite rapid in the sense of smell because receptors are readily fatigued by persistent odors. Newly appearing odors may be detected rapidly, however. It requires only a small amount of a volatile substance to stimulate the olfactory receptors. Inhalation of irritating substances, such as ammonium salts, produces pain through stimulation of the trigeminal nerve; in addition, certain respiratory reflexes are initiated by its odors.

SMELL DISTURBANCES

Anosmia, the loss of smell, is the most frequent disturbance associated with the sense of smell and may accompany such disorders as hypertrophy of nasal

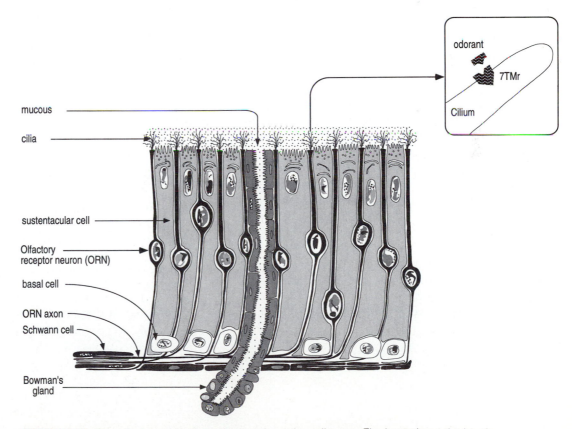

FIGURE 49-15 *The olfactory epithelium, showing the major cell types. The inset shows the location of seven transmembrane (7TMr) odorant receptors on the cilia of the olfactory receptor neurons. (Conn, P.M. Neuroscience in Medicine. Philadelphia: J.B. Lippincott, 1995.)*

mucosa, sinusitis, upper respiratory infections, and allergies. *Hyposmia*, a reduced sense of smell, is most frequently associated with heavy smoking. Facial injuries involving the cribriform plate and certain tumors involving the olfactory groove may result in the loss of smell. Hysteria may be accompanied by anosmia or *hyperosmia* (increased acuity of smell). Olfactory hallucinations and delusions may occur with certain mental illnesses as well as with temporal lobe disorders. Specific smells may precede seizures arising from the uncal region. *Dysosmia* or *parosmia* is a distortion of a smell; it may occur as a result of local nasopharyngeal conditions, such as partial injuries. Age-related changes in smell occur as a result of the decreased number of cells in the olfactory bulb and nasal lining. Years of exposure to smoke and other pollutants also contribute to diminution of the sense of smell in elderly persons.

SMELL ASSESSMENT

The sense of smell can be assessed simply by requesting an individual to identify common aromatic substances, such as coffee, vanilla, and cologne. The person is asked to close his or her eyes and occlude one nostril. Although the person is requested to identify the odor if possible, the ability to do so is less significant than the perception of the odor per se. Therefore, the person is asked to identify the moment at which he or she initially perceives the odor. The procedure is then repeated for the other nostril, and perception is compared.

▼ Chapter Summary

▼ The special senses include vision, hearing, taste, and smell. These senses provide for the ability to perceive the environment and, through transmission to the cerebral cortex, to determine a response.

▼ The eye transmits visual images to the visual area of the occipital lobe of the cerebral cortex. The structures work together to accommodate for distance of objects and to allow the appropriate amount of light to enter the eye.

▼ The visual receptors on the retina are the rods and cones. The cones mediate daylight vision, and the rods work on night vision and are sensitive to movement of objects in the visual field.

▼ Visual defects are very common and include both accommodation defects and refraction defects. More serious disorders include the hemianopsias, scotomas, papilledema, glaucoma, cataracts, detached retina, and retinitis pigmentosa, any of which may lead to blindness.

▼ Hearing is accomplished through the mechanoreceptor called the ear, which is a transducer for sound waves that are sent to the cerebral cortex for interpretation. The auditory cortex allows the individual to recognize tone patterns, analyze characteristics of sound, and localize the origin of the sound.

▼ Hearing loss can occur at any age and results from conduction, sensorineural, or central hearing damage. Loss may be associated with alterations in the vestibular system, which is essential for equilibrium and maintaining the upright position. Vertigo, Meniere disease, nystagmus, and labyrinthine ataxia are associated with vestibular disorders.

▼ Alterations in taste and smell may be caused by environmental factors such as smoking or by central nervous system dysfunction. These senses may be decreased, lost, or altered so that abnormal taste and smell result. Sometimes taste and smell problems occur together.

▼ References

1. Adams, R., and Mauria, V. *Principles of Neurology* (4th ed.). New York: McGraw-Hill, 1989.
2. Carpenter, M., and Sutin, J. *Human Neuroanatomy* (8th ed.). Baltimore: Williams & Wilkins, 1983.
3. Clark, R.G. *Essentials of Clinical Neuroanatomy and Neurophysiology* (6th ed.). Philadelphia: Davis, 1982.
4. Guyton, A.C. *Textbook of Medical Physiology* (8th ed.). Philadelphia: W.B. Saunders, 1991.
5. Hubel, D.H., and Wiesel, T.N. Brain mechanisms of vision. *Sci. Am.* 241:150, 1979.
6. Hudspeth, A.J. The hair cells of the inner ear. *Sci. Am.* 248:59, 1983.
7. Moses, R. *Adler's Physiology of the Eye* (8th ed.). St. Louis: Mosby, 1987.
8. Nauta, W.J., and Feirtag, M. The organization of the brain. *Sci Am* 241:99, 1979.
9. Rose, F.C. *The Eye in General Practice.* Baltimore: University Park Press, 1983.
10. Tortora, G.J. and Grabowski, S. *Principles of Anatomy and Physiology* (7th ed.). New York: HarperCollins, 1993.
11. Walton, J. *Brain's Diseases of the Nervous System* (9th ed.). Oxford: Oxford University Press, 1985.

Chapter 50

Common Adaptations and Alterations in Higher Neurologic Function

Reet Henze

▼ **CHAPTER OUTLINE**

▼ **LEARNING OBJECTIVES**

1 Discuss the major classifications of cerebrovascular disease.
2 Describe the pathologic changes that occur with intracerebral hemorrhage, cerebral thrombosis, and embolism.
3 Locate and discuss cerebral aneurysms and arteriovenous malformations.
4 Differential transient ischemic attacks from a cerebrovascular accident.
5 Relate the clinical manifestations of stroke to the underlying etiologic and pathologic bases.
6 Explain why bleeding is a common complication after initial rupture of an intracerebral aneurysm.
7 Describe the neurologic findings in each of the gradations of ruptured cerebral aneurysms.
8 Discuss the implications of vasospasm with ruptured cerebral aneurysm.
9 Explain why arteriovenous malformations rupture and the significance of the location of the bleeding.
10 Distinguish between Wernicke's aphasia, Broca's aphasia, and global aphasia.
11 Define the disorders of speech: **anarthria, agraphia, alexia**, and **word-deafness**.
12 Discuss the various types of apraxia and agnosia.
13 Discuss the pathophysiology of epilepsy.
14 Differentiate between primary or idiopathic and secondary or symptomatic seizures.
15 Discuss partial versus generalized seizures.
16 Describe changes on the electroencephalogram that correlate with three different types of seizures.

Barbara L. Bullock: PATHOPHYSIOLOGY: ADAPTATIONS AND ALTERATIONS IN FUNCTION, 4th ed.
© 1996 J.B. Lippincott-Raven Publishers

Cerebrovascular diseases (pathologic processes in cerebral blood vessels) lead to hospitalization for more persons than any other neurologic disorder. Cerebrovascular accidents (CVAs) are the third leading cause of death (after heart disease and cancer) in the United States. Major disabilities frequently remain in those who survive the initial assault. Paresis, aphasia, agnosia, and apraxia are among the common associated impairments. Epilepsy is another major neurologic disorder. As a neurologic disease, it ranks second only to CVAs in number of persons affected in the United States.

▼ Cerebrovascular Disease: Pathology and Related Clinical Signs

Cerebrovascular disease results either directly or indirectly, suddenly or over time, from a disruption of cerebral blood flow that causes a variety of brain dysfunctions. The brain does not tolerate anoxia because it has no oxygen reserve. Therefore, permanent cell damage can occur rather rapidly with a disruption of cerebral blood flow. Short periods of hypoxia (15 minutes or less) usually result in reversible neurologic deficits, and those lasting longer can lead to permanent neurologic deficits and cerebral infarction. Those neurologic impairments that result from a sudden disruption of the blood supply to a specific area of the brain are referred to as CVAs or strokes.

Cerebrovascular disease is commonly associated with hypertensive and atherosclerotic disease. Both of these conditions are closely linked with other conditions and risk factors: hypercholesterolemia, arteriovenous malformations (AVMs), arteritis, vasospasm, cigarette smoking, obesity, diabetes mellitus, physical inactivity, emotional stress, and family history of premature atherosclerosis.

As is the case with most neuropathology, the site of a cerebral vascular lesion is more critical in the production of pathologic signs and symptoms than is its pathology. The area of the brain involved depends on the specific cerebral vessel affected. Table 50-1 lists major cerebral arteries and the effects associated with their involvement.

The disruption of cerebral blood flow in cerebrovascular disease may be caused by occlusion of cerebral arteries or by hemorrhage. Occlusive disease results from thrombosis and embolism. Hemorrhagic disease results from intracerebral, subarachnoid, or AVM bleeding into the brain parenchyma or spaces.[3] Whatever the cause, ischemia and eventual necrosis of the brain parenchyma may result. CVAs also can be described according to onset and duration: completed CVA, progressing or evolving CVA, and transient ischemic attack

(TIA). A stroke is said to be completed if the blood supply has been cut off to a portion of the brain and permanent neurologic alterations have followed. Progressing or evolving stroke, usually seen with occlusive disease, progresses over hours or days and finally results in permanent deficits. TIAs are strokes that last from a few minutes to a few hours, and the neurologic deficits resolve.

TABLE 50-1 *Clinical Findings with Occlusion of Major Cerebral Arteries*

Occluded Arteries	Associated Findings
Internal carotid system	Contralateral hemiparesis Dysphasia with dominant side involvement Blindness, visual blurring Agnosia Hemianopia Cranial nerve deficits Contralateral anosognosia Bruit over occluded artery
Middle cerebral artery	Contralateral arm and leg weakness or paralysis Homonymous hemianopia Eye deviation to opposite side Dysphagia or aphasia with dominant side involvement Anosognosia with nondominant hemisphere involvement Contralateral sensory impairment Apraxia with nondominant side involvement
Anterior cerebral artery	Contralateral paralysis of leg, foot, and arm (lesser degree) Bladder incontinence Sensory deficit in leg, foot, toes Akinetic mutism Eye deviation toward affected side Gait impairment Mood disturbance, personality change
Vertebral-basilar system	Variations in level of consciousness Hemianopia Possible quadriplegia Eye muscle paralysis Headache Limb weakness Nystagmus Diplopia Mutism Dysarthria Ataxia Dysphagia Varying sensory deficits (numbness) Vertigo Varying cranial nerve deficits

A TIA causes a temporary episode of neurologic dysfunction as a result of a diminished blood supply to a specific area of the brain, usually from thrombotic origins secondary to atherosclerosis (atheroma). TIAs usually last no longer than 15 minutes, although some may exhibit signs up to 24 hours.

Virtually any cerebral artery may be involved, and symptoms vary according to the area of involvement. They may range from minor focal deficits to major deficits resulting in complete loss of consciousness. Because the same diseased vessel is usually involved, the recurring TIA symptoms are similar with each episode. Common findings with TIAs include transient episodes of contralateral weakness of the face, arms, and legs (hemiparesis) as well as sensory deficits (hemiparesthesias) and visual impairments. Involvement of the ophthalmic artery results in unilateral visual symptoms, known as amaurosis fugax. In this condition, the individual loses sight in one eye for 2 to 3 minutes as a result of a transient ischemia of the retina.

TIAs may be associated with the development of collateral communicating vessels in the intracerebral arterial system that compensate in a short time for the deficits from the occlusion of one arterial source. Nevertheless, many persons who experience a TIA are thought to be at significant risk for strokes at a later time.[1]

Diagnosis of TIAs is based on clinical findings after other conditions such as postural hypotension, Adams-Stokes syndrome, and seizure disorders are ruled out. Angiographic evaluation may be used to locate the pathologic process in the cerebral arteries. Radiopaque substances are injected to outline the cerebral vasculature and identify areas of narrowing or disease.

OCCLUSIVE CEREBROVASCULAR DISEASE

Occlusive cerebrovascular disease results from thrombosis and formation of emboli in the cerebral vessels. The effects of occlusion vary with its extent of involvement, time, and location. In addition, the collateral vessels available to divert the remaining circulation affect the blood flow to a specific area of the brain. Obstruction of the flow to any region rapidly results in cell ischemia, followed by potentially irreversible necrosis and cerebral infarction.

Cerebral Thrombosis

Atherosclerotic thrombosis is the leading cause of CVAs. Ischemic infarction in the brain frequently results from an embolus that has been dislodged from an atherosclerotic plaque. Impediment of the blood flow contributes to formation of emboli. The most common areas of thrombus formation are those at which atheromatous plaques have already resulted in narrowing of the vessels. Such areas most commonly occur at curves and bifurcations. Sites frequently affected are the internal carotid artery in the region of the carotid sinus, the junction of the vertebral and basilar arteries, the bifurcation of the middle cerebral artery, the posterior cerebral artery in the area of the cerebral peduncle, and the anterior cerebral artery in the area of the corpus callosum.[3,8]

Wide variations may be observed in clinical signs resulting from disruption of blood flow to specific regions of the brain. Occlusions of major arteries manifest the clinical findings given in Table 50-1. Obstruction to blood flow may cause infarction to the area supplied by the affected arteries. This type of lesion may be referred to as an atherothrombotic brain infarction.

Brain infarcts are often described as red (hemorrhagic) or white (anemic). In the first few days, pathologic section shows the pale or white infarcts to assume a muddy, mottled appearance that is associated with surrounding tissue edema. After about 10 days, liquefaction of the area becomes evident from the release of neuronal lysosomes and other lytic substances into the brain parenchyma.[4] Scar tissue begins to form at the margins of the necrotic area. The necrotic tissue is removed and replaced by cystic scar tissue. Gliosis (proliferation of glial cells) around the area is characteristic and is followed by polymorphonuclear leukocyte exudation, leading to removal of the necrotic debris. Therefore, characteristic scar tissue is laid down after the acute inflammation subsides.

Red infarcts also cause tissue destruction. Red blood cells are broken down and removed. The necrotic parenchyma undergoes liquefaction, and characteristic scar tissue is formed at the margins of the affected area. Cerebral edema accompanies cerebral infarction and is maximal 3 to 5 days after an acute stroke.[9] Cerebral edema is a major cause of death after acute stroke.

The onset of cerebral thrombosis is usually gradual, with periods of progression and periods of improvement. Progression may occur which is indicated by a more severe neurologic deficit. The deficit may improve or remain the same. The neurologic exam then describes *progressing stroke, TIA,* or *complete stroke.* When it progresses the pattern is apparently caused by spread of the thrombus and is called a *thrombotic stroke in evolution.* The thrombosis causes the cerebral infarction, and it may be associated with a hemorrhage into the brain parenchyma. Symptoms often begin or are noted in the early morning. These may consist of headache, vertigo, mental confusion, aphasia, and focal neurologic signs, which may occur weeks to months before the stroke is completed.

Recovery is variable and depends on the location

and the amount of intracerebral damage. Function in an affected leg usually is recovered before arm and hand function, which may not return at all.

Cerebral Embolism

Cerebral embolism is second only to thrombosis as a cause of stroke. The main source of an embolus is the heart. Heart conditions that predispose an individual to cerebral embolization include atrial fibrillation, bacterial endocarditis, rheumatic endocarditis and the valvular diseases that may follow it, and congenital heart disease.[8] Less common sources of emboli are fat, air, or tumor cell emboli. The embolus frequently lodges in the middle cerebral artery, which is a direct continuation of the carotid artery. Massive brain infarction occurs if a large embolus lodges in a major cerebral vessel. However, large thrombi frequently break into smaller clots that travel to occlude more distal branches.

The onset of embolic infarction is always very sudden, and the effect is immediate. There usually are no warning signs. The clinical features depend on the artery affected and the amount and location of brain infarction (see Table 50-1). Aggressive treatment of the underlying cause must ensue to prevent subsequent episodes.

HEMORRHAGIC CEREBROVASCULAR DISEASE

Cerebrovascular disease resulting from intracranial bleeding is the third leading cause of CVAs. Bleeds may occur in vessels deep within the parenchyma or in those close to the surface of the brain.

Intracerebral Hemorrhage

Hypertension is the major cause of spontaneous bleeding into the brain parenchyma. Continued grossly elevated blood pressure weakens the vessel and eventually causes its rupture. It is thought that microaneurysms called *Charcot-Buchard aneurysms* form at bifurcations of small intracerebral arteries, probably as a result of the sustained hypertension.[6] Common loci of small arterial hemorrhages are the penetrating branches of the middle cerebral artery, the striate arteries (Fig. 50-1). The severity of the hemorrhage is related to the amount of blood extravasated and the region of the brain affected. Intracerebral bleeds tend to occur deep within the brain substance (Fig. 50-2A). The most common areas of bleeding in the brain secondary to hypertension are the putamen and the adjacent internal capsule. These areas account for about 50% of cases.[1, 6] Other potential sites are the caudate nucleus; thalamus; central white matter of the temporal, parietal, and frontal lobes; cerebellum; and pons.

In large bleeds, the extravasation of blood forms a

circular mass that disrupts and compresses surrounding brain tissue, resulting in infarction and tissue necrosis. These hemorrhages can displace midline structures and compress vital centers, leading to coma and, eventually, to death. Commonly, blood seeps into the ventricular system (see Figure 50-2B). In most cases of large hemorrhage, analysis of cerebrospinal fluid reflects the presence of blood. Intracerebral hemorrhages may also be small, single bleeds or have several foci. Some may reflect no obvious neurologic deficits, whereas a large number of small hemorrhages in the parenchyma may result in severe neurologic impairment.

Intracerebral bleeds occur abruptly, and the symptoms evolve rather rapidly. Prodromal symptoms are usually absent. Severe headache occurs fairly consistently. Other symptoms relate to the region of the brain involved. The blood in the parenchyma causes extensive neuronal destruction, and the central area of hemorrhage is often surrounded by small hemorrhages. The blood is treated like foreign material and eventually is broken down, phagocytized by macrophages, and removed from the area. The remaining area is eventually filled with connective tissue and new capillaries.

Ischemia secondary to arterial spasm may follow rupture of the diseased vessels. Blood in the brain parenchyma serves as an irritant to surrounding vessels. The

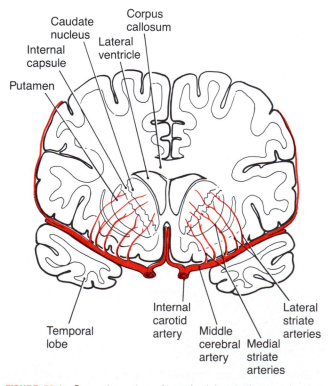

FIGURE 50-1 *Coronal section of cerebral hemispheres, showing striate arterial supply from the middle cerebral artery. (Adapted from: Snell, R.S. Clinical Neuroanatomy for Medical Students (3rd ed.). Boston: Little, Brown, 1992.)*

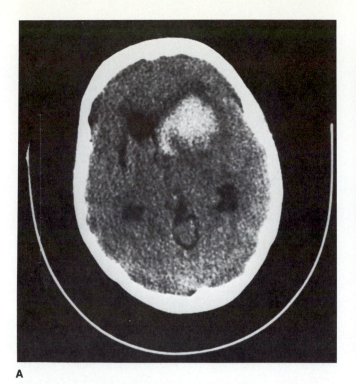

A

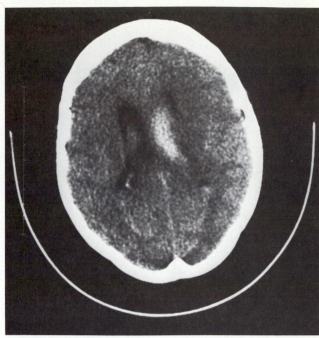

B

FIGURE 50-2   *A. Computed tomography scan, showing large, right hemispheric intracerebral bleed.*
B. Same bleed, showing intraventricular involvement.

most common cause of subarachnoid hemorrhage (bleeding into the ventricles and subarachnoid space) is rupture of an intracerebral aneurysm.

Aneurysms

Cerebral aneurysms are mainly related to developmental defects, and aneurysms of this type account for 95% of aneurysms that rupture.[4] Developmental defects involve a weakness in the middle coat (tunica media) of the vessel that results in a saccular outpouching at the weakened area. These so-called *saccular* or *berry aneurysms* can vary from one to several centimeters in size, usually have a well-defined neck, and originate most often near bifurcations in the anterior vessels of the circle of Willis (Figs. 50-3 and 50-4).[7] Berry aneurysms have the highest frequency of rupture in persons between ages 30 and 60 years, and both sexes are affected equally. Of persons with developmental cerebral aneurysms, about one-fifth demonstrate numerous aneurysms.

Less common than developmental aneurysms are those associated with atherosclerotic degenerative changes of the cerebral vasculature. They are known as fusiform aneurysms and result from weakening of the tunica media secondary to degenerative atherosclerotic processes. The arteries become thin and fibrous, apparently as a result of long-term hypertension. Although fusiform aneurysms of cerebral arteries may occur in some youn-

ger persons, they usually affect those older than 50 years of age.

Cerebral aneurysms can remain silent for many years, often going undetected throughout life and being discovered only on routine postmortem examination. They become evident during life when they rupture or compress adjacent nerve tissue, causing focal cerebral disturbances.

The signs and symptoms of subarachnoid bleeding from a ruptured aneurysm may be localized as a result of the pressure exerted on surrounding tissue. Focal localizing signs are related to the region of the brain involved and may include visual defects, cranial nerve paralysis, hemiparesis, and focal seizures. Generalized signs of subarachnoid bleeding reflect meningeal irritation. They include photophobia, fever, malaise, vomiting, abnormal mentation with disorientation, and nuchal rigidity. If conscious, the patient complains of a severe headache of a different nature from any experienced previously. Transitory unconsciousness or extended coma may accompany bleeding from a ruptured aneurysm. Initial and prolonged coma usually indicates an unfavorable outcome. It is common to assess neurologic findings after a ruptured cerebral aneurysm according to grade (Table 50-2).

The aneurysm decreases in size after rupture, and a fibrin clot forms over the site of the rupture. The person is at risk for a recurrence of bleeding during the first few

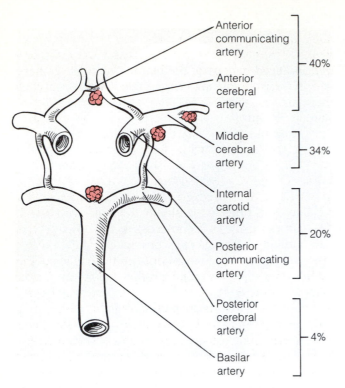

FIGURE 50-3 *Common sites for berry aneurysms in the circle of Willis.*

Anterior communicating artery
Anterior cerebral artery ⎫ 40%

Middle cerebral artery ⎫ 34%

Internal carotid artery
Posterior communicating artery ⎫ 20%

Posterior cerebral artery
Basilar artery ⎫ 4%

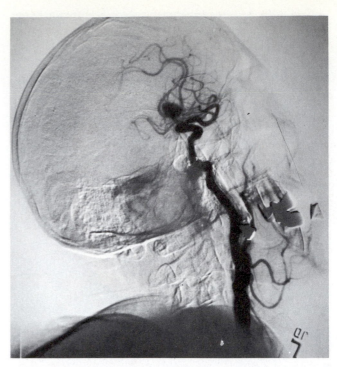

FIGURE 50-4 *Arteriogram showing cerebral aneurysm involving the anterior communicating artery.*

weeks after the initial bleed, during the period of clot lysis. Recurrent bleeding in cerebral aneurysms increases mortality risk considerably.

Diagnosis of ruptured cerebral aneurysm is based on history, clinical examination, lumbar puncture, cerebral angiography, computed axial tomography, and magnetic resonance imaging. Treatment is conservative initially, in an effort to stabilize the pathologic processes. After stabilization has been accomplished, surgical intervention is usually necessary to resolve the aneurysm if its location makes such intervention feasible.

Vasospasm frequently accompanies ruptured cerebral aneurysms. It accounts for 50% of the morbidity and mortality of patients who survive the initial bleed.[5, 6] Cerebral vasospasm is an angiographically demonstrated narrowing of arteries of the circle of Willis. Vasospasm has been shown to develop 3 to 12 days after hemorrhage, with its highest incidence 4 to 8 days after the bleed.[2, 5] Narrowing of the vessel lumen occurs, and the velocity of the blood flow increases. The vessel narrowing may lead to cerebral ischemia, infarction, and clinically evident neurologic deficits. The deficits appear insidiously as cerebral blood flow is decreased and reflect changes in the level of consciousness, speech dysfunction, headache, lethargy, and disorientation in concert with focal motor deficits.

The precise cause of vasospasm is unknown, but it is thought to be related to release of certain intrinsic chemicals associated with lysis of the clot and to release of

other vasoactive mediators. The mediators include calcium ions released from lysed red blood cells, oxygen free radicals from tissue damage, and oxyhemoglobin. These substances, in turn, induce lipid peroxidation.[2, 5] Other vasoactive substances associated with inflammation, such as serotonin, prostaglandins, catecholamines, histamine, and angiotensin, are also thought to contribute to vasospasm.[5, 6]

Vasospasm is diagnosed by patient history, clinical presentation, and cerebral angiography. A relatively new, noninvasive device that detects vasospasm is transcranial Doppler ultrasonography (see p. 965). Cerebral vasospasm is managed with calcium channel blockers as

---

TABLE 50-2 *Grades of Ruptured Cerebral Aneurysms*

Grade	Neurologic Findings
I	Alert and oriented, mild headache, minimal nuchal rigidity, no neurologic deficits
II	Alert and oriented, moderate to severe headache, signs of meningeal irritation, no neurologic deficits
III	Drowsy and confused, minimal focal neurologic deficits, signs of meningeal irritation
IV	Stuporous or unresponsive, major neurologic deficits may be present, mild decerebrate rigidity
V	Coma and decerebrate rigidity

well as with administration of fluid volume and vaso-pressors to maintain perfusion. Surgical intervention for ruptured aneurysm is usually performed early after admission, before vasospasm occurs. If surgery is not accomplished early, it is usually delayed until vasospasm has been reduced.[2]

Arteriovenous Malformations

Vascular malformations usually result from developmental defects of the cerebral veins and arteries in certain localized regions of the brain. These defects have very few distinguishing characteristics with respect to their location. The AVMs may also be secondary to trauma or injury.

The veins in these vascular malformations appear to connect to the arteries without an intermediate capillary bed (Fig. 50-5). The vessel walls are very thin, are dilated from high blood flow, and lack the normal structure of arteries and veins. Because they lack the intermediary capillary bed, they do not supply the brain with blood. These malformations are referred to as AVMs or, less appropriately, as aneurysms or angiomas (Fig. 50-6). They are present most commonly on the surface of the cerebral hemispheres, although they can occur deeper within the cerebral lobes, brain stem, or spinal cord. Although many AVMs are present from birth, they may not become evident until young adulthood or later. Their presence is manifested by symptoms of hemorrhage, seizures, headaches, or focal neurologic deficits. A bruit may be audible over the area of the malformation.

As the very thin walls of these vessels become engorged, the vessels are particularly vulnerable to rupture and bleeding. Bleeding most commonly occurs into the subarachnoid space and, therefore, the symptoms are

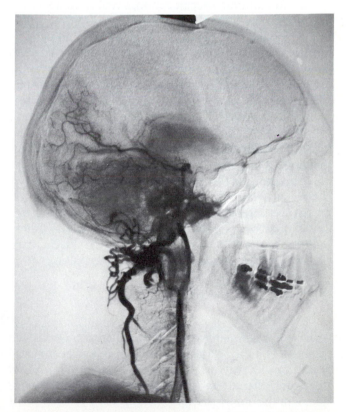

FIGURE 50-5 *Arteriogram showing an arteriovenous malformation that is fed by the vertebral artery and drains into superficial veins and the internal jugular vein.*

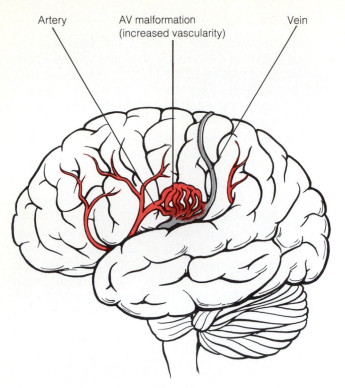

FIGURE 50-6   *Appearance of superficial arteriovenous (AV) malformation. Vessels are dilated and tortuous.*

similar to those observed with ruptured cerebral aneurysms. In addition, specific findings reflect the region of the brain that is involved.

Diagnosis of AVM is based on clinical findings and results of one or more of the following tests: cerebral angiography, lumbar puncture, computed tomography, magnetic resonance imaging, electroencephalography (EEG), and radiology. Treatment consists of surgical ligation and excision of the feeder vessels into the area, if possible. After an AVM has been surgically resected, the blood flow increases to the region of the brain that was previously hypoperfused because of the diversion of large amounts of blood to the malformation. This causes a state of hyperperfusion and has been known to result in hemorrhage in some patients. If the location of the AVM does not permit surgical excision, embolization may be performed to occlude the feeder vessels in an attempt to reduce the blood flow to the AVM.

▼ *Speech Disorders*

Language is defined as audible, articulate human speech produced by the action of the tongue and adjacent vocal cords. *Speech* may be the act of speaking, the result of speaking, the utterance of vocal sounds that convey ideas, or the ability to express thoughts by words. Mechanisms of speech are accomplished through internal symbolization and thought. Language is dependent on

retention, recall, visualization, and the integration of symbols. Speech depends on the interpretation of auditory and visual images, which reach the higher human processes during differing states of consciousness including, to some degree, the lower states of consciousness.

Language is a function primarily of the left cerebral hemisphere. Figure 50-7 shows the approximate location of the speech centers in the brain. The ability to produce language depends on the normal function and integrity of the primary receptive areas in the temporal and occipital lobes and the expressive areas in the inferior part of the frontal lobe of the dominant hemisphere. To speak, one must initially formulate the thought to be expressed, choose appropriate words, and then control the motor activity of the muscles of phonation and articulation. Simultaneously, accurate recording of visual and auditory stimuli is necessary before the significance of the words used can be appreciated. Language and speech can become impaired in many ways.

APHASIA

Aphasia is a neurologic defect in speech. The ability either to comprehend and integrate *receptive language* or to formulate and use *expressive language*, or both, is impaired. The receptive language modalities are *reading*, which requires visual integration and comprehension of printed words, and *listening*, which requires auditory integration and comprehension of verbal words. The expressive language modalities are *writing*, which requires visual-motor formulation and use of printed words, and *speaking*, which requires oral-motor formulation and the use of verbal words. The aphasic person usually has some impairment of all language modalities.

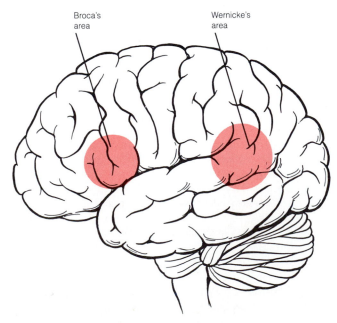

FIGURE 50-7   *Location of speech centers in the brain.*

Aphasia is usually caused by organic disease of the brain involving a lesion in the left cerebral hemisphere. This hemisphere is considered to be dominant in the reception and expression of language in most people. Infrequently, aphasia has occurred in right-sided lesions associated with right-handed persons. However, their right-handedness has sometimes been forced or induced. In left-handed persons, lesions of the left or of the right hemisphere may cause aphasia, but most frequently the left.

If certain portions of the cortex and subcortical associated pathways of the dominant hemisphere are altered by lack of blood supply (loss of oxygen or hemorrhage into the brain tissue), speech patterns become altered, limited, or destroyed, depending on the magnitude of the pathology. Vascular disturbances are the most common cause of aphasia. Infarction, caused by thrombotic embolic occlusion of the middle cerebral artery or the left internal carotid artery, is the cause in the majority of cases and impairs both spoken and written language. TIAs and migraine headaches can trigger transitory speech disorders.

Space-occupying lesions, such as intracerebral hemorrhages, intracranial tumors, and infections, also can cause aphasia. Left hemisphere aphasia results from damage to a specific region of the brain: the first and second temporal gyri, the insula, or the posterior part of the third convolution. Visual and auditory impulses reach the cerebral cortex posteriorly through the occipital lobe and anteroinferiorly through the temporal lobe. Extraction of the semantic value of the auditory and visual message and of the symbolic formation of the expressed message occurs in the posterior portion of the temporal convolutions. The anterior part of the region is necessary for the motor realization of the expressed message. Many cortical areas and association pathways are concerned in the integration of the function of speech.

Many combinations of vascular, neoplastic, and traumatic causes and locations of lesions lead to different language patterns. Classifications have been developed to define prominent characteristics, to localize position and size of cerebral lesions, and to assess the language deficit pattern in each category of aphasia. The primary types of speech disorders include 1) Wernicke's aphasia, which causes disturbances of all language activities except articulation; 2) Broca's aphasia, which involves disturbances in spoken and written language with dysarthria (disorder of articulation); 3) global aphasia; and 4) selective disorders of receptive and expressive activities of spoken or written language.

Wernicke's Aphasia

The posterior one-third of the superior temporal convolution of the dominant hemisphere is called the Wernicke area (see Figure 50-7). The Wernicke area influences the understanding and interpretation of word symbols. Lesions in other areas, particularly in the posterior half of the dominant hemisphere, angular gyrus, and supramarginal gyrus, influence speech function through the involvement of association fibers.

Wernicke's aphasia is an impairment in comprehension of speech and includes central, receptive, cortical, sensory, auditory, semantic, and conduction aphasia. Affected persons have fluent, spontaneous speech with normal rhythm and articulation, but comprehension, repetition, and naming are impaired. These people lack insight into their deficit. Speech appears devoid of meaning despite the fluency and spontaneity. Expression is hindered by difficulty in the choice of words to speak and to write. Repetition, reading aloud, and writing from dictation are deranged. Understanding of spoken language is disturbed. The speech of others is heard but the words are not comprehended. Speech lacks content and contains much meaningless expression. Likewise, the written words lack meaning.

Lesions in the Wernicke area inhibit comprehension in spoken and written language because of their interconnections with the angular gyrus. Lesions of the angular gyrus and posteroinferior part of the parietal lobe may cause acalculia, autotopagnosia, and disorientation for right and left sides (Table 50-3).

Broca's Aphasia

The lesion in Broca's aphasia is located in the caudal part of the inferior frontal gyrus rostral to the motor area of the tongue, pharynx, or larynx, or it may involve the pathways carrying impulses from the temporal lobe to this area (see Figure 50-7). Broca's aphasia includes disorders described as cortical motor, expressive, and verbal aphasias and disorders in expression of spoken language. The person may not be able to utter a word or may have extremely limited speech. The speech is usually nonfluent, slow, and poorly articulated. Small words are frequently omitted from sentences. Simultaneously, the person fully comprehends the spoken word and obeys commands. Efforts to speak are frustrated by inability to find appropriate words. Agraphia, reduction of written language, coexists with aphasia and can be more severe in some persons. Agrammatism, if present in spoken language, is also present in written language (see Table 50-3). Unlike patients with Wernicke's aphasia, those with Broca's aphasia are aware of the problem; this often leads to feelings of frustration and depression.

Global Aphasia

Global aphasia is caused by large lesions involving both Broca and Wernicke areas of the dominant cerebral hemisphere. Commonly, the lesion is an occlusion of the left internal carotid artery or middle cerebral artery.

TABLE 50-3 *Terms Used to Describe Some Disorders of Higher Cortical Function*

Term	Definition
Acalculia	Inability to solve mathematical problems
Agnosia	Loss of comprehension of auditory, tactile, visual, or other sensations although the sensations and the sensory system are intact
Auditory agnosia	Inability to recognize auditory objects
Tactile agnosia	Inability to identify objects by touch
Visual agnosia	Inability to recognize objects seen
Verbal agnosia	Inability to recognize spoken language
Agrammatism	Inability to arrange words in grammatic sequence or to form a grammatic or intelligent sentence
Anosognosia	Lack of awareness of presence of disease (eg, paralysis)
Apraxia	Inability to carry out a voluntary movement although the conductive systems are intact
Constructional apraxia	Inability to construct models (with matchsticks, cubes, etc.), to assemble puzzles, or to draw
Dressing apraxia	Inability to dress or undress
Autotopagnosia	Inability to orient various parts of the body correctly
Dysarthria	Disorder of articulation
Prosopagnosia	Inability to recognize faces and one's own face

Blood supply to the language areas of the brain is almost exclusively through the middle cerebral artery. As the term implies, *global aphasia* affects all aspects of speech. People with global aphasia usually have hemiplegia and are unable to comprehend or speak. At best, they may be able to utter an occasional isolated word or well-known cliche. They are unable to repeat what is said to them and are unable to read and write.

SELECTIVE DISORDERS OF RECEPTIVE OR EXPRESSIVE ACTIVITIES OF SPOKEN AND WRITTEN LANGUAGE

The pure disorders of receptive and expressive speech include anarthria, agraphia, alexia, and word-deafness. In *anarthria*, reading aloud and voluntary speech repetition are disturbed, whereas understanding of spoken and written language and the ability to write remain normal. It usually appears as a sequela of Broca's aphasia. In *agraphia*, all forms of writing are defective. The lesion may be located in the posterior part of the second frontal gyrus. *Alexia* severely impairs reading of words, but reading of letters is less obstructed. Language activities may be normal except for the recognition of written symbols. The lesion is located in the lingual and fusiform gyri. *Word-deafness* is impairment in the understanding of spoken language, repetition, and writing from dictation; all other speech activities are normal. The lesion is in the superior aspect of the temporal lobe.

▼ *Apraxia*

Apraxia is the inability to carry out a voluntary, purposeful, movement, although the conductive systems are intact, indicating cerebral cortical integrative impairment. The person is able to make the individual movements that comprise execution of a certain act but cannot execute the total act. There is no paralysis, ataxia, abnormal movement, or sensory loss.

To execute a skilled movement, one must use a logical routine. First, the verbal command is received at the primary auditory cortex and relayed to the auditory association areas for comprehension. The information is relayed by the association fiber systems to the motor association areas in the premotor cortex of the dominant hemisphere. From the dominant premotor cortex, information is conveyed to the premotor and motor cortices of the nondominant hemisphere to enable the nondominant hand to perform the learned skilled movement.

Apraxia is caused by damage to the association areas or fibers concerned with voluntary motor activity. Lesions in these areas cause impairment in accordance with their locations. Those between the supramarginal gyrus and premotor regions of the dominant parietal lobe may produce bilateral apraxia (see Figure 50-7). They usually also result in an aphasia. Lesions of the dominant premotor association areas may produce bilateral impairment in certain tongue and hand movements. Those of the anterior half of the corpus callosum result in an apraxia of the nondominant hand.

Apraxia of the lips and tongue is fairly common and may occur with lesions of the left supramarginal gyrus or the left motor association cortex. The condition frequently accompanies apraxia of the limbs. Apraxia of the limbs may be revealed as dressing apraxia (inability to dress or undress) or as constructional apraxia (inability to construct models with matchsticks or cubes, to assemble puzzles, or to draw). Specific types of apraxias are summarized in Table 50-4.

The location of lesions producing the various apraxias is somewhat controversial. All forms of apraxia may occur in cases of diffuse brain damage leading to dementia, which suggests that symptoms may be caused by the mass effect of a lesion rather than by its location.

▼ *Agnosia*

Perception occurs when sensory data originating at sensory receptors are forwarded by peripheral and spinal pathways to the primary sensory cortex for analysis and sorting. These data are dispatched to the association areas that contain the memory banks for higher-order interpretation, and there they are translated into codes and symbols of language. This process of recognizing the significance of sensory stimuli is known as *gnosia*. *Agnosia*, impairment of this faculty of recognition, is caused by lesions of the association areas of the cerebral cortex; the primary sensory pathways remain intact. The affected person recognizes objects by one sense and yet does not recognize the same object by another sense.

TYPES OF AGNOSIA

The three types of agnosia are visual agnosia, an inability to recognize objects seen; tactile agnosia, an inability to identify objects by touch; and auditory agnosia, an inability to recognize sounds although auditory sensation is intact. A person with visual agnosia may not recognize a safety pin just by looking at it but can name it instantly if it is placed in the hand. Conversely, a person with tactile agnosia visually identifies the safety pin that he or she was unable to recognize by touch alone.

Visual Agnosia

Visual agnosia is caused by a lesion of the visual association areas. Lesions limited to these areas do not cause blindness. Objects are clearly seen but are not recognized or identified. Visual agnosia is characterized by inability to recognize any object or shape by sight, although it can be recognized through other senses, such as touch or smell. Categories include agnosia for objects, agnosia for colors, and prosopagnosia.

Persons suffering from object agnosia are not able to recognize objects visually. Those with color agnosia are unable to recognize colors, a defect that may be confined to one half of the visual fields (called *hemiagnosia* for colors). Prosopagnosia renders the person unable to recognize faces, sometimes even his or her own face in the mirror. The person is unable to recognize a familiar face but can identify the person as soon as he or she starts to speak.

TABLE 50-4 *Types and Characteristics of Apraxias*

Type of Apraxia	Characteristics	Anatomical Region Involved
Ideational	Inability to grasp the idea required in executing a motor activity	Large areas of the cerebral cortex, especially dominant parietal area
Ideomotor	Inability to perform the motor act required to perform an activity	Dominant hemisphere temporal, frontal, and parietal lobes
Limb-Kinetic	Inability to execute fine motor activity in a single limb	Premotor cortex
Dressing	Inability to dress or groom oneself correctly; may be unilateral, frequently involving the left side	Nondominant parietal lobe
Constructional	Inability to construct objects accurately because of disruption of special relationships	Right or left parietal lobe
Gait	Inability to walk in a smooth, coordinated manner; gait is short and shuffling	Frontal lobe and basal ganglia
Facial	Inability to produce facial movements on command	Dominant hemisphere

Tactile Agnosia

Normal tactile recognition is the ability to identify an object by touch without the help of other sensory information. Feeling movements provide impressions until the object is identified. Lesions of the parietal lobe posterior to the somesthetic area produce tactile agnosia, or the inability to identify objects by touch and feeling. It is often called *astereognosis*. Some previously acquired factual information is lost from the brain's memory stores. Therefore, the person cannot compare present sensory phenomena with past experience.

Auditory Agnosia

Auditory agnosia is the inability to recognize sounds. The auditory sensation is intact. It is often difficult to differentiate auditory agnosia from a sensory aphasia. The first temporal convolution and part of the second temporal convolution of the dominant hemisphere are considered important for auditory recognition.

From the descriptive point of view, auditory agnosia is the inability to recognize familiar concrete sounds, such as animal noises, a sounding bell, or the ticking of a clock (agnosia for nonlinguistic sounds). Other auditory perceptual disorders include verbal agnosia (the inability to recognize spoken language), sensory amusia (the inability to recognize music), and congenital auditory agnosia (primary retardation of speech development, usually associated with mental retardation).

▼ Body Image

Human beings build images of their bodies from sensory impulses received from special senses that provide information on the relations between the body (skin, muscles, bones, and joints) and the external environment. This concept of body image is stored in the association areas of the parietal lobes. Lesions of the nondominant (usually the right) parietal lobe, particularly the inferior parietal lobe, may create abnormalities in concepts of body image. Lack of awareness of the left side of the body despite intact cortical and primary sensation is exhibited. Lack of awareness of hemiparesis may be observed. The person may perceive sensory stimuli that are applied independently to the two sides of the body, but if sensory stimuli are applied bilaterally simultaneously, one stimulus is usually ignored.

GERSTMANN SYNDROME

Lesions of the left (dominant) parietal lobe, particularly of the supramarginal and angular gyrus areas, may produce one or more of a complex of symptoms known as Gerstmann syndrome (bilateral asomatognosia). It includes right-left disorientation, that is, inability to distinguish right from left. Finger agnosia is exhibited by failure to recognize one's fingers in the presence of intact sensation, and it is associated with constructional apraxia. Acalculia (inability to solve mathematical problems) and dyslexia (impairment of the ability to read) are common when the lesion involves the angular gyrus of the dominant hemisphere.

▼ Seizure Disorders

Epilepsy, a general term used synonymously in this chapter with seizure disorders, is characterized by sudden, excessive discharges of electrical energy in neurons. These may occur within a structurally normal or diseased central nervous system. The discharge may trigger a convulsive movement, interrupt sensation, alter consciousness, or lead to some combination of these disturbances. Seizures may originate from diverse factors that are metabolic, toxic, degenerative, genetic, infectious, neoplastic, or traumatic, or from unknown factors.

Seizures may be linked with increased local excitability (epileptogenic focus), reduced inhibition, or a combination of both. Some neurons in focal lesions have been identified as hypersensitive and remain in a state of partial depolarization. Increased permeability of their cytoplasmic membranes makes these neurons susceptible to activation by hyperthermia, hypoglycemia, hyponatremia, hypoxia, repeated sensory stimulation, and even certain phases of sleep. Reduced inhibition may be caused by a lesion of the cortex.

After the intensity of a seizure discharge has progressed sufficiently, it may spread to adjacent cortical, thalamic, or brain stem nuclei, or to other regions of the brain. Excitement feeds back from the thalamus to the primary focus and to other parts of the brain. This process is evidenced by the high-frequency discharge shown on EEG. Within the process, a diencephalocortical inhibition intermittently interrupts the discharge and converts the tonic phase (muscle contraction) to the clonic phase (alternating contraction and relaxation). The discharges become less and less frequent until they cease.

Severe seizures can cause systemic hypoxia; this is accompanied by acidosis from increased lactic acid, which results from respiratory spasms, airway blockage, and the excessive muscular activity that accompanies seizures. An extremely severe, prolonged seizure can cause respiratory arrest or cardiac standstill. Metabolic needs increase markedly during a seizure, causing increased cerebral blood flow, glycolysis, and tissue respiration.

CLASSIFICATION OF SEIZURES

Seizures have been classified according to location of the focus, etiologic basis, and clinical features. The International Classification System listed in Box 50-1 has been adopted worldwide and is used in this chapter. It is based on clinical features and associated EEG findings in seizures that are generalized or partial. *Generalized seizures* have bilaterally symmetric epileptigenic foci originating within deep subcortical diencephalic structures; partial seizures usually begin in a cortical focus but may arise from subcortical structures. Seizures may be *primary* or *idiopathic* if their origin is unknown, or they may be *secondary* or *symptomatic* if a definitive diagnosis is determined.

PARTIAL SEIZURES

Partial seizures arise from a focal area and progress in a manner consistent to the area of irritation. They are characterized by specific, repeated patterns of activity and are of two general types: *simple* or *elementary*, in which consciousness remains unimpaired, and *complex*, in which there is accompanying alteration in consciousness. Partial seizures can have a motor, sensory, or varied complex focus.

Focal Motor Seizures (Jacksonian Seizures)

Focal motor seizures usually originate in the premotor cortex and cause involuntary movements of the contralateral limbs. A common manifestation is the turning of the affected person's head and eyes away from the irritable focus (contraversive movement). This may be the extent of the seizure, or it may start in one portion of the premotor cortex and spread gradually in clonic movements to the adjacent region. The clinical manifestations change accordingly.

Typically, the convulsive movement in jacksonian seizures begins in the distal portion of an extremity and progresses medially. For example, a seizure starting in the foot may move up the leg, down the arm, and to the face; or it may begin in the hand, spread to the face, and then to the leg. This is called *jacksonian march*. The seizure begins with a tonic contraction and rapidly progresses to a clonic movement. The episode may last 20 to 30 seconds without loss of consciousness. Conversely, it may spread to the opposite hemisphere with resultant loss of consciousness, thus becoming a generalized seizure. Despite the greater frequency of focal seizures in young children, the jacksonian march appears most often in adults and adolescents; focal motor seizures may also occur in certain metabolic derangements.

Focal Sensory Seizures

A lesion in the postcentral or precentral convolution of the sensory cortex in the parietal lobe provokes focal sensory seizures. A simple, uniform, tactile, auditory, or visual experience with complaints of numbness, tingling, pins-and-needles sensation, coldness, or a sensation of water running over a portion of the body may be described. This type of seizure usually begins in the lips, fingers, and toes, and remains localized or progresses to adjacent body parts. If the lesion is in the sensory association area, the experience is more complex and may be visual or auditory. If it is visual, sensations of light, darkness, or color may be experienced. If it is auditory, the person may complain of buzzing, roaring in the ears, or hearing voices or words. Consciousness and memory are preserved.

Complex Partial Seizures (Psychomotor)

Temporal lobe structures, the medial surface of the hemispheres, and the limbic system are involved with this disorder. However, certain psychomotor seizures may arise from the frontal lobe. Children, as well as adults, are affected with this form of seizure. The affected person may exhibit bizarre behavior and exaggerated emotionality. These seizures may be characterized by slow, paroxysmal waves in either the anterior or posterior leads of the EEG. Episodic fluctuations in attitude, attention, behavior, or memory occur. The person seems to interact in a purposeful, although inappropriate, manner. Seizures may begin with an olfactory aura or an unpleasant smell or taste. On other occasions, the person may experience hallucinations or perceptual illusions; he or she may perceive strange objects and people as familiar (*deja vu*) or familiar objects and people as strange (*jamais vu*). The person appears to be in a dreamy state and may be unresponsive to vocal stimulation but mechanically performs a task while the seizure is progressing (automatism). These mechanical, abnormal movements and inappropriate speech may also be associated characteristics. Strong epigastric and abdominal sensations commonly occur.

Later, episodic recall is lost, and the person is amnesic to the aberrant behavior. Automatisms, if present, include chewing, smacking, licking of the lips, or clapping of the hands. Less frequently, the head and eyes may turn to one side, or tonic spasms of the limbs may occur. Some psychomotor seizures last about a minute, some may continue for hours, and others may progress to tonic, tonic-clonic, or other forms of generalized seizures.

GENERALIZED SEIZURES

Generalized seizures involve both cerebral hemispheres and commonly result in loss of consciousness, which may vary from a very brief episode to a more prolonged time. Anterograde and retrograde amnesia frequently accompany the loss of consciousness. The most common forms of generalized seizures are petit mal (absence) and grand mal (tonic-clonic). Generalized seizures also include myoclonic and akinetic types.

Absence Seizures (Petit Mal)

These seizures exhibit a characteristic spike-and-wave pattern with 3 cycles per second (cps) on the EEG. The term *absence seizure* is used because the person, although present physically, is absent with respect to higher cortical functions during the episode. The majority of such persons have normal intelligence and have no significant abnormal physical findings on neurologic examination. Onset is usually about 5 years of age, and attacks are most prevalent in childhood. Absence seizures decrease after puberty.

Petit mal seizures are characterized by a loss of awareness that may be accompanied by automatisms, such as flicking of the eyelids, twitching of facial muscles, or staring into space while general postural tone is preserved. They may be precipitated by seeing bright or flashing lights or hearing loud noises, and they may be preceded by hyperventilation. Attacks may recur numerous times during the day. They may last from 5 to 10 seconds, after which consciousness is abruptly restored and the interrupted activity is promptly resumed. Memory may be defective only through the seizure. As the person reaches adolescence, frequency decreases and he or she may develop other types of seizures, usually tonic-clonic.

Tonic-Clonic Seizures (Grand Mal)

Electrical disruption with grand mal seizures originates anywhere in the forebrain and usually engulfs the whole forebrain. The epileptic discharge shows nonfocal changes of high amplitude and rapid synchronous bursts on the EEG. For several hours preceding the seizure, vague prodromal sensations, such as epigastric distress, muscular twitching, or other unnatural sensations, may occur. Commonly, a brief aura, an indication of impending seizure consisting of a specific movement or unnatural sensation, is the last thing the affected person remembers before losing consciousness.

After the aura, if one is present, the person abruptly loses consciousness, falls to the ground, and suffers generalized tonic contractions, followed by clonic contractions of all muscles. Muscle contraction in the tonic phase lasts for a few seconds. The entire body becomes rigid with the arms and legs extended. The jaws become clenched, the head may be retracted, and the eyeballs are rolled backward. As air is forced through the closed vocal cords, the diaphragm contracts, and a loud cry may be emitted. Breathing usually ceases during this time. Movements become jerky in the clonic phase as muscle groups contract and relax. The arms and legs contract and relax forcibly. Breathing becomes noisy and stertorous, and profuse perspiration is noted. Excessive salivation and loss of bladder or bowel sphincter control may also occur.

Contractions become slower, sometimes irregular, and then stop. The entire seizure usually lasts 3 to 5 minutes and is followed by a period of unconsciousness. Spasms of the tongue and jaw may cause biting injuries to the tongue or cheeks. Unconsciousness for the entire seizure is characteristic and may continue up to one-half hour after the episode. As consciousness is regained, the person is often briefly confused, fatigued, and drowsy and complains of muscle soreness. The person has no memory of the seizure attack but usually remembers the aura. In the early part of the postseizure period, there may be reflex signs characteristic of upper motor neuron disorder (see p. 1026). Paralysis may follow the attack for a short time and is described as postconvulsive (*postictal*) or *Todd paralysis*.

Febrile grand mal convulsions are common in children younger than 5 years of age, predominantly in those between 6 months and 3 years of age. These are generalized and of short duration. There is a high familial frequency of this type of seizure, and these children may experience nonfebrile seizures in later life.

Grand mal seizures that follow one another without restoration of consciousness are called *status epilepticus*, or seizures without interruption. These may be of the tonic-clonic nature or of the absence type. Common precipitating factors include abrupt cessation of anticonvulsant medication and alcohol withdrawal. This disorder is serious and produces exhaustion, hypoxia, acidosis, and other metabolic derangements. Hospitalization and prompt pharmacotherapy are urgently required to prevent irreversible brain damage or death.

Myoclonic Seizures

Persons with myoclonic seizures have sudden rapid flexion of the limbs and trunk, singularly or repeatedly, usually with a momentary loss of consciousness. Loud sounds or bright lights may precipitate the episodes. Intentional movement worsens them. These disorders occur with greatest frequency in childhood but may continue after puberty. Bilateral, synchronous 3-cps discharges are seen on EEG during each episode.

Myoclonic spasms occurring in infancy, called *massive spasms*, are first seen at 6 to 9 months of age and continue to age 2 or 3 years. There is usually associated retardation of psychomotor development, and the spasms may be related to other conditions, such as phenylketonuria, perinatal brain damage, pyridoxine deficiency, or tuberous sclerosis. Myoclonic spasms may be generalized or multifocal, and they tend to disappear with growth, but other seizure patterns may emerge. In adults, myoclonic seizures may accompany dementia in conditions such as Creutzfeldt-Jacob disease and in certain acute conditions, such as acute viral encephalitis (see pp. 1069–1070). A benign form of myoclonus has been described that is associated with sudden myoclonic jerks when falling asleep or awakening.

Akinetic Seizures

In these seizures, persons experience sudden loss of consciousness and fall to the ground without contraction or motion. Muscle tone is lost briefly, but resumed almost immediately. A history of infantile spasms and mental retardation is often present.

Infantile Spasms

Characteristically, infantile spasms affect children between the ages of 3 months and 2 years. These seizures may be associated with an unknown metabolic disturbance (primary infantile spasms), or they may be caused by a variety of known degenerative, structural birth injuries or developmental conditions, including amino acid abnormalities, phenylketonuria, and tuberous sclerosis (secondary infantile spasms). The seizures are characterized by flexor spasms of the extremities and frequently are associated with mental retardation.

Lennox-Gastaut Syndrome

The Lennox-Gastaut seizures occurring in childhood are associated with prolonged seizures in a febrile episode of acute encephalitis or encephalopathy. Seizures may recur spontaneously or with subsequent infections and febrile illnesses. These febrile-associated seizures may be compounded with atonic and ataxic spells, tonic seizures, and atypical petit mal and psychomotor seizures. Mental retardation is a common finding with this syndrome.

SECONDARY OR SYMPTOMATIC GENERALIZED SEIZURES

Secondary seizures are caused by some metabolic or structural underlying disorder. Metabolic disturbances can result from conditions such as renal failure, hypoglycemia, hypoxia, hyponatremia, hypernatremia, hypercalcemia, hepatic failure, or withdrawal of drugs. Meningitis and encephalitis in children lead to strong convulsive tendencies. After recovery, there may be residual recurrent generalized, focal, or psychomotor seizures. Many structural lesions are caused by disorders in cerebral blood supply, intracranial tumors, or scarring of the brain. These conditions can produce various types of seizure activity.

ELECTROENCEPHALOGRAPHY IN SEIZURES

The EEG is a sensitive tool for diagnosis and clinical evaluation of epilepsy. Despite its value, the diagnosis of epilepsy should not be based solely on the EEG findings, because some individuals have abnormal EEGs without clinical signs of seizure activity, and a significant number of those exhibiting clinical signs of epilepsy present normal EEGs. It does provide useful information in conditions such as brain abscess, tumor, hematoma, epilepsy, and trauma.

The electrical discharges produced by the brain's electrical activity are called *brain waves* and are recorded by electrodes placed on the surface of the scalp. Because the EEG is a surface recording, it reflects the most superficial activity, especially that of the cerebral cortex. The waves are recorded while the person is awake and resting in a darkened room or with the eyes closed. Movements and external distractions are minimized. During a recording of the brain's waves, the subject may be asked to hyperventilate to stimulate characteristic seizure activity secondary to alkalosis and vasoconstriction. Certain provocative techniques, photic stimulation, and sleep deprivation may be useful in initiating abnormal electrical activity in some persons. EEG recording during sleep may also be useful in detecting abnormalities.

Number of complete cycles of a rhythm in
one second (cps)

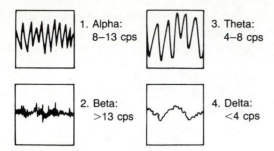

1. Alpha:
   8–13 cps

2. Beta:
   >13 cps

3. Theta:
   4–8 cps

4. Delta:
   <4 cps

FIGURE 50-8 *Frequency of brain waves.*

In normal adults, the dominant activity in the parietal occipital areas occurs at 8 to 13 cps, identified as *alpha rhythm*. In the frontal areas, the dominant activity is of lower amplitude and faster frequency (greater than 13 cps), and is known as *beta rhythm*. Slower frequencies than alpha rhythm are recognized as slow waves. Those at 4 to 8 cps are *theta rhythms*, and those at 1 to 3 cps are *delta rhythms* (Fig. 50-8). Theta waves are considered abnormal sometimes, whereas delta waves are always abnormal EEG waves, indicating injury to brain tissue. Other abnormalities are spikes, high-voltage waves, and asymmetrical frequency and amplitude between the hemispheres. Normal EEG variations occur. Age differences are noted on the EEG (Figs. 50-9 and 50-10). An infant at 13 months has dominant awakened activity of 4 to 5 cps; at age 5 years, 6 to 7 cps; and at age 12 years, 8 to 9 cps (alpha rhythm).

Abnormalities in EEGs are useful in diagnosing epilepsy, particularly if they are recorded during the seizure activity. During petit mal epilepsy, one can observe repetitive, slow, regular, rhythmic outbursts consisting of spike and delta waves at a frequency of 3 Hz (Fig. 50-11). Grand mal epilepsy reflects high-frequency spikes (Fig. 50-12), and temporal lobe seizures may demonstrate spikes or rhythmical outbursts of the slower delta or theta waves. EEGs may be normal between seizures. Brain masses such as tumors, hematomas, and abscesses may demonstrate localized slow-wave (delta) activity. Stupor and coma produce widespread, diffuse slow-wave activity.

Encephalopathy may produce theta waves. Asymmetrical, localized spike and wave patterns are recorded over areas of involvement in partial seizures. In some neurologic degenerative conditions, such as Parkinson disease and muscular dystrophy, the EEG may remain normal.

The EEG is useful in determining brain death. Electrocerebral silence (isoelectric EEG) is indicative of irreversible coma associated with global cerebral ischemia.

▼ Tics or Tourette's Syndrome

Tics are abrupt, unpredictable repetitive movements, sounds, or gestures that last a very short time. Tics are variable in nature and may be jerky (*clonic*) or sustained (*tonic*). Tourette's syndrome is characterized by verbal and motor tics with abnormal behavioral symptoms. The frequency of the tics varies from mild, occasional motor tics to severe, uncontrolled, and disabling motor and phonic tics. Most persons affected have temporary control of the tics for an hour or more. The pathophysiology of tics or Tourette's syndrome is unknown but it is thought to be due to a neurotransmitter abnormality in a portion of the basal ganglia which is functionally linked to the limbic system.[7]

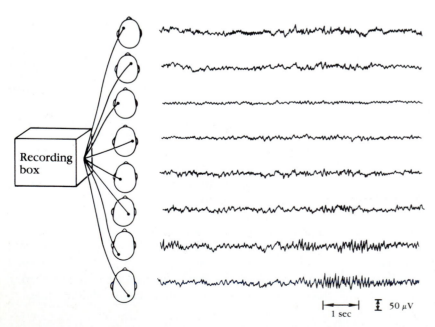

Recording
box

|← 1 sec →| ⊥ 50 μV

FIGURE 50-9 *Normal electroencephalogram in an adult.*

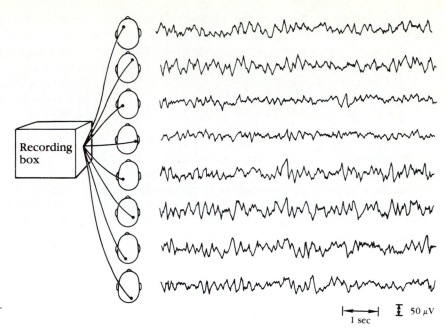

FIGURE 50-10 *Normal electroencephalogram in a child.*

1 sec   50 μV

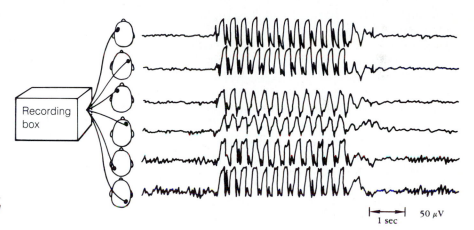

FIGURE 50-11 *Appearance of electroencephalogram during petit mal seizure.*

1 sec   50 μV

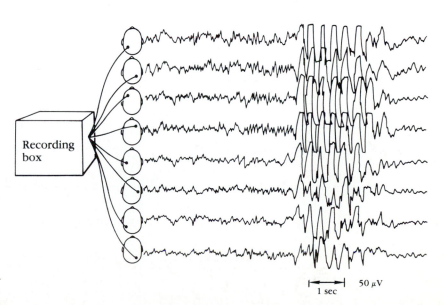

FIGURE 50-12 *Appearance of electroencephalogram during grand mal seizure.*

1 sec   50 μV

Idiopathic tic disorders are more frequently seen in males and may decline after about one year. The onset of tics also may be seen after head injury or stroke. Drugs such as cocaine may be linked to the onset.

▼ *Chapter Summary*

▼ Cerebrovascular disease results from disruption of cerebral blood flow, which decreases the oxygen supply to the brain. The result can be temporary or permanent dysfunction. Temporary dysfunction is commonly described as a transient ischemic attack and usually indicates severe disease in one or more cerebral arteries.

▼ Cerebral thrombosis usually results from a thrombotic occlusion on an atherosclerotic plaque, whereas cerebral embolism may come from a floating thrombus released from the endocardial surface of the heart.

▼ Intracerebral hemorrhage may result from atherosclerosis or from intracranial aneurysm. After an intracerebral hemorrhage has occurred, the brain injury may be increased by vasospasm. Arteriovenous malformations are usually congenital and may rupture into the subarachnoid space.

▼ Speech disorders are mainly described with the term aphasia, which can encompass many different speech problems, depending on which speech center is affected. Apraxia is a term used for inability to carry out a voluntary, purposeful movement; many types have been described.

▼ Agnosia is a term used for inability to recognize through the other senses certain common objects through the other senses.

▼ The term seizure refers to various types of motor and sensory disruptions. Partial seizures do not usually cause loss of consciousness. Generalized seizures may cause loss of consciousness and abnormal motor control (tonic-clonic seizures). Electroencephalograms are helpful in diagnosing seizure activity and many other abnormalities such as tumors, cortical dysfunction, and brain death.

▼ *References*

1. Adams, R., and Maurice, V. *Principles of Neurology* (4th ed.). New York: McGraw-Hill, 1989.
2. Bell, T. LaGrange, K.M., Maier, C.M., and Steinberg, G.K. Transcranial doppler: Correlation of blood velocity measurement with clinical status in subarachnoid hemorrhage. *J. Neurosci. Nurs.* 24:4, 1992.
3. Caplan, L.R. Cerebrovascular disease (stroke). In Stein, J. (ed.). *Internal Medicine* (4th ed.). St. Louis: Mosby, 1994.
4. DeGirolami, U., Frosch, M.P., and Anthony, D.C. The central nervous system. In Cotran, R.S., Kumar, V., and Robbins, S. *Robbins' Pathologic Basis of Disease* (5th ed.). Philadelphia: W.B. Saunders, 1994.
5. Flynn, E. Cerebral vasospasm following intracranial aneurysm rupture: A protocol for detection. *J. Neurosci. Nurs.* 21:5, 1989.
6. Jackson, L. Cerebral vasospasm after intracranial aneurysmal subarachnoid hemorrhage: A nursing perspective. *Heart Lung* 15:14, 1986.
7. Moskowitz, C. Movement disorders. In Barker, E. *Neuroscience Nursing.* St. Louis, Mosby, 1994.
8. Pallett, P., and O'Brien, M. *Textbook of Neurological Nursing.* Boston: Little, Brown, 1985.
9. Wall, M. Cerebral thrombosis: Assessment and nursing management of acute phase. *J. Neurosci. Nurs.* 18:36, 1986.

Chapter 51

Pain

Barbara L. Bullock

▼ LEARNING OBJECTIVES

1 Define **pain** in terms of cause and individual effect.
2 Describe the pain receptors through which pain perception is achieved.
3 Differentiate fast from acute pain and slow from dull pain.
4 Define the purposes of the neospinothalamic and paleospinothalamic tracts.
5 Describe the spinoreticular system.
6 Describe the important chemical transmitters involved in pain modulation.
7 Distinguish between cutaneous pain and deep somatic pain.
8 Explain the gate-control theory.
9 Distinguish between the causes of and the reactions to acute and chronic pain.
10 Discuss the effects of chronic pain on human physiology and psychosocial interactions.
11 Locate the sites of referred pain according to the affected deep organ.
12 Compare intracranial and extracranial headache regarding cause and clinical picture.
13 Define **hyperalgesia, neuralgia**, and **causalgia**.

Pain is a sensation caused by some type of noxious stimulation. It is described with many terms such as mild, severe, chronic, acute, burning, dull, sharp, referred, localized, throbbing, or crushing. Because pain makes a person aware of something that may cause tissue damage, it is considered to be a protective mechanism. Pain is usually perceived as a warning that something is amiss, and it prompts the individual to take some action, such as seeking medical help.

Pain is always subjective in nature. The response to the painful sensation is also subjective and individual, and it is highly influenced by the person's culture, society, race, and sex. Study of the pain response has led to some understanding of the mechanisms by which pain is perceived, mediated, and transported. There is less understanding concerning the highly individual responses to the painful experience. Table 51-1 gives some definitions that are helpful in sorting out the various components of pain perception and response. These help to keep the concept in perspective while indicating the psychological and physiological natures of the phenomenon.

Pain is a signal that an injured (damaged) part of the body needs attention or rest, and the person takes action to decrease the perception of pain.[18] The pain signal may be present to facilitate stillness and allow an injured part to heal.[15] The above concepts are valid for acute, short-term pain but do not help to explain the suffering of long-term or chronic pain. Significant differences exist in pain types and, therefore, in the pain response.

▼ Neurophysiology of Pain

PAIN RECEPTORS AND PATHWAYS

Pain receptors, also called *nociceptors*, are naked nerve endings found in almost every tissue of the body.[5,6] These respond to thermal, chemical, and mechanical stimulation. The degree or amplitude of the stimulation determines whether the perception is pleasurable or painful. The two major types of receptors are the small, myelinated A-delta fibers and the larger, unmyelinated C fibers. The A-delta fibers conduct impulses at a very

TABLE 51-1 *Definitions of Pain*

Term	Definition
Pain	An unpleasant sensory and emotional experience associated with actual or potential tissue damage, or described in terms of such damage
Pain receptor	A primitive, unorganized, weedlike nerve ending with many overlapping branches from receptors above and below it
Afferent pain fibers	Pain-conducting fibers for both fast and slow pain signals; A delta fibers are rapid conducting; C fibers are slow conducting
Epicritic pain	Specific, localized, cutaneous; conducting from a specific skin area, usually referred to as a dermatome
Protopathic pain	Deep somatic and visceral pain conducted through larger, more diffuse pathways, causing a generalized, poorly localized pain
Spinothalamic tracts	Principal pain-conducting pathways in the spinal cord
Reticulospinal tract	Pain-conducting pathway of more diffuse nature, still passing through segments of sympathetic ganglia to the thalamus and cerebral cortex
Pain stimuli	May be detectable injury or may not be known; the stimuli cause a reported pain sensation; the effect depends on the presence of other peripheral stimuli and on CNS activity; stimuli differ in their effectiveness according to changes in the CNS response
Impairment	Loss or abnormality of psychological, physiologic, or anatomic structure or function
Functional limitation	Restriction or inability to perform an activity in the manner considered normal for a human being; includes loss of capabilities caused by inability to integrate physical and psychological function as a result of pain or other impairment
Disability	A disadvantage for an individual person that limits or prevents fulfillment of a normal role
Operational definitions	Considering the presenting complaints in terms of pain sensation and behavior, functional status at work and home, emotional state, and somatic preoccupation

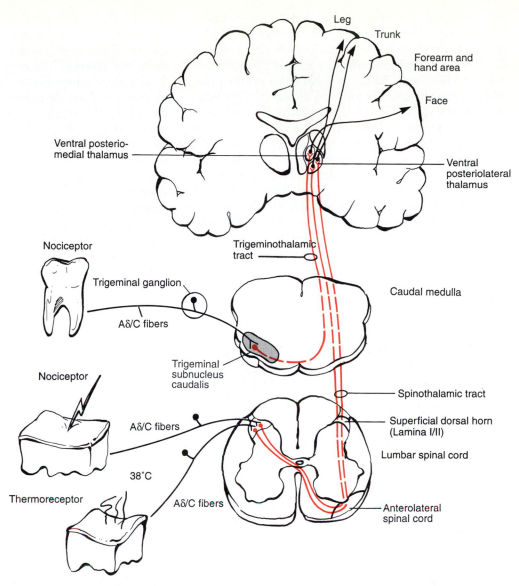

FIGURE 51-1 *Thermoreceptive and nociceptive sensory channels. (Conn, P.M.* Neuroscience in Medicine. *Philadelphia: J.B. Lippincott, 1995.)*

rapid rate and are responsible for transmitting acute sharp pain signals from the peripheral nerves to the spinal cord.[6] The A-delta fibers are activated by thermal and mechanical stimuli.[13] The C fibers transmit sensory input at a much slower rate and probably produce slow, chronic pain. The C fibers respond to thermal, mechanical, and chemical stimulation.[13] Figure 51-1 illustrates the thermoreceptive and nociceptive sensory channels. The usual initiating process for the acute pain response involves a traumatic event (such as cutting the finger), which produces a bright, sudden, sharp pain that is followed in a second or so by a slow, burning, throbbing pain. As the slow pain continues, the pain is usually perceived to be more severe, and after a variable period of time it may be perceived as intolerable.

Pain is perceived when the tolerance at the site is reached and the impulses are sent along the sensory pathway to the dorsal root ganglia, then to the spinal cord, after which they cross over into the spinothalamic tract. *Pain tolerance* refers to that variable period of time of pain endurance before a pain response is initiated. If the pain stimulus is repetitive or continuous, the tolerance for it usually decreases. Pain tolerance is a very individual characteristic and is influenced by family, race, culture, personality, and life situations. *Pain threshold*, on the other hand, is the point at which the noxious stimulus is perceived as pain. Acute painful stimuli, such as following an injury, will be more acutely felt than long-term or chronic pain. The description of the pain therefore is often localized to the acute pain, with later description of other painful sites after the acute pain subsides.

The first-order fibers are the A-delta and C fibers, and they have their cell bodies in the dorsal root ganglia. The cell bodies synapse with the dorsal horns, while the fibers cross the spinal cord, and ascend in the spinothalamic tracts (Fig. 51-2). These tracts form the anterolateral system, and the function appears to be similar to that in the spinothalamic tract, which relays temperature and crude touch signals to the brain.[6] Some axons in the spinothalamic tract ascend to terminate in the thalamus, and some terminate in the reticular formation (RF). From the RF, axons often communicate to the cerebral cortex somatic sensory areas (Fig. 51-3). This system is thought to transmit burning and dull pain. If pain becomes chronic, there may be associated peripheral factors, or the pain may be caused by central nervous system damage or psychological abnormalities in a histologically normal brain.[8]

The dorsal root ganglia are found on the dorsal or posterior root of all spinal nerves and conduct impulses into the spinal cord. The spinal or segmental nerve conducts the epicritic (discriminated, usually acute) pain from a specific area on the skin called a *dermatome*.[7] The dermatomes are described and illustrated on pages 948–951. The dermatomes usually have distinct boundaries, but a ganglion may carry some information from the dermatome immediately above or below it.[7] Deep somatic and visceral pain is usually poorly localized and discriminated. It is also called *protopathic pain* and is not as rigidly related to the nerve roots. It may travel with the autonomic nerve fibers that supply an affected area.[7]

Processing of sensations in the cerebral cortex allows for discriminative, exact, and meaningful interpretation of pain, but this processing is not necessary to the perception of pain.[4] In other words, pain can be experienced

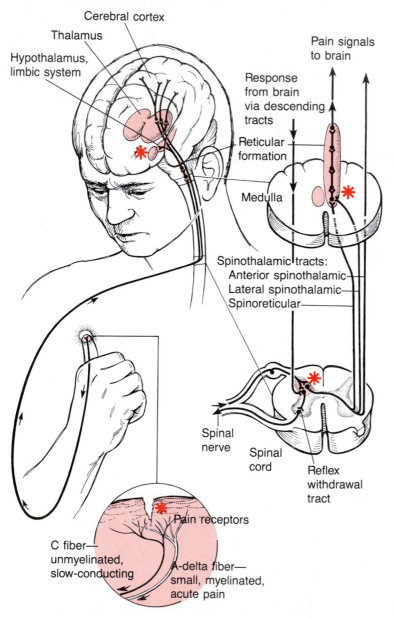

FIGURE 51-2 *Neural pathways of pain.*

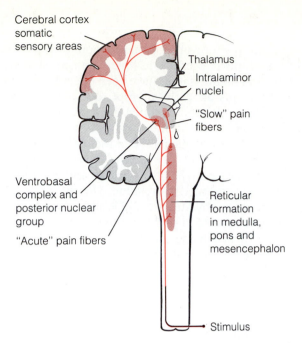

Cerebral cortex somatic sensory areas

Thalamus

Intralaminor nuclei

"Slow" pain fibers

Ventrobasal complex and posterior nuclear group

"Acute" pain fibers

Reticular formation in medulla, pons and mesencephalon

Stimulus

FIGURE 51-3 *Perception of pain may occur in the mesencephalon or in higher cortical levels.*

without precise processing in the cerebral cortex, as has been noted in cases of severe head injury. About three-fourths to nine-tenths of pain fibers terminate in the medulla, pons, and mesencephalon; from these areas, higher-order neurons transmit to the thalamus, hypothalamus, and cerebrum (see Figure 51-3).[6] A small number of acute pain fibers (A-delta fibers) pass directly to the thalamus, and their impulses are then transmitted to the cerebral cortex to precisely localize the pain source. A great number of slow-chronic pain fibers (C fibers) terminate in the reticular formation of the brain stem and excite the reticular activating system (see p. 1023). This system serves the function of arousing and promoting actions to rid the body of the painful stimulus.[4] These C fiber pathways yield a dull, sickening, poorly localized pain. Acute pain may be followed by poorly localized discomfort, such as after stubbing a toe.[10]

Pain response is never simple. Despite extensive research, the mechanism and perception is still not totally understood. The acute response previously described is relatively predictable in that there is a tissue-damaging stimulus that usually provokes a physical as well as a subjective response. The physical response to a pinprick, for example, is reflex withdrawal from the pin, whereas pain from deep tissue damage usually causes tonic muscle contractions and immobility to splint the area.[17] In the pinprick example, the information is projected to the postcentral gyrus, which then allows for cognitive discrimination of the source of tissue injury.

Certain known stimuli produce the response from

nociceptors. These are *prostaglandins, bradykinins, histamines*, and other chemotactic substances that are released by damaged tissue. These substances cause stimulation of the nociceptors, and the pain persists as long as the stimuli are in the tissues. *Substance P*, which is present in synaptic vesicles of the unmyelinated fibers, activates the pain response when it is released after injury. An attempt has been made to link the magnitude of the pain response to the amount of substance P released into the tissues. This view is very poorly substantiated in actual clinical practice, underscoring the fact that the pain response is unique to the individual perceiving it.[3]

ENDOGENOUS PAIN CONTROL SYSTEM

The brain has the capability to control the intensity of pain signals by activation of an endogenous pain control system. This system, illustrated in Figure 51-4, consists of three major parts: the *periaqueductal gray area* of the mesencephalon and upper pons, the *raphe magnus nucleus*, and a *pain inhibitory complex* located in the dorsal horns of the spinal cord.[6] Many of the nerve fibers secrete *enkephalin*, and the fibers originating in the raphe magnus nucleus that terminate in the dorsal horns of the spinal cord secrete *serotonin*. Serotonin acts on another set of local cord neurons that secrete enkephalin.[6] Enkephalins bind to specific receptors and inhibit the release of substance P, thus providing analgesia for

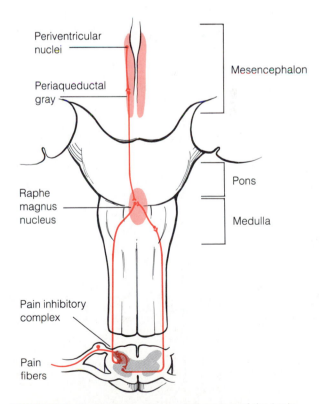

Periventricular nuclei

Periaqueductal gray

Mesencephalon

Pons

Medulla

Raphe magnus nucleus

Pain inhibitory complex

Pain fibers

FIGURE 51-4 *Endogenous pain control system of the brain.*

nociceptive stimulation. The analgesia system can block both fast and slow types of pain signals at the initial entry point to the spinal cord. The central pain control system also includes multiple areas within the brain that have opiate receptors. These areas secrete opiate-like substances, including β-*endorphin, met-enkephalin, leu-enkephalin,* and *dynorphin*. These substances are increased in response to stress, and they serve to increase analgesia.

Therapeutic devices can be used to suppress pain by stimulating large sensory nerve fibers. *Transcutaneous electric nerve stimulation (TENS)* has been used in cases of acute postoperative and severe, persistent pain. It employs a battery-operated portable unit with electrodes that are attached to the skin near the source of pain.[11] Theoretically, the TENS unit works by closing the gates as described by the gate-control theory (see next section). This is achieved by overstimulation of large-diameter sensory neurons to flood the central gates in the spinal cord and block the perception of pain sensation carried by unmyelinated fibers (Fig. 51-5). Counter-irritation (sensory stimulation) has been used for many years to relieve pain. The methods employed include rubbing, massage, heat or cold applications, mildly painful stimuli, electroanalgesia, and even acupuncture.[14]

▼ *Pain Theory*

To explain the universal phenomenon of pain, numerous theories concerning its origin, transmission, perception, and manifestation have been offered. The *specificity theory* was an early attempt to explain all pain physiologically. It simply related the amount of pain to the amount of noxious stimulation and tissue damage. It failed to address chronic pain and individual variations in the pain response. The *pattern theory* related pain intensity to the strength of the stimulus and the summative effect of continued stimulation. The *gate-control theory* was published by Melzack and Wall in 1965. Because its concepts have been usable in treating pain, it is still considered to be reliable, especially in the understanding of the acute pain response.

GATE-CONTROL THEORY

The gate-control theory proposed the presence of neural gating mechanisms at different levels of the central nervous system to account for interactions between pain and other sensory modalities. It combined aspects of the specificity and pattern theories with an explanation for the pain perception and response differences among

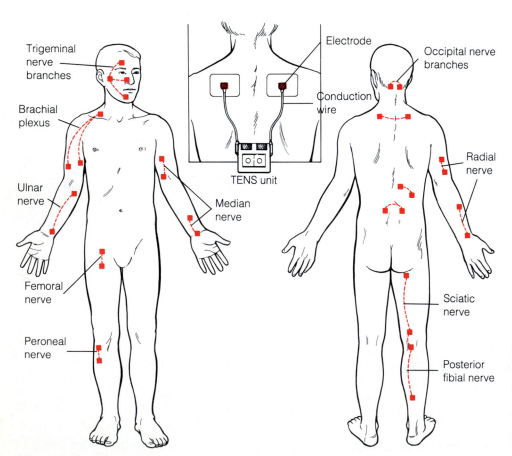

Trigeminal nerve branches

Brachial plexus

Ulnar nerve

Femoral nerve

Peroneal nerve

Electrode

Conduction wire

TENS unit

Median nerve

Occipital nerve branches

Radial nerve

Sciatic nerve

Posterior fibial nerve

FIGURE 51-5 *Transcutaneous electric nerve stimulation (TENS) unit may be placed close to source of pain to activate various nerves. The purpose is to flood the gates in the spinal cord and block the perception of pain. Various sites are used depending on the location of the painful stimulus.*

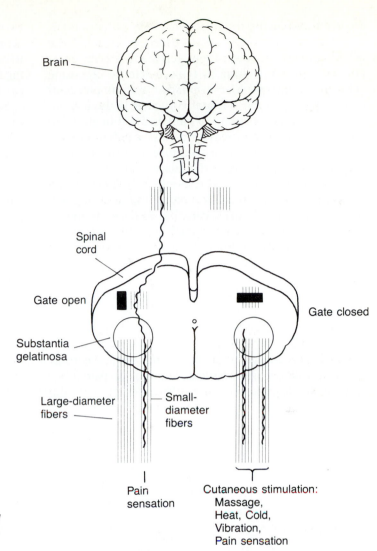

Brain

Spinal
cord

Gate open

Gate closed

Substantia
gelatinosa

Large-diameter
fibers

Small-
diameter
fibers

Pain
sensation

Cutaneous stimulation:
Massage,
Heat, Cold,
Vibration,
Pain sensation

FIGURE 51-6 *Gate-control theory of pain. (Hudak, C.M., and Gallo, B. Critical Care Nursing [6th ed.]. Philadelphia: J.B. Lippincott, 1994.)*

individuals. The gate control theory recognizes three factors concerned with pain transmission and modulation: the arrival of nociceptive stimuli, the effect of other converging peripheral stimuli that may exaggerate or diminish the effect of the nociceptive stimuli, and the presence of central nervous system controls that influence the input.[17, 18]

The theory proposes that peripheral stimulation produces nerve impulses that are projected to a gating mechanism in the spinal cord. Pain impulses are transmitted through small-diameter fibers in the area of the substantia gelatinosa, which can inhibit or facilitate the pain impulses. The substantia gelatinosa acts as a gate-control system to modulate (inhibit) the flow of nerve impulses from peripheral fibers to the central nervous system (Fig. 51-6).[16] There are central transmission or trigger cells (T cells) that act as a central nervous system control to stimulate selective brain processes that influence the gate-control system. If T cell activity is inhibited, the impulse is not transmitted to the brain because

the gate is closed. The T cells activate neural mechanisms in the brain that are responsible for pain perception and response. If pain signals are persistent, the fraction of impulses allowed to pass through the various gates gradually declines. This is partly controlled by the transmitters, enkephalin and serotonin. These transmitters partly regulate the release of substance P, the peptide that conveys pain information.

The *central control system* rapidly activates two cognitive subsystems in the brain. This activation selectively modulates or inhibits peripheral nerve impulses before they are projected to the brain. Specifically, the central control system activates the descending efferent fibers in the brain stem reticular formation and cortex. The central control system regulates activity in the *sensory-discriminative*, *motivational-affective*, and *cognitive-evaluative* systems. These systems determine pain response. The sensory-discriminative system is mediated through the brain stem and cerebral processing centers. It processes pain intensity and strength along with the character of the event producing the experience. The motivational-affective component appears to be mediated through the brain stem and reticular system. It is manifested by emotional features that lead to typical defense or escape behaviors. The cognitive-evaluative system processes pain meaning in the cerebral cortex. It is the learned response to the perception of pain and is thought to be the area where pain modulation may be enhanced. It is this system that interacts with central control activities, such as distraction, fear, and anxiety, and it may intervene between stimulus and response.[12, 16] The activated central control system can inhibit or facilitate pain perception.[18] The mechanism used has to do with unique individuality relating to emotional, cognitive, and attentional factors that influence the perception of the nociceptive stimulus.[18]

two processes. The acute pain problem is similar to the acute illness model, and the chronic pain problem tends to be the disease state itself.[8] In acute illness, the following four features apply: 1) the illness is symptomatic and can be labeled; 2) the illness is caused by external disease agents; 3) the illness is short-term; 4) treatment can cure the problem and eliminate symptoms.[8] Chronic pain does not seem to be a continuation of acute pain but is thought to involve changes in either the peripheral or central nervous systems, or both.[16, 18]

In chronic pain, the assumption that the pain is temporary becomes less believable for the person as each day passes. Secondly, the assumption that treatment will result in a cure is challenged because the pain may continue without an "organic" cause.[8] Many factors enter into the adjustment of persons suffering chronic pain, many of which decrease pain tolerance and interfere with the normal activities of life.

▼ Acute Versus Chronic Pain

The main clinical distinction between acute and chronic pain is primarily based on the duration of the pain problem. Table 51-2 indicates the differences between the

ACUTE PAIN

Acute pain is viewed as a reaction to a stimulus that produces a generalized response. Sympathetic (adrenergic) reactions increase the energy necessary to mo-

---

TABLE 51-2 *Acute Versus Chronic Pain*

Acute	*Chronic*
CHARACTERISTICS	
Limited duration	Prolonged, generally lasting more than 6 months
Purposeful, serves as a sign of impending tissue damage	Serves no useful purpose
Gradually subsides	Often progresses in severity as pathology increases
Can generally localize pain	Localization imprecise; often pain is described as ache or soreness
Behavior usually restless, thrashing, pacing, rubbing body part, grimacing, and other facial expression of pain	Apt to be tired-looking, may or may not have facial expression of pain, often depressed Suffering causes exhaustion of physical and mental capabilities Pain becomes a central life focus Accommodates behavior to pain
Usually signaled by a rise in pulse rate, decrease in blood pressure, and onset of sweating (diaphoresis)	Often has complex history of surgical procedures and therapies and a history of dependence on medications
RESPONSIVENESS TO ANALGESICS	
Usually readily responsive	Less responsive
Tolerance usually does not develop	Tolerance usually develops
Sedative effect of analgesic is an advantage	Sedative effect of analgesic is a disadvantage
Oral or parenteral routes	Usually oral route is employed
Standard doses can be used	Doses must be titrated to needs and level of tolerance of individual
Additional drugs are seldom required to manage pain	Additional drugs are often required to manage pain (tricyclic antidepressants or amphetamine)

Swonger, A., and Matejski, M. *Nursing Pharmacology*. Glenview, Ill.: Scott Foresman, 1988.

bilize an emergency response.[15] The characteristic pain response includes the following:

1. Marked elevation of systolic and diastolic blood pressure
2. Tachycardia
3. Peripheral vasoconstriction
4. Pupillary dilatation
5. Sweating
6. Hyperventilation
7. Inhibition of gastrointestinal motility
8. Increase in muscle tension and hypermotility of muscles
9. Extreme anxiety
10. Hostility
11. Glycogen outpouring from the liver to increase blood sugar

Acute pain sensations and complaints are usually appropriate to the tissue-damaging response. The response may be related to an observable injury that abates after natural healing or medical treatment has been employed. The amount of pain expected is often inferred from the diagnosis of the causative agent.[8] The person may be asked to rate the pain on a numerical or word-association basis. The visual analog scale is used to progress from an anchor of no pain to pain of maximal intensity. The McGill Pain Questionnaire consists of words arranged into classes that describe the pain experience in terms of its sensory quality, affective quality, and overall evaluative quality. This scale has been used to distinguish among pain syndromes. The tool provides information on pain quality and intensity as well as affective components. Figure 51-7 provides a sample of the McGill Pain Questionnaire. Judgments are made concerning the amount of pain to be expected, and the responses of the affected person to treatment measures and analgesia are evaluated.

CHRONIC PAIN

Chronic pain is defined as pain that persists more or less continuously for longer than 6 months. It causes a change in the pattern of physiologic and psychological responses. Although sympathetic nervous system responses predominate in acute pain, they become habitual in the chronic state with an emergence of vegetative signs.[16] These signs include sleep disturbances (delayed onset and frequent awakening), lack of energy, depression, and irritability.[16] Pain tolerance for other, even minor, injuries is lessened. A change in eating habits is often described; weight loss or gain is reported. The vegetative signs may relate to a depletion of central serotonin, which has been shown to cause sleep disturbances, lowered pain tolerance, and depression.[16]

Possible Physiologic Changes

Although none of the physiologic changes of chronic pain has been precisely identified, it is thought that changes after an injury can occur in the nerve terminals,

afferent fibers, and central system. Some of these changes can contribute to chronic pain.[19] Impulse conduction patterns may be changed by injury through sensitization of nerve endings.[18] These nerve endings may suffer changes in structure caused by tissue breakdown products. Also, if there has been severance of a nerve axon, false signals may be sent to the central system as the nerve regenerates and be interpreted as pain. Peripheral nerve damage can cause central change in the dorsal root ganglia, which then are sensitive to circulating adrenalin and mechanical distortion.[19] The neurotransmitters in the substantia gelatinosa may become depleted, causing less resistance to painful input. The C fibers that are intimately involved with slow pain transmission have terminal arbors that innervate some cell regions not normally excited. With damage, these regions may be enlarged. After a nociceptive stimulus is received with a warning event (eg, knowing that a certain movement causes pain), the central system may learn to respond to the expected stimulus as well as to the actual pain stimulus.[18, 19]

Classifying Chronic Pain

To classify chronic pain precisely, the following characteristics are considered: region affected, system affected, pattern or temporal characteristics, time since onset, and suspected cause. These give a pattern and provide the clinician with a basis for prognosis and treatment.[2] Often, however, there is no clear-cut diagnosis or treatment. An operational definition of chronic pain must then be developed in order to deal constructively with the individual problem. The components of an operational definition of chronic pain are pain sensation, pain behavior, functional status at work and home, emotional state, and somatic preoccupation.[2] Each of these is briefly considered here.

PAIN SENSATION. Pain sensation is the actual experience of pain; it includes location, pain quality, and activities that aggravate or cause the pain. Evaluation of this component mainly requires subjective reporting by the person.

PAIN BEHAVIOR. Pain behavior refers to a complex set of expressions that indicate that the person is experiencing pain. These include direct observation and reports by the person.[2] People experiencing chronic pain tend to be less active and have fewer interpersonal interactions than their normal counterparts.[16] The tendency is to solicit more medical interventions and to overuse analgesics and other drugs.[16] The chronic invalid behaviors may involve adopting the sick role, including a preoccupation with the symptom of pain. These patients often are dissatisfied with medical care and are looking for a cure. Conversely, if the medical practitioner cannot discover a pathologic reason for the pain, categorization

McGill Pain Questionnaire

Patient's Name _____ Date _____ Time_____am/pm

PRI: S_____ A_____ E_____ M_____ PRI(T)_____ PPI_____
(1–10)   (11–15)   (16)   (17–20)   (1–20)

1 FLICKERING QUIVERING PULSING THROBBING BEATING POUNDING	**11 TIRING** EXHAUSTING
	12 SICKENING SUFFOCATING
2 JUMPING FLASHING SHOOTING	**13 FEARFUL** FRIGHTFUL TERRIFYING
3 PRICKING BORING DRILLING STABBING LANCINATING	**14 PUNISHING** GRUELLING CRUEL VICIOUS KILLING
4 SHARP CUTTING LACERATING	**15 WRETCHED** BLINDING
5 PINCHING PRESSING GNAWING CRAMPING CRUSHING	**16 ANNOYING** TROUBLESOME MISERABLE INTENSE UNBEARABLE
6 TUGGING PULLING WRENCHING	**17 SPREADING** RADIATING PENETRATING PIERCING
7 HOT BURNING SCALDING SEARING	**18 TIGHT** NUMB DRAWING SQUEEZING TEARING
8 TINGLING ITCHY SMARTING STINGING	**19 COOL** COLD FREEZING
9 DULL SORE HURTING ACHING HEAVY	**20 NAGGING** NAUSEATING AGONIZING DREADFUL TORTURING
10 TENDER TAUT RASPING SPLITTING	**PPI** 0 NO PAIN 1 MILD 2 DISCOMFORTING 3 DISTRESSING 4 HORRIBLE 5 EXCRUCIATING

BRIEF	RHYTHMIC	CONTINUOUS
MOMENTARY	PERIODIC	STEADY
TRANSIENT	INTERMITTENT	CONSTANT

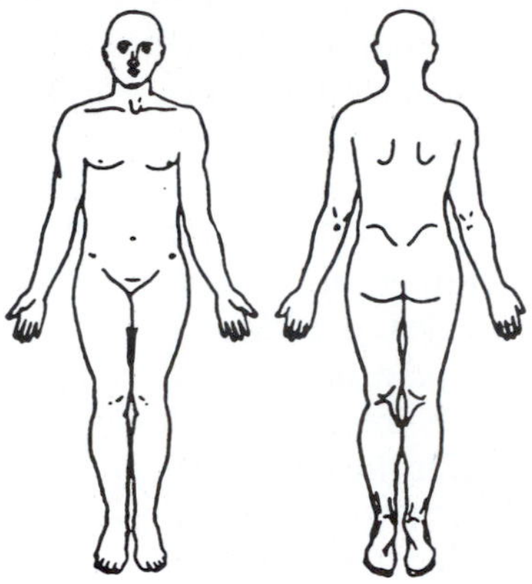

E = EXTERNAL
I = INTERNAL

COMMENTS:

FIGURE 51-7 *The McGill Pain Questionnaire. The numbers of the descriptors in each category are S (subjective), 1–10; A (affective), 11–15; E (evaluate), 16; M (miscellaneous), 17–20. Pain rating index (PRI) is computed by the chosen words. Present pain index (PPI) is the rate of the pain intensity. A descriptor of the nature of the pain is checked, and the pain is located on the figure with E or I for external or internal pain. Comments include response to pain medications. (Melzack, R. The McGill Pain Questionnaire. In Melzack, R. [ed.]. Pain Measurement and Assessment. New York: Raven, 1983.)*

of the pain as psychogenic is an attitude that is frustrating for the one suffering and counterproductive in pain management.

FUNCTIONAL STATUS AT WORK OR HOME. Job performance usually declines because there is increasing preoccupation with the pain sensation. Functional abilities (rather than disabilities) must be assessed to prevent loss of employment or placement on medical disability. In home or interpersonal relationships, loss of control is exhibited by increasing reliance on the sick role to manipulate or tyrannize others.[16] Roles are shifted, and guilt arises in family members who cannot help the person with chronic pain.

EMOTIONAL STATE. Depression is the most common result of chronic pain. Anxiety, fatigue, and irritability also can play a role in enhancing the pain experience. If the pain has a definite source, such as cancer pain, the focus is on the source and the person may not be incapacitated by the pain.

SOMATIC PREOCCUPATION. The term somatic preoccupation refers to heightened sensitivity or selective attention to bodily discomfort.[1] This means that the person may consciously dwell on the pain experience. This preoccupation often results in heightened pain response.

▼ Specific Types of Pain

The material in the previous sections of this chapter has discussed pain that is carried through acute pain fibers and slow pain fibers, as well as the problem of how chronic pain is transmitted. The following section presents some samples of specific types of pain, some of which are mainly acute and some which are chronic. A complete listing of pain-producing conditions is not presented, and the reader is referred to other areas of this text and to the bibliography at the end of the unit for further details.

CUTANEOUS PAIN

Cutaneous pain is usually direct, acute pain that is precisely localized from the skin. The area of nerve segment affected is along a distinct dermatome (see pp. 948–951). The nerve fibers between the dermatomes actually overlap to some extent. For example, T6 stimulus reception results in pain being experienced in the T5, T6, and T7 dermatome areas.[1] The three distinct skin layers produce different pain sensation. The epidermis produces itching and burning pain; the dermis produces localized, superficial pain; and damage in the subcutaneous tissues produces an aching, throbbing pain.[11]

VISCERAL PAIN

Visceral pain tends to be diffuse or poorly localized. Those suffering rarely can precisely localize the pain or identify any potential causative factors. Abdominal pain is an example of this form, and pain that arises from abdominal organs is poorly localized and is often described as dull, gnawing, or burning. The pain is usually induced by stretching or tonic contractions.[10] The feeling of pain requires interpretation by the cerebral cortex; this results from nerves that cross to the opposite side of the cord and ascend in the lateral spinal thalamic tract to the midbrain and thalamus, which transmits the impulses to the cortex. Some visceral pain is *referred* in nature.

REFERRED PAIN

Referred pain is a felt pain sensation that is localized in a part of the body considerably removed from the area actually initiating the pain. Normally, the pain arises in a deep organ and is felt on an area of body surface. Reflex muscular spasm is a common cause of referred pain. The muscle spasm initiates severe back pain, headaches, and other painful reactions.[6]

Visceral or deep organ pain may be produced by ischemia, chemical stimuli, spasm, or overdistention of a hollow viscus such as the gut or gallbladder. The pain may be referred through particular parietal transmission pathways to other areas on the skin and perceived as sharp, burning, often excruciating pain in the distant location.[6] The visceral nerve transmission is usually through slow pain C fibers, and the interconnecting parietal pathways are transmitted through A-delta fibers, which accounts for how these transmissions are perceived. Figure 51-8 shows surface areas of referred pain and their usual source of origin.

Chest pain that arises from cardiac ischemia is discussed in detail on pages 461–462. The pain impulses are conducted through sympathetic nerves to the first four or five thoracic ganglia and to the spinal cord through second, third, fourth, and fifth spinal nerves.[4] The heavy, oppressive substernal pain that is felt may be caused by blood vessel spasm or muscle reaction.[1] Figure 51-9 illustrates a vicious cycle that can be set up and may even persist after cardiac healing.

Esophageal, gastric, and gallbladder pain may all be confused with cardiac pain because of the overlapping areas of referral. Kidney, colon, and small intestine pain may have abdominal areas of referral, whereas uterus and ureter pain often are referred into the groin. Table 51-3 indicates some common referral sites associated with visceral structure damage.

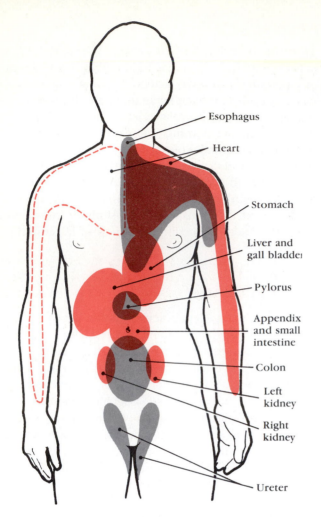

Esophagus

Heart

Stomach

Liver and gall bladder

Pylorus

Appendix and small intestine

Colon

Left kidney

Right kidney

Ureter

FIGURE 51-8 *Typical areas of referred pain from visceral organs.*

TABLE 51-3 *Localization of Referred Pain from Visceral Structure Damage*

Visceral Structure Damage	Area of Skin Experiencing Pain
Diaphragm	Skin of ipsilateral shoulder and outer surface of upper arm
Heart	Dermatomes C3–T8, with resulting pain in left arm and hand, especially in distribution of ulnar nerve; shoulder, back, substernal region, neck, axilla, and jaw; occasionally stomach, with ''indigestion'' symptoms noted
Stomach	Dermatomes T6–T9; chest and substernal region
Ovaries	Dermatome T10; periumbilical
Uterus	Dermatomes S1–S2, sometimes manifesting as pain in lower back
Prostate	Dermatomes T10–T12, manifesting as pain in periumbilical and inguinal areas, tip of penis, and occasionally scrotum
Kidneys	Dermatomes T10–L1; lower back and umbilical area
Rectum	Dermatomes S2–S4; low sacral back pain and sciatic pain in upper thigh or calf on dorsum of leg

Hendler, N. *Diagnosis and Nonsurgical Management of Chronic Pain.* New York: Raven, 1981.

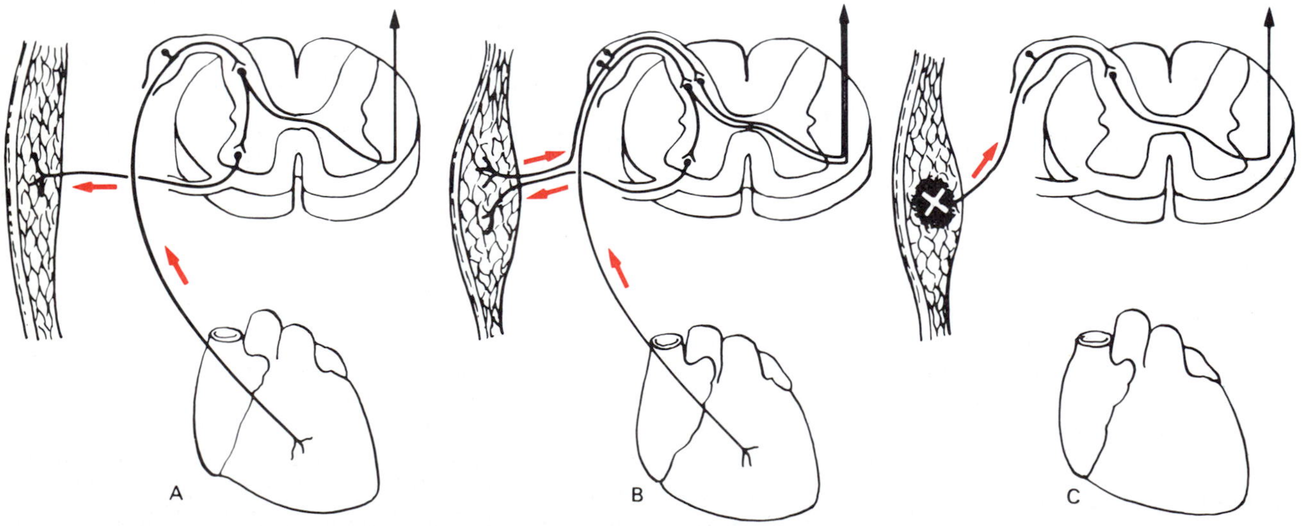

A

B

C

FIGURE 51-9 *Sequence of development of somatic components of cardiac pain.* **A.** *Nociceptive afferent input into dorsal horn causes efferent stimulation of muscles in the chest wall, which leads to muscle spasm.* **B.** *Muscle spasm acts as a new source of noxious input that produces trigger areas, and thus a vicious cycle develops.* **C.** *Nociceptive input from muscle continues after healing of the heart lesion. Injection of trigger areas with a local anesthetic eliminates the pain. (Bonica, J. The Management of Pain [2nd ed.]. Philadelphia: Lea & Febriger, 1990.)*

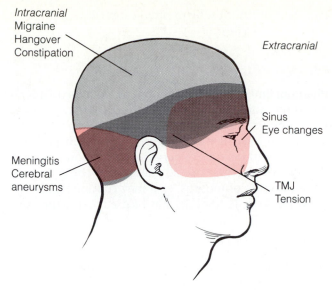

Intracranial
Migraine
Hangover
Constipation

Extracranial

Sinus
Eye changes

Meningitis
Cerebral
aneurysms

TMJ
Tension

FIGURE 51-10 *Areas of headache from different causes. Areas of overlap often make the source of the headache difficult to identify. TMJ, temporomandibular joint.*

HEADACHE

Headaches are an extremely common phenomenon that may result from stimuli inside or outside of the cranium. Figure 51-10 shows areas of headache that result from different causes. Table 51-4 summarizes the causes of headache. Intracranial origins include vascular stretching, meningeal trauma, and low cerebrospinal fluid pressure.[9] Stimulation of pain receptors above the tentorium causes referred headaches to the front half of the head. Those beneath the tentorium cause occipital headaches, which are usually intense in nature.[6] In addition, alcohol is thought to be a direct chemical irritator of the meninges, and constipation probably causes toxic products or circulatory system changes.[6]

Migraine headaches are thought to be caused by vasospasm of certain cerebral arteries that produce intracerebral ischemia, followed by vasodilation and stretching of arterial walls. The precise mechanism of production is unknown, but disturbance in the trigeminal pathways may be a major factor.[6] Table 51-5 describes the characteristics of vascular or migraine headaches.

TABLE 51-4 Causes of Headache

1. Migraine
    Migraine without aura (*common migraine*)
    Migraine with aura (*classic migraine*)
      Familial hemiplegic migraine
      Basilar migraine
      Aura without headache (*migraine equivalent*)
    Ophthalmoplegic migraine
    Retinal migraine
    Childhood periodic syndromes that may be precursors of, or associated with, migraine
    Complications of migraine
      Status migrainosus
      Migrainous infarction
2. Tension-type headache
    Episodic and chronic forms
3. Cluster headache and chronic paroxysmal hemicrania
    Cluster headache (*migrainous neuralgia*, Horton syndrome)
    Episodic and chronic forms
    Chronic paroxysmal hemicrania
4. Miscellaneous headaches unassociated with a structural lesion
    Idiopathic stabbing headache (*ice-pick pains*)
    External compression headache (*swim-goggle headache*)
    Cold stimulus headache (*ice-cream headache*)
    Benign cough headache
    Benign exertional headache
    Headache associated with sexual activity
5. Headache associated with head trauma
    Acute
    Chronic
6. Headache associated with vascular disorders
    Transient ischemic attacks
    Stroke
    Subarachnoid hemorrhage
    Arteritis (*temporal arteritis*)
    Carotid or vertebral artery pain
    Acute pressor reactions (eg, in pheochromocytoma)
7. Headache associated with nonvascular intracranial disorder
    Increased intracranial pressure
    Decreased intracranial pressure (*postlumbar puncture headache*)
    Intracranial infections (meningitis, encephalitis)
    Intracranial neoplasms
8. Headache associated with substances or their withdrawal
    Alcohol
    Vasodilator drugs
    Ergotamine and analgesic abuse
    Caffeine withdrawal
9. Headache associated with noncephalic infection
    Systemic or focal viral and bacterial infections
10. Headache associated with metabolic disorder
    Hypoxia, hypercapnia, hypoglycemia
11. Headache or facial pain associated with disorder of the cranium, neck, eyes, ears, nose, sinuses, teeth, mouth, or other facial or cranial structures
12. Cranial neuralgias, nerve trunk pain, and deafferentiation pain including compression or distortion of cranial nerves and second or third cervical roots, optic neuritis, diabetic neuritis, postherpetic neuralgia, Tolosa-Hunt syndrome, neck–tongue syndrome, and trigeminal neuralgia (*tic douloureux*).

* This summary is based on the classification of headache, cranial neuralgias, and facial pain prepared by the International Headache Society, 1988.
    Kelley, W.N. *Textbook of Internal Medicine* (2nd ed.). Philadelphia: J.B. Lippincott, 1992.

TABLE 51-5 *Characteristics of Vascular or Migraine Headaches*

Characteristics	Description
Onset	Childhood through puberty, plus family history
Location	70–80% temple or forehead Unilateral, spread to occiput, neck, shoulder Whole head; one side more painful
Intensity	Mild to severe
Quality	Throbbing, pulsing
Pattern	Stage I—prodromal (aura); stage II—headache Scintillating scotoma; visual disturbances; paresthesia; dizziness; head noises
Duration	Stage I, 20–30 min; stage II, 12–24 h
Frequency	Several times per day, week, or year
Associated symptoms	Increased urination, nervousness, colitis, abdominal pain, nasal symptoms, dyspepsia, diarrhea, constipation, sweating, exhaustion, pallor, fever, red dull eyes, awaken 3–4 AM
Chronology	3–9% of population; onset as early as age 8 mo; in children females and males are equal; 23% onset before age 40 y; more common in females
Aggravating/easing factors	Menstruation aggravates, contraceptives aggravate Pregnancy eases, tryptophan eases
Precipitating factors	Glare, dust, odors, temperature changes, barometric pressure and humidity changes, stress—physical and psychologic, lack of oxygen, hunger, smoking, decrease in blood serotonin

Mannheimer, J., and Lampe, B. *Clinical Transcutaneous Electrical Nerve Stimulation.* Philadelphia: Davis, 1989.

Headaches of extracranial origin include those associated with nasal sinus disorders or eye changes, and the so-called *tension headache*. Nasal congestion and pressure are caused by infection and congestion of the frontal and maxillary sinuses with pain in the eyes, forehead, and scalp. Eye changes may cause headache as a result of excessive irradiation, eye muscle fatigue, conjunctival irritation, and glaucoma.[6,9] Tension headache is probably the most common kind of headache; it usually is described as a headache resulting from emotional stress or fatigue.[9] Spasms of the neck muscles are thought to be associated because they are attached to the base of the skull. Another common cause of headache is the *temporomandibular joint (TMJ) syndrome*. The pain results from a joint problem in the mandible, usually caused by poor bite. This difficult problem often causes intermittent or chronic headaches.

PHANTOM LIMB PAIN

Phantom limb pain is felt after the amputation of a limb and is not universal to all affected persons. It is characterized by tingling, burning, or intolerable pain in the amputated extremity. It may result from a self-perpetuating, closed-loop type of nervous stimulation similar to that described with chronic chest pain. The pain may remit in weeks or months, or it may continue for years. Nerve blocks or TENS units may be used to stop the pain.

HYPERALGESIA

Hyperalgesia is the term used for an excessively excitable pain pathway. The basic causes include excessive sensitivity of pain receptors (primary hyperalgesia) and facilitation of sensory transmission (secondary hyperalgesia). Primary hyperalgesia results from stimulation of numerous cutaneous receptors, as with sunburned skin. Secondary hyperalgesia frequently results from spinal cord or thalamic lesions.[9] Other terms used for this syndrome are *neuralgia* and *causalgia*.

In neuralgia, a severe, shooting, or throbbing pain results from light or normal stimulation of superficial areas. The pain follows the areas supplied by specific spinal or cranial nerve roots. A common type of neuralgia, trigeminal neuralgia (tic douloureux), causes lightninglike stabs of pain involving the second or third divisions of the trigeminal nerve.[13] Other types of neuralgias include postherpetic neuralgia, which causes shocklike pains along a dermatome after an attack of herpes zoster, and glossopharyngeal neuralgia, which is felt in the tonsils and posterior pharynx.[13]

Causalgia results from actual damage to any of the peripheral nerves. The pain is continuous and is often exacerbated by emotional stress.[13] It is probably generated by excess sympathetic nervous system activity on the already damaged nerves. These syndromes may respond well to sympathetic blockage and early mobilization.[13]

▼ Chapter Summary

▼ Pain is a sensation caused by some type of noxious stimulation. It has many characteristics but is usually perceived as a warning that something is wrong. The response to pain is always subjective and is determined by culture, society, race, gender, and other factors.

▼ Pain receptors are found in most tissues of the body. The responses of these receptors to nociceptive stimulation are conducted through the dorsal root ganglia to the spinal cord and the spinothalamic tract. Synapses in the thalamus or the reticular matter eventually conduct the impulses to the cortex, where the pain is interpreted. There are certain mediators that enhance the pain response and some that help to control the intensity of the pain signals.

▼ The most commonly accepted pain theory is the gate-control theory, which proposes that peripheral stimulation produces nerve impulses that are projected to a gating mechanism in the spinal cord. This gating mechanism can inhibit or facilitate the pain impulses. The central control system rapidly determines the pain response.

▼ Pain can be classified as acute or chronic. Acute pain is a reaction to a stimulus that produces a generalized response with activation of the sympathetic reactions. Chronic pain is pain that persists continuously for longer than 6 months and causes a change in the pattern of physiologic and psychological responses.

▼ Specific types of pain can be either acute or chronic and include cutaneous pain, visceral pain, referred pain, headache, phantom limb pain, and hyperalgesia.

▼ *References*

1. Bonica, J. *The Management of Pain* (2nd ed.). Philadelphia: Lea & Febiger, 1990.
2. Feuerstein, M. Definitions of pain. In Tollison, C.D. *Handbook of Chronic Pain Management*. Baltimore: Williams & Wilkins, 1989.
3. Freeman, M.E. The hypothalamus. In Conn, P.M. *Neuroscience in Medicine*. Philadelphia: J.B. Lippincott, 1995.
4. Ganong, W.F. *Review of Medical Physiology* (16th ed.). Norwalk, Conn.: Appleton & Lange, 1994.
5. Gebhart, G.F. Somatovisceral sensation. In Conn, P.M. *Neuroscience in Medicine*. Philadelphia: J.B. Lippincott, 1995.
6. Guyton, A. *Textbook of Physiology* (8th ed.). Philadelphia: W.B. Saunders, 1991.
7. Hall, J.L. Anatomy of pain. In Tollison, C.D. *Handbook of Chronic Pain Management*. Baltimore: Williams & Wilkins, 1989.
8. Hanson, R.S., and Gerber, R.F. *Coping with Chronic Pain*. New York: Guilford Press, 1990.
9. Lance, J. Approach to the patient with headache. In Kelley, W.N. *Textbook of Internal Medicine* (2nd ed.). Philadelphia: J.B. Lippincott, 1992.
10. Levitt, M.D. Approach to the patient with abdominal pain. In Kelley, W.N. *Textbook of Internal Medicine* (2nd ed.). Philadelphia: J.B. Lippincott, 1992.
11. Mannheimer, J., and Lampe, G. *Clinical Transcutaneous Electrical Nerve Stimulation*. Philadelphia: Davis, 1989.
12. McCaffrey, M., and Beebe, A. *Pain: A Clinical Manual for Nursing Practice*. St. Louis: Mosby, 1989.
13. Moulin, D. Approach to the patient with chronic pain. In Kelley, W.N. *Textbook of Internal Medicine* (2nd ed.). Philadelphia: J.B. Lippincott, 1992.
14. Pinals, R.S. Approach to and management of back and neck pain. In Kelley, W.N. *Textbook of Internal Medicine* (2nd ed.). Philadelphia: J.B. Lippincott, 1992.
15. Sjolund, B., Eriksson, M., and Loese, J. Transcutaneous and implanted electric stimulation of peripheral nerves. In Bonica, J. *The Management of Pain* (2nd ed.). Philadelphia: Lea & Febiger, 1990.
16. Sternbach, R.A. Acute versus chronic pain. In Wall, P., and Melzack, R. *Textbook of Pain* (2nd ed.). Edinburgh: Churchill Livingstone, 1989.
17. Wall, P.D. Introduction. In Wall, P., and Melzack, R. *Textbook of Pain* (2nd ed.). Edinburgh: Churchill Livingstone, 1989.
18. Wall, P.D. The dorsal horn. In Wall, P., and Melzack, R. *Textbook of Pain* (2nd ed.). Edinburgh: Churchill Livingstone, 1989.
19. Whitehead, W., and Kuhn, W. Chronic pain: An overview. In Miller, T.W. *Chronic Pain*. Madison, Conn.: International University Press, 1990.

Chapter 52

Traumatic Alterations in the Nervous System

Reet Henze

▼ CHAPTER OUTLINE

▼ LEARNING OBJECTIVES

1. Distinguish between the two aspects of consciousness.
2. Describe the role of the reticular activating system in modulating consciousness.
3. Explain the basis for alterations in the level of consciousness.
4. Explain the etiologic basis of coma.
5. Contrast coma of metabolic origin with coma of structural injury.
6. Discuss the basis of coma from supratentorial and infratentorial lesions.
7. Describe associated functional disturbances common in comatose persons, including altered motor and pupillary responses, respiratory patterns, and eye movements.
8. Differentiate between upper and lower motor neuron lesions.
9. Explain the various types of skull fractures.
10. Differentiate between cerebral concussion and contusion.
11. Discuss type of injury, early and progressive clinical signs and symptoms, and treatment of epidural hematoma, subdural hematoma, subdural hygroma, subarachnoid hemorrhage, and intracerebral hematoma.
12. Describe the effect produced by cerebral vasospasm associated with subarachnoid hemorrhage.
13. Differentiate between cytotoxic and vasogenic cerebral edema.
14. Discuss how traumatic injury may occur to each of the cranial nerves and the clinical findings associated with these injuries.
15. Discuss the cause of increased intracranial pressure.
16. Discuss the major types of brain shifts that can occur with increased intracranial pressure.
17. Discuss the medical management of increased intracranial pressure.
18. Discuss the mechanisms of spinal cord injury.
19. Explain the morphologic changes associated with irreversible spinal cord damage.
20. Describe functional alterations in relation to the level of spinal cord injury.
21. Explain the basis for spinal shock and the associated clinical findings throughout its course.
22. Discuss the etiologic basis, physiologic changes, and immediate treatment of autonomic dysreflexia.
23. Describe injuries resulting in intravertebral disk herniation.
24. Identify regions of the vertebral column that are most commonly involved in disk herniation.
25. Discuss diagnosis and treatment of intravertebral herniated disk.

Barbara L. Bullock: PATHOPHYSIOLOGY: ADAPTATIONS AND ALTERATIONS IN FUNCTION, 4th ed.
© 1996 J.B. Lippincott-Raven Publishers

Traumatic insults to the nervous system can result in major changes in physiologic functioning and mental processing. Damage secondary to a primary injury of the nervous system, such as cerebral edema and increased intracranial pressure (ICP), can be more devastating than the original injury. Many structural and metabolic processes impinging on the brain lead to alterations in consciousness and varying degrees of brain dysfunction. This chapter begins with a focus on consciousness and its varying levels reflective of clinical findings.

▼ Consciousness

The conscious state of human existence involves complex neural networks that provide for wakefulness and an awareness of self and environment. Two aspects of consciousness are content of consciousness and arousal. The former relates to mental activities such as perception of self and memory, and the latter relates to a state of wakefulness. The levels of function of the nervous system can be roughly related clinically to varying levels of consciousness. In essence, if higher levels no longer function because of various disease or traumatic processes, lower levels can be observed functioning. Content of consciousness activities (mental activities) are carried out at the highest level: the cerebral cortex. The arousal phenomenon arises from a much lower level in the brain stem structures. Within each of the two components of consciousness, there exist varying degrees of function. The structures necessary for consciousness include the intact central structures of the diencephalon and projections from it, the thalamocortical system, and the reticular activating system (RAS) of the brain stem. The cerebral cortex provides perception to the neural basis of consciousness that arises from the lower levels of the brain.[1]

The RAS is important in modulating wakefulness, arousal, and conscious perception of the environment. It arises from the deep structures of the brain and brain stem to project onto the cortex. This portion of the RAS is known as the *ascending reticular activating system*. A portion of the RAS bypasses the thalamus on its projectory route; another part terminates in the specific nuclei of the thalamus and, from these, projects diffusely to the entire cortex. The former is referred to as the nonspecific or diffuse thalamocortical system and the latter as the specific thalamocortical system.[16]

Sensory stimulation is transmitted by the afferent pathways to projection areas on the cerebral cortex by specific and nonspecific thalamic nuclei for conscious perception. Chapter 48 details the important functions of the thalamus in receiving sensory information from various parts of the body and relaying these onto specific areas of the cortex. This relay involves a three-synapse transmission to the projection site on the cortex and is part of the specific thalamocortical system. The nonspecific thalamocortical system, on the other hand, does not project to specific nuclei of the thalamus but bypasses the thalamic region in groups of nuclei, including the midline nuclei, intralaminar nuclei, and reticular thalamic nucleus. Nonspecific system conduction involves a multisynaptic path with indistinct boundaries and numerous interconnections with the specific thalamic nuclei before final projection to widely distributed cortical receiving areas.

During sleep and anesthesia, transmissions of the specific thalamic nuclei remain unchanged, but the nonspecific system becomes suppressed. In normal, wakeful brain functioning, a continuous activating flow from the nonspecific system controls the state of consciousness or wakefulness at any given time. This flow is known as the RAS, and it is driven by a brain stem region known as the *bulboreticular facilitory area*. Acetylcholine is the excitatory neurotransmitter in arousal. As the activating afferent flow diminishes, sleep states ensue. The *reticular inhibitory area* in the lower brain stem is activated during this time and inhibits brain activity in higher regions through secretion of the inhibitory hormone, *serotonin*. Major damage to the RAS results in greatly diminished cortical activation, which affects the conscious state.

Investigators have applied electrical stimulation to different areas of the RAS in an attempt to understand its function better. Electrical stimulation of the upper brain stem portion of the RAS produces immediate waking in the sleeping animal and general activation of the entire central nervous system. In contrast, electrical stimulation of the RAS as it arises from the thalamic nuclei results in more specific activation of the cortex, which allows for mental activities requiring a more direct focus. During sleep, the RAS may be activated by various external and internal stimuli. Some of these are more potent activators than others; for example, pain is a strong activator.

In addition to stimulation of the RAS from the afferent ascending system, stimulation may also descend from all areas of the cerebral cortex and, in turn, further excite the brain stem excitatory areas. Particularly strong stimulation arrives from the cortical motor projection areas. It is well known that activity such as walking wards off sleep that might otherwise overtake a person during sitting or reclining.

▼ Alterations in Consciousness

The most sensitive indicator of brain function is level of consciousness. A wide range of consciousness may be observed, from an alert state to deep coma. Subtle changes that affect diagnosis and management can occur within short time spans. A person with a normal level of consciousness is awake, aware, and interacting appropriately with the environment when not engaged in normal sleep. Alertness; orientation to time, place, and person; and general responses to the surroundings are evaluated frequently in individuals with cerebral neurologic disturbances. A person whose level of consciousness deteriorates from a normal interaction with the environment may lapse slowly or very rapidly to a totally unresponsive state, depending on the underlying neurologic pathology.

Slow deterioration of the level of consciousness reveals different levels of response that can be observed clinically. Subjective observations may be described: the lethargic person is somnolent and drowsy and responds sluggishly to verbal and painful stimuli. Heightened stimuli may be necessary to evoke a response, and the person may drift back into sleep soon after the stimulation. The person may be oriented or may exhibit occasional disorientation. As brain function deteriorates, lethargy becomes stupor. Vigorous and persistent noxious stimuli are necessary to evoke a response, because verbal stimuli usually produce little response. The attention span is very short, and excessive motor responses may be exhibited.

Further deterioration of brain function is reflected in ensuing coma. The first sign is a light coma or semicoma, in which no responses are made to ordinary verbal and tactile stimuli. However, motor responses do occur in a reflexive manner to noxious stimuli. Deepening coma is observed when reflexive motor responses are no longer elicited in response to vigorous noxious stimulation and flaccidity of the extremities predominates. Pupillary, pharyngeal, and corneal responses may be minimal or absent. Thermoregulatory mechanisms become erratic, and respiratory patterns become irregular.

COMA

The importance of an intact and functioning ascending RAS extending from the midbrain to the hypothalamus, the thalamus, and finally the cerebral cortex was discussed in Chapter 48. Disruption of the conscious state is usually related to an etiologic basis of structural, metabolic-toxic, or, uncommonly, psychogenic origin.

A person whose coma results from structural processes has incurred physical damage to the brain, such as a contusion, infection, intracerebral bleeding, tumor, or edema. Coma results from structural causes when damage occurs to both cerebral cortices or the brain stem. Brain expansion, such as that which occurs in the herniation syndromes, may cause secondary damage to the structures necessary for consciousness and result in coma. The distinguishing characteristics of structurally-induced coma are focal signs that reflect the area of the brain involved. Initially, in most cases, these focal signs are unilateral processes, such as hemiparesis and unilateral pupillary dilation. Without intervention, the focal signs may become bilateral.

Toxic or metabolically-induced coma results from ingestion of exogenous nervous system poisons (toxins) or from disease processes that produce endogenous materials that interfere with normal brain metabolism. In contrast to structurally-induced coma, there are usually no asymmetrical body signs in metabolically-induced coma.

Coma can also have psychogenic origins. Psychogenic coma can be differentiated from organic coma by attempting to open one of the affected person's eyelids. Active resistance to eyelid opening occurs with psychogenic coma. With true coma, the eyelid is readily opened, falls back into prior position slowly, and remains slightly open. The cold caloric test (oculovestibular reflex) is another effective means to distinguish between psychogenic and organic coma (see pp. 1028–1029). If nystagmus occurs during the test, the unresponsiveness is psychogenic.[3] Conjugate eye movments are normal, and dysconjugate, asymmetric, or nonexistent eye movements are abnormal. The common causes of coma are summarized in Box 52-1.

BOX 52-1 ▼ Common Etiologic Bases for Coma

Structural Processes
  Supratentorial lesions
    Epidural hematoma
    Tumor
    Infection
    Hemorrhage
    Subdural hematoma
    Contusion
    Edema
  Infratentorial lesions
    Hemorrhage
    Infarction
    Aneurysm
    Tumor
    Contusion
Endogenous Metabolic Processes
  Renal failure (uremia)
  Diabetic ketoacidosis
  Electrolyte imbalances
  Hyperosmolarity
  Acidosis
  Hepatic encephalopathy
  Hypoxia
  Hypercarbia
  Hypoglycemia
Exogenous Toxic Poisons
  Sedative drugs
  Alcohol
Psychogenic Disorders
  Fainting
  Hysteria
  Catatonia

Clinical Findings

Coma has been likened to sleep, and similarities do exist. For example, both states lack conscious behavior, and electroencephalogram recordings tend to show slow rhythms in both. Nevertheless, the differences are striking. People may be aroused from sleep, but those in profound coma cannot be aroused. Eye movements may be lacking in coma as a result of acute neurologic processes, and rapid eye movement sleep patterns are not present. As coma becomes chronic, some people display periods of restlessness that may be equated with sleep-wakefulness cycles.

Supratentorially Induced Coma

Isolated, small lesions of the cerebral hemispheres are not sufficient to cause coma so long as the ascending RAS and its connections to the cortex are intact. With progressively larger hemispheric lesions in regions above the tentorium, behavior becomes dulled until maximum obliteration of the cortex occurs and no content of consciousness is preserved. Supratentorial hemispheric lesions produce coma by enlarging sufficiently to cross midline structures and compress the opposite hemisphere (Fig. 52-1) or by caudal compression of the diencephalon and midbrain. Dangerous manifestations of hemispheric compression include herniations of the diencephalon or uncus through the tentorial notch, which results in aggravating vascular obstruction and accentuation of the ischemia that is already present. Similarly, circulation of cerebrospinal fluid (CSF) is blocked with transtentorial herniation, and the pressure rises in the cranium. Transtentorial herniation is also accompanied by brain stem hemorrhages and ischemia that is thought to be caused by the midbrain and pons stretching the medial branches of the basilar artery.

Infratentorially Induced Coma

Coma as a result of dysfunction or destruction of areas below the tentorium may arise from within the brain stem structures and produce destructive effects directly on the paramedian midbrain-pontine reticular formation. Lesions external to the brain stem may compress the reticular formation and may involve direct invasive destruction or compression of its blood supply, resulting in brain stem ischemia and eventual necrosis. The brain stem may be destroyed by cerebrovascular accident, neoplasm, aneurysms, hematomas, infectious processes, or head trauma.

Lesions external to the brain stem may compress the tegmentum, resulting in damage to the neural tissue. This may compromise the vascular supply and result in ischemia. In addition, the mesencephalic tegmentum may be compressed through an upward herniation of the cerebellum and midbrain through the tentorial notch. This compression results in tissue distortion and vascular obstruction with eventual coma. Expanding lesions of the posterior fossa (cerebellum) are a common cause of upward herniation of structures through the tentorial notch. Downward compression of the brain stem may result from the herniation of the cerebellar tonsils through the foramen magnum. This results in compression and ischemia of the medulla with resultant circulatory and respiratory aberrations.

Functional Disturbances Associated With Coma

Certain clinical alterations in function reflect the level and extent of underlying brain pathology. These include alterations in consciousness, motor responses, respiratory patterns, pupillary responses, and eye movements.

The patient's motor responses may be significant in relation to the extent of pathology and depth of coma. Evaluation of limb movement is a means of assessing asymmetry of function in the nervous system. A consistently justifiable correlation between the level of consciousness and the motor responses cannot always be made, because each of these functions is controlled by separate pathways and stands apart. Nevertheless, lesions at certain levels within the central nervous system result in specific types of motor responses that are readily observable clinically and indicate the region of the pathology.

If no response is elicited to verbal stimuli, other stimuli are used to arouse a response. The responses are significant in that they may indicate the extent of damage by their purposefulness. Purposeful motor responses to noxious stimuli in the comatose person indicate that the sensory pathways and corticospinal pathways are

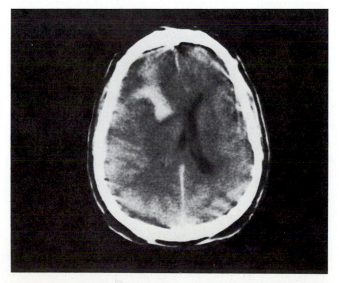

FIGURE 52-1 *Intracerebral bleeding in left frontal lobe (light area). Compression of left lateral ventricle with slight compression of midline structures.*

functioning. An example is an attempt to push the noxious stimulus away. Inappropriate motor responses are stereotyped patterns that commonly indicate the level or region of damage. *Decorticate* and *decerebrate motor responses* are examples of inappropriate involuntary responses that indicate neurological damage below the level of the cerebral cortex (Fig. 52-2).

The decorticate response denotes supratentorial dysfunction, which is commonly observed with the interruption of the corticospinal pathways by lesions of the internal capsule or cerebral hemisphere. It is clinically manifested by a flexion response of the upper extremities and an extension response of the lower extremities. The arms are adducted and in rigid flexion, with the hands rotated internally and fingers flexed. The decerebrate response is elicited in persons with extensive brain stem damage to the midpontine level, and those with large cerebral lesions that compress the lower thalamus and midbrain. Severe metabolic disorders, such as hypoglycemia, hepatic coma, and certain drug intoxications, can diminish brain stem function and induce a decerebrate response. Characteristic musculoskeletal patterns include extension responses of both upper and lower extremities.

Fully expressed, the decerebrate individual exhibits opisthotonos posturing (head extended, body arched) with clenched teeth and arms rigidly extended, adducted, and hyperpronated. The legs are stiffly extended and feet plantar flexed. The extent of the decerebrate response correlates with severity of the pathology. It occasionally appears as wavering back and forth between decorticate and decerebrate postures, reflecting physiologic changes.

Decerebrate responses of the upper extremities together with flaccidity of the lower extremities indicates more extensive brain stem damage, extending even beyond the pons level. In certain persons, asymmetry of abnormal and normal responses may reflect underlying cerebral pathology. For example, a patient may exhibit a unilateral decorticate response, or a decorticate response on one side and a decerebrate response on the other side.

Unilaterally absent motor responses to noxious stimuli indicate interruption in the corticospinal pathways, damage to the RAS at the pontomedullary level, or psychogenic disruption. Hyperreflexia and the presence of the Babinski response support structural lesions of the central nervous system as the origin of the coma. Certain metabolic abnormalities, such as hypoglycemia and uremia, may exhibit the same signs but can be quickly confirmed by laboratory studies.

Paralysis

Paralysis, the loss of voluntary movement, is relatively common with trauma to the nervous system. Lesions involving the corticobulbar and corticospinal tracts are known as *upper motor neuron lesions* and result in *spastic paralysis* (Fig. 52-3A). Lesions involving motor cranial nerves, whose cell bodies are in the brain stem nuclei, and spinal nerves, whose cell bodies are in the anterior horn of the spinal cord, are referred to as *lower motor neuron lesions* and result in *flaccid paralysis* (see Figure 52-3B). Motor and sensory losses may coexist, indicating mixed motor and sensory nerve involvement or involvement of both the anterior and posterior roots.

The activity of the reflex arc provides the muscle with tone. Interruption of the arc, associated with lower motor neuron lesions, results in atony and soft, unresponsive muscle. Voluntary activity and reflex action cannot be elicited if the final common pathway of the lower motor neuron is severed. Deep tendon reflexes are absent also. With lesions of the upper motor neuron, the activity of the reflex arc remains intact, although voluntary control of movement is lost. The pyramidal tract and its collaterals, as well as other descending tracts that influence lower motor neurons, may be involved in the paralysis. The muscle feels hard, is very sensitive to stretch, and is said to be *hypertonic*. Deep tendon reflexes are increased after a period of areflexia that occurs immediately after onset of this type of lesion. The characteristics of upper and lower motor neuron lesions are summarized in Table 52-1.

Pupillary Responses in Altered States of Consciousness

The close anatomic relations of fibers that control pupillary reactions and consciousness provide a valuable guide to the location of the pathologic processes causing coma. Other origins of coma also may be assessed by the pupillary responses, because metabolic aberrations leave

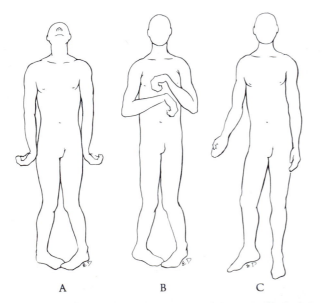

FIGURE 52-2 *Abnormal posturing.* **A.** *Decerebrate posturing.* **B.** *Decorticate posturing.* **C.** *Position in early hemiplegia. (Dossey, B.M., Guzzette, C.E.* Critical Care Nursing *[3rd ed.]. Philadelphia: J.B. Lippincott, 1992.)*

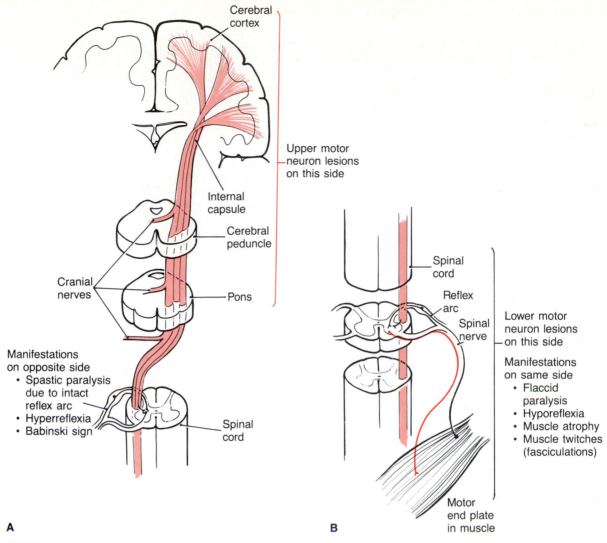

FIGURE 52-3 **A.** *Effect of upper motor neuron lesions.* **B.** *Effect of lower motor neuron lesions.*

little effect on the pupils but certain structural pathology produces distinct changes.

Pupillary responses are regulated by the sympathetic and parasympathetic nervous systems. A balance is normally maintained by the two systems to produce a pupillary aperture appropriate to the prevailing environment. *Mydriasis* (dilation) is produced by the sympathetic nervous system and *miosis* (constriction) by the parasympathetic nervous system. The parasympathetic impulses arrive through the third cranial nerve from the *Edinger-Westphal nuclei* in the midbrain. The sympathetic innervation arrives by a more complex route that originates in the hypothalamus, traverses the brain stem, and travels along with the internal carotid artery into the skull, where it reaches the eye through the filaments of the ophthalmic artery and a division of the fifth cranial nerve. Damage to specific areas of the brain produces characteristic pupillary responses that are valuable for diagnostic purposes (Fig. 52-4).

Pupils' size, position, and response to bright light are observed during assessment of the neurologic status of the comatose patient. Normal response to bright light in a partially darkened room is a brisk constriction of the pupil; other responses may indicate abnormal neurologic processes. In addition, simultaneous constriction normally occurs in the opposite pupil (*consensual reflex*). Pupils normally are at midposition and *conjugate* (equally coupled) at rest. In coma, eyes may exhibit slow, random, roving movements that may be conjugate or dysconjugate. These movements cannot be mimicked voluntarily; hence, they are valuable in differential diagnosis.

Damage to the midbrain results in fixed pupils that are not reactive to light but do fluctuate in size. Pupils that react imply a functioning midbrain, because midbrain lesions usually impinge on both the sympathetic and parasympathetic eye pathways. Lesions affecting the midbrain most commonly result from transtentorial herniation. Other causes include neoplasms and vascular abnormalities affecting the midbrain. Involvement of the sympathetic fibers, either centrally between the hypo-

TABLE 52-1 *Characteristics of Upper Motor Neuron and Lower Motor Neuron Lesions*

Upper Motor Neuron	Lower Motor Neuron
Spastic paralysis	Flaccid paralysis
Hyperreflexia (increased deep tendon reflexes)	Hyporeflexia (decreased deep tendon reflexes)
Unilaterally upgoing great toe (Babinski sign)	Absent or normal plantar response
Minimal or no muscle atrophy	Significant muscle atrophy
Fasciculations absent	Fasciculations present

thalamus and spinal cord or peripherally at the superior cervical ganglion, in the cervical sympathetic chain, or along the carotid artery, results in ipsilateral pupillary constriction, ptosis (drooping eyelid), and anhidrosis (absence of sweat) of the ipsilateral side of the face (*Horner syndrome*). Pupillary light reflex remains intact with hypothalamic damage. The combination of symptoms indicating Horner syndrome with central involvement is significant in that they may lead to progressive neurologic deterioration resulting in transtentorial herniation (see pp. 1041–1043).

Pontine lesions interfere with descending sympathetic pathways and thus produce bilateral small pupils. Pupils in persons with pontine involvement usually react to light, but this response may be difficult to discern without a magnifying glass.

Involvement of the third cranial nerve may be observed in comatose persons if the lesions compress the temporal uncus sufficiently to cause herniation and resultant third nerve compression against the tentorium.

Initially, a unilateral, dilated, nonreactive pupil is observed; this may progress to bilateral involvement with expanding cranial pathology.

In the assessment of pupillary size and reactivity to determine the origin of coma, awareness of certain pharmacologic effects may be useful. Heroin, morphine, and other opiates produce pupils characteristic of pontine lesions; that is, pupils become pinpoint and difficult to assess for light reactivity. Cocaine dilates pupils through interference with norepinephrine absorption by nerve endings. Ingestion of large amounts of atropine or scopolamine results in dilated, nonreactive pupils, which may give a false impression of a structural lesion.

Profound ischemia, usually secondary to severely diminished cardiac output, results in dilated, nonreactive pupils. In rare cases, a tight constriction may be observed. Metabolically-produced coma usually results in pupils that are reactive until the terminal stage; this provides significant data in differential diagnosis of coma.

Eye Reflexes in Altered States of Consciousness

Vestibuloreflex pathways lie near areas controlling consciousness and, therefore, provide for a useful assessment guide. The *oculocephalic reflex* (*doll's head response*) is assessed by briskly rotating the head from side to side with the eyelids held open. In the positive response, eyes deviate conjugatively and oppositely to the head deviation. As the neck is extended, the eyes deviate to a downward gaze; as it is flexed, the eyes deviate to an upward gaze. The presence of the doll's head response indicates an intact brain stem and intact cranial nerves controlling eye movement. The oculocephalic reflex is tested in persons whose voluntary eye responses cannot be tested because of coma. Absence of the doll's head response indicates brain stem dysfunction.

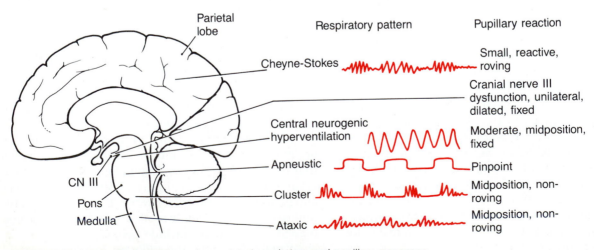

FIGURE 52-4 *Level of lesion/injury and associated respiratory and pupillary responses.*

Oculovestibular reflex (*cold caloric stimulation*) is obtained by introducing cold water slowly into the intact, patent ear canal. Normal response implies that some intact brain stem function is present and is reflected by an intermittent tonic deviation of the eyes to the side of the irrigated ear. The reflex arc for both the oculocephalic and oculovestibular responses consists of the vestibulocochlear nerve (cranial nerve VIII) as the afferent limb and the oculomotor and abducens nerves (cranial nerves III and VI, respectively) as the efferent limb.

Respiratory Patterns in Altered States of Consciousness

Because of the neurologic influences on respiration in various regions of the brain, respiratory patterns observed during coma are useful in diagnosis (see Figure 52-4). *Central neurogenic hyperventilation* is deep, rapid breathing that usually indicates dysfunction in the brain stem tegmentum between the midbrain and pons. It accompanies traumatic brain injury and intracranial hypertension. Respiratory alkalosis is revealed by laboratory findings of low carbon dioxide tension and high pH. *Apneustic* breathing consists of a prolonged inspiratory phase followed by an expiratory pause. This pattern reflects pontine-level damage, usually pontine infarctions secondary to basilar artery occlusions.

Ataxic breathing results from lesions in the RAS of the dorsomedial portion of the medulla and is characteristically a very irregular breathing pattern with irregularly interspersed pauses. The respiratory center tends to be hyposensitive, and minimal depression, with either mild sedation or sleep, may lead to apnea. Usually, persons with ataxic respirations who are apneic secondary to depressant drugs or sleep respond to verbal commands to resume breathing. In severe medullary compression or lesions, ataxic breathing is viewed as a preterminal event.

Cheyne-Stokes respiration consists of a regular crescendo-decrescendo pattern altering with periods of apnea. It reflects bilateral hemispheric dysfunction with a brain stem that is essentially intact. The hemispheric disturbances resulting in Cheyne-Stokes respiration are usually deep within the brain, involving the basal ganglia and internal capsule. This respiratory pattern also accompanies disturbances of metabolic pathogenesis affecting similar cerebral regions, such as occurs with congestive heart failure. Cheyne-Stokes respiration results from an increased sensitivity to carbon dioxide levels, which leads to hyperpnea (increased respiratory rate). The blood carbon dioxide level then falls to below the stimulatory level, resulting in a period of apnea. During the apneic period, the carbon dioxide again accumulates to the respiratory threshold level, and the cyclic hyperpnea and apnea continue.

Cluster breathing, such as *Biot* breathing, which is not associated with a regular pattern, may result from damage in the high medulla or low pons region. Lesions in the low brain stem also may lead to frequent yawning and hiccups. The underlying mechanism for this is not clearly understood.

Occasionally, *posthyperventilation apnea* is observed with diffuse, bilateral central disease. Respirations cease as a result of the drop in partial pressure of carbon dioxide levels caused by a period of hyperventilation, and they return after P_{CO_2} levels normalize.

Clinical Assessments

Accurate neurologic assessment of the person in a coma is crucial for correct treatment and best possible outcome. Initial assessment provides a comparative basis for subsequent observations. Changes in neurologic status are particularly important and may reveal serious pathologic processes within the nervous system. Early detection and intervention for neurologic problems may prevent or minimize potentially devastating outcomes.

The *Glasgow Coma Scale* is an assessment tool that has received wide acceptance in assessing responsiveness to stimuli (Box 52-2). It provides an objective means for making and recording standardized observations with respect to eye opening, verbal responses, and motor responses. The best response in each of these categories is checked at regular time intervals and given a numeric value; the total of these values can range from 3 for complete unresponsiveness to 15 for the normal, healthy response. It also provides a prognostic guide in that persons with a Glasgow Coma Scale score of 7 or below

BOX 52-2 ▼ Glasgow Coma Scale

Eye Opening	
Spontaneously	4
To verbal stimuli	3
To pain	2
Never	1
Best Verbal Response	
Oriented and converses	5
Disoriented and converses	4
Inappropriate words	3
Incomprehensible sounds	2
No response	1
Best Motor Response	
Obeys commands	6
Localizes to pain	5
Flexion withdrawal	4
Flexor posture (decorticate)	3
Extensor posture (decerebrate)	2
No response	1
Total	3–15

usually have a guarded prognosis, and those having a score above 7 have a more favorable prognosis.

▼ *Traumatic Head Injury*

Our highly mechanized society has produced an appalling number of traumatic injuries, most resulting from use of the automobile. Many of these injuries involve the head. The resulting mortality is associated with injury and compression of the brain stem, cerebral contusions and lacerations, large expanding hemispheric lesions, and cerebral edema.

The cranial vault affords protection to the brain by means of the hair, skin, bone, meninges, and CSF. When force is applied, these protective encasements absorb energy that would normally be transmitted to the skull contents. If the force exceeds absorption capacity, it is transmitted to the cranial contents, and tissue damage results. The resultant injury frequently correlates with the amount of force applied to the cranial contents. The effect of head trauma may be direct structural injury (primary injury) or a secondary tissue response (secondary injury).

Head injuries with no obvious external damage but with an intact skull are referred to as *closed head injuries*. In contrast, *open head injuries* may reveal penetration of the scalp, skull, meninges, or brain tissue. Closed head injuries frequently result from sudden acceleration-deceleration accidents (Fig. 52-5). The cranial contents shift to the side opposite the impact within the rigid skull. This is known as the *contrecoup* injury and may lead to contusions and lacerations as the semisolid brain moves over rough projections within the cranial cavity. In addition, the cerebrum may rotate with trauma, resulting in damage to the upper midbrain as well as areas of the frontal, temporal, and occipital lobes. Neck injury is assumed to be present with traumatic head injuries until it is ruled out.

SKULL FRACTURES

A blow to the head may result in one of several types of skull fractures, or a combination of types. Skull fractures may lack significance in themselves unless communication with the brain results and the cranial contents or bone fragments are driven into the neural tissue. These injuries show that a major blow has occurred to the head and potentially severe injury has been incurred by the brain. Skull fractures may be *linear, comminuted, compound*, or *depressed*. The most common linear fractures are simply line fractures without displacement or communication with cranial contents. Comminuted fractures are multiple linear fractures and have the same characteristics. Compound fractures provide communication of the cranial contents with the lacerated scalp

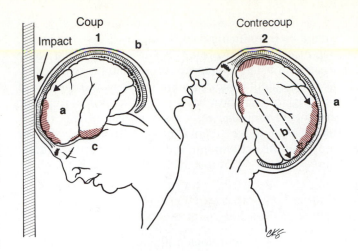

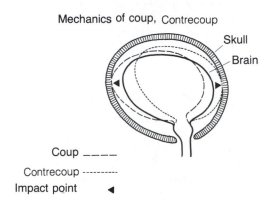

FIGURE 52-5 *Coup and contrecoup head injury after blunt trauma. 1, Coup injury: impact against object; a, site of impact and direct trauma to brain; b, shearing of subdural veins; c, trauma to base of brain. 2. Contrecoup injury: impact within skull; a, site of impact from brain hitting opposite side of skull; b, shearing forces throughout brain. These injuries occur in one continuous motion: the head strikes the wall (coup), then rebounds (contrecoup). (Hudak, C., and Gallo, B. Critical Care Nursing: A Holistic Approach [6th ed.]. Philadelphia: J.B. Lippincott, 1994.)*

and are more serious than linear and comminuted fractures. They require debridement and wound closure within 48 hours. Depressed skull fractures result in deformation of the cranial tissue by bone fragments. They decrease the volume of the cranial cavity and may produce uncal herniation. Venous return may be impeded, and secondary hemorrhages in the midbrain and pons may result. Cranial nerves also may be injured by skull fractures.

Basilar skull fractures involve the base of the skull at the anterior, middle, or posterior fossa and can involve more than one of these regions. Although basilar skull fractures may be difficult to detect on radiographs, they do present some characteristic clinical signs. Fractures of the anterior and middle fossae in association with severe head trauma are more common than those of the posterior fossa. Persons with anterior fossa basilar skull fractures may exhibit periorbital ecchymosis (raccoon eyes), first cranial nerve injury reflecting anosmia, and visual and pupil abnormalities (second and third cranial nerve injuries). The presence of CSF rhinorrhea strongly suggests an anterior fossa basilar skull fracture. The signs of middle fossa basilar skull fractures include CSF otorrhea, hemotympanium, ecchymosis over the mastoid bone (the Battle sign), and facial paralysis (seventh cranial nerve injury). Involvement of the posterior fossa basilar skull may be indicated by signs of medullary failure.

CONCUSSION

Concussions are caused by sudden movement of the brain and result in a diffuse, transient, and reversible injury to the brain. The word concussion means to "shake violently." Damage may occur in many areas, and the extent of involvement is variable, ranging from very mild dysfunction to severe involvement characterized by neurologic dysfunction, unconsciousness, and traumatic amnesia. Involvement of the brain stem, RAS, and certain subcortical areas may result in prolonged unconsciousness. Relatively minor concussions caused by mild blows to the head may lead to transient loss of consciousness owing to temporary physiologic disruption of the RAS. If present, the period of unconsciousness ranges from seconds to as long as a few hours or more in severe cases. No structural injury is sustained, and the process is reversible after neuronal function returns.

Persons suffering concussions are amnesic to the accident and may appear confused for a short period after the accident. Memory loss associated with events before the time of injury is referred to as *retrograde amnesia* and that regarding events after the time of injury are called *antegrade amnesia*. Persons suffering from both retrograde and antegrade amnesia are said to have *traumatic amnesia*. The length of unconsciousness and amnesia is generally proportional to the severity of the concussion. The longer the period of unconsciousness and amnesia, the more severe the injury.

Usually, neurologic signs rapidly return to normal, and further deterioration does not result from the concussion after the initial impact. Headaches and dizziness accompany concussions and may persist for a long period after the injury. Some people also continue to experience problems with attention, anxiety, irritability, memory, judgment, and concentration. These symptoms are referred to as the *postconcussion syndrome*.

CONTUSION

Contusion, or bruising of the brain, occurs as a result of blunt trauma in closed head injuries (see Figure 52-5), and brain tissue destruction occurs at the area of the blow (*coup area*) or at the side opposite the blow (*contrecoup area*). Contrecoup injuries may occur as a result of rapid deceleration (from an impact that stops a moving head) or acceleration (from an object striking a relatively stationary head). The cerebral hemispheres, particularly the basal anterior portions of frontal and temporal lobes and posterior portions of the occipital lobes, are frequently involved because these areas slide over bony irregularities of the base of the skull. Blows to the back of the head may result in contrecoup injuries to frontal and temporal lobes. A variety of neurologic abnormalities may result from *hemispheric contusions*, even though consciousness may be retained. In contrast, *brain stem contusions* result in loss of consciousness from tissue injury to the brain stem RAS. Unconsciousness may last for hours, or the person may never recover consciousness.

Cerebral lacerations involve traumatic disruption in continuity of brain tissue. Cerebral lacerations are inevitably associated with severe head injuries and occur as a result of closed blunt trauma, depressed skull fractures, or penetrating trauma. Frequently, they are accompanied by cerebral contusions and concussions. Clinical findings and recovery depend on the region involved and the extent of tissue injury.

Visible bruising occurs with cerebral contusions because of the petechial hemorrhage that results from the blow to the head. The injured area swells and becomes visibly red and progressively purple owing to venous obstruction and local edema. With large hemorrhages or clusters of small hemorrhages, ICP increases. Electroencephalogram recordings made directly over an area of contusion reveal progressive abnormalities with the appearance of high-amplitude theta and delta waves (see pp. 966–967). Findings from computed axial tomography (CT) or magnetic resonance imaging support the diagnosis of brain contusion. Regional hypoxia and acidosis may result in the contused area and produce hyperemia. Cerebral oxygen consumption is reduced by contusions, and cerebral lactate production is greatly increased, probably because of increased regional hypoxia and the resultant anaerobic metabolism.

Contusions may be partially reversible, depending on the severity of the blow and the amount of tissue injury. Lighter blows usually result in faster recovery. Large contusions and bleeds may require surgical intervention.

VASCULAR INJURIES OF THE BRAIN

Potentially catastrophic intracranial processes may result from hemorrhage into the cranial vault from epidural, subdural, subarachnoid, or intracerebral vascular sources. Persons who are lucid for a period of time after trauma and then begin to deteriorate neurologically are probably suffering from cerebrovascular injury and bleeding into the cranial contents. Bleeding into the rigid cranium results in increased ICP, which is manifested by its localized or generalized effects on the brain (see pp. 1039–1043).

Epidural Hematoma

A serious sequela of head injuries is the epidural hematoma or hemorrhage, which is venous or arterial bleeding into the extradural space that results in compression of the brain toward the opposite side (Fig. 52-6). These bleeds can arise in various regions of the brain. Those occurring in the lateral brain tend to be most severe, running a course more rapid than the other, more slowly developing epidural hematomas in the frontal and occipital areas. A common epidural bleed occurs as the result of middle meningeal artery injury in the parietotemporal area. This bleed is often accompanied by linear fractures of the skull at the temporal region over the middle meningeal artery. As the blood volume increases within the cranium from the lacerated vessel, the brain is subjected to increasing pressure and distortion, which without surgical intervention usually results in a fatal outcome within 24 hours.

The person with a parietotemporal epidural hematoma follows a predictable course. After the initial blow to the head, a lucid interval of varying length follows, although a brief period of unconsciousness often precedes the lucid interval, reflecting the concussive effects of head injury. The lucid interval may vary from 10 to 15 minutes to hours or, rarely, days. During this period, a severe headache often occurs. Progressive loss of consciousness and deterioration in neurologic signs follow as a result of the expanding lesion and extrusion of the medial portion of the temporal lobe through the tentorial opening. *Temporal lobe (uncal) herniation* compresses the brain stem and presents the distinct clinical picture of intracranial hypertension. Deterioration of the level of consciousness results from compression of the brain stem RAS as the temporal lobe herniates on its

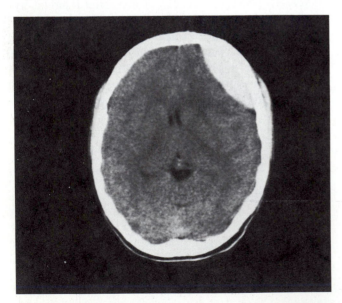

FIGURE 52-6 *Epidural hematoma (light area in well-contained round configuration) in right frontal lobe.*

upper portion. Respirations become deep and labored initially and then shallow and irregular. Contralateral motor deficiencies result from compression of the corticospinal tracts that pass through the brain stem. Distinct ipsilateral pupillary changes can be observed because the nucleus of the third cranial nerve originates in the brain stem and traverses upward through the tentorial opening. Seizures may present at any time during this progressive course. Without surgical intervention, continual bleeding leads to progressive neurologic degeneration, as evidenced by bilateral pupillary dilation, bilateral decerebrate response, and profound coma with irregular respiratory patterns.

Epidural hematomas are identified by the initial clinical picture, CT scans, roentgenograms, and electroencephalographic changes. The CT scans provide the most useful information. If a scanner is unavailable, carotid arteriography is used to outline the hematoma. Radiographs often reveal the linear fracture in the parietotemporal area and displacement of the pineal gland by the hematoma. The scan identifies any abnormal masses and structural shifts within the cranium. Electroencephalographic readings may reveal diffuse slowing in the waves over the hematoma, reflecting compression of the underlying structures. Prompt surgical intervention to ligate the bleeding vessel and evacuate the hematoma can result in recovery with little or no neurologic damage.

Subdural Hematoma

Subdural hematomas are the most commonly encountered meningeal hemorrhages. They occur in *acute, subacute,* and *chronic* forms and may be unilateral or bilateral (Fig. 52-7). Bleeding into the subdural space (between dura mater and arachnoidea mater) as a result of injury to vessels may be from either venous or arterial sources, although the venous source is more common.

Acute subdural hematomas result from severe head injuries and may accompany other manifestations of cerebral trauma, such as contusions and lacerations. They may resemble epidural hematomas in their neurologic deficits and may undergo rapid deterioration without prompt intervention. Symptoms usually appear within 48 hours of injury. The person may be unconscious and rapidly deteriorate, or he or she may be in a lucid state that deteriorates to drowsiness, agitation, stupor, and coma. Signs of brain stem compression are evidenced by a unilaterally dilated pupil and contralateral hemiparesis. Acute subdural hematomas are identified in the same manner as epidural hematomas. Once diagnosed, they constitute a surgical emergency and must be treated promptly. The hematomas can be evacuated through burr holes or by craniotomy. Acute hematomas carry a high mortality, even with surgical intervention.

Subacute subdural hematomas have a better prog-

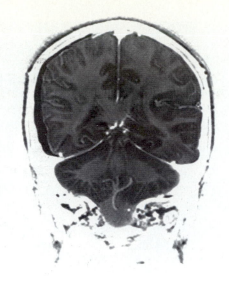

A

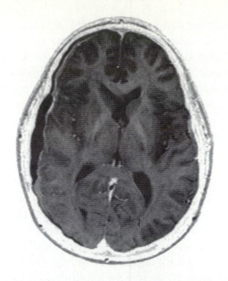

B

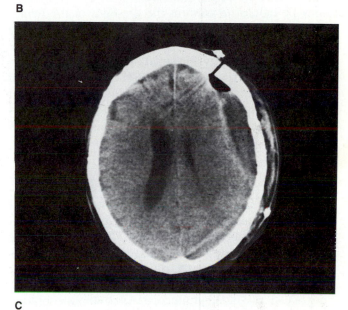

C

FIGURE 52-7 *A. Subdural hematoma coronal view.* **B.** *Subdural hematoma, transverse view.* **C.** *Subdural hematoma recurring after craniotomy (darker area in right frontoparietal region), showing compression of right ventricle.*

nosis because the venous bleeding tends to be slower than in the acute form. Symptoms usually appear within 2 days to 2 weeks after injury. The person is usually lucid after the head injury; this state progressively degenerates to drowsiness, stupor, and coma. The person may stabilize into a coma for a few days and not exhibit the steady deterioration that accompanies the epidural hematomas. The period of stability is followed by a period of fluctuating neurologic signs that progresses to increasing ICP and eventually to a fatal outcome in the absence of surgical intervention. The presence of subacute subdural hematoma is established by the clinical signs, magnetic resonance images, CT scans, or roentgenograms. Early surgical intervention results in an improved prognosis.

Chronic subdural hematomas result from very slow bleeding that is caused by an insignificant injury. This type of injury is most common in infants, in elderly persons, in apparently demented or alcoholic persons, and in those on long-term anticoagulant therapy. Symptoms appear over a wide time span, from 2 weeks to several months after injury. Because the bleeding slowly accumulates as a clot within the subdural space, a period of hemolysis follows. Cerebrospinal fluid is attracted to the lysed blood by osmosis through the arachnoid membrane. The increasing size of the subdural hematoma impinges further on surrounding capillaries, tearing some of them and initiating more bleeding. This increases the osmotic force even further and contributes to the increase in the overall size of the hematoma. An encasing membrane may eventually form around the hematoma and may calcify, or the hematoma may continue its slow bleed and, without proper intervention, produce transtentorial herniation and a fatal outcome.

A person with chronic subdural hematoma may or

may not recall injury to the head. A period of weeks may follow the injury during which the person experiences headache, slowness of thinking, apathy, drowsiness, and confusion. He or she is usually conscious on admission to the hospital and may complain of a generalized dull headache. In the early stages, the person may exhibit some hemiparesis on the contralateral side. As progressive changes develop, focal seizures, papilledema, homonymous hemianopsia, aphasia, and waxing and waning of the level of consciousness may occur.

Chronic subdural hematomas may be identified by the xanthochromic appearance (yellow or straw-colored tinge from hemoglobin breakdown) and the relatively low protein content of the CSF. The electroencephalogram may show increased slow activity in the theta and delta waves with diminished voltage in the region of the hematoma. CT scans, radiographs, and arteriography may be helpful to confirm the presence of the hematoma. Chronic subdural hematomas are usually drained through burr holes. After drainage, a bone flap may be turned to remove any thickened membranes and diminish the possibility of recurrence. Small chronic subdural hematomas may be managed without surgery. With proper intervention, the prognosis for these lesions is considerably better than for the more acute forms of hematoma.

Subdural Hygroma

Subdural hygroma, an excessive collection of fluid under the dura mater, most commonly results from trauma. Tearing of the arachnoid allows CSF to escape into the subdural space. Because of the vascularity of the arachnoid, some vessels are usually damaged, also allowing CSF to mix with blood in the subdural space. This mixing of CSF and blood produces a highly osmotic solution that continues to pull in fluid and slowly expands in size. The diagnosis is confirmed with certainty by burr hole skull opening, although hygromas may be revealed by CT scan and other radiologic procedures. Developing signs and symptoms of subdural hygromas after trauma are very similar to those of chronic subdural hematomas. Symptoms are relieved by drainage of the fluid unless a large collection of fluid-produced neurologic deficits and other pathologic processes is present.

Subarachnoid Hemorrhage

Subarachnoid hemorrhage is bleeding into the subarachnoid space (Fig. 52-8). It may occur spontaneously with a disruption in the vascular integrity, it may accompany cerebral trauma, or, most commonly, it may result from congenital malformations of cerebrovascular beds, such as arteriovenous malformations or cerebral aneurysms (see pp. 995–996). These lesions also may be associated with developmental defects in the media and

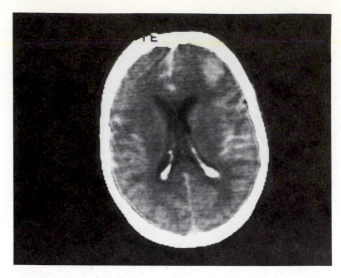

FIGURE 52-8   *Subarachnoid bleeding (light diffuse areas throughout brain).*

elastica of vessels. Bleeding into the subarachnoid space originates from arterial sources, and the blood mixes freely with the circulating CSF, irritating the adjacent central nervous system structures.

The clinical signs in subarachnoid hemorrhage are generalized and in most situations do not focus in the area of involvement; therefore, they are not significant in localizing the site of hemorrhage. They include headache, which is frequently described as severe, violent, or excruciating. Some persons retain consciousness initially, although about half experience a delayed-onset coma. Conscious persons complain of visual disturbances such as photophobia or diplopia and deterioration of vision. Fever, malaise, vomiting, and nuchal rigidity are also possible additional clinical findings. Abnormal mentation with disorientation is not uncommon. The spinal fluid is grossly bloody and exhibits increased pressure. Xanthochromia is noted within a few hours of the bleed and persists for 20 to 30 days. The spinal fluid also shows increased monocytes and protein. Other helpful diagnostic procedures are cerebral angiography and CT scan.

Cerebral vasospasm is a frequent and potentially serious complication associated with subarachnoid hemorrhage. It may accompany hemorrhage resulting from ruptured cerebral aneurysm, trauma, tumor, or arteriovenous malformation to a lesser degree. Cerebral vasospasm is the angiographically demonstrated narrowing of portions of the involved arteries.[9] Symptomatic vasospasm becomes evident about 4 to 12 days after the hemorrhage and usually resolves within 3 weeks. The symptoms include worsening headache, low-grade fever, change in level of consciousness, aphasia, and hemiparesis.[15] The focal deficits are related to the area involved. The exact cause of cerebral vasospasm remains unknown, but it is hypothesized that certain substances that are involved may have spasmogenic properties; these substances include serotonin, prostaglandins, and catecholamines, which are released from platelets and erythrocytes, as well as histamine, oxyhemoglobin, and angiotensin.[15]

Subarachnoid hemorrhage may be treated surgically or conservatively, depending on the general overall condition of the patient. Those who are obtunded and experiencing significant vasospasm are usually not good surgical risks and are treated conservatively with strict bed rest until the condition improves or vasospasm decreases. Recurrence of bleeding is always a possibility, and much of the focus of care is directed at preventing recurrence.

Intracerebral Hematoma

Traumatic disruption of vessels within the cerebral substance may result in neurologic deficits, depending on the location and amount of bleeding. The shearing forces that result from brain movement within the skull frequently lead to laceration of the vessels and hemorrhage into the parenchyma. Common sites of intracerebral bleeding are the frontal and temporal lobes. Those intracerebral hematomas associated with trauma account for a very small percentage of all intracerebral hematomas.

Individuals with intracerebral bleeding may be comatose, or they may have a lucid period before lapsing into a coma. Motor deficits may be present, and decorticate or decerebrate responses may occur. The bleeding site can be identified by CT scan (see Figure 52-1) or by cerebral arteriography. The CSF pressure may be elevated, and the fluid may appear bloody or xanthochromic.

Intracerebral hematomas may be treated by surgical decompression through burr holes or by removal of a bone flap. Surgical evacuation often is impossible because of the location of the hematoma. Even with successful surgical evacuation, neurologic deficits often remain owing to residual effects of the hematoma and trauma. Conservative treatment focuses on minimization of cerebral edema and increased ICP through medications, postural positioning, and supportive therapy.

INITIAL ASSESSMENT AND MANAGEMENT OF HEAD INJURIES

After the initial assurance of an adequate airway, effective respiratory exchange, and absence of acute shock, a careful history is obtained. If possible, the nature of the accident is determined and the lapse of time since the accident is noted. This information may help the clinician to localize of the site of injury and may give some indication of its degree. Neurologic evaluation of the level of consciousness, pupillary responses, motor activity, respiratory patterns, and vital signs is obtained for a baseline assessment. In addition, the head is examined carefully to determine the presence of lacerations, foreign objects, or depressed skull fractures. The ear canals are evaluated for the presence of blood and cerebrospinal fluid. Otoscopic examination of the tympanic membrane is carried out to assess for a bluish coloration (indicating bleeding into the middle ear). The presence of ecchymosis over the mastoid area (*Battle sign*) may indicate a basilar skull fracture. Blood from the ear, if mixed with CSF (*otorrhea*), does not clot and leaves a halo effect at the periphery of the drainage on dressings or pillow. Mixed blood and CSF drained from the nose (*rhinorrhea*) has characteristics similar to those of otorrhea.[14]

Persons with acute head injuries should be treated as if they also have sustained a cervical spine injury until it is proven otherwise. Pain, if present, may be associated with the area of neck injury. However, this is not a totally reliable indicator of the presence of spinal cord injury because pain may not be exhibited and cannot be verified in the unconscious person. Careful palpation of the neck and alignment of the spinous process at the midline of the posterior neck should be done to evaluate for possible cervical cord injury. The neck is immobilized with sandbags, cervical collars, or head straps until cervical radiographs indicate no abnormalities.

Vital signs reflect the status of the head-injured patient and may support the late findings of increased ICP or the presence of shock. Elevated temperature may indicate small brain stem hemorrhages or trauma directly to the thermoregulatory mechanisms of the hypothalamus. Focal seizures may accompany acute head injuries and help to localize the site of the lesion. Observations of the nature and origin of the onset of the seizures are invaluable to the overall assessment of the head-injured patient.

▼ Assessment of Traumatic Disruption to Cranial Nerves

Persons who have suffered a head injury may experience partial or total loss of function of cranial nerves. If the person is conscious, the function of each of the nerves can be assessed briefly. In addition, the integrity of several of the cranial nerves can be assessed grossly in the unconscious patient.

OLFACTORY NERVE

The first cranial nerve extends from the inferior surface of the frontal lobe and mediates the sense of smell. Disruption of the olfactory nerve may accompany acute head injury, particularly in the presence of basilar skull fractures involving the anterior fossa or fractures of the cribriform plate. Nerve filaments may be damaged in contrecoup injuries after trauma to the occipital or parietotemporal region. Other disorders responsible for disruption of the sense of smell (*anosmia*) include upper respiratory infections, rhinitis, tumors, meningitis, and subarachnoid hemorrhages. The first cranial nerve can be assessed simply by requesting the person to close his or her eyes and identify some common odors such as soap, coffee, and alcohol. Each nostril is tested individually, and the person is asked to occlude one nostril while the other is being tested. First cranial nerve function cannot be evaluated in the unconscious patient.

OPTIC NERVE

The second cranial nerve is necessary for vision. Visual impulses originate in the photoreceptors of the retinas and are transmitted by the optic nerve to the optic chiasm and to the various parts of the occipital cortex for recognition and interpretation. Lesions of trauma or intrinsic origin anywhere along these pathways cause specific patterns of visual loss (see Figure 49-3). Damage to the optic nerve usually results from force to the frontal area of the skull. Vision defects may also result from injury to the vessels supplying the optic nerve. Vision loss is maximal immediately after injury. If vision is to be recovered, it may be anticipated within the first month after injury, because optic nerve atrophy begins within this time. Injury to the occipital lobe may also result in impaired vision. However, pupillary light reflexes commonly remain intact in this situation, and prognosis generally is favorable.

Careful clinical evaluation of the visual fields can very significantly aid determination of the site of a lesion. The quadrants of each eye of the cooperative person can be examined individually by superimposing the examiner's eye directly in the visual field of the person. The examiner closes the eye directly across from the person's closed eye. The person is instructed to look directly into the examiner's eye and is asked to signal when he or she first sees the examiner's finger move into the visual field. This test is repeated for each of the four quadrants of each eye: superior, inferior, temporal, and nasal. Assuming the examiner's vision to be normal, the injured person should see the finger at the same time the examiner does. A more rudimentary assessment is simply to ask the person to count the number of fingers the examiner is holding out. An unresponsive or uncooperative person may respond with a blink to a threatened motion toward the head if visual fields are at least partially intact. An unconscious person's ability to perceive light can be assessed during examination of the direct light reflex, because the second cranial nerve forms the afferent nerve for this reflex arc.

A frequently encountered vision disturbance is *homonymous hemianopsia*, in which corresponding halves of bilateral vision are lost. In addition to trauma, cerebral infarctions, tumors, and abscesses can cause homonymous hemianopsia. This defect can be recognized by having the person count all 10 fingers held out by the examiner. Wide turning of the person's head to visualize all fingers may indicate a homonymous hemianopsia.

OCULOMOTOR, TROCHLEAR, AND ABDUCENS NERVES

The third, fourth, and sixth nerves are motor nerves that are usually examined together because of their cooperative function in controlling the movements of the eyes. In addition, the oculomotor nerve innervates the levator palpebrae superioris muscle, which mediates elevation of the eyelids, and the constrictor muscle of the iris, which alters pupillary aperture in accordance with the degree of illumination. The oculomotor nerve serves as the efferent pathway for the direct light reflex. Similarly, convergence and accommodation are mediated by the third nerve. Pupillary responses are more fully discussed in Chapter 49.

The nuclei of the oculomotor nerve are in the midbrain. The axons traverse ventrally to emerge from the midbrain at the level of the tentorial notch and pass through a portion of the cerebral peduncle. At this level, the nerve is particularly vulnerable to compression from other cerebral structures, and its encroachment is reflected by unilateral pupil change on the ipsilateral side.

The third cranial nerve innervates the levator of the eyelid, superior and inferior recti, inferior oblique, and medial rectus. It moves the eyes upward, downward, obliquely, and medially. The nuclei of the trochlear nerve also are in the midbrain caudal to the oculomotor nucleus, and they transmit impulses to the superior oblique muscle to move the eye down and out. The abducens nuclei are in the lower pons below the fourth ventricle floor and control lateral eye movements by innervating the superior, inferior, and medial rectus muscles and the inferior oblique muscle.

Trauma to the frontal region of the skull may cause injury to the third, fourth, and sixth nerves. Brain stem trauma may cause difficulties with conjugate movement, and paralysis of individual nerves may ensue in some individuals. Upward gaze and convergence and lateral eye movements may be interrupted with brain stem lesions. Numerous combinations of third, fourth, and sixth nerve palsies may accompany injuries to the nerves of the superior orbital fissure. Frequently, these injuries are accompanied by diplopia.

To assess extraocular eye movements, the examiner observes the person's eyes for conjugate gaze. They are examined with respect to each other and should be aligned parallel in the visual axis when the person is gazing straight ahead. Extraocular function is evaluated by asking the patient to follow movement of the examiner's finger in six cardinal directions. In the comatose patient, spontaneous eye movement may be observed. Eye movement also may be observed by assessing the oculocephalic reflex (doll's head maneuver).

TRIGEMINAL NERVE

The fifth cranial nerve is a mixed motor and sensory nerve and mediates sensations from over the entire face and scalp to the vertex, the paranasal sinuses, the nasal and oral cavities, and the cornea. The motor component of the fifth nerve innervates the muscles of mastication. The sensory nuclei of the trigeminal nerve are in the gasserian ganglion anterior to the pons, and the motor nuclei arise in the midpons region.

The extracranial portions of the fifth nerve are most frequently involved in traumatic injuries. Scalp wounds or compression fractures of the supraorbital area may sever the supraorbital portion of the fifth nerve. This condition may be identified by the paresthesias, hyperesthesias, and neuralgic pain that linger in the affected scalp and forehead. The infraorbital portion may also be severed, resulting in anesthesia of the affected cheek and upper lip.

Disruption of parts of the fifth nerve may be caused by tumors arising in the posterior fossa or by generalized trauma to the cerebellopontinle region or local trauma to the face. *Tic douloureux*, or *trigeminal neuralgia*, occurs primarily in women in the fifth and sixth decades of life and is manifested by excruciating, unpredictable, paroxysmal pain along part or all of the divisions of the fifth nerve. The cause of this condition remains obscure, but it has been known to be exacerbated by infections, emotional upset, facial movements, and drafts.

The three major divisions of the fifth nerve are the *ophthalmic, maxillary*, and *mandibular*. Each of these divisions is examined for touch perception and discrimination on both sides of the face. With the person's eyes closed, the examiner tests areas with a wisp of cotton and a pin, asking the person to identify which area is being touched. The afferent limb of the corneal reflex is mediated by the fifth cranial nerve. The *corneal reflex* is assessed by stroking the cornea with a wisp of cotton from the side while the person's eyes are turned to the opposite side to avoid an involuntary blink.

The motor component of the fifth nerve is examined by having the person clench the teeth and open the mouth while the examiner palpates the jaw. Deviation occurs to the affected side in the presence of weakness.

Most of the assessment of the fifth cranial nerve requires cooperation by the person; however, a few aspects may be assessed in the comatose patient. The chin can be pushed down and resistance noted. The corneal reflex also can be assessed.

FACIAL NERVE

The seventh cranial nerve is a mixed motor and sensory nerve, although its primary innervation is motor control of the muscles of facial expression. Its sensory component mediates taste perception in the anterior two-thirds of the tongue and innervates the lacrimal and certain salivary glands. The nucleus for the seventh nerve is in the lower pons. Certain cortical innervation of the voluntary movement of the face is transmitted to portions of the seventh nerve nucleus by way of the corticobulbar tract. Some of these axons cross to the contralateral nuclei, and others terminate in the ipsilateral nuclei. High face muscles are innervated by fibers from both contralateral and ipsilateral sides, and the lower muscles are innervated by fibers from the contralateral cortex only. Weakness generated from the effects on the corticobulbar tract are of central (upper motor neuron) origin and causes only contralateral lower face weakness. Ipsilateral weakness of an entire side of the face is of peripheral (lower motor neuron) origin, from a lesion at the nucleus or from the peripheral axon of the seventh nerve.

Dysfunction of the seventh nerve may occur with basilar skull fractures because its location traversing the temporal bone makes it particularly susceptible to injury. Fractures of the petrous portions of the temporal bone may result in injury to the seventh nerve and resultant facial paralysis. In such situations, the prognosis is generally favorable, and function returns with slow recovery that may last for months.

Proximity of the seventh nerve to the middle ear increases the injurious effects of middle ear infections and tumors of that region on the nerve. Central facial paralysis can result from infarctions, lesions, and abscesses of the contralateral cerebral cortex. *Bell's palsy* is an inflammatory response to infections and allergies that affects the seventh nerve within the temporal bone, resulting in ipsilateral facial paralysis.

Assessment of the facial nerve includes examination of facial tone and symmetry, which is done by requesting the person to wrinkle the forehead, smile, whistle, close the eyes, and show the teeth. The sensory component can be assessed by application of sweet, sour, salty, and bitter substances to the appropriate areas of the anterior tongue and by having the person identify the tastes. The mouth is rinsed between applications of the test substances.

The corneal reflex may be assessed in the comatose patient because the efferent limb of the reflex is mediated by the facial nerve. In addition, facial grimacing can be noted in response to noxious stimulation.

VESTIBULOCOCHLEAR NERVE

The eighth cranial nerve is composed of the vestibular and cochlear divisions, the former mediating balance and equilibrium and the latter, hearing. Nuclei of the acoustic nerve are in the lower pons. Traumatic head injury can cause loss of hearing from fractures that extend through the middle ear. Severing of the nerve results in permanent deafness. Hemorrhage into the middle ear also compromises hearing; however, it does carry a prognosis of some recovery of hearing as the blood clot is absorbed. Edema and contusions of the eighth nerve result in hearing impairments that recover with the healing process. Vertigo results from edema or hemorrhage into the labyrinth; it is aggravated by head movement and is associated with nausea and vomiting. Although vertigo may be resolved within 2 or 3 weeks, the person may continue to feel lightheaded and may reveal signs of ataxia for months after the injury. True vertigo results from labyrinthine disease; the classic type is Meniere disease (see p. 984).

Hearing can be assessed simply by covering one of the person's ears and whispering softly near the other. This is repeated for the other ear. Ability to hear whispered sounds is fairly indicative of normal hearing. Should whispering not be audible, further testing is indicated. The vestibular component is investigated primarily through a described history of vertigo, unsteadiness of gait, and nausea. Testing is undertaken on the basis of the presence of the above symptoms. Hearing can be assessed grossly in the comatose patient by observing the response to noise or verbal stimuli. Lack of response may also indicate deep coma. The vestibular component may be assessed by the oculocephalic or oculovestibular reflexes.

GLOSSOPHARYNGEAL AND VAGUS NERVES

The ninth and tenth nerves are anatomically and structurally similar and therefore are examined together. The glossopharyngeal nerve innervates the muscles of the pharynx, the posterior one-third of the taste sensation of the tongue, the sensations of the tonsils, pharynx, and carotid sinuses, and the carotid body. The vagus nerve has widespread innervation of the thoracic and abdominal visceral organs as well as the larynx and pharynx. The nuclei of these nerves are in the medulla. Traumatic injury to the lower brain stem, fractures of the posterior fossa, and vascular injuries at the base of the skull may injure the ninth and tenth nerves. This condition is reflected in dysphagia and a diminished or absent gag reflex.

Assessment of the ninth and tenth cranial nerves involves an initial inspection of the soft palate for symmetry. A gag reflex is elicited with a tongue blade in contact with the posterior oropharynx. Normally, the palate elevates and the pharyngeal muscles contract. The person is asked to swallow water, and the ability to do this without regurgitation is assessed. Speech is observed for signs of abnormal phonation and hoarseness. The gag and swallowing reflexes are routinely assessed in the comatose patient by observing the ability to handle secretions. The presence of this ability indicates gross function of the ninth and tenth cranial nerves.

ACCESSORY NERVE

The eleventh cranial nerve nuclei are in the anterior gray column of the first few segments of the cervical spinal cord and innervate the sternocleidomastoid and trapezius muscles to allow lifting or shrugging of the shoulders, head rotation, and neck extension. Low brain stem injuries and fractures of the posterior fossa and basilar skull may result in injury and paralysis of the eleventh nerve. In addition, trauma to the neck region may result in impairment of the spinal accessory nerve. Weakness on one side may be suggestive of a stroke, whereas bilateral weakness may indicate motor neuron diseases or neuromuscular problems.

The functioning of this motor nerve in innervation of the sternocleidomastoid is evaluated by having the person turn the head toward the shoulder while the examiner puts resistance on the movement and assesses the strength of the muscle. This test is repeated on the other side. The functioning of the trapezius is evaluated by having the person raise the shoulders against the resistance applied by the examiner. Assessment of this cranial nerve requires cooperation, and therefore its integrity cannot be determined in a comatose patient.

HYPOGLOSSAL NERVE

The twelfth cranial nerve is a motor nerve innervating the musculature of the tongue to allow normal articulation and food management in the mouth. Its nucleus is in the floor of the fourth ventricle. The function of the hypoglossal nerve may be jeopardized by trauma to the neck or to the regions described for eleventh nerve injuries. Traumatic lesion may result in unilateral tongue weakness, which is evidenced by deviation of the protruding tongue to the weak side. Bilateral tongue weakness is most commonly associated with disease processes, such as amyotrophic lateral sclerosis and poliomyelitis.

The function of the hypoglossal nerve is evaluated by having the person protrude the tongue and observing for any deviation. The strength of the muscles of the tongue is assessed by the examiner by pushing against the cheek as the person presses outward with the tongue. Notation is made of any difficulty with articulation during conversation. In the comatose patient, one can note the position and movement of the tongue when the mouth is opened. The tongue normally lies in the midline, and deviation to either side is abnormal.

▼ Cerebral Edema

A common and serious sequela of head injury is cerebral edema, wherein the total water content in the brain parenchyma becomes excessive. In addition to head injury, cerebral edema may also occur with intracranial surgery, brain tumors, hypoxemia, infarctions, and infections. Two distinct types have been identified: *cytotoxic* and *vasogenic*.

Cytotoxic cerebral edema reflects cellular dysfunction or injury and occurs secondarily to conditions that result in the accumulation of metabolic waste products associated with cerebral hypoxia. Cytotoxic edema affects primarily the gray matter of the brain. The fluid collection is intracellular within most of the cell components of the brain. The sodium pump is not able to remove accumulating intracellular sodium because of adenosine triphosphate deficiency that results from hypoxia. The accumulated intracellular sodium pulls water into the cell, and waste products of anaerobic metabolism accumulate, rendering the cell dysfunctional. Cytotoxic edema occurs with certain intoxications, hypoxia, some metabolic disorders, and water overload.

Vasogenic edema is caused by damage to or dysfunction in the cerebral blood vessels. The fluid forms intercellularly, and its composition is very similar to plasma. This type of cerebral edema results from increased permeability of the capillary membranes and widening of the junctions between the cells (breakdown of the blood-brain barrier). The widening of these normally tight junctions allows plasma proteins from the blood to pass into the extracellular spaces. Vasogenic edema occurs commonly with trauma, including surgical trauma, contusions, inflammatory processes, neoplasms, and subdural and epidural hematomas.

Alteration in the blood-brain barrier probably occurs in both types of cerebral edema. The mechanism of the alteration is not known, but it may be associated with loss of cerebral autoregulation. As a result of malfunction of the blood-brain barrier, the brain becomes more permeable to molecules that normally do not cross this barrier.

As cerebral edema increases within the nonflexible skull, clinical signs indicate increased ICP and decreased cerebral blood flow. If edema progresses, neurologic function continues to deteriorate because of intracranial shifts or herniations. The signs indicating increased ICP, brain shifts, and herniations are discussed in the following sections.

The morphologic changes in the edematous brain, as seen at surgery or autopsy, are characteristic and striking. The brain appears heavy and boggy. The gyri have lost their normal triangular appearance, and the sulci have been obliterated. Brain sections reveal flattened ventricles and an indiscernible subarachnoid space.[11]

▼ Intracranial Hypertension

Head injuries may lead to increased ICP because of expanding brain volume, increased blood volume, or increased accumulation of CSF. Without treatment, the increased hypertension may compromise neurologic function and life itself. Therefore, early diagnosis and treatment are essential. In addition to trauma, increased ICP accompanies many other neurologic problems and conditions such as tumors, infections, and bleeds.

In the adult, the cranial vault affords a nonflexible encasement around the brain tissue (which makes up 80% of cranial contents) and the extracellular fluid, which is primarily blood and CSF (each making up 10% of contents). Although total intracranial volume varies slightly, ICP remains relatively constant. Transient increases are normal and are associated with activities such as coughing, sneezing, and straining. A small increase in volume of one of the cranial components is compensated normally by a decrease in the volume of another (*Monro-Kellie hypothesis*). Intracranial CSF may be shifted to the subarachnoid space of the spine, and the vascular bed of the brain may be reduced by shifting the blood to areas of less resistance.[7]

A measure of stiffness of the brain, known as *elastance*, indicates the brain's tolerance for increases in volume. Elastance is described by the formula, $E = P/V$, where E = elastance, P = pressure, and V = volume. If elastance is low, then there is volume reserve. High elastance indicates a stiff or tight brain. Intracranial *compliance*, the ability of the cranial contents to adapt to changes in volume, is determined by the volume and rate of displacement of intracranial tissue, blood, and CSF. Compliance (C) is the reciprocal of elastance and can be described by the formula, $C = V/P$; hence, high elastance represents low compliance.

During the period of compensation when the volume-pressure curve is increasing slowly, relatively large intracranial volume increases can be tolerated without significant ICP changes (adequate compliance, low elastance).[4] After the small margin of compensation within the cranium is exhausted, small increases in volume result in large rises in ICP (decreased compliance, high elastance) (Fig. 52-9). Without intervention, decompensation and death ensue.

Clinical indicators of increased ICP, if present, include headache, recurrent vomiting, decreased level of

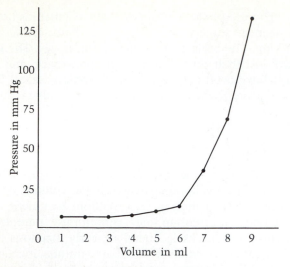

FIGURE 52-9 *Relation between intracranial fluid volume and pressure. The volume of fluid that can be displaced is limited, and if the volume continues to expand, the intracranial pressure is elevated at an increasingly rapid rate. (Dossey, B.M., Guzzette, C.E. Critical Care Nursing [3rd ed.]. Philadelphia: J.B. Lippincott, 1992.)*

consciousness, papilledema, pupillary dilation, peripheral motor changes, and respiratory irregularities. Decreasing pulse, elevated systolic pressure, and widening pulse pressure (Cushing response) are compensatory mechanisms that attempt to maintain cerebral blood flow. The presence of clinical signs indicating brain stem involvement (eg, hypertension, bradycardia, irregular respirations) usually indicates that the person has reached a state of decompensation and has a poor prog-

nosis for recovery. Treatment is most effective while the brain is in a compensatory state, because after compensatory mechanisms have been used up, the pressure within the cranium rises rapidly, inflicting damage to neurons.

Intracranial monitoring provides a reliable means to detect changes in ICP before clinical signs are evident. This is most conveniently done by measuring CSF because pressure is equally transmitted in all directions in fluid.[5] Changes in ICP can be monitored by the use of various devices, some of which are displayed in Figure 52-10. The pressure sensed by these devices is converted to electrical impulses through a transducer. Table 52-2 shows a comparison of the monitoring devices. Common waveform variations associated with intracranial hypertension are demonstrated in Figure 52-11. Normal ICP is less than 13 mm Hg or 200 mm H_2O. Some fluctuations over the narrow normal range are common. Normal intracranial wave patterns are reflective of arterial and respiratory influences (Fig. 52-12).

The pressure in the cranium can rise either abruptly or insidiously. Severely head-injured patients with rapidly increasing ICP and intracranial bleeding frequently have escape of blood into the CSF, which results in an increased osmotic force, thereby increasing CSF volume. Cerebral vasculature increases in size in response to hypercarbia, hypoxia, and acidosis, again contributing to increasing cerebral volume and pressure. In turn, the expansions of tissue and CSF volume commonly associated with increased ICP result in compression of cerebral vessels, decreased cerebral blood flow, and disruption of the blood-brain barrier. Reflexive increase in blood pres-

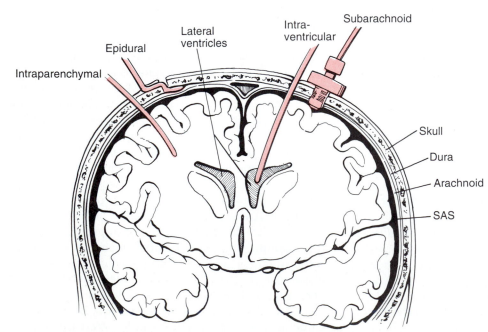

FIGURE 52-10 *Sites for monitoring intracranial pressure. The intraventricular catheter is inserted through a bur hole in the frontal lobe, down into a lateral ventricle near the foramen of Monro. Placement of a probe in the epidural space carries minimal risk for brain infection because the dura remains intact. The subarachnoid bolt is placed in the subarachnoid space (SAS), but it often needs irrigation with saline to remain patent. Intraparenchymal microtransducers can usually be inserted 2 to 3 cm into white matter without complications. (Lyons, M.K., Meyer, F.H. Cerebrospinal fluid physiology and the management of increased intracranial pressure. Mayo Clin Proc 65:684, 1990.)*

TABLE 52-2 *Comparison of Monitoring Devices: Advantages and Disadvantages*

Monitoring Device	Advantages	Disadvantages
Intraventricular catheter (IVC)	Accurate measurement of ICP Allows drainage/sampling of CSF Allows instillation of contrast media Provides reliable evaluating volume, pressure responses	Provides additional site for potential infection Most invasive method for monitoring ICP Must be balanced and recalibrated frequently Catheter can become occluded by blood or tissue
Subarachnoid bolt/screw	Allows sampling of CSF Lower infection rates than with the IVC Quickly and easily placed	Tendency for dampened waveforms Less accurate at high ICP pressures May become occluded by tissue or blood Must be balanced and recalibrated frequently (ie, q4h and whenever the patient is repositioned)
Subdural, extradural catheter/sensor	Least invasive Easily and quickly placed	Increasing baseline drift over time; therefore, accuracy and reliability are questionable Does not provide for CSF sampling
Fiberoptic probe/catheter	Can be placed in subdural or subarachnoid space, in ventricle, or into brain tissue Easily transported Requires zeroing only once (during insertion) Baseline drift to 1 mm Hg/day No irrigation—less risk of infection Less waveform artifact No need to adjust transducer to patient position	Does not provide for CSF sampling Cannot be recalibrated once it is placed Breakage of the fiberoptic cable

CSF, cerebrospinal fluid; *ICP*, intracranial pressure.
Gilliam, E.E. Intracranial hypertension: Advances in intracranial pressure monitoring. *Crit Care Nurs Clin North Am* 2:21, 1990.

sure and decrease in pulse occur as the body attempts to increase cerebral blood flow. The pathologic effects of increased ICP are demonstated in Figure 52-13. Without adequate intervention, the cerebral structures shift, and decompensation is manifested by a decrease in the systemic blood pressure and a rapid, irregular, weak pulse.

INTRACRANIAL SHIFTS (HERNIATION SYNDROMES)

Major brain shifts that can occur in response to expanding cerebral pathology are cingulate herniation, transcalvarial herniation, central transtentorial herniation, uncal herniation, and *cerebellar foramen magnum herniation* (Fig. 52-14). These develop in response to intracranial hypertension in a cranium that is subdivided into compartments by a rather rigid dura mater. The falx cerebri divides the cerebral hemispheres, and the ten-

torium cerebelli divides the cerebrum from the cerebellum. The tentorial notch is the oval-shaped opening in the tentorium cerebelli that allows the passage of nerve tracts and blood vessels. Expanding cerebral pathology in any one of the compartments shifts pressure to a compartment of lesser pressure. The signs and symptoms associated with intracranial shifts depend on the amount of compensation, the compartment involved (ie, supratentorial or infratentorial), and the location of the lesion in that compartment.

Cingulate herniation represents lateral displacement of an expanding cerebral mass that compresses the cingulate gyrus under the falx cerebri, which displaces the internal cerebral vein. This displacement results in compression of the vessel and leads to ischemia and edema, potentially further increasing the ICP.

Transcalvarial herniation occurs with open head injuries in which the brain tissue extrudes through an

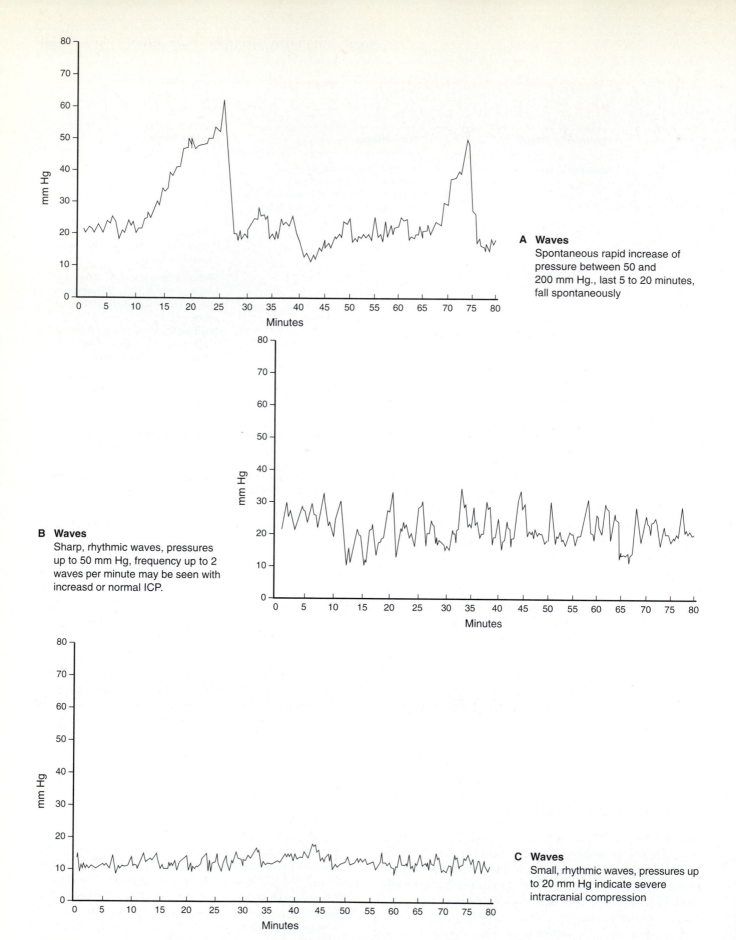

A Waves
Spontaneous rapid increase of pressure between 50 and 200 mm Hg., last 5 to 20 minutes, fall spontaneously

B Waves
Sharp, rhythmic waves, pressures up to 50 mm Hg, frequency up to 2 waves per minute may be seen with increasd or normal ICP.

C Waves
Small, rhythmic waves, pressures up to 20 mm Hg indicate severe intracranial compression

FIGURE 52-11 *Intracranial wave patterns. A, B, C waves indicating variations in intracranial pressure.*

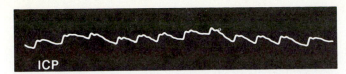

FIGURE 52-12 *Intracranial pressure waveform demonstrating hemo-dynamic and respiratory oscillations. Notice the vascular pressure-type notches in the waveforms and the baseline variations that reflect respirations. (Hudak, C.M., and Gallo, B.M. Critical Care Nursing [6th ed.]. Philadelphia: J.B. Lippincott, 1994.)*

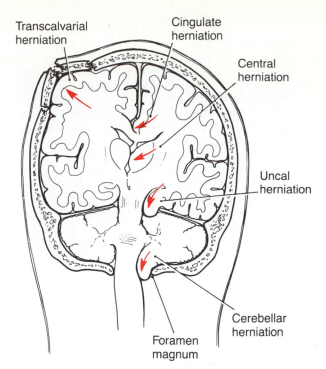

FIGURE 52-14 *Major types of intracranial herniations.*

unstable fractured skull. It is usually associated with increased cerebral mass secondary to edema.

Central transtentorial herniation (a rostral-caudal displacement) may result from supratentorial lesions; however, it is more commonly associated with diffuse increased ICP, as in Reye's syndrome. Pressure is exerted centrally, and downward displacement occurs, encroaching on the diencephalon and midbrain. Cingulate and uncal herniation may precede the central transtentorial herniation. Clinical signs of central transtentorial herniation reflect increasing ICP and include changes in alertness and visual acuity. Papilledema results from optic nerve compression because interference occurs with venous return from the optic disk. As central expansion progresses caudad, brain stem compression is reflected clinically by a further deteriorating level of consciousness. With compression of the corticospinal tract, the Babinski response is elicited and the extremities become rigid and deteriorate to a decorticate or decerebrate posture (see pp. 1025–1026). Early central herniation exhibits pupillary constriction, which leads to moderate dilation without light reflex response as increasing pressure is exerted on the midbrain region. Wide, fixed dilation is a terminal sign. Respiratory patterns initially may be periodic with yawning and sighing interruptions. This changes to a persistent hyperventila-

tion as central compression continues caudad and, in terminal stages, becomes an ataxic pattern before respiratory arrest.

Lesions in the lateral middle fossa or medial part of one temporal lobe result in *uncal herniation*. Crowding in the uncus and hippocampal gyrus at the tentorial notch compresses the third nerve, which results in a unilaterally dilated pupil on the ipsilateral side and contralateral motor defects. In cases in which the uncus compresses and displaces the diencephalon and midbrain to the opposite side, pupillary dilation and motor changes occur opposite the side of the lesion. Without successful intervention after the initial pupillary dilation, neurologic deterioration may progress rapidly to stupor, absence of extraocular movement, hemiplegia, and decerebrate posturing. Terminal stages of uncal herniation resemble those of central herniation.

Cerebellar herniation through the foramen magnum results from expanding lesions of the cerebellum and may involve unilateral or bilateral displacement. Cerebellar foramen magnum herniation and traumatic, rapidly expanding lesions below the tentorium result in brain stem dysfunction with a rapid loss of consciousness and other neurologic deficits indicating severe dysfunction. The dysfunction is caused by the direct effects on the vital centers in the brain stem and the inability of the subtentorial contents to compensate adequately. Motor responses vary from flaccidity to flexor and then to extensor responses. Low brain stem breathing patterns, such as apneustic and ataxic breathing, predominate.

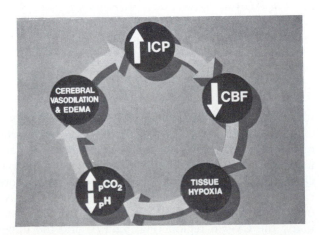

FIGURE 52-13 *Pathological cycle resulting from increased intracranial pressure. CBF, cerebral blood flow; ICP, intracranial pressure. (Source: Hudak, C.M., and Gallo, B.M. Critical Care Nursing [6th ed.]. Philadelphia: J.B. Lippincott, 1994.)*

CASE STUDY 52-1

Curt Schultz is a previously healthy 37-year-old maintenance worker who was in a head-on car accident while on his way home from his sister's birthday celebration. He was the unrestrained driver in a small truck and had no passengers. Curt's truck was severely damaged and required extensive manipulation to get Curt extricated. At the scene, the paramedics found him somewhat dazed but responding appropriately to questions. He had bruises and lacerations about his face and scalp that were bleeding quite profusely. Paramedics noted an area of indented, broken glass on the truck windshield, which they surmised could have been hit by Curt's head. Curt complained of head, neck, and leg pain at the scene.

First vital signs obtained by the paramedics were blood pressure 152/94, pulse 124, respirations 32. Airway, breathing, and circulation were adequate. Other assessments at the scene were as follows:

Level of consciousness—responding slowly, knows own name, uncertain of own address, asks "What happened?" Glasgow Coma Scale score = 13.
Motor activity—moves all extremities, diminished strength, equal handgrasp.
Head—bleeding from head and scalp lacerations, possible depressed region on high forehead.
Pupils—pupils equal and react to light, 6 cm.
Extremities—compound fracture of right thigh, moderate amount of blood noted in seat of truck around right thigh.

After Curt was transported to the local trauma center, the following physical assessment was made on admission:

Level of consciousness—anxious, agitated; knows own name, asks repetitively what happened to him; responds appropriately to command. Glasgow Coma Scale score = 14.
Sensory—complaining of head, neck, leg pain; demanding a pain killer.
Vital signs—blood pressure 148/96, pulse 128, respirations 34.
Pupils—pupils equal and react to light, 5 cm.
Head—multiple bleeding cuts on face and scalp; depressed area on high forehead, bruising around eyes and behind the ears.

Thirty minutes after arrival, the following observations were recorded:

Level of consciousness—difficult to arouse.
Pupils—right pupil 4 cm, reactive to light; left pupil 8 cm, nonreactive.
Motor activity—moving right extremities less than left extremities; right handgrasp much weaker than left; bilateral decortication noted with noxious stimulation.
Vital signs—blood pressure 174/104, pulse 88, respirations 22; respirations appear in clusters interspersed with short periods of apnea. Glasgow Coma Scale score = 7.

1. *What is the apparent mechanism of injury experienced? Based on this, discuss the neurological injuries that could be anticipated with Curt.*
2. *What are primary and secondary brain injuries? What primary and secondary injuries threaten Curt?*
3. *What is a brain concussion, and what are its presenting signs and symptoms? Which of these, if any, are evident in Curt? What long-term changes in function and behavior may be anticipated?*
4. *Discuss the pathological basis and clinical findings of a brain contusion. How is a brain contusion diagnosed? Given the information regarding Curt, is it possible to identify a contused brain with him?*
5. *After controlling for the immediate life-threatening injuries and problems, what are the major concerns in managing Curt's neurologic injuries early after injury? What assessments and interventions should be employed in preventing and minimizing these?*
6. *What is the significance of the bruising around Curt's eyes and behind his ears? What other signs would you look for with this type of injury? What are the potential hazards associated with this type of injury?*
7. *Discuss the pathological significance of the changes in Curt's level of consciousness, pupillary responses, motor responses, and vital signs. What interventions are required?*
8. *Curt has a possible depressed skull fracture. Describe the physical findings associated with depressed skull fractures and the potential hazards to the patient.*

See Appendix G for discussion.

▼ Spinal Cord Injury

Traumatic spinal cord injuries are increasingly common because of the extensive use of the automobile and increased time spent in recreation and sports activities. Figures 52-15 and 52-16 show the relation of spinal cord injury to traumatic events and its incidence in the younger population. Additionally, SCI affects the male population more frequently than females by an 82% to 18% margin.[13] The extent and level of spinal cord injuries vary widely. Whiplash, which occurs in acceleration injuries, may result in very minor discomfort from a mild hyperextension type of cord injuries; on the other hand, total quadriplegia may result from serious spinal cord damage associated with severe fracture dislocations of the cervical vertebral column. Traumatic injury to the spinal cord can occur at any level, although the areas most frequently damaged are the lower cervical spine, particularly the C5–C6 region (Fig. 52-17), and the upper thoracic spine.

Common mechanisms of spinal cord injury from traumatic impact include hyperextension and hyper-

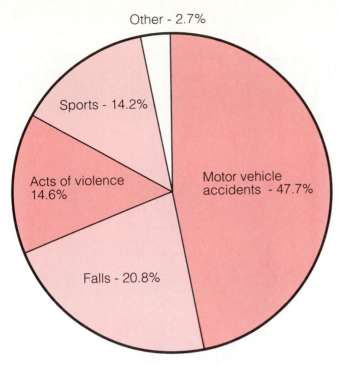

FIGURE 52-15 *Distribution of spinal cord injury by cause. (Stover, S.L., and Fine, P.R.* Spinal Cord Injury: The Facts and Figures. *Birmingham: University of Alabama at Birmingham, 1985.)*

flexion injuries, frequently accompanied by rotational movement, vertical compression, or lateral flexion. Penetrating injuries, such as missile trauma or stab wounds, are commonplace. The resultant spinal cord damage may be transient or permanent, depending on the extent of parenchymal damage. Injuries similar to those that occur to the brain can also occur to the spinal cord, including concussion, contusion, hemorrhage, laceration, and compression. Associated vertebral injuries may lead to spinal cord damage in subluxations (incomplete dislocations), compression fractures (see Figure 45-9), fracture dislocations, and other vertebral injuries. The extent of cord damage in vertebral injuries is related to the degree of bony encroachment or compression on the cord. Severe injuries result in partial or complete functional transection of the spinal cord. These injuries make the person susceptible to immobility, muscle atrophy, bone demineralization, infections, thrombus formation, and skin breakdown.

MORPHOLOGIC CHANGES ASSOCIATED WITH IRREVERSIBLE CORD DAMAGE

Experimentally-induced spinal cord injury in laboratory animals has provided insight into the structural changes that occur at varying times after injury. A force strong enough to result in irreversible total paraplegia causes severe edema and hemorrhage within a few hours, followed by massive necrosis and, finally, parenchymal and

vessel destruction. Immediately after cord injury, focal hemorrhages begin in the gray matter and rapidly increase in size until the entire gray matter is hemorrhagic and necrotic. The hemorrhages in the white matter proximal to the gray matter do not coalesce but are associated with massive edema that envelops all of the white matter. The cord edema frequently spreads to involve surrounding segments. It has been speculated that norepinephrine, which is released in large amounts by the traumatized cord, contributes to the hemorrhagic necrosis caused by direct physical damage.[12] The lesion is progressive for several hours. After the injury, the hemorrhage into the gray matter is present within 15 minutes, and disintegration of the myelin sheath and axonal shrinkage occur within 1 to 4 hours.[4]

FUNCTIONAL ALTERATIONS RELATED TO LEVEL OF INJURY

Cervical spine injuries occurring above the fourth cervical cord segment (C4) may be fatal, because if innervation of the diaphragm and intercostal muscles is obliterated by the injury, the patient dies from respiratory failure.[8] With increasing sophistication of the public in knowledge and technique of cardiopulmonary resuscitation, increasing numbers of these victims arrive at emergency medical facilities. With improved medical technology, life expectancy for these patients has improved significantly.[13] High cervical cord transection results in quadriplegia.

Persons with injuries below the fifth cervical cord

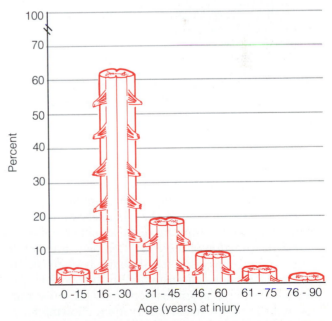

FIGURE 52-16 *Age at Injury. (Stover, S.L., and Fine, P.R.* Spinal Cord Injury: The Facts and Figures. *Birmingham: University of Alabama at Birmingham, 1985.)*

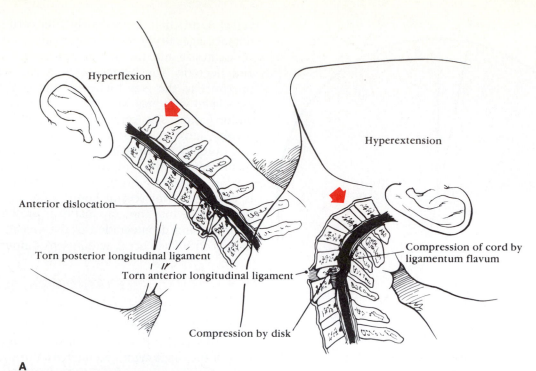

A

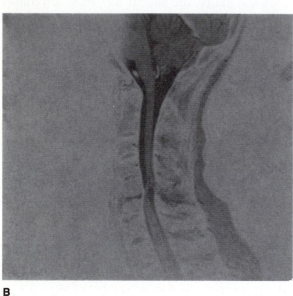

B

FIGURE 52-17 ***A.*** *Mechanisms of spinal injury. (Dossey, B.M., Guzzetta, C.E., and Kenner, C.V., Critical Care Nursing [4th ed.]. Philadelphia: J.B. Lippincott, 1992.)* ***B.*** *Computed tomography scan of cervical injury.*

segment (C5) have full innervation of the sternocleidomastoid, trapezius, and other muscles and, therefore, retain neck, shoulder, and scapula movement. Individuals with lesions at the sixth cervical cord segment (C6) have the function of the shoulder and elbow and partial function of the wrist. Complete innervation of the rotator muscles of the shoulder is retained, and partial innervation is transmitted to the serratus, pectoralis major, and latissimus dorsi muscles. Wrist muscles and the biceps retain innervation, allowing for elbow and wrist flexion.

Persons with injuries at the seventh (C7) and eighth (C8) cord segments exhibit additional elbow, wrist, and

hand function. Innervation is intact to the triceps and common and long finger extensors, enabling elbow extension and flexion and functional, although weak, finger extension and flexion.

Transection injuries to the region of the *thoracic* and *lumbar* cord render the victim paraplegic (Fig. 52-18*A*). Those with high thoracic injury of first thoracic cord segment (T1), retain full innervation of upper extremity musculature. Injuries experienced at the sixth thoracic segment (T6) allow the person to have an increased respiratory reserve because intercostal innervation is intact. Those experiencing 12th thoracic segment (T12) lesions have partial innervation to the lower extremities

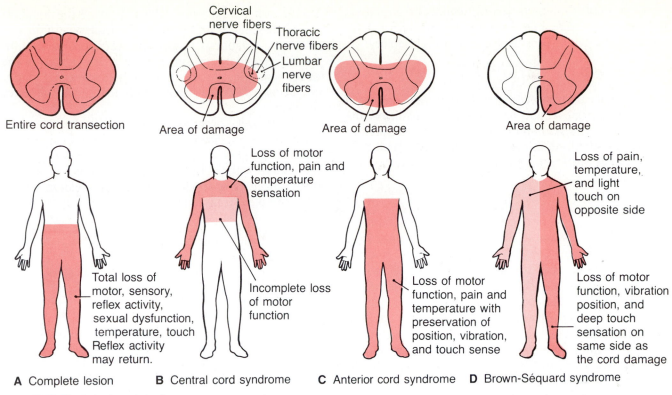

A Complete lesion   **B** Central cord syndrome   **C** Anterior cord syndrome   **D** Brown-Séquard syndrome

FIGURE 52-18 *Spinal cord syndromes.*

and may, in fact, regain ambulation when supported by long-leg braces and assisted by crutches.

Persons who sustain *low lumbar* and *sacral* cord lesions have full innervation to upper extremities and trunk, hip flexors and extensors, knee extensors, and ankle movement. Therefore, these individuals are able to ambulate with minimal supportive devices.

FUNCTIONAL ALTERATIONS RELATED TO INCOMPLETE CORD INJURIES (CORD SYNDROMES)

Central cord syndrome occurs as a result of hyperextension injuries secondary to trauma of the cervical cord. To a lesser extent, it is also associated with disruption in cervical cord blood supply and degenerative processes of the spine (see Figure 52-18*B*). Central cord syndrome symptoms vary with the extent of trauma and edema as well as the specific location. Motor weakness occurs in this syndrome in both upper and lower extremities, although it is usually greater in the upper extremities because more damage occurs to the centrally located cervical tracts that supply the upper extremities. Loss of pain and temperature sensation varies, although greater losses occur in the upper extremities.

In *anterior cord syndrome*, there is damage to the anterior portion of the spinal cord which abolishes motor function, pain, and temperature sensation below the level of the injury. The senses of vibration, touch, and position are retained (see Figure 52-18*C*). The spinothalamic and corticospinal tracts project through this area of the cord, and clinical findings that are associated with disruption of these tracts are produced. Complete motor loss (corticospinal tract) occurs, as well as loss of pain, touch, and temperature sensations (spinothalamic tract) below the level of the lesion. Proprioception, light touch, and vibratory sensations remain intact.[2] Anterior cord syndrome injuries occur as a result of forward dislocation or subluxation of vertebrae, acute intravertebral herniations, flexion injuries, and conditions that compress arteries supplying the anterior spinal cord.[6] This relatively rare injury is usually seen in persons older than 40 years of age.

Brown-Sequard syndrome results from injury to one side of the spinal cord (see Figure 52-18*D*). This may occur as a result of a transverse hemisection secondary to stab or missile injury, trauma resulting in fracture-dislocation of a spinous process, or acute herniated intervertebral disk. The clinical findings reveal ipsilateral paralysis and loss of proprioception, touch, and vibratory sense, in conjunction with contralateral loss of pain and temperature sensation below the level of the lesion. Horner syndrome may accompany Brown-Sequard cord injuries at or above the T1 level. This is supported by findings of ptosis, pupillary constriction, and anhidrosis on the affected side. In this syndrome, the preganglionic sympathetic neurons are involved at the level of injury.[13, 17]

SPINAL CORD TRANSECTION

Total spinal cord transection results in immediate loss of all voluntary movement from the segments below the transection. The skin and other tissues become permanently anesthetized. Initially, reflex activity is abolished; however, it does recover and eventually may become hyperactive.

Spinal Shock

The rapid depression of cord reflex activity after high cord injury (above T6) is referred to as spinal shock or posttransectional areflexia. It results from the interruption of neural pathways to the remainder of the central nervous system. The exact mechanisms causing spinal shock and recovery of reflexes are still elusive. It has been postulated that the excitatory effects of α and γ motoneurons from higher centers on other spinal motoneurons are lost owing to disruption of the descending pathways, and, therefore, inhibitory spinal internuncial neurons become disinhibited, resulting in reduced resting excitability and diminished reflexes. Considerable variability in the duration of spinal shock exists in humans. Some reflexes may reappear as early as 2 or 3 days after transection, and others may not return for 6 weeks or longer. The earliest indicator of resolution of spinal shock is the return of perianal reflexes. Spinal shock is more pronounced in the cord segments surrounding the lesion, and recovery of reflexes usually occurs there last.

In addition to areflexia in spinal shock, clinical signs include unopposed parasympathetic autonomic deficits, which are reflected in hypotension (from loss of vasomotor tone), bradycardia (associated with reflex vagal stimulation), and loss of sweating, piloerection, and body temperature control below the area of injury. The body tends to assume the temperature of the environment (poikilothermia). Because of the depressed vasoconstrictive action below the level of the lesion, patients are susceptible to severe postural hypotension. Bowel and bladder reflexes from the sacrum are inhibited, and control over their functions is temporarily lost during spinal shock. Loss of sensation and flaccid paralysis occur below the transection site. Considerable variation exists in functional capacity after cord injury and, therefore, variation is observed in the extent of spinal shock.

Return of Flexion-Extension Reflexes After Cord Injury

Recovery from spinal shock usually is a long and slow process. The return of stretch and flexion reflexes after severe cord injury is first seen in response to noxious stimulation. An example of this response is the dorsiflexion of the great toe in response to stimulation of the sole of the foot (Babinski's sign). Complications such as infection and malnutrition may delay the return of the flexor responses. As the flexor reflex recovers, it gradually becomes excited more readily from wider areas of the skin.

As recovery progresses after cord injury, flexor reflexes are interspersed with extensor spasms, with ultimate progression to predominantly extensor activity. Individuals with partial cord transection usually exhibit strong extensor spasticity, whereas this seldom occurs with complete transection.

Return of Autonomic Reflexes After Cord Injury

The autonomic spinal reflexes include those that control reflexive action of vasomotor activity, diaphoresis, and emptying of the bladder and rectum. Vasomotor reflexes are abolished below the level of transection during spinal shock, but, with time, tonic autonomic activity returns and wide fluctuations in arterial pressure diminish. Temperature control by the skin is essentially abolished for a time after spinal transection because autonomic innervation for sweating is suppressed.

Reflex emptying of the bladder and rectum does occur in patients with spinal transections after a period of initial atony and increased sphincter tone. Dilation of the bladder with urine eventually overcomes sphincter resistance, and overflow incontinence occurs. With time, spontaneous, brief contractions of the bladder evolve into larger contractions that are accompanied by bladder sphincter opening and brief micturition. Small amounts of urine are voided, with varying amounts of residual urine retained. Sensory stimuli may be used to precipitate micturition, such as tapping on the abdomen, anal stimulation, or stroking of the inner aspect of the upper thigh. Downward manual pressure on the lower abdomen over the bladder (Credé maneuver) is also used to initiate micturition.

Autonomic dysreflexia or *autonomic hyperreflexia* comprises a cluster of symptoms in which many spinal cord autonomic responses are discharging simultaneously and excessively. This syndrome occurs in persons with high spinal cord injuries above the level of the sixth or seventh thoracic cord segment.[10] Its occurrence is highly unpredictable, and it can arise unexpectedly years after the injury. The symptoms occur in response to a specific noxious stimulus, appear quickly, and can lead to life-threatening conditions, such as severe hypertension, seizures, cerebral hemorrhage, and myocardial infarction.[13] Therefore, measures must be taken rapidly to identify the precipitating cause and remove it.

The symptoms of autonomic dysreflexia occur as a result of blockage of the afferent sensory transmissions at the level of the lesion. The transmission in autonomic dysreflexia is caused by a mass discharge that results from stimulation of a large portion of the sympathetic nervous system by sensory receptors. Noxious agents stimulate sensory receptors, which transmit to the spinal cord and ascend the posterior columns and spinothalamic tracts. As the impulses ascend the cord, they reflexively stimulate the neurons of the sympathetic nervous system in the lateral horn of the cord. Because the modulating effects from higher centers are blocked, the sympathetic reflex activity continues unabated, causing arteriolar spasm of the skin, pelvic viscera, and arterioles, and resulting in vasoconstriction.[6] As a result, the person may experience a pounding headache, blurred vision, and severe hypertension that may rise as high as 300 mm Hg systolic. The increased blood pressure distends the carotid sinus and aortic arch baroreceptors, which, in turn, stimulate the vagus nerve to decrease the heart rate and dilate the skin vessels above the level of the lesion in an attempt to lower the blood pressure. The dilated vessels produce flushing and profuse diaphoresis above the level of injury. Because these impulses from higher centers are blocked to the lower body, the vessels remain vasoconstricted and the patient exhibits *cutes anserina* (goose flesh) and pale skin below the lesion. Other symptoms include restlessness, nasal congestion, and nausea.[6, 17]

Precipitating factors leading to autonomic dysreflexia most commonly include bladder and bowel distention or manipulation. Other triggering stimuli include decubitus ulcers, spasticity, stimulation of pain receptors, pressure on the penis, and strong uterine contractions.[13] When the symptoms occur, rapid intervention is necessary to lower the blood pressure. The head of the bed is elevated, because persons with high cord injuries usually have lower blood pressure in the sitting position. The source of stimulation must be found rapidly and removed. If these measures are not successful in reducing hypertension, ganglionic-blocking agents or other antihypertensive drugs are given intravenously.

CASE STUDY 52-2

Josephine is a 47-year-old female who, along with her husband, joined the annual summer cross-country motorcycle trek with the Smithfield Motorcycle Club. One day, shortly after getting on the road again, Josephine was pulling out to pass an automobile when a truck in the third lane pulled over into Josephine's lane and into her motorcycle. Immediately after crashing and hitting the pavement, Josephine attempted to get up, but she instantly fell to the ground and lay motionless. A policeman who happened to be following closely behind the motorcycle group stopped and activated the emergency medical system.

Findings on admission to the emergency room of the local hospital were as follows:

Level of consciousness—alert, oriented, highly anxious, complaining of severe neck pain.
Vital signs—blood pressure 92/48, temperature 97.8°F, pulse 62, respirations 28 and shallow.
Motor and sensory activity—no movement or sensation in lower extremities, flaccid paralysis; exhibits gross arm movements; shoulders seem elevated.
Chest—diminished breath sounds in bases, decreased chest expansion, increased abdominal excursion with breathing.
Extremities—warm to touch; right lower leg is deformed; multiple abrasions and bruises on arms and legs.
Abdomen—no bowel sounds.

The following interventions were done: 1) neck and spine immobilization; 2) large-bore intravenous needle inserted in left antecubital area; 3) magnetic resonance imaging, showing fracture-dislocation at C5; 4) X-ray studies, showing fractured right fibula (cast applied); 5) peritoneal tap (negative); 6) Gardner-Wells tongs with 35-lb weights. Ten days after admission, Josephine had a cervical fusion operation.

Two months after her discharge to the Rehabilitation Hospital, Josephine complained of a severe headache and dizziness. Her blood pressure was 287/126, pulse 62, respirations 32 and shallow.

1. *Discuss the pathophysiological basis and associated clinical findings in terms of respiratory function or dysfunction with Josephine's spinal cord injury.*
2. *What are potential early postinjury hazards for Josephine?*
3. *Discuss the pathological basis of spinal shock. What clinical findings with Josephine support a diagnosis of spinal shock?*
4. *What bowel or bladder changes are anticipated with Josephine early after injury? What interventions are necessary?*
5. *Josephine is prone to a lifetime of physical hazards based on her injury. Discuss these.*
6. *What most likely happened to Josephine at the Rehabilitation Hospital during her hypertensive episode? What could have caused this, and what is its pathological basis? What rapid interventions may be employed? What are the major hazards associated with this condition?*

See Appendix G for discussion.

INTERVERTEBRAL DISK HERNIATION

Intervertebral disks are fibrocartilagenous bodies that are positioned between the vertebrae of the spinal column. They are composed of a central portion, the semigelatinous *nucleus pulposus*, and the fibrous rings, *annulus fibrosus*, that surround it. The nucleus pulposus serves as a medium for transport between the disk and surrounding capillaries and affords shock absorption for the vertebral column. In addition to encasing the nucleus pulposus, the annulus fibrosus also serves as a vertebral shock absorber and allows for vertebral motion. Intervertebral disks and vertebral bodies are joined by longitudinal ligaments—anteriorly by the anterior longitudinal ligament, and posteriorly within the vertebral canal by the posterior longitudinal ligament.

Herniation or rupture of the nucleus pulposus of the intervertebral disk is caused by minor or major trauma in about half of the cases of herniation (Fig. 52-19). In other cases, onset is acute with no history of serious trauma. Sudden straining of the back in an unusual position and lifting while bending forward are frequently reported to be associated with disk herniation. Herniation of the nucleus pulposus produces pain, sensory loss, and paralysis by pressure on the spinal nerve roots or on the spinal cord. The most common herniations occur in the lumbosacral intervertebral disks (L4–L5 and L5–S1); such injuries reflect a clinical picture of sciatica. Herniations of the cervical disks occur occasionally, and those in the thoracic region are rare.

Clinical findings associated with ruptured or herniated disks are related to the size and location of the extruded material. Single nerve roots may be involved in small lesions; however, several roots may be compressed. The spinal cord may be compressed by large, centrally situated cervical disks, and symptoms are reflective of spinal cord tumors or degenerative diseases.

Most *lumbosacral herniations* occur in the interspaces between the fourth or fifth lumbar vertebrae or between the fifth lumbar and the first sacral vertebrae. Sciatic symptoms associated with lumbosacral herniation include pain in the lower back that radiates down the posterior surface of one or both legs. The pain occurs as a result of posterolateral displacement of the disk and compression on the pain sensory pathways of the cord or sensory part of the compressed nerve. In unilateral involvement, scoliosis occurs toward the side opposite the sciatic pain, and movement of the lumbar spine is limited. Paresthesias in the leg or foot are common. Tenderness is experienced on palpation along the course of the sciatic nerve. Motor weakness occurs in a small percentage of cases. Hypoesthesia to touch or pinprick is present in about one-half of cases. A decreased or absent ankle reflex is common with herniation of the lumbosacral disk. Coughing, sneezing, or straining may produce radiation of pain along the course of the sciatic nerve. Symptoms are usually unilateral; however, with large central protrusions, they may be bilateral.

Herniation of the cervical disks occurs most commonly at the level of the fifth through seventh cervical roots. Displacement of the disk in this region causes stiffness of the neck and shoulder pain that radiates down the arm into the hand. Paresthesias may accompany the pain. Weakness and atrophy of the biceps and diminution of the biceps reflex may be present with sixth cervical root damage. Paresthesias and sensory loss in the index finger, weakness of the triceps muscle, and loss of triceps reflex are indicative of involvement of the seventh cervical root. Eighth cervical root compression produces forearm pain along the medial side as well as sensory loss along the medial cutaneous nerve of the forearm and the ulnar nerve distribution in the hand.

Diagnosis and Management

Differential diagnosis must be undertaken if an individual presents with symptoms of herniated disk, because other conditions have similar symptoms, including spinal cord tumors, syringomyelia, spinal arthritis, and other degenerative disk conditions. Radiologic findings supportive of herniated disk show loss of normal curvature of the spine, scoliosis, and narrowing of intervertebral spaces. Diagnosis is most conclusively demonstrated by contrast myelography, which reveals defects in the outline of the subarachnoid space or interruption of the flow of the dye in the presence of herniated disks. In addition, CT scanning or magnetic resonance imaging may be effective for visualization of defective disks. Other diagnostic tools used for a definitive diagnosis include electromyography, diskography, and nerve root infiltration.

Conservative treatment in the acute stage is focused on bed rest, local application of heat, and use of analge-

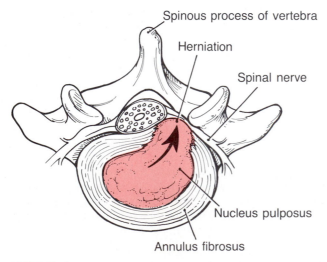

FIGURE 52-19 *Herniated disk with the nucleus pulposus in the spinal root.*

sics. Traction to lower extremities may be applied initially with lumbosacral disk herniations. Cervical halter traction is indicated for cervical disk involvement. With the resolution of the acute stage, the patient is placed in a program of graded exercises to increase muscle strength. Surgical intervention is indicated if conservative modes of treatment fail and progressive neurological defects are evidenced. The goal of surgical removal is the relief of pressure on nerve roots. In addition to the traditional surgical approaches, microsurgical (microdiskectomy) techniques allow removal of the involved tissue through a small incision, resulting in minimal tissue trauma.

▼ Chapter Summary

▼ Maintenance of the conscious state requires the working together of complex neural networks that determine wakefulness and sleep patterns. The reticular activating system is essential in the communication of information from the environment through the brain stem and projection onto the cortex. Alterations in level of consciousness provide a sensitive indicator of brain function. Deterioration of brain function may result in coma, which can be caused by structural or metabolic injury. All of the functions of the body are affected and can be assessed through evaluation of movement, pupillary responses, respiratory patterns, and cognitive responses to stimuli.

▼ Traumatic head injuries include concussion, contusion, and vascular injuries of the brain. The location and magnitude of a bleed determine the clinical picture and ultimate outcome. Some bleeds stop spontaneously, but others must be surgically repaired for life to be maintained.

▼ Traumatic disruption to the cranial nerves is assessed systematically. Damage may be caused by direct trauma or secondarily by edema or hemorrhage in surrounding structures.

▼ Cerebral edema is a reaction of brain tissue to injury; its outcome depends on the ability of the brain to compensate for the injury and the adequacy of treatment. Cerebral edema, bleeding, and other factors can lead to increased intracranial pressure, which can cause shifting of intracranial contents and herniation syndromes.

▼ Spinal cord dysfunction may result from trauma, disk herniation, tumors, or disease of the spinal cord. Functional alterations are related to the level of injury and whether the injury involves complete or partial transection of the cord. After trauma, there is usually a period of spinal shock, and then, depending on the level of the injury, there may be autonomic hyperreflexia, which can be a life-threatening event.

▼ Disk herniation can result from trauma, especially that caused by lifting of heavy objects; it causes pain and dysfunction in the area supplied by the cord segment.

▼ References

1. Adams, R., and Victor, M. *Principles of Neurology* (5th ed.). New York: McGraw-Hill, 1993.
2. Aisen, M. Differential diagnosis of spinal cord disease. In Barclay, L. (ed.). *Clinical Geriatric Neurology*. Philadelphia: Lea & Febiger, 1993.
3. Couldwell, W.T. and Weiss, M.H. Critical care of the neurosurgical patient. In Berk, J.L., and Sampliner, J.E. *Handbook of Critical Care* (3rd ed.). Boston: Little, Brown, 1990.
4. DeGirolami, U., Frosch, M.P., and Anthony, D.C. The central nervous system. In Cotran, R., Kumar, V., and Robbins, S. *Robbins' Pathologic Basis of Disease* (5th ed.). Philadelphia: W.B. Saunders, 1994.
5. Gilliam, E.E. Intracranial hypertension: Advances in intracranial pressure monitoring. *Crit. Care Nurs. Clin. North Am.* 2:21, 1990.
6. Guttierrez, P., Vulpe, M., and Young, R. Spinal cord injury. In Stein, J. (ed.). *Internal Medicine* (4th ed.). St. Louis: Mosby, 1994.
7. Guyton, A. *Textbook of Medical Physiology* (8th ed.). Philadelphia: W.B. Saunders, 1991.
8. Hughes, M.C. Critical care nursing for the patient with a spinal cord injury. *Crit. Care Nurs. Clin. North Am.* 2:33, 1990.
9. Jackson, L. Cerebral vasospasm after an intracranial aneurysmal subarachnoid hemorrhage: A nursing perspective. *Heart Lung* 1:14, 1986.
10. Kidd, P.S. Emergency management of spinal cord injuries. *Crit. Care Nurs. Clin. North Am.* 2:349, 1990.
11. Mergner, W.J., and Trump, B.F. Hemodynamic disorders. In Rubin, E., and Farber, J.L. *Pathology* (2nd ed.). Philadelphia: J.B. Lippincott, 1994.
12. Schwenker, D. Cardiovascular considerations in the critical care phase. *Crit. Care Nurs. Clin. North Am.* 2:363, 1990.
13. Stelling, J. Spinal cord injury. In Howell, E., Widra, L., and Hill, M.G. (eds.), *Comprehensive Trauma Nursing*. Glenview, Ill.: Scott Foresman, 1988.
14. Stewart-Amidei, C., and Hill, M.G. Head Trauma. In E. Howell, L. Widra, and M.G. Hill (eds.), *Comprehensive Trauma Nursing*. Glenview, Ill.: Scott Foresman, 1988.
15. Susi, E.A., and Walls, S.K. Traumatic cerebral vasospasms and secondary head injury. *Crit. Care Nurs. Clin. North Am.* 2:15—D20, 1990.
16. Tortora, G., and Grabowski, S. *Principles of Anatomy and Physiology* (7th ed.). New York: Harper Collins, 1993.
17. Walleck, C.A. Neurologic considerations in the critical care phase. *Crit. Care Nurs. Clin. North Am.* 2:357, 1990.

Chapter 53

Tumors and Infections of the Central Nervous System

Gretchen McDaniel

▼ **CHAPTER OUTLINE**

▼ **LEARNING OBJECTIVES**

1 Identify the tissues from which central nervous system tumors may originate.
2 Describe the classification systems for cranial and spinal tumors.
3 Compare the frequency and malignancy of brain and spinal tumors.
4 Describe central nervous system alterations that lead to focal disturbances and increased intracranial pressure.
5 State what is thought to be the basis for the localized cerebral edema that surrounds brain tumors.
6 Describe central nervous system alterations that lead to the development of papilledema.
7 State the body's compensatory mechanisms for dealing with increased intracranial pressure.
8 Describe the clinical manifestations associated with brain tumors.
9 Discuss the clinical manifestations associated with tumors of the frontal, temporal, parietal, and occipital lobes, the cerebellum, and the brain stem.
10 Discuss the clinical manifestations associated with various types of spinal tumors and with different levels of compression by spinal tumors.
11 Describe techniques used to diagnose brain and spinal tumors.
12 Compare and contrast characteristics of the central nervous system tumors: tissue type, appearance, rate of growth, invasive qualities, central nervous system alterations, and pertinent clinical manifestations.
13 State the two most common primary sites from which metastasis occurs to the brain.
14 State the various routes by which microorganisms reach the central nervous system.
15 List the ways in which viruses gain access to the body.
16 State the ways in which viruses invade the central nervous system.
17 Compare and contrast characteristics of the central nervous system infections: routes of infection, central nervous system alterations, pertinent clinical manifestations, and prognosis.

Barbara L. Bullock: PATHOPHYSIOLOGY: ADAPTATIONS AND ALTERATIONS IN FUNCTION, 4th ed.
© 1996 J.B. Lippincott-Raven Publishers

Tumors of the central nervous system (CNS) and the invasion of this system by infectious organisms are discussed in this chapter. Frequency, alterations within the CNS, resultant clinical manifestations, and relevant diagnostic studies are reviewed. The topic is vast, and the reader is referred to special texts for additional information and study of the subject.

▼ Tumors

GENERAL CONSIDERATIONS

Tumors of the CNS include both benign and malignant neoplasms within the brain and the spinal cord. They can arise from the glial cells, blood vessels and connective tissue, meninges, pituitary gland, or pineal gland (Fig. 53-1). Metastatic tumors from primary sites throughout the body are also encountered within the CNS. With their variety and complexity, classification of intracranial tumors becomes a problem. An abridged version of the World Health Organization's classification of intracranial tumors is presented in Table 53-1.

Intraspinal tumors are classified according to their location in relation to the dura and spinal cord as well as by their histologic type. Extradural lesions are those arising from the extradural space or vertebral bodies. Intradural lesions include both those arising from the blood vessels, meninges, or nerve roots (extramedullary) and those arising from within the substance of the spinal cord itself (intramedullary).

The location, size, and invasive quality of intracranial and intraspinal neoplasms are responsible for certain neurologic symptoms. The destruction and displacement of tissue, in addition to increased intracranial pressure, cause specific symptoms (Fig. 53-2). Advancements in diagnostic techniques, medical therapeutics, and neurosurgical techniques have improved the prognosis for people who have brain tumors. Spinal cord tumors are more easily removed surgically than brain tumors. If the tumor is recognized early and removed, prognosis for a patient with an intraspinal tumor is quite favorable.

PREVALENCE

The prevalence of primary CNS tumors in the United States is approximately 14.7 per 100,000 population. They occur in all age groups and in both sexes. The percent of cases by tumor type and mean age at diagnosis is presented in Table 53-2. In addition, the brain and its coverings are frequently involved by metastatic neoplasm (Table 53-3). Approximately 1% of all autopsied deaths indicate the presence of CNS tumors.[7]

Although intracranial tumors can occur at any age, their frequency seems to be increased in young children and again in the fifth and sixth decades of life. In children, brain tumors are the most common solid tumors and the second most common malignancy after leukemia.[7, 13] The most common brain tumors of childhood include craniopharyngiomas, ependymomas, medulloblastomas, cerebellar astrocytomas, brain stem gliomas, optic path gliomas, and pinealomas. In adults, gliomas account for approximately one-half of all brain tumors.[17] Pituitary adenomas, acoustic neuromas, and meningiomas are prevalent during adulthood and almost completely absent during childhood.

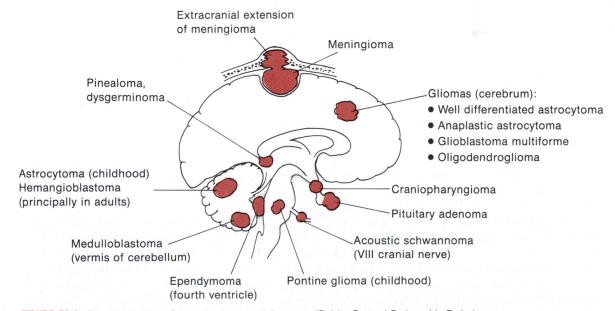

FIGURE 53-1 *The distribution of common intracranial tumors. (Rubin, E., and Farber, J.L. Pathology, [2nd ed.]. Philadelphia: J.B. Lippincott, 1994.)*

TABLE 53-1 *World Health Organization Brain Tumor Classification (Abridged)*

TUMORS OF NEUROEPITHELIAL TISSUE
  Astrocytic tumor
    Astrocytoma
    Pilocytic astrocytoma
    Subependymal giant cell astrocytoma
    Astroblastoma
  Oligodendroglial tumor
    Oligodendroglioma
    Mixed oligoastrocytoma
  Ependymal and choroid plexus tumor
    Ependymoma
      Myxopapillary ependymoma
      Subependymoma
    Choroid plexus papilloma
  Pineal cell tumor
    Pineocytoma
    Pineoblastoma
  Neuronal tumor
    Gangliocytoma
    Ganglioglioma
    Ganglioneuroblastoma
    Neuroblastoma
  Poorly differentiated and embryonic tumor
    Glioblastoma
    Medulloblastoma
    Gliomatosis cerebri

NERVE SHEATH TUMORS
  Neurilemmoma
  Neurofibroma

TUMORS OF MENINGEAL AND RELATED TISSUES
  Meningioma
  Meningeal sarcoma
  Xanthomatous tumor

PRIMARY LYMPHOMA AND BLOOD VESSEL TUMORS
  Hemangioblastoma

GERM CELL TUMORS
  Germinoma
  Embryonal cell carcinoma
  Teratoma

OTHER TUMORS AND TUMOR-LIKE LESIONS
  Craniopharyngioma
  Rathke cleft cyst
  Epidermoid
  Dermoid
  Colloid cyst
  Lipoma
  Choristoma
  Vascular malformations
    Capillary telangiectasia
    Cavernous hemangioma
    Arteriovenous malformation
    Venous malformation

TUMORS OF THE ANTERIOR PITUITARY
  Pituitary adenoma
  Pituitary adenocarcinoma

LOCAL EXTENSION FROM REGIONAL TUMORS
  Glomus jugulare tumor
  Chordoma
  Chondroma
  Chondrosarcoma
  Adenoid cystic carcinoma

METASTATIC TUMORS

UNCLASSIFIED TUMORS

Hoff, J., and Boland, M. Central nervous system. In Greenfield, L. (ed.), *Surgery: Scientific Principles and Practice.* Philadelphia: J.B. Lippincott, 1993.

Intraspinal tumors occur less frequently than those that involve the brain, and they are rare in children. Intraspinal tumors account for approximately 15% of all primary tumors in hospitalized neurosurgical patients.[16] Twenty-five percent of intraspinal tumors are extradural, and they are usually metastatic. Seventy-five percent are intradural. Of these, extramedullary lesions are more common than intramedullary lesions. Extramedullary tumors are usually meningiomas or neurofibromas, and they are easily removed surgically. Intramedullary tumors have the same cellular origins as intracranial tumors and usually infiltrate surrounding tissue. These intramedullary tumors are often gliomas (particularly ependymomas), and they commonly arise from the cauda equina and lumbar areas. Astrocytomas, oligodendrogliomas, glioblastomas, hemangioblastomas, and medulloblastomas occur less frequently and can arise in any of the spinal segments.

ALTERATIONS IN THE CENTRAL NERVOUS SYSTEM CAUSED BY TUMORS

Brain tumors may be benign or malignant with regard to histology and morphology of their cellular components. However, all tumors of the brain are potentially harmful because of their relation to vital structures. Malignant or harmful effects may be produced by histologically benign lesions.

Brain tumors rarely metastasize to extraneural tissue; however, they infiltrate into surrounding nervous

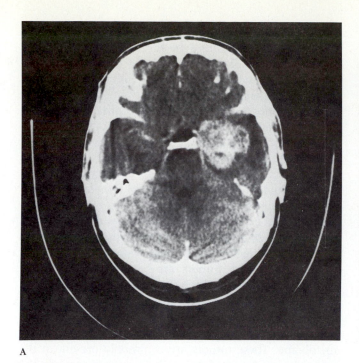

A

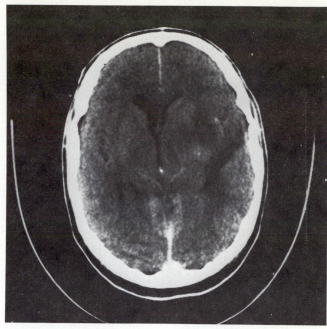

B

FIGURE 53-2 **A.** *Contrast-enhanced computed tomography scan, showing right cerebral metastatic tumor.* **B.** *View of compression and shift of midline structures by the same tumor.*

tissue, into the meninges, or through the ependymal layer into the ventricles. After the tumor gains access to the subarachnoid space or ventricular system, and thus to the cerebrospinal fluid (CSF) pathways, it may spread throughout the entire CNS, including the spinal cord and peripheral nerve roots.[7]

Within the confined space of the skull, a growing tumor alters the normally stable volume of the brain, blood, and CSF. As the mass grows, compression of brain tissue and alterations in blood and CSF circulation lead to focal disturbances and increased intracranial pressure. More specifically, tumor growth can produce any of several alterations. Compression of brain tissue

and invasion of brain parenchyma cause destruction of neural tissue. Blood circulation may be decreased to such an extent that necrosis of brain tissue occurs. Compression, infiltration of neural tissue, and decreased blood supply may also lead to altered neural excitability with resultant seizure activity. Elevation of capillary pressure, caused by compression of venules in the area adjacent to the tumor, is thought to be the basis for the localized cerebral edema that often surrounds the tumor (Fig. 53-3).

As the volume of the intracranial contents is increased, CSF is displaced from the subarachnoid space and ventricles through the foramen magnum to the spi-

TABLE 53-2 *Primary Brain Tumors—Distribution by Tumor Type*

Tumor	Percent of Cases	Mean Age at Diagnosis (years)
Glioblastoma	40	54
Astrocytoma	16	37
Meningioma	18	55
Schwannoma	2	57
Pituitary adenoma	12	39
Lymphoma	2	46
Other	10	—

Laws, E., and Thapar, R. Brain tumors. *CA: Cancer J Clin* 43:264, 1993.

TABLE 53-3 *Metastatic Brain Tumors—Distribution by Primary Cancer* *

Primary Cancer	Percentage of Brain Metastases
Pulmonary	50
Breast	15
Gastrointestinal	8
Genitourinary	6
Melanoma	6
Unknown Primary	10
Other	5

* Annual U.S. incidence: 80,000–100,000 cases

Laws, E., and Thaper, R. Brain tumors. *CA: Cancer J Clin* 43:264, 1993.

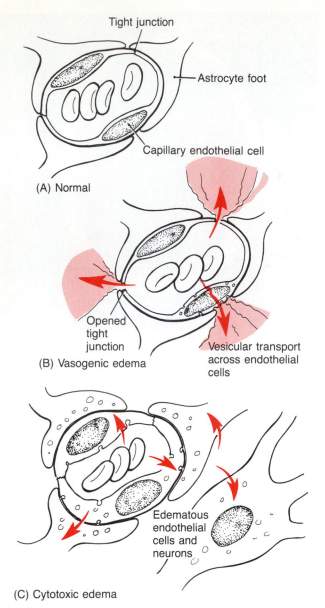

FIGURE 53-3 *Development of cerebral edema as a response to tumor pressure. **A.** Normal astrocyte. 1**B.** Vasogenic edema. **C.** Cytotoxic edema. Both B and C may be seen with tumor infiltration.*

cranial blood volume. These compensatory mechanisms may take days or months to be effective and therefore are not useful with rapidly developing intracranial pressure.[17] Untreated increased intracranial pressure can cause brain herniation (Fig. 53-4).

Alterations as a result of intraspinal tumors are largely caused by compression of the spinal cord, interference with circulation, and pressure on veins or arteries. Ischemia of cord segments occurs, as well as edema below the level of compression. Extradural spinal tumors usually result from extraneural metastases, particularly from the breast or lung, and cause rapid compression of the spinal cord. Hemorrhage caused by metastases, as well as vertebral column collapse, adds to the compressive effects of extradural tumors.

Extramedullary tumors are basically of two types, neurofibromas and meningiomas, and they are usually benign. Neurofibromas grow in the nerve root and often form an hourglass-like expansion that extends into the extradural space. Meningiomas grow from the arachnoid membrane. These tumors are commonly present in the posterolateral aspect of the cord. They often result in the Brown-Sequard syndrome, owing to compressive damage to one-half of the spinal cord (see pp. 1047–1048).

As mentioned previously, intramedullary tumors are histologically the same as intracranial tumors. These lesions damage sensory fibers that cross each other in the center of the cord. They also destroy neurons. There

nal subarachnoid space. The CSF is also displaced through the optic foramen to the perioptic subarachnoid space. With elevations in CSF pressure, particularly in the perioptic subarachnoid space, venous drainage from the optic nerve head and retina is impaired. This is manifested by papilledema or choked disk. Growth of the mass may also obstruct CSF circulation from the lateral ventricles to the subarachnoid space with resultant hydrocephalus.

Rapid development of any of these situations causes a life-threatening increase in intracranial pressure. Compensatory mechanisms exist and include decreased parenchymal cell numbers, decreased intracellular fluid contents, decreased CSF volume, and decreased intra-

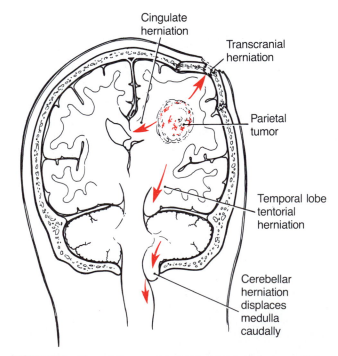

FIGURE 53-4 *Mass shifts associated with a parietal lobe tumor. There is cingulate displacement toward the opposite side. The temporal lobe herniates through the tentorium causing brain stem compression. Cerebellar herniation into the foramen magnum displaces the medulla caudally. Transcranial herniation toward the skull is seen.*

often is an association between intramedullary tumors and syringomyelia.[1]

CLINICAL MANIFESTATIONS

The symptoms produced by intracranial tumors are extremely variable and depend on characteristics of the neoplasm, invasive qualities, location, and rate of growth. Because these tumors eventually give rise to an increase in intracranial pressure, three symptoms may occur: headache, vomiting, and papilledema. Additionally, changes in mental function and seizures often occur as a result of CNS tumors (Table 53-4).

Headache is a common symptom of intracranial tumors. Early in the course of tumor growth, headache is thought to result from local displacement and traction of pain-sensitive structures within the skull—cranial nerves, arteries, veins, and venous sinuses. As the tumor grows, the pain is reflective of generalized increased intracranial pressure. The headache is usually temporary, although it may be severe, dull or sharp, and intermittent. It is usually most severe on awakening and tends to improve throughout the day. Typically, it is aggravated by stooping, coughing, or straining to have a bowel movement. In general, the headache has little localizing value with regard to tumor site.

Vomiting is also experienced by many individuals with intracranial tumors, particularly those who suffer from tumors of the posterior fossa. It is a result of stimulation of the emetic center in the medulla. Vomiting associated with tumors is not necessarily preceded by nausea and is not related to ingestion of food. It often occurs before breakfast and is frequently projectile.

Papilledema may not be present in the early stages of tumor growth but occurs as intracranial pressure increases. In some persons, papilledema does not develop even after the intracranial pressure becomes greatly elevated. Hemorrhages may be seen around the optic disk in association with papilledema. Complaints of blurred vision and halos around lights with enlargement of a blind spot and fleeting moments of dimmed vision (amaurosis fugax) may be elicited.

Local effects of intracranial tumors occur as a result of irritation, destruction, or compression of neural tissue in the location of the tumor. Generally speaking, supratentorial lesions give rise to paralysis, seizures, memory loss, visual field defects, and impairment in consciousness; infratentorial lesions give rise to cranial nerve dysfunction and ataxia.

Frontal lobe tumors cause disturbed mental status, speech disturbances, generalized or focal seizures, hemiparesis, and ataxia. Mental symptoms are manifested by progressive apathy, mild dementia with impairment of memory and intellect, decreased judgment, altered social adaptation, labile emotions, and depression. Aphasia or apraxia may occur if the left or dominant

frontal lobe is affected. Pressure on motor areas produces hemiparesis and may result in jacksonian seizures, which may progress to generalized seizures. The unsteady gait associated with frontal lobe tumors may resemble cerebellar ataxia.

Involvement of the dominant temporal lobe may cause sensory aphasia, which begins with difficulty in naming objects. The person has difficulty comprehending the spoken word and speaks in jargon. Tinnitus occurs as a result of irritation to the adjacent cortex or temporal auditory receptor. Anterior temporal lobe tumors cause visual field changes that may progress to complete hemianopsia. Psychomotor seizures may occur.

Parietal lobe involvement may include motor-sensory focal seizures, agnosia, hypoesthesia (decreased sensitivity to touch), paresthesia, and dyslexia. Visual defects may also occur. Tumors of the parietal lobe in the dominant hemisphere may result in difficulty comprehending language; those in the nondominant hemisphere parietal lobe may interfere with awareness of contralateral body parts.

Involvement of the occipital lobe may produce visual field disturbances in the form of homonymous hemianopsia and quadratic defects. This may be associated with visual agnosia (loss of comprehension of visual sensation) on the dominant side, hallucinations, and convulsive seizures that are preceded by an aura.

Cerebellar tumors produce disturbances in equilibrium and coordination. The specific disorder depends on the location and size of the tumor. Disorders of movement may include nystagmus, adiadochokinesia (inability to make rapid alternative movements), asynergia (incoordination of muscle groups), dysmetria (abnormal force of muscular movements), intention tremor, and deviation from a line of movement. Hypotonia may be present. Speech disturbances may be observed, with tendency toward staccato or scanning speech. Papilledema often occurs with a cerebellar tumor. Cerebellar tumors may exert pressure on the brain stem and result in cranial nerve deficits.

Brain stem involvement produces varied effects. There is increasing paralysis of the cranial nerves, with paralysis of eye movements, loss of facial sensation, and difficulty swallowing. Motor deficits reflect involvement of the descending and ascending motor tracts. Lesions of the hypothalamus may produce diabetes insipidus, obesity, disturbances of temperature regulation, and somnolence. Parinaud syndrome, which is often associated with tumors in the pineal gland or the midbrain, involves impairment of upward gaze and convergent nystagmus.

Clinical manifestations associated with spinal cord tumors depend on the type of lesion and the level at which the lesion occurs (Table 53-5). Generally speaking, a soft, slow-growing mass causes gradual compres-

(text continues on page 1060)

TABLE 53-4 *Intracranial Tumor Syndromes*

Principal Symptoms	Tumor Location	Tumor Types	Principal Symptoms	Tumor Location	Tumor Types
"Dementia"/ personality change	Frontal lobe	Glioblastoma multiforme Anaplastic glioma Astrocytoma Oligodendroglioma Lymphoma Metastasis Meningioma		Leptomeningeal	Acute leukemia Non-Hodgkin lymphoma Carcinoma Sarcoma
	Corpus callosum	Glioblastoma multiforme Anaplastic glioma Astrocytoma Oligodendroglioma Lymphoma	Hemiparesis, hemisensory, hemianopsia	Cerebral hemi-sphere	Glioblastoma multiforme Anaplastic glioma Astrocytoma Oligodendroglioma Lymphoma Metastasis
	Multiple sites	Metastasis Lymphoma	Headache, gait ataxia	Bifrontal/corpus callosum	Glioblastoma multiforme Anaplastic glioma Astrocytoma Oligodendroglioma Lymphoma Meningioma
Headaches, vomit-ing, papilledema	Frontal lobe	Glioblastoma multiforme Anaplastic glioma Astrocytoma Oligodendroglioma Metastasis		Posterior fossa	Medulloblastoma Cerebellar astrocytoma Ependymoma Hemangioblastoma Metastasis
	Temporal lobe (nondominant)	Glioblastoma multiforme Anaplastic glioma Astrocytoma Oligodendroglioma Ganglioglioma Meningioma Metastasis		Leptomeningeal	Acute leukemia Non-Hodgkin lymphoma Carcinoma Sarcoma
	Intraventricular (third, lateral)	Ependymoma Pineal tumors Germ cell tumors Meningioma Choroid plexus papilloma Colloid cyst Craniopharyngioma Neurocytoma	Headache, cranial neuropathy	Subfrontal	Meningioma
				Sellar/suprasellar	Pituitary adenoma Craniopharyngioma Meningioma, Dermoid/Epidermoid Metastasis Optic nerve glioma Chordoma

Location	Tumor types	Clinical features	Location	Tumor types
Posterior fossa	Medulloblastoma Cerebellar astrocytoma Ependymoma Hemangioblastoma Metastasis		Parasellar	Pituitary adenoma Meningioma Metastasis
Cerebellopontine angle	Acoustic neuroma Meningioma Ependymoma Choroid plexus papilloma Dermoid/epidermoid Metastasis Chordoma Paraganglioma Brain-stem glioma	Seizures	Brain stem Cerebral hemisphere	Brain stem glioma Metastasis Glioblastoma multiforme Anaplastic glioma Astrocytoma Oligodendroglioma Lymphoma Metastasis Meningioma
Clivus/base of skull	Chordoma Paraganglioma Meningioma Metastasis Sarcoma (skull)	Parinaud syndrome	Pineal region	Pineal tumor Germ cell tumor Ependymoma Astrocytoma Meningioma Choroid plexus papilloma Metastasis
Leptomeningeal	Acute leukemia Non-Hodgkin lymphoma Carcinoma Sarcoma			
Sellar/suprasellar (Headache, endocrinopathy)	Pituitary adenoma Craniopharyngioma Germ cell tumor Hypothalamic glioma Metastasis			

Kelley, W.N. (ed.). *Textbook of Internal Medicine* (2nd ed.). Philadelphia: J.B. Lippincott, 1992.

TABLE 53-5 *Common Symptoms of Spinal Cord Tumors*

Symptom	Description
Pain in spine, neck, back	Usually gradual in onset; may occur suddenly with sudden movement or injury; aggravated by Valsalva maneuver; nocturnal pain predominates because of recumbency (patient may prefer to sleep upright)
Radicular pain	Occurs in the distribution of segmental innervation; aggravated by movement that alters anatomic relationships; causes diagnostic confusion (T8) root involvement may be misinterpreted as ulcer disease)
Medullary referred pain	Shooting or burning over peripheral areas; often bilateral; not influenced by Valsalva maneuver; appears at different sites
Motor disturbances	Motor deficits are caused by lesions of the pyramidal or corticospinal tracts, causing spasticity and increased reflexes and spastic gait; weakness may present as a limp in the guise of muscle stiffness or rigidity
Nonspecific sensory disturbances	Numbness; tingling; coldness

McQuat, F. The insidious spinal cord tumor. *J. Neurosurg. Nurs.* 13:18, 1981.

sion of the spinal cord with gradually increasing neurologic signs. Malignant and metastatic tumors cause rapid compression of the spinal cord and destruction of the neural tissue.

Extradural tumors usually result from metastasis from primary tumor sites. Local, dull pain is often the first symptom; it is intensified with movements of the spine. Later, because of rapid growth, the spinal cord becomes compressed and severe pain occurs. Early signs of cord compression include loss of joint position sense, loss of vibration sense, and spastic weakness below the level at which the lesion occurs. Without surgical removal of the tumor, irreversible damage may occur, including irreversible paraplegia.

Extramedullary lesions, primarily neurofibromas and meningiomas, are usually benign and early in their growth involve the periphery of the cord. There is pain in the back and along the spinal roots. The pain is worse at night and is aggravated by movement or straining. Posteriorly situated tumors produce sensory losses, including paresthesias and loss of proprioceptive sense. Sensory loss first occurs below the level of the lesion. Anterior compression of the cord causes severe motor dysfunctions. Lateral cord compression may produce the Brown-Sequard syndrome, in which there is ipsilateral motor weakness and deep sensory loss, as well as contralateral loss of pain and temperature perception below the level of the lesion. Early diagnosis and surgical removal produce good prognoses.

Intramedullary tumors tend to be more benign histologically, are slow growing, and have a more benign course than similar intracranial tumors. There is usually a dull, aching pain in the area of the lesion. A dissociated sensory loss occurs in which there is a bilateral loss of pain and temperature sense that extends through all involved segments. However, the senses of touch, motion, position, and vibration are usually preserved. Intramedullary tumors may extend through several spinal cord segments, making surgical removal difficult.

The various levels at which spinal cord tumors may cause compression are the foramen magnum, the cervical region, the thoracic region, the lumbosacral region, and the cauda equina. A summary of signs and symptoms of common root lesions appears in Table 53-6. A tumor in the area of the foramen magnum compresses intracranial contents, nerve roots, and the spinal cord. This causes suboccipital pain. Dermatomes C2 and C3 are compressed, which produces weakness of the head and neck. As the tumor extends into the intracranial cavity, increased pressure is produced, as well as pressure on the cerebellum and cranial nerve nuclei.

Tumors in the cervical region produce motor and sensory losses in the shoulders, arms, and hands. Bicep, tricep, and brachioradial tendon reflexes may be lost, and varying motor and sensory deficits of the upper extremities arise if the lesion occurs in the lower cervical region. High cervical tumors compress the diaphragmatic nerves and result in paralysis of the diaphragm. Thoracic lesions may produce pain and tightness across the chest and abdomen. Lower-extremity paresthesias may develop with the loss of abdominal reflexes if the lesion is in the lower thoracic area. Paralysis of the intercostal muscles results at the involved region.

Upper lumbar lesions cause hip flexion weakness,

lower leg spasticity, loss of knee–jerk reflexes, brisk ankle reflexes, and bilateral Babinski signs. With extensive involvement of the high lumbar cord, movement and sensation are lost in the lower limbs. Sensory deficits result in the area of the perineum. Lower lumbar and upper sacral lesions cause weakness of perineal, calf, and foot muscles. There is often loss of the Achilles reflex. Lower sacral lesions cause sensation losses in the buttocks and perianal area. Bladder and bowel control may be impaired. Lesions in the cauda equina region cause impotence and loss of sphincter control; pain in the sacral and perineal areas often radiates to the legs.

DIAGNOSIS

The first basic step in the diagnosis of CNS tumors is a detailed history and careful neurologic examination. Second, neuroimaging techniques are performed. The computed axial tomography (CT) is the screening procedure of choice because it is noninvasive and nonpainful. It involves the use of a computer which, because of various absorptive characteristics of brain tissue, blood, CSF, cyst fluid, and tumors, can process numerous high-speed films to produce a pictorial print of transverse sections of the body. Magnetic resonance imaging produces views of the brain in successive layers within a powerful magnetic field. Images are clear and more precisely identified than with CT scanning (see p. 964).

Lumbar puncture is rarely indicated but may be performed to examine the CSF. In the presence of tumors, this test usually reveals a normal CSF glucose level, an elevated protein level, and sometimes tumor cells. Because of the danger of brain herniation, lumbar puncture is not performed if there is obvious evidence of increased intracranial pressure. Electroencephalography and nuclear scanning are of little diagnostic value if used alone but support other diagnostic measures. Pneumoencephalography and ventriculography are obsolete tests.

Angiography detects displacement of vessels from their normal position because of tumor growth. It also provides information concerning the intrinsic vasculature of the tumor. The procedure may be useful in planning for surgery, particularly in the presence of vascular tumors.[9]

Evaluation of somatosensory evoked potentials is a neurodiagnostic test used to localize sensory deficits. This test evaluates the functions of sensory pathways from a peripheral nerve to the sensory cortex. The examiner electrically stimulates the relevant nerve and records afferent activity at various levels. Brain tumors may cause delays in sensory pathway conduction as a result of brain tissue compression and abnormal vascularization.[5]

Finally, to make a diagnosis, tumor histology must be determined. This usually requires surgery and examination of tumor tissue.

TABLE 53-6 *Symptoms and Signs of Common Root Lesions*

Root	Location of Pain	Sensory Loss	Reflex Loss	Weakness and Atrophy
C5	Lower neck, tip of shoulder, arm	Deltoid area (inconsistent)	Biceps	Shoulder abductors, biceps
C6	Lower neck, medial scapula, arm, radial side of forearm	Radial side of hand, thumb, index finger	Biceps	Biceps
C7	Lower neck, medial scapula, precordium, arm, forearm	Index finger, middle finger	Triceps	Triceps
C8	Lower neck, medial arm and forearm, ulnar side of hand, fourth and fifth fingers	Ulnar side of hand, fourth and fifth fingers		Intrinsic hand muscles
L4	Low back, anterior and medial thigh	Anterior thigh	Quadriceps	Quadriceps
L5	Low back, lateral thigh, lateral leg, dorsum of foot, great toe	Great toe, medial side of dorsum of foot, lateral leg, and thigh		Toe extensors, ankle dorsiflexors, and evertors
S1	Low back, posterior thigh, posterior leg, lateral side of foot, heel	Lateral foot, heel, posterior leg	Achilles	Ankle dorsiflexion and plantar flexion

Simpson, J., and Magee, K. *Clinical Evaluation of the Nervous System.* Boston: Little, Brown, 1970.

TUMORS OF NEUROEPITHELIAL TISSUE (GLIOMAS)

The glial cells, which provide support and protection for nerve cells, include astrocytes, oligodendroglial cells, and ependymal cells. Gliomas, as a group, comprise 40% to 60% of primary brain tumors in adults.[11] Approximately 8,000 people are diagnosed with gliomas each year in the United States.[8] The tumors are named and classified according to cell type: astrocytomas, oligodendrogliomas, and ependymomas. Gliomas can invade any area of the CNS and are infiltrating by nature. They also may spread from one area of the brain or spinal cord to another.

Astrocytomas

Astrocytomas develop from astrocytes. These spider-shaped or star-shaped cells infiltrate brain tissue and are frequently associated with cysts of various sizes. Their invasive nature usually makes surgical removal difficult. An exception is the pilocytic astrocytoma, which grows in the cerebellum and optic nerve and has a good prognosis after removal.[6]

Astrocytomas have varying degrees of malignancy. Some are well-differentiated and grow slowly for many years but may become more anaplastic over time and are classified as anaplastic astrocytomas and glioblastomas. Gross inspection usually reveals poorly defined, gray-white, infiltrative masses that enlarge and distort underlying CNS tissue. The initial symptom often is a focal or generalized seizure. Headaches, mental disturbances, and signs of increased intracranial pressure may develop several years later.

Other astrocytomas are very poorly differentiated, anaplastic tumors that have a rapid rate of growth. On gross inspection, they are large, infiltrative lesions. The tumor's prognosis is dismal; death occurs within months to a few years after diagnosis.

Glioblastomas

Glioblastomas are extremely malignant, highly vascular tumors that often arise from undifferentiated astrocytomas (Fig. 53-5). The appearance on gross inspection varies according to the region of the brain in which it arises, the degree of necrosis, and the presence of hemorrhage. Glioblastomas grow very rapidly, are invasive, and are resistant to various combinations of surgery, radiotherapy, and chemotherapy. Tissue necrosis and brain edema are characteristic, and prognosis is poor. Ninety percent of those with these tumors die within 2 years after diagnosis.[6] Giant-cell glioblastoma and gliosarcoma are varieties of glioblastoma.[1]

Oligodendrogliomas

Oligodendrogliomas arise from oligodendroglia, which are neuroglia with vinelike processes that are scattered throughout the CNS. The frontal lobe is the most common site for this tumor (40% to 70% of cases).[2] Gross examination usually reveals well-defined, gray, globular masses that may contain cystic foci, calcifications, and hemorrhagic areas.[16] These tumors are similar in behavior to astrocytomas in that they usually grow slowly. However, rapid growth sometimes occurs, and these tumors may imitate the glioblastomas. Differentiation may be made only on histologic examination. Oligo-

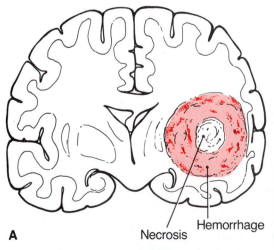
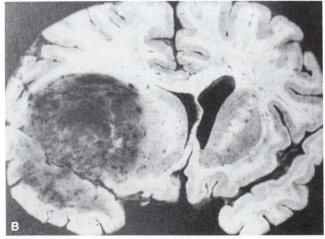

FIGURE 53-5 **A.** *Well-defined tumor compresses adjacent cerebral tissue.* **B.** *Large mass has displaced ventricles and cerebral midline structures. (Source: Adams, J. and Graham, D. An Introduction to Neuropathology [2nd ed.]. London: Churchill-Livingstone, 1994)*

dendrogliomas also have a tendency to form focal calcifications.

Ependymomas

Ependymal cells line the ventricular walls and form the central canal in the spinal cord. These tumors occur more commonly in children and adolescents than in adults.[1] Usually, cranial ependymomas appear as fairly well-defined masses that grow by expansion.[6] Ependymomas tend to form small canals (rosettes) within the tumor. The tumor cells also align themselves around blood vessels (pseudorosettes). Those that arise from ependymal cells lining the walls of the ventricular system fill and obstruct the ventricles and invade adjacent tissue. This can obstruct CSF passage and lead to the development of hydrocephalus. The most common site of ependymomas is the fourth ventricle.

Ependymomas that arise within the spinal cord represent a large percentage of intraspinal gliomas. Symptoms are related to the spinal level at which they occur. The location of these tumors often makes them inaccessible to removal by surgery. Even though they grow slowly, the prognosis is poor and death occurs within a few years.

Variants of ependymomas include subependymomas and myxopapillary ependymomas. Subependymomas arise from neuroglial tissue beneath the ependymal lining and are composed of astrocytic and ependymal elements. These small, hard, lobular tumors rarely grow large enough to cause symptoms. Myxopapillary ependymomas are composed mostly of ependymal cells arising almost exclusively in the filum terminale.

Pineal Cell Tumors

Pinealomas are rare tumors composed of large epithelial cells present in the adult pineal gland. Cell differentiation divides pinealomas into pinealocytomas and pinealoblastomas. Pinealomas cause symptoms by compressing the aqueduct of Sylvius, which causes hydrocephalus and increased intracranial pressure. Treatment may include a combination of surgery, atrioventricular shunt, and radiotherapy. Choroid plexus papillomas are rare tumors that occur primarily in children. Gross inspection reveals well-defined, cauliflower-like, papillary masses that often protrude into the fourth ventricle.[7, 16] Although histologically benign, they may cause intraventricular bleeding, papilledema, hydrocephalus, and increased intracranial pressure. Treatment includes surgery followed by radiotherapy.

TUMORS OF NEURONAL ORIGIN

Cerebral neuroblastomas arise in precursor cells of neurons. Gross examination reveals well-defined, gray, granular masses that may contain areas of necrosis, hemorrhage, and cysts.[6] Neuroblastomas are rare and usually occur during the first decade of life. Their rate of growth is rapid, and they commonly recur after surgery.

Gangliogliomas are very rare tumors composed of neuroglial tissue. Gross inspection reveals well-defined masses with granular surfaces. Calcifications and small cysts may be present within the mass. These tumors are most common in children and young adults. If the location permits surgical excision, the prognosis is good.

TUMORS OF EMBRYONIC ORIGIN

Medulloblastomas arise predominantly from primitive cells in the cerebellum. They have the potential to develop along neuronal or neuroglial lines. Gross inspection usually reveals fairly well-demarcated, gray-white masses with indistinct edges.[6] Medulloblastomas occur almost exclusively in children and account for approximately 20% of pediatric brain tumors.[13] This tumor type has been found in adults in rare situations up to the sixth decade of life. They most frequently affect males. They are highly malignant, grow rapidly, and infiltrate throughout the subarachnoid space with resultant widespread meningeal foci. The CSF pathways become blocked, and signs of increased intracranial pressure develop. These tumors are associated with increasing ataxia, headaches, and forceful vomiting. The prognosis is dismal, but combinations of surgery, radiotherapy, and chemotherapy can prolong survival.

TUMORS OF THE MENINGES

Meningiomas are primary tumors arising from the meninges (Fig. 53-6). They are most common in females and occur usually in the seventh decade of life.[16] These tumors make up approximately 15% of all primary intra-

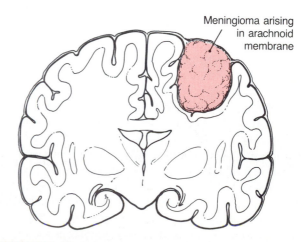

Meningioma arising in arachnoid membrane

FIGURE 53-6 *Meningioma.*

cranial tumors.[1] Meningeal constituents that may be involved include arachnoid cells, fibroblasts, and blood vessels. Gross inspection tends to reveal tough, gray-white, irregular to round, lobular masses.[6] Meningiomas are quite vascular and are seen readily on radioisotope scans. They are usually well-circumscribed and encapsulated and press into surrounding tissue. The tumors may penetrate adjacent bone, but widespread infiltration of surrounding nervous tissue is not common. Most of these tumors are benign and grow slowly, so that initial symptoms may be overlooked. As they continue to grow, symptoms include seizures, headache, visual impairment, hemiparesis, and aphasia. If they are diagnosed early and are in an area accessible to surgery, complete excision is possible and a good prognosis results. There is a 20% recurrence rate if these tumors are not completely resected.[15] Prognosis of meningiomas largely depends on the location of the tumor.[7]

TUMORS OF THE PITUITARY GLAND

Pituitary adenomas are a special group of nervous system tumors that produce neurologic signs and symptoms if they put pressure on the hypothalamus, optic chiasm, third ventricle, or medial temporal lobe. The initial symptoms are hormonal disturbances or visual field defects. Table 53-7 presents hormonal tests for the detection of pituitary tumors. These tumors arise from the three cell types in the anterior pituitary: basophil cells, which stain blue; eosinophil cells, which stain red; and chromophobe cells, which do not stain. Although pituitary tumors have usually been classified according to cell type, it is more accurate to identify them as functioning (secreting a hormone) or nonfunctioning (nonsecreting). However, they usually contain a predominant cell type. Most often, the chromophobe cells give rise to these tumors (see p. 693). Prognosis depends on the success of treatment, which may include irradiation, hypophysectomy, or hormone replacement. Treatment is considerably more successful if the tumor is still confined to the sella.

Adrenocorticotropic hormone–producing pituitary adenomas are primarily composed of basophil cells and are usually so small that adjacent tissue is not compressed. They have powerful effects, however, because of hypersecretion of adrenocorticotropic hormone, which is one of several mechanisms that produce Cushing syndrome. Symptoms of Cushing syndrome include weakness, emotional lability, moon face, obesity of the torso, hypertension, salt and water retention, diabetes mellitus, glycosuria, osteoporosis, skin striae over the abdomen, hirsutism, and amenorrhea (see pp. 701–702).

Pituitary adenomas inducing gigantism and acromegaly are primarily composed of acidophilic cells; they are

small and rather slow-growing. They cause an increase in the output of growth hormone. If they develop before bone growth is complete, gigantism results. Tumor development after bone growth has stopped produces the clinical picture called *acromegaly*. These adenomas may grow to such size that they press on the optic chiasm, causing complete or partial bitemporal hemianopsia or other visual disturbances.

Nonsecreting pituitary adenomas are the most common pituitary tumors and are composed primarily of chromophobe cells. Although these cells have no known special function, tumors arising from them are rather large and produce symptoms by compressing the pituitary gland, optic chiasm, hypothalamus, and adjacent brain tissue. These tumors usually produce hypopituitarism. Signs and symptoms include a sallow ap-

TABLE 53-7 *Hormonal Tests for Detection of Pituitary Adenomas*

Hormone	Test
Prolactin	Serum prolactin level Chlorpromazine- or TRH-provocative tests L-dopa suppression
Somatotropin	Serum GH level Glucagon L-dopa Glucose suppression Somatomicid C
Adrenocorticotropin	Serum cortisol Urinary steroids Metyrapone test Dexamethasone suppression
Gonadotropin	Serum FSH LH Estradiol Testosterone GnRH stimulation
Thyrotropin	TSH T_4 TRH
Vasopressin	Urine and serum osmolality after water restriction for deficiency of hormone; without water restriction for excess of hormone

BUN, blood urea nitrogen; FSH, follicle-stimulating hormone; GH, growth hormone; GnRH, gonadotropin-releasing hormone; LH, luteinizing hormone; T_4, thyroxine; TRH, thyrotropin-releasing hormone; TSH, thyroid-stimulating hormone.

Adams, R., and Victor, J.M. *Principles of Neurology* (5th ed.). New York: McGraw-Hill, 1993.

pearance, loss of body hair, weakness, amenorrhea, loss of sexual desire, low basal metabolism, hypoglycemia, hypotension, and electrolyte disturbances. As the tumor presses on the optic chiasm, bitemporal hemianopsia is produced and blindness may result (see pp. 692–693).

TUMORS OF THE CRANIAL AND PERIPHERAL NERVES AND NERVE ROOTS

Neurilemomas (schwannomas) and neurofibromas arise from cells that ensheath cranial nerves, peripheral nerves, cauda equina, and nerve roots. The three types of cells within the nerve sheaths are *Schwann cells, perineural cells,* and *fibroblasts* in the epineurium and endoneurium. Although the three cells are similar morphologically, Schwann cells are usually the primary source of tumors.

Neurilemmomas are tumors that arise from the Schwann cells and occur on any of the nerves or nerve roots. The tumors are firm, circumscribed, well-encapsulated, and white to gray.[5] Many lesions may be present on the same nerve or throughout the body. They often involve the vestibulocochlear division of the acoustic (eighth) cranial nerve (acoustic neuroma), most frequently at the cerebellopontile angle, or where the acoustic nerve enters the internal auditory meatus. Bilateral involvement of the acoustic nerve occurs in von Recklinghausen neurofibromatosis, type 2.

Acoustic neuromas produce the following symptoms because of position or disruption in function: impaired hearing; tinnitus; vertigo; balance and coordination difficulties; ataxia; loss of caloric vestibular reactivity with horizontal nystagmus; palsies of the third, fifth, and seventh cranial nerves; and signs of increased intracranial pressure as the normal flow of CSF is obstructed. Complete surgical removal is usually attempted to prevent recurrence of the tumor, but this often produces cranial nerve dysfunctions, such as deafness or facial paralysis.

Neurofibromas arise primarily from Schwann cells and fibroblasts and generally tend to be multiple and encapsulated. Gross examination reveals enlargement of the affected nerve or nerve root. Numerous tumors are often present, especially in association with the hereditary disease, von Recklinghausen neurofibromatosis.

PRIMARY LYMPHOMA AND BLOOD VESSEL TUMORS

Hemangioblastomas are neoplasms made up of an aggregation of blood vessels that may also be cystic. These arise most commonly in the cerebellum but may occur in the cerebrum. Symptoms include ataxia, dizziness, and signs of increased intracranial pressure. Because erythropoietin is often secreted from these tumors, polycythemia may be exhibited. If the cerebellar cyst can be opened and the hemangioblastomatous nodule excised, the prognosis is good. A combination of cerebellar hemangioblastoma in association with cysts of the kidneys and pancreas, together with angiomatosis of the retinae, is known as *von Hippel–Lindau syndrome*. This disease is inherited as a dominant trait.[7]

OTHER TUMORS AND TUMORLIKE LESIONS

Dermoids

Dermoids may occur anywhere in the CNS but frequently arise in the ventricular system. They may obstruct the third ventricle, the aqueduct of Sylvius, or the fourth ventricle. Dermoids contain skin appendages and are often accompanied by overlying bone and skin defects.

Craniopharyngiomas (Rathke Pouch Tumors)

Craniopharyngiomas are tumors derived from the Rathke pouch, a pouch in the embryonic membrane that develops into the anterior lobe of the pituitary. They are most often located above the sella turcica. This tumor is encapsulated and grows as a solid mass or, more often, as a cyst. The cyst often contains thick, brown, oily fluid and often has some degree of calcification. Rupture of the cystic fluid into the subarachnoid space may cause recurrent bouts of "sterile" meningitis or, in some cases, bacterial meningitis. As the craniopharyngioma grows, pressure is applied to the pituitary gland, the optic chiasm, and, sometimes, the base of the brain. Erosion of the sella wall may occur. Symptoms most commonly occur in children and young adults and reflect signs and symptoms of pituitary hypofunction, hydrocephalus, visual disturbances, and diabetes insipidus. Surgical removal is possible if the site is accessible.

Arteriovenous Malformations

These malformations consist of abnormal collections of blood vessels in which arteries join veins directly rather than through capillaries. The majority of angiomas are in the posterior half of the cerebral hemispheres. The abnormal vessels are present at birth and enlarge with the passage of time. Symptoms may not occur for years, although manifestations are often noted between 10 and 30 years of age. As the vessels grow, they may compress the normal brain, and weak walls may bleed into the cerebral or subarachnoid spaces. Mortality associated with the first hemorrhage is about 10%.[16] Recurrence of hemorrhage is a constant danger, and various modes of treatment have been used. Symptoms vary according to the region of involvement and the size of the malformation. In some cases, there are no clinical symptoms and the malformation is found only on autopsy.

GERM CELL TUMORS

Germinomas are the most common germ cell tumors usually found in the pineal and hypothalamic region. Teratomas, which are more common in children, are rare germ cell tumors found in the pineal region. As a result of embryonic displacement, the more differentiated teratomas may contain cartilage and bone.

CHORDOMAS

Chordomas are rare, congenital, malignant tumors that are derived from remnants of the primitive notochord. They are jellylike, gray-pink growths and grow near the sella turcica, at the base of the brain, or in the cervical or the sacrococcygeal areas. These tumors erode the bone and invade the dura. Total surgical removal is impossible because of their highly invasive nature. Symptoms of congenital tumors usually develop within the first 10 years of life and depend on the size and location of the lesion.

METASTATIC TUMORS

Metastases most commonly occur from primary sites in the lungs (45%) and breast (20%), but neoplasms of the gastrointestinal tract, genitourinary tract, bone, thyroid gland, and nasal sinuses can also metastasize to the brain and spinal cord.[7] Metastatic tumors are usually solid, circumscribed masses that are surrounded by vasogenic edema. They may be solitary tumors or multiple small masses scattered throughout the CNS. Signs and symptoms vary with the location, size, and number of lesions. Intracranial metastases most often appear in individuals who already have symptoms of far-advanced cancers, but occasionally they produce the initial symptoms. Even with combinations of surgery, radiotherapy, and chemotherapy, prognosis is poor.

▼ *Infections*

GENERAL CONSIDERATIONS

Central nervous system tissue is not immune to viral, bacterial, or other infections. The infections usually arise initially in another region of the body. Organisms can

---

CASE STUDY 53-1

Mrs. M is a 35-year-old teacher who is married and has one child. She has enjoyed good health except for having a tonscillectomy at age 8. Mrs. M began experiencing early morning headaches about 6 months before her initial visit to her family physician. Episodes of nausea and vomiting prompted Mrs. M's visit. During her check-up, Mrs. M stated that she thought she was losing her mind because her husband had been noticing a difficulty in her ability to name objects and had complained about her irritability and mood swings. Also, she had noticed ringing in her right ear. Mrs. M was scheduled for further neurologic testing. While awaiting the tests, she had a seizure.

Mrs. M was given a detailed neurologic examination that revealed the presence of papilledema. Also, neuroimaging studies were performed. The results of a computed axial tomography scan revealed a poorly demarcated mass causing expansion of the right temporal lobe. Magnetic resonance imaging confirmed these results and additionally revealed the presence of cerebral edema. Eventually Mrs M was diagnosed with astrocytoma.

1. *What type of brain tumor is an astrocytoma?*
2. *Isn't Mrs. M too young to have an astrocytoma?*
3. *Is Mrs. M exhibiting symptoms of a brain tumor?*
4. *Why are computed tomography and magnetic resonance imaging useful techniques for diagnosis of a brain tumor?*
5. *What is the treatment and prognosis for Mrs. M?*

See Appendix G for discussion.

---

gain access to the CNS in several ways: 1) by spread from adjacent structures, such as nasal sinuses, skull, or middle ear; 2) by entrance through penetrating wounds; and 3) through the bloodstream. After infectious organisms enter the CNS, they can spread rapidly by way of the CSF, leading to widespread, devastating results. There are six potential sites for CNS infections: bone, extradural space, subdural space, subarachnoid space, intracerebral areas, and intraventricular sites (Fig. 53-7). Diagnosis of any CNS infections depends on evidence of the infective organism, together with changes in pressure, glucose level, and protein level in the CSF. Magnetic resonance imaging may provide evidence of focal inflammatory disease. The CNS alterations and clinical manifestations vary according to the type of infection.

VIRAL INFECTIONS

Viruses may gain access to the body orally, through the respiratory system, by animal or mosquito bites, or across the placenta to the fetus. Once inside the body,

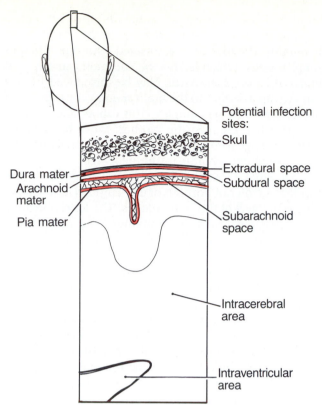

FIGURE 53-7 *There are six potential sites for CNS infections: bone (skull), extradural space, subdural space, subarachnoid space, intracerebral area, intraventricular area.*

they make their way to the CNS through the hematogenous route by the cerebral capillaries and the choroid plexus. Other entry routes include the peripheral nerves and, possibly, penetration of the olfactory mucosa.[2] Within the CNS, viruses apparently affect specific, susceptible cells, and the pathologic effects are considerably different. Damage to the CNS may be caused by direct viral invasion of cells with subsequent lysis (acute encephalitis); by selective lysis with resulting demyelination (progressive multifocal leukoencephalopathy); by immune responses to viral antigens (acute disseminated encephalomyelitis); and, in some cases, by cellular destruction without apparent inflammatory or immune response. Viruses can also remain latent in cells for months or years until circumstances trigger acute infections (see pp. 278–282). Innumerable viruses are known to invade the nervous system, and only a representative sample of the most frequently encountered viruses is presented in the following section.

Acute Encephalitis

Encephalitis is a general term that encompasses infections of the brain parenchyma in which a wide range of symp-

toms is manifested. Although encephalitis may be caused by bacteria, rickettsia, parasites, or fungi, viral infections are most common. Presented in Box 53-1 are a variety of causes of viral encephalitis and virus-related acute encephalopathies. Symptoms include headache, high fever, confusion, convulsions, and restlessness that progresses to stupor and coma. There may also be focal CNS impairments, such as hemiparesis, asymmetry of tendon reflexes, Babinski sign, involuntary movements, ataxia, and difficulty in speaking or understanding. Brain stem involvement may be manifested by facial weakness or ocular palsies. Analysis of CSF usually reveals increased numbers of lymphocytes, normal to slightly increased pressure, slightly increased protein level, normal glucose level, and normal chloride level. A comatose state may persist for days, weeks, or months after the acute infection. Residual effects may include behavior and personality changes, mental deterioration, parkinsonism, paralysis, and persistent seizures. The

---

BOX 53-1 ▼ Causes of Viral Encephalitis and Virus-Related Acute Encephalopathies

Viral encephalitis
  Sporadic
    Mumps
    Herpes simplex viruses
    Lymphocytic choriomeningitis virus
    Cytomegalovirus
    Epstein–Barr virus
    Adenovirus
    Rabies
  Epidemic
    Arboviruses (St. Louis, Eastern, Western, California, Venezuelan equine, Colorado tick fever)
    Enteroviruses (coxsackievirus and echoviruses)
Postinfectious encephalomyelitis
  Measles
    Varicella
    Mumps
    Rubella
    Influenza
  Viral infections in immunocompromised patients
    Cytomegalovirus
    Herpes simplex viruses
    Enteroviruses
    Adenoviruses
    Measles
    JC virus (progressive multifocal leukoencephalopathy)
    Human immunodeficiency viruses (HIV)
  Virus-associated encephalopathy
    Reye syndrome

Weiner, L.P. Viral encephalitis. In Johnson, R.T. (ed.), *Current Therapy in Neurologic Disease 3.* Philadelphia: B.C. Decker, 1990.

specific signs and symptoms that predominate depend on the causative organism. A wide variety of viruses cause encephalitis, and a discussion of the more common ones follows.

ARTHROPOD-BORNE VIRAL ENCEPHALITIS. The large group of viruses called *arboviruses*, after their arthropod vectors, commonly cause encephalitis. The organisms seem to occur in certain geographic locations and during certain seasons, especially in summer and early fall, when mosquitoes are biting. Except for tick-borne arboviruses, all of these viruses have vertebrate hosts with mosquito vectors. The principal site of infection in humans is the brain parenchyma. Clinical manifestations of the different arboviruses are similar; however, they may vary with age of the afflicted person. For example, onset of fever and convulsions is most abrupt in children.

Eastern equine encephalitis, occurring primarily in the eastern United States, is an infrequent cause of encephalitis. It is the most serious of the arboviruses because it causes extensive destruction of the cerebral cortex and white matter. In about 1 of every 19 affected persons there is clinical evidence of encephalitis caused by this virus, and among those persons, mortality is close to 80%.[6] Those who survive often have residual effects that include blindness, deafness, mental retardation, emotional disorders, and hemiplegia. The greatest change in CSF is the presence of large numbers of polymorphonuclear leukocytes.

Western equine encephalitis may involve the upper spinal cord as well as large portions of the brain. It is most common in the western region of the United States. Fever, stupor, dizziness, confusion, and headache are common symptoms. Mortality is lower than with eastern equine encephalitis. Postencephalitic parkinsonism is a common sequela of this type of encephalitis.

St. Louis encephalitis is a milder form of the disease and may involve both the brain and spinal cord. It occurs primarily in the central and western United States. Prominent meningeal involvement accompanies St. Louis encephalitis. Other findings include fever, athetosis, drowsiness or stupor, tremors, and, more commonly, seizures. Any age group may develop this infection, and recovery is usually good.

California encephalitis affects children more frequently than adults. Its onset is insidious, and its signs include headache, fever, vomiting, mental confusion, seizures, and stupor that may deteriorate to coma. Although recovery from the acute episode is common, residual learning difficulties, emotional lability, and seizures may remain as long-term problems.

HERPES SIMPLEX. Herpes simplex virus is the cause of a very serious and common form of encephalitis that can produce illness in any age group. This type of encephalitis has been reported in all parts of the world. Most frequently, the disease is associated with type I herpes simplex virus, which is also the common cause of oral mucosal lesions. The virus may be introduced from a primary lip infection to the brain stem by the trigeminal nerve. Type II herpes simplex virus causes genital infection. If it is present in the mother, it can be acquired during passage through an infected birth canal and produces acute encephalitis in the neonate.[2]

Alterations in the CNS are more common in the medial and inferior portions of the temporal lobes and in the orbital gyri of the frontal lobes. The lesions include hemorrhagic necrosis, inflammation, and perivascular infiltrates (Fig. 53-8). The CSF reveals increased pressure, increased protein level, increased number of lymphocytes, and the presence of red cells because of the hemorrhagic nature of the lesions. Serologic tests and brain biopsy confirm a diagnosis of herpes simplex encephalitis. Clinical manifestations include acute onset with headache, fever, convulsions, confusion, stupor, and coma, in addition to focal disturbances related to lesions in specific portions of the temporal and frontal lobes. After a diagnosis of herpes simplex virus is made, treatment with acyclovir is instituted.[18]

RABIES. Clinical cases of rabies in human beings are rare, but if the disease becomes established, it is almost always fatal. This dreaded viral disease can affect anyone who has sustained a bite through the skin by a rabid animal (usually dogs, cats, bats, foxes, raccoons, or skunks). Its incubation period varies from 14 days to 3 months. Survival of inoculated victims depends on specific postexposure prophylaxis.

The virus makes its way from the wound to the CNS through the peripheral nerves, producing degenerative changes in these neurons. Alterations in the CNS include brain edema, neuron degeneration, and vascular congestion. Inflammatory reactions seem to be greatest in the basal nuclei, midbrain, and medulla. The spinal cord, sympathetic ganglia, and dorsal root ganglia may also be involved. Negri bodies, which are oval-shaped, eosinophilic, cytoplasmic inclusions, are a characteristic histologic feature of rabies.

Clinical manifestations occur in stages, beginning with generalized malaise, apathy, fever, and headache. These general symptoms, together with pain and numbness in the area of the wound, are diagnostic of the illness in its early stage. Within 24 to 72 hours, an excitement phase occurs. It is marked by extreme fear, violent spasms of the larynx when swallowing that lead to hydrophobia, and dysphagia, which leads to salivation with frothing from the mouth. Heightened sensitivity to external stimuli can produce localized twitching and generalized seizures. Facial numbness, dysarthria,

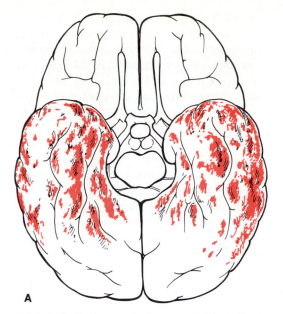
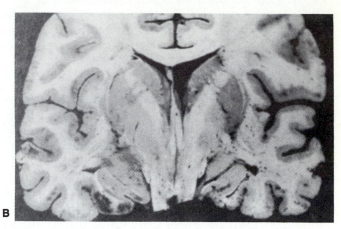

FIGURE 53-8 *Herpes simplex encephalitis.* **A.** *The temporal lobes are preferentially involved by a hemorrhagic, necrotizing inflammation.* **B.** *Infiltration seen throughout white matter. (Adams, J. and Graham, D. An Introduction to Neuropathology [2nd ed.]. London: Churchill-Livingstone, 1994)*

hallucinations, and a confusional psychosis accompany this phase. Finally, there are alternating periods of stupor and mania, high fever, flaccid paralysis, coma, and respiratory failure. Death usually occurs from respiratory center failure within 2 to 7 days after the onset of neurologic symptoms.

Slow Virus Diseases

Unlike the acute encephalitides, the slow virus diseases go through a long latent period, lasting from months to years, before they manifest symptoms. After symptoms have appeared, these diseases tend to progress at a slower pace. Two general types of slow infections exist: 1) true slow virus infections, including subacute sclerosing panencephalitis, progressive multifocal leukoencephalopathy, and progressive rubella panencephalitis; and 2) unconventional agent infections (spongiform encephalopathies), which include Creutzfeldt-Jakob disease and kuru.[1] The former are caused by known, conventional viruses; the latter are caused by still unidentified agents that have some resemblance to viruses but do not produce an immune reaction in the host.

SUBACUTE SCLEROSING PANENCEPHALITIS. This illness usually occurs in children and is related to a prior infection by the measles virus. Granular regions, areas of focal destruction, and proliferation of neuroglial cells are present in the CNS. The CSF reveals an increased protein level, an increased gamma globulin fraction, and a high level of measles antibody. There is also evidence of measles antigen in neurons and glial cells. Bursts of high-voltage and sharp waves are noted on electroenceph alographic examination. The illness occurs in stages over several years. Initially, personality changes occur; intellectual deterioration, seizures, ataxia, and visual disturbances follow; and finally, rigidity, progressive unresponsiveness, and signs of autonomic dysfunction cause death within a few months or 1 to 3 years.

PROGRESSIVE MULTIFOCAL LEUKOENCEPHALOPATHY. This condition most often occurs in middle-aged persons who have chronic debilitating diseases such as rheumatoid arthritis, acquired immune deficiency syndrome (AIDS), or neoplastic disease, and in those who are receiving immunosuppressive therapy. Opportunistic viruses, such as Creutzfeldt-Jakob virus or simian virus 40, cause CNS alterations, including widespread demyelinization of white matter, particularly of the cerebral hemispheres, the brain stem, the cerebellum, and, rarely, the spinal cord. The CSF usually remains normal. Diagnosis of lesions may be facilitated by CT scanning.[2] Symptoms of progressive multifocal leukoencephalopathy include hemiparesis, visual field defects, aphasia, ataxia, dysarthria, confusion, and eventually coma. Death occurs within 3 to 20 months after onset of symptoms.

PROGRESSIVE RUBELLA PANENCEPHALITIS. This type of encephalitis, associated with rubella of either congenital or childhood origin, appears after a long latent period and continues on a progressive course. Initial symptoms are subtle changes in behavior and intellectual performance. Seizures arise in association with progressive mental deterioration, motor incoordination, and spasticity; mutism, quadriplegia, and ophthalmoplegia mark the terminal stages of the disease. Progressive rubella panencephalitis seems to affect the white matter primarily, destroying nerve cells and attracting lymphocytes and mononuclear cells.

SUBACUTE SPONGIFORM ENCEPHALOPATHY. Subacute spongiform encephalopathy, also known as Creutzfeldt-Jakob disease or transmissible viral dementia, is a rare, rapidly progressive disease that usually occurs in late middle age. It produces CNS alterations mainly in the cerebral and cerebellar cortices and occasionally in the basal ganglia. Alterations include neural degeneration, gliosis, and a spongelike condition in affected areas. Although serologic studies and CSF are normal, there is usually an associated, distinctive electroencephalographic pattern of diffuse nonspecific slowing, which changes to sharp waves or spikes on an increasingly flat background.[2]

The early clinical manifestations include personality changes, memory loss, visual abnormalities (distortions of shape, decreased visual acuity), and delirium. These symptoms are followed rapidly by dementia, myoclonic contractions, dysarthria, and ataxia, which eventually give way to stupor and coma, although myoclonic contractions continue. To date there is no effective treatment. Death usually occurs within 1 to 2 years after onset of symptoms.

KURU. Kuru, the first slow viral infection documented in humans, occurs in the Fore natives of Papua, New Guinea. The disease is associated with cannibalism in this tribe. Although the CNS alterations are similar to those associated with subacute spongiform encephalopathy, in kuru the spongelike conditions are more prominent in the corpus striatum and cerebellum.[18] Clinical manifestations include progressive cerebellar ataxia, shivering tremors, abnormal extraocular movement, incontinence, progression to complete immobility, and dementia in the terminal stage. After the onset of symptoms, death usually occurs within 3 to 6 months.

Human Immunodeficiency Virus Type 1

All parts of the CNS may be involved in the course of infection by the human immunodeficiency virus type 1 (HIV-1). One or more neurologic syndromes have been reported in approximately 40% of persons who have AIDS (see pp. 336–346).[4] Neurologic complaints are the initial symptoms in 10% of all AIDS patients. Nervous system involvement may result from primary HIV infection, secondary to immunosuppression, or both. The major neurologic complications associated with HIV-1 infection are presented in Table 53-8.

DIRECT NEUROLOGIC EFFECTS OF HIV-1. People initially infected with the HIV-1 virus may develop *acute aseptic meningitis* as a result of CNS response to viral invasion. A mild lymphocytic pleocytosis and modest CSF protein elevation may occur.[1] Clinical manifestations include headache, cranial neuropathies, and symptoms associated with meningeal irritation and transient encephalopathies.

HIV-1 encephalopathy and *encephalitis* have been described as the most common neurologic pathologies associated with AIDS. One-third of AIDS patients develop these conditions early in the course of the disease, and two-thirds develop them late in the illness.[2] Also known as *AIDS dementia complex*, HIV encephalopathy occurs as a result of direct HIV invasion of the CNS through infected macrophages or through the blood-brain barrier by endothelial cells.[4] CT scan or magnetic resonance imaging reveals mild to moderate brain atrophy and white matter changes (Fig. 53-9). Examination of CSF reveals pleocytosis and an elevated protein level. Many microscopic changes have been described in HIV dementia.

TABLE 53-8 *Major Neurologic Complications of HIV-1 Infection*

Direct Effects of HIV-1	Opportunistic Processes
Acute aseptic meningitis	Cryptococcal meningitis*
Chronic pleocytosis	Toxoplasmosis*
HIV-1 encephalopathy*	CMV retinitis/encephalitis*
Vacuolar myelopathy	Other CNS opportunistic infections*
Predominantly sensory neuropathy	Herpes group radiculitis
Inflammatory demyelinating polyneuropathy	Progressive multifocal leukoencephalopathy*
Mononeuritis multiplex	Primary CNS lymphoma*
Myopathy	Systemic lymphoma*
	Neurosyphilis

* AIDS-defining condition.

AIDS, acquired immunodeficiency syndrome; *CNS*, central nervous system; *CMV*, cytomegalovirus; *HIV*, human immunodeficiency virus.

McArthur, J. Neurologic diseases associated with HIV-1 infection. In Johnson, R.T. (ed.), *Current Therapy in Neurologic Disease 3.* Philadelphia: B.C. Decker, 1990.

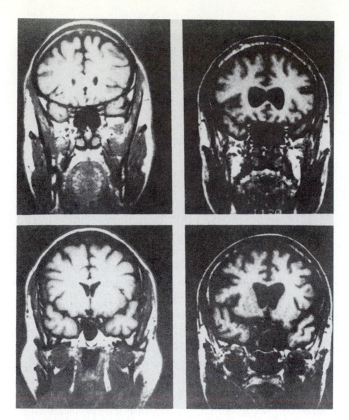

FIGURE 53-9 *Atrophy in HIV dementia: MRI. Patient with severe HIV dementia showing central and cortical atrophy on the right with age-matched control on the left. (Source: Appel, S. Current Neurology. St. Louis: C. V. Mosby, 1994).*

Recommended terminology for HIV-associated CNS neuropathy is presented in Table 53-9. The correlation between pathologic changes and the clinical features of progressive dementia in AIDS remains somewhat unclear.[12]

In adults, clinical manifestations include progressive dementia with memory loss, disorientation, intellectual impairment, mood changes, psychotic behavior, leg weakness, seizures, and headache. In infants and children, manifestations of HIV encephalopathy include developmental delays, cognitive deterioration, corticospinal tract signs, or microencephaly. Temporary improvement in dementia may occur with administration of zidovudine. However, there is rarely improvement in persons with far-advanced dementia.[12]

OPPORTUNISTIC PROCESSES OF THE CNS ASSOCIATED WITH HIV-1. A number of opportunistic processes involving the CNS affect AIDS patients (see Table 53-8). These processes reflect the underlying immune deficiency produced by HIV and destruction of CD4 lymphocytes by this virus. During the course of the AIDS illness, multiple opportunistic processes may occur concurrently, complicating diagnosis and treatment.

The most common and treatable intracranial focal complication is *cerebral toxoplasmosis*. The obligate intracellular protozoan, *Toxoplasma gondii*, produces multiple inflammatory and necrotic abscesses throughout the cerebral hemispheres, especially in the basal ganglia.

TABLE 53-9 *Recommended Terminology for HIV-Associated CNS Disease*

New Name	Old Name	Definition
HIV encephalitis	Giant cell encephalitis, multi-nucleated cell encephalitis, sub-acute encephalitis	Multiple disseminated foci of microglia, macrophages, MNGCs. If MNGCs not present, HIV antigen or nucleic acids demonstrated by immunocytochemistry or in situ hybridization
HIV leukoencephalopathy	Diffuse myelin pallor, progressive diffuse leukoencephalopathy	Diffuse damage to white matter with myelin loss, reactive astrogliosis, macrophages and MNGCs, or detectable HIV antigen or nucleic acids
Diffuse poliodystrophy	Subacute encephalitis	Diffuse reactive astrogliosis and microglial activation involving cerebral gray matter. NOTE: This term designates diffuse pathology of cortical and subcortical gray matter structures that may underlie neuronal loss or changes in synaptic or dendritic anatomy
Vacuolar myelopathy	Vacuolar myelopathy	Multiple areas of spinal cord involved by vacuolar myelin changes with intravacuole macrophages

CNS, central nervous system; *HIV*, human immunodeficiency virus; *MNGC*, multinucleated giant cells.
McArthur, J., and Harrison, M. HIV-Asociated dementia. In Appel, S. (ed.), *Current Neurology*, St. Louis: Mosby, 1994.

These abnormalities are revealed on CT and magnetic resonance imaging studies. CSF reveals an elevated protein level, a decreased glucose level, and pleocytosis. Long-term suppressive therapy is required with clindamycin and pyrimethamine.

Cryptococcus neoformans, a yeast, is the most common fungal infection, affecting the CNS in 6% to 11% of AIDS patients.[4] Clinical manifestations are typical of meningitis symptoms and include headache, neck stiffness, fever, altered mentation, and nausea. Actual culture isolation of the cryptococci may be possible from the CSF. Treatment with flucytosine and itraconazole has shown promise as primary therapy and for maintenance.

Encephalitis in AIDS patients can also be produced by *cytomegalovirus* (CMV) and *human papovavirus*, which cause progressive multifocal leukoencephalopathy. Cytomegalovirus causes infection in the retina and visual loss in 20% of AIDS patients.[12] Progressive multifocal leukoencephalopathy is evident initially as a progressive accumulation of focal neurologic deficits; this complication develops in approximately 2% of people with AIDS.

Additional opportunistic infections include *herpes zoster* and *neurosyphilis*. Herpes zoster radiculitis occurs in 5% to 10% of AIDS patients.[1] Treatment may not be required unless cervical or lumbar dermatomes are involved and produce severe myeloradiculitis with permanent motor deficits. Although neurosyphilis is not strictly an opportunistic infection, it has been suggested that the course of syphilis is accelerated in AIDS patients.[12] Also, there appears to be an increase in the frequency of syphilitic meningitis and of meningovascular syphilis in AIDS patients.

It has been suggested that, in addition to opportunistic infections, primary CNS lymphomas develop in 5% of AIDS patients. Unifocal or multifocal lesions are present on CT scans. Clinical manifestations include focal neurologic dysfunction with dementia, confusion, or lethargy. Radiotherapy is used to reduce tumor size and manage symptoms.

Aseptic Meningitis Complex (Benign Viral Meningitis)

Aseptic meningitis complex, or benign viral meningitis, is a general name for disorders in which there is evidence of meningeal irritation although pyogenic organisms, parasites, or fungi are not present in the CSF. Lymphocytes are commonly present in the CSF in people with aseptic meningitis. A virus is thought to be the causative agent, and the following viruses have been found in more than one-third of the persons with aseptic meningitis complex: mumps, herpes simplex, coxsackievirus, lymphocytic choriomeningitis virus, and ECHO virus. It has also been recognized that HIV may produce an acute aseptic meningitis with an infectious mononucleosis-like clinical picture.[2] The symptoms are mild, and most patients recover from these illnesses without significant residual effects.

Viruses Acquired Congenitally

Viruses are capable of crossing the placenta to reach the fetus, especially during the first trimester of pregnancy. They often produce devastating effects on the fetus. Although it is possible for many types of viruses to infect the fetus, the most common ones are *rubella* and *CMV*.

Congenital rubella infection is often acquired during the first 10 weeks of gestation. The virus invades the brain of the fetus and contributes to the establishment of severe mental retardation, seizures, and motor defects. Other manifestations may include low birth weight, abnormally small eyeballs, pigmentary retinal degeneration, glaucoma, cloudy cornea, cataracts, neurocochlear deafness, enlarged liver and spleen, jaundice, and patent ductus arteriosus or intraventricular septal defects.[2] These severe effects are preventable by ensuring that women receive the rubella vaccine before they become pregnant. Congenital rubella syndrome has been reduced by 96% in the United States as a result of immunization programs.[3]

Cytomegaloviruses usually infect the fetus early in the first trimester of pregnancy, and they may produce cerebral malformation. Later, even if the brain is normally formed, CMV may produce inflammatory necrosis in various parts of the brain. Nervous system effects of this infection include mental defects, convulsions, microcephaly, and often hydrocephalus. Other manifestations include enlarged liver and spleen, jaundice, melena, hematemesis, and petechiae.[2] CMV affects approximately 3,000 children annually in the United States.[18] Whether a fetus has been infected by CMV cannot be determined until birth (and in some cases, several years later) because the infection is not apparent in pregnant women.

Myelitis

The word myelitis refers to inflammation of the spinal cord. Poliomyelitis and herpes zoster are the two principal types of myelitis.

POLIOMYELITIS. Since the advent of the Salk vaccine in 1955 and the oral Sabin vaccine in 1958, cases of paralytic poliomyelitis are uncommon in the United States. The synonym for poliomyelitis is *infantile paralysis*; however, the disease occurs in all age groups. The disease is known to occur throughout the world, and peak frequency is during the summer months. Approximately 15 cases are reported each year in the United States.[2] In one of 100 infected persons the virus invades the CNS and replicates in the spinal neurons or brain stem.[6] The human intestinal tract is the main viral reservoir for this ribonucleic acid virus, which infects through the fecal-oral route. Incubation lasts from 1 to 3 weeks. The virus then penetrates intestinal walls, invades the bloodstream, and is carried throughout the body.

Alterations in the CNS include destruction of nerve cells, cellular infiltration, edema, and severe inflammatory processes that produce tissue necrosis and hemorrhages. Although the entire CNS may be involved, the predominant site of alterations is the anterior horn of the spinal cord. Examination of CSF usually shows no evidence of the virus during the clinical disease; however, the protein level is elevated, the glucose level is normal, and the number of lymphocytes is increased. Most persons infected with the virus experience no symptoms, or only a vague illness, because of the failure of the virus to invade the CNS. Even after CNS invasion, clinical effects range from a mild, nonparalytic form of the disease to a severe, paralytic form. This variation in symptoms is related to the severity of the inflammatory response and to the degree to which nerve cells are injured.

Nonparalytic poliomyelitis produces general symptoms of fever, headache, listlessness, anorexia, nausea, vomiting, sore throat, and aching muscles. At this point, the disease may be resolved. With increasing irritability, restlessness, muscle tenderness and spasms, neck and back pain, and neck stiffness, Kernig and Brudzinski signs, the paralytic form of the disease is often imminent.

Paralytic poliomyelitis is often divided into three types: *spinal, bulbar,* and *encephalitic.* This division is primarily useful as a descriptive mechanism, because these types are often combined during the course of the disease. Spinal involvement may include muscle weakness with fasciculations, diminished reflexes in association with progressive abdominal and limb muscle weakness, eventual paralysis (the level varying among different age groups), and muscle atrophy. Bulbar involvement impairs the ability to swallow, disturbs respiration and vasomotor control, and progressively slows respirations. Cyanosis and hypertension may occur, followed by hypotension and circulatory collapse. Mortality is as high as 75% if there is accompanying paralysis of phrenic and intercostal muscles.[2] Involvement of the high brain stem and hypothalamus produces encephalitic symptoms that include restlessness, confusion, and anxiety initially, progressing to stupor and coma.[2]

A *postpolio syndrome* has been recently described and refers to neurologic changes years after resolution of the initial polio infection. It is characterized by progressive muscular weakness in previously affected muscle groups. There is no current evidence of persistence of the polio virus in the motor neurons or that re-activation of the virus has caused the syndrome. The cause of the syndrome, 25 to 35 years after the initial illness, is thought to be due to gradual deterioration of motor neurons.[6]

HERPES ZOSTER (SHINGLES). Herpes zoster infection, caused by the varicella zoster virus, occurs most commonly in adulthood, particularly with advancing age, and in persons with underlying systemic diseases, such as the leukemias or lymphomas. The development of this illness is not completely understood. It is thought that herpes zoster infection represents a reactivation of varicella virus that persists in the nerve ganglia after a primary infection with chickenpox. Herpes zoster is not communicable, except possibly to people who have not had chickenpox.[2] People who have herpes zoster infection usually have a past history of chickenpox. Nervous system alterations include congested, edematous, and hemorrhagic dorsal root ganglia. There is also disintegration of ganglion cells. Painful, vesicular skin eruptions, which harbor varicella zoster virus, are associated with involvement of the corresponding dorsal root ganglion or gasserian ganglion. The dermatomes most commonly involved are T5 through T10; however, any dermatome may be involved. In some cases, accompanying sensory losses and motor palsies occur. Although most patients recover, the process is often slow and painful. The pain may persist for months or even years.

Postinfectious and Postvaccinal Diseases

Acute disseminated (postinfectious) encephalomyelitis, acute inflammatory polyradiculoneuropathy (Guillain-Barré syndrome), and Reye syndrome often occur during or shortly after viral infection or, rarely, after vaccinations for smallpox, rabies, or typhoid. These conditions often require individual susceptibility to the virus or viral effects.

ACUTE DISSEMINATED (POSTINFECTIOUS) ENCEPHALO-MYELITIS. Postinfectious encephalomyelitis develops 2 to 4 days after a rash and is thought to be an autoimmune response to myelin that is triggered by a virus.[6] Demyelination occurs in the region of the brain stem and spinal cord. In addition, the meninges are infiltrated by inflammatory cells. Clinical manifestations include headaches, stiffness of the neck, lethargy, and eventually coma. Some 10% to 20% of affected persons die in the acute phase of the illness.[2] Neurologic residual effects are severe in those who survive.

ACUTE INFLAMMATORY POLYNEUROPATHY (GUILLAIN-BARRÉ SYNDROME). This syndrome is thought to be the result of an autoimmune reaction triggered by a virus in the peripheral nerves. Nervous system alterations include inflammatory infiltrate around vessels throughout the cranial and spinal nerves, demyelination, and axon destruction. The CSF reveals an elevated protein level and pleocytosis. Clinical manifestations include proximal and distal weakness or paralysis of extremities, hypotonia, areflexia, pain, and paresthesias. Weakness that progresses to total motor paralysis of respiratory muscles can result in death. Autonomic dysfunction may occur with resultant sudden fluctuations in blood pressure and heart rate, orthostatic hypotension, and cessation of sweating. Persons who survive the acute phase of the disease usually recover completely; however, some have residual motor or reflex deficits.

REYE SYNDROME. Reye syndrome seems to occur after infections with viruses such as influenza B and varicella, although the relation between the virus and the pathologic changes that ensue is not understood. Whether the condition results from the viral infection or from treatment with aspirin is under investigation. The probability is high that the syndrome is produced in concert with aspirin ingestion.[6] Many factors, including genetic and environmental components, apparently function together in the production of this catastrophic disorder. It occurs predominantly in children between 6 months and 15 years of age.[6] It is characterized by the onset of acute encephalopathy 10 days to 2 weeks after a viral infection. Cerebral edema is produced, as well as fatty changes in the liver and renal tubules. The disease is also characterized by hypoglycemia, increased serum aminotransferases, and serum ammonia levels. Clinical manifestations include persistent vomiting, delirium, seizures, stupor, and eventual coma. Respiratory distress, tachypnea, and apnea are prominent features in infants. Full-blown disease with encephalopathy and liver involvement carries a 40% to 60% mortality rate, but these figures appear to be improving because of earlier diagnosis and supportive treatment. The initiation of treatment before the coma occurs has reduced associated fatality to 5% to 10%.[2]

BACTERIAL INFECTIONS

Pyogenic Infections

The brain and its coverings can be infected by pyogenic (pus-forming) microorganisms. The most common organisms that are responsible for bacterial infections are normally harbored in the nasopharynx. Bacteria enter the CNS by spread from adjacent cranial structures, through the bloodstream. In a few cases, the infection is iatrogenic, for example, from a lumbar puncture or contaminated scalpel. It is frequently difficult to determine the exact entry route of the organism. Within the CNS, the effects of pyogenic microorganisms may be disastrous.

BACTERIAL MENINGITIS (LEPTOMENINGITIS). The leptomeninges and subarachnoid space are primary targets for invasion by pyogenic microorganisms. After an infection enters any part of the subarachnoid space, it spreads quickly throughout CSF pathways in the brain and spinal cord. An inflammatory reaction is set up in the pia and arachnoid and in the ventricles. Any microorganisms that enter the body can cause meningitis. However, some bacteria are more prominent and seem to be more prevalent in certain age groups. Pneumococcus organisms are commonly cultured in very young persons and in adults older than 40 years of age, *Escherichia coli* in the neonatal period, *Haemophilus influenzae* in infants and young children, and *Neisseria meningitidis* in adolescents and young adults. Fifty percent of the cases in infants and young children are attributed to *H. influenzae*.[14] Spinal fluid cultures usually reveal the causative agent.

Meningococcal infections develop more rapidly and distinctly than other forms of meningitis. They may occur singularly or in epidemics where overcrowding exists. The organism is spread by droplet infection from those who harbor the meningococcus in their nasal passages. Disease onset is heralded by a distinctive petechial or purpuric rash. A particularly disastrous event (Waterhouse-Friderichsen syndrome) may occur after any bacterial meningitis, although it is most commonly associated with fulminant meningococcemia. This condition is manifested by overwhelming bacteremia, adrenocortical necrosis, and vasomotor collapse. *H. influenzae* meningitis commonly follows ear and upper respiratory infections in the young. Pneumococcal meningitis can be related to prior infections in the lungs, nasal sinuses, and heart valves.

Alterations occurring with the various bacterial infections include swelling and congestion of the brain and spinal cord, as well as exudate within the subarachnoid space (Fig. 53-10). In severe cases, inflammatory cells can occlude vessels that penetrate the brain, resulting in areas of necrosis. The CSF reveals elevated protein, decreased glucose, decreased chloride, elevated pressure, and the presence of large numbers of leukocytes.

Clinical manifestations of acute pyogenic meningitis are fever, headache, pain with eye movement, photophobia, neck and back stiffness, positive Kernig and Brudzinski signs, generalized convulsions, drowsiness, and confusion. Focal signs may be observed with some bacterial infections as a result of occlusion of vessels and regional brain necrosis. Stupor, followed by coma and death, may occur without prompt and adequate treatment. Residual effects are also a danger because of the destruction or fibrotic thickening of the meningeal frame-

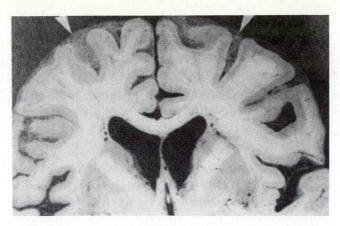

FIGURE 53-10 *Acute meningitis. There is a thick layer of pus in the subarachnoid space (arrows). (Source: Adams, J. and Graham, D. An Introduction to Neuropathology [2nd ed.]. London: Churchill-Livingstone, 1994)*

work. Potential residual effects include optic arachnoiditis, meningomyelitis, and chronic meningoencephalitis with hydrocephalus. Again, with prompt diagnosis and antibiotic therapy, these residual effects are less common than they once were.

BRAIN ABSCESS. Approximately one-half of all brain abscesses are secondary to infection in the nasal cavity, middle ear, or mastoid cells. The remaining cases result from a primary focus of infection elsewhere in the body, particularly in the lungs or pleura, the heart, or the distal bones (Fig. 53-11). Streptococci, staphylococci, and pneumococci are often the causative organisms. A small proportion (about 10%) of cases result from infection introduced through compound skull fractures or intracranial operations.[2]

An abscess occurs after an inflammation, caused by an invading organism, liquefies and begins to accumulate leukocytes. A fibrous capsule is formed in an effort to contain the pus. As the abscess expands, nerve tissue is compressed and destroyed. Chronic inflammation and pronounced edema surround the abscess (Fig. 53-12). The CSF reveals a normal glucose level, an increased protein level, and an increased leukocyte count. The CSF pressure is often moderately elevated early in the abscess formation and markedly elevated in the later stages. If the abscess ruptures into the subarachnoid space or ventricles, organisms can be cultured from CSF. Other diagnostic techniques that may be used are skull films, CT scans, electroencephalography, and ventriculography.

The most common initial clinical manifestation is headache; other symptoms are similar to those produced by growing masses within the brain. The increased intracranial pressure and focal complaints related to the location of the abscess are important. In

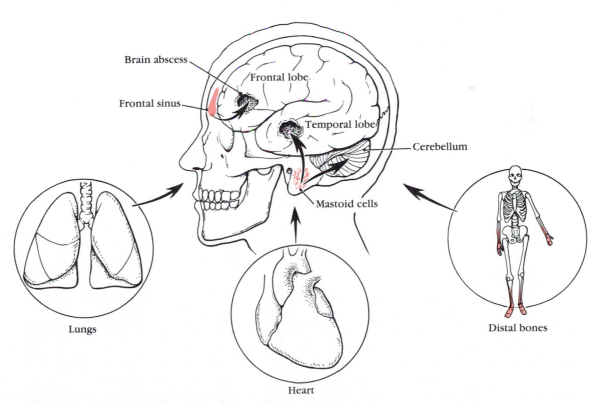

FIGURE 53-11 *Origins and locations of cerebral abscesses.*

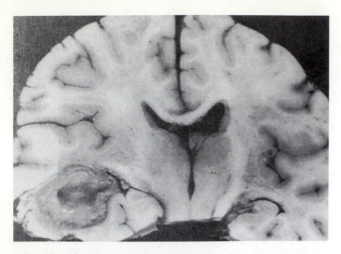

FIGURE 53-12 *Cerebral abscess. There is an encapsulated abscess in the left temporal lobe secondary to chronic suppurative otitis media. (Source: Adams, J. and Graham, D. An Introduction to Neuropathology [2nd ed.]. London: Churchill-Livingstone, 1994)*

addition, a brain abscess can rupture and lead to other complications, such as sinus thrombosis, ventriculitis, or meningitis. Mortality from brain abscesses has been greatly reduced owing to successful combinations of antibiotic therapy and surgery.

SUBDURAL EMPYEMA. The term *empyema* refers to pus in a body cavity; thus, subdural empyema is a suppurative process in the subdural space. It usually occurs between the dura's inner surface and the outer surface of the arachnoid. The most common causative organisms are streptococci or bacteroides; less often, *Staphylococcus aureus, E. coli*, and pseudomonas are the causative agents.[2] Infective organisms usually travel to the subdural space by spread from thrombophlebitis or by erosion through bone or dura from the frontal sinuses, ethmoid sinuses, middle ear, or mastoid cells. Exudate is present on the undersurface of the dura. As the empyema grows, pressure is applied to the underlying cerebral hemisphere. Thrombophlebitis of cerebral veins that are near the subdural empyema can contribute to ischemic necrosis of the cortex. The CSF reveals elevated pressure, increased protein, a normal glucose level, and an increased number of lymphocytes.

Many affected persons have a history of chronic mastoiditis or sinusitis. Clinical manifestations indicating that the infection has spread to the subdural space include fever, general malaise, a localized headache that becomes generalized, associated vomiting, and neck stiffness. As the empyema enlarges, focal neurologic signs, lethargy, and coma develop. Prognosis depends on the success of surgery and antibiotic therapy, as well as the extent to which neurologic deficits have occurred.

Tuberculous Infections

Tuberculous meningitis and tuberculomas of the brain and spinal cord are usually secondary to a tuberculous focus in another part of the body. With the recent resurgence of tuberculosis, the frequency of tuberculous meningitis and tuberculomas of the brain and cord may also be increased.

TUBERCULOUS MENINGITIS. Tuberculous meningitis occurs in areas of high tuberculosis prevalence, primarily in young children. In low-frequency areas, it occurs mostly in the elderly population as a result of reactivation of dormant organisms. Tuberculous meningitis is caused by *Mycobacterium tuberculosis*. This condition has a slower onset and a more chronic course than pyogenic meningitis.

The base of the brain and the spinal cord become compressed by shaggy, necrotic, fibrinous, yellow exudate. There may also be large areas of caseation and tiny tubercles around the blood vessels.[2] The CSF reveals increased pressure, elevated protein and decreased glucose levels (but not as low as values observed in pyogenic meningitis), and the presence of polymorphonuclear leukocytes and lymphocytes. With careful technique in obtaining a specimen, tubercle bacilli may be recovered from CSF.

Clinical manifestations depend on the chronicity of the disease and the extent of pathologic processes. In general, adults have headache, fever, lethargy, confusion, neck stiffness, positive Kernig and Brudzinski signs, weight loss, and night sweats. Young children often experience vomiting, irritability, and seizures.

Due to the slow onset of this illness, neurologic damage may be present before treatment is sought. Then, even though the person survives, there may be lasting effects, such as recurrent seizures, retarded intellectual development, mental disturbances, visual disturbances, deafness, and hemiparesis.

TUBERCULOMAS OF BRAIN AND SPINAL CORD. Tuberculomas (tuberculous granulation masses), although rare in the United States, constitute from 5% to 30% of all intracranial space-occupying lesions in underdeveloped countries.[2] Tuberculomas are single or multiple and contain a core of caseation necrosis surrounded by a fibrous capsule. Within the brain and spinal cord, they produce neurologic effects similar to those of other expanding intracranial and intraspinal lesions. The CSF reveals an increased level of protein and a small number of lymphocytes. Tuberculomas of the brain and spinal cord have been known to calcify while still small, before any neurologic changes have occurred. These small calcifications are often found at autopsy.

Tuberculous infection may affect the spinal cord in a number of ways, causing spinal block. Evidence of spinal root disease may be the result of invasion of the underlying parenchyma by inflammatory meningeal exudate. Compression by an epidural mass of granulation tissue produces spinal symptoms and Pott paraplegia.[2]

Neurosyphilis

The frequency of neurosyphilis (tertiary stage of syphilis) has decreased in the last several decades as a result of prompt diagnosis and treatment of early syphilis. The overall frequency of syphilis is increasing, however, particularly in young persons.

Treponema pallidum, a spirochete, is a spiral, motile organism that causes syphilis. After this organism is introduced into the body, it usually invades the CNS within 3 to 18 months. Neurosyphilis, unless treated, is progressive in most affected persons and includes several forms: asymptomatic neurosyphilis, meningovascular syphilis, general paresis, and tabes dorsalis (see pp. 1163–1164).

Meningitis is the initial event in all forms of neurosyphilis, but the severity of symptoms varies among the different forms, and the infection may remain asymptomatic for several years. The CSF is the most accurate, sensitive indicator that an active neurosyphilitic infection is present. Serologic tests are positive: the VDRL (Veneral Disease Research Laboratory) slide test, the Kolmer test, the fluorescent treponemal antibody absorption test, and the treponema immobilization test. Changes in CSF also include an increased protein level; increased presence of lymphocytes, plasma cells, and mononuclear cells; and an abnormal colloidal gold curve.

ASYMPTOMATIC NEUROSYPHILIS.   As the name *asymptomatic neurosyphilis* implies, there are usually no physical signs or symptoms of the meningitis. This form of the disease is recognized by the changes in CSF and serologic test results, which are the same as in the symptomatic form. Treatment prevents further development of the disease.

MENINGOVASCULAR NEUROSYPHILIS. This form of neurosyphilis commonly develops 6 to 7 years after the original infection. The CNS alterations include infiltration of meninges and blood vessels with plasma cells and lymphocytes, inflammation of arteries, and fibrosis that leads to occlusion of vessels. The vascular lesions are referred to as Heubner arteritis. Miliary gummas may also be seen in the meninges. Clinical manifestations are similar to those of low-grade meningitis, cerebrovascular accident, or mental derangement. Without treatment, neurologic deficits continue to progress.

GENERAL PARESIS.   This form of neurosyphilis usually develops 15 to 20 years after the original infection. Early treatment of syphilis has decreased the incidence of general paresis. In this form of neurosyphilis, the parenchyma of the brain is involved owing to the presence of spirochetes. There is a diffuse destruction of cortical neurons and a proliferation of astrocytes. Plasma cells and lymphocytes accumulate around blood vessels. The clinical manifestations are those of progressive mental and physical deterioration. Initially, slight memory loss, changes in behavior, and decreased ability to reason occur. Later, the patient develops a severe dementia with elaborate delusional systems and disregard for moral and social standards. Physically, he or she experiences dysarthria, tremor of the tongue and hands, myoclonic jerks, muscular hypotonia, hyperactive tendon reflexes, Babinski signs, seizures, and Argyll Robertson pupils. Without treatment, the prognosis is poor and death occurs in a few years.

TABES DORSALIS.   Tabes dorsalis, like general paresis, occurs many years after the onset of infection. This form of neurosyphilis is also uncommon now because of improved, early treatment with penicillin. The CNS alterations include degeneration of the posterior columns, fibrosis around the posterior roots, and destruction of proprioceptive fibers in the radicular nerves. These changes produce various symptoms, the most common being ataxia. Other features of this type of neurosyphilis are lightning pains (sudden sharp pains lasting only a portion of a second), ataxia resulting from sensory defects, and urinary incontinence. Visceral symptoms include vomiting and bouts of sharp epigastric pain that extend around the body. Other clinical manifestations may include Argyll Robertson pupils, Charcot joints (from repeated injury to insensitive joints), absence of vibration sense and deep tendon reflexes, and a positive Romberg sign. The Romberg sign is the inability to maintain balance with the eyes closed and the feet together. Although treatment with penicillin can arrest the disease process, residual effects, such as urinary incontinence, lightning pains, visceral crises, and Charcot joints, may persist indefinitely.

Lyme Disease (Lyme Borreliosis)

Lyme disease is caused by the spirochete *Borrelia burgdorferi,* which is transmitted to humans by the ixodid deer tick. In the United States, Lyme disease is the most common vector-borne disease and is increasing in frequency. The incidence in the United States has increased from 226 cases in 1980 to more than 7,000 cases in 1989–1990.[9] The increased incidence is thought to be caused by the resurgence of the deer population, the spread of tick vectors to new areas, and the spread of suburban populations into once rural areas.[10] The disease typically occurs in the warmer months (May through August), and 25% to 50% of the cases are reported in children younger than 16 years of age.[9] The diagnosis is based on the clinical symptoms and the results of serologic studies for immunoglobulin G antibodies to *Borrelia.*

The disease is multisystem, with neurological manifestations developing in 10% to 15% of the cases after an interval of 1 to 6 months. Neurologic involvement is manifest as meningitis, meningoencephalitis with severe headache, cranial nerve palsies (especially cranial nerve VII), polyradiculoneuropathy, mononeuropathy multiplex, an neuropathy resembling Guillain-Barré syndrome, or myelopathy. Late neurologic manifestations include a syndrome resembling multiple sclerosis.[9] The treatment includes a variety of antibiotics with intravenous penicillin or ceftriaxone, which is used in treating the neurologic aspects of the disease.

Disorders Caused by Bacterial Exotoxins

Bacterial exotoxins can have powerful effects on the CNS and can result in life-threatening motor problems. The major diseases produced by these toxins are tetanus, diphtheria, and botulism.

TETANUS. *Clostridium tetani* produces tetanus after contaminating penetrating wounds or the umbilical cord of the newborn with spores. These anaerobic, spore-forming bacilli produce two exotoxins: a tetanolysin and a tetanospasmin. Neurotoxic effects are produced by tetanospasmin. Most of the toxin enters the peripheral endings of motor neurons from the bloodstream, travels up the fibers to the spinal cord and brain stem, and crosses the synaptic cleft to the inhibitory neurons, where it prevents the release of glycine. Glycine is a neuromuscular transmitter secreted mainly in the synapses of the spinal cord; it acts as an inhibitor. The action of tetanospasmin is through an affinity for the sympathetic nervous system, the medullary centers, the anterior horn cells of the spinal cord, and the motor end plates in skeletal muscle. It produces uninhibited motor responses, which lead to the typical muscle spasm.

The incubation period varies from several days to several months. Usually, symptoms occur within 2 weeks after wound contamination. The initial manifestation is usually difficulty opening the jaw (trismus); thus, the synonym *lockjaw.* There is generalized muscle stiffness with eventual muscle spasms (tetanic seizures or convulsions). These convulsions are very painful and can occur spontaneously or in response to the slightest stimuli.

Facial spasms produce a characteristic sardonic smile (risus sardonicus). Contractions of back muscles produce a forward arching of the back (opisthotonos). Spasms of glottal, laryngeal, and respiratory muscles cause difficulty in breathing and often lead to death from asphyxia. In established clinical cases of tetanus, overall mortality is 50%.[2] The toxin is not able to cross the blood-brain barrier, which accounts for the normal mentation in these patients.[6] The disease is prevented with active immunization with tetanus toxoid. Also, prompt administration of antitoxin may prevent progression of symptoms.

DIPHTHERIA. *Corynebacterium diphtheriae* produces an acute infection: diphtheria. Although open wounds in any part of the body can provide entry for this organism, the usual portal of entry is the oral cavity. The incubation period is 1 to 7 days. During this time, the organism becomes established and proliferates at the site of implantation, usually the throat and trachea. The bacteria produce exotoxin that is absorbed by the blood and carried to the CNS and heart. Early general manifestations of the disease are fever, sore throat, chills, and malaise. Local neurologic manifestations occur within 5 to 12 days and include vomiting, dysphagia, possible cranial nerve involvement, and nasal voice due to palatal paralysis. Blurred vision and loss of accommodation occur in the second or third week owing to ciliary paralysis. Between the fifth and sixth weeks, weakness and paralysis of the extremities may occur. Most neurologic disturbances disappear slowly, and patients usually improve completely if respiratory obstruction or cardiac failure does not supervene. The disease is prevented by immunization; prompt administration of antitoxin may prevent clinical manifestations.

BOTULISM. *Clostridium botulinum* can contaminate and produce exotoxins in foods such as fruits, vegetables, and meats that are kept for long periods of time without refrigeration. After ingestion, the toxin resists gastric digestion, is absorbed by the blood, and then travels to the nervous system. The botulinum toxin acts only on the presynaptic endings of neuromuscular junctions and autonomic ganglia. It prevents the release of acetylcholine and causes symptoms resembling those of myasthenia gravis. The result is a descending form of paralysis from the cranial nerves downward. Symptoms occur within 12 to 36 hours after ingestion of the contaminated food.[2] Neural symptoms may or may not be preceded by nausea and vomiting. The affected person may develop cranial nerve palsies, blurred vision, diplopia, ptosis, strabismus, hoarseness, dysarthria, dysphagia, vertigo, deafness, constipation, and progressive muscle weakness. Tendon reflexes may be absent. Sensation remains intact, and the person is conscious throughout the illness. Even with prompt administration of *C. botulinum* antitoxins, death occurs in about 15% of cases because of paralysis of respiratory muscles and respiratory infections. Those who survive usually recover completely with effective supportive care over a long, slow course.[6]

FUNGAL INFECTIONS

Fungi infect the CNS less commonly than bacteria and viruses. Their effects can be similar to those of bacterial infection but more difficult to treat. Fungal infections can produce brain abscesses, meningitis, meningoencephalitis, and thrombophlebitis of vessels within the CNS. Like other infections, fungal infections of the CNS are usually secondary to a primary source of infection elsewhere in the body. In addition, they may be a complication of another disease process, such as cancer, or they may be related to use of immunosuppressant drugs.

Fungi usually spread to the CNS through the bloodstream. In the CNS, they cause an inflammatory reaction, and a purulent exudate involves the meninges. In some cases, invasion of vessel walls results in vasculitis and thrombosis with subsequent nervous tissue infarction. The process develops slowly over days or weeks. Clinical manifestations are similar to those of tuberculous meningitis. Hydrocephalus is often a related complication. The CSF reveals elevated pressure, increased protein level, decreased glucose level, moderate pleocytosis (increased number of lymphocytes), and often the isolation of the infective organism. Many types of fungi can invade the CNS. The most common infections are candidiasis, cryptococcosis, coccidioidomycosis, and mucormycosis.

CANDIDIASIS. *Candida albicans* is a fungus normally present in the oral cavity, in the gastrointestinal tract, and in the female vagina. It normally does not cause symptoms unless the host is immunocompromised or the normal protective barriers to infection are breached. Disseminated candidiasis in the CNS may appear as meningitis, with lymphocytes found in the CSF. Candidiasis in the eye is called *Candida* endophthalmitis; it affects the retina and may lead to blindness.

CRYPTOCOCCOSIS (TORULOSIS). Common in soil and bird droppings, cryptococci are the most frequent cause of fungal infection of the CNS. The fungus is transmitted to humans through the respiratory tract. Cryptococcosis, which usually arises secondary to a pulmonary infection, produces cysts and granulomas in the cortex and occasionally in the deep white matter and basal ganglia. These cysts contain large numbers of organisms. *Cryptococcus neoformans* is recovered from spinal fluid. Mortality, even in the absence of preexisting diseases (lymphomas and Hodgkin disease), is almost 40%.[2] Clinical features are similar to those of subacute meningitis or encephalitis.

COCCIDIOIDOMYCOSIS. *Coccidioides immitis* produces a relatively mild, flulike illness involving the respiratory organs. Common in the southwestern United States, coccidioidomycosis may become a chronic, diffuse, granulomatous disease that spreads throughout the body. The meninges and CSF may become involved, with resultant pathologic and clinical manifestations similar to those of tuberculous meningitis. If the meninges become involved, treatment is difficult. Amphotericin B is the only effective drug; even with this treatment, the disease is often fatal.

MUCORMYCOSIS. Mucormycosis, also called zygomycosis or phycomycosis, is a rare opportunistic infection occurring in very debilitated persons that is caused by fungi of the order Mucorales. One of the primary sites of invasion is the nasal sinuses. From the nasal sinuses, the organism may spread along invaded vessels to periorbital tissue and the cranial vault. Nervous tissue infarctions occur as a result of vascular occlusion. Once the organism has invaded the brain, prognosis is very poor.

PROTOZOAL INFECTIONS

Malaria

Plasmodium vivax produces the most common form of malaria. This organism does not actually invade brain tissue, but the parasitized red blood cells block microcirculation, which leads to tissue hypoxia and ischemic necrosis. The vessel blockage within the brain leads to glial necrosis, which causes drowsiness, confusion, and seizures. Quinine is used for treatment and is helpful unless the cerebral symptoms are far advanced.

Plasmodium falciparum produces a form of malaria that has more severe symptoms. The parasite fills capillaries, and Dürck nodes (small foci of necrosis surrounded by glia) are present in brain tissue. The CSF reveals elevated pressure and contains leukocytes. Clinical manifestations include focal neurologic signs, headache, seizures, aphasia, cerebellar ataxia, hemiplegia, hemianopsia, and, eventually, coma. Cerebral malaria caused by *P. falciparum* is usually rapidly fatal.

Toxoplasmosis

Toxoplasma gondii produces an infection that is either acquired or congenital. The organism is acquired either congenitally, by eating raw beef, or by contact with cat feces. Acquired toxoplasmosis rarely produces clinical effects. In clinical cases, the white and gray matter contain necrotic lesions that harbor *T. gondii*. Symptoms are similar to those of meningoencephalitis. Acquired toxoplasmosis is often observed in persons with AIDS. Congenital toxoplasmosis causes much destruction of the neonatal brain. Signs of infection are fever, rash, seizures, and enlarged liver and spleen, which may be present at birth. Slow psychomotor development becomes evident early in life. In some cases, clinical manifestations of the illness are not present for days, weeks, or months. These clinical effects include hydrocephalus, retardation, cerebral calcification, and chorioretinitis.

Amebiasis

Infection with amoebae may be acquired by swimming in lakes or ponds. The causative organisms are usually of the *Naegleria* genus, and there is a prevalence of cases in the southeastern United States. The CNS alterations include abscesses in the cortex and purulent exudate involving the meninges. The CSF findings are similar to those of bacterial meningitis. The disease is rapidly progressive, and the symptoms include nausea, vomiting, fever, neck stiffness, focal neurologic signs, seizures, and, eventually, coma. This illness is usually fatal within a week of onset because of resistance of *Naegleria* to treatment.

Trypanosomiasis

Several strains of *Trypanosoma brucei* produce African sleeping sickness, which is transmitted by the tsetse fly. Two epidemiologic patterns are described: Gambian (middle and west African) and Rhodesian (east African). The Rhodesian type is more severe, with intercurrent infections and myocarditis dominating the clinical picture. Within 2 years after infection with the Gambian form, trypanosomes produce meningoencephalitis, with thickening of the meninges and cerebral edema. Symptoms range from somnolence to convulsions and coma. Mortality depends on the effectiveness of treatment and the degree of CNS involvement.

Trypanosoma cruzi produces Chagas disease in Central and South America, and rarely in North America. The organism is transmitted by biting bugs commonly called assassin bugs. Chagas disease is either acute or chronic. The acute form is prevalent in children and produces fever, enlarged liver and spleen, myocardial involvement with congestive failure, and, eventually, involvement of the lungs, meninges, and brain. Months or years after an acute attack, the chronic form may develop with subsequent meningoencephalitis. Pentavalent arsenicals have shown some success in the treatment of both types of trypanosomiasis.

Trichinosis

Trichinella spiralis enters the body when raw or insufficiently cooked pork is eaten. Within 2 to 3 days, early symptoms of the disease are apparent. The symptoms are mainly caused by the invasion of muscle by larvae, which produces mild gastroenteritis, muscle weakness, and tenderness. Three to 6 weeks after ingestion, larvae invade the nervous system. Lymphocytic and mononuclear infiltration of the meninges occurs, as does focal gliosis. Symptoms of CNS involvement include headache, confusion, neck stiffness, seizures, and, occasionally, coma. Although trichinosis is usually not fatal, seizures and neurologic deficits may continue indefinitely.

METAZOAL INFECTIONS

Cysticercosis

Ingestion of encysted eggs of the pork tapeworm, *Taenia solium*, produce cysticercosis. This disease is most common in South American countries. The larvae spread throughout the body and develop cysts in any body tissue. Cystic nodules within the brain produce symptoms similar to those of brain tumors. Jacksonian seizures are common manifestations. Prognosis depends on the extent of neurologic damage and the effectiveness of therapy with praziquantel, an anthelminthic agent.

Echinococcosis (Hydatid Disease)

Hydatid disease is caused by the ingestion of larvae of the canine tapeworm, *Echinococcus granulosus*. The larvae invade the liver, lungs, bones, and, less frequently, the brain. The larvae become encysted and are at first microscopic. However, within 5 or more years, the cysts may grow to massive sizes of 10 cm or more.[6] Within the brain, symptoms are similar to those associated with brain tumors. The amount of local destruction throughout the body determines the prognosis.

RICKETTSIAL INFECTIONS

Rickettsial infections are relatively rare in the United States. They are caused by microorganisms that are obligate intracellular parasites that multiply only within living cells of susceptible hosts. Their cycle involves an animal reservoir and an insect vector (eg, ticks, fleas, lice, mites). The cycle of epidemic typhus involves only lice and human beings. Major rickettsial diseases include epidemic (primary) typhus, which is louse-borne; murine (endemic) typhus, flea-borne; scrub typhus or tsutsugamushi fever, mite-borne; Rocky Mountain spotted fever, tick-borne; and Q fever, tick-borne and airborne. Within the CNS, rickettsial diseases can produce lesions in the gray and white matter. Focal gliosis, together with mononuclear leukocytes, produces characteristic typhus nodules.

All the rickettsial diseases except Q fever have similar pathologic and clinical effects. A 3- to 18-day incubation period ends with the abrupt onset of high fever, chills, headache, and weakness, followed by a generalized macular rash. During the second week after the onset of fever, the CNS becomes involved, producing apathy, dullness, intermittent episodes of delirium, and, eventually, stupor and coma. Occasionally, in untreated cases, focal neurologic manifestations and optic neuritis occur. The CSF may be completely normal. Q fever is not accompanied by a rash and produces symptoms similar to those of a low-grade meningitis. Mortality from typhus is greatest during epidemics. Early antibiotic therapy has reduced fatality rates to less than 10% for typhus and 5% for Rocky Mountain spotted fever.[2] Fatalities are rarely associated with scrub typhus or Q fever.

▼ Chapter Summary

▼ Tumors of the CNS, which can be either benign or malignant, arise from the glial cells, blood vessels, meninges, pituitary, or pineal gland. They may arise in the brain or spinal column.

▼ Brain tumors rarely metastasize but do infiltrate surrounding nervous tissue and cause a displacement of intracranial contents and increased intracranial pressure. The clinical signs of tumors relate to their location and rate of growth. Common manifestations include headache, motor and speech disturbances, visual and equilibrium disturbances, and any of the signs of increased intracranial pressure.

▼ Spinal cord tumors cause effects according to their level and size.

▼ Infections of the CNS can be caused by viruses, bacteria, fungi, protozoa, metazoa, and rickettsia. They can cause encephalitis, which is infection of the brain parenchyma, or meningitis, which is infection of the covering of the brain. Some organisms affect the spinal cord or dermatomes. Some organisms cause brain abscess, and some cause a subdural empyema. The type of clinical picture seen depends on the type of organism and its ability to produce disease.

▼ References

1. Adams, J., and Graham, D. *An Introduction to Neuropathology* (2nd ed.). London: Churchill Livingstone, 1994.
2. Adams, R., and Victor, M. *Principles of Neurology* (5th ed.). New York: McGraw-Hill, 1993.
3. Bale, J.F. Viral infection. In Johnson, R.T. (ed.), *Current Therapy in Neurologic Disease 3*. Philadelphia: B.C. Decker, 1990.
4. Beckham, M.M. Neurologic manifestations of AIDS. *Crit. Care Nurs. Clin. North Am.* 2:29, 1990.
5. Berkshire, J., and Watson-Evans, H. Meningioma: A nursing perspective. *J. Neurosci. Nurs.* 21:233, 1989.
6. Cotran, R.S., Kumar, V., and Robbins, S.L. *Robbins' Pathologic Basis of Disease* (5th ed.). Philadelphia: W.B. Saunders, 1994.
7. Davidson, G. Nervous system. In Walker, J. (ed.), *Pathology of Human Disease*. Philadelphia: Lea & Febiger, 1989.
8. Dropcho, E.J. Glioma. In Johnson, R.T. (ed.), *Current Therapy in Neurologic Disease 3*. Philadelphia: B.C. Decker, 1990.
9. Guberman, A. *An Introduction to Clinical Neurology*. Boston: Little, Brown, 1994.
10. Jacobs, R. Infectious diseases: Spirochetal. In Tierney, L., McPhee, S., and Papadakis, M. (eds.). *Current Medical Diagnosis and Treatment* (23rd ed.). Norwalk, Conn.: Appleton & Lange, 1994.
11. Laws, E., and Thapar, K. Brain tumors. *CA: Cancer J. Clin.* 43:5 1993.
12. McArthur, J., and Harrison, M. HIV-associated dementia. In Appel, S. (ed.), *Current Neurology*. St. Louis: Mosby, 1994.
13. Phillips, P.C. Brain tumors in children. In Johnson, R.T. (ed.), *Current Therapy in Neurologic Disease 3*. Philadelphia: B.C. Decker, 1990.
14. Prendergast, V. Bacterial meningitis update. *J. Neurosci. Nurs.* 19:2, 1987.
15. Ransohoff, J., Koslow, M., and Cooper, P. Cancer of the central nervous system and pituitary. In Holleb, A., et al. (eds.), *American Cancer Society Textbook of Clinical Oncology*. Atlanta, Ga.: American Cancer Society, 1991.
16. Russel, D., and Rubinstein, L. *Pathology of Tumors of the Nervous System* (5th ed.). Baltimore: Williams & Wilkins, 1989.
17. Schwartz, S.I. (ed.). *Principles of Surgery* (6th ed.). New York: McGraw-Hill, 1994.
18. Weiner, L.P. Viral encephalitis. In Johnson, R.T. (ed.), *Current Therapy in Neurologic Disease 3*. Philadelphia: B.C. Decker, 1990.

Chapter 54

Degenerative and Chronic Alterations in the Nervous System

Reet Henze

▼ CHAPTER OUTLINE

Paralyzing Developmental or Congenital
*   Disorders*
Spina Bifida
Syringomyelia
Hydrocephalus
    Pseudotumor Cerebri
Cranial Malformations
Cerebral Palsy
Disorders Characterized by
*   Progressive Weakness or Paralysis*

Myasthenia Gravis
Subacute Combined Degeneration of the Cord
Guillain-Barré Syndrome (Acute Inflammatory
    Polyneuropathy)
Multiple Sclerosis
Amyotrophic Lateral Sclerosis
Disorders Characterized by
*   Abnormal Movements*
Parkinson Disease
Drug-Induced Dyskinesias and Dystonias

Torticollis
Huntington Disease
Disorders Characterized by
*   Memory and Judgment Deficits*
Atherosclerotic Dementia
Alzheimer Disease
Pick Disease
Neurosyphilis
Chapter Summary

▼ LEARNING OBJECTIVES

1 Differentiate between primary and secondary disabilities.
2 Identify examples of developmental, congenital, and degenerative alterations in the nervous system.
3 Explain why the site of a neurologic alteration has a greater impact on the production of clinical signs
   than does the nature of the lesion.
4 Identify examples of congenital and developmental alterations in the motor areas of the brain and cord.
5 Identify examples of developmental and degenerative alterations in the upper voluntary motor areas of the nervous system
   leading to progressive weakness, tremor, or spastic paralysis.
6 Contrast upper and lower motor neuron paralysis.
7 Describe alterations in the lower voluntary motor areas of the nervous system leading to transient or permanent sensory or motor
   changes, or flaccid paralysis.
8 Describe the structural basis for signs and symptoms of bulbar palsy.
9 Explain the physiologic basis for medical treatment of muscle weakness and fatigue related to inadequate transmission of impulses
   across the myoneural junction.
10 Describe pathologic changes in the extrapyramidal motor system that result in the loss of normal automatic
   or spontaneous body movements.
11 Describe pathologic changes in the extrapyramidal system that result in the generation or facilitation of abnormal movements.
12 Identify examples of structural alterations that affect higher cerebral functions, such as memory and judgment.
13 Discuss known and theorized pathological bases of progressive degeneration in memory and judgment.

Barbara L. Bullock: PATHOPHYSIOLOGY: ADAPTATIONS AND ALTERATIONS IN FUNCTION, 4th ed.
© 1996 J.B. Lippincott-Raven Publishers

A *primary disability* is a structural and functional alteration that results directly from a pathologic process. Primary disabilities are caused by congenital disorders, genetic disorders, injuries, or diseases, and, unlike cardiovascular or skeletal disorders, they usually are referred to in terms of the functional, rather than the structural, alteration. For example, terms such as "spastic quadriplegia" and "right homonymous hemianopsia" are more frequently used than such "phrases as demyelination of the . . . tracts" or "anoxia of the. . . branch of the . . . nerve."

One reason for referring to primary neurologic alterations in functional terms is that often the nature of the lesion is hard to identify early in the course of the disease. Also, the description of the dysfunction helps to pinpoint the site of the lesion, even if it does not give much evidence as to its nature. The location of changes in the nervous system determines the clinical signs and symptoms regardless of whether the lesion that interrupts the generation or transmission of nerve impulses is developmental, infectious, degenerative, vascular, neoplastic, or traumatic. A lesion that interrupts the pyramidal tracts in the brain or cord may produce spastic paralysis whether it is caused by neuronal anoxia or an inborn metabolic defect in the nerve cells. Similarly, an imbalance between the neurotransmitters in the basal ganglia results in abnormalities of movement whether it is caused by degeneration of dopamine-releasing neurons after carbon monoxide poisoning or by the dopamine-blocking or -binding effects of phenothiazine drugs.

The degenerative and other neurologic disorders selected as examples in this chapter share common signs and symptoms because they cause structural or chemical alterations in common locations in the brain. Because their causes vary greatly, their treatments and prognoses are quite different, even if initial symptoms seem similar.

Secondary disabilities are caused by restrictions or conditions imposed because of the presence or treatment of primary neurologic disability. These secondary conditions may arise from forced inactivity, such as a muscle contracture that occurs in a paralyzed limb. They also may arise from injury; for example, when a paralyzed extremity is not properly supported, its weight may cause subluxation of the associated joint. Most of the secondary disabilities associated with primary neurologic disease are progressive, and they can be threatening to function and to life, even if the primary disorder is resolved. Secondary disabilities often are as preventable as they are crippling.

Organic disease of the nervous system usually is long-term and does not always end with recovery. If a person does recover from a neurologic disease, full function may not be regained, even though the causative agent has been eliminated. This is the case, for example, with neurosyphilis. Residual primary damage or secondary disabilities can linger or become permanent.

Even if recovery is possible or if the disorder is self-limiting (eg, Guillain-Barré syndrome), it usually takes considerable time for full function to return.

▼ *Paralyzing Developmental or Congenital Disorders*

Developmental disorders occur if neurologic structures fail to develop to full size or mature function, or if they develop abnormally. Their causes usually are not known. Congenital diseases are those present at birth; clinically, the classification includes diseases of apparent genetic origin and those that occur during fetal life as a result of infection, anoxia, malnutrition, or some other traumatic or toxic factor.

SPINA BIFIDA

Spina bifida is a developmental disorder of the vertebral arches. During embryogenesis, the bony arch of the canal fails to close completely. If this is the only defect, it is called *spina bifida occulta* because there are no signs of neurologic deficit to signify its presence. The bony defect is identifiable only by radiography or palpation. The site of the lesion may be marked by dimpling and wisps of hair on the skin surface. The cause of this defect is unknown, although various theories link it with prenatal infection, prenatal drug usage, folate deficiency in early gestation, or heredity.[10] Spina bifida occulta may occur with no clinical signs or symptoms. It is possible for late signs such as persistent or intermittent enuresis (the most common symptom), late walking, or even chronic cold feet to be traced to a previously undetected lesion.

Spina bifida often is associated with a defect in the closure of the neural tube (Fig. 54-1). This can range from a closed but dilated central cord canal (*syringomyelocele*) to a sac protruding through the bony defect that contains meninges (*meningocele*) or, more commonly, a protruding sac that includes elements of the spinal cord (*meningomyelocele*). These sacs may leak cerebrospinal fluid (CSF) if the skin covering is incomplete. Other defects, such as abnormal neural tissue or a fistula, may be associated with this type of spina bifida. In the occipital area, brain elements may protrude through a defect in the skull; this impairment is referred to as an *encephalocele*.

Several forms of spina bifida can be diagnosed in utero by amniocentesis and ultrasonography or at birth by the presence of the sac protruding through the defect in the vertebral arch. If the sac is a meningocele, it is possible for the infant to show no signs of neurologic deficit, although hydrocephalus may occur after surgical repair. The meningomyelocele is accompanied by signs

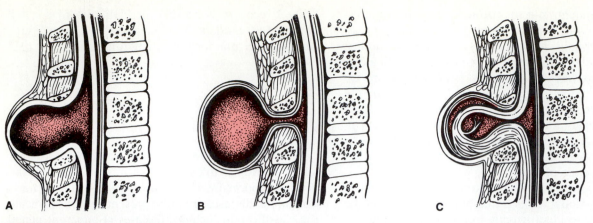

FIGURE 54-1 *Types of spina bifida.* **A.** *Syringomyelocele.* **B.** *Meningocele.* **C.** *Meningomyelocele.*

of neurologic damage, the extent of which depends on the size and level of the lesion and the presence of dysplastic neural tissue. If the defect occurs in the lumbosacral area, flaccid paralysis of the lower limbs and absence of sensation below the level of the lesion usually are present. Sphincter control also is affected in both bowel and bladder. These neurologic deficits occur because the defect and abnormal tissue often involve all or most of the lumbosacral spinal cord together with the nerve roots entering and exiting in the lumbosacral area. Alteration in blood supply because of pressure, trauma, or infection also may contribute to the interruption of the reflex arcs in the area. If the tip end of the conus terminalis is intact, some external bowel sphincter control may be present because of an intact reflex arc.[27] The frequency of accompanying mental retardation with severe developmental spinal defects is high.

Prognosis for life and function are excellent with spina bifida occulta and after surgical repair of a meningocele, especially in the absence of hydrocephalus. Surgical repair commonly is undertaken with serious developmental spinal defects to avoid the dangerous complication of ascending meningitis. About 50% of children who survive surgical treatment for meningomyelocele reach adulthood, and some may learn to walk with braces and crutches. The primary disabilities of meningomyelocele may be resolved, but complications result from secondary disabilities, especially immobility.

SYRINGOMYELIA

Syringomyelia refers to the development of a *syrinx*, which is an abnormal cleft or cavity in cord tissue.[10] The cause of primary syringomyelia remains unknown, although considerable attention has been given to its origin as a congenital neural tube defect. Unlike spina bifida, syringomyelia is characterized by the onset of progressive motor symptoms in the adult. Weakness and spastic paralysis and alterations in sensory function may

progress steadily or intermittently throughout the remainder of life. These symptoms are similar to those of some spinal cord tumors.

Syringomyelia is considered to be a developmental disorder that involves enlargement of affected segments of the spinal cord and development of tubular fluid cavities. It may be a developmental defect that involves disruption of CSF flow through the outlets of the fourth ventricle. It is present throughout embryogenesis but does not become symptomatic until the normally microscopic central canal of the spinal cord balloons and forms fluid-filled cavities in the nervous tissue of the cord itself (Fig. 54-2). A pathologic cavity caused by retained CSF, called a syrinx, results; thus, the name syringomyelia.

Syringomyelia may occur in association with other developmental defects such as spina bifida, Chiari malformation, and hydrocephalus. Secondary syringomyelia may accompany tumors, infections, trauma, bleeding, and infarction in the central nervous system. Signs and symptoms of syrinx formation normally occur after 30 years of age, although they may begin at any age. The nature of the clinical signs depends on the level and size of the cavities and which structures are affected. The syrinx typically develops from the center of the cord outward, in the direction of the dorsal gray horns (Fig. 54-3). Because pain and temperature fibers cross immediately in the cord and are relayed by the cells in the dorsal gray horns of the cord, the loss of these sensations with analgesia, thermoanesthesia, and preservation of the touch sensation are early signs of the onset of syringomyelia. Accompanying these early signs are weakness and wasting of hands and arms. If the syrinx spreads anteriorly toward the anterior horn cells, signs of lower motor neuron damage with small-muscle atrophy occur. Signs and symptoms develop asymmetrically at first, but cord compression may become so severe that complete paraplegia results.

The lower cervical and upper thoracic areas of the cord most commonly develop syrinx-related alterations.

If the brain stem is affected initially or by extension, the condition is termed *syringobulbia*. Characteristic symptoms of medullary involvement, resulting from cranial nerve damage, include weakness of facial and palatal muscles, laryngeal palsy, wasting and weakness of the tongue, loss of pain and temperature sensation, and onset of trigeminal pain. Dizziness may occur. Severe involvement of the medulla oblongata may be lethal.

In primary syringomyelia, the CSF remains normal unless its circulation becomes obstructed. The protein content is high in CSF of syringomyelia associated with tumor growth. The cord enlarges in the area of syrinx formation, and signs and symptoms may be suggestive of spinal cord tumor, multiple sclerosis, or amyotrophic lateral sclerosis. Later, manifestations of poorly healed, painless injuries with trophic skin lesions confirm the diagnosis of syringomyelia.

Clinical manifestations may be stationary for years, or slow progression may lead to death from brain stem involvement or from secondary problems such as extensive decubitus ulcers, renal infection, and pneumonia. Symptomatic treatment is aimed at preventing lethal and crippling secondary disabilities. If attempted early in primary syringomyelia, surgical decompression of the medulla and fourth ventricle by removal of the posterior rim of the foramen magnum has yielded promising results in arresting and, occasionally, reversing the sensory losses. Some patients with associated hydrocephalus benefit from ventriculoperitoneal shunting. If the outlets in the fourth ventricle are occluded, they are opened, and the central canal may be aspirated at the time of surgery.

HYDROCEPHALUS

The word *hydrocephalus* refers to an increased quantity of CSF within the ventricles of the cerebrum. If CSF pressure is normal or only sporadically increased with gradual cortical atrophy, the symptoms begin slowly and relate to memory and judgment deficits, speech disor-

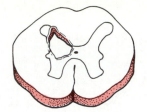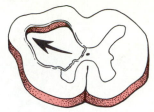

FIGURE 54-3 *Development of a syrinx from the center outward into the dorsal gray horns.*

ders, alterations in gait, some spasticity, incontinence, and the signs of progressive dementia. If the pressure is elevated because of excess formation, faulty circulation, or inadequate reabsorption of CSF, the symptoms are more abrupt in onset and more severe.

The most common cause of hydrocephalus is obstruction to the flow of CSF (Fig. 54-4). In the fetus or neonate, the obstruction may result from cerebellar dysplasia, tumor, subarachnoid hemorrhage, or infectious or developmental abnormalities of the cerebellar tonsils, medulla, cerebral aqueduct, or fourth ventricle. In the older person, the obstruction may be caused by trauma, infection, or tumor. If the obstruction is within the CSF pathways, the disorder is classified as *noncommunicating* or *obstructive hydrocephalus*. If CSF can gain access to the subarachnoid space and is then not absorbed by the arachnoid villi, it is classified as a *communicating hydrocephalus*. This type of hydrocephalus may be associated with postmeningitic or posthemorrhagic states. Excess formation of CSF is rare and may be caused by choroid plexus tumors. Noncommunicating hydrocephalus caused by faulty circulation or obstruction results in enlargement of the ventricular system. This eventually leads to signs of increased intracranial pressure in adults and to bulging fontanelles and an enlarged head in infants. The treatment of choice is the removal of the obstruction. Prognosis depends on the cause and severity of the obstruction and on the timing and effectiveness of the treatment.

Clinical manifestations of hydrocephalus depend on the age and rapidity of onset and the nature and success of the treatment. A newborn infant who exhibits a grossly enlarged head, widely separated cranial sutures, and protruding eyes usually has irreversible signs of prolonged pressure, such as blindness from optic atrophy, paralysis, and mental retardation. In other infants, rapidly increasing head circumference, feeding problems, irritability, delayed motor skills, high-pitched cry, and turned down (setting-sun) eyes are signs of progressive hydrocephalus (Fig. 54-5). Because cerebral expansion is permitted by the open sutures and fontanelles in infancy, classic signs of increasing intracranial pressure, such as headache, vomiting, and altered vital signs, usually are minimal or absent. In older children or adults whose cranial sutures have closed, headache and vomit-

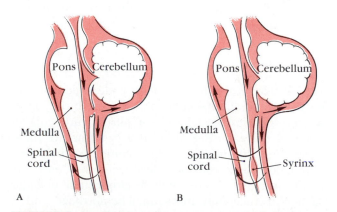

FIGURE 54-2 *Syringomyelia.* **A.** *Normal circulation.* **B.** *Presence of syrinx in the spinal column.*

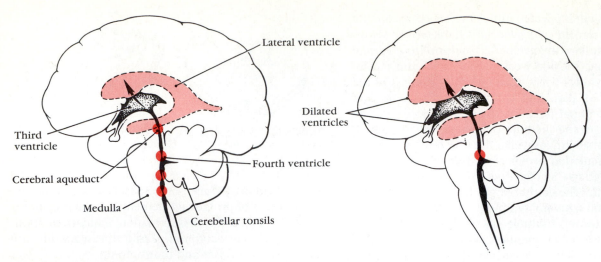

FIGURE 54-4 Schematic representation of areas of possible obstruction to spinal fluid and resulting ventricular enlargement.

ing often are early signs, and they develop with much less trapping of CSF and greater increases in CSF.

Diagnosis is based on clinical observation of head circumference increase in infants and on demonstration of dilated ventricles. Magnetic resonance imaging or computed tomography often demonstrates the ventricular dilatation and the cause. In the absence of these modalities, a combination of skull films, angiography, and air studies can identify hydrocephalus.

Pseudotumor Cerebri

A condition that most frequently occurs in young, obese women, pseudotumor cerebri is related to hydrocephalus and is associated with CSF increases.[14] Intracranial pressure is greatly elevated, usually to 250 to 400 mm H_2O, and may be as high as 600 mm H_2O. Persons with this benign intracranial hypertension have headache and papilledema. Focal signs and other neurologic deficits usually are absent. Treatment focuses on serial lumbar punctures to drain CSF and maintain intracranial

pressure near normal. In many instances, these individuals recover after repeated lumbar punctures have restored the balance of CSF formation and absorption.

CRANIAL MALFORMATIONS

Arrested brain growth is the cause of the cranial malformation called *microcephaly vera*, or small head. Premature suture closure, frequently associated with microcephaly, results from arrested brain growth and is not a cause of it. This is an inherited defect of an autosomal recessive or sex-linked gene. There is no treatment for the severe mental retardation of microcephaly, which often is accompanied by cerebral palsy or seizure activity. *Craniostenosis* is early closure and ossification of one or more of the sutures in the skull that occurs before brain growth is arrested. Early recognition and immediate surgery to create artificial sutures are necessary to decompress the brain and to limit the extent of neurologic damage caused by increasing intracranial pressure. If treatment is absent or delayed, this pressure can cause exophthalmos, optic atrophy, seizures, and mental retardation.

CEREBRAL PALSY

The term *cerebral palsy* includes a wide variety of nonprogressive brain disorders that occur during intrauterine life, during delivery, or during early infancy. Cerebral palsy, by definition, is a syndrome of motor disabilities, although it may be accompanied by mental retardation or seizure disorders, or both. Causes are many and include cerebral developmental disorders such as microcephaly, intracranial hemorrhage, and cerebral anoxia, as well as poisoning by toxins such as excessive bilirubin in the blood (kernicterus). Prenatal

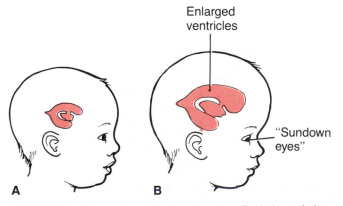

FIGURE 54-5 **A.** Normal cephalic shape in infant. **B.** Hydrocephalus with characteristic "sun-set" or "sun-down" eyes.

factors include infection with rubella, nutritional deficiency, and blood factor incompatibility. Asphyxia can produce cerebral palsy either prenatally or during labor or delivery. Intrapartum production of cerebral palsy also may be related to anesthesia or various metabolic disturbances. Postpartum development of cerebral palsy is relatively uncommon but may develop after central nervous system infections, asphyxia, or head trauma.[5]

Clinical manifestations of cerebral palsy depend on the areas of the brain that have sustained damage. Three main groups have been described according to the dominant signs (Table 54-1). The *paralytic cerebral palsies* are caused by damage to the cortical motor cells and the pyramidal tracts in the brain. These typically are manifested as spastic diplegias, quadriplegias, or hemiplegias. The *dyskinetic cerebral palsies* are caused by damage to the extrapyramidal system and are characterized by abnormal movements of an athetoid, choreiform, or dystonic nature (see pp. 1093–1094). The *ataxic cerebral palsies* indicate cerebellar damage, and they typically involve incoordination and gait disturbances. Mixed cerebral palsy can combine any of the these clinical presentations.

Symptoms are present and nonprogressive from birth or early infancy, and diagnosis usually is made early in the preschool years. Treatment is aimed at preventing crippling secondary disabilities and providing special education to ensure the greatest possible function.

▼ Disorders Characterized by Progressive Weakness or Paralysis

Progressively paralyzing neurologic disorders affect the pyramidal system of the brain or cord, or the final common pathway between the cord and the muscle. They can result from dietary deficiencies, autoimmune disorders, genetic defects, or infectious diseases, and they can be idiopathic. If the reflex arc remains intact, the usual sign is a spastic paresis or paralysis with normal or hyperactive reflexes. If the lower motor neuron or final common pathway is interrupted, the result is flaccid paralysis with diminished or absent reflexes. If the damage is spread throughout the motor system, as in amyotrophic lateral sclerosis, spasticity is present until the final common pathway is interrupted, after which characteristic flaccidity and atrophic wasting of muscles predominate. Prognosis and treatment depend on the nature of the disease and the availability and use of treatment.

Myasthenia gravis is a chronic voluntary muscle disorder that destroys the acetylcholine (ACh) receptors of the neuromuscular junction. The result of this destruction is

---

TABLE 54-1 *Types and Clinical Manifestations of Cerebral Palsies*

Type	Percentage	Clinical Manifestations
Spastic, paralytic diplegia	50	Spasticity predominates, especially in the legs. Mental retardation occurs only in a small percentage. Walking is delayed, and the gait is stiff and awkward, often with crossing of the legs, called scissors gait. Lower legs often are splayed outward and feet are flexed. Speech may be markedly impaired or unaffected. Sphincter control is usually attained but delayed.
Quadriplegia	30	Spasticity of all four extremities is common. Often associated with marked retardation. Children are nonambulatory and attain little or no speech or sphincter control.
Hemiplegia	10	Spasticity and control affect one side of the body. The clinical picture varies according to associated mental retardation. Two-thirds to three-fourths have normal intelligence. Seizures are common with one-third.
Dyskinetic CP Ataxic CP	10	Dyskinetic CP exhibits elements of extrapyramidal system dysfunction. Abnormal movements (choreoathetotic) may predominate, increase or decrease as the child grows older. Mental retardation is frequent. Ataxic CP indicates cerebellar damage and ataxic gait; incoordination is characteristic. Either dyskinetic or ataxic CP may be associated with other forms and is difficult to clearly differentiate. If it can be clearly identified, it is classified as mixed CP. Mixed CP may refer to any combination of the clinical manifestations.

CP, cerebral palsy.

impairment of nerve impulse passage (Fig. 54-6). Myasthenia gravis most commonly occurs in young adults, and it progresses with remissions and exacerbations. It is characterized by activity-induced abnormal muscle fatigability. The fatigue results in typical drooping of eyelids (ptosis) and jaw, nasal voice, slurred speech, and weakness of the proximal extremities; all symptoms worsen during the day but improve with rest or with the use of anticholinesterase drugs, such as neostigmine. Muscle fibers eventually may degenerate, and weakness, especially of the muscles of the head, neck, trunk, and limbs, may become irreversible. Hyperplasia of the thymus frequently is associated, and about 12% of persons with myasthenia gravis have a thymoma (benign thymic tumor).[9] Reflexes may remain normal or reflect fatigue, decreasing with each repeated test. There appears to be no sensory alteration.

Several primary muscle disorders cause clinically similar fatigue in the muscles, but only myasthenia gravis responds to anticholinesterase drugs. Myasthenia gravis involves progressive failure of impulse conduction at the neuromuscular junction.[21] Myasthenic crisis, a severe exacerbation of the disease, is associated with severe muscle weakness, respiratory insufficiency, and great difficulty in swallowing. These symptoms are associated with insufficient anticholinesterase drug therapy. It is an autoimmune disease, with cellular and humoral factors that contribute to the disease. The triggering mechanism for the autoimmune response remains elusive. Circulating ACh-receptor antibodies have been identified that link themselves to receptor sites in the voluntary muscles, damaging and blocking the receptors. In some cases, aggregates of lymphocytes are present in the muscles and other organs. Postsynaptic membrane abnormalities cause the muscles to become less responsive to nerve impulses. ACh is less effective in producing the desired depolarization in the affected muscles, and muscle contractions become less effective with each rapidly succeeding nerve impulse.[21]

The observed relation between myasthenia gravis and rheumatoid arthritis, systemic lupus erythematosus, and disorders of the thyroid, such as thyroiditis and thyrotoxicosis, is believed to be based on a common disturbance of the immune system, expressed in different ways. The nature of these disturbances is not fully understood, nor is their relation clear. Many experts postulate that genetic characteristics may constitute risk factors for autoimmune disorders such as myasthenia gravis, thyroiditis, and even diabetes mellitus.[21]

During the early active stage of myasthenia gravis, after the characteristic remissions and exacerbations have begun but before muscle atrophy sets in, some patients respond well to surgical removal of the thymus. Many believe that early thymectomy may decrease the level of autoimmune activity before much permanent damage is sustained by the ACh-receptor sites in the voluntary muscles. Plasmapheresis is another method of treatment aimed at removing anti ACh-receptor antibodies from the blood to decrease the autoimmune activity.[21] Steroids usually are given to suppress the production of antibodies. Other immunosuppressive drugs, such as azathioprine, have been beneficial in some cases. Anticholinesterase drugs are administered to prevent the breakdown of the ACh at the myoneural junction. Too much anticholinesterase drug activity may produce skeletal muscle weakness that resembles the myasthenic defect.[17] Additional clinical signs include nausea, vomiting, gastrointestinal irritability, bradycardia, diarrhea, pallor, miosis, and excessive salivation. This response is known as *cholinergic crisis*, and it is hard to differentiate clinically from myasthenic crisis, or disease exacerbation.[17] Most persons who are in a crisis state are treated for cholinergic crisis, withdrawn from the anticholinesterase drugs, and maintained on assisted respiration until the type of crisis can be identified.

The course of myasthenia gravis is variable. Some people do not develop any symptoms other than the initial ocular muscle fatigue and weakness. Others who

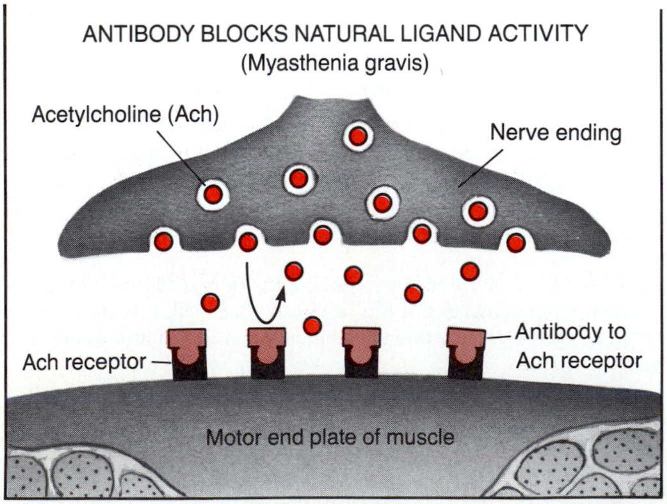

ANTIBODY BLOCKS NATURAL LIGAND ACTIVITY
(Myasthenia gravis)

Acetylcholine (Ach)

Nerve ending

Ach receptor

Antibody to Ach receptor

Motor end plate of muscle

FIGURE 54-6 *Antireceptor antibody. Inhibition of synaptic transmission in myasthenia gravis leads to profound muscle weakness. (Rubin, E., and Farber, J.L. Pathology, [2nd ed.]. Philadelphia: J.B. Lippincott, 1994.)*

exhibit more generalized symptoms respond well to standard treatment for years. A small percentage suffer the acute, fulminating disease accompanied by muscle atrophy with poor response to all treatment. It may first manifest itself during pregnancy or with surgical procedures requiring general anesthesia. Death from myasthenia gravis usually occurs within the first 5 to 10 years of onset, when the disease is most acute. Lethal crises do not usually occur until late in the disease, and the damage sustained tends to remain constant or to be compensated for by other muscles. Death that occurs after many years usually is caused by the secondary problem of immobility, which leads to pneumonia.

Myasthenic mothers can pass the antibodies to their infants through the placenta. These infants may experience spontaneous recovery from the myasthenia symptoms within 1 to 3 months, or they may persist with the disease for their lifetime.

SUBACUTE COMBINED DEGENERATION OF THE CORD

Vitamin B_{12} deficiency, which usually occurs as part of pernicious anemia, can lead to degeneration of the white matter in the lateral and posterior spinal, peripheral polyneuropathy, and slight cerebral atrophy (see also pp. 1090–1091). Neurologic manifestations begin gradually and usually are accompanied by the classic megaloblastic anemia. Unusual sensations such as tingling, numbness, and pain often are the first symptoms of neurologic degeneration. These paresthesias are followed by motor signs of weakness and incoordination. The paresthesias and motor signs both tend to begin in the lower limbs and move to the upper limbs and trunk as the disease spreads up the posterior and lateral cord. With progressive and untreated degeneration of the cord, sensory ataxia and either spastic paralysis with hyperactive reflexes or flaccid paralysis with absent reflexes may occur in all four limbs, with the most pronounced symptoms in the lower limbs. If degeneration is confined to the posterior columns, incoordination is predominant. If it is more lateral, weakness and paralysis are most characteristic. The nature of the paralysis is influenced by the presence or absence of peripheral neuropathy and the status of the reflex arc. In addition to these motor signs, there may be optic atrophy or nystagmus if the second or third cranial nerve is affected. The other cranial nerves seldom are affected. Cerebral atrophy may result in impaired memory, confusion, paranoid behavior, irritability, and depression.

The damaged peripheral nerves eventually regenerate, with improvement in sensory symptoms, coordination, and reflexes, but spasticity and signs of cerebral atrophy are not likely to disappear, because central nervous system damage is not reversible. Early diagnosis is important, because the condition is treatable and reversible if symptoms have been present for only a short

duration. Clinically similar disorders, such as neurosyphilis and multiple sclerosis, must be ruled out by gastric acid evaluation, blood tests for megaloblastic anemia, and bone marrow evaluation for abnormalities of red cells. Serum B_{12} may be evaluated, or tests may be made of vitamin B_{12} absorption using radioactive vitamin B_{12}.

GUILLAIN-BARRÉ SYNDROME (ACUTE INFLAMMATORY DEMYELINATING POLYNEUROPATHY)

An acute, often postinfectious polyneuritis, Guillain-Barré syndrome, may be caused by an allergic response or some type of hypersensitivity reaction. The specific triggering mechanism for this disturbance in the immune response remains unknown, but the lymphocytes become sensitized and begin to destroy myelin.[9] The onset usually occurs a few days or weeks after a febrile illness, vaccination, injury, or surgery. Guillain-Barré syndrome has no predilection for age group, sex, or race; if an infectious cause (most often respiratory or gastrointestinal) can be demonstrated, it usually is viral. The syndrome also has occurred after immunizations.

Demyelination and degeneration of the myelin sheath and axon occur in the segmental peripheral nerves and the anterior and posterior spinal nerve roots. Cranial nerve involvement, especially involvement of cranial nerve VII (facial), is commonly observed. Lymphocytes and macrophages infiltrate the myelin sheath initially, and later, if disease progression continues, the axon itself is involved.[9] Inflammation, edema, and damaged nerves result in both sensory and motor dysfunction.

The initial clinical symptom is general bilateral weakness, first manifested by difficulty in walking. These symptoms become progressive and are accompanied by paresthesias (numbness and tingling) and, possibly, pain in the back. The symptoms begin in the lower extremities and progress symmetrically in an ascending manner to involve the muscles of the trunk, upper extremities, and cranial nerves. Complete flaccid paralysis may or may not occur. Maximum manifestations of the disease occur in about 1 to 2 weeks, although the rate of spread varies. In severe cases, total paralysis develops rapidly, and serious respiratory involvement requires ventilatory support. Sensory involvement is usually less profound than the motor involvement. Changes in proprioception and vibratory sense are the most commonly observed sensory deficits, but deficits in light touch, pinprick, muscle sensitivity, and temperature sensations may occur.

Variant autonomic dysfunctions may occur: postural hypotension, tachycardia, dysrhythmias, diaphoresis, urinary retention and other manifestations. Reflexes normally are diminished or lost, but they occasionally remain normal, even with severe muscle weakness. If the onset of flaccid paralysis is sudden and symmetric and it is accompanied by sensory changes, diagnosis of Guillain-Barré syndrome can be made by clinical observation and history alone. Muscle atrophy is not common but may occur if axon loss is severe. Electrodiagnostic studies show slowing of nerve conduction in most affected persons. CSF protein level becomes markedly elevated after the first few days of illness, whereas the cell count remains negative (albuminocytologic dissociation).[9]

If death occurs, it usually is caused by respiratory arrest, pneumonia or pulmonary emboli. For survivors of respiratory problems, the prognosis for eventual recovery of function is good. The paralysis may stop as insidiously as it started. The return of motor function occurs in a descending manner, at a slower rate than the ascending onset of symptoms. Eighty-five percent of patients make a complete recovery in 4 to 6 months, but others may have severe residual disabilities. The rate of recovery depends on the extent of neural and axonal regeneration required. Treatment with steroids, adrenocorticotropic hormone, or other immunosuppressant drugs may or may not be beneficial in altering the course of the disease. Plasmapheresis is used to remove the offending antibodies. This treatment seems to be most effective early in the course of the disease.

MULTIPLE SCLEROSIS

Multiple sclerosis (MS) is a relatively common chronic and progressive inflammatory, demyelinating disease of the central nervous system. The peripheral nervous system remains uninvolved. It is estimated that 250,000 to 350,000 people are affected with MS in the United States.[18] It results in diverse manifestations of neurologic alteration. Its basic cause or causes are unknown, but it probably is an autoimmune disorder influenced by a genetic susceptibility. The possibility that a latent viral infection precipitates the disease has been investigated without success.[8] Dietary deficiencies and acute viral infections also have been studied as causative agents. Stress and trauma seem to play a role in precipitating the onset of MS or in exacerbating the symptoms. MS is most common in colder climates, and onset usually occurs in persons between the ages of 20 and 40 years. Women have a higher incidence than men.[10] The incidence of MS is much higher in people of European origin, and much lower among Orientals, Africans, and Native Americans.[1,10] The incidence in close family members is at least five times that of the general population; this fact has led to speculation that exposure to a pathogenetic agent or inherited susceptibility to the disease may be involved. If one of a set of identical twins has MS, there is a 50% chance that the other will develop some evidence of MS.[8]

The disease normally begins rather suddenly with the occurrence of a set of focal symptoms of visual disturbance or of motor dysfunction in one or two limbs. The causative lesion or plaque is present predominantly in the white matter of the central nervous system, and the myelin sheaths that normally act as insulation around nerve fibers are lost. Loss of myelin slows, blocks, or distorts transmission of nerve impulses. Inflammatory edema around the plaques contributes to early acute symptoms. During the course of the disease, some of the myelinated fibers may regenerate, and associated symptoms may disappear. Gliosis eventually occurs in the lesions; scar tissue replaces myelin and may replace the axis cylinders themselves, leading to permanent disability. From this gliosis comes the term *sclerosis*, meaning induration or scarring. Oligodendrocytes disappear, and astrocytes proliferate.[28]

Initial symptoms may be transient, and often they are followed by complete, or nearly complete, recovery as the myelin is replaced. Periods of remission are common. Later alterations become permanent, with remissions and exacerbations limited to new symptoms superimposed on a baseline of disability. This permanence in symptoms is caused by gradual disruption and destruction of the nerve cells themselves, even though this is initially a disease of the myelin sheath rather than of the cells.[1] If the lesions are predominantly in the pyramidal tracts of the cerebrum or spinal cord, the symptoms are motor. If they affect the lateral spinothalamic or posterior tracts of the cord, sensory changes are noted. Weakness or spastic paralysis of the limbs and sphincters with hyperactive reflexes is common. Sexual dysfunction, with impotence in men and alteration in vaginal sensations in women, is a common and disturbing aspect of sensorimotor changes. Paresthesias such as pain, numbness, and tingling may be noted in the limbs or the face. Emotional changes may range from emotional lability to sustained euphoria or severe depression.[1,8]

Brain stem lesions often contribute to emotional lability and also produce symptoms of cranial nerve injury. The optic, oculomotor, trochlear, and abducens nerves and the vestibular branch of the auditory nerve are especially common sites of damage. Visual signs and symptoms range from nystagmus, to diplopia, to visual dimness, to patchy or complete blindness.[28] Optic neuritis with visual loss, eye movement pain, and swelling of the optic disc is the initial presentation in 17% of cases.[11] Pupillary abnormalities may be noted. Dizziness may be mild, or it may be severe and associated with nausea and vomiting. Speech may be difficult because of spastic weakness of facial and speech muscles. Dysphagia makes eating difficult and increases the danger of aspiration. Cerebellar lesions also affect speech, producing slurred, uncoordinated articulation. Other signs, such as intention tremor of the hands, head tremor, and staggering gait, are indicative of cerebellar lesions.

Although early clinical manifestations may be limited to effects of alteration in the cerebellar area, the brain stem, or the cerebrum, late MS usually affects all parts of the central nervous system. The classic triad that Charcot described in 1868, which occurs late in the disease, includes nystagmus, intention tremor, and speech disorders.[3] Spastic paraplegia, incontinence, and extreme emotional lability also are typical of the late stages of MS.

The diagnosis is based on history, clinical features, observation of the pattern of remission and exacerbation of symptoms, and ruling out of other diseases such as subacute combined degeneration of the cord (see p. 1089). Studies of antibodies in the blood or CSF often show gamma globulin abnormalities in those with established MS. The most consistent CSF finding is the presence of increased amounts of oligoclonal bands of immunoglobulin G (normally less than 5 mg/dL).[8] These bands are characteristic of MS but may also occasionally be seen in other central nervous system illnesses such as syphilis and lupus erythematosus.[8] Other changes in the CSF are inconsistent and nonspecific.

Other evaluative data to support the diagnosis of MS may be acquired with studies of evoked responses or with computed tomography or magnetic resonance imaging scans. Evoked-potential testing involves an electrophysiologic measurement in which a stimulus is delivered and its transit through the nervous system is timed. The common tests are the visual, brain stem auditory, and somatosensory evoked responses. More than 80% of cases of persons with chronic relapsing or chronic progressive MS have an abnormal response.[8] Computed tomography scans are often negative in MS, showing only hypodense lesions and some cerebral atrophy. Magnetic resonance imaging scans are usually positive, with the plaque-like lesions clearly visible.[8]

The prognosis varies from progression to death in less than 6 months (acute MS) to a benign course for more than 20 years without shortening or alteration of productive life. Fulminant cases that are fatal within weeks to months show intense inflammatory response in the lesions.[1] Even if the patient survives to old age, the last years may be spent as a spastic paraplegic, with visual disorders, incontinence, dysarthria, and lack of emotional control. Death often is caused by secondary disorders such as pneumonia or septic decubitus ulcers.

Treatment of MS usually is supportive for the symptoms exhibited and focused on prevention of complications. Special high-vitamin or low-fat diets have failed to consistently influence the course of the disease. Immunosuppression through the use of plasma exchange, steroids, azathioprine, and cyclophosphamide has provided encouraging results.[8]

AMYOTROPHIC LATERAL SCLEROSIS

Amyotrophic lateral sclerosis (ALS, or Lou Gehrig disease) is a primary neurologic disease that affects motor function and results in alterations of gait and paralysis. Respiratory muscles are weakened and eventually paralyzed. It is a noninflammatory disease of the upper and lower motor neurons, with demyelination secondary to axon degeneration. Unlike MS, which classically is characterized by remissions and exacerbations, ALS usually steadily progresses to death within 2 to 6 years of diagnosis.[15] Premature aging of nerve cells as a result of some environmental or genetic factor, nutritional deficiencies, heavy-metal poisoning, an autoimmune response, metabolic defects, and even a dormant virus have all been identified as possible causes or contributors to ALS.[26] Familial autosomal dominant patterns account for 5% to 10% of total cases, and the gene is located on chromosome 21q.[10, 28]

Loss of the motor cells in the cerebral cortex can result in signs of upper motor neuron damage, with weakness or spastic paralysis and hyperactive reflexes. Muscle involvement is asymmetrically distributed. This is especially likely to occur in the lower limbs. Damage to cranial nerves in the medulla produces signs of *bulbar palsy* of either the spastic or flaccid type. Bulbar palsy refers to weakness or paralysis of the muscles supplied by the motor cranial nerves. Commonly, upper and lower motor neuron damage are mixed in ALS. Lower motor signs predominate in the upper extremities, and upper motor signs predominate in the lower extremities. When reflexes are interrupted, muscles atrophy secondary to denervation and loss of muscle tone. In these areas, diminished reflexes or flaccid paralysis occurs. Muscle atrophy often is present in the upper limbs and tongue.

Degeneration may occur anywhere within the pyramidal system, in the anterior motor cells of the spinal cord, or in the ventral nerve roots. It is most severe in the cervical cord and characteristically does not affect peripheral nerves. The muscle fasciculations or twitching frequently seen in the upper limbs or tongue are thought to be caused by accumulating excessive neurotransmitter at the myoneural junction rather than by abnormal spontaneous discharges of degenerating nerve cells.

The onset of ALS usually occurs after age 50, and it is twice as prevalent in men as in women. One common early sign if the brain stem is involved may be muscle fasciculations of the tongue. Fasciculations, which also may be seen in the hands or upper limbs, are small local muscle contractions that occur if a muscle is tapped or moved passively. Whenever the brain stem is affected, slurred speech and weakness of the palate and facial muscles may occur. Reflexes may be normal, hyperactive, or diminished, depending on whether there is lower motor neuron damage (Box 54-1). If lower motor neuron damage is present, muscle wasting occurs in the tongue and other muscles. Swallowing eventually is affected, and speech may become unintelligible.

Weakness and clumsiness are first noted in the distal portions of the upper limbs, and wasting of the muscles of the hand is characteristic. Sexual dysfunction, such as impotence, is an early sign; bowel and bladder sphincters usually are not affected until late in the disease. Lower-extremity function is retained longer than upper-extremity function, but as the disease progresses, the latter also is lost. Characteristically, there is no sensory alteration in ALS, and intellectual function is retained until death. Paralysis of the trunk and respiratory muscles occurs late in the course of the disease if bulbar palsy does not cause death first. Death often is caused by pneumonia or respiratory failure.[2]

Diagnosis is based on characteristic clinical signs, such as upper limb weakness, wasting of hand muscles, and muscle fasciculations. Disorders such as syringomyelia, cord tumors, and neurosyphilis may cause similar clinical signs, but they usually have pain and sensory changes associated with them. The absence of muscle atrophy and lack of muscle response to edrophonium hydrochloride rule out a diagnosis of myasthenia gravis. Biopsy of muscle and electromyography show denervation atrophy in ALS. Prognosis is worst if the brain stem is affected first. Life expectancy is best if the degeneration remains confined to the lower motor neurons of the middle and lower spinal cord. Affected persons seldom survive longer than 10 years after onset, but death can occur within a year. Treatment is symptomatic, with no beneficial effects from antiinflammatory and immunosuppressive drugs.

▼ *Disorders Characterized by Abnormal Movements*

Abnormal movements often indicate alterations in the extrapyramidal motor system. This system is not clearly understood, so the relation of the pathology and structural alterations to the clinical manifestations is not clear. Abnormal movements often result from alterations and reflect a disturbance in the balance between the excitatory and inhibitory neurotransmitters in the basal ganglia. The neurotransmitters involved apparently are dopamine, ACh, and gamma-aminobutyric acid (GABA). The basal ganglia most often affected are the four that make up the corpus striatum: caudate, putamen, globus pallidus, and claustrum. In some disorders, such as early parkinsonism, conscious effort can temporarily suppress these movements, but typically they return if the person relaxes or is distracted.

The abnormal movements that result are of different types and may be painful or incapacitating. They range from the fine, rhythmic quivering tremor to the violent, irregular jerking or twisting movements of *ballismus*. *Dyskinesias*, or alterations in voluntary muscle movement, and *dystonias*, or alterations in muscle tone (eg, rigidity), are both classified as abnormalities of movement. *Fixed* or *intermittent muscle spasms*, such as are characteristic of torticollis, may be included unless they are caused by muscle rather than nerve damage. *Choreas* are irregular muscle twitchings that may become so severe that they contribute to death from exhaustion. *Athetosis*, or athetoid movements, are slow, repeated, purposeless muscle movements that may affect the digits only or the entire body.

There are many causes of extrapyramidal dysfunction. Cerebral anoxia or trauma in utero or during delivery can produce an athetoid cerebral palsy, spastic cerebral palsy, or both. The characteristic tremors of parkinsonism may be produced by therapy with the major tranquilizers of the phenothiazine family or by carbon monoxide poisoning. The exhausting muscle twitchings of chorea may be caused by a genetic defect or an infectious disease. As with all neurologic disorders, abnormal movements give more clues about which structures are damaged than about what has damaged them. Therefore, a complete physical examination and a thorough family history may be more important than laboratory test results in identifying the source of the problem.

PARKINSON DISEASE

Parkinson disease, also known as paralysis agitans or idiopathic parkinsonism, is a common, chronic degenerative disease of the late middle age and elderly populations. The triggering mechanism for Parkinson disease remains elusive. Various theories abound for its pathogenesis, including metabolic and viral origins. The disease occurs in persons between 50 and 80 years of age, with onset of symptoms most commonly at about age 60. Parkinson disease is an extrapyramidal disorder of the basal ganglia.

The basal ganglia include the caudate nucleus, the putamen, and the globus pallidus. The subthalamic nucleus and substantia nigra, together with the basal ganglia and the motor neurons of the spine, form the extrapyramidal system (see pp. 950–951). The extrapyramidal motor system helps to maintain an upright posture, muscle tone, and coordination. It regulates some of the automatic movements in expressions and walking that produce smooth motion.[4]

Dopamine is one of the chemical transmitters in the brain that is stored in the cells of the basal ganglia. It is depleted in Parkinson disease, particularly in the substantia nigra and corpus striatum. The clinical signs apparently arise from progressive degeneration of the pigmented cells of the substantia nigra (Fig. 54-7).[10, 28] The underlying cause of this cellular destruction is unknown. It has been suggested that 80% depletion of dopamine has occurred before clinical signs of parkinsonism become evident.[4] Dopamine-containing neurons project to the corpus striatum through fibers called the nigrostriatal pathway. In the corpus striatum, dopamine and Ach are important in controlling complex movements. Dopamine acts as an inhibitory transmitter, and Ach acts as an excitatory transmitter. Coordinated voluntary motor activity occurs as a result of a balance between the excitatory cholinergic and inhibitory dopaminergic secretions. With dopamine depletion in Parkinson disease, the classic triad of parkinsonism appears: tremors, rigidity, and bradykinesia (slow movement). The striatal cells, under the predominance of Ach, initiate action potentials more rapidly because the counterbalance of dopamine is decreased or absent.

In addition to tremors, rigidity, and bradykinesia, Parkinson disease is characterized by a masklike facial expression and infrequent blinking, which are caused by diminished automatic movements. Speech is quiet and monotonous. Writing tends to be small, leading to an undecipherable trail. Cognitive and perceptual abilities reflect deterioration in memory and problem-solving in many affected persons. Spontaneous, automatic movements, such as swinging of the arms when walking, also diminish and cease. The body posture becomes stooped, with apparent flexion of the limbs. The characteristic gait progresses with small, shuffling steps that pick up speed as the patient travels. Increasing muscle rigidity in both extensor and flexor muscles may cause jerky or spastic movements. Rather than losing voluntary function, the person finds it increasingly difficult to initiate voluntary acts (akinesia), and the actions tend to be slow and clumsy.

The tremors of parkinsonism commonly occur in the hands initially and then progress to involve the ankles, head, or mouth. The tremors are most prominent during rest. They can be suppressed with conscious effort for brief periods and usually disappear with sleep. If the index finger and thumb are both involved, the tremors may be described as "pill-rolling." Intention tremors, or tremors that occur during the performance of a precise movement, may also be present. Both resting and intention tremors worsen under emotional stress, although extreme provocation may result in the quick, efficient performance of complex motor functions. Other symptoms, such as heat intolerance, excessive salivation, dysphagia, diaphoresis, constipation, and urinary incontinence, result from autonomic nervous system dysfunction. Intellectual deterioration and dementia are common after Parkinson disease becomes advanced.[3]

Drug-induced parkinsonism, which is caused by dopamine binding or blocking by drugs such as chlorpromazine, usually disappears after the drug is withdrawn or decreased. Symptoms that result from a discrete episode of cerebral anoxia or trauma, such as carbon monoxide poisoning or head injury, may stabilize. Most cases of idiopathic Parkinson disease are characterized by progressive disability until death occurs from secondary problems such as pneumonia 10 or more years after onset of the disease. Diagnosis is based on signs and symptoms and on ruling out of other diseases associated with muscle rigidity or tremors, such as multiple sclerosis and neurosyphilis.[16] Treatment focuses on restoring the balance between dopaminergic and cholinergic activity through pharmacologic intervention.

DRUG-INDUCED DYSKINESIAS AND DYSTONIAS

The major tranquilizers have many effects on the extrapyramidal nervous system. Besides the drug-induced parkinsonian syndrome, which usually occurs early in therapy, there may be a number of other effects, some of which are reversible and some permanent. Dyskinesias are rhythmic, involuntary movements such as chewing

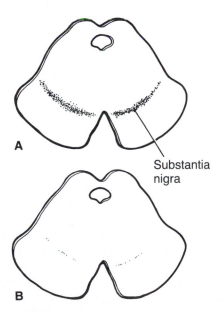

FIGURE 54-7 *Changes of Parkinson disease.* **A.** *Normally substantia nigra of middle brain is clearly demarcated.* **B.** *Little to no substantia nigra can be seen in advanced parkinsonism.*

or smacking. Dystonias are painful, distorted movements of the face, head, or limbs. Variation exists in severity of dystonias.

Dyskinesias and dystonias can occur alone or in association with more typically parkinsonian symptoms soon after major tranquilizer therapy is begun. Chronic tardive dyskinesia is a combination of dyskinesia and dystonia that is related to long-term administration of the neuroleptic drugs. Persistent dyskinesia may occur even after discontinuation of the drug, but it may improve spontaneously over a period of months.[24] *Akathisia*, or restlessness in the muscles, is more difficult to treat and may require dosage reduction or a change in drugs.[24]

Dyskinesias and dystonias also may occur during therapy with levodopa. They usually disappear as the drug is decreased. If the symptoms appear before the tremors of parkinsonism are under control, the increased dosage of levodopa needed to control the tremors may lead to intolerable dyskinesias or dystonias. However, if the dosage is decreased to eliminate the dystonias, the tremors may become much worse.

Dyskinesias that occur late in a tranquilizer therapy or after the drug has been discontinued (tardive dyskinesias) may be evidence of permanent, irreversible change in the extrapyramidal nervous system. This change may be in the dopamine receptors themselves.

TORTICOLLIS

Torticollis, or wryneck, is an intermittent or sustained dystonic contraction of the cervical muscles on one side of the neck caused by hysteria, drug therapy, or organic neurologic disease. It may occur as one of the painful dystonias in early phenothiazine therapy or, rarely, it may accompany primary parkinsonism. If it occurs in association with primary or secondary parkinsonism, it may be caused by a relative increase in cholinergic activity in the brain associated with a striatal dopamine deficiency.

The angle of head rotation depends on which muscles are affected; the affected muscles often hypertrophy in response to the constant or frequent powerful muscle contractions. The muscles most commonly involved are the scalene, sternocleidomastoid, and trapezius. The spasm may occur suddenly and painfully, which is characteristic of the drug-induced dystonias and hysteria. The contraction also can occur slowly. Primary muscle fibrosis after trauma and abnormalities of the cervical spine must be ruled out as the cause of this disorder. If major tranquilizers are being used, reduction in dose or anticholinergic therapy may prove useful. Psychotherapy or relaxation therapy may be helpful for hysterical torticollis. If the cause is a lesion in the corpus striatum, the prognosis for cure is poor.[29] In severe cases, the only successful treatment is to transect the upper anterior cervical roots and spinal accessory nerves.

HUNTINGTON DISEASE

Huntington disease, or Huntington chorea, is an inherited autosomal dominant disorder characterized by a progressive degeneration of the cerebral cortex and of the basal ganglia, particularly the caudate nucleus and putamen. In addition to the dramatic choreiform movements for which it is named, there is progressive deterioration of higher intellectual functions, such as memory and judgment, to the point of severe dementia and death. This relatively uncommon inherited disease has its onset of symptoms between 35 and 50 years of age.[13] Its genetic marker has been traced to a defect on chromosome 4.

In Huntington chorea, the neurotransmitter GABA is markedly reduced in the involved areas of the brain. ACh also seems to be reduced, resulting in an imbalance among the three transmitters—GABA, ACh, and dopamine. If dopamine predominates, chorea results, indicating heightened dopamine sensitivity of the striated receptors.[13] If chorea is the major motor symptom, degenerative lesions are especially common in the caudate. In those occasional persons in whom rigidity and tremors predominate, lesions seem to be more likely in the putamen. In many cases of Huntington chorea, lesions are common throughout the corpus striatum and in the thalamus as well.[29] As is usual with extrapyramidal disorders, the full significance of these lesions is not totally understood.

It is believed that GABA is an inhibitory transmitter whose major function is inhibition of target pathways.[25] Degeneration of these neurons causes increasingly violent choreiform movements in the face, neck, and arm, which may be the first signs of neurologic disease. In addition to the chorea or, less commonly, widespread muscle rigidity and tremors, dementia develops that is characterized by impulsiveness, paranoia, neurosis, emotional outbursts, loss of judgment and memory, irritability or apathy, delusions or hallucinations, and suicidal tendencies. The dementia seems to result from atrophy of the cerebral cortex, especially over the frontal and parietal lobes.[29]

If a family history of Huntington chorea exists, diagnosis is made by this history and by confirming physical examination. With a negative family history, diseases such as neurosyphilis must be ruled out. Huntington chorea normally progresses to death from pneumonia or heart failure in 10 to 20 years. No treatment is known to have an effect on the progression of the disease. Drugs that stimulate GABA and ACh synthesis have proved ineffective in treatment of this disease.

▼ Disorders Characterized by Memory and Judgment Deficits

The term dementia refers to an organically caused syndrome of cognitive impairment. There is widespread deterioration in the cerebral cortex, especially in the frontal lobes. Characteristically, decreasing quality of judgment, loss of abstract thinking and reasoning, and diminished memory are accompanied by emotional changes ranging from apathy to lability. There are many causes of dementia, but there is no theory for the cause or pathophysiology of most of these diseases.[3] The examples presented here have been selected because dementia is the prime symptom and because the syndrome demonstrates similarity to vascular, infectious, and other types of lesions. No cures exist, but, in some cases, the pathologic process may be arrested with subsequent therapy for residual problems.

ATHEROSCLEROTIC DEMENTIA

Cerebral atherosclerosis can contribute to the development of transient ischemic attacks or cerebrovascular accidents of a focal nature (see Chap. 50). Cerebral atherosclerosis also can produce the symptoms of dementia secondary to diffuse, small cerebral infarctions and widespread cerebral anoxia. About 13% of dementias are attributed to cerebral atherosclerosis.[4] The term *senile dementia* may be used for the results of diffuse cerebral atherosclerosis; it usually refers to a condition of decreasing intellectual capability with increasing disorientation and emotional lability in the aged person. The disorder most frequently seems to be caused by a decreasing blood supply and cerebral anoxia resulting in cortical degeneration. Sensory deprivation and overmedication among the institutionalized elderly population may be contributing factors to the progression of senile dementia.

ALZHEIMER DISEASE

A common, slowly progressive cerebral degeneration characterized by dementia, Alzheimer disease appears most commonly in individuals older than 65 years of age. The cause of Alzheimer disease remains unknown. Extensive research has been conducted in an attempt to better understand this devastating disease, and a variety of theories have been proposed for its etiological basis. Among these are invasion by slow viruses, ACh deficiency, aluminum excess, autoimmune responses, genetic predisposition, amyloid protein deposition, and vascular changes.[6, 10]

The slow virus theory proposes that a yet unknown unconventional virus with an incubation period of many years infects the individual and causes progressive pathology in the brain. The slow virus theory has been hypothesized based on the findings of an identified slow virus invasion in two other dementias, kuru and Creutzfeldt-Jakob disease, where the pathological changes in the brain are similar to those found in Alzheimer disease.

Research studies have shown that the level of ACh in the cerebral cortex and hippocampus in patients with Alzheimer disease is dramatically lower than in comparable healthy individuals.[7] Pharmaceutical agents that interfere with ACh levels in the brain have produced temporary interference with cognition in healthy persons that is similar to the cognitive impairments seen in people with Alzheimer disease. Excess of certain substances in the brains of these patients has been studied. Aluminum, one of these substances, has been shown to induce neurofibrillary tangles in animal brains, but they differ in appearance and location from those found in Alzheimer-affected brains.[19] The finding of excessive aluminum in the brains of Alzheimer patients remains puzzling, but there is no conclusive evidence that it has a toxic impact on the brain or that it has accumulated as a result of the progressive changes in the brain.

An autoimmune theory proposes that persons with Alzheimer disease have developed antibodies against their own brain tissue, resulting in an attack on the brain parenchyma. It has been speculated that the neuron changes normally associated with aging stimulate some antibody formation, but that these antibodies are generally contained outside of the brain tissue by the blood-brain barrier.[10] The antibodies are thought to be increased and not contained by the blood-brain barrier in patients with Alzheimer disease.

Yet another causative theory is the accumulation of amyloid protein fragments in the brain of affected persons. The Alzheimer-affected brain contains large numbers of amyloid-bearing neuritic plaques in areas that are critical to cognition (the cortex and hippocampus). These senile plaque formations are amyloid β-protein deposits and are associated with degeneration of surrounding neurons.[23] The amyloid β-protein findings have also helped explain the genetic basis of Alzheimer disease. Researchers have identified that the β-amyloid depositions can arise directly as a result of a genetic mutation that, in turn, can initiate some forms of Alzheimer disease.[23] The precursor to the β-amyloid protein is encoded by the gene located on chromosome 21. This is a particularly interesting finding in that the people with Down syndrome present an extra chromosome 21, and many of these persons develop Alzheimer disease in their fourth decade. Increased amyloid β-protein depositions are common in those with familial Alzheimer disease; the condition may also take forms other than the chromosome 21 form, with its genesis traced to various genetic defects.[23]

It was speculated for decades that Alzheimer disease results from insufficient oxygenation of the brain as a result of arteriosclerotic changes in the blood vessels. This theory has been discarded because there are no consistent findings to support it. However, changes in the blood-brain barrier may play some role in Alzheimer disease in that entrance is afforded to substances not ordinarily allowed entrance. Finally, the cerebral vasculature of patients with Alzheimer disease contains amyloid proteins that interfere with normal nutrient exchange and blood-brain barrier activity.

Pathologic changes include cortical degeneration, which is most marked in frontal, temporal, and parietal lobes. Extensive convolutional atrophy of the brain with enlargement of the ventricular system is seen.[10] Characteristic degeneration includes a decrease in neurons that is most pronounced in regions of the brain that are responsible for cognition, memory, and other thought processes. Neurons accumulate as characteristic fiberlike strands, known as *neurofibrillary tangles*. The blood vessels contain and are surrounded by amorphous aggregates of protein. In addition, deposits of cellular debris and amyloid (neuritic plaques) are present throughout the brain. Finally, there is marked reduction in the production of neurotransmitters, particularly ACh.[29] There seems to be a direct correlation between the degree of dementia and the loss of ACh in the brain.

Early symptoms are insidious and include loss of memory, carelessness about personal appearance, emotional disturbances that progress to complete disorientation, severe deterioration in speech, incontinence, and stereotyped, repetitive movements. Memory impairment is related to loss of neurons in the hippocampus and a decrease in ACh receptors in the forebrain.[20] Depression is common as the persons recognizes the cognitive decline that is occurring. Progression to severe dementia is relentless and occurs over a period of 5 to 10 years, although the rate of progression varies. Terminally, the person loses all cognitive ability and cannot perceive, think, speak, or move.[12] Death results from secondary causes such as septic decubitus ulcers, dehydration, and pneumonia. Because there is no definitive diagnostic test for Alzheimer disease, the diagnostic workup should include a thorough physical examination, neurological workup, and psychiatric evaluation. Diagnosis is usually made after other conditions that can cause dementia have been ruled out. No treatment at this time seems to have a significant effect on the course of the disease.

PICK DISEASE

Pick disease, a degenerative neurologic disease of the fourth and fifth decades, is thought to be passed on by an autosomal dominant gene. It affects women more than

men and may occur in families.[3] The clinical picture is similar to that of Alzheimer disease. Degeneration occurs, with atrophy of the frontal and temporal lobes. The first three cortical layers are most severely involved, and the gyri are so dramatically atrophied as to give this area of the brain the appearance of a dried walnut. The unaffected cells frequently swell, and they contain cytoplasmic filamentous inclusions known as *Pick bodies*.[3]

In contrast to Alzheimer disease and Huntington chorea, the initial signs and symptoms of Pick disease reflect personality changes that elude the person's awareness. The behavioral deterioration is evidenced by disinterest in surroundings, irritability, forgetfulness, confusion, cognitive sluggishness, apathy, and dementia. As the disease progresses, language deteriorates to echolalia (parrotlike repetition of words), stereotyped words and phrases, incomprehensible jargon, and, finally, mutism. Motor deterioration begins with gait disturbances, weakness, and rigidity and progresses to flexion contractions and paraplegia. Computed tomography scans show lobar atrophy, but the electroencephalogram is often normal until very late in the course of the disease.[12] There is no known effective treatment of Pick disease. Supportive and symptomatic treatment is the mainstay of care. Death occurs after a 2- to 10-year course.[3]

NEUROSYPHILIS

Neurosyphilis, seldom seen now in industrialized cultures, is thought to be caused by the spirochete, *Treponema pallidum*. This organism reaches the nervous system during the second stage of a syphilitic infection, and its accompanying neurologic symptoms may not appear for months or years. If neurologic symptoms appear within a few years of the initial infection, they tend to be focal and to respond well to antibiotic therapy. If the onset of neurologic symptoms is delayed, the earliest signs reveal widespread pathology and do not respond as well to therapy.

In the second stage of syphilis, the symptoms of neurosyphilis are transient and vague, including headache and intermittent pains in the trunk and limbs. Rarely, acute meningitis or encephalitis occurs and may result in seizures or coma.[29] A few years after this early stage, inflammation of arterial walls and meningitis often occur, occasionally manifesting a communicating hydrocephalus. Symptoms of the vascular pathology and meningitis include seizures, headache, anxiety, and signs of cranial nerve damage, such as palsies, neuralgia, dizziness, and deafness.[29]

Blood tests for syphilis usually are positive in secondary and early tertiary neurosyphilis. The CSF is positive for *T. pallidum*, and the serum protein level and mononuclear cell count are elevated. These tests, used to confirm the diagnosis of neurosyphilis and to monitor the response to antibiotic therapy, indicate success when the cell count falls, the protein content decreases, and changes eventually occur in the VDRL (Venereal Disease Research Laboratory) test.

General paresis develops about 20 years after the initial infection, and the spirochetes seem to invade the brain parenchyma and cord tissue rather than stay in the meninges and blood vessels. As a result, lesions are spread diffusely over the cerebral cortex, the basal ganglia, and, sometimes, the cerebellar cortex. Early symptoms include impaired memory and concentration. Later, characteristic personal carelessness, impulsiveness, incontinence, and signs of both receptive and expressive aphasia develop. Seizures are common, as are irregular and miotic pupils. The reaction of the pupils to light is diminished or absent, even though they may accommodate to distance changes; this condition is called *Argyll Robertson pupils*, and it signifies midbrain damage. It is especially suggestive of neurosyphilis, although similar pupil changes may be seen in other disorders, such as alcoholic polyneuropathy. Because of damage to the cortical motor cells and pyramidal tracts, voluntary motor function decreases and reflexes become hyperactive; if the cord is invaded, however, reflexes may diminish or disappear. The untreated end result of general paresis usually is a bedridden, incontinent, confused, hallucinating person who is susceptible to all the secondary problems of immobility. Penicillin and erythromycin are curative for syphilis, and no tolerance to the drugs appears to be developed by the organism.

▼ Chapter Summary

▼   Degenerative and chronic alterations in the nervous system can be caused by developmental, congenital, autoimmune, postinfectious, and unknown conditions. The diseases may be progressive and cause increasing disability or they may improve after the causative factor is removed.

▼   Developmental and congenital disorders include such conditions as spina bifida, syringomyelia, hydrocephalus, and cerebral palsy. These conditions are more frequently seen in the younger person and often cause disability immediately after birth.

▼   Disorders characterized by progressive weakness or paralysis include some autoimmune and probable autoimmune conditions such as myasthenia gravis and multiple sclerosis. A postinfectious syndrome, Guillain-Barré, is a demyelinating condition that usually occurs after a viral infection, with increasing paralysis that ascends and then descends with little or no residual disability.

▼   Disorders characterized by abnormal movements include Parkinson disease and several much less common conditions. Parkinson disease is caused by decrease in dopamine stores in the basal ganglia of the brain.

▼   Disorders characterized by memory and judgment deficits include atherosclerotic dementia and Alzheimer disease, which are very common problems, especially in elderly persons. Other conditions that can cause dementia may be related to viral or bacterial infection.

▼ References

1. Antel, J.P., and Arnasan, B.G. Demyelinating Diseases. In Wilson, J., et al. (eds.), *Harrison's Principles of Internal Medicine* (12th ed.). New York: McGraw-Hill, 1991.
2. Barker, E., and Hobdell, R. Neuromuscular disorders. In Barker, E. *Neuroscience Nursing*. St. Louis: Mosby, 1994.
3. Beal, M.F., Richardson, E.P., and Martin, J.B. Degenerative diseases of the nervous system. In Wilson, J., et al. (eds.), *Harrison's Principles of Internal Medicine* (12th ed.). New York: McGraw-Hill, 1991.
4. Bunting, L., and Fitzsimmons, B. Degenerative disorders. In Barker, E., *Neuroscience Nursing*. St. Louis: Mosby, 1994.
5. Caviness, V.S. Neurocutaneous syndromes and other developmental disorders of the central nervous system. In Wilson, J., et al. (eds.), *Harrison's Principles of Internal Medicine* (12th ed.). New York: McGraw-Hill, 1991.
6. Cohen, A.D. *The Brain in Human Aging*. New York: Springer-Verlag, 1988.
7. Davis, P. Neurotransmitters and neuropeptides in Alzheimer's disease. In Katzman, R., (ed.). *Biological Aspects of Alzheimer's Disease*. Cold Spring Harbor, N.Y.: Cold Spring Harbor Laboratory, 1983.
8. Dawson, D. Demyelinating diseases. In Stein, J., (ed.). *Internal Medicine* (4th ed.). St. Louis: Mosby, 1994.
9. De Girolami, U.D., Anthony, D.C., and Forsch, M.P. Peripheral nerve and skeletal muscle. In Cotran, R., Kumar, V., and Robbins, S. *Robbins' Pathologic Basis of Disease* (5th ed.). Philadelphia: W.B. Saunders, 1994.
10. De Girolami, U.D., Frosch, M.P., and Anthony, D.C. The central nervous system. In Cotran, R., Kumar, V., and Robbins, S. *Robbins' Pathologic Basis of Disease* (5th ed.). Philadelphia: W.B. Saunders, 1994.
11. Ebers, G.C. Demyelinating diseases. In Kelley, W.N. (ed.), *Textbook of Internal Medicine* (2nd ed.). Philadelphia: J.B. Lippincott, 1992.
12. Folstein, M.F., and Ross, C. Cognitive impairment in the elderly. In Kelley, W.N. (ed.), *Textbook of Internal Medicine* (2nd ed.). Philadelphia: J.B. Lippincott, 1992.
13. Govan, A.D.T., Macfarlane, P.S., and Callander, R. *Pathology Illustrated* (3rd ed.). New York: Churchill Livingstone, 1991.
14. Johanson, C.E. Ventricles and cerebrospinal fluid. In Conn, P.M. *Neuroscience in Medicine*. Philadelphia: J.B. Lippincott, 1995.
15. Lannon, M., et al. Comprehensive care of the patient with Parkinson's disease. *J. Neurosurg. Nurs.* 18:121, 1986.
16. Logigian, E.L. Disease of peripheral nerve and motor neurons. In Stein, J. (ed.), *Internal Medicine* (4th ed.). St. Louis: Mosby, 1994.

17. McKenry, L.M., and Salerno, E. *Mosby's Pharmacology in Nursing*. St. Louis: Mosby Year Book, 1992.
18. Miller, C.M., and Hens, M. Multiple sclerosis: A literature review. *J. Neurosci. Nurs.* 25:3, 1993.
19. Reisberg, B. (ed.). *Brain Failure: An Introduction to Current Concepts of Senility*. New York: Free Press, 1981.
20. Rodnitzky, R.L. Clinical correlation: Dementia and abnormalities of cognition. In Conn, P.M. *Neuroscience in Medicine*. Philadelphia: J.B. Lippincott, 1995.
21. Rodnitzky, R.L. Clinical correlation: Myasthenia gravis. In Conn, P.M. *Neuroscience in Medicine*. Philadelphia: J.B. Lippincott, 1995.
22. Rodnitzky, R.L. Clinical correlation: Peripheral neuropathy. In Conn, P.M. *Neuroscience in Medicine*. Philadelphia: J.B. Lippincott, 1995.
23. Selkoe, D.J. Amyloid protein and Alzheimer's disease. *Sci. Am.* 265:5, 1991.
24. Sudarsky, L.R. Parkinsonism and movement disorders. In Stein, J. (ed.), *Internal Medicine* (4th ed.). St. Louis: Mosby, 1994.
25. Sundberg, D.K. Chemical messenger systems. In Conn, P.M. (ed.), *Neuroscience in Medicine*. Philadelphia: J.B. Lippincott, 1995.
26. Tandon, R., and Bradley, W.G. Amyotrophic lateral sclerosis. Pt. 2: Etiopathogenesis *Ann. Neurol.* 18:419, 1985.
27. Vigliarolo, D. Managing bowel incontinence in children with meningomyelocele. *Am. J. Nurs.* 80:105, 1980.
28. Vogel, F.S., and Bouldin, T.W. The nervous system. In Rubin, E., and Farber, J.L. *Pathology* (2nd ed.). Philadelphia: J.B. Lippincott, 1994.
29. Walton, J.N. *Brain's Diseases of the Nervous System* (9th ed.). New York: Oxford University Press, 1985.

▼ Unit Bibliography

Adams, J.H., and Graham, D.I. *An Introduction to Neuropathology* (2nd ed.). New York: Churchill Livingstone, 1994.
Adams, R., and Maurice, V. *Principles of Neurology* (5th ed.). New York: McGraw-Hill, 1993.
Appel, S.H., et al. Amyotrophic lateral sclerosis. *Arch. Neurol.* 3:234, 1986.
Barker, E. *Neuroscience Nursing*. St. Louis: Mosby Year Book, 1994.
Barnett, H.J.M. *Stroke: Pathophysiology, Diagnosis, and Management* (2nd ed.). New York: Churchill Livingstone, 1992.
Bastragel-Mason, P.J. Neurodiagnostic testing in critically ill adults. *Crit. Care Nurs.* 12:5, 1992.
Beekham, M.M. Neurologic manifestations of AIDS. *Crit. Care Nurs. Clin. North Am.* 2:29, 1990.
Bell, T.E., LaGrange, K.M., Maier, C.M., et al. Transcranial Doppler: Correlation of blood velocity measurement with clinical status in subarachnoid hemorrhage. *J. Neurosci. Nurs.* 24:4, 1992.
Bonica, J. *The Management of Pain* (2nd ed.). Philadelphia: Lea & Febiger, 1990.
Cohen, G.D. *The Brain in Human Aging*. New York: Springer-Verlag, 1988.
Conn, P.M. *Neuroscience in Medicine*. Philadelphia: J.B. Lippincott, 1995.
Cormack, D.H. *Essential Histology*. Philadelphia: J.B. Lippincott, 1993.
Cotran, R.S., Kumar, V., and Robbins, S.L. *Robbins' Pathologic Basis of Disease* (5th ed.). Philadelphia: W.B. Saunders, 1994.
Dalession, D.J., and Silberstein, S.D. *Wolff's Headache and Other Head Pain* (6th ed.). New York: Oxford University Press, 1993.

Damasio, A.R., and Damasio, H. Brain and language. *Sci. Am.* 267:3, 1992.
Ebersole, P., and Hess, P. *Toward Health Aging: Human Needs and Nursing Response* (4th ed.) St. Louis: Mosby, 1994.
Fischbach, G. Mind and brain. *Sci. Am.* 267:50, 1992.
Flynn, E.P. Cerebral vasospasm following intracranial aneurysms rupture: A protocol for detection. *J. Neurosci. Nurs.* 21:6, 1989.
Ganong, W.F. *Review of Medical Physiology* (16th ed.). Norwalk, Conn.: Appleton & Lange, 1994.
Garner, A., Klintworth, A.K. *Pathobiology of Ocular Disease: A Dynamic Approach*. New York: Dekker, 1994.
Germon, K. Interpretation of ICP pulse waves to determine intracerebral compliance. *J Neurosci Nurs* 20:6, 1988.
Guberman, A. *An Introduction to Clinical Neurology*. Boston: Little, Brown, 1994.
Guyton, A.C. *Textbook of Medical Physiology* (8th ed.). Philadelphia: W.B. Saunders, 1991.
Hanneman, E. Brain resuscitation. *Heart Lung* 15:3, 1986.
Hanson, R.S., and Gerber, R.F. *Coping with Chronic Pain*. New York: Guilford Press, 1990.
Hartmann, A., Yatsu, F., and Kuschusky, W. *Cerebral Ischemia and Basic Medical Treatment*. New York: Springer-Verlag, 1994.
Hickey, J. *The Clinical Practice of Neurological and Neurosurgical Nursing* (4th ed.). Philadelphia: J.B. Lippincott, 1994.
Hooshmad, H. *Chronic Pain: Reflex, Symptomis Dystrophy, Prevention and Management*. Boca Raton, Fla.: CRC Press, 1993.
Hudspeth, A. The hair cells of the inner ear. *Sci Am* 248:54, 1983.
Jackson, L. Cerebral vasospasm after intracranial aneurysmal subarachnoid hemorrhage: A nursing perspective. *Heart Lung* 15:14, 1986.
Jankovic, J., and Tolosa, E. *Parkinson's Disease and Movement Disorders*. Baltimore: Urban & Schwarzenberg, 1988.
Johnson, R.T. *Current Therapy in Neurologic Disease 3*. Philadelphia: B.C. Decker, 1990.
Kelley, W.N. (ed.). *Textbook of Internal Medicine* (2nd ed.) Philadelphia: J.B. Lippincott, 1992.
Leverenz, J., and Sumi, S. Parkinson's disease in patients with Alzheimer's. *Arch. Neurol.* 7:662, 1986.
Mannheimer, J., and Lampe, G. *Clinical Transcutaneous Electrical Nerve Stimulation*. Philadelphia: Davis, 1989.
March, K. Transcranial doppler sonography: Noninvasive monitoring of intracranial vasculature. *J. Neurosci. Nurs.* 22:113, 1990.
Marshall, S.B., Marshall, L.F., Vos, H.R., et al. *Neuroscience Critical Care: Pathophysiology and Patient Management*. Philadelphia: W.B. Saunder, 1990.
McArthur, J., and Harrison, M. HIV-associated dementia. In Appel, S. (ed.). *Current Neurology*. St. Louis: Mosby, 1994.
McCaffrey, M., and Beebe, A. *Pain: A Clinical Manual for Nursing Practice*. St. Louis: Mosby, 1989.
Miller, T.W. *Chronic Pain*. Madison, Conn.: International University Press, 1990.
Moses, R. (ed.). *Adler's Physiology of the Eye* (7th ed.). St. Louis: Mosby, 1981.
Oertel, L.B. The dilemma of cerebral vasospasm treatment. *J. Neurosurg. Nurs.* 17:1, 1985.
Packer, L., Prilipko, L., and Cristen, Y. *Free Radicals in the Brain: Aging, Neurological and Mental Disorders*. New York: Springer-Verlag, 1992.
Perkin, G. *Basic Neurology*. Chichester, Engl.: Elles Harwood, 1986.
Richmond, T. A critical care challenge: The patient with a cervical spinal cord injury. *Focus* 12:23, 1985.
Rubin, E., and Farber, J.L. *Pathology* (2nd ed.). Philadelphia: J.B. Lippincott, 1994.
Salzman, S.K., and Faden, A.I. *The Neurobiology of CNS Trauma*. New York: Oxford University Press, 1994.
Schwartz, S.I. *Principles of Surgery* (6th ed.). New York: McGraw-Hill, 1994.

Schwartzkroin, P.A. *Epilepsy: Modes, Mechanisms, and Concepts.* New York: Cambridge University Press, 1993.

Selkoe, D.J. Amyloid protein and Alzheimer's disease. *Sci. Am.* 265:5, 1991.

Standler, N. *A Short Course in Pathology.* New York: Churchill Livingstone, 1994.

Tollison, C.D. *Handbook of Chronic Pain Management.* Baltimore: Williams & Wilkins, 1989.

Wald, M. Cerebral thrombosis: Assessment and nursing management of the acute phase. *J. Neurosci. Nurs.* 18:36, 1986.

Wall, P., and Melzack, R. *Textbook of Pain* (2nd ed.). Edinburgh: Churchill Livingstone, 1989.

Walter, J. *Pathology of Human Disease.* Philadelphia: Lea & Febiger, 1989.

Walton, J. *Brain's Diseases of the Nervous System* (6th ed.). Oxford: Oxford University Press, 1985.

Wang, C., et al. Brain injury due to head trauma. *Arch. Neurol.* 6:570, 1986.

Weisberg, L. Subdural empyema. *Arch. Neurol.* 5:49, 1986.

Wilson, J., et al. (eds.). Harrison's Principles of Internal Medicine (12th ed.). New York: McGraw-Hill, 1991.

Zeki, S. The visual image in mind and brain. *Sci. Am.* 267:3, 1992.

Reproduction

UNIT 16 discusses reproductive physiology and the common pathologic problems associated with both the male and the female reproductive systems. Chapter 55 provides an overview of normal and altered male reproductive function. A discussion of normal and altered female reproductive function is presented in Chapter 56. Included in both chapters are an overview of the anatomy and physiology of each system and laboratory and diagnostic aids in the examination of these systems. Chapter 57 presents a discussion of those sexually transmitted diseases that affect reproductive function.

The reader is encouraged to use the learning objectives as a study guide outline. The unit bibliography gives direction for further research.

Chapter 55

Normal and Altered Male Reproductive Function

Sharron P. Schlosser

▼ **CHAPTER OUTLINE**

▼ **LEARNING OBJECTIVES**

1. Describe the development and function of the male sex organs.
2. List three functions of the male reproductive system.
3. Discuss spermatogenesis.
4. List and discuss the factors involved in determining male fertility.
5. List and discuss the stages of male response in the sex act.
6. Distinguish between erection, emission, and ejaculation in the sex act.
7. Identify the functions of testosterone.
8. Describe the production and degradation of testosterone.
9. Discuss the influence of the hypothalamus and anterior pituitary on the production of testosterone and spermatogenesis.
10. Briefly describe three diagnostic tests used to determine alterations in male reproductive function.
11. Distinguish between prostatitis, benign prostatic hyperplasia, and carcinoma of the prostate.
12. Discuss the staging of prostatic carcinoma.
13. Define **phimosis, paraphimosis, hypospadias, epispadias, balanitis, priapism, hydrocele, varicocele, torsion of testis, cryptorchidism, orchitis**, and **epididymitis**.
14. Describe the four types of testicular germ cell tumors.
15. List and describe the three major stages of testicular tumors.
16. Discuss the possible influence on male offspring of in utero exposure to diethylstilbestrol.

Barbara L. Bullock: PATHOPHYSIOLOGY: ADAPTATIONS AND ALTERATIONS IN FUNCTION, 4th ed.
© 1996 Lippincott-Raven Publishers

Reproductive function is an integral facet of the human being. Survival of the species depends on proper functioning of the reproductive system. Alterations in male function may be disturbing if they represent a threat to reproductive function and a man's self-image. Alterations can occur in any reproductive organ at any age. This chapter provides an overview of both normal and altered male reproductive function, including congenital anomalies, infections, and cancers. It also includes the diagnostic aids for abnormalities.

▼ Anatomy

The male reproductive system includes both essential and accessory organs (Fig. 55-1). The essential organs are the testes, which produce sperm; accessory organs

include the epididymis, vas deferens, seminal vesicles, ejaculatory ducts, prostate gland, and urethra. The supporting structures of the scrotum, penis, and spermatic cords also are considered accessory organs.

SCROTUM

The scrotum is a saclike structure suspended between the penis and anus in the perineal area. It is composed of fascial connective tissue and contains smooth muscle, known as dartos fascia, and two lateral compartments. The testes are located within these compartments, and the left testis usually is lower than the right one. In the mature male, the scrotum is covered with sparse hair and is darker than adjacent skin. It is sensitive to touch, temperature, pain, and pressure.

The scrotum functions to protect and support the

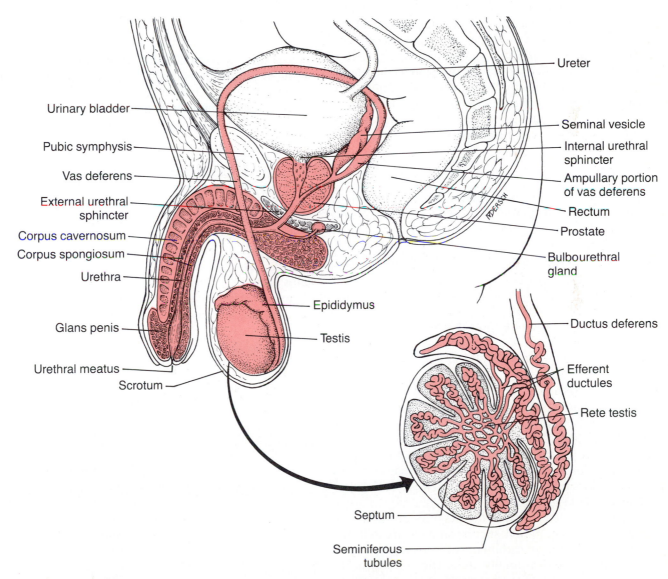

FIGURE 55-1 *Organs of the male reproductive system. (Reeder, S.J., Martin, L.L. and Koniak, D. Maternity Nursing [17th ed.]. Philadelphia: J.B. Lippincott, 1992.)*

testes and sperm. The cremaster, a thin skeletal muscle, and the dartos contract when cold to draw the testes closer to the body. When warm, the muscles relax, allowing the testes to drop away from the body. This process permits the testes to maintain a more constant environmental temperature, which is about 3°F lower than normal body temperature. If the environmental temperature is too high, spermatogenesis is impaired.

TESTES

The testes are two ovoid glands suspended in the scrotum by attachment to both scrotal tissue and spermatic cords. The testes measure 4 to 5 cm in length by 2 to 3 cm in diameter and weigh 10 to 15 g. The testes consist of two layers of tissue—the tunica vaginalis and the tunica albuginea. The tunica vaginalis is a thin, serous covering acquired from the peritoneum during descent. The tunica albuginea is a tough, fibrous membrane that encapsulates the testes. Extensions of the tunica albuginea divide the testes into lobules. Each lobule contains *seminiferous tubules* and *interstitial cells of Leydig*. The seminiferous tubules function as the site for spermatogenesis. Sertoli cells, located in the walls of the tubules, serve to produce and secrete nutrients for spermatogonia in the tubules. Testosterone, the male hormone, is secreted by the interstitial cells.

EPIDIDYMIS

The epididymis is a tortuous genital duct, about 6 m in length, that connects the testis and vas deferens and serves as a passageway for spermatozoa. It is located on top of the testis and is divided into three parts: the head, which is connected to the testis; the body; and the tail, which is continuous with the vas deferens (Fig. 55-2). Sperm are stored in the epididymis up to 2 weeks. During this time, they mature, develop the power of motility, and become capable of fertilizing an ovum.

VAS DEFERENS

The vas deferens is an uncoiled, fibromuscular tube or duct that is about 45 cm long and 2.5 mm thick. This duct ascends from the tail of the epididymis in the scrotum into the abdomen, where it passes over the bladder. On the posterior end of the bladder, the duct enlarges into the ampulla of the vas deferens and joins with the duct from the seminal vesicle to form the ejaculatory duct (Fig. 55-3).

The vas deferens stores the majority of the sperm. During the storage period, sperm metabolism continues, and large amounts of carbon dioxide are produced and secreted into the surrounding fluid. The resulting acidic pH inhibits activity of the sperm during storage. When stimulated, the sympathetic nerves from the pelvic

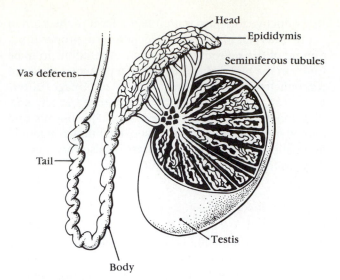

FIGURE 55-2 *The vas deferens in relation to the tubules of the testis and epididymis.*

plexus cause peristaltic contractions of the muscular layer and result in emission of stored sperm into the ejaculatory ducts. On release to the exterior, the sperm again exhibit the power of motility.[5]

SEMINAL VESICLES

The seminal vesicles are two saclike structures about 5 cm long, lined with secretory epithelium, and located directly behind the urinary bladder (see Figure 55-3). They produce a viscous, alkaline, yellowish fluid that makes up a large part of the seminal fluid volume. This fluid is rich in fructose, an energy source for sperm metabolism. Fluid from the seminal vesicles also contains citric acid, five amino acids, and prostaglandins. Sympathetic stimulation produces contractions of the seminal vesicles and emission of the contents.

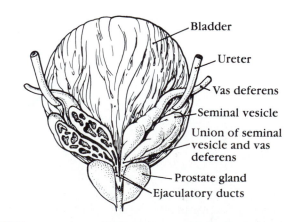

FIGURE 55-3 *Union of the seminal vesicles with the vas deferens and entrance into the prostate gland.*

EJACULATORY DUCTS

The ejaculatory ducts, two short tubes about 2 cm in length, are formed by union of the ampullae of the vas deferens and the ducts of the seminal vesicles. The ejaculatory ducts descend through the prostate gland and terminate in the prostatic urethra, where sperm and secretions from the seminal vesicles and prostate are emitted.

PROSTATE GLAND

The prostate gland is a walnut-sized gland about 4 cm in diameter and 3 cm thick, weighing about 20 g. It is located just below the bladder and surrounds the ejaculatory duct and about 2.5 cm of the urethra. The gland is divided into five lobules by the urethra and the ejaculatory duct. Its primary function is to secrete a thin, milky, alkaline fluid that constitutes a large part of the seminal fluid volume. This fluid is discharged into the urethra during emission and helps to neutralize the acidic fluids of the male urethra and female vagina. In addition, the prostate gland secretes acid phosphatase (PAP) and prostate-specific antigen (PSA), which can be used in assessment of prostatic function.

URETHRA

The urethra is the terminal portion of the seminal fluid passageway. It is about 18 to 20 cm long and is divided into three areas: the prostatic urethra, the membranous urethra, and the penile urethra. The prostatic urethra is the proximal portion and is about 2.5 cm in length. The membranous urethra is the shortest and central section; it measures 0.5 cm and contains the external sphincter. The distal portion is the longest at about 15 cm and constitutes the penile urethra.

BULBOURETHRAL GLANDS

The bulbourethral (Cowper) glands are two pea-sized, brownish glands located just below the prostate. These glands are about 1 cm in diameter and drain into the urethra. On sexual stimulation, these glands secrete a clear, viscous, alkaline fluid that lines the urethra, neutralizes the pH, and lubricates the tip of the penis in preparation for intercourse.

PENIS

The penis is a long, cylinder-like structure covered by a loose layer of skin. It consists of the body and the glans. The body contains three compartments of erectile tissue: two corpora cavernosa and the corpus spongiosum (see Figure 55-1). The corpora cavernosa are large and parallel to each other. The corpus spongiosum is smaller, is located lower than the corpora cavernosa, and contains the urethra. Distally, the corpus spongiosum expands to form the glans penis. In the uncircumcised male, a fold of loose skin, the prepuce, covers the glans. The erectile tissue is spongelike and contains large venous sinuses interspersed with arteries and veins. Sexual stimulation results in dilation of the arteries and arterioles and distention of the cavernous spaces with blood. Filling of the erectile tissue results in erection of the penis. The penis serves two functions: it contains the urethra, which is the passageway for urine, and it is the male organ of copulation.

▼ Male Reproductive Functions

The male reproductive system serves three primary functions: spermatogenesis, performance of the sex act, and hormonal regulation of male sexual function.

SPERMATOGENESIS

The seminiferous tubules of the newborn male's testes contain primitive sex cells called *spermatogonia*. They are located in two to three layers in the outer border of the tubular epithelium (Fig. 55-4). At puberty (about age 13), spermatogenesis begins in all the seminiferous tubules as a result of stimulation by the adenohypophysial (anterior pituitary) gonadotropic hormones (see pp. 682–683).

During spermatogenesis, a series of meiotic divisions occurs. The primary spermatocyte divides into two secondary spermatocytes, which subsequently divide and produce four spermatids (Fig. 55-5). During this process, each cell retains one of each pair of 23 chromosomes. Of the 23 chromosomes, one is the sex chromosome. In the process of spermatid production, each cell loses most of its cytoplasm and elongates into a sperm, which consists of a head, a neck, a body, and a tail (Fig. 55-6). The head is formed after nuclear material rearranges and the cell membrane contracts around it. This part of the sperm fertilizes the ovum, and the tail portion provides rapid motility.

FERTILITY

Male fertility depends on the quantity of semen ejaculated, the number of sperm per milliliter, and the motility and morphology of the sperm. The seminal fluid ejaculated with each coitus averages 400 million sperm in a fluid volume of about 3 mL. If the number of sperm in each milliliter drops below 20 to 50 million, *infertility* (defined as the inability to conceive after 12 months of adequate exposure in unprotected intercourse) or *sterility* (absolute inability to conceive) frequently results. The acrosome on the head of the sperm produces

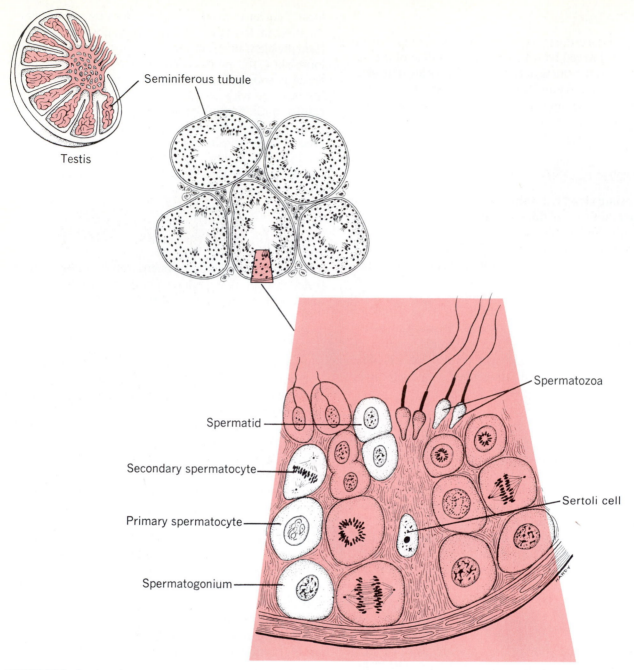

FIGURE 55-4 *Section of a seminiferous tubule, showing stages of spermatogenesis. (Reeder, S.J., Martin, L.L. and Koniak, D. Maternity Nursing [17th ed.]. Philadelphia: J.B. Lippincott, 1992.)*

the enzymes *hyaluronidase* and several proteinases. It is believed that these enzymes are necessary to remove the outer cell layers of the ovum. Only one sperm is responsible for the actual fertilization (Fig. 55-7).

MALE FUNCTION IN THE SEX ACT

With respect to sexual behavior, human beings differ from all other living creatures. In animals, for example, sex drive and behavior are instinctual and depend on

hormones. With humans, the initiation of the sex act may begin through physical or mental stimulation (see Flowchart 55-1). Erotic thoughts and dreams may produce erection and ejaculation in the male.

The most important area of sexual stimulation in the male is the glans penis. Sexual sensations produced by the massage of intercourse pass through the pudendal nerve, into the sacral portion of the spinal cord, and on to the cerebrum. Physical stimulation also may occur with touching of the anal epithelium, perineum, or scrotum.

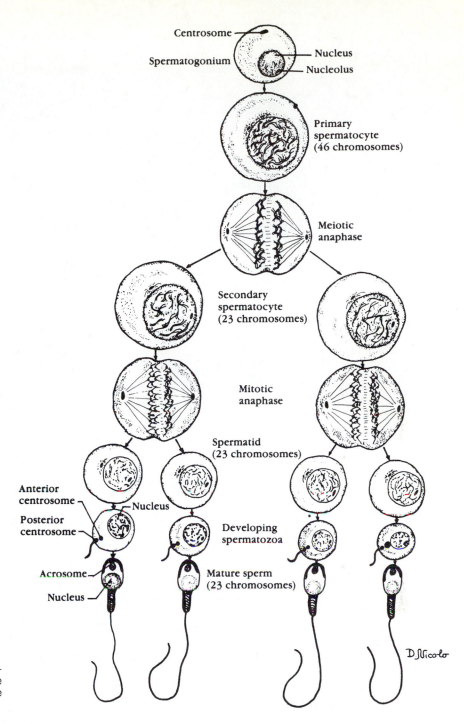

FIGURE 55-5 *Maturation of male reproductive cells. (Miller, M.A., and Brooten, D.A. The Childbearing Family: A Nursing Perspective [2nd ed.]. Boston: Little, Brown, 1983.)*

These sexual sensations enter the pudendal nerve from the perineal and scrotal nerves and then enter the sacral portion of the spinal cord to be transmitted to the cerebrum.

The first effect of sexual stimulation is *erection* of the penis. The penis normally is flaccid because of constriction of the arterioles that supply its vascular spaces (Fig. 55-8). Sexual arousal results in a stimulation of parasympathetic nerves and inhibition of sympathetic nerves to the arterioles. As a result, the penile arterioles dilate and the veins constrict. Blood is forced into the vascular spaces and erectile tissue. The blood flow, under pressure, produces a ballooning effect of the erectile tissue and results in a hard, elongated penis. During this first stage of the male sexual response, parasympathetic stimulation results in discharge of lubricating fluid, primarily from the bulbourethral glands.

The second stage involves two processes: *emission* and *ejaculation* (Flowchart 55-2). Emission is initiated when sympathetic impulses are emitted by reflex centers in the spinal cord and pass to the smooth muscle of the

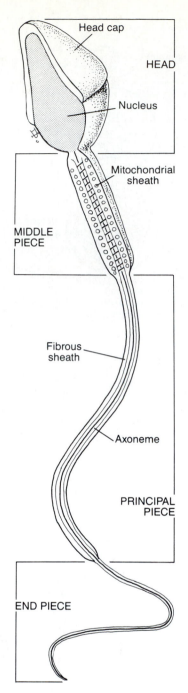

FIGURE 55-6 *Main parts of a spermatozoon. (Cormack, D.H., Essential Histology. Philadelphia: J.B. Lippincott, 1993.)*

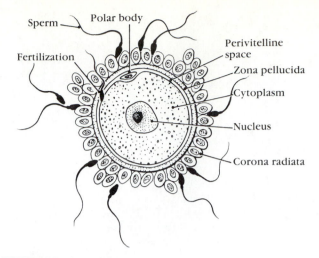

FIGURE 55-7 *Fertilization of an ovum.*

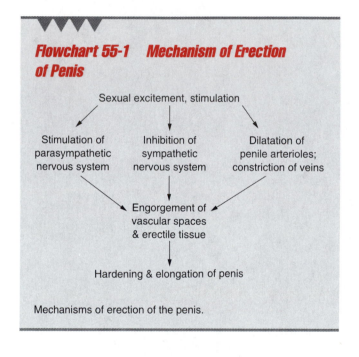

Flowchart 55-1   Mechanism of Erection of Penis

Sexual excitement, stimulation

Stimulation of parasympathetic nervous system

Inhibition of sympathetic nervous system

Dilatation of penile arterioles; constriction of veins

Engorgement of vascular spaces & erectile tissue

Hardening & elongation of penis

Mechanisms of erection of the penis.

genital ducts, producing contractions and forcing the sperm and seminal fluid into the internal urethra. Filling of the internal urethra then initiates impulses that result in contractions of the skeletal muscle at the base of the penis. During these contractions, the sphincter at the base of the bladder constricts, preventing the expulsion of urine, as seminal fluid and sperm are expelled through the external urethral orifice. This ejaculation represents a parasympathetic response and culminates the sex act for the male.

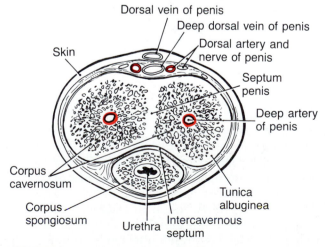

FIGURE 55-8 *Vascular supply and interior structures of the penis.*

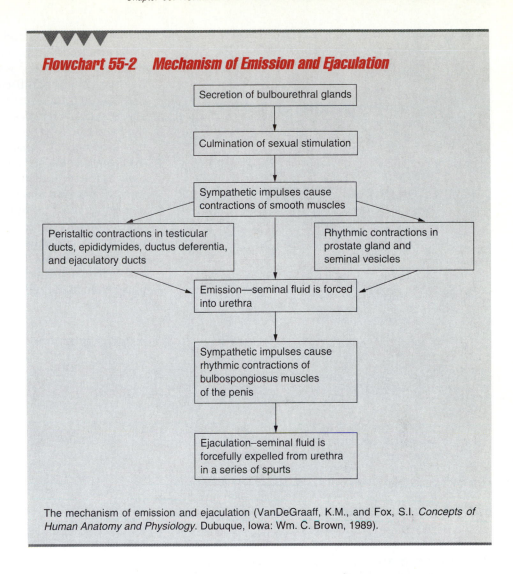

Flowchart 55-2   Mechanism of Emission and Ejaculation

Secretion of bulbourethral glands

↓

Culmination of sexual stimulation

↓

Sympathetic impulses cause contractions of smooth muscles

Peristaltic contractions in testicular ducts, epididymides, ductus deferentia, and ejaculatory ducts

Rhythmic contractions in prostate gland and seminal vesicles

Emission—seminal fluid is forced into urethra

↓

Sympathetic impulses cause rhythmic contractions of bulbospongiosus muscles of the penis

↓

Ejaculation–seminal fluid is forcefully expelled from urethra in a series of spurts

The mechanism of emission and ejaculation (VanDeGraaff, K.M., and Fox, S.I. *Concepts of Human Anatomy and Physiology.* Dubuque, Iowa: Wm. C. Brown, 1989).

HORMONAL REGULATION OF MALE SEXUAL FUNCTION

Male sexual function is regulated by a complex feedback mechanism that involves hormones secreted by the hypothalamus, anterior pituitary, and testes.

Hypothalamus and Pituitary

The hypothalamus secretes two gonadotropin-releasing factors: follicle-stimulating hormone–releasing factor (FSH-RF) and luteinizing hormone–releasing factor (LH-RF). As Flowchart 55-3 shows, when secreted by the hypothalamus, these releasing factors are conducted through the blood flow channels, called the hypothalamic-ohypophysial portal system, to the pituitary.

Elevated levels of FSH-RF and LH-RF stimulate the anterior pituitary to secrete two sex hormones: follicle-stimulating hormone (FSH) and luteinizing hormone (LH), which is also referred to as interstitial cell-stimulating hormone (ICSH). ICSH then stimulates

Leydig cells to produce testosterone. A rise in the blood level of testosterone provides negative feedback to the hypothalamus and anterior pituitary, thus reducing the levels of FSH-RF and LH-RF from the hypothalamus and inhibiting the pituitary's response to these gonadotropin-releasing factors. A drop in FSH-RF and LH-RF stimulates a reduction in the secretion of FSH and ICSH. A drop in the ICSH then inhibits secretion of testosterone. As testosterone levels drop, the hypothalamus and anterior pituitary are again triggered to secrete ICSH (Flowchart 55-4). It also is believed that the testes are responsible for the secretion of inhibin, a polypeptide hormone. This hormone seems to inhibit production of FSH without affecting the production of LH.

FSH is responsible for conversion of spermatogonia into sperm, and ICSH stimulates the production of testosterone. Without FSH, spermatogenesis does not occur, and without testosterone, the sperm do not mature. The secretion of FSH and ICSH is controlled not only by testosterone but also by FSH-RF and LH-RF. Stress and emotions affect secretory function of the hypothalamus

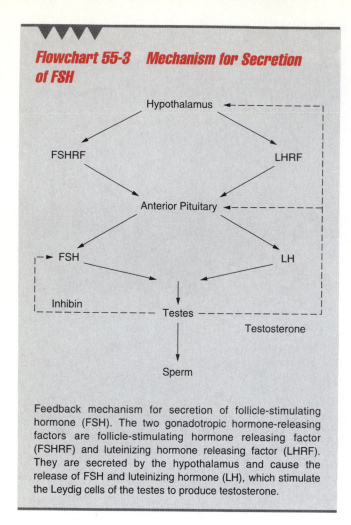

Flowchart 55-3   Mechanism for Secretion of FSH

Feedback mechanism for secretion of follicle-stimulating hormone (FSH). The two gonadotropic hormone-releasing factors are follicle-stimulating hormone releasing factor (FSHRF) and luteinizing hormone releasing factor (LHRF). They are secreted by the hypothalamus and cause the release of FSH and luteinizing hormone (LH), which stimulate the Leydig cells of the testes to produce testosterone.

and usually decrease secretion of the releasing factors. During fetal life, the production of human chorionic gonadotropin (HCG) also is important in the development of male sex organs. HCG possesses properties that are similar to those of ICSH; it stimulates the interstitial cells in the fetal testes to produce testosterone, which is then responsible for the development of the male organs.

Male Sex Hormones

The male sex hormones, also known as androgens, are secreted primarily by the *interstitial cells of Leydig* in the testes and in smaller amounts by the adrenals. The testosterone released by these cells circulates in the bloodstream for only 15 to 30 minutes before it is either fixed in tissues to perform intracellular functions or degraded by the liver. After testosterone enters the cells, it is converted to *dihydrotestosterone*. Dihydrotestosterone combines with nuclear protein and promotes messenger ribonucleic acid synthesis, which then enhances cellular protein production. Testosterone not fixed in tissues is converted in the liver into androsterone and dehydroepiandrosterone. These forms are conjugated into glu-

curonides or sulfates and are excreted in bile or urine as 17-ketosteroids, as shown in Flowchart 55-5. The inactivation process for testosterone accounts for the ineffectiveness of oral administration of this hormone.

Testosterone controls development of male secondary sex characteristics, regulates metabolism, affects fluid and electrolyte balance, and inhibits anterior pituitary secretion of gonadotropins. The influence of testosterone on male secondary sex characteristics begins as early as the second month of embryonic life, when HCG from the placenta stimulates production of small amounts of testosterone. This testosterone is thought to affect the development of the penis, scrotum, prostate gland, seminal vesicles, and genital ducts in the fetus. During childhood, virtually no testosterone is produced until puberty, at which time secretion rapidly increases. After puberty and continuing until maturity at about age 20,

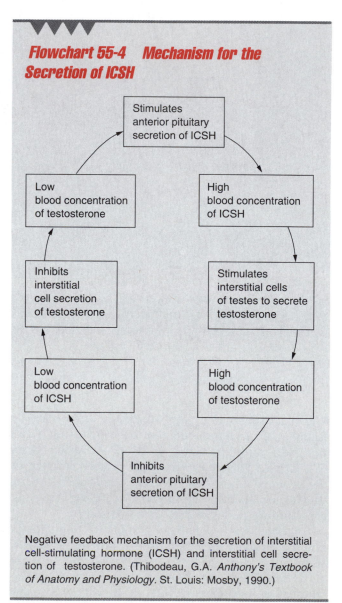

Flowchart 55-4   Mechanism for the Secretion of ICSH

Negative feedback mechanism for the secretion of interstitial cell-stimulating hormone (ICSH) and interstitial cell secretion of testosterone. (Thibodeau, G.A. *Anthony's Textbook of Anatomy and Physiology.* St. Louis: Mosby, 1990.)

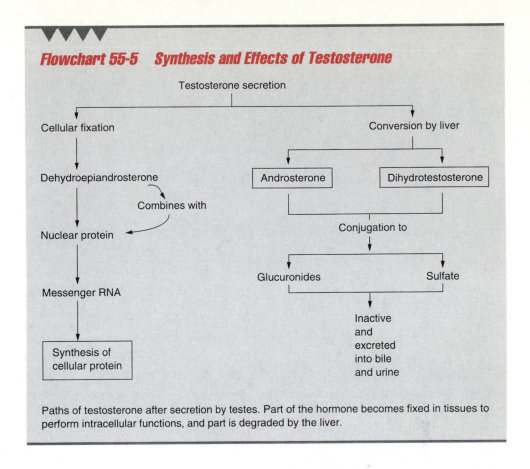

Flowchart 55-5   Synthesis and Effects of Testosterone

Paths of testosterone after secretion by testes. Part of the hormone becomes fixed in tissues to perform intracellular functions, and part is degraded by the liver.

testosterone stimulates enlargement of the penis, scrotum, and testes.

Testosterone also stimulates protein anabolism, which is directly responsible for virilization of the male. The secondary sex characteristics—muscular development and strength; hair growth on the face, axillae, and chest; bone growth; and deepening of the voice—are manifestations of this process. In affecting bone growth, testosterone also functions in early uniting of the epiphyses and shafts of long bones, which stops the growth process. The basal metabolic rate increases under the influence of this hormone.

Testosterone secondarily increases retention of sodium, potassium, calcium, and water. The hormone levels can affect the fluid balance by influencing iron retention by the kidneys. By this method the body retains substances necessary to effect the anabolic process. High levels of testosterone inhibit secretion of gonadotropins by the anterior pituitary.

▼ Physical, Laboratory, and Diagnostic Tests

Physical examination, computed tomographic scanning, ultrasonography, and laboratory evaluation are all important in the assessment of male reproductive function.

These assessments aid diagnosis of infectious disorders, infertility, and neoplastic disease. Physical examination detects redness, swelling, discharge, and abnormal masses; laboratory evaluation centers on testicular function, cultures, and serology testing. Primary laboratory studies include measurement of testosterone secretion, examination of seminal fluid, serology, and cultures for infectious disorders.

PHYSICAL EXAMINATION

The physical examination includes inspection and palpation of the external genitalia and a rectal examination. After visual examination of the external genitalia, the examiner palpates the scrotal contents for abnormal masses. A rectal examination is performed to detect the size and texture of the prostate as well as the presence and location of masses. Prostatic massage also may be performed to obtain a sample of prostatic secretions.

TESTOSTERONE MEASUREMENT

Testosterone, a 19-carbon hormone that affects the development of male sex characteristics, degrades into androsterone and dehydroepiandrosterone, which can be measured as *17-ketosteroids*. About one-third of 17-ketosteroid excretions in the male can be attributed to testosterone and its products.

TABLE 55-1 *Normal Hormone Levels*

Hormone	Age	Blood	Urine
Testosterone			
Male	Adult	0.3–1.0 g/dL (average = 0.7)	47–156 g/24 h (average = 70)
	Adolescent	0.10 g/dL	
Female	All ages	0–0.1 g/dL (average = 0.04)	0–15 g/24 h (average = 6)
17-Ketosteroids			
Male and female	All ages	25–125 g/dL	
Male	10 y		1–4 mg/24 h
	20–30 y		6–26 mg/24 h
	50 y		5–18 mg/24 h
	70 y		2–10 mg/24 h
Female	10 y		1–4 mg/24 h
	20–30 y		4–14 mg/24 h
	50 y		3–9 mg 24 h
	70 y		1–7 mg/24 h
Chorionic gonadotropin			
Male			0

Testosterone levels, measured directly, are particularly helpful in assessing hypogonadism, impotence, cryptorchidism, and pituitary gonadotropin functions in the male. Male hypogonadism and Klinefelter syndrome can be associated with a decreased testosterone level.

In women, testosterone measurement may assist in the diagnosis of ovarian and adrenal tumors. Adrenal neoplasms, benign and malignant ovarian tumors, adrenogenital syndrome, and Stein-Leventhal syndrome with virilization frequently are associated with an increased testosterone level. Table 55-1 depicts normal laboratory values for testosterone production; these values may vary slightly from institution to institution.

Levels of 17-ketosteroids may be high in testicular tumors and adrenal cortical hyperplasia. Before puberty, spermatogenesis seldom occurs as a result of testosterone production.

SEMEN EXAMINATION

Semen examination is of particular importance in evaluation of infertility. Seminal fluid for examination is best collected through masturbation, which provides a complete specimen of ejaculate. This method also protects sperm morphology and motility, which may be affected by rubber condoms.

Both the sperm and the quantity of fluid are examined. Semen viscosity and morphology and motility of the sperm are assessed. The normal sperm count varies widely. Most authorities consider the presence of 50 million sperm per milliliter or more to be normal; however, pregnancies have been documented with lower levels. The normal volume of ejaculate is 3 to 5 mL. Infertility has been associated with both lower and higher volumes.

The morphology and motility of sperm may be factors in infertility even if the count is normal. High percentages of inactive or abnormally formed sperm are associated with infertility. Viscosity of seminal fluid may vary. Initially thick, the fluid must liquefy to allow normal motility of the sperm. This liquefaction usually is complete in 15 to 20 minutes. Normal semen test results are summarized in Table 55-2.

TISSUE BIOPSY

Testicular biopsy may be indicated if the semen examination reveals no sperm or to aid in the diagnosis of testicular atrophy. If a testicular tumor is suspected, biopsy usually is performed only after orchiectomy, to prevent dissemination of the tumor cells. Tissue biopsy is also helpful in diagnosis of cancer of the penis or prostate. A needle biopsy of suspicious prostate tissue can be obtained through either the perineal or transrectal route.

TABLE 55-2 *Semen Examination*

Test	Normal Results
Sperm count	50–60 million/mL or more
Volume	3–6 mL
Morphology	60% of sperm motile; 50% of normal morphology
Liquefaction	Complete in 15–20 min
pH	7.2–7.8
Leukocyte count	0–2000/mL

TRANSRECTAL ULTRASONOGRAPHY

Transrectal ultrasonography is a relatively new procedure used in the diagnosis of prostate cancer. It involves the use of ultrasonic waves from a rectal probe to produce an image of the prostate. A major limitation of this modality is the lack of consensus regarding appropriate transrectal ultrasonography criteria for malignancy. Although not considered an effective screening device for detection of prostate cancer, it is useful as a guide for accurate needle puncture during biopsy.[7]

PROSTATE-SPECIFIC ANTIGEN

Prostate-specific antigen (PSA) is a glycoprotein which is normally found only in the epithelial cells of the prostate gland. Thus, it is specific to prostate tissue, not prostate cancer, and can be elevated in prostatic hypertrophy and prostatitis. Transrectal ultrasonography and prostate biopsy also may produce an elevation of the PSA, and values may be affected for 2 to 3 weeks after these procedures.[4] The PSA is most effective in early detection if used in combination with digital rectal examination. PSA levels are especially helpful in monitoring of patients after treatment of malignancy and in detection of recurrent malignant disease as well as early detection. The American Cancer Society now recommends that men 50 years and older have a PSA test annually.[1]

Interpretation of PSA values is dependent on the laboratory test performed.[8] Values at or about 4 ng/mL are considered to be within normal limits for the Hybritech Tandem-R test, which is used by more than 95% of laboratories.[4,8] A PSA value greater than 5 ng/mL indicates the need for referral to a urologist; a biopsy is recommended if the PSA value is 10 ng/mL. A PSA value of 4.1 to 5.0 ng/mL should be confirmed with a repeat test. If the value continues to be greater than 4.0 ng/mL, the patient is referred for further evaluation.[4]

▼ Alterations in Male Function

PENIS

Alterations in the penis and penile function can be divided into those alterations related to congenital anomalies and those that affect the adult. Congenital and childhood alterations include phimosis and paraphimosis, hypospadias, and epispadias. Adult alterations include Peyronie disease, priapism, balanitis, and carcinoma.

Phimosis and Paraphimosis

Phimosis is a condition in which the prepuce is too narrow or stenosed to retract over the glans penis. In more severe cases, urinary flow may be obstructed. It frequently is congenital, but it may occur after infection or injury. If manual retraction is unsuccessful in treating the condition, surgical intervention is indicated. If untreated, this condition predisposes the man to secondary infection, scarring, and perhaps cancer because secretions and smegma accumulate under the prepuce and cannot be cleaned away. Forcible retraction of the foreskin may lead to constriction, swelling, and pain of the glans penis. Circumcision may be performed to correct the problem.

Paraphimosis occurs when the foreskin is retracted behind the corona of the glans. Impaired blood flow results in edema of the glans. Surgical intervention is indicated if manual correction fails.

Hypospadias

At about 7 to 8 weeks' gestation, the embryo develops a genital tubercle and two genital swellings. In the male fetus, the genital tubercle develops into the penis. The two swellings develop into two folds (urethral and scrotal), which descend and fuse. This fusion closes the urethra in the penis and forms the scrotum. Failure of these folds to fuse on the ventral side results in the congenital anomaly of hypospadias. The urethral orifice is located on the under side of the penis from close to the normal opening all the way to the perineum (Fig. 55-9). The foreskin on the ventral side usually is absent.

The condition also is associated with undescended testes and chordee. Chordee occurs when a fibrous band of tissue replaces the normal skin and produces a ventral curvature of the penis. If the anomaly is so severe that the infant's sex is questionable, chromosomal studies are initiated. Surgical repair is aimed at straightening the penis and forming a urethra that terminates as centrally as possible.

Epispadias

Epispadias, a rare congenital anomaly, results from failure of the dorsal side of the penis to fuse. The urethral

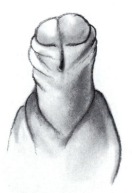

FIGURE 55-9 *Hypospadias is a congenital displacement of the urethral meatus to the inferior surface of the penis. A groove from the actual urethral meatus to its normal location on the tip of the glans. (Bates, B. A Guide to Physical Examination and History Taking [6th ed.]. Philadelphia: J.B. Lippincott, 1995.)*

opening is located on this surface rather than in the center. The urethral opening may be found just behind the glans, or it may extend the length of the penis if associated with exstrophy of the bladder. Surgical repair is aimed at establishing a normally functioning urethra and penis.

Balanitis

Balanitis is an inflammation of the glans penis. It most frequently occurs in uncircumcised males who exercise poor hygiene. It also may result from venereal disease. Clinical manifestations include redness, swelling, pain, and purulent drainage. Infection may cause adhesions and scarring. Cultures and sensitivity tests are performed to diagnose the infective organism and initiate appropriate antibiotic therapy. Circumcision may be indicated in uncircumcised males.

Peyronie's Disease

Peyronie's disease is a condition characterized by the formation of fibrous plaques on the dorsal side of the penis (Fig. 55-10). It also is accompanied by penile curvature and pain during erection. It frequently is associated with Dupuytren contracture of the hand tendons. The condition is found primarily in middle-aged and older men.

Priapism

Priapism refers to prolonged, persistent penile erection in the absence of sexual stimulation. The condition is extremely painful and may last from hours to several days. The cause is unknown; however, it has been associated with leukemia and sickle cell anemia. Surgical intervention within the first few hours provides drainage from the corpora cavernosa and helps to prevent impotence.

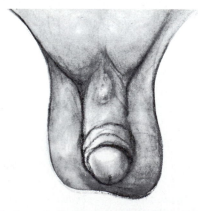

FIGURE 55-10 *Peyronie disease. In Peyronie disease, there are palpable, nontender, hard plaques just beneath the skin, usually along the dorsum of the penis. The patient complains of crooked, painful erections. (Bates, B. A Guide to Physical Examination and History Taking [6th ed.]. Philadelphia: J.B. Lippincott, 1995.)*

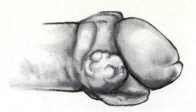

FIGURE 55-11 *Carcinoma of the penis. Carcinoma may present as an indurated nodule or ulcer that usually is nontender. Limited almost completely to men who are not circumcised in childhood, it may be masked by the prepuce. Any persistent penile sore must be considered suspicious. (Bates, B. A Guide to Physical Examination and History Taking [6th ed.]. Philadelphia: J.B. Lippincott, 1995.)*

Penile Carcinoma

Penile carcinoma (Fig. 55-11), a rare condition that tends to progress slowly, includes two neoplastic lesions: carcinoma in situ, or Bowen disease, and invasive carcinoma. Carcinoma in situ appears as a smooth, red lesion with a well-demarcated border. There also is the potential for conversion to invasive squamous cell carcinoma. Surgical excision is the treatment of choice. Prophylactic treatment may include radiation and administration of 5-fluorouracil.

Invasive squamous cell carcinoma primarily affects the prepuce and glans. The lesion appears as a small, gray, crusted papule that gradually enlarges and produces necrotic ulceration in the center. Larger lesions that involve the shaft of the penis or the inguinal nodes may require penile resection or amputation. A summary of the staging and tissue involvement is provided in Table 55-3.

Radiation therapy and chemotherapy are used increasingly as palliative and curative treatments. Early circumcision seems to prevent development of the squamous cell carcinoma, whereas chronic infection and infection from the human papillomavirus increase the risk of penile carcinoma.

SCROTUM, TESTES, AND EPIDIDYMIS

Hydrocele

A hydrocele is an accumulation of clear or straw-colored fluid within the tunica vaginalis sac that encloses the testis (Fig. 55-12). It is the most common cause of scrotal

TABLE 55-3 *Staging of Penile Carcinoma*

Stage	Involvement
I	Glans or prepuce
II	Shaft of penis
III	Inguinal lymph nodes (operable)
IV	Inguinal lymph nodes (inoperable)
	Metastasis

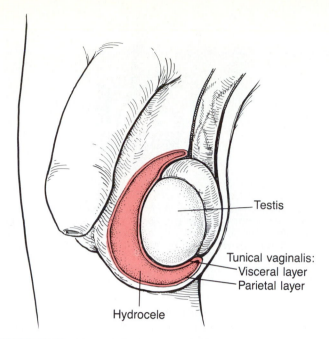

FIGURE 55-12   *A hydrocele is a nontender, fluid-filled mass that occupies space in the tunica vaginalis.*

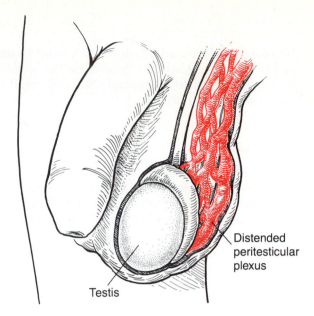

FIGURE 55-13   *A varicocele is varicose veins on the spermatic cord. It appears and feels like a "bag of worms" in the area.*

enlargement.[2] It frequently develops without a known cause, but it may occur after epididymitis, orchitis, injury, or neoplasm. In the neonate, it results from late closure of the tunica vaginalis. The condition may be asymptomatic or may cause pain or tension in the scrotal sac. Treatment may include aspiration or incision if the hydrocele is large or uncomfortable or if the testis cannot be palpated. Transillumination provides a differential diagnosis between hydrocele and solid testicular masses.

Varicocele

Varicocele most often occurs in young men between the ages of 15 and 25. It refers to the abnormal dilation of the venous plexus of the testis, and it is most often found on the left side. Occurrence on the right side is strongly suggestive of a tumor obstructing a vein above the scrotum. Palpation reveals dilated and tortuous veins, often described as a "bag of worms" (Fig. 55-13). Clinically, the primary concern relates to potential infertility. Both motility and number of sperm are decreased because of the increased warmth created by vascular engorgement. The condition usually is asymptomatic, but the man may complain of a dragging sensation or dull pain in the scrotum. Scrotal support is the treatment of choice. Surgical ligation of the internal spermatic vein is reserved for severe conditions or if an increased sperm count is desired.

Torsion of the Testis

Torsion of the testis (Fig. 55-14), an infrequent cause of testicular enlargement, primarily occurs during adoles-

cence. It may occur spontaneously or after physical exercise. This condition results from rotation of the testis within the tunica vaginalis, which cuts off the blood supply to the testis. With twisting of the spermatic cord and testis, venous obstruction results in vascular engorgement and sometimes extravasation of blood into the scrotal sac. The first symptom usually is sudden onset of severe pain in the testicular area. It is unrelieved by rest or scrotal support and may radiate into the groin.

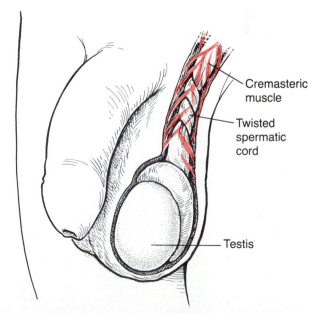

FIGURE 55-14   *Torsion or twisting of the testis on the spermatic cord causes an acutely painful and swollen organ with retraction upward in the scrotum.*

Other manifestations include scrotal edema, testicular tenderness, and perhaps nausea and vomiting. If the torsion cannot be reduced, surgical intervention to untwist the spermatic cord and immobilize the testis is indicated. Untreated torsion of the testis may result in atrophy, abscess, or infertility.

Cryptorchidism

During fetal development, the testes form in the abdomen and normally descend into the scrotum during the last trimester of pregnancy. Incomplete or maldescent of the testis results in cryptorchidism. The testis may remain in the abdomen or be arrested in the inguinal canal, in the low pelvis, or high in the scrotum (Fig. 55-15). It may be unilateral or bilateral; unilateral

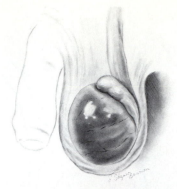

FIGURE 55-16 *Acute orchitis. An acute, inflamed testis is painful, tender, and swollen. The testis may be difficult to distinguish from the epididymis. The scrotum may be reddened. Look for evidence of postpubertal mumps or other, less common infectious causes. (Bates, B. A Guide to Physical Examination and History Taking [6th ed.]. Philadelphia: J.B. Lippincott, 1995.)*

cryptorchidism is somewhat more common on the right.[2] Retractile testis refers to a testis that normally descends into the scrotum but occasionally is pulled back into the inguinal canal. Ectopic testis is one that descends to the wrong area, such as the perineum.

The cause of cryptorchidism is unknown; however, it has been associated with a shortened spermatic cord, testosterone deficiencies, narrowed inguinal canal, and adhesions of the pathway. It is necessary to correct the condition if sterility is to be avoided, because after puberty, the undescended testes atrophy progressively. Spermatogenesis decreases, and the cells may be replaced by collagenous fibrous tissue. Because there is a direct relation between cryptorchidism and testicular cancer, surgical placement in the scrotum is recommended.

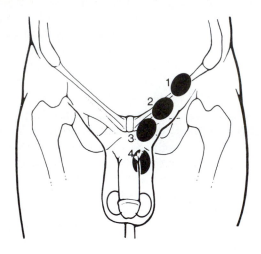

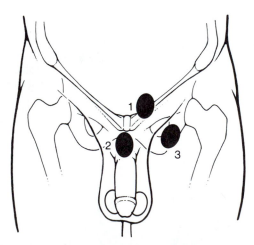

FIGURE 55-15 *Cryptorchidism. **A.** Incomplete descent of a testis may involve four separate regions: 1, in the pelvic cavity; 2, in the inguinal canal; 3, at the superficial inguinal ring; and 4, in the upper scrotum. **B.** An ectopic testis may be 1, in the superficial fascia of the anterior pelvic wall; 2, at the root of the penis; or 3, in the perineum. (VanDeGraaff, K.M., and Fox, S.I. Concepts of Human Anatomy and Physiology. Dubuque, Iowa: Wm. C. Brown, 1989.)*

Orchitis

Orchitis, inflammation of the testes, may be acquired as an ascending infection of the genital tract, through lymphatic spread, or as a complication of mumps, because the mumps virus is excreted through the urine. Infection may be bilateral or unilateral, and it is most often caused by ascending bacteria, including *Staphylococcus*, *Streptococcus*, *Escherichia coli*, *Klebsiella pneumoniae*, and *Pseudomonas aeruginosa*. Orchitis, as a complication of mumps, occurs in about 18% of men with mumps and primarily affects adults.[2]

Clinical manifestations include severe testicular pain, swelling, chills, and fever (Fig. 55-16). On examination, the testis appears swollen and tender with a swollen and red scrotum. Complications, including hydrocele and abscess, may result in sterility or impotence. Treatment includes bed rest, scrotal support, warm compresses, and antibiotics, if indicated. Analgesics may be indicated for relief of pain. Surgical intervention may be indicated for drainage of the hydrocele. Abscess formation usually requires surgical removal of the testis.

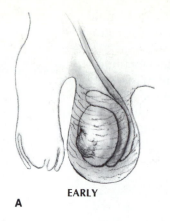
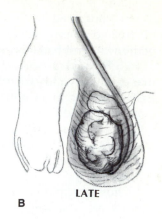

EARLY A B **LATE**

FIGURE 55-17 *Tumor of the testis.* **A.** *Early. A tumor of the testis usually appears as a painless nodule. It does not transilluminate. Any nodule within the testis must raise the suspicion of cancer.* **B.** *Late. As a testicular neoplasm grows and spreads, it may seem to replace the entire organ. The testis characteristically feels heavier than normal. (Bates, B. A Guide to Physical Examination and History Taking [6th ed.]. Philadelphia: J.B. Lippincott, 1995.)*

Testicular Tumors

With the exception of leukemia and lymphoma, testicular tumors are the most common cancer in men between 20 and 34 years of age (Fig. 55-17).[3] These tumors are predominantly malignant, often metastasize before diagnosis, and arise from germ cells.[3] The benign tumors usually arise from the interstitial cells of Leydig or Sertoli cells.

Although several classifications have been used with testicular cancer, the most frequently used one was proposed by the Armed Forces Institute of Pathology and modified by the World Health Organization. This classification proposes two groups based on histologic pattern type: 1) those tumors with one histologic pattern type present and 2) those tumors with more than one histologic pattern type present. Tumors of a single histologic pattern type can be further classified into seminoma and nonseminomatous tumors. Table 55-4 provides a summary of this classification with the associated appearance, incidence, and sites of metastasis.

Seminomas are the most common tumors and appear as gray-white, fleshy masses. Most seminomas remain localized until late in the course of the disease, when metastases occur to regional and aortic lymph nodes. Because of their sensitivity to irradiation, pure seminomas confined to the testis with no apparent metastases or elevated biochemical markers are best treated with this modality after operation. Even if retroperitoneal metastasis of less than 5 cm is confirmed by lymphangiography or CT scanning, radiation therapy is the treatment of choice.

Elevated (HCG) and α-fetoprotein (AFP) levels indicate need for more extensive histologic studies in an effort to identify syncytiotrophoblastic cells and nonseminoma germ cells. Elevated levels usually indicate presence of nonseminoma cells, even if their presence

TABLE 55-4 *Classification of Testicular Germ Cell Tumors*

Classification	Appearance	Incidence (%)	Metastases
SINGLE HISTOLOGIC PATTERN		60	
Seminoma	Large, gray, white fleshy mass	40	Regional aortic lymph nodes
Nonseminomas Embryonal carcinoma	Small, gray, white nodule	10–20	Lymph nodes, liver, lungs, bones
Choriocarcinoma	Small, gray; frequently not palpable; contains both cytotrophoblast and syncytiotrophoblastic cells	1	Organ by way of bloodstream
Teratoma	Variable	10	Lymphatic
MULTIPLE HISTOLOGIC PATTERN		40	
Teratocarcinoma (teratoma and embryonal carcinoma or yolk sac tumor)			
Seminoma plus others			
Choriocarcinoma plus others			
Any other combination			

is not confirmed by histologic findings, and should be treated appropriately with chemotherapy, retroperitoneal lymphadenectomy, or both.

Embryonal carcinomas are highly malignant tumors that exhibit a wide variety of cell types and may secrete HCG. They occur in both adults and children. Small, gray-white nodules are formed, which usually do not invade the entire testis. Metastasis to the lymph nodes, liver, lungs, and bones is frequent. Yolk sac tumors repeat the development of a yolk sac, and these tumors secrete AFP.

Choriocarcinomas are small, gray tumors that frequently are not palpable. Characteristically, they produce both cytotrophoblastic and syncytiotrophoblastic cells identical to those formed in the placenta. These cells secrete HCG, which, when found, aids in the diagnosis of choriocarcinoma. Early, distant metastasis usually causes death within a year of diagnosis.

Teratoma and teratocarcinoma are tumors with various cellular types. Teratomas are composed of tissues normally derived from the primary germ layers (ectoderm, mesoderm, endoderm) of the embryo. Teratocarcinoma contains both embryonal carcinoma and teratoma cells. Metastases normally follow the lymphatic system but may involve many other structures.

The exact cause of testicular cancer has not been determined. Predisposing factors that seem to contribute to its development include cryptorchidism, genetic influence, age, and race. The genetic influence is evidenced by a higher incidence in brothers and by contralateral tumors in unilateral cryptorchidism. Testicular cancer more frequently occurs in Caucasian men than in African American men. The incidence of testicular cancer decreases with age.

The most frequent symptom of a testicular tumor is painless enlargement of the testis. On examination, the mass does not transilluminate, and lymphadenopathy may be noted. The affected male may complain of a feeling of heaviness or a dull ache. Gynecomastia is associated with tumors that produce HCG and estrogen. Low back pain may be associated with retroperitoneal lymph node involvement. Other symptoms may be present that vary with the site of metastasis.

Diagnosis and staging are based on physical examination, protein biochemical markers in serum, CT scanning, and biopsy after removal of the entire testis (Table 55-5). In addition to manual palpation of the tumor, two protein biochemical markers in serum are especially beneficial in diagnosing and staging of testicular tumors. These markers are the β subunit of HCG and AFP. Tumors with trophoblastic elements are responsible for the β subunit of HCG, although this marker may be present even if these elements are apparently absent. Levels of AFP are elevated in about 60% of men with nonseminomatous germ cell tumors.

Treatment varies with the type and stage of disease and includes surgery, radiation, and chemotherapy, either alone or in various combinations. Pure seminomas without evidence of metastasis usually are treated with radiation. In the United States, nonseminomatous tumors most often are treated with orchiectomy, retroperitoneal resection, or chemotherapy. The most commonly used chemotherapeutic agents include vinblastine, bleomycin, cisplatin, dactinomycin, doxorubicin, and cyclophosphamide. Various combinations of these drugs are being used in cancer treatment centers across the nation.

Prognosis depends on the histologic type of the tumor, stage of disease, and use of appropriate therapy. Pure seminoma in the earlier stages is associated with a cure rate as high as 100%. Metastatic disease of a differing histologic type, not sensitive to radiation, usually accounts for failure. The cure rate associated with stages I and IIa nonseminomatous tumors is 95% or greater. Because of the progress made in recent years in treatment, persons with stage IIb or III disease now see a cure rate of 80% to 90%.[3]

Epididymitis

Epididymitis occurs if disease-producing organisms in the urine, urethra, prostate gland, or seminal vesicles spread to the epididymis (Fig. 55-18). Acute epididy-

TABLE 55-5 *Staging of Testicular Cancer*

Stage	Involvement
I	Testis
II	Primary regional retroperitoneal lymph nodes
IIa	Metastases usually <5 cm
IIb	Metastases >5 cm
III	Visceral metastases below diaphragm; metastases above diaphragm; persistent biologic marker elevation after orchiectomy

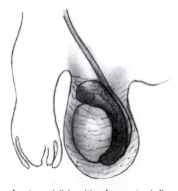

FIGURE 55-18 *Acute epididymitis. An acute, inflamed epididymis is tender and swollen, and may be difficult to distinguish from the testis. The scrotum may be reddened, and the vas deferens also may be inflamed. Epididymitis chiefly occurs in adults. Coexisting urinary tract infection or prostatitis supports the diagnosis. (Bates, B. A Guide to Physical Examination and History Taking [6th ed.]. Philadelphia: J.B. Lippincott, 1995.)*

mitis may result from sexually transmitted organisms, *Pseduomonas aeruginosa*, or enteric bacteria. The most common sexually transmitted organisms are *Neisseria gonorrhoeae* and *Chlamydia trachomatis*. It also may occur as a complication of prostatectomy. Symptoms include pain, chills, fever, and malaise, with scrotal swelling so great that it interferes with ambulation and produces congestion of the testes. Necrosis and fibrosis may occlude the genital ducts and result in sterility. Treatment includes bed rest, scrotal elevation, sitz baths, hot or cold applications, and antibiotics appropriate for the organism.

PROSTATE

The prostate gland maintains its normal size until about age 50. At this point, in some men, it begins to decrease in size. This atrophy is associated with a decrease in testosterone level and usually produces no symptoms. Other alterations in prostate function normally occur in adult life and involve an enlargement of the prostate gland. These conditions include prostatitis, benign prostatic hyperplasia, and carcinoma.

Prostatitis

Prostatitis, inflammation of the prostate gland, usually results from ascending infection of the urethra; it also may result from descending infection from the bladder or kidneys; hematogenous spread from the teeth, the skin, or the gastrointestinal or respiratory system; or lymphogenous spread from rectal bacteria. This condition occurs in three forms: acute bacterial, chronic bacterial, and chronic abacterial.

Acute bacterial prostatitis is caused by the same organisms that produce urinary tract infections. The most frequent causative organism is *E. coli*, which ascends from the urethra. Manifestations of acute bacterial prostatitis include chills and fever, dysuria, urinary frequency and urgency, and hematuria. It also may be associated with suprapubic, perineal, or scrotal pain and purulent urethral discharge. On rectal examination, the prostate is enlarged, tender, and warm. The seminal vesicles also may be palpable, because infection of these organs frequently accompanies prostatitis. Urinalysis may be positive for blood and pus cells. Urine cultures aid in diagnosis of the specific organism. Although prostate massage can aid in identification of the organism, it should be used judiciously, because it can precipitate bacteremia. Catheterization, if performed on a man with acute prostatitis, may be responsible for spreading the inflammation into the bladder. Appropriate antibiotics, analgesics, and sitz baths, if instituted early, usually resolve the condition. The infection may become chronic if it is not adequately treated.

Chronic bacterial prostatitis may represent a continuation of acute prostatitis that did not completely respond to antibiotics. Some men are asymptomatic, with diagnosis occurring on routine urinalysis. Clinical manifestations in others include low-grade fever, dull perineal pain, nocturia, and dysuria. Inflammatory cells and bacteria usually are found in prostatic secretions. The infection may be resistant to antibiotics because the antibiotics do not adequately penetrate the prostate.

Abacterial prostatitis is the most common form of prostatitis.[2] Symptoms are mild and include low back pain and urinary frequency and urgency with rectal, urethral, or perineal discomfort. Physical examination usually reveals a nontender prostate with normal urine and prostate fluid. Evidence of inflammation (ie, lymphocytes) may be present. Chronic abacterial prostatitis may be related to excessive alcohol or caffeine intake.

Benign Prostatic Hyperplasia (BPH)

Benign prostatic hyperplasia (BPH), enlargement of the prostate, is a common condition that affects most men after age 50. As many as 95% of men older than 70 years of age are affected.[2] Hyperplasia occurs and produces large, fairly discrete nodules located in the median and lateral lobes. Enlarging nodules compress the prostatic portion of the urethra, producing symptoms of urinary obstruction (Fig. 55-19).

Before the 1990s, treatment for BPH was surgical. However, nonsurgical treatment now includes the administration of α-1-sympathetic blockers and 5-α-reductase inhibitors.[4,6] The α-1-sympathetic blockers reduce urethral restriction and improve voiding by reducing smooth muscle tone around the bladder neck and prostate. Prostate bulk is reduced, with resultant improvement in voiding, by the administration of 5-α-reductase inhibitors, including finasteride. These drugs block the production of 5-α-dihydrotestosterone, the physiologically active form of testosterone, without lowering testosterone levels. The use of these medications may have an impact on diagnosis and treatment of prostate cancer, because cancer is often diagnosed at time of treatment for benign prostatic hyperplasia.[4] Because of the obstructive nature of BPH, the pathogenesis and clinical manifestations are discussed on pages 648–649.

Cancer of the Prostate

The American Cancer Society estimated an incidence of 106,000 new cases of prostate cancer in 1990. Excluding skin cancer, prostate cancer is the most common cancer in men.[1] It also is the second leading cause of cancer deaths in men.[1] Prostate cancer primarily occurs in men older than 50 years of age, with a peak incidence at about age 75.

The usual form of prostate cancer is adenocarcinoma. One system for grading the adenocarcinoma is based on degrees of differentiation (well-differentiated, moderately well-differentiated, and poorly differenti-

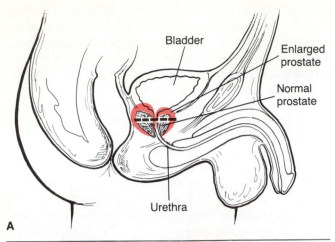

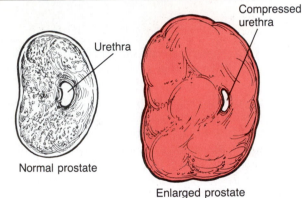

Cross-section of prostate gland

FIGURE 55-19 ***A.*** *Location of the prostate gland.* ***B.*** *Comparison of the normal prostate gland with the enlarged prostate seen in benign prostatic hyperplasia.*

ated). Tumors that are poorly differentiated are more invasive. The major system currently being used, however, is the Gleason or Veterans Administration system.[7] This system describes five grades of tumor, based on architectural characteristics. The predominant and the next most prevalent architectural characteristics are described. A score of 1 to 5 is given to each pattern, and the scores are then added for the final grade. A score of 1 represents a tumor with well-differentiated, circumscribed, uniform glands; a grade of 4 or 5 reflects tumors with less glandular differentiation, invasive patterns, and diffuse single-cell infiltration. Combined scores of 2 to 4 represent well-differentiated tumors with a good prognosis. Combined scores of 8 to 10 represent poorly-differentiated tumors with a poor prognosis.

The disease most often occurs in the posterior lobe; hard, fixed nodules can be palpated on rectal examination. In the early stages, it produces no symptoms. For this reason, metastasis is common, with the most frequent sites being bones, lungs, lymph nodes, and liver. Early symptoms are those of urethral obstruction; by this time, metastasis is usually present.

Based on inconclusive data, risk factors associated with increased incidence of prostate cancer include age, race, genetic predisposition, hormonal influences, venereal disease, and environmental factors (dietary fat and chemical carcinogens). As noted previously, the incidence of prostate cancer increases with age. It occurs more often in African Americans than in Caucasians. Research studies indicate that, among environmental factors, dietary fat may be important. The incidence of prostate cancer among Japanese and Polish men is very low. If these men immigrate to parts of the world that have a higher incidence, their chance of developing prostate cancer increases.[7]

Probably the most beneficial of all diagnostic tools is the digital rectal examination. It should be performed during annual examinations in all men older than 40 years of age. Because most tumors arise in the posterior lobe, palpation usually is easy. Additional diagnostic studies include prostate ultrasonography, measurement of acid phosphatase and alkaline phosphatase levels, biopsy of detectable lesions of the posterior lobe, and CT scanning (or radiography of the spine and pelvis if computed tomography is unavailable). Cystoscopy and lymphangiography also aid in diagnosis of the extent of the disease. Additionally, the American Cancer Society now recommends that all men 50 years of age or older have a PSA test annually (see p. 1113). The combination of digital rectal examination and PSA is probably the most effective means of early detection.

As in other forms of cancer, disease staging becomes important in determining appropriate therapy. Although a number of staging classifications have been proposed, the tumor-node-metastasis (TNM) staging classification for cancer of the prostate is summarized in Table 55-6.[2]

Treatment depends on the stage of the disease and the patient's age and symptoms. Options include surgery or radiation therapy, or both; hormones; and chemotherapy. Hormonal therapy with estrogens is aimed at decreasing testosterone levels. Gonadotropin-releasing hormone analogues may be used to decrease production of pituitary gonadotropin and testicular androgens. These analogues have an associated decrease in the risk of cardiovascular disease and thromboembolism. The 5-year survival rate is 92% after diagnosis of a localized lesion is made. The overall 5-year survival rate for all stages has increased to 78%.[1]

EXPOSURE TO DIETHYLSTILBESTROL (DES)

The use of diethylstilbestrol (DES) in the treatment of threatened spontaneous abortion rapidly increased from the late 1940s through the 1960s. The effects of in utero exposure of the female fetus to this drug had been known and publicized for years before evidence associating certain reproductive anomalies with in utero exposure of the male fetus to DES began to emerge in the late

TABLE 55-6 *Staging of Prostate Cancer*

Stage	Occurrence (%)	Involvement
PRIMARY CANCER		
T1	5–10	Rectal examination reveals no palpable tumor
a		Microscopic examination—≤3 foci of carcinoma
b		Microscopic examination—>3 foci of carcinoma
T2	20	Tumor limited to gland
a		Diameter <1.5 cm; surrounded by normal tissue on at least 3 sides
b		Diameter >1.5 cm; involves more than 1 lobe
T3	40–45	Tumor not fixed; invasion of prostatic apex into or beyond the prostatic capsule, bladder neck, or seminal vesicles
a		
b		
T4		Fixed or adjacent structures
REGIONAL LYMPH NODES*		
N0		Pelvic lymph nodes not involved
N1		Single pelvic node ≤2 cm
N2		1 lymph node, >2 but <5 cm
N3		Pelvic lymph node >5 cm or multiple nodes <5 cm
DISTANT METASTASIS		
M0		No known distant metastasis
M1		Distant or lymph node outside pelvis

* Staging based on histologic examination.

1970s. Reported anomalies involve the urethra, epididymis, testes, and semen. Urethral anomalies include meatal stenosis and hypospadias. More specifically, exposure to DES has been associated with low sperm counts, abnormally-shaped sperm, and decreased volume of ejaculate. Congenital anomalies in males include undescended or underdeveloped testes, testicular cysts, and abnormal meatal openings.

▼ Chapter Summary

▼ The male reproductive system includes the testes, which produce sperm, and the accessory organs, which include the epididymis, vas deferens, seminal vesicles, ejaculatory ducts, prostate gland, urethra, scrotum, penis, and spermatic cords.

▼ The primary functions of the male reproductive system are spermatogenesis, performance of the sex act, and hormonal regulation of male sexual function.

▼ Diagnostic tests for altered male reproductive function include physical examination, testosterone measurement, and semen examination. In addition, other alterations of the male sex organs may be identified by tissue biopsy, transrectal ultrasonography, and measurement of prostate-specific antigen.

▼ Alterations in male function affect the penis, scrotum, testes, epididymis and prostate gland. These can include congenital anomalies, infections and inflammations, obstructions, and cancers of the male sex organs.

▼ References

1. American Cancer Society. *Cancer Facts & Figures—1990*. Atlanta: American Cancer Society, 1990.
2. Cotran, R.S., Kumar, V., and Robbins, S.L. *Robbins' Pathologic Basis of Disease* (5th ed.). Philadelphia: W.B. Saunders, 1994.
3. Garnick, M.B., Krane, R.J., Scully, R.E., et al. Cancer of the testis. In American Cancer Society Massachusetts Division, *Cancer Manual* (8th ed.) Boston: American Cancer Society, 1990.
4. Greco, K.E., and Blank, B. Prostate-specific antigen: The new early detection test for prostate cancer. *Nurse Pract.* 18:30, 33–34, 37–38, 1993.
5. Guyton, A.C. *Textbook of Medical Physiology* (8th ed.). Philadelphia: W.B. Saunders, 1991.
6. Holdcroft, C. Finasteride for benign prostatic hyperplasia. *Nurse Pract.* 18:57–58, 1993.
7. Shipley, W.U., Meares, E.M., Schwartz, J.H., et al. Cancer of the prostate. In American Cancer Society Massachusetts Division, *Cancer Manual* (8th ed.). Boston: American Cancer Society, 1990.
8. Wozniak-Petrofsky, J. The significance of prostatic-specific antigen in men with prostate disease. *Geriatr. Nurs.* 14:150, 1993.

Chapter 56

Normal and Altered Female Reproductive Function

Sharron P. Schlosser

▼ **LEARNING OBJECTIVES**

1 Describe the development and function of the female sex organs.
2 Compare the functions of estrogen, progesterone, prolactin, and prostaglandins.
3 Discuss the three phases of the menstrual cycle, including hypothalamic and pituitary influence.
4 Describe the phases involved in the female response in the sex act.
5 Describe oogenesis, fertilization, and implantation.
6 Define **menopause** and discuss the physiologic basis for the associated symptoms.
7 Define the various diagnostic tests used in diagnosis of female reproductive alterations.
8 Describe the clinical manifestations of endometriosis and its pathologic basis.
9 Distinguish between primary and secondary dysmenorrhea.
10 Discuss the role of prostaglandins in dysmenorrhea.
11 Define **dysfunctional uterine bleeding**.
12 Distinguish between primary and secondary amenorrhea.
13 Compare and contrast the forms of vaginitis with respect to causative organisms, clinical manifestations, and diagnostic studies.
14 Distinguish between cervical erosion and eversion.
15 Define **toxic shock syndrome** and give its clinical manifestations.
16 Compare and contrast uterine fibroids and endometrial cancer.
17 Distinguish between functional ovarian cysts, benign neoplastic tumors of the ovary, and ovarian cancer.
18 Compare and contrast the three types of trophoblastic disease.
19 Discuss the sequential process of cellular proliferation of cervical cancer.
20 Describe the effects of diethylstilbestrol administration on mothers and offspring.
21 Describe the staging systems of cancer of the ovary, breast, cervix, and endometrium.
22 Describe the pathology and clinical manifestations of breast cancer.

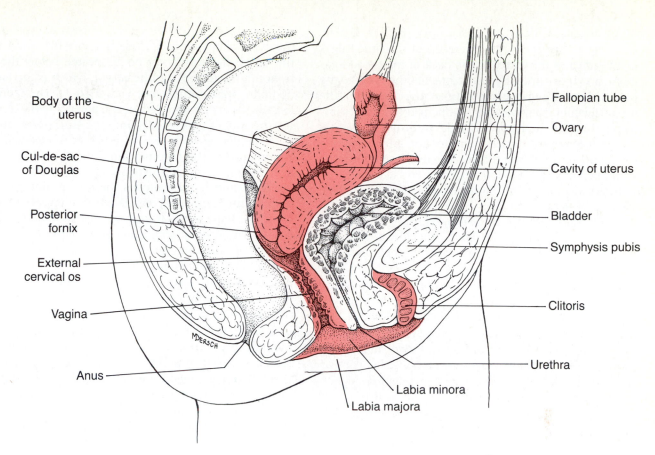

FIGURE 56-1 *Female reproductive system, as seen in sagittal section. (Reeder, S.J., Martin, L.L. and Koniak, D. Maternity Nursing [17th ed.]. Philadelphia: J.B. Lippincott, 1992.)*

For many women, the ability to conceive and bear children is an essential part of being a woman, and alterations in this function represent a threat to body image and self-concept. Alterations may occur in all reproductive organs and at any age. This chapter provides an overview of the anatomy and physiology fundamental to understanding alterations in female reproduction as well as a discussion of these alterations.

▼ *Anatomy*

The female reproductive organs include both essential and accessory organs (Figs. 56-1 and 56-2). The essential organs are the ovaries, which produce ova. The accessory organs include the fallopian tubes, uterus, and vagina, which serve as ducts; Bartholin, Skene, and mammary glands; and external genitalia.

OVARIES

The ovaries are two nodular, ovoid glands located on either side of the uterus. Each ovary is 3.5 cm long, 2 cm wide, and 1 cm thick and is attached by three ligaments:

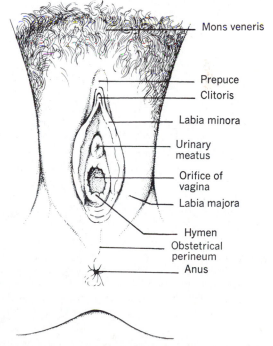

FIGURE 56-2 *External genitalia of the female. (Reeder, S.J., Martin, L.L. and Koniak, D. Maternity Nursing [17th ed.]. Philadelphia: J.B. Lippincott, 1992.)*

mesovarium, ovarian, and suspensory (Fig. 56-3). The mesovarium ligament, an extension of the broad ligament, attaches the ovary to the back of the broad ligament, and the ovarian ligament attaches the ovary to the uterus. The suspensory ligament is an extension of the broad ligament beyond the fallopian tubes, and it attaches the ovary to the pelvic wall. The broad ligament is an extension of the parietal peritoneum, and it supports the fallopian tubes and uterus. The ovaries perform the vital functions of ovulation and hormone secretion. The pituitary regulation of these functions is discussed on pages 678–684.

The ovary consists of four layers: the germinal epithelium, the tunica albuginea, the cortex, and the medulla (Fig. 56-4). The germinal epithelium is the covering on the outer portion of the ovary. The tunica albuginea is a layer of collagenous connective tissue just below the germinal epithelium. The cortex is composed of fine areolar stroma, blood vessels, and follicles containing ova at various stages of development. The medial portion of the ovary is the hilum, where nerves and blood vessels enter the ovary. It is composed of connective tissue and hilar cells, which secrete steroid hormones. The inner portion is the medulla, which is composed of stroma or connective tissue, smooth muscle, blood and lymph vessels, and nerves.

UTERUS

The uterus is a hollow, pear-shaped, highly muscular organ that, in the nonpregnant state, is 7 cm long, 5 cm wide, and 2.5 cm in diameter. It consists of three parts: the dome-shaped fundus, located above the entrance of the tubes; the corpus, or body, located below the entrance of the tubes; and the cervix, which is the lowest and narrowest portion (see Figure 56-3). The uterus is located posterior to the bladder and anterior to the rectum. It is essential in menstruation, pregnancy, and labor.

The uterine walls are composed of three layers: the endometrium, the myometrium, and the peritoneum, also known as the perimetrium (see Figure 56-3). The endometrium is the mucous membrane lining of the body of the uterus. It consists of three layers of tissue: stratum compactum, stratum spongiosum, and stratum basale. The *stratum compactum* is the surface layer and consists of partially ciliated simple columnar epithelium. The *stratum spongiosum* is the spongy middle layer of loose connective tissue. Both the stratum compactum and the stratum spongiosum slough during menstruation and after delivery. The *stratum basale* is the dense inner layer that attaches to the myometrium. The myometrium is the thick middle layer that consists of three layers of smooth-muscle fibers supported by connective tissue. This layer blends into the endometrium and provides great strength for the uterus. The myometrial layer is thickest in the fundus, which allows for more force during the contractions of labor, aiding in delivery. The third layer of the uterine wall, the peritoneum, consists of a thin, serous membrane covering almost all of the uterus. On the anterior surface, the peritoneum is reflected onto the bladder below the internal os of the cervix.

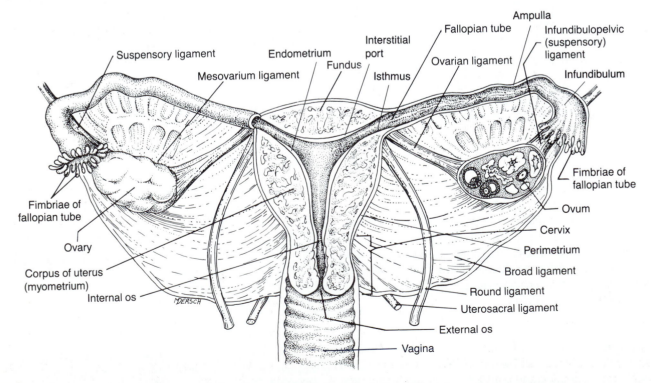

FIGURE 56-3 *Anterior view of the uterus and related structures. (Reeder, S.J., Martin, L.L., and Koniak, D. Maternity Nursing [17th ed.]. Philadelphia: J.B. Lippincott, 1992.)*

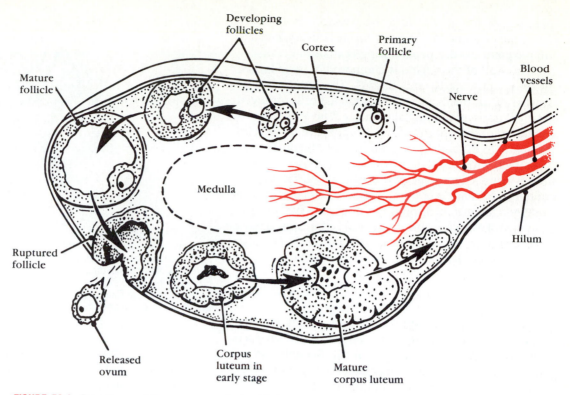

FIGURE 56-4   *Four layers of the ovary: germinal epithelium, tunica albuginea, cortex, and medulla.*

The uterus is mainly supported by the levator ani muscles and eight ligaments, which include two broad ligaments, two uterosacral ligaments, and a posterior, an anterior, and two round ligaments. The broad ligaments are continuations of the parietal peritoneum that extend from the walls and floor of the pelvis to the lateral walls of the uterus. The uterosacral ligaments also are extensions of the peritoneum. They connect the uterus and sacrum by extending from the pelvic floor around the rectum to the sacrum. The round ligaments are fibromuscular cords that extend from the upper outer portion of the uterus through the inguinal canals and terminate in the labia majora. The outer ligaments are extensions of the peritoneum (see Figure 56-3).

Two of these ligaments are of particular importance because of the pouches they form. The posterior ligament forms the rectouterine pouch (or cul-de-sac of Douglas) as it extends from the posterior surface of the uterus to the rectum (see Figure 56-1). This is the lowest point of the pelvic cavity. The anterior ligament forms the uterovesical pouch as it extends from the anterior uterus to the posterior bladder. This pouch is not as deep as the rectouterine pouch.

FALLOPIAN TUBES

The fallopian tubes are slender, muscular tubes about 10 cm in length and 0.7 cm in diameter. They are located in the folds of the broad ligaments and attached at the upper outer angles of the uterus. These structures are the passageway through which the ova travel to the uterus and are the normal site for conception.

The fallopian tubes consist of four sections: interstitial section, isthmus, ampulla, and infundibulum (see Figure 56-3). The interstitial section is short and narrow and lies within the muscular wall of the uterus. The isthmus is the straight part with a thick, muscular wall and narrow lumen. It is adjacent to the uterus and is the usual site for tubal ligation. The ampulla, the longest and widest section, is thin-walled with a highly folded lining. The wide distal opening near the ovary is the infundibulum, or fimbriated end. Through muscular action, the fimbriae wave back and forth to create a current that moves ova toward the infundibulum.

Three histologic layers compose the wall of the fallopian tube: serous, muscularis, and mucosa. The serous layer is the outer, lubricative layer formed by part of the visceral peritoneum. The muscularis layer consists of two layers of smooth muscle whose peristaltic contractions aid in movement of the ovum through the tube. The mucosa layer is the inner lining and consists of ciliated columnar cells.

VAGINA

The vagina is a musculomembranous canal located anterior to the rectum and posterior to the urethra. It is about 9 cm long and extends upward from the vulva to the midpoint of the cervix. It is the passageway both for menstrual flow and for the fetus during delivery, and it is the recipient for the penis during sexual intercourse.

The wall of the vagina is composed of three layers: mucosal, muscularis, and fibrous. The mucosal layer consists of stratified squamous epithelial cells arranged in small, transverse folds called rugae. The muscularis is composed of smooth muscle and connective tissue with the ability to distend. The fibrous layer is the outer layer that attaches to the pelvic organs. It is composed of dense fibrous connective tissue and elastic fibers. The vagina contains no glands, but the epithelial cells of the mucosa undergo changes in response to estrogen. Without the influence of estrogen, the epithelium is thin and consists almost entirely of basal cells. The mucosal cells also contain a considerable amount of glycogen.

BARTHOLIN GLANDS

The Bartholin (or greater vestibular) glands are two bean-shaped, mucus-secreting glands located on each side of the vaginal orifice (Fig. 56-5). Secretion is increased during sexual excitement and moistens the inner surface of the labia in preparation for intercourse. The duct may become obstructed or infected, particularly by gonococci, and a Bartholin cyst or abscess may be formed (Fig. 56-6).

SKENE GLANDS

Skene glands are tiny, mucus-secreting glands located just posterior to the external urethral meatus (see Figure 56-2). The mucus from the Skene glands, together with

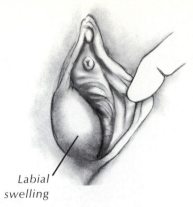

Labial swelling

FIGURE 56-6 *Inflammation of Bartholin gland. Inflammation of Bartholin glands may be acute or chronic. Causes include gonococci, Chlamydia trachomatis, and other organisms. Acutely, it appears as a tense, hot tender abscess. Look for pus coming out of the duct or erythema around the duct opening. Chronically, a nontender cyst occupies the posterior labium. It may be large or small. (Bates, B. A Guide to Physical Examination and History Taking [6th ed.]. Philadelphia: J.B. Lippincott, 1995.)*

mucus from glands in the urethra, keeps the urethral opening moist and lubricated. The Skene glands also are susceptible to infection by gonococci, which are difficult to eradicate from this location.

BREASTS

The breasts, which contain the mammary glands, are two skin glands located over the pectoral muscles between the second and sixth ribs. The breasts extend from the lateral sternum to the anterior borders of the axillae. The portion of the breast that extends upward and laterally to the axilla, called the breast tail, and lies in proximity to blood and lymph vessels. The breasts are attached by a layer of connective tissue. Each breast consists of a nipple and surrounding areola, lobes, ducts, and fibrous and fatty tissue (Fig. 56-7). The function of the breast is to secrete milk to nourish the newborn infant.

The nipple, a cylindric projection near the center of the breast, is located approximately in the fourth intercostal space. It is surrounded by a pigmented, circular area, the areola, and is perforated by ductal openings. Sexual stimulation results in engorgement and muscle contraction, which causes the nipple to become erect.

The mature female breast is made up of 15 to 20 lobes arranged around the nipple. Each lobe is further composed of a number of lobules. Inside each lobule are the alveoli, which contain both myoepithelial and acinar cells. The acinar cells are secretory cells in lactation, and the myoepithelial cells contract to force milk into the ducts. Each lobule is drained by intralobular ducts that empty into the lactiferous duct. These ducts dilate into a reservoir, called the lactiferous sinus or ampulla, just before they open in the nipple. Lobes and ducts are

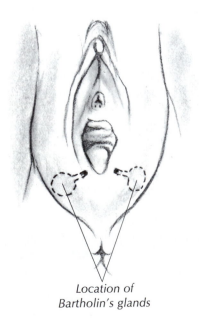

Location of Bartholin's glands

FIGURE 56-5 *Location of Bartholin glands. (Bates, B. A Guide to Physical Examination and History Taking [6th ed.]. Philadelphia: J.B. Lippincott, 1995.)*

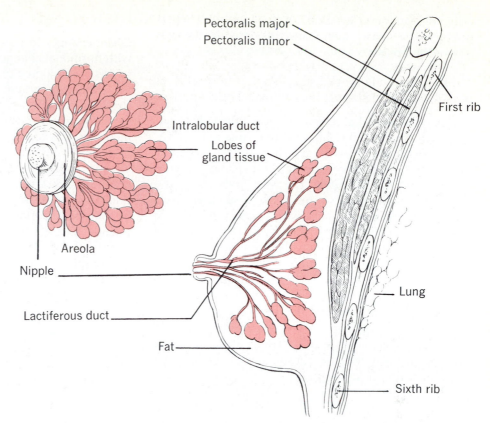

FIGURE 56-7 *Glandular tissue and ducts of the mammary gland. (Reeder, S.J., Martin, L.L. and Koniak, D. Maternity Nursing [17th ed.]. Philadelphia: J.B. Lippincott, 1992.)*

separated by fibrous tissue. Fatty tissue contributes to breast size.

Lymph drainage of the breast is important, especially in breast cancer. Lymph vessels normally follow the lactiferous ducts and eventually drain into the central axillary nodes (Fig. 56-8). This creates drainage of the superficial, areolar, and glandular parts of the breast. Blood is supplied by branches of the thoracic artery.

During puberty, breast development is controlled by estrogen and progesterone. Estrogen stimulates deposits of adipose tissue and growth of the glands and ducts, and progesterone stimulates development of the secreting

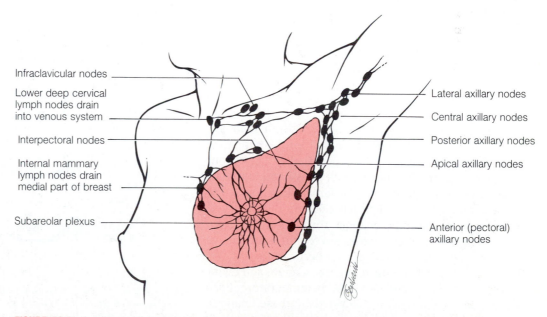

FIGURE 56-8 *Lymphatic drainage of the breast. (Smeltzer, S.C. and Bure, B.G. Brunner and Suddarth's Textbook of Medical Surgical Nursing [7th ed.]. Philadelphia: J.B. Lippincott, 1992.)*

cells. Pregnancy and lactation are associated with hypertrophy of the breasts; menopause may produce an atrophy of the breasts.

EXTERNAL GENITALIA

The external genitalia, commonly called the vulva, consists of the mons pubis, labia majora, labia minora, clitoris, urinary meatus, vaginal orifice, and vestibule (see Figure 56-2). Sometimes the Bartholin glands are considered part of the vulva. The *mons pubis* is a subcutaneous pad of adipose connective tissue that covers the symphysis. It is covered with coarse pubic hair at puberty. The *labia majora* consists of two prominent longitudinal folds of pigmented skin that extend down and back from the mons pubis. They are 7 to 8 cm in length and 2 to 3 cm wide. The labia majora are composed of areolar and adipose tissue as well as extensive lymph vessels, and they are covered on the outside with hair. Both sebaceous and sweat glands are contained within the labia majora. On the inside, the labia majora are smooth and moist. The labia majora are synonymous with the scrotum in the male.

The *labia minora* are two smaller, thin folds that lie within the labia majora. They extend down and back from the clitoris. The labia minora contain no hair but are rich in sebaceous glands. The *clitoris* is a small, rounded projection, highly sensitive to touch. It is 5 to 6 mm long and 6 to 8 mm wide. The clitoris is composed of erectile tissue and is synonymous in origin with the penis. The *vestibule* is an almond-shaped flat area that extends from the clitoris to the fourchette. It is bordered by the labia minora, and contains openings to the urethral orifice, vaginal orifice, Bartholin glands, and Skene glands.

▼ Female Reproductive Functions

Female reproductive functions, which begin with puberty and end with menopause, fall into two phases: 1) preparation of the body for conception and gestation; and 2) gestation. The specific functions include the reproductive cycle, production of female hormones, the sex act, and gestation. The female reproductive cycle involves many periodic changes throughout the span from menarche to menopause. Successful reproductive function depends on changes that occur in the ovaries, endometrium, myometrium, breasts, vagina, and endocrine glands and on changes in body temperature. Even the woman's emotions are affected by these changes. Various organs respond differently to the changes, but all can be related to the menstrual cycle.

HYPOTHALAMIC INFLUENCE

Cyclic changes in the female reproductive cycle begin with hormonal changes initiated by the hypothalamus, which is considered to be part of both the nervous and the endocrine systems. Both physical and emotional stressors can affect menstrual regularity through nervous control of the hypothalamus. Depending on the messages it receives, the hypothalamus then secretes hormones called *releasing* or *inhibiting factors*, which act directly on the pituitary gland (Flowchart 56-1). Neurosecretory substances that are secreted by the hypothalamus and transported through the hypothalamic-hypophyseal portal system to the anterior pituitary include follicle-stimulating hormone (FSH) releasing factor, luteinizing hormone (LH) releasing factor, and luteotropic hormone inhibiting factor. These factors act on the anterior pituitary to control the gland's secretion. *Oxytocin*, secreted by the posterior pituitary, increases

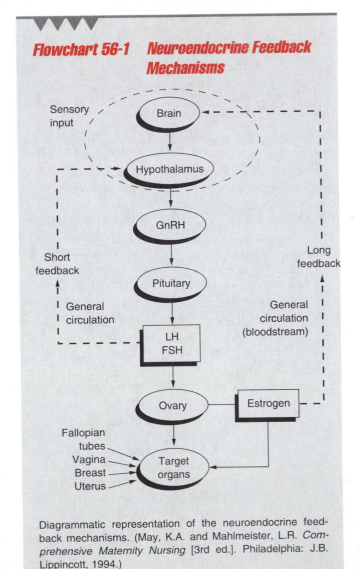

Flowchart 56-1 Neuroendocrine Feedback Mechanisms

Diagrammatic representation of the neuroendocrine feedback mechanisms. (May, K.A. and Mahlmeister, L.R. *Comprehensive Maternity Nursing* [3rd ed.]. Philadelphia: J.B. Lippincott, 1994.)

uterine contractions during labor and moves milk from breast glands to nipples during suckling.

PITUITARY INFLUENCE

The anterior pituitary secretes two hormones that directly influence reproductive function: follicle-stimulating hormone (FSH) and luteinizing hormone (LH). Together with estrogen and progesterone, FSH and LH act directly on the ovaries to control ovulation. The release of FSH and LH is regulated by feedback effects of estrogen and progesterone on the hypothalamus (see flowchart). Additionally, the anterior pituitary secretes *prolactin*, also called luteotropic hormone. Prolactin acts on the breasts to control lactation after delivery. The release of prolactin is prevented by the prolactin inhibiting factor, which is controlled by high levels of estrogen or progesterone. Suckling and low estrogen levels stimulate prolactin production.

MENSTRUAL CYCLE

The menstrual cycle involves regular changes that are repeated about every 28 days. This process varies in individual women but has three phases: menstrual, proliferative, and secretory. The proliferative and secretory phases are separated by ovulation (Fig. 56-9).

Menstrual Phase

The menstrual phase begins with the onset of the menses and lasts about 5 days. Average blood loss is 30 to 150 mL, although the amount varies widely. During the menstrual phase, the blood levels of both estrogen and progesterone are low. This phase also involves degeneration and sloughing of the stratum compactum and most of the stratum spongiosum.

Proliferative Phase

The proliferative phase follows the menstrual phase and is accompanied by changes in the endometrium, myometrium, and ovaries. The cyclic changes in these organs result from fluctuation in gonadotropin and estrogen levels. Changes in the endometrium and myometrium are primarily controlled by blood levels of estrogen. With increasing levels of estrogen, the endometrium thickens as the endometrial cells and arterioles grow longer and more coiled. The water content of the endometrium and contractions of the myometrium also increase. These changes in the endometrium and myometrium prepare the uterus for implantation of the fertilized ovum.

Changes in the ovaries occur in what is referred to as the follicular phase. This ovarian phase encompasses both the menstrual and the proliferative phases of the menstrual cycle. Low levels of estrogen in the menstrual phase signal the production of FSH by the anterior pituitary. In the ovaries, FSH production then stimulates the primary follicles. At that time, a number of follicles begin to mature. Soon only one, the *graafian follicle*, begins to dominate, and the others recede. This follicle gradually moves to the surface of the ovary (see Figure 56-9). The follicle contains the ovum and is surrounded by a layer of granulosa cells, which are further surrounded by specialized cells called the *theca interna* and *theca externa*. Estrogen is secreted by the theca interna, and the granulosa cells supply nutrition for the ovum.

As the follicle enlarges, fluid begins to collect inside, pushing the ovum to one side. It is surrounded on the outside by granulosa cells called the cumulus oophorus. A clear membrane also develops and surrounds the ovum. This inner surrounding is termed the zona pellucida. Outside the zona pellucida and inside the cumulus oophorus is a single layer of cells called the corona radiata. While these changes are occurring within the follicle, the anterior pituitary begins gradual secretion of LH, which stimulates the follicles to increase estrogen production. High levels of estrogen then signal the hypothalamus to stop producing FSH releasing factor. Production of LH continues, resulting in a surge of LH that triggers ovulation within 1 to 24 hours. At ovulation, the mature ovum is extruded from the ovary with both the zona pellucida and corona radiata surrounding it.

Ovulation

Ovulation divides the proliferative and secretory phases of the menstrual cycle and usually occurs 14 days before the onset of the next menstrual cycle. It may be accompanied by low abdominal pain, termed *mittelschmerz*. The escape of fluid or blood from the follicle is believed to produce peritoneal irritation that causes the pain. Ovulation also is accompanied by changes in cervical mucus. Cervical mucus increases in amount as it becomes clear and thin. Under the influence of high estrogen levels, it forms a ferning pattern when allowed to dry on a slide (Fig. 56-10).

Oogenesis

Unlike spermatogenesis, which continuously produces many sperm, oogenesis is the cyclic production of single ova. Immediately before ovulation, the primary oocyte undergoes its first meiotic division, resulting in a secondary oocyte that contains 23 chromosomes and most of the cytoplasm. A second body is formed, and it is referred to as the first polar body. This first polar body receives 23 chromosomes but little cytoplasm. The secondary oocyte then undergoes a second meiotic division. Both cells again contain 23 chromosomes, but only one receives the majority of cytoplasm. This cell is the *mature ovum*, and the second cell is known as the second polar

1. Low level of estrogen in menstrual phase signals hypothalamus to secrete GRF, which stimulates the anterior pituitary to produce FSH.

2. FSH stimulates follicles in ovary to mature. One follicle becomes dominant and grows to become the graafian follicle.

3. Cells surrounding the ovum in the follicle secrete estrogen. High levels of estrogen result in the thickening of the endometrium.

4. Anterior pituitary releases a surge of LH, which facilitates ovulation.

5. LH also influences the development of the corpus luteum from the remnants of the graafian follicle.

6. The corpus luteum secretes large amounts of progesterone and some estrogen, which act on the endometrium, causing the vessels to lengthen and coil and the glands to expand and secrete.

7. If the ovum is not fertilized, the corpus luteum degenerates, resulting in decreasing estrogen and progesterone levels.

8. Decreased hormone levels result in blood vessels constriction in the endometrium. Without a supply of nutrients the tissue degenerates and sloughs away.

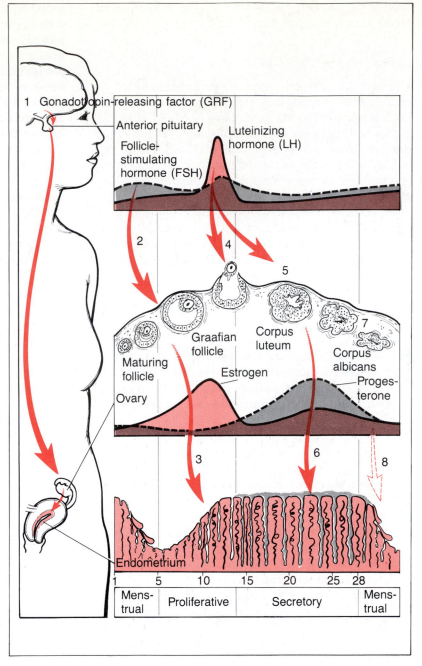

FIGURE 56-9 *Phases of the menstrual cycle*

body. Meiosis is arrested at this phase if fertilization does not occur. Fig. 56-11 shows the maturation of one ovum.

Secretory Phase

The secretory phase begins with ovulation, and is characterized by formation of the corpus luteum in the ovary, production of progesterone and estrogen, secretory changes in the endometrium, and decreased contractions in the myometrium. This phase of the menstrual cycle corresponds with the luteal phase in the ovary.

During the luteal phase, the follicle walls collapse with some hemorrhage into the cavity, forming a corpus hemorrhagia. Under the influence of LH, the granulosa cells hypertrophy, take on a yellow color, and become known as luteal cells. This golden body, the corpus luteum, continues to function for about 7 to 8 days. Its primary function is to secrete progesterone and some estrogen. These hormones initiate the negative feedback loop to the hypothalamus and pituitary gland that prevents further ovulation within the cycle. In the absence of fertilization, luteal cells begin to degenerate, causing a decrease

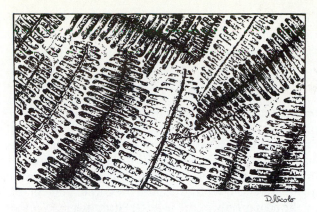

FIGURE 56-10 *Fern pattern seen on microscopic examination of cervical mucus at midcycle in normal menstruating women. (Miller, M.A., and Brooten, D.A. The Childbearing Family: A Nursing Perspective [2nd ed.]. Boston: Little, Brown, 1983.)*

in estrogen and progesterone levels. The corpus luteum eventually is converted into the corpus albicans, which moves to the center of the ovary and finally disappears.

The production of progesterone by the corpus luteum leads to secretory changes in the endometrium that create a favorable environment for pregnancy. Increase in the endometrium at this time is believed to be caused by swelling from increased water content rather than cellular proliferation. The endometrium becomes more vascular, with coiled spiral arteries located close to the surface. The changes produce a thick, succulent environment, rich in glycogen and ideal for implantation of the fertilized ovum. Progesterone also is associated with a decrease in myometrial contractions. In addition, women may notice fluid retention, breast tenderness and fullness, moodiness, and premenstrual tension from the high levels of progesterone. Increased levels of progesterone also cause an increase in basal body temperature during the secretory phase of the menstrual cycle. This characteristic of progesterone provides the basis for basal temperature studies for women with fertility problems.

In the absence of fertilization and implantation, progesterone secretion falls, which is a signal for the beginning of a new cycle. Degenerated endometrium sloughs, the hypothalamus begins to secrete releasing factors, and the cycle begins again.

PRODUCTION OF FEMALE HORMONES

Estrogen and progesterone are the two primary female hormones. Others are androgen, prolactin, and the prostaglandins.

Estrogen

Estrogen is a general term for a class of hormones predominantly present in the female. It is a steroid hormone

primarily secreted by the ovaries and by the placenta during pregnancy, with a small amount being secreted by the adrenal cortices. There are a number of natural estrogens, but only three are potent enough to produce physiologic effects: estradiol, estrone, and estriol. The major estrogen, estradiol, is the most potent (12 times greater than estrone), but the ovaries secrete about four times more estrone. Both estradiol and estrone can be identified in venous blood from the ovary, and estriol is oxidized mainly in the liver from estradiol and estrone.

After being secreted by the ovaries, estradiol and estrone either enter cells to perform their functions or are oxidized principally in the liver to estriol. Estrogens are inactivated in the liver through conjugation with sulfuric acid and glucuronic acid. The glucuronides and sulfates are then excreted in the bile. Estrogens in extracellular fluids are primarily in the form of estroprotein, another

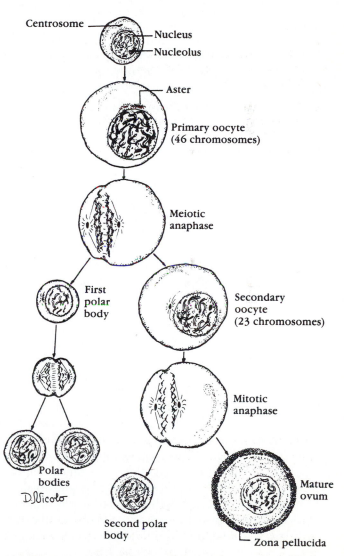

FIGURE 56-11 *Maturation of female reproductive cells, resulting in formation of one mature ovum. (Source: Miller, M.A. and Brooten, P.A. The Childbearing Family: A Nursing Perspective [2nd ed.]. Boston: Little, Brown, 1993.)*

metabolite produced in the liver. This inactivation process accounts for the ineffectiveness of the natural estrogens when they are administered orally. Conditions that depress liver function also may be associated with increased estrogen levels because of the absence of the inactivation process.

In the clinical setting, two other forms of estrogen may be used: synthetic and conjugated. The synthetic estrogens are of particular importance because of their potency when administered orally. Estrogen affects cell proliferation and development of the female secondary sex characteristics as well as the menstrual cycle.

Throughout childhood, small quantities of estrogen are produced, but at puberty, the levels greatly increase. As a result of estrogen influence, the sex organs, including external genitalia, breasts, ovaries, fallopian tubes, uterus, and vagina, increase in size. Vaginal epithelium thickens and differentiates into layers that increase the resistance of the vagina to injury and infection. The epithelium also increases its glycogen levels. Estrogens also affect the fat deposits in the vulva and mons pubis, growth of the pelvis, and distribution of axillary and pubic hair. The onset of puberty is associated with a rapid growth rate in the female. Estrogens cause early uniting of the epiphyses and shafts of the long bones, causing female growth to cease earlier than male growth. They also affect calcium and phosphate retention, which is important in menopause, when estrogen levels are greatly reduced.

Estrogens influence the skin and capillary walls. With increased levels of estrogen, the skin becomes soft, smooth, and thicker than that of a child. It also is more vascular. For this reason, women may bleed more when cut or note increased skin warmth. In addition, the capillary walls become stronger. When estrogen levels are low, there is a greater tendency toward bruising.

Progesterone

Progesterone often is considered the hormone of pregnancy because of its effect on the endometrium and myometrium. It is produced almost exclusively by the corpus luteum in the nonpregnant female and by the placenta during pregnancy. Chemically, natural progesterone is similar to estrogen. It is less potent than estrogen and is secreted in larger amounts. Shortly after secretion, it is degraded to pregnanediol and excreted in this form in the urine. In addition to its uterine effects, progesterone affects the breasts. Whereas estrogen is responsible for breast growth, progesterone is responsible for maturation of lobules and alveoli, so that they may become secretory when stimulated by prolactin.

Androgens

Female androgens are secreted in small amounts by the adrenal glands and ovaries. In disruptions of female function, the amount of secretions can become significant and result in masculine hair distribution, acne, and deepening of the voice.

Prolactin

Prolactin is a protein hormone secreted by the anterior pituitary. Its release is stimulated by suckling during breastfeeding and by low estrogen levels. High estrogen and progesterone levels trigger the release of prolactin inhibiting factor from the hypothalamus, thus preventing its secretion. Prolactin stimulates production of milk by the acinar cells in the alveoli. Pituitary gland tumors can cause milk production, even in the absence of pregnancy.

Prostaglandins

Prostaglandins are a group of potent lipids that function as local hormones. They are considered important in reproductive physiology. Prostaglandins have been separated into three groups: prostaglandins A, E, and F (PGA, PGE, and PGF). Each group exerts different actions on systems of the body. Prostaglandins are synthesized from phospholipids in various body tissues.[22] Phospholipase A, an enzyme, is responsible for liberation of essential fatty acids from the phospholipids. The essential fatty acids are then converted to PGE or PGF by prostaglandin synthetase. As Flowchart 56-2 shows, PGA is produced by additional metabolism of PGE. Prostaglandins are degraded primarily in the lungs soon after they enter the circulation. For this reason, their actions seem to be mainly local.

Although there are many prostaglandins, only PGE_2 and PGF_2 primarily affect reproduction. Both have been identified in endometrial tissue, where they exert a stimulating effect on the uterus.[28] Levels of prostaglandins vary with the phases of the menstrual cycle with much higher levels of PGE_2 during menses and higher PGF_2 during midluteal and menses (Table 56-1). Elevated levels of PGE_2 and PGF_2 have been identified as a possible factor in primary dysmenorrhea. PGE_2 is administered to induce uterine contractions for intrauterine fetal death, missed abortion, and hydatidiform mole.

FEMALE RESPONSE IN THE SEX ACT

The female response in the sex act is a normal physiologic process. Although each woman has different levels of response, the physiologic events of response occur in an orderly sequence: excitation, plateau, orgasm, and resolution (Fig. 56-12).

Excitation begins with either physical or emotional stimulation. The first response to sexual stimulation is vaginal lubrication. This is a result of vasodilatation and congestion and can occur within 10 to 30 seconds of stimulation. Transudation of fluid, not secretion, ac-

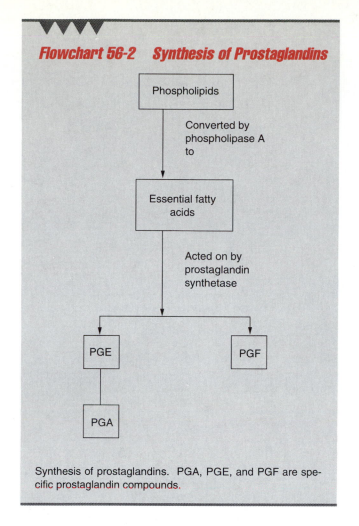

Flowchart 56-2   Synthesis of Prostaglandins

Phospholipids

Converted by phospholipase A to

Essential fatty acids

Acted on by prostaglandin synthetase

PGE   PGF

PGA

Synthesis of prostaglandins. PGA, PGE, and PGF are specific prostaglandin compounds.

counts for lubrication, because the vagina contains no secretory glands. Other characteristics of the excitement phase include engorgement and enlargement of the labia, clitoris, and uterus; enlargement and ballooning of the vagina; elevation of the uterus and cervix; and nipple erection. Blood pressure and pulse increase, and the "sex flush" may appear as a measleslike rash on epigastrium, chest, and throat.

The plateau phase is reached as sexual arousal is increased. Characteristics of this phase include retraction of the clitoris against the symphysis, narrowing of the vaginal opening, increased length and diameter of the vagina, deep red coloring of the labia minora, and complete elevation of the uterus. Breast size may increase in the plateau phase, and the sex flush may spread over the shoulders, inner surface of arms, and perhaps abdomen, back, and thighs. Respiratory rate also increases late in the plateau phase.

During orgasm, vasocongestion reaches its maximum and stimulates the reflex stretch mechanism. As a result, rhythmic contractions occur in the clitoris, the uterus, the outer one-third of the vagina, and perhaps the rectal sphincter. Rhythmic contractions also may be noted in the arms, legs, abdomen, and buttocks.

During resolution, the final phase of sexual response, the body returns to its preexcitement phase. Within 10 to 15 seconds, the clitoris returns to normal and normal color returns to the labia minora. Ten to 15 minutes are required for the vagina to return to normal, and the cervical os remains open for about 30 minutes. Unlike the male, who experiences a refractory period during

TABLE 56-1 *Normal Hormone Levels*

Hormone	Blood	Urine
Pregnanediol		
Male		<1.5 mg/24 h
Female		
Proliferative phase		0.5–1.5 mg/24 h
Luteal phase		2–7 mg/24 h
Postmenopausal		0.2–1.0 mg/24 h
Estrogens (total)		
Male		4–25 µg/24 h
Female		4–60 µg/24 h with increase in pregnancy
Prolactin	<20 ng/mL	
Progesterone		
Proliferative phase	<1.0 ng/mL	
Luteal phase	<2.0 ng/mL	
Follicle-stimulating hormone		6–50 mouse uterine units/24 h
Luteinizing hormone		
Proliferative phase	<70 mIU/mL	
Luteal phase	>70 mIU/mL	
Estriol		10–20 mg/24 h

Excitement Stage

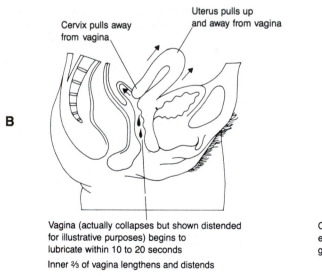

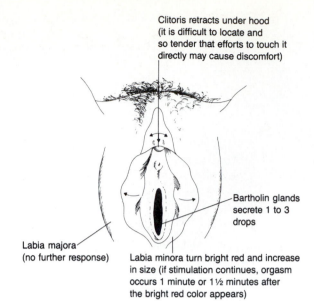

Plateau Stage

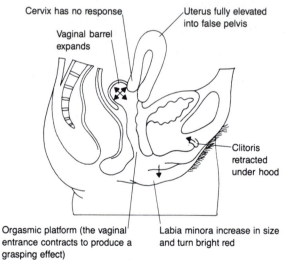

FIGURE 56-12 *Female sexual response cycle.* **A.** *Changes in external genitalia.* **B.** *Changes in internal genitalia. (Reeder, S.J., Martin, L.L. and Koniak, D. Maternity Nursing [17th ed.]. Philadelphia: J.B. Lippincott, 1992.)*

resolution when he is incapable of sexual stimulation, some women are capable of several orgasms without dropping below the plateau phase. Resolution then follows the last orgasm.

GESTATION

Gestation begins with fertilization of the ovum and continues throughout the development of the fetus. A concise discussion of the biophysical development of reproduction as a basis for discussion of the alterations in normal pregnancy is provided in Chapter 5.

MENOPAUSE

Menopause, the cessation of menstruation, marks the final phase of female reproductive function. The transition or gradual change in ovarian function is termed *climacteric*. The average age of menopause for women in the United States is 50 years. Menopause is complete after the woman has experienced no menstrual periods for 1 year. In some women, menopause occurs abruptly with complete cessation of menstruation after normal periods. In others, gradual cessation is characterized by decreased amounts of bleeding with monthly cycles,

Orgasm Stage

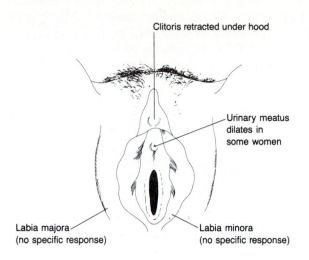

Clitoris retracted under hood

Urinary meatus dilates in some women

Labia majora (no specific response)

Labia minora (no specific response)

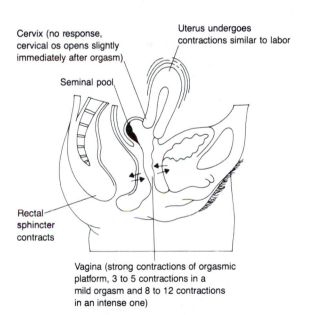

Cervix (no response, cervical os opens slightly immediately after orgasm)

Uterus undergoes contractions similar to labor

Seminal pool

Rectal sphincter contracts

Vagina (strong contractions of orgasmic platform, 3 to 5 contractions in a mild orgasm and 8 to 12 contractions in an intense one)

Resolution Stage

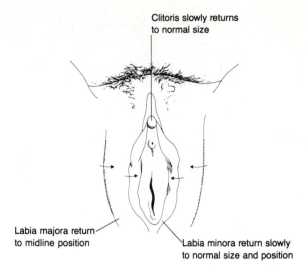

Clitoris slowly returns to normal size

Labia majora return to midline position

Labia minora return slowly to normal size and position

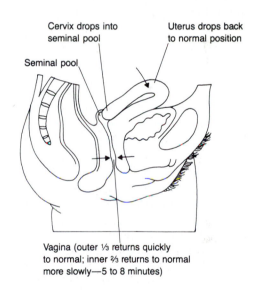

Cervix drops into seminal pool

Uterus drops back to normal position

Seminal pool

Vagina (outer ⅓ returns quickly to normal; inner ⅔ returns to normal more slowly—5 to 8 minutes)

FIGURE 56-12   (continued)

periods of amenorrhea, and, finally, complete cessation of normal periods. Menopause is accompanied by decreased estrogen levels and reversal in estrogen forms. The production of all estrogens by the ovaries decreases. The primary estrogen in menopause is estrone, which is derived from androstenedione and fat conversion.

Menopause frequently is associated with other physiologic changes and symptoms. These include hot flashes, changes in reproductive organs, cardiovascular disease, osteoporosis, and nervousness and psychological problems.[22] The most common symptom is hot flashes. These begin as a feeling of warmth in the chest and progress upward over the neck and face. They may be accompanied by flushing of the skin in these areas and profuse diaphoresis. The exact cause has not been determined, but they appear to be related to estrogen withdrawal.

Changes in reproductive organs include atrophy of the labia; dryness and thinning of vaginal walls; decreased support of bladder, rectum, and uterus; and decreased size of the uterus and cervix. These changes are all associated with lower estrogen levels and account for such complaints as dyspareunia, stress incontinence, and vaginal itching and burning. Evidence supports increased frequency of hypertension, stroke, and heart disease after menopause.[30] Decreased estrogen levels also are linked to osteoporosis and increased bone fragility. Estrogen administration has been shown to halt the process in young women who undergo surgical removal of the ovaries.

Psychological symptoms associated with menopause include nervousness, depression, headache, insomnia, decreased sex drive, memory loss, vertigo, and a feeling of worthlessness and hopelessness. No connection has been identified between these symptoms and estrogen levels; therefore, basic personality and cultural influences are of more importance in determining treatment.

▼ Laboratory and Diagnostic Aids

GYNECOLOGIC EXAMINATION

The most important of all diagnostic tools available is the physical examination. Gynecologic examination of the female reproductive system involves three steps: external examination, speculum examination, and bimanual examination. External examination includes inspection and palpation of the breasts, palpation of the abdomen, and inspection of the external genitalia. With these procedures, one can detect masses, redness, and swelling or lesions of the breasts and external genitalia.

The speculum examination allows for visualization of the cervix and vaginal wall and detection of redness, lesions, swelling, or unusual discharge. Specimens for laboratory tests, including Papanicolaou (Pap) smear, wet smear, gonorrhea cultures, and biopsies, also may be collected at this time.

The final step is the bimanual examination, in which the uterus, ovaries, and fallopian tubes are palpated. It also usually involves either a rectal or a rectovaginal examination by which the examiner is able to palpate such pelvic structures as the posterior surface of the uterus, the uterosacral ligaments, and the cul-de-sac of Douglas.

HORMONE LEVELS

Both bioassay and chemical methods are available for determining ovarian hormone levels. These tests are time-consuming, difficult to perform or to standardize, and expensive. Therefore, most of the studies to detect hormone levels are indirect.

Progesterone

Progesterone is a steroid that is degraded shortly after secretion. Most of this degradation occurs in the liver, with the major end product being pregnanediol. Because pregnanediol is excreted in the urine, its rate of excretion can be used to estimate progesterone formation. This estimation must be done by chemical means because pregnanediol exerts no progesteronic effects. Results are difficult to standardize, but the generally accepted normal values are summarized in Table 56-1. Increased levels of progesterone may be associated with luteal cysts of the ovary, arrhenoblastoma of the ovary, and hyperadrenocorticism. Decreased levels may occur in amenorrhea, threatened abortion, fetal death, and toxemia of pregnancy.

Indirect methods of determining progesterone levels include endometrial biopsy and basal body temperature. An endometrial biopsy is useful in determining the stage of the menstrual cycle and, therefore, the level of hormone production. In studying basal body temperature charts, a sustained rise of 1°F implies that ovulation has taken place and that progesterone secretion is adequate.

Estrogen

One useful laboratory test in the study of estrogen levels is measurement of 24-hour urinary estriol excretion. Because estriol is produced by the placenta, it represents both fetal and placental activity. A significant drop (40% less than the mean of three previous values) may indicate that the fetus is in jeopardy, because urinary estriol excretion increases as pregnancy progresses. Incomplete 24-hour urine specimens and pyelonephritis have been known to affect the results. Normal findings are 10 to 20 mg/24 h.

Changes in cervical mucus and epithelial cells of the vagina are good indicators of estrogen production. Cervical mucus undergoes definite changes in response to estrogen and progesterone production. Spinnbarkeit and ferning are two characteristics of cervical mucus that can easily be studied. Spinnbarkeit refers to the elasticity of cervical mucus at the time of ovulation, which allows the examiner to draw it out into a long, thin thread of 15 to 20 cm. During minimal estrogen production, threads reach only 1 to 2 cm.

Ferning refers to the pattern created when cervical mucus dries under the influence of estrogen (see Figure 56-10). It occurs when sodium chloride in the mucus crystallizes. Estrogen secretion increases the sodium chloride content of cervical mucus, whereas progesterone decreases it. Therefore, the level of estrogen without progesterone determines the presence of a ferning pattern. This pattern is fullest and most complete at the time of ovulation.

Vaginal smears also are useful in determining estrogen levels because the vaginal cells undergo cyclic changes. Estrogen thickens the vaginal epithelium. Glucose excretion also corresponds to estrogen secretion. Both are highest at the time of ovulation.

SMEARS

Papanicolaou Smear

A specimen for Pap smear is best collected from the cervical canal and the squamocolumnar junction near the external os during the speculum examination. Dry cotton swabs are used to collect cervical canal secretions, and a small wooden spatula is used for the squamocolumnar specimen (Fig. 56-13). The specimen is then transferred to a glass slide, where it is fixed for staining and microscopic examination. The primary purpose of a Pap smear is to screen for abnormal cervical cells and indicate the need for more extensive testing.

The high rate of false-negative reports associated with the earlier reporting systems led to the development, in 1988, of a new nomenclature for reporting Pap smear findings. This system, known as the Bethesda system (TBS I), was revised in 1991 (TBS II).[24] Currently, the Bethesda system is being used by more than 80% of the cytology laboratories in the United States.[24] The TBS system uses three areas of classification: adequacy of specimen, general categorization, and descriptive diagnosis. Each category reflects three subcategories. The adequacy of specimen is classified as satisfactory for evaluation; unsatisfactory for evaluation; or satisfactory for evaluation but limited by, for example, atrophy and inflammation.[24] For general categorization, specimens are described as within normal limits, as having benign cellular changes, or as having epithelial cell abnormalities. Subcategories for the descriptive diagnosis include benign cellular changes (infection and re-active changes), epithelial cell abnormalities with low-grade and high-grade squamous intraepithelial lesions, and glandular cell abnormalities.[24]

The new system has resulted in about 10% of Pap smears being classified as abnormal.[25] Based on individual patient age and history, follow-up may include repeat smears, colposcopy, biopsy, and endocervical curettage. The American Cancer Society recommends that women 18 to 20 years of age have an annual Pap smear until at least three negative tests have been obtained.[18] Sexually active women younger than this age should also have annual Pap smears. The American College of Obstetrics and Gynecology continues to recommend annual tests for most women, owing to the difficulty in determination of women at high risk for cervical cancer.[18]

Wet Smear

Wet smears are especially beneficial in diagnosing the cause of vaginitis. In this procedure, a specimen of vaginal discharge is placed on a slide, mixed with a drop of saline solution or potassium hydroxide, and examined under the microscope for *Candida*, *Trichomonas*, or other organisms. It is not conclusive for gonorrhea.

BIOPSY

Endometrial Biopsy

To take an endometrial biopsy, a curet is inserted through the cervix, placed against the uterine wall, and slowly withdrawn. It is best to repeat the procedure on different walls of the uterus to obtain enough tissue to represent a major portion of the uterus. Endometrial biopsy is especially useful in evaluation of dysfunctional bleeding. It may be helpful in diagnosis of endometrial cancer, but there is a chance that scattered growths may be missed. Another use for endometrial biopsy is in infertility studies. It is best performed just before the onset of menses, or day 22 of the menstrual cycle. It can interfere with pregnancy if conception has occurred.

Cervical Biopsy

A punch biopsy instrument is used in the physician's office to obtain samples of cervical tissue. This can aid in more precise diagnosis of questionable lesions. It also is helpful in removal of small polyps.

Cone Biopsy

Cone biopsy, also referred to as conization, involves removal of a cone-shaped specimen of cervical tissue, any visible lesions, and tissue specimens of the squamocolumnar junction and cervical canal. It may be used as follow-up to Pap smear or punch biopsy.

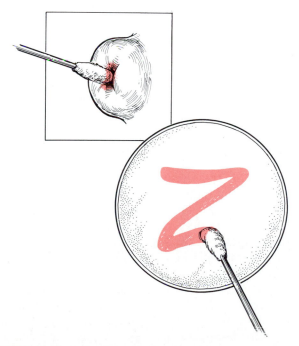

FIGURE 56-13 *Method for obtaining Pap smear.*

Open Breast Biopsy

Breast biopsy is surgical intervention to remove a lump. A frozen section can be examined for immediate classification; more extensive pathologic studies require additional time.

Needle Biopsy

The physician inserts a needle into a breast lesion and aspirates its contents. This procedure may be performed in the office and is followed up as necessary.

Vulvar Biopsy

Punch biopsy forceps can be used to obtain vulvar tissue. The gross appearance frequently is normal, and staining procedures must be used to identify pathology.

RADIOGRAPHY

Hysterosalpingography

Hysterosalpingography is a radiographic examination of the uterus and fallopian tubes. A small cannula is inserted through the cervix, and radiopaque dye is injected into the uterus and fallopian tubes. Filling of the uterus and tubes can be observed on the fluoroscopy screen. Spot films also may be made. Hysterosalpingography is especially useful for observing the size and shape of the uterus and tubes and any tubal obstruction.

Mammography

Mammography is a radiologic examination of the breasts. It is useful to detect early lesions that cannot be palpated and to determine the exact location of deep tumors. It may be useful in predicting cancer. With the refinement of this procedure, radiation exposure is minimal, and it is now considered safe for routine screening. The American Cancer Society recommends a baseline mammogram on all women between 35 and 40 years of age, routine mammograms every 2 years between ages 40 and 49, and annual examinations for women 50 years of age or older. For women at increased risk for breast cancer, mammography may be initiated on an annual basis at 40 years of age.

OTHER PROCEDURES

Colposcopy

The colposcope is a binocular diagnostic instrument that provides a magnified (19–20X) view of the cervix and vaginal walls. It is mounted on a tripod and makes no contact with the patient. Colposcopy is useful to follow up abnormal results of Pap smears, to identify abnormal areas for biopsy, and to examine lesions on the vulva. Colposcopy also is recommended in follow up of women whose mothers took diethylstilbesterol (DES) during pregnancy; it also may be used for women with dyspareunia and bleeding with intercourse. Each procedure involves the following five observations: vascular pattern, color tone, intercapillary distance, borderline versus normal tissue, and surface pattern.[28]

Laparoscopy and Culdoscopy

Both laparoscopy and culdoscopy are surgical procedures that allow the physician to visualize the pelvic area through a lighted tube. The procedures are performed to observe the condition and position of the various organs and the presence of any scarring, endometrial tissue, or infection. A tubal ligation also may be performed through the laparoscope.

Hysteroscopy

Hysteroscopy is an office procedure that can be used in follow up to hysterosalpingography findings of abnormal uterine contour or in treatment of certain uterine fibroids and polyps.[32] This procedure allows the physician to visualize the inner portion of the uterus and to collect a biopsy specimen from any abnormal area.

Ultrasonography

Ultrasonography, also referred to as sonography, is a noninvasive technique that is particularly useful in providing pictures of soft tissues of the body. Little preparation is necessary for pelvic ultrasonography except that the woman must have a full bladder. The bladder, distended with 200 to 400 mL of urine, is used as a reference point and to displace the pelvic organs for better visualization. Overdistention can distort the findings.

An ultrasound transducer serves as both a transmitter and a receiver. It converts an electrical signal into ultrasound energy, which is transmitted into the body and then reflected from tissues of different densities. These reflections of ultrasound energy are then received by the transducer and converted again to electrical energy for recording. The procedure is painless and takes about 5 to 30 minutes to complete.

Ultrasonography has become a valuable diagnostic tool in both obstetrics and gynecology. In obstetrics, it is especially useful to confirm pregnancy, to establish or confirm dates or placental location, to rule out large or small size for gestational age, to determine fetal position, and to detect hydrops. Gynecologists use ultrasonography to assist in the diagnosis of uterine malformation, hydatidiform mole, tumors, ovarian masses, pelvic inflammatory disease, tubal malformations, and pelvic abscess or hematoma.

The newest development in sonographic technology involves the use of a transvaginal probe. This procedure allows the physician to obtain immediate imaging information in the office whenever pelvic pathology is suspected. Although more data are available on the use of transvaginal imaging in uterine cancer, the procedure may also be helpful in evaluating for cervial and ovarian cancer.[40]

Schiller's Test

The Schiller's test is a simple procedure that involves painting the cervix with Schiller solution or a similar iodine solution. A normal cervix, which contains glycogen, appears mahogany brown from absorption of the iodine. Abnormal areas that contain no glycogen remain a light brown. The primary usefulness of the test is to locate exact areas for biopsy (Fig. 56-14).

Cultures

Cultures are most helpful in the diagnosis of the specific organism responsible for an infection. A specimen is collected from the infection site with a sterile cotton swab and immediately placed in an appropriate medium. The specimen is then incubated and checked for growth and sensitivity. If gonorrhea is suspected, special precautions should be undertaken to ensure an anaerobic environment. Special media also may be used to reduce growth of other bacteria.

Thermography

Thermography is the photographic display of infrared rays from skin temperature over the breast. Skin temperature is elevated in breast cancer because of increased blood flow in the tumor area. This procedure does not always detect early cancers, and false-positive results are common.

Rubin Test

In the Rubin test, carbon dioxide is injected through a cannula into the uterus. If one or both fallopian tubes are open, the woman feels referred shoulder pain. The value of this test is to determine the patency of at least one tube.

Huhner Test

The Huhner test, also called the postcoital test, is an examination of cervical mucus. Ideally, it is performed during ovulation and within several hours of intercourse. Cervical mucus is collected with an eyedropper or cotton swab and examined under a microscope. It is a simple procedure used in screening for infertility because the examiner can note the characteristics of the cervical mucus as well as the number and activity of sperm present.

▼ Alterations in Female Function

MENSTRUAL PROBLEMS

Endometriosis

Endometriosis refers to the abnormal location of endometrial tissue. Two types of endometriosis, internal and external, are described. *Internal endometriosis*, or adenomyosis, refers to the location of aberrant endometrial tissue within the myometrium. *External endometriosis* refers to the location of endometrial tissue outside the uterus. Sites for external endometriosis include the outer surface or perimetrium of the uterus, fallopian tubes, ovaries (most common site), bladder and rectal surfaces, uterine ligaments, cul-de-sac, rectovaginal septum, appendix, and bowel. Aberrant tissue also may be found in laparotomy scars, vulva, vagina, and umbilicus (Fig. 56-15). In this chapter, the term *adenomyosis* is used to refer to the internal condition and *endometriosis* is used to refer to the external condition.

Endometriosis is characterized by functional aberrant endometrium that responds to hormonal stimulation as normal uterine endometrium does. This tissue grows and thickens under cyclic hormonal influence; as estrogen and progesterone are withdrawn, it reacts with bleeding. Early lesions appear as tiny red-blue spots

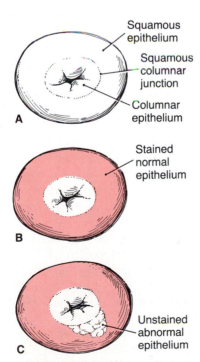

FIGURE 56-14 *Schiller's test.* **A.** *Normal appearance of unstained cervix.* **B.** *Appearance of stained epithelium in normal cervix.* **C.** *Abnormal area does not pick up the stain.*

Squamous epithelium

Squamous columnar junction

Columnar epithelium

A

Stained normal epithelium

B

Unstained abnormal epithelium

C

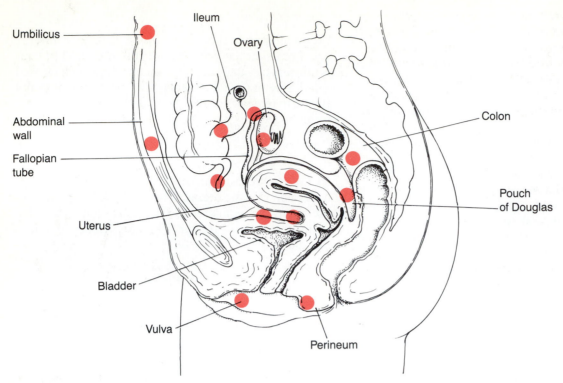

FIGURE 56-15 *Sites of endometriosis. (Rubin, E., and Farber, J.L. Pathology [2nd ed.]. Philadelphia: J.B. Lippincott, 1994.)*

surrounded by puckered scar tissue. Larger masses may form if the smaller lesions coalesce. These usually are located on the serosal layer of the involved organs. In the ovaries, lesions may take the form of *endometriomas*, cystic lesions lined with functioning endometrium. Bleeding within the cysts results in thick, chocolate-colored fluid: thus, the term *chocolate cysts* (Fig. 56-16). Adhesions result when bleeding occurs into the peritoneal cavity, leading to fixation of involved pelvic structures.

It has been estimated that this condition affects five

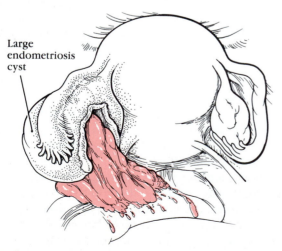

FIGURE 56-16 *Endometriosis with cyst formation.*

million women.[3] Of those women diagnosed with endometriosis, 30% to 50% are infertile. Of women who are infertile, it is estimated that 25% to 50% have evidence of endometriosis.[15] Statistics indicate that more than 50% of teenagers experiencing diagnostic laparoscopy for pelvic pain suffer from endometriosis.[4] Recent data also indicate that endometriosis may be accompanied by reduced bone density.[16]

The exact cause of endometriosis is unknown, but two primary theories are accepted: retrograde menstruation and metaplasia.[28] The *retrograde menstruation* theory, known as the Samson theory, states that during menstruation, endometrial tissue is regurgitated through the fallopian tubes into the pelvic cavity, where it implants. The *metaplasia* theory suggests that the undifferentiated coelomic epithelia of the embryo remain dormant until menarche. This tissue then begins to respond to estrogen and progesterone in a way that is similar to that of other endometrial tissue.

Clinical manifestations depend on the location of lesions. The most common symptom is low abdominal or pelvic pain associated with the menstrual period, such as backache and cramps beginning just before or with the onset of menses. The pain increases throughout menstruation and subsides afterward. It is commonly described as a dull, bearing-down type of pain. Its cause is irritation from hemorrhage of the aberrant tissue or from distention. A chocolate cyst may rupture with signs of acute abdomen. Dyspareunia reflects uterine involvement, dysuria reflects bladder involvement, and pain on defecation occurs with rectal involvement. Sterility or infertility may result from extensive scarring of the ovaries and tubes.

In addition to the mechanical factors of scarring and adhesions that contribute to infertility, other aspects being studied are peritoneal, immunologic, and ovulatory factors; abnormalities of fertilization; and early pregnancy loss.[15] The association of toxic effects of prostaglandins, macrophages, and macrophage byproducts may contribute to the scarring and infertility problem.

No specific laboratory test is available for diagnosis of endometriosis. Physical examination may reveal small nodular masses on pelvic organs that enlarge during menstruation and seldom are movable. Laparoscopy and exploratory surgery are the most beneficial because they allow direct visualization of the lesions.

Treatment is medical or surgical and depends on the woman's symptoms, age, and childbearing desires. The most effective treatment, removal of both ovaries, is not a viable option for those desiring future pregnancy.[16] In early endometriosis, treatment consists of analgesia and regular follow-up care. As the condition progresses and symptoms become more severe, surgery is indicated. It is aimed at removing as much endometrial tissue as possible while preserving the uterus and ovaries. Medical treatment may include the administration of drugs, including gonadotropin-releasing hormone agonists, Danazol (an androgen preparation), high-dose progestins, and the progestin-estrogen oral contraceptive pill, which prevent ovulation or produce a pseudopregnancy.[16]

In adenomyosis, endometrial tissue has invaded the myometrium. The invasion may be diffuse or localized, and it results in an enlarged uterus (Fig. 56-17). This buried endometrium usually is nonfunctional. Symptoms include menorrhagia, dyspareunia, dysmenorrhea, and generalized pelvic discomfort. The usual treatment is hysterectomy, which is indicated by symptoms.

Premenstrual Syndrome

Premenstrual syndrome (PMS) is a term used to cover collectively the discomforts noted before the onset of menses. The symptoms vary with individuals but most frequently include headache, breast tenderness, abdominal heaviness and bloating, edema, weight gain, backache, nervous irritability, mood changes, crying spells, depression, insomnia, and anxiety. These symptoms worsen 7 to 10 days before menses and subside when the menstrual flow is well established, usually within 2 days. This classic pattern of PMS has been differentiated from premenstrual magnification, which is characterized by medium to high symptom severity after menses and a high level of severity premenstrually.[36] Although the exact cause of PMS has not been identified, proposed

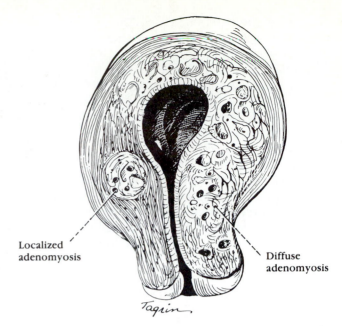

FIGURE 56-17 *Appearance of adenomyosis of the uterus. It can be localized or diffuse.*

Localized adenomyosis

Diffuse adenomyosis

theories include: 1) decreased β-endorphin levels during the luteal phase of the menstrual cycle; 2) decreased serotonin and platelet uptake of serotonin; 3) progesterone withdrawal; 4) hormonal fluid retention; 5) increased prolactin levels; 6) abnormal prostaglandin metabolism; 7) hypothalamic-pituitary-adrenal dysregulation; 8) hypoglycemia; and 9) thyroid dysfunction.[10]

Premenstrual syndrome affects 3% to 5% of women, and diagnosis is based on daily records of symptoms and their severity.[41] Additionally, various laboratory tests should be done to rule out medical problems. Treatment is symptomatic and varies with individuals. The most frequently used treatments include vitamins, diuretics, dietary restriction of sodium and carbohydrates, exercise, tranquilizers, and sedatives.

Dysmenorrhea

Dysmenorrhea may occur as a single entity or as part of the premenstrual syndrome. Dysmenorrhea means painful menstruation, commonly referred to as cramps. There are two types of dysmenorrhea: primary and secondary. *Secondary dysmenorrhea* is caused by organic pelvic disease such as cancer of the uterus, bladder, or intestinal tract. The term *primary dysmenorrhea* refers to painful menses unrelated to an obvious physical cause. It usually begins with the establishment of the ovulatory cycle. Spasmodic primary dysmenorrhea usually is characterized by sharp cramping sensations during the first day or two of menses. It may improve as cycles are reestablished after pregnancy. Congestive primary dysmenorrhea frequently occurs in association with premenstrual syndrome. It is characterized by a dull, aching pain before the onset of menses. The cause of primary dysmenorrhea remains unknown. One theory attributes it to the secretion of prostaglandins, especially PGE_2, which have a stimulating effect on uterine muscle. The nausea, vomiting, and diarrhea associated with dysmenorrhea also have been attributed to prostaglandins. Other possible factors include acute anteflexion of the uterus, estrogen—progesterone imbalance, and hypersensitivity to pain (Fig. 56-18).

The most common treatments include hormones, analgesics, prostaglandin synthetase, optimum health maintenance, and psychotherapy. Hormonal therapy is aimed at preventing ovulation, because anovulatory cycles seldom are painful. Antiprostaglandins, such as aspirin, indomethacin, naproxen, and ibuprofen, may be administered before the onset of menses to inhibit prostaglandin synthesis. The drugs not only inhibit prostaglandin synthesis but also block its action. Mild analgesics also may be administered.

Abnormal Uterine Bleeding

Abnormal uterine bleeding is the most common reason women visit the gynecologist and the leading indication for dilatation and curettage.[37] It is defined as a cycle

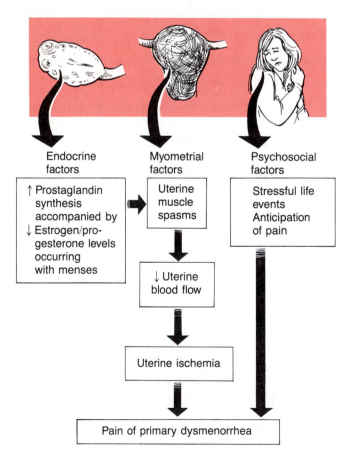

FIGURE 56-18 *Causes of pain in primary dysmenorrhea.*

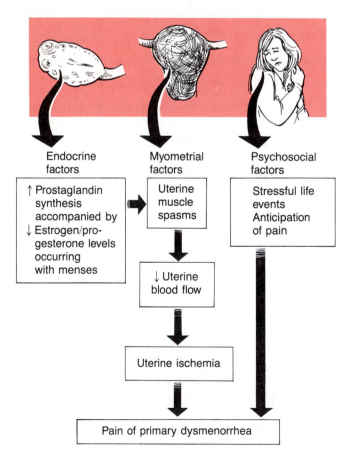
Endocrine factors — ↑ Prostaglandin synthesis accompanied by ↓ Estrogen/progesterone levels occurring with menses

Myometrial factors — Uterine muscle spasms → ↓ Uterine blood flow → Uterine ischemia

Psychosocial factors — Stressful life events Anticipation of pain

Pain of primary dysmenorrhea

TABLE 56-2 *Terminology Associated with Abnormal Uterine Bleeding*

Term	Definition
Metrorrhagia or intermenstrual bleeding	Bleeding between periods
Menorrhagia or hypermenorrhea	Excessive menstrual flow
Polymenorrhea	Abnormally frequent menstrual bleeding
Oligomenorrhea	Abnormally infrequent menses
Hypomenorrhea	Deficient menstrual flow
Amenorrhea	Absence of menstrual flow
Perimenopausal bleeding	Irregular bleeding before menopause
Postmenopausal bleeding	Bleeding that occurs 1 or more years after menopause

length of less than 21 days, bleeding lasting more than 7 days, or blood loss exceeding 80 mL.[44] This condition usually is a symptom of some underlying disease process rather than a disease entity itself. Terms used to describe abnormal uterine bleeding are defined in Table 56-2.

The many causes of abnormal uterine bleeding can be grouped into four major categories: 1) complications of pregnancy; 2) organic lesions; 3) constitutional diseases; and 4) true dysfunctional uterine bleeding. Complications of pregnancy include abortion, trophoblastic disease, and ectopic pregnancy. Organic lesions include conditions associated with pelvic diseases, such as infections, tumors, and polyps. Constitutional diseases are conditions such as hypertension, blood dyscrasias, and hormonal dysfunction. No pelvic disease is present, but symptoms are reflected through abnormal uterine bleeding. The last category represents abnormal bleeding associated with endocrine dysfunction.

DYSFUNCTIONAL UTERINE BLEEDING. The term *dysfunctional uterine bleeding* refers to abnormal bleeding that is the result of endocrine dysfunction. Fifty percent of dysfunctional uterine bleeding occurs in women older than age 40 years, and 20% occurs in adolescents younger than age 20 years.[37] It often is associated with absence of ovulation, but it also is seen in ovulatory cycles. In anovulatory cycles, no corpus luteum is formed, no progesterone is produced, and no secretory changes occur in the endometrium. The endometrium becomes hyperplastic. As estrogen levels decrease from degenerating follicles, withdrawal bleeding occurs. Dysfunctional uterine bleeding occasionally results from inadequate production of progesterone after ovulation.

Psychogenic uterine bleeding may be included in dysfunctional uterine bleeding after both organic and constitutional causes have been ruled out. The influence of emotional stimulation on the hypothalamus and the resultant influence on the gonadotropic hormones are discussed in Chapter 36. Emotions also may directly affect the uterine blood vessels and produce bleeding.

Diagnosis is made after a complete and thorough menstrual history. Physical examination reveals pelvic lesions and aids in the diagnosis of constitutional diseases. Laboratory studies include thyroid function, complete blood count, blood sugars, and coagulation profile to rule out blood dyscrasias. Studies to determine the presence of ovulation include measurements of estrogen, prolactin, LH, FSH, and progesterone levels, endometrial biopsy, and spinnbarkeit and ferning studies of cervical mucus. During the climacteric, both cytologic studies and biopsy are important to rule out cancer.

Treatment for dysfunctional uterine bleeding may be medical or surgical. Medical treatment includes the use of nonsteroidal antiinflammatory agents to inhibit prostaglandins; antifibrinolytics; and hormones (Danazol, gonadotropin-releasing hormone analog, high-dose estrogens, oral contraceptives, and progestins). Surgical treatment includes dilatation and curretage, endometrial ablation, and hysterectomy.[44] The use of Lupron, a gonadotropin-releasing hormone analog, to suppress the endometrium before ablation improves the results of this operative procedure.

AMENORRHEA. Amenorrhea is not a disease entity. It may indicate a serious condition, or it may be completely normal, as in pregnancy. *Primary amenorrhea* refers to a failure to begin menstrual cycles. *Secondary amenorrhea* occurs after a variable period of normal function. Causes of amenorrhea may be physiologic, anatomic, genetic, endocrinologic, constitutional, or psychogenic. Physiologic causes include pregnancy, lactation, menopause, and adolescence. Anatomic factors include congenital anomalies, hysterectomy, and endometrial destruction. Genetic factors include Turner syndrome and hermaphroditism. Dysfunction of the hypothalamus, pituitary, ovary, thyroid, or adrenal glands also may produce amenorrhea. Malnutrition, obesity, drug addiction, diabetes, and anemia are all constitutional problems that can prevent menstrual periods. Psychogenic factors include psychosis and anorexia nervosa. Menstrual dysfunction also is seen in athletes as a result of physical and emotional stress, changes in body composition and weight, and alteration in hormonal secretions. Specific diagnostic tools, in addition to history and physical examination, include thyroid function studies, serum prolactin level, buccal smear, skull radiography, progesterone challenge test, and hormone values.

REPRODUCTIVE TRACT INFECTIONS
Atrophic Vaginitis

Atrophic vaginitis refers to inflammation of the atrophied epithelium in postmenopausal women. It produces an irritating vaginal discharge with pruritus, swelling, and secondary dyspareunia and dysuria. Red strawberry spots may be seen on the vaginal wall. Bleeding may occur from trauma to the thin epithelium, but cancer must be ruled out as its cause. Estrogen therapy is used to convert the epithelium to the more normal, thick, stratified, squamous layer.

Cervicitis

Cervicitis refers to inflammation of the cervix, which may be acute or chronic. Acute cervicitis usually occurs with other acute reproductive tract infections. Causative organisms include *Gonococcus, Staphylococcus,* and *Streptococcus* species and *Escherichia coli.* Speculum examination reveals an edematous, congested cervix with purulent discharge. Symptoms may include dyspareunia, backache, dull pain in the lower abdomen, and urinary frequency and urgency. Pain may be noted on palpation. Cultures and smears identify the causative organism, and appropriate antibiotic therapy is then instituted.

Many women exhibit some form of chronic cervicitis. It may occur after acute infection, childbirth trauma, or abortion. The cervical canal is primarily affected, but there are no characteristic findings of the cervix. The only symptom may be a mucopurulent vaginal discharge or, occasionally, paracervical or low back pain. Abnormal bleeding is rare and often indicates cervical cancer. Physical examination may reveal cervical erosions, cervical eversions, or nabothian cysts.

Cervical erosion refers to an area of the surface of the cervix in which the surface epithelium is partially or totally absent (Fig. 56-19A). It appears red and raw. Columnar cells are more likely to exhibit this characteristic than squamous cells, and they are not as curable. *Cervical eversion* refers to a portion of the cervix in which columnar epithelium of the cervical canal extends outward (see Figure 56-19B). The characteristic squamocolumnar junction is then located along the outer edge of the lesion. Eversion most commonly occurs in women who are taking oral contraceptives, young women who have never been pregnant, and daughters of women who took DES during pregnancy. There is an increase in mucoid secretions. In an attempt to repair the eversion, the squamous cells begin to grow inward. As this invasion progresses, the mucus-secreting glands are obliterated. Their secretions are then trapped beneath the epithelium, producing *nabothian cysts.* These cysts are filled with normal mucus, are not infected, and produce no symptoms.

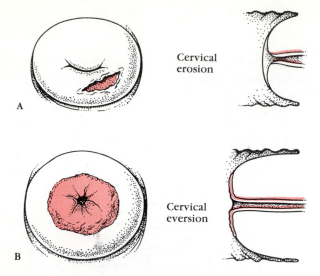

Cervical erosion

Cervical eversion

FIGURE 56-19 **A.** *Cervical erosion.* **B.** *Cervical eversion.*

The primary concern in diagnosing cervicitis is screening for cervical cancer because the lesions are not easily differentiated by the naked eye. In addition to cultures, Pap smear, colposcopy, and biopsy are the most important screening aids.

Silver nitrate, douches, and antibiotics are relatively ineffective methods of treatment because of the depth of the lesions. Small areas may be treated with thermal cautery or cryosurgery. Entire areas are treated in depth; healing and reepithelialization then take place. The sloughing cervical tissue produces an annoying discharge that may be treated with antibiotic creams for 7 to 10 days. Complete healing may take 6 to 8 weeks.

Toxic Shock Syndrome

Toxic shock syndrome (TSS) is an entity first recognized and reported in 1978. It is caused by a toxin produced by the *Staphylococcus aureus* bacteria. Although the condition most often affects menstruating women younger than 30 years of age who use tampons, its incidence has increased in nonmenstruating women, men, and children.[11] In menstruating women, the risk is greatest among those using superabsorbent tampons. Cases of nonmenstrual TSS have been linked to barrier contraceptives, intravenous drug use, burns, insect bites, surgical wounds, nonsurgical wounds, postpartum and gynecologic infections, vagintis, and lung abscesses. It has also been seen immediately after influenza.[11,45]

The link with tampons is most interesting because the unused tampons of women who develop TSS contained no *S. aureus.*[9] Two theories support the tampon link. One states that bacteria are nourished by carboxymethyl cellulose, which is present in many tampons.[9] The other theory indicates that conditions for bacterial growth are improved through the use of superabsorbent

tampons. Clinical manifestations of TSS include elevated temperature, which is sudden in onset; vomiting and diarrhea; and an erythematous macular rash that is present especially on the palms and soles. The sunburnlike rash progresses to peeling of palms and soles about 10 days later. Renal dysfunction may develop, with decreased urine output. Hypotension and shock may develop. Laboratory studies usually reveal elevated blood urea nitrogen, serum creatinine, bilirubin, and creatine phosphokinase levels. Additional complications associated with TSS include disseminated intravascular coagulation, adult respiratory distress syndrome, and acidosis. Box 56-1 summarizes criteria for diagnosis.

Treatment varies, depending on the extent of symptoms. It may include antibiotics (penicillinase-resistant penicillin) or cephalosporins, intravenous colloid to prevent fluid loss from blood vessels, ventilation therapy, heparin, blood transfusion, and correction of acid-base imbalance.

Pelvic Inflammatory Disease

Pelvic inflammatory disease (PID) is a general term used to refer to any infection of the upper reproductive tract

---

BOX 56-1 ▼ Toxic Shock Syndrome Case Definition

Fever (temperature ≥38.9°C or 102°F)
Rash (diffuse macular erythroderma)
Desquamation, 1–2 wk after onset of illness, particularly of palms and soles
Hypotension (systolic blood pressure ≤90 mm Hg for adults or less than fifth percentile by age for children <16 years old, or orthostatic syncope)
Involvement of three or more of the following organ systems:
Gastrointestinal (vomiting or diarrhea at onset of illness)
Muscular (severe myalgia or creatine phosphokinase level ≥2 × ULN)
Mucous membrane (vaginal, oropharyngeal, or conjunctival) hyperemia
Renal (BUN or Cr ≥2 × ULN or ≥5 white blood cells/high-power field—in the absence of a urinary tract infection)
Hepatic (total bilirubin, SGOT, or SGPT ≥2 × ULN)
Hematologic (platelets ≤100,000/μL)
Central nervous system (disorientation or alterations in consciousness without focal neurologic signs when fever and hypotension are absent)
Negative results on the following tests, if obtained:
Blood, throat, or cerebrospinal fluid cultures
Serologic tests for Rocky Mountain spotted fever, leptospirosis, measles

BUN, blood urea nitrogen; *Cr,* creatinine; *SGOT,* serum glutamic-oxaloacetic transaminase; *SGPT,* serum glutamic-pyruvic transaminase; *ULN,* upper limits of normal.
Centers for Disease Control. *MMWR Morb Mortal Wkly Rep* 29:442, 1980.

(above the cervix). More precise terms such as endometritis, endoparametritis, salpingitis, oophoritis, and pelvic peritonitis indicate specific areas of involvement (Fig. 56-20). Common causes of PID include *Gonococcus*, Staphylococcus, and *Streptococcus* species, and *Chlamydia trachomatis* (see Chap. 57). It often occurs after delivery or abortion and in women who use intrauterine devices as a means of contraception. Emerging data also indicate that there is an increased risk among cigarette smokers.[42]

Symptoms include the sudden onset of severe pelvic pain, chills and fever, nausea, vomiting, and a heavy, purulent vaginal discharge with foul odor. Vaginal bleeding also may be present. It may result in scarring and obstruction of the fallopian tubes. One of the most important diagnostic tools in PID is a complete and thorough history. Specific information of most importance relates to previous reproductive tract infection, delivery, abortion, pelvic surgery, onset of pain, date of last menses, sexual history, and type of contraceptive used. Specific diagnostic tests include cultures of any discharge, complete blood count, and possibly ultrasound studies if pelvic abscess is suspected.

Medical regimen depends on the cause, acuteness, and extent of the infection. Hospitalization with bed rest and appropriate intravenous antibiotics may be indicated. Analgesics may be ordered for pain. Removal of an intrauterine device is indicated if one is present. Surgical drainage usually is recommended for an abscess. The importance of follow-up care cannot be overemphasized. Untreated or inadequately treated PID may result in infertility or sterility.

BENIGN CONDITIONS OF THE FEMALE REPRODUCTIVE TRACT

Uterine Fibroids

Uterine fibroids, also referred to as *leiomyomas, myomas,* or *fibromyomas,* are second only to pregnancy as the most common cause of uterine enlargement. Twenty percent to 50% of women between 30 and 50 years of age have some evidence of these growths. Fibroids are masses of muscle and connective tissue that are stimulated by estrogen, thereby increasing in size with pregnancy and decreasing in size with menopause. Diagnosis most often is made on the basis of physical examination. Ultrasonography, radiography, hysteroscopy, and dilatation and curettage may aid in the diagnosis. The tumors occur singly or in groups, and they vary from the size of a pea to that of an apple or a cantaloupe. They are firm, smooth, and spheric. Sectioning of a fibroid tumor reveals a pinkish white, whorled, and lined muscle bundle.

Position in the uterine wall determines the classification of fibroids (Fig. 56-21). Intramural or interstitial tumors are present in central portions of the uterine wall; these are the most common. Submucosal tumors are located between the endometrium and the uterine lining. Projection into the uterine cavity with subsequent distortion and enlargement of the endometrium may cause excessive menstrual bleeding and habitual abortion. Subserous fibroids lie beneath the serous lining of the uterus and project outward into the abdominal cavity. If a subserous tumor extends outward on a stalk, it is said to be *pedunculated.*

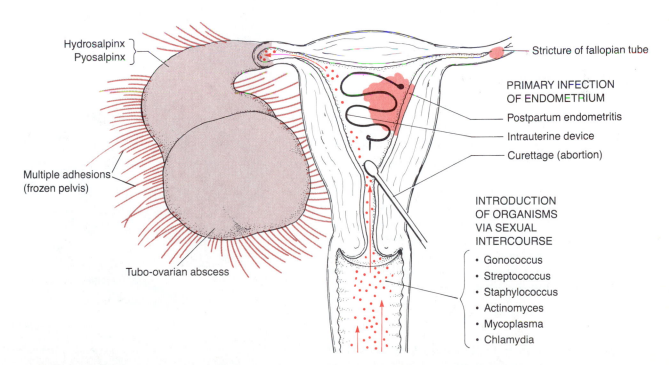

Hydrosalpinx
Pyosalpinx

Multiple adhesions
(frozen pelvis)

Tubo-ovarian abscess

Stricture of fallopian tube

PRIMARY INFECTION
OF ENDOMETRIUM

Postpartum endometritis

Intrauterine device

Curettage (abortion)

INTRODUCTION
OF ORGANISMS
VIA SEXUAL
INTERCOURSE

- Gonococcus
- Streptococcus
- Staphylococcus
- Actinomyces
- Mycoplasma
- Chlamydia

FIGURE 56-20 *Pelvic inflammatory disease. (Rubin, E., and Farber, J.L. Pathology [2nd ed.]. Philadelphia: J.B. Lippincott, 1994.)*

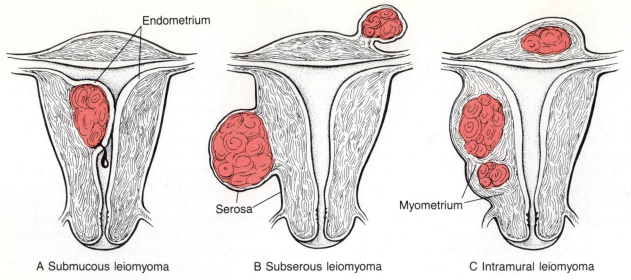

Endometrium

Serosa

Myometrium

A Submucous leiomyoma   B Subserous leiomyoma   C Intramural leiomyoma

FIGURE 56-21 *Appearance of uterine fibroids.*

Many fibroids are asymptomatic. As they enlarge, the woman may experience excessive or prolonged bleeding during regular monthly cycles, urinary frequency, constipation, abdominal fullness, low abdominal pain, dysmenorrhea, and infertility. Abnormal bleeding usually occurs with submucous tumors because of the increased amount of endometrium to build and slough. Enlargement of fibroids can produce pressure on the bladder, urethra, rectum, or nerves. Infertility and habitual abortion most frequently occur with submucous tumors because of distortion of the endometrium and uterine cavity. Enlarging fibroids have been known to interfere with delivery of a full-term fetus.

The course of treatment is determined by age, parity, symptoms, and condition of the woman and by size and location of tumors. No treatment is necessary for asymptomatic patients. Women who are approaching menopause usually are observed at regular intervals, because withdrawal of estrogen results in a stationary or decreasing size of the fibroids. Hysteroscopic surgery may be most beneficial for women with submucosal myomas, whereas hysterectomy may be indicated for the woman who does not want additional children.[32] It is advisable to delay surgery in the woman who is anemic. The administration of gonadotropin-releasing hormone agonist usually produces amenorrhea, which allows spontaneous recovery from the anemia. Intramural tumors also may shrink during this time.

Functional Ovarian Cysts

Functional ovarian cysts are the result of normal ovarian function, and account for more than 50% of ovarian enlargements (Fig. 56-22). A functional follicular cyst results if a maturing follicle fails to rupture an ovum. Instead, it continues to enlarge and produce estrogen. A corpus luteum cyst occurs when the corpus luteum fails to degenerate normally; it continues to grow and produce progesterone. Functional ovarian cysts ordinarily produce no symptoms. They may be noted on periodic examination, and they usually disappear after the next

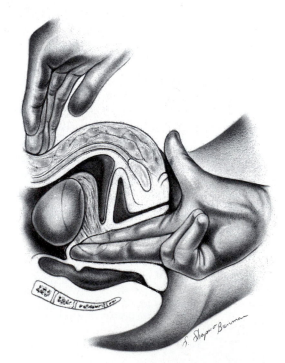

FIGURE 56-22 *Ovarian cysts and tumors may be detected as adnexal masses on one or both sides. Later they grow up out of the pelvis. Cysts tend to be smooth and compressible; tumors are often nodular. Uncomplicated cysts and tumors are usually not tender. (Source: Bates, B. A Guide to Physical Examination and History Taking [6th ed.]. Philadelphia: J.B. Lippincott, 1995.)*

menstrual cycle. If a functional cyst ruptures, it may tear an ovarian vessel. Intraperitoneal bleeding occurs, and the extent of symptoms is related to the amount of hemorrhage. With excessive bleeding, abdominal pain may be severe in onset, requiring hospitalization and surgery.

Benign Neoplastic Tumors of the Ovaries

Benign neoplasms are more important than functional cysts, although they occur less frequently. They may grow to be quite large and secrete hormones. Classification is by cellular origin: germ cell, germinal epithelium, gonadal stroma, or nonspecialized stroma. Three of the most common benign neoplasms are cystic teratomas or dermoid cysts, serous cystadenomas, and mucinous cystadenomas.

Dermoid cysts represent about 15% to 20% of all ovarian neoplasms. They arise from germ cells and are most common in women who are between 18 and 35 years of age. The tumor is gray and smooth and contains tissue from all three germ layers—commonly skin, hair, and sebaceous glands.

Benign serous cystadenomas arise from germinal epithelium and, with mucinous cystadenomas, account for about 50% of benign ovarian neoplasms. They most frequently affect women between the ages of 40 and 50. The tumors may be unilateral or bilateral. They are pearly gray, lobulated, and filled with a clear, yellow fluid that becomes brown if there is bleeding in the cyst. *Psammoma bodies*, which are small, calcified granules, may be present in the cell wall. Papillary serous cystadenomas may develop into cancers.

Mucinous cystadenomas also arise from germinal epithelium and usually are unilateral. Most are larger than serous cystadenomas, contain no psammoma bodies, and contain thick, straw-colored fluid.

Most ovarian tumors are asymptomatic and are noted on routine pelvic examination. After they are enlarged enough to produce pressure, the woman may complain of pain on defecation, dyspareunia, heaviness, and sterility. Increased enlargement may result in abdominal distention, dyspnea, and anorexia. Menstrual irregularities, masculinization, and feminization may occur if hormones are produced. Complications include rupture, hemorrhage, possible infection, and torsion of pedicle cyst. The treatment of choice is surgical removal, because the tumors increase in size and may undergo malignant changes.

Benign Breast Alterations

The two most common benign breast alterations are fibrocystic disease and fibroadenoma. Fibrocystic disease is the most common of all female breast lesions, affecting 50% of women of childbearing age. The peak incidence is noted at about 40 years of age.[38] It is a benign neoplasm that consists of proliferative ductal epithelium and fibrous stroma. Characteristically, the lesion becomes nodular from fibrous thickening. It may be tender, especially before menstruation, and may exhibit cystic formation. Complaints of dull, heavy pain and a sense of fullness that increases before menstruation are characteristic. The nodule most often is located in the upper outer quadrant of the breast.

Fibrocystic disease tends to follow a progressive course of three stages.[38] The first stage occurs in young women from the late teen years to the early 30s. At this time, there is tenderness and fullness but minimal lumpiness during the week before menstruation. The second stage appears in women in their mid-30s and 40s. Nodules may be noted, causing the woman to see a physician. Discomfort is greater and occurs for a longer period. During the third stage, lesions appear suddenly and are painful. Biopsy often is implemented to differentiate this lesion from breast cancer.

The exact cause is unknown, but it is thought to result from abnormal or exaggerated response of breast tissue to cyclic hormonal stimulation. Methylxanthines, which include caffeine, also have been implicated as a possible cause. These substances are responsible for inhibiting an enzyme that breaks down cyclic adenosine monophosphate (cAMP).[38] As a result, cAMP levels rise. Levels of cAMP also have been found to be higher in women with fibrocystic disease.

Medical management of fibrocystic disease includes administration of oral contraceptives and progestins. Danazol and bromocriptine therapy have been used to obtain subjective relief of symptoms.[38]

The second most common benign breast tumor is fibroadenoma. Physical examination reveals a well-outlined, solid, firm lump that moves freely. It most often occurs in the upper outer quadrant of the breast in women between 15 and 40 years of age. It is the most common breast lesion in the adolescent female. The cause of this condition is unknown, but estrogen stimulation is suspected because it primarily occurs in younger women and seldom after menopause. Treatment is surgical removal of the lump. Recurrence is common.

PREMALIGNANT AND MALIGNANT CONDITIONS

Gestational Trophoblastic Neoplasms

The term *gestational trophoblastic neoplasms* refers to three complications of uterine pregnancy: hydatidiform mole, invasive mole, and choriocarcinoma. Hydatidiform mole usually is benign with malignant potential, whereas choriocarcinoma is a highly aggressive cancer. Staging of gestational trophoblastic neoplasms is reflected in Table 56-3. Findings from clinical examination, initial levels of

TABLE 56-3 *Staging System for Gestational Trophoblastic Tumors*

Stage	Description
I	Localized to uterus
II	Involves vagina, pelvic structures, or both
III	Involves lungs, with or without vaginal or pelvic spread
IV	Involves distant organs

human chorionic gonadotropin (HCG) before treatment, chest radiography, pelvic ultrasonography, and brain and liver scans provide the basis for this staging system.[19]

HYDATIDIFORM MOLE. The incidence of hydatidiform mole is approximately 1 in every 1,500 live births in the United States.[19] The incidence is higher in Asia and Mexico.[20] Approximately 15% of patients with molar pregnancy develop a nonmetastatic gestational trophoblastic tumor, and about 5% develop metastatic disease.[19] This condition represents a malformation of the placenta. It is characterized by absence of embryo development; conversion of the chorionic villi into marked vesicles with clear, thick, sticky fluid; and production of HCG. Molar pregnancies are classified as partial or complete, based on morphology, chromosomal pattern, and histopathology.[5] Complete moles usually reflect one of two chromosomal patterns: 46 XX, or 46 XY. The 46 XX pattern results from the fertilization of an anuclear empty ovum by a 23 X sperm that subsequently duplicates itself. This pattern occurs in approximately 90% of complete moles. The 46 XY pattern occurs in 6% to 10% of complete moles when two sperm fertilize an anuclear empty ovum. All chromosomes come from the father in both patterns.[6, 19]

Clinical manifestations of complete moles include intermittent bleeding, excessive increase in uterine size, no evidence of fetal development, and markedly elevated HCG levels. The woman may experience intermittent bleeding after amenorrhea. A dark brown vaginal discharge may be accompanied by passage of watery fluid that contains characteristic vesicles. Even by the 16th to 20th week, no fetal heart tones are heard and no fetal movement is felt; ultrasonography reveals no fetal skeleton. Levels of HCG are higher than those associated with normal pregnancy. Hyperemesis gravidarum, bilateral ovarian cysts, and toxemia of pregnancy before the 24th week also have been observed with hydatidiform mole.

In contrast, the partial mole reflects a triploid chromosomal pattern (69 XXY or 69 XYY) to which both parents contribute, with the paternal contribution being doubled.[20] The partial mole is characterized by embryonic or fetal tissue as well as chorionic villi swelling. Most women present with signs and symptoms of incomplete or missed abortion. No fetal heart tones are heard, and the size of the uterus usually is appropriate for gestational age.[5]

Diagnostic tools include suction curettage, histologic studies, measurement of HCG levels, and ultrasonography. Histologic studies can be performed on tissue that is passed spontaneously or obtained from dilatation and curettage. Curettage scrapings usually include both superficial and deep tissue to determine invasiveness. Ultrasonography reveals a characteristic pattern of hydatidiform mole, which helps in differentiation (Fig. 56-23).

Treatment of choice is evacuation of the uterus as soon as possible after diagnosis. Possible means for evacuation of uterine contents include dilatation and curettage, suction curettage, and hysterectomy. After evacuation, HCG levels (especially the β subunit) are initially checked every week, until levels are less than 5 mIU/dL for three consecutive weeks, and then monthly for at least six consecutive months. During this time levels should remain less than 5 mIU/dL.[19] Pregnancy should be avoided during the entire follow-up period. HCG levels ordinarily return to normal within a week or so. About 50% of those whose HCG levels are still elevated at 4 weeks develop choriocarcinoma, unless chemotherapy is instituted. Chemotherapy may be instituted if

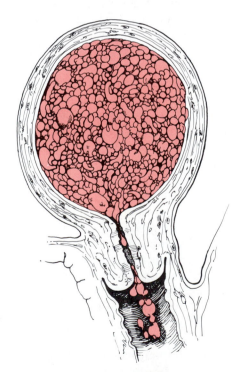

FIGURE 56-23 *Hydatidiform mole. (Reeder, S.J., Martin, L.L., and Koniak, D. Maternity Nursing [17th ed.]. Philadelphia: J.B. Lippincott, 1992.)*

HCG levels rise, plateau and stabilize, or if metastatic disease occurs. Chemotherapeutic agents include the folic acid antagonists methotrexate and dactinomycin.

INVASIVE MOLE. The diagnosis of invasive mole is made if HCG levels remain elevated in the absence of pregnancy and metastasis. It is characterized by the presence of chorionic villi deep within the myometrium. Penetration of the uterine wall with rupture and hemorrhage is possible. Curettage may not be successful in removing the lesion because of the depth of invasion. Chemotherapy with methotrexate or actinomycin D usually is initiated. Levels of HCG are measured weekly until normal levels are maintained for three consecutive weeks; thereafter, they are measured at monthly intervals for 1 year.

CHORIOCARCINOMA.   Choriocarcinoma is a rare, malignant tumor of the trophoblast that most commonly occurs in the uterus. It affects 1 in 40,000 to 70,000 pregnancies in the United States.[13] It primarily affects women younger than 20 or older than 40 years of age. It is characterized by sheets of immature cells (cytotrophoblasts and syncytiotrophoblasts) that invade the uterine wall and produce necrosis and hemorrhage. Chorionic villi are not present. Choriocarcinoma may occur in the ovaries. The only symptom noticed may be a bloody, brownish discharge associated with irregular bleeding or continual bleeding after a delivery or abortion. The first symptoms frequently are related to metastasis. Because the most common site of metastasis is the lung, hemoptysis may be the first complaint. Other metastatic sites include the vagina, brain, liver, oral cavity, and kidneys. Levels of HCG remain markedly elevated. A poor prognosis is associated with metastases to liver and central nervous system.[19]

Chemotherapy is the treatment of choice if metastases have occurred. Methotrexate with folinic acid and actinomycin D are administered sequentially if there is low risk for drug resistance. Patients considered to be at high risk for drug resistance include those with central nervous system and liver metastases, patients with HCG levels greater than 100,000 IU/dL, and those in whom it has been more than 4 months since pregnancy. Before the use of chemotherapeutic agents, the prognosis for a woman with choriocarcinoma was extremely grim, with death occurring within 1 to 2 years. The cure rate now approaches 100% for those who have metastatic disease with favorable features.[19] Prognosis continues to be directly related to the degree of metastasis, duration of disease, and HCG titer.

Exposure to Diethylstilbestrol

DES, the first synthetic estrogen, was released in the 1940s. It was used to prevent miscarriage, to suppress lactation after delivery, and as hormonal therapy for dysfunctional uterine bleeding after menopause. In the late 1960s, it became linked with adenocarcinoma of the vagina, vaginal adenosis, squamous cell carcinoma of the cervix and vagina, and cervical dysplasia, as well as congenital abnormalities of both male and female offspring and impaired sperm production in males exposed in utero.

Cancer of the vagina is a rare condition that occurs most commonly in women older than 50 years of age. It usually is the squamous cell type, but adenocarcinoma has been identified in a number of adolescent girls whose mothers received DES during pregnancy. Vaginal adenosis is a benign condition in which the transformation zone of the squamocolumnar junction extends over the vaginal portion of the cervix and may involve the vaginal walls. This condition is extremely common in daughters of mothers who took DES and may predispose them to adenocarcinoma. A question also arises as to whether adenosis may progress to squamous cell cancer of the cervix or vagina. Additionally, DES has been associated with congenital anomalies, including cervical anomalies such as collars, hoods, and ridges and altered fallopian tube structure. Based on hysterosalpingography findings, the most common uterine anomaly is a T-shaped uterus.[29]

Lowered fertility rates have been identified in both male and female offspring of mothers who took DES. Irregular or infrequent menstrual periods as well as increased incidence of incompetent cervix have been associated with in utero exposure of females to DES. There also is an increased rate of spontaneous abortion and premature delivery in women exposed to DES.

The most important factors in treatment of DES problems are identification of those exposed and follow-up care every 6 to 12 months. Children of women known or suspected to have had DES exposure should have regular examinations beginning at puberty. Routine procedures should include Pap smears and colposcopy. Precancerous cell changes can be found early and appropriate therapy initiated. Reproductive tract surgery should be used cautiously in women exposed to DES because of the increased risk of cervical stenosis. Controversy continues over the use of cerclage procedures in an attempt to decrease spontaneous abortion caused by incompetent cervix.[29]

Endometrial Carcinoma

Endometrial cancer currently accounts for about 7% of all cancers in the female and has surpassed cervical cancer in incidence.[14] An estimated 31,000 cases of uterine cancer, most endometrial, occurred in 1994, with an estimated 5,900 deaths.[1] It primarily affects postmenopausal women, with peak occurrence in women older than 50 years of age.[1] Experimental evidence has linked endometrial cancer with ingestion of exogenous estrogens. Endogenous estrogen production unbalanced by progesterone may contribute to its frequency in early menopause. However, evidence indicates a decreased risk of endometrial cancer if estrogen therapy is supplemented with progesterone for 2 weeks of each cycle. Additional factors that seem to increase the risk of endometrial cancer include early menarche, late menopause, tamoxifen, history of infertility, anovulation, nulliparity, obesity, diabetes, and hypertension. Demographics indicate a higher incidence in urban, white, and Jewish women.[14]

In many cases, malignant changes are preceded by abnormal cell maturation. Cystic hyperplasia, a condition related to unopposed estrogen stimulation, is considered only weakly precancerous, but atypical hyperplasia represents a pathologic form of hyperplasia usually considered to be premalignant. Adenomatous hyperplasia has been known to occur both spontaneously and as a result of estrogen drugs. If adenomatous hyperplasia is associated with the administration of estrogen, the estrogen should be discontinued and a curettage is performed. If atypical adenomatous hyperplasia persists, treatment may include progestin or hysterectomy. Treatment with progestin is followed by curettage.[7] If untreated, the process progresses to an in situ lesion in which the cells are larger and more disoriented. Nuclei may be present in different locations with varying size and staining characteristics. About 85% of endometrial cancer is adenocarcinoma. Cells may be well differentiated or so undifferentiated that no glandular pattern is evident.

Metastasis occurs first to the cervix and myometrium and later involves the vagina, pelvis, and lungs. Increased risk of vaginal recurrence, myometrial invasion, and nodal spread is associated with poorly differentiated tumor patterns. Staging or extension of the lesion from the site of origin and grading of cellular differentiation of endometrial cancer are possible only after removal of the uterus and subsequent pathologic studies. Therefore, grading is of little value in determining initial therapy. The grades of endometrial cancer are I through III, with grade I representing well-differentiated cells and grade III, undifferentiated.

The staging process varies within institutions and parts of the nation. The Federation Internationale de Gynecologic et Obstetrique has adopted a system of five major stages (Table 56-4). Other staging procedures divide the disease into fewer stages: stages I and II with confinement to the uterus, and stage III limited to pelvic spread. The staging and grading procedures are most important in determining appropriate therapy, which includes surgery, radiation, or a combination. Progestation therapy or local irradiation may be used in patients with advanced, incurable disease in an effort to control pain and bleeding. Response rate depends largely on progesterone receptor status, with a response rate of

---

TABLE 56-4 *Stages of Endometrial Carcinoma as Devised by FIGO*

Stage	Description
0	Carcinoma in situ
I	Tumor confined to the corpus uteri
II	Tumor involves both the corpus and the cervix
III	Tumor extends outside the uterus, but not outside the true pelvis
IV	Tumor involves bladder or rectum, or extends outside the true pelvis

FIGO, Federation Internationale de Gynecologic et Obstetrique.

80% in patients who are progesterone receptor-positive. A response rate of only 20% is associated with patients who are receptor-negative.[7] Progesterone therapy, after it is instituted, should be continued indefinitely, because recurrences after discontinued therapy may not respond to medication. Chemotherapy is used less frequently but may include doxorubicin, cyclophosphamide, and cisplatin. Response rates vary from 30% to 60% with short durations, from 4 to 10 months.[7]

The first sign of endometrial cancer is abnormal uterine bleeding. It may range from light, irregular bleeding with intermenstrual spotting to heavy, prolonged periods if it occurs before menopause. After menopause, any bleeding should be suspicious. Another early sign may be marked leukorrhea. Both signs reflect erosion and ulceration of the endometrium. Later signs include cramping, pelvic discomfort, lower abdominal or bladder pressure, bleeding after intercourse, and swollen lymph nodes. The most important diagnostic tool is probably dilatation and curettage, because it allows the most comprehensive study. Routine Pap smears have limited usefulness unless metastasis has occurred. Both endometrial biopsy and washing may reveal abnormal endometrial tissue.

The American Cancer Society reports an overall 5-year survival rate of 83% with endometrial cancer.[1] This survival rate rises to 94% if it is diagnosed in the early stages and to about 100% if it is discovered in the precancerous stage. If diagnosed with endometrial cancer in a regional stage, about 69% of patients survive for 5 years.

Cervical Cancer

The American Cancer Society reports that the incidence of cervical cancer mortality has stabilized.[14] Cervical cancer usually occurs between the ages of 30 and 50 in women who 1) have a history of early age at first intercourse; 2) are of low socioeconomic status; 3) are black; 4) received DES during pregnancy; 5) have had many sexual partners; or 6) are multiparous.[1] Additional risk factors include cigarette smoking and certain sexually transmitted diseases, especially genital herpes and human papillomavirus (see pp. 1166–1167).[1,31] Chronic cervicitis and unrepaired cervical lacerations also seem to predispose to cancer.

Cancer of the cervix normally is of the squamous cell type, and it represents a sequential process of cellular proliferation. It usually begins in the transformation zone of the squamocolumnar junction as a basal cell hyperplasia (Fig. 56-24). As the hyperplasia extends toward the surface, it becomes known as dysplasia, which refers to the disorderly cellular arrangement in the upper layers of the epithelium. The nuclei of these cells are enlarged and stain darkly. Some cells may be multinucleated. The number of atypical cells determines the classification: mild, moderate, or severe.

The next stage in the sequential process is carcinoma in situ. This stage represents an involvement of the entire epithelial cell layer and is referred to as intraepithelial neoplasm. The term *cervical intraepithelial neoplasia* refers to all dysplasia and carcinoma in situ, because the potential for progression and metastasis exists.

There are three forms of invasive cervical cancer: fungating, ulcerative, and infiltrative. The fungating tumor is a nodular thickening of the epithelium that may project above the mucosa. The ulcerative lesion represents a sloughing necrosis of the central portion of the tumor. Infiltrative invasion represents downward growth into the stroma. As metastasis continues, there is spread to the bladder, rectum, and lymph nodes; the lungs, bones, and liver eventually may be involved. The slow process of metastasis is believed to occur as long as 10 to 30 years after the precursor of carcinoma in situ.[4] In more rapidly growing lesions, invasion can occur in 3 to 4 years.

Because early cervical cancer is asymptomatic, early diagnosis and staging of the lesion are essential (Table 56-5). Routine Pap smears have probably done more

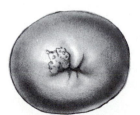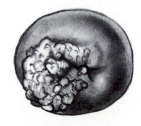

FIGURE 56-24 *Carcinoma of the cervix usually begins at or near the cervical os. It often has a hard, granular surface that bleeds easily. In later stages, an extensive, irregular, cauliflower-type growth may develop. Early carcinomas are clinically indistinguishable from ectropions and may even be present in a cervix that appears normal. (Bates, B. A Guide to Physical Examination and History Taking [6th ed.]. Philadelphia: J.B. Lippincott, 1995.)*

TABLE 56-5 *FIGO Recommendations for Staging Cervical Cancer*

Stage	Description
0	Carcinoma in situ
I	Carcinoma limited to the cervix
II	Carcinoma extends beyond the cervix and involves the upper two thirds of the vagina
III	Carcinoma involves the lower one third of the vagina and has become fixed to the pelvic wall
IV	Carcinoma involves the rectum or bladder, or extends beyond the true pelvis

FIGO, Federation Internationale de Gynecologic et Obstetrique.

than any other diagnostic tool to detect early cervical cancer. Early cervical intraepithelial neoplasia also can be detected by Pap smears. Histologic confirmation is obtained through colposcopy, cervical biopsy, and conization.

Laser surgery, electrocautery, and cryosurgery are procedures aimed at treating the neoplasia or removing the lesion in early-stage cancer. Total hysterectomy, radical hysterectomy, radiation therapy, or pelvic exenteration may be indicated as the extent of cancer increases. The 5-year survival rate with cervical cancer continues to be less than that with endometrial cancer. The American Cancer Society reports an overall survival rate of 67% for patients with cervical cancer.[1] The survival rate increases significantly with localized disease (90%).

Ovarian Cancer

Although ovarian cancer accounts for only 4% of all cancers among women, it is the most lethal of all cancers affecting the female reproductive system.[1] This lethality has been attributed to the lack of an effective screening tool for early detection and lack of diagnosis of early symptoms.[8] Epithelial tumors of the ovary affect women primarily between ages 40 and 70 years, whereas germ cell ovarian tumors occur in younger women.

Before diagnosis, the woman may note vague complaints of bladder or bowel dysfunction, including stomach ache, flatus, and distention. The presence of these complaints, especially in middle-aged women without a definitive diagnosis may indicate the need for further study. The most common sign is abdominal enlargement. Ovarian cancer should be suspected in any postmenopausal woman with ovarian enlargement and in any woman, regardless of age, with an ovarian mass larger than 5 cm. Palpation of the ovaries after menopause is abnormal and another indication for further study. Because there are no obvious signs or symptoms until the tumor has spread, early detection is by chance and during routine examination.

Several serum markers also are helpful in diagnosing suspected ovarian cancer. These markers include CA-125, carcinoembryonic antigen (CEA), HCG, and α-fetoprotein. Measurement of CA-125 uses a monoclonal antibody to detect antigens in the blood; although not specific for ovarian carcinoma, CA-125 is elevated in 85% of women with advanced ovarian cancer. This marker is not elevated in mucinous cancers, however.[2] HCG and α-fetoprotein levels aid in diagnosis of germ cell tumors. Other diagnostic aids include chest radiography, computed tomographic scanning of the abdomen and pelvis, ultrasonography, and liver function and renal function tests.

The risk of ovarian cancer increases with age. There also is increased risk associated with nulliparity, breast cancer, and family history of ovarian cancer. Although additional research is needed to confirm the relation, preliminary data indicate potential links with talcum powder and diets high in animal fat.[8] Decreased risk of ovarian cancer has been associated with an increased number of pregnancies, birth control pills, tubal sterilization, and perhaps hysterectomy.[1, 8, 21, 23]

The World Health Organization has classified ovarian tumors as epithelial tumors, malignant germ cell tumors, and sex cord or stromal tumors. Figure 56-25 shows the classification of ovarian neoplasms based on cell of origin. Common epithelial cancers account for almost 90% of ovarian tumors, and the other two types account for 5% each. Epithelial tumors are further divided into different forms (Table 56-6). Prognosis is more favorable for more well-differentiated tumors.

Staging of ovarian tumors is based on criteria established by Federation Internationale de Gynecologic et Obstetrique and provides the basis for determining treatment.[2] An abbreviated form of this staging appears in Table 56-7. Clinical evidence for the staging is obtained during clinical examination and surgery.

Initial treatment in any woman with ovarian cancer is surgical hysterectomy and bilateral salpingo-oophorectomy with omentectomy. Stage Ia ovarian cancer, which is well-differentiated and confined to the ovary, usually requires no further treatment. Adjuvant therapy should be considered for all other women with stage I and stage II disease. Adjuvant therapy may include single-agent alkylating chemotherapy or intraperitoneal therapy.[2] Treatment of germ cell tumors, which occur unilaterally and in girls and young women, is aimed at preserving fertility. Unilateral oophorectomy is the primary treatment for stage I disease. Adjuvant

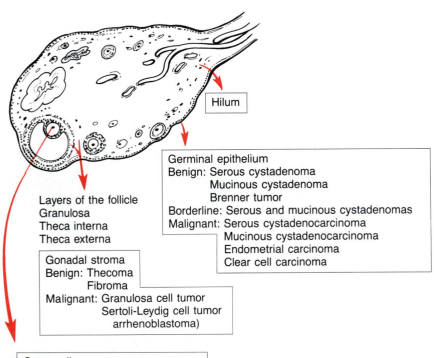

Hilum

Layers of the follicle
Granulosa
Theca interna
Theca externa

Germinal epithelium
Benign: Serous cystadenoma
Mucinous cystadenoma
Brenner tumor
Borderline: Serous and mucinous cystadenomas
Malignant: Serous cystadenocarcinoma
Mucinous cystadenocarcinoma
Endometrial carcinoma
Clear cell carcinoma

Gonadal stroma
Benign: Thecoma
Fibroma
Malignant: Granulosa cell tumor
Sertoli-Leydig cell tumor
arrhenoblastoma)

Germ cell
Benign: Dermoid cyst (teratoma)
Malignant: Dysgerminosa
Endodermal sinus
tumor
Choriocarcinoma
Embryonal carcinoma

FIGURE 56-25 *Classification of ovarian neoplasms based on cell of origin. (Adapted from Rubin, E. and Farber, J.L.* Pathology *[2nd ed.]. Philadelphia: J.B. Lippincott, 1994.)*

TABLE 56-6 *WHO Classification of Ovarian Cancer*

EPITHELIAL	
Serous	Microscopic appearance similar to epithelium of fallopian tube
Endometroid	Microscopic appearance similar to epithelium of endometrium
Clear cell	Variation of endometrioid with clear cells
Mucinous	Microscopic appearance similar to endocervical epithelium
MALIGNANT GERM CELL	
Dysgerminoma	Large cells resembling primitive germ cells
Yolk sac tumor	Microscopic appearance similar to yolk sac
Immature teratoma	Mature and immature tissue from endoderm, mesoderm, ectoderm of embryo
SEX CORD–STROMAL	
Granulosa cell	Appearance similar to granulosa cells of developing follicle

WHO, World Health Organization.

chemotherapy includes the use of vincristine—dactinomycin—cyclophosphamide and vinblastine—bleomycin—cisplatin. Dysgerminomas are highly sensitive to radiation and are treated with radiation therapy.

The American Cancer Society reports a 5-year survival rate with ovarian cancer of only 41%.[1] With early diagnosis and treatment, the survival rate may approach 88%. Survival rate associated with regional metastasis is 36% compared with only 17% with distant metastasis.

Breast Cancer

The most common site of cancer in women continues to be the breast. Breast cancer is second only to lung cancer as a cause of death from cancer in women. The condition

TABLE 56-7 *Accepted Staging Classification for Ovarian Cancer*

Stage	Description
I	Tumor limited to one or both ovaries
II	Tumor involves one or both ovaries with pelvic extension
III	Tumor growth with widespread intraperitoneal metastasis
IV	Tumor growth involves metastasis outside the peritoneal cavity

occurs only rarely in men but strikes about 1 in 8 women.[17] The frequency of breast cancer increases with age, with the greatest incidence occurring in women over age 50. Personal or family history of breast cancer, especially in a mother or sister, greatly increases one's chances of developing breast cancer. Race is another important factor: although the incidence of breast cancer is greater in white women, the rate of mortality is higher among black women. This difference probably reflects the disease stage at diagnosis between the two groups. Nulliparas, women who deliver their first term pregnancy after age 30, and women with late menopause (after age 45) are at increased risk for breast cancer. Although findings are inconclusive and need additional study, obesity, high-fat diet, oral contraceptives, and estrogen replacement may influence the risk of developing breast cancer. A controversial risk factor is the association with moderate alcohol consumption (approximately two drinks per day).[39]

Breast cancer usually is discovered by the woman herself. She notes a single lump that is painless, nontender, and movable. It most frequently is found in the upper outer quadrant (Fig. 56-26). The tumor may arise in either the ducts or lobules, and may be either infiltrating or noninfiltrating. As the condition progresses, the tumor becomes adherent to the pectoral muscles and fixed. Dimpling and retraction of the skin and nipple may develop. Peau d'orange skin may be noted, with

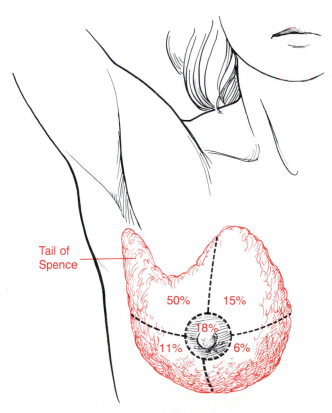

Tail of Spence

FIGURE 56-26 *Sites of breast tumors.*

dimpling that resembles the skin of an orange in the area of tumor involvement. Breast distortion or change in breast contour may be observed, as may axillary adenopathy. Nipple discharge that is unilateral and serous may indicate intraductal papilloma or chronic cystic mastopathy. Definitive diagnosis should be made, because nipple discharge may occur in breast cancer. Biopsy of any persistent dermatitis on nipple or areola is made to rule out Paget disease.

The most common histologic types are ductal and lobular. The infiltrating ductal type is the most common, accounting for about 70% of breast cancers. Approximately 10% of breast cancers are infiltrating lobular carcinomas. Prognosis is similar for both.[39] Other histologic types include tubular, medullary, papillary, and mucinous carcinomas. Although these types are uncommon, their prognosis is better than that of infiltrating ductal or lobular carcinomas.[39] Primary metastatic sites include lymph nodes, lungs, bones, liver, and pleura, although metastasis may occur anywhere (Fig. 56-27).

The increased use of screening mammography has contributed to increased identification of ductal carcinoma in situ. In this lesion, also referred to as intraductal carcinoma, all malignant cells are located within the ducts, and there is no invasion of breast tissue. The appearance on mammogram is that of microcalcifications.[39] The probability that this condition will progress to an invasive cancer is unknown.

Breast self-examination is widely taught for detection of lumps in the breast, and it should be done on a monthly basis by all women older than 18 years of age. In addition, all women between 18 and 35 years of age should have breast examinations performed by a professional at least every 3 years. Professional examination should be done annually in women older than 40 years of age. Ultrasonography is especially helpful in differentiating cystic lesions from solid masses. However, the only effective technique for locating nonpalpable lesions is mammography. The American Cancer Society and National Cancer Institute recommend that a baseline mammogram be obtained on all women between 35 and 39 years of age. Women between 40 and 49 years of age should have a mammogram at least every 2 years, or annually if they are at high risk. All women 50 years of age or older should have a mammogram on an annual basis.[1]

Definitive diagnosis is necessary whenever a breast mass is identified. Needle aspiration usually is sufficient if benign cysts are suspected. Nonpalpable areas of density or microcalcifications identified by mammography can be localized by use of fine wire placement for biopsy. Definitive diagnosis can be made by excision and biopsy of the mass.

After a cancer has been diagnosed, all patients should be screened for metastasis before implementation of a specific treatment regimen. Screening techniques may include bone scans, liver function studies, chest radiography, and determination of alkaline phosphatase, serum calcium, and phosphorus levels. However, the single most important prognostic screen in breast cancer is the status of the lymph nodes, with node-negative patients having the best prognosis.

Additional screening measures used to determine the appropriate therapy include tumor study for estrogen and progesterone receptor protein levels, serum marker levels, and flow cytometry. Estrogen and progesterone receptor protein levels are helpful in determining the prognosis as well as predicting response to hormonal therapy. Levels vary in premenopausal and postmenopausal women. Table 56-8 reflects values and their meaning in premenopausal women. Because these values increase with age, postmenopausal women may demonstrate levels as high as 200 fmol/mg. Studies indi-

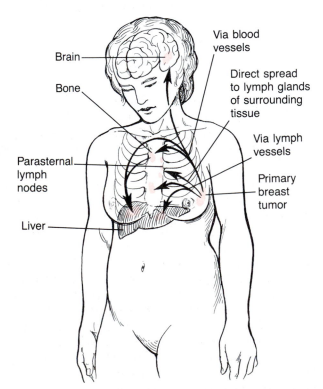

FIGURE 56-27 *Sites for metastasis of cancer of the breast.*

TABLE 56-8 *Estrogen and Progesterone Receptor Protein Values*

Values	Interpretation
<3 fmol/mg	Negative
3–10 fmol/mg	Suggestive, borderline
>10 fmol/mg	Positive

cate that the prognosis is better in those patients with receptor-positive tumors. Researchers believe that receptor-positive tumors also are more susceptible to hormonal therapy with tamoxifen.

The two serum markers used to determine therapy in breast cancer are CEA and cystic disease protein. CEA levels greater than 10 mg/mL and cystic disease protein values greater than 150 mg/mL provide presumptive evidence of recurrent disease or metastasis to distant organs. Flow cytometry analysis provides information on tumor DNA index (ploidy) and the percentage of cells in S phase. This procedure is being used in clinical areas across the nation in an attempt to identify women at high risk for breast cancer.

One of the newer techniques used to evaluate patients with breast cancer is thymidine labeling. This test requires viable tumor tissue and may be especially valuable to determine patients at risk for relapse. Researchers have found that even patients with negative nodes run a greater risk of relapse if they have a high thymidine-labeling index.[35] A test to measure oncogene amplification is showing potential for differentiating patients who will do well from those likely to suffer recurrence.[35,39]

Staging of breast cancer is based on the tumor-node-metastasis classification. In this process, the tumor is evaluated for size and extent of involvement in surrounding tissue and lymph nodes as well as distant metastasis. The summary of this process presented in Table 56-9 is modified from the American Cancer Society staging.[39] No standard has been established regarding the number of nodes involved for positive versus negative grading (Fig. 56-28).

The treatment for breast cancer is highly individualized. Most women with early disease are given the option of either lumpectomy with radiation or total mastectomy. Axillary node resection should accompany both procedures. Results of follow-up screening then can be used to determine the need for adjuvant chemotherapy or hormonal therapy. Lumpectomy without radiation is associated with a failure rate greater than 30% and should not be considered a viable alternative.[39] Chemotherapy and tamoxifen can decrease the risk of relapse or recurrent disease even if nodes are negative. Therefore, the decision regarding adjuvant therapy should be made only after thorough discussion with the patient regarding the chance of relapse without treatment, expected decrease in risk associated with the therapy, and expected side effects of therapy.[39] Tamoxifen is less toxic than the chemotherapy but should be taken for 5 years. The most frequently used chemotherapeutic drugs include doxorubicin, cyclophosphamide, methotrexate, 5-fluorouracil, prednisone, and vincristine. Combination chemotherapy includes the use of cyclophosphamide and 5-fluorouracil combined with either doxorubicin or methotrexate and the use of all five drugs together.

TABLE 56-9 *Staging of Breast Cancer*

Stage	Class	Description
0	TIS	Carcinoma in situ including Paget disease without tumor
	N0	No palpable axillary nodes
	M0	No evident metastasis
I	T1	Tumor 2 cm or less
	N0	No palpable axillary nodes
	M0	No evident metastasis
II	T0	No palpable tumor
	T1	Tumor 2 cm or less
	T2	Tumor less than 5 cm
	N1	Palpable axillary nodes with histologic evidence of breast cancer
	M0	No evidence of metastasis
III	T3	Tumor more than 5 cm; may be fixed to muscle or fascia
	N1 or N2	Fixed nodes
	M0	No evidence of metastasis
IV	T4	Tumor any size with fixation to chest wall or skin; presence of edema, including peau d'orange; ulceration; skin nodules; inflammatory carcinoma
	N3	Supraclavicular or intraclavicular nodes or arm edema
	M1	Distant metastasis present or suspected

Modified from American Cancer Society Staging, 1990.

The American Cancer Society reports a 93% survival rate after 5 years for breast cancer that is still localized at diagnosis. The survival rate drops to 72% with regional spread and to only 18% with distant metastases.[1]

Vulvar Cancer

The incidence of vulvar cancer is increasing, with about 1.8 per 100,000 women being affected.[34] This increased incidence is believed to be the result of improved attention to and diagnosis of obvious lesions and chronic pruritus of the vulva. Obvious lesions and chronic pruritus that do not respond promptly to local therapy should be biopsied to aid in early diagnosis. Historically, vulvar cancer has been considered to be a disease that primarily affects women between 50 and 60 years of age, with at least 30% of cases being diagnosed in women 70 years of age or older.[34] However, the incidence of vulvar intraepithelial neoplasia has increased greatly in women younger than 40 years of age, which suggests that a venereally transmitted agent such as the human papillomavirus may be a predisposing factor. Additional risk factors associated with vulvar cancer include chronic vulvar inflammation and smoking.

A. Stage 1
  • Tumor mass small, less than 2 centimeters
  • Tumor localized
  • No lymph node involvement

B. Stage 2
  • Tumor mass may be up to 5 centimeters
  • Axillary lymph nodes may be involved

C. Stage 3
  • Tumor mass larger than 5 centimeters
  • Edema of overlying skin
  • May have ulceration of skin
  • Tumor solidly fixed to chest wall
  • Lymph node involvement may also include infraclavicular and supraclavicular nodes

D. Stage 4
  • More extensive signs of breast involvement
  • Evidence of distant metastases to bone, lungs, brain, liver, or kidney
  • Frequent parasternal lymph node involvement
  • Arm edema from lymphatic involvement

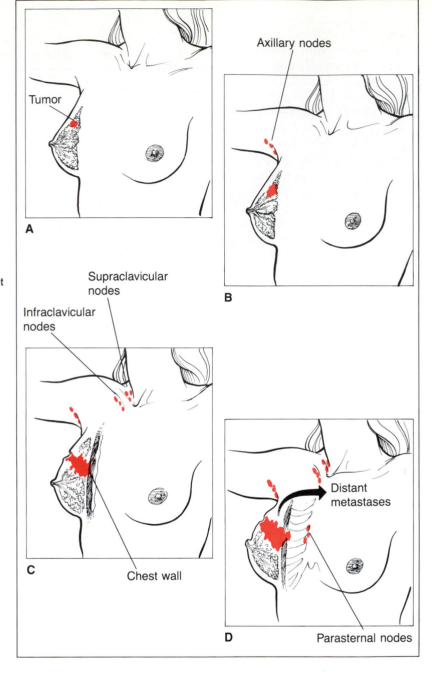

FIGURE 56-28   *Staging of breast cancer.*

Vulval intraepithelial neoplasia may appear as white, red, blue, or brown pigmented lesions. The lesions may occur singly or as multiple papules or macules (Fig. 56-29). Lesions also may be found on perianal skin. Most often, the patient is asymptomatic. If symptoms are present, they include complaints of pruritus and vulvar burning.

There are basically three types of vulvar cancer: squamous cell carcinoma, malignant melanoma, and Paget disease of the vulva.[18] Squamous cell carcinoma is the most common. Growth tends to be slow, with orderly spread to regional lymph nodes. Tumors involving the vagina, urethra, perineum, or anus may spread directly to deep pelvic nodes.[18] The second most common vulvar cancer is malignant melanoma, which appears as blue or black lesions on the vulva. Paget disease of the vulva is characterized by a diffuse lesion tht extends to the posterior fourchette and into the anus.[18] Diagnosis is based on biopsy findings. A hand magnifying lens or the lens of the colposcope may be helpful in identifying biopsy sites.

Treatment choices include local excision, laser vaporization, cryotherapy, and electrocautery. In cases of local invasion, local excision is the treatment of choice.

CASE STUDY 56-1

Ann Jones is a 47-year-old white female. She is married and has one daughter, age 20 years, currently in college. LeAn was born when Ann was 27 years old. Pregnancy, labor, and delivery were uneventful. Ann has generally experienced good health, with the exception of a hysterectomy and oophorectomy that were performed at age 45 for metrorrhagia and menorrhagia. Exogenous estrogen (Premarin, 0.625 mg daily) is the only medication taken on a regular basis. As a nurse, she knows the importance of routine health maintenance and has practiced health promotion, including routine breast self-examination, for many years. She is a nonsmoker and consumes alcohol socially. Physical examination reveals a well-developed, white female who presents with no complaints at this time. Vital signs are blood pressure 124/76, heart rate 76, respirations 18, height 157.5 cm (62 in), weight 67.5 kg (150 lb). Blood chemistry profile results are all within normal limits. Blood cholesterol is 160. Family history indicates that Ann's mother died of breast cancer at 55 years of age, only 2.5 years after initial diagnosis; she experienced no other health problems. Ann's father is a smoker and suffers from emphysema and heart disease. She has two brothers, both living and well.

Mammography reveals a small, suspicious calcification in the upper outer quadrant of the right breast. Comparison with previous mammograms indicates that this is a change from previous findings. Palpation fails to identify any abnormality. Based on family history, a biopsy is performed, which indicates that the mass is 1 cm in diameter and malignant. Surgical options are discussed, including 1) lumpectomy with radiation and 2) modified radical mastectomy with no anticipated follow-up needed.

1. *Which history and physical examination finding indicated the need for biopsy?*
2. *What was the basis for her treatment options?*

One week later, Ann enters the hospital for a lumpectomy to be followed by 6 weeks of radiation therapy. She is discharged 3 days after operation following an uneventful postoperative recovery period. The initial pathology report indicates carcinoma in situ with negative nodes. Computed tomography scan indicates no evidence of metastasis. Therefore, radiation therapy is begun about 7 days after operation. Completed tumor studies indicate that the tumor was estrogen-receptor positive and that there is a high probability of recurrence. After consultation with an oncologist, the decision is made to institute prophylactic chemotherapy followed by tamoxifen. Chemotherapy is to be initiated on completion of the radiation.

3. *What factors resulted in revision of Ann's anticipated treatment plan?*
4. *What stage would Ann's cancer have been in at the time of initial diagnosis?*

Five years after initial diagnosis, Ann is doing well with no evidence of metastasis or recurrence.

See Appendix G for discussion.

There is no consensus regarding the management of vulvar cancer. With more and more younger women being affected, there is growing concern for conservative treatment that limits anatomic deformity, preserves psychosexual function, promotes a positive self-image, and at the same time provides adequate treatment of the cancer. The Gynecologic Oncology Group has concluded that treatment for vulvar cancer must be determined on an individual basis.[26] Factors to consider in determining individual treatment include depth of invasion, midline location, histologic grade, and vascular space involvement. Treatment regimens include surgery with and without node resection, radiation therapy, and chemotherapy. Chemotherapeutic agents used include 5-fluorouracil, cisplatin, and carboplatin. Radiation therapy may include intracavitary radium or external radiation.[26]

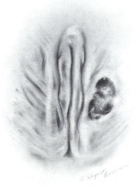

FIGURE 56-29 *An ulcerated or raised red vulvar lesion in an elderly woman may indicate vulvar carcinoma. (Bates, B. A Guide to Physical Examination and History Taking [6th ed.]. Philadelphia: J.B. Lippincott, 1995.)*

▼ *Chapter Summary*

▼ The female reproductive system provides the structures necessary to conceive and bear children. The structures include the ovaries, which produce the ova, and the accessory structures, which provide a place for the fertilized ovum to become an embryo and then a fetus. These include the uterus and fallopian tubes.

▼ The female reproductive functions begin with puberty and end with menopause. These include two phases, preparation for conception and actual gestation. The process requires a hormonal integration that includes the hypothalamus, the pituitary, the ovaries, and the target organs.

▼ Preparation for conception involves the menstrual cycle, which has three phases: menstrual, proliferative, and secretory. Conception involves the female sexual response, fertilization, implantation, and growth of the fetus.

▼ Many tests are used to diagnose alterations in the female reproductive system. These include hormone levels, smears, biopsies, and radiographic procedures, among others.

▼ Alterations in female function include menstrual problems, infections, and benign and malignant processes.

▼ Menstrual problems include endometriosis, premenstrual syndrome, dysmenorrhea, and abnormal uterine bleeding. These conditions are very common and may require medical or surgical treatment.

▼ Infections of the reproductive tract may develop from sexually transmitted diseases or from the implantation of organisms that overcome the normal defenses of the system.

▼ Benign conditions include uterine fibroids, ovarian cysts and tumors, and benign breast alterations, such as fibrocystic disease.

▼ Malignant and premalignant conditions include gestational neoplasms, DES exposure, and endometrial, cervical, ovarian, breast, and vulvar cancers. The incidence of endometrial cancer is increasing, and diagnostic and treatment methods are improving. Cervical cancers have an excellent prognosis if routine screening tests are performed. Ovarian cancer is not as frequently seen, but it has a much poorer prognosis owing to difficulties in diagnosing it before metastasis has occurred. Breast cancer is experienced by one out of nine women; treatment is improving depending on the stage at which it is detected. Vulvar cancer is much less common and occurs most often in elderly women.

▼ References

1. American Cancer Society. *Cancer Facts and Figures—1994.* Atlanta: American Cancer Society, 1994.
2. Ball, H.G., Bell, D.A., and Griffin, T.W. Cancer of the ovary. In American Cancer Society Massachusetts Division, *Cancer Manual* (8th ed.). Boston: American Cancer Society, 1990.
3. Ballweg, M.L. Public testimony to the U.S. Senate Committee on Labor and Human Resources, Subcommittee on Aging, May 5, 1993.
4. Berger, G.S. How many women are affected by endometriosis? *Contemp. OB/GYN* 38(10):47–60, 1993.
5. Berkowitz, R.S., Goldstein, D.P., and Bernstein, M.R. Partial molar pregnancy: A separate entity. *Contemp. OB/GYN* 31(6):99, 1988.
6. Berkowitz, R.S., Goldstein, D.P., and Bernstein, M.R. Updated approach to complete molar pregnancy. *Contemp. OB/GYN* 38(7):78–84, 1993.
7. Berkowitz, R.S., Young, R.H., and Tak, W.K. Cancer of the female genital tract: Cancer of the endometrium. In American Cancer Society Massachusetts Division, *Cancer Manual* (8th ed.). Boston: American Cancer Society, 1990.
8. Burcks, J.A. Ovarian cancer: The most lethal gynecologic malignancy. *Nurs. Clin. North Am.* 27:835–845, 1992.
9. Centers for Disease Control. Follow-up on toxic-shock syndrome. *MMWR* 29:441, 1980.
10. Chuong, C.J., Pearsall-Otey, L.R., and Rosenfield, B.L. Revising treatments for premenstrual syndrome. *Contemp. OB/GYN* 39(1):66–76, 1994.
11. Colbry, S.L. A review of toxic shock syndrome: The need for education still exists. *Nurse Pract.* 17(9):39–43, 1992.
12. Collins-Hattery, A.M., and Blumberg, B.D. S phase index and ploidy prognostic markers in node negative breast cancer: Information for nurses. *Oncol. Nurs. Forum* 18:59–62, 1991.
13. Cotran, R.S., Kumar, V., and Robbins, S.L. *Robbins' Pathologic Basis of Disease* (5th ed.). Philadelphia: W.B. Saunders, 1994.
14. Curry, S.L., and Kelly, S. Cancer of the female genital tract: Overview. In American Cancer Society Massachusetts Division, *Cancer Manual* (8th ed.). Boston: American Cancer Society, 1990.
15. Damario, M.A., and Rock, J.A. Exploring causes of infertility associated with endometriosis. *Contemp. OB/GYN* 38(Special issue, Sept. 15), 1993.
16. Chestnut, C.H. III. Endometriosis therapy: What impact on bone mass? *Contemp. OB/GYN* 38(10):62–74, 1993.
17. Ellerhorst-Ryan, J.M., and Goeldner, J. Breast cancer. *Nurs. Clin. North Am.* 27:821–833, 1992.
18. Fuller, A.F. Jr., Young, R.H., and Tak, W.K. Cancer of the female genital tract: Cancer of the cervix, vulva, and vagina. In American Cancer Society Massachusetts Division, *Cancer Manual* (8th ed.). Boston: American Cancer Society, 1990.
19. Goldstein, D.P. Gestational trophoblastic neoplasms. In American Cancer Society Massachusetts Division. *Cancer Manual* (8th ed.). Boston: American Cancer Society, 1990.
20. Gorrie, T.M., McKinney, E.S., and Murray, S.S. Complications of pregnancy. In Murray, S.S. *Foundations of Maternal Newborn Nursing.* Philadelphia: W.B. Saunders, 1994.
21. Grimes, D.A. Primary prevention of ovarian cancer. *JAMA* 270:2855–2856, 1993.
22. Guyton, A.C. *Textbook of Medical Physiology* (8th ed.). Philadelphia: W.B. Saunders, 1991.
23. Hankinson, S.E., et al. Tubal ligation, hysterectomy, and risk of ovarian cancer: A prospective study. *JAMA* 270:2813–2818, 1993.
24. Herbst, A.L., Jones, H. III, Reid, R., et al. Interpreting the new Bethesda classification system. *Contemp. OB/GYN* 38(8):88–107, 1993.
25. Jones, H. III, Noller, K., Reid, R., et al. Managing patients with low-grade Pap smears. *Contemp. OB/GYN* 38(11):82–94, 1993.
26. Karlan, B.Y., and Lagasse, L.D. Conservative manage-

ment of vulvar cancer. *Contemp. OB/GYN* 35(6):27, 1990.

27. King, M.C., Rowell, S., and Love, S.M. Inherited breast and ovarian cancer: What are the risks? What are the choices? *JAMA* 269:1975–1980, 1993.

28. Kistner, R.W. *Gynecology: Principles and Practice* (4th ed.). Chicago: Year Book Medical Publishers, 1986.

29. Levy, M.J., and Stillman, R.J. Reproductive surgery and the DES uterus. *Contemp. OB/GYN* 35(2):97, 1990.

30. London, R.S., and Hammond, C.B. The climacteric. In Scott, J.R., et al. (eds.), *Danforth's Obstetrics and Gynecology* (7th ed.). Philadelphia: J.B. Lippincott, 1994.

31. Lovejoy, M.N. Precancerous and cancerous cervical lesions: The multicultural "male" risk factor. *Oncol. Nurs. Forum* 21:497–504, 1994.

32. March, C.M. Hysteroscopic resection of submucous myomas. *Contemp. OB/GYN* 35(2):59, 1990.

33. Markman, M. Value of intraperitoneal therapy for ovarian Ca. *Contemp. OB/GYN* 39(1):52–74, 1994.

34. McLachlin, C.M., and Crum, C.P. Precursors and pathogenesis of vulvar squamous Ca. *Contemp. OB/GYN* 39(5): 11–25, 1994.

35. Merkel, D.E. Prognostic markers in early breast cancer. *Contemp. OB/GYN* 39(1):34–51, 1994.

36. Mitchell, E.S., Woods, N.F., and Lentz, M.J. Differentiation of women with three perimenstrual symptom patterns. *Nurs. Res.* 43:25–30, 1994.

37. Murata, J.M. Abnormal genital bleeding and secondary amenorrhea: Common gynecological problems. *J. Obstet. Gynecol. Neonatal Nurs.* 19:26, 1990.

38. Norwood, S.L. Fibrocystic breast disease: An update and review. *J. Obstet. Gynecol. Neonatal Nurs.* 19:116, 1990.

39. Osteen, R.T., et al. Cancer of the breast. In American Cancer Society Massachusetts Division. *Cancer Manual* (8th ed.). Boston: American Cancer Society, 1990.

40. Patsner, B. Office transvaginal sonography: Uterine cancer applications. *Contemp. OB/GYN* 38(Special issue, June 15):11–20, 1993.

41. Reid, R.L. Premenstrual syndrome. *N. Engl. J. Med.* 324: 1208–1210, 1991.

42. Scholes, D., Daling, J.R., and Stergachis, A.S., Current cigarette smoking and risk of acute pelvic inflammatory disease. *Am. J. Public Health* 82:1352–1355, 1992.

43. Slattery, M.L., Robison, L.M., Schuman, K.L., et al. Cigarette smoking and exposure to passive smoke are risk factors for cervical cancer. *JAMA* 261:1593, 1989.

44. Valle, R.F. Assessing new treatments for dysfunctional uterine bleeding. *Contemp. OB/GYN* 39(4):43–60, 1994.

45. Woods, S.L., and Jackson, B. The human immunodeficiency virus and nonmenstrual toxic shock syndrome: A female case presentation. *Nurse Pract.* 19(1):68–71, 1994.

Chapter 57

Sexually Transmitted Diseases

Sharron P. Schlosser

▼ CHAPTER OUTLINE

▼ LEARNING OBJECTIVES

1 Identify the causative organism for each of the sexually transmitted diseases.
2 Discuss the clinical manifestations of each sexually transmitted disease.
3 Identify the three most prevalent sexually transmitted diseases.
4 Discuss the impact of each sexually transmitted disease on the fetus or neonate.
5 Discuss the appropriate diagnostic aids and treatment for each sexually transmitted disease.

Barbara L. Bullock: PATHOPHYSIOLOGY: ADAPTATIONS AND ALTERATIONS IN FUNCTION, 4th ed.
© 1996 J.B. Lippincott-Raven Publishers

Sexually transmitted diseases (STDs) represent a major health problem facing people throughout the world. The term STD refers to the increasing number of conditions so classified by the Centers for Disease Control. These diseases include conditions caused by bacterial pathogens, viruses, fungi, protozoa, and parasites (Table 57-1).

Primary STDs in terms of morbidity and mortality in the United States include gonorrhea, chlamydia, chancroid, syphilis, genital herpes, hepatitis B, cytomegalovirus, and human papillomavirus (condylomata acuminata).[1] Additional STDs impacting reproductive function if not treated include granuloma inguinale, lymphogranuloma venereum, trichomonal vaginitis, candidiasis, and *Haemophilus vaginalis* vaginitis. Conditions are discussed in this chapter based on the classifications reflected in Table 57-1 and as they affect both men and women.

Another group of conditions considered to be STDs are those infections caused by enteric pathogens. These organisms are believed to be transmitted by oral-anal sexual contact, and include *Shigella*, *Entamoeba histo-* *lytica*, and *Giardia lamblia*. The Centers for Disease Control also recognizes scabies, pediculosis pubis, *Campylobacter*, and shigellosis as sexually transmitted diseases. More information on these infections can be found in Chapter 14; hepatitis B is discussed on pages 828–829. The human immunodeficiency virus (HIV) is a sexually transmitted viral infection that is increasing in epidemic proportions in the United States and also worldwide. A complete discussion of HIV is found on pages 336–346.

▼ Bacterial Sexually Transmitted Diseases

GONORRHEA

The most frequently reported STD in the United States is gonorrhea.[1] It ranks second in prevalence among STDs and continues to occur in epidemic proportions. The overall incidence of gonorrhea has decreased 29% in

---

TABLE 57-1 *Sexually Transmitted Diseases*

Disease	Organism	Morphology
BACTERIAL		
Gonorrhea	*Neisseria gonorrhoeae*	Gram-negative diplococcus
Syphilis	*Treponema pallidum*	Spirochete
Chancroid	*Haemophilus ducreyi*	Gram-negative bacillus
Granuloma inguinale	*Donovania granulomatis*	Gram-negative bacillus
Lymphogranuloma venereum	*Chlamydia*	
Chlamydia	*Chlamydia trachomatis*	
Vaginitis	*Haemophilus vaginalis*	Gram-negative bacillus
Shigellosis	*Shigella*	Gram-negative aerobic, bacillus
VIRAL		
Genital herpes	Herpesvirus hominis type 2	DNA present
Condylomata acuminata	Human papillomavirus	DNA present
Acquired immune deficiency syndrome	Human immunodeficiency virus	RNA retrovirus
Cytomegalovirus	Cytomegalovirus	DNA present
Hepatitis B	Hepatitis B	DNA type
FUNGAL		
Candidiasis	*Candida albicans*	Yeast-like cells
PROTOZOAN		
Trichomoniasis	*Trichomonas vaginalis*	Flagellate
Amebiasis	*Entamoeba histolytica*	Anaerobic motile trophozoite (active); cyst transmission
Giardiasis	*Giardia lamblia*	Flagellate
PARASITIC		
Scabies	*Sarcoptes scabiei*	
Pediculosis pubis	*Phthirius pubis*	

males and 24% in females, but this decrease has not been reflected among blacks or adolescents.[18] The primary concerns in the treatment of gonorrhea are the frequent coexistence of chlamydia infections, often unrecognized, and the increasing number of antibiotic-resistant strains.[1]

The causative organism in gonorrhea is *Neisseria gonorrhoeae*, which is a gram-negative diplococcus. This organism thrives in the warm, moist environment of mucous membranes. It may spread rapidly during menstruation because of the favorable environment produced by the blood. It does not survive well outside the body. The organism exhibits increasing resistance to penicillin. In addition to sexual transmission, it can be contracted by the fetus during delivery or by people who have skin breaks that come in contact with contaminated discharge. It may occur in the throat, eyes, or rectum as the result of oral-anal or anal-genital sexual contact or by contamination during the birth process.

Women who contract gonorrhea often are asymptomatic. If symptoms are present, they may include green or yellow vaginal discharge, dysuria, urinary frequency, pruritus, and a red, swollen vulva. Rectal discharge may be seen with rectal infection. The Skene and Bartholin glands may be involved. The most severe complication of gonorrhea is pelvic inflammatory disease, which results in increased incidence of ectopic pregnancy and infertility (Fig. 57-1).

In the symptomatic male, urethritis occurs 2 to 10 days after exposure. At this time, a purulent discharge from the urethral meatus is noted. The discharge is clear

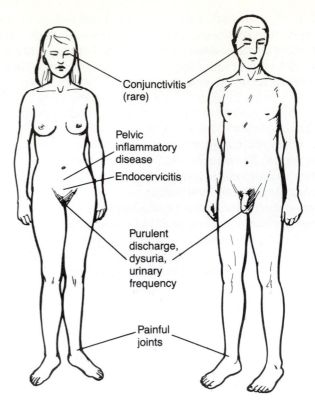

FIGURE 57-2 *Clinical manifestations and complications of untreated gonorrhea.*

at first but soon becomes white or even green. It may be accompanied by itching, burning, and pain around the meatal opening, especially during voiding. In the absence of prompt treatment, infection is likely to spread to involve the prostate, seminal vesicles, and epididymis. With chronic or prolonged infection, abscesses, tissue destruction, and scarring may result. Urethral strictures can lead to hydronephrosis, and epididymitis can cause sterility. Other complications that may occur from gonococcal bacteremia include suppurative arthritis, acute bacterial endocarditis, and suppurative meningitis. Figure 57-2 illustrates the clinical manifestations and complications that may be seen in the infected woman and man.

Conclusive diagnosis must be made on the basis of cultures because there are no serology tests for diagnosis. Culture media usually contain antibiotics to inhibit growth of other bacteria, and they are placed in an atmosphere of increased carbon dioxide. Bacterial growth should be apparent within 24 to 48 hours if gonorrheal organisms are present.

Treatment with ceftriaxone plus doxycycline is instituted immediately.[1] A follow-up culture should be done in 3 to 7 days to document eradication of the organism. In people who are sensitive to penicillin or with gonococcal strains that are resistant to penicillin, other antibiotics may be used. Sexual partners should be treated

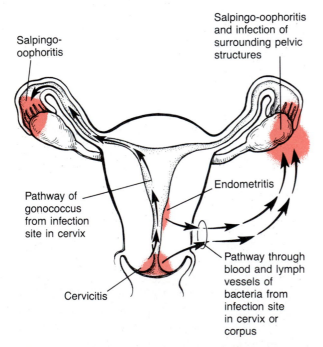

FIGURE 57-1 *Complications of gonorrhea in the female reproductive tract: cervicitis, endometritis, salpingo-oophoritis, and surrounding pelvic infection.*

concurrently, and intercourse should be avoided until repeat cultures indicate a cure. Single infection with the gonococcus organism does not confer immunity. Current recommendations also include concurrent screening and treatment for chlamydia.[1]

SYPHILIS

Syphilis occurs less frequently than gonorrhea but is a more serious condition. The incidence of syphilis declined from the 1950s until 1985, when it reached an all-time low.[1] From 1986 to 1991, there was a dramatic increase in the number of cases reported.[17] The greatest increase was seen among blacks, hispanics, and females.[1] Two factors contributing to this increase in U.S. urban populations were increased used of crack cocaine, and exchange of sex for drugs.[8]

The causative organism in syphilis is the spirochete *Treponema pallidum*. Because of its size, the spirochete is visible only with darkfield microscopy. It is sensitive to both drying and temperature, and it normally enters the skin through moist mucous membranes. It also has been known to enter through breaks in the skin. Transmission may be through sexual contact, by personal contact, or from an infected mother to her unborn fetus.

The course of syphilis progresses in four stages: primary, secondary, latent, and tertiary. Within 24 hours after the spirochete has entered, it spreads throughout the body. Primary syphilis develops after an incubation period of 10 days to 3 months. The first symptom, a chancre, appears at the site of entry (Fig. 57-3). The chancre usually is a painless, red, hardened lesion that may resemble a pimple and often is accompanied by regional lymphadenopathy (Fig. 57-4*A* and *B*). Because the affected person feels well, the infection may go undetected at this stage, and results of serology tests are normal. The infection site and the blood are highly contagious at this time. The chancre usually disappears

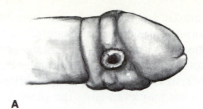

A

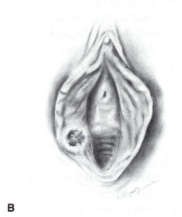

B

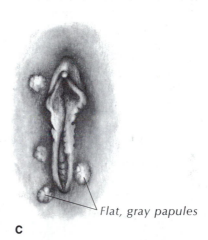

Flat, gray papules

C

FIGURE 57-4 *A. Syphilitis chancre. **B.** Syphilitic chancre on vulva. **C.** Secondary syphilis. (Bates, B. A Guide to Physical Examination and History Taking [6th ed.]. Philadelphia: J.B. Lippincott, 1995.)*

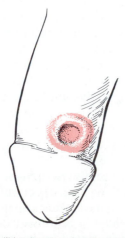

FIGURE 57-3 *Syphilitic chancre. A patient with primary syphilis displays a rounded, raised penile chancre, with central ulceration.*

within 2 to 6 weeks, with or without treatment. Diagnosis is based on identification of the spirochete from the ulceration.

The second stage appears at variable times up to 6 months later. It begins with the development of a generalized, usually maculopapular rash, especially on the palms and soles. Other lesions may be follicular, pustular, or scaling. Large elevated plaques, termed condylomata lata (wartlike, flattened areas), develop on the genitalia (see Figure 57-4C). Secondary syphilis also may be characterized by fever, headaches, loss of appetite, sore mouth, and alopecia. Generalized lymphadenopathy, hepatitis, and nephrosis may occur. Spirochetes are present in all lesions, especially condylomata lata. Syphilis in this stage remains highly contagious, and spirochetes may even cross the placenta to an unborn baby. About 4 to 12 weeks after the beginning of the second stage, all symptoms disappear and the disease enters a latent period. Results of serology tests at this time usually are positive. The course of the disease is variable at this stage. After the latent period, syphilis may be cured spontaneously, remain latent permanently, relapse, or enter the fourth stage.

After a period of years, the condition progresses to tertiary syphilis and eventually is no longer contagious. Fifty percent of those with tertiary syphilis remain symptom-free; however, results of serology tests may remain positive, and the spirochetes can affect an unborn fetus if an infected woman becomes pregnant. For the other infected people, the disease progresses and develops into late clinical syphilis, which can affect any body part (Fig. 57-5). Chronic inflammation of bones and joints may occur. Gummas, large necrotic areas, may develop in the liver, bones, and testes, producing a nodular pattern of cirrhosis, joint destruction, and enlargement resembling a tumor. Gummatous lesions

in the central nervous system are rare, but meningovascular syphilis commonly causes infiltration of the meninges and blood vessels by lymphocytes and plasma cells.[9] Neurosyphilis involves the loss of cortical neurons because of the large number of spirochetes throughout the brain parenchyma. The effect of neurosyphilis is dementia and behavioral changes that progress to psychotic behavior and ataxic paresthesias. Finally, losses of position, deep pain, and temperature sensation occur. The average interval from infection to symptomatic neurosyphilis is 20 to 30 years.

Infection with *T. pallidum* confers immunity on the infected person. Both syphilitic reagin and treponemal immobilizing serum antibodies are produced after 1 to 4 months. Treponemal immobilizing antibodies are specific and probably account for the active immunity. Syphilitic reagin is the basis for both complement fixation and flocculation diagnostic tests. Diagnosis for syphilis is based on microscopic examination and testing of tissue and serum. Darkfield microscopy involves wet-mount specimen preparation from moist lesions. If immediate examination of smears is not available, the direct fluorescent antibody test for *T. pallidum* is an alternative. This test involves fixation and staining of material in preparation for shipment to lab facilities.[6] Silver stains aid in detection of the *T. pallidum* organism. Serology tests aid in diagnosis of syphilis after the antigen-antibody reaction has occurred. Serology tests include the VDRL (Venereal Disease Research Laboratory) and rapid plasma reagin tests, both being nontreponemal tests. Treponemal tests include fluorescent treponemal antibody absorption and the microhemagglutination assay for *T. pallidum* antibodies.[6]

Penicillin continues to be the drug of choice for treating people with syphilis. It must be given in doses appropriate to the stage of disease. In individuals with known sensitivity to penicillin, treatment may include doxycycline, tetracycline, or erythromycin.[6] Because of its teratogenic effect, tetracycline should not be administered to pregnant women; in these cases, the treatment of choice becomes erythromycin. Treatment should be initiated at any point of diagnosis during pregnancy to prevent additional damage to the fetus. Transplacental transmission of the disease leads to death or extensive infection in the infant. Eyes, liver, teeth, and lungs can be affected, leading to dysfunction of the organs in the infant.

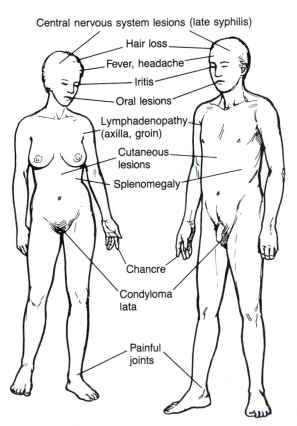

FIGURE 57-5 *Clinical manifestations and complications of untreated syphilis.*

CHANCROID

Chancroid is an acute disease process that produces a soft chancre or shallow, ragged ulcer after an incubation period of up to 10 days. This condition is prevalent worldwide, especially in Southeast Asia, Africa, and South America. It is caused by the gram-negative bacillus *Haemophilus ducreyi*. Within 3 to 5 days after exposure, a maculopapular lesion appears on the penis or vulva. This lesion progresses to pustular lesions and eventually to sloughing of the skin. This process results in a painful ulcer 1 to 3 cm in diameter. Self-inoculation with the causative organism results in the appearance of numerous lesions. Inguinal lymph nodes become swollen and tender. Suppuration from lymph nodes and the necrotic chancre occurs. Gram staining of exudate, culture, and biopsy aid in diagnosis. Good hygiene and treatment with azithromycin, erythromycin, ceftriaxone, or sulfisoxazole (Gantrisin) and allow healing in 2 to 4 weeks.

GRANULOMA INGUINALE

Granuloma inguinale (donovanosis) is a chronic disease process caused by the gram-negative bacillus *Calymmatobacterium granulomatis*. It begins as a papule and progresses to a spreading, necrotic ulcer with extensive scarring. It has a low degree of infectivity and progressively involves the skin and lymphatics of the groin and inguinal areas. Smears and biopsy aid in identification of Donovan bodies and differentiation from other STDs. Antibiotic treatment with tetracycline usually results in complete healing. Gentamicin and chloramphenicol also have been used in treatment of granuloma inguinale.

LYMPHOGRANULOMA VENEREUM

Lymphogranuloma venereum, which is caused by a strain of *Chlamydia* organisms, is rare in the United States. It is characterized by a small, painless papule or vesicle that appears after an incubation period of less than 3 weeks. Spontaneous healing usually occurs after several days. Within 2 to 8 weeks, painful lymphatic involvement occurs with possible obstruction. Malaise, fever, and headache may be noted. In addition to history and physical examination, aspiration of lymph for complement fixation and skin test with Frei antigen may be performed to confirm the diagnosis. Treatment of lymphogranuloma venereum includes erythromycin, doxycycline, and sulfisoxazole.

BACTERIAL VAGINITIS

This vaginitisis is probably caused by an aerobic bacteria. It was previously termed *Gardnerella* vaginitis. It is thought to be spread through sexual contact, and elimination of the infection requires treatment of both sexual partners. The most outstanding symptom is a thin, heavy, gray discharge with the presence of only mild irritation. There is an unpleasant musty or fishy genital odor. Diagnosis is presumptive with a saline wet mount which will reveal "clue cells" (epithelial cells with striped borders). Also, the presence of fishy odor is made

through a sniff or "whiff" test.[3] Ampicillin or tetracycline may be administered orally for systemic effect. Milder cases may be treated with sulfonamide creams or suppositories such as sulfathiazole, sulfisoxazole, or nitrofurazone. Metronidazole also may be used.

CHLAMYDIA TRACHOMATIS

Chlamydia are the most common sexually transmitted organisms in the United States today.[1, 18] Precise data on prevalence and incidence of this disease are not available owing to the lack of a comprehensive national surveillance system. However, the number of states with mandatory reporting legislation has increased from 18 in 1987 to 36 in 1991.[18] It has been observed most often in the younger population, especially in sexually active adolescents. People considered to be at increased risk for chlamydial infection include those who have more than one current sex partner, have a history of multiple partners, are 15 to 24 years of age, are using a nonbarrier contraceptive, or are from lower socioeconomic status.

The causative organism in chlamydial infections is *Chlamydia trachomatis*, an intracellular bacterial parasite. Physical examination with cultures and Papanicolaou smears aids in ruling out herpes, gonorrhea, and other conditions. Clinical diagnosis often is based on documentation of urethritis with discharge or symptoms of cervicitis after gonorrhea has been ruled out. Gram staining may indicate the presence of polymorphonuclear leukocytes. Definitive diagnosis of chlamydial infection is based on tissue culture. Preferred sites for screening specimens are the male urethra and the female endocervix.[7] This time-consuming and expensive technique requires meticulous care in transporting the specimen to a laboratory equipped to perform the examination.

To avoid the problems associated with chlamydia cultures, two nonculture tests have been developed. These tests are the Chlamydiazyme enzyme immunoassay and the Microtract direct fluorescent antibody test. The Chlamydiazyme test depends on an antigen-antibody reaction to detect the presence of chlamydia lipopolysaccharide and therefore detects *Chlamydia psittaci* and *Chlamydia pneumoniae*.[7] The Microtract test detects the presence of major outer membrane protein for *Chlamydia trachomatis* as well as chlamydia lipopolysaccharide. Specimens are collected, placed on a slide, and fixed before being transported to the laboratory. A fluorescence microscope is used to read the stained and incubated slide. Positive screening results should be followed by additional testing. Follow up may include culture, a second nonculture test to detect a different antigen or nucleic acid sequence, or use of an unlabeled "blocking" antibody or "competitive" probe to confirm the positive results.[7]

Other tests are available that provide more limited information. These tests include nucleic acid hybridization tests (DNA probes); a rapid chlamydia test that detects all three species; and the leukocyte esterase test. The leukocyte esterase test uses a urine specimen to detect enzymes produced by polymorphonuclear leuko-cytes.[7] It has been suggested that this test be considered during routine examination in asymptomatic, sexually active adolescent and young adult males.[2]

The most outstanding symptoms, if any are present, involve the genitourinary system. In women, these symptoms include lower abdominal pain, vaginal dis-charge, dysuria, urinary frequency, and vaginal bleed-ing. Discharge, if present, may be heavy with a fishy odor. The discharge is gray-white and creamy and usu-ally is not accompanied by itching or irritation. Exam-ination of the cervix, the most common site of female infection, may reveal congestion, mucopurulent dis-charge, or ectopy. Acute salpingitis, conjunctivitis, and repeated sore throats may be noted in women. If left untreated, the infection can result in pelvic inflamma-tory disease with salpingitis, infertility, and even sterility. Chlamydia infection also has been associated with in-creased incidence of ectopic pregnancy. Chronic infec-tion may result if appropriate therapy fails to eradicate the organisms, if inappropriate drugs are used, if the prescribed dose is inadequate, or if the duration of treat-ment is inappropriate.[21] The presence of chlamydia infec-tion during pregnancy has been associated with preterm delivery, intrauterine growth retardation, premature rupture of membranes, and perinatal mortality.[4]

In men, the presence of chlamydia organisms can result in often asymptomatic urethritis and epididymi-tis.[10] Emerging data also indicate a possible link between chlamydia infection and male infertility.[12]

A child can acquire the disease through contact with an infected birth canal during delivery. The disease in the neonate may cause conjunctivitis or pneumonia. Pro-phylactic treatment of the newborn child with erythro-mycin ophthalmic ointment helps to prevent neonatal conjunctivitis.[13]

Chlamydia infections usually are controlled with antibiotics, including doxycycline or azithromycin. Al-ternative treatment includes ofloxacin, erythromycin, or sulfisoxazole. Erythromycin should be used to treat the disease during pregnancy.[7] Treatment of chlamydial in-fection also requires treatment of the sexual partner. Lack of treatment in the partner may result in reinfection of the patient.

▼ Viral Sexually Transmitted Diseases

GENITAL HERPES

Genital herpes, one of the most common of the primary STDs, is a highly contagious condition caused by the herpesvirus hominis (HVH) type 2, one of the herpes simplex viruses. Type 1 refers to the common cold sore or fever blister that primarily occurs above the waist. There are two forms: primary and recurrent. After incubation of 3 to 7 days, HVH type 2 produces single or multiple vesicles greater than 1 mm in diameter that rupture spontaneously after 24 to 72 hours. These vesicles are accompanied by redness and swelling. After rupture of the vesicles, painful, reddened ulcers develop that even-tually scab, heal, and disappear. The primary attack usually lasts for 3 to 4 weeks before the virus becomes dormant in the nerve cells. Sores reappear whenever the virus is triggered to multiply. Factors known to trigger outbreak of symptoms include colds, fever, severe sun-burn, menstruation, gastrointestinal upset, and stress. Recurrent attacks produce less edema and inflamma-tion, and lesions usually disappear in 7 to 10 days. An estimated 80% or more of infected people experience recurrences at least once a year.

The first attack of genital herpes usually is the worst and is characterized by small, extremely painful blisters. Before the appearance of blisters, the affected person may notice a tingling or burning sensation, possibly followed by intense itching. In the male, lesions of 0.5 to 1.5 cm are present on the glans penis, prepuce, buttocks, and inner thighs (Fig. 57-6). In the female, 90% of the lesions appear on the cervix. Contamination of other body parts may lead to lesions on the thighs, buttocks, and fingers. Secondary infection may occur after the blisters rupture. In both sexes, the initial infection may

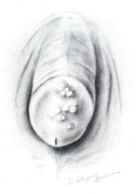

A

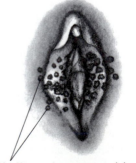

Shallow ulcers on red bases

B

FIGURE 57-6 *A. Genital herpes on penis. B. Genital herpes on vulva. (Bates, B. A Guide to Physical Exam-ination and History Taking [6th ed.]. Philadelphia: J.B. Lippincott, 1995.)*

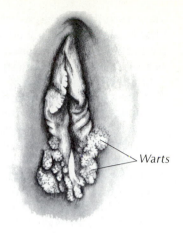

Warts

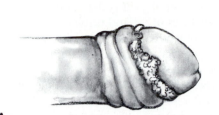

FIGURE 57-7 *A. Venereal wart (condyloma acuminatum) on penis. B. Venereal wart on vulva. (Bates, B. A Guide to Physical Examination and History Taking [6th ed.]. Philadelphia: J.B. Lippincott, 1995.)*

A

B

be accompanied by fever, swelling, enlarged painful lymph nodes, and, in the male, dysuria. Fever and enlarged lymph nodes are less likely to occur with subsequent attacks. Infected people should be cautioned that shedding of the virus may occur even in the absence of symptoms.[5]

There is no known cure for herpes. Several agents have been used with varying success in the treatment of lesions. These include iodine solutions, chloroform, immunotherapy, bacillus Calmette-Guérin vaccine, nitrous oxide, ether, and photoinactivation with a light-sensitive dye and fluorescent light. The only effective antiviral drug in the United States is acyclovir (Zovirax). Alone it is inactive, but in contact with the virus, it is converted to an active form by an enzyme, thymidine kinase, produced by the virus. It hastens healing and decreases transmissibility but has no effect on recurrence.

Herpes infection can be painful and annoying to the affected adult, but it can represent a life-threatening situation to an unborn fetus. This disease can produce abortion or premature delivery. Genital herpes is highly contagious when the vesicles rupture, and delivery through an infected vagina increases the chance that the infection will be passed to the infant.[3] Herpes infection in a newborn can produce brain damage or death. Although the accepted standard is cesarean delivery for women with their first clinical attack of herpes, the practice of cesarean delivery in women with a history of active herpes is being questioned.[16] Another primary concern for women with herpesvirus is the increased risk of cervical cancer. It is now suspected that herpes may be a factor in the development of cervical and vulvar cancer.

HUMAN PAPILLOMAVIRUS

Condylomata acuminata, referred to as venereal warts, are caused by the *human papillomavirus*. Infection often coexists with other STDs such as *Trichomonas, Monilia,* and gonorrhea. The incubation period between infection and development of the lesions is 1 to 3 months. The characteristic cauliflower-like lesions (Fig. 57-7) are estrogen-dependent and are located on the introitus, vulva, or rectum. These lesions may be associated with heavy vaginal discharge, foul odor, and bleeding. Anyone with external growths should be examined for lesions within the vagina, cervix, or rectum. Women with a history of infection caused by human papillomavirus are at increased risk for cancer of the cervix, vulva, and vagina. A relation also has been established between both penile and anal cancer and papillomavirus infection.[13]

Diagnosis is based on clinical appearance or history of sexual contact with an infected person. Biopsy may be performed to rule out vulvar tumors, and a VDRL test may be performed to rule out the condylomata lata found in secondary syphilis.

Treatment for human papillomavirus is aimed at removal of the lesion, not eradication of the virus. Condylomata acuminata lesions are treated with podophyllin (20% to 25%) in tincture of benzoin. This solution should be applied to all lesions at weekly intervals until the lesions are resolved. Podophyllin is a corrosive solution, and should be washed off within 2 to 4 hours of the initial application. Length of application may be increased with subsequent treatments, provided there is no adverse effect. Petroleum jelly may be used to protect the surrounding normal tissue. Cautery, cryotherapy, carbon dioxide laser surgery, or 5-fluorouracil cream may be used, depending on the size of the lesions. Radiation therapy may be indicated. For lesions measuring more than 1.5 to 2 cm, surgical excision, cryotherapy, or cautery usually is used. Concurrent treatment of sexual partners may help to prevent recurrence.

HUMAN IMMUNODEFICIENCY VIRUS

The multiplicity of transmission routes has contributed to the controversy over the status of HIV and the clinical manifestations of acquired immune deficiency syndrome (AIDS) as an STD. This syndrome, has received much medical attention since it was first identified in

1979. Although more extensive discussion of the pathophysiology of HIV infection, including AIDS, is found on pages 336–346, a brief discussion of its sexual transmission and the impact of AIDS on pregnancy and the neonate is provided here.

The increased number of reproductive-age women infected with HIV has resulted in an increased number of infected infants. As many as 85% of reported cases of HIV infection in women occur in women of reproductive age.[15] Data regarding HIV infection and pregnancy continue to emerge. These data indicate that the infection can be spread to infants during pregnancy, during childbirth, or after delivery.[15] The only certain way to prevent complications associated with HIV or its spread to an infant is to avoid pregnancy or terminate the pregnancy, and these are not viable options for some women. These women may not have been successful in preventing conception, may not choose to terminate the pregnancy for personal reasons, or may be diagnosed at a time when termination is not an option because of the length of the gestation.[15]

Although the pregnant woman who is HIV-positive may be asymptomatic, symptoms that are present are the same as those normally associated with early symptomatic HIV disease or late symptomatic HIV disease (AIDS). The symptoms of early symptomatic HIV disease include fatigue, weight loss, shortness of breath, headache, nasal stuffiness, persistent diarrhea, night sweats, chronic cough, genital ulcers, and enlargement of the liver, spleen, and lymph nodes.[10] Late symptomatic HIV disease includes infections with opportunistic organisms, especially *Pneumocystis carinii*, and certain malignancies (see pp. 343–345). Manifestations of the disease in infants may include failure to thrive; diarrhea; enlarged lymph nodes, liver, and spleen; candidiasis in the mouth; and developmental delays.[17]

Although several techniques are being researched to help diagnose AIDS in neonates, no simple, inexpensive method is presently available. Even the results of enzyme immunoassay studies and the Western blot technique are not reliable because of the presence of immunoglobulin G antibody acquired from the mother during pregnancy.[15] The most common laboratory finding is an elevated gamma globulin level, but decreased levels have also been noted.[15]

Throughout pregnancy, labor, and delivery, care should be taken to avoid infant contact with seropositive maternal blood. This includes avoidance of internal fetal monitoring and fetal scalp blood sampling. Care in handling the neonate should be taken by health care workers, and universal precautions should be practiced by those potentially in contact with blood, vaginal secretions, and amniotic fluid.

▼ Fungal Sexually Transmitted Disease

CANDIDIASIS

Candidiasis is a vaginal infection produced by the fungus *Candida albicans*. It also is referred to as moniliasis, thrush, and yeast infection, and it is not always caused by sexual transmission. The organism normally is present on the skin and in the digestive tract, and it may colonize the vagina of some asymptomatic women. Symptoms arise if there is an overgrowth of the organism, which most frequently occurs during pregnancy, after antibiotic therapy, in diabetics, and in women taking oral contraceptives. Infection results from decreased resistance to endogenous flora or from direct mucosal contact (especially sexual contact) with lesions in others. Infants may become infected at delivery and develop thrush. In pregnant women and those taking oral contraceptives, estrogen levels are high, resulting in high glycogen levels that produce a favorable environment for fungal growth. It is believed that systemic antibiotics also suppress the normal bacterial flora in the vagina, and in diabetics the vaginal environment is "sweeter," both of which encourage fungal growth.

The yeast infection produces a heavy, white, cottage cheese–like discharge that is odorless. Complaints of severe itching, dysuria, dyspareunia, and perineal burning are common. The vulva appears erythematous and inflamed (Fig. 57-8). Speculum examination may reveal

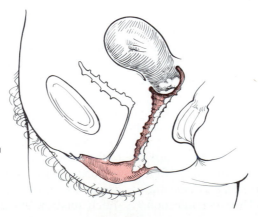

Discharge—may be thin but characteristically thick, white and curdy

Vaginal mucosa—in severe cases, red and inflamed

Cervix—may show patches of discharge

Vulva—often reddened, itchy and swollen

Urethra—no infection

Bartholin gland—no infection

FIGURE 57-8 Monilia *(Candidal)*

white plaques on the vaginal wall. Diagnosis is confirmed by wet smear examination with potassium hydroxide.

Antifungal preparations such as nystatin, miconazole, and clotrimazole are the treatments of choice. These medications are used as topical drugs and are inserted into the vagina, where they exert a local action on the organism. Absorption is poor from the skin and mucous membranes in the vagina. In the past, gentian violet swabs and suppositories were used, but they produce staining and sometimes allergic reactions. Taking lactobacillus tablets and eating yogurt may be helpful in restoring the normal bacterial flora after antibiotic therapy. Correction of any abnormally high blood glucose levels in the diabetic is essential to control of the disease. Treatment of the male partner may be necessary to break the reinfection cycle.

▼ Protozoal Sexually Transmitted Disease

TRICHOMONAL VAGINITIS

Trichomoniasis is a vaginal infection caused by the single-celled protozoan, *Trichomonas vaginalis* (Fig. 57-9). The organism may remain dormant for extended periods and prefers a basic vaginal pH. It has been identified in the male urethra and prostate, so sexual contact serves as a frequent source of reinfection for the female. The frequency of *Trichomonas* infection is highest in women with many sexual partners. The organism produces an

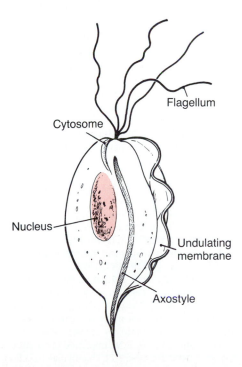

FIGURE 57-9 *Microscopic appearance of Trichomonas vaginalis organism.*

intense itching and burning of the vulva and vagina. It is accompanied by a moderate to profuse discharge that is thin, frothy, and greenish yellow to greenish white with a foul odor. Examination of the cervix may reveal small, deep, red spots referred to as strawberry spots. Microscopic examination of a wet smear reveals a one-celled protozoan with four flagellae. Cultures seldom are done to confirm the diagnosis.

The treatment of choice is a trichomonacidal drug, metronidazole. It is effective in eradicating the organism in 90% of cases. It may be accompanied by severe side effects and should be used only after confirmed diagnosis of *Trichomonas*. Side effects of metronidazole include leukopenia, nausea, diarrhea, headache, and alcohol intolerance. The drug has been found to produce cancer in mice and birth defects in guinea pigs and mice. Therefore, its use is avoided in pregnant women or in those suspected of being pregnant. Alternative treatment includes AVC cream or suppositories, Aci-Jel, and iodoquinol. Again, treatment of the male partner may be necessary to prevent the reinfection cycle.

▼ Chapter Summary

▼ Sexually transmitted diseases include a variety of infectious diseases that are primarily transmitted through sexual contact. Most of the organisms can be transmitted by other routes as well. The organisms that can cause sexually transmitted diseases include some bacteria, viruses, fungi, protozoa, and parasites. Most of the sexually transmitted diseases can be treated, and complications are rare if they are treated early in the course of the disease.

▼ Gonorrhea and syphilis are common bacterial sexually transmitted diseases. Untreated syphilis is more serious than gonorrhea and can cause neurosyphilis 20 to 30 years after infection. Other bacterial sexually transmitted diseases include chancroid, granuloma inguinale, chlamydia, and lymphogranuloma inguinale.

▼ Chlamydia are the most common sexually transmitted organisms in the United States. Chlamydia infection must be differentiated from gonorrhea infection and treated to prevent multiple complications.

▼ Virally transmitted sexually transmitted diseases include genital herpes, human papillomavirus, and human immunodeficiency virus. Herpes produces painful lesions that are highly contagious and in the newborn can produce brain damage or death. It is also linked with cervical and vulvar cancer. Human immunodeficiency virus infection produces the deadly acquired immunodeficiency syndrome, fully discussed in Chapter 17.

▼ The most common fungal sexually transmitted disease is candidiasis, which is commonly seen as a nonsexually transmitted disease in women who are diabetic, pregnant, or taking oral contraceptives.

▼ Trichomoniasis is a common vaginal infection caused

by protozoan infection. It produces a profuse vaginal discharge that is very irritating to the tissues of the vagina.

▼ References

1. Alexander, L.L. Sexually transmitted diseases: Perspectives on this growing epidemic. *Nurse Pract.* 17(10):31–42, 1992.
2. Aronson, M.D., and Phillips, R.S. Screening young men for chlamydial infection. *JAMA* 270:2097–2098, 1993.
3. Bates, B. *A Guide to Physical Examination and History Taking* (6th ed.). Philadelphia: J.B. Lippincott, 1995.
4. Blackburn, L.S. Effective treatment of *Chlamydia trachomatis* infection during pregnancy to prevent perinatal and infant complications. *Nurse Pract.* 17(5):56–60, 1992.
5. Brock, B.V., Selke, S., Benedetti, J., et al. Frequency of asymptomatic shedding of herpes simplex virus in women with genital herpes. *JAMA* 263:418, 1990.
6. Buckley, H.B. Syphilis: A review and update of this "new" infection in the 90s. *Nurse Pract.* 17(8):25–32, 1992.
7. Centers for Disease Control. Recommendations for the prevention and management of *Chlamydia trachomatis* infections. *MMWR* 42(RR–12):1–39, 1993.
8. Centers for Disease Control. Selective screening to augment syphilis casefinding—Dallas, 1991. *MMWR* 42:424–427, 1991.
9. Cotran, R.S., Kumar, V., and Robbins, S.L. *Robbins' Pathologic Basis of Disease* (5th ed.). Philadelphia: W.B. Saunders, 1994.
10. Fekety, S.E. Managing the HIV-positive patient and her newborn in a CNM service. *J. Nurse Midwifery* 34:253–258, 1989.
11. Genc, M., Ruusuvaara, L., and Mardh, P. An economic evaluation of screening for *Chlamydia trachomatis* in adolescent males. *JAMA* 270:2057–2064, 1993.
12. Greendale, G.A. The relationship of *Chlamydia trachomatis* infection and male infertility. *Am. J. Public Health* 83:996–1001, 1993.
13. Hess, D.L. Chlamydia in the neonate. *Neonatal Network* 12(3):9–12, 1993.
14. Palefsky, J.M., Gonzales, J., Greenblatt, R.M., et al. Anal intraepithelial neoplasia and anal papillomavirus infection among homosexual males with group IV HIV disease. *JAMA* 263:2911, 1990.
15. Porcher, F.K. HIV-infected pregnant women and their infants: Primary health care implications. *Nurse Pract.* 17(11):46–54, 1992.
16. Randolph, A.G., Washington, A.E., and Prober, C.G. Cesarean delivery for women presenting with genital herpes lesions: Efficacy, risks and costs. *JAMA* 270:77–82, 1993.
17. Scott, G.B., Clinical manifestations of HIV infection in children. *Pediatric Ann.* 17:365–370, 1988.
18. United States Department of Health and Human Services. *Healthy People 2000. National Health Promotion and Disease Prevention Objectives.* DHHS Pub. No. (PHS) 91-50212, Washington, D.C.: U.S. Government Printing Office, 1991.
19. Webster, L.A., and Rolfs, R.T. Surveillance for primary and secondary syphilis—U.S. 1991. *MMWR* 42(SS-3):13–19, 1993.
20. Webster, L.A., Greenspan, J.R., Nakashima, A.K., et al. An evaluation of surveillance for *Chlamydia trachomatis* infections in U.S., 1987–1991. *MMWR* 42(SS-3):21–27, 1993.
21. Workowski, K.A. Long term eradication of *Chlamydia trachomatis* genital infection after antimicrobial therapy. *JAMA* 270:2071–2075, 1993.

▼ Unit Bibliography

Alexander, L.L. Sexually transmitted diseases: Perspectives on this growing epidemic. *Nurse Pract.* 17(10):31–42, 1992.
American Cancer Society. *Cancer Facts and Figures—1994.* Atlanta: American Cancer Society, 1994.
Armsden, G.C., and Lewis, F.M. Behavioral adjustment and self-esteem of school-age children of women with breast cancer. *Oncol. Nurs. Forum* 21:39–45, 1994.
Aronson, M.D., and Phillips, R.S. Screening young men for Chlamydial infection. *JAMA* 270:2097–2098, 1993.
Arvin, A., Corey, L, and Hirschman, S. Benefit from today's antivirals. *Contemp. OB/GYN* 38(9):58–75, 1993.
Baron, R.H. Dispelling the myths of pregnancy-associated breast cancer. *Oncol. Nurs. Forum* 21:507–512, 1994.
Bast, R., Fenoglio-Preiser, C.M., Ozer, H., et al. Clinical applications of tumor markers. *Contemp. OB/GYN* 38(11):59–72, 1993.
Bates, B. *A Guide to Physical Examination and History Taking* (5th ed.). Philadelphia: J.B. Lippincott, 1991.
Belsky, D.H., Hediger, M.L., and Scholl, T.O. Hormone replacement therapy: Use routine endometrial sampling. *Contemp. OB/GYN* 38(11):46–56, 1993.
Berger, G.S. How many women are affected by endometriosis? *Contemp. OB/GYN* 38(10):47–56, 1993.
Berkowitz, R.S., Goldstein, D.P., and Bernstein, M.R. Updated approach to partial molar pregnancy: A separate entity. *Contemp. OB/GYN* 38(7):78–84, 1993.
Blackburn, L.S. Effective treatment of *Chlamydia trachomatis* infection during pregnancy to prevent perinatal and infant complications. *Nurse Pract.* 17(5):56–60, 1992.
Brock, B.V., Selke, S., Benedetti, J., et al. Frequency of asymptomatic shedding of herpes simplex virus in women with genital herpes. *JAMA* 263:418, 1990.
Brown, L.W., and Williams, R.D. Culturally sensitive breast cancer screening programs for older black women. *Nurse Pract.* 19(3):21–35, 1994.
Brucks, J.A. Ovarian cancer: The most lethal gynecologic malignancy. *Nurs. Clin. North Am.* 27:835–845, 1992.
Buckley, H.B. Syphilis: A review and update of this "new" infection of the '90s. *Nurse Pract.* 17(8):25–32, 1992.
Burnhill, M.S. Clinician's guide to counseling patients with chronic vaginitis. *Contemp. OB/GYN* 35(1):37, 1990.
Champion, V.L. Instrument refinement for breast cancer screening behaviors. *Nurs. Res.* 42:139–143, 1993.
Chuong, C.J., Pearsall, K.J., Otey, L.R., et al. Revising treatments for premenstrual syndrome. *Contemp. OB/GYN* 39(1):66–76, 1994.
Chow, J.M., Yonekura, M.L., Richwald, G.A., et al. The association between *Chlamydia trachomatis* and ectopic pregnancy: A matched-pair, case-control study. *JAMA* 263:3164, 1990.
Cohen, I., Veille, J., and Calkins, B.M. Improved pregnancy outcome following successful treatment of chlamydial infection. *JAMA* 263:3160, 1990.

Colbry, S.L. A review of toxic shock syndrome: The need for education still exists. *Nurse Pract.* 17(9):39–43, 1992.

Colditz, G.A. Family history, age, and risk of breast cancer: Prospective data from the nurses' health study. *JAMA* 270: 338–343, 1993.

Collins-Hattery, A.M., and Blumberg, B.D. S phase index and ploidy prognostic markers in node negative breast cancer: Information for nurses. *Oncol. Nurs. Forum* 18:59–62, 1991.

Cotran, R.S., Kumar, V., and Robbins, S.L. *Robbins' Pathologic Basis of Disease* (5th ed.). Philadelphia: W.B. Saunders, 1994.

Crum, C.P. Koilocytosis in Pap smears: How useful a finding? *Contemp. OB/GYN* 38(7):66–77, 1993.

Damario, M.A., and Rock, J.A. Exploring causes of infertility associated with endometriosis. *Contemp. OB/GYN* 38(Special issue, Sept. 15), 1993.

DeCherney, A.H., Dawood, M.Y., and Chesnut, C.H., Endometriosis therapy: What impact on bone mass? *Contemp. OB/GYN* 38(10): 62–74, 1993.

Deitch, D.V., and Smith, J.E. Symptoms of chronic vaginal infection and microscopic condyloma in women. *J. Obstet. Gynecol. Neonatal Nurs.* 19:133, 1990.

Ellerhorst-Ryan, J.M., and Goeldner, J. Breast cancer. *Nurs. Clin. North Am.* 27:821–833, 1992.

Engelking, C. New approaches: Innovations in cancer prevention, diagnosis, treatment, and support. *Oncol. Nurs. Forum* 21:62–71, 1994.

Epstein, J.I., Walsh, P.C., Carmichael, M., et al. Pathologic and clinical findings to predict tumor extent of nonpalpable (stage T1c) prostate cancer. *JAMA* 271:368–374, 1994.

Gelfand, M.M. Treating menopausal symptoms with estrogen and androgen preparations. *Contemp. OB/GYN* 39(5):31–36, 1994.

Golfarb, H.A. Removing uterine fibroids laparoscopically. *Contemp. OB/GYN* 39(2):50–72, 1994.

Gompel, C., and Silverberg, S.G. *Pathology in Gynecology and Obstetrics.* Philadelphia: J.B. Lippincott, 1994.

Greendale, G.A. The relationship of *Chlamydia trachomatis* infection and male infertility. *Am. J. Public Health* 83:996–1001, 1993.

Grimes, D.A. Primary prevention of ovarian cancer. *JAMA* 270:2855–2856, 1993.

Guyton, A.C. *Textbook of Medical Physiology* (8th ed.). Philadelphia: W.B. Saunders, 1991.

Harger, J.H. Genital herpes infections. *Contemp. OB/GYN* 35(5):83, 1990.

Harris, J.R., Hellman, S., Henderson, I.C., et al. *Breast Diseases* (2nd ed.). Philadelphia: J.B. Lippincott, 1991.

Herbst, A.L., Jones, H. III, Reid, R., et al. Interpreting the new Bethesda classification system. *Contemp. OB/GYN* 38(8):88–107, 1993.

Hess, D.L. Chlamydia in the neonate. *Neonatal Network* 12(3):9–12, 1993.

Higgs, D.J. The patient with testicular cancer: Nursing management of chemotherapy. *Oncol. Nurs. Forum* 17:243, 1990.

Hillard, P.A., and Rebar, R.W. Abnormal uterine bleeding needs a special approach. *Contemp. OB/GYN* 35(5):51, 1990.

Hoskins, W.J., Perez, C.A., and Young, R.C. *Principles and Practice of Gynecologic Oncology.* Philadelphia: J.B. Lippincott, 1992.

Jones, H. III, Noller, K., Reid, R., et al. Managing patients with low-grade Pap smears. *Contemp. OB/GYN* 38(11):82–94, 1993.

Jones, K.D., and Lehr, S.T. Vulvodynia: Diagnostic techniques and treatment modalities. *Nurse Pract.* 19(4):34–46, 1994.

Karlan, B.Y., and Lagasse, L.D. Conservative management of vulvar cancer. *Contemp. OB/GYN* 35(6):27, 1990.

Kerlikowske, K. Positive predictive value of screening mammography by age and family history of breast cancer. *JAMA* 270: 2444–2450, 1993.

King, M.C., Rowell, S., and Love, S.M. Inherited breast and ovarian cancer: What are the risks? What are the choices? *JAMA* 269: 1975–1980, 1993.

Ko, J.H., and Fu, Y.S. Flow cytometry in gynecologic cancer: Current status. *Contemp. OB/GYN* 39(Special issue, April 15):41–56, 1994.

Kurman, R.J. Interim guidelines for management of abnormal cervical cytology. *JAMA* 271:1866–1869, 1994.

Lilley, L.L. Impact of radiation on prostate cancer. *Geriatr. Nurs.* 12: 174–177, 1991.

Lovejoy, N.C. Precancerous and cancerous cervical lesions: The multicultural "male" risk factor. *Oncol. Nurs. Forum* 21:497–504, 1994.

Martin, J.P. Male cancer awareness: Impact of an employee education program. *Oncol. Nurs. Forum* 17:59, 1990.

Mason, D.R. Erectile dysfunctions: Assessment and care. *Nurse Pract.* 14(12):23, 1989.

Merkel, D.E. Prognostic markers in early breast cancer. *Contemp. OB/GYN* 39(1):34–51, 1994.

Mitchell, E.S., Woods, N.F., and Lentz, M.J. Differentiation of women with three perimenstrual symptom patterns. *Nurs. Res.* 43:25–30, 1994.

Mock, V. Body image in women treated for breast cancer. *Nurs. Res.* 42:153–157, 1993.

Murata, J.M. Abnormal genital bleeding and secondary amenorrhea: Common gynecological problems. *J. Obstet. Gynecol. Neonatal Nurs.* 19:26, 1990.

Nielsen, B., Miaskowski, C., McCoy, C., et al. The development and implementation of standards of care in a breast cancer screening program. *Oncol. Nurs. Forum* 18:67–72, 1991.

Norwood, S.L. Fibrocystic breast disease: An update and review. *J. Obstet. Gynecol. Neonatal Nurs.* 19:116, 1990.

Nuovo, G.J., and Pedemonte, B.M. Human papillomavirus types and recurrent cervical warts. *JAMA* 263:1223, 1990.

Pierce, P.F. Deciding on breast cancer treatment: A description of decision behavior. *Nurs. Res.* 42:22–28, 1993.

Porcher, F.K. HIV infected pregnant women and their infants: Primary health care implications. *Nurse Pract.* 17(11):46–54, 1992.

Randolph, A.G., Washington, A.E., and Prober, C.G. Cesarean delivery for women presenting with genital herpes lesions: Efficacy, risks and costs. *JAMA* 270:77–82, 1993.

Reid, R.L. Premenstrual syndrome. *N. Engl. J. Med.* 324:1208–1210, 1991.

Roy, M. VIN—Latest management approaches. *Contemp. OB/GYN* 31(5):170, 1988.

Rutledge, D.N. Effects of age on lump detection accuracy. *Nurs. Res.* 41:306–308, 1992.

Schaffer, S.D., and Philput, C.B. Predictors of abnormal cervical cytology: Statistical analysis of human papillomavirus and cofactors. *Nurse Pract.* 17(3):46–50, 1992.

Schiffman, M.H. Latest HPV findings: Some clinical implications. *Contemp. OB/GYN* 38(10):27–40, 1993.

Scholes, D., Daling, J.R., and Stergachis, A.S. Current cigarette smoking and risk of acute pelvic inflammatory disease. *Am. J. Public Health* 82:1352–1355, 1992.

Sciarra, J.J. *Gynecology and Obstetrics.* Philadelphia: J.B. Lippincott, 1995.

Scott, J., DiSaia, P.J., Hammond, C. *Danforth's Obstetrics and Gynecology* (7th ed.). Philadelphia: J.B. Lippincott, 1994.

Shafer, M., et al. Evaluation of urine-based screening strategies to detect *Chlamydia trachomatis* among sexually active asymptomatic young males. *JAMA* 270:2065–2070, 1993.

Shangold, M., Rebar, R.W., Wentz, A.C., et al. Evaluation and management of menstrual dysfunction in athletes. *JAMA* 263:1665, 1990.

Shingleton, H.M., and Orr, J.W. *Cancer of the Cervix.* Philadelphia: J.B. Lippincott, 1994.

Speroff, L. Breast cancer and postmenopausal hormone therapy. *Contemp. OB/GYN* 35(1):71, 1990.

Valle, R.F., Assessing new treatments for dysfunctional uterine bleeding. *Contemp. OB/GYN* 39(4):43–60, 1994.

Ward, S.E. Patients' reactions to completion of adjuvant breast cancer therapy. *Nurs. Res.* 41:362–366, 1992.

Waxman, E.S. Sexual dysfunction following treatment for prostate cancer: Nursing assessment and interventions. *Oncol. Nurs. Forum* 20:1567–1571, 1993.

Whitman, S. An intervention to increase breast and cervical cancer screening in low-income African-American women. *Family and Community Health* 17(1):56–63, 1994.

Woods, S.L., and Jackson, B. The human immunodeficiency virus and nonmenstrual toxic shock syndrome: A female case presentation. *Nurse Pract.* 19(1):68–71, 1994.

Workowski, K.A. Long-term eradication of *Chlamydia trachomatis* genital infection after antimicrobial therapy. *JAMA* 270:2071–2075, 1993.

Yoder, L.H. The epidemiology of ovarian cancer: A review. *Oncol. Nurs. Forum* 17:411, 1990.

Appendix A

Recommended Daily Dietary Allowances for Women (Nonpregnant)

	Ages			
	11–14	*15–18*	*19–22*	*23–50*
Energy, kcal	2200	2100	2100	2000
Protein, g	46	46	44	44
Vitamin A, RE	800	800	800	800
IU	4000	4000	4000	4000
Vitamin D, μg	10	10	7.5	5
Vitamin E, Q-TE	8	8	8	18
Ascorbic acid, mg	50	60	60	60
Niacin, mg	15	14	14	13
Riboflavin, mg	1.3	1.3	1.3	1.2
Thiamin, mg	1.1	1.1	1.1	1.0
Vitamin B_6, mg	1.8	2.0	2.0	2.0
Folacin, μg	400	400	400	400
Vitamin B_{12}, μg	3	3	3	3
Calcium, mg	1200	1200	800	800
Phosphorus, mg	1200	1200	800	800
Iodine, μg	150	150	150	150
Iron, mg	18	18	18	18
Magnesium, mg	300	300	300	300
Zinc	15	15	15	15

Source: Food and Nutrition Board, Committee on Dietary Allowances, National Research Council. *Recommended Dietary Allowances* (9th ed.). Washington, D.C.: National Academy of Sciences, 1980.

Appendix *B*

Recommended Daily Dietary Allowances for Pregnant and Lactating Women

	Ages				Differences for Lactation
	11–14	*15–18*	*19–22*	*23–50*	
Energy, kcal	2500	2400	2400	2300	+200
Protein, g	76	76	74	74	−10
Vitamin A, RE	1000	1000	1000	1000	+200
IU	5000	5000	5000	5000	+1000
Vitamin D, μg	15	15	12.5	10	same
Vitamin E, Q-TE	10	10	10	10	+1
Ascorbic acid, mg	70	80	80	80	+20
Niacin, mg	17	16	16	15	+3
Riboflavin, mg	1.6	1.6	1.6	1.5	+0.2
Thiamin, mg	1.5	1.5	1.5	1.4	+0.1
Vitamin B_6, mg	2.4	2.6	2.6	2.6	−0.1
Folacin, μg	800	800	800	800	−300
Vitamin B_{12}, μg	4	4	4	4	same
Calcium, mg	1600	1600	1200	1200	same
Phosphorus, mg	1600	1600	1200	1200	same
Iodine, μg	175	175	175	175	+25
Iron, mg	18+	18+	18+	18+	+6
Magnesium, mg	450	450	450	450	same
Zinc	20	20	20	20	+5

Source: Food and Nutrition Board, Committee on Dietary Allowances, National Research Council. *Recommended Dietary Allowances* (9th ed.). Washington, D.C.: National Academy of Sciences, 1980.

Appendix C

Average Heights and Weights by Age and Sex: U.S. Health Examination Study 1960–62

Age (Yrs.)	Males Height (In.)	Males Weight (Lbs.)	Females Height (In.)	Females Weight (Lbs.)
18–24	68.7	160	63.8	129
25–34	69.1	171	63.7	136
35–44	68.5	172	63.5	144
45–54	68.2	172	62.9	147
55–64	67.4	166	62.4	152
65–74	66.9	160	61.5	146
75–79	65.9	150	61.1	138

Based on a nationwide probability sample of 7710 persons. Averages and fiftieth percentiles were quite equal. Both secular trends and aging changes are mirrored by such measures as the three-inch difference in height of younger and older males.

Source: Public Health Service Publication 1000, Series 11, No. 8, Washington, D.C.: Government Printing Office, 1965.

Appendix D

Age (years) and Sex Group	Weight[b]		Height[b]		Protein	Fat-Soluble Vitamins			
						Vita-min A	Vita-min D	Vita-min E	Vita-min K
	kg	lb	cm	in					
					gm	µg RE[c]	µg[d]	mg α-TE[a]	µg
INFANTS									
0.0–0.5	6	13	60	24	13	375	7.5	3	5
0.5–1.0	9	20	71	28	14	375	10	4	10
CHILDREN									
1–3	13	29	90	35	16	400	10	6	15
4–6	20	44	112	44	24	500	10	7	20
7–10	28	62	132	52	28	700	10	7	30
MALES									
11–14	45	99	157	62	45	1000	10	10	45
15–18	66	145	176	69	59	1000	10	10	65
19–24	72	160	177	70	58	1000	10	10	70
25–50	79	174	176	70	63	1000	5	10	80
51+	77	170	173	68	63	1000	5	10	80
FEMALES									
11–14	46	101	157	62	46	800	10	8	45
15–18	55	120	163	64	44	800	10	8	55
19–24	58	128	164	65	46	800	10	8	60
25–50	63	138	163	64	50	800	5	8	65
51+	65	143	160	63	50	800	5	8	65
pregnant					60	800	10	10	65
lactating									
1st 6 months					65	1300	10	12	65
2nd 6 months					62	1200	10	11	65

[a] The allowances, expressed as average daily intakes over time, are intended to provide for individual variations among most normal persons as they live in the United States under usual environmental stresses. Diets should be based on a variety of common foods in order to provide other nutrients for which human requirements have been less well defined. Revised 1989. Designed for the maintenance of good nutrition of practically all healthy people in the United States.

[b] Weights and heights of Reference Adults are actual medians for the U.S. population of the designated age, as reported by NHANES II. The median weights and heights of those under 19 years of age were taken from P.V.V. Hamil, T.A. Drizd, C.L. Johnson, R.B. Reed, A.F. Roche, and W.M. Moore: Physical growth. National Center for Health Statistics Percentiles. Am. J. Clin. Nutr. 32:607, 1979. The use of these figures does not imply that the height-to-weight ratios are ideal.

Water-Soluble Vitamins							Minerals						
Vitamin C	Thiamin	Riboflavin	Niacin	Vitamin B_6	Folate	Vitamin B_{12}	Calcium	Phosphorus	Magnesium	Iron	Zinc	Iodine	Selenium
——— mg ———			mg NE[f]	mg	——— µg ———		——————— mg ———————					——— µg ———	
30	0.3	0.4	5	0.3	25	0.3	400	300	40	6	5	40	10
35	0.4	0.5	6	0.6	35	0.5	600	500	60	10	5	50	15
40	0.7	0.8	9	1.0	50	0.7	800	800	80	10	10	70	20
45	0.9	1.1	12	1.1	75	1.0	800	800	120	10	10	90	20
45	1.0	1.2	13	1.4	100	1.4	800	800	170	10	10	120	30
50	1.3	1.5	17	1.7	150	2.0	1200	1200	270	12	15	150	40
60	1.5	1.8	20	2.0	200	2.0	1200	1200	400	12	15	150	50
60	1.5	1.7	19	2.0	200	2.0	1200	1200	350	10	15	150	70
60	1.5	1.7	19	2.0	200	2.0	800	800	350	10	15	150	70
60	1.2	1.4	15	2.0	200	2.0	800	800	350	10	15	150	70
50	1.1	1.3	15	1.4	150	2.0	1200	1200	280	15	12	150	45
60	1.1	1.3	15	1.5	180	2.0	1200	1200	300	15	12	150	50
60	1.1	1.3	15	1.6	180	2.0	1200	1200	280	15	12	150	55
60	1.1	1.3	15	1.6	180	2.0	800	800	280	15	12	150	55
60	1.0	1.2	13	1.6	180	2.0	800	800	280	10	12	150	55
70	1.5	1.6	17	2.2	400	2.2	1200	1200	320	30	15	175	65
95	1.6	1.8	20	2.1	280	2.6	1200	1200	355	15	19	200	75
90	1.6	1.7	20	2.1	260	2.6	1200	1200	340	15	16	200	75

[c] Retinol equivalents. 1 retinol equivalent = 1 µg retinol or 6 µg β-carotene. See text for calculation of vitamin A activity of diets as retinol equivalents.

[d] As cholecalciferol. 10 µg cholecalciferol = 400 IU of vitamin D.

[e] α-Tocopherol equivalents. 1 mg d-α tocopherol = 1 α-TE. See text for variation in allowances and calculation of vitamin E activity of the diet as α-tocopherol equivalents.

[f] 1 NE (niacin equivalent) is equal to 1 mg of niacin or 60 mg of dietary tryptophan.

Food and Nutrition Board, National Academy of Sciences—National Research Council Recommended Dietary Allowances (RDAs)[c]

Height, cm	Body Mass Index, kg/m²													
	19.0	20.0	21.0	22.0	23.0	24.0	25.0	26.0	27.0	28.0	29.0	30.0	35.0	40.0
	Body Weight, kg													
140.0	37.2	39.2	41.2	43.1	45.1	47.0	49.0	51.0	52.9	54.9	56.8	58.8	68.6	78.4
142.0	38.3	40.3	42.3	44.4	46.4	48.4	50.4	52.4	54.4	56.5	58.5	60.5	70.6	80.7
144.0	39.4	41.5	43.5	45.6	47.7	49.8	51.8	53.9	56.0	58.1	60.1	62.2	72.6	82.9
146.0	40.5	42.6	44.8	46.9	49.0	51.2	53.3	55.4	57.6	59.7	61.8	63.9	74.6	85.3
148.0	41.6	43.8	46.0	48.2	50.4	52.6	54.8	57.0	59.1	61.3	63.5	65.7	76.7	87.6
150.0	42.8	45.0	47.3	49.5	51.8	54.0	56.3	58.5	60.8	63.0	65.3	67.5	78.8	90.0
152.0	43.9	46.2	48.5	50.8	53.1	55.4	57.8	60.1	62.4	64.7	67.0	69.3	80.9	92.4
154.0	45.1	47.4	49.8	52.2	54.5	56.9	59.3	61.7	64.0	66.4	68.8	71.1	83.0	94.9
156.0	46.2	48.7	51.1	53.5	56.0	58.4	60.8	63.3	65.7	68.1	70.6	73.0	85.2	97.3
158.0	47.4	49.9	52.4	54.9	57.4	59.9	62.4	64.9	67.4	69.9	72.4	74.9	87.4	99.9
160.0	48.6	51.2	53.8	56.3	58.9	61.4	64.0	66.6	69.1	71.7	74.2	76.8	89.6	102.4
162.0	49.9	52.5	55.1	57.7	60.4	63.0	65.6	68.2	70.9	73.5	76.1	78.7	91.9	105.0
164.0	51.1	53.8	56.5	59.2	61.9	64.6	67.2	69.9	72.6	75.3	78.0	80.7	94.1	107.6
166.0	52.4	55.1	57.9	60.6	63.4	66.1	68.9	71.6	74.4	77.2	79.9	82.7	96.4	110.2
168.0	53.6	56.4	59.3	62.1	64.9	67.7	70.6	73.4	76.2	79.0	81.8	84.7	98.8	112.9
170.0	54.9	57.8	60.7	63.6	66.5	69.4	72.3	75.1	78.0	80.9	83.8	86.7	101.2	115.6
172.0	56.2	59.2	62.1	65.1	68.0	71.0	74.0	76.9	79.9	82.8	85.8	88.8	103.5	118.3
174.0	57.5	60.6	63.6	66.6	69.6	72.7	75.7	78.7	81.7	84.8	87.8	90.8	106.0	121.1
176.0	58.9	62.0	65.0	68.1	71.2	74.3	77.4	80.5	83.5	86.7	89.8	92.9	108.4	123.9
178.0	60.2	63.4	66.5	69.7	72.9	76.0	79.2	82.4	85.5	88.7	91.9	95.1	110.9	126.7
180.0	61.6	64.8	68.0	71.3	74.5	77.8	81.0	84.2	87.5	90.7	94.0	97.2	113.4	129.6
182.0	62.9	66.2	69.6	72.9	76.2	79.5	82.8	86.1	89.4	92.7	96.1	99.4	115.9	132.5
184.0	64.3	67.7	71.1	74.5	77.9	81.3	84.6	88.0	91.4	94.8	98.2	101.6	118.5	135.4
186.0	65.7	69.2	72.7	76.1	79.6	83.0	86.5	89.9	93.4	96.9	100.3	103.8	121.1	138.4
188.0	67.2	70.7	74.2	77.8	81.3	84.8	88.4	91.9	95.4	99.0	102.5	106.0	123.7	141.4
190.0	68.6	72.2	75.8	79.4	83.0	86.6	90.3	93.9	97.5	101.1	104.7	108.3	126.4	144.4
192.0	70.0	73.7	77.4	81.1	84.8	88.5	92.2	95.8	99.5	103.2	106.9	110.6	129.0	147.5
194.0	71.5	75.3	79.0	82.8	86.6	90.3	94.1	97.9	101.6	105.4	109.1	112.9	131.7	150.0
196.0	73.0	76.8	80.7	84.5	88.4	92.2	96.0	99.9	103.7	107.6	111.4	115.2	134.5	153.7
198.0	74.5	78.4	82.3	86.2	90.2	94.1	98.0	101.9	105.9	109.8	113.7	117.6	137.2	156.8
200.0	76.0	80.0	84.0	88.0	92.0	96.0	100.0	104.0	108.0	112.0	116.0	120.0	140.0	160.0

[a] Each entry gives the body weight in kilograms (kg) for a person of a given height and body mass index.
[b] Desirable body mass index range in relation to age (from Bray[7]).

Age Group, y	Body Mass Index, kg/m²	Age Group, y	Body Mass Index, kg/m²
19–24	19–24	45–54	22–27
25–34	20–25	55–64	23–28
35–44	21–26	65 +	24–29

Source: G.A. Bray, D.S. Gray, Obesity, Part 1. Pathogenesis. West Med J 149:429. 1988.

Appendix *F*

SUMMARY OF CARDIAC DYSRHYTHMIAS

Normal cardiac conduction (illustrated below) involves the passage of the pacemaking impulse from the SA node to the AV node to the bundle of His, bundle branches, Purkinje fibers, and ventricular muscle. This transcribes wave forms that are described as P, QRS, and T with intervals P-R, QRS, and Q-T. Since ECG paper is divided into segments with small blocks being 0.04 seconds in time and the larger blocks being 0.2 second in time, these intervals can be timed. The normal P-R interval is 0.12 to 0.20 seconds and the normal QRS is 0.06 to 0.1 second in time. The normal cardiac rate is 60 to 100 beats or QRS complexes per minute.

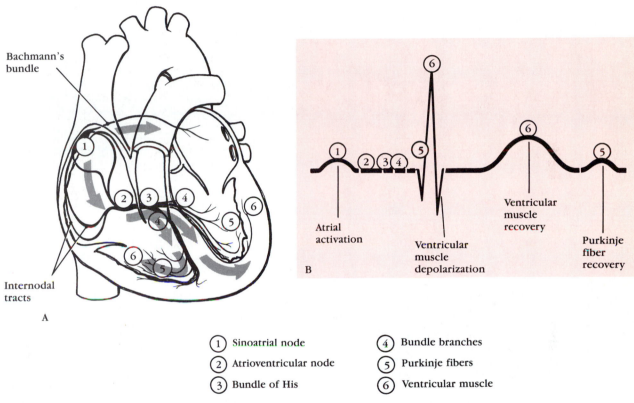

① Sinoatrial node	④ Bundle branches
② Atrioventricular node	⑤ Purkinje fibers
③ Bundle of His	⑥ Ventricular muscle

FIGURE F1 *A. Normal cardiac conduction. B. Correlation of electrical events of the heart and ECG tracing.*

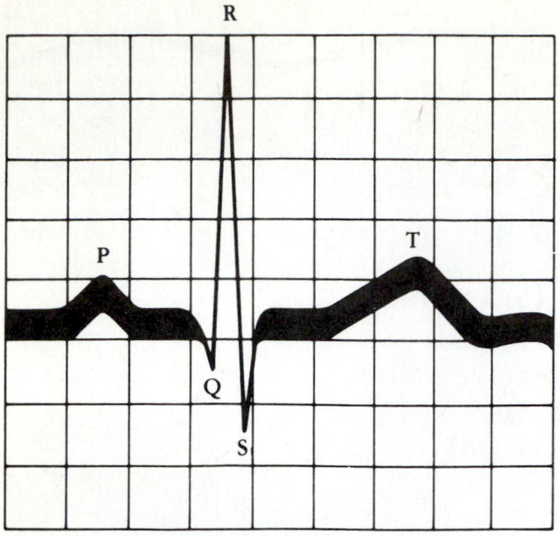

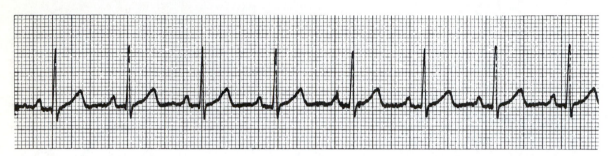

FIGURE F2   *The normal electrocardiogram from lead II. Each small square represents 0.04 seconds on the horizontal plane. Measurements are made of time required for impulses to pass through different portions of the conduction system. The P wave indicates SA node initiaiton of the impulse. The QRS indicates ventricular depolarization and the T wave reflects ventricular repolarization. The P-R interval is from the beginning of the P wave to the beginning of the QRS and normally is 0.12 to 0.2 seconds. The QRS is normally 0.06 to 0.1 seconds.*

FIGURE F3

NORMAL SINUS RHYTHM
Rhythm: regular
Rate: 60–100
P-R interval: – .12 to 0.20 seconds
QRS: 0.06–0.10 seconds

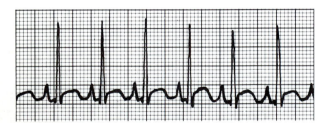

FIGURE F4

SINUS TACHYCARDIA
Rhythm: regular
Rate: 100 to 160
P-R interval: 0.12–0.20 seconds
QRS: normal

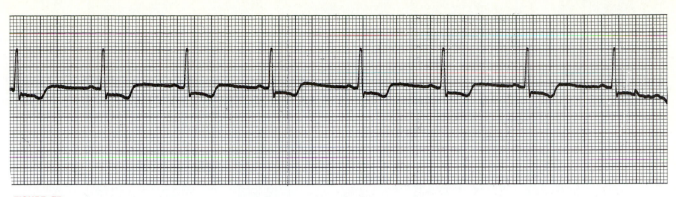

FIGURE F5

SINUS BRADYCARDIA
Rhythm: regular
Rate: less than 60
P-R interval: normal
QRS: normal

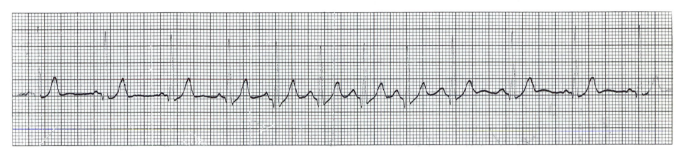

FIGURE F6

SINUS ARRHYTHMIA (DYSRHYTHMIA)
Rhythm: irregular, rate increases with inspiration, slows with expiration
Rate: less than 100
P-R interval: normal
QRS: normal

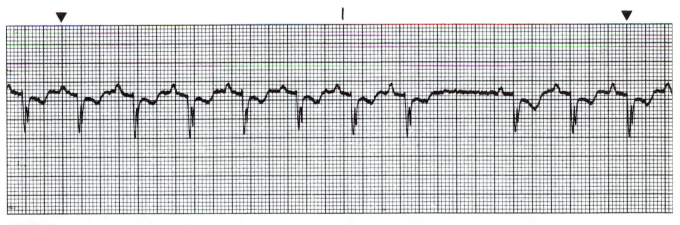

FIGURE F7

SINUS ARREST, PAUSE, OR EXIT BLOCK
Rhythm: irregular, due to the depression of sinus node activity. May be varying lengths of time of loss of atrial stimulation. Sometimes an escape rhythm form the AV node will cause a ventricular beat.
Rate: Slows conduction during the time of the arrest
P-R: normal except during the sinus depression
QRS: normal
(Source: Hudak, CM, and Gallo, B.M. *Critical Care Nursing,* [7th ed.] Philadelphia: J.B. Lippincott, 1994.)

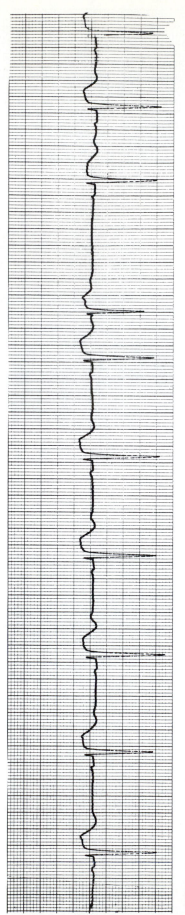

FIGURE F8

PREMATURE ATRIAL CONTRACTIONS (PACs)

Rhythm: irregular due to the origination of a beat outside the normal conduction system (ectopic).

Rate: does not interfere with the normal sinus rate, except for PACs

P-R: P wave is abnormal and interval may be slight shortened in ectopic beat

QRS: normal

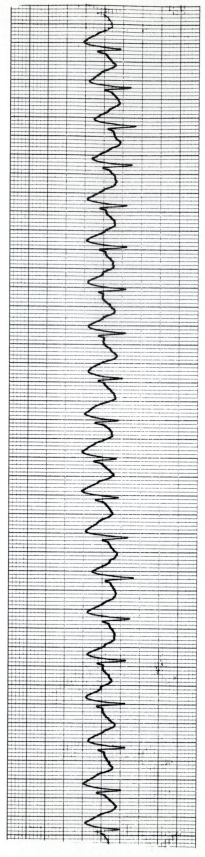

FIGURE F9

ATRIAL TACHYCARDIA

Rhythm: regular

Rate: 160 to 250 beats per minute

P-R: usually initiated by a PAC, is a run of 6 or more. P waves are abnormal

QRS: normal

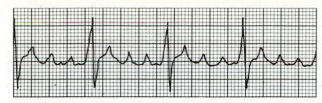

FIGURE F10

ATRIAL FLUTTER
Rhythm: usually regular
Rate: ventricular rate responds to the amount of atrial block
P-R: P waves are replaced by flutter waves which occur at a rate of 250 to 350 per minute. The ventricles block at a ratio of 2:1 to 4:1
QRS: normal
(**Source:** Hudak, CM, and Gallo, B.M. *Critical Care Nursing,* [7th ed.] Philadelphia: J.B. Lippincott, 1994.)

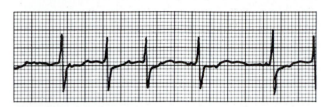

FIGURE F11

ATRIAL FIBRILLATION
Rhythm: irregularly irregular
Rate: variable. Usually rapid on initiation of rhythm. Decreases when controlled by medication
P-R: no P waves are seen, replaced by an irregular wavy baseline. The atria are fibrillating due to impulses arising at a rate grater than 350. The ventricles respond when the AV node is stimulated to threshold and can receive the impulse.
QRS: normal
(**Source:** Hudak, CM, and Gallo, B.M. *Critical Care Nursing,* [7th ed.] Philadelphia: J.B. Lippincott, 1994.)

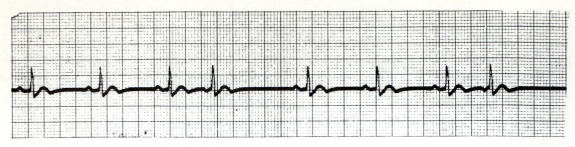

FIGURE F12

PREMATURE JUNCTIONAL CONTRACTIONS
Rhythm: irregular
Rate: does not interfere with the underlying sinus rhythm except during the junctional beat.
P-R: usually shortened. The P wave is conducted in a retrograde fashion in junctional beat
QRS: normal
(**Source:** B.H. **Yee and** S.I. **Zorb,** *Cardiac Critical Care Nursing.* Boston: Little, Brown, 1986.)

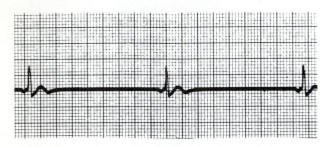

FIGURE F13

JUNCTIONAL ESCAPE RHYTHM
Rhythm: regular
Rate: 40 to 60 beats per minute
P-R: usually shortened. P waves may be retrograde prior to QRS or
following it.
QRS: normal
(**Source:** B.H. **Yee and** S.I. **Zorb,** *Cardiac Critical Care Nursing.* Boston: Little, Brown, 1986.)

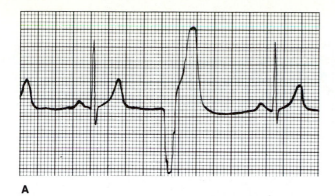

A

Ventricular premature contraction.

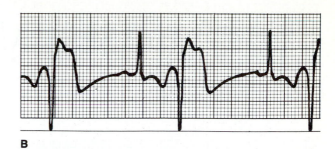

B

Ventricular bigeminy. (Every other beat is a VPB.)

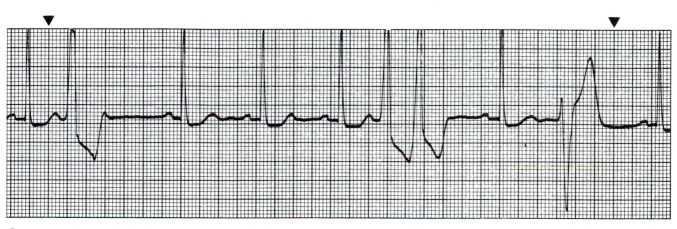

C

Multiformed VPBs.

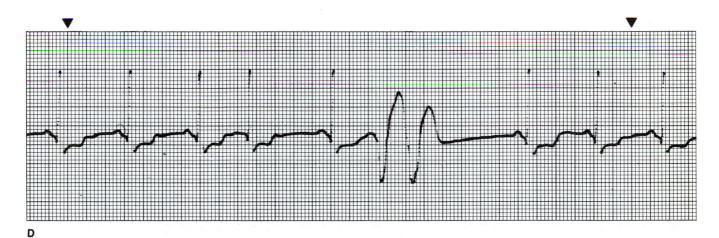

D

Couplet (two VPBs in a row).

FIGURE F14

PREMATURE VENTRICULAR CONTRACTIONS (PVCs) or VENTRICULAR PREMATURE BEATS (VPBs)
Rhythm: irregular
Rate: variable. Only interrupts the cycle of the ectopic, ventricular contraction
P-R: normal in sinus beats, not measurable in PVC
QRS: wide, bizarre, greater than 0.12 seconds
(Source: Hudak, CM, and Gallo, B.M. *Critical Care Nursing,* [7th ed.] Philadelphia: J.B. Lippincott, 1994.)

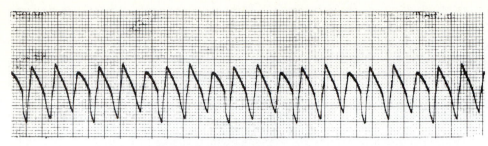

A

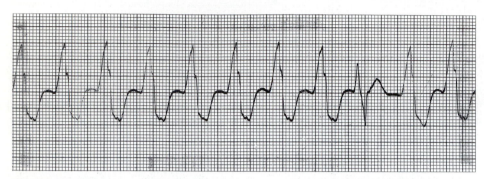

B

FIGURE F15

VENTRICULAR TACHYCARDIA
Rhythm: regular or slightly irregular
Rate: 120 to 250 beats per minute
P-R: not measurable
QRS: wide, bizarre, greater than 0.12 seconds. More than 3 PVCs in a row is called ventricular tachycardia
(Source: B.H. Yee and S.I. Zorb, *Cardiac Critical Care Nursing.* Boston: Little, Brown, 1986.)

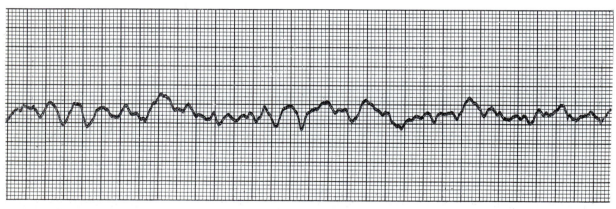

FIGURE F16

VENTRICULAR FIBRILLATION
Rhythm: irregular
Rate: not measurable
P-R: not measurable
QRS: not measurable, replaced by an irregular wavy baseline. No coordinated electrical or mechanical activity in the ventricle, no cardiac output.

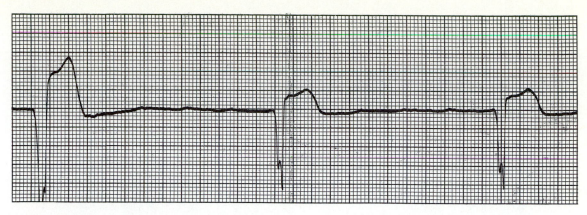

FIGURE F17

IDIOVENTRICULAR RHYTHM
Rhythm: usually regular
Rate: 20 to 40 beats per minute
P-R: not measurable
QRS: wide, bizarre, greater than 0.12 seconds. Considered to be an escape rhythm and is often seen terminally. In reperfusion of the myocardium, this rhythm may be seen and is usually called accelerated idioventricular rhythm because it occurs at a rate to 60 to 110 per minute.

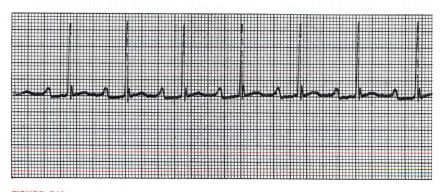

FIGURE F18

FIRST DEGREE ATRIOVENTRICULAR HEART BLOCK
Rhythm: regular
Rate: normal
P-R: prolonged, greater than 0.20 seconds, indicates a delay of conduction at the AV node
QRS: normal

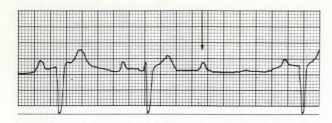

A

Second-degree block—Mobitz I (Wenckebach). The arrow indicates the nonconducted P wave in this sequence.

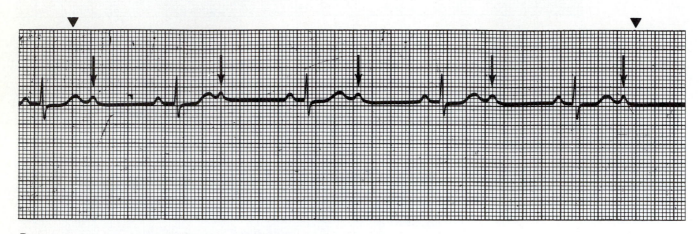

B

Second-degree block—Mobitz II. Arrows denote blocked P wave (2:1 block).

FIGURE F19

SECOND DEGREE ATRIOVENTRICULAR HEART BLOCK
Rhythm: depends on the type. Mobitz Type I (Wenckebach) irregular, Mobitz Type II regular or irregular.
Rate: varies but usually slower than normal
P-R: Mobitz Type I has gradual lengthening of the P-R interval until one P wave is blocked and a beat is dropped. Mobitz Type II has a constant P-R in the beats that are conducted. It may occur in regular sequence of 2:1, 3:1, etc. block or occasional P waves may not be conducted.
QRS: usally normal
(**Source:** Hudak, CM, and Gallo, B.M. *Critical Care Nursing,* [7th ed.] Philadelphia: J.B. Lippincott, 1994.)

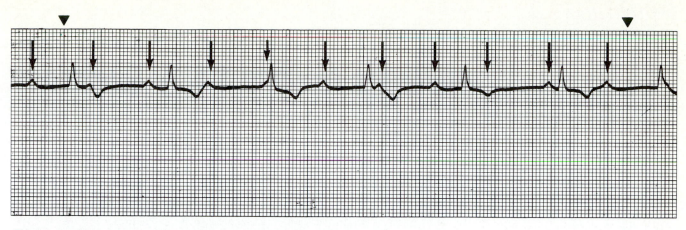

Third-degree block (complete AV block). Arrows denote P waves. Note the lack of relationship between the atria (P wave) and ventricles (QRS).

FIGURE F20

THIRD DEGREE ATRIOVENTRICULAR HEART BLOCK
Rhythm: regular
Rate: usually less than 40 ventricular beats, atrial rate is normal
P-R: no relationship between the P waves and the QRS. Indicate that there is a complete block at the AV node or lower.
QRS: normal or prolonged.
(**Source:** Hudak, CM, and Gallo, B.M. *Critical Care Nursing,* [7th ed.] Philadelphia: J.B. Lippincott, 1994.)

Appendix G

Answers to Case Study Questions

CASE STUDY ANSWERS CHAPTER 4

1. Maternal age greater than 40 years and paternal age greater than 55 years increases the risk for having a child with Down syndrome.

2. The facial appearance of the child is characteristic with flat facial profile, upslanting of the eyes, small nose, and palpebral fissures. A simian crease in the hand is found in 50% of persons with Down syndrome.

3. The genetic defect results when nondisjunction of chromosome 21 occurs at meiosis, producing one gamete with an extra chromosome and one gamete with no chromosome.

Union of the 24-chromosome gamete with a normal sperm produces a 47-chromosome zygote, trisomy 21. Sex-linked trisomies may also be seen.

4. A variable degree of mental retardation is common in these children who have an average intelligence quotient of 50. Retarded growth and increased incidence of cardiac defects all also common.

5. The continuing cyanosis after birth may result from cyanotic intracardiac defects, especially tetralogy of Fallot which is discussed on page 493.

CASE STUDY ANSWERS CHAPTER 9

1. This is probably a disorder of excessive somnolence (DOES) that results from obstructive apnea. The obesity, constant sleepiness, snoring, nighttime restlessness, and nodding off during sedentary periods are characteristic of this form of sleep disorder.

2. A sleep log or sleep lab might be used to diagnose the problem.

3. The condition begins with progressive relaxation of the muscles of the chest, diaphragm, and throat causing airway obstruction for as long as 30 seconds. The individual continues to attempt to breathe with chest and abdominal movements

until the breath is strong enough to relieve the obstruction. Airway constriction causes the snoring. This condition would interrupt both REM and nonREM sleep.

4. DOES results from the effects of sleep pattern interruption. DIMS results from multiple factors that affect the inability to initiate and maintain sleep. Disorders of the sleep-wake cycle occur when the normal sleep cycle is interrupted, such as working night shifts or traveling by air across multiple time zones. Dysfunctions associated with sleep or arousal include a diverse group of disturbances that may result from illnesses or may result in sleep walking or bedwetting.

CASE STUDY ANSWERS CHAPTER 11

1. Metabolic alkalosis is indicated. There is compensation in the P_{CO_2} to 48 which occurs because of respiratory retention of CO_2 which is acid.

2. Metabolic alkalosis results from the retention of alkali over acid and may be seen with vomiting, ingestion of bases, or administration of sodium bicarbonate (such as during a cardiac arrest resuscitation procedure). Metabolic acidosis results from the excessive production or retention of acid over base and alteration of the normal 1:20 ratio of carbonic acid to bicarbonate. Respiratory alkalosis results from the respiratory excretion of CO_2 through hyperventilation. Respiratory acidosis results

from the retention of CO_2 due to hypoventilation.

3. The sodium excess is probably the result of the ingestion of excess sodium bicarbonate (baking soda). Hypokalemia is usually seen with alkalosis because the kidneys are retaining hydrogen and excreting potassium in its place to try to compensate for the alkalotic state.

4. Severe clinical signs of apathy, mental confusion, weakness, muscle cramps, and dizziness are common.

5. Prevention of this form of metabolic alkalosis requires education of the patient and providing some other form of relief for her indigestion that would not alter the acid-base balance.

CASE STUDY ANSWERS CHAPTER 12

1. Hypoalbuminemic malnutrition or stressed starvation is indicated. Five percent of dextrose in water contains only 170 calories per liter. No intravenous protein has been given and clear liquids administered orally do not provide adequate calories or protein to provide for basal needs, much less the needs for a reparative process.

2. In stressed starvation, the neuroendocrine control mechanisms are altered and increased levels of glucagon cause an increase in blood glucose. This hypermetabolism stimulates insulin release, but insulin resistance in the tissues allows hyperglycemia to persist. Gluconeogenesis from proteins occurs and proteins are lost. Lipolysis occurs but ketones are not utilized for brain metabolism as they are in marasmus. The main calorie source is protein and the administration of intravenous dextrose prevents ketoadaptation. Skeletal muscle is catabolized to provide energy sources. The liver, which normally produces albumin and other essential proteins, produces acute phase reactants such as interleukin. Alterations in the serum levels of the proteins can be used to assess the degree of nutritional depletion. Hypoalbuminemia alters wound healing and makes nutritional repletion difficult. Obese individuals often suffer greatly from this type of starvation and it is not recognized because of their physical size.

3. Severe protein depletion is indicated with the albumin level of 2 g/dL or less.

4. Clinical manifestations include decreased wound strength, poor wound healing, altered coagulation, decreased immune response, and interstitial edema. Loss of muscle tone and increased incidence of infections are commonly seen. In marasmic individuals, there is a reduction in body weight but also a preservation of serum proteins and immune competence at the expense of the muscles and visceral protein. Kwashiorkor is evidenced by a low ratio of protein to calories with dermatitis and hair changes. Body weight may not change but protein is deficient.

5. Changes in the plasma levels of the branched-chain amino acids may be seen in repletion before albumin changes. Adequate protein must be given for repletion and to provide a source for anabolism.

CASE STUDY ANSWERS CHAPTER 13

1. Hypovolemic shock due to blood loss is indicated. The patient could have sustained a hemothorax in the area of the fractured ribs or he might have peritoneal bleeding from splenic rupture or other organ damage. The abdominal tenderness supports bleeding in the abdominal area. Decreased breath sounds may indicate a hemothorax or pneumothorax. The pale appearance and profuse perspiration are typical manifestations of the compensation by the sympathetic system.

2. Hemorrhagic shock results from direct blood loss. Both cells and plasma are lost to the central circulation. Distributive shock results from vasodilation of the arteriolar bed and loss of effective, not actual, blood volume. Cardiogenic shock results from failure of the heart to sustain adequate cardiac output. The decreased blood volume in hypovolemic shock leads to decreased venous return causing decreased cardiac output. The decreased blood pressure initiates the sympathetic response of tachycardia and vasoconstriction. The renin-angiotensin-aldosterone system enhances the vasoconstriction and through sodium retention causes an increase in blood volume. There is inadequate tissue perfusion that, when it persists, causes anoxic cell injury, anaerobic glycolysis, metabolic acidosis, renal failure, and cardiac depression. The compensatory mechanisms are instituted in order to return the body to the homeostatic state until erythrocytes can be produced to replace those lost and restore oxygenation.

3. The Swan-Ganz readings indicate hypovolemia with a decreased pulmonary artery pressure and especially a wedge pressure which is markedly decreased.

4. The initial treatment is to administer fluids, especially volume expanders, to raise the blood pressure. It is critical to identify the source of the hemorrhage. Depending on the amount of blood lost, blood transfusions may be given. Hemothorax requires the insertion of a chest tube. Peritoneal lavage may reveal intraperitoneal hemorrhage which requires surgery to identify the source and stop the hemorrhage.

CASE STUDY ANSWERS CHAPTER 15

1. Wound healing begins with the acute inflammatory reaction that follows injury and hemostasis. Wound healing may cause the scarring response that requires initial wound closure, remodeling, and definitive scar. There is a vascular phase and a cellular reaction that clears the area of foreign debris. The wound can be repaired through simple resolution, regeneration, and/or repair by scar.

2. The example indicates a breakdown in the healing process that results from infection and resultant poor wound closure. The base of the wound appears to have closed. The wound must heal by second intention from the base upwards.

3. The area must be cleared of infection and devitalized tissue. The obese individual often has a decreased blood supply which is necessary for healing. Nutritional balance must be adequate to provide the resources for a strong tensile wound. Early indications of healing include bright red granulation tissue that bleeds easily and exudate that is cleared from the wound.

4. Delay in healing may result from infection, the decreased blood supply in fatty tissue, altered nutritional status, and possibly the age of the patient.

5. Appropriate treatment includes open wound care that allows the wound to heal from the base upwards, providing adequate nutrition and fluids, and promoting and maintaining adequate blood pressure.

CASE STUDY ANSWERS CHAPTER 17

1. In 1993 the Centers for Disease Control and Prevention (CDC) included under Clinical Category B the presence of vulvovaginal candidiasis which is persistent, frequent, or poorly responsive to treatment in women with laboratory evidence of HIV infection. It is important to rule out diabetes mellitus through the use of a fasting blood sugar test. A positive HIV-antibody test will confirm the diagnosis of symptomatic HIV disease in women with persistent vulvovaginal candidiasis.

2. The incubation time is the time elapsed between infection with the HIV and the diagnosis of AIDS-related symptoms. The incubation time for HIV may be as long as 12 years. During this time, HIV replicates and increases in number in the infected person. Infected persons will be able to transmit the virus whether or not they are symptomatic.

3. Seroconversion time is the time that the immune system requires to produce an antibody titer that is sufficiently high to be detected by antibody tests such as the ELISA or the Western Blot analysis. In the majority of cases, this time is 6 to 12 weeks. This concept should not be confused with that of incubation time. The ELISA is a screening test, and all persons who test positive must be confirmed by a diagnostic test such as the Western Blot analysis. The combination of two ELISAs and a Western Blot analysis yield a high level of accuracy (99%) in detecting HIV-infected persons.

4. Acute retroviral syndrome (ARS) probably represents the first efforts of the immune system in combating an HIV infection. ARS is expressed by mononucleosis-like symptoms (or influenzalike) that occur between 2 and 4 weeks after exposure. Symptoms will usually disappear in a few days. A diffuse rash may accompany this symptoms complex, and may persist for 7 to 10 days. It is believed that a large percentage of infected persons experience these manifestations. However, because of its similarity to an influenza attack, many cases go unnoticed or unreported.

5. Three modes of transmission have been identified: unprotected sexual activity, blood-to-blood contact, and vertical (mother-to-child) transmission. The absence of transmission by casual contact has been well documented among family members of infected persons, health care providers, etc. If one believes the statement made by Ms. H. that her husband was the only sex partner she ever had, then her only risk factor was unprotected sexual activity with her husband. Considering his extramarital sexual relationships, he was probably the source of her HIV infection. An incubation time of approximately 5 years falls within the norm as range for HIV disease.

Assuming that Ms. H. acquired the virus from her husband before conceiving her daughter, the child would be at risk of being infected through vertical transmission. Every child born to an HIV-infected mother carries a 25% to 35% risk of being born infected, either through transplacental or intrapartum infection. The remaining 65% to 75% escape infection probably because of low maternal virus load. Because one does not know when Ms. H. became infected, her daughter either was born to an uninfected woman or escaped infection if her mother was already infected.

6. One of the consequences of HIV infection is a progressive loss of helper T cells, also referred to as T4 cells, which are very important cells in the regulation and modulation of immune function. Through the secretion of specialized lymphokines (such as interleukin 2), T4 cells are directly responsible for regulation of cell-mediated immune response, and indirectly, for antibody secretion by B cells. Loss of T4 cells will result in a compromised immune system and will eventually render the host unable to oppose a series of opportunistic infections and malignancies. One of the major causes of morbidity and mortality among HIV-infected individuals is *Pneumocystic carinii* pneumonia (PCP). Progressive loss of T4 cells will greatly predispose HIV-infected persons to develop PCP. This is especially true for individuals with a T4 cell count that reaches below 200 cells/mm^3, at which point prophylaxis against PCP should be instituted.

7. AZT is one of four currently approved antiretroviral agents in the United States. All agents act by blocking reverse transcription and arresting virus replication within infected cells. As such, AZT does not act directly on free viruses, which means that an infected person must remain in treatment for the duration of his or her lifespan. Any drug with such a requirement should have minimal (or tolerable) side effects. The major toxicity of AZT is to the bone marrow, resulting in anemia in many cases. In situations in which treatment with AZT becomes the only option, drugs that increase hematopoiesis may be used in conjunction with the antiretroviral agents. Another limitation of AZT is its limited efficacy. The earlier a person begins AZT treatments, the sooner it may have to be discontinued, as it loses its efficacy between 18 and 30 months of use. Until recently, this represented a serious life-threatening limitation. However, the development of other antiretroviral agents may allow for combination or sequential drug protocols, much like those used in cancer therapy.

8. Psychosocial interventions include safer sex practices including the correct use of latex condoms. Maintaining an active lifestyle and decisions regarding disclosure of HIV status are essential. Identifying personal support systems and decisions relating to future care of the dependent child must be made. Health care costs are major and must be discussed before major expenses are incurred. Support groups and HIV clinics can aid the patient during the progression of the disease.

CASE STUDY ANSWERS CHAPTER 18

1. Type I: Immediate hypersensitivity with anaphylactic shock is indicated.

2. Antigen-specific allergic reactions are usually mediated primarily by IgE interactions with mast cells. The shock reaction occurs with a large systemic reaction in an individual who has been previously sensitized to the allergen. The mast cells release histamine and other mediators, causing increased vascular permeability and bronchoconstriction. The itching sensation is due to the hives that appear on the surface of the skin usually first at the site of the bee sting. Angioneurotic edema follows which results from the vasodilatation and swelling around the eyes. Acute anxiety, pruritus, dyspnea, wheezing, and hypotension are all physiologic manifestations of the effect of the interaction.

3. Epinephrine is an effective bronchodilator for the bronchospasm. The hydrocortisone blocks the effects of the interaction. Benadryl, an antihistamine drug, also is often given. The epinephrine response is immediate and together with the hydrocortisone may be life saving.

4. Avoidance of areas where the patient could be stung may decrease the risk. Most highly allergic individuals are taught to carry a "bee sting" kit and are taught to administer the drugs immediately after being stung.

CASE STUDY ANSWERS CHAPTER 20

1. Chronic myelogenous leukemia (CML) is the same as chronic myelocytic leukemia. It is characterized by granulocytic cells that cause a marked elevation in the leukocyte count. The chromosome marker, Ph1 (Philadelphia) is found in 90% of cases. CML is diagnosed by well-differentiated leukemic cells that are granulocytic. The spleen becomes very enlarged. The course of the disease is slowly progressive for about 3 years and then it can enter an accelerated phase that terminates in an acute leukemia. In comparison to acute myelocytic leukemia, the cells are more mature and proliferate more slowly. The white blood cell (WBC) count is very high with CML, from 50,000 to 500,000/µL.

2. The clinical marker for CML is the Philadelphia chromosome.

3. Anemia, bleeding, and opportunistic infections are late developing due to crowding out of the normal erythrocytes, platelets, and lymphocytes by the large number of myelocytes which in themselves do not function well. The opportunistic organisms can be any that normally do not cause infection in the immune-competent individual.

4. The accelerated phase is heralded by rapid onset of anemia, hemorrhages, and often a DIC-type syndrome. The most common cause of death is infection resulting from marrow failure. Anorexia, weight loss, and weakness progress rapidly. Central nervous system (CNS) manifestations may result from leukemic infiltration of the meninges, CNS, and cranial nerves and these include headache and visual disturbances. Bone pain and hepatosplenomegaly are results of infiltration of the area with leukemic cells.

5. Chemotherapy, especially with oral alkylating agents, may decrease the WBC count and improve the condition for a period of time. Median survival is still only 3 to 4 years. Irradiation may be used for the splenomegaly or for bone marrow pain to decrease leukemic infiltration. Chemotherapy often causes neutropenia, stomatitis, and nausea and vomiting which may increase the risk for infection and enhance the cachexia noted in the disease.

CASE STUDY ANSWERS CHAPTER 23

1. Risk factors include obesity, smoking, elevated serum cholesterol with low levels of high-density lipoprotein (HDL) cholesterol, and high stress levels related to recent unemployment.

2. The probable diagnosis is acute anterior myocardial infarction (MI).

3. Acute anterior MI is usually caused by thrombosis of the left coronary artery, especially the left anterior descending. The area of the heart affected is susceptible to increased irritability and this resulted in the ventricular fibrillation and the PVCs seen later. Also, contractility of the heart is impaired and may produce left heart failure and cardiogenic shock. Infarction of the myocardium must be replaced by scar tissue which requires a period of 6 to 8 weeks during which other complications can result.

4. The cholesterol level is markedly elevated and the HDL cholesterol is very low, indicating a very high risk for atherogenesis. The CPK elevation may partly be due to resuscitation and release of this enzyme from muscle; the CPK-MB is very significant for myocardial damage and signifies a large area of infarction. The 12-lead ECG reveals acute injury in the anterior and anteroseptal portions of the heart. These changes will resolve to Q waves within 36 to 48 hours.

5. Ventricular fibrillation is the most common cause of death in persons with MI. The damaged area of the heart is irritable and sets up a focus that causes PVCs, ventricular tachycardia, and ventricular fibrillation. Defibrillation has been shown to be the most effective emergency treatment for ventricular fibrillation.

6. The chest tightness is the early sign of ischemic pain. The heart responds to lack of oxygen by a sensation of pain. This sensation may radiate through nerve roots to the shoulder, arm, back, neck, jaw, or even stomach.

7. A therapeutic plan requires patient cooperation with diet changes, weight loss, exercise, cessation of smoking, and an attempt at stress reduction. Medication regimens must be followed. A support group such as a cardiac rehabilitation program may assist Mr. Dow in adhering to a plan.

CASE STUDY ANSWERS CHAPTER 24

1. Acute bacterial endocarditis (ABE) with mitral and aortic insufficiency is indicated.

2. Ms. Jones' clinical history of IV drug abuse and the sudden onset of the symptoms support the diagnosis of ABE. Blood cultures can be used to isolate the organism responsible. The loud systolic and diastolic murmurs would support mitral and aortic insufficiency, but an echocardiogram and a left heart catheterization would be more definitive.

3. Acute bacterial endocarditis is most frequently caused by *Staphylococcus aureus*, an organism of high virulence that frequently resides on contaminated needles. The organisms cause sepsis and attach to the endocardial lining forming large, septic vegetations that are friable and embolize through the arterial circuit. The vegetations settle on the cardiac valves and

invade the leaflets, causing destruction and incomplete closure of the valves. Large insufficiency alters blood flow so that the symptoms of heart failure can rapidly result.

4. Without treatment, the prognosis for this condition is very poor. With treatment, prognosis is good if life-style changes are made.

5. Treatment includes antibiotic therapy given intravenously. Emergency valve replacement is often performed to prevent death from congestive heart failure. Recurrence can be prevented by drug abuse therapy, prophylactic administration of antibiotics before any invasive procedure, improvement of the nutritional status, and anticoagulation therapy if artificial valves were placed. Major teaching and compliance are necessary for improvement of the prognosis.

CASE STUDY ANSWERS CHAPTER 25

1. Left heart failure (LHF) with pulmonary edema is indicated.

2. Coarse rales in all lung fields, a loud gallop rhythm, dyspnea, ashen color, orthopnea, and respiratory rate all support LHF with pulmonary edema. The pulmonary artery catheter data indicate elevation in pressures, especially the wedge pressure which is at the accepted level for pulmonary edema. Cardiac output is decreased and compensation occurs through tachycardia and vasoconstriction.

3. Oxygen is used to improve oxygen saturation and decrease the extreme dyspnea. Morphine decreases anxiety, respirations, and causes vasodilation (especially venous) which decreases the preload on the heart.

4. LHF results when the left ventricle cannot sustain an adequate cardiac output for the needs of the body. The sympathetic system is activated causing vasoconstriction, tachycardia, and increased cardiac contractility. The renal system conserves the fluid volume through the activation of renin which causes vasoconstriction and release of aldosterone which

causes the retention of sodium. All of these factors increase the cardiac workload. As the left ventricle cannot pump all of its contents forward, blood dams back into the left atrium, the pulmonary capillary system, and when it reaches a critical level begins to move into the interstitial spaces between the capillaries and the alveoli. Oxygen has difficulty traversing this fluid and oxygen availability decreases. The fluid begins to fill the alveoli causing coughing up of clear, frothy sputum. As the pressure builds in the pulmonary system, the right ventricle is trying to pump its contents forward and gradually it, too, is unable to empty properly. The venous pressure then elevates.

5. Support measures include diuretics to remove the excess fluid overload. Drugs to strengthen the cardiac contractility may be used (ie, dobutamine). Drugs to reduce afterload and systemic vascular resistance may be used to decrease the oxygen needs of the heart (ie, nitroprusside). If the clinical condition worsens, respiratory support and ventilation may be necessary to improve oxygenation.

CASE STUDY ANSWERS CHAPTER 27

1. Atherosclerotic lesions probably begin with the fatty streak composed of lipid droplets deposited on the intima of arteries. As the lesion expands, smooth muscle cells migrate into the intima. The atherosclerotic lesion is composed of fatty

and fibrofatty material that protrudes into the artery and compromises blood flow. The altered intimal surface initiates the intrinsic coagulation system and the final obstruction is usually due to a clot. Hemorrhage into the plaque itself may also occur.

2. Collateral circulation involves opening small arterial channels which may help to sustain blood flow to the area for a time. In many cases, the blood flow is impaired but gangrene does not occur because of the collateral circulation.

3. The symptom of intermittent claudication occurs because of inadequate circulation to the limb usually during exercise. Gradually less and less exercise will produce the uncomfortable squeezing, aching pain. It is relieved by rest when the circulation is restored to the limb. Loss of pulses usually indicates occlusion of the main vessels as does the loss of color of the extremity.

4. Smoking has been closely associated with the acceleration of atherosclerotic changes. It enhances atheroma development and often causes spasm of the affected vessels. The carbon

monoxide and nicotine in tobacco smoke are related to development of the disease.

5. Doppler studies use ultrasound waves to evaluate flow through both veins and arteries. The proximal and distal pressures of the suspected lesion are auscultated to determine the pressure gradient and it is compared with the systemic blood pressure. The femoral arteriogram requires the use of contrast media injected into the artery and it shows the exact location of the lesion, the amount of obstruction, the presence of collateral circulation, and the vessels open below the lesion.

6. A femoral popliteal bypass operation usually involves the use of a piece of saphenous vein which is inserted above the lesion and bypassed around the obstructed area, being inserted in the open vessel below the lesion.

CASE STUDY ANSWERS CHAPTER 29

1. Tuberculosis (TB) typically causes an encapsulated tubercle in which the organism may or may not be killed. The lifetime risk of developing active TB following exposure is 5% to 10% in the healthy individual whereas it is 50% or greater in the HIV-positive individual. Reactivation of dormant infection is the usual cause and is seen in circumstances that depress the immune system.

2. TB is transmitted by means of aerosolized droplet nuclei when a person with active infection speaks, coughs, laughs, or sneezes. It is most readily spread in overcrowded conditions, with persons who practice poor hygiene and are undernourished. These individuals often seek and receive inadequate health care, including inadequate or incomplete drug therapy and follow-up. Measures to prevent this tragedy include improved health care and education about the importance of drug therapy and follow-up. Improved nutrition and living conditions could decrease the incidence. Of greatest concern is the spread of multiple drug-resistant TB which has apparently developed because of inadequate therapy.

3. TB develops when the affected individual inhales the organism from an infected person. The small size of the organism causes it to be deposited in the lung periphery. In the immunocompetent individual the organism becomes surrounded by leukocytes and inflammation results. The macrophages replace the leukocytes which may carry live organisms

away from the primary site. The macrophages engulf the organism and join together to form a giant ring around the cells. Within this giant cell, caseous necrosis develops and the surrounding ring contains activated T lymphocytes. The resulting tubercle may contain live organisms that are walled away from the body. Later, the tubercle may break down for a number of reasons, and the infection may spread throughout the lung tissue and lymphatic system. Bones, meninges, and other organs may become affected. The cause of death is usually respiratory failure.

4. In the HIV-infected individual, the immune system is compromised and the infection may progress unchecked to systemic proliferation affecting multiorgans. The presence of severe pulmonary symptoms along with unusual systemic symptoms should alert the health care provider to the possibility of TB. Sputum cultures will often confirm the diagnosis.

5. The treatment protocol for TB includes use of multiple drugs that can kill the organism. Combination drug therapy may be used if drug-resistant TB is suspected. Treatment must continue for an adequate time to kill the organism. Interfering factors in this case possibly include life-style factors that would prevent him or her from initiating and maintaining a treatment protocol. Treatment is often less effective when the individual has significant immune suppression which might be suggested by the x-ray pattern compatible with *Pneumocystis carinii*.

CASE STUDY ANSWERS CHAPTER 33

1. Damage to the kidney structures occurs gradually in many cases. Often there is no reported history of disease at all, just the gradual onset of renal failure.

2. This case illustrates a probable immune-mediated glomerular disease. It could be a result of poststreptococcal glomerulonephritis which would be unusual because the original disease occurred in childhood. This could be any of the chronic forms of glomerulonephritis or nephropathy. In any case, the result is chronic glomerulonephritis which is a slowly

progressive condition that may exhibit both nephrotic and nephritic characteristics.

3. The glomeruli become scarred and may be obliterated. The glomeruli and renal capsule are infiltrated with inflammatory cells. Vascular sclerosis contributes to the hypertension that is usually associated. Progressive renal dysfunction occurs and nephrons are progressively lost. Retention of nitrogenous wastes, loss of protein in the urine, hypertension, and water balance problems gradually occur.

4. Delaying the chronic renal failure resulting from this condition can be promoted by preventing infection, maintaining adequate nutritional balance, decreasing the protein intake, and maintaining fluid intake and output.

5. Treatment is not needed in early insufficiency. Dietary treatment and prevention of infection can be used during renal insufficiency and early chronic renal failure. In end-stage renal failure, hemodialysis may be the only chronic form of treatment if surgical transplantation is not possible.

CASE STUDY ANSWERS CHAPTER 35

1. Acute renal failure due to ischemic tubular necrosis is the probable diagnosis. Nephrotoxic tubular necrosis also could be the result of the ingestion of drugs.

2. Low blood pressure leads to decreased renal perfusion. The drugs and alcohol consumed can cause nephrotoxic damage. Oliguria followed by anuria may result. Impaired renal function causes the retention of nitrogenous wastes and potassium as well as other electrolytes. Tubular obstruction may result from swelling and necrosis of the tubular cells. The course varies with the duration of the renal insult. In the initiating stage, the initial insult is produced, the maintenance stage is characterized by oliguria and electrolyte imbalances; recovery is characterized by gradual increase of urine output with diuresis and early loss of electrolytes and water. Return of the ability to concentrate urine occurs gradually and recovery does not always occur.

3. The level of the serum potassium could cause cardiac dysrhythmias and cardiac arrest. Some method to lower the serum potassium is essential. This could include potassium ion exchange resins, hemodialysis, or peritoneal dialysis.

4. The outcome depends on the success of the treatment for the electrolyte imbalances and the restoration of adequate blood pressure. Ms. Jones is young and has a greater potential for recovery than an elderly person might. Renal function may be totally restored or renal insufficiency or chronic renal failure may be the ultimate outcome.

5. Treatment options include potassium-decreasing drugs, hemodialysis, or peritoneal dialysis to help restore a more normal fluid and electrolyte balance. Fluid intake may be limited and dietary restriction of protein may be prescribed if the problem persists when Ms. Jones is able to take a diet. If Ms. Jones is anuric, she could become fluid overloaded without fluid restriction. Restriction of protein decreases the amount of nitrogenous wastes that the kidneys must excrete.

CASE STUDY ANSWERS CHAPTER 38

1. Graves' disease is a multisystem disorder that includes hyperthyroidism, diffuse thyroid enlargement, infiltrative ophthalmopathy, infiltrative dermopathy, and lymphoid hyperplasia in any combination. The thyroid gland is enlarged two to three times normal size, usually symmetric. Exophthalmos or bulging eyes due to increased retroorbital pressure is common and may be accompanied by infiltration of the eyes. Periorbital edema is common. Infiltrative dermopathy is commonly called pretibial myxedema causing barklike appearance of the skin due to accumulation of hyaluronic acid in the interstitial spaces forming a boggy and nonpitting edema. The lymphoid hyperplasia is probably related to the autoimmune component of this disease.

2. The autoimmune component occurs when the T lymphocytes become sensitized to antigens within the thyroid gland and stimulate B lymphocytes to make antibodies to the antigens. The immunoglobulin identified called long-acting thyroid stimulator (LATS) has all of the functions of thyroid-stimulating hormone. Another antoantibody has been found which binds to TSH receptor sites and results in thyroid hypersecretion.

3. Graves' disease occurs more frequently in family members so it tends to support the diagnosis.

4. The exophthalmos is a distinguishing feature of this disease and supports the autoimmune nature of the condition.

5. Irritability and fidgeting are manifestations of the effect of the excessive hormone secretion. The weight loss and hot feelings are also signs of excessive thyroid hormones.

6. Pretibial myxedema causes a nonpitting, boggy edema of the pretibial of one or both legs. It may be mild or severe and is believed to closely relate to immunologic disruption and be a result of the immunologic reaction.

CASE STUDY ANSWERS CHAPTER 39

39-1

1. Mrs. Miller is obese, is over 40, and has a family history of diabetes.

2. *Clinical*

Manifestations	Pathophysiology
Weakness	Electrolyte imbalance, potassium loss, and dehydration.
Polyuria	Glucose acts as an osmotic diuretic, pulls water from the tissues, and causes excessive urination.
Polydipsia (excessive thirst)	Water loss from frequent urination and dehydration causes thirst.

Reddened area on toe/ long-term respiratory infection	Poor response to infection is related to poor circulation, leading to poor healing.
Visual changes	Changes in microvascular and retinopathies lead to blurred vision.
Sweet breath	The breakdown of free fatty acids and their excretion from lungs as compensatory mechanism cause an acetone breath.
Numbness in extremities	Membrane thickening, plaque formation, and decreased peripheral circulation along with myelin changes contribute to altered sensations.

3. Hyperglycemia, which occurs in varying degrees, is responsible for the long-term complications (retinopathy, neuropathy, nephropathy, and vascular disease) of diabetes mellitus. In both types there is an absolute or relative lack of insulin.

In IDDM there is destruction of the beta cells. This is accompanied by islet cell antibodies (ICA). There also is excess alpha cell functioning (glucagon). The mechanism is related to a combination of environmental and immune factors which are influenced by genetic susceptibility. NIDDM is characterized by some beta cell functioning. There are changes in islet cells. Genetic susceptibility combined with obesity are major factors in the incidence.

4. This test provides an accurate indicator of the person's average blood glucose. It measures the amount of glucose in the bloodstream by measuring the combination of glucose with hemoglobin as the RBCs circulate. Because the destruction and formation of RBCs is ongoing, the glycosylated hemoglobin value reflects blood sugar levels for approximately 120 days before the test. It is useful in diagnosing, monitoring control, and evaluating success of treatment.

39-2

1. Alcohol abuse and biliary disease are the major risk factors for pancreatitis. In urban areas alcoholism is the major cause.

2. Clinical manifestations include: Pain: edema that causes distention of the pancreatic capsule; pancreatic autodigestion from enzymes; local peritonitis from enzyme release into the peritoneal area

Nausea/vomiting: decreased intestinal motility and pain trigger nausea and vomiting

Vascular and cardiac dysfunction: release of vasoactive substances which cause capillary permeability, vasodilation, and hypotension

Jaundice: obstruction of the common bile duct from edema

Pleural effusion: extension of inflammatory process

Hyperglycemia: damage to islet cells

3. The precise mechanism that triggers the sequence of enzymatic activity is unknown. A variety of factors such as viral infections, trauma, and drugs have been implicated.

4. Exactly how the enzymes are activated remains unclear, but trypsin is believed to play a major role.

5. A *pseudocyst* is an encapsulated collection of debris, tissue, fluid, blood, and high enzyme content. Pseudocysts are usually within or adjacent to the pancreas. Pseudocysts may resolve or may become infected. A *pancreatic abscess* is a collection of necrotic tissue and a suppurative process.

6. The elevation of the serum lipase and both the serum and urine amylase levels gives certainty to the diagnosis along with other clinical findings. Damage to acinar cells of the pancreas causes release of amylase. Amylase is cleared by the kidney and is found in elevated levels in pancreatic disease. Lipase, like amylase, is secreted by the pancreas and appears in the serum following damage to the acinar cells.

39-3

1. Her current respiratory infections, failure to thrive, and steatorrhea are part of the clinical picture of CF. Laboratory findings of elevated sweat chlorides, absence of trypsin in duodenal aspirations, and low fat retention coefficient are characteristic of CF. The finding of atelectasis on x-ray along with a positive family history of CF offer further support of a diagnosis of CF.

2. The inheritance pattern is autosomal recessive. Both parents carry the gene. Therefore, with each pregnancy, there is a 25% risk that a child will have CF, a 50% risk that a child will carry the trait, and a 25% chance that a child will neither carry the trait or have the disease.

Two main types of testing, direct and indirect, can be used to identify carriers and diagnose CF. Prenatal diagnosis is done by amniocentesis or chorionic villi sampling (CVS). Chromosomal studies are done to identify the CF gene.

3. Dysfunction of the exocrine glands is the pathological mechanism in CF. Although CF is a multisystem disorder, the respiratory system and pancreas of the gastrointestinal system are primarily affected.

Pulmonary involvement is the most significant aspect of CF. Large amounts of thickened secretions produced by the bronchial mucous glands along with decreased ciliary motility lead to chronic secretion retention. Obstruction with thick mucus predisposes the lungs to infection. Chronic inflammation also leads to bronchiectasis, airtrapping, and obstructive pulmonary disease.

In the pancreas, obstruction of the pancreatic ducts with thick mucus blocks the flow of pancreatic enzymes which lead to degeneration and fibrosis of the pancreas. With deficiencies of pancreatic enzymes, there is inadequate breakdown of proteins and fats. Malabsorption of nutrients occurs and results in nutritional abnormalities.

4. Progression of pulmonary disease follows chronic infection. Fibrosis with poor oxygen and carbon dioxide exchange results in changes in pulmonary vasculature, pulmonary hypertension, and eventually cor pulmonale (right-sided failure).

5. Inadequate pancreatic enzymes lead to poor fat absorption, resulting in frothy, fatty, and foul-smelling stools.

6. In persons with the CF gene, there is a defect in chloride conductions across epithelia. In a sweat electrolyte test, sweat is induced by electrical current (iontophoresis), collected, and analyzed for sodium and chloride content. This test is specific for CF.

7. Persons with CF have thick mucus which obstructs the pancreatic ducts. Therefore, the pancreatic enzymes are decreased or absent from the duodenum. Contents of the duodenum are aspirated and enzyme content is determined.

8. Obstruction of pancreatic ducts by mucous plugs prevents enzymes which break down fats from entering the intestine. Without the enzymes, there is fat malabsorption, resulting in large, frothy, and foul-smelling stools. A 72-hour collection would reflect fat absorption. Large amounts of fat in feces is called steatorrhea.

9. Advances in molecular genetic testing for CF offer a basis for risk counseling for family members with a history of CF.

CASE STUDY ANSWERS CHAPTER 41

1. The colon cancer is in the left descending colon because it could undergo direct biopsy. The symptoms of melena, diarrhea, and constipation are common with left-sided lesions.

2. The carcinoembryonic antigen (CEA) is almost always positive with widespread metastases. It can be used to gauge the effectiveness of therapy. Normal levels of CEA are less than 2.5 ng/mL and may be elevated in nonmalignant inflammation of the gastrointestinal tract. Mr. Fry's CEA is markedly elevated, indicating probable metastasis.

3. Metastasis is due to invasion of surrounding channels especially lymphatic, peritoneum, and venous channels. Distant metastasis areas include the liver, lungs, bones, and brain.

4. The stage is difficult to determine without pathology reports, but one would think that it was at least Stage B2 which involves tumors invading the serosa without lymph node metastasis.

5. Table 41-4 lists nine recommendations for lowering the risk of colorectal cancer.

CASE STUDY ANSWERS CHAPTER 43

1. Laënnec's cirrhosis or alcoholic cirrhosis of the liver often produces esophageal varices and hemorrhoids. These may rupture into the esophagus causing the loss of large quantities of blood into the stomach. Severity of bleeding is increased due to high portal pressures and the low levels of clotting factors produced by the liver.

2. Fatty infiltration of the hepatocytes causes (eventually) liver cell necrosis and inflammation. Scar formation follows with shrinking of the size of the liver and destruction of the hepatocytes. Portal hypertension and ascites result from obstruction to blood flow. Ascites is further enhanced by decreased albumin levels resulting from the inability of the cells to produce albumin. Biliary obstruction and inability of the cells to conjugate bilirubin lead to jaundice. Coagulation defects result from the deficiency of factor formation by the liver. Palmar erythema and spider nevi are due to hyperestrogenemia and/or clotting disturbances. Serum ammonia levels are enhanced by the liver dysfunction and the breakdown of red blood cells in the gastrointestinal tract following the bleeding episode.

3. Low-protein diets are prescribed to decrease nitrogenous loads which can cause onset of hepatic encephalopathy. These may decrease the serum ammonia and other nitrogenous substances that the liver cannot metabolize.

4. Alcohol induces metabolic changes in the liver that lead to fatty infiltration and eventually scarring. This decreases the functional reserve of the liver and produces inability of the hepatocytes to function. Early changes include coagulation defects and liver enlargement. Alcoholic liver disease follows long-term ingestion of 80 g/day of ethanol but this amount is markedly decreased in susceptible individuals.

5. With abstinence from alcohol, liver function tests may return nearly to normal. Fifty percent of individuals with significant cirrhosis die within 5 years, but this can be markedly altered by abstinence from alcohol. Death may be due to hepatic encephalopathy, liver failure, infection, gastrointestinal bleeding, or hepatocellular carcinoma.

ANSWERS TO CASE STUDIES CHAPTER 45

1. Gout is indicated.

2. When body fluids are supersaturated with uric acid, monosodium urate crystals precipitate in the joints. This causes acute arthritis when the synovial joints are affected. It may be primary or secondary and may be due to overproduction of uric acid, retention of uric acid due to renal malfunction, or both mechanisms. The mass of urate crystals with its surrounding inflammation is called a tophus.

3. Potential complications include joint deformity, pain from continual inflammation, and spreading of tophi formation from joints to many locations, including the heart valves and aorta.

4. Gout attacks are associated with overeating, alcoholism, obesity, hypertriglyceridemia, and family history of the disease.

5. Life-style adjustments that can decrease the number of attacks include modification of diet by eating less-rich foods, decrease in or abstinence from alcohol, stress reduction, weight loss, and regular use of drugs that inhibit uric acid production.

CASE STUDY ANSWERS CHAPTER 47

1. Family history (genetically determined) and environmental factors are causative factors.

2. It is a disease of epidermal proliferation with sharply defined erythematous plaques covered by silvery white, loosely adherent scales. It is usually distributed over the knees, elbows, scalp, and lumbosacral skin. Nails may be involved with pitting and dimpling. It may be associated with arthritis or, rarely, pustular lesions that can spread and be fatal.

3. Exacerbating factors include local trauma, overexposure to the sun, infection, stress, and physical illness.

4. Control of the disease is improved by avoiding local skin injury, infection, and stress, maintaining good nutrition, and avoiding excessive weight gain.

CASE STUDY ANSWERS CHAPTER 50

1. Cerebral aneurysms can result from developmental defects or as a result of arteriosclerotic degenerative changes associated with aging. The fact that Barbara is relatively young would lead one to believe that her aneurysm is associated with developmental defects. Furthermore, Barbara is in the age range where developmental cerebral aneurysms make their existence known. Developmental aneurysms appear as a result of a weakened area in the vessel, frequently in areas of bifurcation of vessels. The weakened area results in an outpouching that has a well-defined neck. These are commonly referred to as berry aneurysms and are most frequently found in the region of the circle of Willis. Many ruptured cerebral aneurysms appear in the anterior communicating arteries of the circle of Willis such as those that presented in Barbara.

2. Ruptured cerebral aneurysms are diagnosed based on the patient's history and presenting signs and symptoms. If the patient is conscious, he or she usually complains of a severe headache, unlike any experience before. A CT scan or MRI, lumbar puncture, and cerebral angiography provide definitive diagnosis of a ruptured cerebral aneurysm. The early signs and symptoms supporting the diagnosis of ruptured cerebral aneurysms in Barbara include the sudden severe headache associated with physical exertion (though this may not always be seen in association with physical exertion, it frequently is), sudden loss of consciousness, disorientation, and confusion upon regaining consciousness, complaint of neck pain, difficulty expressing herself, and vomiting.

3. Barbara is drowsy and exhibits periods of confusion. She complains of a headache and neck pain, both of which could indicate meningeal irritation. She has mild neurological deficits. These findings in Barbara are consistent with a Grade III ruptured cerebral aneurysm.

4. Barbara has strong potential to develop cerebral vasospasm and this generally occurs within 3 to 10 days after the bleed. It is preferable to accomplish the ligation of the aneurysm while there is little or no vasospasm as patients in vasospasm tend to be more unstable, making conditions less than ideal for surgical intervention. Therefore, if possible, the clipping of Barbara's aneurysm is accomplished early.

5. Barbara, in all likelihood, is experiencing cerebral vasospasm. The change in clinical status in this timeframe is consistent with cerebral vasospasm. This is a common sequela with cerebral bleeds and ruptured cerebral aneurysms. Cerebral vasospasm is a narrowing of cerebral arteries commonly seen within 3 to 12 days after a cerebral bleed. With the narrowing of the artery, velocity of the blood flow to this area of the brain is increased. The narrowing of the vessel can result in ischemia and infarction of the brain distal to the area of spasm. The disruption in normal blood flow is reflected by neurological deficits corresponding to the ischemic regions of the brain.

Although the precise cause of vasospasm is not known with certainty, there are several theories about its cause. Prominent among these is that there is a release of intrinsic chemicals associated with lysis of the clot as well as accumulation of other vasoactive mediators. These include substances such as calcium ions, oxygen-free radicals, oxyhemoglobin, serotonin, prostaglandins, catecholamines, histamine, and angiotensin.

6. Cerebral vasospasm is diagnosed by patient history and patient clinical presentation. Cerebral angiography is used to confirm vasospasm. Transcranial Doppler ultrasonography is a useful noninvasive beside diagnostic tool that monitors cerebral blood flow and the changes in blood flow associated with cerebral vasospasm.

CASE STUDY ANSWERS CHAPTER 52

52-1

1. Curt seems to have suffered a sudden acceleration-deceleration injury as evidenced by the circumstances of the accident (severe damage to the truck, broken glass in windshield). The picture here seems to reflect a coup-contrecoup injury where there is injury not only at the site of impact (coup), but also at the opposite side of impact (contrecoup) as the buoyant brain shifts within the rigid skull.

2. Primary injuries are those that result from the physical insult to the brain and generally entail structural injury to the cranial contents. Secondary injuries result from the primary injury as the brain tissue responds to that insult. The primary injuries that threaten Curt's brain are contusions and lacerations as the brain shifts over the rough ridges within the cranial cavity. These injuries may be quite extensive and involve large areas of the cerebrum and brain stem. Brain stem injuries are associated with rotation of the cerebrum and usually result in loss of consciousness which Curt did not exhibit at this time. Therefore, Curt has probably had only cerebral hemispheric involvement. The nature of Curt's injury also makes him a good candidate for a cervical cord injury. The secondary injuries that could be anticipated with Curt include cerebral bleeds, cerebral edema, and increased intracranial pressure.

3. A concussion is a diffuse, transient, and reversible injury to the brain caused by a sudden blow to the head. It is a violent shaking of the brain that results in temporary changes in neuronal firing. Concussions range from very mild to quite severe interruptions in brain function. Some individuals experience very transitory changes in the level of consciousness, whereas others may be rendered unconscious for much longer. Usually the individual who has suffered a concussion is amnesic to the event that caused the concussion. Other than the amnesia to the event, the individual will not present with significant neurological deficits. Supporting data that might indicate that Curt experienced a concussion was the fact that he was "somewhat dazed" at the scene of the accident, self-oriented, and unaware of what happened to him. No other neurological deficits are noted early postinjury. One could anticipate potential problems with Curt's attention span, memory, anxiety, and irritability on a longer term basis after this accident.

4. Contusion is a bruising of the brain as a result of a blow to the head. It usually is associated with structural damage to the parenchyma of the brain including small hemorrhages, edema, local acidosis, and changes in the EEG. In acceleration-deceleration injuries, the bruising may occur in the coup and contrecoup areas of the blow to the brain. Because there are bony irregularities within the cranium, it is not uncommon to see cerebral lacerations associated with cerebral contusions. Neurological deficits vary with severity of injury and area of brain or brain stem involved. They frequently include changes in the level of consciousness and motor-sensory alterations.

Diagnosis of brain contusions is based on the mechanism of injury, clinical presentation, and CT or MRI findings. EEG recordings over the contused area show abnormal waves. Though early after admission Curt does not present specific neurological signs supporting a contusion, a brain contusion in Curt at this point probably can be assumed based on the mechanism of injury and later deteriorating neurological findings. Additionally, the depressed area in the high forehead area may indicate a possible underlying brain contusion.

5. Major concerns postinjury would be extension of the primary injuries and development of secondary injuries. Curt could very well have an associated neck injury given the circumstances of the accident. Therefore, neck immobilization is a critical intervention until this potential injury is ruled out. Additional potential problems for Curt include cerebral bleed, cerebral edema, increased intracranial pressure, and seizures. An awareness for their potential development and astute neurological assessment are essential. All neurological complications of head injury cannot be prevented, but their detection and early intervention can prevent/minimize permanent neurological deficits

6. The findings of bruising around the eyes (periorbital ecchymosis or raccoon eyes) and behind the ears, on the mastoid bone area (Battle's sign) suggest basilar skull fracture. There is a suggestion of involvement of both anterior and middle fossa skull with Curt. In addition to the periorbital ecchymosis and mastoid region bruising, anterior fossa involvement may reveal cranial nerve I, II, or III abnormalities as well as CSF rhinorrhea. CSF otorrhea, hemotympanium, VII cranial nerve deficits, and Battle's sign suggest a break in the integrity of the skull and put Curt at risk for intracranial infection.

7. The change in the level of consciousness with Curt most likely resulted from an expanding cerebral lesion that has encroached on the reticular activating fibers. The reticular activating system is diffusely distributed in the cerebral hemispheres and brain stem. Its connections between higher and lower centers travel through the tentorial opening, a region that is frequently compressed as cranial contents shift medially with increasing intracranial pressure. Likewise, fibers controlling pupillary responses and voluntary movement travel through the tentorial opening and, therefore, corresponding alteration in function would be noted. Changes in vital signs indicate compensatory responses in an attempt to maintain cerebral blood flow. The most important intervention at this time is to notify the physician immediately of the clinical changes as Curt requires surgical intervention to ligate the bleeding vessel(s).

8 Depressed skull fractures are fractures that denote bony displacement into the brain parenchyma. They may result in secondary bleeds and increased intracranial pressure. The findings evident with depressed skull fractures relate to the region of the brain involved and the extent of brain tissue involvement. Hazards associated with depressed skull fractures may include increased intracranial pressure, brain tissue injury, alterations in venous return, secondary hemorrhages, and intracranial infections.

52-2

1. Josephine has spinal cord trauma that involves injury at the C5 level. This is one of the more commonly injured areas of the spinal cord. If sufficient injury has occurred to the spinal cord, the individual will be rendered quadriplegic. Josephine would retain neck, shoulder, and scapula movement as the innervation to the sternocleidomastoid muscle is intact. It would be anticipated that sensory perception is obliterated below the area innervated through the fifth cervical segment.

Respiratory innervation is mediated through the diaphragmatic nerve that evolves from C3 to C4 and through the intercostal nerves that evolve from the T1 to T12 region. Josephine's injury is above the thoracic spinal cord and, therefore, she has lost the intercostal innervation for respirations. However, Josephine's diaphragmatic innervation is intact as her injury is slightly below the level of the origin of diaphragmatic innervation. Therefore she has limited respiratory muscle function.

2. Josephine is at risk for developing spinal cord edema which could extend the cord injury and result in respiratory arrest. Josephine's cord injury is at level C5. Should the cord edema ascend to include C4 or higher the only remaining respiratory muscle innervation may be obliterated. Other postinjury hazards for Josephine include the autonomic nervous

system changes associated with spinal shock, gastrointestinal, bladder, and bowel atony, and emboli secondary to venous pooling associated with peripheral vasodilation.

3. Spinal shock results from a high spinal cord injury (above T6) where sympathetic nervous system innervation is obliterated and unopposed parasympathetic innervation from higher areas predominates. The modulation of sympathetic-parasympathetic innervation is inhibited by the cord lesion. In addition to flaccid paralysis and areflexia, the resulting findings associated with spinal shock relate autonomic nervous system deficits. Unopposed parasympathetic nervous system results in hypotension, bradycardia, loss of sweating, piloerection, and poikilothermia (ambient temperature regulation). Additionally, bowel and bladder reflexes are lost during spinal shock. Clinical signs supporting spinal shock in Josephine include BP 92/48, T 97.8, P 62, flaccid paralysis, and bowel atony.

4. A period of spinal shock or postinjury areflexia ensure for a period of time. Organized neural pathways are interrupted and reflex responses are inhibited below the level of the lesion. Bowel and bladder reflexes originate in the sacral regions and, therefore, are inhibited and conscious control over their function is lost. Therefore, Josephine may need a Foley catheter inserted initially and assistance with bowel evacuation.

5. Josephine is prone to hazards of immobility due to major motor-sensory losses. The most significant of these include skin breakdown, infections, muscle atrophy, bone demineralization, and thrombus formation.

6. Josephine most likely suffered an episode of autonomic dysreflexia or autonomic hyperreflexia. This is an exaggerated response of the sympathetic nervous system in individuals with high spinal cord injuries (above T6). A mass sympathetic discharge occurs in response to a specific noxious stimulus. This discharge occurs as a result of stimulation of sensory receptors which, in turn, transmit to the spinal cord and continue ascending in the spinal cord via posterior columns and spinothalamic tracts and reflexively stimulate the sympathetic nervous system neurons in the lateral areas of the cord. The parasympathetic modulation from higher centers is blocked by the injury and the sympathetic nervous system effect continues unabated, resulting in arteriolar spasm and vasoconstriction below the level of the lesion. This results in severe hypertension, headache, and visceral changes. The high blood pressure is sensed by the higher centers and the parasympathetic system is stimulated and results in bradycardia, and vasodilation above the level of the lesion. As a result, the individual presents with flushing and diaphoresis above the level of the lesion and pale skin with gooseflesh below the level of injury. The individual will be very anxious, restless, and may experience nausea.

A cause of autonomic dysreflexia in Josephine could be a full bladder or bowel. A quick intervention that might be employed with Josephine is to quickly raise the head of the bed to obtain some postural hypotension. Then it is important to look for the underlying cause and eliminate it. Major hazards associated with this exaggerated sympathetic response are cerebral hemorrhage and myocardial infarction.

CASE STUDY ANSWERS CHAPTER 53

1. An astrocytoma is a tumor of neuroepithelial tissue (glioma). Glial cells are the supporting cells of the brain. These spider-shaped or star-shaped cells infiltrate brain tissue and are frequently associated with cysts of various sizes. Their invasive nature usually makes surgical removal difficult.

2. According to Law (1993), reference in chapter list, the average age at diagnosis of a person found to have an astrocytoma is 37 years. Prognostic factors in patients with astrocytomas of the brain are more favorable when the age of the patient is less than 40 years of age.

3. Because brain tumors eventually give rise to an increase in intracranial pressure, the three symptoms of brain tumors that often occur are headache, vomiting and papilledema. Headache is a common symptom of intracranial tumors believed to be a result from local displacement and traction of pain-sensitive structures within the skull-cranial nerves, arteries, veins, and venous sinuses. As the tumor grows, the pain is reflective of generalized increased intracranial pressure. The headache may be dull and is usually temporary. It is generally most severe on awakening and tends to improve throughout the day. The headache may be aggravated by stooping, coughing, or straining to have a bowel movement.

Vomiting is also experienced by many persons with intracranial tumors. Vomiting associated with tumors is not necessarily preceded by nausea and is not related to ingestion of food. It often occurs before breakfast and is frequently projectile.

Papilledema (edema of the optic disk) occurs as intracranial pressure increases. Visual symptoms of brain tumors, such as blurring and enlarged blind spot, are associated with papilledema.

In addition to these symptoms, a person who has a brain tumor may experience seizures, changes in mental function, and personality changes. The involvement of Mrs. M.'s dominant temporal lobe produced sensory aphasia, which begins with difficulty in naming objects. Also, the individual has difficulty comprehending the spoken work and speaks in jargon. Tinnitus occurs as a result of irritation to the adjacent cortex or temporal auditory receptor.

4. The CT scan is the screening procedure of choice because it is noninvasive and nonpainful. It involves the use of a computer, which because of various absorptive characteristics of brain tissue, blood, CSF, cyst fluid, and tumors, can process numerous high-speed films to produce a pictorial print of transverse sections of the brain. The MRI views the brain in successive layers within a powerful magnetic field. An MRI also allows for the assessment of physiology, such as reactions to the tumor—cerebral edema—as well as the nature and extent of blood flow.

5. Mrs. M. will most likely undergo biopsy and radical excision if possible. Following excision and biopsy report, radiotherapy and chemotherapy may be indicated. Often these tumors are not radiosensitive.

Prognosis is variable as astrocytomas have varying degrees of malignancy. Some are well differentiated and grow slowly for many years but may become more anaplastic over time.

Other astrocytomas are very poorly differentiated, anaplastic astrocytomas, and have a rapid rate of growth and poor prognosis.

Also, Mrs. M.'s prognosis is more favorable because she is younger than 40 years old.

CASE STUDY ANSWERS CHAPTER 55

The following findings indicated need for biopsy:

1. First-degree relative (mother) with history of breast cancer

Changes in mammogram from previous findings

Overweight, white female

Somewhat controversial and lacking consistent data, alcohol consumption, and hormone replacement therapy.

Additional factors for concern are birth of only one child when she was 27 years old.

2. It was a small tumor with negative nodes, and no obvious metastasis

3. It was a positive estrogen-receptor tumor and probability of recurrence.

4. It would be classified as stage 0—tissue report of tumor 1-cm in diameter, in situ, and no node involvement. There was no evident metastasis.

Index

Pathophysiology: Adaptations and Alterations in Function, Fourth Edition
Self-Study Disk Instructions

This electronic self-study program has been designed for use with an IBM or IBM-compatible computer and requires DOS version 3.0 or higher, 512KB RAM, a 3.5 inch disk drive, and a CGA graphics card or better.

To start the program, insert the diskette in your disk drive, type "a:" (or the appropriate letter for your disk drive—usually a or b), and press the <Enter> key. At the prompt (A:\> or B:\>), type "go" and press the <Enter> key to start the program.

This self-study program enables you to answer approximately 350 questions in a manner similar to the way you will take the NCLEX examination. As in the NCLEX, all questions in this program are multiple choice. To answer the questions, you will need to use only the up and down arrow keys and the <Enter> key. Use the arrow keys to highlight the answer you wish to select and press <Enter> to make the selection. Instructions are provided at the bottom of the screen.

The Main Menu of the program looks like this:

Instructions
Choose a Test
Review Results
Quit

Highlight your choice using the arrow keys and press <Enter> to select it.

Selecting the **Instructions** option will display an instructions screen.

Selecting the **Choose a Test** option will provide you with a list of 15 tests, each corresponding to a unit in *Pathophysiology*. To begin taking a test, use the arrow keys to highlight the name of the Test you wish to take and press the <Enter> key.

After you have selected a topic, you will be asked if you wish to take the test in *Study Mode* or *Test Mode*. To select a mode, press the <Alt> key at the same time as the underlined letter in your choice (<Alt>S for *Study Mode*, <Alt>T for *Test Mode*).

Study Mode lets you know immediately if the answer you selected was correct and provides you with feedback for correct and incorrect choices. If you select an incorrect answer, try again until you find the correct answer.

If you select *Test Mode*, you will be given the options of having the test timed (press <Alt>I), having the screen display the time remaining (press <Alt>R), and having the screen display the number of questions remaining in the test (press <Alt>Q). While in *Test Mode*, you will not receive immediate feedback on your answers. When you have answered all the questions, or when time has expired, you will be shown how many questions you have answered correctly.

After seeing your test results in *Test Mode*, you will have the options of printing the results of the test (press <Alt>P), reviewing the questions again in *Study Mode* (press <Alt>S), or returning to the main menu (press <Alt>M).

If you choose to review the question in *Study Mode*, you will see all the questions in that particular test again. The questions you answered correctly will be indicated with a check mark in front of the question number. All questions without a check mark were either answered incorrectly or not answered. In this mode, you will receive instant feedback on the answers you select.

The results for each test taken in a single session are temporarily stored in memory. Choosing the **Review Results** option from the Main Menu will show you the results for any test you have taken during this session.

Selecting the **Quit** option from the Main Menu will end the session and return you to DOS.

Pathophysiology: Adaptations and Alterations in Function, Fourth Edition
Self-Study Disk Instructions

This electronic self-study program has been designed for use with an IBM or IBM-compatible computer and requires DOS version 3.0 or higher, 512KB RAM, a 3.5 inch disk drive, and a CGA graphics card or better.

To start the program, insert the diskette in your disk drive, type "a:" (or the appropriate letter for your disk drive—usually a or b), and press the <Enter> key. At the prompt (A:\> or B:\>), type "go" and press the <Enter> key to start the program.

This self-study program enables you to answer approximately 350 questions in a manner similar to the way you will take the NCLEX examination. As in the NCLEX, all questions in this program are multiple choice. To answer the questions, you will need to use only the up and down arrow keys and the <Enter> key. Use the arrow keys to highlight the answer you wish to select and press <Enter> to make the selection. Instructions are provided at the bottom of the screen.

The Main Menu of the program looks like this:

Instructions
Choose a Test
Review Results
Quit

Highlight your choice using the arrow keys and press <Enter> to select it.

Selecting the **Instructions** option will display an instructions screen.

Selecting the **Choose a Test** option will provide you with a list of 15 tests, each corresponding to a unit in *Pathophysiology*. To begin taking a test, use the arrow keys to highlight the name of the Test you wish to take and press the <Enter> key.

After you have selected a topic, you will be asked if you wish to take the test in *Study Mode* or *Test Mode*. To select a mode, press the <Alt> key at the same time as the underlined letter in your choice (<Alt>S for *Study Mode*, <Alt>T for *Test Mode*).

Study Mode lets you know immediately if the answer you selected was correct and provides you with feedback for correct and incorrect choices. If you select an incorrect answer, try again until you find the correct answer.

If you select *Test Mode*, you will be given the options of having the test timed (press <Alt>I), having the screen display the time remaining (press <Alt>R), and having the screen display the number of questions remaining in the test (press <Alt>Q). While in *Test Mode*, you will not receive immediate feedback on your answers. When you have answered all the questions, or when time has expired, you will be shown how many questions you have answered correctly.

After seeing your test results in *Test Mode*, you will have the options of printing the results of the test (press <Alt>P), reviewing the questions again in *Study Mode* (press <Alt>S), or returning to the main menu (press <Alt>M).

If you choose to review the question in *Study Mode*, you will see all the questions in that particular test again. The questions you answered correctly will be indicated with a check mark in front of the question number. All questions without a check mark were either answered incorrectly or not answered. In this mode, you will receive instant feedback on the answers you select.

The results for each test taken in a single session are temporarily stored in memory. Choosing the **Review Results** option from the Main Menu will show you the results for any test you have taken during this session.

Selecting the **Quit** option from the Main Menu will end the session and return you to DOS.